肿瘤组织病理学诊断
Diagnostic Histopathology of Tumors

（第3版）

下卷

注　意

　　医学在不断进步。虽然标准安全措施必须遵守，但由于新的研究和临床实践在不断拓展我们的知识，在治疗和用药方面做出某种改变也许是必需或适宜的。建议读者核对本书所提供的每种药品的生产厂商的最新产品信息，确认推荐剂量、服用方法与时间及相关的禁忌证。确定诊断、决定患者的最佳服药剂量和最佳治疗方式以及采取适当的安全预防措施是经治医师的责任，这有赖于他（她）们的个人经验和对每一位患者的了解。在法律允许的范围内，对于因与本书所包含的资料相关而引起的任何人身损伤或财产损失，出版商和编著者均不承担任何责任。

出版者

肿瘤组织病理学诊断

Diagnostic Histopathology of Tumors

（第3版）

下卷

主编 Christopher D.M. Fletcher
主译 回允中

北京大学医学出版社
Peking University Medical Press

图书在版编目（CIP）数据

肿瘤组织病理学诊断：第3版／（美）弗莱彻（Fletcher,C.D.M.）著；回允中译.
—北京：北京大学医学出版社，2009
　书名原文：Diagnostic Histopathology of Tumors, Third Edition
　ISBN 978-7-81116-794-8

Ⅰ.肿…Ⅱ.①弗…②回…Ⅲ.肿瘤—诊断学：组织学（生物）：病理学　Ⅳ.R730.4

中国版本图书馆CIP数据核字（2009）第062721号

北京市版权局著作权合同登记号：图字：01-2007-4610

Diagnostic Histopathology of Tumors, 3rd edition
Christopher D.M. Fletcher
ISBN-13: 978-0-443-07434-9
ISBN-10: 0-443-07434-8

Copyright © 2007, Elsevier Limited. All rights reserved.

Authorized Simplified Chinese translation from English language edition published by the Proprietor.
978-981-272-068-9
981-272-068-5

Elsevier (Singapore) Pte Ltd.
3 Killiney Road, #08-01 Winsland House I, Singapore 239519
Tel: (65) 6349-0200, Fax: (65) 6733-1817
First Published 2009
2009年初版

Simplified Chinese translation Copyright © 2009 by Elsevier (Singapore) Pte Ltd and Peking University Medical Press. All rights reserved.

Published in China by Peking University Medical Press under special agreement with Elsevier (Singapore) Pte Ltd. This edition is authorized for sale in China only, excluding Hong Kong SAR and Taiwan. Unauthorized export of this edition is a violation of the Copyright Act. Violation of this Law is subject to Civil and Criminal Penalties.

本书简体中文版由北京大学医学出版社与Elsevier (Singapore) Pte Ltd.在中国境内（不包括香港特别行政区及台湾）协议出版。本版仅限在中国境内（不包括香港特别行政区及台湾）出版及标价销售。未经许可之出口，是为违反著作权法，将受法律之制裁。

肿瘤组织病理学诊断（第3版）

主　　译：	回允中
出版发行：	北京大学医学出版社（电话：010-82802230）
地　　址：	(100191)北京市海淀区学院路38号 北京大学医学部院内
网　　址：	http://www.pumpress.com.cn
E-mail：	booksale@bjmu.edu.cn
印　　刷：	北京画中画印刷有限公司
经　　销：	新华书店
责任编辑：	马联华　畅晓燕　陈奋　李海燕　　责任校对：杜悦　　责任印制：郭桂兰
开　　本：	889mm×1194mm 1/16　印张：61　字数：2092千字
版　　次：	2009年8月第1版　2009年8月第1次印刷
书　　号：	ISBN 978-7-81116-794-8
定　　价：	1550.00元（上下卷）

版权所有，违者必究
（凡属质量问题请与本社发行部联系退换）

目录

著者名单		xi
译校者名单		xv
主译的话		xvii
著者前言		xix

上卷

1 绪言 1
Christopher D.M. Fletcher

2 心脏和心包肿瘤 7
Anton E. Becker

3 脉管肿瘤 41
Eduardo Calonje 和 Christopher D.M. Fletcher

4 上呼吸道肿瘤 83
　第一部分　鼻腔、副鼻窦和鼻咽 83
　Bruce M. Wenig
　第二部分　喉和气管 150
　Ben Z. Pilch

5 肺和胸膜肿瘤 181
Cesar A. Moran 和 Saul Suster

6 口腔肿瘤 215
The late D. Gordon MacDonald 和
Paul M. Speight

7 涎腺肿瘤 239
Wah Cheuk 和 John K.C. Chan

8 食管和胃肿瘤 327
Fiona Campbell、Gregory Y. Lauwers 和
Geraint T. Williams

9 小肠和大肠（包括肛门部）肿瘤 379
Jeremy R. Jass

10 肝、胆囊和胆管肿瘤 417
Sanjay Kakar 和 Linda D. Ferrell

11 胰腺外分泌肿瘤 463
Günter Klöppel 和 David S. Klimstra

12 泌尿道肿瘤 485
John N. Eble 和 Robert H. Young

13 女性生殖道肿瘤 567
　第一部分　卵巢、输卵管 567
　　　　　　以及阔韧带和圆韧带
　Charles F. Zaloudek
　第二部分　子宫内膜 652
　George L. Mutter 和 Tan A. Ince
　第三部分　胎盘肿瘤和妊娠 672
　　　　　　滋养细胞疾病
　Christopher P. Crum、Yonghee Lee 和
　David R. Genest
　第四部分　子宫肌层 683
　Marisa R. Nucci
　第五部分　宫颈 697
　Marisa R. Nucci、Kenneth R. Lee 和
　Christopher P. Crum
　第六部分　阴道 719
　Marisa R. Nucci
　第七部分　外阴 730
　Marisa R. Nucci

14 男性生殖道肿瘤 749
Jae Y. Ro、Mahul B. Amin、Kyu-Rae Kim 和
Alberto G. Ayala
　第一部分　前列腺和精囊 749
　第二部分　睾丸和睾丸周围组织 812
　第三部分　阴茎和阴囊 861

15 腹膜肿瘤 881
Philip B. Clement

16 乳腺肿瘤 903
Ian O. Ellis、Sarah E. Pinder 和 Andrew H.S. Lee

下卷

17	垂体肿瘤 M. Beatriz S. Lopes	971	
18	甲状腺与甲状旁腺肿瘤 John K.C. Chan	997	
	第一部分　甲状腺	997	
	第二部分　甲状旁腺	1080	
19	肾上腺肿瘤 Ernest E. Lack	1099	
20	胰腺内分泌肿瘤 Günter Klöppel 和 Philipp U. Heitz	1123	
21	淋巴网状系统肿瘤	1139	
	第一部分　淋巴结 John K.C. Chan	1139	
	第二部分　脾 Wah Cheuk 和 John K.C. Chan	1289	
	第三部分　胸腺 Wah Cheuk 和 John K.C. Chan	1315	
22	造血系统肿瘤 Jeffery L. Kutok	1363	
23	皮肤肿瘤 Daniel J. Santa Cruz	1423	
24	软组织肿瘤 Christopher D.M. Fletcher	1527	
25	骨关节系统肿瘤 K. Krishnan Unni 和 Carrie Y. Inwards	1593	
26	中枢神经系统肿瘤 M. Beatriz S. Lopes 和 Scott R. VandenBerg	1653	
27	周围神经外胚层肿瘤 Christopher D.M. Fletcher	1733	
28	自主神经系统（包括副神经节）肿瘤 Ernest E. Lack	1763	
29	眼和眼附属器肿瘤 Robert Folberg	1781	
30	耳肿瘤 Leslie Michaels	1813	
31	肿瘤诊断中的电子显微镜检查 Bruce Mackay	1831	
32	分子遗传学技术在诊断和预后中的应用 Janina A. Longtine 和 Jonathan A. Fletcher	1861	
	索引		

Yonghee Lee MD
Associate Professor of Pathology
Pochon CHA University College of Medicine
Bundang CHA General Hospital
Kyonggi-do, Korea

Janina A. Longtine MD
Chief, Molecular Diagnostics
Department of Pathology
Brigham & Women's Hospital;
Associate Professor of Pathology
Harvard Medical School
Boston, MA, USA

M. Beatriz S. Lopes MD
Professor of Pathology and Neurological Surgery
Department of Pathology - Neuropathology
University of Virginia School of Medicine
Charlottesville, VA, USA

The late D. Gordon MacDonald BDS PhD FRCPath FDSRCPS(G)
Formerly Professor in Oral Pathology and Honorary Consultant
Department of Oral Medicine & Pathology
Glasgow Dental Hospital
Glasgow, UK

Bruce Mackay MD PhD
Emeritus Professor of Pathology
University of Texas MD Anderson Cancer Center
Missouri City, TX, USA

Leslie Michaels MD FRCPath FRCP(C) FCAP
Professor Emeritus
Department of Histopathology
Royal Free and UCL Medical School
London, UK

Cesar A. Moran MD
Professor of Pathology, Director of Thoracic Pathology and Deputy Chairman
Department of Pathology
The University of Texas
MD Anderson Cancer Center
Houston TX, USA

George L. Mutter MD
Associate Professor of Medicine
Harvard Medical School;
Pathologist, Division of Women's and Perinatal Pathology
Department of Pathology
Brigham and Women's Hospital
Boston, MA, USA

Marisa R. Nucci MD
Associate Pathologist
Divisions of Women's and Perinatal Pathology and Surgical Pathology
Department of Pathology
Brigham and Women's Hospital;
Assistant Professor of Pathology
Harvard Medical School
Boston, MA, USA

Ben Z. Pilch MD
Associate Pathologist
Massachusetts General Hospital;
Associate Professor of Pathology
Harvard Medical School
Boston, MA, USA

Sarah E. Pinder MBChB FRCPath
Consultant Breast Pathologist
Histopathology Department
Addenbrooke's NHS Trust
Cambridge, UK

Jae Y. Ro MD PhD
Professor of Pathology
Department of Pathology
The Methodist Hospital
Weill Medical College of Cornell University
Houston, TX, USA

Daniel J. Santa Cruz MD
Cutaneous Pathology
WCP Laboratories Inc.
St Louis, MO, USA

Paul M. Speight BDS FDSRCPS(Glas) PhD FRCPath FDS RCS(Edin)
Professor of Oral and Maxillofacial Pathology
Department of Oral and Maxillofacial Pathology
School of Clinical Dentistry
University of Sheffield
Sheffield, UK

Saul Suster MD
Professor and Vice Chair
Director of Anatomic Pathology
The Ohio State University Hospital
Columbus, OH, USA

K. Krishnan Unni MB BS
Professor of Pathology and Orthopedics and
Consultant, Division of Anatomic Pathology and
Division of Orthopedic Oncology
Mayo Clinic College of Medicine
Rochester, MN, USA

Scott R. VandenBerg MD PhD
Professor of Pathology and Neurological Surgery
University of California School of Medicine,
San Francisco
San Francisco, CA, USA

Bruce M. Wenig MD
Chairman
Department of Pathology and Laboratory Medicine
Beth Israel Medical Center;
Professor of Pathology
Albert Einstein College of Medicine
New York, NY, USA

Geraint T. Williams BSc MD MRCR FRCP(Lond) FRCPath FMedSci
Professor of Pathology
Department of Pathology
Wales College of Medicine
Cardiff University
Cardiff, UK

Robert H. Young MD FRCPath
Director of Surgical Pathology
Department of Anatomic Pathology
Massachusetts General Hospital
Boston, MA, USA

Charles F. Zaloudek MD
Professor of Pathology
Department of Pathology
University of California, San Francisco
San Francisco, CA, USA

译校者名单

北京大学人民医院病理科

回允中　阚　秀　戴　林　沈丹华　谢大鹤　钱利华　鲍冬梅　陈定宝
孙昆昆　郑红芳　刘芳芳　王功伟　张晓波　高松源

北京大学临床肿瘤医院暨北京市肿瘤防治研究所病理科

薛卫成　刘毅强　时云飞　李香菊　董　彬　孙　宇　李忠武

哈尔滨医科大学第二附属医院病理科

杜金荣　韩丽姝　陈英准　李莹杰　韩桂萍　张艳梅　姜　影

大连医科大学

病理学教研室　　唐建武　李连宏　孙　雷
附属第一医院　　关宏伟
附属第二医院　　王莉芬

昆明医学院病理学教研室

王　芳　季语祝　沈　勤　庄利萍　郭　君　唐　莹　卜亚军

吉林大学第二医院病理科

高洪文

主译的话

Dr. Fletcher 主编的《肿瘤组织病理学诊断》（Diagnostic Histopathology of Tumors）一书自1995年首次出版以来，已两度再版，其第3版的中文译本即将与广大病理医生及相关临床医生见面。这是我主译的第七部诊断病理学巨著。十多年来，我为主译这些病理学巨著付出了许多，当然也从中学到了很多，获益匪浅。病理学涉及面很广，很多人感到知识匮乏，解决这个问题的必由之路就是"天天读"，除此以外没有捷径，这是病理学界许多同仁的共识。

《肿瘤组织病理学诊断》是一部好书——是一部按器官系统论述肿瘤组织病理学诊断的教科书。同其他病理学巨著一样，其每一章节均是从成百上千篇参考文献中提取精华撰写而成，是千千万万科学工作者常年辛勤劳动的结晶，这样的教科书自然具有权威性。我20年前的一篇个案报告竟然也被收入其中，作为参考文献引用（见本书377页参考文献416），就是一个很好的例证。

不断更新的教科书是你我永远的老师。值此《肿瘤组织病理学诊断》第3版中文版即将面世之际，我想在这里再次强调"请书会诊"（Textbook Consultation）的重要性。"请人会诊"（Human Consultation）固然重要，但在某种程度上，"请书会诊"似乎更为重要，尤其是在诊断有分歧的病例，无疑是可以选择的正确方法。对此，我想以高度富于细胞的子宫平滑肌瘤（highly cellular leiomyoma）为例说明这个问题。高度富于细胞的子宫平滑肌瘤是一种必须与子宫内膜间质肿瘤鉴别的、比较少见的子宫间叶性肿瘤。由于不太熟悉或根本不知道有这样一种疾病存在，"请人会诊"时诊断意见往往出入很大，不但不能解决问题，有时反而会令人无所适从。争论的焦点无非是：其是来源于平滑肌还是来源于子宫内膜间质，是良性肿瘤还是恶性肿瘤。高度富于细胞的子宫平滑肌瘤的组织学表现由于与子宫内膜间质肿瘤的组织学表现非常相似，容易被误诊为子宫内膜间质肿瘤。但是仔细观察会发现，其具有几个与子宫内膜间质肿瘤明显不同的特征（本书第684页仅寥寥数语就将此描述得清清楚楚），了解这些诊断和鉴别诊断要点，就不难做出正确诊断。此时，"请书会诊"不仅可以解决诊断问题，还能免除一些无谓的纷争。此外，千万不要忘记，在免疫组织化学染色不支持组织形态学诊断时，不能根据一个看似异常的免疫染色结果（尤其是阴性结果）来否定一个明确的形态学诊断，这是组织病理学诊断的重要原则之一。

毋庸置疑，病理医生在肿瘤诊断方面起着无与伦比的作用。由于所有肿瘤诊断均应采用严格的组织学标准，可以想见，在病理学诊断领域说"我说是就是"（金口玉言）的时代将一去不复返了！（The days of saying "It is what it is because I say it is" are gone! 见本书绪言部分）。诊断标准多数来源于经典的教科书，读书是为了实践，事实证明，读书可以明显提高病理学诊断水平。因此，我深切希望本书能为提高肿瘤组织病理学诊断水平做出应有的贡献。

本书的译者们为本书的出版付出了艰辛的劳动，在此表示深切的谢意。主译水平有限，错误在所难免，敬请读者批评指正。

北京大学人民医院 病理科
北京五洲女子医院 病理科

回允中
2009-03-26

著者前言

在本书第 2 版出版与第 3 版出版的 7 年间隔中，传统的形态学和免疫组织化学检查仍是卓越的、最可靠的和成本-效果最好的方法，诊断和预后评估仍然依靠它们做出，在多数情况下，肿瘤如何适当切除的决定也主要经由它们做出。在诸如分子遗传学诊断、基因表达谱和蛋白组学（proteomics）等更昂贵的现代技术可以应用的今天，当各种检查所得结果差异更大时——不仅在发达地区和发展中（或不发达的）地区之间（达到骇人听闻的程度），甚至在不同的发达国家或地区之间——在某种程度上，这些"传统"技术和解读方法的作用再一次得到认证。而上面提到的许多新技术也已经实现它们应用于临床的承诺。

的确，现在分子诊断的作用已经稳固确立。近些年来，分子诊断技术不断扩展，包括：敏感性试验，如在乳腺癌和结肠癌；神经胶质肿瘤的预测；追踪残留的微小疾病的更敏感方法，特别是在恶性淋巴造血系统肿瘤。分子诊断的这种广泛而又重要的作用在新的第 3 版全书中均有所反映，并且在 Janina Longtine 和 Jonathan Fletcher 撰写的第 32 章进行了特别讨论。也许最高层面的分子学进展是基于可重复的相关靶分子的确认的合理的靶向治疗不断增加。值得注意的是，这些靶分子多数是通过免疫组织化学检查（如 HER2/neu、c-kit 和 EGFR）确认的，至少开始时是这样的。然而，由于常常发生治疗对抗且不清楚对抗机制，为了选择最佳治疗方法，可能需要更多地依靠突变分析。近几年来，由于注意力已经集中到酪氨酸激酶上，一些持乐观态度的人希望：通过广泛筛选某种特定肿瘤的"着丝粒"（kinome），可以确认适当的激活靶点或易于干预的信号通路。在可预知的将来，这种技术还不太可能广泛应用，因此，在更好地了解治疗改变的相关性和激酶过表达或激活的真正机制之前，最好还是加以小心。

值得注意的是，从表面上看，肿瘤形态学分类和预测方法的进展步伐并没有明显减慢，而是继续发展并更加精确，这有助于不断提高解剖病理学的价值。这些进展多数已被收录在新版 WHO 分类中，后者在过去 5 年左右的时间中已经陆续发布。另外，与临床或治疗有关的"新的"肿瘤类型（或亚型）不断得到认可，形式上是各种各样的。本书第 3 版已根据这些新的信息进行了修订，有些章节是重新撰写的，特别是有关肝胆系统肿瘤、女性生殖道、造血系统和眼（及其附属器）章节的许多内容。

一如既往，所有的错误或遗漏都是我这个编者的责任。在这里，我首先要深深地感谢各位著者，他们对本书倾注了极大的热情，并为本书提供了大量高质量的素材。其次还要深深地感谢我的杰出的秘书 Kathleen Radzikowski，我还要感谢 Elsevier 的"主要负责人员"Michael Houston、Sheila Black 和 Bryan Potter，感谢他们的辛勤工作和大力支持。

Christopher D.M. Fletcher
Boston，2006
回允中译

垂体肿瘤
Tumors of the pituitary gland

M. Beatriz S. Lopes 著

董 彬　孙昆昆　薛卫成 译

引言	971
垂体的解剖学和组织学	972
垂体腺瘤	973
垂体癌	974
垂体腺瘤的发病机制	975
术中会诊和标本处理	977
腺瘤的类型	978
其他肿瘤和炎症性病变	989
其他病变	993

引言　Introduction

垂体与蝶鞍区肿瘤大约占所有脑肿瘤的10%～15%[1]。蝶鞍区可发生多种肿瘤，反映了其解剖学的复杂性。表17.1列出了最常见的鞍区和鞍旁肿瘤，最常见者是垂体腺瘤，这是一种源于腺垂体细胞的良性上皮性肿瘤。事实上，在神经外科临床实践中，垂体腺瘤属第三大常见的颅内肿瘤，仅次于胶质瘤和脑膜瘤[1]。在作者单位，垂体腺瘤大约占蝶鞍病变的75%（表17.2）。垂体腺瘤主要累及21～60岁的女性，但事实上它可发生于各年龄组[2]。垂体腺瘤很少累及儿童，儿童垂体腺瘤常常是功能性腺瘤，并且更具有侵袭性。在美国，黑人垂体腺瘤的发生率（1.2/100 000人-年）略高于白人（0.9/100 000人-年）[1]。在尸检病人中，10%～15%可偶然发现垂体腺瘤[3-5]。

表17.1　垂体和蝶鞍区肿瘤及瘤样病变

1. 垂体前叶肿瘤
   - 垂体腺瘤
   - 垂体癌
   - 梭形细胞嗜酸细胞瘤
2. 垂体后叶肿瘤
   - 神经节细胞瘤
   - 垂体后叶星形细胞瘤-垂体细胞瘤
   - 颗粒细胞肿瘤
   - Langerhans细胞组织细胞增生症
3. 非垂体来源的肿瘤
   - 颅咽管瘤
   - 脑膜瘤
   - 脊索瘤和软骨瘤
   - 生殖细胞肿瘤
   - 转移性肿瘤
4. 囊性病变
   - Rathke 裂囊肿
   - 蛛网膜囊肿
   - 表皮样/皮样囊肿
5. 炎症性病变
   - 淋巴细胞性垂体炎
   - 肉芽肿性垂体炎
   - 结节病

表17.2　垂体腺瘤及蝶鞍区其他病变的发病率——Virginia大学，1992—2002

病变	发病率（%）
垂体腺瘤	74
Rathke裂囊肿（RCC）	5
颅咽管瘤	4
垂体卒中	2
囊肿（除RCC外）	2
炎症性病变	1
转移癌	1
脑膜瘤	1
难以归类的病变	1
正常垂体[a]	9

[a] 大多数病例临床怀疑为腺瘤

除肿瘤之外，垂体还可以发生多种非肿瘤性病变，需要与垂体肿瘤进行鉴别。本章仅讨论鞍区最常见且较为独特的病变。

垂体的解剖学和组织学

成人垂体呈豆形，位于颅底蝶鞍区一个小的骨性腔室内。腺体大小约13mm×9mm×6mm，重量大约为0.6g，根据性别的不同略有差异（0.4～0.9g）[6]，女性稍重于男性，特别是妊娠期和哺乳期的妇女更明显[7]。

垂体通常分为两部分：垂体前叶（又称腺垂体）和垂体后叶（又称神经垂体）（参见Page的综述[8]）。垂体前叶最大，约占垂体的75%～80%，由以下三部分构成：（1）远侧部；（2）中间部；（3）结节部。腺垂体属上皮来源，源自口腔外胚层的内褶——Rathke囊。垂体后叶来源于神经系统，源自第三脑室底外凸处。神经垂体由垂体柄（又称漏斗部）和神经部构成，该部分将垂体与大脑直接连在一起。

垂体表面覆盖着自颅底延伸而来的硬脑膜，硬脑膜分为两层：一层衬覆于蝶鞍底；另一层在垂体柄水平形成鞍膈。垂体被许多重要的解剖学结构所包绕。垂体侧面是海绵窦，内含颈内动脉、静脉丛以及第Ⅲ、Ⅳ、Ⅴ和Ⅵ对颅神经。垂体上方是视神经交叉和视束，下方则是蝶骨和蝶窦。

垂体前叶有多种不同的细胞类型和功能（图17.1至17.3）。许多新近发现的转录因子以多步骤、严格控制的方式参与了垂体前叶的组织发生（参见Page的综述[8]）。Rathke囊至少产生6种垂体特异性细胞。其中5种属功能性细胞，根据所产生的激素进行命名(图17.3)：

1. 生长激素细胞产生生长激素（GH）
2. 催乳素细胞产生催乳素（PRL）
3. 促肾上腺皮质激素细胞产生促肾上腺皮质激素（ACTH）
4. 促甲状腺激素细胞产生促甲状腺激素（TSH）
5. 促性腺激素细胞产生卵泡刺激素（FSH）和黄体生成素（LH）

在垂体的组织发生过程中，这5种细胞的分化反映了各自的激素控制基因的一过性表达[9-14]。垂体前叶的第6种细胞是滤泡星形细胞（folliculostellate cell），它是一种特殊的支持细胞，具有吞噬和分泌生长因子等多种功能[15-17]。

镜下，垂体前叶呈明确的腺泡样结构，网织纤维染

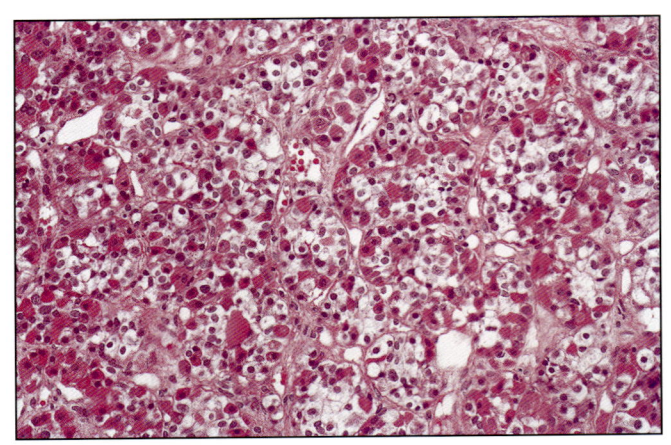

图17.1　正常垂体前叶的组织学表现。HE染色显示正常垂体具有多种细胞类型。在同一个腺泡中，嗜碱、嗜酸和嫌色细胞混杂存在。

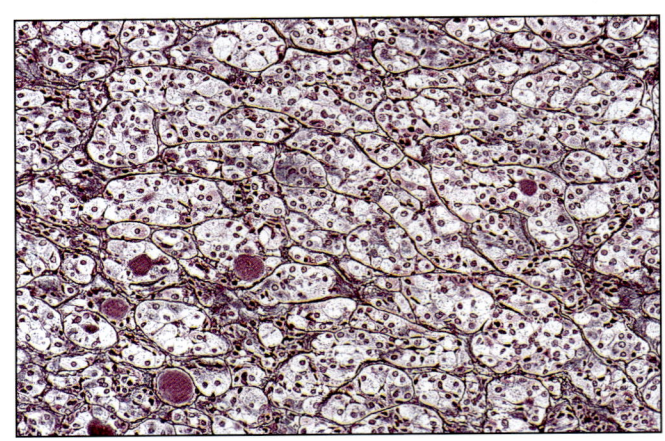

图17.2　网织纤维染色可见在正常垂体腺泡周围包绕着纤细的网织纤维网。注意腺泡的大小有差别。

色可清楚地显示（图17.2）。每个腺泡均由不同的激素分泌细胞混合组成（图17.1）。然而，不同类型的细胞在腺体内的位置具有选择性。生长激素细胞数目最多，主要位于腺体侧翼。促肾上腺皮质激素细胞占腺垂体细胞总数的10%～15%，主要位于中央裂，在垂体后叶前方。催乳素细胞可见于垂体前叶各部分，而促性腺激素细胞则广泛分布在整个腺体中，没有明显的聚集部位。促甲状腺激素细胞不足腺垂体细胞总数的5%，主要位于垂体前叶中央裂中前方的小片区域中[6]。

垂体后叶（神经垂体）是由网状交织的轴突和神经纤维以及一种被称为垂体后叶细胞（pituicyte）的特殊胶质细胞构成。垂体后叶细胞形态学呈拉长的单极或双极细胞，胞浆延伸呈单个或多个突起。垂体后叶细胞呈

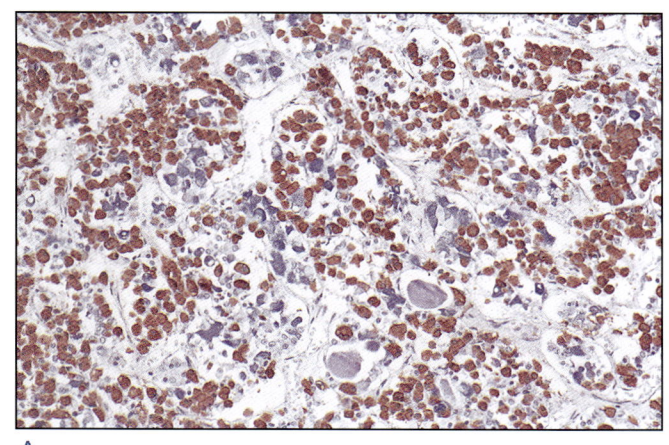

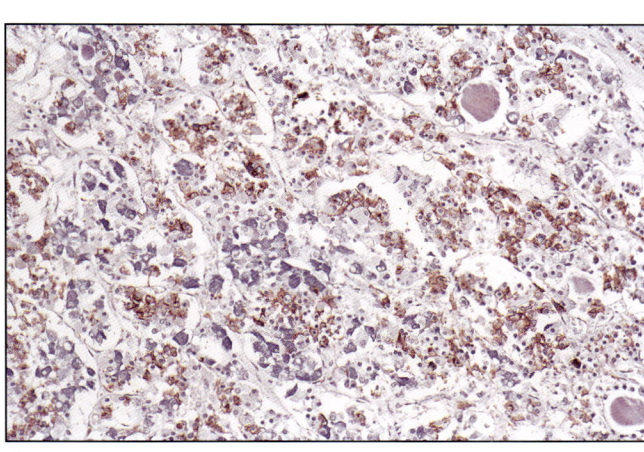

图17.3 单个腺泡中不同的细胞群体。(A) 生长激素阳性细胞是正常垂体的最大群体。(B) 正常垂体中的促肾上腺皮质激素阳性细胞。(C) 正常垂体中的催乳素阳性细胞。

胶质纤维酸性蛋白（GFAP）强阳性，类似于中枢神经系统其他区域的胶质细胞，垂体后叶细胞的突起延伸到邻近的结缔组织或血管壁。

需特别指出的是垂体后叶会发生*嗜碱性细胞浸润*现象。浸润的嗜碱性细胞呈 ACTH 免疫反应阳性，随着年龄的增长出现在垂体前叶和后叶交界处。虽然属于正常生理过程，没有临床意义，但是重要的是不要将它误认为嗜碱性细胞腺瘤侵及垂体后叶。

垂体腺瘤　Pituitary adenomas

分类

过去曾提出多种垂体腺瘤的分类方法。最初的形态学分类是由 Cushing 于 1912 年提出[18]，目前多采用肿瘤形态学与患者临床内分泌表现相结合的分类方法。随着肿瘤诊断现代技术的应用，通过对照肿瘤的内分泌活性、形态学特征、免疫组化特点以及超微结构表现，数十年来我们获得了大量有关腺垂体肿瘤的病理生物学知识。大多数实验室现在仍然采用临床形态学分类，不仅有助于进一步了解垂体腺瘤的细胞遗传学，而且也有助于我们识别临床表现相似的不同肿瘤类型。近年来，出现了许多可用于垂体肿瘤的分子学新技术。在垂体腺瘤的实验室研究中，原位杂交和其他分子技术的使用，使我们能够多方面地了解这些肿瘤的内分泌学特点及其细胞功能。尽管目前这些技术主要用于科研，但是它们在常规诊断中的运用也为期不远。

垂体腺瘤的临床分为两大类：根据是否出现内分泌症状，分为临床功能性腺瘤和临床无功能性腺瘤。大部分腺瘤属于功能性肿瘤，包括分泌 PRL、GH、ACTH 的肿瘤[19]（表17.3）。但是，大约 1/3 的垂体腺瘤既无临床表现，也无激素分泌过多的生化证据[20]。这些临床无功能性腺瘤通常仅出现局部肿块所致的症状，诸如头痛、颅神经功能缺陷（包括视野紊乱），以及由于垂体柄受压所致的轻度高催乳素血症（所谓的*垂体柄效应*）。

根据肿瘤的大小及其大体解剖学特点，腺瘤可分为微腺瘤（肿瘤直径 <1cm）和大腺瘤（肿瘤直径 > 1cm）(图17.4)。巨大腺瘤(肿瘤直径 > 4cm)很罕见。大腺瘤易于出现持续性鞍上延伸、大体浸润和复发。在临床实践中，最常采用的是 Hardy 提出的影像学分类[21]。

形态学上，垂体腺瘤有多种分类方法。主要依据病理医师所采用的形态学方法。因不能识别具体的腺瘤类型，那些根据嗜酸性、嗜碱性和嫌色性等染色特点作为主要分类原则的做法目前已过时。垂体腺瘤具有多种不同的生长方式（弥漫性、乳头状、梁状等）（图17.5），可出现在任何一型垂体腺瘤中。尽管这些组织学特点无预后意义，但是对各种病变的识别有助于垂体腺瘤的鉴

表17.3	各类垂体腺瘤的发生频率：Virginia大学，1992—2002年（共计1184例）
垂体腺瘤类型	病变所占比例（%）
PRL-分泌腺瘤	15
GH-分泌腺瘤	17
GH和PRL共分泌腺瘤	2
ACTH分泌腺瘤[a]	29
促性腺激素腺瘤	17
裸细胞腺瘤	19
TSH-分泌腺瘤	1

[a] 包括无症状的促肾上腺皮质激素细胞腺瘤。

PRL：催乳素；GH：生长激素；ACTH：促肾上腺皮质激素；TSH：促甲状腺激素。

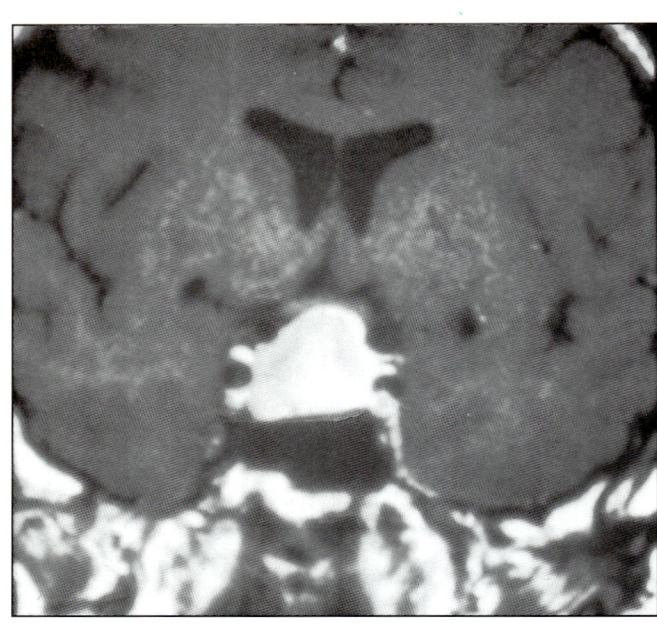

图17.4 垂体腺瘤。核磁共振T1相增强后显示一个大的腺瘤压迫视神经交叉。

别诊断。通过免疫组化可以获得肿瘤所分泌激素的有用信息[22]。虽然免疫组化是一种好的分类方法，但它仍无法鉴别出许多有临床预后意义的特殊肿瘤亚型。为了进行更为精确的分类，需要分析腺瘤的超微结构[23]。这里所讨论的垂体腺瘤的不同类型是根据免疫组化表型和最重要的超微结构特征来分类的。本章将遵循WHO最近颁布的垂体肿瘤分类标准[24]。

垂体腺瘤和癌的侵袭性与增殖潜能

垂体腺瘤或呈膨胀性生长（图17.6），或向邻近结构侵袭（图17.7和17.8）。前者肿瘤通常较小，边界清晰，且局限于蝶鞍区。侵袭性腺瘤则生长迅速，并可播散至邻近组织，如蝶窦、海绵窦（图17.7），某些病例亦可播散至大脑[25,26]。

从垂体腺瘤发展成侵袭性较强肿瘤的机制尚不完全清楚，在绝大多数肿瘤中，尚未证实从良性腺瘤至侵袭性腺瘤和癌是一种连续性增生过程。垂体腺瘤出现局部侵犯和侵及邻近结构似乎与其组织学特点无关。侵袭性腺瘤不一定出现肿瘤侵袭的组织学特点，例如多形性、核异型性和核分裂象增多等表现。虽然临床上功能性腺瘤和无功能性腺瘤均可表现为侵袭性腺瘤，但是大体侵犯（gross invasion）仍多见于功能性腺瘤[25,26]。另一方面，侵袭性和肿瘤大小有关，大腺瘤发生侵袭的几率高于微腺瘤[26]。

垂体腺瘤的增殖活性研究是用来鉴别侵袭性与惰性（良性）垂体腺瘤的辅助手段（图17.9）[27-31]。这些研究表明，大多数肿瘤生长较为缓慢，多数增殖指数低于3%。临床上功能性腺瘤的增殖指数明显高于无功能腺瘤[26,28]。侵袭性腺瘤和垂体癌的增殖指数明显高于非侵袭性腺瘤[27,29]。虽然这些数据表明，Ki-67（MIB1）的表达与垂体肿瘤的侵袭性之间存在密切关系，但仍未发现增殖指数与肿瘤复发之间存在明显关系[28,30,31]。因此，建议将核分裂活性高和（或）Ki-67标记指数高的垂体腺瘤诊断为*非典型腺瘤*，需要密切随访[32]。

垂体癌 Pituitary carcinomas

垂体癌非常少见，不足所有垂体肿瘤的1%。垂体癌的确诊主要依据出现脑脊髓或系统性转移[32]。多数病例具有内分泌功能，其中最常见的是分泌PRL的肿瘤，其次是分泌ACTH的肿瘤[33,34]。无功能癌较为罕见[35]。许多垂体癌的初始病程与良性垂体腺瘤没有差别。随着病程进展，出现多次局部复发，之后是转移播散。少数情况下，某些垂体癌的行为提示一开始就是恶性。近期的研究表明几乎所有的垂体癌最初都表现为侵袭性大腺瘤，形态学有非典型性，核分裂活性高，增殖指数高[34]。此外，与垂体腺瘤不同，垂体癌常表现p53蛋白的过表达（见下文）[34]。目前，识别这些侵袭性较高的肿瘤成为病理医生的一种挑战。

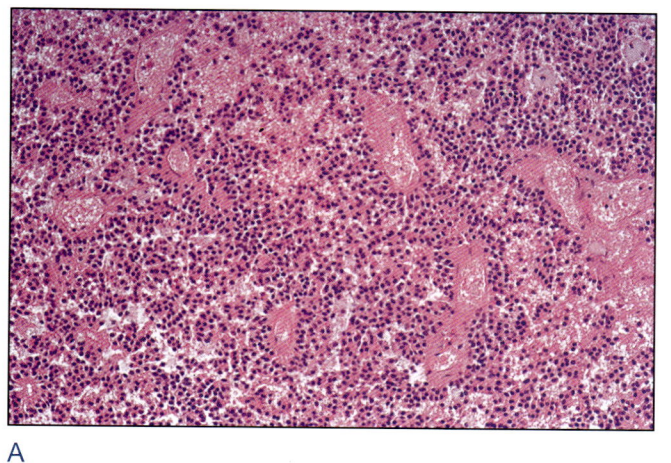

A

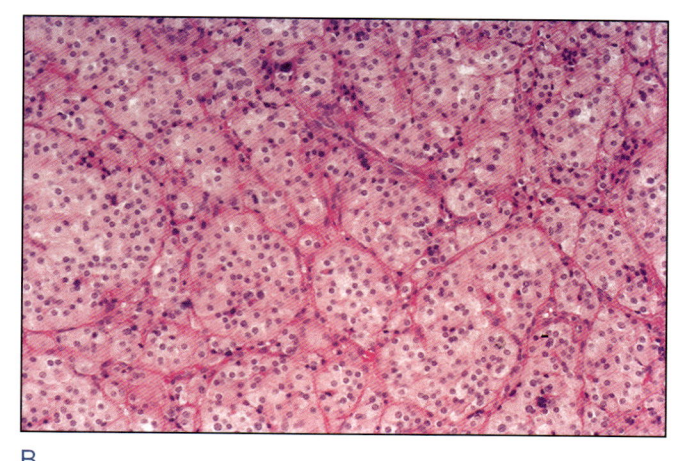

B

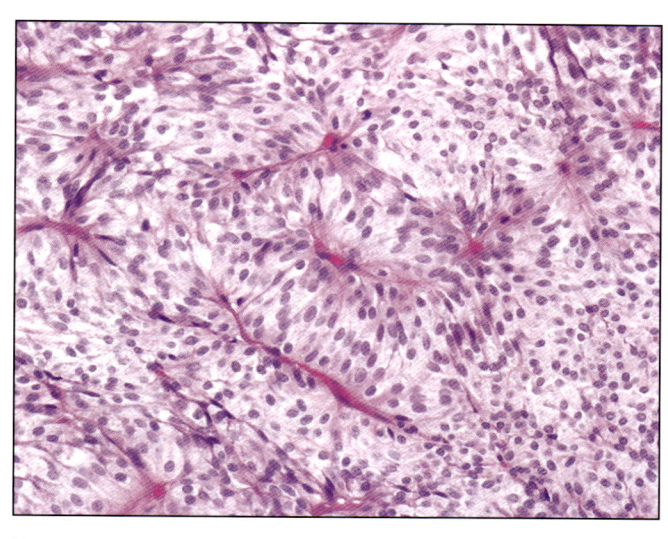

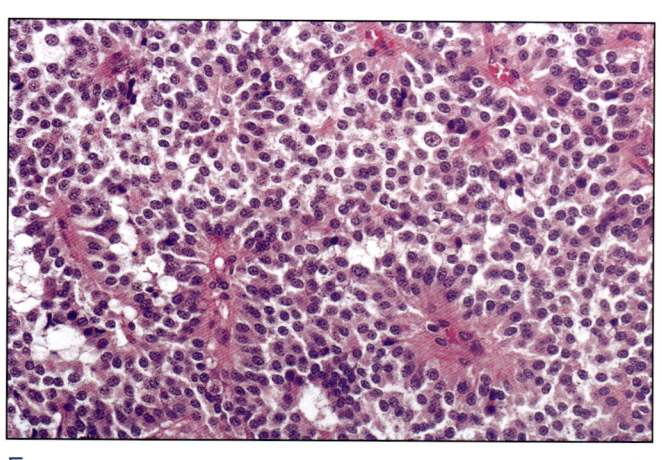

C

D

E

图17.5 垂体腺瘤可出现多种组织学生长形态。（A）乳头状生长；（B）腺泡状生长；（C）梁状生长；（D）梭形细胞形态；（E）乳头状垂体腺瘤的高倍观。

垂体腺瘤的发病机制

尽管进行了较为详尽的研究，但是目前对于人类垂体肿瘤的发病机制和演进过程所知甚少。垂体腺瘤的发生似乎是一个多因素、多步骤过程，其中内分泌因素、遗传易感性和特定的体细胞突变可能均参与了这一过程。在大量垂体腺瘤中通过 X 染色体失活分析发现大多数肿瘤均为单克隆起源[36-39]。

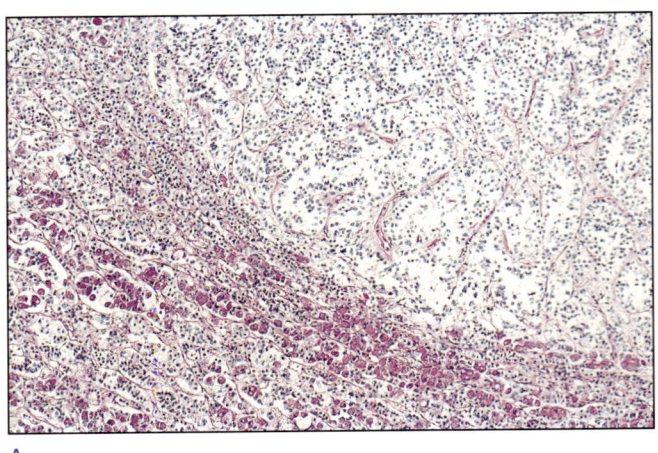
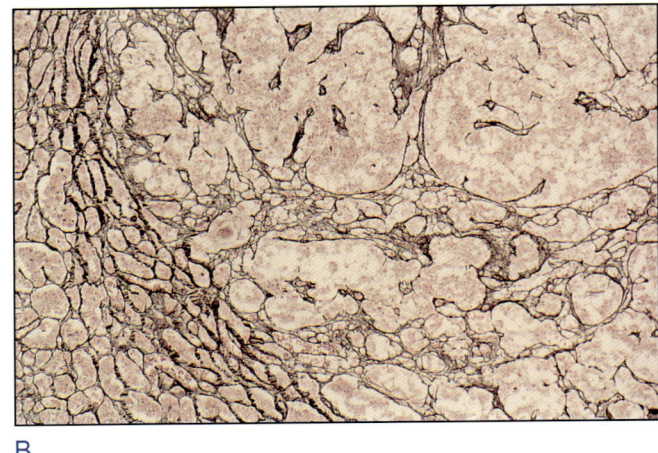

图17.6 垂体腺瘤压迫残留垂体。（A）过碘酸-Schiff(PAS)染色显示腺瘤比正常垂体的细胞成分单一。（B）网织纤维染色显示：与邻近的正常腺体比较，腺瘤的网织纤维崩解。

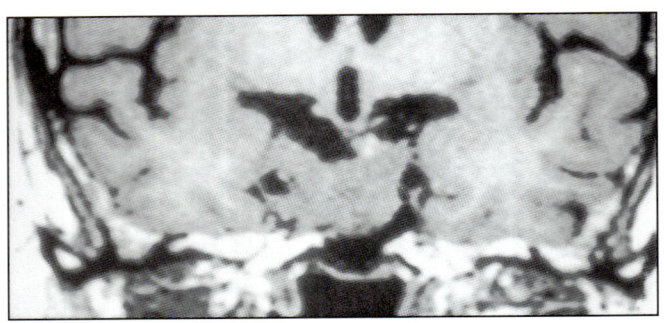

图17.7 侵袭性垂体腺瘤。核磁共振T1相增强后显示垂体腺瘤侵及海绵窦。

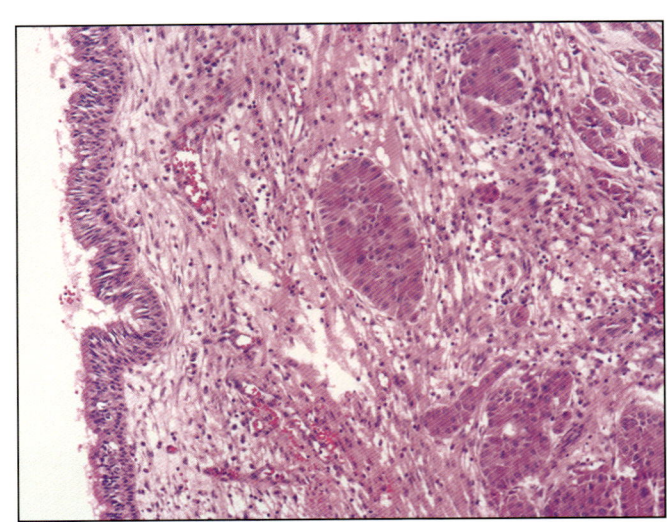

图17.8 垂体腺瘤侵及垂体邻近结构。侵袭性腺瘤侵及黏膜下窦。

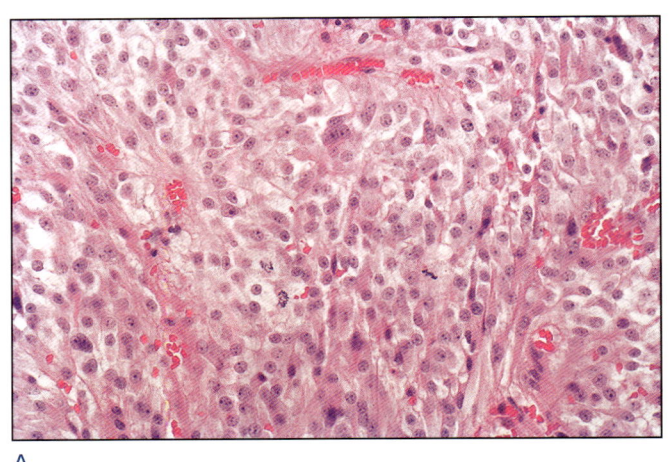
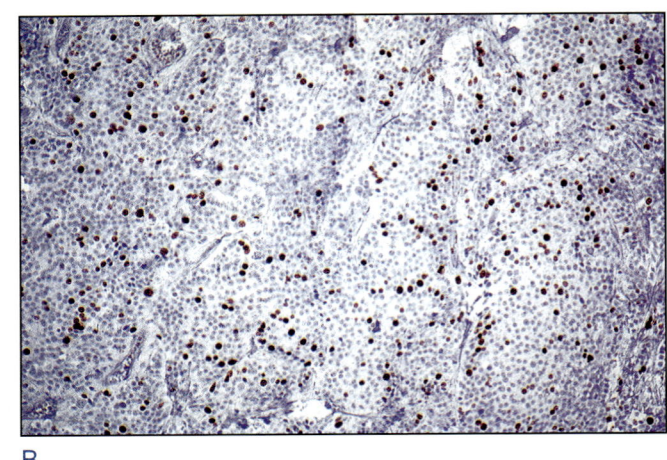

图17.9 垂体腺瘤的增殖潜能。（A）本例为复发的促肾上腺皮质激素分泌腺瘤，HE染色易见核分裂象。（B）Ki-67免疫组化显示高增殖指数。

至今，垂体腺瘤中可见两种具有明显特征的遗传学异常。第一种与染色体11q13上的肿瘤抑制基因等位缺失有关，也就是MEN1的遗传学缺陷[40]。MEN1综合征患者的11q13缺失存在于垂体腺瘤中[41,42]，也常见于甲状旁腺增生和胰腺内分泌肿瘤等其他病症中。仅有3%的垂体腺瘤患者具有MEN1背景，且尚未发现MEN1基因在散发性垂体腺瘤中起主要作用。虽然10%~20%的散发性垂体腺瘤患者存在11q13的杂合性缺失，提示该部位可能存在肿瘤抑制基因[41-45]，但MEN1的体细胞突变率非常低（大约2%）[46]。以上发现提示MEN1基因似乎在散发性垂体腺瘤中不起主要作用。

垂体腺瘤中第二种常见的基因突变是gsp癌基因突变，这是一种G蛋白α亚单位的点突变（$G_s\alpha$）[47,48]。在生长激素细胞中，$G_s\alpha$是腺苷酸环化酶的刺激蛋白，与细胞膜上的生长激素释放激素（GH-releasing hormone，GHRH）受体偶联。GHRH诱导GH基因转录，导致GH的产生、分泌以及生长激素细胞的增殖。突变的$G_s\alpha$蛋白抑制了三磷酸鸟苷的活性，使腺苷酸环化酶系统保持连续的开启状态，类似于细胞膜上的GHRH激素信号效应。gsp突变可见于大约40%的GH分泌腺瘤[43,48-50]。虽然与没有gsp突变的GH分泌肿瘤相比，具有gsp突变的GH分泌腺瘤在临床和生化检查上有所不同，但这些肿瘤在形态学上并无差异[50]。gsp癌基因突变在其他垂体肿瘤亚型中很少见，仅见于10%的临床无功能垂体腺瘤和5%的促肾上腺皮质激素细胞腺瘤中[50]。gsp基因的激活性突变也见于McCune-Albright综合征，该综合征的特点是生长激素细胞的增生以及骨组织中出现多处纤维性异型增生[51]。

还有许多癌基因和肿瘤抑制基因可能在垂体肿瘤的发生过程中起作用。垂体肿瘤转化基因（pituitary tumor-transforming gene，PTTG）转录一种可在有丝分裂、细胞转化以及DNA修复和基因调控过程中发挥作用的多功能蛋白。在人类中已发现三种同源基因：（1）位于染色体5q33上的PTTG1；（2）位于染色体4p12上的PTTG2；（3）位于染色体8q22上的PTTG3[52]。在包括垂体在内的绝大多数正常人体组织中，PTTG蛋白表达水平均较低。然而，在包括垂体腺瘤在内的多种实体瘤中，其表达则较高[53]。PTTG表达可见于包括功能性和无功能性腺瘤在内的各种垂体腺瘤亚型[54-56]。通过细胞周期依赖激酶所致的PTTG磷酸化、与生长因子（特别是纤维母细胞生长因子2）的相互作用以及刺激血管生成等多种机制，PTTG参与了垂体肿瘤的始动和演进过程[56]。

在3例远处转移的垂体癌[51,57]和1例侵袭性催乳素瘤中[58]检测到了H-ras原癌基因的点突变。

肿瘤抑制基因TP53突变是人类癌症中最常见的遗传学改变。但是，TP53基因突变在垂体肿瘤的发生过程中似乎未起到重要作用。在功能性腺瘤、无功能腺瘤、垂体癌及其转移灶中，均未发现TP53基因突变和染色体17p缺失[57,59]。然而，采用针对TP53基因产物的免疫组化研究表明，在许多高度侵袭性腺瘤和癌中，可以见到p53蛋白的过表达，提示可能有基因突变之外的其他机制参与了蛋白的过表达[60]。p53蛋白过表达在某些复发性和侵袭性腺瘤中的意义仍不明确。

通过对大量腺瘤的检测，均未发现肿瘤抑制基因RB的突变[61,62]。但是，在某些高侵袭性腺瘤和垂体癌中，可以见到RB的等位基因缺失[63]。综上所述，这些结果提示虽然PTTG、H-ras、RB以及TP53基因点突变并未直接参与垂体肿瘤的发生，但这些癌基因和抑癌基因可能在垂体癌的进展和转移过程中发挥了重要作用。

通过异常的自分泌和旁分泌机制，许多生长因子和下丘脑营养因子也参与了垂体肿瘤的生长维持（参见Lloyd等的综述[32]）。

术中会诊和标本处理
Intraoperative consultation and specimen handling

在外科手术开始前，即应对垂体腺瘤进行评估。必须由病理医师、内分泌医师、神经放射学医师及神经外科医师共同组成一个工作密切相关的团队，才能确保正确地获取标本并对临床病理关系进行充分评估。术中会诊诊断垂体腺瘤的价值有限。尽管术中会诊能正确识别腺瘤组织，但它却不能确定腺瘤的亚型，也不能明确手术切缘的情况和肿瘤的侵犯程度。较之冰冻切片，细胞学涂片或印片可以更好地反映细胞学细节。腺瘤通常比正常垂体细胞成分更为单一（图17.10）。此外，涂片和印片也能显示乳头和钙化等组织排列。更重要的是，涂片可以避免小标本在冰冻过程中出现的假象。

正确的组织固定和处理对于获取可靠的病理结果至关重要。应在手术室接收新鲜标本（图17.11）。组织碎块应当适当固定以备必要的超微结构检查，剩余的标本应立即进行甲醛溶液固定，用于常规石蜡包埋和切片。如果组织较多，可冻存一部分以备进一步的生物化学和分子学研究。除了HE染色切片外，还应同时进行连续切片用于网织纤维银染和所分泌垂体激

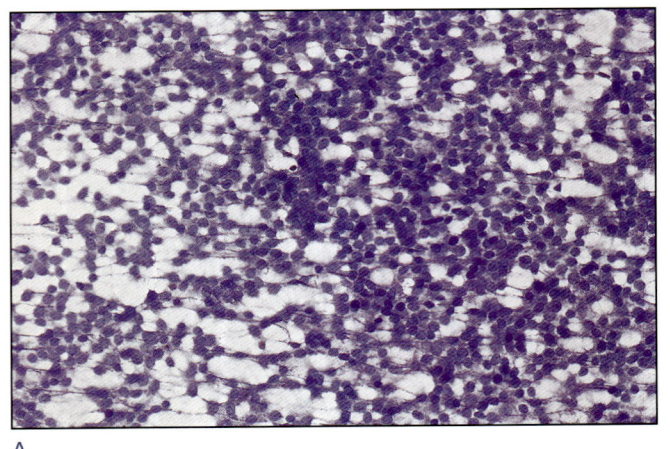

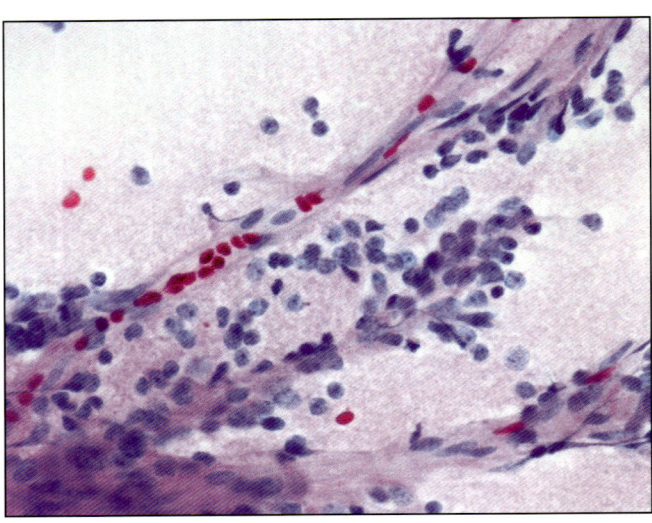

图17.10 垂体腺瘤的术中印片。（A）垂体腺瘤的术中印片Morris染色显示颗粒性背景中均匀的细胞成分。（B）印片上容易看到乳头状结构。

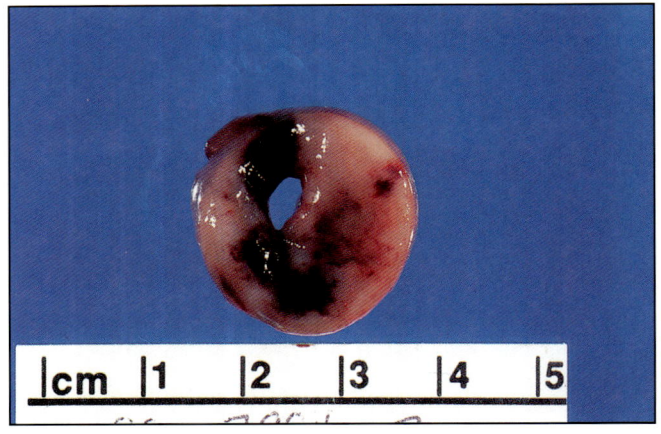

图17.11 大腺瘤的大体图像显示质软、褐色的垂体腺瘤。常可见由于手术操作造成的局灶急性出血区。

素的免疫组化染色。在大型医院或研究机构，应该常备完整的垂体分泌激素的抗体谱系。这一谱系包括GH、PRL、ACTH、β-LH、β-FSH、β-TSH和糖蛋白α亚单位（α-SU）。由于经济条件所限，许多实验室可能仅根据临床背景，选择某些抗体进行免疫染色。虽然免疫组化可针对细胞贮存的相应激素发生反应，但它与激素合成水平和功能未必有关。电镜在腺瘤评估中起重要作用。许多与诊断有关的形态学特点仅在超微结构分析中可以见到（参见下文不同的肿瘤亚型）。

腺瘤的类型

催乳素分泌腺瘤
Prolactin-secreting adenomas

催乳素分泌肿瘤，亦称催乳素瘤，占功能性垂体腺瘤的近80%和全部垂体腺瘤的40%～50%[64,65]。但是，由于此类肿瘤易于通过多巴胺激动剂进行药物控制，需行外科手术进行治疗的催乳素瘤已越来越少。在本研究所里，催乳素瘤占肿瘤标本的15%（表17.3）。大多催乳素瘤为微腺瘤，好发于生育年龄妇女，常表现为闭经、溢乳和不孕[64]。大腺瘤（肿瘤>1cm）仅发生于30%的高催乳素血症妇女[66]。相反，在男性和老年女性，催乳素瘤多为大腺瘤，症状多为头痛、神经功能障碍以及视力减退[67]。在男性，阳痿和性欲减退是高催乳素血症的常见症状。在垂体腺瘤，出现持续性高催乳素血症和神经影像学改变，即可以确诊催乳素瘤[2,64]。

在光镜下，肿瘤细胞大小中等，胞浆嫌色性或轻度嗜酸性，核呈椭圆形，位于细胞中央，可见小核仁（图17.12）。大约10%～20%的病例可见不同程度的钙化，有时可以非常明显，形成所谓的"垂体石"（图17.13）[68]。催乳素瘤亦可产生淀粉样物质，形成小的透明小体。钙化和淀粉样小体并非催乳素瘤所特有，但较之其他垂体腺瘤更常见[68,69]。

免疫组化染色显示明确的PRL阳性。染色形态很有特征，位于核周部，呈点状分布（图17.14）。某些作者将这种免疫反应形态命名为"Golgi"模式，反映出激素主要位于Golgi复合体中[68]。

目前，大多数采用手术治疗的催乳素瘤患者，术前均进行不同程度的多巴胺激动剂治疗。因此，大部分手术标本中可见药物产生的形态学影响。这些药物造成催乳素细胞萎缩，导致肿瘤缩小[64]。肿瘤细胞变小，胞浆收缩，核浓染[70,71]。此外，长期用药可导致不同程度的

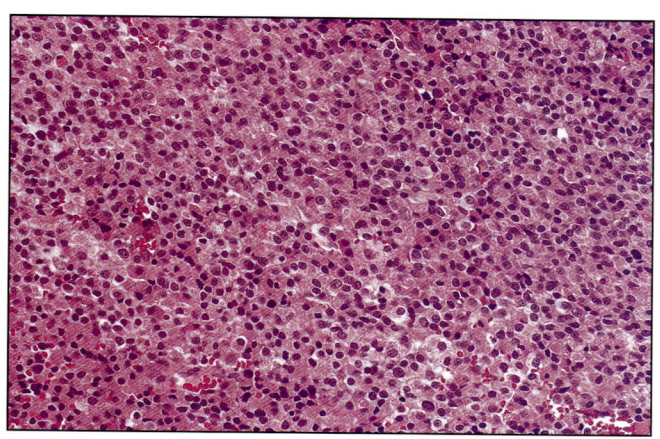

图17.12 催乳素（PRL）分泌腺瘤。PRL细胞腺瘤显示嫌色性胞浆，核位于中央，染色质细腻。

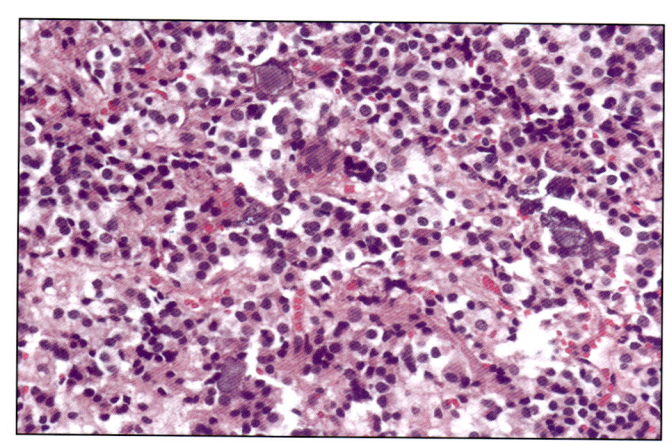

图17.13 催乳素（PRL）分泌腺瘤。这些肿瘤中常可见到微小钙化。

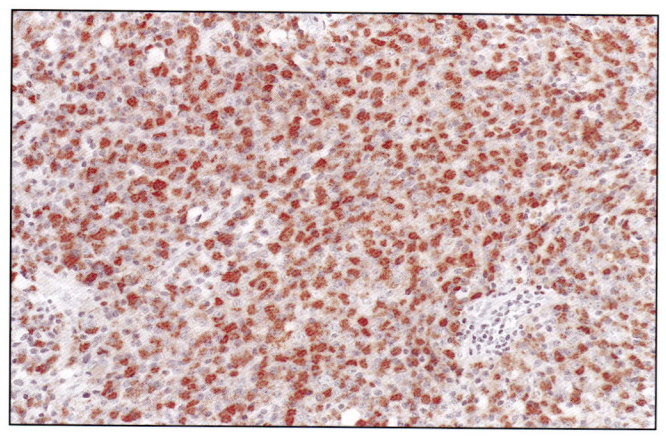

图17.14 催乳素（PRL）分泌腺瘤。核周区常可见特有的PRL免疫反应阳性。

血管周和肿瘤间质纤维化（图17.15）。

催乳素瘤的超微结构很具有特征性[19]。PRL细胞腺瘤可分为致密颗粒型和稀疏颗粒型。稀疏颗粒型PRL细胞腺瘤是最常见的肿瘤类型，类似于正常垂体中正在分泌催乳素的细胞。腺瘤细胞的特点是具有明显的粗面内质网、明显的高尔基复合体和少量小的（150~300nm）分泌颗粒（图17.16）。此类肿瘤的典型表现是错位胞外分泌（misplaced exocytosis），也就是颗粒从细胞侧面外泌。依靠电镜诊断PRL细胞腺瘤存在争议，因为区分这两种腺瘤亚型并无临床价值[72]。

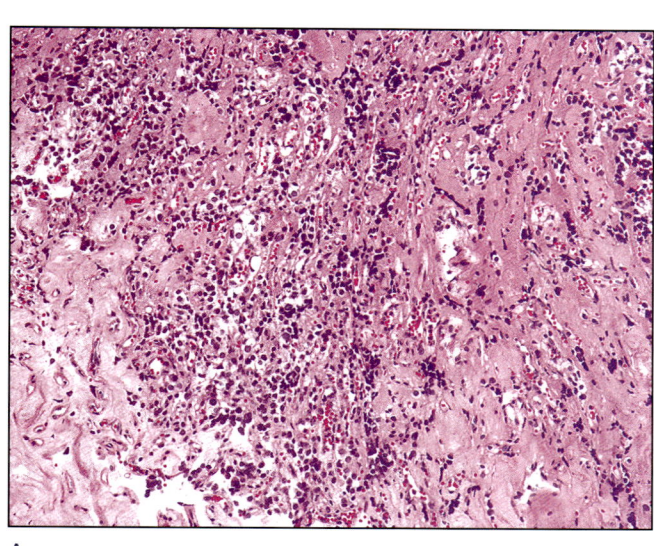

A

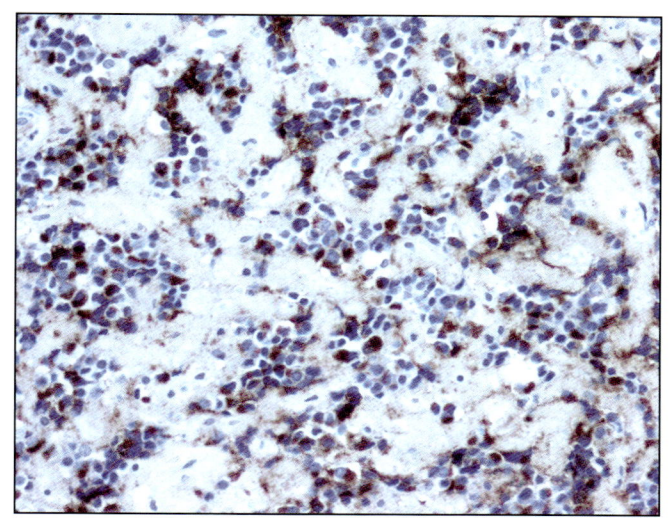

B

图17.15 催乳素（PRL）分泌腺瘤。（A）经药物治疗后，PRL细胞腺瘤显示肿瘤细胞萎缩和间质纤维化。（B）虽然经过了治疗，肿瘤细胞中仍可见局灶的PRL免疫反应性。

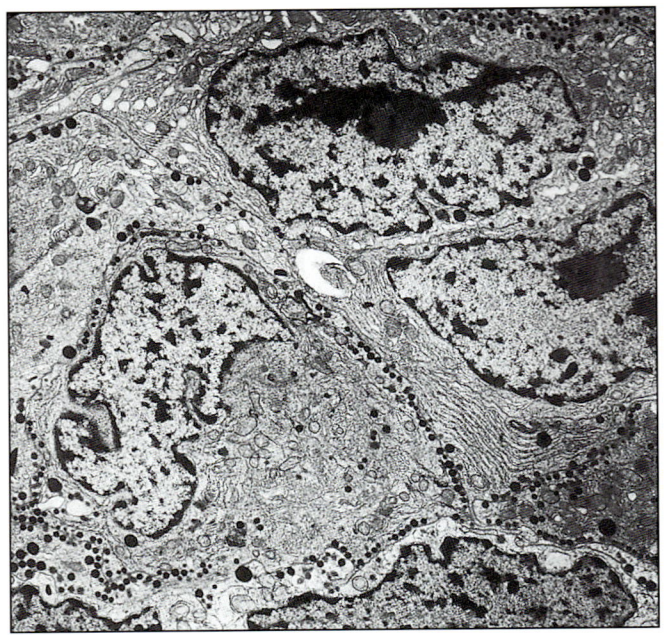

图17.16 催乳素（PRL）分泌腺瘤的超微结构。稀疏颗粒型PRL细胞腺瘤中可见明显的粗面内质网和高尔基复合体，以及散在的分泌颗粒。

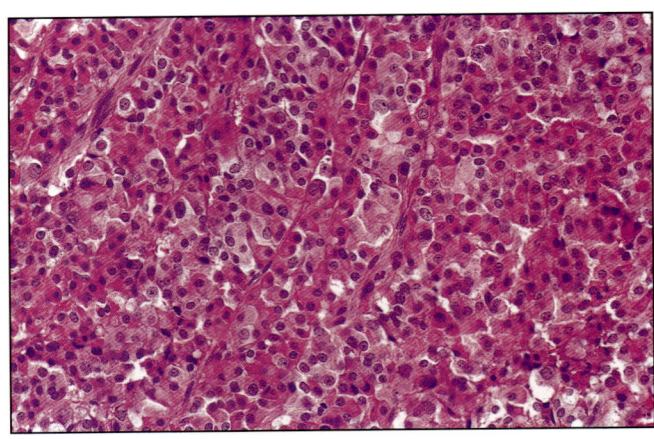

图17.17 生长激素（GH）分泌腺瘤。GH细胞腺瘤显示嗜酸性、颗粒状胞浆，核位于中央，有明显的核仁。

生长激素分泌腺瘤
Growth hormone-secreting adenomas

大约20%的垂体腺瘤显示与GH分泌有关的临床或免疫组化证据。GH分泌腺瘤常伴有血浆GH和胰岛素样生长因子I（IGF-I）的高水平，并可有肢端肥大和巨人症的症状和体征[2]。肢端肥大症的发生无性别差异，平均诊断年龄是40～45岁。症状通常进展缓慢，至诊断时的平均病程大约为7～10年[73]。少数情况下，GH的过度分泌可导致巨人症，主要见于儿童和青少年骨骺闭合前发生该病的情况。大多数肢端肥大症患者初诊时表现为大腺瘤，多数出现鞍上扩张和鞍旁浸润[74]。因而，有巨大肿瘤的患者也常出现包括头痛和视野缺陷在内的肿瘤膨胀所致的继发症状。大约30%～50%的病人可出现PRL和GH联合分泌，导致高催乳素血症的症状和体征[74,75]。GH/PRL混合分泌型肿瘤将在下一章节中讨论。

在HE染色切片，GH分泌腺瘤呈嗜酸性或嫌色性。这种组织形态的不同反映了胞浆中分泌颗粒数量的不同。在嗜酸性腺瘤中，细胞胞浆中颗粒相对较多，超微结构水平可见大量的分泌颗粒（图17.17）。细胞核多位于中央，呈椭圆形，有明显的核仁。常见细胞核多形性和多核细胞。在分泌颗粒较少的肿瘤，即所谓的稀疏颗粒型GH细胞腺瘤中（见下文），胞浆呈嫌色性，细胞核偏心（图17.18）。胞浆中可见核旁嗜酸性结构，即出

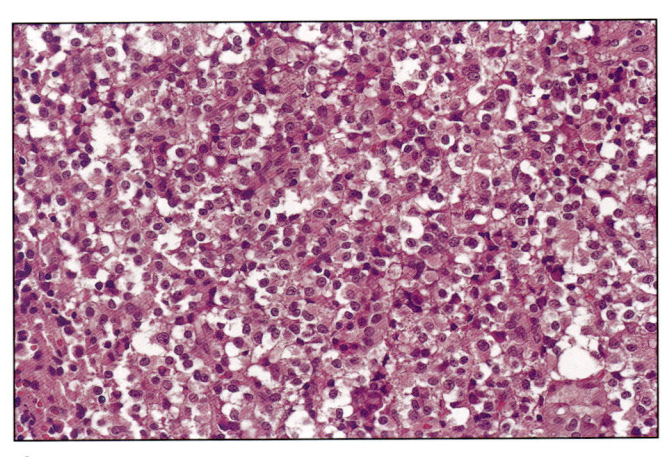

A

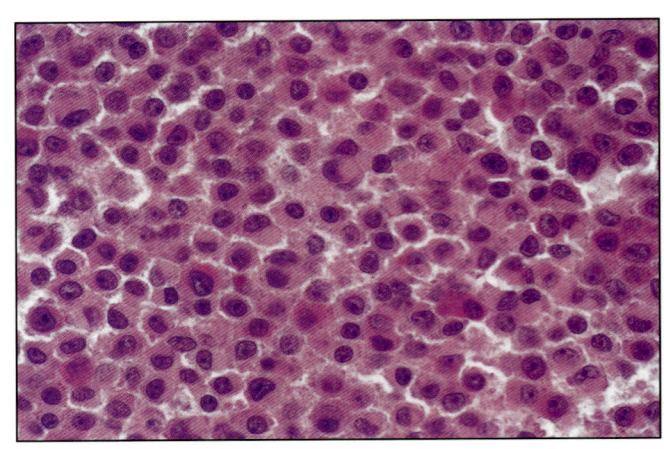

B

图17.18 生长激素（GH）分泌腺瘤。（A）呈嫌色性外观的GH细胞腺瘤。（B）高倍镜下可见稀疏颗粒型GH细胞腺瘤核周的"纤维性小体"。

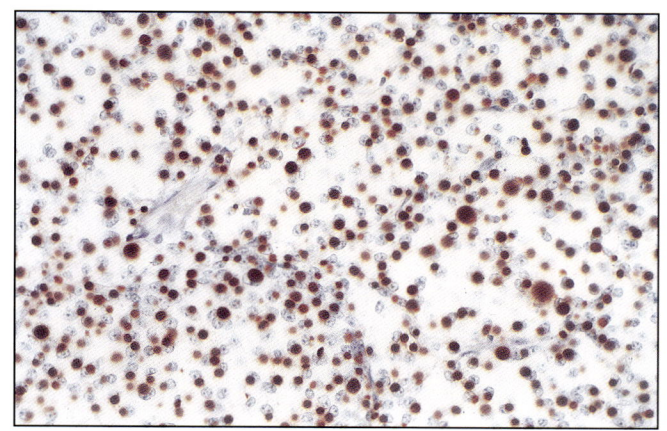

图17.19 生长激素分泌腺瘤。在稀疏颗粒型肿瘤中，细胞角蛋白免疫组化染色显示核周"纤维性"小体。

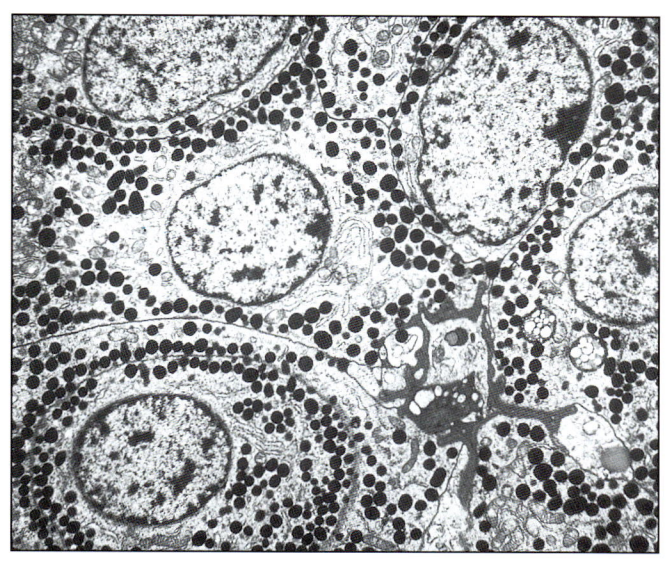

图17.20 生长激素（GH）分泌腺瘤的超微结构。本例为致密颗粒型GH细胞腺瘤，可见分化成熟的细胞器及丰富的大分泌颗粒。

现所谓的"纤维性小体"。这些结构在超微结构水平表现为中间丝和微管聚集。

免疫组化染色显示不同程度的GH阳性反应。在嗜酸性腺瘤，肿瘤弥漫表达GH，占据整个肿瘤细胞胞浆。在大多数嗜酸性腺瘤，GH阳性弥漫分布于整个肿瘤中。相反，在嫌色性肿瘤，GH染色多呈局灶性，阳性表达主要局限于核周区，与催乳素瘤中所见的Golgi模式相似。此外，在稀疏颗粒腺瘤中，其"纤维性"小体多呈细胞角蛋白强阳性表达（图17.19）[76]。许多GH分泌腺瘤可出现其他垂体激素继发性阳性表达[74,77]。可见局灶性PRL免疫组化阳性表达，尽管患者并未在临床或生化检查上见到高催乳素血症证据。同样，在许多GH分泌腺瘤中可出现糖蛋白激素β-FSH、β-LH、α-SU的免疫阳性反应，偶尔可见β-TSH的阳性反应。除了特征明显的混合性GH/PRL分泌腺瘤（见下文）之外，大多数此类病例的多种激素分化不产生临床症状。

GH细胞腺瘤分两个亚型，致密颗粒型和稀疏颗粒型腺瘤，通过超微结构分析很容易区分[19]。致密颗粒型GH细胞腺瘤由类似于垂体正常生长激素细胞的腺瘤细胞构成（图17.20），其特点是有发育完善的粗面内质网系统、明显的Golgi复合体和大量的分泌性大颗粒（300～600nm）。稀疏颗粒型GH细胞腺瘤不同于非肿瘤性生长激素细胞（图17.21）。此类细胞仅有中等量的粗面内质网和Golgi膜，并有少量的小分泌颗粒（100～250nm）。此类腺瘤最明显的特征是出现"纤维性小体"，这些小体由中间丝和管状滑面内质网构成。

通过电镜区分两类GH细胞腺瘤并非完全必要。因为根据光镜特征和辅助性免疫组化染色即可对二者进行区分。加入细胞角蛋白免疫组化染色即可证实"纤维性小体"的存在。区分这两种GH细胞腺瘤亚型的临床意义目前仍有争议。较致密颗粒型GH细胞腺瘤而言，稀

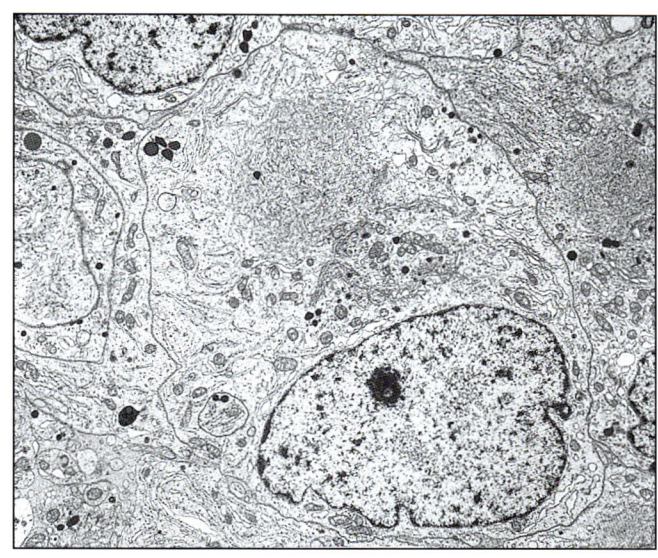

图17.21 生长激素（GH）分泌腺瘤的超微结构。图例所示为一稀疏颗粒型GH细胞，可见少量的分泌颗粒及特征性的"纤维性小体"。

疏颗粒型GH细胞腺瘤似乎更具侵袭性生物学行为[78,79]。作者所在单位对随诊的90例肢端肥大症患者的研究表明，虽然这两种GH分泌腺瘤亚型的治愈率和生存期无明显差异，但稀疏颗粒型腺瘤较易出现局部浸润[74]。

同催乳素瘤一样，采用长效生长抑素类似物[主要是奥曲肽(octreotide)]对肢端肥大症进行药物内分泌治疗已非常普遍[2,80]。这些药物可能会改变GH分泌腺瘤

的形态；其中最常见的是出现不同程度的血管周及间质纤维化[81,82]。在超微结构水平，可见分泌颗粒的大小/数目增加和溶酶体激活。与溴隐亭(bromocriptine)效应不同，这些治疗后的肿瘤较少见到因粗面内质网和Golgi膜退化所致的细胞体积缩小。

混合性 GH-PRL 分泌腺瘤
Mixed GH/PRL-secreting adenomas

如前所述，很大一部分GH分泌腺瘤也同时分泌PRL。在本单位，大约一半的手术切除GH分泌腺瘤患者同时出现肢端肥大症和高催乳素血症[74]。这组腺瘤可分为三种形态学不同的肿瘤亚型，它们均可同时见到GH和PRL的分泌：混合性GH细胞/PRL细胞腺瘤(the mixed GH-cell/PRL-cell adenoma)、催乳素生长激素细胞腺瘤（mammosomatotroph cell adenoma）和嗜酸性干细胞腺瘤(acidophilic stem cell adenoma)[74,83-86]。该肿瘤分类是建立在对肿瘤组织进行详尽的免疫组化和超微结构检查基础之上，这种划分具有临床及预后意义。与嗜酸性干细胞腺瘤相比，混合性GH细胞/PRL细胞腺瘤和催乳素生长激素细胞腺瘤的生长较为缓慢[84,86]。根据我们的经验，这些混合型肿瘤比单纯的GH分泌腺瘤更具侵袭性，手术治愈率较低[74]。由于这些肿瘤类型具有特点，下面将对每种亚型分别讨论。

混合性 GH 细胞 /PRL 细胞腺瘤
Mixed GH-cell/PRL-cell adenoma

混合性GH细胞/PRL细胞腺瘤的显著临床特点是肢端肥大症，而高催乳素血症的症状和体征通常不明显。形态学与GH分泌腺瘤相似，呈嗜酸性或嫌色性外观（图17.22A）。免疫组化染色显示强度和分布不同的GH和PRL共表达（图17.22B,C）。两种细胞或呈小团灶状分布，或呈弥散性分布。在超微结构水平，此类腺瘤呈双态性，由两类不同的细胞群，即颗粒密度不同的GH细胞和PRL细胞构成（图17.22D）[84,85]。

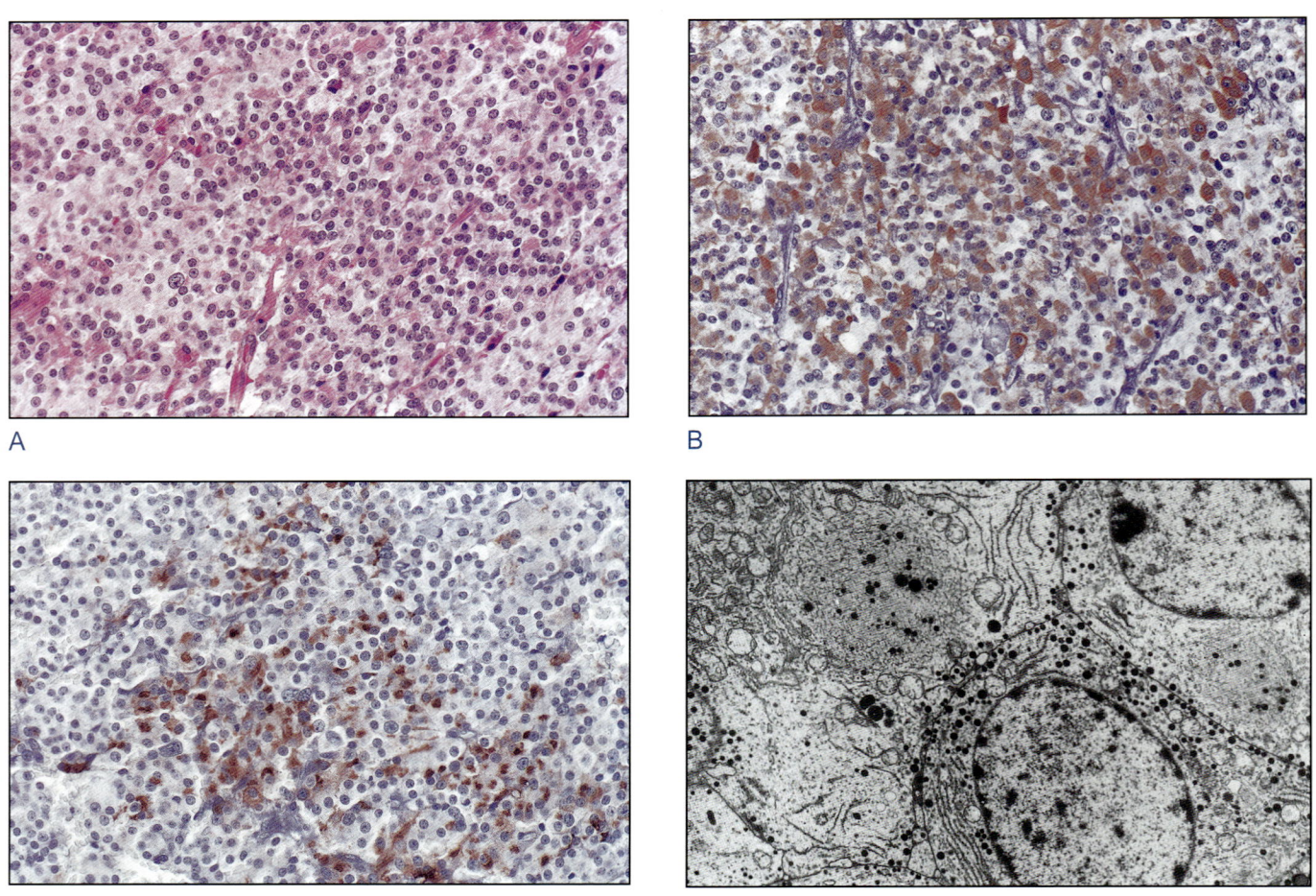

图17.22 混合性生长激素(GH)细胞/催乳素(PRL)细胞腺瘤。（A）HE染色切片无法鉴别混合性GH/PRL腺瘤与GH腺瘤，细胞呈嗜酸性或嫌色性。在不同的细胞群中，肿瘤细胞分别呈GH（B）和PRL（C）阳性表达。（D）超微结构检查证实该肿瘤由两种细胞群构成，分别是PRL细胞（底部）和稀疏颗粒型GH细胞（上部）。注意GH细胞胞浆中的纤维性小体结构。

催乳素生长激素细胞腺瘤
Mammosomatotroph cell adenoma

这类罕见的产生 GH/PRL 的肿瘤不足垂体腺瘤总数的 2%,大约占肢端肥大症相关性肿瘤的 8%[87,88]。与混合型 GH 细胞/PRL 细胞腺瘤相似,这些肿瘤也出现循环中 GH 水平增高和肢端肥大症;而高催乳素血症则较为少见。在组织学上,此类肿瘤 HE 染色呈嗜酸性,免疫组化显示在同一肿瘤细胞胞浆中同时出现 GH 和 PRL 阳性表达(图 17.23A-C)。免疫双标和免疫电镜技术亦证实上述所见[87]。超微结构分析表明,此类肿瘤为高分化腺瘤,由兼备 GH 和 PRL 细胞特点的单形细胞群构成(图 17.23D)[86,87]。肿瘤细胞与致密颗粒型 GH 细胞相似,但其分泌颗粒大小不等(200~2000nm)。可见特征性的颗粒外泌和分泌物的细胞外沉积,这一特点与 PRL 细胞分化一致。

嗜酸性干细胞腺瘤
Acidophilic stem cell adenoma

这种混合型腺瘤亚型极为少见[84,89]。以我们的经验,此类腺瘤仅占 GH/PRL 分泌肿瘤的一小部分[74]。与上述两种亚型不同,此类肿瘤患者多伴有不同程度的高催乳素血症[84]。肢端肥大症较少见,GH 水平多为正常。肿瘤大多为生长迅速的大腺瘤,具有侵袭性特点。由于多数患者具有高催乳素血症的临床特点,注意不要误诊为偏良性的催乳素瘤。光镜下,嗜酸性干细胞腺瘤呈嫌色性,伴局部嗜酸性变。同一细胞胞浆内可见 PRL 和少量 GH 免疫反应性。确诊该腺瘤亚型,需做电镜检

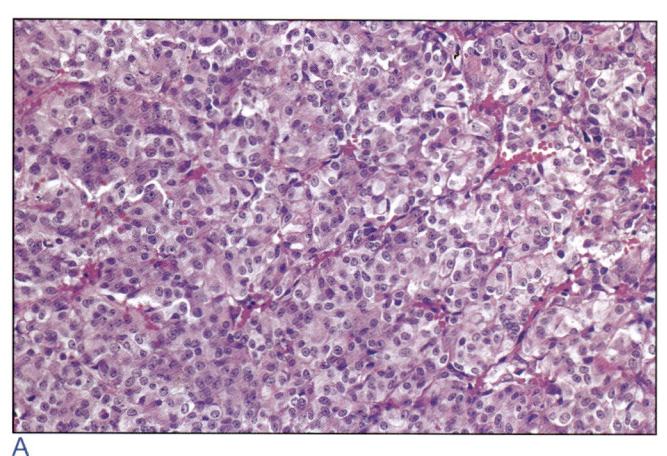

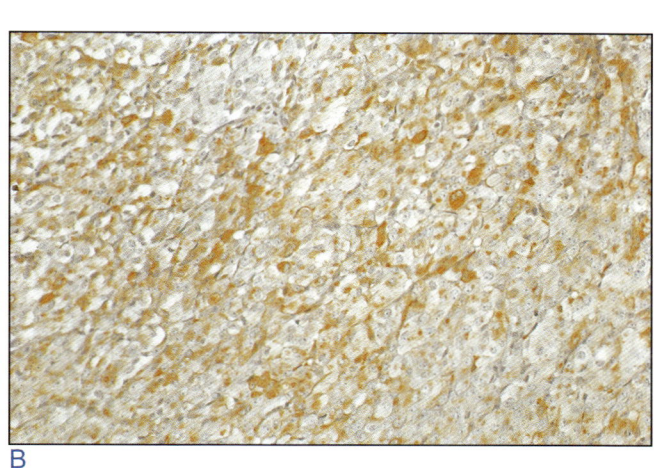

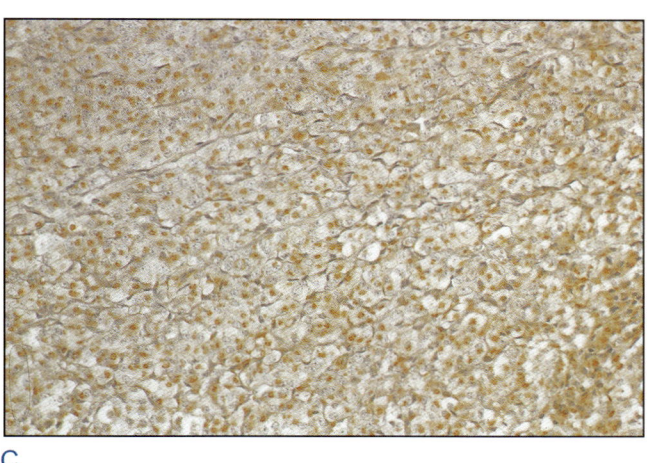

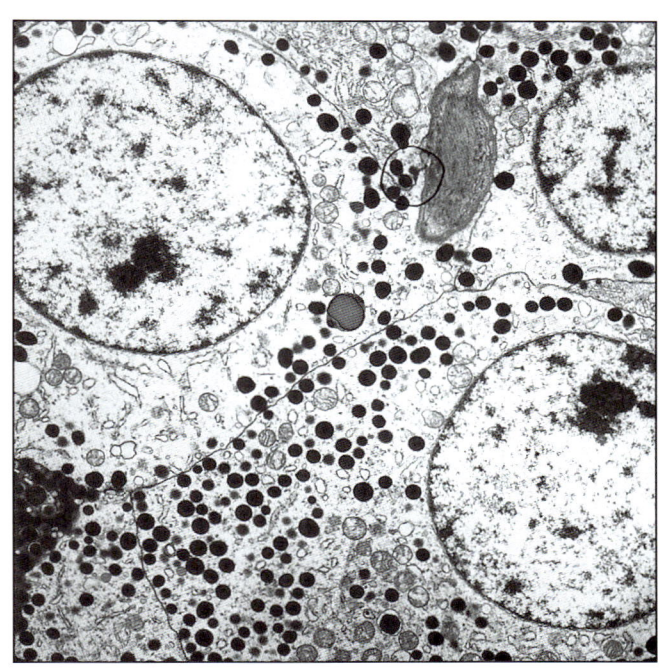

图 17.23 催乳素生长激素细胞腺瘤。(A)与混合性生长激素(GH)细胞/催乳素(PRL)细胞腺瘤相似,催乳素生长激素细胞腺瘤的组织学外观无明显特征。免疫组化显示,GH(B)和 PRL(C)染色阳性同时出现于同一细胞群中。(D)此类肿瘤超微结构所见以单一细胞群为特征,显示大量的分泌颗粒和错位的胞外分泌(圆圈标注)。

查[19,84,89]。电镜下显示发育不成熟的单一细胞群，类似稀疏颗粒型 GH 细胞和 PRL 细胞。多数病例可出现引起嗜酸性变的巨大线粒体。

ACTH 分泌腺瘤
ACTH-secreting adenoma

内源性 Cushing 综合征可由下述两种机制造成[2,90]：

1. ACTH-依赖型，由于垂体 ACTH 分泌过度或存在异位 ACTH 分泌肿瘤。
2. ACTH-非依赖型，由肾上腺肿瘤或其他自主性肾上腺疾病所引起的肾上腺皮质激素自分泌所致。

ACTH 依赖型 Cushing 综合征约占内源性病例的 85%，其中 80% 由垂体 ACTH 分泌腺瘤所致。仅有少数 ACTH 依赖型 Cushing 综合征患者是由分泌促肾上腺皮质激素释放激素（CRH）的肿瘤（主要是类癌）引起[91,92]。习惯上将垂体 ACTH-依赖性疾病称为"Cushing 病"。

ACTH 分泌腺瘤主要由两种亚型构成：

1. 与 Cushing 病或 Nelson 综合征有关的内分泌活性肿瘤[2,93]。
2. 临床无功能肿瘤，也就是所谓的静默型促肾上腺皮质激素细胞腺瘤[94-97]。

与 Cushing 病有关的 ACTH 分泌腺瘤大约占所有腺瘤的 10%～15%。个别情况下，促肾上腺皮质激素细胞增生也可导致 Cushing 病。但是，无论从临床还是病理角度，对这一现象的认识均有分歧。Cushing 病可见于各年龄组，其发病高峰在 30～40 岁之间，女性好发，女性与男性的比例为 8:1[2]。儿童中罕有 Cushing 病发生，其临床过程较凶险，治愈率亦低于成人[98,99]。与成人病例相反，发生于青春期前儿童的 Cushing 病男性比女性常见[100]。

绝大多数 ACTH 分泌腺瘤属微腺瘤，其中 15% 在外科手术时发现有侵犯[25]。尽管多数腺瘤发生于垂体中线部位，亦即所谓的黏液部（mucoid wedge），位于侧翼和后部等邻近垂体后叶的情况也不少见。

ACTH 分泌腺瘤的 HE 染色多呈嗜碱性，PAS 染色强阳性。胞浆呈明显颗粒状，胞核大，染色质粗糙，可见明显核仁。可出现一定程度的核多形性（图 17.24）。细胞边界清晰，彼此呈"铺砖样"排列。乳头状结构常见。有时亦可见腺瘤呈嫌色性形态，胞浆颗粒不明显。

偶尔，束状透明带环绕胞浆，形成"靶细胞"样外观，这种情况即所谓的 Crooke 透明变（hyaline change）（图 17.25）。这些透明带是由细胞角蛋白中间丝积聚所致，似乎是血浆促肾上腺皮质激素水平过高对垂体细胞

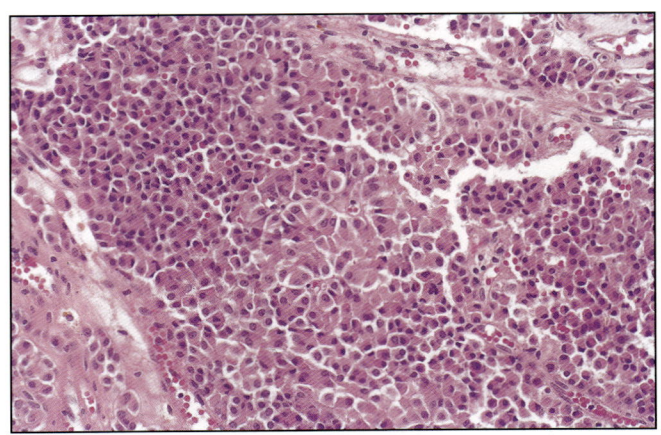

图 17.24　促肾上腺皮质激素细胞腺瘤。由大细胞构成，胞浆呈多角形、嫌色性，并有较大的多形核。有时可见细胞的"铺砖样"排列。

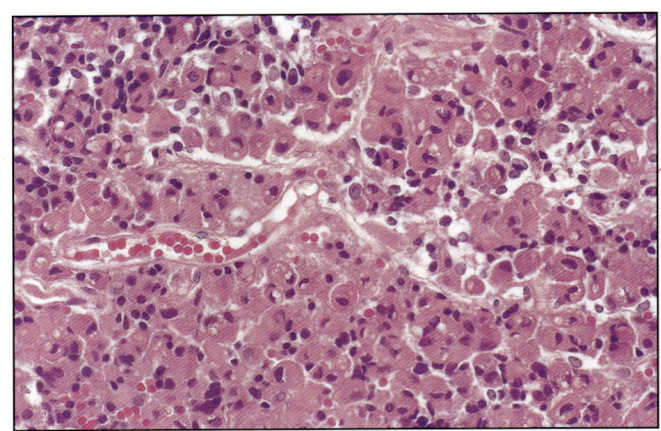

图 17.25　促肾上腺皮质激素细胞腺瘤。胞浆中可见由透明带积聚所形成的特征性 Crooke 透明变(hyaline change)。

的直接影响[101]。Crooke 透明变亦可见于 Cushing 病或其他病理性、医源性肾上腺皮质功能亢进患者的正常垂体。显示广泛透明变的促肾上腺皮质激素细胞腺瘤（即所谓的 Crooke 细胞腺瘤），似乎更易发生局部侵犯和复发[101a]。

发生 Nelson 综合征（特点为皮质激素分泌增多，常规 X 线检查无垂体病变证据，以致实施不恰当的肾上腺切除，之后发现有垂体腺瘤）的腺瘤，其组织学改变与 Cushing 病相关腺瘤类似，但无中间丝积聚，不出现 Crooke 透明变（图 17.26）[19]。

免疫组化研究显示肿瘤中存在不同程度的 ACTH 免疫阳性表达（图 17.27）。此外，还可见到与阿片促黑激素皮质素原（proopiomelanocortin, POMC）前体分子有关的其他肽类，包括 β-促脂素、β-内啡肽以及 α-黑素细胞刺激激素[102]。在临床实践中，这些相关肽类的存在远不如 ACTH 重要。

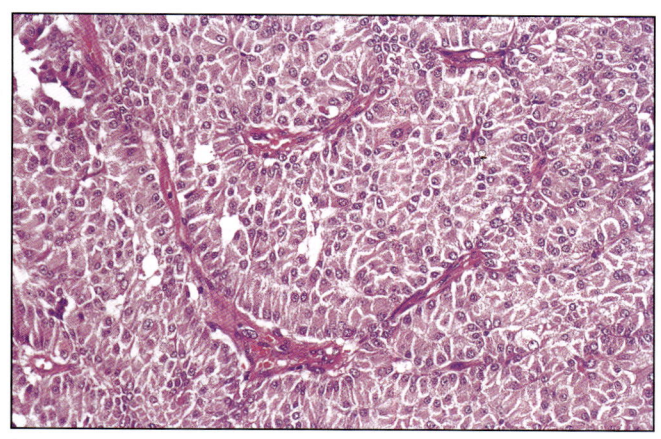

图17.26 Nelson综合征腺瘤。在Nelson综合征患者中，促肾上腺皮质激素细胞腺瘤与Cushing病患者的腺瘤具有相同的组织学外观和免疫组化表现。但在超微结构水平，此类病变缺乏中间丝的积聚。

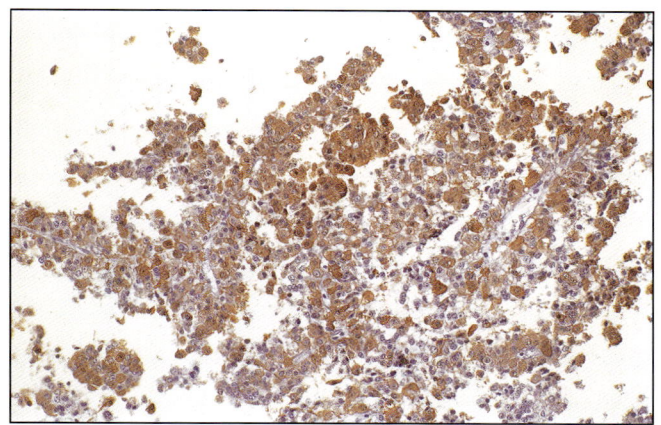

图17.27 促肾上腺皮质激素(ACTH)-细胞腺瘤。在此乳头状促肾上腺皮质激素细胞腺瘤中，ACTH免疫组化染色呈强阳性。

ACTH分泌腺瘤的超微结构特点是细胞分化良好，类似正常促肾上腺皮质激素细胞[19]。表现为发育成熟的细胞器，包括粗面内质网、滑面内质网、明显的Golgi复合体和大量的大分泌颗粒（250～700nm）。分泌颗粒的形状各异（泪滴状、球形、心形），电子密度也各不相同。在Cushing病患者的腺瘤中，成束的中间丝靠近细胞核，形成易识别的大环。功能性ACTH细胞腺瘤的超微结构分析并不十分必要，因为组织学和免疫组化研究足以提供正确诊断。

静默型"促肾上腺皮质激素细胞"腺瘤 Silent "corticotroph" adenomas

此腺瘤亚型以ACTH及其相关肽类的免疫反应阳性为特征，而患者既不出现Cushing病的临床体征，也不出现反映ACTH分泌过量的血浆水平改变。因而，这些静默型腺瘤的准确评估，必须依靠详尽的形态学、免疫组化检查和超微结构分析。由于静默型腺瘤属临床无功能腺瘤，因此绝大多数是大腺瘤，临床上常表现为肿块压迫的症状和体征。这些腺瘤的特点是容易发生出血和卒中，大约1/3的患者可出现这一症状[96]。

静默型促肾上腺皮质激素细胞腺瘤有两种亚型[103]。静默1型促肾上腺皮质激素细胞腺瘤的形态学与Cushing病的功能性促肾上腺皮质激素细胞腺瘤无法区分[19,103]。但是，与Cushing病患者相比，该腺瘤更多见于老年人。如上所述，此类腺瘤无论在光镜还是超微结构水平，均与伴Cushing病的促肾上腺皮质激素细胞腺瘤相同。

静默2型"促肾上腺皮质激素细胞"腺瘤的形态学不同于促肾上腺皮质激素细胞腺瘤[19,103]。此类腺瘤组织学呈嫌色性或轻度嗜碱性，更类似于典型的无功能裸细胞腺瘤（见下文）。免疫组化显示有ACTH和POMC-相关肽类的活性表达。超微结构特点不如经典型或静默1型促肾上腺皮质激素细胞腺瘤典型，但是分泌颗粒的形态具有促肾上腺皮质激素细胞的特征。

尚未发现可引发静默型促肾上腺皮质激素细胞腺瘤的正常细胞表型。据推测，静默1型肿瘤可能源自垂体后叶的嗜碱性细胞，其形态类似于垂体前叶的促肾上腺皮质激素细胞[19]。

促性腺激素分泌（促性腺激素细胞）腺瘤 Gonadotropin-secreting (gonadotroph) adenomas

传统上认为，分泌促性腺激素、FSH和LH的垂体腺瘤属于少见肿瘤。与其他具有分泌活性的肿瘤不同，促性腺激素细胞腺瘤通常不引起激素生成过量的临床综合征。此类肿瘤的激素产量不高，因而很难检测到激素水平过高的现象。随着现代实验室技术的出现，许多以前被归类为无功能的垂体腺瘤，已被证实产生促性腺激素或其亚单位[104-107]。基于这些研究结果，促性腺激素细胞腺瘤可能占临床无功能腺瘤的一大部分，占整个垂体腺瘤的大约20%（表17.3）。

促性腺激素细胞腺瘤主要好发于50～60岁或更年长者，男性发病率稍高于女性[107]。通常此类腺瘤主要表现为临床无功能性肿瘤，多数症状是局部肿瘤压迫引起。包括视力障碍、头痛、垂体功能减退、性欲丧失和颅神经麻痹。超过70%的垂体促性腺激素细胞腺瘤患者以视野缺损为首发症状，这是由于肿瘤向鞍上延伸，压迫视神经交叉所致。促性腺激素细胞腺瘤的临床和生化诊断标准已在别处讨论[107]。

光镜下，多数促性腺激素细胞腺瘤具有嫌色性胞

腺瘤的类型

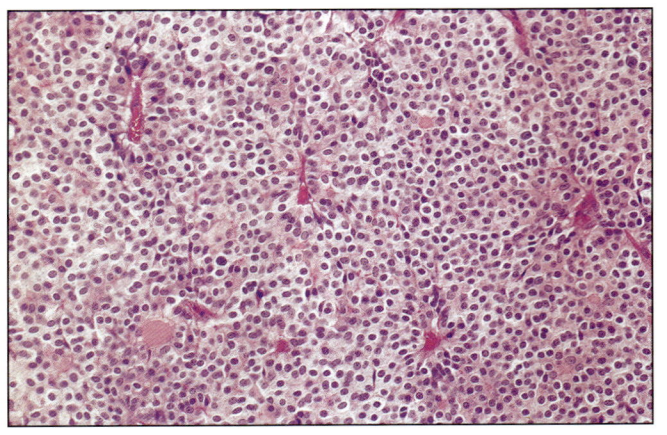

图17.28 促性腺激素分泌腺瘤。细胞呈嫌色性，具有乳头状排列特点。

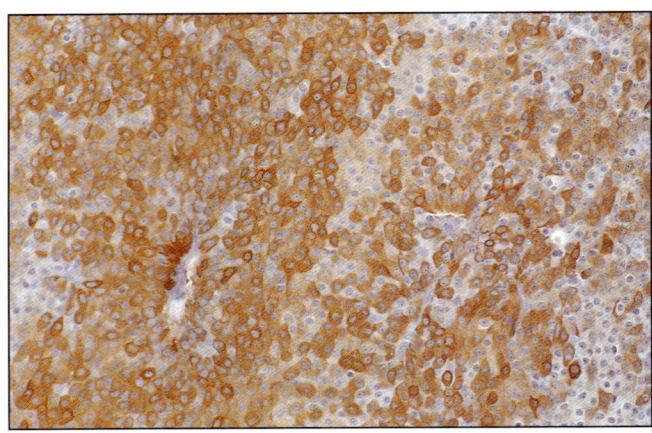

图17.29 促性腺激素分泌腺瘤。此乳头状排列的腺瘤呈卵泡刺激素免疫反应强阳性。注意免疫阳性细胞集中在血管周围。

浆，细胞核染色质细腻（图 17.28）。肿瘤细胞可呈弥漫性排列，亦常见明确的乳头状排列。乳头状结构的特点是拉长的胞浆突起向血管延伸，类似于围绕血管的假菊形团结构。免疫组化显示肿瘤具有不同程度的 β-FSH、β-LH、α-SU 阳性表达或这三种激素的联合表达（图17.29）[105,106,108]。免疫阳性细胞可散布于整个腺瘤中，但通常成簇分布。较之其他糖蛋白而言，β-FSH 的免疫组化阳性表达更为常见，且染色强度较强，分布较广[108]。

超微结构水平，促性腺激素细胞腺瘤的特点是细胞细长有极向，含有少量的小 (50～200nm) 分泌颗粒（图17.30）。在胞浆中，分泌颗粒分布不均匀，通常沿胞膜分布。目前提出了促性腺激素细胞腺瘤的性别相关分类法[109]。多数女性腺瘤患者显示 Golgi 复合体典型的空泡样变，致使其 Golgi 复合体呈蜂窝状外观。

在促性腺激素细胞腺瘤中，β-FSH 和（或）β-LH 的免疫活性及其超微结构分化程度与临床症状学之间的关系还所知甚少。尽管根据糖蛋白免疫反应将肿瘤归入促性腺激素细胞腺瘤的做法具有科研价值，但对此类患者的临床处理并无不同。多数患者目前均按"临床无功

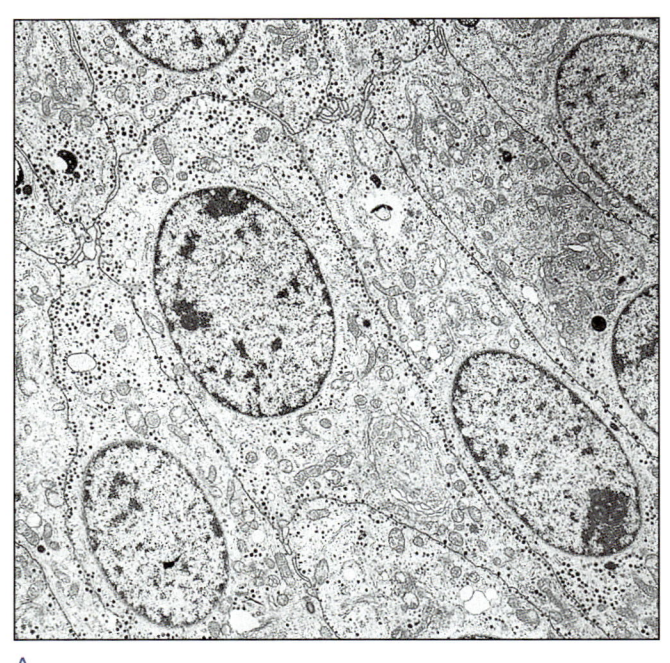

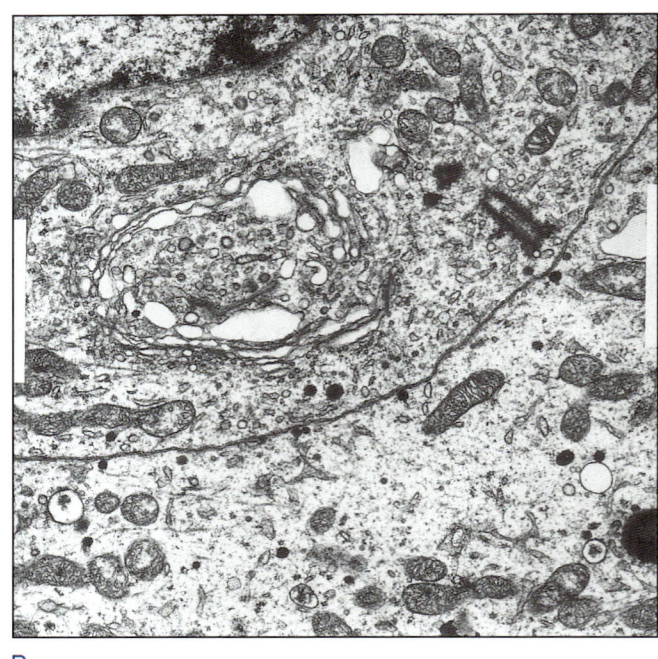

图17.30 促性腺激素分泌腺瘤的超微结构。（A）促性腺激素细胞腺瘤通常分化良好，由具有极性的长形细胞构成，分泌颗粒小，主要分布于胞浆周围。（B）促性腺激素细胞腺瘤具有明显的Golgi复合体。

能腺瘤"进行治疗，其目的是恢复视力，保持垂体功能和防止复发[2]。

裸细胞腺瘤和嗜酸细胞瘤
Null-cell adenoma and oncocytomas

大约 20% 的腺瘤无论是临床还是免疫组化方面均无产生激素的证据（表17.3）[110]。"裸细胞腺瘤"的命名很大程度上是基于此类肿瘤缺乏特定分化的超微结构特点[111]。裸细胞腺瘤发生的临床环境与促性腺激素细胞腺瘤相似，也表现为肿块所致的症状和体征[107]。本病好发于绝经后女性和老年男性，裸细胞腺瘤发现时多为大腺瘤。较小的肿瘤则是在核磁共振检查时偶然发现。

光镜下，裸细胞腺瘤多呈嫌色性（图17.31）。与促性腺激素细胞腺瘤相似，此类肿瘤细胞亦呈弥散性分布和（或）呈明显的乳头状排列。在一部分病例，可见嗜酸细胞变性（oncocytic degeneration），因而，又称为嗜酸性裸细胞腺瘤（嗜酸细胞瘤）[112]。此类肿瘤对任何垂体激素的免疫反应均可呈阴性（"免疫阴性"腺瘤），或呈局灶性 β-FSH、β-LH 和（或）α-SU 弱阳性表达。细胞培养发现裸细胞腺瘤偶尔有糖蛋白激素基因的一过性表达，并可分泌少量此类激素，因而可以出现糖蛋白类激素免疫反应[112-114]。在超微结构水平，裸细胞腺瘤的细胞器发育不完全，仅见少量的小分泌颗粒（图17.32）[19,111]。在发生嗜酸细胞变性时，可出现大量的线粒体。

裸细胞腺瘤的细胞发生机制尚不清楚。由于许多裸细胞腺瘤可有局灶性 β-FSH、β-LH 和（或）α-SU 的免疫阳性表达，与促性腺激素细胞腺瘤存在相当大的重叠。因此，裸细胞腺瘤与促性腺激素细胞腺瘤的鉴别标准还存在争议[72,115]。但在超微结构水平，裸细胞腺瘤相

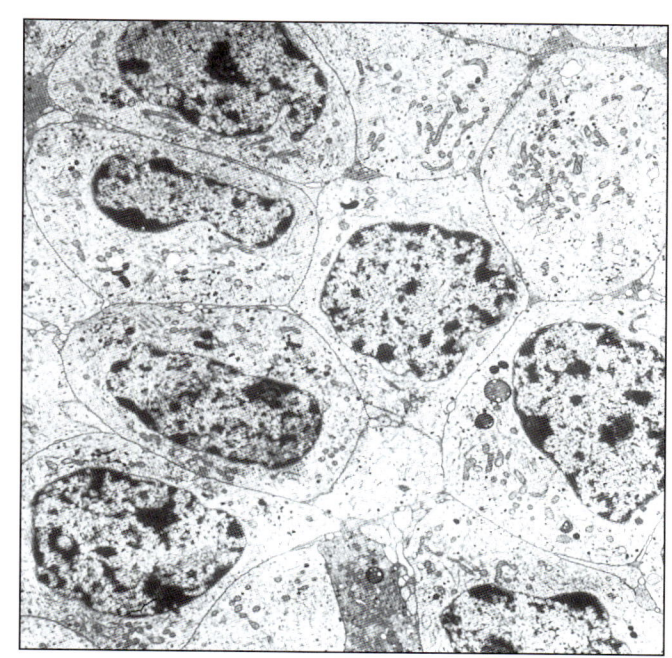

图17.32 裸细胞腺瘤的超微结构。裸细胞腺瘤由分化较差的细胞构成，含有少量小分泌颗粒。

对缺乏合成性细胞器，不同于正常、成熟的促性腺激素细胞。这两种肿瘤可能源自相同的前体细胞，可以形成分化较好的促性腺激素细胞和分化较差的细胞。如前所述，鉴别这两种腺瘤类型几乎没有任何临床意义。

最近发现，还有一类独特而少见的嗜酸细胞肿瘤亚型，即梭形细胞嗜酸细胞瘤[115a-c]。此类病变要与垂体后叶的星形细胞瘤鉴别，其特点是细胞呈梭形，富含线粒体，S-100 和 EMA 免疫反应阳性，但 GFAP 和神经内分泌标记多为阴性。人们推测，此类罕见的肿瘤可能源于滤泡 - 星形细胞（folliculo-stellate cell）[115a]。

TSH 分泌腺瘤
TSH-secreting adenomas

TSH 分泌腺瘤或促甲状腺激素细胞腺瘤是最少见的垂体腺瘤（表17.3）[116-118]。此类肿瘤可伴有 TSH 水平异常增高和甲状腺功能亢进症，但亦可见于甲状腺功能低下或正常的患者[116,119,120]。大多数肿瘤属侵袭性大腺瘤。

光镜下，促甲状腺激素细胞腺瘤常呈嫌色性。腺瘤通常由细长形、多角形或不规则形的细胞构成，具有长的胞浆突起（图17.33）[117]。免疫组化检查常发现胞浆中出现不同程度的 TSH 阳性表达。α-SU 染色亦通常为阳性。电镜下，细胞中等分化，只有少数粗面内质网和 Golgi 复合体[19]。分泌颗粒较小（100~200nm），圆形，电子密度均匀，常沿细胞膜排列。如临床表现和 TSH

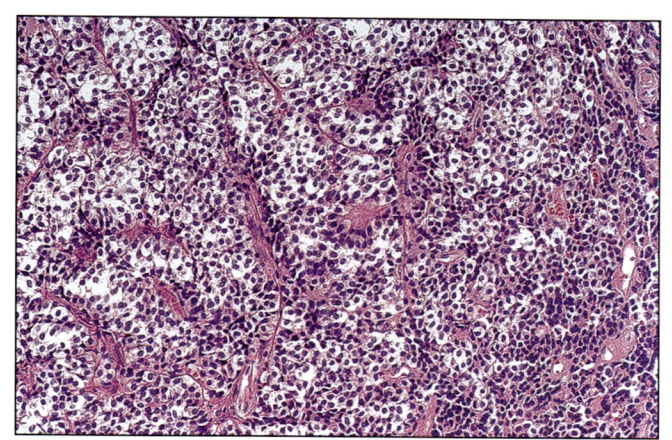

图17.31 裸细胞腺瘤。裸细胞腺瘤可呈多种组织学外观。大多表现为弥漫排列的嫌色细胞。

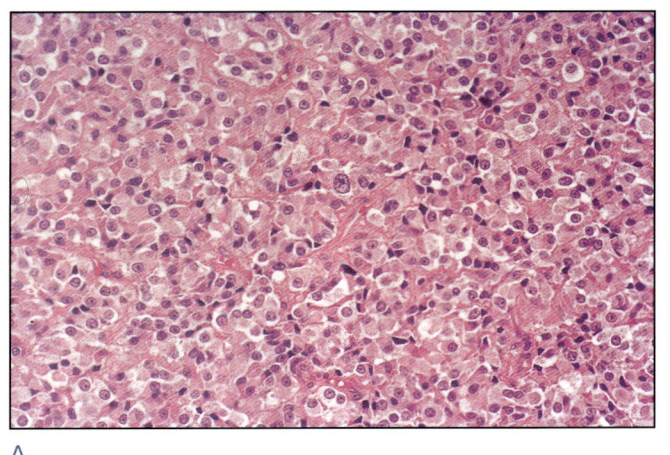 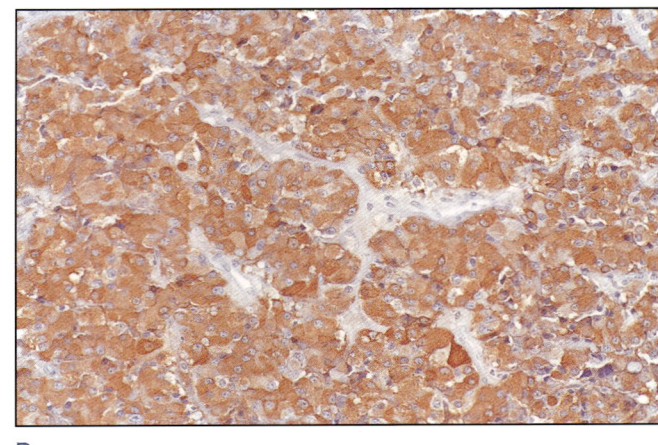

图17.33 促甲状腺激素(TSH)分泌腺瘤。（A）促甲状腺激素细胞腺瘤大多由多角形细胞构成，细胞核位于中央，有明显的核仁。（B）此类肿瘤TSH免疫阳性反应的变化范围很大。在该病例中，绝大部分肿瘤细胞呈TSH强阳性表达。

免疫组化检查不能确立TSH分泌腺瘤诊断，此时，只能借助于电镜表现做出适当的诊断。

多激素分泌腺瘤 Plurihormonal adenomas

多激素分泌腺瘤属罕见腺瘤，可以出现一种以上的垂体激素免疫反应性，与垂体前叶正常的细胞发生和发展无关。由于此类肿瘤非常罕见，其临床特点尚不明确。然而，多数文献报道的病例均有肿瘤压迫症状。多激素分泌腺瘤既可以是单形性腺瘤，也可以是多形性腺瘤。单形性多激素分泌腺瘤由分泌两种或两种以上激素的单一细胞组成；而多形性多激素分泌腺瘤则由两种或两种以上形态不同的细胞群组成。

虽然多激素分泌腺瘤可以出现任何激素组合，但是，下列激素组合不包括在内：（1）GH、PRL和TSH组合；（2）FSH和LH组合。因为在GH分泌腺瘤和促性腺激素细胞腺瘤中，这几种激素本身即常为联合表达（参见上文）[121]。已有FSH与GH，或者是PRL与TSH联合表达的报道[121]。个别情况下，多激素分泌腺瘤可出现ACTH免疫阳性反应。目前还发现一种罕见的促肾上腺皮质激素细胞腺瘤亚型，该肿瘤可同时表达α-SU，多数病例显示复发和侵袭性生物行为[122]。

垂体卒中 Pituitary apoplexy

垂体卒中主要由肿瘤梗死和出血所致，表现为腺瘤迅速增大。多数病例表现为急性临床过程，常需神经外科急诊手术治疗[2,123]。卒中亦可呈亚急性临床进程，表现为腺瘤内出血、坏死或囊性变[123-125]。虽然各

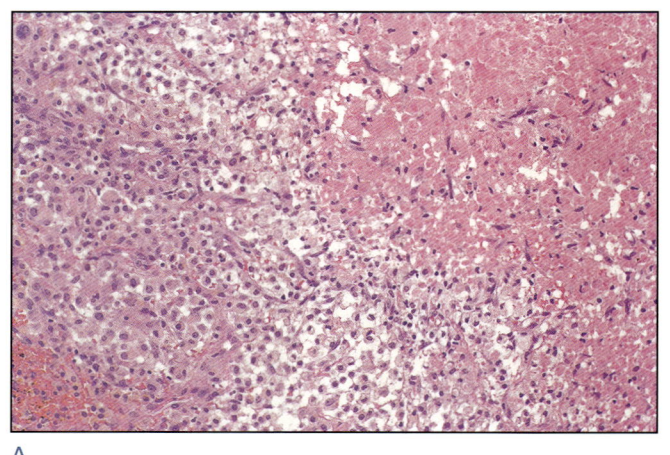 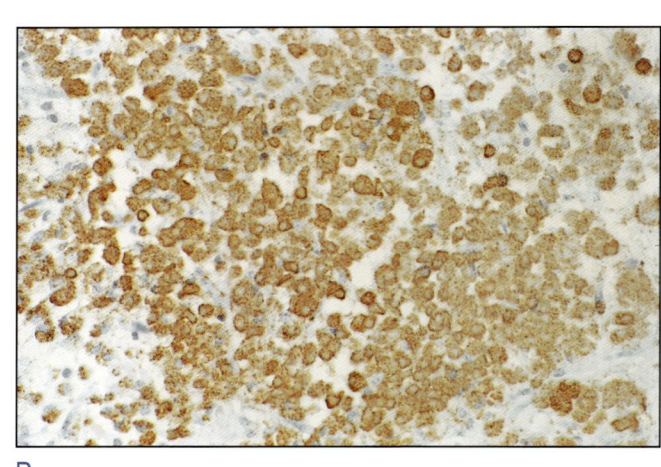

图17.34 垂体卒中。（A）垂体腺瘤显示广泛坏死，伴有巨噬细胞浸润。（B）尽管出现广泛坏死，本例静默型促肾上腺皮质激素细胞腺瘤仍可见促肾上腺皮质激素的免疫阳性表达。

种免疫类型的垂体腺瘤均可能出现卒中,但是无功能性大腺瘤尤其容易发生梗死。如前所述,其中一种是静默型促肾上腺皮质激素细胞腺瘤(见上文)。手术标本主要由出血和坏死的肿瘤构成(图17.34)。可通过异常的网织纤维网和局灶垂体激素免疫反应识别出来。

其他肿瘤和炎症性病变
Other tumors and inflammatory lesions

垂体后叶神经节细胞瘤
Gangliocytoma of the posterior pituitary

源自垂体后叶的神经节细胞瘤较为罕见。最近,有一份55例病人的文献综述[126]。绝大多数神经垂体的神经节细胞瘤是神经节细胞瘤和垂体腺瘤的混合体,即所谓的混合性神经节细胞瘤-垂体腺瘤(mixed gangliocytoma-pituitary adenoma)。某些研究人员也采用垂体腺瘤-垂体前叶神经元迷芽瘤(pituitary adenoma-adenohypophyseal neuronal choristoma, PANCH)这一名称[127]。这些肿瘤与神经内分泌功能紊乱有关,临床上大多表现为肢端肥大症,有文献报道少数病例可表现为Cushing病和高催乳素血症[126,128-130]。患者的临床、生化和影像学表现均无法与其他表现为肢端肥大症或Cushing病的病例进行区分。混合性神经节细胞瘤-垂体腺瘤是在对肿瘤进行形态学分析时发现的。激素不活跃肿瘤也有报道[128]。

组织学上,该病变由腺瘤和成熟的神经节细胞成分混合构成,不同细胞成分之间无明确分界(图17.35)。两种细胞成分的比例变化范围很大。神经节细胞通常较大,锥形神经元嵌入不同程度的神经毡样

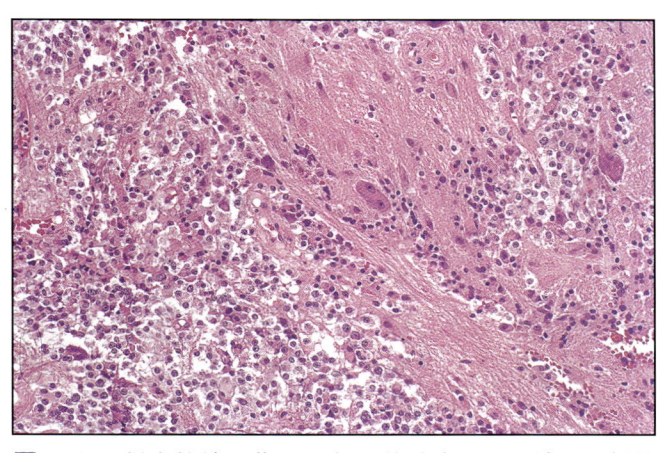

图17.35 混合性神经节细胞瘤/垂体腺瘤。显示神经毡样基质中混杂有神经节细胞和腺瘤细胞。注意图中的双核神经节细胞。

基质中。这些细胞可通过神经元相关蛋白(如神经丝蛋白、突触素)免疫组化,以及银浸染识别出来(图17.36)。肿瘤中见不到神经胶质成分,进一步证明肿瘤单纯的神经节衍化。腺瘤成分由嫌色或略嗜酸性的细胞组成,排列成大小不等的巢。根据腺瘤所分泌激素的不同,可出现GH、PRL、ACTH和糖蛋白免疫反应性。

关于蝶鞍神经节细胞肿瘤的起源有许多种学说。其中两种学说与该肿瘤组织学发生有关。第一种学说是下丘脑神经元异位到蝶鞍区,并因此产生下丘脑释放因子,进而刺激腺瘤增生。支持性证据是某些肿瘤的神经元成分具有下丘脑神经元的形态学特点,含有GHRH、CRH和GnRH等释放因子[129,131]。第二种学说是神经元成分来源于稀疏颗粒型腺瘤细胞的神经元分化。该理论的依据来自GH分泌肿瘤的电镜和免疫组化研究[127],在一例混合性肿瘤中,见到处于神经元和腺垂体细胞之间的

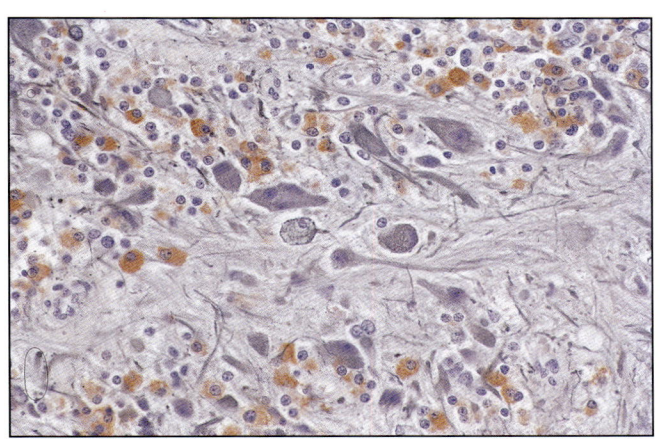

A

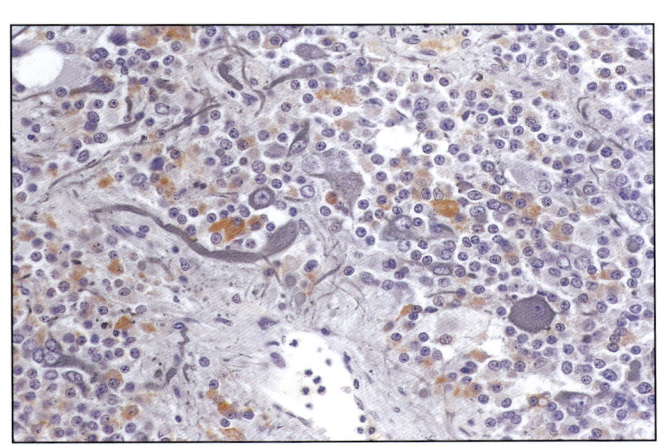

B

图17.36 混合性神经节细胞瘤/垂体腺瘤。(A, B)免疫组化双标记染色显示腺瘤细胞呈生长激素阳性(棕色),而神经节细胞呈神经丝阳性(灰色)。

中间细胞。

垂体后叶星形细胞瘤——垂体细胞瘤
Astrocytoma of the posterior pituitary–pituicytoma

垂体后叶可发生一种特殊亚型的低级别星形细胞瘤。尽管报道的例数尚少[132,133]，但有关此类肿瘤的综合分析已经发表[134]。这些星形细胞瘤也称为垂体细胞瘤（pituicytoma）或漏斗瘤（infundibuloma），被认为源于垂体细胞（垂体后叶内固有的胶质细胞）[135]，因此得名垂体细胞瘤。

垂体细胞瘤的临床表现主要取决于肿瘤大小和对邻近结构的压迫效应。大部分患者表现为视觉症状和垂体功能减退体征。某些病人可出现尿崩症。

肿瘤由排列成束的细长的毛细胞样星形细胞构成，与毛细胞型星形细胞瘤相似（图17.37）。然而，多数肿瘤缺少毛细胞型星形细胞瘤典型的双相结构，不出现Rosenthal纤维和嗜酸性颗粒小体[134]。通常肿瘤细胞呈波形蛋白和S-100蛋白免疫阳性表达。GFAP强阳性表达可出现于许多病例（图17.38），但在另一些病例，其表达可为局灶性甚或缺如[134]。其MIB-1标记指数通常较低[134]。

由于罕见，有关垂体后叶星形细胞瘤的准确临床行为目前尚无定论。但是多数报道的病例表现出低级别肿瘤的生物学行为，次全切除后有复发倾向[134]。

颗粒细胞瘤 Granular cell tumor

颗粒细胞瘤发生于垂体柄或垂体后叶，通常于成人尸检时偶然发现[136]。个别情况下肿瘤可引发临床症状，目前文献中仅有60例此类肿瘤的报道[137-139]。症状与肿瘤的大小和肿块效应有关，主要表现为视力障碍和垂体功能减退。此外，表现为尿崩症和脑室内出血的肿瘤也有文献报道[137,140]。鞍区颗粒细胞瘤也称为神经垂体的迷芽瘤、颗粒细胞垂体细胞瘤、颗粒细胞肌母细胞瘤。

鞍区颗粒细胞瘤的形态类似于外周神经系统颗粒细胞瘤（参见第27章）。肿瘤由多角形大细胞构成，胞浆富含抗淀粉酶的PAS染色阳性颗粒，胞核呈圆形，染色质细腻，核仁大小均匀（图17.39）。电镜下可见其胞浆富含大量溶酶体，致使其胞浆呈颗粒样外观。

神经垂体颗粒细胞瘤之来源目前尚不清楚。与外周神经系统颗粒细胞瘤不同，只有少数蝶鞍区颗粒细胞瘤呈S-100蛋白阳性[141]。同样，少数病例GFAP阳性，提示神经垂体颗粒细胞瘤可能源于垂体细胞[141]。多数肿瘤可见神经元特异性烯醇化酶和巨噬细胞/溶酶体标志物CD68的免疫阳性表达。

颗粒细胞瘤通常属生长缓慢的良性肿瘤，仅有少数

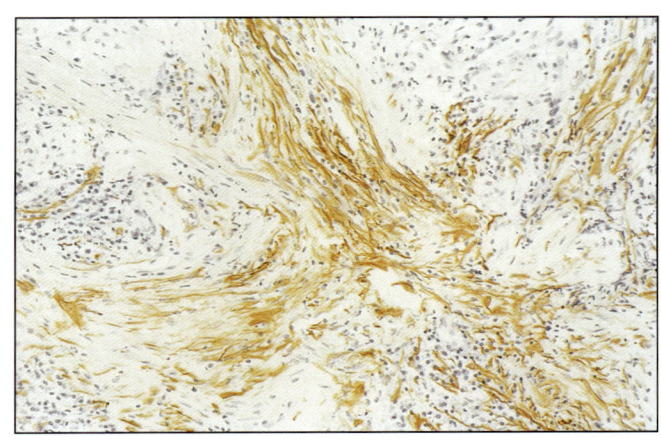

图17.38 垂体后叶星形细胞瘤。肿瘤细胞强表达胶质纤维酸性蛋白。

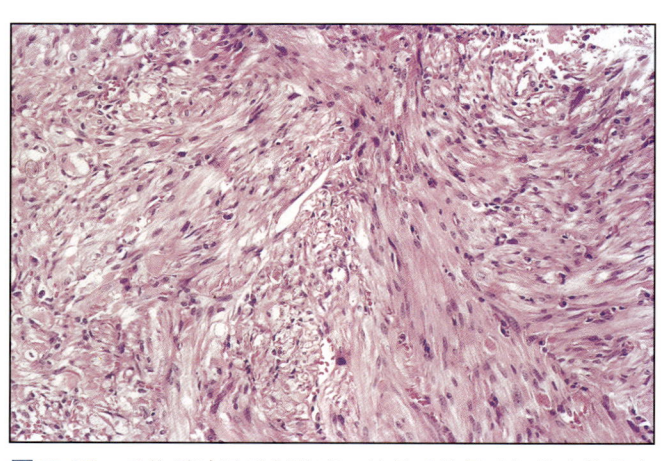

图17.37 垂体后叶星形细胞瘤。神经垂体星形细胞瘤的特点是呈束状排列的细长纤维性细胞。高倍镜下，可见肿瘤细胞的毛细胞性、纤维性特点。

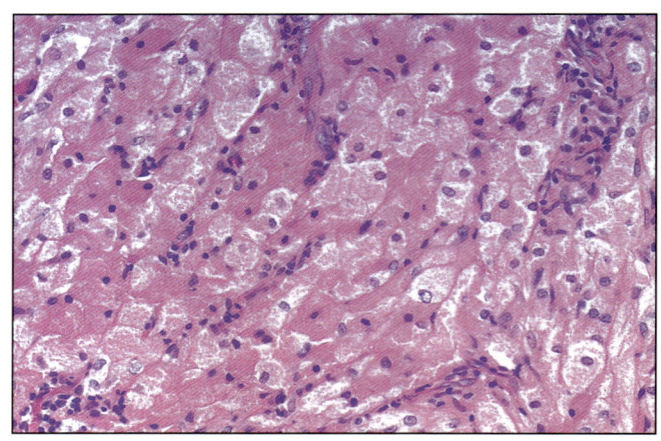

图17.39 垂体柄颗粒细胞瘤，其组织学类似于其他部位的颗粒细胞瘤。以颗粒状胞浆和中心胞核的大细胞为特征。

病例可出现侵袭性临床行为[138,139]。

颅咽管瘤 Craniopharyngioma

颅咽管瘤占所有颅内肿瘤的1%~2%，大约占鞍区肿瘤的10%。大部分好发于儿童和青少年，少数亦可发生于老年患者[142,143]。儿童颅咽管瘤患者通常表现为内分泌异常，例如生长迟缓和尿崩症[142,143]。而在成年人，则多表现为肿块的压迫效应，出现视力缺陷和垂体功能减退等症状。此外，垂体柄受压也可引起轻度催乳素水平升高。大部分颅咽管瘤位于鞍上，尽管肿瘤可存在鞍内部分，某些甚至完全发生于鞍膈下[142]。若肿瘤较大，则可向鞍旁区域甚或向脑实质内生长[144]。

颅咽管瘤的组织发生与Rathke裂囊肿有关，二者均源于垂体始基。尽管大多数颅咽管瘤与Rathke裂囊肿显著不同，已有报道发现个别肿瘤同时具有这两种病变的特点[145]。组织学上，颅咽管瘤表现为复杂的具有上皮性生长特点的生长模式（图17.40）。有关颅咽管瘤组织学形态的更详尽描述，请参见第26章。

Rathke裂囊肿 Rathke's cleft cyst

Rathke裂是Rathke囊的残余，是垂体前叶的胚胎发生始基。在正常垂体中，它表现为垂体前叶和后叶交界处的上皮性内衬。Rathke裂囊肿多于尸检时偶然发现，很少引起症状，约占鞍区手术病变的5%（表17.2）[146]。若囊肿持续增大，可出现临床症状。有症状的囊肿通常≥1cm，主要是由于压迫邻近结构所致，临床表现包括视力失调、垂体功能减退或尿崩症[147-150]。

组织学上，Rathke裂囊肿内衬纤毛立方上皮，伴有数目不等的柱状细胞和杯状细胞（图17.41）。此外，偶尔出现腺垂体细胞。鳞状细胞化生并不少见，主要见于陈旧性出血和炎症浸润的病例[146]。脓肿形成属罕见并发症[149]。对于囊肿壁破裂或发炎的病例，复发性Rathke裂囊肿并不少见[148,150]。

鞍区很少发生其他囊肿性病变，包括皮样囊肿、表皮样囊肿以及蛛网膜囊肿。

炎症性垂体炎 Inflammatory hypophysitis

炎症性垂体炎是垂体的少见疾病，以炎症细胞局灶或弥漫浸润并最终破坏垂体为特征[151,152]。准确的发病率尚不知晓。虽然大部分患者采用药物治疗，但该病所致的垂体增大和肿块效应会导致手术干预和腺体切

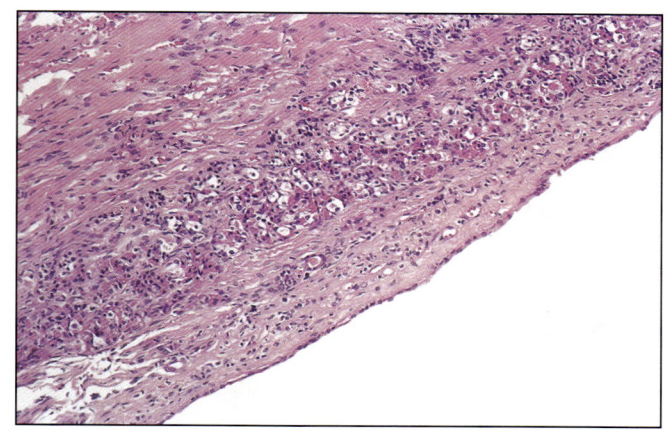

A

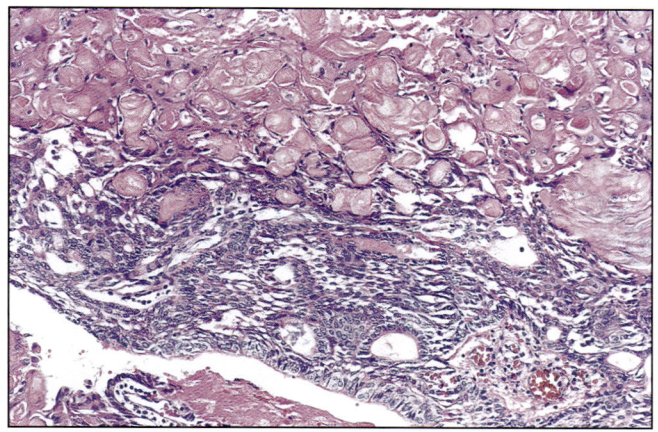

图17.40 颅咽管瘤通常显示成釉细胞瘤形态，其特点是复层上皮伴有栅栏状排列的基底细胞。可有角化和微囊性改变。

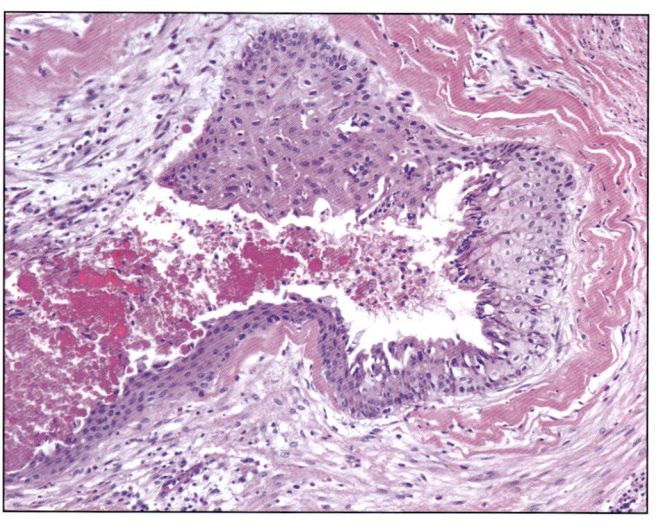

B

图17.41 Rathke裂囊肿。（A）Rathke裂囊肿表现为垂体附近的单层立方上皮囊肿。（B）Rathke裂囊肿发生的鳞状细胞化生并不少见。

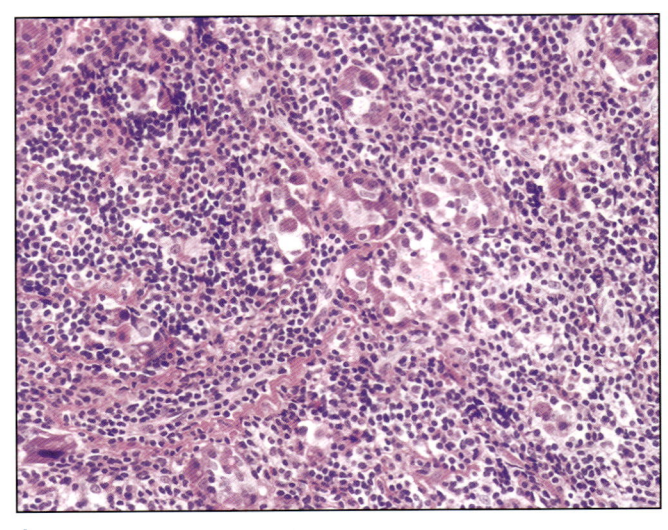 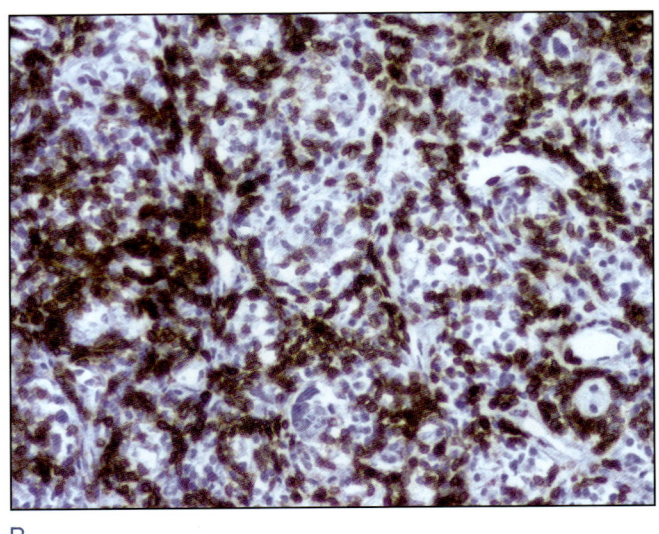

图17.42 淋巴细胞性垂体炎。（A）淋巴细胞性垂体炎的特点是在垂体前叶腺体中出现淋巴细胞和浆细胞浸润。（B）CD3免疫染色勾画出弥漫性淋巴细胞浸润。

除[153]。除此类病变外，垂体还可发生继发性垂体炎，此时或有明确的致病因素（细菌、病毒和真菌），或患有其他全身系统性病变，例如结节病。

组织学上，炎症性垂体炎分为三类：（1）淋巴细胞性垂体炎；（2）肉芽肿性垂体炎；（3）黄瘤性垂体炎[153]。最常见的是淋巴细胞性和肉芽肿性垂体炎，我们将在下文进行讨论。

淋巴细胞性垂体炎　Lymphocytic hypophysitis

淋巴细胞性垂体炎属少见疾病，主要好发于妊娠晚期或产后妇女[2]。本病男性罕见[154-156]。患者可表现为垂体增大所引起的症状和（或）部分垂体功能减退或全垂体功能减退症状[153,156]。由于垂体柄受压，血浆PRL水平可轻度升高。某些病人亦可表现为尿崩症，这表明炎症性病变可能已波及到垂体后叶和垂体柄[156,157]。此时，即可采用漏斗神经垂体炎（infundibular neurohypophysitis）这一术语。神经影像学显示垂体增大，常出现鞍上延伸证据[153,158]。

手术切除标本通常呈黄色，大体检查质硬，明显不同于质软的腺瘤。组织学上，淋巴细胞性垂体炎的特点是垂体前叶出现淋巴细胞和浆细胞浸润（图17.42）。偶尔可见生发中心。此外还可见到成簇的上皮样组织细胞，但不出现结构完整的肉芽肿。本病晚期的特点为垂体实质萎缩，出现不同程度的纤维化和残留的淋巴组织（图17.43）。

多条线索均提示本病属于自身免疫性疾病[155,159]，某些病例可检测到直接对抗垂体细胞的抗体。20%的病例伴有其他内分泌性或免疫性疾病（参见Thodou等的

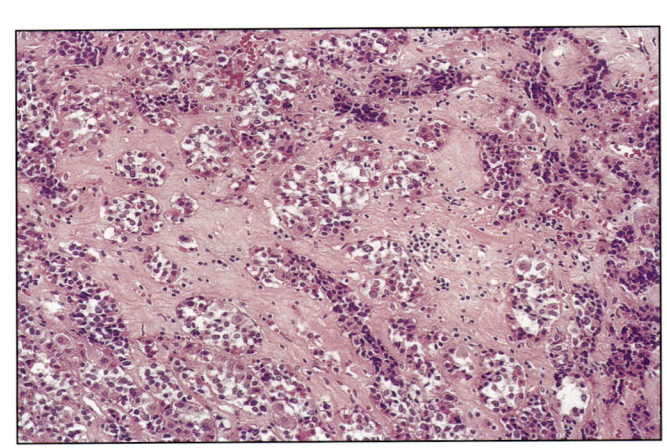

图17.43 淋巴细胞性垂体炎。垂体炎晚期出现实质萎缩、间质纤维化和局灶炎细胞浸润。

综述[156]）。许多病人采用皮质类固醇治疗有效，尽管某些患者仍需手术缓解压迫症状并采用激素替代疗法治疗垂体功能减退[153,160]。Tashiro等对淋巴细胞性垂体炎和其他炎症性疾病的临床、影像学和病理学等方面的一系列表现进行了全面的综述[152]。

巨细胞肉芽肿性垂体炎　Giant-cell granulomatous hypophysitis

巨细胞肉芽肿性垂体炎是发生于垂体的一类罕见的特发性慢性炎症性疾病[152,158,160]。与淋巴细胞性垂体炎不同，巨细胞肉芽肿性垂体炎同妊娠无关，亦无性别倾向[153,158]。此病好发于中老年妇女，而淋巴细胞性垂体炎则好发于较年轻的女性。肉芽肿性垂体炎主要影响垂体前叶，大部分患者表现为垂体功能减退[160]。

组织学上，巨细胞肉芽肿性垂体炎之特点是形态完好的非干酪样肉芽肿，伴不同程度的淋巴细胞浸润（图17.44）。可出现某种程度的实质纤维化。某些肉芽肿性疾病，包括结节病和Langerhans细胞组织细胞增生症，倾向于累及垂体后叶和下丘脑（图17.45）。因此，临床诊断时要排除特异性肉芽肿性疾病和诸如结核之类的感染性疾病。

其他病变 Miscellaneous lesions

许多肿瘤和疾病均可累及鞍区（表17.1）。这些肿瘤源自硬脑膜和蝶鞍的覆盖物（脑膜瘤和所谓的脑膜血管外皮细胞瘤），也可以来自骨性结构（如脊索瘤、软骨瘤和软骨肉瘤）[161-167]。蝶骨的浆细胞瘤（图17.46A）

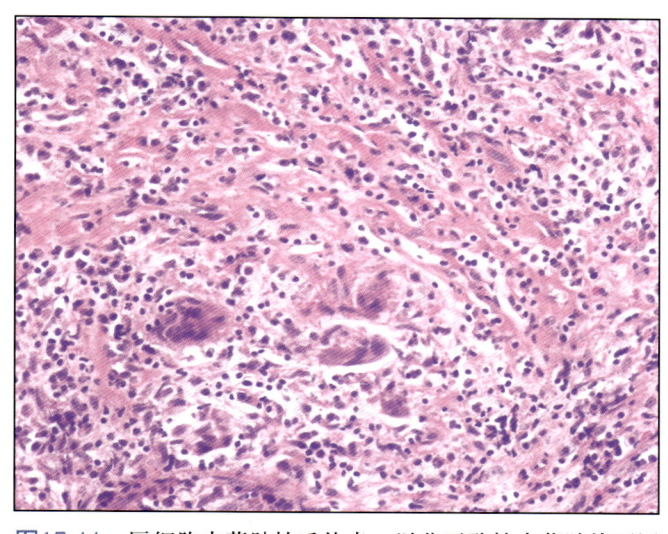

图17.44　巨细胞肉芽肿性垂体炎。以非干酪性肉芽肿伴不同程度的淋巴细胞浸润为特征。

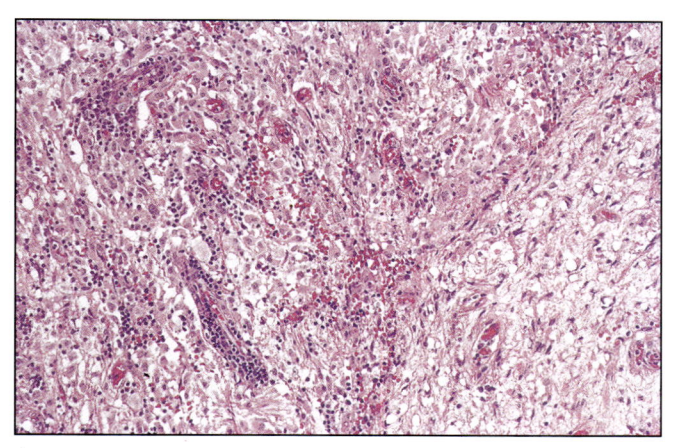

A

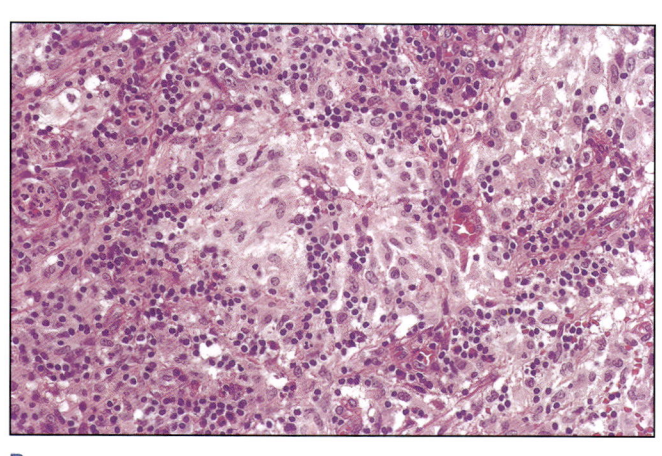

B

图17.45　Langerhans细胞组织细胞增生症。（A）Langerhans细胞组织细胞增生症侵及垂体后叶（左图）。（B）增生的上皮样组织细胞与淋巴细胞和嗜酸性粒细胞混杂在一起。

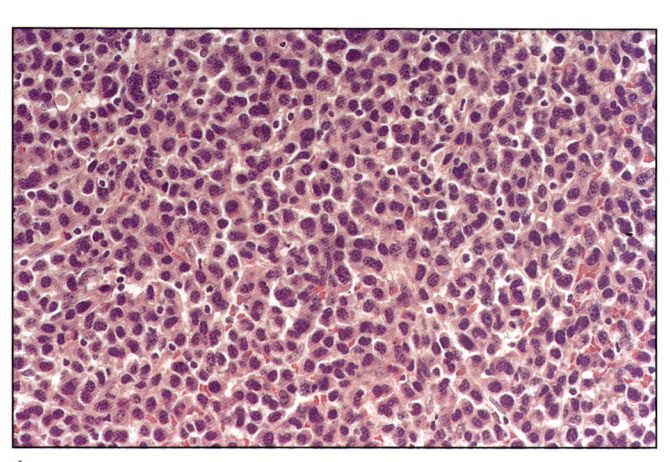

A

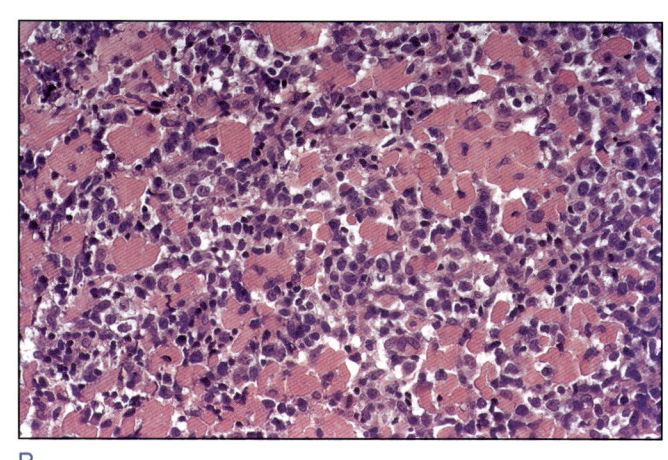

B

图17.46　（A）浆细胞瘤侵及垂体。（B）大B细胞淋巴瘤侵及垂体。

可侵及蝶鞍，形成与垂体腺瘤相似的影像学改变，并可引发垂体功能减退症状，有时甚至由于垂体柄受压而出现轻度高催乳素血症[167]。淋巴瘤亦可累及垂体（图17.46B）。

垂体转移性肿瘤约占外科切除标本的1%（表17.2），在尸检中发现转移癌的情况较多[168,169]。较之垂体前叶而言，垂体后叶更容易出现转移癌。多数转移至垂体的肿瘤不产生症状，若出现临床表现则最常见的是尿崩症，主要是垂体后叶和垂体柄受到侵犯所致[169]。其中，最常见的原发病灶是乳腺癌（图17.47）和肺癌。

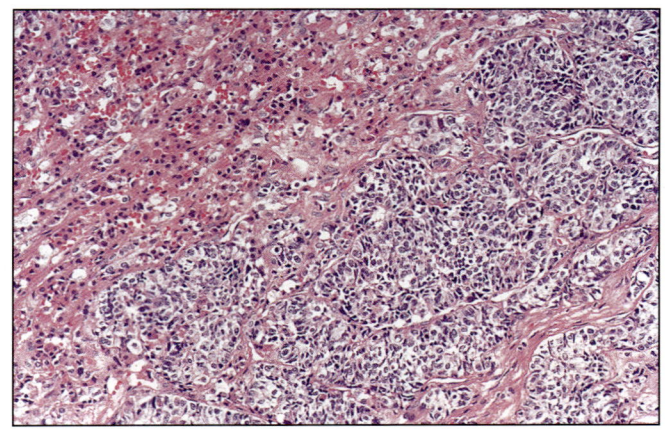

图17.47 乳腺癌转移至垂体。

参考文献

1. CBTRUS 2002 Statistical report: primary brain tumors in the United States, 1995–1999. Central Brain Tumor Registry of the United States. Available online at: www.cbtrus.org
2. Thorner M O, Vance M L, Laws E R Jr et al. 1998 The anterior pituitary. In: Wilson J D, Foster D W, Kronenberg H M et al. (eds) Williams textbook of endocrinology. W B Saunders, Philadelphia, p 249–340
3. Parent A D, Bebin J, Smith R R 1981 Incidental pituitary adenomas. J Neurosurg 54: 228–231
4. Kontogeorgos G, Kovacs K, Horvath E et al. 1991 Multiple adenomas of the human pituitary. A retrospective autopsy study with clinical implications. J Neurosurg 74: 243–247
5. Ezzat S, Asa S L, Couldwell W T et al. 2004 The prevalence of pituitary adenomas. A systematic review. Cancer 101: 613–619
6. Lloyd R V 1993 Embryology and anatomy of the pituitary gland. In: Lloyd R V (ed) Surgical pathology of the pituitary gland. W B Saunders, Philadelphia, p 1–17
7. Scheithauer B W, Sano T, Kovacs K et al. 1990 The pituitary gland in pregnancy: a clinicopathologic and immunohistochemical study of 69 cases. Mayo Clin Proc 65: 461–474
8. Page R B 1994 The anatomy of the hypothalamo–hypophysial complex. In: Knobil E, Neil J D (eds) The physiology of reproduction, 2nd edn. Raven Press, New York, p 1527–1619
9. Scully K M, Rosenfeld M G 2002 Pituitary development: regulatory codes in mammalian organogenesis. Science 295: 2231–2235
10. Asa S L, Kovacs K, Lazlo F A et al. 1986 Human fetal adenohypophysis: histologic and immunocytochemical analysis. Neuroendocrinology 43: 308–316
11. Asa S L, Kovacs K, Singer W 1991 Human fetal adenohypophysis: morphological and functional analysis in vitro. Neuroendocrinology 53: 562–572
12. Dubois P M, Hemming F J 1991 Fetal development and regulation of pituitary cell types. J Electron Microsc Tech 19: 2–20
13. Simmons D M, Voss J W, Ingraham H A et al. 1990 Pituitary cell phenotypes involve cell-specific Pit-1 mRNA translation and synergistic interactions with other classes of transcription factors. Genes Dev 4: 695–711
14. Japon M A, Rubinstein M, Low M J 1994 In situ hybridization analysis of anterior pituitary hormone gene expression during fetal mouse development. J Histochem Cytochem 42: 1117–1125
15. Marin F, Stefaneanu L, Kovacs K 1991 Folliculo-stellate cells of the pituitary. Endocr Pathol 2: 180–192
16. Horvath E, Kovacs K 2002 Folliculo-stellate cells of the human pituitary: a type of adult stem cell? Ultrastruct Pathol 26: 219–28
17. Inoue K, Mogi C, Ogawa S et al. 2002 Are folliculo-stellate cells in the anterior pituitary gland supportive cells or organ-specific stem cells? Arch Physiol Biochem 110: 50–53
18. Cushing H 1912 The pituitary body and its disorders. J B Lippincott, Philadelphia
19. Horvath E, Kovacs K 1991 The adenohypophysis. In: Kovacs K, Asa S L (eds) Functional endocrine pathology. Blackwell Scientific Publications, Boston, p 245–281
20. Snyder P J 1993 Clinically nonfunctioning pituitary adenomas. Endocrinol Metab Clin North Am 22: 163–175
21. Hardy J 1969 Transsphenoidal microsurgery of the normal and pathological pituitary. Clin Neurosurg 16: 185–217
22. Kovacs K, Horvath E 1986 Tumors of the pituitary gland. In: Atlas of tumor pathology, series 2, fascicle 21. Armed Forces Institute of Pathology, Washington
23. Horvath E, Kovacs K 1992 Ultrastructural diagnosis of human pituitary adenomas. Microsc Res Tech 20: 107–135
24. DeLellis R A, Lloyd R V, Heitz P U et al. (eds) 2004 World Health Organization classification of tumours. Pathology and genetics of tumours of endocrine organs. IARC Press, Lyon
25. Scheithauer B W, Kovacs K, Laws E R Jr et al. 1986 Pathology of invasive pituitary tumors with special reference to functional classification. J Neurosurg 65: 733–744
26. Meij B P, Lopes M B S, Ellegala D B et al. 2002 The long-term significance of microscopic dural invasion in 354 patients with pituitary adenomas treated with transsphenoidal surgery. J Neurosurg 96: 195–208
27. Thapar K, Kovacs K, Scheithauer B W et al. 1996 Proliferative activity and invasiveness among pituitary adenomas and carcinomas: an analysis using the MIB-1 antibody. Neurosurg 38: 99–107
28. Jaffrain-Rea M L, Di Stefano D, Minniti G et al. 2002 A critical reppraisal of MIB-1 labeling index significance in a large series of pituitary tumours: secreting versus non-secreting adenomas. Endocr Rel Cancer 9: 103–113
29. Schreiber S, Saeger W, Ludecke D K 1999 Proliferation markers in different types of clinically non-secreting pituitary adenomas. Pituitary 1: 213–220
30. Losa M, Franzin A, Mangili F 2000 Proliferation index of non-functioning pituitary adenomas: correlations with clinical characteristics and long-term follow-up results. Neurosurgery 47: 1313–1318
31. Hentschel S J, McCutcheon E, Moore W et al. 2003 p53 and MIB-1 immunohistochemistry as predictors of the clinical behavior of non-functioning pituitary adenomas. Can J Neurol Sci 30: 215–219
32. Lloyd R V, Kovacs K, Young W F Jr et al. 2004 Pituitary tumours: Introduction. In: DeLellis R A, Lloyd R V, Heitz P U et al. (eds) World Health Organization classification of tumours. Pathology and genetics of tumours of endocrine organs. IARC Press, Lyon, p 10–13
33. Lübke D, Saeger W 1995 Carcinomas of the pituitary: definition and review of the literature. Gen Diagn Pathol 141: 81–92
34. Pernicone P J, Scheithauer B W, Sebo T J et al. 1997 Pituitary carcinoma: a clinicopathologic study of 15 cases. Cancer 79: 804–812
35. Roncaroli F, Scheithauer B W, Young W F et al. 2003 Silent corticotroph carcinoma of the adenohypophysis. A report of five cases. Am J Surg Pathol 27: 477–486
36. Alexander J M, Biller B M K, Bikkal H et al. 1990 Clinically nonfunctioning pituitary tumors are monoclonal in origin. J Clin Invest 86: 336–340
37. Herman V, Fagin J, Gonsky R et al. 1990 Clonal origin of pituitary adenomas. J Clin Endocrinol Metab 71: 1427–1433
38. Clayton R N, Farrell W E 2001 Clonality of pituitary tumours: more complicated than initially envisaged? Brain Pathol 11: 313–327
39. Herman V, Melmed S 1991 Clonality of endocrine tumors. Endocrinol Pathol 2: 61–63
40. Bystrom C, Larsson C, Bloomberg C et al. 1990 Localization of the MEN1 gene to a small region within chromosome 11q13 by deletion mapping in tumors. Proc Natl Acad Sci USA 87: 1968–1972
41. Bale A J, Norton J A, Wong E L et al. 1991 Allelic loss on chromosome 11 in hereditary and sporadic tumors related to familial multiple endocrine neoplasia type 1. Cancer Res 51: 1154–1157
42. Thakker R V, Pook M A, Wooding C et al. 1993 Association of somatotrophinomas with loss of allelles on chromosome 11 and with *gsp* mutations. J Clin Invest 91: 2815–2821
43. Boggild M D, Jenkinson S, Pistorello et al. 1994 Molecular genetic studies of sporadic pituitary hormones. J Clin Endocrinol Metab 78: 387–392
44. Bates A S, Farrell W E, Bicknell E J et al. 1997 Allelic deletion in pituitary adenomas reflects aggressive biological activity and has potential value as a prognostic marker. J Clin Endocrinol Metab 82: 818–824
45. Prezant T R, Levine J, Melmed S 1998 Molecular characterization of the MEN1 tumor suppressor gene in sporadic pituitary tumors. J Clin Endocrinol Metab 83: 1388–1391

46. Wrocklage C, Gold H, Hackl W 2002 Increased menin expression in sporadic pituitary adenomas. Clin Endocrinol 56: 589–594
47. Vallar L, Spada A, Giannattasio G 1987 Altered G_s and adenylate cyclase activity in human GH-secreting pituitary adenomas. Nature 330: 566–568
48. Clementi E, Malgaretti N, Meldolesi J et al. 1990 A new constitutively activating mutation of the G_s protein a subunit-*gsp* oncogene is found in human pituitary tumours. Oncogene 5: 1059–1061
49. Spada A, Arosio M, Bochicchio D et al. 1990 Clinical, biochemical, and morphological correlates in patients bearing growth hormone-secreting pituitary tumors with or without constitutively active adenylyl cyclase. J Clin Endocrinol Metab 71: 1421–1426
50. Lania A, Mantovani G, Spada A 2003 Genetics of pituitary tumors: focus on G-protein mutations. Exp Biol Med 228: 1004–1017
51. Weinstein L S, Shuhua Y, Warner D R et al. 2001 Endocrine manifestations of stimulatory G protein a-subunit mutations and the role of genomic imprinting. Endocr Rev 22: 675–705
52. Pei L, Melmed S 1997 Isolation and characterization of a pituitary tumor-transforming gene (PTTG). Mol Endocrinol 11: 433–441
53. McCabe C J, Heaney A P 2003 Pituitary tumour transforming gene in endocrine cancer. Clin Endocrinol 58: 673–682
54. Saez C, Japon M A, Ramos-Morales F et al. 1999 hpttg is over-expressed in pituitary adenomas and other primary epithelial neoplasias. Oncogene 18: 5473–5476
55. Zhang X, Horwitz G A, Heaney A P et al. 1999 Pituitary tumor transforming gene expression in human pituitary adenomas. J Clin Endocrinol Metab 84: 761–767
56. McCabe C J, Khaira J S, Boelaert K et al. 2003 Expression of pituitary tumour transforming gene (PTTG) and fibroblast growth factor-2 in human pituitary adenomas: relationship to clinical tumour behavior. Clin Endocrinol 58: 141–150
57. Herman V, Drazin N Z, Gonsky R et al. 1993 Molecular screening of pituitary adenomas for gene mutations and rearrangements. J Clin Endocrinol Metab 77: 50–55
58. Karga H J, Alexander J M, Hedley-Whyte E T et al. 1992 *Ras* mutation in human pituitary tumors. J Clin Endocrinol Metab 74: 914–919
59. Levy A, Hall L, Yeudall W A et al. 1994 p53 gene mutations in pituitary adenomas: rare events. Clin Endocrinol 47: 809–814
60. Thapar K, Scheithauer B W, Kovacs K et al. 1996 p53 expression in pituitary adenomas and carcinomas: correlation with invasiveness and tumor growth fractions. Neurosurgery 38: 765–771
61. Cryns V L, Alexander J M, Klibanski A et al. 1993 The retinoblastoma gene in human pituitary tumors. J Clin Endocrinol Metab 77: 644–646
62. Zhu J, Leon S P, Beggs A H et al. 1994 Human pituitary adenomas show no loss of heterozygosity at the retinoblastoma gene locus. J Clin Endocrinol Metab 78: 922–927
63. Pei L, Melmed S, Scheithauer B et al. 1995 Frequent loss of heterozygosity at the retinoblastoma susceptibility gene (RB) locus in aggressive pituitary tumors: evidence for a chromosome 13 tumor suppressor gene other than RB. Cancer Res 55: 1613–1616
64. Thorner M O 2002 Hyperprolactinemia. In: Besser GM, Thorner MO (eds) Comprehensive clinical endocrinology. Mosby, Edinburgh, p 73–84
65. Serri O, Chik C L, Ur E et al. 2003 Diagnosis and management of hyperprolactinemia. CMAJ Canad Med Assoc J 169: 575–581
66. Randall R V, Laws E R Jr, Abboud C F et al. 1983 Transsphenoidal microsurgical treatment of prolactin-producing pituitary adenomas. Results in 100 patients. Mayo Clin Proc 58: 108–121
67. Thapar K, Laws E R Jr 1995 Pituitary tumors. In: Kaye A H, Laws E R Jr (eds) Brain tumors. An encyclopedic approach. Churchill Livingstone, Edinburgh, p 759–773
68. Horvath E, Kovacs K 1986 Pathology of prolactin cell adenomas of the human pituitary. Semin Diagn Pathol 3: 4–17
69. Landolt A M, Kleihues P, Heitz P U 1987 Amyloid deposits in pituitary adenomas. Arch Pathol Lab Med 111: 453–458
70. Tindall G T, Kovacs K, Horvath E et al. 1982 Human prolactin-producing adenomas and bromocriptine: a histological, immunocytochemical, ultrastructural and morphometric study. J Clin Endocrinol Metab 55: 1178–1183
71. Kovacs K, Stefaneanu L, Horvath E et al. 1991 Effect of dopamine agonist medication on prolactin producing adenomas: a morphological study including immunocytochemistry, electron microscopy and in situ hybridization. Virchows Arch A Pathol Anat Histopathol 418: 439–446
72. Kovacs K, Scheithauer B W, Horvath E et al. 1996 The World Health Organization classification of adenohypophysial neoplasms: a proposed five-tier scheme. Cancer 78: 502–510
73. Melmed S 1995 Acromegaly. In: Melmed S (ed) The pituitary. Blackwell Science, Cambridge, MA, p 413–442
74. Kreutzer J, Vance M L, Lopes M B S et al. 2001 Surgical management of GH-secreting pituitary adenomas: an outcome study using modern remission criteria. J Clin Endocrinol Metab 86: 4072–4077
75. Shimon I, Melmed S 1997 Acromegaly. Differential diagnosis and treatment. In: Wierman M E (ed) Contemporary endocrinology, vol 3. Diseases of the pituitary: diagnosis and treatment. Human Press, Totowa, p 135–152
76. Neumann P E, Goldman J R, Horoupian D S et al. 1985 Fibrous bodies in growth hormone-secreting adenomas contain cytokeratin filaments. Arch Pathol Lab Med 109: 505–508
77. Scheithauer B W, Kovacs K, Randall R V et al. 1986 Pathology of excessive production of growth hormone. Clin Endocrinol Metab 15: 655–681
78. Kovacs K, Horvath E 1986 Pathology of growth hormone-producing tumors of the human pituitary. Semin Diagn Pathol 3: 18–33
79. Yamada S, Aiba T, Sano T et al. 1993 Growth hormone producing pituitary adenomas: correlations between clinical characteristics and morphology. Neurosurgery 33: 20–27
80. Vance M L, Harris A G 1991 Long term treatment of 189 acromegalic patients with the somatostatin analog octreotide. Results of the International Multicenter Acromegaly Study Group. Arch Intern Med 151: 1573–1578
81. Beckers A, Kovacs K, Horvath E et al. 1991 Effect of treatment with octreotide on the morphology of growth hormone-secreting pituitary adenomas: study of 24 cases. Endocrinol Pathol 2: 123–131
82. Ezzat S, Horvath E, Harris A G et al. 1994 Morphological effects of octreotide on growth hormone-producing pituitary adenomas. J Clin Endocrinol Metab 79: 113–118
83. Corenblum B, Sirek A M, Horvath E et al. 1976 Human mixed somatotrophic and lactotrophic pituitary adenomas. J Clin Endocrinol Metab 42: 857–863
84. Horvath E, Kovacs K, Singer W et al. 1981 Acidophil stem cell adenoma of the human pituitary: clinico-pathological analysis of 15 cases. Cancer 47: 761–771
85. Lloyd R V, Gikas R V, Chandler W F 1983 Prolactin and growth hormone-producing pituitary adenomas: an immunohistochemical and ultrastructural study. Am J Surg Pathol 7: 251–260
86. Horvath E, Kovacs K, Killinger D W et al. 1983 Mammosomatotroph cell adenoma of the human pituitary: a morphologic entity. Virchows Arch A Pathol Anat Histopathol 398: 277–289
87. Felix I A, Horvath E, Kovacs K et al. 1986 Mammosomatotroph adenoma of the pituitary associated with gigantism and hyperprolactinemia. A morphological study including immunoelectron microscopy. Acta Neuropathol 71: 76–82
88. Maartens N F, Lopes M B S, Ellegala D et al. 2001 Clinicopathological features and outcome in patients with mammosomatotroph adenomas [abstract]. Endocr Pathol 12: 226
89. Horvath E, Kovacs K, Smyth H S et al. 1988 A novel type of pituitary adenoma: morphological features and clinical correlations. J Clin Endocrinol Metab 66: 1111–1118
90. Magiakou M A, Chrousos G P 1994 Diagnosis and treatment of Cushing disease. In: Imura H (ed) The pituitary gland, 2nd edn. Raven, New York, p 391–508
91. Carey R M, Varma S K, Drake C R Jr et al. 1984 Ectopic secretion of corticotropin-releasing factor as a cause of Cushing's syndrome. N Engl J Med 311: 13–20
92. Auchus R J, Mastorakos G, Friedman T C et al. 1994 Corticotropin-releasing hormone production by a small cell carcinoma in a patient with ACTH-dependent Cushing syndrome. J Endocrinol Invest 17: 447–452
93. Kemink S A G, Smals A G H, Hermus A R M M et al. 1997 Nelson's syndrome: a review. Endocrinologist 7: 5–9
94. Lloyd R V, Fields K, Jin L et al. 1990 Analysis of endocrine active and clinically silent corticotropic adenomas by in situ hybridization. Am J Pathol 137: 479–488
95. Scheithauer B W, Jaap A L, Horvath E et al. 2000 Clinically silent corticotroph tumors of the piuitary gland. Neurosurgery 47: 723–730
96. Webb K M, Laurent J L, Okonkwo D et al. 2003 Clinical characteristics of silent corticotrophic adenomas and creation of an internet-accessible database to facilitate their multi-institutional study. Neurosurgery 53: 1076–1085
97. Lopez J A, Kleinschmidt-DeMasters B K, Sze C-I et al. 2004 Silent corticotroph adenomas: further clinical and pathological observations. Hum Pathol 35: 1137–1147
98. Leinung M C, Kane L A, Scheithauer B W et al. 1995 Long term follow-up of transsphenoidal surgery for the treatment of Cushing's disease in childhood. J Clin Endocrinol Metab 80: 2475–2479
99. Storr H L, Plowman P N, Carroll P V et al. 2003 Clinical and endocrine responses to pituitary radiotherapy in pediatric Cushing's disease: an effective second-line treatment. J Clin Endocrinol Metab 88: 34–37
100. Storr H L, Isidori A M, Monson J P et al. 2004 Prepubertal Cushing's disease is more common in males, but there is no increase in severity at diagnosis. J Clin Endocrinol Metab 89: 3818–3820
101. Neumann P E, Horoupian D S, Goldman J E et al. 1984 Cytoplasmic filaments of Crooke's hyaline change belong to the cyokeratin class: an immunocytochemical and ultrastructural study. Am J Pathol 116: 214–222
101a. George D H, Scheithauer B W, Kovacs K et al. 2003 Crooke's cell adenoma of the pituitary: an aggressive variant of corticotroph adenoma. Am J Surg Pathol 27: 1330–1336
102. Stefaneanu L, Kovacs K, Horvath E et al. 1991 In situ hybridization study of proopiomelanocortin (POMC) gene expression in human pituitary corticotrophs and their adenomas. Virchows Arch [A] 419: 107–113
103. Horvath E, Kovacs K, Killinger D W et al. 1980 Silent corticotropic adenomas of the human pituitary gland: a histologic, immunocytologic and ultrastructural study. Am J Pathol 98: 617–638
104. Jameson J L, Klibanski A, Black P M et al. 1987 Glycoprotein hormone genes are expressed in clinically nonfunctioning pituitary adenomas. J Clin Invest 80: 1472–1478
105. Kontogeorgos G, Kovacs K, Horvath E et al. 1993 Null cell adenomas, oncocytomas, and gonadotroph adenomas of the human pituitary: an immunocytochemical and ultrastructural analysis of 300 cases. Endocrinol Pathol 4: 20–27

106. Young W F, Scheithauer B W, Kovacs K et al. 1996 Gonadotroph adenoma of the pituitary gland: a clinicopathologic analysis of 100 cases. Mayo Clin Proc 71: 649–656
107. Snyder P J 1997 Gonadotroph and other clinically nonfunctioning pituitary adenomas. In: Arnold A (ed) Endocrine neoplasms. Kluwer Academic, Norwell, p 57–72
108. Sano T, Yamada S 1994 Histologic and immunohistochemical study of clinically non-functioning pituitary adenomas: special reference to gonadotropin-positive adenomas. Pathol Int 44: 697–703
109. Horvath E, Kovacs K 1984 Gonadotroph adenomas of the human pituitary: sex-related fine structural dichotomy. A histologic, immunohistochemical, and electron microscopic study of 30 tumors. Am J Pathol 117: 429–440
110. Asa S L, Kovacs K 1992 Clinically non-functioning human pituitary adenomas. Can J Neurol Sci 19: 228–235
111. Kovacs K, Horvath E, Ryan N et al. 1980 Null cell adenoma of the human pituitary. Virchows Arch [A] 387: 165–174
112. Yamada S, Asa S L, Kovacs K 1988 Oncocytomas and null cell adenomas of the human pituitary: morphometric and in vitro functional comparison. Virchows Arch [A] 413: 333–339
113. Asa S L, Gerrie B M, Singer W et al. 1986 Gonadotropin secretion in vitro by human pituitary null cell adenomas and oncocytomas. J Clin Endocrinol Metab 62: 1011–1019
114. Saccomanno K, del Alamo P G, Bassetti M et al. 1993 In vitro detection of glycoprotein production and secretion by human nonfunctioning pituitary adenomas. J Endocrinol Invest 16: 109–115
115. Sano T, Yamada S, Ozawa Y et al. 2003 Endocrine surgical pathology: lesson from pituitary cases that are discordant between clinical and pathologic diagnosis. Endocrinol Pathol 14: 151–157
115a. Roncaroli F, Scheithauer B W, Cenacchi G et al. 2002 Spindle cell oncocytoma of the adenohypophysis: a tumor of folliculostellate cells? Am J Surg Pathol 26: 1048–1055
115b. Kloub O, Perry A, Tu P H, Lipper M, Lopes M B 2005 Spindle cell oncocytoma of the adenohypophysis: report of two recurrent cases. Am J Surg Pathol 29: 247–253
115c. Dahiya S, Sarkar C, Hedley-Whyte E T et al. 2005 Spindle cell oncocytoma of the adenohypophysis: report of two cases. Acta Neuropathol 110: 97–99
116. Greenman Y, Melmed S 1995 Thyrotropin-secreting pituitary tumors. In: Melmed S (ed) The pituitary. Blackwell Science, Cambridge, MA, p 546–558
117. Girod C, Trouillas J, Claustrat B 1986 The human thyrotropic adenoma: pathologic diagnosis in five cases and critical review of the literature. Semin Diagn Pathol 3: 58–68
118. Mindermann T, Wilson C B 1993 Thyrotropin-producing pituitary adenomas. J Neurosurg 79: 521–527
119. Beck-Peccoz P, Brucker-Davis F, Persani L et al. 1996 Thyrotropin-secreting pituitary tumors. Endocrinol Rev 17: 610–638
120. Samuels M H 1997 Thyrotropin-secreting pituitary tumors. In: Wierman M E (ed) Contemporary endocrinology, vol 3. Diseases of the pituitary: diagnosis and treatment. Human Press, Totowa, p 295–304
121. Horvath E, Lloyd R V, Kovacs K et al. 2004 Plurihormonal adenoma. In: DeLellis R A, Lloyd R V, Heitz P U et al. (eds) 2004 World Health Organization classification of tumours. Pathology and genetics of tumours of endocrine organs. IARC Press, Lyon, p 35
122. Berg K K, Scheithauer B W, Felix I et al. 1990 Pituitary adenomas that produce adrenocorticotropic hormone and alpha-subunit: clinicopathological, immunohistochemical, ultrastructural, and immunoelectron microscopic studies in nine cases. Neurosurgery 26: 397–403
123. Randeva H S, Schoebel J, Byrne J et al. 1999 Classical pituitary apoplexy: clinical features, management and outcome. Clin Endocrinol 51: 181–188
124. Ebersold M J, Laws E R Jr, Scheithauer B W et al. 1983 Pituitary apoplexy treated by transsphenoidal surgery: a clinicopathological and immunohistochemical study. J Neurosurg 58: 315–319
125. Ahmed M, Rifai A, Al-Jurf M et al. 1989 Classical pituitary apoplexy: presentation and follow-up of 13 patients. Horm Res 31: 125–132
126. Geddes J F, Jansen G H, Robinson S F et al. 2000 'Gangliocytomas' of the pituitary: a heterogeneous group of lesions with differing histogenesis. Am J Surg Pathol 24: 607–613
127. Horvath E, Kovacs K, Scheithauer B W et al. 1994 Pituitary adenoma with neuronal choristoma (PANCH): composite lesion or lineage infidelity? Ultrastruct Pathol 18: 565–574
128. Towfighi J, Salam M M, McLendon R E et al. 1996 Ganglion cell-containing tumors of the pituitary gland. Arch Pathol Lab Med 120: 369–377
129. Asa S L, Scheithauer B W, Bilbao J M et al. 1984 A case for hypothalamic acromegaly: a clinico-pathological study of six patients with hypothalamic gangliocytomas producing growth hormone-releasing factor. J Clin Endocrinol Metab 58: 796–802
130. Li J Y, Racadot O, Kujas M et al. 1989 Immunocytochemistry of four mixed pituitary adenomas and intrasellar gangliocytomas associated with different clinical syndromes: acromegaly, amenorrhea-galactorrhea, Cushing's disease and isolated tumoral syndrome. Acta Neuropathol 77: 320–328
131. Saeger W, Puchner M J A, Lüdecke D K 1994 Combined sellar gangliocytoma and pituitary adenoma in acromegaly or Cushing's disease: a report of 3 cases. Virchows Arch [A] 425: 93–99
132. Rossi M L, Bevan J S, Esiri M M et al. 1987 Pituicytoma (pilocytic astrocytoma). Case report. J Neurosurg 67: 768–772
133. Hurley T R, D'Angelo C M, Clasen R A et al. 1994 Magnetic resonance imaging and pathological analysis of a pituicytoma: case report. Neurosurgery 35: 314–317
134. Brat D J, Scheithauer B W, Staugaitis S M et al. 2000 Pituicytoma. A distinctive low-grade glioma of the neurohypophysis. Am J Surg Pathol 24: 362–368
135. Hatton G I 1988 Pituicytes, glia, and control of terminal secretion. J Exp Biol 139: 67–79
136. Boecher-Schwarz H G, Fries G, Bornemann A et al. 1992 Suprasellar granular cell tumor. Neurosurgery 31: 751–754
137. Schlachter L B, Tindall G T, Pearl G S 1980 Granular cell tumor of the pituitary gland associated with diabetes insipidus. Neurosurgery 6: 418–421
138. Schaller B, Kirsch E, Tolany M et al. 1998 Symptomatic granular cell tumor of the pituitary gland: case report and review of the literature. Neurosurgery 42: 166–170
139. Vogelgesang S, Junge M H, Pahnke J et al. 2002 August 2001: Sellar/suprasellar mass in a 59-year-old woman. Brain Pathol 12: 135–136
140. Graziani N, Dufour H, Ficarella-Branger D et al. 1995 Suprasellar granular-cell tumour, presenting with intraventricular haemorrhage. Br J Neurosurg 9: 97–102
141. Nishioka H 1993 Immunohistochemical study of granular cell tumors and granular pituicytes of the neurohypophysis. Endocrin Pathol 4: 140–145
142. Laws E R Jr, Thapar K 1994 The diagnosis and management of craniopharyngioma. Growth Genet Horm 10: 6–11
143. Laws E R Jr 1997 Craniopharyngioma: transsphenoidal surgery. Curr Ther Endocrinol Metab 6: 35–38
144. Young S C, Zimmerman R A, Nowell M A et al. 1987 Giant cystic craniopharyngiomas. Neuroradiology 29: 468–473
145. Russell D S, Rubinstein L J 1989 Pathology of tumours of the nervous system, 5th edn. Edward Arnold, London, p 695–704
146. Midha R, Jay V, Smyth H S 1991 Transsphenoidal management of Rathke's cleft cysts. A clinicopathological review of 10 cases. Surg Neurol 35: 446–454
147. Ersahin Y, Ozdamar N, Demirtas E et al. 1995 A case of Rathke's cleft cyst presenting with diabetes insipidus. Clin Neurol Neurosurg 97: 317–320
148. Mukherjee J J, Islam N, Kaltsas G et al. 1997 Clinical, radiological and pathological features of patients with Rathke's cleft cysts: tumors that may recur. J Clin Endocrinol Metab 82: 2357–2362
149. Bognar L, Szeifert G T, Fedorcsak I et al. 1992 Abscess formation in Rathke's cleft cyst. Acta Neurochir 117: 70–72
150. Yamamoto M, Jimbo M, Ide M et al. 1993 Recurrence of symptomatic Rathke's cleft cyst: a case report. Surg Neurol 39: 263–268
151. Cheung C C, Ezzat S, Smyth H S et al. 2001 The spectrum and significance of primary hypophysitis. J Clin Endocrinol Metab 86: 1048–1053
152. Tashiro T, Sano T, Xu B et al. 2002 Spectrum of different types of hypophysitis: a clinicopathologic study of hypophysitis in 31 cases. Endocrinol Pathol 13: 183–195
153. Leung G K K, Lopes M B S, Thorner M O et al. 2004 Primary hypophysitis: a single-center experience in 16 cases. J Neurosurg 101: 262–271
154. Supler M L, Mickle J P 1992 Lymphocytic hypophysitis: report of a case in a man with contrasting cavernous sinus involvement. Surg Neurol 37: 472–476
155. Lee J H, Laws E R Jr, Guthrie B L et al. 1994 Lymphocytic hypophysitis: occurrence in two men. Neurosurgery 34: 159–163
156. Thodou E, Asa S I, Kontogeorgos G et al. 1995 Lymphocytic hypophysitis: clinicopathologic findings. J Clin Endocrinol Metab 80: 2302–2311
157. Imura H, Nakao K, Shimatsu A et al. 1993 Lymphocytic infundibuloneurohypophysitis as a cause of central diabetes insipidus. N Engl J Med 329: 683–689
158. Scanarini M, d'Avella D, Rotilio A et al. 1989 Giant-cell granulomatous hypophysitis: a distinct clinicopathological entity. J Neurosurg 71: 681–686
159. Barbaro D, Loni G 2000 Lymphocytic hypophysitis and autoimmune thyroid disease. J Endocrinol Invest 23: 339–340
160. Honegger J, Fahlbusch R, Bornemann A et al. 1997 Lymphocytic and granulomatous hypophysitis: experience with nine cases. Neurosurgery 40: 713–723
161. McKeever P E, Blaivas M, Sima A A F 1993 Neoplasms of the sellar region. In: Lloyd R V (ed) Surgical pathology of the pituitary gland. W B Saunders, Philadelphia, p 141–210
162. Thodou E, Kontogeorgos G, Scheithauer B W et al. 2000 Intrasellar chordomas mimicking pituitary adenoma. J Neurosurg 92: 976–982
163. Isaacs R S, Donald P F 1995 Sphenoid and sellar tumors. Otolaryngol Clin North Am 28: 1191–1229
164. Raco A, Bristot R, Domeniucci M et al. 1999 Meningiomas of the tuberculum sellae. J Neurosurg Sci 43: 253–262
165. Samii M, Tatagiba M, Monteiro ML 1996 Meningiomas involving the parasellar region. Acta Neurochir [Suppl] 65: 63–65
166. Kinjo T, al-Mefty O, Ciric I 1995 Diaphragma sellae meningiomas. Neurosurgery 36: 1082–1092
167. Smith M V, Laws E R Jr 1994 Magnetic resonance imaging measurements of pituitary stalk compression and deviation in patients with nonprolactin-secreting intrasellar and parasellar tumors: lack of correlation with serum prolactin levels. Neurosurgery 34: 834–839
168. Jin L, Lloyd R V 1993 Metastatic neoplasms to the pituitary gland. In: Lloyd R V (ed) Surgical pathology of the pituitary gland. W B Saunders, Philadelphia, p 137–140
169. Sioutos P, Yen V, Arbit E 1996 Pituitary gland metastases. Ann Surg Oncol 3: 94–99

甲状腺与甲状旁腺肿瘤
Tumors of the thyroid and parathyroid glands

18

第一部分

甲状腺　The thyroid gland

John K. C. Chan 著
孙 宇　李忠武　薛卫成 译

甲状腺		黏液表皮样癌	1037
正常甲状腺	997	显示C细胞分化的肿瘤	1038
甲状腺肿瘤：概述	997	显示滤泡和C细胞分化的肿瘤	1046
甲状腺肿瘤的诊断	1000	甲状腺的胸腺及相关性鳃囊肿瘤	1047
滤泡或化生上皮肿瘤	1000	淋巴造血细胞肿瘤	1049
乳头状癌	1000	间叶性肿瘤及其他肿瘤	1052
滤泡性肿瘤（滤泡性腺瘤和滤泡癌），包括Hurthle细胞肿瘤	1015	甲状腺不常见肿瘤及瘤样病变	1054
		甲状腺转移性恶性肿瘤	1055
未分化（间变性）癌	1029	甲状腺肿瘤诊断中的实际问题	1055
低分化甲状腺癌	1033	甲状腺病变的细针穿刺细胞学	1061
柱状细胞癌	1036	甲状腺肿瘤的术中冰冻切片诊断	1062

正常甲状腺
The normal thyroid gland

甲状腺为双叶状器官，位于颈前上段气管前方。胚胎上起源于原始咽基，并在发育中的舌下生长。成人正常甲状腺重 15～40 克。组织学上，由含类胶质的滤泡构成，滤泡内衬胞核一致、圆形、深染的立方上皮。滤泡上皮合成甲状腺激素（甲状腺素、三碘甲状腺原氨酸），在机体代谢调节中起重要作用。

被认为来源于后鳃体的滤泡旁 C 细胞构成甲状腺的一小部分。滤泡旁 C 细胞呈多角形或梭形，胞浆透明或浅染，单个或成群分布于滤泡基底膜或滤泡间隙内。常规显微镜下难以识别，降钙素免疫组化染色能很好地显示滤泡旁 C 细胞，因为降钙素是滤泡旁 C 细胞最重要的激素产物。滤泡旁 C 细胞并非均匀分布于甲状腺内，而是沿着假定的中轴局限于甲状腺侧叶的中、上 1/3 的实质中。

甲状腺肿瘤：概述
Thyroid tumors: an overview

甲状腺癌相当常见，年发病率介于 (0.5～10)/100 000 之间。最常见的肿瘤及其发病率列于表 18A.1。由 2004 世界卫生组织（WHO）分类修订而来的甲状腺肿瘤分类列于表 18A.2[1]。根据监测、流行病学和最终结果（SEER）的研究，主要甲状腺癌10年相对生存率如下：乳头状癌，0.98；滤泡癌，0.92；髓样癌，0.80；未分化癌，0.13[2]。

原发性甲状腺癌(primary thyroid cancers)的一般情况

- 乳头状癌是最常见的组织学类型。
- 除血管肉瘤外，甲状腺肿瘤的女性患者是男性的2～4倍[3]。女性通常预后略好。

甲状腺肿瘤：概述

表18A.1　甲状腺主要原发性恶性肿瘤的大致发病比例

肿瘤类型	发病比例（%）
乳头状癌	70~85
滤泡癌	5~10
髓样癌	5
恶性淋巴瘤	4~5
未分化癌	2~5
低分化（岛状）癌	0.4~10

- 分化较好的肿瘤通常发生于比较年轻的病人，而分化较差的肿瘤发生于年龄较大的病人。低、中和高度恶性肿瘤的平均发病年龄分别为40、50和60岁（表18A.3）。
- 相同类型的肿瘤，40岁以下的年轻病人通常比年老病人预后好[2]。
- 除了年龄，原发瘤的大小和肿瘤分期（有无甲状腺外侵犯及转移）通常是最重要的预后因素[2]。甲状腺肿瘤的TNM分期系统列于表18A.4和18A.5。这种TNM分期的特殊之处在于它同时考虑病人的年龄和肿瘤的类型，但是它的临床重要性已得到证实[4-6]。

儿童甲状腺癌(thyroid cancers in children)的特征[7-12]

- 在儿童，乳头状癌也是最常见的组织学类型。
- 在儿童，已知的促进甲状腺癌发生的唯一因素是放射线，如切尔诺贝利（Chernobyl）核事件。
- 甲状腺内的癌通常为多灶性癌。
- 大多数病人表现为颈部肿块，60%~80%有可触及的淋巴结。不管最初的手术范围多大，后者复发的危险性高[13]。
- 与成人相比，儿童甲状腺癌生物学上更具侵袭性，甲状腺外扩散更常见，淋巴结或远处转移发生率较高。肺转移率约为10%。复发率为10%~35%。然而，其预后很好，死亡率只有2.6%。

表18A.2　原发性甲状腺肿瘤的分类，根据WHO分类（2004）修订

组别	肿瘤
甲状腺滤泡或化生上皮肿瘤	滤泡性腺瘤（包括Hurthle细胞腺瘤和玻璃样变梁状肿瘤） 滤泡癌（包括Hurthle细胞癌） 　　微小浸润 　　广泛浸润 乳头状癌 柱状细胞癌（乳头状癌柱状细胞亚型） 黏液表皮样癌 伴嗜酸细胞增多的硬化性黏液表皮样癌 黏液癌 低分化甲状腺癌，包括岛状癌 未分化（间变性）癌（包括鳞状细胞癌和癌肉瘤）
显示C细胞分化的肿瘤	髓样癌
显示滤泡和C细胞分化的肿瘤	碰撞瘤：滤泡/乳头状癌和髓样癌 混合性髓样和滤泡细胞癌
显示胸腺或相关鳃囊分化的肿瘤	异位胸腺瘤 伴胸腺样分化的梭形上皮肿瘤 显示胸腺样成分的癌或甲状腺内胸腺癌
淋巴细胞肿瘤	恶性淋巴瘤 浆细胞瘤
甲状腺内甲状旁腺肿瘤	甲状旁腺腺瘤 甲状旁腺癌
间叶性和其他肿瘤	良性和恶性间叶肿瘤，如孤立性纤维瘤、平滑肌瘤、外周神经鞘瘤、血管肉瘤 副神经节瘤 畸胎瘤

表18A.3	原发性甲状腺癌的行为分组	
肿瘤行为分组	病种	主要死因
低度恶性	乳头状癌	局部疾病
	微小浸润型滤泡癌	远处转移
	黏膜相关淋巴组织型结外边缘区B细胞淋巴瘤	远处转移
中度恶性	广泛浸润型滤泡癌	远处转移
	低分化甲状腺癌	远处转移
	髓样癌	远处转移
	弥漫大B细胞淋巴瘤	远处转移
高度恶性	未分化癌	局部疾病和远处转移
	血管肉瘤	局部疾病和远处转移

表18A.4	甲状腺肿瘤的TNM分期 (International Union Against Cancer,第6版)		
分期	定义	分期	定义
原发肿瘤(T)[a]		间变性(未分化)癌(均属于T4)	
TX	原发肿瘤无法评估	T4a	甲状腺内(任何大小),手术可切除
T0	无原发肿瘤证据	T4b	甲状腺外(任何大小),手术不能切除
T1	肿瘤局限于甲状腺,最大径≤2cm		
T2	肿瘤局限于甲状腺,最大径>2cm但≤4cm		
T3	肿瘤最大径>4cm,局限在甲状腺内;或任何大小肿瘤伴轻微的甲状腺外扩散(例如:扩散到胸骨舌骨肌或甲状腺周围软组织)	区域淋巴结(N)[b]	
		NX	区域淋巴结无法评估
		N0	区域淋巴结无转移
		N1	区域淋巴结有转移
T4a	任何大小的肿瘤扩散到甲状腺被膜外并侵袭皮下组织、喉、气管、食管或喉返神经	N1a	转移到Ⅵ区(气管前、气管旁和喉前/Delphian)淋巴结
T4b	肿瘤侵袭到椎体前筋膜或纵隔血管,或包裹颈动脉	N1b	转移到单侧、双侧或对侧颈淋巴结或上纵隔淋巴结
		远处转移(M)	
		MX	远处转移无法评估
		M0	无远处转移
		M1	有远处转移

[a]对于多灶性肿瘤(m),肿瘤大小的分类由最大结节的直径决定。
[b]区域淋巴结指颈部和上纵隔淋巴结。

Sobin LH, Wittekind C International Union Against Cancer (UICC) © 2002 TNM classification of Malignant Tumors, 6th edition. John Wiley & Sons, Inc., New York, USA. Reprinted with permission of John Wiley & Sons, Inc.

切尔诺贝利核事件相关性甲状腺癌的特征[14-21]
Features of Chernobyl nuclear accident-associated thyroid cancer

- 1986年4月26日在切尔诺贝利发生的核事件提供了大量有关放射性碘泄漏与甲状腺癌发生的自然病史信息。
- 与以前相比,切尔诺贝利周围地区甲状腺癌的发生率按照距离的不同,增加了6～500倍。最大病例数发生在甲状腺放射剂量≥0.5Gy的区域。
- 核事件后,甲状腺癌发生的潜伏期相对较短,平均6～7年。核事件发生时<5岁或尚未出生(in utero)的个体占大多数。
- 诊断时年龄常≤14岁,发病年龄小于与核事故无关的散发性儿童甲状腺癌。
- 大多数病例为乳头状癌(～95%),常显示滤

表18A.5	甲状腺肿瘤分期（International Union Against Cancer，第6版）	
分期	<45岁	≥45岁
乳头状癌或滤泡癌		
I	任何T，任何N，M0	T1，N0，M0
II	任何T，任何N，M1	T2，N0，M0
III	–	T3，N0，M0
		T1/T2/T3，N1a，M0
IVA	–	T4a，任何N，M0
		T1/T2/T3，N1b，M0
IVB	–	T4b，任何N，M0
IVC	–	任何T，任何N，M1
髓样癌	–	与乳头状癌/滤泡癌分期相同
	所有病例	
未分化癌[a]		
IVA	T4a，任何N，M0	
IVB	T4b，任何N，M0	
IVC	任何T，任何N，M1	

[a] 未分化癌的所有病例属于IV期。
(After Sobin LH, Wittekind C 2002 TNM classification of malignant tumors, 6th edn. Wiley, New York.)

泡性、实性或混合性滤泡性/乳头状/实性结构，不同于典型的散发性儿童乳头状癌结构。与散发病例相比，其RET/PTC（尤其RET/PTC3）基因重排率较高。
- 肿瘤一经发现即表现为较强的侵袭性，如甲状腺外扩散、静脉浸润、淋巴结转移。
- 淋巴细胞性甲状腺炎和抗甲状腺过氧化物酶抗体的出现较之散发病例更常见。

甲状腺肿瘤的诊断
Diagnosis of thyroid tumors

对于大多数甲状腺肿瘤，单靠形态学即可做出诊断。然而，对于形态特殊的甲状腺肿瘤或髓样癌的诊断，免疫组化是必不可少的。比较有用的抗体列于表18A.6(图18A.1)[22-27]。尽管有些抗体，如HBME-1、galectin-3或双肽基氨基肽酶IV（dipeptidyl aminopeptidase IV），被认为有助于区分甲状腺恶性肿瘤和良性病变，但由于经常出现假阳性和假阴性，其价值有限[28-33]。电镜很少用于甲状腺肿瘤的诊断。尽管对于甲状腺肿瘤分子遗传学的理解不断提高，分子研究到目前为止仍未用于常规

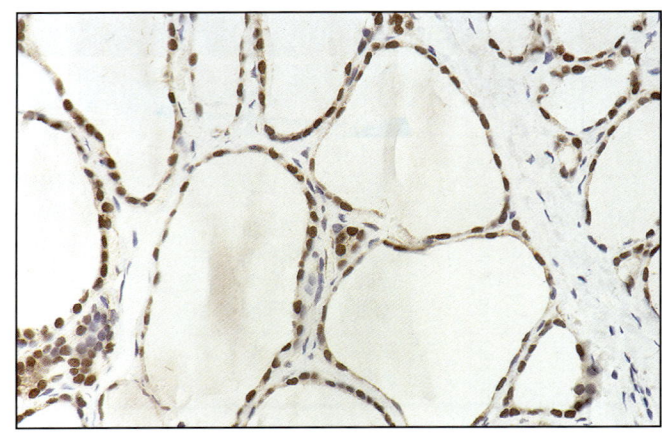

图18A.1　正常甲状腺。甲状腺滤泡上皮呈TTF-1核阳性。

诊断。

正如其他内分泌器官肿瘤，甲状腺肿瘤出现细胞核非典型性并不等同于恶性。实际上，出现在内分泌器官内的非典型、深染细胞核更可能是对过度刺激的反应，而不意味着具有恶性潜能。例如在桥本甲状腺炎和激素生成不良中，常出现一些核多形性孤立细胞。

本章首先讨论乳头状癌，因为这种肿瘤是根据细胞学特征来准确定义的，只有当缺乏乳头状癌细胞学特征时，才能做出滤泡性肿瘤的诊断。由于滤泡性腺瘤和滤泡癌是密切相关且需要病理医师加以鉴别的疾病，将它们放在一起讨论是合理的。一些临床研究将乳头状癌和滤泡癌归在"分化性甲状腺癌"的范围内[34]，这一做法是不合理的，因为它们在临床、组织学和生物学上迥然不同（表18A.7）[35-39]。RNA/DNA显微芯片研究已清楚显示这些肿瘤显示明显不同的基因表达谱，乳头状癌过表达CITED1、claudin-10和胰岛素样生长因子结合蛋白6（IGFBP-6）；滤泡癌低表达IGFBP-6和(或)CAV-1和CAV-2[40]。

滤泡或化生上皮肿瘤
Tumors of follicular or metaplastic epithelium

乳头状癌　Papillary carcinoma

定义

乳头状癌被定义为一种"显示滤泡细胞分化证据并具有独特细胞核特征的恶性上皮性肿瘤"[1]。也就是说，诊断的关键是核的特征（详见下文），并不要求出现浸润性生长[41-44]。

表18A.6　对甲状腺肿瘤诊断有用的抗体

抗体	特异性	甲状腺肿瘤的反应性	诊断注意事项或特殊的诊断价值
甲状腺球蛋白	330-kDa糖基化蛋白，是甲状腺滤泡上皮分化的特异性标志物。滤泡上皮和类胶质依功能状态而呈不同程度染色。	滤泡性腺瘤(癌) 乳头状癌 低分化癌 柱状细胞癌 滤泡-滤泡旁细胞癌 (未分化癌呈阴性)	如果染色仅见于肿瘤的周边部分，可能是周围甲状腺的甲状腺球蛋白扩散造成的人工假象。 甲状腺球蛋白对于确定转移性肿瘤来源于甲状腺是很有价值的。
降钙素	滤泡旁C细胞标志物	髓样癌 滤泡-滤泡旁细胞癌	转移性肿瘤降钙素阳性强烈支持甲状腺原发，尽管其他肿瘤有时降钙素阳性，如喉神经内分泌癌
TTF-1	38-kDa核蛋白，介导甲状腺特异性基因转录，表达于甲状腺滤泡和滤泡旁C细胞以及肺泡细胞。	滤泡性肿瘤 乳头状癌 低分化甲状腺癌 髓样癌 (未分化癌常为阴性)	非鳞状细胞肺癌和肺外小细胞癌常为阳性
嗜铬素或突触素	高度敏感和特异的广谱神经内分泌标志物。甲状腺滤泡旁C细胞阳性，而滤泡上皮细胞阴性。	髓样癌 副神经节瘤 甲状腺内甲状旁腺肿瘤 转移性神经内分泌肿瘤	当降钙素染色不确定时，支持髓样癌的诊断
细胞角蛋白	上皮标志物	各种甲状腺滤泡上皮肿瘤 髓样癌 胸腺-鳃囊相关肿瘤 甲状腺内甲状旁腺肿瘤 转移癌	对区别副神经节瘤（阴性）和其他神经内分泌肿瘤（阳性）有用。 潜在缺陷：浆细胞瘤和血管肉瘤偶尔细胞角蛋白阳性。
白细胞共同抗原(CD45)	白细胞特异性标志物	淋巴瘤 白血病	对于检测"未分化"甲状腺肿瘤有用，注意浆细胞瘤可能为阴性
S-100	正常甲状腺滤泡上皮，尤其Hurthle细胞不同程度地表达S-100	许多不同类型的甲状腺肿瘤呈不同程度的S-100阳性	除用于证实副神经节瘤的支持细胞，在甲状腺肿瘤诊断中没有特殊价值。S-100阳性的支持细胞也见于遗传性髓样癌
甲状旁腺素	甲状旁腺细胞的特异标志物	甲状腺内甲状旁腺肿瘤	对证实肿瘤来源于甲状旁腺最有帮助

临床特征

乳头状癌可累及任何年龄组，以女性多见（表18A.7）[45-49]。多数患者表现为无痛性甲状腺或颈部包块，而一些病人以淋巴结转移为首发症状，在同侧甲状腺内常能发现隐匿的原发瘤（图18A.2）。囊性转移容易出现问题，因为在临床或组织学上容易误诊为鳃裂囊肿或良性囊肿（图18A.3）[50,51]。少数乳头状癌发生于甲状舌管，通常为偶然发现[52]。

表18A.7	甲状腺分化型癌的重要特征	
	乳头状癌	滤泡癌
发生率	较常见（占所有甲状腺癌的70%以上）	较少见（占所有甲状腺癌的10%以下）
性别	女性居多（男:女，1:2.5）	女性居多（男:女，1:2.5～1:4）
年龄	年龄范围广，平均43岁	微小浸润型：平均48岁；广泛浸润型：平均55岁
临床表现	生长缓慢的甲状腺肿块；偶然发现；颈部淋巴结转移	生长缓慢的甲状腺结节；少数表现为快速生长的甲状腺肿块或远处转移
大体表现	常呈浸润性，质硬，颗粒状	有包膜的肉质肿块。广泛浸润型可见浸润和卫星结节
甲状腺内分布	常见多灶性病变(20%～87.5%)	通常单发
组织学诊断依据	典型的核特征（重叠的毛玻璃样核、核沟、核内假包涵体）。浸润不是诊断的必备条件	滤泡性肿瘤必须有血管和(或)包膜浸润；缺乏乳头状癌的核特征
扩散方式	局部浸润；淋巴管扩散，40%的病例出现淋巴结转移；远处转移罕见，最常见肺转移	局部扩散很少超出甲状腺被膜；淋巴结转移不常见；主要通过血行转移（尤其广泛浸润型），骨和肺是常见部位
生物学行为	惰性；可发生远期复发；长期随访癌相关死亡率仅为6.5%	累积死亡率：微小浸润型3%；广泛浸润型32%
分子学发病机制	*BRAF*突变；*RET*或*TRK*与伴侣基因*PTC*融合；*RAS*癌基因突变（?）	*RAS*癌基因突变；*PAX8/PPARγ*融合

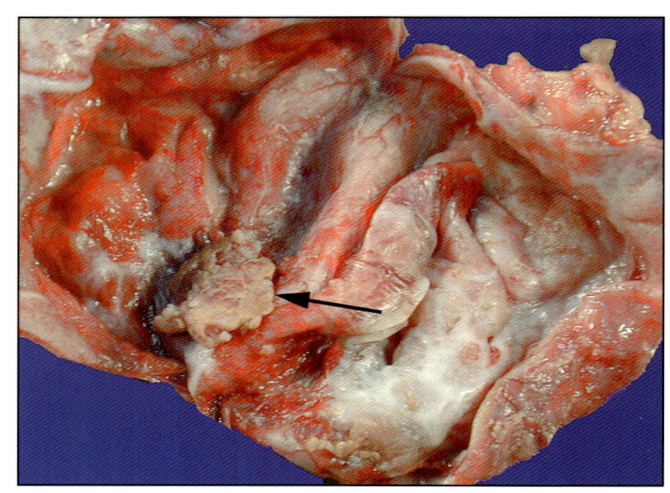

图18A.2 乳头状癌的颈淋巴结囊性转移。病人表现为颈部大囊肿。切开后腔面光滑或小梁状，可见乳头状突起（箭头）。

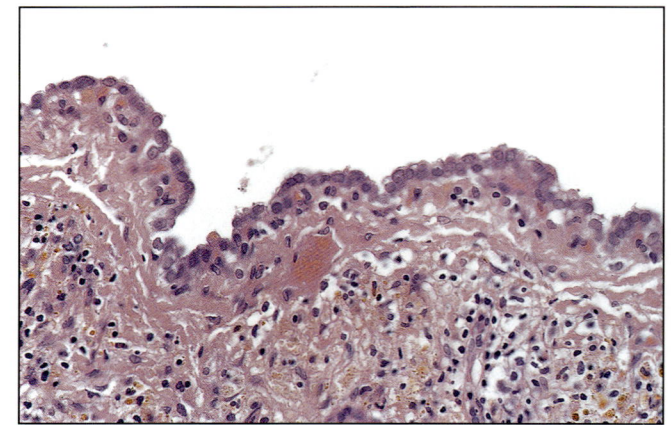

图18A.3 乳头状癌颈淋巴结囊性转移。囊壁由残存淋巴细胞和纤维组织组成，被覆立方（某些区域为扁平）上皮。乳头状癌的核特征在被覆上皮中不明显，因此会毫无怀疑地误诊为良性囊肿或鳃裂囊肿。

病因学及易感因素

头颈部放射治疗史、来自核事件（如切尔诺贝利事件）或原子弹（如广岛原子弹爆炸的幸存者）的辐射暴露、桥本甲状腺炎、家族性腺瘤性息肉病及Cowden病均增加乳头状癌的危险性[15,53-55]。一些伴常染色体显性遗传的家族性病例已有报道，即所谓的家族性非髓样甲状腺癌；一些病例以微小癌居多[56-60]。

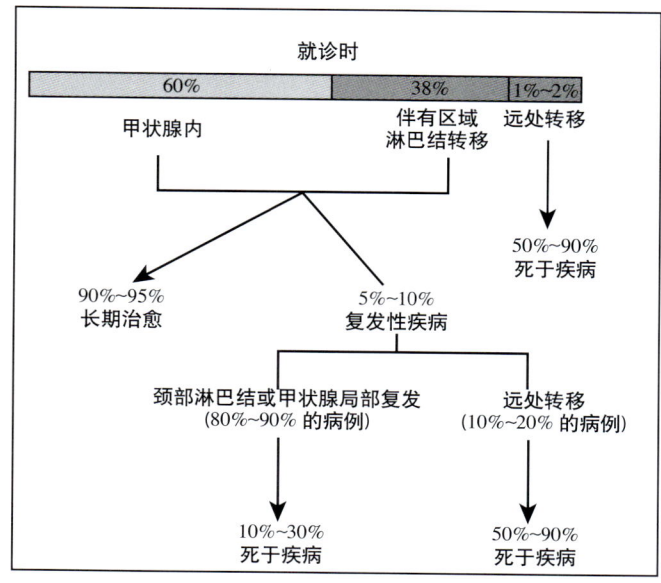

图18A.4 甲状腺乳头状癌的自然发展史流程图。

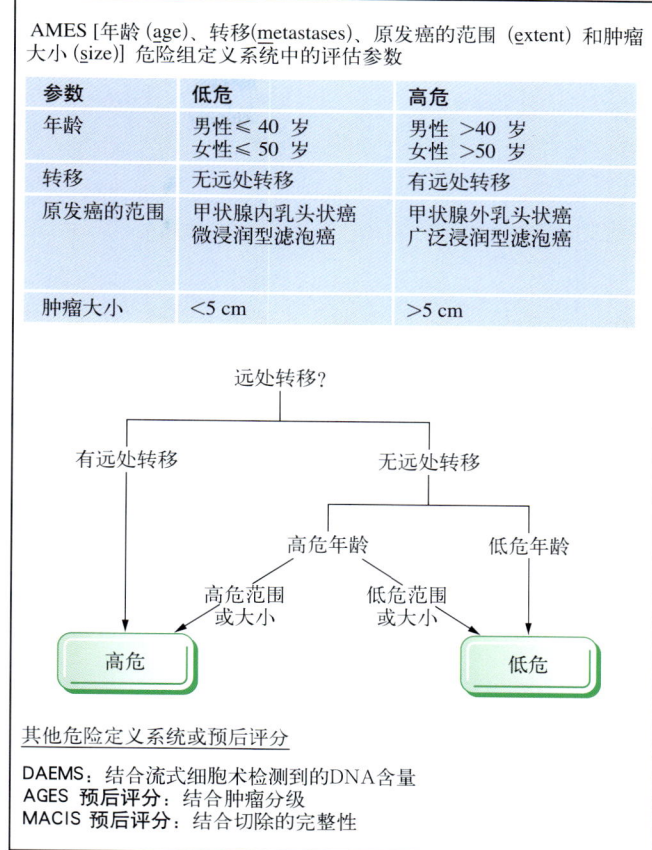

图18A.5 高分化甲状腺癌（乳头状癌和滤泡癌）的危险分组。

临床行为及治疗

乳头状癌是一种惰性肿瘤，长期预后极好。它的自然病史描述于图18A.4。根据Mayo医院的长期随访研究发现，癌相关死亡率仅为6.5%[47]。乳头状癌倾向于局部浸润（甲状腺实质、甲状腺周围软组织，少数可以侵及气管）和局部淋巴结转移（好转移于颈正中和同侧颈部淋巴结）[61]。治疗后，残存甲状腺、颈部软组织或颈淋巴结可发生局部复发。远处转移不常见（9%～14%），通常发生在疾病晚期[36,62-64]。复发可发生在初诊20～30年后[65]。风险评估系统（risk assignment system）现在被广泛用于指导治疗（图18A.5）[66-68]。

关于乳头状癌治疗方法的选择没有一致意见。由于常常多灶性发生，传统上推荐的治疗方法是全甲状腺切除[69]，现在该方法仍被许多外科医生和肿瘤学家所推荐以减少复发和死亡率[70-72]。然而，一些研究已表明，单侧甲状腺切除术或全叶切除术对于无明显肿瘤残留的低危病人具有相同的效果[47,63,73-79]。术后通常给予抑制剂量的甲状腺素。术后放射性碘治疗的作用也存在争议，尽管一些研究证实放射性碘治疗不能改善预后（至少对于低危病人），而另一些研究表明能减少局部复发率[47,63,76,80-83]。然而，对于高危病人标准的治疗包括全甲状腺切除、放射性碘和抑制性甲状腺素。淋巴结切除术适用于淋巴结有转移或肿瘤出现甲状腺外浸润时[84]。前哨淋巴结切除和预防性正中淋巴结切除的价值仍不能确定[85-89]。

大体表现

乳头状癌通常呈浸润性生长，边界不清，质硬（图18A.6）。灰白色，由于乳头的出现而呈颗粒状（图18A.7）。由于出现沙粒体和钙化，切面有沙砾感。多灶性病变常见（～65%）；尽管传统上认为源于腺体内转移，分子学研究提示每个病灶为独立的肿瘤[41,48,90-96]。少数情况下肿瘤界清，有包膜。主要或完全由滤泡组成的乳头状癌切面更有肉质感。

组织学表现

细胞学特征 乳头状癌的细胞核通常较大，密集，卵圆形，毛玻璃样（类似"孤儿安妮"的眼睛），具有核沟，并含有明显的小核仁[43]。细胞拥挤导致细胞核重叠排列（图18A.8）。有时，细胞核可呈现一种"凹陷"或杯状形态（图18A.8A）。

毛玻璃改变指细胞核看上去发空，含有少量边集的尘状染色质（图18A.8B），被认为是甲醛固定产生的人工假象，因为此现象在冰冻切片或细胞学标本中并不明显[97-99]。在石蜡切片中，可见于80%以上的乳头状癌[97,100]。然而，这一特征并非乳头状癌特有，良

乳头状癌

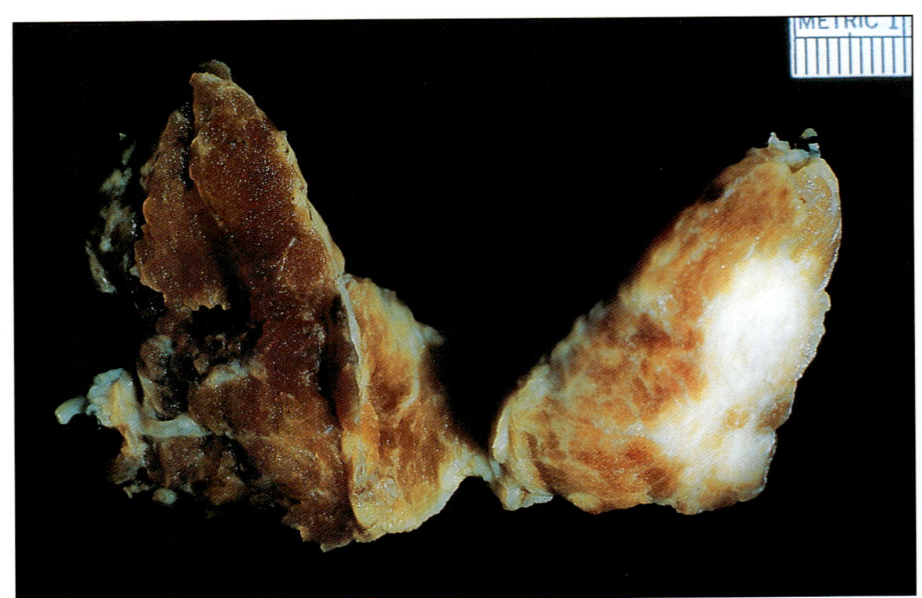

图18A.6 乳头状癌大体标本，以边界不清及硬化为特征。

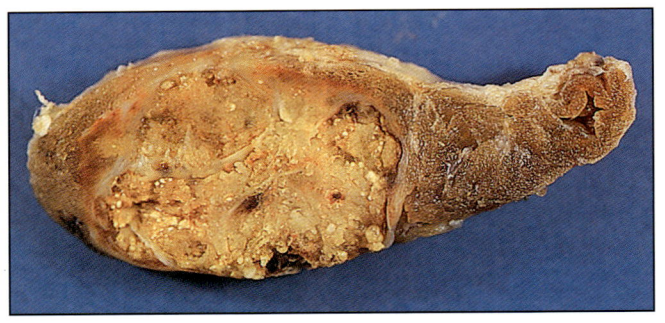

图18A.7 乳头状癌。切面可见肿瘤呈粗糙颗粒状突起，其中散在窄小的囊性间隙。这种特征性外观是由于发育不良的乳头突入囊腔所致，黄色斑点代表大的沙粒体和钙化灶。

性病变如结节性增生、滤泡性腺瘤、Graves 病及桥本甲状腺炎都可见局灶透明核[100]。

乳头状癌的另一特征是核沟，由核膜折叠形成（图18A.8B）[100]。见于几乎所有乳头状癌，至少局灶可见核沟。核沟在细胞涂片中很清楚[101-103]。然而，核沟也并非特有的诊断特征，因为它还可见于实性细胞巢、某些滤泡性肿瘤（尤其是 Hurthle 细胞型）、玻璃样变小梁腺瘤、低分化甲状腺癌和非甲状腺来源的腺癌[43,100,104,105]。

由胞浆内陷形成的核内假包涵体，表现为淡染、有膜包绕的空泡。为乳头状癌典型特征而非专有特征，通常仅见于一小部分肿瘤细胞（图 18A.8A）[100,105-107]。

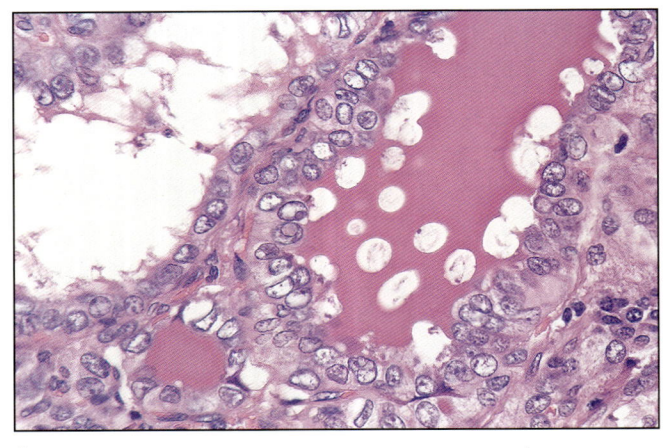

A

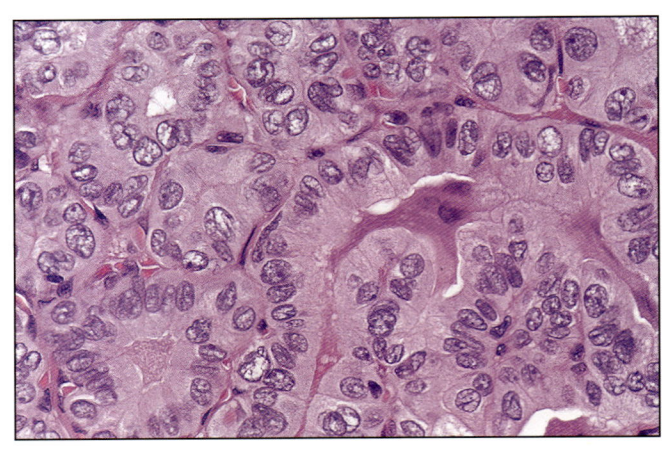

B

图18A.8 乳头状癌特征性的细胞核。（A）核卵圆形、毛玻璃样或浅染，核拥挤、重叠。有些核内可见假包涵体。一个核（左下视野）呈部分"凹陷"表现。（B）核卵圆形、浅染、有深核沟。核缺乏极向。可见小核仁。在滤泡腔内有一个多核组织细胞，这种现象在乳头状癌中并不少见。

一些乳头状癌的上述核特征不明显或只局灶分布。核不呈毛玻璃样，而只是浅染或呈均匀分布的细染色质。偶尔，核染色质粗，多形性明显。在这些病例，乳头状癌的诊断更多地依赖于结构特点以及寻找更具有诊断性核特征的病灶。

分裂象通常缺乏或罕见。然而，在一些高度浸润性肿瘤或复发病例，分裂象易见[108-110]。

肿瘤细胞呈多角形或立方形，但可变扁，呈圆顶状、鞋钉样或柱状。胞浆轻度嗜酸至双嗜性，但可嗜酸或透明（图18A.8）[109,111-114]。有时可见胞浆黏液（图18A.9）[115,116]。大约一半病例发生鳞状分化；与乳头状癌典型的核特征丧失有关（图18A.10）。

结构特征 乳头状癌通常呈浸润性生长（图18A.11），然而有些肿瘤界清，甚至有包膜。有研究表明，浸润程度与淋巴结转移率成正比[117]。一些肿瘤显示囊性变，在淋巴结转移灶中尤其常见（图18A.3）。淋巴扩散并不少见。

乳头通常具有分支（图18A.12），伴有纤细的纤维血管轴心。然而，乳头也可宽大，轴心由纤维细胞、水肿或玻璃样变的组织构成，内含泡沫状巨噬细胞、脂肪细胞或小的肿瘤性滤泡（图18A.12B）[118-120]。有时，可形成由微乳头构成的细胞簇（图18A.9）。

滤泡常常存在。滤泡大小、形状不同，通常拉长或形状不规则，内含深染的类胶质（图18A.13）。有些滤泡较大，因含类胶质而明显扩张。常见滤泡内出血。滤泡与乳头常发生复杂性混合，产生一种复杂的管-乳头结构（图18A.13B）。较少见的结构包括微腺体、花环样、筛状、管网状、小梁状和实性（图18A.14）[43,121]。

间质（stroma） 乳头状癌常伴有丰富的硬化性间质，可以表现为钙化或骨化（图18A.11）[122,123]。致密的玻璃样纤维化是区分乳头状癌（89%）与滤泡癌（18%）的一个有用的特征[122]。细胞丰富的结缔组织增生性间质可出现在浸润癌前缘[41]。通常有成片淋巴细胞、浆细胞和巨噬细胞浸润。

46%的病例在滤泡腔和乳头中会出现胞浆深染的多核组织细胞（图18A.8B）。由于在良性病变和其他类型肿瘤中极其少见，这些细胞具有诊断价值[124]。

沙粒体为层状钙化结构，出现在一半的病例中[41,125]。它们出现在乳头轴心、纤维间质或肿瘤细胞内（图18A.12A）。在甲状腺，它们实际上就能确定乳头状癌的诊断[108]。一旦在甲状腺内发现沙粒体，就应仔细寻找乳头状癌灶。在Hurthle细胞肿瘤和玻璃样变小梁腺瘤中常见的类胶质钙化不同于沙粒体，它们全部位于滤泡腔内。

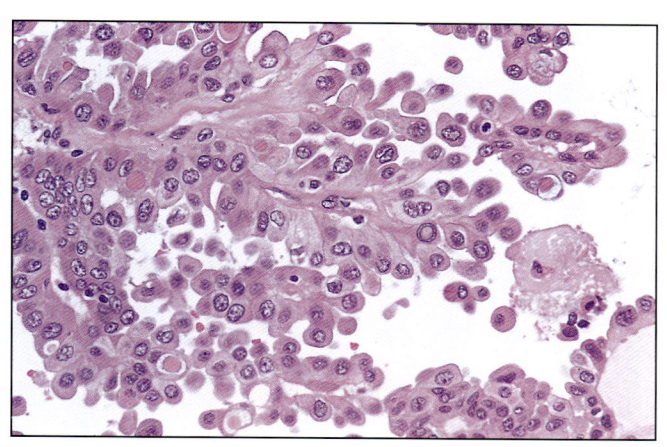

图18A.9 乳头状癌伴细胞簇形成（微乳头）。可见核内假包涵体。一些细胞有胞浆黏液空泡。

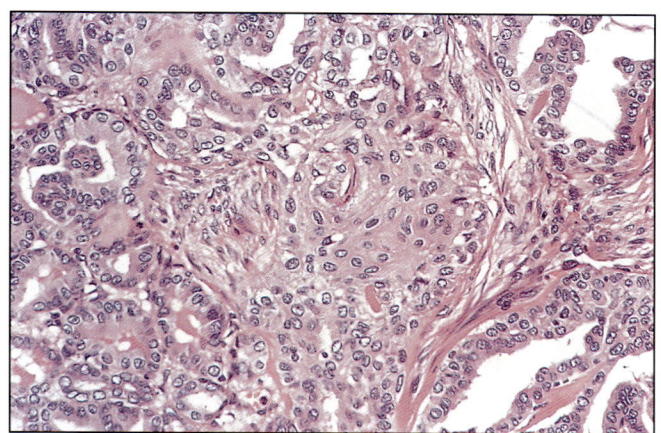

图18A.10 乳头状癌鳞状化生。注意鳞状成分中核形态温和。

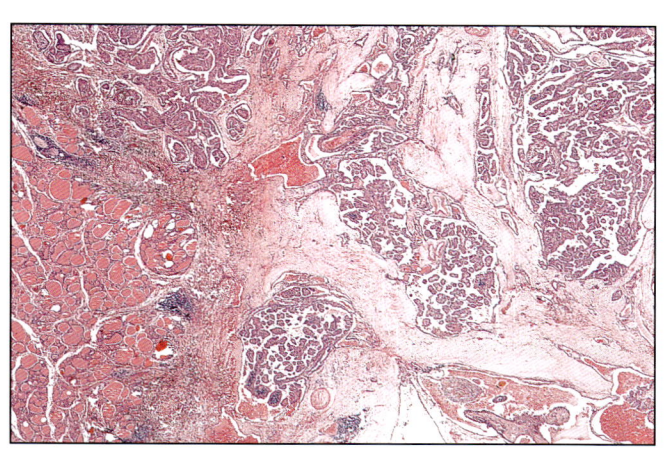

图18A.11 典型的乳头状癌。注意浸润性生长方式、硬化和分支状乳头结构。

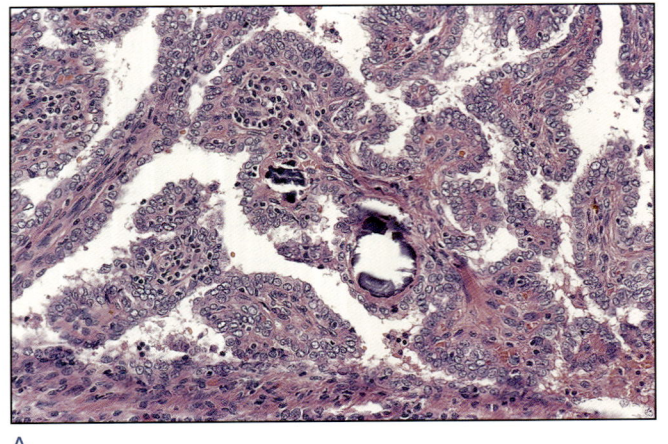

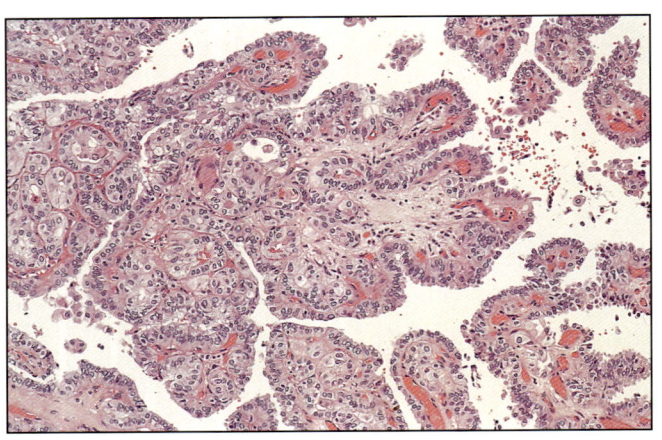

图18A.12 乳头状癌。（A）分支状乳头有纤细的纤维血管轴心，内见沙粒体。（B）此处描述的巨乳头较少见。

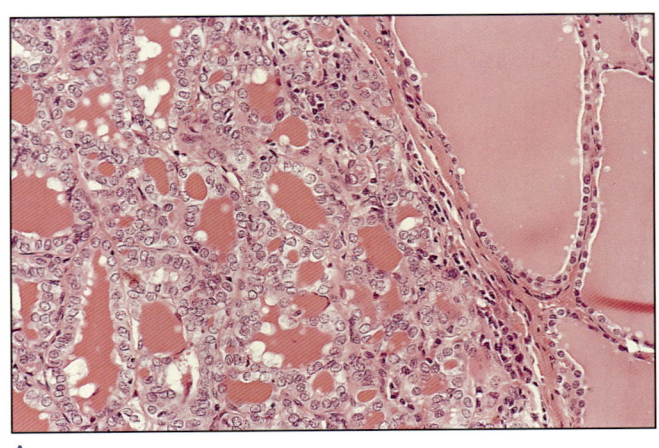

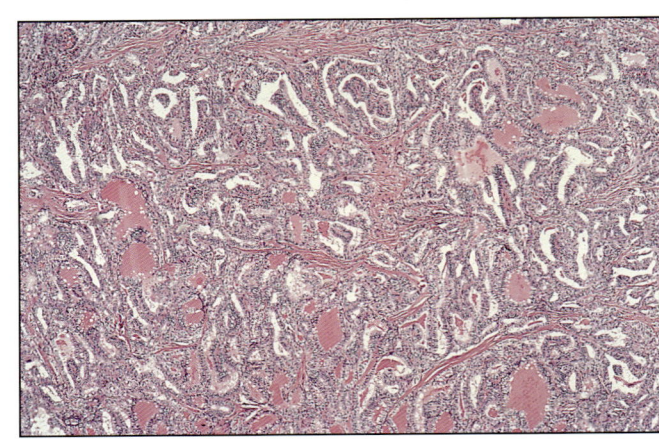

图18A.13 乳头状癌。（A）滤泡常见。与右侧残存甲状腺比较，滤泡伸长，充满深染类胶质。（B）复杂的管状乳头结构常见。

乳头状癌的亚型
Variants of papillary carcinoma

乳头状癌的许多亚型已有描述。这些亚型并非相互排斥，因为某个肿瘤可满足多种亚型的描述。大多数只是形态上的亚型，不具有预后重要性。高细胞型、弥漫硬化型、弥漫滤泡型、实性型、小梁状和去分化型在生物学上更具有侵袭性，而包膜内型预后较好。

滤泡亚型（Follicular variant） 指全部或几乎完全由滤泡组成的乳头状癌[126]。多数呈侵袭性生长（图18A.15），有些位于包膜内（所谓的Lindsay瘤）。滤泡大小、形状不一，滤泡常常拉长，形状不规则，乳头状结构不充分，类胶质常常深染，边缘呈锯齿状（图18A.15B）[127]。可出现沙粒体和硬化。诊断依靠乳头状癌典型的核特征。临床行为与经典的乳头状癌无差别[128,129]。

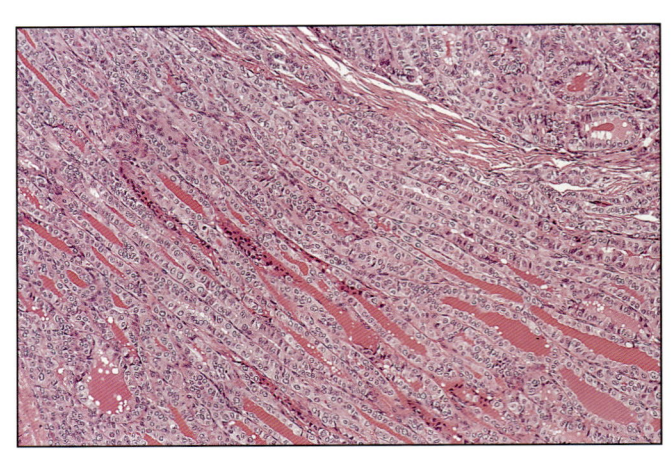

图18A.14 由明显伸长的滤泡和小梁组成的乳头状癌。

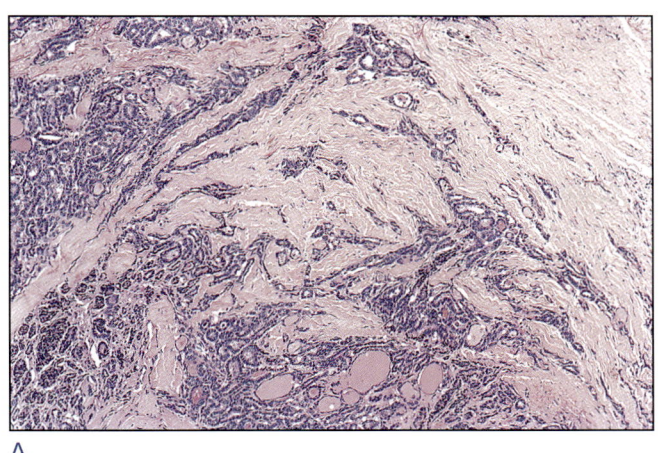
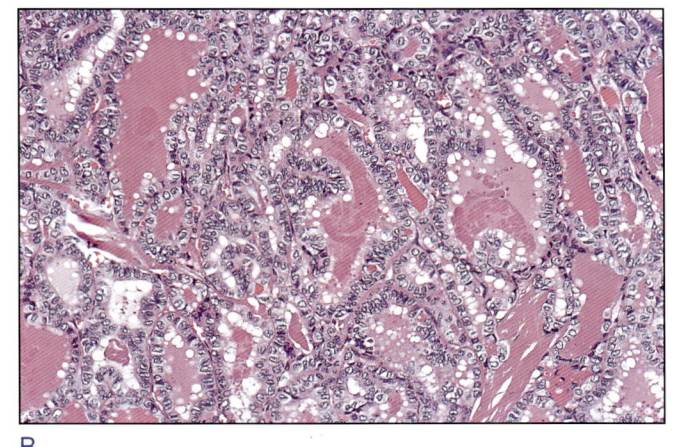

图18A.15 乳头状癌，滤泡亚型。（A）大多数滤泡亚型乳头状癌呈浸润性生长伴硬化性间质。（B）滤泡伸长，可见发育不全的乳头。类胶质常深染，呈扇贝形。

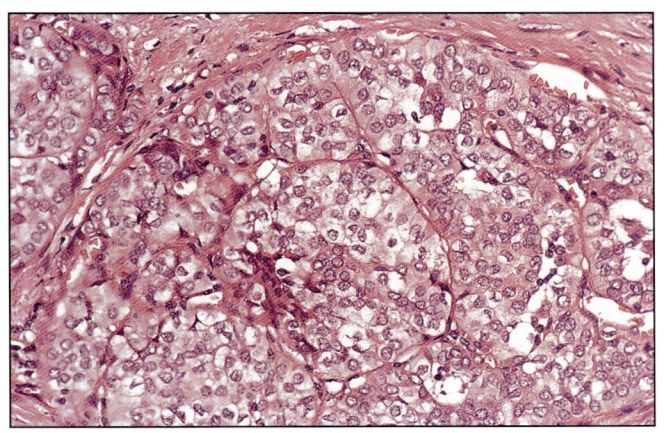

图18A.16 乳头状癌，实性亚型。肿瘤呈岛屿状、片状分布，由纤细的血管分隔。核特征与典型的乳头状癌无差别。

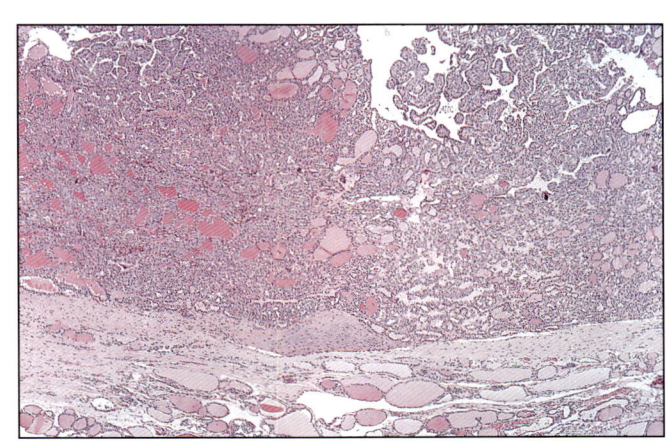

图18A.17 乳头状癌，包膜内亚型。此肿瘤由乳头和滤泡组成。

实性亚型（Solid variant） 指具有50%以上实性生长方式的乳头状癌[41,48,63,130]。圆形或不规则的肿瘤细胞岛常被纤细的纤维血管分隔，具有乳头状癌核的特征（图18A.16）。没有肿瘤坏死[131]。该类型在核事件相关性甲状腺乳头状癌中所占比例较高。与普通的乳头状癌相比，其远处转移的频率稍高，预后稍差[131]。主要的鉴别诊断是低分化癌（核较深染，核分裂象常见）和髓样癌（点彩状染色质，降钙素阳性）。

包膜内亚型（Encapsulated variant） 此型占乳头状癌的4%～14%[36,63,109,132,133]。纤维性包膜可能显示或不显示肿瘤浸润（图18A.17），但淋巴结转移可能发生在无包膜或血管浸润的情况下。那些完全由滤泡组成的病例与滤泡性腺瘤（癌）难以鉴别。与经典型乳头状癌相比，病人较年轻，较少出现压迫症状，淋巴结转移率低（12%～38%）。预后极好，治疗后所有病人无病生存[75,132-134]。

弥漫硬化亚型（Diffuse sclerosing variant） 该型常累及儿童和年轻成人，表现为双侧或单侧弥漫性甲状腺肿胀[108]。血清抗甲状腺球蛋白或抗微粒体抗体可阳性，更类似甲状腺炎[135-137]。大多数（但并非所有）研究表明此型生物学上较经典型乳头状癌更具侵袭性，表现为更高的淋巴结转移率（几乎100%）和频繁的远处转移[136-144]。然而，经过充分的治疗，死亡率与经典型相似，大概与病人年轻有关。

甲状腺实质被白色坚硬的组织弥漫替代，切面有沙砾感。典型的组织学特征包括[135,142,145,146]：
- 弥漫累及一叶或两叶（图18A.18A）
- 硬化
- 重度淋巴浆细胞浸润
- 丰富的沙粒体

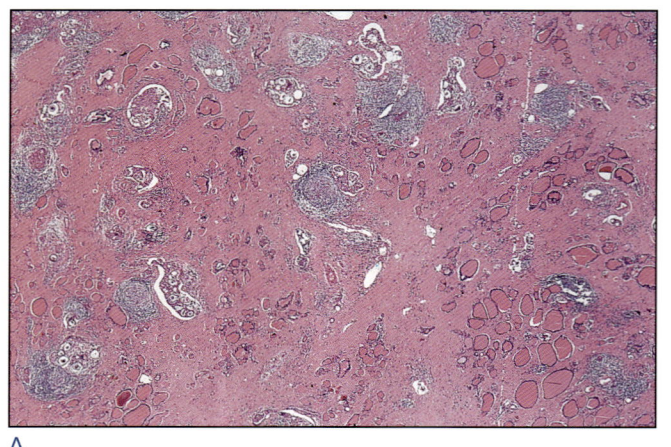

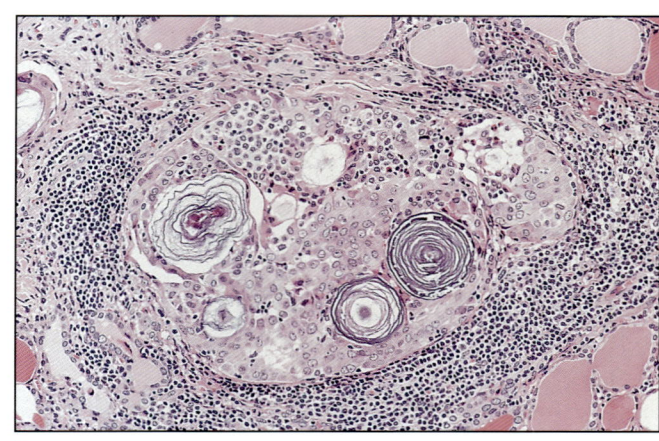

图18A.18 乳头状癌，弥漫硬化亚型。（A）甲状腺显示弥漫、广泛纤维化，淋巴细胞浸润及多个小的肿瘤细胞岛，给人以甲状腺炎的印象。（B）肿瘤细胞常呈鳞状上皮样，沙粒体丰富。

- 分散的乳头状癌小岛，伴明显的鳞状或鳞样分化（图18A.18B），尽管有时还可见到一个独立的肿块
- 广泛的淋巴细胞浸润

常有大量 S-100 蛋白阳性的树突状细胞散布于肿瘤中。早期广泛的淋巴浸润被看作是导致这种特殊组织学形态的关键因素。在初检时，组织学类似于甲状腺炎。然而，沙粒体的出现以及组织切片中由于钙化小体刀切困难引起的刀痕提示可能存在乳头状癌，需要进一步寻找分散的小的肿瘤细胞岛。然而，乳头状癌特征性的核特点通常在鳞状分化区丧失。

弥漫滤泡亚型（Diffuse follicular variant） 这是一种罕见的乳头状癌的浸润形式。发生于年轻病人（平均年龄21.3岁），特征是全甲状腺弥漫受累，不形成可辨认的结节，完全或主要为滤泡生长方式，无纤维化[147-149]。因为滤泡较大甚至呈囊性，与胶样腺瘤样甲状腺肿鉴别困难（图18A.19）。注意观察核的特征，尤其是较小的滤泡，临床特征（如转移的证据）对于诊断必不可少。此型转移至淋巴结（87.5%）、肺（75%）和骨（25%）的几率较高。由于对放射性碘治疗反应极好加之患者年轻，预后仍然很好。

高细胞亚型（Tall cell variant） 在新版WHO分类中，此型的诊断标准较以前严格，定义由"大多数肿瘤细胞高度是宽度的二倍"变更为"细胞高度至少是宽度的三倍"（图 18A.20）[37,43,91,150-152]。与经典型乳头状癌相比，高细胞亚型显示如下特征[37,43,91,150,151,153-156]：
- 年龄稍大（平均 50～57 岁）

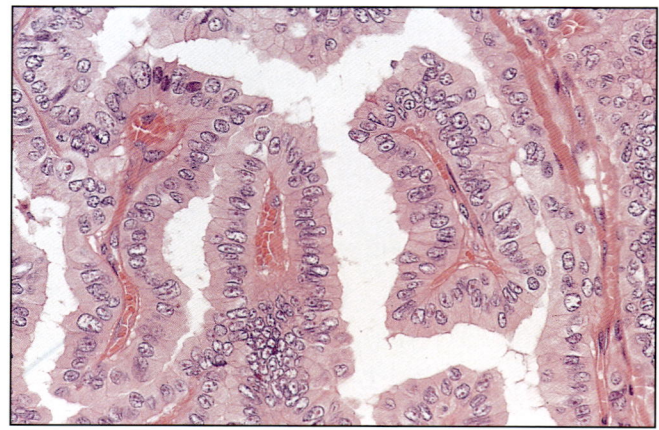

图18A.19 乳头状癌，弥漫滤泡亚型。注意完全为滤泡生长方式伴轻微硬化。与结节性甲状腺肿鉴别困难。(Courtesy of Dr. J. Soares, Lisbon, Portugal.)

图18A.20 乳头状癌，高细胞亚型。细胞柱状，胞浆嗜酸性、颗粒状，但核与典型的乳头状癌无差别。

- 肿瘤较大
- 更容易向甲状腺外扩展（42%～82%）
- 更具侵袭性（复发率18%～58%；死亡率9%～25%）

一些病例去分化形成梭形细胞鳞癌或未分化癌[157-159]。

高细胞亚型常显示 LeuM1(CD15)、上皮膜抗原、c-Met 以及与乳头状癌侵袭相关的标志物强阳性[151,160]。与经典型（11%）相比，高细胞型 p53 阳性率（61%）较高，但与预后无关[155]。约 1/3 病例显示 *RET/PTC* 易位，选择性地累及 *RET/PTC3*。体外研究表明，*RET/PTC3* 较 *RET/PTC1* 更具潜在的促有丝分裂作用，这或许能解释高细胞亚型的临床侵袭性[161]。

高细胞亚型常富于乳头及高度浸润性。呈典型乳头状癌特征的核大多位于基底。胞浆丰富，因线粒体堆积而呈嗜酸性。有时可观察到胞浆（尤其是核下）局灶透明[162]。此型需与柱状细胞癌鉴别，后者的被覆细胞更高，细胞核更长、假复层、深染。

尽管高细胞亚型比经典乳头状癌更具侵袭性，复发或死亡率几乎仅见于 III 期或 IV 期病人[155]。因此，分期在决定预后方面可能比组织学类型更重要[163]。即使高细胞的形态学被忽略，对病人来说或许不存在真正的伤害，因为疾病的侵袭特征很容易被识别，如体积大和甲状腺外扩散。

柱状细胞亚型(Columnar cell variant)　见柱状细胞癌（第 1036 页）。

嗜酸细胞亚型[Oxyphilic (oncocytic, Hurthle cell) variant]　该病变主要由因线粒体积聚而呈丰富嗜酸胞浆的细胞组成（图 18A.21）[109,164]。可能因线粒体气球样变引起胞浆部分或全部透明[112]。具有典型的乳头状癌细胞核，尽管可能深染，核仁明显[165,166]。生物学行为及分子特征与经典型乳头状癌无差别[166-169]。与 Hurthle 细胞滤泡性肿瘤的鉴别极为重要（见滤泡性肿瘤章节中

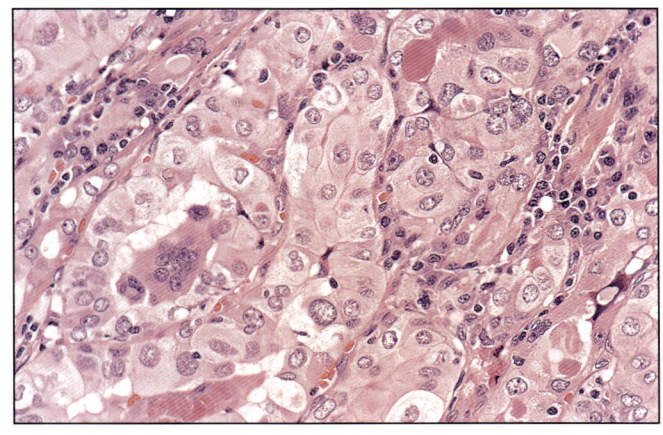

图18A.21　乳头状癌，嗜酸细胞亚型。肿瘤细胞具有丰富的嗜酸性颗粒状胞浆，但细胞不"高"。此例细胞核中度异型性，符合所谓的"异型性明显"，有些研究者认为该特征与预后差相关。左侧视野滤泡腔中可见多核巨细胞。

Hurthle 细胞腺瘤/腺癌部分）[168,169]。

Warthin 瘤样亚型(Warthin tumor-like variant)　少数乳头状癌类似于涎腺的 Warthin 瘤，呈乳头状生长，乳头轴心伴有大量淋巴浆细胞浸润。乳头被覆细胞常常嗜酸性，可为高细胞（图 18A.22）[170-175]。报道为"高细胞乳头状癌伴广泛淋巴细胞浸润"的病例可能代表这一亚型[176]。间质中淋巴细胞表型与慢性淋巴细胞性甲状腺炎相似。

透明细胞亚型(Clear cell variant)　少数乳头状癌病例因糖原积聚而显示广泛的透明胞浆。在那些混合有嗜酸细胞的病例，透明细胞改变局限于细胞的顶部，由线粒体气球样变造成[111,112,114,177,178]。

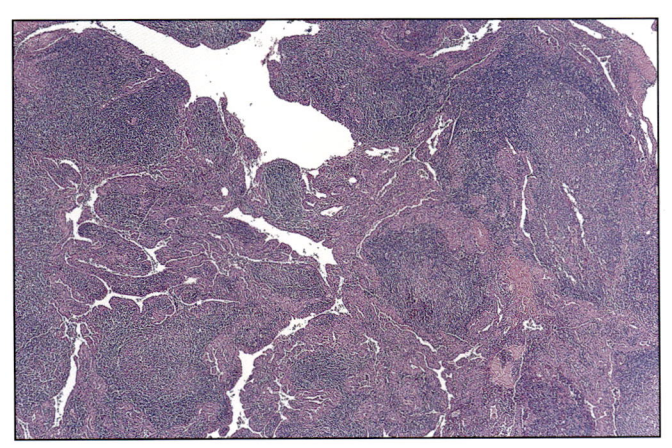
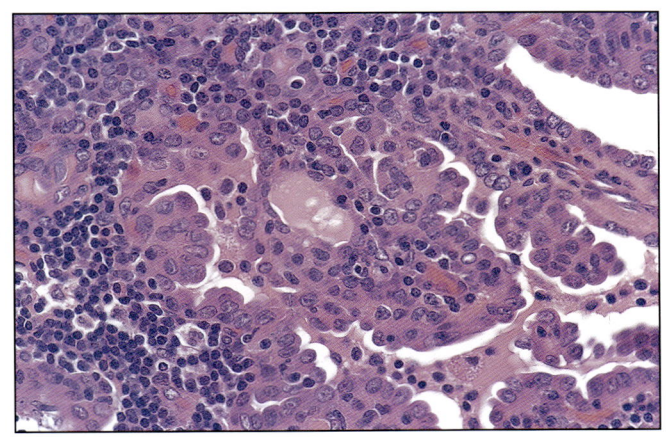

图18A.22　乳头状癌，Warthin瘤样亚型。（A）乳头被覆嗜酸细胞，含淋巴间质，类似涎腺的Warthin瘤。（B）乳头被覆的肿瘤细胞呈嗜酸性。

乳头状癌

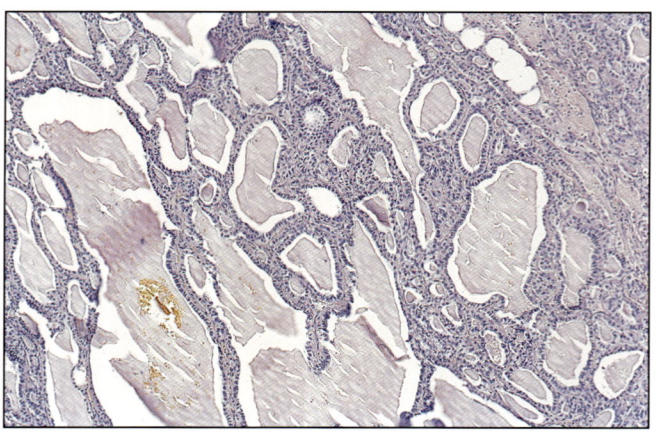

图18A.23 乳头状癌，巨滤泡亚型。主要由充满类胶质的大滤泡组成，似胶样结节。

巨滤泡亚型（Macrofollicular variant） 指50%以上的区域由大滤泡组成的肿瘤[179-183]。此型可能被误诊为结节性甲状腺肿或巨滤泡性腺瘤，但注意到核的特征将会做出正确的诊断（图18A.23）。巨滤泡的被覆细胞变扁，因而可能不显示乳头状癌的特征性核。所以，最好以较小的滤泡判断。偶尔可以发生去分化形成未分化癌[182]。

小梁亚型（Trabecular variant） 此型显示超过50%的肿瘤呈梁状生长。肿瘤细胞立方或柱状，在长直的小梁内垂直排列（图18A.14）。这些肿瘤常相对较大，具有侵袭性。单因素和多因素分析表明此型预后较差[184]。有些作者认为这种形态是乳头状癌的一种低分化亚型[185]。

筛状-桑葚样亚型（包括FAP相关性甲状腺癌） [Cribriform-morular variant (including FAP-associated thyroid carcinoma)] 这是一种罕见类型（新版WHO分类中称为"筛状型"），以明显的筛状结构为特征，散在鳞状分化（桑葚样）岛，其细胞核内常有轻度嗜酸性、均质、含生物素的包涵体（图18A.24）[186-188]。紧密排列的滤泡、乳头和小梁常混合存在。特点是腔内缺乏类胶质。肿瘤细胞柱状、立方状或扁平。核染色质丰富，但局灶总可见典型的乳头状癌的核特征。有些肿瘤细胞肥胖，梭形，排列成束状或漩涡状。肿瘤常界清，甚至有包膜，伴或不伴包膜及血管浸润。易被误诊为高细胞乳头状癌、柱状细胞癌或玻璃样变小梁状腺瘤或腺癌。

此型乳头状癌可散发（常为孤立性）或发生于家族性腺瘤性息肉病（常为多中心）[189]。实际上，发生于家族性腺瘤性息肉病（FAP）患者的多数甲状腺癌属于这一组织类型[190-193]。女性明显多见（男女比例为1:17），诊断时的平均年龄为27.7岁，有时先于FAP的诊断[192,194]。此型诊断的意义是提示临床医生警惕与FAP的相关性[189]。

肿瘤常显示乳头状癌的特征性*RET/PTC*重排[193,195]。在FAP相关病例，*APC*基因主要发生胚系突变（有时伴体细胞突变）；在一些散发病例，*APC*基因通过体细胞突变受累[193,194,196-198]。ß-catenin基因（*CTNNB1*）外显子3发生体细胞突变，导致ß-catenin移位到细胞核内，是该类型独特而普遍的发现（图18A.25），提示这一分子改变在筛状-桑葚样亚型的形态发生和发展中具有重要作用[199,200]。

伴脂肪瘤样间质的乳头状癌（papillary carcinoma with lipomatous stroma） 在少数病例，脂肪细胞散在分布于乳头状癌内[118-120,201,202]。

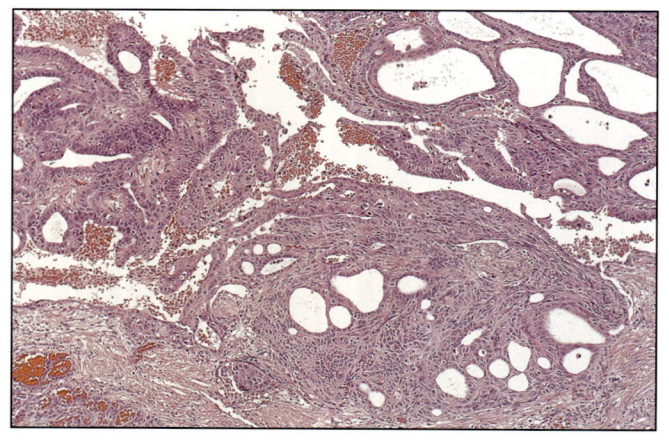
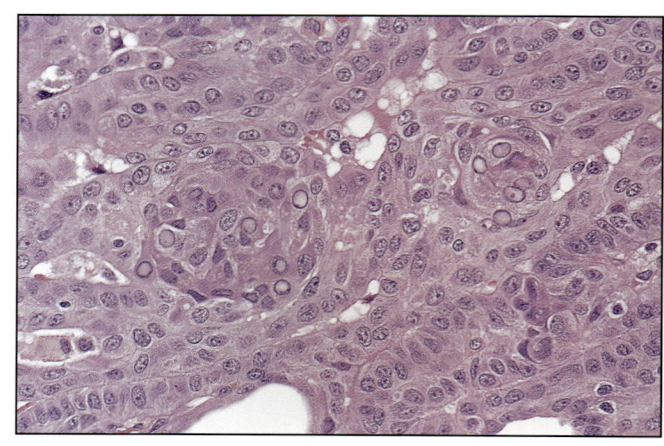

图18A.24 乳头状癌，筛状-桑葚样亚型。（A）显示典型的混合性结构特征，筛状结构、滤泡、实性桑葚样和乳头（左上角）的复杂混合。（B）组成桑葚体的细胞核含有均匀、嗜酸性、富于生物素的包涵体。桑葚体外的一些细胞核具有乳头状癌特征性核沟。

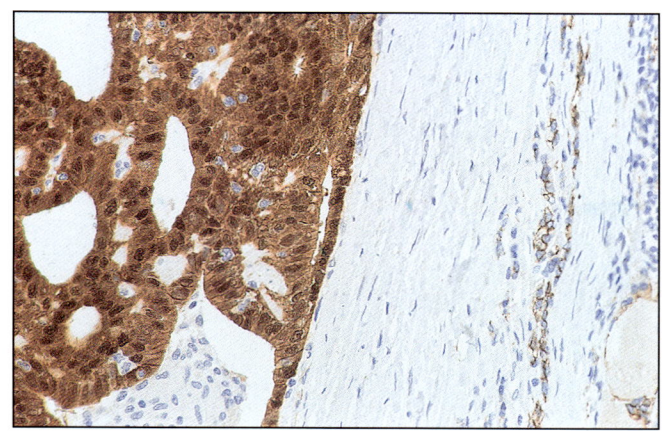

图18A.25 乳头状癌，筛状-桑葚样亚型。ß-catenin染色显示异常核着色。与正常甲状腺滤泡上皮内ß-catenin的膜着色形成对比（右侧）。

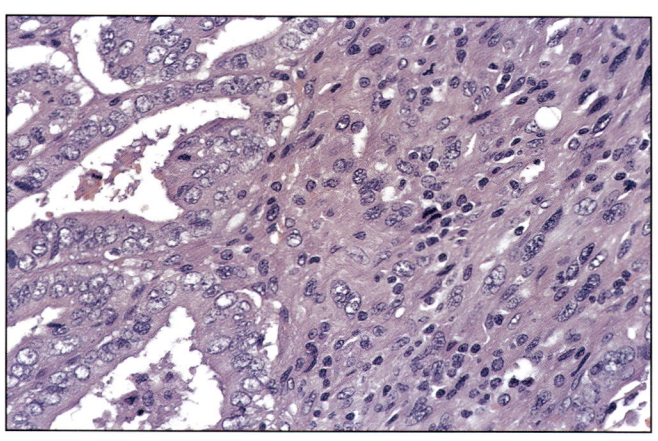

图18A.27 去分化乳头状癌。左侧为乳头状癌；右侧的间变性癌主要由具有多形性核的肥胖梭形细胞组成。

伴丰富结节性筋膜炎样间质的亚型 (variant with exuberant nodular fasciitis-like stroma) 少数情况下，乳头状癌伴有丰富的结节性筋膜炎或纤维瘤病样反应性间质，其病变的肿瘤本质可能被掩盖（图18A.26A）[203-210]。间质由梭形细胞组成，位于有外渗红细胞的含血管的纤维黏液基质中（图18A.26B）。梭形细胞为肌纤维母细胞，可能是间质对浸润性肿瘤的过度反应。间质与肿瘤的相互作用可能导致特殊的组织学结构，让人联想到乳腺的纤维腺瘤、叶状肿瘤或纤维囊肿病。肿瘤巢可以很分散、不明显。所报道的呈黏液瘤样改变的乳头状癌病例可能是此型的极端形式[211]。

伴梭形细胞化生的亚型 (variant with spindle cell metaplasia) 少数乳头状癌病例会出现梭形肿瘤细胞，所占比例多少不一[212, 213]。形态温和的梭形细胞形成短束状，与乳头状癌成分融合。报道为"乳头状癌梭形细胞转化"的病例可能是一种去分化乳头状癌而不是此类型[214]。

去分化乳头状癌 (Dedifferentiated papillary carcinoma) 是指乳头状癌与未分化或低分化甲状腺癌并存的情形（图18A.27）[24]。后一成分可出现于乳头状癌发生或复发时。这种转化可发生于原发灶或转移灶[108,175,215]。由于高级别成分的存在，预后差，除非未分化成分仅占整个肿瘤的一小部分[64,216-219]。

微小癌（乳头状微小肿瘤）
Microcarcinoma (papillary microtumor)

"隐匿乳头状癌"这一术语曾被用来指偶然发现的肿瘤或小肿瘤，引起许多混乱。1988年WHO分类建议以"微小乳头状癌"替代这一术语，其定义为<1 cm的肿瘤[220]。即使发生淋巴结和罕见的远处转移，其预后极好，

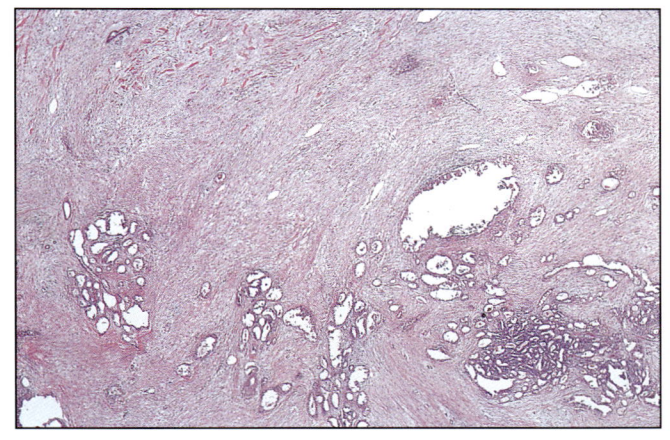

A   B

图18A.26 伴丰富结节性筋膜炎样间质的乳头状癌。（A）丰富的间质将肿瘤分割成数个小叶。（B）间质由位于纤维黏液基质中的梭形细胞组成。

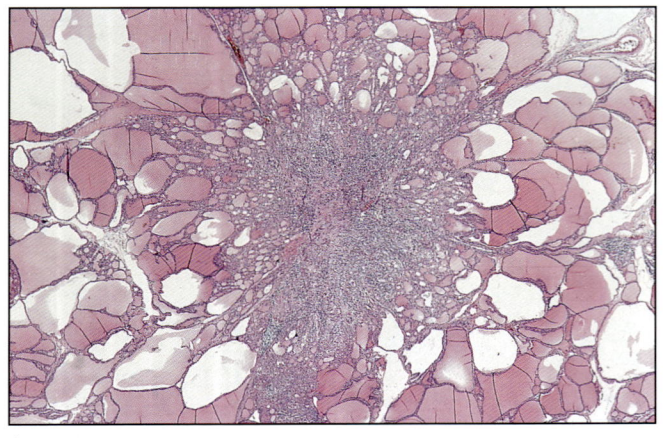
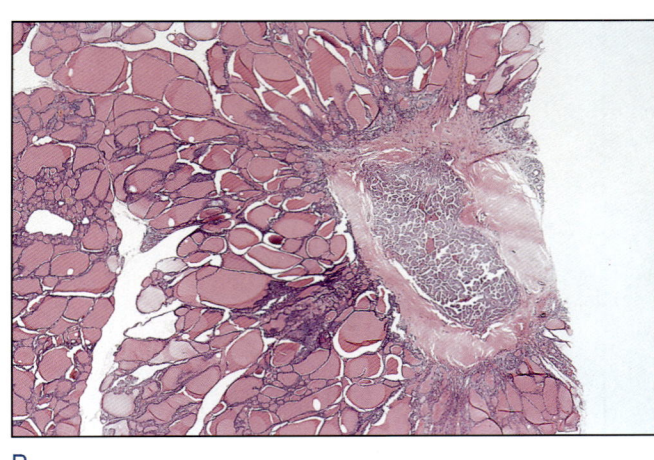

图18A.28　潜在乳头状癌。（A）具有星状外观和轻度硬化。（B）显示明显硬化和包膜。

因而有单独识别的价值[47,221-226]。一组 90 例的甲状腺微小癌，平均随访 17.3 年，所有病人健在，即使其中有些病人在发病时已有颈部淋巴结转移[227]。少数转移淋巴结＞ 3 cm，且无包膜的微小乳头状癌病人预后不良[228]。2004 年的 WHO 分类，微小乳头状癌的定义变严格，只包括偶然发现的＜ 1 cm 的乳头状癌，而不包括有临床表现的体积小的乳头状癌。

为避免混乱，采用前列腺癌中的命名方式比较合适：隐匿 (occult) 乳头状癌是继转移性肿瘤发现后在甲状腺中发现的癌；潜在 (latent) 乳头状癌是在甲状腺切除 / 腺叶切除标本或尸检中偶然发现的癌。隐匿和潜在乳头状癌可以是微小癌，也可以不是微小癌。

据报道不同国家潜在乳头状癌的发病率变化很大，芬兰（35.6%）和日本 (17.9%～28.4%) 最高，瑞士（1.2%）最低[229-231]。大多数研究报道的发病率在 5%～10%[43,229,232-238]。差别较大的原因可能是由于诊断标准和检查技术不同，但也可能与遗传因素有关。大多数潜在乳头状癌发生于青春期后，其后发生率并不随年龄增长而增加[231,239-241]。因而，这些潜在性肿瘤绝大多数处于静止状态，而不发展为临床明显的疾病[108,235,242]。此外，女性发病不占优势以及其与普通乳头状癌的发病率缺乏相关性均提示潜在乳头状癌的生物学行为不同于临床症状明显的乳头状癌[231]。不管是腺叶切除还是整个甲状腺切除标本，偶然发现的潜在乳头状癌无需额外治疗。病理报告中指出其良性的生物学行为十分重要。考虑到极好的预后以及避免过诊断，Porto 提案建议将其更名为"乳头状微小肿瘤"以取代其恶性称谓[243]。

大多数潜在乳头状癌体积小，以滤泡结构为主。最常见类型是浸润型，常伴有硬化，呈星形外观（图 18A.28）。另一类型为局限型，聚集的肿瘤性滤泡与周围滤泡和谐共处但形态截然不同，可有轻度硬化或无硬化（图 18A.29）[225]。少数病例具有包膜（图 18A.28B）[244]。这些微小癌有时在同一腺叶呈多灶性分布 (23%)，并可累及另一叶(17%)[227]。可发生区域淋巴结转移(16%)，但常为微转移，即使不切除也会保持休眠状态[227]。

免疫组织化学

乳头状癌显示广谱细胞角蛋白、甲状腺球蛋白、TTF-1 阳性，而神经内分泌标志物阴性（表 18A.7）。

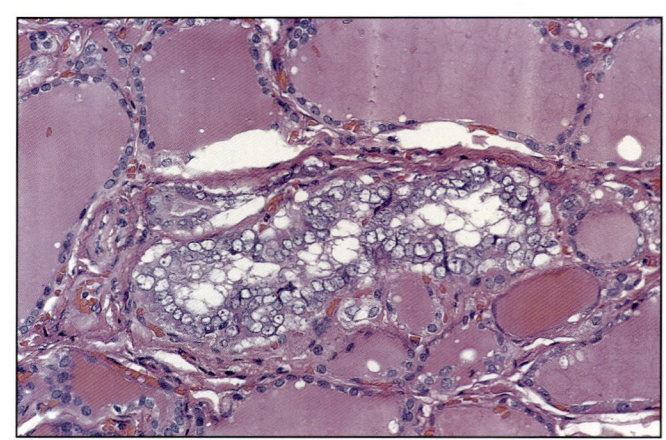

图18A.29　潜在乳头状癌。这一偶然发现的乳头状癌病灶由一些滤泡组成，不伴有硬化。注意密集的空泡状细胞核，与周围正常滤泡明显不同。

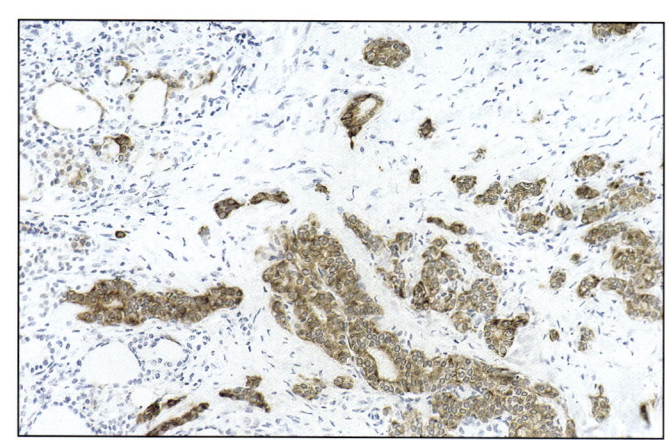

图18A.30 乳头状癌。细胞角蛋白19阳性。

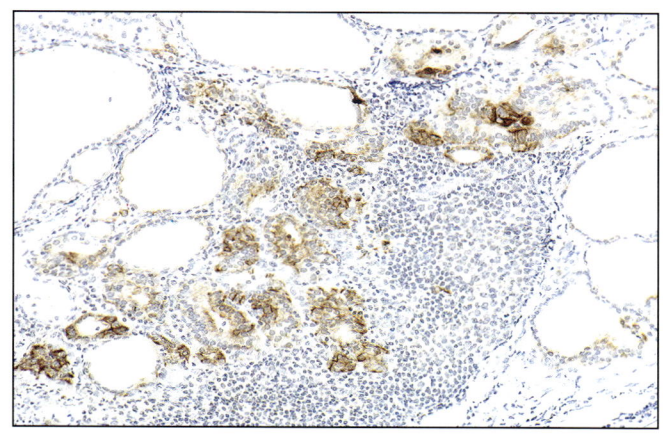

图18A.31 甲状腺炎。在甲状腺炎等反应性病变中，甲状腺滤泡上皮也表达细胞角蛋白19。

在鳞状分化区，甲状腺球蛋白和TTF-1染色常丧失。甲状腺球蛋白的免疫染色有助于判断原发灶未知的转移是否来源于甲状腺，也能判断淋巴结内的囊性结构是甲状腺乳头状癌囊性转移还是其他良性囊肿。

在乳头状癌与良性甲状腺病变（例如核透明或浅染的滤泡性病变）及其他甲状腺肿瘤的鉴别诊断中，许多标志物如高分子量细胞角蛋白（34ßE12、细胞角蛋白1）、细胞角蛋白19、galectin-3、间皮相关抗体HBME-1、Leu7(CD57)、CITED1、纤维连接蛋白-1、CD15(LeuM1)、CD44或血小板源性生长因子的单一或联合表达有一定价值，但这些标志物并非完全特异，即使在典型的乳头状癌染色可呈灶状或微弱阳性（图18A.30）[30,31,245-267]。此外，正常滤泡、非肿瘤性病变（尤其是甲状腺炎）和良性甲状腺肿瘤可局灶阳性（图18A.31）。

细胞遗传学和分子特征

乳头状癌中发现三条相互独立的分子通路，这些肿瘤分子分类显示相似而独特的基因表达谱[268-271]：

1. 8%~60%的病例（大约30%~40%成人病例）因染色体内倒转或染色体易位引起原癌基因*RET*或*TRK*的激活[3,35,272-288]。有趣的是，以*RET/PTC*反转录病毒载体转染原代培养的人甲状腺上皮细胞，细胞核会发生改变，包括核形不规则及出现常染色体，表明遗传学改变可能是乳头状癌特征性核的基础[289]。至于*RET/PTC*是否存在于非肿瘤性甲状腺组织，如桥本甲状腺炎和良性结节仍存在争议[290,292]。
2. 大约40%的病例发生*BRAF*突变。
3. *ras*突变选择性地发生于滤泡亚型。

*RET*基因（关于此基因的具体描述见甲状腺髓样癌部分）的酪氨酸激酶区可与许多在甲状腺上皮细胞中表达的基因融合，如*PTC1* inv(10)(q11.2q21)、*PTC2* t(10;17)(q11.2;q23)、*PTC3* 10q11.2同臂内倒位、*PTC4*和*PTC5*[293-296]。融合使RET蛋白形成二聚体，导致酪氨酸激酶能够不依赖配体而激活[295,297-299]。*RET/PTC1*融合最常见，其次为*RET/PTC3*[3,35,275-288,300]。*RET/PTC*基因融合频率较常见于儿童和年轻病人（50%~60%）、切尔诺贝利事件相关乳头状癌（60%~80%，*RET/PTC3*最常见）、儿童期接受过放射线治疗的病人（60%~70%，*RET/PTC1*最常见）[281,286,287,301-305]。*RET/PTC*融合也与疾病的局部进展、淋巴结转移、低增殖活性和去分化倾向低存在相关性[94,270,286,306-309]。*RET/PTC1*与乳头结构为主的乳头状癌和乳头状微小癌相关；*RET/PTC3*与高细胞和实性亚型相关[161,287,296]；*RET/PTC*融合未见于滤泡性肿瘤、低分化癌或未分化癌。

少数情况下，编码神经生长因子受体的*TRK*基因，通过1q23-24上染色体重排而受到许多不相关基因的调控，如*NTRK1/TPM3*（原肌球蛋白基因）、*NTRK1/TPR*、*NTRK1/TAG*[272,277,278,281,307,310,311]。

BRAF属于RAF蛋白激酶家族，在RAS/RAF/MEK/MAPK通路的信号传导中起中心作用，介导细胞的生长、分化和生存[312]。*BRAF*基因在1799位点核苷酸的错义突变（以前错误地认为是1796位点），由胸腺嘧啶（T）转换为腺嘌呤（A），导致谷氨酸替代缬氨酸（V600E突变，以前错误地认为是V599E），发生在29%~69%的乳头状癌病例[268,270,271,312-317]。*BRAF* V600E突变较少见于儿童和年轻人的乳头状癌（0~13%）[312,315,318,319]。*BRAF*突变较常见于典型乳头状癌、高细胞型、Warthin瘤样型和嗜酸细胞型，但罕见于滤泡亚型。BRAF突变对预后的意义存在争议；一些研究报道伴V600E突变的乳头状癌与侵袭性特征，如年龄较大、甲状腺外扩展、分期高（III和IV期）、淋巴结转移及肿瘤复发有关[270,320,321]，而另一些研究没有证明任何预后关系[268,319]。1/3～1/2的未分化癌和0～13%的低分化癌可检测到BRAF突变，但在滤泡性肿瘤和髓样癌中无突变。因此至少一些未分化癌似乎由乳头状癌转化而来[322,323]。

Ras基因突变（N-ras和H-ras最常见，累及第61密码子）见于大约15%的乳头状癌，所有阳性病例均为滤泡亚型（见下文）[270,296]。少部分滤泡亚型（7%）显示不同于V600E的BRAF突变，在密码子601（K601E）由谷氨酸代替赖氨酸[319,324]。

有关目前所诊断的"乳头状癌滤泡亚型"(follicular variant of papillary carcinoma) 本质的争议

乳头状癌滤泡亚型的分子改变与经典乳头状癌明显不同，即缺少RET易位，BRAF V600E突变率很低以及出现一定比例的ras突变或PAX8/PPARγ易位，频率类似于滤泡性腺瘤或滤泡癌（表18A.8）。这一点实际上与甲状腺滤泡性腺瘤/滤泡癌中所见相同。如文献所述，有ras突变的乳头状癌其核特征不明显，缺乏甲状腺外扩散，淋巴结转移率较低[270]。这些都与典型的滤泡性腺瘤/滤泡癌一致，而与乳头状癌不同。作者认为目前许多诊断为包膜内滤泡亚型的乳头状癌病例实际上是被误诊（过诊）为乳头状癌的滤泡性腺瘤（癌）[325,326]。

乳头状癌的预后因素

乳头状癌的各种预后因素中，年龄、肿瘤大小和分期最重要。810例乳头状癌病人平均随访20年，低危组（n=403）、中危组（n=313）和高危组（n=94）的生存率分别为99%、83%和43%[78]。

- 年龄。40岁以下的病人死亡率非常低[47,48,65,78,80,82,221,327-332]。
- 性别。大多数研究报道男性预后较差[78,82,165,328,331-336]。
- 肿瘤大小。乳头状癌死亡风险随原发瘤的大小而增加[47]。小于1～1.5 cm的肿瘤预后非常好[47,219,221,337]，而大于4 cm的肿瘤预后差[78,336]。
- 分期。甲状腺外扩散是指甲状腺周围软组织受累，表明预后不良。而某些略有（显微镜下）甲状腺外扩散的病例，预后与没有甲状腺外扩散的病例相似[47,76,78,329,332,338]。食管或气管浸润与特别不利的结局相关（10年生存率为63%）[339]。一旦有远处转移，预后明显变差[340]。淋巴结转移的预后重要性存在争议，一些研究表明淋巴结转移对生存无影响，而另一些研究证实对生存有负面影响[47,78,80,327,330-332,341-344]。然而，如果淋巴结转移出现包膜外扩散则增加远处转移的危险性，预后较差[345]。
- 肿瘤包膜。肿瘤有包膜者预后较好[63,132,134]。
- 组织学亚型。没有证据表明乳头状癌中滤泡和乳头的比例会影响预后[63,64,346]。高细胞型、弥漫硬化型、弥漫滤泡型、实性型、梁状型和去分化型更具侵袭性。
- 肿瘤切除的完整性。肿瘤切除不完整会增加复发的危险性[67,347]。
- 其他报道的需进一步确认的预后因素如下：
  - 组织学特征。多因素分析发现组织学分级高（核异型、坏死和/或血管浸润）预后差[348,349]。细胞异型性明显（细胞复层排列，细胞及核的大小、形状明显不同，染色质分布不均匀）和梁状生长方式与较差的预后有关[184,185,334,335]。间

表18A.8	乳头状癌和滤泡性肿瘤的各种分子改变频率		
	滤泡性腺瘤或癌（%）	经典乳头状癌（%）	乳头状癌滤泡亚型(%)
RET/PTC易位	0	26～28	3
BRAF突变	0	53～75（V600E）	0～7（K601E）
RAS突变	18～53	0	25～47
PAX8/PPARγ易位	滤泡性腺瘤：4～33 滤泡癌：45～63		38

质有骨形成预后较好[123]。周围甲状腺呈慢性甲状腺炎背景是有利的预后因素[331]。

- 免疫组化表达：LeuM1 阳性（预后较差）[350]，上皮膜抗原阳性（远处转移或死亡率较高）[351]，p53 阳性（预后较差或无影响）[352,353]，E-cadherin 阴性（预后较差）[354]，RB 蛋白低水平表达（预后较差）[355]，S-100 阳性的组织细胞密度高（预后较好）[356]。
- 浸润大血管（预后较差）[63,341]。
- DNA 倍体：多倍体（预后较差）[357]；非整倍体（大于 60 岁的病人预后较差，并与甲状腺外肿瘤扩散有关）[123,358]。

鉴别诊断

- 伴有乳头状结构的各种病变（见*甲状腺肿瘤诊断中的实际问题*部分，第 1055 页）。
- 伴有滤泡结构的各种病变（见*甲状腺肿瘤诊断中的实际问题*部分，第 1056 页）。
- 伴有实性结构的各种病变，对于实性亚型（见*甲状腺肿瘤诊断中的实际问题*部分，第 1060 页）。

滤泡性肿瘤（滤泡性腺瘤和滤泡癌），包括Hurthle细胞肿瘤
Follicular neoplasms (follicular adenoma and follicular carcinoma), including Hurthle cell neoplasms

定义

滤泡性腺瘤和滤泡癌分别指显示滤泡细胞分化但缺乏乳头状癌诊断特征的甲状腺良性和恶性上皮肿瘤[220,359,360]。毫无疑问，滤泡癌是肿瘤。组织化学和分子学研究已证明，用严格的形态学标准诊断的滤泡性腺瘤，尤其当有边界清楚的纤维性包膜时，是克隆性病变，从而支持滤泡性腺瘤是肿瘤性而不是增生性结节[361-365]。

临床特征

过去，滤泡癌占所有原发性甲状腺癌的 10%～20%[366]，近年来由于早期乳头状癌的检出增加以及乳头状癌滤泡亚型的诊断方法放宽，其发病率已降至 5%～10%[367,368]。在地方性甲状腺肿发病区，滤泡癌的发病率较高，碘缺乏可能是主要的致病因素，因为在饮食中补碘后该地区的滤泡癌发病率下降[53]。少数情况下，滤泡癌可发生于已有的滤泡性腺瘤基础上[369]。激素生成障碍、辐射和 Cowden 病易发生滤泡癌[55,370,371]。少数滤泡性肿瘤病例是遗传性非髓样甲状腺癌综合征的一部分。此综合征的一种少见形式以多发性嗜酸性肿瘤为特征；受累基因（*TCO*）已定位于染色体 19p13.2[372-375]。

滤泡性腺瘤（Follicular adenoma）　滤泡性腺瘤大多数发生于 20～50 岁的成人，但任何年龄均可受累。女性更常见（男女比 1:6）。大多数病人表现为各阶段孤立性甲状腺结节。碘扫描时腺瘤通常不摄取碘（冷结节），但少数可为热结节并引起甲状腺功能亢进（所谓毒性腺瘤）。滤泡性腺瘤为良性，可通过腺叶切除术治愈。

滤泡癌（Follicular carcinoma）　与滤泡性腺瘤相比，滤泡癌的平均发病年龄较大（表 18A.7 和 18A.9）。大多数病人表现为甲状腺肿块，11% 的病人以远处转移为首发症状，如骨痛、骨折或软组织内有搏动感的肿块[62,132,366,376]。与乳头状癌相反，主要播散方式是血行（易累及骨和肺）而非淋巴道转移[369]。转移及存活几率很大程度上取决于局部病变的范围，也就是要判定是微浸润型还是广泛浸润型（见表 18A.9）。图 18A.32 描述了滤泡癌的自然发展史。令人惊讶的是，一些以转移为首发症状的病人，甲状腺切除后仍然难以明确恶性诊断，

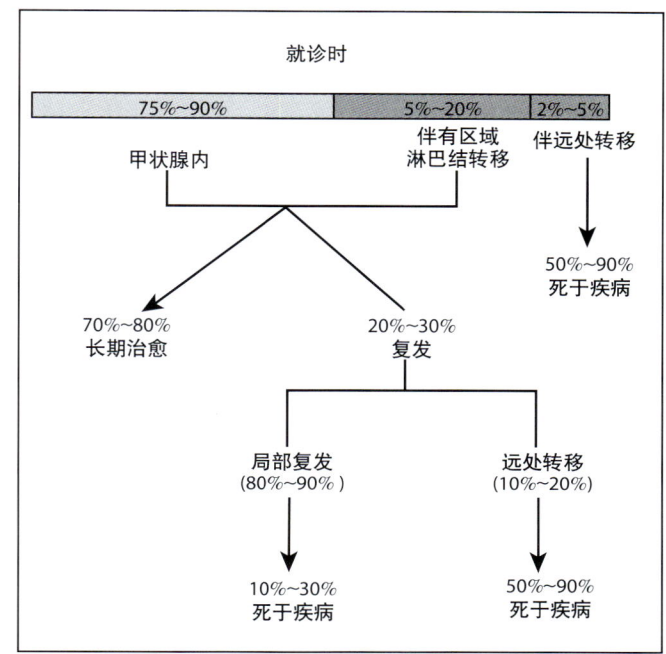

图18A.32　滤泡癌的自然发展史流程图。

表18A.9 滤泡癌的分类

	微小浸润			广泛浸润 (明显浸润)
	仅包膜浸润	有限的血管浸润 (<4)	广泛的血管浸润 (≥4)	
诊断标准	有包膜的肿瘤伴组织学检查可识别的微小浸润			伴邻近甲状腺和(或)血管的广泛浸润
	仅包膜浸润,无血管浸润	少于4个血管浸润±包膜浸润	超过4个血管浸润±包膜浸润	
就诊平均年龄		较年轻（47~50岁）		较老（53~59岁）
局部复发	无	罕见	罕见	有
区域淋巴结转移	无	罕见	罕见	常见（13%~24%）
远处转移	0	罕见(5%),远期	有时	常见(29%~69%)，尤其转移到肺、骨、脑、肝
临床结局	疾病相关死亡~0%	预后极好，长期死亡率低（3%~5%）	预后稍差，累积死亡率为18%	预后差，长期死亡率为30%~50%
治疗	腺叶切除	腺叶切除或次全甲状腺切除±抑制剂量的甲状腺素	全甲状腺切除，放射性碘和抑制剂量的甲状腺素	全甲状腺切除，放射性碘和抑制剂量的甲状腺素

表现为滤泡性肿瘤无血管浸润，只有不明确的包膜浸润。

大体表现

滤泡性腺瘤和微浸润滤泡癌均有包膜，除后者包膜较厚外，大体上两者通常难以区分。大小1~10cm。实性、肉质感、黄褐色至浅棕色，有时有光泽（图18A.33）。可发生继发性改变，如出血、囊性变。广泛浸润型滤泡癌缺乏完整的包膜，且于肿瘤主体外见明显的浸润，扩张的血管内可见癌栓。

组织学表现

滤泡性肿瘤几乎总是被覆纤维性包膜，滤泡癌的包膜较滤泡性腺瘤厚。然而，对于一些广泛浸润的滤泡癌没有明确的包膜。肿瘤由紧密排列的滤泡、小梁或实性片块组成；少数情况下局灶可有乳头状结构。肿瘤细胞呈立方或矮柱状，含深染或浅染圆形核，核仁不明显，有些肿瘤的细胞核有多形性（图18A.34至18A.36）。在形态一致的细胞核中常见散在增大的深染核。除一些广泛浸润性滤泡癌外，核分裂象少见。胞浆嗜酸或透明。

对于一个具体病例，组织学结构可完全一致或不同。主要由大滤泡、正常大小滤泡或小滤泡组成的肿瘤，分别称为大滤泡型、正常滤泡型和小滤泡型（胎儿型）（图18A.34B）。呈梁状（实性）排列的肿瘤称为梁状或胚胎型（图18A.35）。

肿瘤中，纤细的毛细血管位于滤泡和细胞岛之间，但在常规组织学切片中常不明显（图18A.34A）。常见出血、含铁血黄素沉积、硬化、水肿、坏死及囊性变等继发改变。淀粉样变少见[377]。

滤泡癌转移灶的形态与原发瘤相似，形态可以非常温和以致类似于正常甲状腺组织（图18A.37）。

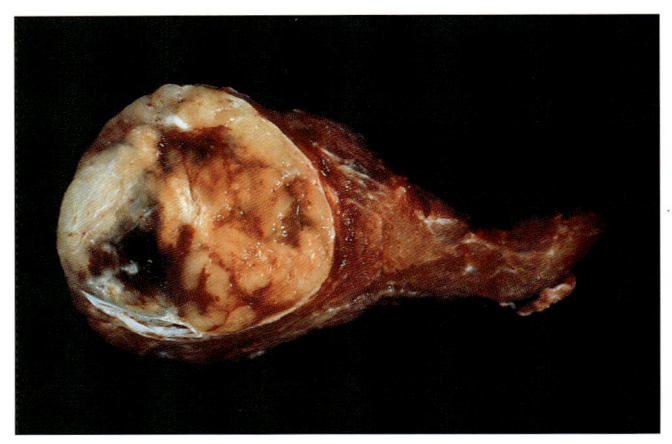

图18A.33 滤泡性腺瘤的大体标本。注意非常薄的纤维性包膜和肉样外观。微小浸润性滤泡癌也会有相同表现。

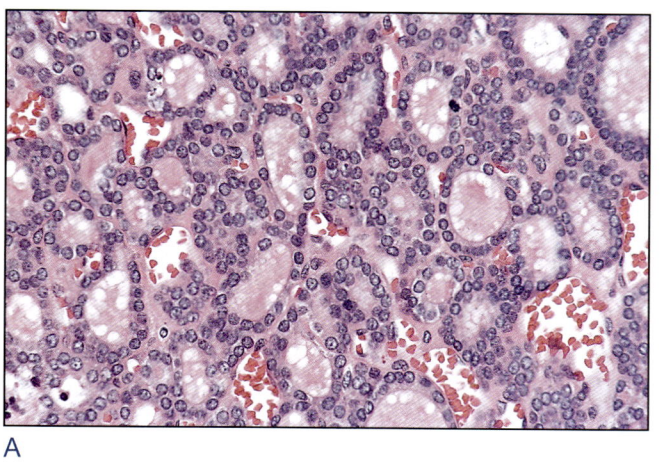

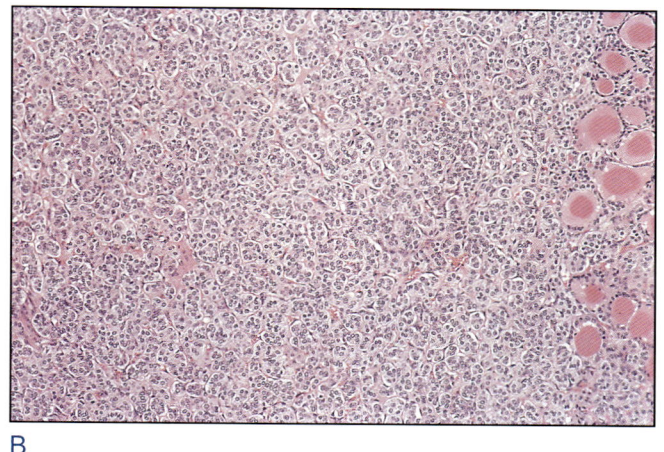

图18A.34 滤泡性腺瘤的结构特征。（A）肿瘤由中等大小的滤泡组成，其内衬细胞具有规则的圆形核。滤泡间的毛细血管常不明显。（B）由小滤泡和小梁组成的肿瘤。

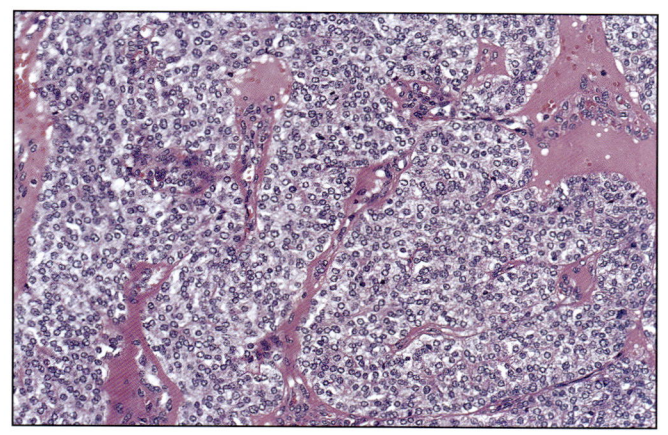

图18A.35 滤泡性腺瘤。显示实性生长方式，被纤细的纤维血管间隔分开。使人怀疑为髓样癌。此时免疫组化对于判定滤泡或滤泡旁分化必不可少。

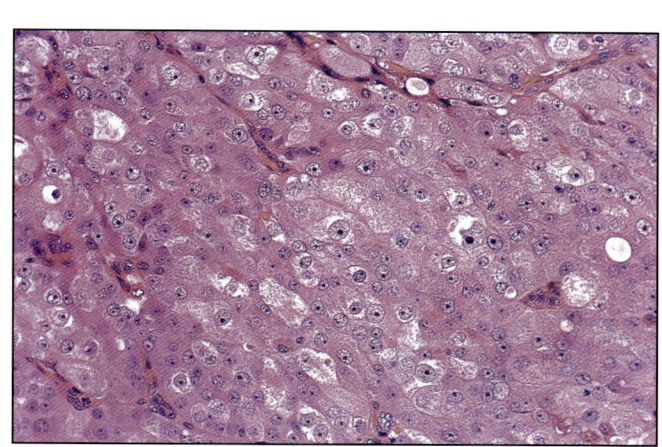

图18A.36 滤泡癌。此例核异型性明显。肿瘤表现为实性和梁状生长方式。

滤泡癌(follicular carcinoma)与滤泡性腺瘤(follicular adenoma)的鉴别标准

滤泡性肿瘤缺乏乳头状癌的特征性结构，区分癌与腺瘤的唯一标准是滤泡癌具有血管和(或)包膜侵犯，这意味着可靠区分两者需要在肿瘤与甲状腺交界处仔细检查[220]。尽管出现以下特征很可能是滤泡癌（图

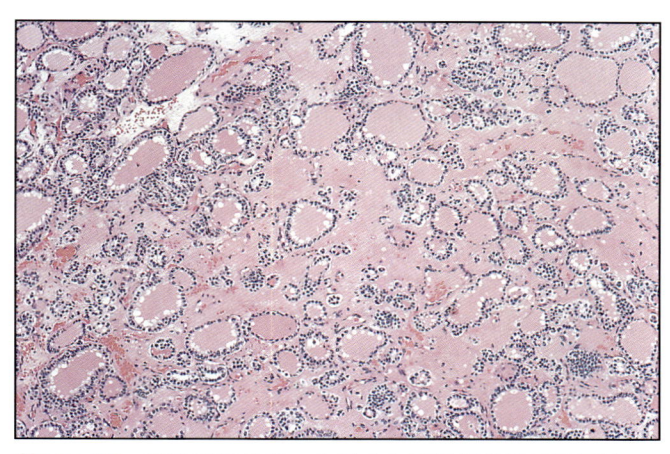

图18A.37 滤泡癌骨转移。实际上与正常甲状腺无法区分。

滤泡性肿瘤

18A.34B 和 18A.35），如果经仔细的组织学取材未发现浸润证据，仍要将它们称为滤泡性腺瘤：

- 厚的纤维性包膜
- 细胞密集，具有实性、梁状或微滤泡生长方式
- 弥漫的核异型性
- 核分裂象易见

由于微小浸润性滤泡癌预后极好（表18A.9），浸润标准必须严格把握以避免过诊断[378-383]。

血管浸润（vascular invasion） 受累血管必须位于纤维性包膜或包膜外（图18A.38和18A.39），血管内肿瘤细胞团表面需被覆内皮细胞（图18A.39B）[384]。只有当肿瘤细胞团粘附于血管壁伴血栓形成时，可以不要求肿瘤细胞岛被覆内皮细胞。对于轻微突向包膜薄壁血管内的滤泡团，如果深切和进一步取材都没有明确的血管浸润，可不予考虑（图18A.40）。肿瘤岛周围的收缩假象也与血管浸润相似，但裂隙没有内皮细胞被覆（图18A.41）。有时，在包膜血管内可见与血管轮廓不一致、边界凹凸不平且无内皮细胞被覆的不规则肿瘤细胞团，是由标本切割过程中的人工移位造成的，不应认为是血管浸润（图18A.42）[384]。

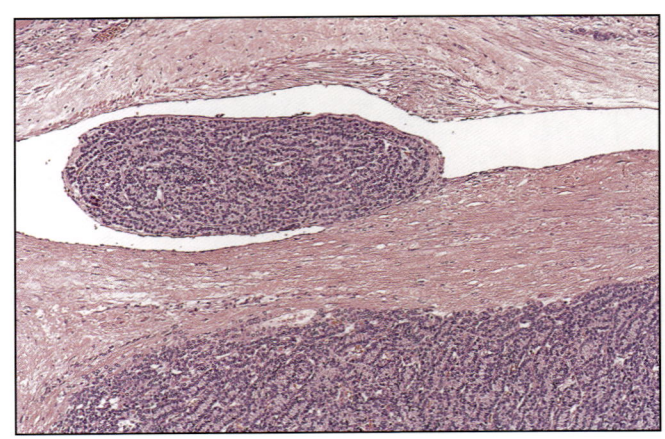

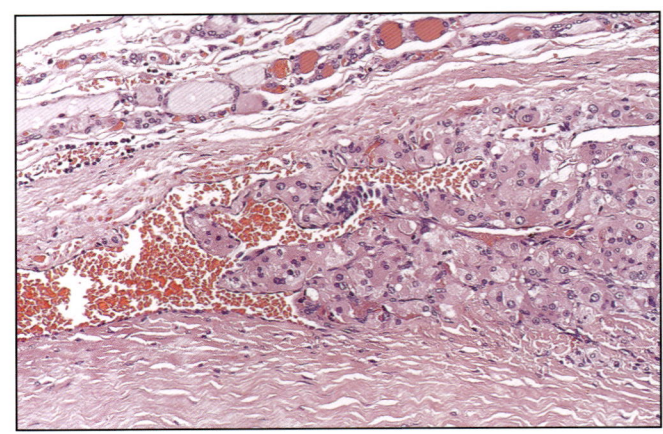

图18A.39 显示血管浸润的滤泡癌。（A）厚的纤维包膜内出现血管腔内息肉状瘤栓，肿瘤粘附于血管壁，但不是识别血管浸润的必要标准。（B）位于腔内的肿瘤栓子被覆内皮细胞。

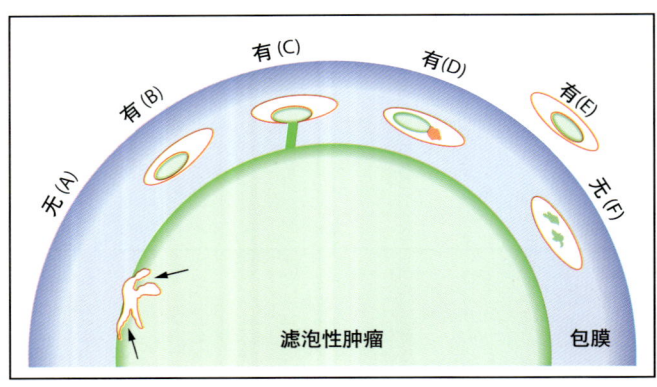

图18A.38 判断滤泡性肿瘤有无血管浸润的示意图。(A)肿瘤突入完全位于肿瘤内的血管不构成血管浸润。(B)肿瘤栓子位于包膜血管腔内，且被覆内皮细胞，符合血管浸润的标准。(C)有时，肿瘤侵犯纤维性包膜，并突入包膜血管腔内。其表面被覆血管内皮，符合血管浸润的标准。(D)尽管血管内肿瘤岛不被覆内皮细胞，但伴有纤维蛋白血栓，也符合血管浸润。(E)肿瘤包膜外血管内出现被覆内皮细胞的肿瘤岛为血管浸润。(F)肿瘤被人为带入血管腔，表现为血管腔内不规则肿瘤碎片，无内皮细胞被覆，不伴有纤维蛋白血栓。

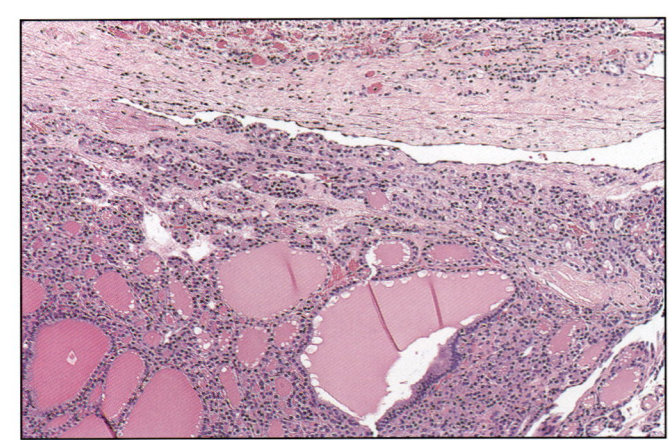

图18A.40 滤泡性腺瘤。仅看到肿瘤性滤泡突向血管内侧，不足以诊断血管浸润。

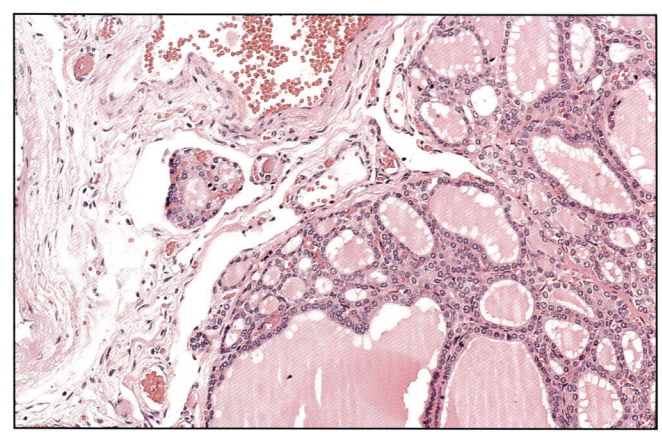

图18A.41 滤泡性腺瘤中的假血管浸润。左侧的细胞岛由收缩间隙围绕。小岛和间隙表面均无内皮细胞被覆。

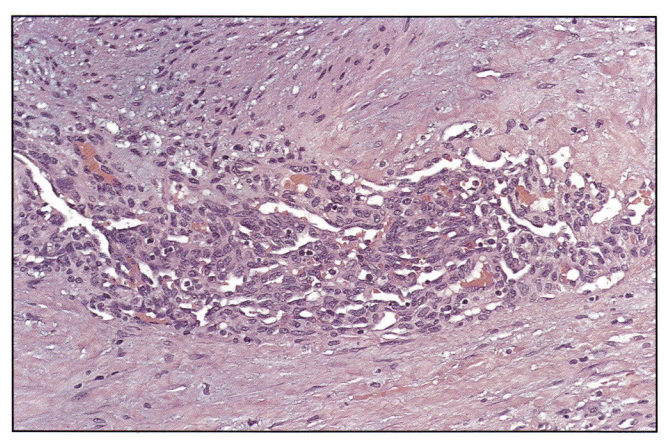

图18A.43 伴包膜血管内皮细胞增生的滤泡性肿瘤，类似于血管浸润。血管内皮增生产生不规则裂隙。

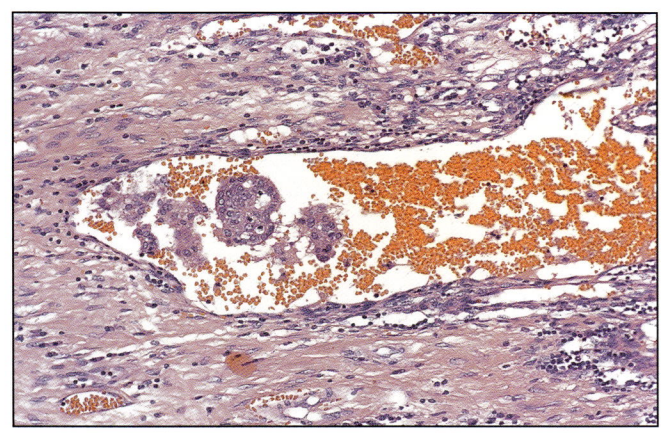

图18A.42 滤泡性肿瘤。包膜血管腔内可见许多肿瘤碎片。因形状不规则，无血管内皮被覆，且缺乏血栓，不满足血管浸润诊断标准。

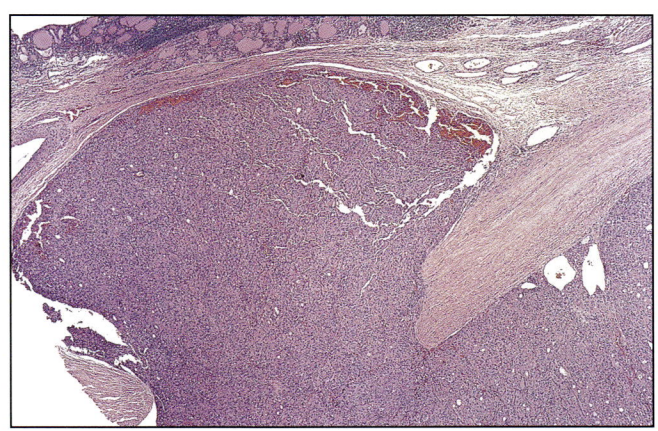

图18A.44 显示包膜浸润的滤泡癌。肿瘤已完全穿透厚的纤维包膜，即超过包膜的外轮廓。

与血管浸润类似的罕见情况是包膜血管的内皮细胞增生。仔细观察会发现血管内息肉状病变由肥胖的梭形内皮细胞和周细胞组成，与肿瘤性滤泡上皮细胞截然不同（图18A.43）。尽管血管内皮增生本身不构成血管浸润，但是这种情况下要仔细取材、检查以发现真正的血管浸润[385,386]。

包膜浸润 (Capsular invasion) 必须完全穿透纤维包膜；即瘤巢必须超过包膜的外轮廓假想线（图18A.44）[337,359,366,383,384]。评估包膜浸润时遇到的问题由图18A.45（或图18A.46）来解释。经广泛取材仔细评估后，仍缺乏完全包膜侵犯的肿瘤不应诊断为癌[387]，尽管一些作者认为不完全包膜侵犯足以诊断滤泡癌[388,389]。一个主要鉴别诊断是由细针穿刺引起的包膜破裂（图18A.47）。

血管浸润和包膜浸润实际上密切相关。显示血管浸润的肿瘤常出现包膜浸润。瘤巢常侵入或穿透包膜并直接延伸进入血管。

滤泡癌的分类
Categories of follicular carcinoma

滤泡癌诊断后，进一步分类很重要（表18A.9）[49,130,220,337,341,384,390-394]。

微小浸润滤泡癌 (Minimally invasive follicular carcinoma) 大体上可见包膜，只有组织学上可见局灶包膜（血管）浸润（图18A.39和18A.44）。应按照下面的具体标准继续分类。

- 除近期的一项研究外[397]，仅有包膜浸润的肿瘤实际上无转移风险[390,395,396]。

滤泡性肿瘤

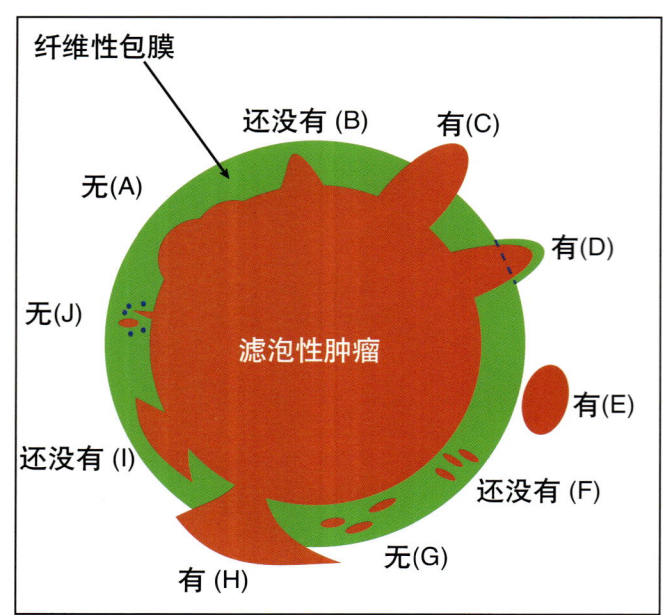

部位	主要特征	是否为包膜浸润？
A	突入包膜内侧	不是。这是滤泡性腺瘤的常见特征
B	瘤巢扎入包膜但未侵透	还不够。因为这一特征提示浸润，应深切并补充取材
C	瘤巢已侵过包膜的外轮廓	是。这显示包膜的完全侵犯
D	瘤巢已侵过包膜外轮廓假想线，但仍被薄的纤维包膜包绕	是
E	富于细胞的卫星结节，细胞结构特征与肿瘤主体相似	是。这一现象源于未切到包膜浸润点
F	有些滤泡垂直于包膜排列	还不够。因为这一特征提示浸润，应深切并补充取材
G	有些滤泡平行排列于包膜	不是。这可能不是一个积极的浸润，而是滤泡陷入纤维化的包膜
H	蘑菇形瘤巢已完全侵透纤维包膜	是
I	蘑菇形瘤巢侵入但未侵透包膜	还不够。因为这一特征提示浸润，应深切并补充取材
J	纤维性包膜内退变的肿瘤性滤泡（小浸润巢），伴有一些淋巴细胞和噬铁组织细胞	不是。代表先前细针穿刺造成的包膜破裂

图18A.45 说明滤泡性肿瘤有无包膜浸润的示意图。图示描述一被纤维性包膜（绿色）包绕的滤泡性肿瘤（红色），以及可能发生的各种情况。

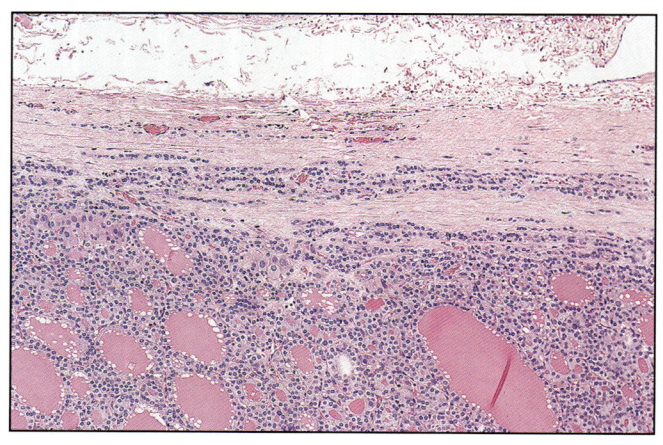

图18A.46 滤泡性腺瘤。包膜中出现与胶原纤维平行的受挤压的滤泡，不要认为是包膜浸润。

- 血管浸润<4个血管的肿瘤，转移率低（~5%）[390]。
- 血管浸润≥4个血管的肿瘤，转移风险较高，大约为18%。有些研究将这些病例与广泛浸润性滤泡癌归为一组[220,390,398,399]。

由于预后好，对低风险病人行一叶甲状腺切除±抑制性甲状腺素治疗已足够（见图18A.5的风险分组）[62,73,74,132,384,400,401]，然而有些研究者建议对所有病人行甲状腺全切术[57,71,72]。甲状腺全切除和放射性碘治疗应用于高风险病人；全甲状腺切除的目的是切除所有可能与残存或转移的滤泡癌竞争吸收放射性碘的正常甲状腺组织[337]。

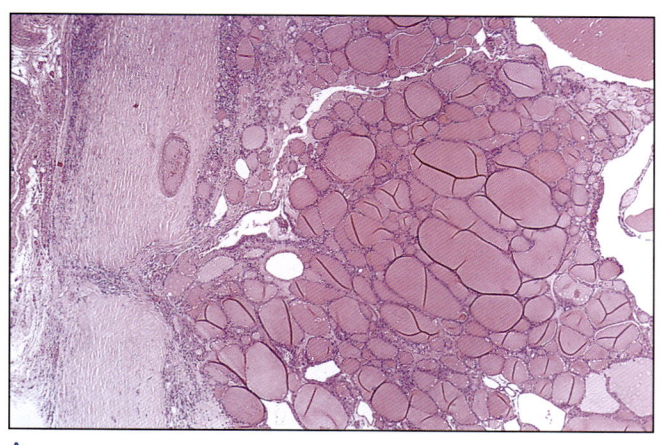
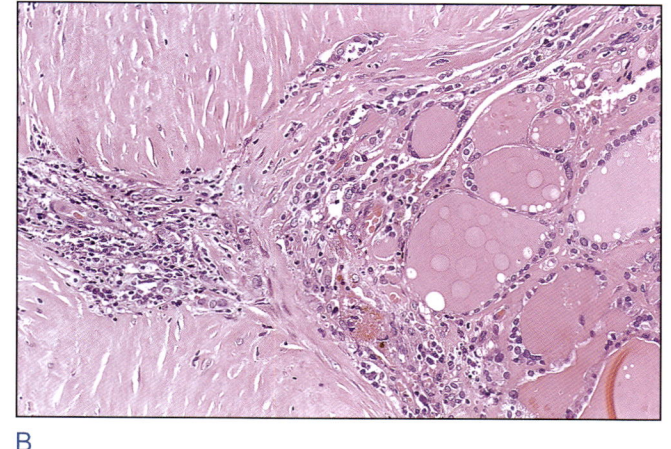

图18A.47 滤泡性腺瘤，显示细针穿刺引起的包膜破裂，类似于包膜浸润。（A）小团肿瘤组织进入厚的纤维包膜。（B）高倍镜下，瘤巢周围见慢性炎症细胞浸润和含铁血黄素沉积，一些滤泡细胞变性。

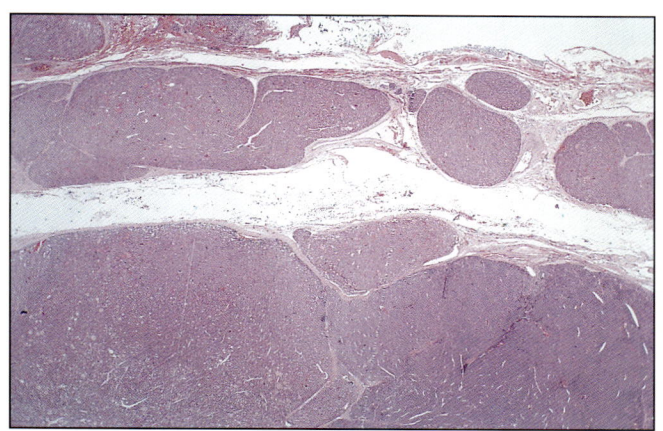

图18A.48 广泛浸润性滤泡癌。注意肿瘤主体以外明显的浸润。

广泛浸润性滤泡癌（widely invasive follicular carcinoma）表现为甲状腺实质和血管的弥漫浸润，常无完整包膜（图18A.48）。文献报道的很大比例的"广泛浸润性滤泡癌"实际为低分化（岛状）癌。发病时，区域淋巴结和远处转移分别见于7%和29%～66%的病例[49,390,402]。经随访发现更多的病人将发生淋巴结和远处转移，尤其易转移至骨和肺[390,402]。一项长期随访研究发现，29%的病人死于疾病，41%带病生存，只有22%无病生存[402]。肿瘤侵袭颈部软组织对生存不利（6年死亡率为53%，而局限于甲状腺内的癌为28%）[380,390,400,403,404]。广泛浸润性癌是侵袭性肿瘤，需行甲状腺全切、放射性碘和抑制性甲状腺素治疗。

滤泡性病变(follicular lesions)的诊断需多少蜡块(blocks)？如何取材最好？

理想状态是将整个标本取材进行组织学检查以鉴别滤泡癌和腺瘤[405]。然而，这样做不切实际，尤其是较大的肿瘤。有些作者推荐最少10个蜡块[406]。图18A.49描述了甲状腺肿瘤病理国际研讨会推荐的方法[384]。大多数蜡块应从肿瘤的外周部分包括与正常甲状腺交界处取材，而不是从中心部分取材。应通过最大径将结节一分为二，再放射状切成楔形组织块进行组织切片检查[405]。

滤泡性肿瘤的亚型
Variants of follicular neoplasm

玻璃样变梁状腺瘤（副神经节瘤样腺瘤）和癌 [Hyalinizing trabecular adenoma (paraganglioma-like adenoma) and carcinoma] 玻璃样变梁状腺瘤是滤泡性腺瘤的少见亚型，可被误诊为副神经节瘤、髓样癌或乳头状癌[104,407-411]。与慢性淋巴细胞性甲状腺炎有关[408,411]。Carney等报道的11例经平均10年的随访均未复发或转移[104]。其他组报道的病例有相似的良性过程[412]。玻璃样变梁状结构并非为滤泡性肿瘤所特有，可局灶见于胶样结节、甲状腺炎和经典乳头状癌[413-415]。

玻璃样变梁状癌罕见，与玻璃样变梁状腺瘤鉴别之处在于有无血管和(或)包膜浸润[416-418]。然而，有些报道的病例可能是FAP相关性乳头状癌的筛状-桑葚样亚型[416]。

玻璃样变梁状腺瘤的特征是呈长波纹卷曲的梁状和束状排列，细胞细长或多角形伴轻度嗜酸性胞浆（图18A.50）。细长的肿瘤细胞垂直于小梁排列。常见散在

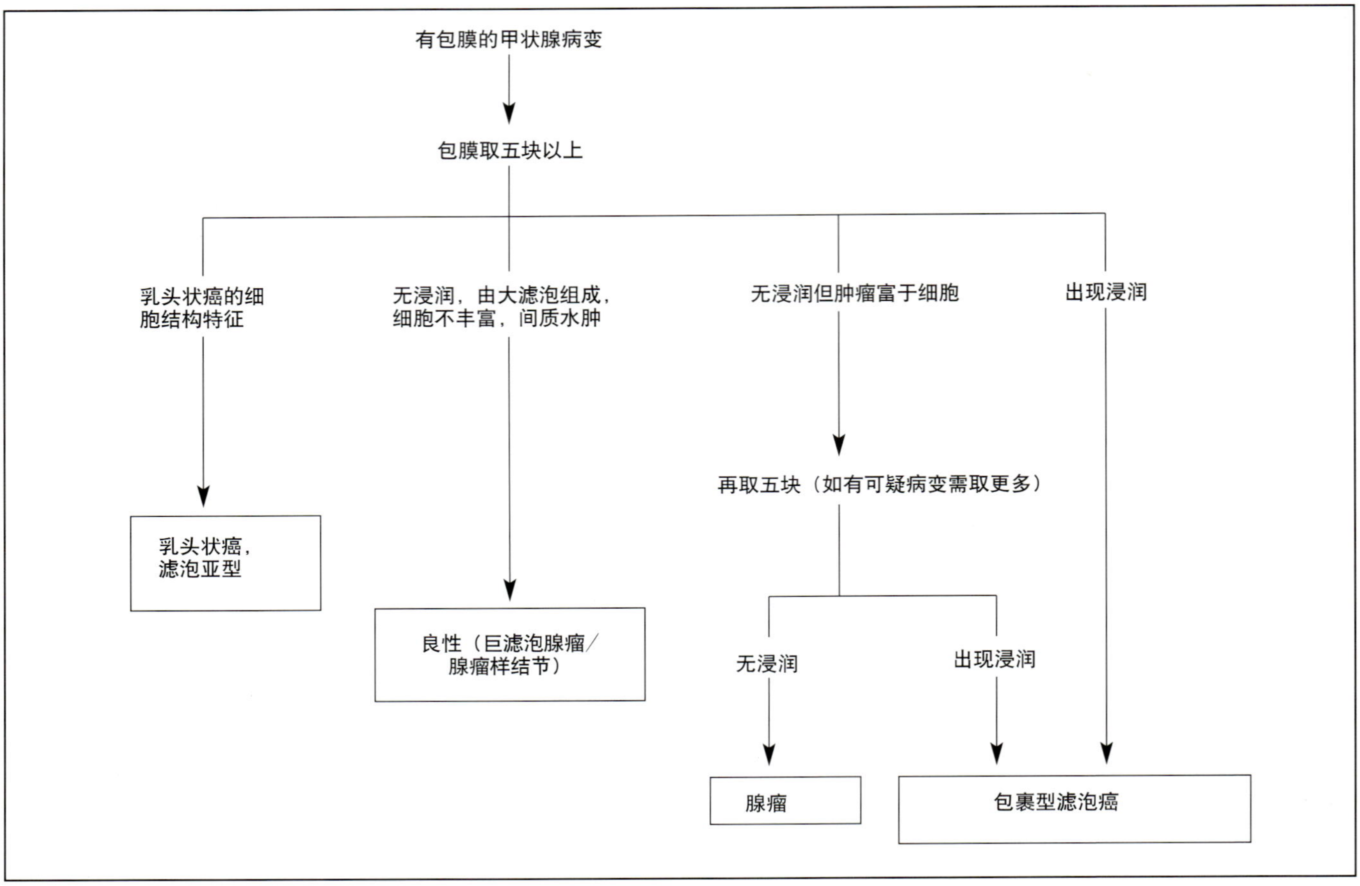

滤泡性肿瘤

```
                    有包膜的甲状腺病变
                           ↓
                      包膜取五块以上
          ┌────────────┬─────────────┬────────────┐
          ↓            ↓             ↓            ↓
    乳头状癌的细     无浸润，由大滤泡组成，  无浸润但肿瘤富于细胞   出现浸润
    胞结构特征       细胞不丰富，间质水肿
                                      ↓
                               再取五块（如有可疑病变需取更多）
                                   ┌──────┴──────┐
                                   ↓             ↓
          ↓              ↓       无浸润         出现浸润
      乳头状癌，       良性（巨滤泡腺瘤/
      滤泡亚型        腺瘤样结节）
                                   ↓             ↓            ↓
                                  腺瘤         包裹型滤泡癌
```

图18A.49　推荐的滤泡性病变取材方法。

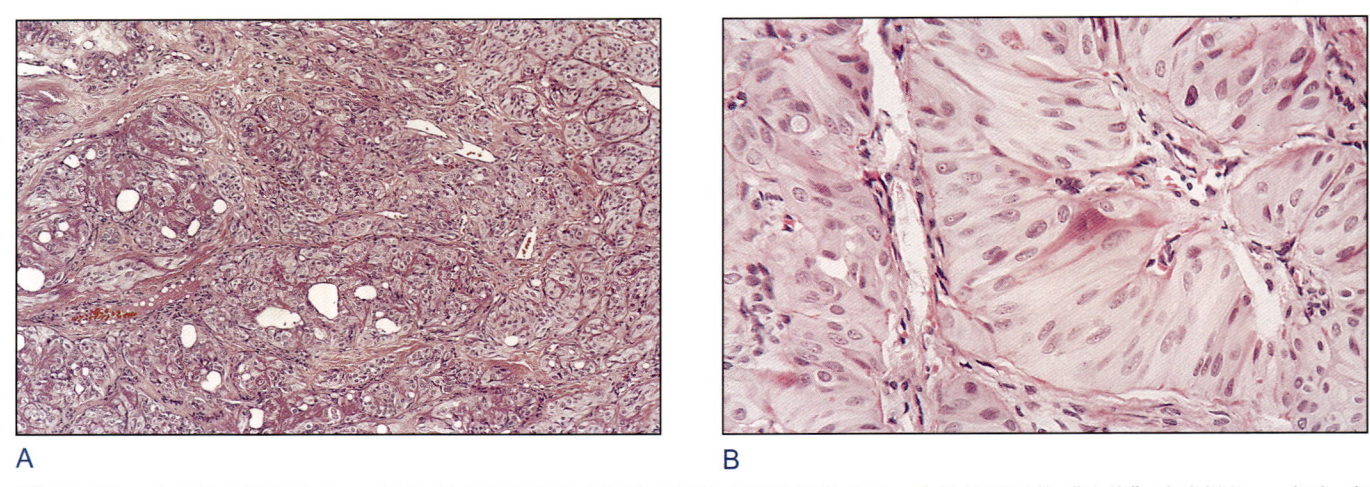

图18A.50　玻璃样变梁状腺瘤。（A）波纹状卷曲的小梁及穿插的小囊腔是其特征。左侧见明显的"块状"玻璃样物。（B）瘤细胞垂直于小梁排列。注意核沟、假包涵体和核周空晕。

的微囊和较大的囊腔，代表发育不良或真正的滤泡。核卵圆形，染色质细腻，可见一定程度的多形性。核沟、假包涵体和核周空晕常见（图18A.50B）。胞浆内有独特的黄色小体，常位于核周，浅黄色球形，有折光性，5μm大小；周围是透明空晕，超微结构显示为巨大的溶酶体（图18A.51）[419]。纤细的纤维血管间质玻璃样变，有时表现为与瘤细胞混合存在的块状嗜酸性沉积物。可见与发育不良型滤泡相关的钙化性类胶质。肿瘤显示甲状腺球蛋白阳性，局限于微囊和滤泡。因少数髓样癌在组织学上与其有相似之处，应做免疫组织化学染色加

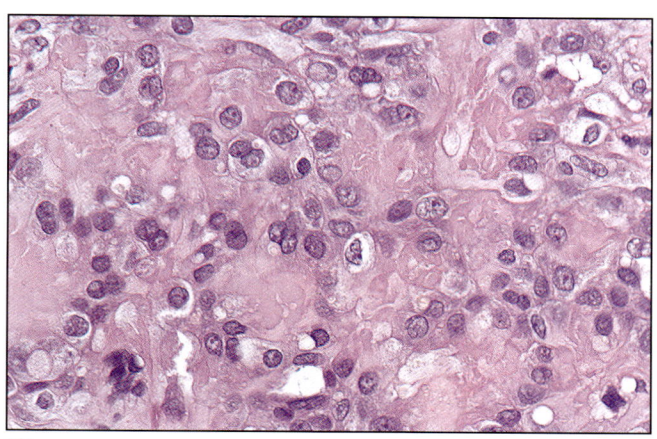

图18A.51 玻璃样变梁状腺瘤。一些细胞中可见核旁黄色小体，绕以透明空晕。

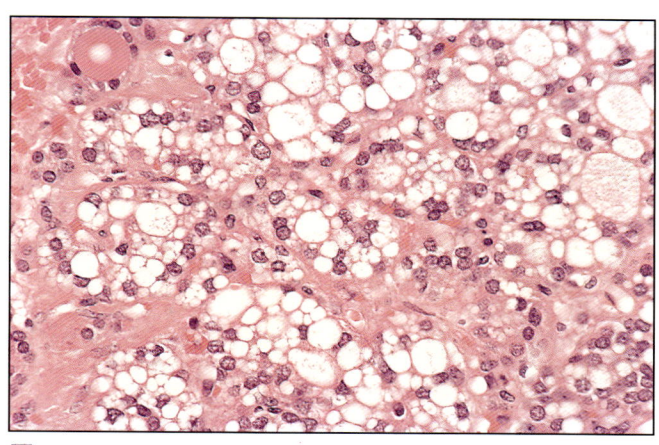

图18A.52 印戒细胞腺瘤。注意空泡状胞浆和核偏位。(Courtesy of Dr. I. T. M. Kung, Melbourne, Australia.)

以鉴别[420]。曾报道的嗜铬素免疫反应[408]未得到进一步的证实[412]。玻璃样变梁状腺瘤胞浆常显示独特的MIB-1(Ki67)颗粒状胞浆染色及胞膜染色，甲状腺肿瘤的其他类型无此特征[412,421,422]。

玻璃样变梁状腺瘤（癌）的分类存在争议。基于以下特点，一些作者认为是乳头状癌的一种少见的包膜内亚型：

- 在一些病例与典型的乳头状癌混合或共存；
- 在一些典型的乳头状癌中，局灶可见玻璃样变梁状肿瘤样区域；
- 核特征与乳头状癌明显相似；
- 至少部分病例的免疫组织化学表达与乳头状癌相似（如高分子量角蛋白、细胞角蛋白19、基底膜沉积物）；
- 在一定比例的病例中，证实有 *RET/PTC* 易位[411,412,415,417,423-426]。

然而，一些研究并未发现玻璃样变梁状腺瘤表达高分子量细胞角蛋白和细胞角蛋白19[427]。galectin-3 表达频率明显低于乳头状癌（40%：83%）[422]。某些已证实有 *RET/PTC* 易位的玻璃样变梁状肿瘤，其诊断的可靠性已遭到怀疑[422]。在玻璃样变梁状腺瘤未发现乳头状癌另一特征性分子特征——*BRAF* 突变[426]。由于肿瘤的本质存在分歧，新版 WHO 分类采用非正式名称"玻璃样变梁状肿瘤"进行命名[428]。

印戒细胞腺瘤／癌（Signet-ring cell adenoma/carcinoma） 病变可见明确的胞浆空泡，将核挤向一侧（图18A.52）[429-432]。胞浆空泡染色常显示为黏液物质，且甲状腺球蛋白阳性。超微结构上，对应于被覆微绒毛的细胞内腔。印戒细胞改变可为局灶或弥漫性，与充

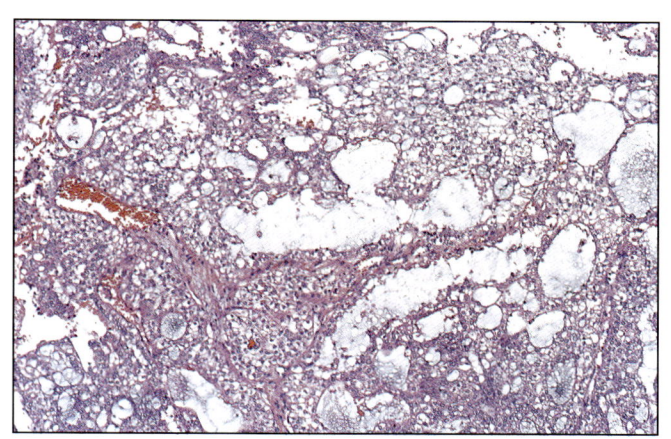

图18A.53 滤泡癌，黏液亚型。肿瘤的特征为出现充满黏液物质的多囊性间隙。某些区域有较大的黏液池。此例诊断癌的依据是有血管浸润（未显示）。

满细胞外黏液的微囊间隙混合存在。

黏液亚型（Mucinous variant） 此型见丰富的细胞外碱性黏液物质沉积，常伴有微囊、网状或多囊性生长方式[433]。也可出现一些大的黏液池（图18A.53）。有些病例肿瘤上皮可见印戒细胞改变。

透明细胞滤泡性肿瘤，包括富脂腺瘤（Clear cell follicular neoplasm, including lipid-rich adenoma） 透明细胞改变可发生于许多甲状腺肿瘤（滤泡性肿瘤、乳头状癌、髓样癌、甲状腺内甲状旁腺肿瘤、转移性肾细胞癌）以及正常或增生的甲状腺（表18A.10）。其产生机制包括线粒体的气球样变、脂质堆积（富脂腺瘤）[111,434,435]、糖原堆积或细胞内甲状腺球蛋白沉积[111,113]。

透明细胞滤泡性肿瘤由滤泡、小梁或实性片块组成（图18A.54）；血管／包膜浸润是区分癌和腺瘤的唯一标

表18A.10 甲状腺透明细胞肿瘤的鉴别诊断

病名	透明细胞特征	其他特征	诊断性免疫组化标志物
伴透明细胞的乳头状癌	胞浆透明是由于糖原堆积或超微结构可见的囊泡形成。胞浆常呈纤细网状	其他区域常见乳头状癌的典型特征（如乳头、伸长的滤泡、拥挤而浅染或毛玻璃核）	甲状腺球蛋白阳性 TTF-1阳性
柱状细胞癌（某些病例）	胞浆透明限于核下区，常形成空泡	明显的乳头及核假复层；核深染	甲状腺球蛋白阳性 TTF-1阳性
透明细胞滤泡腺瘤/癌或Hurthle细胞腺瘤/癌	透明胞浆常呈细颗粒状或细网状；细胞膜通常不易碎。有些病例细胞呈印戒细胞表现	局灶出现滤泡。有些病例有Hurthle细胞成分	甲状腺球蛋白阳性 TTF-1阳性
髓样癌透明细胞亚型	胞浆透明	别处常见髓样癌的典型特征；可见淀粉样物	甲状腺球蛋白阴性 降钙素阳性 TTF-1阳性
甲状腺内甲状旁腺腺瘤/癌	水样透明胞浆及易碎的细胞膜	纤细的血管。透明细胞常与具有双嗜性或嗜酸性胞浆的细胞混合	甲状腺球蛋白阴性 甲状旁腺激素阳性 TTF-1阴性
转移性肾细胞癌	水样透明胞浆及易碎的细胞膜	明显的纤细血管。局灶见一些腺腔；腺腔内可见出血	甲状腺球蛋白阴性 TTF-1阴性 降钙素阴性 甲状旁腺激素阴性 CD10或RCC(gp200)阳性

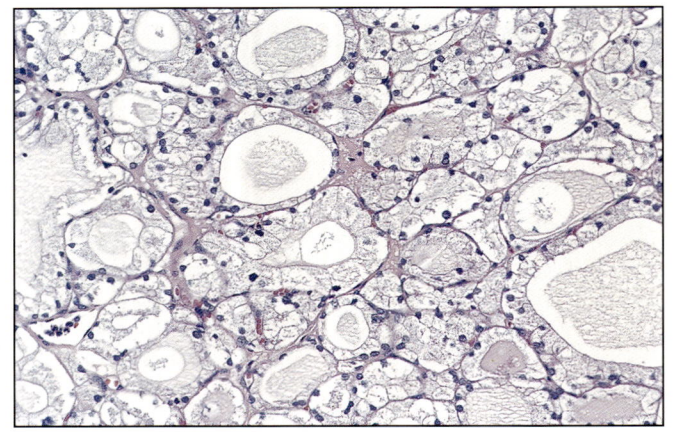

图18A.54 滤泡性腺瘤，透明细胞亚型。胞浆不是水样透明，而是呈细网状。

准。如果对分化有疑问，甲状腺球蛋白和TTF1免疫染色可确诊。

滤泡性腺瘤伴乳头状增生（滤泡性腺瘤的乳头状亚型）[Follicular adenoma with papillary hyperplasia (papillary variant of follicular adenoma)] 这是主要发生于儿童和青少年的良性肿瘤[436,437]。有包膜，部分囊性，由乳头和滤泡构成（图18A.55）。核圆形、深染，规则地排列于细胞基底部。缺乏乳头状癌的核特征。腔内巨噬细胞和滤泡上皮常见含铁血黄素沉积。

热腺瘤（Hot adenoma） 少数滤泡性腺瘤功能亢进，自主产生甲状腺素。放射性碘扫描为"热"结节。有些热腺瘤形态上与普通滤泡性腺瘤无法区分，但有些由具有乳头状内折被覆高立方细胞的滤泡组成，与Graves病中的滤泡相似（图18A.56）。一些热腺瘤中检测到编码促甲状腺素受体和刺激性G蛋白α亚单位的基因激活性体突变，这种改变也见于少数滤泡癌[3,364,438-442]。

伴脂肪瘤样间质或软骨化生的滤泡性肿瘤（Follicular neoplasm with lipomatous stroma or cartilaginous metaplasia） 罕见的腺脂肪瘤[甲状腺脂肪瘤(thyrolipoma)]是含有散在成熟脂肪细胞的滤泡性腺瘤[443,444]。更为少见的是，脂肪细胞可见于滤泡癌中[119]。滤泡性腺瘤中可出现的间叶成分包括脂肪、纤维组织、平滑肌、软骨和骨，已有报道可显示广泛软骨样化生的滤泡性腺瘤[445,446]。

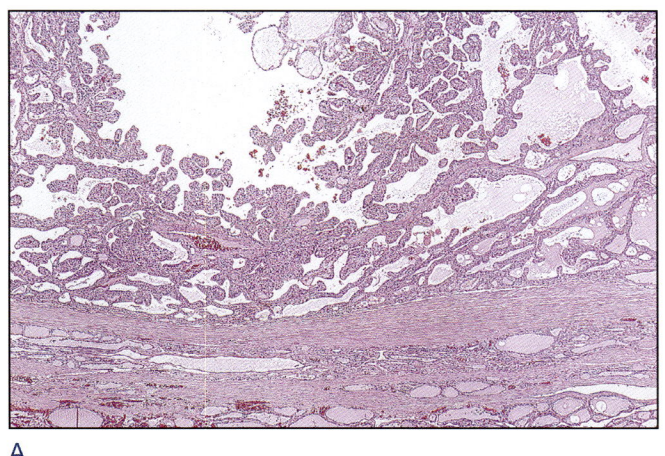
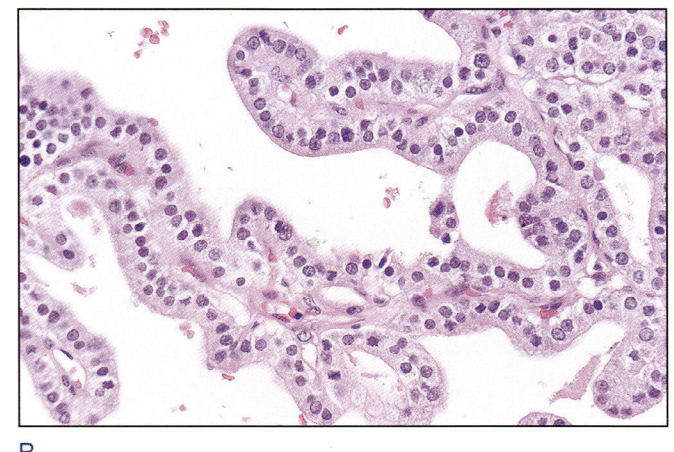

A

B

图18A.55 滤泡性腺瘤伴乳头状增生。（A）包膜内肿瘤具有复杂的乳头。（B）衬覆乳头的矮柱状细胞含规则的、位于基底的深染圆形核。

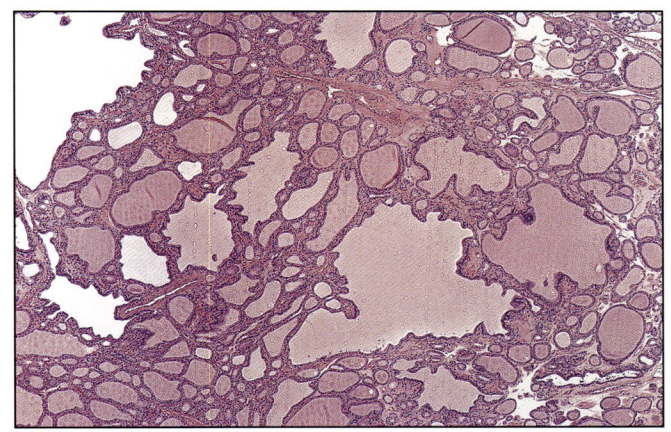

图18A.56 高功能滤泡性腺瘤（毒性腺瘤）。滤泡有短粗的乳头状突起，与Graves病中的滤泡相似。

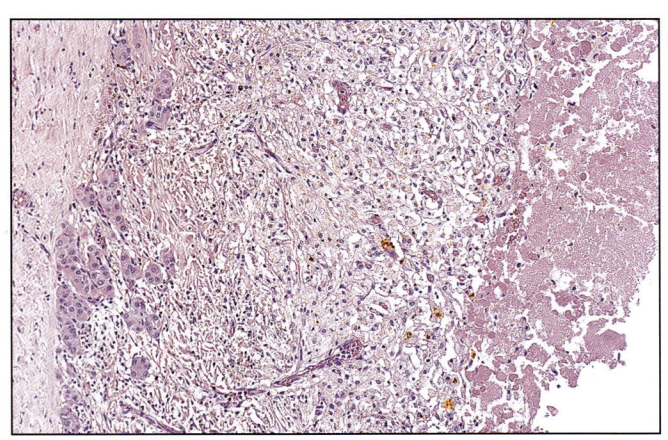

图18A.57 细针穿刺后发生梗死的Hurthle细胞腺瘤。右侧可见坏死的细胞残影。中间显示针对坏死的组织细胞反应，左侧可见薄层存活细胞。

细针穿刺后发生梗死的滤泡性肿瘤(Infarcted follicular neoplasm following fine needle aspiration) 有时滤泡性肿瘤细针穿刺后，会发生部分或完全梗死，在Hurthle细胞肿瘤中尤其常见[447-450]。根据穿刺与切除之间的时间间隔，可有凝固性坏死、出血、巨噬细胞聚集及不同程度的纤维肉芽组织机化（图18A.57）。在一些病例边缘仍可有薄层肿瘤存活。有趣的是，完全梗死的滤泡癌中浸润的细胞巢常存活。梗死的原因可能是出血引起病灶内压力增高，导致包膜内肿瘤的血供不足。梗死可产生以下诊断问题：

- 难以辨别肿瘤的真正性质；
- 过度增生的肉芽组织（具有泡状核的肥胖间质细胞）和混杂的巨噬细胞可误诊为未分化癌（图18A.58）。

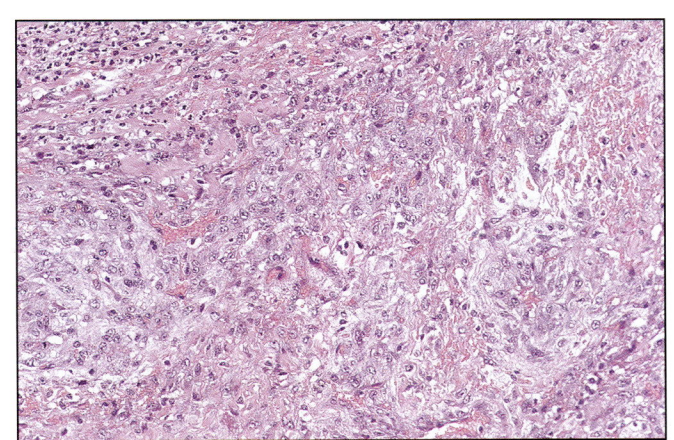

图18A.58 伴梗死后过度修复改变的Hurthle细胞腺瘤。梗死周围的肉芽组织含有肥胖的梭形细胞，其核有一定异型性，可误诊为未分化癌。

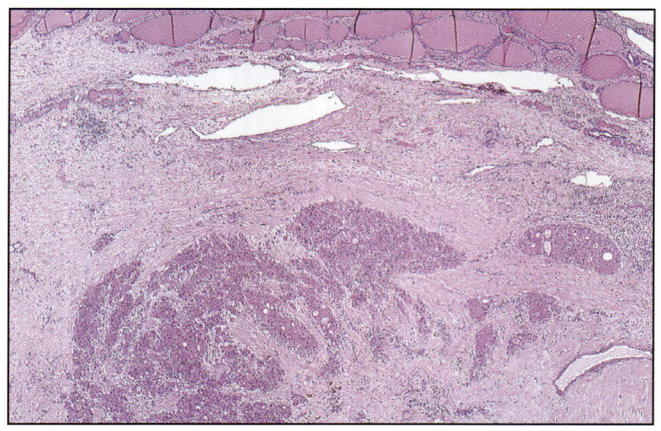

图18A.59　Hurthle细胞腺瘤，梗死后硬化。肿瘤不完全梗死后产生的纤维组织将残留肿瘤分割成不规则小岛，产生假浸润结构。

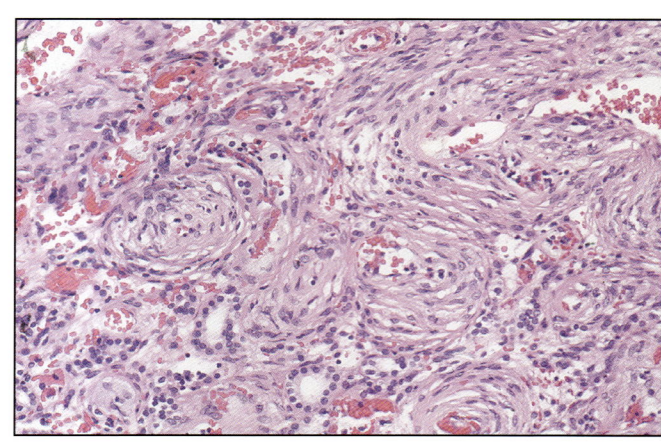

图18A.60　滤泡性腺瘤伴梭形细胞化生。病灶有稀薄的包膜，主要由肥胖的梭形细胞组成，围绕血管形成漩涡状。部分梭形细胞与滤泡融合（左下角）。

随后的纤维化可将残留肿瘤分割成不规则的小岛，产生假浸润结构（图18A.59）。
- 梗死周围残留的肿瘤可表现出明显的反应性核异型，导致误诊为高级别癌。滤泡扩张也可产生血管肉瘤样形态。

伴梭形细胞化生的滤泡性腺瘤（Follicular adenoma with spindle cell metaplasia）　罕见情况下，滤泡性腺瘤含有数量不等的肿瘤性梭形细胞，形成短束状或围绕血管呈漩涡状（图18A.60）。细胞角蛋白、甲状腺球蛋白、TTF-1阳性证实梭形细胞的化生性质[213]。

非典型腺瘤（Atypical adenoma）　显示普遍的核异型性、巨细胞或特殊组织学结构（如梭形细胞束），但经仔细取材仍缺乏血管/包膜浸润的滤泡性腺瘤被称为非典型腺瘤（图18A.61）[451]。长期的随访研究已证明非典型腺瘤具有良性临床经过[390,406,451]。

伴奇异核的滤泡性腺瘤（Follicular adenoma with bizarre nuclei）　此型为另外一种有代表性的滤泡性腺瘤，含有散在的核奇异深染的巨细胞[37,452]。

Hurthle 细胞腺瘤/癌
Hurthle cell adenoma/carcinoma

病理特征　Hurthle(oncocytic、oxyphilic、Askanazy)肿瘤的组成细胞具有丰富的嗜酸性胞浆，因线粒体积聚而呈颗粒状(图18A.62)。与所有富于线粒体的肿瘤一样，大体上呈亮棕色。因线粒体的气球样变，细胞浆可以部分或完全透明（图18A.62B）。细胞排列成小滤泡、梁状、

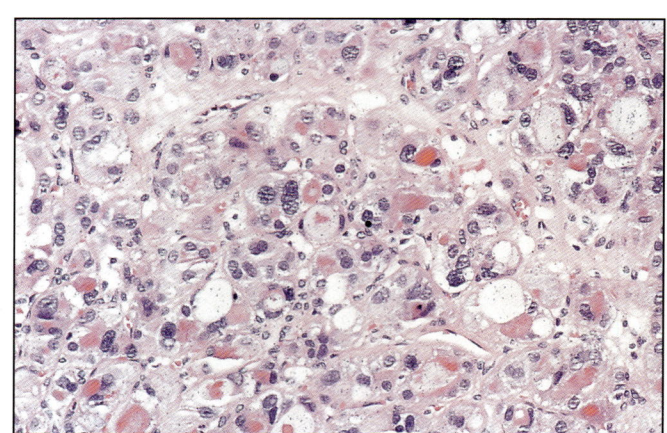

图18A.61　非典型腺瘤。可见高度异型的细胞核。经广泛取材未发现浸润。

实性片状或乳头状（图18A.63）。类胶质可钙化，类似于沙粒体（图18A.63B）。核圆形，染色质颗粒状或粗糙，核仁明显。偶尔可见核沟。通常可见散在的大细胞核和某种程度的核多形性。Hurthle 细胞肿瘤被认为是滤泡性肿瘤的一个亚型，而不是一个独立的疾病，因其与常见的滤泡性肿瘤有形态连续性：一些滤泡性肿瘤仅局灶可见 Hurthle 细胞，或单个肿瘤细胞呈不完全的 Hurthle 细胞改变[359,369]。

大多数 Hurthle 细胞肿瘤为孤立性，少数病例为多灶或双侧性[453]。Hurthle 细胞肿瘤易自发或于细针穿刺后发生梗死。

临床特征和行为　20世纪70年代及80年代初期的研究认为，Hurthle 细胞肿瘤为潜在恶性，不管组织学有无浸润均应积极治疗[453-456]，最近许多令人信服的研

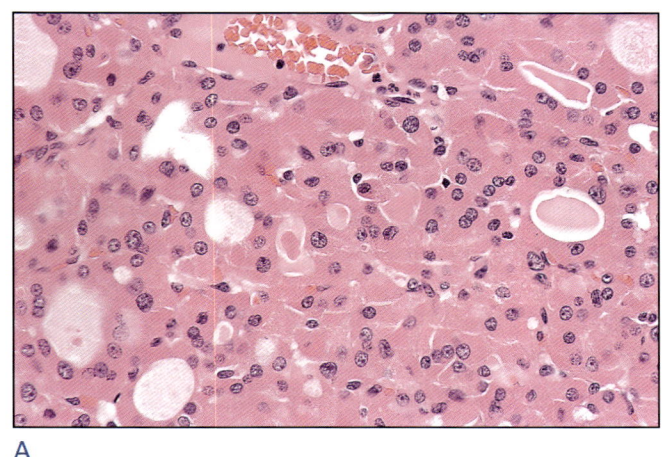
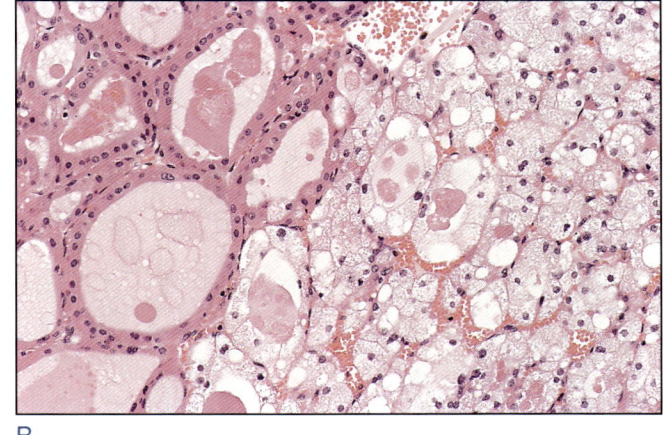

图18A.62　Hurthle细胞腺瘤。（A）注意嗜酸性颗粒状胞浆及相当大的细胞核。（B）局灶透明细胞改变是一常见现象。

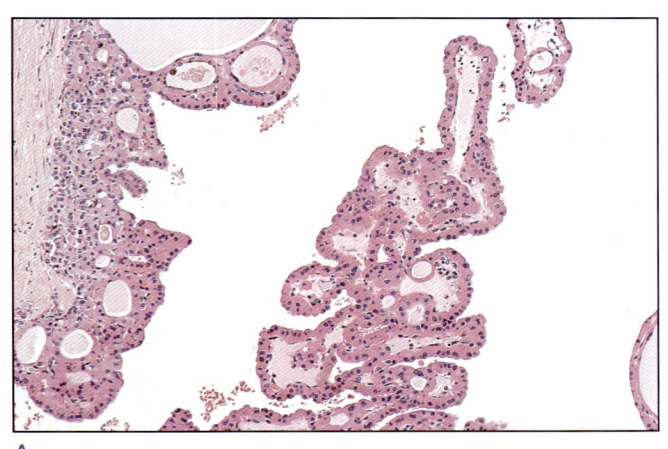
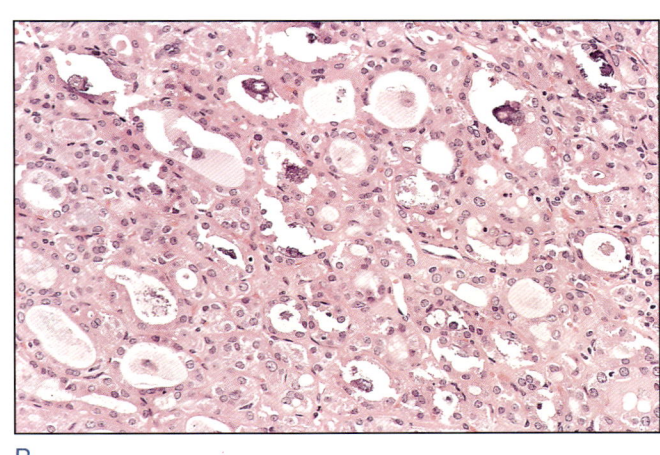

图18A.63　Hurthle细胞腺瘤。（A）局灶乳头形成。（B）常见钙化的类胶质，可被误诊为沙粒体。

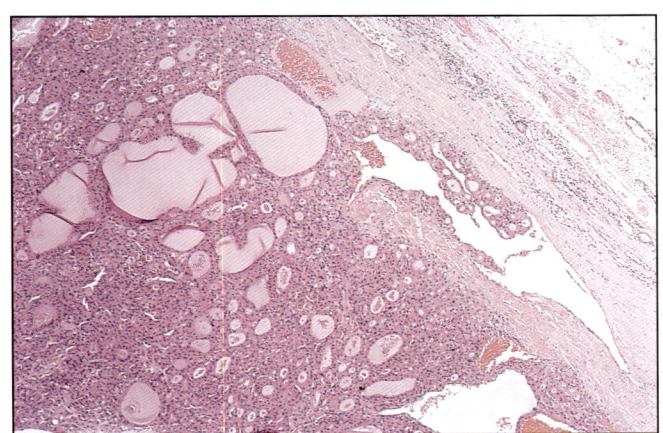

图18A.64　有血管浸润的Hurthle细胞癌（右侧）。

究表明组织学特征能准确地预测Hurthle细胞肿瘤的行为（图18A.64）[366,378,379,382,387,403,453,457-465]。无浸润的肿瘤可行结节切除或腺叶切除，而浸润性病例（癌）需行全甲状腺切除和放射治疗，这些肿瘤可局部复发，发生区域淋巴结或远处转移（尤其转移到骨和肺）[366,382,387,464,466]。与非Hurthle细胞滤泡性肿瘤相比，Hurthle细胞肿瘤的恶性频率较高（35%）[379-382,467,468]。≥4 cm的Hurthle细胞肿瘤与恶性强相关[467]。与Hurthle细胞腺瘤相比，Hurthle细胞癌易发生于较大年龄组（癌患者51.0岁，腺瘤患者43.1岁），并且体积较大（癌大小4.3 cm，腺瘤大小2.9 cm）[465]。

有时，恶性潜能不确定的Hurthle细胞肿瘤用于描述显示某些不确定浸润特征的病例；随访发现此类病人生存良好，因而这些肿瘤最好简单归类为Hurthle细胞腺瘤[387,469]。DNA倍体无法区分Hurthle细胞腺瘤和癌[470,471]，但在Hurthle细胞癌，非整倍体较二倍体更具侵袭性。

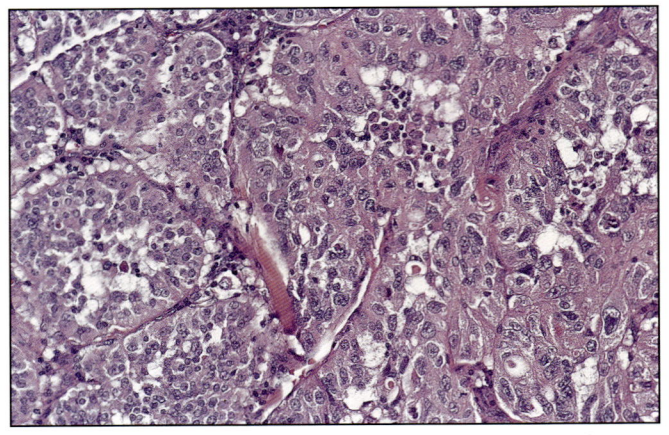

图18A.65 Hurthle细胞癌，所谓的低分化型。肿瘤呈实性生长方式。具有多形性核的大嗜酸性细胞位于右侧，小的嗜酸性细胞位于左侧。

Hurthle 细胞癌的总死亡率约为30%～70%[366,382,387]。老年、肿瘤体积大（>4 cm）及广泛血管浸润与预后较差相关[399,465,469]。与普通的滤泡癌相比，Hurthle 细胞癌通常放射性碘吸收不满意；较常发生甲状腺外扩展、局部复发及淋巴结转移；总体来说，更具侵袭性[369,380,387,404,465,472]。然而，当根据浸润范围对比两组时，许多差别不明显[369,473]。Papotti 等发现肿瘤75%以上的区域出现实性或梁状结构（大细胞或小细胞亚型），表明为预后较差的低分化亚型（图18A.65）。此型病人30%死于疾病或出现复发，而不属于低分化亚型的病例死亡率为2.5%[474]。

免疫组化在滤泡性肿瘤诊断中的作用

除非肿瘤具有特殊的形态特征，如明显的纤维血管间隔、印戒细胞、透明细胞或玻璃样变梁状结构，通常不需要做免疫组化。肿瘤的滤泡本质可通过甲状腺球蛋白或TTF-1阳性加以证实。Hurthle 细胞肿瘤也通常着染S-100蛋白[475]。

已对多种抗体在鉴别滤泡癌和滤泡性腺瘤的潜在价值方面进行研究，但到目前为止仍没有可靠的指标。

- 内皮标志物染色因常不稳定，不能有效地检测血管浸润[476-478]。含肿瘤巢的血管可缺乏染色，尽管有令人满意的内部阳性对照。
- 各种肿瘤标志物，如癌胚抗原（CEA）、癌基因产物（ras p21、c-myc）、细胞周期依赖性激酶抑制蛋白（p27）、增殖标志物（Ki67）、表皮生长因子、P-糖蛋白及HMGI(Y)(high-mobility group I)蛋白均没有帮助[479-485]。
- 尽管一些抗体，如组织多肽抗原、二肽基氨基肽酶 IV、Leu-7、甲状腺过氧化物酶（MoAb 47）、HBME-1、galectin-3、基质金属蛋白酶-2、基质金属蛋白酶-7及环氧合酶-2被报道在滤泡性腺瘤和滤泡癌表达不同[28,30,31,422,486-496]，但是尚不足以在常规诊断中应用。

滤泡性腺瘤(follicular adenoma)和滤泡癌(follicular carcinoma)存在根本差异吗？

在细胞结构、组织形态、免疫表型、DNA 倍体或分子改变方面，滤泡性腺瘤和滤泡癌没有显著差异[497-501]。27%的腺瘤可为非整倍体，而随访超过5年，病人仍很好[502]。而且，微滤泡腺瘤的 ras 癌基因表达率几乎与滤泡癌一样高[3,480,503,504]。

如果人们接受某些滤泡性腺瘤实际上是"原位"癌[383,500,505]，那么上述结果有意义。当对滤泡癌伴混合性腺瘤及原位癌进行比较时，很难找到明确的区分指标。从治疗角度而言，识别这些缺乏转移潜能的隐藏的原位癌并不重要。目前，组织学评价仍是区分滤泡癌和滤泡性腺瘤的金标准。

细胞遗传学和分子特征

滤泡性肿瘤有两条主要的、不重叠的分子通路。

- 源于 t(2;3)(q13;p15) 的 PAX8/PPARγ 融合发生于大约一半的滤泡癌和10%的滤泡性腺瘤。有趣的是，Hurthle 细胞肿瘤无此基因融合[506]。PAX8 编码一种在甲状腺发生和分化过程中起重要作用的转录因子，而 PPARγ 编码一种过氧物酶体增殖-活化受体。除一些"乳头状癌的滤泡亚型"之外，在其他甲状腺肿瘤中未发现此基因融合[296,507]。有 PAX8/PPARγ 基因融合的滤泡癌倾向于发生明显浸润，是二倍体或近二倍体并伴频繁的染色体丢失[508]。
- ras 基因激活点突变在滤泡性腺瘤和滤泡癌中发生率均相当高，表明 ras 突变为肿瘤发生的早期事件[3,38]。N-ras 突变发生于17%的滤泡性腺瘤和50%的滤泡癌，最常累及第61位密码子，导致CAA（谷氨酰胺）改变为CGA（精氨酸）；这一突变发生于0%的乳头状癌和25%的未分化癌[504]。H-ras 第12位密码子突变发生于33%的滤泡性腺瘤，71%的非典型腺瘤，33%的滤泡癌[509]。K-ras 突变较少见[504,510]。有 ras 突变的肿瘤倾向于伴染色体获得的非整倍体[324]。

Cowden疾病基因——PTEN的半合子丢失发生于26%的滤泡性腺瘤，但在滤泡癌罕见[511]。因基因扩增导致 BRAF 基因拷贝数增加或7号染色体拷贝数增加发生于16%～45%的滤泡性或Hurthle细胞肿瘤；这组滤泡癌与缺乏BRAF扩增的肿瘤相比，似乎更常发生广泛浸润（67% versus 18%）[512]。

滤泡癌的预后因素

滤泡癌的临床结局常可通过危险性分组来预测（图 18A.5，见第 1003 页）[404]。低危、中危和高危组病人的 20 年生存率分别为 97%、87% 和 49%[404]。自然病史描述于图 18A.32，见第 1015 页。

- 微小浸润型（仅包膜浸润、血管浸润或广泛血管浸润）明显不同于广泛浸润型（表 18A.9）。
- 转移：发病时已远处转移是极为不利的预后因素[340,366,387,390,395,403,404,513]。骨转移尤其不好[514]。据报道淋巴结转移对预后无明显影响[343,404]或者有不利影响[513]。
- 年龄：小于 30～40 岁的病人比年龄较大的病人预后好得多[332,337,366,387,390,400,403,404,513,515]。
- 性别：一些研究表明，男性预后较差[332,387,400,513]。
- 组织学类型：组织形态与预后的关系不确定[366,387,390]。有些研究显示，与非 Hurthle 细胞滤泡癌相比，Hurthle 细胞癌侵袭性较强[366,369,404]、较弱[390]或相似[217,473]。75% 以上区域呈实性或梁状结构的病例预后较差[474]。
- 肿瘤大小：超过 3.5～6 cm 的肿瘤预后较差[337,387,404,513,515]。
- 据报道需要证实的预后因素：
  - 滤泡癌中 DNA 非整倍体的预后意义存在争议。尽管有些研究表明非整倍体滤泡癌较二倍体滤泡癌更致命，另一些研究没有发现它的独立预后意义[498,499,516]。
  - E-cadherin 表达缺乏与预后较差相关[354]。
  - p53 出现异常可能增加转移的机会[474,517]。

鉴别诊断

- 胶样（腺瘤样）结节。滤泡性腺瘤与腺瘤样结节的鉴别存在困难，有时是主观的，但就治疗而言，不是非常重要。
- 桥本甲状腺炎和激素生成障碍。有时，桥本甲状腺炎或激素生成障碍甲状腺肿中的多发增生结节，使人担心可能为广泛浸润性滤泡癌。这些病灶缺乏血管浸润，不同结节的细胞密度和滤泡大小不同。
- 甲状腺内甲状旁腺肿瘤。发生在甲状腺内的甲状旁腺肿瘤可类似于微滤泡甲状腺肿瘤、透明细胞甲状腺肿瘤和 Hurthle 细胞肿瘤。见甲状腺内甲状旁腺肿瘤部分（第 1054 页）。临床信息（高钙血症）和甲状旁腺激素的免疫组化染色可解决鉴别诊断问题。
- 髓样癌。髓样癌的腺样、嗜酸细胞和玻璃样小梁亚型可类似于滤泡性肿瘤。显著纤维血管间隔的出现总应该想到髓样癌的可能性。所以，任何表现"特殊"的滤泡性肿瘤，应检查更多的组织，寻找髓样癌更具诊断性的区域，并应做免疫组化检查。
- 乳头状癌。在滤泡性肿瘤中常见浅染、透明的核，尤其在固定欠佳的中心部分。最重要的是不要将这样的核改变误认为是乳头状癌。（见*甲状腺肿瘤诊断中的实际问题*部分，第 1055 页）

未分化（间变性）癌
Undifferentiated (anaplastic) carcinoma

临床特征

未分化癌占甲状腺癌的 2%～5%[24,518-521]。然而，在地方性甲状腺肿流行区，如阿尔卑斯山地区可高达 30%～40%，近几十年来由于碘的补充，未分化癌的发生率已下降[522,523]。辐射是另一可能的病因[53,524]。

未分化癌在女性（男：女比例为 1:1.1 至 1:2）和年龄较大者（平均年龄 70 岁）更常见[24,26,519,525-527]。表现如下[24,218,518,519,524]：

- 长期甲状腺肿的病人近期甲状腺快速增大（最常见）
- 无甲状腺肿的病人，甲状腺肿物快速生长
- 复发性高分化甲状腺癌病人近期快速生长
- 局部或远处发生转移的肿瘤

患者常伴有声嘶、吞咽困难和呼吸困难[24]。少数情况下肿瘤能产生粒细胞集落刺激因子，引起明显的白细胞增多[528]。

肿瘤常表现为早期广泛浸润以致大约一半的病例不能手术。区域淋巴结和远处转移（最常转移至肺和骨）常见。尽管进行了积极治疗，大多数病人于 1 年内死亡，中位生存时间仅 4 个月[529-535]。5 年生存率为 3.6%～10%。尽管紫杉醇（paclitaxel）似乎有希望，但化学治疗并没有明显提高生存率[536,537]。化学耐药可能由于多药耐药相关蛋白和较少见的 P-糖蛋白过表达所致[538,539]。少数存活者常小于 60 岁，肿瘤相对较小（< 5～6 cm），能被完全切除，并辅以放疗和（或）化疗[218,520,521,527,529,533,540]。

大体表现

肿瘤广泛取代甲状腺实质，常浸润邻近软组织和器官如喉、气管、咽和食管。呈肉样，灰白色，常见坏死和出血。平均大小 6.4 cm[527]。

组织学表现

尽管组织学特征变化不定，梭形和巨细胞癌形象地描述了这一高度多形性和浸润性肿瘤的突出特征

（图 18A.66）[24,218]。肿瘤细胞上皮样，大的多角形或圆形细胞呈束状和片状排列（图 18A.67）；偶尔局部可见鳞状分化[372]。一些肿瘤主要或全部呈肉瘤样，类似于纤维肉瘤、恶性纤维组织细胞瘤、血管外皮细胞瘤、血管肉瘤或横纹肌肉瘤（图 18A.67B）。细长或肥胖的梭形细胞排列成交叉束状或无规则排列，细胞核中到重度异型性。核分裂象可见，凝固性坏死常较广泛。

常见显著的炎症表现，中性粒细胞最为突出；在一些肿瘤细胞浆内甚至可见中性粒细胞聚集。常见淋巴管血管浸润。肿瘤浸润血管壁常使管腔消失，是未分化甲状腺癌一个常见的特征（图 18A.68）[24]。

充分取材的病例中，50%～89% 可见分化型甲状腺癌或低分化甲状腺癌[24,216,218,518,531,541,542]，表明未分化癌通常由分化型癌（常为静止性）发生"去分化"形成。非整倍体分化型甲状腺癌更容易"去分化"[541]。

"小细胞型"未分化癌实际上近来已无报道。过去诊断的病例重新分类如下[24,218,518,543-547]：

- 恶性淋巴瘤（大多数病例）。
- 淀粉样物稀少的髓样癌。
- 低分化（岛状）癌。
- 转移性小细胞癌。
- 真正的甲状腺小细胞癌[546,547]，十分罕见，常有神经内分泌分化。更为可取的是将这些病例命名为小细胞神经内分泌癌，而不包括在甲状腺未分化癌内。

未分化癌的形态变异
Morphologic variants of undifferentiated carcinoma

血管瘤样型 (Angiomatoid variant)　　以不规则、相互

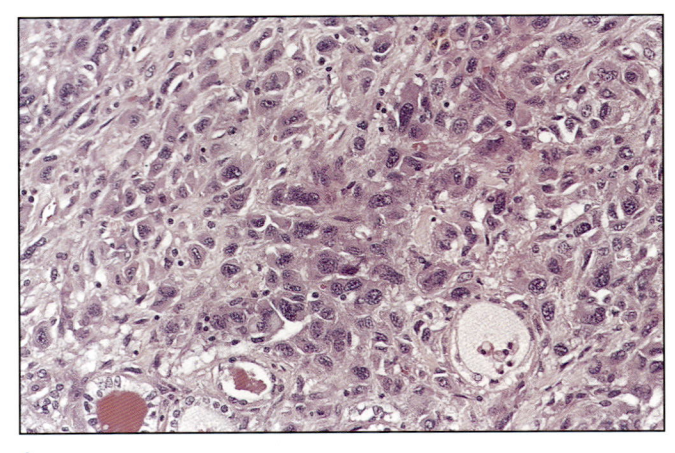

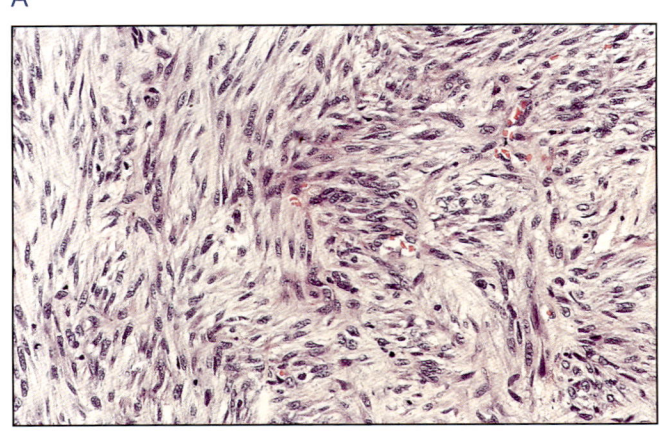

图18A.67　未分化癌。（A）此例以排列成片状的多角形大细胞为主，细胞核高度多形性。（B）此例以梭形细胞为主，伴核多形性，类似肉瘤。同一病例通常可见两种细胞类型。

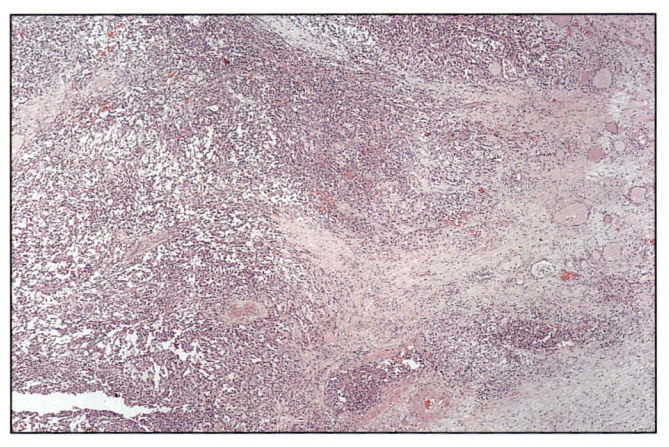

图18A.66　广泛浸润甲状腺实质和血管（下方）的未分化癌。

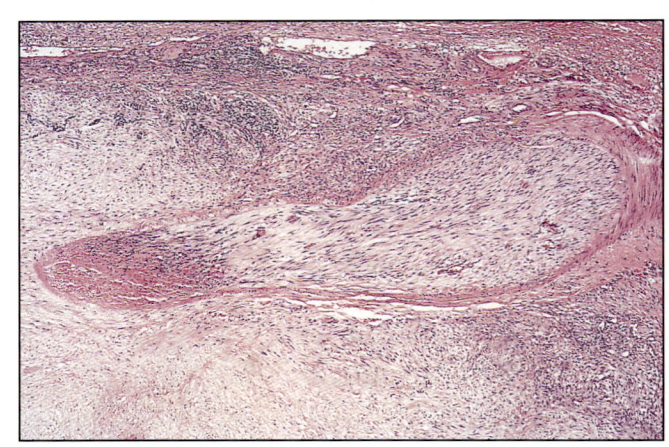

图18A.68　未分化癌。常见血管内膜和肌壁浸润，是此型肿瘤的典型特征。

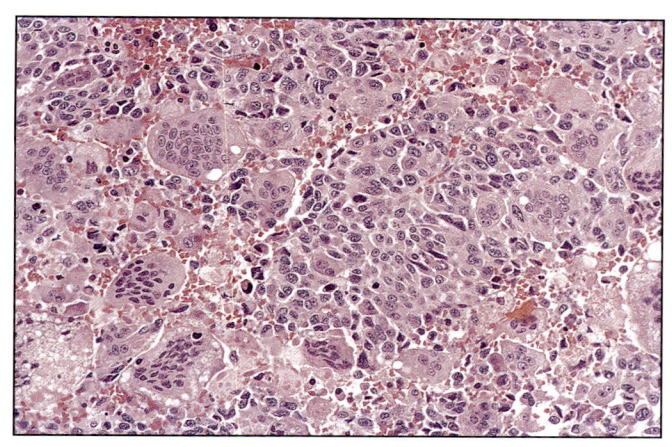

图18A.69 未分化癌，破骨细胞亚型。破骨巨细胞散在于多形性肿瘤细胞中。这些巨细胞是反应性组织细胞，不属于肿瘤细胞。

吻合的衬覆肿瘤细胞的裂隙为特征，裂隙内可含有血，类似血管肉瘤。

破骨细胞型 (Osteoclastic variant) 大量非肿瘤性破骨巨细胞（组织细胞）散在分布于未分化癌中（图18A.69）[548-550]。

横纹肌样型 (Rhabdoid variant) 特征为大的卵圆形肿瘤细胞伴奇异核，核仁突出，胞浆丰富、嗜酸性，内含丝状核旁包涵体[551-553]。

淋巴上皮瘤样癌 (Lymphoepithelioma-like carcinoma) 特征为片状、巢状癌组织与大量小淋巴细胞和浆细胞混合[554]。与伴胸腺样成分的癌（CASTLE）的不同之处在于缺乏叶状生长结构，常见凝固性坏死和CD5阴性。

寡细胞型 (Paucicellular variant) 此型因组织学与Riedel甲状腺炎相似而难以诊断。是一种细胞稀少的浸润性肿瘤，伴有致密硬化、梗死（常误认为硬化，但可通过血管残影加以识别），局灶可见轻度核异型的梭形细胞和少量淋巴细胞（图18A.70）。梭形细胞侵及血管致管腔消失及细胞角蛋白阳性可支持诊断[555-557]。

癌肉瘤 (Carcinosarcoma) 罕见，未分化癌中可见肿瘤性软骨、骨或骨骼肌[558,559]。

腺鳞癌 (Adenosquamous carcinoma) 是一种伴局灶

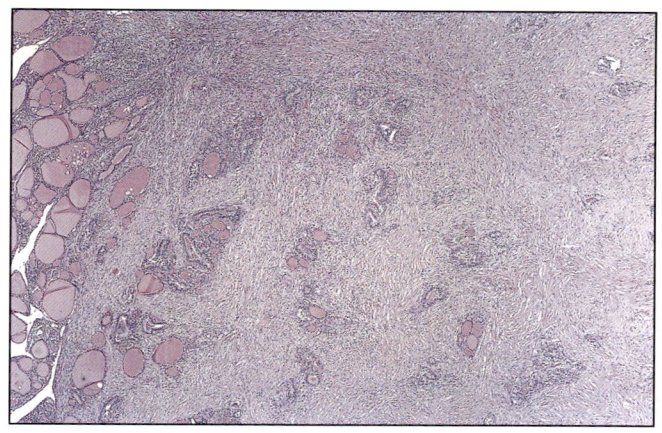

A

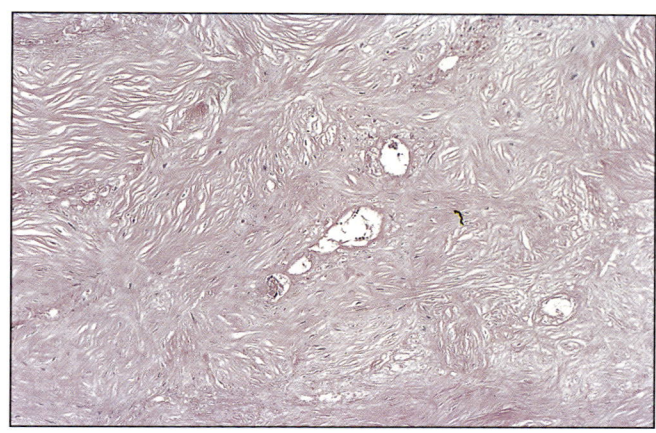

B

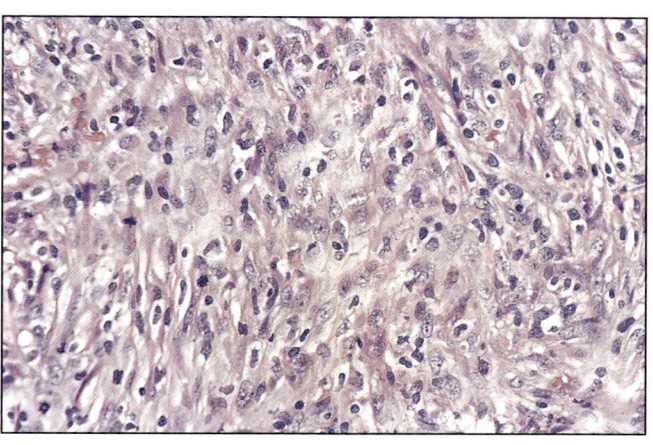

C

图18A.70 未分化癌，寡细胞亚型。（A）这种浸润性病变不同于普通未分化癌之处在于细胞很少，加之散在的淋巴细胞，类似于Riedel甲状腺炎。（B）这个区域看上去类似硬化，实际上是梗死区，血管残影可作为依据。（C）在周边区域，肌纤维母细胞样梭形细胞具有轻度核异型性，偶见核分裂象。这些实际上是间变癌的肿瘤细胞，细胞角蛋白强阳性（未显示）。在其他区域，梭形细胞阻塞血管腔，这是未分化癌的特征。

未分化（间变性）癌

黏液产生的鳞状细胞癌[560]。

鳞状细胞癌（Squamous cell carcinoma） 甲状腺的鳞状细胞癌是完全由鳞状细胞成分组成的高度致命的肿瘤[518,560-567]。由于临床特征或行为与未分化癌无法区分以及某些病例中可见分化性癌成分[159,561,568,569]，作为未分化癌的亚型更为合适。一些病例呈甲状腺球蛋白或TTF-1局灶阳性[570]。在确诊原发性甲状腺鳞状细胞癌之前，必须除外以下可能性：
- 累及甲状腺的转移性鳞状细胞癌。
- 邻近肿瘤（如喉癌）直接侵犯甲状腺。
- 类似鳞状细胞癌的发展缓慢的肿瘤：乳头状癌伴鳞状分化；黏液表皮样癌；伴嗜酸性粒细胞增多的硬化性黏液表皮样癌；CASTLE。

免疫组织化学

尽管命名为癌，并非所有的病例都能在免疫组化或超微水平显示出上皮分化的确切证据[571]。然而，这并不影响实际工作，因为符合未分化癌形态特征的肿瘤呈侵袭性生长。

47%～100%的病例细胞角蛋白阳性[24,519,526,572,573]。如果抗原修复技术充分，且几种角蛋白抗体联合应用，阳性率可达90%[26]。约50%的病例上皮膜抗原阳性[26,519,526]，50%～100%的病例波形蛋白阳性[526,572]。甲状腺球蛋白和TTF-1几乎总是阴性，除非出现分化性甲状腺癌成分[26,27,519,544,574]。降钙素和神经内分泌标志物阴性[24,519]。一些病例VIII因子相关抗原局灶阳性[573]，可能反映局灶内皮分化。

表皮生长因子受体（EGFR）通常阳性，可能是EGFR抑制剂治疗的潜在靶标[575-577]。

细胞遗传学和分子特征

P53在各型甲状腺癌的阳性率如下：滤泡癌15%；乳头状癌10%；低分化癌40%；未分化癌70%[578-580]。这些发现表明 *p53* 基因异常在分化性癌向未分化癌的转化中起重要作用[531,578-585]。

ß-catenin基因突变常见（61%），造成蛋白定位于核，可能激活转录而有助于肿瘤形成和侵袭[586]。其他常见的遗传性变化包括3p13-14、7p22-pter、8q22-qter获得、9q34-qter获得/扩增、11q13获得、5q11-31、16p、18q丢失[587-591]。cDNA显微芯片分析发现许多基因过表达或低表达[592]。

一些病例中发现 *BRAF* 突变、*RET/PTC* 融合基因或 *ras* 突变，支持长期以来的观察，即一些未分化癌是由乳头状癌或滤泡癌进展而来[296,551,593-596]。

鉴别诊断

- 肉瘤。甲状腺原发肉瘤无疑存在，但实际上任何"肉瘤样"肿瘤首先应认为是未分化癌，除非有其他足够证据[24]。这种区分并非很重要，因为都属于行为凶险的甲状腺多形性恶性肿瘤。
- 乳头状癌实性型。乳头状癌实性区具有典型乳头状癌的核特征，缺乏未分化癌的怪异核和常见的核分裂。
- 低分化（岛状）癌。低分化甲状腺癌通常细胞排列规则，形成岛状并伴有微滤泡，细胞较小，核一致，甲状腺球蛋白阳性。
- 胸腺相关肿瘤。
- 大细胞淋巴瘤。淋巴瘤粘聚性差。浆细胞样胞浆或滤泡腔内充满肿瘤细胞支持淋巴瘤的诊断。免疫组化很容易鉴别（表18A-6）。
- 转移癌。必须进行临床病理联系来区分原发或转移性未分化癌。如果大量肿瘤位于淋巴管或血管内应怀疑转移癌。如果分化性甲状腺癌与未分化癌相伴随支持原发癌。
- 甲状旁腺癌。诊断线索为出现透明细胞和混合细胞类型，缺乏核分裂象。
- Riedel甲状腺炎。寡细胞型未分化癌不应误诊为Riedel甲状腺炎，后者预后好。如出现以下特征，强烈提示未分化癌：梗死；一些病灶有细胞非典型性；血管被增生的梭形细胞阻塞；与邻近组织离散；细胞角蛋白阳性（图18A.71）。
- 血管肉瘤。

与甲状腺血管肉瘤的疾病分类学关系
The nosologic relationship with angiosarcoma of the thyroid

尽管有些研究者认为甲状腺的血管肉瘤就是未分化癌[597,598]，现在已明确甲状腺存在原发性血管肉瘤[522,572,599,600]。然而，未分化癌和血管肉瘤似乎是具有相似病因的相互重叠的疾病（表18A.11）[572,573,601,602]。

实际上将伴有血管瘤样特征的多形性甲状腺肿瘤称为未分化癌或血管肉瘤并不重要，因为两者预后都很差。然而，当免疫组化和(或)超微结构证明有明确的内皮分化时，应诊断为血管肉瘤[522,572,599]（见第1052页）。

甲状腺"复合性未分化癌-血管肉瘤"有可能起源于原始细胞，因为有些肿瘤根本无分化（细胞角蛋白阴性的未分化癌），有些显示明确的上皮分化（未分化癌），有些显示明确的内皮分化（血管肉瘤），有些显示中间

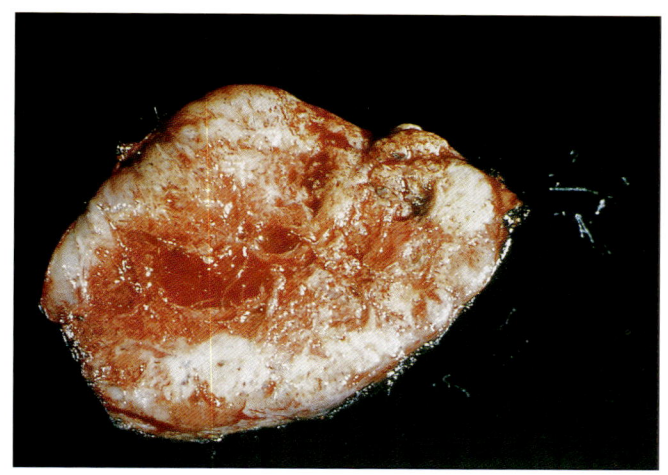

图18A.71 低分化甲状腺癌的大体标本。肿瘤呈肉样，有出血、坏死。

特征（血管瘤样未分化癌）[602-604]。

低分化甲状腺癌
Poorly differentiated thyroid carcinoma

定义

低分化甲状腺癌显示有限的滤泡细胞分化证据，形态学和生物学特征介于分化型和未分化型甲状腺癌之间[158,185,542,605-608]。大多数肿瘤呈岛状生长方式，被称为"岛状癌 (insular carcinoma)"[542]或"原始细胞癌 (primordial cell carcinoma)"[605]。Tscholl-Ducommun & Hedinger 报道的病例可能是岛状癌的例证[165]。然而，Sakamoto 等[185]报道的低分化癌中，并不是所有病例都代表目前所接受的概念，因为这些作者将所有伴实性、梁状或硬化性生长结构的滤泡癌或乳头状癌均归入此范围中[608]。

低分化甲状腺癌的完整形态谱尚待定义[608]。因岛状癌是最具特征的一组，以下将详细讨论。

临床特征

岛状癌患者通常为中老年，平均年龄 53～58.4 岁[49,402,542,605]。女性较男性更常受累（男女比例为 1:2）。病人观察到甲状腺肿块约 1～17 年。少数病人表现为骨转移。发现时常呈局部进展性，59% 有甲状腺外扩散[402]。发病时，明显淋巴结和远处转移分别占 16%～48% 和 12%～44%[402,542]。

治疗后，63% 的病例仍发生复发或转移[402,542,605]。疾病的整个过程中，淋巴结转移发生在大约60%的病例，远处转移（尤其到骨和肺）发生在大约70%的病例[49]。结合四组随访数据，27% 的病人死于疾病，31% 带病生存，只有 37% 无病生存[158,402,542,605]。因很大比例带病生存的病人最终死于肿瘤，长期死亡率接近 50%。死因通常因为转移，而不是无法控制的复发。年龄大、肿瘤体积大、甲状腺外扩散和淋巴结转移与预后差相关。出现未分化癌预示预后极差[158]。

全甲状腺切除外加放射性碘和抑制性甲状腺素是最基本的治疗[542]。对放射性碘摄取好[609]。由于预后差，

表18A.11 甲状腺未分化癌与血管肉瘤的异同点	
相似点	**不同点**
二者均常见于甲状腺肿流行的阿尔卑斯山区，由于预防性碘治疗的使用而发病率下降（未分化癌从37%降至24%；血管肉瘤从7.1%降至4.3%）。	未分化癌以女性居多，而血管肉瘤以男性多。
二者均主要发生于老年人，有长期的甲状腺肿背景。	未分化癌常伴有分化性甲状腺癌，而血管肉瘤并非如此。
二者均可很快引起死亡。	
形态学相似。	
免疫组织化学表现相似。	
二者常为波形蛋白阳性	
未分化癌可表达内皮标志物	
血管肉瘤可表达细胞角蛋白（0～75%）	

低分化甲状腺癌

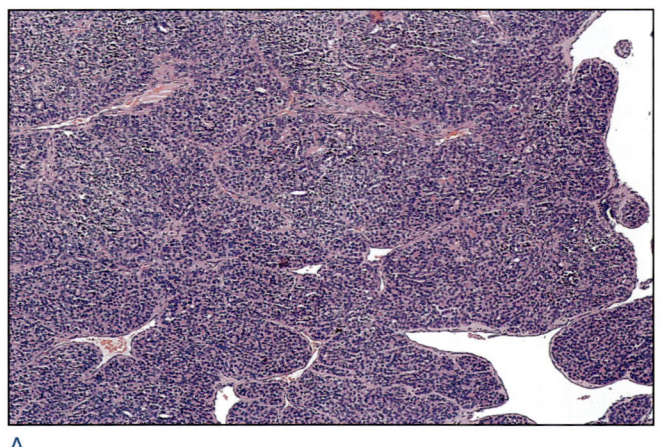

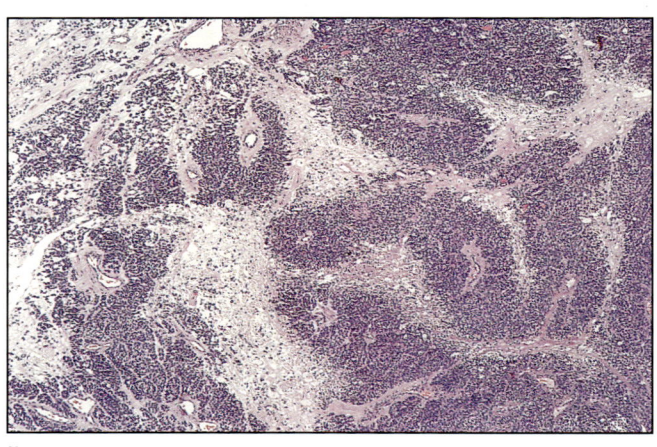

图18A.72 低分化甲状腺癌。（A）大的实性肿瘤细胞岛，间隔以小滤泡。（B）明显的坏死导致"血管外皮细胞瘤样"表现。

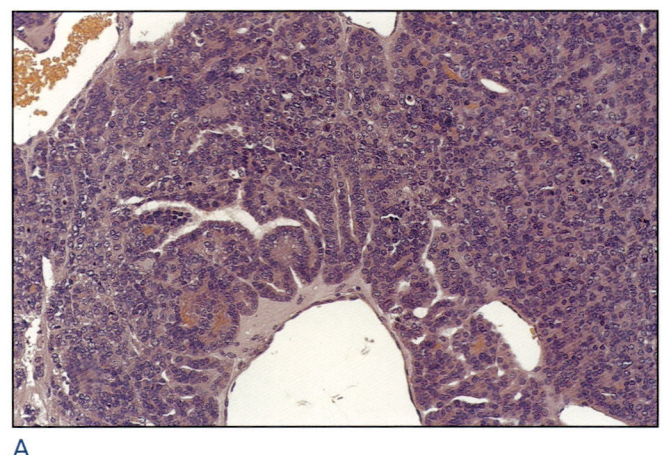

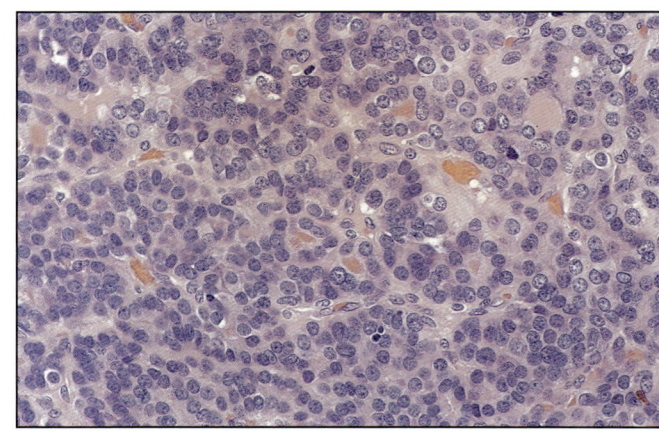

图18A.73 岛状癌。（A）实性生长的肿瘤内，局灶常见彩带样结构。（B）肿瘤细胞小，核浆比高，核深染圆形。散在充满类胶质的间隙，代表发育不良的滤泡。

也可进行外部放疗和化学治疗。

大体表现

肿瘤有部分包膜或呈浸润性生长。实性、质硬，切面灰白；出血、坏死常见（图18A.71）。

组织学表现

岛状癌以大的实性巢状生长，常间隔以数量不等的发育不良小滤泡（图18A.72）。细胞巢周围常见人工收缩。肿瘤也常呈弥漫片状、梁状、彩带样和乳头状生长（图18A.73A）。可有似淀粉样变的硬化间质。坏死常见，导致血管外皮细胞瘤样表现（图18A.72B）。血管浸润常见[542,610]。

肿瘤细胞相对小，一致，圆形深染或泡状核，核仁不明显（图18A.73B）[605]。胞浆少。核分裂活性不定，但总能发现。某些病例，可有少量典型乳头状癌和滤泡癌成分（图18A.74）。

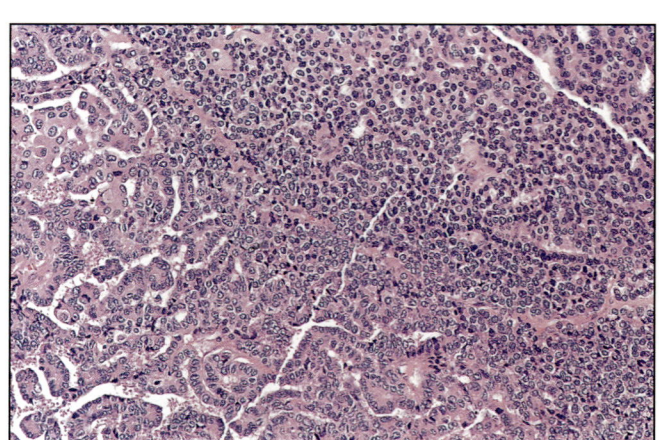

图18A.74 此例低分化甲状腺癌可见乳头状癌成分（右下角）。

有些低分化甲状腺癌不符合上述的岛状癌组织学标准，由较大细胞组成或形成梁状、实性或局灶滤泡的结构[605,611]。

免疫组织化学

甲状腺球蛋白阳性，但局限于发育不良的滤泡和孤立的细胞，以核旁小球的形式出现[542,605,612]。TTF-1 常阳性[25]。降钙素阴性。低分化甲状腺癌 bcl-2 的阳性率(84.2%) 较未分化癌（13.6%）高，有助于两者的鉴别[613]。与分化型甲状腺癌相比，细胞周期依赖性激酶抑制蛋白 p27 表达下降而 Ki67 指数升高[606,614]。

分子学特征

低分化甲状腺癌 p53 的阳性表达率 (41% ～ 53%) 介于分化型甲状腺癌 (11% ～ 14%) 和未分化癌 (64% ～ 83%) 之间，表明至少在一定比例的病例中，p53 的突变介导分化型甲状腺癌向低分化癌转化[578,613]。未分化癌中常见的分子改变，ß-catenin 基因 CTNNB1 的突变出现在 25% 的病例[296]。

一部分低分化甲状腺癌有 ras 基因点突变 (18% ～ 27%)，表明与滤泡癌有关[296,402,510]。BRAF 基因突变不常见，除非出现乳头状癌成分[322,615,616]。

鉴别诊断

- 髓样癌。低分化甲状腺癌的生长方式及淀粉样硬化，使其看上去像髓样癌。髓样癌可通过较明显的血管、颗粒状胞浆和点彩状染色质加以识别。甲状腺球蛋白和降钙素染色可将两者加以鉴别（表 18A.6）。
- 乳头状癌实性亚型。
- 未分化甲状腺癌。低分化癌缺乏未分化癌明显的核多形性和较多的分裂象，并且可见发育不良的滤泡及甲状腺球蛋白阳性。

与其他甲状腺癌的关系

与未分化癌快速致命的病程不同，低分化甲状腺癌在多年后才引起死亡（平均生存 3.9 年）。由于低分化甲状腺癌的甲状腺外扩散和淋巴结转移率高以及在某些病例中出现乳头状癌成分，因此将其看做一种独立的疾病，而不是简单地归为"低分化滤泡癌"[49]。然而，低分化甲状腺癌明显与滤泡癌或乳头状癌密切相关，在一些病例可见相互移行(图 18A.74)。使用低分化甲状腺癌命名，避免将其硬性归入乳头状癌或滤泡癌范畴。

低分化癌通常直接发生，也可以由分化性甲状腺癌通过反复复发或同时存在转化而来[24,524]。它们也可以在最初或复发时转化为未分化癌（图 18A.75）。

有些研究者将低分化甲状腺癌一词用于具有实性、梁状或硬化性生长结构的分化性甲状腺癌或高细胞乳头状癌和柱状细胞癌（低分化乳头状癌）[474,617]。尽管这

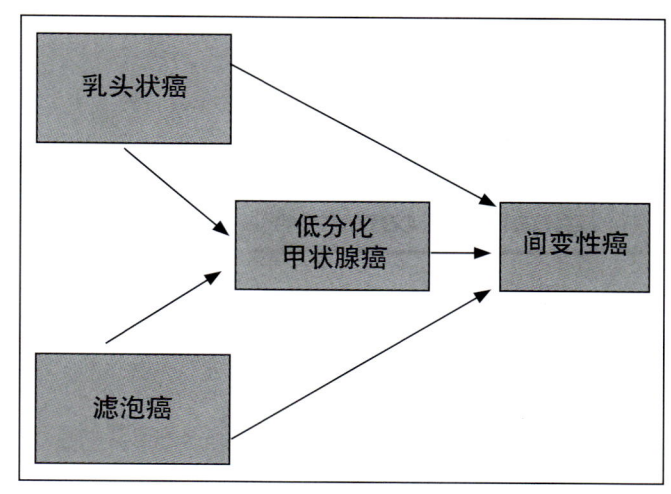

图18A.75　分化性甲状腺癌、低分化癌和间变性癌之间的关系。

些肿瘤比起典型的分化性甲状腺癌更具侵袭性，但可通过其他已知的预后因素，如甲状腺外扩散和肿瘤分期预测它们的侵袭过程，所以将它们归入乳头状癌和滤泡癌的范畴更为合适。

分化性甲状腺癌 (differentiated thyroid carcinoma) 中出现岛状癌 (insular carcinoma) 成分预后会更差吗？

有些研究显示分化性甲状腺癌中即使含少量低分化癌成分也会使预后变差[610,618]。对 44 例伴岛状癌成分的甲状腺癌(30 例滤泡癌和 14 例乳头状癌)进行研究发现，46% 死于疾病，5% 带病生存，49% 无病生存。多因素分析，岛状癌成分的出现是乳头状癌或滤泡癌的一个独立的凶险预后因素[619]。

然而，另一项研究发现岛状癌成分不影响滤泡癌或乳头状癌的结局[620]。对 41 例伴有局灶或以岛状癌为主的甲状腺癌（17 例乳头状癌，24 例滤泡癌）进行分析发现，41% 的肿瘤局限于甲状腺内，35% 局部扩散，24% 远处转移。14% 的病人死于疾病，21% 带病生存。岛状癌的范围与肿瘤分期、随访状态或倍体无相关性。相反，分期和病人年龄影响结局。

这些矛盾的结果难以得出一致结论，但如何定义岛状癌可能是导致这些差别的原因。实际中，如果岛状癌成分出现于其他典型的乳头状或滤泡癌中，病理报告中应指出预后可能更差。然而，如果岛状癌成分少，且局

限于包膜内病变，可能不会对分化性癌的结局产生不利影响。

柱状细胞癌
Columnar cell carcinoma

临床特征

Evans 首先报道，柱状细胞癌是比分化型甲状腺癌更具侵袭性的一种罕见的甲状腺肿瘤[621]。最初的研究发现，病人发生远处转移并于 20～23 个月死于肿瘤。最近的研究发现，只有明显浸润性生长的病例呈侵袭性过程，而有包膜的肿瘤预后好。

浸润性柱状细胞癌男性多见（男：女比例为 9:6），平均年龄 55 岁[621-631]。远处（肺和脊柱）及区域淋巴结转移率高。死亡率高；13 例随访病例中，10 例在 7 个月至 10.5 年死于疾病，3 例带病生存 27 个月至 9 年。

另一方面，有包膜的肿瘤以女性占明显优势（男：女比例为 1:18）[622,630,632-634]。平均年龄 42.7 岁。18 例随访病例中，16 例存活 2～22 年且身体健康，1 例带病生存 4 年，1 例死于无关疾病。

组织学表现

浸润性肿瘤常表现为甲状腺外扩散。有包膜的肿瘤可有包膜浸润，有时有血管浸润。

柱状细胞癌以混合性乳头、复杂腺体、筛状和实性结构为特征（图 18A.76）。乳头和腺体被覆高柱状细胞，

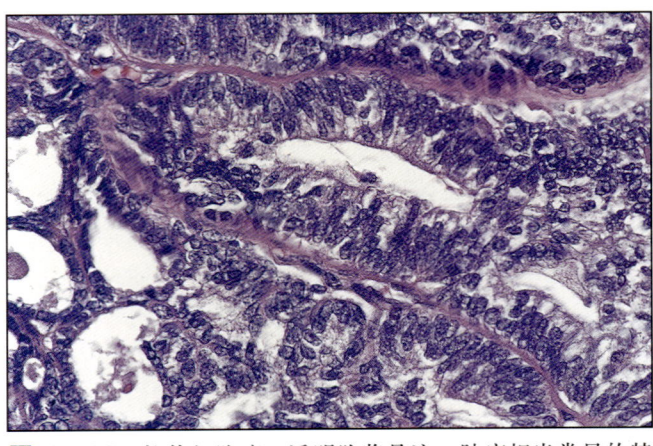

图18A.77　柱状细胞癌。透明胞浆是这一肿瘤相当常见的特征，与早分泌期子宫内膜相似。

核呈假复层排列、深染、卵圆形或梭形（图 18A.76）。可出现核下空泡及透明胞浆（图 18A.77）。实性区细胞常较小，多角形。也可见梭形细胞束。肿瘤细胞甲状腺球蛋白阳性。

柱状细胞癌不同于乳头状癌的高细胞亚型，柱状细胞更高、核深染、呈明显假复层排列，胞浆缺乏嗜酸性改变。简单地讲，柱状细胞癌组织学上类似于结直肠癌或子宫内膜样腺癌，而高细胞乳头状癌更像典型的乳头状癌。

有关柱状细胞癌本质的争议

有人认为柱状细胞癌是一种独特的疾病，另一些人（包括新版 WHO 分类）认为其结构与乳头状癌相似，

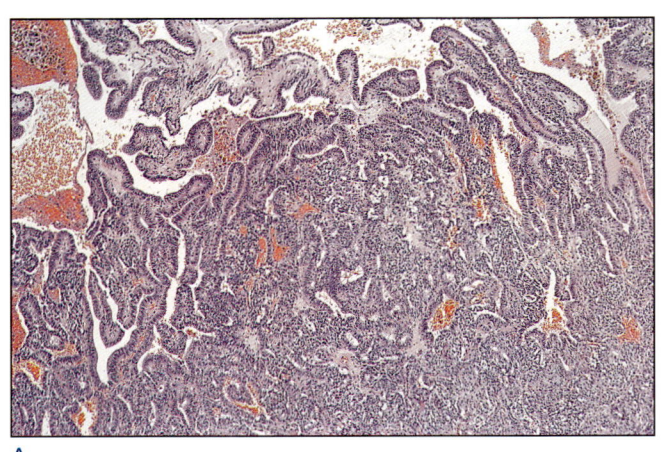

A

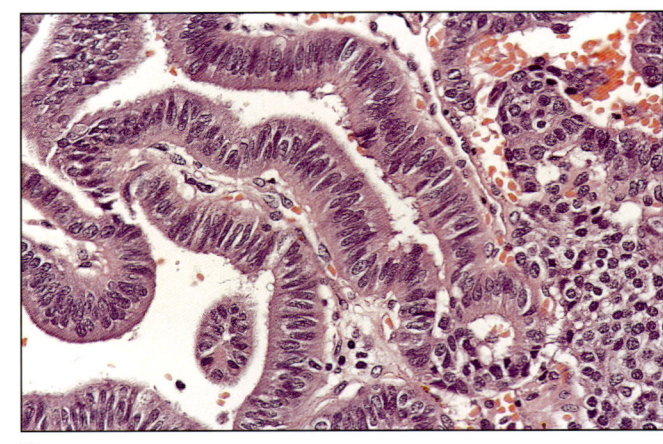

B

图18A.76　柱状细胞癌。（A）混合性乳头、管状和实性结构。（B）乳头被覆高柱状细胞，核呈假复层排列。实性区（右侧）细胞常较小。

少数病例与高细胞乳头状癌共存（混合），因而是乳头状癌的一种亚型[152,627,629,630,635,636]。与乳头状癌的筛状-桑葚亚型和FAP相关性甲状腺癌在形态上有重叠。实际上，Evans报道的一例发生在FAP病人的柱状细胞癌可能为FAP相关性筛状-桑葚样乳头状癌[633]。

黏液表皮样癌
Mucoepidermoid carcinoma

临床特征

原发性黏液表皮样癌是一种罕见的、含表皮样和黏液成分的低度恶性肿瘤[637]。文献报道大约24例（不包括伴嗜酸细胞增多的硬化性黏液表皮样癌，在下文论述）[638-651]。男：女比例为9：15，年龄范围为10～67岁，平均37.9岁。病人表现为甲状腺肿块，约20%的病例有甲状腺外扩散。尽管淋巴结转移常见（14/23），远处转移则罕见（3/23）。18例随访病人中，14例健康存活6个月至22年，2例于诊断后5～12年发生转移，1例术后死亡，1例13个月后死亡（此例病人肿瘤含未分化癌成分）。

组织学表现

肿瘤边界不清，由位于硬化背景中的细胞岛组成。一些肿瘤细胞为鳞状，而另一些含有胞浆黏液。可见筛状结构，腺腔拉长，含类胶质样物。偶尔可见乳头。核深染或浅染；轻到中度多形性。较大细胞岛内常见粉刺

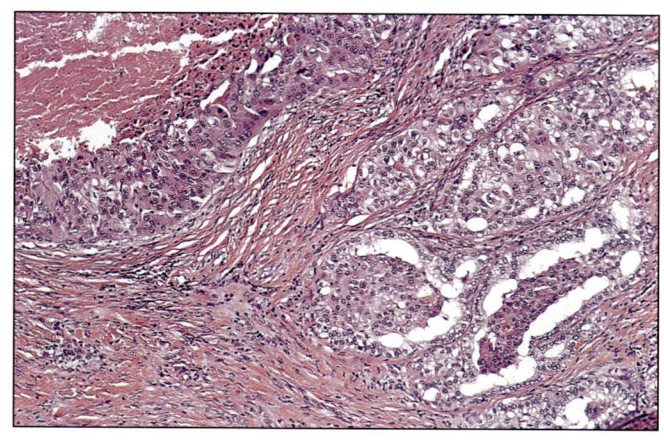

图18A.79 显示由典型的乳头状癌（右下）逐渐转化为黏液表皮样癌（左上）的病例。

样坏死（图18A.78），也可形成沙粒体。甲状腺球蛋白和TTF-1局灶阳性[637,645]。

与其他甲状腺肿瘤的组织发生关系

Harach推测甲状腺黏液表皮样癌起源于后鳃体（实性细胞巢）[652]。一些病例可能起源于甲状舌管[646]。然而，多数学者认为黏液表皮样癌是乳头状癌的一种罕见的化生亚型，原因是有相似的发病统计，乳头状癌具有化生潜能，可有硬化，偶尔形成乳头、沙粒体，发展缓慢，淋巴结转移率高；这些特征与涎腺的黏液表皮样癌不同。在一些病例中，典型的乳头状癌可与黏液表皮样癌混合存在，支持以上的观点（图18A.79）[644,645,647-650]。

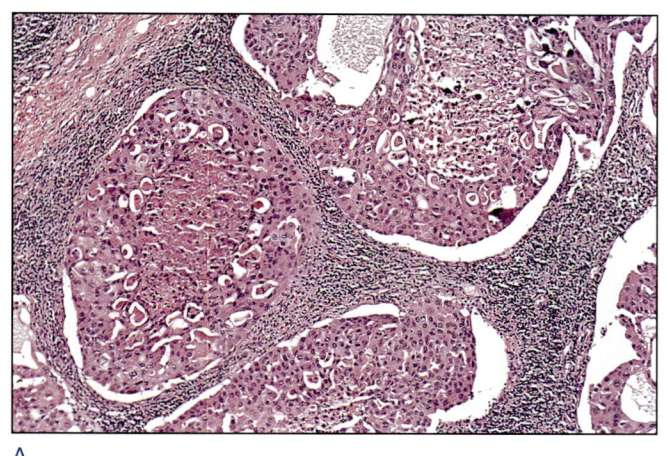

A

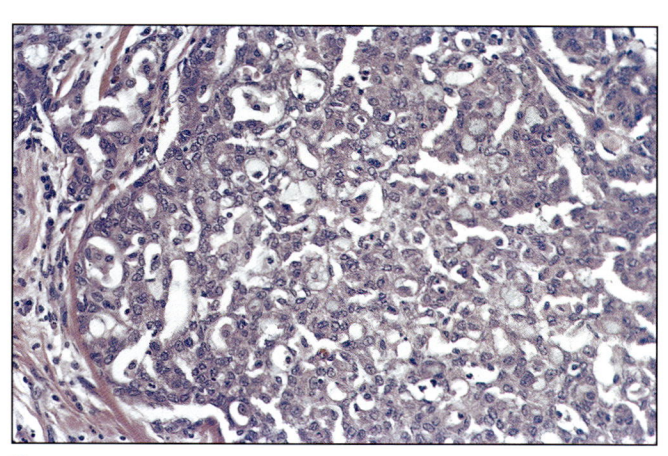

B

图18A.78 黏液表皮样癌。（A）鳞状肿瘤细胞岛内散在充满黏液的空隙。注意典型的粉刺样坏死和偶尔出现的沙粒体。（B）实性肿瘤岛被一些不规则的小囊腔所分割，黏液分泌细胞散布其间。黏液表皮样癌的细胞核常常温和。

伴嗜酸细胞增多的硬化性黏液表皮样癌
Sclerosing mucoepidermoid carcinoma with eosinophilia

临床特征

伴嗜酸细胞增多的硬化性黏液表皮样癌是一种罕见的低度恶性肿瘤，发生于桥本甲状腺炎（大多数为纤维型）背景上，可能起源于化生的鳞状上皮[653,654]。是一种不同于黏液表皮样癌的病变。发生于成人，平均年龄54.9岁。女性明显占优势（男：女比例为1:16）[646,653,655-660]。大多数病人表现为生长缓慢的甲状腺肿块。甲状腺外扩散发生于大约一半的病例，淋巴结转移发生于1/3的病例。随访3个月至9年，约一半的病人无病生存，一半有局灶或远处扩散[654]。

病理学

肿瘤通常呈浸润性，常见甲状腺外扩散。由位于硬化性间质中的相互吻合的细胞索和巢组成，伴有嗜酸性粒细胞和小淋巴细胞浸润（图18A.80A）。肿瘤细胞多角形，核轻到中度异型性，核仁明显。瘤巢内常见鳞状分化灶和小黏液池（图18A.80B）。也可见到因细胞分离产生的假血管瘤样结构。少数情况下可见透明细胞岛[661]。常见神经浸润和血管腔消失。

肿瘤细胞角蛋白阳性，甲状腺球蛋白和降钙素阴性。约一半的病例TTF-1阳性[661]。

鉴别诊断

此型肿瘤与更富于浸润性的未分化癌或鳞状细胞癌的鉴别最为重要。后者呈更弥漫的片状或大的岛状生长，核异型更明显，核分裂和坏死常见；如果出现炎症成分，通常是中性粒细胞而不是嗜酸性粒细胞。还需与甲状腺的旺炽性鳞状化生 (florid squamous metaplasia) 鉴别，后者缺乏细胞异型性和真正的浸润性质。

黏液癌 Mucinous carcinoma

甲状腺的原发性黏液癌相当罕见，仅有4例报道[662-665]。其中两例存活15个月和8年，另两例分别于8个月和2年后因皮肤、肺或骨转移而死亡。Deligdisch等报道的1例不是黏液癌，而是伴黏液产生的滤泡癌[436]。组织学上，黏液癌与其他部位的胶样癌相似。在3例研究中，2例甲状腺球蛋白阳性。

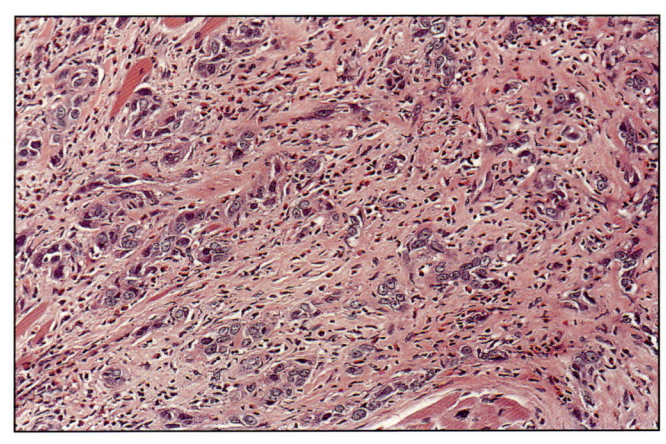

A

B

图18A.80 伴嗜酸细胞增多的硬化性黏液表皮样癌。（A）肿瘤细胞条索浸润于富含嗜酸性粒细胞的硬化性间质中。（B）有些肿瘤细胞岛可见角化和黏液池。

显示C细胞分化的肿瘤
Tumors showing C-cell differentiation

甲状腺髓样癌
Medullary thyroid carcinoma

定义

甲状腺髓样癌是一种显示滤泡旁C细胞分化的恶性肿瘤[666]。特征性地分泌降钙素，但也可产生许多其他的肽类物质。迄今为止，无对应的良性肿瘤描述。实际上，根据Huss & Mendelsohn的研究，20%的有包膜的髓样癌在发生时已有淋巴结转移[420]。

临床特征

发病人口特征见表18A.12[667-679]。多数患者表现为甲状腺肿块、吞咽困难、声嘶或颈淋巴结肿大[680]。约

表18A.12 甲状腺髓样癌（MTC）的不同临床形式

	散发性MTC	遗传性MTC[a]		
		家族性MTC	MEN2A	MEN2B
诊断时的平均年龄	44～50	45～55	25～35	10～20
男:女比例	1:1.4		1:1.1	
遗传模式	无	常染色体显性遗传		
综合征中的其他成分	无	无	嗜铬细胞瘤（40%～60%），甲状旁腺增生（10%～30%）。变异型：皮肤苔藓样淀粉样变性或先天性巨结肠病	嗜铬细胞瘤（40%～60%），黏膜神经瘤，Marfan综合征样表现
肿瘤双侧发生率（%）	0～32	92～98		
背景中C细胞增生	通常缺乏	通常出现		
诊断时淋巴结转移（%）	40～50	10～20	14	38
诊断时远处转移（%）	12	0	0～3	20
行为	预后居中；肿瘤相关死亡率约为30%	最缓慢；肿瘤相关死亡率约为0%	相对缓慢；肿瘤相关死亡率为0～17%	以前认为最具侵袭性，但最近的研究没有证实这一观察
RET原癌基因的胚系突变	无	累及外显子10、11、13或14的突变	累及外显子10或11的突变（外显子13突变罕见）	多数是累及外显子16（密码子918）的单一类型突变，ATG→ACG（甲硫氨酸→苏氨酸）

MEN2A：多发性内分泌肿瘤2A型；MEN2B：多发性内分泌肿瘤2B型；MTC：甲状腺髓样癌。
[a]尽管使用遗传性这一术语，可能没有阳性家族史；可能是新突变的结果

20%～40%的病人有腹泻[668]。少数病例由于促肾上腺皮质激素（ACTH）的分泌产生Cushing综合征[681,682]。偶尔，肿瘤因血清CEA无法解释地升高而被发现。

大约70%～80%的髓样癌为散发性（多数为单侧），20%～30%为遗传性（伴高外显率和不定表达的常染色体显性遗传）[667,669,679]，特征是发病年龄早、多中心和双侧肿瘤，并伴有C细胞增生（表18A.12）[668-675,683-685]。髓样癌的各种遗传形式由RET基因的胚系突变引起（图18A.81）[676-678]。

在一些中心，对有结节性甲状腺疾病的病人常规筛查降钙素，可早期发现散发性髓样癌[686,687]。在一组研究中[688]，63%的甲状腺切除病人发现有髓样癌（主要为女性），而其余只有C细胞增生（全部为男性

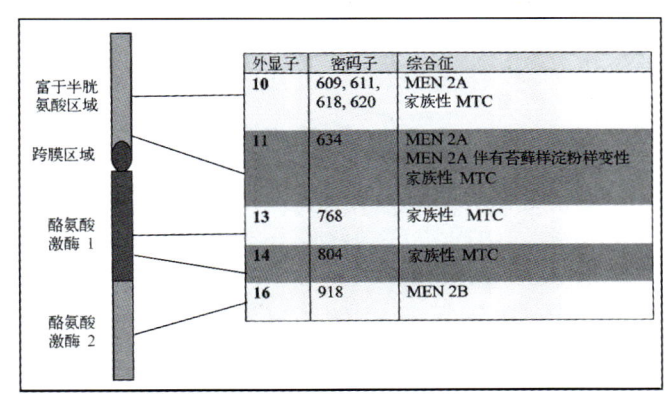

图18A.81 RET原癌基因产物结构、胚系突变的常见部位以及与临床综合征关系的示意图。MEN：多发性内分泌肿瘤；MTC：甲状腺髓样癌。

病人）。在前一组，37.5% 的病人伴发 C 细胞增生。因此，C 细胞增生是遗传性髓样癌特征性而非特异性表现。

临床行为

髓样癌确诊时的分期如下：I 期，21%；II 期，21%；III 期，47%；IV 期，12%[689]。肿瘤有转移至颈部淋巴结（1/3 ~ 2/3）和上纵隔的倾向[668,680,690]。治疗后 1/3 局部复发[680]。在疾病晚期，可转移至其他部位，如肺、肝、肾上腺和骨，尽管确诊时 8% 的病人已发生远处转移[690]。5 年、10 年、15 年的生存率分别为 65% ~ 87%、51% ~ 78% 和 65%[667,680,691-693]，表明此型肿瘤发展缓慢，通常不会很快致命。然而，髓样癌诊断 10 年后，仍有较高的死亡率[693]。肿瘤局限于甲状腺内的病人，长期生存率为 95%[690]。即使出现远处转移，病人仍可生存多年。髓样癌放疗不敏感，充分的外科清除（全甲状腺切除术）是主要的治疗手段[694,695]。

大体表现

髓样癌常界清，尽管小肿瘤（< 7 mm）更常为浸润性[696,697]。少数情况下有完整的包膜。肿瘤质硬、灰白、棕褐或红棕色。常位于侧叶中 1/3，是 C 细胞密度最高的区域[674]。较大的肿瘤可见出血和中心坏死[698]。

组织学表现

髓样癌典型的组织学表现为多角形或肥胖的梭形细胞排列成片状、巢状或不规则细胞岛，间隔以纤细的纤维血管分隔（图 18A.82）[699,700]。脉管较乳头状癌或滤泡癌更明显。偶尔可见漩涡状、梁状、假乳头状、菊形团、管状、微腺样或筛状结构（图 18A.83）[669,697]。细胞解离和间质水肿很常见（图 18A.84）。细胞核圆形或卵圆形，典型的含有细的点彩状染色质和明显的核仁（图 18A.85）。核多形性常不明显，分裂象少见。胞浆细颗粒状。约 50% 的病例有胞浆黏液[116,701]，少数情况下肿瘤细胞可呈印戒细胞表现[702]。淋巴管浸润很常见[697]。

80% ~ 85% 的病例[698]可见淀粉样物，数量不恒定，为粉染的无定形物，形成小球或大块沉积物（图 18A.84）。可有钙化或异物巨细胞反应。

甲状腺髓样癌的变异型
Variants of medullary thyroid carcinoma

髓样癌有许多组织学亚型，大多数不具有预后意义，只是会造成诊断上的问题，但幸运的是，通过仔细观察，常能找到部分典型的髓样癌区域。如果出现淀粉样物也是诊断的重要线索。

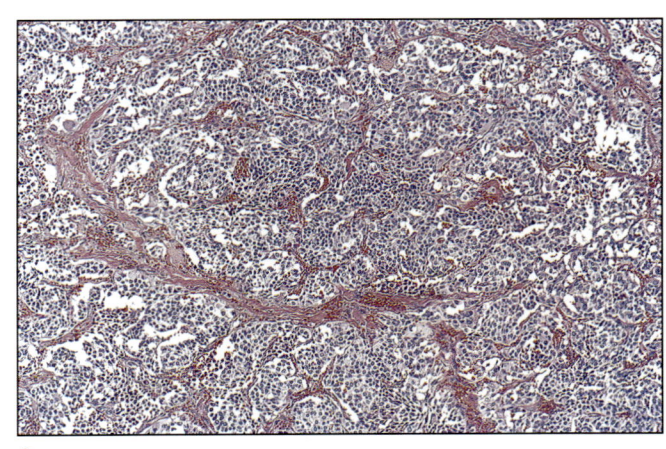

A

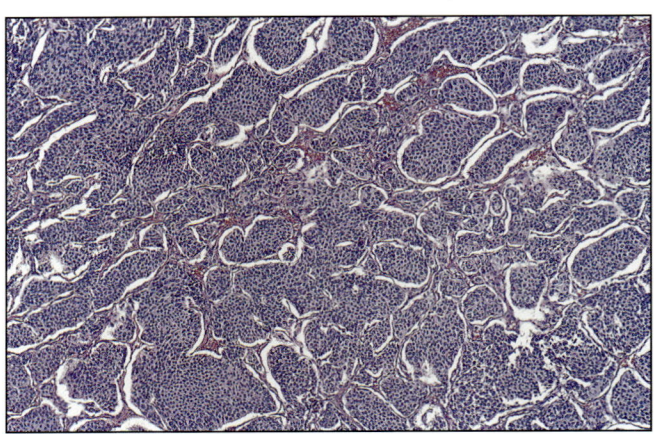

B

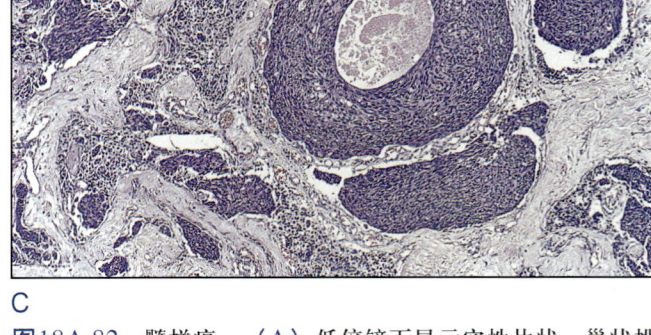

C

图18A.82 髓样癌。（A）低倍镜下显示实性片状、巢状排列的肿瘤细胞，被纤细的纤维血管间隔分隔。（B）此例瘤巢排列紧密，类似副神经节瘤。（C）较少见的是肿瘤呈不规则岛状和片状生长，被丰富的纤维间质隔开。

腺样/滤泡型（Glandular/follicular） 髓样癌可形成空心腺体/小管或含嗜酸性分泌物的滤泡（图 18A.86）。腺腔缘由于神经内分泌颗粒的积聚而呈深嗜酸性颗粒

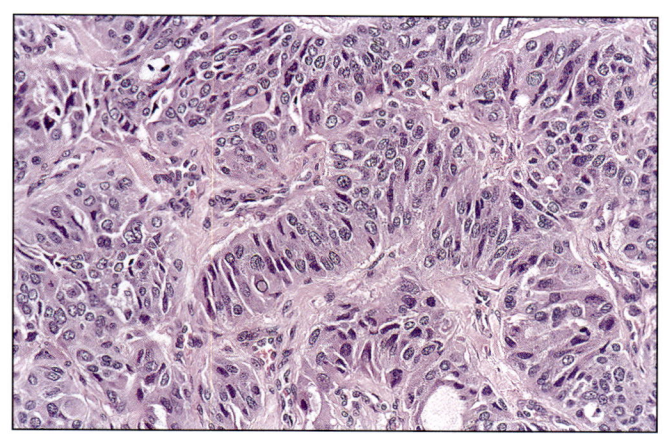

图18A.83 呈明显梁状生长形态的髓样癌。

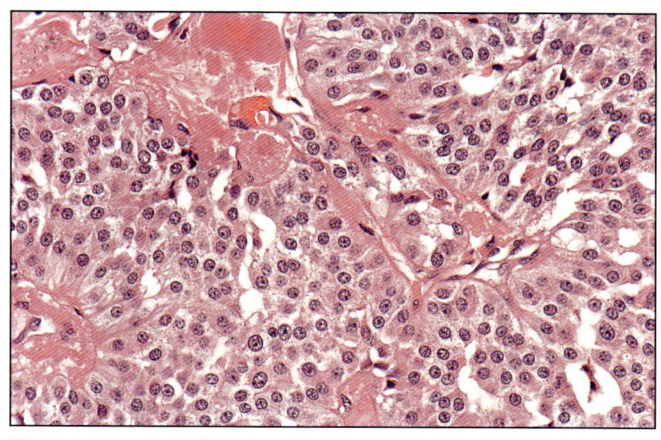

图18A.85 典型髓样癌。肿瘤细胞核规则，染色质细，胞浆呈细颗粒状。

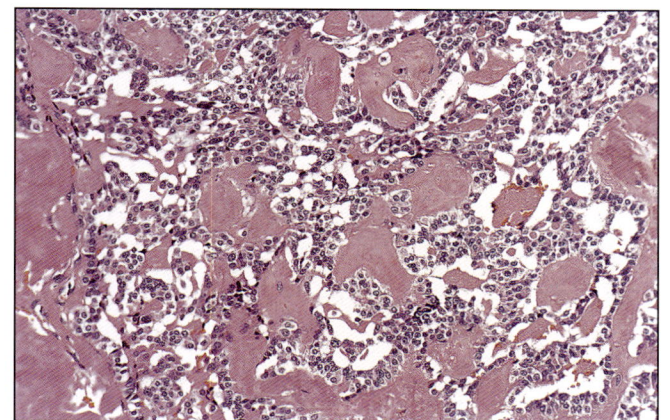

图18A.84 髓样癌。此视野可见两个典型特征：丰富的淀粉样物和肿瘤细胞解离。

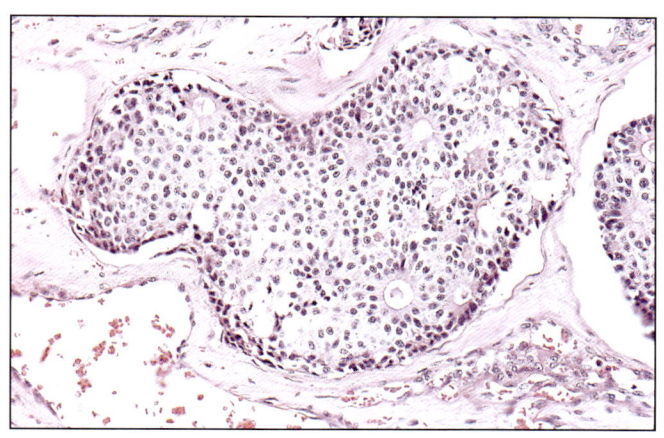

A

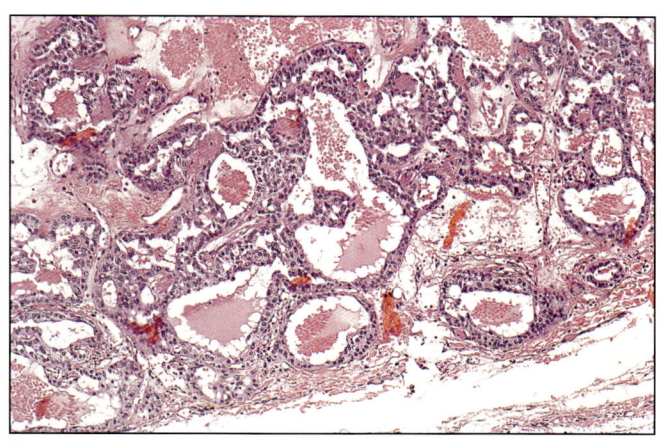

B

图18A.86 髓样癌。（A）有小管/滤泡形成。注意管腔周围的胞浆颗粒更突出。（B）肿瘤具有含分泌物的滤泡，类似于滤泡性肿瘤。

状，这一特征通过嗜铬素免疫染色容易见到，靠近腔面的染色更强[703,704]。此型可通过点彩状染色质、细的颗粒状胞浆、纤细的纤维血管间隔和降钙素阳性与滤泡性肿瘤鉴别。与低分化（岛状）甲状腺癌的鉴别可能困难，免疫组化染色可解决这一问题。

嗜酸型（Oxyphilic） 髓样癌胞浆内线粒体的堆积可导致明显的嗜酸性表现，可呈局灶或弥漫分布（图18A.87）[700,705,706]。偶尔出现的实性、梁状和滤泡结构可进一步增加与Hurthle细胞腺瘤/癌的相似性。正确诊断的线索是具有明显的纤维血管间隔和出现典型髓样癌灶（并非一定能发现）。

巨细胞（间变）型[Giant cell(anaplastic)] 在其他方面典型的髓样癌，局灶可见伴有奇异核和核假包涵体的大细胞[707-709]。然而，核分裂象少见（图18A.88）。并不确定这些肿瘤是否更具有侵袭性，但许多报道的病例是致命的[698]。

透明细胞型（Clear cell） 罕见情况下，髓样癌可全部或部分由透明细胞组成[710,711]。

显示C细胞分化的肿瘤

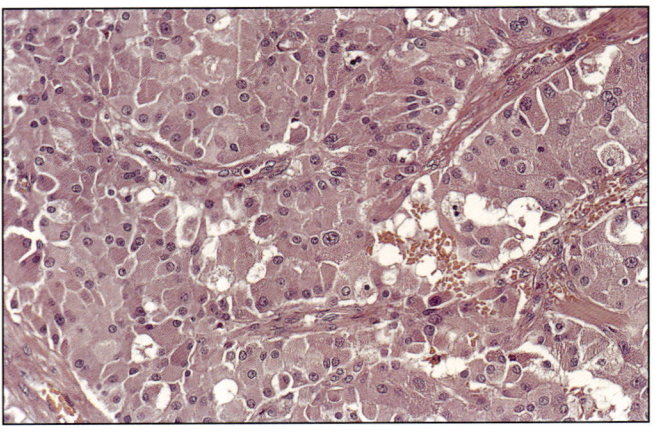

图18A.87 髓样癌，嗜酸型。肿瘤细胞大，含丰富的嗜酸性颗粒状胞浆。注意典型的纤细脉管。

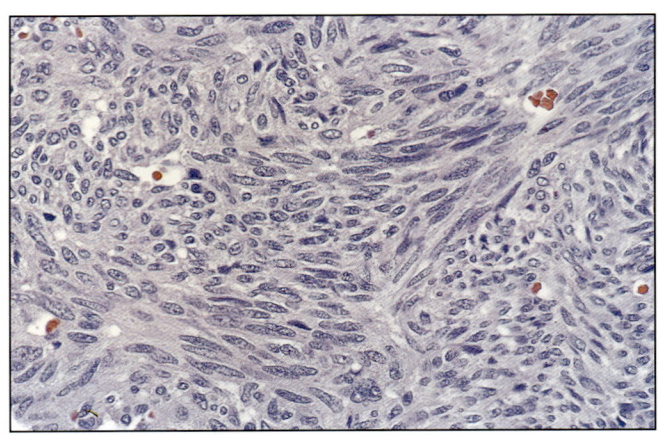

图18A.89 髓样癌，梭形细胞型。肿瘤形成相互交叉的梭形细胞束，类似间叶性肿瘤。

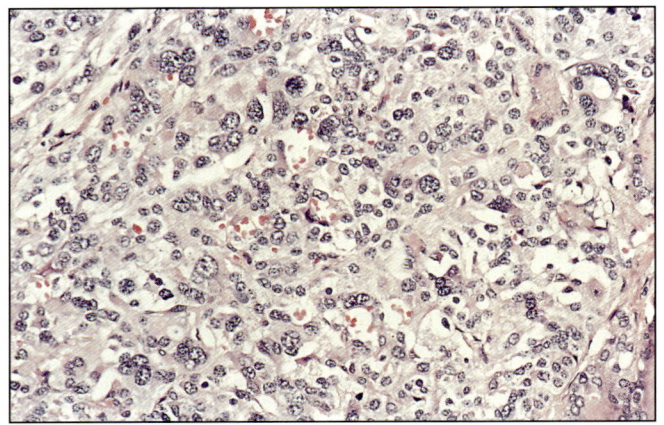

图18A.88 髓样癌，巨细胞型。可见大的奇异核细胞，但未见核分裂象。

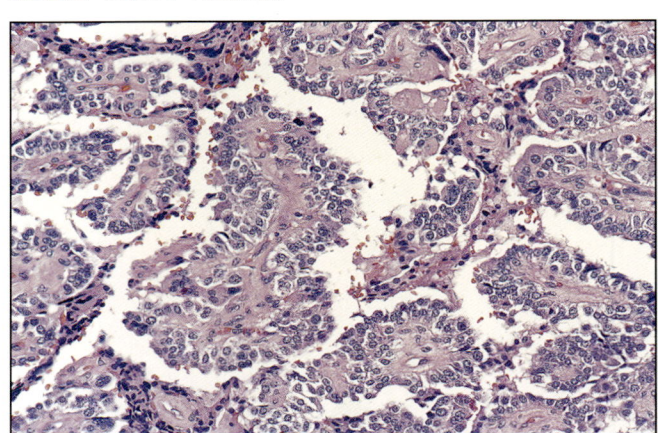

图18A.90 髓样癌，乳头型。乳头大多数是由细胞解离形成的假乳头，因为它们表面起伏不平。

梭形细胞型（Spindle cell） 梭形细胞在髓样癌并不少见，但有些髓样癌几乎全部由肥胖或细长的梭形细胞排列成相互交叉的束状、漩涡状和巢状，类似于间叶性肿瘤（图18A.89）。

色素型（Pigmented） 髓样癌的罕见病例会伴有黑色素沉积[712-714]。

鳞状（Squamous） 偶尔，髓样癌可显示局灶鳞状分化[705,715]。

乳头状（Papillary） 组织断裂形成的假乳头以及罕见的真乳头可见于髓样癌（图18A.90）[716]。可通过核的特征与乳头状癌鉴别。此型被认为预后较好，但由于例数太少而不能得出确切结论[704]。

假血管肉瘤样（Pseudoangiosarcomatous） 一些病例因明显的细胞解离和病灶内出血而产生裂隙样结构，类似于血管肉瘤[717]。

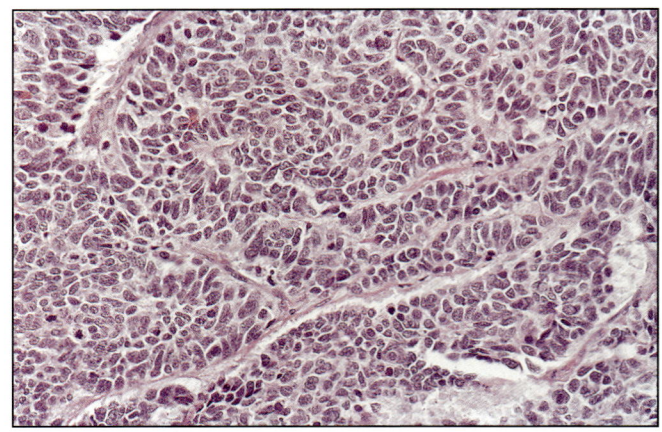

图18A.91 髓样癌，小细胞型。与肺小细胞癌有明显相似之处。

小细胞型（Small cell） 罕见的髓样癌由排列成片状和巢状的小细胞组成，组织学上与肺小细胞癌相似（图18A.91）。在一些病例，典型的髓样癌病灶可见[708]。这些是倾向于广泛播散的高度侵袭性肿瘤。除非在多发性内分泌肿瘤2型（MEN2）的背景下，诊断髓样癌是困难的。免疫组化最有帮助。降钙素可能阴性，但CEA和神经内分泌标志物常阳性。

神经母细胞瘤样（Neuroblastoma-like） 有时，可有纤维间质和菊形团，类似神经母细胞瘤[718]。

玻璃样变小梁腺瘤样（Hyalinizing trabecular adenoma-like） 少数髓样癌，形态与玻璃样变小梁腺瘤难以区分，缺少淀粉样物[420]。免疫组化对于证实诊断必不可少。

类癌样（Carcinoid-like） 有些髓样癌表现出类似前肠、中肠或后肠类癌的组织学特征，肿瘤细胞岛、小梁或腺体由玻璃样变的纤维间质分隔。可有典型的髓样癌成分。这样的病例可被误诊为滤泡性肿瘤或转移性类癌[719]。

副神经节瘤样（Paraganglioma-like） 肿瘤呈巢状结构，类似副神经节瘤。散在分布着 S-100 阳性支持细胞样树突状细胞[714]。

微小髓样癌（潜伏癌）[Medullary microcarcinoma (latent carcinoma)] 甲状腺切除标本或尸检中偶然可以发现 < 1 cm 的散发性髓样癌[233,720-722]。不伴有临床症状时，预后极好[722]。

免疫组织化学

髓样癌典型的免疫表型为细胞角蛋白、广谱神经内分泌标志物、降钙素、CEA 和 TTF-1 阳性。免疫组化有重要的诊断意义，髓样癌（20%～30%的病例为遗传性）的诊断应做免疫组化加以证实。

大多数病例降钙素阳性（图 18A.92）[715,723-725]。通常呈强染色，几乎所有细胞均着色。降钙素少的髓样癌比降钙素多者侵袭性更强[715,726]。许多其他肽类在髓样癌中有不同的表达率，如降钙素基因相关肽（CGRP）、生长抑素、ACTH、β-内啡肽、5-羟色胺、胃泌素、组胺酶、阿片肽和胃泌素释放肽[727,728]。这些标志物的染色很少用于诊断，尽管少数髓样癌 CGRP 阳性，降钙素阴性[729]。

88%～100% 的病例癌胚抗原阳性[700,711,715,725,730]。随着特异性单克隆抗体的使用，CEA 对甲状腺髓样癌的诊断特异性大大提高。即使降钙素和其他神经内分泌标志物或肽类阴性，CEA 免疫反应可支持家族性髓样癌或 MEN 中髓样癌（大多数为低分化小细胞型）的诊断[698]。

S-100 阳性支持细胞在发生于 MEN 或家族性髓样癌的肿瘤中较散发性肿瘤更常见（62.5% versus 9.3%）[731]。这也导致与副神经节瘤有某些免疫表型的重叠，除了髓样癌细胞角蛋白阳性，而副神经节瘤阴性[732]。

电子显微镜

有膜包绕的电子致密颗粒大小 100～300nm[711]。单个细胞内颗粒的大小不同。粗面内质网和高尔基体常丰富。

分子特征

RET 原癌基因，位于染色体 10q11.2，在髓样癌的发生中起重要作用。*RET* 基因由 21 个外显子组成，编码一种受体酪氨酸激酶，其由半胱氨酸丰富的膜外区、跨膜区和细胞内酪氨酸激酶成分组成（图 18A.81）。*RET* 基因的胚系突变发生于 MEN2 和家族性甲状腺髓样癌的病人。发生在 MEN2A 和家族性髓样癌的突变，因形成二聚体而激活受体，发生在 MEN2B 的突变引起酪氨酸激酶底物特异性的改变[733-735]。大多数突变累及细胞外半胱氨酸丰富区的五个半胱氨酸密码子之一，导致半胱氨酸被另一种氨基酸替代。密码子 634，尤其 TGC → CGC（半胱氨酸→精氨酸）转换在 MEN2A 最常受累[736,737]。

散发性髓样癌 *RET* 基因的体细胞点突变发生于 26%～69% 的病例，最常累及外显子 16 的 918 密码子（ATG → ACG）[737-741]。

临床-分子相关性

伴有嗜铬细胞瘤和甲状旁腺疾病的 MEN2A，几乎所有突变发生于密码子 634。在缺乏嗜铬细胞瘤的 MEN2A 和家族性髓样癌，密码子 609、611、618 和 620 更常受累[733]。伴外显子 13 的 790/791 密码子突变的 MEN2A 侵袭性较弱[742]。几乎所有 MEN2B 有相似的突变：外显子 16 的 918 密码子 ATG → ACG（甲硫氨酸→苏氨酸）[736,737,743]。

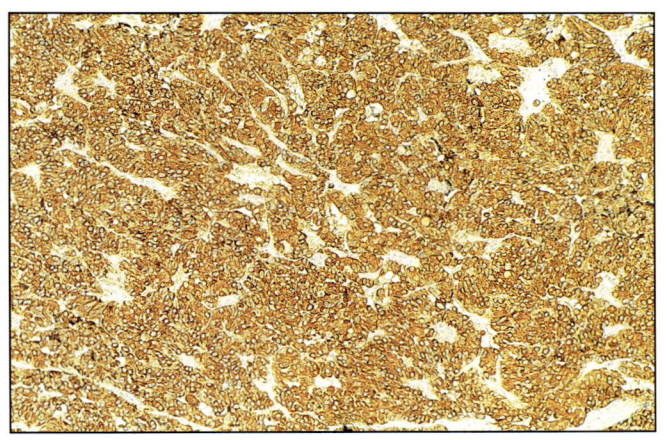

图18A.92 髓样癌。所有肿瘤细胞降钙素强阳性。在髓样癌的诊断中，免疫组化证实是必要的。

预后因素

多因素分析，年龄和分期是最重要的独立因素[667,690-693]。

- 分期。疾病分期是最重要的单一预后因素；尤其就诊时即出现淋巴结转移预后更差（10年生存率由86%～95%降至46%～55%)[332,669,679,680,690,692,694,715,744]。对侧颈部或纵隔淋巴结受累与远处转移有关[745]。远处转移与预后差相关[695]。甲状腺外浸润具有较高的复发风险，肿瘤浸润到颈部软组织与疾病进展和生存降低有关[692,695,744]。
- 年龄。超过45～60岁的病人预后相当差[332,667,669,679,680,690,692,694,715,746]。
- 性别。女性预后较好[332,692,715]，但多因素分析显示这一因素不具有预后意义[690,691]。
- MEN2A的髓样癌较散发性髓样癌预后好，而MEN2B的髓样癌预后较差[669,683,693,747,748]。但在一项研究中，经多因素分析发现这一因素不具有预后意义[667]。
- 经筛查发现的小肿瘤预后极好，治愈率为94.7%[675,679,686,693,696]。大于1 cm的肿瘤是不利的预后因素[693]。
- 生物化学治疗成功者预示生存好（10年生存率为98%，而生物化学治疗不成功者为70%）[691,744]。
- 预后差的组织学特征包括核分裂多（每25个高倍视野超过1个）、小细胞亚型[708]、坏死[696,697,708,746,749]、鳞状化生[746]和缺乏淀粉样物[692,693]。
- 降钙素表达少的髓样癌（少于50%的肿瘤细胞阳性）较降钙素多的髓样癌预后差[746,750-752]。有时，肿瘤发生时降钙素多，在复发时降钙素变少。
- 已报道的需进一步证实的预后因素如下：
  - CD15/LeuM1 强表达提示局部复发和死亡的风险较高[753,754]。
  - 嗜铬素B 或 bcl-2 低表达更具侵袭性[755,756]。
  - 已报道 N-myc 表达增加是不利的预后因素[757]。
  - 微血管计数高与较差的预后有关[758]。
  - 非整倍体肿瘤较二倍体肿瘤更具侵袭性[693,715,759,760]。

鉴别诊断

- 低分化（岛状）甲状腺癌。
- 玻璃样变小梁腺瘤。长的起伏的小梁在髓样癌中非常罕见[669]，核特征（核沟、假包涵体、核周空晕）支持玻璃样变小梁腺瘤的诊断。
- 副神经节瘤（见下文）。
- 转移性神经内分泌癌（见下文）。
- Hurthle 细胞肿瘤（显示嗜酸性变的病例）。
- 未分化癌。怪异和高度非典型的细胞（但核分裂不常见）可见于其他方面表现典型的髓样癌；这些肿瘤不应误诊为未分化癌。
- 甲状旁腺肿瘤。淀粉样物罕见于甲状旁腺肿瘤[761]。免疫组化在与髓样癌的鉴别中有帮助。

C细胞增生作为遗传性髓样癌(hereditary medullary carcinoma)的指征及定义问题

通常建议在所有髓样癌病例中寻找C细胞增生，若有则为遗传性髓样癌，需筛查家族成员（图18A.93）。因形态学不能可靠地识别C细胞，需做降钙素或广谱神经内分泌标志物染色。然而，关于C细胞增生的概念无一致意见。各种研究所采用的弥漫性C细胞增生的标准包括："含20个以上C细胞的细胞团"[762]；"100倍放大倍数的一个低倍视野内有50个以上C细胞"[763,764]；"与年龄、性别匹配的对照组（每个低倍视野少于10个C细胞）比较，C细胞的大小和数目增加"（图18A.94）[765]。观察发现以上定义的"C细胞增生"的标准也能出现在正常个体（尤其在老年人和实性细胞巢周围）[764,766]、甲状腺非髓样肿瘤周围（如滤泡性腺瘤和淋巴瘤）[763,767]以及甲状腺炎中[763,764,766,767]，使问题更加复杂化。

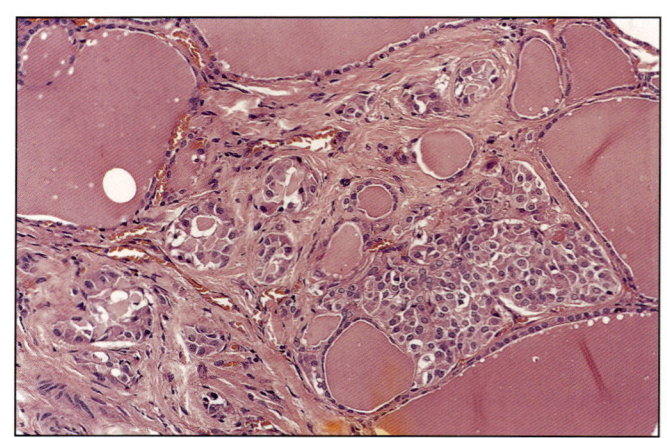

图18A.93 多发性内分泌肿瘤2A型（MEN2A）病人髓样癌旁的结节性C细胞增生。一些甲状腺滤泡被具有轻度核非典型性的C细胞所替代。此型C细胞增生也被称为肿瘤性C细胞增生，在常规的显微镜下易识别，罕见于MEN2以外。

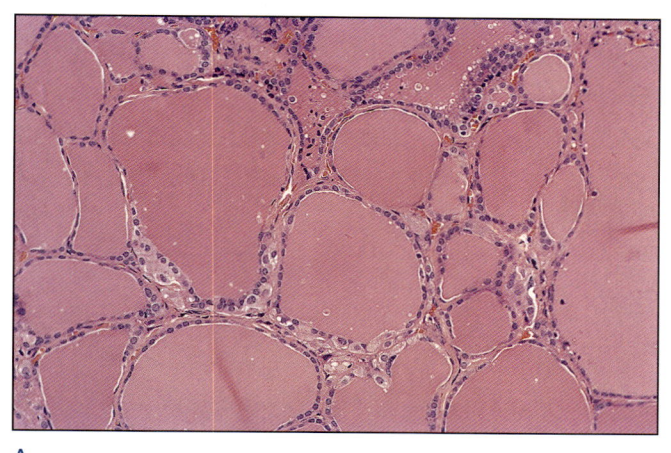
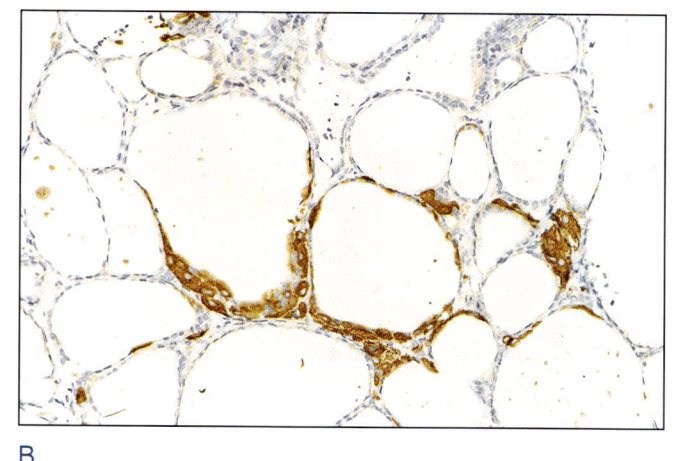

图18A.94 多发性内分泌肿瘤2A型（MEN2A）病人髓样癌旁的弥漫型C细胞增生。（A）除常有大量浅染胞浆外，难以识别出增生的C细胞。（B）相应区域降钙素染色显示C细胞，多位于滤泡的基底膜内。此型C细胞增生与正常个体的所谓生理性C细胞增生难以鉴别，或与MEN2以外的各种甲状腺病变相关。

结节型或肿瘤型C细胞增生的定义为"滤泡腔被实性聚集的C细胞完全占据"（图18A.93）[765,768]。当出现结节状聚集时，毫无疑问C细胞发生了增生，但与微小髓样癌或髓样癌的甲状腺内扩散鉴别困难[684,751]。与肿瘤主体比较，细胞核通常较小，染色质结构不同，胞浆浅染。McDermott等发现Ⅳ型胶原（基底膜）的免疫染色有帮助：被连续的基底膜完全包裹的病变是证实位于滤泡内（结节性C细胞增生）；而基底膜缺损或伴有基底膜再生的病例，提示为髓样癌[769]。

遗传型髓样癌的诊断

检测遗传型髓样癌最可靠的方法是分子分析[770,771]。大多数遗传性病例有*RET*原癌基因胚系突变，即突变不仅见于肿瘤细胞，也见于体内所有细胞。*RET*基因的常见突变位点见于图18A.81。识别*RET*基因胚系突变的重要性在于需要注意病人综合征中其他成分的发展（表18A.12），以及筛查家族成员以便携带者做预防性甲状腺切除。

可以从外周血白细胞或石蜡包埋非肿瘤组织中提取DNA进行*RET*原癌基因胚系突变分析。运用聚合酶链反应扩增多个外显子，然后进行DNA测序以检测突变。此外，可做单链构象多态性或异源双链技术检测异常条带以筛查突变（图18A.95）。可疑突变的性质可通过直接DNA测序或使用限制性核酸内切酶剪切检测已知的突变部位而进一步证实。

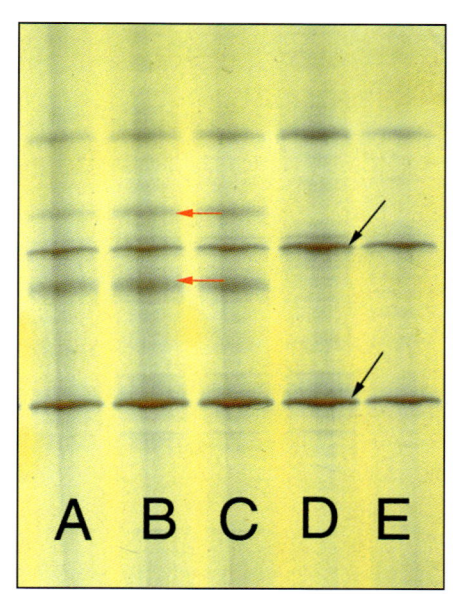

图18 A.95 *RET*基因外显子11的聚合酶链反应扩增产物的单链构象分析（电泳胶银染色）。D道为正常个体；黑箭头指示对应*RET*基因DNA链的两条带。B道为一例已知的多发性内分泌肿瘤2A型（MEN2A），有密码子634突变；两条异常条带（红箭头）提示突变。A道为MEN2A可疑病例；异常条带提示*RET*突变。C道为前者的哥哥，结果提示携带*RET*基因的胚系突变。E道为前者的姐姐，结果提示其未受影响。

筛查散发性髓样癌病人的 *RET* 突变也具有价值，因为1.5%～23%的病例证实有 *RET* 基因的胚系突变[733,737,740,772-775]。

*RET*基因胚系突变患者预防性甲状腺切除标本中的病理所见

经筛查有 *RET* 基因胚系突变（germline mutation）的家族成员通常建议行预防性甲状腺切除。C细胞增生到髓样癌的进展存在年龄相关性，进展速度受所累及的密码子影响[748,776-778]。因为较小的髓样癌可以治愈，并且可以发生在儿童期，所以应尽早实施手术。MEN2A患者要在6岁前而MEN2B患者要在半岁前实施手术[779-784]。如果血清降钙素水平升高或患者大于10岁，需要考虑淋巴结切除[780,785]。手术是安全的，尽管可能有并发症如持久的甲状旁腺功能低下（6.7%）以及单侧喉返神经麻痹（1.3%）[785]。

在一项包括75例有 *RET* 基因胚系突变的儿童和青少年（<20岁）的预防性甲状腺切除标本中，61%（46例）的病例为髓样癌，最小的患者仅4岁，其中6.5%的病例有淋巴结转移（3/46）。其余病例（39%）仅见C细胞增生[785]。96%的病人生物化学治疗有效。单独降钙素水平检测不能区分髓样癌和单纯的C细胞增生。

显示滤泡和C细胞分化的肿瘤
Tumors showing both follicular and C-cell differentiation

混合性滤泡-滤泡旁癌的出现产生了相当大的影响，因为它对滤泡细胞和滤泡旁C细胞起源不同的传统概念提出挑战[786]。文献报道的混合性滤泡-滤泡旁癌至少包括两种情况：碰撞瘤和真正的滤泡-滤泡旁癌。

碰撞瘤 Collision tumor

碰撞瘤由两种可识别的甲状腺癌类型组成：

1. 滤泡癌＋髓样癌[787-790]。
2. 乳头状癌＋髓样癌[786,787,790-793]。

两种成分可彼此邻近或相互混合。这些肿瘤的生物学行为了解甚少，但可能由更具侵袭性的成分决定。

真正的滤泡-滤泡旁癌（所谓的中间型分化性癌）
True follicular–parafollicular carcinoma (so-called differentiated carcinoma of intermediate type)

定义

滤泡-滤泡旁癌（混合性髓样和滤泡细胞癌）是非常罕见的肿瘤，表现为滤泡和滤泡旁成分的复杂混合[794-797]。尽管两种成分可能起源于共同的干细胞，大多数病例显示双重起源[797]。有趣的是，滤泡成分有时是非肿瘤成分[798]。

病理学

肿瘤通常无包膜。常表现为伴混合性滤泡结构的髓样癌[796]。其他病例呈实性、巢状和（或）筛状生长伴混合性滤泡，以及绕以纤维间隔的致密多角形细胞巢或小梁（图18A.96）[794,799-801]。偶尔，可见淀粉样物。超微结构证实有含神经内分泌颗粒的细胞、滤泡细胞、中间型细胞和未分化细胞（indifferent cell）[794]。

根据定义，所有病例均表达甲状腺球蛋白（滤泡和筛状区最明显，有时表达于实性区）和降钙素（实性区最明显）[794,797]。尽管在一些病例可见两种激素共表达的细胞，多数病例中甲状腺球蛋白阳性细胞和降钙素阳性细胞是分开的。

如能在转移部位证实滤泡和滤泡旁成分，诊断较简单。如果肿瘤限于甲状腺内，必须除外伴非肿瘤性甲状腺滤泡的典型髓样癌，换句话说，滤泡-滤泡旁癌中的滤泡应位于肿瘤深部，且被覆核增大、深染的细胞[796]。

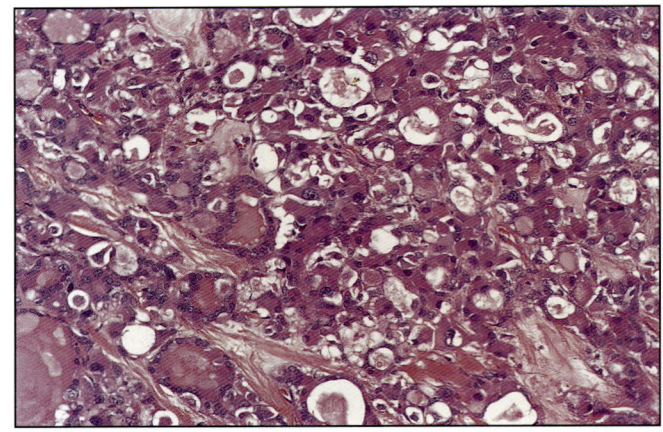

图18A.96 滤泡-滤泡旁癌。实性生长的多角形细胞（降钙素阳性）与小滤泡（甲状腺球蛋白阳性）混合。

临床行为

这些肿瘤通过淋巴和血行扩散，比起分化性甲状腺癌更具侵袭性。18 例病人中，6 例转移，4 例于术后 1 个月至 15 年死于肿瘤[794]。另一方面，Holm 等的研究发现，髓样癌成分表达甲状腺球蛋白者较阴性患者预后好[802]。然而，不同研究中的肿瘤不具有可比性；Ljungberg 等报道的肿瘤看起来像中分化滤泡癌，而 Holm 等报道的肿瘤形态上是典型的髓样癌。

甲状腺的胸腺及相关性鳃囊肿瘤
Thymic and related branchial pouch tumors of the thyroid

甲状腺发生的胸腺及相关性鳃囊肿瘤可能源于甲状腺内偶然出现的隔离胸腺组织或鳃囊衍生物。这些少见的肿瘤包括异位胸腺瘤、伴胸腺样分化的梭形上皮肿瘤（SETTLE）和 CASTLE[803]。

异位胸腺瘤　Ectopic thymoma

临床和病理学特征

肿瘤的组织学类似于纵隔胸腺瘤（见第 21 章），可发生于甲状腺内或附着于甲状腺上[803,804]。多数病人是中年妇女，表现为孤立的甲状腺结节。肿瘤有包膜，呈拼图样分叶（图 18A.97A）。由数量不等的浅染肥胖或梭形上皮细胞和小淋巴细胞混合组成（图 18A.97B）。除 1 例外，所有呈良性生物学行为[805,806]。

鉴别诊断

上皮细胞丰富的胸腺瘤可误诊为未分化癌；可通过有包膜、独特的小叶结构以及缺乏明显的核非典型性加以识别。

淋巴细胞丰富的肿瘤可误诊为恶性淋巴瘤，但可通过小叶结构、大细胞的粘附性生长方式（血管周围和纤维间隔旁最明显）、核膜薄以及浅染大细胞胞浆界限不清加以鉴别。鉴别困难病例，细胞角蛋白免疫染色对凸显上皮成分有用。

伴胸腺样分化的梭形上皮肿瘤
Spindle epithelial tumor with thymus-like differentiation

临床特征

SETTLE 也被称为伴黏液囊肿的甲状腺内梭形细胞肿瘤，有时被报道为"甲状腺胸腺瘤"或"甲状腺畸胎瘤"，是一种发生于年轻人（4～59 岁，平均 18 岁）的罕见肿瘤[803,807-820]。男性为主（男：女比例为 1.5:1）。病人通常表现为无痛性甲状腺肿块。

肿瘤的生物学行为不可预测，有远期发生远处转移的趋势（随访 5 年以上为 70%），最常转移至肺[803,821]。即使发生转移，这一发展缓慢的肿瘤仍保持持久性病程。

病理学

肿瘤平均大小 3.6 cm。界清或浸润性，硬化性间质将肿瘤分割成不完整的小叶。肿瘤富于细胞，以网状梭形细胞束与上皮性条索、小管或乳头紧密混合为特征（图 18A.98A）。梭形细胞核伸长、温和、染色质细；核分裂

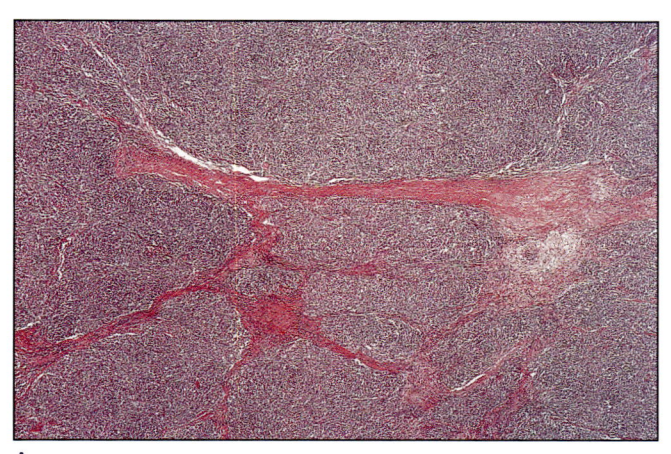

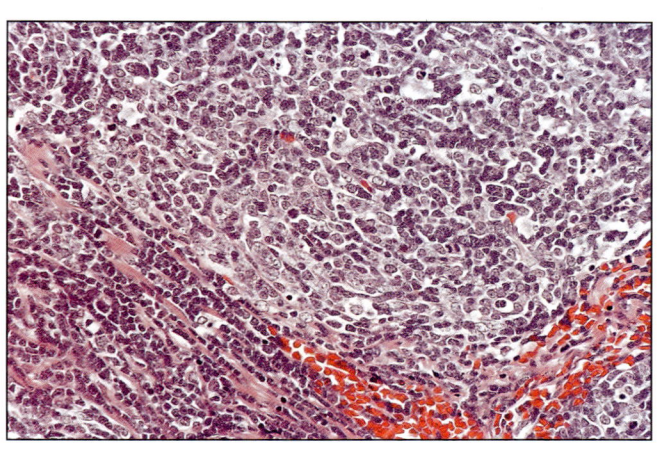

图18A.97　甲状腺内异位胸腺瘤。（A）注意胸腺瘤典型的拼图样小叶。（B）较大的淡染细胞为上皮细胞，而较小的深染细胞是淋巴细胞。

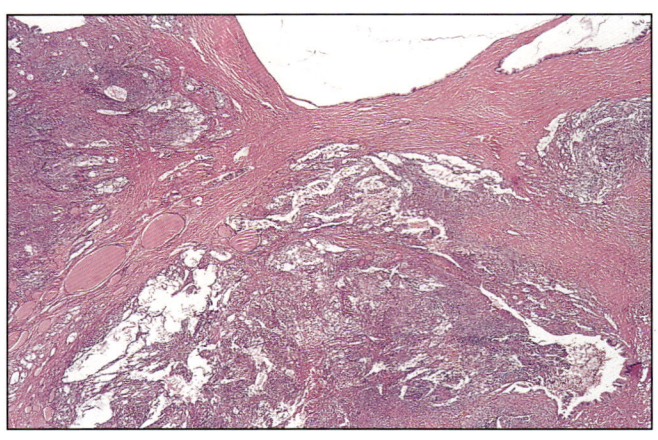
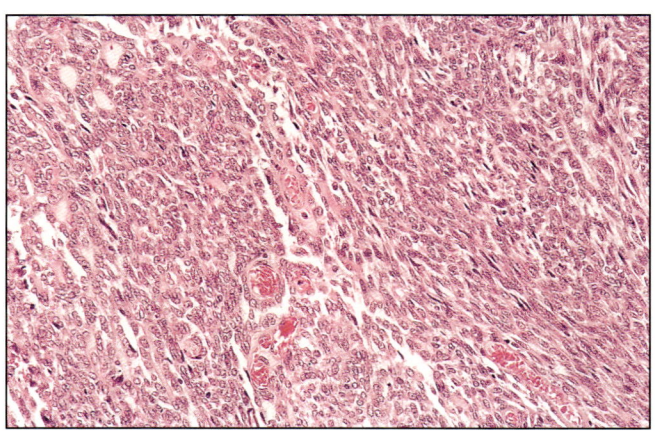

图18A.98 甲状腺内伴胸腺样分化的梭形上皮肿瘤。(A) 硬化性条索将肿瘤分成不规则结节状。视野下方可见网状排列的梭形细胞。上方可见被覆黏液上皮的囊肿。(B) 紧密排列的、温和的梭形细胞与上皮样小管混合(左侧)。

不常见(图18A.98B)。一些病例可见被覆黏液或呼吸型上皮的分散的腺性结构。罕见情况下,可能有局灶鳞状分化、明显的核分裂或局灶坏死[815,817]。也有几乎全部由梭形细胞组成的单相型结构[814]。淋巴细胞稀少或缺如。

少数情况下,甲状腺内被覆纤毛上皮的黏液囊肿出现在肿瘤旁,提示SETTLE可能起源于这些鳃囊残余[813]。目前,没有充足的证据支持肿瘤来源于胸腺。

免疫组化、超微结构和鉴别诊断

细胞角蛋白阳性以及超微结构可见张力丝和桥粒,证明肿瘤为上皮性。最重要的是不要将这一发展缓慢的肿瘤误诊为快速致命的甲状腺未分化癌和不成熟畸胎瘤。该肿瘤的形态与滑膜肉瘤相似,但不同于后者之处在于细胞角蛋白普遍阳性,偶尔出现黏液或呼吸性上皮,缺乏SYT/SSX易位。

伴胸腺样成分的癌
Carcinoma with thymus-like element

临床特征

CASTLE最初被Miyauchi等描述为"甲状腺内胸腺瘤",组织学上类似于胸腺癌而不是胸腺瘤[803,822-830]。主要累及中老年人(平均年龄48.5岁),表现为甲状腺肿块。肿瘤通常累及甲状腺下极和邻近的甲状腺外组织。1/3~1/2的病例发生区域淋巴结转移。肿瘤病程长,常见远期局部复发。大多数病人术后和(或)放射治疗后长期生存,然而个别病例可能侵袭性较强[831]。

病理学

大体上,肿瘤为边界清楚、质硬、分叶状、灰褐色肿块。组织学主要以推挤性方式浸润甲状腺。不同大小、轮廓光滑的瘤细胞小叶或瘤细胞索被宽大的细胞性纤维间隔分隔(图18A.99)。肿瘤细胞或界限模糊、核泡状、核仁明显;或呈胞界较清楚的鳞样表现。有些肿瘤细胞呈梭形。肿瘤岛常被纤细的纤维血管间隔分割。肿瘤细胞和纤维间隔有数量不等的淋巴细胞和浆细胞浸润。

免疫组织化学和遗传学研究

肿瘤细胞表达细胞角蛋白和p63,不表达甲状腺球蛋白、降钙素和TTF-1[832]。少数肿瘤细胞神经内分泌标志物阳性。像胸腺癌一样,CD5和CD117常为阳性[833,834]。这种表现与附近发现的异位胸腺组织均说明肿瘤为异位性(甲状腺内)胸腺癌。然而,也有人认为起源于实性细胞巢[832]。浸润的淋巴细胞表现为成熟T和B细胞混合,不同于胸腺瘤的未成熟T细胞。肿瘤EB病毒阴性[835]。

鉴别诊断

最重要的是要与更具侵袭性的未分化癌(包括淋巴上皮瘤样癌)或鳞状细胞癌鉴别。鉴别特征包括:
- 推挤性浸润边缘
- 由致密纤维性间隔产生的小叶结构
- 凝固性坏死缺乏或少见
- CD5和CD117阳性

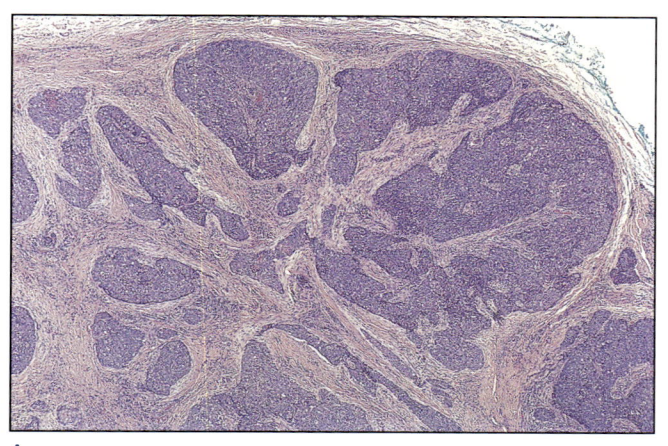

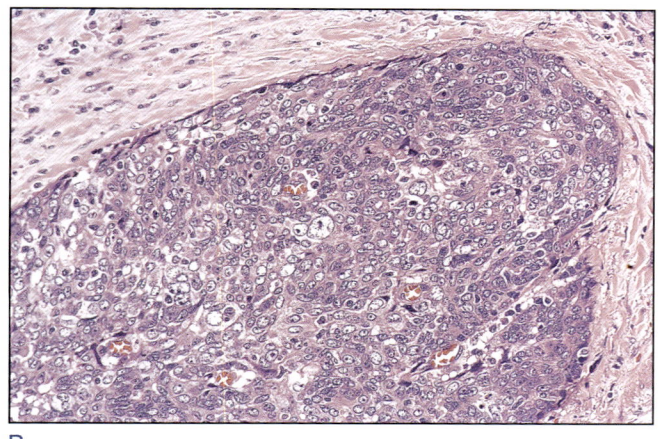

图18A.99 伴胸腺样成分的癌。(A) 肿瘤具有宽阔的浸润性前缘,由被致密纤维间隔分隔的肿瘤细胞岛组成,类似于胸腺癌或胸腺瘤。(B) 肿瘤由鳞状细胞岛组成。此例淋巴细胞和浆细胞较少,其他病例慢性炎症细胞可以丰富。

淋巴造血细胞肿瘤
Tumors of hematolymphoid cells

恶性淋巴瘤 Malignant lymphoma

临床特征

甲状腺原发淋巴瘤仅占所有结外淋巴瘤的2.5%~3%,占所有甲状腺恶性肿瘤的4%~5%[836]。许多过去诊断为"小细胞未分化癌"的病例实际上为恶性淋巴瘤[837]。

甲状腺淋巴瘤更常发生于女性(男:女比例为1:2.5),主要见于但不局限于中老年人(平均年龄59~68岁)[838-848]。淋巴瘤常发生于桥本甲状腺炎或淋巴细胞性甲状腺炎基础上[838,842,847,848]。

临床表现可以非常不同:

- 快速增大的甲状腺肿块,可伴吞咽困难或声嘶,与未分化癌难以区分;症状主要见于大B细胞淋巴瘤患者[848]。
- 缓慢生长的甲状腺结节或多结节性甲状腺肿。
- 甲状腺逐渐弥漫增大,类似甲状腺炎。
- 长期桥本甲状腺炎病人发生的甲状腺肿块。
- 甲状腺切除标本中偶然发现,主要是结外边缘区B细胞淋巴瘤(黏膜相关淋巴组织型,MALT)[838,849,850]。

有些病人可能有甲状腺功能低下[843]。肿瘤可位于甲状腺内或侵出甲状腺。区域淋巴结可受累。总体5年生存率是50%~77%[839,840,842,848,851-855]。一些病例可复发于胃肠道,可解释为淋巴细胞异常"归巢"于其他黏膜部位[838,856]。

大体表现

淋巴瘤在甲状腺内形成边界不清、质韧或质软的肿块。切面凸起,鱼肉样,浅棕色,质地均匀,坏死可有可无。大小从<1 cm到>14 cm[841]。

甲状腺原发淋巴瘤(primary thyroid lymphoma)的组织学亚型

甲状腺原发霍奇金淋巴瘤极为罕见[857]。弥漫大B细胞淋巴瘤(超过70%)和MALT型结外边缘区B细胞淋巴瘤(包括较早文献所报道的中心母细胞-中心细胞淋巴瘤、免疫细胞瘤及中间性淋巴细胞淋巴瘤)占绝大多数病例[838,845,858]。滤泡性淋巴瘤很少发生于甲状腺[859-861]。少数血管内淋巴瘤病和T细胞淋巴瘤,包括一些表达γδT细胞受体的淋巴瘤已有报道[860,862-865]。

黏膜相关淋巴组织型(MALT)结外边缘区B细胞淋巴瘤
Extranodal marginal zone B-cell lymphoma of MALT type

这些发展缓慢的肿瘤与发生在胃或涎腺的同类肿瘤相似,播散前会长时间局限于甲状腺内[859,866,867]。预后极好,但发生大细胞转化时预后变坏(见第21章)[849]。对放疗反应敏感[868]。

反应性淋巴滤泡常散布于弥漫浸润的淋巴瘤细胞中。淋巴瘤细胞呈中心细胞样,核轻度不规则折叠,深染,胞浆淡染,胞浆量可多可少(图18A.100)。常浸润甲状腺滤泡,使其扩张而形成淋巴上皮病变(图18A.100B)[838,849]。可发生反应性淋巴滤泡植入,类似滤泡性淋巴瘤(图18A.101)[849,869]。常混有含Dutcher

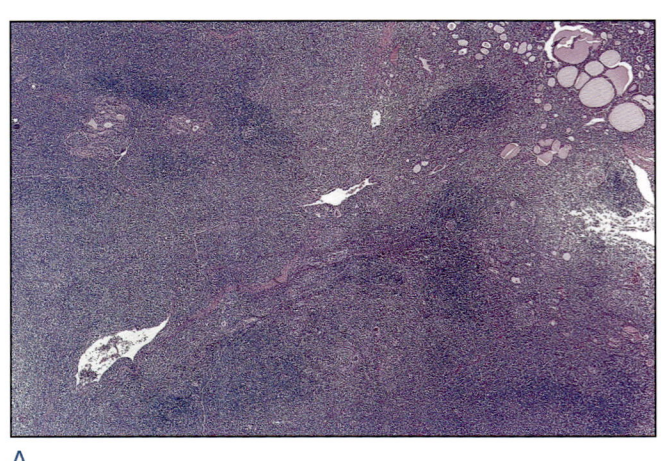
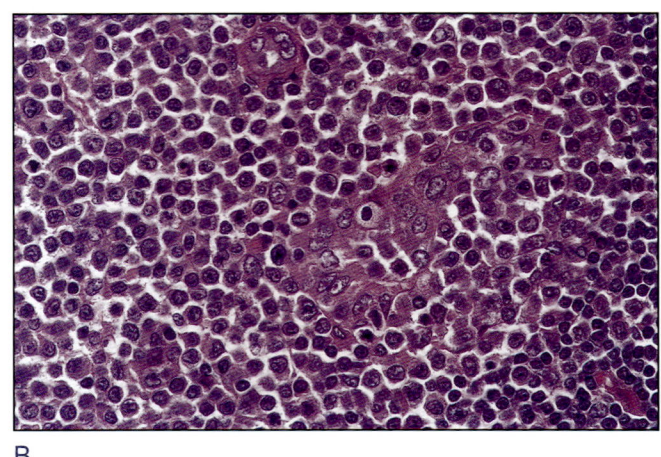

图18A.100 黏膜相关淋巴组织型结外边缘区B细胞淋巴瘤。（A）甲状腺内淋巴细胞呈广泛破坏性浸润。低倍镜下，淡染区与深染区交替，使染色成斑驳状，此为结外边缘区B细胞淋巴瘤的特征。由不同种类的细胞组成：小淋巴细胞、浆细胞和单核样B细胞。（B）中心可见淋巴上皮病变。淋巴瘤细胞浸润引起甲状腺滤泡扩张，轮廓模糊。淋巴瘤细胞核折叠，胞浆呈浆细胞样。

小体或胞浆免疫球蛋白包涵体的浆细胞[848]。区域淋巴结呈现滤泡周或弥漫受累。

淋巴瘤细胞B细胞标志物阳性，但CD5、CD10、CD23和cyclinD1阴性[859,866]。浆细胞和部分中心细胞样细胞表达免疫球蛋白。重链常为IgG型[849,851]。约50%的病例显示新近描述的染色体易位 t(3;14)(p14.1;q32) 伴 FOXP1/IGH 融合；而从未发现在其他部位的结外边缘区B细胞淋巴瘤所报道的 API2/MALT1、MALT1/IGH、IGH/bcl-10 易位，表明不同部位的MALT淋巴瘤形成的分子通路不同（见第21章）[870-873]。

弥漫大B细胞淋巴瘤 Diffuse large B-cell lymphoma

此型肿瘤可原发（de novo）或由黏膜相关淋巴组织型结外边缘区B细胞淋巴瘤转化而来[839,840,842,852,874]。

弥漫浸润的淋巴瘤细胞破坏甲状腺组织（图18A.102）。细胞核圆形、泡状，核仁明显，有中等量双嗜性胞浆（图18A.102B）。可见多核或怪异的瘤细胞。单个瘤细胞常浸润甲状腺滤泡，取代滤泡上皮或阻塞滤泡腔[839,841,860,875]。有时可见血管侵犯[839,841]。瘤细胞表达白细胞共同抗原和B细胞标志物。

滤泡性淋巴瘤 Follicular lymphoma

主要发生于妇女，平均年龄50岁[861]。常显示2级或3级肿瘤性滤泡。由于淋巴上皮病变明显和滤泡扩张，可能与结外边缘区B细胞淋巴瘤有明显的组织相似性。肿瘤细胞CD20、CD10和bcl-6阳性。甲状腺原发滤泡性淋巴瘤常缺少bcl-2蛋白表达或bcl-2基因重排。

预后因素

- 组织学类型。尽管一些研究未发现组织学类型与预后相关[838,840,842,843,876]，现有证据表明黏膜相关淋巴组织型结外边缘区B细胞淋巴瘤较弥漫大B细胞淋巴瘤的预后好得多[839,868,874]。按照AFIP的研究结果，前者5年疾病特异性生存率为100%，而

图18A.101 黏膜相关淋巴组织型结外边缘区B细胞淋巴瘤。淋巴滤泡由单一细胞组成，类似于滤泡性淋巴瘤。然而，这是由于淋巴瘤细胞植入已存在的反应性增生滤泡而引起，不是肿瘤性滤泡。

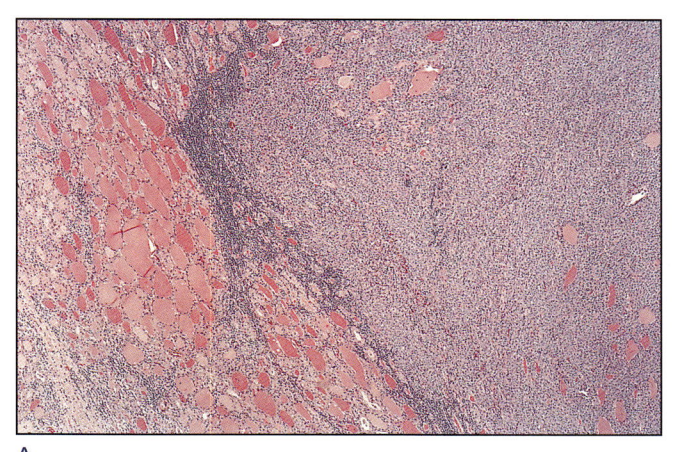

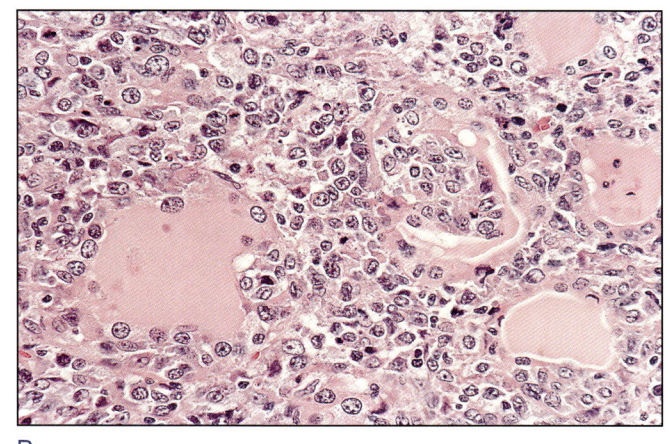

图18A.102 甲状腺弥漫大B细胞淋巴瘤。（A）淋巴瘤细胞弥漫浸润，破坏甲状腺组织。（B）淋巴瘤细胞呈中心母细胞样。浸润甲状腺滤泡，形成腔内"栓子"。

后者为71%～78%(取决于有无MALT淋巴瘤成分)[848]。甲状腺原发滤泡性淋巴瘤的预后也很好[861]。

- 局部疾病的范围。大多数研究发现甲状腺外扩散预后差，5年生存率为40%，而甲状腺内肿瘤为85%[839-842,845,848]。
- 许多研究表明，颈部或纵隔淋巴结受累是不利的预后因素[840,841,848,854]。
- 一些研究发现年龄大（超过60～65岁）与预后差相关[839,840,855]。
- 其他已知的与预后差相关的特征：
  - 大于10 cm[839,845]
  - 血管浸润[841,848]
  - 坏死[841]

鉴别诊断

- 桥本或淋巴细胞甲状腺炎。伴明显炎症细胞反应的桥本甲状腺炎与结外边缘区B细胞淋巴瘤（可能发生于甲状腺炎）的鉴别极其困难[849]。以下的组织学表现提示淋巴瘤：
  - 密集的淋巴组织浸润（可为局灶性）
  - 宽阔的中心细胞样细胞或透明细胞带（单核样B细胞）
  - 明显的淋巴上皮病变

淋巴瘤的诊断可通过免疫染色证实（成片的CD20阳性B细胞，B细胞CD43异常表达或轻链限制性）。

- 未分化癌。细胞缺乏粘附性及肿瘤细胞阻塞滤泡腔强烈支持淋巴瘤。免疫组化染色较容易鉴别（表18A.6）。

甲状腺浆细胞瘤
Plasmacytoma of the thyroid

临床特征

甲状腺原发浆细胞瘤不常见[841,877]。病人常为中老年人，男性患者略多。大多数表现为缓慢增大的甲状腺肿块。有些病例可伴有桥本甲状腺炎[878]。与其他部位的髓外浆细胞瘤一样，预后好。由于临床行为相似，被认为是黏膜相关淋巴组织型结外边缘区B细胞淋巴瘤伴明显浆细胞分化的极端形式[879]。

病理学

大多数病例全部由看上去成熟的浆细胞组成，而一些病例浆细胞分化较差，伴大的多形性核和明显的核仁（间变性浆细胞瘤）。

鉴别诊断

- 浆细胞瘤需与浆细胞肉芽肿（炎性假瘤）鉴别，表现为更多的炎细胞混合和纤维母细胞增生[880,881]。证实浆细胞为克隆性的免疫球蛋白染色对于鉴别诊断最有帮助。
- 浆细胞瘤不同于恶性淋巴瘤之处是由单一的浆细胞组成，CD20阴性。

朗格汉斯细胞组织细胞增生症
Langerhans cell histiocytosis

临床特征

朗格汉斯细胞组织细胞增生症是朗格汉斯细胞的克

隆性增生。可为只累及甲状腺的单一病灶或为播散性疾病的一部分。

发病年龄范围广（平均 37 岁），无性别倾向[882-890]。常因其他疾病而切除的甲状腺或在尸检中偶然发现，偶尔表现为巨大肿块，临床上像甲状腺癌。局限于甲状腺内者，预后非常好，但伴有系统性疾病的患者预后差。

病理表现

甲状腺内朗格汉斯细胞可呈片状或广泛浸润，伴或不伴甲状腺外扩散。朗格汉斯细胞核扭曲，有核沟，核膜薄，胞浆量中等，嗜酸性。常侵入甲状腺滤泡上皮并破坏滤泡。偶尔可见多核组织细胞散在分布。混有多少不等的嗜酸性粒细胞，有时形成嗜酸性脓肿。一些病例可被误诊为甲状腺未分化癌。免疫组化 S-100、CD1a 和 langerin 染色可证实诊断。

间叶性肿瘤及其他肿瘤
Mesenchymal tumors and other tumors

血管肉瘤　Angiosarcoma

临床特征

在较早的文献中，血管肉瘤常被称为血管内皮瘤，比较少见[600]。碘缺乏是可能的病因，因为在阿尔卑斯山地区更为流行[600]。主要见于老年（平均 66 岁），男性略占优势（男：女比率为 1.2∶1）[522]。病人表现为突然出现的颈部肿块，可引起吞咽和呼吸困难，常发生于长期的甲状腺肿基础上。一些有发热，而另一些表现为远处转移。常见转移扩散，肺、胸膜、淋巴结、肾上腺、胃肠道和骨为好发部位[522]。甲状腺血管肉瘤极具侵袭性，中位生存时间仅 3.5 个月。少数生存者全部为缺乏甲状腺外扩散的小肿瘤[891]。

大体表现

肿瘤通常表现为单一结节，中心有一个充满凝固性或液态血液的腔，边缘是一层"橡胶玻璃样物（rubber hyaline）"，与包绕的灰白肿瘤组织混合。常见坏死和出血[522]。

组织学表现

组织学特征类似于软组织低分化血管肉瘤，是一种多形性肿瘤，血管形成区域表现为不规则血管裂隙、相互吻合的腔隙或不连续的胞浆空泡（图 18A.103）。上皮样血管肉瘤是一种形态学亚型，特征为多角形肿瘤性内皮细胞，胞浆丰富嗜酸性、玻璃样，具有明显双嗜性或嗜碱性核仁的泡状核（图 18A.104）[891-894]。

免疫组织化学

各种内皮细胞标志物阳性，如 CD31、CD34 和Ⅷ因子相关抗原[572,573]，偶尔细胞角蛋白阳性[892]。

鉴别诊断

- 未分化癌 [见未分化（间变性）癌，考虑到形态学与生物学行为与血管肉瘤有一定程度重叠，第 1033 页]
- 细针穿刺后甲状腺滤泡上皮的反应性血管改变或假血管肉瘤样改变。

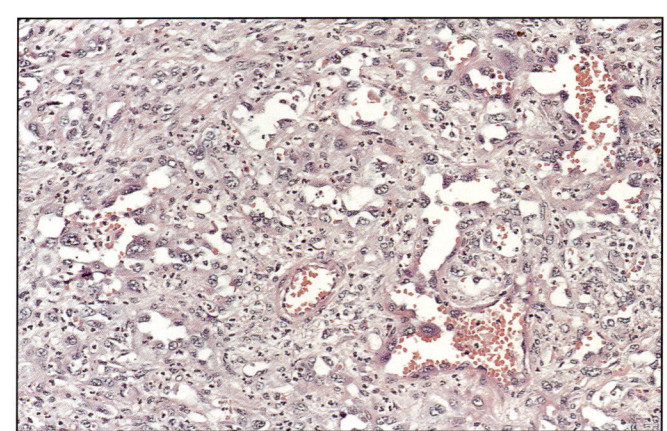

图18A.103　甲状腺血管肉瘤。吻合的腔隙被覆高度非典型性细胞。（Courtesy of Dr. L. Ma, Hong Kong.）

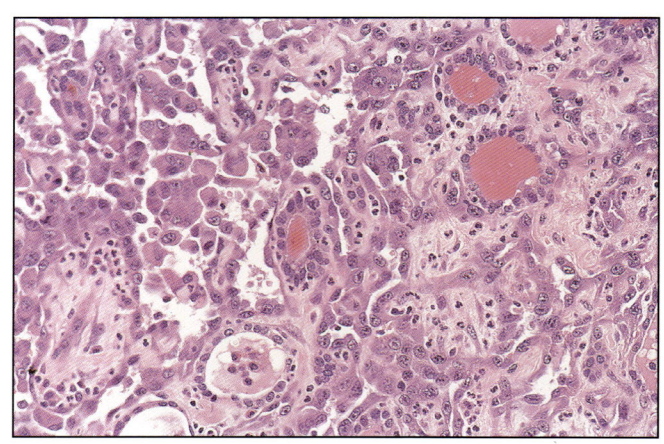

图18A.104　甲状腺上皮样血管肉瘤。上皮样的瘤细胞以及由吻合血管腔隙形成的管状乳头状结构与腺癌极为相似。

- 甲状腺肿内自发的反应性内皮增生（Masson瘤）[895]。
- 伴嗜酸细胞增多的硬化性黏液表皮样癌（假血管瘤样结构）。

孤立性纤维瘤　Solitary fibrous tumor

临床特征

孤立性纤维瘤的形态与胸膜和胸膜外同类肿瘤相似（见第24章），很少原发于甲状腺[896-900]。所有病人为成人，女性多见。目前为止，报道的病例均为良性[900]，但将来可能会遇到具有恶性行为的病例。

病理学

孤立性纤维瘤通常界清，边缘可见锯齿状浸润或陷入的甲状腺滤泡。多细胞区与寡细胞区交替存在，伴有随意分布的良性梭形或星形细胞，与纤细或粗大的胶原纤维密切相邻（图18A.105）。肿瘤细胞胞浆少。常见血管外皮细胞瘤样结构。以夹杂成熟脂肪细胞为特征的脂肪细胞亚型已有描述[901]。瘤细胞CD34、CD99、bcl-2和波形蛋白阳性，但细胞角蛋白和S-100阴性[900,902]。

平滑肌肿瘤　Smooth muscle tumor

甲状腺平滑肌肿瘤极为罕见，恶性数量超过良性[903]。平滑肌瘤有包膜，局限于甲状腺，大小1.5～3.5cm。无细胞异型性、坏死和核分裂[903]。外科切除可以治愈。

平滑肌肉瘤发生于年龄较大的病人，常较大，1.9～12 cm。与未分化癌相反，肿瘤与长期存在的甲状腺肿或甲状腺肿瘤无关。疾病早期发生肺和其他部位的转移，大多数病人2年内死亡[903-907]。已报道一例发生于先天性免疫缺陷儿童的EB病毒相关性平滑肌肉瘤[908]。组织学上，肿瘤由核分裂活跃、胞浆嗜酸性的非典型梭形细胞束组成。常见坏死、出血、浸润性生长和甲状腺外扩散。需做平滑肌表型的免疫组化和（或）超微结构检查以证实诊断，尤其在与未分化癌的鉴别中。

外周神经鞘瘤　Peripheral nerve sheath tumor

发生于甲状腺的神经鞘瘤极为罕见[883]。Schwannoma细胞瘤为良性，而恶性外周神经鞘瘤具有高度侵袭性，早期即发生播散[883,909]。

副神经节瘤　Paraganglioma

临床特征

发生于甲状腺的副神经节瘤罕见，被认为起源于喉下副神经节，有时位于甲状腺包膜内。在20例已报道的病例中，19例为女性，大多为40～60岁[242,910-913]。病人表现为颈部肿块，有些有高血压史。少数病例可发生于遗传性副神经节瘤综合征[912]。肿瘤界清，或局部延伸入邻近的喉或气管。14名随访病人在术后5个月到8年健康存活。无复发或转移。

病理学和免疫组化

多数肿瘤大小约2 cm，尽管偶尔可能10 cm[242,914]。具有细颗粒胞浆的卵圆形细胞（广谱神经内分泌标志物阳性，细胞角蛋白、甲状腺球蛋白和降钙素阴性）组成泡巢状结构，绕以一层不明显的支持细胞（S-100和胶质纤维酸性蛋白阳性）（图18A.106）。散在的肿瘤细胞核增大、深染或奇异形，导致错误地诊断为恶性。肿瘤血管丰富，间质水肿、玻璃样变或硬化。

鉴别诊断

由于形态上与玻璃样变小梁腺瘤和髓样癌有重叠，应做免疫组化证实诊断（见表18A.6）。出现梁状结构、胶样物质或真正的腺腔不可能诊断为副神经节瘤。

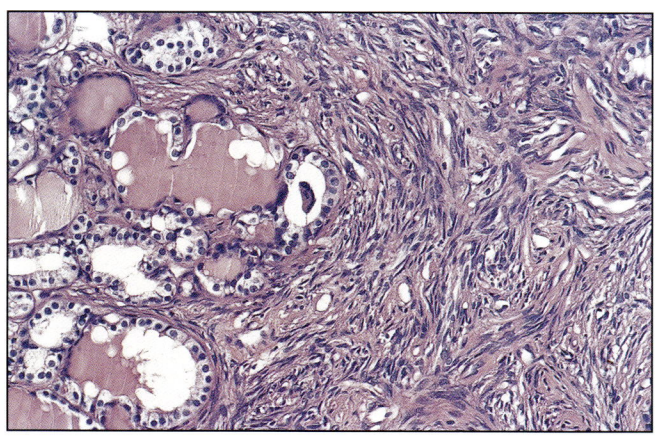

图18A.105　甲状腺孤立性纤维瘤。周边可见一些内陷的甲状腺滤泡。肿瘤由纤细胶原纤维和良性梭形细胞混合组成。

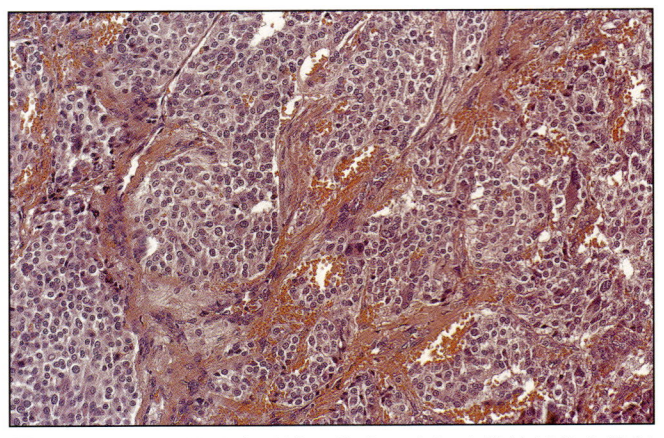

图18A.106　甲状腺内副神经节瘤。瘤细胞巢被纤维血管间隔分隔。形态与髓样癌鉴别困难。

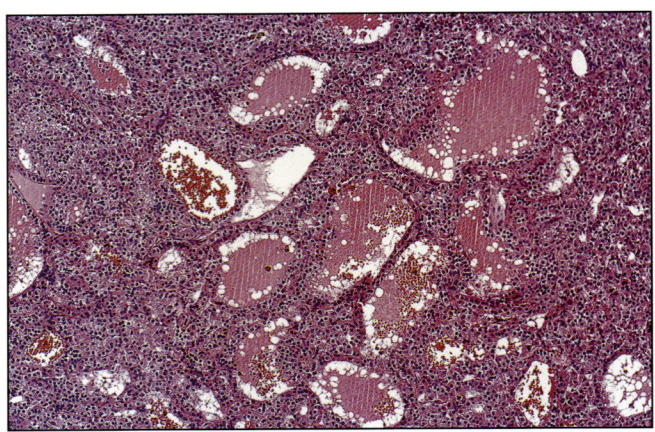

图18A.107　甲状腺内甲状旁腺腺瘤。滤泡的出现可误诊为甲状腺滤泡性肿瘤。

畸胎瘤　Teratoma

新生儿和婴儿甲状腺畸胎瘤
Thyroid teratoma in neonates and infants

发生在死婴、新生儿或婴儿的甲状腺畸胎瘤通常体积大、多囊性，引起呼吸或喂养困难[915-918]。未成熟畸胎瘤比成熟畸胎瘤更常见，由各胚层的未成熟组织组成。神经外胚层组织可能明显。尽管一些病例会引起呼吸道阻塞，肿瘤不发生播散，外科切除后预后极好[917,918]。

儿童和成人甲状腺畸胎瘤
Thyroid teratoma in children and adults

发生于儿童和成人的甲状腺畸胎瘤临床上通常高度恶性[918-922]。病人为中、青年，女性明显多见。常见局部复发、颈淋巴结转移和肺转移。对化疗和放疗的反应常短暂，大多数病人1年内死亡，有些病例经积极的化疗和手术可以长期生存[923,924]。

组织学上，常为未成熟畸胎瘤（大多数3级），伴明显的原始神经外胚层组织。神经组织的出现是与未分化癌鉴别的重要的提示性组织学特征。

甲状腺内甲状旁腺肿瘤
Intrathyroid parathyroid tumor

因为甲状旁腺紧邻或有时完全包埋在甲状腺中，甲状旁腺肿瘤表现为甲状腺内肿瘤并不令人惊奇[925,926]。甲状旁腺癌也可直接侵入甲状腺，临床上相似于原发性甲状腺癌。常误诊为滤泡性腺瘤、滤泡癌或未分化癌，因为根本没有考虑到甲状旁腺的可能性，而且偶尔出现的滤泡样结构增加了与原发性甲状腺肿瘤的相似性（图18A.107）。

以下为提示甲状旁腺肿瘤的组织学线索：

- 混合细胞类型（透明细胞、嗜酸细胞、轻度嗜碱细胞）
- 具有大量水样透明胞浆和清晰细胞膜的细胞
- 细胞膜清楚的嗜酸性细胞（与Hurthle细胞膜不清相反）
- 大量的纤细血管
- 沿纤细纤维血管轴呈栅栏状排列的细胞核
- 核分裂象少见的"未分化甲状腺癌"

甲状旁腺激素阳性而甲状腺球蛋白阴性可证实诊断。

甲状腺不常见肿瘤及瘤样病变
Unusual and uncommon tumors and tumor-like lesions of the thyroid

甲状腺可发生白血病[927,928]、霍奇金淋巴瘤[857]、Rosai-Dorfman病[929,930]、炎性假瘤（浆细胞肉芽肿）[880]和淋巴上皮囊肿[931,932]。报道发生于甲状腺的罕见肿瘤包括滤泡树突状细胞肿瘤[933]、多形性腺瘤[934]、一种不常见的混合瘤[935]、软骨瘤性错构瘤[936]、玻璃样细胞肿瘤（玻璃样梁状腺瘤的亚型）[937]、纤维瘤病[938]、颗粒细胞瘤[939,940]、横纹肌瘤、纤维肉瘤[941,942]、血管外皮细胞瘤（婴儿肌纤维瘤病？）[943,944]、滑膜肉瘤[945]、脂肪瘤[946]、脂肪肉瘤[947]、软骨肉瘤（化生性未分化癌？）[948]、骨肉瘤（化生性未分化癌？）[949]、血管瘤[950]、淋巴管瘤[951]、上皮样血管内皮瘤[952]和小细胞神经内分泌癌[546]。

甲状腺转移性恶性肿瘤
Metastatic malignant neoplasms in thyroid

甲状腺作为恶性肿瘤系统性转移的组成部分

除被邻近癌（如喉癌）浸润之外，甲状腺常被晚期癌症的转移性肿瘤所累及，因为甲状腺富于淋巴管和血管[953]。诊断上很少引起问题，因为甲状腺内的转移灶通常较小而且其他部位已经有明显广泛的转移性疾病[954]。转移可发生于原发性肿瘤诊断后10多年以后[955]。易转移至甲状腺的肿瘤为肺癌（通常是腺癌）、乳腺癌、恶性黑色素瘤和肾细胞癌[954-957]。罕见情况下，沙粒体可出现在甲状腺内的转移性腺癌，需与甲状腺乳头状癌相鉴别[958]。

甲状腺转移作为肿瘤的首发表现

少数情况下，转移性肾细胞癌可表现为甲状腺结节，或发生于已知肾原发性肿瘤的病人（平均间隔9.4年），或作为隐匿性肾细胞癌的首发表现（约1/3）[111,954,959]。尽管大多数病人发展为播散性疾病（在甲状腺发现病变后平均4.9年），约1/3的病人在手术切除后存活或无疾病迹象却死亡[959]。转移性肾细胞癌组织学上可被误诊为各种伴透明细胞的原发性甲状腺肿瘤。支持前者诊断的特征包括多病灶、细胞膜易碎、胞浆水样透明、窦状血管、腺腔内新鲜出血，免疫组化甲状腺球蛋白或TTF-1阴性[1111]。

起源于支气管或腹腔内的转移性神经内分泌癌（类癌和非典型类癌）可首先表现为甲状腺肿瘤，可为孤立性或多发性结节[960]。甲状腺内的转移性肿瘤常被误诊为髓样癌，只有经过随访才逐渐显明原发肿瘤。神经内分泌癌呈巢状、缎带样、岛状、玫瑰花结样和片状生长，伴有纤维血管间质。不支持髓样癌的特征包括主要在裂隙中生长，缺乏C细胞增生，多发病灶，上皮下细胞球形突入甲状腺滤泡内，以及缺乏淀粉样物。血清降钙素水平不高，降钙素和CEA免疫组化阴性。

甲状腺肿瘤诊断中的实际问题

免疫组化研究的局限性

目前，尚无免疫组化或分子标志物能可靠地将乳头状癌或滤泡癌与它们的良性对应物区分开来（见乳头状癌免疫组化部分，第1012页）。形态学评估仍然是甲状腺癌诊断的金标准[556]。

乳头状病变：诊断方法
Papillary lesion: approach to diagnosis

问题

单独出现乳头不足以诊断乳头状癌，因为许多甲状腺病变可出现乳头。必须考虑细胞学（核特征）和生长方式（乳头结构和其他结构形态）。

主要鉴别诊断

- 乳头状癌
- 结节性甲状腺肿
- 滤泡性腺瘤亚型（滤泡性腺瘤伴乳头状增生、毒性滤泡性腺瘤、伴乳头的Hurthle细胞腺瘤/癌）
- 柱状细胞癌
- 髓样癌，乳头状亚型
- 甲状腺功能亢进
- 桥本甲状腺炎

诊断方法

结节性甲状腺肿和滤泡性腺瘤伴乳头状增生中的乳头通常较宽，轴心内含有滤泡（图18A.55和图18A.108），尽管也可出现纤细的分支状乳头。最重要的是，柱状被覆细胞具有规则、不拥挤、位于基底的圆形深染细胞核，类似穿在线上的珠子，这与乳头状癌拥挤的、极向紊乱的浅染核形成鲜明对照。

甲状腺功能亢进、桥本甲状腺炎和毒性滤泡性腺瘤的乳头不分支、短而粗、突出于滤泡腔内，且缺乏明确的纤维血管轴心（图18A.56）[44]。尽管在桥本甲状腺炎常见透明核，但缺乏明确的乳头状癌核特征。

乳头可见于柱状细胞癌和髓样癌（图18A.76），但缺乏乳头状癌的核特征。而且，髓样癌中的乳头多为假乳头，其表面高低不平，是由细胞解离形成的（图18A.90）。

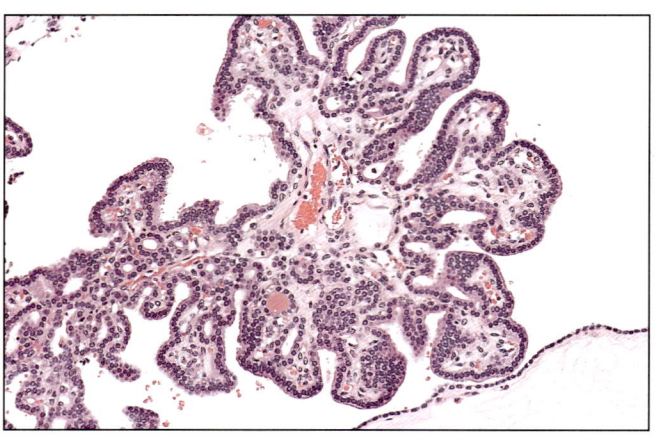

图18A.108 结节性甲状腺肿的巨乳头。注意乳头较宽，细胞呈柱状，细胞核深染位于基底。

Hurthle 细胞腺瘤（癌）常含有较少的乳头成分。乳头通常不分支，细胞核不拥挤（图 18A.63）。然而，偶尔可见核沟。滤泡腔内的钙化类胶质不应误诊为沙粒体。

有包膜的滤泡性病变：诊断方法
Encapsulated cellular follicular-patterned lesion: approach to diagnosis

鉴别诊断

- 腺瘤样 / 增生结节
- 滤泡性腺瘤（包括 Hurthle 细胞腺瘤）
- 滤泡癌（包括 Hurthle 细胞癌）
- 乳头状癌，具有包膜的滤泡亚型
- 髓样癌，滤泡 / 管状亚型
- 甲状腺内甲状旁腺腺瘤

主要诊断问题

评价的关键特征为是否出现乳头状癌特征性的核。另外，需评价生长方式、间质的性质及背景甲状腺的情况。例如，明显的纤维血管间隔应考虑到髓样癌和甲状旁腺肿瘤的可能性。

髓样癌的滤泡 / 管状亚型不应引起诊断上的问题（图 18A.86），因在其他区域常有髓样癌的诊断特征，如特征性的纤维血管间隔、淀粉样物、点彩状染色质和颗粒状胞浆（图 18A.82）。可疑甲状旁腺肿瘤的特征在甲状腺内甲状旁腺肿瘤章节讨论（第 1054 页）。

滤泡癌和滤泡性腺瘤的鉴别依靠在前者找到血管和（或）包膜浸润。腺瘤样结节和滤泡性腺瘤在形态上没有明确的鉴别标准[961]。然而，只要没有浸润，结节被定义为哪一种无关紧要。通常认为支持滤泡性腺瘤的特征包括：

- 孤立结节而不是多发结节
- 有明显的纤维包膜
- 膨胀性生长
- 包膜内外滤泡的细胞结构特征不同

当有一些浅染或透明细胞核时，乳头状癌滤泡亚型和滤泡性腺瘤 / 癌的鉴别是最困难的。因为有些乳头状癌可不显示全部的细胞核特征，而滤泡性腺瘤 / 癌局灶可见透明核或核沟（图 18A.109）。

乳头状癌包膜内滤泡亚型(encapsulated follicular variant of papillary carcinoma) 及滤泡性腺瘤(follicular adenoma)的诊断方法

尽管乳头状癌浸润性（非包膜内）滤泡亚型的诊断可重复性相当高[962]，乳头状癌核特征不明显的包膜内滤泡病灶的诊断可重复性很低[961,963]。很明显，不同病理学家诊断乳头状癌滤泡亚型的标准不同。

保守诊断被证明是合理的，因为即使过低诊断为"滤泡性腺瘤"，包膜型乳头状癌的预后非常好（术后无复发或转移），以致于不会对病人造成伤害。所以，如果有任何的不确定性，宁可诊断良性[44,325,962]，有些争论是由目前的法律诉讼所引起的[964]。

呈滤泡结构的肿瘤诊断为乳头状癌的条件是细胞必须显示典型的乳头状癌核特征，细胞核典型到可作为教科书插图的程度。这些严格的标准列于表 18A.13（图 18A.8 和 18A.15）。如果透明核限于肿瘤中心而周围缺乏，最可能是滤泡性腺瘤或腺瘤样结节固定延迟形成的人工假象。正如在乳头状癌中所讨论的，近年来乳头状癌滤泡亚型有被过度诊断的倾向。

有时，被覆包膜的某些区域看起来似乳头状癌，而另一些区域显示深染圆形核。有两种可能的解释。

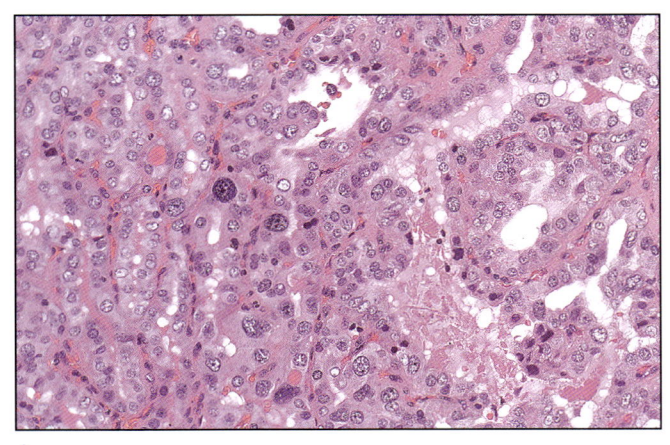 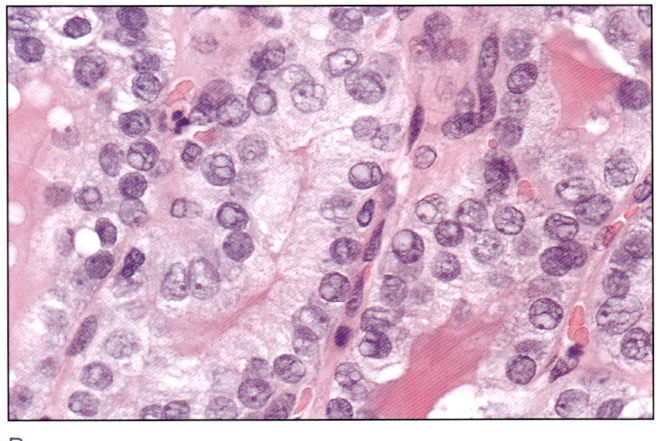

图18A.109 具有类似乳头状癌特征或人工假象的滤泡性腺瘤。（A）滤泡被覆细胞核淡染。核圆形而非卵圆形，无明显的拥挤和核沟。散在的大的深染核在乳头状癌不常见。（B）核空泡人工假象，与核假包涵体的区别在于缺乏清晰的核膜。

表18A.13 有包膜滤泡性肿瘤中乳头状癌的诊断标准[a]	
主要标准	次要标准
核卵圆形而不是圆形	发育不良的乳头
核拥挤、重叠（表现为无极性的"上下交错"的细胞核）	主要为拉长的或不规则形滤泡
	深染的类胶质
浅染或透明的染色质（毛玻璃样），明显的核沟	核假包涵体
沙粒体	滤泡腔内多核组织细胞

[a] 乳头状癌诊断的严格标准是至少三条主要标准或两条主要标准加至少四条次要标准

1. 整个肿瘤为乳头状癌，只在某些病灶核特征不明显。
2. 发生于滤泡性腺瘤中的乳头状癌。如果典型的乳头状癌成分在腺瘤内形成膨胀性肿块或与构成腺瘤的滤泡有明显的过渡，需考虑这种情况（图18A.110）。

乳头状癌包膜内滤泡亚型及滤泡癌(follicular carcinoma)的诊断方法

有些呈滤泡结构的肿瘤明显为恶性，出现了包膜和（或）血管浸润。主要鉴别诊断为滤泡癌和乳头状癌包膜内滤泡亚型。因为已明确诊断为癌，问题不如前一

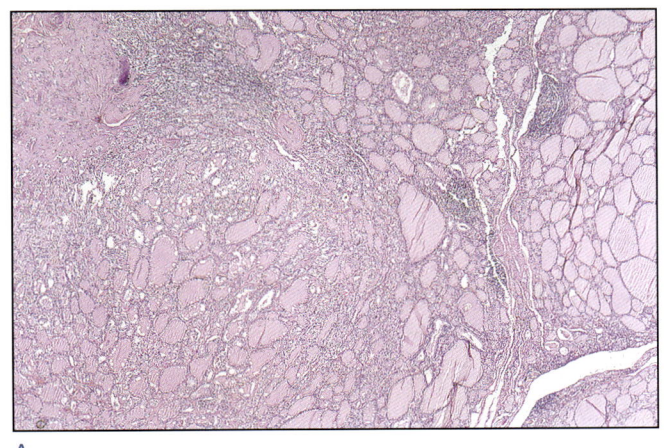 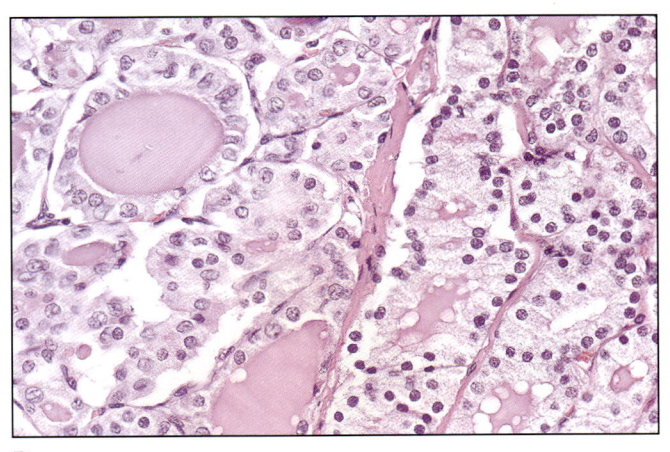

图18A.110 滤泡性腺瘤并发乳头状癌。（A）左侧视野可见有薄层包膜的细胞丰富的肿瘤，显示形态上不同的膨胀性结节。（B）右侧视野为原本存在的腺瘤，滤泡被覆一致、深染、圆形核的细胞。左侧视野为界限清楚的继发性乳头状癌，伴较大、浅染、拥挤及有核沟的细胞核。

节尖锐。与前一节一样，只有当乳头状癌的核特征明显时，才可做出乳头状癌包膜内滤泡亚型的诊断（表18A.13）。

替代性命名

导致过诊断为乳头状癌包膜内滤泡亚型的一个重要因素是法律纠纷，因此为了避免漏掉恶性，病理学家诊断的标准较松。然而，实际的风险很低，因为包膜型乳头状癌几乎从不产生不利的后果。

为了避免乳头状癌的过诊断，对于具有交界性核特征的肿瘤，切尔诺贝利病理专家组已提出一些名称，见图18A.111[965]。当一个有包膜的滤泡性肿瘤显示某些但不明确的乳头状癌核特征时，如果没有明确的包膜和血管浸润，诊断为"不能确定恶性潜能的高分化甲状腺肿瘤"；如果有明确的包膜或血管浸润，诊断为"高分化甲状腺癌，非特指型"（图18A.112）。

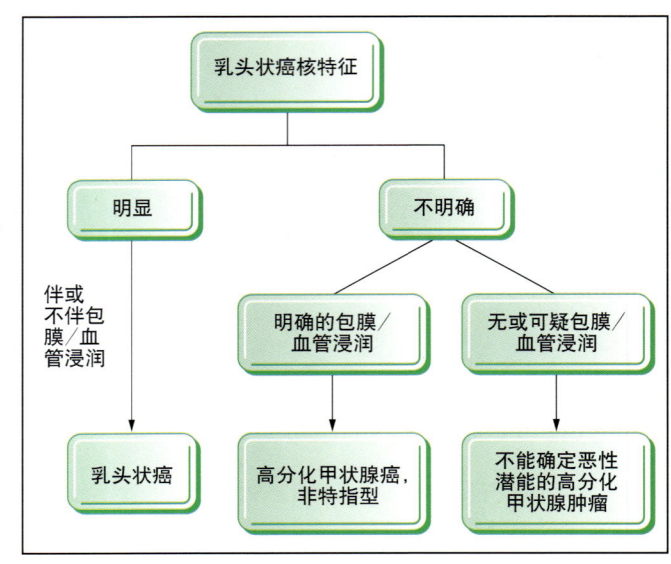

图18A.111 有包膜甲状腺滤泡肿瘤的命名，由切尔诺贝利病理专家组提出。

含淡染/透明核的滤泡群：乳头状癌的最低诊断标准

问题

实际上，透明核作为一种非特异性特征出现在多种良性和恶性甲状腺病变中，可以局灶或广泛，只根据淡染或透明核而诊断乳头状癌是不正确的。有时，细胞核会出现不明原因的淡染和空泡，特征为核内出现多个边缘缺少染色质颗粒的"空洞"（图18A.109B）。

诊断方法

与邻近的甲状腺细胞核进行比较，有助于区分含淡染或透明核的滤泡群性质。细胞核与周围滤泡表现正常的核逐渐过渡强烈支持良性病变而非乳头状癌（图18A.113）。反之，与周围良性部分比较，异常病灶细胞核形态的突然改变（常为核增大）支持乳头状癌的诊断，当然淡染核至少应密集，一些细胞核可见核沟（图18A.29）。如果核特征令人信服，即使病灶由一个滤泡组成，也应诊断为乳头状癌，也就是说，没有最低的大小要求（图18A.29）。

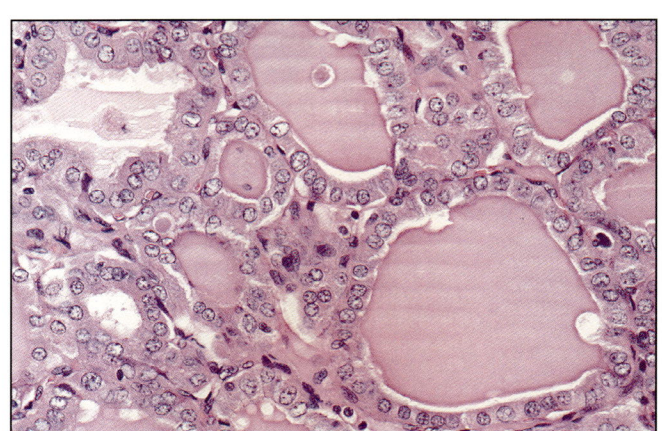

图18A.112 不能确定恶性潜能的高分化肿瘤。这是一个有包膜的滤泡性肿瘤，无包膜或血管浸润证据。显示一些乳头状癌核特征，如浅染和轻度极性紊乱。然而，核为圆形而非卵圆形，核沟不常见。按照切尔诺贝利病理专家组的提议，将伴有不明确乳头状癌核特征的肿瘤命名为"不能确定恶性潜能的高分化肿瘤"。

多发性细胞丰富的滤泡性结节：广泛浸润性癌或多结节性甲状腺肿？

主要鉴别诊断

- 多发性结节性甲状腺肿
- 广泛浸润性滤泡癌
- 激素生成障碍性甲状腺肿

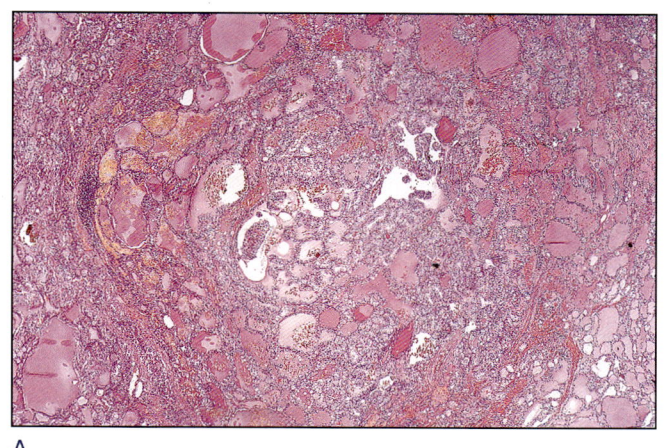 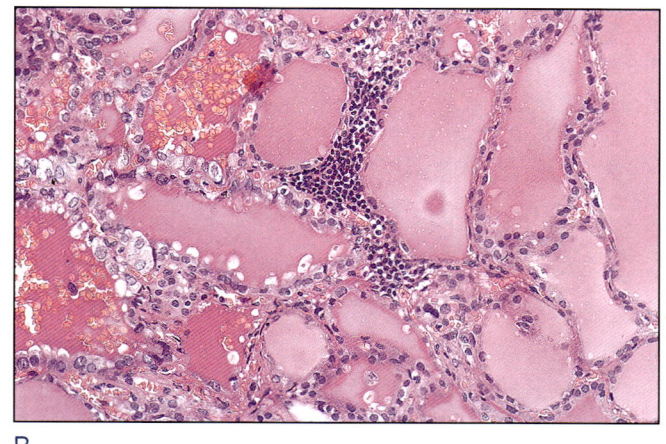

图18A.113 伴透明核的增生性病变。（A）由含透明核的滤泡组成的病灶，可疑为乳头状癌。（B）异常滤泡（左侧）逐渐过渡到正常滤泡（右侧）支持良性病变。

- 结节性桥本甲状腺炎
- 乳头状癌，滤泡亚型

诊断方法

最重要的是评价细胞学。如果出现典型的乳头状癌核特征，应诊断为乳头状癌滤泡亚型。此外，需要鉴别诊断的是广泛浸润性滤泡癌与多发性细胞性腺瘤样结节（如多结节性甲状腺肿、结节性桥本甲状腺炎或激素生成障碍）。支持后者（良性）的特征是：

- 没有广泛浸润性滤泡癌中常能见到的血管浸润
- 不同的结节中细胞组成和滤泡大小不同
- 小结节显然不是来自大结节的"出芽"浸润

结节性甲状腺肿　Nodular goiter

结节性甲状腺肿是外科病理中最常遇到的甲状腺病变。尽管临床上结节可表现为孤立性，然而在超声或病理检查中常见其他背景结节。当有多个结节时，称为多结节性甲状腺肿较合适。结节性甲状腺肿最常由不同大小的含类胶质的扩张滤泡组成（胶样结节）（图18A.114）。中心通常有一些明显隆起或含子滤泡的巨滤泡。被覆巨滤泡的细胞呈立方或柱状，核黑色、圆形，位于基底部。继发性改变如纤维化、出血、囊性变常见。一些结节细胞丰富（腺瘤样结节），由小滤泡或小梁组成，被覆普通细胞或嗜酸细胞，类似于滤泡性肿瘤或乳头状癌滤泡亚型。

结节性桥本甲状腺炎
Nodular Hashimoto thyroiditis

长期的桥本甲状腺炎可形成由紧密排列的小滤泡组成的结节，大多数被覆嗜酸（Hurthle）细胞。结节的多

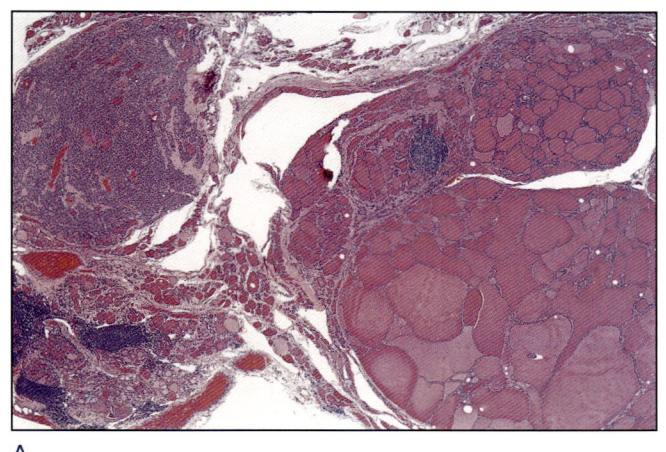 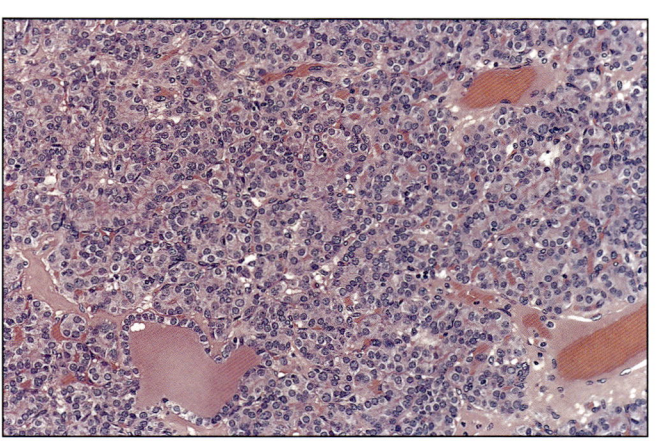

图18A.114 结节性甲状腺肿。（A）此视野可见两个结节；右侧的结节主要是含类胶质的扩张大滤泡，而左侧的结节则富于细胞。（B）左侧结节由微滤泡和小梁组成，此视野与滤泡性腺瘤或滤泡癌无法鉴别。

样性和孤立的多形性核的频繁出现可导致误诊为 Hurthle 细胞癌。如果出现硬化会造成包膜浸润的错觉。然而，没有血管浸润。

激素生成障碍性甲状腺肿
Dyshormonogenetic goiter

激素生成障碍是由甲状腺激素合成遗传性缺陷引起的一种疾病[310]。病人表现为先天性甲状腺功能低下或早期发生甲状腺肿。甲状腺呈不对称增大、多结节，可重达600g。结节常显示丰富的细胞，呈混合性微滤泡、小梁和实性生长方式；可见核非典型性（大的深染细胞核和泡状核）；结节周围纤维化明显；因而可能被误诊为滤泡癌（图18A.115）[966]。通常，不同结节中细胞的多少和结构也不一样，滤泡小，常缺乏类胶质[967]。

伴梁状生长方式的肿瘤
Tumor with trabecular growth pattern

主要鉴别诊断

- 玻璃样变小梁腺瘤/癌
- 髓样癌
- 滤泡性（Hurthle细胞）腺瘤/癌
- 乳头状癌

诊断方法

玻璃样变小梁腺瘤/癌和乳头状癌有相似的核特征：淡染、卵圆形核、核沟及假包涵体常见。支持玻璃样变小梁腺瘤/癌的结构特征为：

- 是波浪状小梁而不是笔直的小梁
- 玻璃样变与小梁相伴，常有大块的嗜酸性沉积物形成
- 胞浆内可见黄色小体

如果缺乏乳头状癌核特征，主要考虑为滤泡性肿瘤和髓样癌。后者的特征是具有明显的纤维血管间隔，常见淀粉样物和颗粒状染色质。

实性生长的浸润性肿瘤
Invasive tumor with solid growth

主要鉴别诊断

- 滤泡癌
- 乳头状癌，实性亚型
- 黏液表皮样癌
- 低分化甲状腺癌
- 未分化癌
- 髓样癌
- CASTLE
- 甲状旁腺癌
- 转移癌
- 恶性淋巴瘤

诊断方法

对于一个呈实性生长的浸润性甲状腺肿瘤，最重要的是不要将生长缓慢的肿瘤（如滤泡癌、实性型乳头状癌、黏液表皮样癌、CASTLE、甲状旁腺癌）误诊为侵袭性较强的未分化癌或大细胞淋巴瘤。这些生长缓慢的肿瘤（除CASTLE外）细胞核常相对温和，而CASTLE可通过肿瘤巢光滑的轮廓以及主要呈推挤性浸润加以识别。

支持甲状旁腺癌诊断的特征在甲状腺内甲状旁腺肿瘤章节内讨论，见第1054页。肿瘤细胞浸润甲状腺滤泡上皮及堵塞滤泡腔是恶性淋巴瘤的常见特征，而血管闭塞是未分化甲状腺癌高度特异的特征。横向纤维血管间隔、细胞解离和淀粉样物（如果出现）是髓样癌的诊断特征。

梭形细胞甲状腺肿瘤
Thyroid tumors with spindle-shaped cells

主要鉴别诊断

- 髓样癌
- 非典型性滤泡性腺瘤（伴梭形细胞）

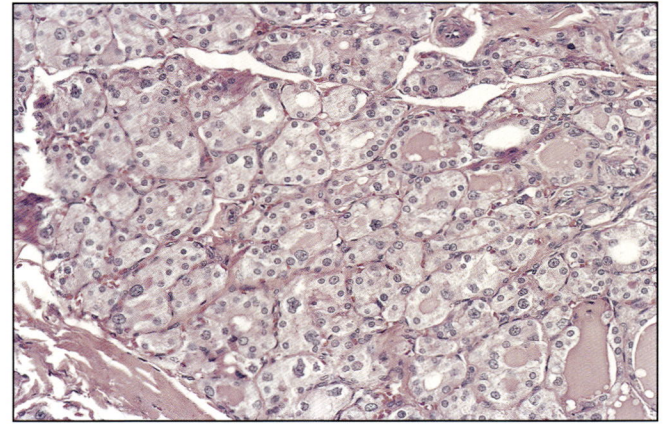

图18A.115 激素生成障碍性甲状腺肿。滤泡小，常缺乏类胶质。有散在增大、深染的细胞核。

- 滤泡性肿瘤伴梭形细胞化生
- 乳头状癌：
  - 伴梭形细胞化生
  - 伴结节性筋膜炎样间质
  - 筛状-桑葚亚型
- 未分化癌
- SETTLE
- 各种良性和恶性间叶肿瘤

诊断方法

许多甲状腺的上皮性肿瘤有显著的肿瘤性梭形细胞成分。但可根据肿瘤其他区域典型的组织学特征做出诊断。例如，梭形细胞如果出现在筛状-桑葚型乳头状癌中，其量相对少且出现于腔内缺乏类胶质的筛状结构中。

未分化癌和肉瘤中的梭形细胞多形性明显，易于诊断。当有明显的纤细的纤维血管间隔时，应首先考虑髓样癌。甲状腺的滑膜肉瘤样肿瘤最可能是SETTLE，以胞浆稀少的梭形细胞束、局部常与腺样结构融合为特征。在伴结节性筋膜炎或纤维瘤病特征的间叶性增生中，应仔细寻找潜在的乳头状癌。

乳头状癌或滤泡性腺瘤中的梭形细胞化生，尤其是成为肿瘤的主要成分时，可以使诊断极为困难。梭形细胞形态温和，至少在一些病灶与肿瘤性滤泡或乳头混合（图18A.60）。细胞角蛋白、甲状腺球蛋白和TTF-1阳性可证实其化生本质。

嗜酸细胞（Hurthle细胞）丰富的甲状腺肿瘤
Thyroid tumors rich in oncocytes (Hurthle cells)

主要鉴别诊断

- Hurthle细胞腺瘤/癌
- 乳头状癌的嗜酸细胞、Warthin瘤样和高细胞亚型
- 髓样癌嗜酸细胞亚型
- 结节性甲状腺肿伴嗜酸（Hurthle）细胞腺瘤样结节
- 桥本甲状腺炎中的嗜酸性结节

诊断方法

嗜酸（Hurthle）细胞是充满线粒体的大细胞，胞浆嗜酸性、颗粒状。因为这些细胞可见于各种甲状腺反应性病变（如老年人甲状腺、桥本甲状腺炎和腺瘤样结节）和甲状腺肿瘤中，富于嗜酸细胞病变的诊断应基于疾病本身而不是这些细胞。嗜酸细胞核常增大伴泡状染色质、核仁明显，甚至可见散在的奇异深染细胞核。

髓样癌嗜酸细胞亚型很少全部由嗜酸细胞组成，在一些病灶常与典型髓样癌混合，因而能做出正确诊断。乳头状癌Warthin瘤样型和高细胞型因前者独特的细胞结构特征及后者明显的乳头状生长方式而易于诊断。

嗜酸细胞结节在结节性甲状腺肿和桥本甲状腺炎中常为多发，而在Hurthle细胞腺瘤/癌中常为孤立性。乳头状癌嗜酸细胞型与Hurthle细胞腺瘤/癌的鉴别更加困难。前者可能不出现乳头，而后者常见。在Hurthle细胞腺瘤/癌中常见钙化的类胶质，可能被误认为沙粒体（乳头状癌特征）。此外，某些Hurthle细胞腺瘤/癌显示核沟或核内包涵体，与乳头状癌在形态上有重叠。诊断乳头状癌嗜酸细胞型，必须表现出广泛的与非嗜酸细胞型一样的核特征（表18A.13），只是由于胞浆丰富使得核拥挤不明显。然而，有些作者对乳头状癌的诊断标准较松[169]。Hurthle细胞癌通过包膜和（或）血管浸润与Hurthle细胞腺瘤区别。

富于透明细胞的甲状腺肿瘤
Thyroid tumors rich in clear cells

参考第1024页表18A.10。

甲状腺病变的细针穿刺细胞学
Fine needle aspiration cytology of thyroid lesions

细针穿刺细胞学在甲状腺肿瘤处理中的作用

细针穿刺细胞学广泛用于甲状腺肿物的筛查及诊断[968-970]。最大的价值是发现携带有甲状腺肿瘤的病人进行早期手术治疗，而对细针穿刺细胞学显示良性结构（如囊肿或胶样结节）的病人进行随访[971]。讨论甲状腺肿瘤的细胞学细节已超出本章的范围。简而言之，穿刺细胞学常能正确诊断乳头状癌，因为此型肿瘤的诊断大部分依靠细胞学细节。因为在针吸材料中不能识别包膜或血管浸润，因此不能区分滤泡性腺瘤和滤泡癌，只能笼统诊断为滤泡性肿瘤。当细胞性胶样结节（腺瘤样结节）与滤泡性肿瘤不能明确区分时，诊断为滤泡性病变是合适的。髓样癌和未分化癌的细胞学诊断常是可能的，

细针穿刺引起的形态学改变

细针穿刺可有以下组织学改变[448,450]：
- 组织损伤。细针穿过的区域形成线性出血道或不规则血肿。邻近的甲状腺滤泡可发生损伤、部分破坏或坏死。少数情况下，出血很广泛以致整个病灶实际上转变成一个血肿，而妨碍了正确的组织学诊断。
- 修复性改变。血肿机化伴肉芽组织形成、慢性炎症细胞浸润、含铁血黄素沉积及纤维瘢痕形成。
- 组织损伤或修复可产生以下反应性细胞学改变：
  - 修复性组织可以很丰富，类似 Kaposi 肉瘤或其他肉瘤；"术后梭形细胞结节"用于表述这种病变[972]。
  - 丰富的、Masson 瘤样反应可导致误诊为血管肉瘤。
  - 组织损伤或梗死区周围残存的滤泡表现出反应性非典型性，如核增大、核仁明显，可被误诊为高级别癌。有时，这些反应性滤泡相互吻合，滤泡内可见出血，呈血管肉瘤样表现（图18A.116）[450,973,974]。
- 肿瘤梗死。Hurthle 细胞肿瘤尤其容易发生梗死，可能是由于线粒体丰富的肿瘤细胞对能量要求较高所致（图18A.57）[447]。因此难以对肿瘤进行诊断或分类。肿瘤梗死可伴有旺盛的修复性反应，可被误诊为未分化癌。

- 上皮移位。肿瘤纤维包膜穿刺部位可有上皮移位。这一现象（包膜破坏）有可能被误认为包膜浸润（滤泡癌）（图 18A.47）。
- 针道肿瘤种植。为非常罕见但有记载的现象[975]。

甲状腺肿瘤的术中冰冻切片诊断
Intraoperative frozen section diagnosis of thyroid tumors

术中冰冻切片诊断的价值

近年来，随着细针穿刺的广泛应用，术中冰冻切片诊断甲状腺病变的使用已减少[976-981]。尽管 Mayo Clinic 报道甲状腺的术中冰冻切片诊断准确率高而且经济，恶性诊断率达到78%[982]，大多数科室认为冰冻切片诊断的延迟率和假阴性率很高[983-987]。

实际上术中冰冻切片的有效性有赖于先前的细针穿刺诊断，总结如下[981,988]：
- 穿刺诊断"明确恶性"：不需要做冰冻诊断。
- 穿刺诊断"滤泡性病变"、"滤泡性肿瘤"或"Hurthle 细胞肿瘤"：冰冻诊断的价值有限或无价值。
- 穿刺诊断"可疑为癌"：冰冻切片最有助于判定良恶性。

术中诊断标本的处理

通常，依照甲状腺标本的大体检查，诊断就可明确。切面呈颗粒状的浸润性肿瘤几乎毫无疑问地为乳头状癌，取一块足够。孤立性、有包膜、肉质感的肿瘤通常为滤泡性腺瘤或微小浸润性滤泡癌；如果未见明显浸润，从包膜区取一块足够用于冰冻诊断。取多块组织做冰冻切片只会拖延报告，且由于冰冻产生的人工假象影响之后的诊断。对于术中诊断，鉴别滤泡性腺瘤和微小浸润性滤泡癌并不那么重要，因为在大多数病例实施腺叶切除术就足够了。

术中细胞学涂片对于甲状腺病灶的评估也是有帮助的，尤其是对乳头状癌和髓样癌的核特征识别。

冰冻切片的主要诊断类别

- 浸润性乳头状病变：乳头状癌，少数情况下是柱状细胞癌。
- 细胞较少、以大滤泡为主的滤泡性病变：良性（胶

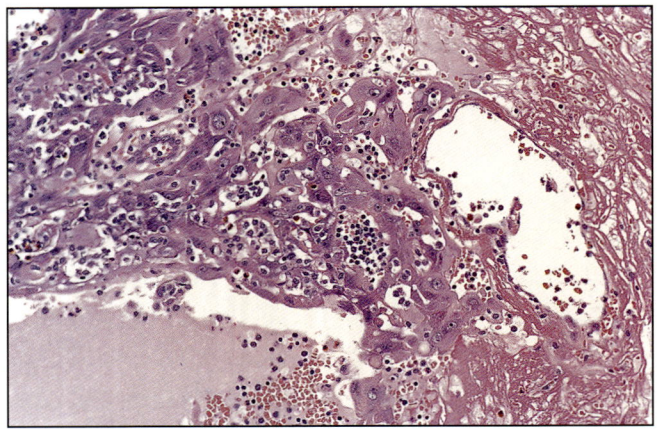

图18A.116 滤泡性腺瘤伴细针穿刺相关的上皮损伤。出血灶周围的甲状腺滤泡细胞相互吻合，显示非典型性，看上去类似血管肉瘤或高级别癌。

样结节或巨滤泡腺瘤）。

- 有包膜的富于细胞的滤泡性病变，冰冻切片上未见浸润：滤泡性肿瘤，依靠石蜡切片做出最终诊断（腺瘤或癌）；如果印片显示乳头状癌的核特征，则为乳头状癌滤泡亚型（或者如果核特征不十分明确，则为滤泡性肿瘤可疑乳头状癌）。
- 伴明确包膜或血管浸润的滤泡性病变：滤泡癌（大部分病例为广泛浸润型；微小浸润型很少于术中冰冻切片确诊）。
- 其他：髓样癌、淋巴瘤、未分化癌。

标本的进一步处理

标本固定后，需进一步取材进行组织学检查。对已一分为二有包膜的肿瘤而言，由于切面隆起，难以获得平行于原切面且带包膜的组织块。在剩余的半个肿块中行放射状切割更为可取，这样能更全面地评估肿瘤包膜。

参考文献

1. DeLellis R A, Williams E D 2004 Thyroid and parathyroid tumours: introduction. In: DeLellis R A, Lloyd R V, Heitz P U et al. (eds) Pathology and genetics. Tumours of endocrine organs. World Health Organization classification of tumours. IARC Press, Lyon, p 49–56
2. Gilliland F D, Hunt W C, Morris D M et al. 1997 Prognostic factors for thyroid carcinoma. A population-based study of 15,698 cases from the Surveillance, Epidemiology and End Results (SEER) program 1973–1991. Cancer 79: 564–573
3. Schlumberger M J 1998 Papillary and follicular thyroid carcinoma. N Engl J Med 338: 297–306
4. Brierley J D, Panzarella T, Tsang R W et al. 1997 A comparison of different staging systems predictability of patient outcome. Thyroid carcinoma as an example. Cancer 79: 2414–2423
5. Gemsenjager E, Heitz P U, Martina B 1997 Selective treatment of differentiated thyroid cancer. World J Surg 21: 546–551
6. Sobin L H, Wittekind C 2002 UICC: TNM classification of malignant tumours, 6th edn. Wiley, New York
7. Feinmesser R, Lubin E, Segal K et al. 1997 Carcinoma of the thyroid in children – a review. J Pediatr Endocrinol Metab 10: 561–568
8. Farahati J, Bucsky P, Parlowsky T et al. 1997 Characteristics of differentiated thyroid carcinoma in children and adolescents with respect to age, gender, and histology. Cancer 80: 2156–2162
9. Massimino M, Gasparini M, Ballerini E et al. 1995 Primary thyroid carcinoma in children: a retrospective study of 20 patients. Med Pediatr Oncol 24: 13–17
10. Giuffrida D, Scollo C, Pellegriti G et al. 2002 Differentiated thyroid cancer in children and adolescents. J Endocrinol Invest 25: 18–24
11. Landau D, Vini L, A'Hern R et al. 2000 Thyroid cancer in children: the Royal Marsden Hospital experience. Eur J Cancer 36: 214–220
12. Chow S M, Law S C, Mendenhall W M et al. 2004 Differentiated thyroid carcinoma in childhood and adolescence – clinical course and role of radioiodine. Pediatr Blood Cancer 42: 176–183
13. Borson-Chazot F, Causeret S, Lifante J C et al. 2004 Predictive factors for recurrence from a series of 74 children and adolescents with differentiated thyroid cancer. World J Surg 28: 1088–1092
14. Abelin T, Averkin J I, Egger M et al. 1994 Thyroid cancer in Belarus post-Chernobyl: improved detection or increased incidence? Soz Praventivmed 39: 189–197
15. Furmanchuk A W, Averkin J I, Egloff B et al. 1992 Pathomorphological findings in thyroid cancers of children from the Republic of Belarus: a study of 86 cases occurring between 1986 ("post-Chernobyl") and 1991. Histopathology 21: 401–408
16. Nikiforov Y, Gnepp D R 1994 Pediatric thyroid cancer after the Chernobyl disaster. Pathomorphologic study of 84 cases (1991–1992) from the Republic of Belarus. Cancer 74: 748–766
17. Nikiforov Y E, Heffess C S, Korzenko A V et al. 1995 Characteristics of follicular tumors and nonneoplastic thyroid lesions in children and adolescents exposed to radiation as a result of the Chernobyl disaster. Cancer 76: 900–909
18. Nikiforov Y, Gnepp D R, Fagin J A 1996 Thyroid lesions in children and adolescents after the Chernobyl disaster: implications for the study of radiation tumorigenesis. J Clin Endocrinol Metab 81: 9–14
19. Pacini F, Vorontsova T, Demidchik E P et al. 1997 Post-Chernobyl thyroid carcinoma in Belarus children and adolescents: comparison with naturally occurring thyroid carcinoma in Italy and France. J Clin Endocrinol Metab 82: 3563–3569
20. Tronko M D, Bogdanova T I, Komissarenko I V et al. 1999 Thyroid carcinoma in children and adolescents in Ukraine after the Chernobyl nuclear accident, statistical data and clinicomorphologic characteristics. Cancer 86: 149–156
21. Rybakov S J, Komissarenko I V, Tronko N D et al. 2000 Thyroid cancer in children of Ukraine after the Chernobyl accident. World J Surg 24: 1446–1449
22. Smith S A, Hay I D, Goellner J R et al. 1988 Mortality from papillary thyroid carcinoma. A case-control study of 56 lethal cases. Cancer 62: 1381–1388
23. Woodruff J M, Huvos A G, Erlandson R A et al. 1985 Neuroendocrine carcinomas of the larynx. A study of two types, one of which mimics thyroid medullary carcinoma. Am J Surg Pathol 9: 771–790
24. Carcangiu M L, Steeper T, Zampi G et al. 1985 Anaplastic thyroid carcinoma. A study of 70 cases. Am J Clin Pathol 83: 135–158
25. Bejarano P A, Nikiforov Y E, Swenson E S et al. 2000 Thyroid transcription factor-1, thyroglobulin, cytokeratin 7, and cytokeratin 20 in thyroid neoplasms. Appl Immunohistochem Mol Morphol 8: 189–194
26. Miettinen M, Franssila K O 2000 Variable expression of keratins and nearly uniform lack of thyroid transcription factor 1 in thyroid anaplastic carcinoma. Hum Pathol 31: 1139–1145
27. Katoh R, Kawaoi A, Miyagi E et al. 2000 Thyroid transcription factor-1 in normal, hyperplastic, and neoplastic follicular thyroid cells examined by immunohistochemistry and nonradioactive in situ hybridization. Mod Pathol 13: 570–576
28. Kotani T, Asada Y, Aratake Y et al. 1992 Diagnostic usefulness of dipeptidyl aminopeptidase IV monoclonal antibody in paraffin-embedded thyroid follicular tumours. J Pathol 168: 41–45
29. Gonzalez-Campora R, Galera-Ruiz D, Armas-Padron J R et al. 1998 Dipeptidyl aminopeptidase IV in the cytologic diagnosis of thyroid carcinoma. Diagn Cytopathol 19: 4–8
30. Sack M J, Astengo-Osuna C, Lin B T et al. 1997 HBME-1 immunostaining in thyroid fine-needle aspirations: a useful marker in the diagnosis of carcinoma. Mod Pathol 10: 668–674
31. Miettinen M, Karkkainen P 1996 Differential reactivity of HBME-1 and CD15 antibodies in benign and malignant thyroid tumours. Preferential reactivity with malignant tumours. Virchows Arch 429: 213–219
32. Tang A C, Raphael S J, Lampe H B et al. 1996 Expression of dipeptidyl aminopeptidase IV activity in thyroid tumours: a possible marker of thyroid malignancy. J Otolaryngol 25: 14–19
33. Umeki K, Tanaka T, Yamamoto I et al. 1996 Differential expression of dipeptidyl peptidase IV (CD26) and thyroid peroxidase in neoplastic thyroid tissues. Endocr J 43: 53–60
34. Cady B, Rossi R 1988 An expanded view of risk-group definition in differentiated thyroid carcinoma. Surgery 104: 947–953
35. Bongarzone I, Butti M G, Coronelli S et al. 1994 Frequent activation of ret protooncogene by fusion with a new activating gene in papillary thyroid carcinomas. Cancer Res 54: 2979–2985

36. Franssila K O 1973 Is the differentiation between papillary and follicular thyroid carcinoma valid? Cancer 32: 853–864
37. Rosai J, Carcangiu M L, DeLellis R A 1992 Tumors of the thyroid gland. Atlas of tumor pathology, series 3, fascicle 5. Armed Forces Institute of Pathology, Washington, DC
38. Wright P A, Lemoine N R, Mayall E S et al. 1989 Papillary and follicular thyroid carcinomas show a different pattern of ras oncogene mutation. Br J Cancer 60: 576–577
39. Chow S M, Law S C, Au S K et al. 2002 Differentiated thyroid carcinoma: comparison between papillary and follicular carcinoma in a single institute. Head Neck 24: 670–677
40. Aldred M A, Huang Y, Liyanarachchi S et al. 2004 Papillary and follicular thyroid carcinomas show distinctly different microarray expression profiles and can be distinguished by a minimum of five genes. J Clin Oncol 22: 3531–3539
41. Carcangiu M L, Zampi G, Rosai J 1985 Papillary thyroid carcinoma: a study of its many morphologic expressions and clinical correlates. Pathol Annu 20: 1–44
42. Hedinger C, Williams E D, Sobin L H 1989 The WHO histological classification of thyroid tumors: a commentary on the second edition. Cancer 63: 908–911
43. Chan J K 1990 Papillary carcinoma of thyroid: classical and variants. Histol Histopathol 5: 241–257
44. Rosai J, Carcangiu M L 1987 Pitfalls in the diagnosis of thyroid neoplasms. Pathol Res Pract 182: 169–179
45. Beaugie J M, Brown C L, Doniach I et al. 1976 Primary malignant tumours of the thyroid: the relationship between histological classification and clinical behaviour. Br J Surg 63: 173–181
46. Hirabayashi R N, Lindsay S 1961 Carcinoma of the thyroid gland: a statistical study of 390 patients. J Clin Endocrinol Metab 21: 1596–1610
47. McConahey W M, Hay I D, Woolner L B et al. 1986 Papillary thyroid cancer treated at the Mayo Clinic, 1946 through 1970: initial manifestations, pathologic findings, therapy, and outcome. Mayo Clin Proc 61: 978–996
48. Meissner W A, Adler A 1958 Papillary carcinoma of the thyroid, a study of the pattern in 226 patients. Arch Pathol 66: 518–525
49. Collini P, Sampietro G, Rosai J et al. 2003 Minimally invasive (encapsulated) follicular carcinoma of the thyroid gland is the low-risk counterpart of widely invasive follicular carcinoma but not of insular carcinoma. Virchows Arch 442: 71–76
50. Verge J, Guixa J, Alejo M et al. 1999 Cervical cystic lymph node metastasis as first manifestation of occult papillary thyroid carcinoma: report of seven cases. Head Neck 21: 370–374
51. al-Talib R K, Wilkins B S, Theaker J M 1992 Cystic metastasis of papillary carcinoma of the thyroid – an unusual presentation. Histopathology 20: 176–178
52. Fernandez J F, Ordonez N G, Schultz P N et al. 1991 Thyroglossal duct carcinoma. Surgery 110: 928–934
53. Williams E D 1979 The aetiology of thyroid tumours. Clin Endocrinol Metab 8: 193–207
54. Plail R O, Bussey H J, Glazer G et al. 1987 Adenomatous polyposis: an association with carcinoma of the thyroid. Br J Surg 74: 377–380
55. Eng C, Parsons R 1998 Cowden syndrome. In: Vogelstein B, Kinzler K W (eds) The genetic basis of human cancer. McGraw-Hill, New York, p 519–525
56. Burgess J R, Duffield A, Wilkinson S J et al. 1997 Two families with an autosomal dominant inheritance pattern for papillary carcinoma of the thyroid. J Clin Endocrinol Metab 82: 345–348
57. Loh K C 1997 Familial nonmedullary thyroid carcinoma: a meta-review of case series. Thyroid 7: 107–113
58. Kraimps J L, Bouin-Pineau M H, Amati P et al. 1997 Familial papillary carcinoma of the thyroid. Surgery 121: 715–718
59. Lupoli G, Vitale G, Caraglia M et al. 1999 Familial papillary thyroid microcarcinoma: a new clinical entity. Lancet 353: 637–639
60. Foulkes W D, Kloos R T, Harach H R et al. 2004 Familial non-medullary thyroid cancer. In: DeLellis R A, Lloyd R V, Heitz P U et al. (eds) Pathology and genetics. Tumours of endocrine organs. World Health Organization classification of tumours. IARC Press, Lyon, p 257–261
61. Gimm O, Rath F W, Dralle H 1998 Pattern of lymph node metastases in papillary thyroid carcinoma. Br J Surg 85: 252–254
62. Shaha A R, Shah J P, Loree T R 1997 Differentiated thyroid cancer presenting initially with distant metastasis. Am J Surg 174: 474–476
63. Carcangiu M L, Zampi G, Pupi A et al. 1985 Papillary carcinoma of the thyroid. A clinicopathologic study of 241 cases treated at the University of Florence, Italy. Cancer 55: 805–828
64. Lindsay A 1969 Papillary thyroid carcinoma revisited. In: Hedinger C E (ed) Thyroid cancer. Springer-Verlag, Berlin, p 29–32
65. Tubiana M, Schlumberger M, Rougier P et al. 1985 Long-term results and prognostic factors in patients with differentiated thyroid carcinoma. Cancer 55: 794–804
66. Cady B 1998 Papillary carcinoma of the thyroid gland: treatment based on risk group definition. Surg Oncol Clin North Am 7: 633–644
67. Hay I D, Bergstralh E J, Goellner J R et al. 1993 Predicting outcome in papillary thyroid carcinoma: development of a reliable prognostic scoring system in a cohort of 1779 patients surgically treated at one institution during 1940 through 1989. Surgery 114: 1050–1057
68. Sanders L E, Cady B 1998 Differentiated thyroid cancer: reexamination of risk groups and outcome of treatment. Arch Surg 133: 419–425
69. Harness J K, McLeod M K, Thompson N W et al. 1988 Deaths due to differentiated thyroid cancer: a 46-year perspective. World J Surg 12: 623–629
70. Chen H, Udelsman R 1998 Papillary thyroid carcinoma: justification for total thyroidectomy and management of lymph node metastases. Surg Oncol Clin North Am 7: 645–663
71. Wax M K, Briant T D 1992 Completion thyroidectomy in the management of well-differentiated thyroid carcinoma. Otolaryngol Head Neck Surg 107: 63–68
72. Lerch H, Schober O, Kuwert T et al. 1997 Survival of differentiated thyroid carcinoma studied in 500 patients. J Clin Oncol 15: 2067–2075
73. Shah J P, Loree T R, Dharker D et al. 1993 Lobectomy versus total thyroidectomy for differentiated carcinoma of the thyroid: a matched-pair analysis. Am J Surg 166: 331–335
74. Van Nguyen K, Dilawari R A 1995 Predictive value of AMES scoring system in selection of extent of surgery in well differentiated carcinoma of thyroid. Am Surg 61: 151–155
75. Vickery A L Jr. 1983 Thyroid papillary carcinoma. Pathological and philosophical controversies. Am J Surg Pathol 7: 797–807
76. Vickery A L Jr., Wang C A, Walker A M 1987 Treatment of intrathyroidal papillary carcinoma of the thyroid. Cancer 60: 2587–2595
77. Hoie J, Stenwig A E, Brennhovd I O 1988 Surgery in papillary thyroid carcinoma: a review of 730 patients. J Surg Oncol 37: 147–151
78. Shaha A R, Shaha J P, Loree T R 1996 Risk group stratification and prognostic factors in papillary carcinoma of thyroid. Ann Surg Oncol 3: 534–538
79. Loree T R 1995 Therapeutic implications of prognostic factors in differentiated carcinoma of the thyroid gland. Semin Surg Oncol 11: 246–255
80. Beenken S, Guillamondegui O, Shallenberger R et al. 1989 Prognostic factors in patients dying of well-differentiated thyroid cancer. Arch Otolaryngol Head Neck Surg 115: 326–330
81. Busnardo B, Girelli M E, Rubello D et al. 1989 Favorable long term results in patients with small differentiated thyroid cancer not treated with radioiodine. Tumori 75: 57–59
82. Mazzaferri E L 1987 Papillary thyroid carcinoma: factors influencing prognosis and current therapy. Semin Oncol 14: 315–332
83. Chow S M, Law S C, Mendenhall W M et al. 2002 Papillary thyroid carcinoma: prognostic factors and the role of radioiodine and external radiotherapy. Int J Radiat Oncol Biol Phys 52: 784–795
84. Noguchi S, Murakami N, Yamashita H et al. 1998 Papillary thyroid carcinoma: modified radical neck dissection improves prognosis. Arch Surg 133: 276–280
85. Goropoulos A, Karamoshos K, Christodoulou A et al. 2004 Value of the cervical compartments in the surgical treatment of papillary thyroid carcinoma. World J Surg 28: 1275–1281
86. Gemsenjager E, Perren A, Seifert B et al. 2003 Lymph node surgery in papillary thyroid carcinoma. J Am Coll Surg 197: 182–190
87. Arch-Ferrer J, Velazquez D, Fajardo R et al. 2001 Accuracy of sentinel lymph node in papillary thyroid carcinoma. Surgery 130: 907–913
88. Chow T L, Lim B H, Kwok S P 2004 Sentinel lymph node dissection in papillary thyroid carcinoma. ANZ J Surg 74: 10–12
89. Fukui Y, Yamakawa T, Taniki T et al. 2001 Sentinel lymph node biopsy in patients with papillary thyroid carcinoma. Cancer 92: 2868–2874
90. Segal K, Friedental R, Lubin E et al. 1995 Papillary carcinoma of the thyroid. Otolaryngol Head Neck Surg 113: 356–363
91. Hawk W A, Hazard J B 1976 The many appearances of papillary carcinoma of the thyroid. Cleve Clin Q 43: 207–215
92. Katoh R, Sasaki J, Kurihara H et al. 1992 Multiple thyroid involvement (intraglandular metastasis) in papillary thyroid carcinoma. A clinicopathologic study of 105 consecutive patients. Cancer 70: 1585–1590
93. Russell W D, Ibanez M L, Clark R L et al. 1963 Thyroid carcinoma: classification, intraglandular dissemination, and clinicopathologic study based upon whole organ section of 80 glands. Cancer 11: 1425–1460
94. Sugg S L, Ezzat S, Rosen I B et al. 1998 Distinct multiple RET/PTC gene rearrangements in multifocal papillary thyroid neoplasia. J Clin Endocrinol Metab 83: 4116–4122
95. Shattuck T M, Westra W H, Ladenson P W et al. 2005. Independent clonal origins of distinct tumor foci in multifocal papillary thyroid carcinoma. N Engl J Med 352: 2406–2412
96. McCarthy R P, Wang M, Jones T D et al. 2006 Molecular evidence for the same clonal origin of multifocal papillary thyroid carcinomas. Clin Cancer Res 12: 2414–2418
97. Hapke M R, Dehner L P 1979 The optically clear nucleus. A reliable sign of papillary carcinoma of the thyroid? Am J Surg Pathol 3: 31–38
98. Kraemer B B 1987 Frozen section diagnosis and the thyroid. Semin Diagn Pathol 4: 169–189
99. Kiyono T, Katagiri M, Harada T 1994 The incidence of ground glass nuclei in thyroid diseases. Thyroidology 6: 43–48
100. Chan J K, Saw D 1986 The grooved nucleus. A useful diagnostic criterion of papillary carcinoma of the thyroid. Am J Surg Pathol 10: 672–679
101. Deligeorgi-Politi H 1987 Nuclear crease as a cytodiagnostic feature of papillary thyroid carcinoma in fine-needle aspiration biopsies. Diagn Cytopathol 3: 307–310
102. Gould E, Watzak L, Chamizo W et al. 1989 Nuclear grooves in cytologic preparations. A study of the utility of this feature in the diagnosis of papillary carcinoma. Acta Cytol 33: 16–20

103. Shurbaji M S, Gupta P K, Frost J K 1988 Nuclear grooves: a useful criterion in the cytopathologic diagnosis of papillary thyroid carcinoma. Diagn Cytopathol 4: 91–94
104. Carney J A, Ryan J, Goellner J R 1987 Hyalinizing trabecular adenoma of the thyroid gland. Am J Surg Pathol 11: 583–591
105. Scopa C D, Melachrinou M, Saradopoulou C et al. 1993 The significance of the grooved nucleus in thyroid lesions. Mod Pathol 6: 691–694
106. Glant M D, Berger E K, Davey D D 1984 Intranuclear cytoplasmic inclusions in aspirates of follicular neoplasms of the thyroid. A report of two cases. Acta Cytol 28: 576–580
107. Oyama T 1989 A histopathological, immunohistochemical and ultrastructural study of intranuclear cytoplasmic inclusions in thyroid papillary carcinoma. Virchows Arch A Pathol Anat Histopathol 414: 91–104
108. Vickery A L, Carcangiu M L, Johannessen J V 1985 Papillary carcinoma. Semin Diagn Pathol 2: 90–100
109. Hazard J B 1968 Nomenclature of thyroid tumors. In: Young S, Inman D R (eds) Thyroid neoplasia. Academic Press, London, 3–37
110. Sobrinho-Simoes M, Sambade C, Nesland J M 1989 Tall cell papillary carcinoma (Letter). Am J Surg Pathol 13: 79–80
111. Carcangiu M L, Sibley R K, Rosai J 1985 Clear cell change in primary thyroid tumors. A study of 38 cases. Am J Surg Pathol 9: 705–722
112. Dickersin G R, Vickery A L Jr., Smith S B 1980 Papillary carcinoma of the thyroid, oxyphil cell type, "clear cell" variant: a light- and electron-microscopic study. Am J Surg Pathol 4: 501–509
113. Schroder S, Bocker W 1986 Clear-cell carcinomas of thyroid gland: a clinicopathological study of 13 cases. Histopathology 10: 75–89
114. Variakojis D, Getz M L, Paloyan E et al. 1975 Papillary clear cell carcinoma of the thyroid gland. Hum Pathol 6: 384–390
115. Chan J K, Tse C C 1988 Mucin production in metastatic papillary carcinoma of the thyroid. Hum Pathol 19: 195–200
116. Mlynek M L, Richter H J, Leder L D 1985 Mucin in carcinomas of the thyroid. Cancer 56: 2647–2650
117. Mai K T, Perkins D G, Yazdi H M et al. 1998 Infiltrating papillary thyroid carcinoma: review of 134 cases of papillary carcinoma. Arch Pathol Lab Med 122: 166–171
118. Bruno R, Ciancia E M, Pingitore R 1989 Thyroid papillary adenocarcinoma: lipomatous-type. Virchows Arch A Pathol Anat Histopathol 414: 371–373
119. Gnepp D R, Ogorzalek J M, Heffess C S 1989 Fat-containing lesions of the thyroid gland. Am J Surg Pathol 13: 605–612
120. Vestfrid M A 1986 Papillary carcinoma of the thyroid gland with lipomatous stroma: report of a peculiar histological type of thyroid tumour. Histopathology 10: 97–100
121. Chan J K, Loo K T 1990 Cribriform variant of papillary carcinoma. Arch Pathol Lab Med 114: 622–624
122. Isarangkul W 1993 Dense fibrosis. Another diagnostic criterion for papillary thyroid carcinoma. Arch Pathol Lab Med 117: 645–646
123. Yamashita H, Noguchi S, Murakami N et al. 1993 DNA ploidy and stromal bone formation as prognostic indicators of thyroid papillary carcinoma in aged patients: a retrospective study. Acta Pathol Jpn 43: 22–27
124. Guiter G E, DeLellis R A 1996 Multinucleate giant cells in papillary thyroid carcinoma. A morphologic and immunohistochemical study. Am J Clin Pathol 106: 765–768
125. Johannessen J V, Sobrinho-Simoes M 1980 The origin and significance of thyroid psammoma bodies. Lab Invest 43: 287–296
126. Chen K T, Rosai J 1977 Follicular variant of thyroid papillary carcinoma: a clinicopathologic study of six cases. Am J Surg Pathol 1: 123–130
127. Rosai J, Zampi G, Carcangiu M L 1983 Papillary carcinoma of the thyroid. A discussion of its several morphologic expressions, with particular emphasis on the follicular variant. Am J Surg Pathol 7: 809–817
128. Zidan J, Karen D, Stein M et al. 2003 Pure versus follicular variant of papillary thyroid carcinoma: clinical features, prognostic factors, treatment, and survival. Cancer 97: 1181–1815
129. Passler C, Prager G, Scheuba C et al. 2003 Follicular variant of papillary thyroid carcinoma: a long-term follow-up. Arch Surg 138: 1362–1366
130. Woolner L B 1971 Thyroid carcinoma: pathologic classification with data on prognosis. Semin Nucl Med 1: 481–502
131. Nikiforov Y E, Erickson L A, Nikiforova M N et al. 2001 Solid variant of papillary thyroid carcinoma: incidence, clinical-pathologic characteristics, molecular analysis, and biologic behavior. Am J Surg Pathol 25: 1478–1484
132. Schroder S, Bocker W, Dralle H et al. 1984 The encapsulated papillary carcinoma of the thyroid. A morphologic subtype of the papillary thyroid carcinoma. Cancer 54: 90–93
133. Moreno A, Rodriguez J M, Sola J et al. 1996 Encapsulated papillary neoplasm of the thyroid: retrospective clinicopathological study with long term follow up. Eur J Surg 162: 177–180
134. Evans H L 1987 Encapsulated papillary neoplasms of the thyroid. A study of 14 cases followed for a minimum of 10 years. Am J Surg Pathol 11: 592–597
135. Chan J K, Tsui M S, Tse C H 1987 Diffuse sclerosing variant of papillary carcinoma of the thyroid: a histological and immunohistochemical study of three cases. Histopathology 11: 191–201
136. Hayashi Y, Sasao T, Takeichi N et al. 1990 Diffuse sclerosing variant of papillary carcinoma of the thyroid. A histopathological study of four cases. Acta Pathol Jpn 40: 193–198
137. Fujimoto Y, Obara T, Ito Y et al. 1990 Diffuse sclerosing variant of papillary carcinoma of the thyroid. Clinical importance, surgical treatment, and follow-up study. Cancer 66: 2306–2312
138. Albareda M, Puig-Domingo M, Wengrowicz S et al. 1998 Clinical forms of presentation and evolution of diffuse sclerosing variant of papillary carcinoma and insular variant of follicular carcinoma of the thyroid. Thyroid 8: 385–391
139. Carcangiu M L, Bianchi S 1989 Diffuse sclerosing variant of papillary thyroid carcinoma. Clinicopathologic study of 15 cases. Am J Surg Pathol 13: 1041–1049
140. Carcangiu M L, Bianchi S, Rosai J 1987 Diffuse sclerosing papillary carcinoma: report of 8 cases of a distinctive variant of thyroid malignancy (Abstract). Lab Invest 56: 10A
141. Soares J, Limbert E, Sobrinho-Simoes M 1989 Diffuse sclerosing variant of papillary thyroid carcinoma. A clinicopathologic study of 10 cases. Pathol Res Pract 185: 200–206
142. Schroder S, Bay V, Dumke K et al. 1990 Diffuse sclerosing variant of papillary thyroid carcinoma. S-100 protein immunocytochemistry and prognosis. Virchows Arch A Pathol Anat Histopathol 416: 367–371
143. Chow S M, Chan J K, Law S C et al. 2003 Diffuse sclerosing variant of papillary thyroid carcinoma – clinical features and outcome. Eur J Surg Oncol 29: 446–449
144. Lam A K, Lo C Y 2006 Diffuse sclerosing variant of papillary carcinoma of the thyroid: a 35-year comparative study at a single institution. Ann Surg Oncol 13: 176–181
145. Gomez-Morales M, Aneiros J, Alvaro T et al. 1989 Langerhans' cells and prognosis of thyroid carcinoma (Letter). Am J Clin Pathol 91: 628–629
146. Gomez-Morales M, Alvaro T, Munoz M et al. 1991 Diffuse sclerosing papillary carcinoma of the thyroid gland: immunohistochemical analysis of the local host immune response. Histopathology 18: 427–433
147. Sobrinho-Simoes M, Soares J, Carneiro F 1990 Diffuse follicular variant of papillary carcinoma of the thyroid: report of eight cases of a distinct aggressive type of thyroid tumor. Surg Pathol 3: 189–203
148. Mizukami Y, Nonomura A, Michigishi T et al. 1995 Diffuse follicular variant of papillary carcinoma of the thyroid. Histopathology 27: 575–577
149. Ivanova R, Soares P, Castro P et al. 2002 Diffuse (or multinodular) follicular variant of papillary thyroid carcinoma: a clinicopathologic and immunohistochemical analysis of ten cases of an aggressive form of differentiated thyroid carcinoma. Virchows Arch 440: 418–424
150. Johnson T L, Lloyd R V, Thompson N W et al. 1988 Prognostic implications of the tall cell variant of papillary thyroid carcinoma. Am J Surg Pathol 12: 22–27
151. Ostrowski M L, Merino M J 1996 Tall cell variant of papillary thyroid carcinoma: a reassessment and immunohistochemical study with comparison to the usual type of papillary carcinoma of the thyroid. Am J Surg Pathol 20: 964–974
152. LiVolsi V A, Albores-Saavedra J, Asa S L et al. 2004 Papillary carcinoma. In: DeLellis R A, Lloyd R V, Heitz P U et al. (eds) Pathology and genetics. Tumours of endocrine organs. World Health Organization classification of tumours. IARC Press, Lyon, p 57–66
153. Terry J H, St John S A, Karkowski F J et al. 1994 Tall cell papillary thyroid cancer: incidence and prognosis. Am J Surg 168: 459–461
154. Machens A, Holzhausen H J, Lautenschlager C et al. 2004 The tall-cell variant of papillary thyroid carcinoma: a multivariate analysis of clinical risk factors. Langenbecks Arch Surg 389: 278–282
155. Ruter A, Dreifus J, Jones M et al. 1996 Overexpression of p53 in tall cell variants of papillary thyroid carcinoma. Surgery 120: 1046–1050
156. Ruter A, Nishiyama R, Lennquist S 1997 Tall-cell variant of papillary thyroid cancer: disregarded entity? World J Surg 21: 15–20
157. Bronner M P, LiVolsi V A 1991 Spindle cell squamous carcinoma of the thyroid: an unusual anaplastic tumor associated with tall cell papillary cancer. Mod Pathol 4: 637–643
158. van den Brekel M W, Hekkenberg R J, Asa S L et al. 1997 Prognostic features in tall cell papillary carcinoma and insular thyroid carcinoma. Laryngoscope 107: 254–259
159. Kleer C G, Giordano T J, Merino M J 2000 Squamous cell carcinoma of the thyroid: an aggressive tumor associated with tall cell variant of papillary carcinoma. Mod Pathol 13: 742–746
160. Nardone H C, Ziober A F, LiVolsi V A et al. 2003 c-Met expression in tall cell variant papillary carcinoma of the thyroid. Cancer 98: 1386–1393
161. Basolo F, Giannini R, Monaco C et al. 2002 Potent mitogenicity of the RET/PTC3 oncogene correlates with its prevalence in tall-cell variant of papillary thyroid carcinoma. Am J Pathol 160: 247–254
162. Monteagudo C, Ain K, Merino M 1990 Mixed forms of tall cell thyroid carcinoma: a clinicopathologic and immunohistochemical study (Abstract). Lab Invest 62: 69A
163. Perez Montiel D, Cantu De Leon D F, Morrison C et al. 2006 Clinical significance of tall cell morphology in papillary thyroid carcinoma: clinicopathologic study of 92 cases (Abstract). Mod Pathol 19: 96A
164. Sobrinho-Simoes M A, Nesland J M, Holm R et al. 1985 Hurthle cell and mitochondrion-rich papillary carcinomas of the thyroid gland: an ultrastructural and immunocytochemical study. Ultrastruct Pathol 8: 131–142
165. Tscholl-Ducommun J, Hedinger C E 1982 Papillary thyroid carcinomas. Morphology and prognosis. Virchows Arch Pathol Anat 396: 19–39
166. Beckner M E, Heffess C S, Oertel J E 1995 Oxyphilic papillary thyroid carcinomas. Am J Clin Pathol 103: 280–287
167. Berho M, Suster S 1997 The oncocytic variant of papillary carcinoma of the thyroid: a clinicopathologic study of 15 cases. Hum Pathol 28: 47–53

168. Sobrinho-Simoes M, Maximo V, Castro I V et al. 2005 Hurthle (oncocytic) cell tumors of thyroid: etiopathogenesis, diagnosis and clinical significance. Int J Surg Pathol 13: 29–35
169. Asa S L 2004 My approach to oncocytic tumours of the thyroid. J Clin Pathol 57: 225–232
170. Apel R L, Asa S L, LiVolsi V A 1995 Papillary Hurthle cell carcinoma with lymphocytic stroma. "Warthin-like tumor" of the thyroid. Am J Surg Pathol 19: 810–814
171. Vera-Sempere F J, Prieto M, Camanas A 1998 Warthin-like tumor of the thyroid: a papillary carcinoma with mitochondrion-rich cells and abundant lymphoid stroma. A case report. Pathol Res Pract 194: 341–347
172. Baloch Z W, LiVolsi V A 2000 Warthin-like papillary carcinoma of the thyroid. Arch Pathol Lab Med 124: 1192–1195
173. Ludvikova M, Ryska A, Korabecna M et al. 2001 Oncocytic papillary carcinoma with lymphoid stroma (Warthin-like tumour) of the thyroid: a distinct entity with favourable prognosis. Histopathology 39: 17–24
174. D'Antonio A, De Chiara A, Santoro M et al. 2000 Warthin-like tumour of the thyroid gland: RET/PTC expression indicates it is a variant of papillary carcinoma. Histopathology 36: 493–498
175. Lam K Y, Lo C Y, Wei W I 2005 Warthin tumor-like variant of papillary thyroid carcinoma: a case with dedifferentiation (anaplastic changes) and aggressive biological behavior. Endocr Pathol 16: 83–89
176. Ozaki O, Ito K, Mimura T et al. 1996 Papillary carcinoma of the thyroid. Tall-cell variant with extensive lymphocyte infiltration. Am J Surg Pathol 20: 695–698
177. Asanuma K, Sugenoya A, Ohashi T et al. 1998 Pure clear cell papillary thyroid carcinoma with chronic thyroiditis: report of a case. Surg Today 28: 464–466
178. Civantos F, Albores-Saavedra J, Nadji M et al. 1984 Clear cell variant of thyroid carcinoma. Am J Surg Pathol 8: 187–192
179. Nakamura T, Moriyama S, Nariya S et al. 1998 Macrofollicular variant of papillary thyroid carcinoma. Pathol Int 48: 467–470
180. Albores-Saavedra J, Gould E, Vardaman C et al. 1991 The macrofollicular variant of papillary thyroid carcinoma: a study of 17 cases. Hum Pathol 22: 1195–1205
181. Albores-Saavedra J, Housini I, Vuitch F et al. 1997 Macrofollicular variant of papillary thyroid carcinoma with minor insular component. Cancer 80: 1110-1116
182. Lugli A, Terracciano L M, Oberholzer M et al. 2004 Macrofollicular variant of papillary carcinoma of the thyroid: a histologic, cytologic, and immunohistochemical study of 3 cases and review of the literature. Arch Pathol Lab Med 128: 54–58
183. Fadda G, Fiorino M C, Mule A et al. 2002 Macrofollicular encapsulated variant of papillary thyroid carcinoma as a potential pitfall in histologic and cytologic diagnosis. A report of three cases. Acta Cytol 46: 555–559
184. Mizukami Y, Noguchi M, Michigishi T et al. 1992 Papillary thyroid carcinoma in Kanazawa, Japan: prognostic significance of histological subtypes. Histopathology 20: 243–250
185. Sakamoto A, Kasai N, Sugano H 1983 Poorly differentiated carcinoma of the thyroid. A clinicopathologic entity for a high-risk group of papillary and follicular carcinomas. Cancer 52: 1849–1855
186. Cameselle-Teijeiro J, Chan J K 1999 Cribriform-morular variant of papillary carcinoma: a distinctive variant representing the sporadic counterpart of familial adenomatous polyposis-associated thyroid carcinoma? Mod Pathol 12: 400–411
187. Yamashita T, Hosoda Y, Kameyama K et al. 1992 Peculiar nuclear clearing composed of microfilaments in papillary carcinoma of the thyroid. Cancer 70: 2923–2928
188. Tsang W Y, Chan J K 1993 Peculiar nuclear clearing composed of microfilaments in papillary carcinoma of the thyroid (Letter). Cancer 72: 300.
189. Tomoda C, Miyauchi A, Uruno T et al. 2004 Cribriform-morular variant of papillary thyroid carcinoma: clue to early detection of familial adenomatous polyposis-associated colon cancer. World J Surg 28: 886–889
190. Harach H R, Williams G T, Williams E D 1994 Familial adenomatous polyposis associated thyroid carcinoma: a distinct type of follicular cell neoplasm. Histopathology 25: 549–561
191. Cetta F, Toti P, Petracci M et al. 1997 Thyroid carcinoma associated with familial adenomatous polyposis. Histopathology 31: 231–236
192. Perrier N D, van Heerden J A, Goellner J R et al. 1998 Thyroid cancer in patients with familial adenomatous polyposis. World J Surg 22: 738–742
193. Soravia C, Sugg S L, Berk T et al. 1999 Familial adenomatous polyposis-associated thyroid cancer: a clinical, pathological, and molecular genetics study. Am J Pathol 154: 127–135
194. Cetta F, Pelizzo M R, Curia M C et al. 1999 Genetics and clinicopathological findings in thyroid carcinomas associated with familial adenomatous polyposis. Am J Pathol 155: 7–9
195. Cetta F, Chiappetta G, Melillo R M et al. 1998 The ret/ptc1 oncogene is activated in familial adenomatous polyposis-associated thyroid papillary carcinomas. J Clin Endocrinol Metab 83: 1003–1006
196. Iwama T, Konishi M, Iijima T et al. 1999 Somatic mutation of the APC gene in thyroid carcinoma associated with familial adenomatous polyposis. Jpn J Cancer Res 90: 372–376
197. Cameselle-Teijeiro J, Ruiz-Ponte C, Loidi L et al. 2001 Somatic but not germline mutation of the APC gene in a case of cribriform-morular variant of papillary thyroid carcinoma. Am J Clin Pathol 115: 486–493
198. Kameyama K, Mukai M, Takami H et al. 2004 Cribriform-morular variant of papillary thyroid carcinoma: ultrastructural study and somatic/germline mutation analysis of the APC gene. Ultrastruct Pathol 28: 97–102
199. Xu B, Yoshimoto K, Miyauchi A et al. 2003 Cribriform-morular variant of papillary thyroid carcinoma: a pathological and molecular genetic study with evidence of frequent somatic mutations in exon 3 of the beta-catenin gene. J Pathol 199: 58–67
200. Ishigaki K, Namba H, Nakashima M et al. 2002 Aberrant localization of beta-catenin correlates with overexpression of its target gene in human papillary thyroid cancer. J Clin Endocrinol Metab 87: 3433–3440
201. Akslen L A, Maehle B O 1997 Papillary thyroid carcinoma with lipomatous stroma (Letter). Am J Surg Pathol 21: 1256–1257
202. Bisi H, Longatto Filho A, de Camargo R Y et al. 1993 Thyroid papillary carcinoma lipomatous type: report of two cases. Pathologica 85: 761–764
203. Chan J K, Carcangiu M L, Rosai J 1991 Papillary carcinoma of thyroid with exuberant nodular fasciitis-like stroma. Report of three cases. Am J Clin Pathol 95: 309–314
204. Michal M, Chlumska A, Fakan F 1992 Papillary carcinoma of thyroid with exuberant nodular fasciitis-like stroma. Histopathology 21: 577–579
205. Mizukami Y, Nonomura A, Matsubara F et al. 1992 Papillary carcinoma of the thyroid gland with fibromatosis-like stroma. Histopathology 20: 355–357
206. Terayama K, Toda S, Yonemitsu N et al. 1997 Papillary carcinoma of the thyroid with exuberant nodular fasciitis-like stroma. Virchows Arch 431: 291–295
207. Acosta J, Rodriguez J M, Sola J et al. 1998 Nodular fasciitis-type papillary thyroid carcinoma. Presentation of a new case. Eur J Surg Oncol 24: 80–81
208. Mizukami Y, Kurumaya H, Kitagawa T et al. 1995 Papillary carcinoma of the thyroid gland with fibromatosis-like stroma: a case report and review of the literature. Mod Pathol 8: 366–370.
209. Toti P, Tanganelli P, Schurfeld K et al. 1999 Scarring in papillary carcinoma of the thyroid: report of two new cases with exuberant nodular fasciitis-like stroma. Histopathology 35: 418–422
210. Inaba M, Umemura S, Satoh H et al. 2002 Papillary carcinoma with fibromatosis-like stroma: a report of two cases. Endocr Pathol 13: 219–225
211. Ostrowski M A, Moffat F L, Asa S L et al. 1989 Myxomatous change in papillary carcinoma of the thyroid, a morphologic subtype of the papillary thyroid carcinoma. Surg Pathol 2: 249–256
212. Woenckhaus C, Cameselle-Teijeiro J, Ruiz-Ponte C et al. 2004 Spindle cell variant of papillary thyroid carcinoma. Histopathology 45: 424–427
213. Vergilio J, Baloch Z W, LiVolsi V A 2002 Spindle cell metaplasia of the thyroid arising in association with papillary carcinoma and follicular adenoma. Am J Clin Pathol 117: 199–204
214. Brandwein-Gensler M S, Wang B Y, Urken M L 2004 Spindle cell transformation of papillary carcinoma: an aggressive entity distinct from anaplastic thyroid carcinoma. Arch Pathol Lab Med 128: 87–89
215. Kawahara E, Ooi A, Oda Y et al. 1986 Papillary carcinoma of the thyroid gland with anaplastic transformation in the metastatic foci. An immunohistochemical study. Acta Pathol Jpn 36: 921–927
216. Spires J R, Schwartz M R, Miller R H 1988 Anaplastic thyroid carcinoma. Association with differentiated thyroid cancer. Arch Otolaryngol Head Neck Surg 114: 40–44
217. Tollefsen R H, DeCosse J J, Hutter R V P 1964 Papillary carcinoma of the thyroid: a clinical and pathological study of 20 fatal cases. Cancer 17: 1035–1044
218. Aldinger K A, Samaan N A, Ibanez M et al. 1978 Anaplastic carcinoma of the thyroid: a review of 84 cases of spindle and giant cell carcinoma of the thyroid. Cancer 41: 2267–2275
219. Rodriguez J M, Moreno A, Parrilla P et al. 1997 Papillary thyroid microcarcinoma: clinical study and prognosis. Eur J Surg 163: 255–259
220. Hedinger C, Williams E D, Sobin L H 1988 Histological typing of thyroid tumors. WHO international histological classification of tumors, 2nd end. Springer-Verlag, Berlin
221. Ito J, Noguchi S, Murakami N et al. 1980 Factors affecting the prognosis of patients with carcinoma of the thyroid. Surg Gynecol Obstet 150: 539–544
222. Chen K T 1989 Minute (less than 1 mm) occult papillary thyroid carcinoma with metastasis (Letter). Am J Clin Pathol 91: 746
223. Kasai N, Sakamoto A 1987 New subgrouping of small thyroid carcinomas. Cancer 60: 1767–1770
224. Laskin W B, James L P 1983 Occult papillary carcinoma of the thyroid with pulmonary metastases. Hum Pathol 14: 83–85
225. Sampson R J, Key C R, Buncher C R et al. 1971 Smallest forms of papillary carcinoma of the thyroid. A study of 141 microcarcinomas less than 0.1 cm in greatest dimension. Arch Pathol 91: 334–339
226. Strate S M, Lee E L, Childers J H 1984 Occult papillary carcinoma of the thyroid with distant metastases. Cancer 54: 1093–1100
227. Rassel H, Thompson L D, Heffess C S 1998 A rationale for conservative management of microscopic papillary carcinoma of the thyroid gland: a clinicopathologic correlation of 90 cases. Eur Arch Otorhinolaryngol 255: 462–467
228. Sugitani I, Yanagisawa A, Shimizu S et al. 1998 Clinicopathologic and immunohistochemical studies of papillary thyroid microcarcinoma presenting with cervical lymphadenopathy. World J Surg 22: 731–737
229. Fukunaga F H, Yatani R 1975 Geographic pathology of occult thyroid carcinomas. Cancer 36: 1095–1099

230. Harach H R, Franssila K O, Wasenius V M 1985 Occult papillary carcinoma of the thyroid. A "normal" finding in Finland. A systematic autopsy study. Cancer 56: 531–538
231. Sampson R J 1977 Prevalence and significance of occult thyroid cancer. In: DeGroot L J, Frohman L A, Kaplan D L (eds) Radiation-associated thyroid carcinoma. Grune & Stratton, New York, p 137–153
232. Arellano L, Ibarra A 1984 Occult carcinoma of the thyroid gland. Pathol Res Pract 179: 88–91
233. Bondeson L, Ljungberg O 1981 Occult thyroid carcinoma at autopsy in Malmo, Sweden. Cancer 47: 319–323
234. Fukunaga F H, Lockett L J 1971 Thyroid carcinoma in the Japanese in Hawaii. Arch Pathol 92: 6–13
235. Lang W, Borrusch H, Bauer L 1988 Occult carcinomas of the thyroid. Evaluation of 1,020 sequential autopsies. Am J Clin Pathol 90: 72–76
236. Ludwig G, Nishiyama R H 1976 The prevalence of occult papillary thyroid carcinoma in 100 consecutive autopsies in an American population. Lab Invest 34: 320–321
237. Ottino A, Pianzola H M, Castelletto R H 1989 Occult papillary thyroid carcinoma at autopsy in La Plata, Argentina. Cancer 64: 547–551
238. Sobrinho-Simoes M A, Sambade M C, Goncalves V 1979 Latent thyroid carcinoma at autopsy: a study from Oporto, Portugal. Cancer 43: 1702–1706
239. Mills S E, Allen M S Jr. 1986 Congenital occult papillary carcinoma of the thyroid gland. Hum Pathol 17: 1179–1181
240. Komorowski R A, Hanson G A 1988 Occult thyroid pathology in the young adult: an autopsy study of 138 patients without clinical thyroid disease. Hum Pathol 19: 689–696
241. Franssila K O, Harach H R 1986 Occult papillary carcinoma of the thyroid in children and young adults. A systemic autopsy study in Finland. Cancer 58: 715–719
242. LaGuette J, Matias-Guiu X, Rosai J 1997 Thyroid paraganglioma: a clinicopathologic and immunohistochemical study of three cases. Am J Surg Pathol 21: 748–753
243. Rosai J, LiVolsi V A, Sobrinho-Simoes M et al. 2003 Renaming papillary microcarcinoma of the thyroid gland: the Porto proposal. Int J Surg Pathol 11: 249–251
244. Schroder S, Pfannschmidt N, Bocker W et al. 1984 Histopathologic types and clinical behaviour of occult papillary carcinoma of the thyroid. Pathol Res Pract 179: 81–87
245. Cheifetz R E, Davis N L, Robinson B W et al. 1994 Differentiation of thyroid neoplasms by evaluating epithelial membrane antigen, Leu-7 antigen, epidermal growth factor receptor, and DNA content. Am J Surg 167: 531–534
246. Lucas S D, Ek B, Rask L et al. 1997 Aberrantly expressed cytokeratin 1, a tumor-associated autoantigen in papillary thyroid carcinoma. Int J Cancer 73: 171–177
247. Miettinen M, Kovatich A J, Karkkainen P 1997 Keratin subsets in papillary and follicular thyroid lesions. A paraffin section analysis with diagnostic implications. Virchows Arch 431: 407–413
248. Raphael S J, McKeown-Eyssen G, Asa S L 1994 High-molecular-weight cytokeratin and cytokeratin-19 in the diagnosis of thyroid tumors. Mod Pathol 7: 295–300
249. Raphael S J, Apel R L, Asa S L 1995 Brief report: detection of high-molecular-weight cytokeratins in neoplastic and non-neoplastic thyroid tumors using microwave antigen retrieval. Mod Pathol 8: 870–872
250. Khan A, Baker S P, Patwardhan N A et al. 1998 CD57 (Leu-7) expression is helpful in diagnosis of the follicular variant of papillary thyroid carcinoma. Virchows Arch 432: 427–432
251. Loy T S, Darkow G V, Spollen L E et al. 1994 Immunostaining for Leu-7 in the diagnosis of thyroid carcinoma. Arch Pathol Lab Med 118: 172–174
252. Chhieng D C, Ross J S, McKenna B J 1997 CD44 immunostaining of thyroid fine-needle aspirates differentiates thyroid papillary carcinoma from other lesions with nuclear grooves and inclusions. Cancer 81: 157–162
253. Ross J S, del Rosario A D, Sanderson B et al. 1996 Selective expression of CD44 cell-adhesion molecule in thyroid papillary carcinoma fine-needle aspirates. Diagn Cytopathol 14: 287–291
254. van Hoeven K H, Kovatich A J, Miettinen M 1998 Immunocytochemical evaluation of HBME-1, CA 19-9, and CD-15 (Leu-M1) in fine-needle aspirates of thyroid nodules. Diagn Cytopathol 18: 93–97
255. Papotti M, Rodriguez J, Pompa R D et al. 2005 Galectin-3 and HBME-1 expression in well-differentiated thyroid tumors with follicular architecture of uncertain malignant potential. Mod Pathol 18: 541–546
256. Pisani T, Vecchione A, Giovagnoli M R 2004 Galectin-3 immunodetection may improve cytological diagnosis of occult papillary thyroid carcinoma. Anticancer Res 24: 1111–1112
257. Xu X C, el-Naggar A K, Lotan R 1995 Differential expression of galectin-1 and galectin-3 in thyroid tumors. Potential diagnostic implications. Am J Pathol 147: 815–822
258. Prasad M L, Pellegata N S, Kloos R T et al. 2004 CITED1 protein expression suggests papillary thyroid carcinoma in high throughput tissue microarray-based study. Thyroid 14: 169–175
259. Prasad M L, Pellegata N S, Huang Y et al. 2005 Galectin-3, fibronectin-1, CITED-1, HBME1 and cytokeratin-19 immunohistochemistry is useful for the differential diagnosis of thyroid tumors. Mod Pathol 18: 48–57
260. Casey M B, Lohse C M, Lloyd R V 2003 Distinction between papillary thyroid hyperplasia and papillary thyroid carcinoma by immunohistochemical staining for cytokeratin 19, galectin-3, and HBME-1. Endocr Pathol 14: 55–60
261. Cvejic D, Savin S, Petrovic I et al. 2005 Galectin-3 expression in papillary microcarcinoma of the thyroid. Histopathology 47: 209–214
262. Lloyd R V 2001 Distinguishing benign from malignant thyroid lesions: galectin 3 as the latest candidate. Endocr Pathol 12: 255–257
263. Shin E, Chung W Y, Yang W I et al. 2005 RET/PTC and CK19 expression in papillary thyroid carcinoma and its clinicopathologic correlation. J Korean Med Sci 20: 98–104
264. Erkilic S, Aydin A, Kocer N E 2002 Diagnostic utility of cytokeratin 19 expression in multinodular goiter with papillary areas and papillary carcinoma of thyroid. Endocr Pathol 13: 207–211
265. Erkilic S, Kocer N E 2005 The role of cytokeratin 19 in the differential diagnosis of true papillary carcinoma of thyroid and papillary carcinoma-like changes in Graves' disease. Endocr Pathol 16: 63–66
266. Sahoo S, Hoda S A, Rosai J et al. 2001 Cytokeratin 19 immunoreactivity in the diagnosis of papillary thyroid carcinoma: a note of caution. Am J Clin Pathol 116: 696–702
267. Yano Y, Uematsu N, Yashiro T et al. 2004 Gene expression profiling identifies platelet-derived growth factor as a diagnostic molecular marker for papillary thyroid carcinoma. Clin Cancer Res 10: 2035–2043
268. Liu R T, Chen Y J, Chou F F et al. 2005 No correlation between BRAFV600E mutation and clinicopathological features of papillary thyroid carcinomas in Taiwan. Clin Endocrinol (Oxf) 63: 461–466
269. Giordano T J, Kuick R, Thomas D G et al. 2005 Molecular classification of papillary thyroid carcinoma: distinct BRAF, RAS, and RET/PTC mutation-specific gene expression profiles discovered by DNA microarray analysis. Oncogene 24: 6646–6656
270. Adeniran A J, Zhu Z, Gandhi M et al. 2006 Correlation between genetic alterations and microscopic features, clinical manifestations, and prognostic characteristics of thyroid papillary carcinomas. Am J Surg Pathol 30: 216–222
271. Frattini M, Ferrario C, Bressan P et al. 2004 Alternative mutations of BRAF, RET and NTRK1 are associated with similar but distinct gene expression patterns in papillary thyroid cancer. Oncogene 23: 7436–7440
272. Pierotti M A, Vigneri P, Bongarzone I 1998 Rearrangements of RET and NTRK1 tyrosine kinase receptors in papillary thyroid carcinomas. Recent Results Cancer Res 154: 237–247
273. Smanik P A, Furminger T L, Mazzaferri E L et al. 1995 Breakpoint characterization of the ret/PTC oncogene in human papillary thyroid carcinoma. Hum Mol Genet 4: 2313–2318
274. Santoro M, Carlomagno F, Hay I D et al. 1992 Ret oncogene activation in human thyroid neoplasms is restricted to the papillary cancer subtype. J Clin Invest 89: 1517–1522
275. Williams G H, Rooney S, Thomas G A et al. 1996 RET activation in adult and childhood papillary thyroid carcinoma using a reverse transcriptase-n-polymerase chain reaction approach on archival-nested material. Br J Cancer 74: 585–589
276. Lam A K, Montone K T, Nolan K A et al. 1998 Ret oncogene activation in papillary thyroid carcinoma: prevalence and implication on the histological parameters. Hum Pathol 29: 565–568
277. Delvincourt C, Patey M, Flament J B et al. 1996 Ret and trk proto-oncogene activation in thyroid papillary carcinomas in French patients from the Champagne-Ardenne region. Clin Biochem 29: 267–271
278. Kitamura Y, Minobe K, Nakata T et al. 1999 Ret/PTC3 is the most frequent form of gene rearrangement in papillary thyroid carcinomas in Japan. J Hum Genet 44: 96–102
279. Santoro M, Dathan N A, Berlingieri M T et al. 1994 Molecular characterization of RET/PTC3: a novel rearranged version of the RET proto-oncogene in a human thyroid papillary carcinoma. Oncogene 9: 509–516
280. Lee C H, Hsu L S, Chi C W et al. 1998 High frequency of rearrangement of the RET protooncogene (RET/PTC) in Chinese papillary thyroid carcinomas. J Clin Endocrinol Metab 83: 1629–1632
281. Bongarzone I, Fugazzola L, Vigneri P et al. 1996 Age-related activation of the tyrosine kinase receptor protooncogenes RET and NTRK1 in papillary thyroid carcinoma. J Clin Endocrinol Metab 81: 2006–2009
282. Zou M, Shi Y, Farid N R 1994 Low rate of ret proto-oncogene activation (PTC/retPTC) in papillary thyroid carcinomas from Saudi Arabia. Cancer 73: 176–180
283. Tallini G, Ghossein R A, Emanuel J et al. 1998 Detection of thyroglobulin, thyroid peroxidase, and RET/PTC1 mRNA transcripts in the peripheral blood of patients with thyroid disease. J Clin Oncol 16: 1158–1166
284. Mayr B, Potter E, Goretzki P et al. 1998 Expression of Ret/PTC1, -2, -3, -delta3 and -4 in German papillary thyroid carcinoma. Br J Cancer 77: 903–906
285. Mayr B, Potter E, Goretzki P et al. 1999 Expression of wild-type ret, ret/PTC and ret/PTC variants in papillary thyroid carcinoma in Germany. Langenbecks Arch Surg 384: 54–59
286. Soares P, Fonseca E, Wynford-Thomas D et al. 1998 Sporadic ret-rearranged papillary carcinoma of the thyroid: a subset of slow growing, less aggressive thyroid neoplasms? J Pathol 185: 71–78
287. Nikiforov Y E, Rowland J M, Bove K E et al. 1997 Distinct pattern of ret oncogene rearrangements in morphological variants of radiation-induced and sporadic thyroid papillary carcinomas in children. Cancer Res 57: 1690–1694
288. Sugg S L, Ezzat S, Zheng L et al. 1999 Oncogene profile of papillary thyroid carcinoma. Surgery 125: 46–52

289. Fischer A H, Bond J A, Taysavang P et al. 1998 Papillary thyroid carcinoma oncogene (RET/PTC) alters the nuclear envelope and chromatin structure. Am J Pathol 153: 1443–1450
290. Wirtschafter A, Schmidt R, Rosen D et al. 1997 Expression of the RET/PTC fusion gene as a marker for papillary carcinoma in Hashimoto's thyroiditis. Laryngoscope 107: 95–100
291. Elisei R, Romei C, Vorontsova T et al. 2001 RET/PTC rearrangements in thyroid nodules: studies in irradiated and not irradiated, malignant and benign thyroid lesions in children and adults. J Clin Endocrinol Metab 86: 3211–3216
292. Nikiforov Y E 2002 RET/PTC rearrangement in thyroid tumors. Endocr Pathol 13: 3–16
293. Sozzi G, Bongarzone I, Miozzo M et al. 1994 A t(10;17) translocation creates the RET/PTC2 chimeric transforming sequence in papillary thyroid carcinoma. Genes Chromos Cancer 9: 244–250
294. Minoletti F, Butti M G, Coronelli S et al. 1994 The two genes generating RET/PTC3 are localized in chromosomal band 10q11.2. Genes Chromos Cancer 11: 51–57
295. Fugazzola L, Pierotti M A, Vigano E et al. 1996 Molecular and biochemical analysis of RET/PTC4, a novel oncogenic rearrangement between RET and ELE1 genes, in a post-Chernobyl papillary thyroid cancer. Oncogene 13: 1093–1097
296. Nikiforov Y E 2004 Recent developments in the molecular biology of the thyroid. In: Lloyd RV (ed) Endocrine pathology: differential diagnosis and molecular advances. Humana Press, Totowa
297. Klugbauer S, Demidchik E P, Lengfelder E et al. 1998 Molecular analysis of new subtypes of ELE/RET rearrangements, their reciprocal transcripts and breakpoints in papillary thyroid carcinomas of children after Chernobyl. Oncogene 16: 671–675
298. Klugbauer S, Demidchik E P, Lengfelder E et al. 1998 Detection of a novel type of RET rearrangement (PTC5) in thyroid carcinomas after Chernobyl and analysis of the involved RET-fused gene RFG5. Cancer Res 58: 198–203
299. Bongarzone I, Butti M G, Fugazzola L et al. 1997 Comparison of the breakpoint regions of ELE1 and RET genes involved in the generation of RET/PTC3 oncogene in sporadic and in radiation-associated papillary thyroid carcinomas. Genomics 42: 252–259
300. Nakazawa T, Kondo T, Kobayashi Y et al. 2005 RET gene rearrangements (RET/PTC1 and RET/PTC3) in papillary thyroid carcinomas from an iodine-rich country (Japan). Cancer 104: 943–951
301. Klugbauer S, Lengfelder E, Demidchik E P et al. 1995 High prevalence of RET rearrangement in thyroid tumors of children from Belarus after the Chernobyl reactor accident. Oncogene 11: 2459–2467
302. Fugazzola L, Pilotti S, Pinchera A et al. 1995 Oncogenic rearrangements of the RET proto-oncogene in papillary thyroid carcinomas from children exposed to the Chernobyl nuclear accident. Cancer Res 55: 5617–5620
303. Pisarchik A V, Ermak G, Demidchik E P et al. 1998 Low prevalence of the ret/PTC3r1 rearrangement in a series of papillary thyroid carcinomas presenting in Belarus ten years post-Chernobyl. Thyroid 8: 1003–1008
304. Bounacer A, Wicker R, Schlumberger M et al. 1997 Oncogenic rearrangements of the ret proto-oncogene in thyroid tumors induced after exposure to ionizing radiation. Biochimie 79: 619–623
305. Learoyd D L, Messina M, Zedenius J et al. 1998 RET/PTC and RET tyrosine kinase expression in adult papillary thyroid carcinomas. J Clin Endocrinol Metab 83: 3631–3635
306. Miki H, Kitaichi M, Masuda E et al. 1999 ret/PTC expression may be associated with local invasion of thyroid papillary carcinoma. J Surg Oncol 71: 76–81
307. Bongarzone I, Vigneri P, Mariani L et al. 1998 RET/NTRK1 rearrangements in thyroid gland tumors of the papillary carcinoma family: correlation with clinicopathological features. Clin Cancer Res 4: 223–228
308. Tallini G, Santoro M, Helie M et al. 1998 RET/PTC oncogene activation defines a subset of papillary thyroid carcinomas lacking evidence of progression to poorly differentiated or undifferentiated tumor phenotypes. Clin Cancer Res 4: 287–294
309. Musholt T J, Musholt P B, Khaladj N et al. 2000 Prognostic significance of RET and NTRK1 rearrangements in sporadic papillary thyroid carcinoma. Surgery 128: 984–993
310. Kopp P, Jameson J L 1998 Thyroid disorders. In: Jameson J L (ed) Principles of molecular medicine. Humana Press, Totowa, p 459–473
311. Beimfohr C, Klugbauer S, Demidchik E P et al. 1999 NTRK1 re-arrangement in papillary thyroid carcinomas of children after the Chernobyl reactor accident. Int J Cancer 80: 842–847
312. Ciampi R, Nikiforov Y E 2005 Alterations of the BRAF gene in thyroid tumors. Endocr Pathol 16: 163–172
313. Cohen Y, Xing M, Mambo E et al. 2003 BRAF mutation in papillary thyroid carcinoma. J Natl Cancer Inst 95: 625–627
314. Fukushima T, Takenoshita S 2005 Roles of RAS and BRAF mutations in thyroid carcinogenesis. Fukushima J Med Sci 51: 67–75
315. Powell N, Jeremiah S, Morishita M et al. 2005 Frequency of BRAF T1796A mutation in papillary thyroid carcinoma relates to age of patient at diagnosis and not to radiation exposure. J Pathol 205: 558–564
316. Smyth P, Finn S, Cahill S et al. 2005 ret/PTC and BRAF act as distinct molecular, time-dependant triggers in a sporadic Irish cohort of papillary thyroid carcinoma. Int J Surg Pathol 13: 1–8
317. Trovisco V, Vieira de Castro I, Soares P et al. 2004 BRAF mutations are associated with some histological types of papillary thyroid carcinoma. J Pathol 202: 247–251
318. Rosenbaum E, Hosler G, Zahurak M et al. 2005 Mutational activation of BRAF is not a major event in sporadic childhood papillary thyroid carcinoma. Mod Pathol 18: 898–902
319. Trovisco V, Soares P, Preto A et al. 2005 Type and prevalence of BRAF mutations are closely associated with papillary thyroid carcinoma histotype and patients' age but not with tumour aggressiveness. Virchows Arch 446: 589–595
320. Xing M, Westra W H, Tufano R P et al. 2005 BRAF mutation predicts a poorer clinical prognosis for papillary thyroid cancer. J Clin Endocrinol Metab 90: 6373–6379
321. Kim K H, Kang D W, Kim S H et al. 2004 Mutations of the BRAF gene in papillary thyroid carcinoma in a Korean population. Yonsei Med J 45: 818–821
322. Soares P, Trovisco V, Rocha A S et al. 2004 BRAF mutations typical of papillary thyroid carcinoma are more frequently detected in undifferentiated than in insular and insular-like poorly differentiated carcinomas. Virchows Arch 444: 572–576
323. Begum S, Rosenbaum E, Henrique R et al. 2004 BRAF mutations in anaplastic thyroid carcinoma: implications for tumor origin, diagnosis and treatment. Mod Pathol 17: 1359–1363
324. Sobrinho-Simoes M, Preto A, Rocha A S et al. 2005 Molecular pathology of well-differentiated thyroid carcinomas. Virchows Arch 447: 787–793
325. Chan J K 2002 Strict criteria should be applied in the diagnosis of encapsulated follicular variant of papillary thyroid carcinoma. Am J Clin Pathol 117: 16–18
326. Wreesmann V B, Ghossein R A, Hezel M et al. 2004 Follicular variant of papillary thyroid carcinoma: genome-wide appraisal of a controversial entity. Genes Chromos Cancer 40: 355–364
327. Woolner L B, Beahrs O H, Black B M et al. 1968 Thyroid carcinoma: general considerations and follow-up data on 1181 cases. In: Young S, Inman D R (eds) Thyroid neoplasia. Academic Press, London, p 51–76
328. Salvesen H, Njolstad P R, Akslen L A et al. 1992 Papillary thyroid carcinoma: a multivariate analysis of prognostic factors including an evaluation of the p-TNM staging system. Eur J Surg 158: 583–589
329. Bellantone R, Lombardi C P, Boscherini M et al. 1998 Prognostic factors in differentiated thyroid carcinoma: a multivariate analysis of 234 consecutive patients. J Surg Oncol 68: 237–241
330. Noguchi S, Murakami N, Kawamoto H 1994 Classification of papillary cancer of the thyroid based on prognosis. World J Surg 18: 552–557
331. Kashima K, Yokoyama S, Noguchi S et al. 1998 Chronic thyroiditis as a favorable prognostic factor in papillary thyroid carcinoma. Thyroid 8: 197–202
332. Bhattacharyya N 2003 A population-based analysis of survival factors in differentiated and medullary thyroid carcinoma. Otolaryngol Head Neck Surg 128: 115–123
333. Frauenhoffer C M, Patchefsky A S, Cobanoglu A 1979 Thyroid carcinoma: a clinical and pathologic study of 125 cases. Cancer 43: 2414–2421
334. Tennvall J, Biorklund A, Moller T et al. 1985 Prognostic factors of papillary, follicular and medullary carcinomas of the thyroid gland. Retrospective multivariate analysis of 216 patients with a median follow-up of 11 years. Acta Radiol Oncol 24: 17–24
335. Tennvall J, Biorklund A, Moller T et al. 1986 Is the EORTC prognostic index of thyroid cancer valid in differentiated thyroid carcinoma? Retrospective multivariate analysis of differentiated thyroid carcinoma with long follow-up. Cancer 57: 1405–1414
336. Kakudo K, Tang W, Ito Y et al. 2004 Papillary carcinoma of the thyroid in Japan: subclassification of common type and identification of low risk group. J Clin Pathol 57: 1041–1046
337. Schroder S, Pfannschmidt N, Dralle H et al. 1984 The encapsulated follicular carcinoma of the thyroid. A clinicopathologic study of 35 cases. Virchows Arch A Pathol Anat Histopathol 402: 259–273
338. Ito Y, Tomoda C, Uruno T et al. 2006 Prognostic significance of extrathyroid extension of papillary thyroid carcinoma: massive but not minimal extension affects the relapse-free survival. World J Surg 30: 780–786
339. McCaffrey T V, Bergstralh E J, Hay I D 1994 Locally invasive papillary thyroid carcinoma: 1940–1990. Head Neck 16: 165–172
340. Zohar Y, Strauss M 1994 Occult distant metastases of well-differentiated thyroid carcinoma. Head Neck 16: 438–442
341. Franssila K O 1975 Prognosis in thyroid carcinoma. Cancer 36: 1138–1146
342. Yasumoto K, Miyagi C, Nakashima T et al. 1996 Papillary and follicular thyroid carcinoma: the treatment results of 357 patients at the National Kyushu Cancer Centre of Japan. J Laryngol Otol 110: 657–662
343. Hughes C J, Shaha A R, Shah J P et al. 1996 Impact of lymph node metastasis in differentiated carcinoma of the thyroid: a matched-pair analysis. Head Neck 18: 127–132
344. Scheumann G F, Gimm O, Wegener G et al. 1994 Prognostic significance and surgical management of locoregional lymph node metastases in papillary thyroid cancer. World J Surg 18: 559–567
345. Yamashita H, Noguchi S, Murakami N et al. 1997 Extracapsular invasion of lymph node metastasis is an indicator of distant metastasis and poor prognosis in patients with thyroid papillary carcinoma. Cancer 80: 2268–2272
346. Tielens E T, Sherman S I, Hruban R H et al. 1994 Follicular variant of papillary thyroid carcinoma. A clinicopathologic study. Cancer 73: 424–431
347. Andersen P E, Kinsella J, Loree T R et al. 1995 Differentiated carcinoma of the thyroid with extrathyroidal extension. Am J Surg 170: 467–470

348. Akslen L A 1993 Prognostic importance of histologic grading in papillary thyroid carcinoma. Cancer 72: 2680–2685
349. Akslen L A, LiVolsi V A 2000 Prognostic significance of histologic grading compared with subclassification of papillary thyroid carcinoma. Cancer 88: 1902–1908
350. Schroder S, Schwarz W, Rehpenning W et al. 1987 Prognostic significance of Leu-M1 immunostaining in papillary carcinomas of the thyroid gland. Virchows Arch A Pathol Anat Histopathol 411: 435–439
351. Yamamoto Y, Izumi K, Otsuka H 1992 An immunohistochemical study of epithelial membrane antigen, cytokeratin, and vimentin in papillary thyroid carcinoma. Recognition of lethal and favorable prognostic types. Cancer 70: 2326–2333
352. Goldenberg J D, Portugal L G, Wenig B L et al. 1998 Well-differentiated thyroid carcinomas: p53 mutation status and microvessel density. Head Neck 20: 152–158
353. Godballe C, Asschenfeldt P, Jorgensen K E et al. 1998 Prognostic factors in papillary and follicular thyroid carcinomas: p53 expression is a significant indicator of prognosis. Laryngoscope 108: 243–249
354. von Wasielewski R, Rhein A, Werner M et al. 1997 Immunohistochemical detection of E-cadherin in differentiated thyroid carcinomas correlates with clinical outcome. Cancer Res 57: 2501–2507
355. Omura K, Nagasato A, Kanehira E et al. 1997 Retinoblastoma protein and proliferating-cell nuclear antigen expression as predictors of recurrence in well-differentiated papillary thyroid carcinoma. J Clin Oncol 15: 3458–3463
356. Schroder S, Schwarz W, Rehpenning W et al. 1988 Dendritic/Langerhans cells and prognosis in patients with papillary thyroid carcinomas. Immunocytochemical study of 106 thyroid neoplasms correlated to follow-up data. Am J Clin Pathol 89: 295–300
357. Hamming J F, Schelfhout L J, Cornelisse C J et al. 1988 Prognostic value of nuclear DNA content in papillary and follicular thyroid cancer. World J Surg 12: 503–508
358. Stern Y, Lisnyansky I, Shpitzer T et al. 1997 Comparison of nuclear DNA content in locally invasive and noninvasive papillary carcinoma of the thyroid gland. Otolaryngol Head Neck Surg 117: 501–503
359. Sobrinho-Simoes M, Asa S L, Kroll T G et al. 2004 Follicular carcinoma. In: DeLellis R A, Lloyd R V, Heitz P U et al. (eds) Pathology and genetics. Tumours of endocrine organs. World Health Organization classification of tumours. IARC Press, Lyon, p 67–72
360. Chan J K C, Hirokawa M, Evans H L et al. 2004 Follicular adenoma. In: DeLellis R A, Lloyd R V, Heitz P U et al. (eds) Pathology and genetics. Tumours of endocrine organs. World Health Organization classification of tumours. IARC Press, Lyon, p 98–103
361. Hicks D G, LiVolsi V A, Neidich J A et al. 1990 Clonal analysis of solitary follicular nodules in the thyroid. Am J Pathol 137: 553–562
362. Thomas G A, Williams D, Williams E D 1989 The clonal origin of thyroid nodules and adenomas. Am J Pathol 134: 141–147
363. Chung D H, Kang G H, Kim W H et al. 1999 Clonal analysis of a solitary follicular nodule of the thyroid with the polymerase chain reaction method. Mod Pathol 12: 265–271
364. Krohn K, Fuhrer D, Holzapfel H P et al. 1998 Clonal origin of toxic thyroid nodules with constitutively activating thyrotropin receptor mutations. J Clin Endocrinol Metab 83: 130–134
365. Kim H, Piao Z, Park C et al. 1998 Clinical significance of clonality in thyroid nodules. Br J Surg 85: 1125–1128
366. Crile G Jr., Pontius K I, Hawk W A 1985 Factors influencing the survival of patients with follicular carcinoma of the thyroid gland. Surg Gynecol Obstet 160: 409–413
367. DeMay R M 2000 Follicular lesions of the thyroid. W(h)ither follicular carcinoma? Am J Clin Pathol 114: 681–683
368. LiVolsi V A, Asa S L 1994 The demise of follicular carcinoma of the thyroid gland. Thyroid 4: 233–236
369. Evans H L, Vassilopoulou-Sellin R 1998 Follicular and Hurthle cell carcinomas of the thyroid: a comparative study. Am J Surg Pathol 22: 1512–1520
370. Harach H R, Soubeyran I, Brown A et al. 1999 Thyroid pathologic findings in patients with Cowden disease. Ann Diagn Pathol 3: 331–340
371. LiVolsi V A, Baloch Z W 1999 Determining the diagnosis and prognosis of thyroid neoplasms: do special studies help? Hum Pathol 30: 885–886
372. Katoh R, Sakamoto A, Kasai N et al. 1989 Squamous differentiation in thyroid carcinoma. With special reference to histogenesis of squamous cell carcinoma of the thyroid. Acta Pathol Jpn 39: 306–312
373. Canzian F, Amati P, Harach H R et al. 1998 A gene predisposing to familial thyroid tumors with cell oxyphilia maps to chromosome 19p13.2. Am J Hum Genet 63: 1743–1748
374. McKay J D, Thompson D, Lesueur F et al. 2004 Evidence for interaction between the TCO and NMTC1 loci in familial non-medullary thyroid cancer. J Med Genet 41: 407–412
375. Maximo V, Botelho T, Capela J et al. 2005 Somatic and germline mutation in GRIM-19, a dual function gene involved in mitochondrial metabolism and cell death, is linked to mitochondrion-rich (Hurthle cell) tumours of the thyroid. Br J Cancer 92: 1892–1898
376. Lo C Y, Lorentz T G, Wan K Y 1995 Follicular carcinoma of the thyroid gland in Hong Kong Chinese. Br J Surg 82: 1095–1097
377. Valenta L J, Michel-Bechet M, Mattson J C et al. 1977 Microfollicular thyroid carcinoma with amyloid rich stroma, resembling the medullary carcinoma of the thyroid (MCT). Cancer 39: 1573–1586
378. LiVolsi V A 1993 Current concepts in follicular tumors of the thyroid. Monogr Pathol 35: 118–137
379. Gosain A K, Clark O H 1984 Hurthle cell neoplasms. Malignant potential. Arch Surg 119: 515–519
380. Watson R G, Brennan M D, Goellner J R et al. 1984 Invasive Hurthle cell carcinoma of the thyroid: natural history and management. Mayo Clin Proc 59: 851–855
381. Evans H L 1984 Follicular neoplasms of the thyroid. A study of 44 cases followed for a minimum of 10 years, with emphasis on differential diagnosis. Cancer 54: 535–540
382. Bronner M P, LiVolsi V A 1988 Oxyphilic (Askanazy/Hurthle cell) tumors of the thyroid: microscopic features predict biologic behavior. Surg Pathol 1: 137–150
383. Schmid K W, Farid N R 2006 How to define follicular thyroid carcinoma? Virchows Arch 448: 385–393
384. Franssila K O, Ackerman L V, Brown C L 1985 Follicular carcinoma. Semin Diagn Pathol 2: 101–122
385. Baloch Z W, LiVolsi V A 1998 Intravascular Kaposi's-like spindle cell proliferation of the capsular vessels of follicular-derived thyroid carcinomas. Mod Pathol 11: 995–998
386. Tse L L, Chan I, Chan J K 2001 Capsular intravascular endothelial hyperplasia: a peculiar form of vasoproliferative lesion associated with thyroid carcinoma. Histopathology 39: 463–468
387. Carcangiu M L, Bianchi S, Savino D et al. 1991 Follicular Hurthle cell tumors of the thyroid gland. Cancer 68: 1944–1953
388. LiVolsi V A, Baloch Z W 2004 Follicular neoplasms of the thyroid: view, biases, and experiences. Adv Anat Pathol 11: 279–287
389. Heffess C S, Thompson L D 2001 Minimally invasive follicular thyroid carcinoma. Endocr Pathol 12: 417–422
390. Lang W, Choritz H, Hundeshagen H 1986 Risk factors in follicular thyroid carcinomas. A retrospective follow-up study covering a 14-year period with emphasis on morphological findings. Am J Surg Pathol 10: 246–255
391. Lang W, Georgii A 1982 Minimal invasive cancer in the thyroid. Clin Oncol 1: 527–537
392. Crile G Jr., Hawk W A 1971 Carcinomas of the thyroid. Cleve Clin Q 38: 97–104
393. Lo C Y, Chan W F, Lam K Y et al. 2005 Follicular thyroid carcinoma: the role of histology and staging systems in predicting survival. Ann Surg 242: 708–715
394. Brennan M D, Bergstralh E J, van Heerden J A et al. 1991 Follicular thyroid cancer treated at the Mayo Clinic, 1946 through 1970: initial manifestations, pathologic findings, therapy, and outcome. Mayo Clin Proc 66: 11–22
395. van Heerden J A, Hay I D, Goellner J R et al. 1992 Follicular thyroid carcinoma with capsular invasion alone: a nonthreatening malignancy. Surgery 112: 1130–1136
396. Thompson L D, Wieneke J A, Paal E et al. 2001 A clinicopathologic study of minimally invasive follicular carcinoma of the thyroid gland with a review of the English literature. Cancer 91: 505–524
397. D'Avanzo A, Treseler P, Ituarte P H et al. 2004 Follicular thyroid carcinoma: histology and prognosis. Cancer 100: 1123–1129
398. Collini P, Sampietro G, Pilotti S 2004 Extensive vascular invasion is a marker of risk of relapse in encapsulated non-Hurthle cell follicular carcinoma of the thyroid gland: a clinicopathological study of 18 consecutive cases from a single institution with a 11-year median follow-up. Histopathology 44: 35–39
399. Ghossein R A, Hiltzik D H, Carlson D L et al. 2006 Prognostic factors of recurrence in encapsulated Hurthle cell carcinoma of the thyroid gland: a clinicopathologic study of 50 cases. Cancer 106: 1669–1676
400. Rossi R L, Nieroda C, Cady B et al. 1985 Malignancies of the thyroid gland. The Lahey Clinic experience. Surg Clin North Am 65: 211–230
401. Brooks J R, Starnes H F, Brooks D C et al. 1988 Surgical therapy for thyroid carcinoma: a review of 1249 solitary thyroid nodules. Surgery 104: 940–946
402. Pilotti S, Collini P, Mariani L et al. 1997 Insular carcinoma: a distinct de novo entity among follicular carcinomas of the thyroid gland. Am J Surg Pathol 21: 1466–1473
403. Jorda M, Gonzalez-Campora R, Mora J et al. 1993 Prognostic factors in follicular carcinoma of the thyroid. Arch Pathol Lab Med 117: 631–635
404. Shaha A R, Loree T R, Shah J P 1995 Prognostic factors and risk group analysis in follicular carcinoma of the thyroid. Surgery 118: 1131–1136
405. Yamashina M 1992 Follicular neoplasms of the thyroid. Total circumferential evaluation of the fibrous capsule. Am J Surg Pathol 16: 392–400
406. Lang W, Georgii A, Stauch G et al. 1980 The differentiation of atypical adenomas and encapsulated follicular carcinomas in the thyroid gland. Virchows Arch Pathol Anat 385: 125–141
407. Sambade C, Sarabando F, Nesland J M et al. 1989 Hyalinizing trabecular adenoma of the thyroid (case of the Ullensvang course). Hyalinizing spindle cell tumor of the thyroid with dual differentiation (variant of the so-called hyalinizing trabecular adenoma). Ultrastruct Pathol 13: 275–280
408. Katoh R, Jasani B, Williams E D 1989 Hyalinizing trabecular adenoma of the thyroid. A report of three cases with immunohistochemical and ultrastructural studies. Histopathology 15: 211–224
409. Bronner M P, LiVolsi V A, Jennings T A 1988 PLAT: paraganglioma-like adenoma of the thyroid. Surg Pathol 1: 383–389

410. Schmid K W, Mesewinkel F, Bocker W 1996 Hyalinizing trabecular adenoma of the thyroid – morphology and differential diagnosis. Acta Med Austriaca 23: 65–68
411. Chetty R, Beydoun R, LiVolsi V A 1994 Paraganglioma-like (hyalinizing trabecular) adenoma of the thyroid revisited. Pathology 26: 429–431
412. Papotti M, Riella P, Montemurro F et al. 1997 Immunophenotypic heterogeneity of hyalinizing trabecular tumours of the thyroid. Histopathology 31: 525–533
413. Chan J K C, Tse C C H, Chiu H S 1990 Hyalinizing trabecular adenoma-like lesion in multinodular goiter. Histopathology 16: 611–614
414. Li M, Rosai J, Carcangiu M L 1995 Hyalinizing trabecular adenoma of the thyroid: a distinct tumor type or a pattern of growth? Evaluation of 28 cases (Abstract). Mod Pathol 8: 54A
415. Fonseca E, Nesland J M, Sobrinho-Simoes M 1997 Expression of stratified epithelial-type cytokeratins in hyalinizing trabecular adenomas supports their relationship with papillary carcinomas of the thyroid. Histopathology 31: 330–335
416. Molberg K, Albores-Saavedra J 1994 Hyalinizing trabecular carcinoma of the thyroid gland. Hum Pathol 25: 192–197
417. Gonzalez-Campora R, Fuentes-Vaamonde E, Hevia-Vazquez A et al. 1998 Hyalinizing trabecular carcinoma of the thyroid gland: report of two cases of follicular cell thyroid carcinoma with hyalinizing trabecular pattern. Ultrastruct Pathol 22: 39–46
418. McCluggage W G, Sloan J M 1996 Hyalinizing trabecular carcinoma of thyroid gland. Histopathology 28: 357–362
419. Rothenberg H J, Goellner J R, Carney J A 1999 Hyalinizing trabecular adenoma of the thyroid gland: recognition and characterization of its cytoplasmic yellow body. Am J Surg Pathol 23: 118–125
420. Huss L J, Mendelsohn G 1990 Medullary carcinoma of the thyroid gland: an encapsulated variant resembling the hyalinizing trabecular (paraganglioma-like) adenoma of thyroid. Mod Pathol 3: 581–585
421. Hirokawa M, Shimizu M, Manabe T et al. 1995 Hyalinizing trabecular adenoma of the thyroid: its unusual cytoplasmic immunopositivity for MIB1. Pathol Int 45: 399–401
422. Lloyd R V 2002 Hyalinizing trabecular tumors of the thyroid: a variant of papillary carcinoma? Adv Anat Pathol 9: 7–11
423. Li M, Carcangiu M L, Rosai J 1997 Abnormal intracellular and extracellular distribution of basement membrane material in papillary carcinoma and hyalinizing trabecular tumors of the thyroid: implication for deregulation of secretory pathways. Hum Pathol 28: 1366–1372
424. Cheung C C, Boerner S L, MacMillan C M et al. 2000 Hyalinizing trabecular tumor of the thyroid: a variant of papillary carcinoma proved by molecular genetics. Am J Surg Pathol 24: 1622–1626
425. Papotti M, Volante M, Giuliano A et al. 2000 RET/PTC activation in hyalinizing trabecular tumors of the thyroid. Am J Surg Pathol 24: 1615–1621
426. Salvatore G, Chiappetta G, Nikiforov Y E et al. 2005 Molecular profile of hyalinizing trabecular tumours of the thyroid: high prevalence of RET/PTC rearrangements and absence of B-raf and N-ras point mutations. Eur J Cancer 41: 816–821
427. Hirokawa M, Carney J A, Ohtsuki Y 2000 Hyalinizing trabecular adenoma and papillary carcinoma of the thyroid gland express different cytokeratin patterns. Am J Surg Pathol 24: 877–881
428. Carney J A, Volante M, Papotti M et al. 2004 Hyalinizing trabecular tumour. In: DeLellis R A, Lloyd R V, Heitz P U et al. (eds) Pathology and genetics. Tumours of endocrine organs. World Health Organization classification of tumours. IARC Press, Lyon, p 104–105
429. Gherardi G 1987 Signet ring cell 'mucinous' thyroid adenoma: a follicle cell tumour with abnormal accumulation of thyroglobulin and a peculiar histochemical profile. Histopathology 11: 317–326
430. Mendelsohn G 1984 Signet-cell-simulating microfollicular adenoma of the thyroid. Am J Surg Pathol 8: 705–708
431. Rigaud C, Peltier F, Bogomoletz W V 1985 Mucin producing microfollicular adenoma of the thyroid. J Clin Pathol 38: 277–280
432. Alsop J E, Yerbury P J, O'Donnell P J et al. 1986 Signet-ring cell microfollicular adenoma arising in a nodular ectopic thyroid. A case report. J Oral Pathol 15: 518–519
433. Deligdisch L, Subhani Z, Gordon R E 1980 Primary mucinous carcinoma of the thyroid gland: report of a case and ultrastructural study. Cancer 45: 2564–2567
434. Schroder S, Husselmann H, Bocker W 1984 Lipid-rich cell adenoma of the thyroid gland. Report of a peculiar thyroid tumour. Virchows Arch A Pathol Anat Histopathol 404: 105–108
435. Toth K, Peter I, Kremmer T et al. 1990 Lipid-rich cell thyroid adenoma: histopathology with comparative lipid analysis. Virchows Arch A Pathol Anat Histopathol 417: 273–276
436. Vuitch F, Leavitt A 1990 Papillary variant of follicular adenoma of thyroid (Abstract). Mod Pathol 3: 104A
437. Mai K T, Landry D C, Thomas J et al. 2001 Follicular adenoma with papillary architecture: a lesion mimicking papillary thyroid carcinoma. Histopathology 39: 25–32
438. Porcellini A, Ciullo I, Pannain S et al. 1995 Somatic mutations in the VI transmembrane segment of the thyrotropin receptor constitutively activate cAMP signalling in thyroid hyperfunctioning adenomas. Oncogene 11: 1089–1093
439. Porcellini A, Ciullo I, Laviola L et al. 1994 Novel mutations of thyrotropin receptor gene in thyroid hyperfunctioning adenomas. Rapid identification by fine needle aspiration biopsy. J Clin Endocrinol Metab 79: 657–661
440. Pinducciu C, Borgonovo G, Arezzo A et al. 1998 Toxic thyroid adenoma: absence of DNA mutations of the TSH receptor and Gs alpha. Eur J Endocrinol 138: 37–40
441. Tonacchera M, Chiovato L, Pinchera A et al. 1998 Hyperfunctioning thyroid nodules in toxic multinodular goiter share activating thyrotropin receptor mutations with solitary toxic adenoma. J Clin Endocrinol Metab 83: 492–498
442. Esapa C, Foster S, Johnson S et al. 1997 G protein and thyrotropin receptor mutations in thyroid neoplasia. J Clin Endocrinol Metab 82: 493–496
443. Hjorth L, Thomsen L B, Nielsen V T 1986 Adenolipoma of the thyroid gland. Histopathology 10: 91–96
444. Laforga J B, Vierna J 1996 Adenoma of thyroid gland containing fat (thyrolipoma). Report of a case. J Laryngol Otol 110: 1088–1089
445. Wolvos T A, Chong F K, Razvi S A et al. 1985 An unusual thyroid tumor: a comparison to a literature review of teratomas. Surgery 97: 613–617
446. Visona A, Pea M, Bozzola L et al. 1991 Follicular adenoma of the thyroid gland with extensive chondroid metaplasia. Histopathology 18: 278–279
447. Kini S R, Miller J M 1986 Infarction of thyroid neoplasms following aspiration biopsy (Abstract). Acta Cytol 30: 591
448. Chan J K, Tang S K, Tsang W Y et al. 1996 Histologic changes induced by fine-needle aspiration. Adv Anat Pathol 3: 71–90
449. Jones J D, Pittman D L, Sandes L R 1985 Necrosis of thyroid nodules after fine needle aspiration. Acta Cytol 29: 29–31
450. LiVolsi V A, Merino M J 1994 Worrisome histologic alterations following fine-needle aspiration of the thyroid (WHAFFT). Pathol Annu 29(part 2): 99–120
451. Hazard J B, Kenyon R 1954 Atypical adenoma of the thyroid. Arch Pathol 58: 554–563
452. Rosai J 1996 Ackerman's surgical pathology, 8th edn. Mosby, St. Louis
453. Flint A, Lloyd R V 1990 Hurthle-cell neoplasms of the thyroid gland. Pathol Annu 25(part 1): 37–52
454. Thompson N W, Dunn E L, Batsakis J G et al. 1974 Hurthle cell lesions of the thyroid gland. Surg Gynecol Obstet 139: 555–560
455. Gundry S R, Burney R E, Thompson N W et al. 1983 Total thyroidectomy for Hurthle cell neoplasm of the thyroid. Arch Surg 118: 529–532
456. Miller R H, Estrada R, Sneed W F et al. 1983 Hurthle cell tumors of the thyroid gland. Laryngoscope 93: 884–888
457. Rosen I B, Luk S, Katz I 1985 Hurthle cell tumor behavior: dilemma and resolution. Surgery 98: 777–783
458. Heppe H, Armin A, Calandra D B et al. 1985 Hurthle cell tumors of the thyroid gland. Surgery 98: 1162–1165
459. Arganini M, Behar R, Wu T C et al. 1986 Hurthle cell tumors: a twenty-five-year experience. Surgery 100: 1108–1115
460. Caplan R H, Abellera R M, Kisken W A 1984 Hurthle cell tumors of the thyroid gland. A clinicopathologic review and long-term follow-up. JAMA 251: 3114–3117
461. Gonzalez-Campora R, Herrero-Zapatero A, Lerma E et al. 1986 Hurthle cell and mitochondrion-rich cell tumors. A clinicopathologic study. Cancer 57: 1154–1163
462. Saull S C, Kimmelman C P 1985 Hurthle cell tumors of the thyroid gland. Otolaryngol Head Neck Surg 93: 58–62
463. Bondeson L, Bondeson A G, Ljungberg O et al. 1981 Oxyphil tumors of the thyroid: follow-up of 42 surgical cases. Ann Surg 194: 677–680
464. Wasvary H, Czako P, Poulik J et al. 1998 Unilateral lobectomy for Hurthle cell adenoma. Am Surg 64: 729–732
465. Lopez-Penabad L, Chiu A C, Hoff A O et al. 2003 Prognostic factors in patients with Hurthle cell neoplasms of the thyroid. Cancer 97: 1186–1194
466. Grant C S, Barr D, Goellner J R et al. 1988 Benign Hurthle cell tumors of the thyroid: a diagnosis to be trusted? World J Surg 12: 488–495
467. Chen H, Nicol T L, Zeiger M A et al. 1998 Hurthle cell neoplasms of the thyroid: are there factors predictive of malignancy? Ann Surg 227: 542–546
468. Hillman N, Hardisson D, Herranz L et al. 1997 Hurthle cell tumors. Ann Med Int 148: 434–439
469. Erickson L A, Jin L, Goellner J R et al. 2000 Pathologic features, proliferative activity, and cyclin D1 expression in Hurthle cell neoplasms of the thyroid. Mod Pathol 13: 186–192
470. Bronner M P, Clevenger C V, Edmonds P R et al. 1988 Flow cytometric analysis of DNA content in Hurthle cell adenomas and carcinomas of the thyroid. Am J Clin Pathol 89: 764–769
471. Ryan J J, Hay I D, Grant C S et al. 1988 Flow cytometric DNA measurements in benign and malignant Hurthle cell tumors of the thyroid. World J Surg 12: 482–487
472. Tollefsen H R, Shah J P, Huvos A G 1975 Hurthle cell carcinoma of the thyroid. Am J Surg 130: 390–394
473. Haigh P I, Urbach D R 2005 The treatment and prognosis of Hurthle cell follicular thyroid carcinoma compared with its non-Hurthle cell counterpart. Surgery 138: 1152–1157
474. Papotti M, Torchio B, Grassi L et al. 1996 Poorly differentiated oxyphilic (Hurthle cell) carcinomas of the thyroid. Am J Surg Pathol 20: 686–694
475. Abu-Alfa A K, Straus F H II, Montag A G 1994 An immunohistochemical study of thyroid Hurthle cells and their neoplasms: the roles of S-100 and HMB-45 proteins. Mod Pathol 7: 529–532
476. Stephenson T J, Griffiths D W, Mills P M 1986 Comparison of Ulex europaeus I lectin binding and factor VIII-related antigen as markers of vascular endothelium in follicular carcinoma of the thyroid. Histopathology 10: 251–260

477. Gonzalez-Campora R, Montero C, Martin-Lacave I et al. 1986 Demonstration of vascular endothelium in thyroid carcinomas using *Ulex europaeus* I agglutinin. Histopathology 10: 261–266
478. Harach H R, Jasani B, Williams E D 1983 Factor VIII as a marker of endothelial cells in follicular carcinoma of the thyroid. J Clin Pathol 36: 1050–1054
479. Davila R M, Bedrossian C W, Silverberg A B 1988 Immunocytochemistry of the thyroid in surgical and cytologic specimens. Arch Pathol Lab Med 112: 51–56
480. Johnson T L, Lloyd R V, Thor A 1987 Expression of ras oncogene p21 antigen in normal and proliferative thyroid tissues. Am J Pathol 127: 60–65
481. Johnson T L, Lloyd R V, Burney R E et al. 1987 Hurthle cell thyroid tumors. An immunohistochemical study. Cancer 59: 107–112
482. Mizukami Y, Nonomura A, Hashimoto T et al. 1991 Immunohistochemical demonstration of epidermal growth factor and c-myc oncogene product in normal, benign and malignant thyroid tissues. Histopathology 18: 11–18
483. Erickson L A, Jin L, Wollan P C et al. 1998 Expression of p27kip1 and Ki-67 in benign and malignant thyroid tumors. Mod Pathol 11: 169–174
484. Loy T S, Gelven P L, Mullins D et al. 1992 Immunostaining for P-glycoprotein in the diagnosis of thyroid carcinomas. Mod Pathol 5: 200–202
485. Chiappetta G, Tallini G, De Biasio M C et al. 1998 Detection of high mobility group I HMGI(Y) protein in the diagnosis of thyroid tumors: HMGI(Y) expression represents a potential diagnostic indicator of carcinoma. Cancer Res 58: 4193–4198
486. Tuccari G, Barresi G 1990 Tissue polypeptide antigen in thyroid tumours of follicular cell origin: an immunohistochemical re-evaluation for diagnostic purposes. Histopathology 16: 377–381
487. Ghali V S, Jimenez E J, Garcia R L 1992 Distribution of Leu-7 antigen (HNK-1) in thyroid tumors: its usefulness as a diagnostic marker for follicular and papillary carcinomas. Hum Pathol 23: 21–25
488. De Micco C, Ruf J, Chrestian M A et al. 1991 Immunohistochemical study of thyroid peroxidase in normal, hyperplastic, and neoplastic human thyroid tissues. Cancer 67: 3036–3041
489. Cho Mar K, Eimoto T, Tateyama H et al. 2006 Expression of matrix metalloproteinases in benign and malignant follicular thyroid lesions. Histopathology 48: 286–294
490. Choi Y L, Kim M K, Suh J W et al. 2005 Immunoexpression of HBME-1, high molecular weight cytokeratin, cytokeratin 19, thyroid transcription factor-1, and E-cadherin in thyroid carcinomas. J Korean Med Sci 20: 853–859
491. Ito Y, Yoshida H, Tomoda C et al. 2005 Galectin-3 expression in follicular tumours: an immunohistochemical study of its use as a marker of follicular carcinoma. Pathology 37: 296–298
492. de Matos P S, Ferreira A P, de Oliveira Facuri F et al. 2005 Usefulness of HBME-1, cytokeratin 19 and galectin-3 immunostaining in the diagnosis of thyroid malignancy. Histopathology 47: 391–401
493. Garcia-Gonzalez M, Abdulkader I, Boquete A V et al. 2005 Cyclooxygenase-2 in normal, hyperplastic and neoplastic follicular cells of the human thyroid gland. Virchows Arch 447: 12–17
494. Ito Y, Yoshida H, Tomoda C et al. 2005 HBME-1 expression in follicular tumor of the thyroid: an investigation of whether it can be used as a marker to diagnose follicular carcinoma. Anticancer Res 25: 179–182
495. Mehrotra P, Okpokam A, Bouhaidar R et al. 2004 Galectin-3 does not reliably distinguish benign from malignant thyroid neoplasms. Histopathology 45: 493–500
496. Haynik D M, Prayson R A 2005 Immunohistochemical expression of cyclooxygenase 2 in follicular carcinomas of the thyroid. Arch Pathol Lab Med 129: 736–741
497. Nafe R, Fritsch R S, Sondah B et al. 1992 Histomorphometry in paraffin sections of thyroid tumors. Pathol Res Pract 188: 1042–1048
498. Backdahl M, Wallin G, Akensten U et al. 1989 Nuclear DNA measurements in follicular thyroid adenomas. Eur J Surg Oncol 15: 125–129
499. Hruban R H, Huvos A G, Traganos F et al. 1990 Follicular neoplasms of the thyroid in men older than 50 years of age. A DNA flow cytometric study. Am J Clin Pathol 94: 527–532
500. Schurmann G, Mattfeldt T, Feichter G et al. 1991 Stereology, flow cytometry, and immunohistochemistry of follicular neoplasms of the thyroid gland. Hum Pathol 22: 179–184
501. Oyama T, Vickery A L Jr., Preffer F I et al. 1994 A comparative study of flow cytometry and histopathologic findings in thyroid follicular carcinomas and adenomas. Hum Pathol 25: 271–275
502. Joensuu H, Klemi P, Eerola E 1986 DNA aneuploidy in follicular adenomas of the thyroid gland. Am J Pathol 124: 373–376
503. Lemoine N R, Mayall E S, Wyllie F S et al. 1989 High frequency of ras oncogene activation in all stages of human tumorigenesis. Oncogene 4: 159–164
504. Oyama T, Suzuki T, Hara F et al. 1995 N-ras mutation of thyroid tumor with special reference to the follicular type. Pathol Int 45: 45–50
505. Vasko V V, Gaudart J, Allasia C et al. 2004 Thyroid follicular adenomas may display features of follicular carcinoma and follicular variant of papillary carcinoma. Eur J Endocrinol 151: 779–786
506. Nikiforova M N, Biddinger P W, Caudill C M et al. 2002 PAX8-PPARγ rearrangement in thyroid tumors. RT-PCR and immunohistochemical analysis. Am J Surg Pathol 26: 1016–1023
507. Nikiforova M N, Lynch R A, Biddinger P W et al. 2003 RAS point mutations and PAX8-PPAR gamma rearrangement in thyroid tumors: evidence for distinct molecular pathways in thyroid follicular carcinoma. J Clin Endocrinol Metab 88: 2318–2326
508. Castro P, Eknaes M, Teixeira M R et al. 2005 Adenomas and follicular carcinomas of the thyroid display two major patterns of chromosomal changes. J Pathol 206: 305–311
509. Bouras M, Parvaz P, Berger N et al. 1995 Ha-ras oncogene (codon 12) mutation in thyroid carcinogenesis: analysis of 60 benign and malignant thyroid tumors. Ann Biol Clin 53: 549–555
510. Manenti G, Pilotti S, Re F C et al. 1994 Selective activation of ras oncogenes in follicular and undifferentiated thyroid carcinomas. Eur J Cancer 7: 987–993
511. Dahia P L, Marsh D J, Zheng Z et al. 1997 Somatic deletions and mutations in the Cowden disease gene, PTEN, in sporadic thyroid tumors. Cancer Res 57: 4710–4713
512. Ciampi R, Zhu Z, Nikiforov Y E 2005 BRAF copy number gains in thyroid tumors detected by fluorescence in situ hybridization. Endocr Pathol 16: 99–105
513. Segal K, Arad A, Lubin E et al. 1994 Follicular carcinoma of the thyroid. Head Neck 16: 533–538
514. Marcocci C, Pacini F, Eliseri R et al. 1989 Clinical and biologic behavior of bone metastasis from differentiated thyroid carcinoma. Surgery 106: 960–966
515. Schmidt R J, Wang C A 1986 Encapsulated follicular carcinoma of the thyroid: diagnosis, treatment and results. Surgery 100: 1068–1076
516. Joensuu H, Klemi P, Eerola E et al. 1986 Influence of cellular DNA content on survival in differentiated thyroid cancer. Cancer 58: 2462–2467
517. Sapi Z, Lukacs G, Sztan M et al. 1995 Contribution of p53 gene alterations to development of metastatic forms of follicular thyroid carcinoma. Diagn Mol Pathol 4: 256–260
518. Rosai J, Saxen E A, Woolner L 1985 Undifferentiated and poorly differentiated carcinoma. Semin Diagn Pathol 2: 123–126
519. LiVolsi V A, Brooks J J, Arendash-Durand B 1987 Anaplastic thyroid tumors. Immunohistology. Am J Clin Pathol 87: 434–442
520. Nel C J, van Heerden J A, Goellner J R et al. 1985 Anaplastic carcinoma of the thyroid: a clinicopathologic study of 82 cases. Mayo Clin Proc 60: 51–58
521. Tan R K, Finley R K III, Driscoll D et al. 1995 Anaplastic carcinoma of the thyroid: a 24-year experience. Head Neck 17: 41–47
522. Egloff B 1983 The hemangioendothelioma of the thyroid. Virchows Arch A Pathol Anat Histopathol 400: 119–142
523. Bacher-Stier C, Riccabona G, Totsch M et al. 1997 Incidence and clinical characteristics of thyroid carcinoma after iodine prophylaxis in an endemic goiter country. Thyroid 7: 733–741
524. Kapp D S, LiVolsi V A, Sanders M M 1982 Anaplastic carcinoma following well-differentiated thyroid cancer: etiological considerations. Yale J Biol Med 55: 521–528
525. Nishiyama R H, Dunn E L, Thompson N W 1972 Anaplastic spindle-cell and giant-cell tumors of the thyroid gland. Cancer 30: 113–127
526. Venkatesh Y S, Ordonez N G, Schultz P N et al. 1990 Anaplastic carcinoma of the thyroid. A clinicopathologic study of 121 cases. Cancer 66: 321–330
527. Kebebew E, Greenspan F S, Clark O H et al. 2005 Anaplastic thyroid carcinoma. Treatment outcome and prognostic factors. Cancer 103: 1330–1335
528. Yazawa S, Toshimori H, Nakatsuru K et al. 1995 Thyroid anaplastic carcinoma producing granulocyte-colony-stimulating factor and parathyroid hormone-related protein. Intern Med 34: 584–588
529. Kobayashi T, Asakawa H, Umeshita K et al. 1996 Treatment of 37 patients with anaplastic carcinoma of the thyroid. Head Neck 18: 36–41
530. Passler C, Scheuba C, Prager G et al. 1999 Anaplastic (undifferentiated) thyroid carcinoma (ATC). A retrospective analysis. Langenbecks Arch Surg 384: 284–293
531. Lo C Y, Lam K Y, Wan K Y 1999 Anaplastic carcinoma of the thyroid. Am J Surg 177: 337–339
532. Lu W T, Lin J D, Huang H S et al. 1998 Does surgery improve the survival of patients with advanced anaplastic thyroid carcinoma? Otolaryngol Head Neck Surg 118: 728–731
533. Haigh P I, Ituarte P H, Wu H S et al. 2001 Completely resected anaplastic thyroid carcinoma combined with adjuvant chemotherapy and irradiation is associated with prolonged survival. Cancer 91: 2335–2342
534. Lam K Y, Lo C Y, Chan K W et al. 2000 Insular and anaplastic carcinoma of the thyroid: a 45-year comparative study at a single institution and a review of the significance of p53 and p21. Ann Surg 231: 329–338
535. Are C, Shaha A R 2006 Anaplastic thyroid carcinoma: biology, pathogenesis, prognostic factors, and treatment approaches. Ann Surg Oncol 13: 453–464
536. Ain K B 1998 Anaplastic thyroid carcinoma: behavior, biology, and therapeutic approaches. Thyroid 8: 715–726
537. Asakawa H, Kobayashi T, Komoike Y et al. 1997 Chemosensitivity of anaplastic thyroid carcinoma and poorly differentiated thyroid carcinoma. Anticancer Res 17: 2757–2762
538. Sugawara I, Arai T, Yamashita T et al. 1994 Expression of multidrug resistance-associated protein (MRP) in anaplastic carcinoma of the thyroid. Cancer Lett 82: 185–188
539. Yamashita T, Watanabe M, Onodera M et al. 1994 Multidrug resistance gene and P-glycoprotein expression in anaplastic carcinoma of the thyroid. Cancer Detect Prev 18: 407–413

540. Nilsson O, Lindeberg J, Zedenius J et al. 1998 Anaplastic giant cell carcinoma of the thyroid gland: treatment and survival over a 25-year period. World J Surg 22: 725–730
541. Galera-Davidson H, Bibbo M, Dytch H E et al. 1987 Nuclear DNA in anaplastic thyroid carcinoma with a differentiated component. Histopathology 11: 715–722
542. Carcangiu M L, Zampi G, Rosai J 1984 Poorly differentiated ("insular") thyroid carcinoma. A reinterpretation of Langhans' "wuchernde Struma." Am J Surg Pathol 8: 655–668
543. Burt A, Goudie R B 1979 Diagnosis of primary thyroid carcinoma by immunohistological demonstration of thyroglobulin. Histopathology 3: 279–286
544. Ralfkiaer N, Gatter K C, Alcock C et al. 1985 The value of immunocytochemical methods in the differential diagnosis of anaplastic thyroid tumours. Br J Cancer 52: 167–170
545. Myskow M W, Krajewski A S, Dewar A E et al. 1986 The role of immunoperoxidase techniques on paraffin embedded tissue in determining the histogenesis of undifferentiated thyroid neoplasms. Clin Endocrinol 24: 335–341
546. Eusebi V, Damiani S, Riva C et al. 1990 Calcitonin free oat-cell carcinoma of the thyroid gland. Virchows Arch A Pathol Anat Histopathol 417: 267–271
547. Wolf B C, Sheahan K, DeCoste D et al. 1992 Immunohistochemical analysis of small cell tumors of the thyroid gland: an Eastern Cooperative Oncology Group study. Hum Pathol 23: 1252–1261
548. Cibull M L, Gray G F 1978 Ultrastructure of osteoclastoma-like giant cell tumor of thyroid. Am J Surg Pathol 2: 401–405
549. Silverberg S G, DeGiorgi L S 1973 Osteoclastoma-like giant cell tumor of the thyroid. Report of a case with prolonged survival following partial excision and radiotherapy. Cancer 31: 621–625
550. Gaffey M J, Lack E E, Christ M L et al. 1991 Anaplastic thyroid carcinoma with osteoclast-like giant cells. A clinicopathologic, immunohistochemical, and ultrastructural study. Am J Surg Pathol 15: 160–168
551. Lai M L, Faa G, Serra S et al. 2005 Rhabdoid tumor of the thyroid gland: a variant of anaplastic carcinoma. Arch Pathol Lab Med 129: e55–e57
552. Sumida T, Hamakawa H, Imaoka M et al. 2001 A case of submandibular malignant rhabdoid tumor transformed from papillary thyroid carcinoma. J Oral Pathol Med 30: 443–447
553. Chetty R, Govender D 1999 Follicular thyroid carcinoma with rhabdoid phenotype. Virchows Arch 435: 133–136
554. Dominguez-Malagon H, Flores-Flores G, Vilchis J J 2001 Lymphoepithelioma-like anaplastic thyroid carcinoma: report of a case not related to Epstein–Barr virus. Ann Diagn Pathol 5: 21–24
555. Wan S K, Chan J K, Tang S K 1996 Paucicellular variant of anaplastic thyroid carcinoma. A mimic of Reidel's thyroiditis. Am J Clin Pathol 105: 388–393
556. Chan J K C, Tsang W Y W 1995 Endocrine malignancies that may mimic benign lesions. Semin Diagn Pathol 12: 45–63
557. Canos J C, Serrano A, Matias-Guiu X 2001 Paucicellular variant of anaplastic thyroid carcinoma: report of two cases. Endocr Pathol 12: 157–161
558. Blasius S, Edel G, Grunert J et al. 1994 Anaplastic thyroid carcinoma with osteosarcomatous differentiation. Pathol Res Pract 190: 507–510
559. Carda C, Ferrer J, Vilanova M et al. 2004 Anaplastic carcinoma of the thyroid with rhabdomyosarcomatous differentiation: a report of two cases. Virchows Arch 446: 46–51
560. Bakri K, Shimaoka K, Rao U et al. 1983 Adenosquamous cell carcinoma of the thyroid after radiotherapy for Hodgkin's disease. Cancer 52: 465–470
561. Harada T, Katagiri M, Tsukayama C et al. 1989 Squamous cell carcinoma with cyst of the thyroid. J Surg Oncol 42: 136–143
562. Huang T Y, Assor D 1971 Primary squamous cell carcinoma of the thyroid gland: a report of four cases. Am J Clin Pathol 55: 93–98
563. Huang T Y, Lin S G 1986 Primary squamous cell carcinoma of the thyroid. Indiana Med 79: 763–764
564. Sarda A K, Bal S, Arunabh et al. 1988 Squamous cell carcinoma of the thyroid. J Surg Oncol 39: 175–178
565. Simpson W J, Carruthers J 1988 Squamous cell carcinoma of the thyroid gland. Am J Surg 156: 44–46
566. Shimaoka K, Tsukada Y 1980 Squamous cell carcinomas and adenosquamous carcinomas originating from the thyroid gland. Cancer 46: 1833–1842
567. Theander C, Loden B, Berglund J et al. 1993 Primary squamous carcinoma of the thyroid – a case report. J Laryngol Otol 107: 1155–1158
568. Harada T, Shimaoka K, Katagiri M et al. 1994 Rarity of squamous cell carcinoma of the thyroid: autopsy review. World J Surg 18: 542–546
569. Lam K Y, Lo C Y, Liu M C 2001 Primary squamous cell carcinoma of the thyroid gland: an entity with aggressive clinical behaviour and distinctive cytokeratin expression profiles. Histopathology 39: 279–286
570. Booya F, Sebo T J, Kasperbauer J L et al. 2006 Primary squamous cell carcinoma of the thyroid: report of ten cases. Thyroid 16: 89–93
571. Hayashi Y, Tokuoka S 1979 Anaplastic carcinoma of the thyroid gland, an ultrastructural study of four cases. Acta Pathol Jpn 29: 119–133
572. Totsch M, Dobler G, Feichtinger H et al. 1990 Malignant hemangioendothelioma of the thyroid. Its immunohistochemical discrimination from undifferentiated thyroid carcinoma. Am J Surg Pathol 14: 69–74
573. Eckert F, Schmid U, Gloor F et al. 1986 Evidence of vascular differentiation in anaplastic tumours of the thyroid – an immunohistological study. Virchows Arch A Pathol Anat Histopathol 410: 203–215
574. Albores-Saavedra J, Nadji M, Civantos F et al. 1983 Thyroglobulin in carcinoma of the thyroid: an immunohistochemical study. Hum Pathol 14: 62–66
575. Schiff B A, McMurphy A B, Jasser S A et al. 2004 Epidermal growth factor receptor (EGFR) is overexpressed in anaplastic thyroid cancer, and the EGFR inhibitor gefitinib inhibits the growth of anaplastic thyroid cancer. Clin Cancer Res 10: 8594–8602
576. Nobuhara Y, Onoda N, Yamashita Y et al. 2005 Efficacy of epidermal growth factor receptor-targeted molecular therapy in anaplastic thyroid cancer cell lines. Br J Cancer 92: 1110–1116
577. Ensinger C, Spizzo G, Moser P et al. 2004 Epidermal growth factor receptor as a novel therapeutic target in anaplastic thyroid carcinomas. Ann N Y Acad Sci 1030: 69–77
578. Dobashi Y, Sakamoto A, Sugimura H et al. 1993 Overexpression of p53 as a possible prognostic factor in human thyroid carcinoma. Am J Surg Pathol 17: 375–381
579. Holm R, Nesland J M 1994 Retinoblastoma and p53 tumour suppressor gene protein expression in carcinomas of the thyroid gland. J Pathol 172: 267–272
580. Soares P, Cameselle-Teijeiro J, Sobrinho-Simoes M 1994 Immunohistochemical detection of p53 in differentiated, poorly differentiated and undifferentiated carcinomas of the thyroid. Histopathology 24: 205–210
581. Matias-Guiu X, Villanueva A, Cuatrecasas M et al. 1996 p53 in a thyroid follicular carcinoma with foci of poorly differentiated and anaplastic carcinoma. Pathol Res Pract 192: 1242–1249
582. Dobashi Y, Sugimura H, Sakamoto A et al. 1994 Stepwise participation of p53 gene mutation during dedifferentiation of human thyroid carcinomas. Diagn Mol Pathol 3: 9–14
583. Pollina L, Pacini F, Fontanini G et al. 1996 bcl-2, p53 and proliferating cell nuclear antigen expression is related to the degree of differentiation in thyroid carcinomas. Br J Cancer 73: 139–143
584. Ito T, Seyama T, Mizuno T et al. 1992 Unique association of p53 mutations with undifferentiated but not with differentiated carcinomas of the thyroid gland. Cancer Res 52: 1369–1371
585. Shahedian B, Shi Y, Zou M et al. 2001 Thyroid carcinoma is characterized by genomic instability: evidence from p53 mutations. Mol Genet Metab 72: 155–163
586. Garcia-Rostan G, Tallini G, Herrero A et al. 1999 Frequent mutation and nuclear localization of beta-catenin in anaplastic thyroid carcinoma. Cancer Res 59: 1811–1815
587. Roque L, Soares J, Castedo S 1998 Cytogenetic and fluorescence in situ hybridization studies in a case of anaplastic thyroid carcinoma. Cancer Genet Cytogenet 103: 7–10
588. Hemmer S, Wasenius V M, Knuutila S et al. 1999 DNA copy number changes in thyroid carcinoma. Am J Pathol 154: 1539–1547
589. Komoike Y, Tamaki Y, Sakita I et al. 1999 Comparative genomic hybridization defines frequent loss on 16p in human anaplastic thyroid carcinoma. Int J Oncol 14: 1157–1162
590. Wreesmann V B, Ghossein R A, Patel S G et al. 2002 Genome-wide appraisal of thyroid cancer progression. Am J Pathol 161: 1549–1556
591. Kadota M, Tamaki Y, Sekimoto M et al. 2003 Loss of heterozygosity on chromosome 16p and 18q in anaplastic thyroid carcinoma. Oncol Rep 10: 35–38
592. Onda M, Emi M, Yoshida A et al. 2004 Comprehensive gene expression profiling of anaplastic thyroid cancers with cDNA microarray of 25 344 genes. Endocr Relat Cancer 11: 843–854
593. Nikiforov Y E 2004 Genetic alterations involved in the transition from well-differentiated to poorly differentiated and anaplastic thyroid carcinomas. Endocr Pathol 15: 319–328
594. Asakawa H, Kobayashi T 2002 Multistep carcinogenesis in anaplastic thyroid carcinoma: a case report. Pathology 34: 94–97
595. Begum S, Rosenbaum E, Henrique R et al. 2004 BRAF mutations in anaplastic thyroid carcinoma: implications for tumor origin, diagnosis and treatment. Mod Pathol 17: 1359–1363
596. Stringer B M, Rowson J M, Parkar M H et al. 1989 Detection of the H-RAS oncogene in human thyroid anaplastic carcinomas. Experientia 45: 372–376
597. Klinck G H 1969 Hemangioendothelioma and sarcoma of the thyroid. In: Hedinger C E (ed) Thyroid cancer. Springer-Verlag, Berlin, p 60–64
598. Meissner W A, Warren S 1969 Tumors of the thyroid gland. Atlas of tumor pathology, series 2, fascicle 4. Armed Forces Institute of Pathology, Washington, DC
599. Ruchti C, Gerber H A, Schaffner T 1984 Factor VIII-related antigen in malignant hemangioendothelioma of the thyroid: additional evidence for the endothelial origin of this tumor. Am J Clin Pathol 82: 474–480
600. Eusebi V 2004 Angiosarcoma. In: DeLellis R A, Lloyd R V, Heitz P U et al. (eds) Pathology and genetics. Tumours of endocrine organs. World Health Organization classification of tumours. IARC Press, Lyon, p 113–114
601. Hedinger C 1981 Geographic pathology of thyroid diseases. Pathol Res Pract 171: 285–292
602. Mills S E, Gaffey M J, Watts J C et al. 1994 Angiomatoid carcinoma and 'angiosarcoma' of the thyroid gland. A spectrum of endothelial differentiation. Am J Clin Pathol 102: 322–330

603. Mills S E, Stallings R G, Austin M B 1986 Angiomatoid carcinoma of the thyroid gland. Anaplastic carcinoma with follicular and medullary features mimicking angiosarcoma. Am J Clin Pathol 86: 674–678
604. Ritter J H, Mills S E, Nappi O et al. 1995 Angiosarcoma-like neoplasms of epithelial organs: true endothelial tumors or variants of carcinoma? Semin Diagn Pathol 12: 270–282
605. Papotti M, Botto Micca F, Favero A et al. 1993 Poorly differentiated thyroid carcinomas with primordial cell component. A group of aggressive lesions sharing insular, trabecular, and solid patterns. Am J Surg Pathol 17: 291–301
606. Tallini G, Garcia-Rostan G, Herrero A et al. 1999 Downregulation of p27KIP1 and Ki67/Mib1 labeling index support the classification of thyroid carcinoma into prognostically relevant categories. Am J Surg Pathol 23: 678–685
607. Sobrinho-Simoes M, Albores-Saavedra J, Tallini G et al. 2004 Poorly differentiated carcinoma. In: DeLellis R A, Lloyd R V, Heitz P U, et al. (eds) Pathology and genetics. Tumours of endocrine organs. World Health Organization classification of tumours. IARC Press, Lyon, p 73–76
608. Rosai J 2004 Poorly differentiated thyroid carcinoma: introduction to the issue, its landmarks, and clinical impact. Endocr Pathol 15: 293–296
609. Bal C, Padhy A K, Panda S et al. 1993 "Insular" carcinoma of thyroid. A subset of anaplastic thyroid malignancy with a less aggressive clinical course. Clin Nucl Med 18: 1056–1058
610. Flynn S D, Forman B H, Stewart A F et al. 1988 Poorly differentiated ("insular") carcinoma of the thyroid gland: an aggressive subset of differentiated thyroid neoplasms. Surgery 104: 963–970
611. Hiltzik D, Carlson D L, Tuttle R M et al. 2006. Poorly differentiated thyroid carcinoma defined on the basis of mitoses and necrosis. A clinicopathologic study of 58 patients. Cancer 106: 1286–1295
612. Pietribiasi F, Sapino A, Papotti M et al. 1990 Cytologic features of poorly differentiated 'insular' carcinoma of the thyroid, as revealed by fine-needle aspiration biopsy. Am J Clin Pathol 94: 687–692
613. Pilotti S, Collini P, Del Bo R et al. 1994 A novel panel of antibodies that segregates immunocytochemically poorly differentiated carcinoma from undifferentiated carcinoma of the thyroid gland. Am J Surg Pathol 18: 1054–1064
614. Resnick M B, Schacter P, Finkelstein Y et al. 1998 Immunohistochemical analysis of p27/kip1 expression in thyroid carcinoma. Mod Pathol 11: 735–739
615. Nikiforova M N, Kimura E T, Gandhi M et al. 2003 BRAF mutations in thyroid tumors are restricted to papillary carcinomas and anaplastic or poorly differentiated carcinomas arising from papillary carcinomas. J Clin Endocrinol Metab 88: 5399–5404
616. Fugazzola L, Mannavola D, Cirello V et al. 2004 BRAF mutations in an Italian cohort of thyroid cancers. Clin Endocrinol (Oxf) 61: 239–243
617. Nishida T, Katayama S, Tsujimoto M et al. 1999 Clinicopathological significance of poorly differentiated carcinoma. Am J Surg Pathol 23: 205–211
618. Decaussin M, Bernard M H, Adeline P et al. 2002. Thyroid carcinomas with distant metastases. A review of 111 cases with emphasis on the prognostic significance of an insular component. Am J Surg Pathol 26: 1007–1015
619. Sasaki A, Daa T, Kashima K et al. 1996 Insular component as a risk factor of thyroid carcinoma. Pathol Int 46: 939–946
620. Ashfaq R, Vuitch F, Delgado R et al. 1994 Papillary and follicular thyroid carcinomas with an insular component. Cancer 73: 416–423
621. Evans H L 1986 Columnar-cell carcinoma of the thyroid. A report of two cases of an aggressive variant of thyroid carcinoma. Am J Clin Pathol 85: 77–80
622. Ferreiro J A, Hay I D, Lloyd R V 1996 Columnar cell carcinoma of the thyroid: report of three additional cases. Hum Pathol 27: 1156–1160
623. Sobrinho-Simoes M, Nesland J M, Johannessen J V 1988 Columnar-cell carcinoma. Another variant of poorly differentiated carcinoma of the thyroid. Am J Clin Pathol 89: 264–267
624. Mizukami Y, Nonomura A, Michigishi T et al. 1994 Columnar cell carcinoma of the thyroid gland: a case report and review of the literature. Hum Pathol 25: 1098–1101
625. Berends D, Mouthaan P J 1992 Columnar-cell carcinoma of the thyroid. Histopathology 20: 360–362
626. Gaertner E M, Davidson M, Wenig B M 1995 The columnar cell variant of thyroid papillary carcinoma. Case report and discussion of an unusually aggressive thyroid papillary carcinoma. Am J Surg Pathol 19: 940–947
627. Akslen L A, Varhaug J E 1990 Thyroid carcinoma with mixed tall-cell and columnar-cell features. Am J Clin Pathol 94: 442–445
628. Genton C Y, Dutoit M, Portmann L et al. 1998 Pathologic fracture of the femur neck as first manifestation of a minute columnar cell carcinoma of the thyroid gland. Pathol Res Pract 194: 861–863
629. Shimizu M, Hirokawa M, Manabe T 1999 Tall cell variant of papillary thyroid carcinoma with foci of columnar cell component. Virchows Arch 434: 173–175
630. Wenig B M, Thompson L D, Adair C F et al. 1998 Thyroid papillary carcinoma of columnar cell type: a clinicopathologic study of 16 cases. Cancer 82: 740–753
631. Hirokawa M, Shimizu M, Fukuya T et al. 1998 Columnar cell carcinoma of the thyroid: MIB-1 immunoreactivity as a prognostic factor. Endocr Pathol 9: 31–34
632. Hui P K, Chan J K, Cheung P S et al. 1990 Columnar cell carcinoma of the thyroid. Fine needle aspiration findings in a case. Acta Cytol 34: 355–358
633. Evans H L 1996 Encapsulated columnar-cell neoplasms of the thyroid. A report of four cases suggesting a favorable prognosis. Am J Surg Pathol 20: 1205–1211
634. Fukunaga M, Shinozaki S, Miyazawa Y et al. 1997 Columnar cell carcinoma of the thyroid. Pathol Int 47: 489–492
635. Putti T C, Bhuiya T A, Wasserman P G 1998 Fine needle aspiration cytology of mixed tall and columnar cell papillary carcinoma of the thyroid. A case report. Acta Cytol 42: 387–390
636. Smith A E, Couch M, Argani P 1998 Pathologic quiz case 1. Papillary thyroid carcinoma (PTC), combined tall cell and columnar variants. Arch Otolaryngol Head Neck Surg 124: 1170–1172
637. Cameselle-Teijeiro J, Wenig B, Sobrinho-Simoes M et al. 2004 Mucoepidermoid carcinoma. In: DeLellis R A, Lloyd R V, Heitz P U et al. (eds) Pathology and genetics. Tumours of endocrine organs. World Health Organization classification of tumours. IARC Press, Lyon, p 82–83
638. Franssila K O, Harach H R, Wasenius V M 1984 Mucoepidermoid carcinoma of the thyroid. Histopathology 8: 847–860
639. Katoh R, Sugai T, Ono S et al. 1990 Mucoepidermoid carcinoma of the thyroid gland. Cancer 65: 2020–2027
640. Rhatigan R M, Roque J L, Bucher R L 1977 Mucoepidermoid carcinoma of the thyroid gland. Cancer 39: 210–214
641. Mizukami Y, Matsubara F, Hashimoto T et al. 1984 Primary mucoepidermoid carcinoma in the thyroid gland. A case report including an ultrastructural and biochemical study. Cancer 53: 1741–1745
642. Harach H R, Day E S, de Strizic N A 1986 Mucoepidermoid carcinoma of the thyroid. Report of a case with immunohistochemical studies. Medicina 46: 213–216
643. Tanda F, Massarelli G, Bosincu L et al. 1990 Primary mucoepidermoid carcinoma of the thyroid gland. Surg Pathol 3: 317–324
644. Bondeson L, Bondeson A G, Thompson N W 1991 Papillary carcinoma of the thyroid with mucoepidermoid features. Am J Clin Pathol 95: 175–179
645. Sambade C, Franssila K, Basilio-de-Oliveirz C 1990 Mucoepidermoid carcinoma of the thyroid revisited. Surg Pathol 3: 271–280
646. Wenig B M, Adair C F, Heffess C S 1995 Primary mucoepidermoid carcinoma of the thyroid gland: a report of six cases and a review of the literature of a follicular epithelial-derived tumor. Hum Pathol 26: 1099–1108
647. Arezzo A, Patetta R, Ceppa P et al. 1998 Mucoepidermoid carcinoma of the thyroid gland arising from a papillary epithelial neoplasm. Am Surg 64: 307–311
648. Viciana M J, Galera-Davidson H, Martin-Lacave I et al. 1996 Papillary carcinoma of the thyroid with mucoepidermoid differentiation. Arch Pathol Lab Med 120: 397–398
649. Miranda R N, Myint M A, Gnepp D R 1995 Composite follicular variant of papillary carcinoma and mucoepidermoid carcinoma of the thyroid. Report of a case and review of the literature. Am J Surg Pathol 19: 1209–1215
650. Cameselle-Teijeiro J, Febles-Perez C, Sobrinho-Simoes M 1995 Papillary and mucoepidermoid carcinoma of the thyroid with anaplastic transformation: a case report with histologic and immunohistochemical findings that support a provocative histogenetic hypothesis. Pathol Res Pract 191: 1214–1221
651. Cameselle-Teijeiro J, Febles-Perez C, Sobrinho-Simoes M 1997 Cytologic features of fine needle aspirates of papillary and mucoepidermoid carcinoma of the thyroid with anaplastic transformation. A case report. Acta Cytol 41(4 suppl): 1356–1360
652. Harach H R 1985 A study on the relationship between solid cell nests and mucoepidermoid carcinoma of the thyroid. Histopathology 9: 195–207
653. Chan J K, Albores-Saavedra J, Battifora H et al. 1991 Sclerosing mucoepidermoid thyroid carcinoma with eosinophilia. A distinctive low-grade malignancy arising from the metaplastic follicles of Hashimoto's thyroiditis. Am J Surg Pathol 15: 438–448
654. Chan J K C, LiVolsi V A, Bondeson L et al. 2004 Sclerosing mucoepidermoid carcinoma with eosinophilia. In: DeLellis R A, Lloyd R V, Heitz P U et al. (eds) Pathology and genetics. Tumours of endocrine organs. World Health Organization classification of tumours. IARC Press, Lyon, p 84
655. Sim S J, Ro J Y, Ordonez N G et al. 1997 Sclerosing mucoepidermoid carcinoma with eosinophilia of the thyroid: report of two patients, one with distant metastasis, and review of the literature. Hum Pathol 28: 1091–1096
656. Geisinger K R, Steffee C H, McGee R S et al. 1998 The cytomorphologic features of sclerosing mucoepidermoid carcinoma of the thyroid gland with eosinophilia. Am J Clin Pathol 109: 294–301
657. Chung J, Lee S K, Gong G et al. 1999 Sclerosing mucoepidermoid carcinoma with eosinophilia of the thyroid glands: a case report with clinical manifestation of recurrent neck mass. J Korean Med Sci 14: 338–341
658. Cavazza A, Toschi E, Valcavi R et al. 1999 Sclerosing mucoepidermoid carcinoma with eosinophilia of the thyroid: description of a case. Pathologica 91: 31–35
659. Baloch Z W, Solomon A C, LiVolsi V A 2000 Primary mucoepidermoid carcinoma and sclerosing mucoepidermoid carcinoma with eosinophilia of the thyroid gland: a report of nine cases. Mod Pathol 13: 802–807
660. Solomon A C, Baloch Z W, Salhany K E et al. 2000 Thyroid sclerosing mucoepidermoid carcinoma with eosinophilia: mimic of Hodgkin disease in nodal metastases. Arch Pathol Lab Med 124: 446–449

661. Albores-Saavedra J, Gu X, Luna M A 2003 Clear cells and thyroid transcription factor I reactivity in sclerosing mucoepidermoid carcinoma of the thyroid gland. Ann Diagn Pathol 7: 348–353
662. Diaz-Perez R, Quiroz H, Nishiyama R H 1976 Primary mucinous adenocarcinoma of thyroid gland. Cancer 38: 1323–1325
663. Sobrinho-Simoes M, Stenwig A E, Nesland J M et al. 1986 A mucinous carcinoma of the thyroid. Pathol Res Pract 181: 464–471
664. Sobrinho-Simoes M A, Nesland J M, Johannessen J V 1985 A mucin-producing tumor in the thyroid gland. Ultrastruct Pathol 9: 277–281
665. Cruz M C, Marques L P, Sambade C C et al. 1991 Primary mucinous carcinoma of the thyroid gland. Surg Pathol 4: 266–273
666. Williams E D 1966 Histogenesis of medullary carcinoma of the thyroid. J Clin Pathol 19: 114–118
667. Raue F, Kotzerke J, Reinwein D et al. 1993 Prognostic factors in medullary thyroid carcinoma: evaluation of 741 patients from the German Medullary Thyroid Carcinoma Register. Clin Invest 71: 7–12
668. Williams E D 1979 Medullary carcinoma of the thyroid. In: DeGroot L J (ed) Endocrinology. Grune & Stratton, New York, p 777–792
669. Saad M F, Ordonez N G, Rashid R K et al. 1984 Medullary carcinoma of the thyroid. A study of the clinical features and prognostic factors in 161 patients. Medicine (Baltimore) 63: 319–342
670. Rosenberg-Bourgin M, Gardet P, de Sahb R et al. 1989 Comparison of sporadic and hereditary forms of medullary thyroid carcinoma. Henry Ford Hospital J 37: 141–143
671. Donovan D T, Levy M L, Frust E J 1989 Familial cutaneous lichen amyloidosis in association with MEN2A: a new variant. Henry Ford Hospital J 37: 147–150
672. Sobol H, Narod S A, Schuffenecker I et al. 1989 Hereditary medullary thyroid carcinoma: genetic analysis of three related syndromes. Henry Ford Hospital J 37: 109–111
673. Farndon J R, Leight G S, Dilley W G 1986 Familial medullary thyroid carcinoma without associated endocrinopathies: a distinct clinical entity. Br J Surg 73: 278–281
674. Wolfe H J, DeLellis R A 1981 Familial medullary thyroid carcinoma and C cell hyperplasia. Clin Endocrinol Metab 10: 351–365
675. Carney J A, Sizemore G W, Hayles A V 1979 C-cell disease of the thyroid gland in multiple endocrine neoplasia, type 2b. Cancer 44: 2173–2183
676. Mulligan L M, Kwok J B, Healey C S et al. 1993 Germ-line mutations of the RET proto-oncogene in multiple endocrine neoplasia type 2A. Nature 363: 458–460
677. Mulligan L M, Eng C, Healey C S et al. 1994 Specific mutations of the RET proto-oncogene are related to disease phenotype in MEN 2A and FMTC. Nat Genet 6: 70–74
678. Hofstra R M, Landsvater R M, Ceccherini I et al. 1994 A mutation in the RET proto-oncogene associated with multiple endocrine neoplasia type 2B and sporadic medullary thyroid carcinoma. Nature 367: 375–376
679. Kebebew E, Ituarte P H, Siperstein A E et al. 2000 Medullary thyroid carcinoma: clinical characteristics, treatment, prognostic factors, and a comparison of staging systems. Cancer 88: 1139–1148
680. Chong G C, Beahrs O H, Sizemore G W et al. 1975 Medullary carcinoma of the thyroid gland. Cancer 35: 695–704
681. Hijazi Y M, Nieman L K, Medeiros L J 1992 Medullary carcinoma of the thyroid as a cause of Cushing's syndrome: a case with ectopic adrenocorticotropin secretion characterized by double enzyme immunostaining. Hum Pathol 23: 592–596
682. Mure A, Gicquel C, Abdelmoumene N et al. 1995 Cushing's syndrome in medullary thyroid carcinoma. J Endocrinol Invest 18: 180–185
683. Kakudo K, Carney J A, Sizemore G W 1985 Medullary carcinoma of thyroid. Biologic behavior of the sporadic and familial neoplasm. Cancer 55: 2818–2821
684. Carney J A, Sizemore G W, Hayles A B 1978 Multiple endocrine neoplasia, type 2b. Pathobiol Annu 8: 105–153
685. Gimm O, Morrison C D, Suster S et al. 2004 Multiple endocrine neoplasia type 2. In: DeLellis R A, Lloyd R V, Heitz P U et al. (eds) Pathology and genetics. Tumours of endocrine organs. World Health Organization classification of tumours. IARC Press, Lyon, p 211–217
686. Henry J F, Denizot A, Puccini M et al. 1998 Latent subclinical medullary thyroid carcinoma: diagnosis and treatment. World J Surg 22: 752–756
687. Rieu M, Lame M C, Richard A et al. 1995 Prevalence of sporadic medullary thyroid carcinoma: the importance of routine measurement of serum calcitonin in the diagnostic evaluation of thyroid nodules. Clin Endocrinol (Oxf) 42: 453–460
688. Kaserer K, Scheuba C, Neuhold N et al. 1998 C-cell hyperplasia and medullary thyroid carcinoma in patients routinely screened for serum calcitonin. Am J Surg Pathol 22: 722–728
689. Modigliani E 1994 Medullary thyroid carcinoma. Curr Ther Endocrinol Metab 5: 112–117
690. Girelli M E, Nacamulli D, Pelizzo M R et al. 1998 Medullary thyroid carcinoma: clinical features and long-term follow-up of seventy-eight patients treated between 1969 and 1986. Thyroid 8: 517–523
691. Modigliani E, Cohen R, Campos J M et al. 1998 Prognostic factors for survival and for biochemical cure in medullary thyroid carcinoma: results in 899 patients. The GETC Study Group. Groupe d'Etude des Tumeurs a Calcitonine. Clin Endocrinol (Oxf) 48: 265–273
692. Scopsi L, Sampietro G, Boracchi P et al. 1996 Multivariate analysis of prognostic factors in sporadic medullary carcinoma of the thyroid. A retrospective study of 109 consecutive patients. Cancer 78: 2173–2183
693. Bergholm U, Bergstrom R, Ekbom A 1997 Long-term follow-up of patients with medullary carcinoma of the thyroid. Cancer 79: 132–138
694. Rossi R L, Cady B, Meissner W A et al. 1980 Nonfamilial medullary thyroid carcinoma. Am J Surg 139: 554–560
695. Fuchshuber P R, Loree T R, Hicks W L Jr. et al. 1998 Medullary carcinoma of the thyroid: prognostic factors and treatment recommendations. Ann Surg Oncol 5: 81–86
696. Bigner S H, Cox E B, Mendelsohn G et al. 1981 Medullary carcinoma of the thyroid in the multiple endocrine neoplasia IIA syndrome. Am J Surg Pathol 5: 459–472
697. Ibanez M L 1974 Medullary carcinoma of the thyroid gland. Pathol Annu 9: 263–290
698. Albores-Saavedra J, LiVolsi V A, Williams E D 1985 Medullary carcinoma. Semin Diagn Pathol 2: 137–146
699. Hazard J B 1977 The C cells (parafollicular cells) of the thyroid gland and medullary thyroid carcinoma. A review. Am J Pathol 88: 213–250
700. Uribe M, Fenoglio-Preiser C M, Grimes M et al. 1985 Medullary carcinoma of the thyroid gland. Clinical, pathological, and immunohistochemical features with review of the literature. Am J Surg Pathol 9: 577–594
701. Zaatari G S, Saigo P E, Huvos A G 1983 Mucin production in medullary carcinoma of the thyroid. Arch Pathol Lab Med 107: 70–74
702. Golouh R, Us-Krasovec M, Auersperg M et al. 1985 Amphicrine-composite calcitonin and mucin-producing carcinoma of the thyroid. Ultrastruct Pathol 8: 197–206
703. Harach H R, Williams E D 1983 Glandular (tubular and follicular) variants of medullary carcinoma of the thyroid. Histopathology 7: 83–97
704. Sambade C, Baldaque-Faria A, Cardoso-Oliveira M et al. 1988 Follicular and papillary variants of medullary carcinoma of the thyroid. Pathol Res Pract 184: 98–107
705. Dominguez-Malagon H, Delgado-Chavez R, Torres-Najera M et al. 1989 Oxyphil and squamous variants of medullary thyroid carcinoma. Cancer 63: 1183–1188
706. Harach H R, Bergholm U 1988 Medullary (C cell) carcinoma of the thyroid with features of follicular oxyphilic cell tumours. Histopathology 13: 645–656
707. Kakudo K, Miyauchi A, Ogihara T et al. 1978 Medullary carcinoma of the thyroid. Giant cell type. Arch Pathol Lab Med 102: 445–447
708. Mendelsohn G, Baylin S B, Bigner S H et al. 1980 Anaplastic variants of medullary thyroid carcinoma: a light-microscopic and immunohistochemical study. Am J Surg Pathol 4: 333–341
709. Bussolati G, Monga G 1979 Medullary carcinoma of the thyroid with atypical patterns. Cancer 44: 1769–1777
710. Landon G, Ordonez N G 1985 Clear cell variant of medullary carcinoma of the thyroid. Hum Pathol 16: 844–847
711. Holm R, Sobrinho-Simoes M, Nesland J M et al. 1985 Medullary carcinoma of the thyroid gland: an immunocytochemical study. Ultrastruct Pathol 8: 25–41
712. Marcus J N, Dise C A, LiVolsi V A 1982 Melanin production in a medullary thyroid carcinoma. Cancer 49: 2518–2526
713. Beerman H, Rigaud C, Bogomoletz W V et al. 1990 Melanin production in black medullary thyroid carcinoma (MTC). Histopathology 16: 227–233
714. Ikeda T, Satoh M, Azuma K et al. 1998 Medullary thyroid carcinoma with a paraganglioma-like pattern and melanin production: a case report with ultrastructural and immunohistochemical studies. Arch Pathol Lab Med 122: 555–558
715. Schroder S, Bocker W, Baisch H et al. 1988 Prognostic factors in medullary thyroid carcinomas. Survival in relation to age, sex, stage, histology, immunocytochemistry, and DNA content. Cancer 61: 806–816
716. Kakudo K, Miyauchi A, Takai S et al. 1979 C cell carcinoma of the thyroid-papillary type. Acta Pathol Jpn 29: 653–659
717. Papotti M, Sapino A, Abbona G et al. 1995 Pseudoangiosarcomatous features in medullary carcinoma of the thyroid. Report of two cases. Int J Surg Pathol 3: 29–34
718. Harach H R, Bergholm U 1992 Small cell variant of medullary carcinoma of the thyroid with neuroblastoma-like features. Histopathology 21: 378–380
719. Harach H R, Bergholm U 1993 Medullary carcinoma of the thyroid with carcinoid-like features. J Clin Pathol 46: 113–117
720. Mizukami Y, Kurumaya H, Nonomura A et al. 1992 Sporadic medullary microcarcinoma of the thyroid. Histopathology 21: 375–377
721. White I L, Vimadalal S D, Catz B et al. 1981 Occult medullary carcinoma of thyroid: an unusual clinical and pathologic presentation. Cancer 47: 1364–1368
722. Guyetant S, Dupre F, Bigorgne J C et al. 1999 Medullary thyroid microcarcinoma: a clinicopathologic retrospective study of 38 patients with no prior familial disease. Hum Pathol 30: 957–963
723. Butler M, Khan S 1986 Immunoreactive calcitonin in amyloid fibrils of medullary carcinoma of the thyroid gland. An immunogold staining technique. Arch Pathol Lab Med 110: 647–649
724. Krisch K, Krisch I, Horvat G et al. 1985 The value of immunohistochemistry in medullary thyroid carcinoma: a systematic study of 30 cases. Histopathology 9: 1077–1089
725. Lloyd R V, Sisson J C, Marangos P J 1983 Calcitonin, carcinoembryonic antigen and neuron-specific enolase in medullary thyroid carcinoma. Cancer 51: 2234–2239
726. Schmid K W, Fischer-Colbrie R, Hagn C et al. 1987 Chromogranin A and B and secretogranin II in medullary carcinomas of the thyroid. Am J Surg Pathol 11: 551–556

727. Bostwick D G, Null W E, Holmes D et al. 1987 Expression of opioid peptides in tumors. N Engl J Med 317: 1439–1443
728. Takami H, Bessho T, Kameya T 1988 Immunohistochemical study of medullary thyroid carcinoma: relationship of clinical features to prognostic factors in 36 patients. World J Surg 12: 572–579
729. Sikri K L, Varndell I M, Hamid Q A et al. 1985 Medullary carcinoma of the thyroid. An immunocytochemical and histochemical study of 25 cases using eight separate markers. Cancer 56: 2481–2491
730. Schroder S, Kloppel G 1987 Carcinoembryonic antigen and nonspecific cross-reacting antigen in thyroid cancer. An immunocytochemical study using polyclonal and monoclonal antibodies. Am J Surg Pathol 11: 100–108
731. Matias-Guiu X, Machin P, Pons C et al. 1998 Sustentacular cells occur frequently in the familial form of medullary thyroid carcinoma. J Pathol 184: 420–423
732. Kimura N, Nakazato Y, Nagura H et al. 1990 Expression of intermediate filaments in neuroendocrine tumors. Arch Pathol Lab Med 114: 506–510
733. Ponder B A J 2002 Multiple endocrine neoplasia type 2. In: Vogelstein B, Kinzler K W (eds) The genetic basis of human cancer, 2nd edn. McGraw-Hill, New York, p 501–513
734. Komminoth P 1997 The RET proto-oncogene in medullary and papillary thyroid carcinoma. Molecular features, pathophysiology and clinical implications. Virchows Arch 431: 1–9
735. Lloyd R V 1995 RET proto-oncogene mutations and rearrangements in endocrine diseases. Am J Pathol 147: 1539–1544
736. Mulligan L M, Marsh D J, Robinson B G et al. 1995 Genotype-phenotype correlation in multiple endocrine neoplasia type 2: report of the International RET mutation consortium. J Intern Med 238: 343–346
737. Komminoth P, Kunz E K, Matias-Guiu X et al. 1995 Analysis of RET protooncogene point mutations distinguishes heritable from nonheritable medullary thyroid carcinomas. Cancer 76: 479–489
738. Eng C, Mulligan L M, Smith D P et al. 1995 Mutation of the RET protooncogene in sporadic medullary thyroid carcinoma. Genes Chromos Cancer 12: 209–212
739. Bugalho M J, Frade J P, Santos J R et al. 1997 Molecular analysis of the RET proto-oncogene in patients with sporadic medullary thyroid carcinoma: a novel point mutation in the extracellular cysteine-rich domain. Eur J Endocrinol 136: 423–426
740. Romei C, Elisei R, Pinchera A et al. 1996 Somatic mutations of the ret protooncogene in sporadic medullary thyroid carcinoma are not restricted to exon 16 and are associated with tumor recurrence. J Clin Endocrinol Metab 81: 1619–1622
741. Marsh D J, Learoyd D L, Andrew S D et al. 1996 Somatic mutations in the RET proto-oncogene in sporadic medullary thyroid carcinoma. Clin Endocrinol (Oxf) 44: 249–257
742. Gimm O, Niederle B E, Weber T et al. 2002 RET proto-oncogene mutations affecting codon 790/791: a mild form of multiple endocrine neoplasia type 2A syndrome? Surgery 132: 952–959
743. Eng C, Mulligan L M 1997 Mutations of the RET protooncogene in the multiple endocrine neoplasia type 2 syndromes, related sporadic tumors, and Hirschsprung disease. Hum Mutat 9: 97–109
744. Brierley J, Tsang R, Simpson W J et al. 1996 Medullary thyroid cancer: analyses of survival and prognostic factors and the role of radiation therapy in local control. Thyroid 6: 305–310
745. Machens A, Holzhausen H J, Dralle H 2006 Contralateral cervical and mediastinal lymph node metastasis in medullary thyroid cancer: systemic disease? Surgery 139: 28–32
746. Franc B, Rosenberg-Bourgin M, Caillou B et al. 1998 Medullary thyroid carcinoma: search for histological predictors of survival (109 proband cases analysis). Hum Pathol 29: 1078–1084
747. Norton J A, Froome L C, Farrell R E et al. 1979 Multiple endocrine neoplasia type IIb: the most aggressive form of medullary thyroid carcinoma. Surg Clin North Am 59: 109–118
748. Ashworth M 2004 The pathology of preclinical medullary thyroid carcinoma. Endocr Pathol 15: 227–232
749. Williams E D, Brown C L, Doniach I 1966 Pathological and clinical findings in a series of 67 cases of medullary carcinoma of the thyroid. J Clin Pathol 19: 103–113
750. Ruppert J M, Eggleston J C, deBustros A et al. 1986 Disseminated calcitonin-poor medullary thyroid carcinoma in a patient with calcitonin-rich primary tumor. Am J Surg Pathol 10: 513–518
751. Saad M F, Ordonez N G, Guido J J et al. 1984 The prognostic value of calcitonin immunostaining in medullary carcinoma of the thyroid. J Clin Endocrinol Metab 59: 850–856
752. Mendelsohn G, Wells S A Jr., Baylin S B 1984 Relationship of tissue carcinoembryonic antigen and calcitonin to tumor virulence in medullary thyroid carcinoma. An immunohistochemical study in early, localized, and virulent disseminated stages of disease. Cancer 54: 657–662
753. Schroder S, Schwarz W, Rehpenning W et al. 1988 Leu-M1 immunoreactivity and prognosis in medullary carcinomas of the thyroid gland. J Cancer Res Clin Oncol 114: 291–296
754. Langle F, Soliman T, Neuhold N et al. 1994 CD15 (LeuM1) immunoreactivity: prognostic factor for sporadic and hereditary medullary thyroid cancer? Study Group on Multiple Endocrine Neoplasia of Austria. World J Surg 18: 583–587
755. Viale G, Roncalli M, Grimelius L et al. 1995 Prognostic value of bcl-2 immunoreactivity in medullary thyroid carcinoma. Hum Pathol 26: 945–950
756. Scopsi L, Sampietro G, Boracchi P et al. 1998 Argyrophilia and chromogranin A and B immunostaining in patients with sporadic medullary thyroid carcinoma. A critical appraisal of their prognostic utility. J Pathol 184: 414–419
757. Roncalli M, Viale G, Grimelius L et al. 1994 Prognostic value of N-myc immunoreactivity in medullary thyroid carcinoma. Cancer 74: 134–141
758. Fontanini G, Vignati S, Pacini F et al. 1996 Microvessel count: an indicator of poor outcome in medullary thyroid carcinoma but not in other types of thyroid carcinoma. Mod Pathol 9: 636–641
759. el-Naggar A K, Ordonez N G, McLemore D et al. 1990 Clinicopathologic and flow cytometric DNA study of medullary thyroid carcinoma. Surgery 108: 981–985
760. Ekman E T, Bergholm U, Backdahl M et al. 1990 Nuclear DNA content and survival in medullary thyroid carcinoma. Swedish Medullary Thyroid Cancer Study Group. Cancer 65: 511–517
761. Ordonez N G, Ibanez M L, Samaan N A et al. 1983 Immunoperoxidase study of uncommon parathyroid tumors. Report of two cases of nonfunctioning parathyroid carcinoma and one intrathyroid parathyroid tumor-producing amyloid. Am J Surg Pathol 7: 535–542
762. Emmersten K, Erno H, Henriques U et al. 1983 C-cells for differentiation between familial and sporadic medullary thyroid carcinoma. Dan Med Bull 30: 353–356
763. Albores-Saavedra J, Monforte H, Nadji M et al. 1988 C-cell hyperplasia in thyroid tissue adjacent to follicular cell tumors. Hum Pathol 19: 795–799
764. Santensanio G, Iafrate E, Partenzi A et al. 1997 A critical reassessment of the concept of C-cell hyperplasia of the thyroid – a quantitative immunohistochem study. Appl Immunohistochem 5: 160–172
765. DeLellis R A, Wolfe H J 1981 The pathobiology of the human calcitonin (C)-cell: a review. Pathol Annu 16: 25–52
766. Chan J K C, Tse C C H 1989 Solid cell nest-associated C-cells: another possible explanation for "C-cell hyperplasia" adjacent to follicular cell tumors (Letter). Hum Pathol 10: 498
767. Baschieri L, Castagna M, Fierabracci A et al. 1989 Distribution of calcitonin- and somatostatin-containing cells in thyroid lymphoma and in Hashimoto's thyroiditis. Appl Pathol 7: 99–104
768. Perry A, Molberg K, Albores-Saavedra J 1996 Physiologic versus neoplastic C-cell hyperplasia of the thyroid: separation of distinct histologic and biologic entities. Cancer 77: 750–756
769. McDermott M B, Swanson P E, Wick M R 1995 Immunostains for collagen type IV discriminate between C-cell hyperplasia and microscopic medullary carcinoma in multiple endocrine neoplasia, type 2a. Hum Pathol 26: 1308–1312
770. Wohllk N, Cote G J, Evans D B et al. 1996 Application of genetic screening information to the management of medullary thyroid carcinoma and multiple endocrine neoplasia type 2. Endocrinol Metab Clin North Am 25: 1–25
771. Frilling A, Dralle H, Eng C et al. 1995 Presymptomatic DNA screening in families with multiple endocrine neoplasia type 2 and familial medullary thyroid carcinoma. Surgery 118: 1099–1103
772. Guyetant S, Josselin N, Savagner F et al. 2003. C-cell hyperplasia and medullary thyroid carcinoma: clinicopathological and genetic correlations in 66 consecutive patients. Mod Pathol 16: 756–763
773. Eng C, Mulligan L M, Smith D P et al. 1995 Low frequency of germline mutations in the RET proto-oncogene in patients with apparently sporadic medullary thyroid carcinoma. Clin Endocrinol (Oxf) 43: 123–127
774. Shirahama S, Ogura K, Takami H et al. 1998 Mutational analysis of the RET proto-oncogene in 71 Japanese patients with medullary thyroid carcinoma. J Hum Genet 43: 101–106
775. Erdogan M F, Gursoy A, Ozgen G et al. 2005 Ret proto-oncogene mutations in apparently sporadic Turkish medullary thyroid carcinoma patients: Turkmen study. J Endocrinol Invest 28: 806–809
776. Machens A, Niccoli-Sire P, Hoegel J et al. 2003 Early malignant progression of hereditary medullary thyroid cancer. N Engl J Med 349: 1517–1525
777. Machens A, Holzhausen H J, Thanh P N et al. 2003 Malignant progression from C-cell hyperplasia to medullary thyroid carcinoma in 167 carriers of RET germline mutations. Surgery 134: 425–431
778. Gimm O, Ukkat J, Niederle B E et al. 2004 Timing and extent of surgery in patients with familial medullary thyroid carcinoma/multiple endocrine neoplasia 2A-related RET mutations not affecting codon 634. World J Surg 28: 1312–1316
779. Lallier M, St-Vil D, Giroux M et al. 1998 Prophylactic thyroidectomy for medullary thyroid carcinoma in gene carriers of MEN2 syndrome. J Pediatr Surg 33: 846–848
780. Hinze R, Holzhausen H J, Gimm O et al. 1998 Primary hereditary medullary thyroid carcinoma – C-cell morphology and correlation with preoperative calcitonin levels. Virchows Arch 433: 203–208
781. van Heurn L W, Schaap C, Sie G et al. 1999 Predictive DNA testing for multiple endocrine neoplasia 2: a therapeutic challenge of prophylactic thyroidectomy in very young children. J Pediatr Surg 34: 568–571
782. Sanso G E, Domene H M, Garcia R et al. 2002 Very early detection of RET proto-oncogene mutation is crucial for preventive thyroidectomy in multiple endocrine neoplasia type 2 children: presence of C-cell malignant disease in asymptomatic carriers. Cancer 94: 323–330
783. Skinner M A, Moley J A, Dilley W G et al. 2005 Prophylactic thyroidectomy in multiple endocrine neoplasia type 2A. N Engl J Med 353: 1105–1113

784. Niccoli-Sire P, Murat A, Rohmer V et al. 2003 When should thyroidectomy be performed in familial medullary thyroid carcinoma gene carriers with non-cysteine RET mutations? Surgery 134: 1029–1036
785. Dralle H, Gimm O, Simon D et al. 1998 Prophylactic thyroidectomy in 75 children and adolescents with hereditary medullary thyroid carcinoma: German and Austrian experience. World J Surg 22: 744–750
786. Lax S F, Beham A, Kronberger-Schonecker D et al. 1994 Coexistence of papillary and medullary carcinoma of the thyroid gland – mixed or collision tumour? Clinicopathological analysis of three cases. Virchows Arch 424: 441–447
787. Gonzalez-Campora R, Lopez-Garrido J, Martin-Lacave I et al. 1992 Concurrence of a symptomatic encapsulated follicular carcinoma, an occult papillary carcinoma and a medullary carcinoma in the same patient. Histopathology 21: 380–382
788. Sobrinho-Simoes M 1993 Mixed medullary and follicular carcinoma of the thyroid. Histopathology 23: 287–289
789. Pfaltz M, Hedinger C E, Muhlethaler J P 1983 Mixed medullary and follicular carcinoma of the thyroid. Virchows Arch A Pathol Anat Histopathol 400: 53–59
790. Parker L N, Kollin J, Wu S Y et al. 1985 Carcinoma of the thyroid with a mixed medullary, papillary, follicular, and undifferentiated pattern. Arch Intern Med 145: 1507–1509
791. Apel R L, Alpert L C, Rizzo A et al. 1994 A metastasizing composite carcinoma of the thyroid with distinct medullary and papillary components. Arch Pathol Lab Med 118: 1143–1147
792. Albores-Saavedra J, Gorraez de la Mora T, de la Torre-Rendon F et al. 1990 Mixed medullary–papillary carcinoma of the thyroid: a previously unrecognized variant of thyroid carcinoma. Hum Pathol 21: 1151–1155
793. Pastolero G C, Coire C I, Asa S L 1996 Concurrent medullary and papillary carcinomas of thyroid with lymph node metastases. A collision phenomenon. Am J Surg Pathol 20: 245–250
794. Ljungberg O 1992 Biopsy pathology of the thyroid and parathyroid. Chapman & Hall, London
795. Burt A D, MacGuire J, Lindop G B et al. 1987 Mixed follicular–parafollicular carcinoma of the thyroid. Scott Med J 32: 50–51
796. Papotti M, Bussolati G, Komminoth P et al. 2004 Mixed medullary and follicular cell carcinoma. In: DeLellis R A, Lloyd R V, Heitz P U et al. (eds) Pathology and genetics. Tumours of endocrine organs. World Health Organization classification of tumours. IARC Press, Lyon, p 92–93
797. Papotti M, Negro F, Carney J A et al. 1997 Mixed medullary-follicular carcinoma of the thyroid. A morphological, immunohistochemical and in situ hybridization analysis of 11 cases. Virchows Arch 430: 397–405
798. Volante M, Papotti M, Roth J et al. 1999 Mixed medullary–follicular thyroid carcinoma. Molecular evidence for a dual origin of tumor components. Am J Pathol 155: 1499–1509
799. Ljungberg O, Ericsson U B, Bondeson L et al. 1983 A compound follicular–parafollicular cell carcinoma of the thyroid: a new tumor entity? Cancer 52: 1053–1061
800. Ljungberg O, Bondeson L, Bondeson A G 1984 Differentiated thyroid carcinoma, intermediate type: a new tumor entity with features of follicular and parafollicular cell carcinoma. Hum Pathol 15: 218–228
801. Mizukami Y, Nonomura A, Michigishi T et al. 1996 Mixed medullary-follicular carcinoma of the thyroid gland: a clinicopathologic variant of medullary thyroid carcinoma. Mod Pathol 9: 631–635
802. Holm R, Sobrinho-Simoes M, Nesland J M et al. 1987 Medullary thyroid carcinoma with thyroglobulin immunoreactivity. A special entity? Lab Invest 57: 258–268
803. Chan J K, Rosai J 1991 Tumors of the neck showing thymic or related branchial pouch differentiation: a unifying concept. Hum Pathol 22: 349–367
804. Lewis J E, Wick M R, Scheithauer B W et al. 1987 Thymoma, a clinicopathologic review. Cancer 60: 2727–2743
805. Chan J K C, Cheuk W, Dorfman D M et al. 2004 Ectopic thymoma. In: DeLellis R A, Lloyd R V, Heitz P U et al. (eds) Pathology and genetics. Tumours of endocrine organs. World Health Organization classification of tumours. IARC Press, Lyon, p 112
806. Kwon Y, Hong E K, Koo H L et al. 2006 Clinicopathological and immunohistochemical studies of thymic-related tumours in thyroid gland: report of five cases. Histopathology 48: 312–315
807. Murao T, Nakanishi M, Toda K et al. 1979 Malignant teratoma of the thyroid gland in an adolescent female. Acta Pathol Jpn 29: 109–117
808. Levey M 1976 An unusual thyroid tumor in a child. Laryngoscope 86: 1864–1868
809. Weigensberg C, Dalsley H, Asa S L et al. 1990 Thyroid thymoma in childhood. Endocrinol Pathol 1: 123–127
810. Harach H R, Saravia Day E, Franssila K O 1985 Thyroid spindle-cell tumor with mucous cysts. An intrathyroid thymoma? Am J Surg Pathol 9: 525–530
811. Kingsley D P E, Elton A, Bennett M H 1968 Malignant teratoma of the thyroid, case report and a review of the literature. Br J Cancer 22: 7–11
812. Hofman P, Mainguene C, Michiels J F et al. 1995 Thyroid spindle epithelial tumor with thymus-like differentiation (the "SETTLE" tumor). An immunohistochemical and electron microscopic study. Eur Arch Otorhinolaryngol 252: 316–320
813. Saw D, Wu D, Chess Q et al. 1997 Spindle epithelial tumor with thymus-like element (SETTLE), a primary thyroid tumor. Int J Surg Pathol 4: 169–174
814. Chetty R, Goetsch S, Nayler S et al. 1998 Spindle epithelial tumour with thymus-like element (SETTLE): the predominantly monophasic variant. Histopathology 33: 71–74
815. Kirby P A, Ellison W A, Thomas P A 1999 Spindle epithelial tumor with thymus-like differentiation (SETTLE) of the thyroid with prominent mitotic activity and focal necrosis. Am J Surg Pathol 23: 712–716
816. Cheuk W, Chan J K C, Dorfman D M et al. 2004 Spindle cell tumour with thymus-like differentiation. In: DeLellis R A, Lloyd R V, Heitz P U et al. (eds) Pathology and genetics. Tumours of endocrine organs. World Health Organization classification of tumours. IARC Press, Lyon, 94–95
817. Xu B, Hirokawa M, Yoshimoto K et al. 2003 Spindle epithelial tumor with thymus-like differentiation of the thyroid: a case report with pathological and molecular genetics study. Hum Pathol 34: 190–193
818. Erickson M L, Tapia B, Moreno E R et al. 2005 Early metastasizing spindle epithelial tumor with thymus-like differentiation (SETTLE) of the thyroid. Pediatr Dev Pathol 8: 599–606
819. Abrosimov A Y, LiVolsi V A 2005 Spindle epithelial tumor with thymus-like differentiation (SETTLE) of the thyroid with neck lymph node metastasis: a case report. Endocr Pathol 16: 139–143
820. Raffel A, Cupisti K, Rees M et al. 2003 Spindle epithelial tumour with thymus-like differentiation (SETTLE) of the thyroid gland with widespread metastases in a 13-year-old girl. Clin Oncol (R Coll Radiol) 15: 490–495
821. Cheuk W, Jacobson A A, Chan J K 2000 Spindle epithelial tumor with thymus-like differentiation (SETTLE): a distinctive malignant thyroid neoplasm with significant metastatic potential. Mod Pathol 13: 1150–1155
822. Asa S L, Dardick I, Van Nostrand A W et al. 1988 Primary thyroid thymoma: a distinct clinicopathological entity. Hum Pathol 19: 1463–1467
823. Kakudo K, Mori I, Tamaoki N et al. 1988 Carcinoma of possible thymic origin presenting as a thyroid mass: a new subgroup of squamous cell carcinoma of the thyroid. J Surg Oncol 38: 187–192
824. Miyauchi A, Kuma K, Matsuzuka F et al. 1985 Intrathyroidal epithelial thymoma: an entity distinct from squamous cell carcinoma of the thyroid. World J Surg 9: 128–135
825. Miyauchi A, Ishikawa H, Maedea M 1989 Intrathyroid epithelial thymoma: a report of six cases with immunohistochemical and ultrastructural studies. Endocrinol Surg 6: 289–295
826. Mizukami Y, Kurumaya H, Yamada T et al. 1995 Thymic carcinoma involving the thyroid gland: report of two cases. Hum Pathol 26: 576–579
827. Watanabe I, Tezuka F, Yamaguchi M et al. 1996 Thymic carcinoma of the thyroid. Pathol Int 46: 450–456
828. Attaran S Y, Omrani G H, Tavangar S M 1996 Lymphoepithelial-like intrathyroidal thymic carcinoma with foci of squamous differentiation. Case report. APMIS 104: 419–423
829. Damiani S, Filotico M, Eusebi V 1991 Carcinoma of the thyroid showing thymoma-like features. Virchows Arch A Pathol Anat Histopathol 418: 463–466
830. Da J, Shi H, Lu J 1999 [Thyroid squamous-cell carcinoma showing thymus-like element (CASTLE): a report of eight cases.] Zhonghua Zhong Liu Za Zhi 21: 303–304
831. Cheuk W, Chan J K C, Dorfman D M et al. 2004 Carcinoma showing thymus-like differentiation. In: DeLellis R A, Lloyd R V, Heitz P U et al. (eds) Pathology and genetics. Tumours of endocrine organs. World Health Organization classification of tumours. IARC Press, Lyon, p 96–97
832. Reimann J D R, Dorfman D M, Nose V 2006 Carcinoma showing thymus-like differentiation of the thyroid (CASTLE): a comparative study. Evidence of thymic differentiation and solid cell nest origin. Am J Surg Pathol 30: 994–1001
833. Dorfman D M, Shahsafaei A, Miyauchi A 1998 Intrathyroidal epithelial thymoma (ITET)/carcinoma showing thymus-like differentiation (CASTLE) exhibits CD5 immunoreactivity: new evidence for thymic differentiation. Histopathology 32: 104–109
834. Berezowski K, Grimes M M, Gal A et al. 1996 CD5 immunoreactivity of epithelial cells in thymic carcinoma and CASTLE using paraffin-embedded tissue. Am J Clin Pathol 106: 483–486
835. Shek T W, Luk I S, Ng I O et al. 1996 Lymphoepithelioma-like carcinoma of the thyroid gland: lack of evidence of association with Epstein–Barr virus. Hum Pathol 27: 851–853
836. Freeman C, Berg J W, Cutler S J 1972 Occurrence and prognosis of extranodal lymphomas. Cancer 29: 252–260
837. Burt A D, Kerr D J, Brown I L et al. 1985 Lymphoid and epithelial markers in small cell anaplastic thyroid tumours. J Clin Pathol 38: 893–896
838. Anscombe A M, Wright D H 1985 Primary malignant lymphoma of the thyroid – a tumour of mucosa-associated lymphoid tissue: review of seventy-six cases. Histopathology 9: 81–97
839. Aozasa K, Inoue A, Tajima K et al. 1986 Malignant lymphomas of the thyroid gland. Analysis of 79 patients with emphasis on histologic prognostic factors. Cancer 58: 100–104
840. Burke J S, Butler J J, Fuller L M 1977 Malignant lymphomas of the thyroid: a clinical pathologic study of 35 patients including ultrastructural observations. Cancer 39: 1587–1602
841. Compagno J, Oertel J E 1980 Malignant lymphoma and other lymphoproliferative disorders of the thyroid gland. A clinicopathologic study of 245 cases. Am J Clin Pathol 74: 1–11
842. Devine R M, Edis A J, Banks P M 1981 Primary lymphoma of the thyroid: a review of the Mayo Clinic experience through 1978. World J Surg 5: 33–38

843. Rasbach D A, Mondschein M S, Harris N L et al. 1985 Malignant lymphoma of the thyroid gland: a clinical and pathologic study of twenty cases. Surgery 98: 1166–1170
844. Woolner L B, McConahey W M, Beahrs O H et al. 1966 Primary malignant lymphoma of the thyroid. Review of forty-six cases. Am J Surg 111: 502–523
845. Singer J A 1998 Primary lymphoma of the thyroid. Am Surg 64: 334–337
846. Pledge S, Bessell E M, Leach I H et al. 1996 Non-Hodgkin's lymphoma of the thyroid: a retrospective review of all patients diagnosed in Nottinghamshire from 1973 to 1992. Clin Oncol 8: 371–375
847. Hamburger J I, Miller J M, Kini S R 1983 Lymphoma of the thyroid. Ann Intern Med 99: 685–693
848. Derringer G A, Thompson L D, Frommelt R A et al. 2000 Malignant lymphoma of the thyroid gland: a clinicopathologic study of 108 cases. Am J Surg Pathol 24: 623–639
849. Hyjek E, Isaacson P G 1988 Primary B cell lymphoma of the thyroid and its relationship to Hashimoto's thyroiditis. Hum Pathol 19: 1315–1326
850. Oertel J E, Heffess C S 1987 Lymphoma of the thyroid and related disorders. Semin Oncol 14: 333–342
851. Mizukami Y, Michigishi T, Nonomura A et al. 1990 Primary lymphoma of the thyroid: a clinical, histological and immunohistochemical study of 20 cases. Histopathology 17: 201–209
852. Rosen I B, Sutcliffe S B, Gospodarowicz M K et al. 1988 The role of surgery in the management of thyroid lymphoma. Surgery 104: 1095–1099
853. Tennvall J, Cavallin-Stahl E, Akerman M 1987 Primary localized non-Hodgkin's lymphoma of the thyroid: a retrospective clinicopathological review. Eur J Surg Oncol 13: 297–302
854. Belal A A, Allam A, Kandil A et al. 2001 Primary thyroid lymphoma: a retrospective analysis of prognostic factors and treatment outcome for localized intermediate and high grade lymphoma. Am J Clin Oncol 24: 299–305
855. DiBiase S J, Grigsby P W, Guo C et al. 2004 Outcome analysis for stage IE and IIE thyroid lymphoma. Am J Clin Oncol 27: 178–184
856. Stone C W, Slease R B, Brubaker D et al. 1986 Thyroid lymphoma with gastrointestinal involvement: report of three cases. Am J Hematol 21: 357–365
857. Wang S A, Rahemtullah A, Faquin W C et al. 2005. Hodgkin's lymphoma of the thyroid: a clinicopathological study of five cases and review of the literature. Mod Pathol 18: 1577–1584
858. Aozasa K, Inoue A, Yoshimura H et al. 1986 Intermediate lymphocytic lymphoma of the thyroid. An immunologic and immunohistologic study. Cancer 57: 1762–1767
859. Isaacson P G 1990 Lymphomas of mucosa-associated lymphoid tissue (MALT). Histopathology 16: 617–619
860. Skacel M, Ross C W, Hsi E D 2000 A reassessment of primary thyroid lymphoma: high-grade MALT-type lymphoma as a distinct subtype of diffuse large B-cell lymphoma. Histopathology 37: 10–18
861. Bacon C M, Diss T C, Ye H et al. 2005 Follicular lymphoma of the thyroid gland (Abstract). Mod Pathol 18(suppl 1): 222A
862. Coltrera M D 1999 Primary T-cell lymphoma of the thyroid. Head Neck 21: 160–163
863. Abdul-Rahman Z H, Gogas H J, Tooze J A et al. 1996 T-cell lymphoma in Hashimoto's thyroiditis. Histopathology 29: 455–459
864. Yamaguchi M, Ohno T, Kita K 1997 Gamma/delta T-cell lymphoma of the thyroid gland (Letter). N Engl J Med 336: 1391–1392
865. Shanks J H, Harris M, Howat A J et al. 1997 Angiotropic lymphoma with endocrine involvement. Histopathology 31: 161–166
866. Isaacson P G 1997 Lymphoma of the thyroid gland. Curr Top Pathol 91: 1–14
867. Thieblemont C, Bastion Y, Berger F et al. 1997 Mucosa-associated lymphoid tissue gastrointestinal and nongastrointestinal lymphoma behavior: analysis of 108 patients. J Clin Oncol 15: 1624–1630
868. Laing R W, Hoskin P, Hudson B V et al. 1994 The significance of MALT histology in thyroid lymphoma: a review of patients from the BNLI and Royal Marsden Hospital. Clin Oncol (R Coll Radiol) 6: 300–304
869. Isaacson P G, Androulakis-Papachristou A, Diss T C et al. 1992 Follicular colonization in thyroid lymphoma. Am J Pathol 141: 43–52
870. Streubel B, Vinatzer U, Lamprecht A et al. 2005 T(3;14)(p14.1;q32) involving IGH and FOXP1 is a novel recurrent chromosomal aberration in MALT lymphoma. Leukemia 19: 652–658
871. Ye H, Gong L, Liu H et al. 2005 MALT lymphoma with t(14;18)(q32;q21)/IGH-MALT1 is characterized by strong cytoplasmic MALT1 and BCL10 expression. J Pathol 205: 293–301
872. Streubel B, Simonitsch-Klupp I, Mullauer L et al. 2004 Variable frequencies of MALT lymphoma-associated genetic aberrations in MALT lymphomas of different sites. Leukemia 18: 1722–1726
873. Ye H, Liu H, Attygalle A et al. 2003 Variable frequencies of t(11;18)(q21;q21) in MALT lymphomas of different sites: significant association with CagA strains of H. pylori in gastric MALT lymphoma. Blood 102: 1012–1018
874. Maurer R, Taylor C R, Terry R et al. 1979 Non-Hodgkin's lymphoma of the thyroid, a clinicopathological review of 29 cases applying the Lukes–Collins classification and an immunoperoxidase method. Virchows Arch A 383: 293–317
875. Bateman A C, Wright D H 1993 Epitheliotropism in high-grade lymphomas of mucosa-associated lymphoid tissue. Histopathology 23: 409–415
876. Pedersen R K, Pedersen N T 1996 Primary non-Hodgkin's lymphoma of the thyroid gland: a population based study. Histopathology 28: 25–32
877. Aozasa K, Inoue A, Yoshimura H et al. 1986 Plasmacytoma of the thyroid gland. Cancer 58: 105–110
878. Kovacs C S, Mant M J, Nguyen G K et al. 1994 Plasma cell lesions of the thyroid: report of a case of solitary plasmacytoma and a review of the literature. Thyroid 4: 65–71
879. Hussong J W, Perkins S L, Schnitzer B et al. 1999 Extramedullary plasmacytoma. A form of marginal zone cell lymphoma? Am J Clin Pathol 111: 111–116
880. Yapp R, Linder J, Schenken J R et al. 1985 Plasma cell granuloma of the thyroid. Hum Pathol 16: 848–850
881. Mizukami Y, Nonomura A, Michigishi T et al. 1996 Pseudolymphoma of the thyroid gland. A case report. Pathol Res Pract 192: 166–169
882. Thompson L D 1996 Langerhans cell histiocytosis isolated to the thyroid gland. Eur Arch Otorhinolaryngol 253: 62–65
883. Thompson L D R, Wenig B M, Adair C F et al. 1996 Peripheral nerve sheath tumors of the thyroid gland, a series of four cases and a review of the literature. Endocr Pathol 7: 309–318
884. Tsang W Y, Lau M F, Chan J K 1994 Incidental Langerhans' cell histiocytosis of the thyroid. Histopathology 24: 397–399
885. Coode P E, Shaikh M U 1988 Histiocytosis X of the thyroid masquerading as thyroid carcinoma. Hum Pathol 19: 239–241
886. Wang W S, Liu J H, Chiou T J et al. 1997 Langerhans' cell histiocytosis with thyroid involvement masquerading as thyroid carcinoma. Jpn J Clin Oncol 27: 180–184
887. Kitahama S, Iitaka M, Shimizu T et al. 1996 Thyroid involvement by malignant histiocytosis of Langerhans' cell type. Clin Endocrinol (Oxf) 45: 357–363
888. Foulet-Roge A, Josselin N, Guyetant S et al. 2002 Incidental Langerhans cell histiocytosis of thyroid: case report and review of the literature. Endocr Pathol 13: 227–233
889. Saiz E, Bakotic B W 2000 Isolated Langerhans cell histiocytosis of the thyroid: a report of two cases with nuclear imaging-pathologic correlation. Ann Diagn Pathol 4: 23–28
890. Elliott D D, Sellin R, Egger J F et al. 2005 Langerhans cell histiocytosis presenting as a thyroid gland mass. Ann Diagn Pathol 9: 267–274
891. Maiorana A, Collina G, Cesinaro A M et al. 1996 Epithelioid angiosarcoma of the thyroid. Clinicopathological analysis of seven cases from non-Alpine areas. Virchows Arch 429: 131–137
892. Eusebi V, Carcangiu M L, Dina R et al. 1990 Keratin-positive epithelioid angiosarcoma of thyroid. A report of four cases. Am J Surg Pathol 14: 737–747
893. Lamovec J, Zidar A, Zidanik B 1994 Epithelioid angiosarcoma of the thyroid gland. Report of two cases. Arch Pathol Lab Med 118: 642–646
894. Goh S G, Chuah K L, Goh H K et al. 2003 Two cases of epithelioid angiosarcoma involving the thyroid and a brief review of non-Alpine epithelioid angiosarcoma of the thyroid. Arch Pathol Lab Med 127: E70–E73
895. Sapino A, Papotti M, Macri L et al. 1995 Intranodular reactive endothelial hyperplasia in adenomatous goitre. Histopathology 26: 457–462
896. Taccagni G, Sambade C, Nesland J et al. 1993 Solitary fibrous tumour of the thyroid: clinicopathological, immunohistochemical and ultrastructural study of three cases. Virchows Arch A Pathol Anat Histopathol 422: 491–497
897. Cameselle-Teijeiro J, Varela-Duran J 1995 CD34 and thyroid fibrous tumor (Letter). Am J Surg Pathol 19: 1096
898. Cameselle-Teijeiro J, Varela-Duran J, Fonseca E et al. 1994 Solitary fibrous tumor of the thyroid. Am J Clin Pathol 101: 535–538
899. Kie J H, Kim J Y, Park Y N et al. 1997 Solitary fibrous tumour of the thyroid. Histopathology 30: 365–368
900. Rodriguez I, Ayala E, Caballero C et al. 2001 Solitary fibrous tumor of the thyroid gland: report of seven cases. Am J Surg Pathol 25: 1424–1428
901. Cameselle-Teijeiro J, Manuel Lopes J, Villanueva J P et al. 2003 Lipomatous haemangiopericytoma (adipocytic variant of solitary fibrous tumour) of the thyroid. Histopathology 43: 406–408
902. Sobrinho-Simoes M, Cameselle-Teijeiro J 2004 Solitary fibrous tumour. In: DeLellis R A, Lloyd R V, Heitz P U et al. (eds) Pathology and genetics. Tumours of endocrine organs. World Health Organization classification of tumours. IARC Press, Lyon, p 118
903. Thompson L D, Wenig B M, Adair C F et al. 1997 Primary smooth muscle tumors of the thyroid gland. Cancer 79: 579–587
904. Kawahara E, Nakanishi I, Terahata S et al. 1988 Leiomyosarcoma of the thyroid gland. A case report with a comparative study of five cases of anaplastic carcinoma. Cancer 62: 2558–2563
905. Iida Y, Katoh R, Yoshioka M et al. 1993 Primary leiomyosarcoma of the thyroid gland. Acta Pathol Jpn 43: 71–75
906. Chetty R, Clark S P, Dowling J P 1993 Leiomyosarcoma of the thyroid: immunohistochemical and ultrastructural study. Pathology 25: 203–205
907. Ozaki O, Sugino K, Mimura T et al. 1997 Primary leiomyosarcoma of the thyroid gland. Surg Today 27: 177–180
908. Tulbah A, Al-Dayel F, Fawaz I et al. 1999 Epstein–Barr virus-associated leiomyosarcoma of the thyroid in a child with congenital immunodeficiency: a case report. Am J Surg Pathol 23: 473–476
909. Andrion A, Bellis D, Delsedime L et al. 1988 Leiomyoma and neurilemoma: report of two unusual non-epithelial tumours of the thyroid gland. Virchows Arch A Pathol Anat Histopathol 413: 367–372
910. Heffess C S, Adair F F, Wenig B M 1995 Paragangliomas of the thyroid gland (Abstract). Int J Surg Pathol 2(suppl): 188

911. Corrado S, Montanini V, De Gaetani C et al. 2004 Primary paraganglioma of the thyroid gland. J Endocrinol Invest 27: 788–792
912. Zantour B, Guilhaume B, Tissier F et al. 2004 A thyroid nodule revealing a paraganglioma in a patient with a new germline mutation in the succinate dehydrogenase B gene. Eur J Endocrinol 151: 433–438
913. Vodovnik A 2002 Fine needle aspiration cytology of primary thyroid paraganglioma. Report of a case with cytologic, histologic and immunohistochemical features and differential diagnostic considerations. Acta Cytol 46: 1133–1137
914. de Vries E J, Watson C G 1989 Paraganglioma of the thyroid. Head Neck 11: 462–465
915. Bale G F 1950 Teratoma of the neck in the region of the thyroid gland, a review of the literature and report of four cases. Am J Pathol 26: 565–580
916. Fisher J E, Cooney D R, Voorhess M L et al. 1982 Teratoma of thyroid gland in infancy: review of the literature and two case reports. J Surg Oncol 21: 135–140
917. Riedlinger W F, Lack E E, Robson C D et al. 2005 Primary thyroid teratomas in children: a report of 11 cases with a proposal of criteria for their diagnosis. Am J Surg Pathol 29: 700–706
918. Thompson L D, Rosai J, Heffess C S 2000 Primary thyroid teratomas: a clinicopathologic study of 30 cases. Cancer 88: 1149–1158
919. Kimler S C, Muth W F 1978 Primary malignant teratoma of the thyroid: case report and literature review of cervical teratomas in adults. Cancer 42: 311–317
920. Hajdu S I, Hajdu E O 1967 Malignant teratoma of the neck. Arch Pathol 83: 567–570
921. Bowker C M, Whittaker R S 1992 Malignant teratoma of the thyroid: case report and literature review of thyroid teratoma in adults. Histopathology 21: 81–83
922. Buckley N J, Burch W M, Leight G S 1986 Malignant teratoma in the thyroid gland of an adult: a case report and a review of the literature. Surgery 100: 932–937
923. Ueno N T, Amato R J, Ro J J et al. 1998 Primary malignant teratoma of the thyroid gland: report and discussion of two cases. Head Neck 20: 649–653
924. Chen J S, Lai G M, Hsueh S 1998 Malignant thyroid teratoma of an adult: a long-term survival after chemotherapy. Am J Clin Oncol 21: 212–214
925. Sawady J, Mendelsohn G, Sirota R L et al. 1989 The intrathyroidal hyperfunctioning parathyroid gland. Mod Pathol 2: 652–657
926. de la Cruz Vigo F, Ortega G, Gonzalez S et al. 1997 Pathologic intrathyroidal parathyroid glands. Int Surg 82: 87–90
927. Neiman R S, Barcos M, Berard C et al. 1981 Granulocytic sarcoma, a clinicopathologic study of 61 biopsied cases. Cancer 48: 1426–1437
928. Naylor B 1959 Secondary lymphoblastoma involvement of the thyroid gland. Arch Pathol 67: 432–438
929. Foucar E, Rosai J, Dorfman R 1990 Sinus histiocytosis with massive lymphadenopathy (Rosai–Dorfman disease): review of the entity. Semin Diagn Pathol 7: 19–73
930. Larkin D F P, Dervan P A, Munnelly J et al. 1986 Sinus histiocytosis with massive lymphadenopathy simulating subacute thyroiditis. Hum Pathol 17: 321–324
931. Ryska A, Vokurka J, Michal M et al. 1997 Intrathyroidal lymphoepithelial cyst. A report of two cases not associated with Hashimoto's thyroiditis. Pathol Res Pract 193: 777–781
932. Louis D N, Vickery A L Jr., Rosai J et al. 1989 Multiple branchial cleft-like cysts in Hashimoto's thyroiditis. Am J Surg Pathol 13: 45–49
933. Galati L T, Barnes E L, Myers E N 1999 Dendritic cell sarcoma of the thyroid. Head Neck 21: 273–275
934. Lange M J 1974 Pleomorphic adenoma of the thyroid containing salivary gland cells with pseudocartilage and myoepithelial cells. Int Surg 59: 178–179
935. Suzuki S, Kasashima F, Nakanishi I et al. 1999 An unusual case of benign thyroid tumour consisting of epithelial and nonepithelial components. Virchows Arch 434: 235–239
936. Chahal A S, Subramanyam C S V, Bhattacharjea A K 1975 Chondromatous hamartoma of the thyroid gland, report of a case. Aust N Z J Surg 45: 30–31
937. Ward J V, Murray D, Horvath E et al. 1982 Hyaline cell tumor of thyroid with massive accumulation of cytoplasmic microfilaments (Abstract). Lab Invest 46: 88A
938. Samsi A B, Shah H K, Vaidya A et al. 1992 Fibromatosis of thyroid gland (a case report). J Postgrad Med 38: 36–37
939. Mahoney C P, Patterson S D, Ryan J 1995 Granular cell tumor of the thyroid gland in a girl receiving high-dose estrogen therapy. Pediatr Pathol Lab Med 15: 791–795
940. Baloch Z W, Martin S, Livolsi V A 2005 Granular cell tumor of the thyroid: a case report. Int J Surg Pathol 13: 291–294
941. Sichel J Y, Wygoda M, Dano I et al. 1996 Fibrosarcoma of the thyroid in a man exposed to fallout from the Chernobyl accident. Ann Otol Rhinol Laryngol 105: 832–834
942. Shin W Y, Aftalion B, Hotchkiss E et al. 1979 Ultrastructure of a primary fibrosarcoma of the human thyroid gland. Cancer 44: 584–591
943. Dictor M, Elner A, Andersson T et al. 1992 Myofibromatosis-like hemangiopericytoma metastasizing as differentiated vascular smooth-muscle and myosarcoma. Myopericytes as a subset of "myofibroblasts." Am J Surg Pathol 16: 1239–1247
944. Ostrowski M L, Cartwright J J, Maldonada J E et al. 1995 Hemangiopericytoma of the thyroid: an unusual spindle cell lesion. Int J Surg Pathol 2: 311–318
945. Kikuchi I, Anbo J, Nakamura S et al. 2003 Synovial sarcoma of the thyroid. Report of a case with aspiration cytology findings and gene analysis. Acta Cytol 47: 495–500
946. Leiva S F, Navachia D, Nigro N et al. 2004 Lipoma in the thyroid? J Pediatr Endocrinol Metab 17: 1013–1015
947. Andrion A, Gaglio A, Dogliani N et al. 1991 Liposarcoma of the thyroid gland. Fine-needle aspiration cytology, immunohistology, and ultrastructure. Am J Clin Pathol 95: 675–679
948. Tseleni-Balafouta S, Arvanitis D, Kakaviatos N et al. 1988 Primary myxoid chondrosarcoma of the thyroid gland. Arch Pathol Lab Med 112: 94–96
949. Ohbu M, Kameya T, Wada C et al. 1989 Primary osteogenic sarcoma of the thyroid gland: a case report. Surg Pathol 2: 67–72
950. Pickleman J R, Lee J F, Straus F H et al. 1975 Thyroid hemangioma. Am J Surg 129: 331–333
951. Gardner D F, Frable W J 1989 Primary lymphangioma of the thyroid gland. Arch Pathol Lab Med 113: 1084–1085
952. Siddiqui M T, Evans H L, Ro J Y et al. 1998 Epithelioid haemangioendothelioma of the thyroid gland: a case report and review of literature. Histopathology 32: 473–476
953. Shimaoka K, Sokal J E, Pickren J W 1962 Metastatic neoplasms of the thyroid. Cancer 15: 557–565
954. Ivy H K 1984 Cancer metastatic to the thyroid: a diagnostic problem. Mayo Clin Proc 59: 856–859
955. Nakhjavani M K, Gharib H, Goellner J R et al. 1997 Metastasis to the thyroid gland. A report of 43 cases. Cancer 79: 574–578
956. McCabe D P, Farrar W B, Petkov T M et al. 1985 Clinical and pathologic correlations in disease metastatic to the thyroid gland. Am J Surg 150: 519–523
957. Lam K Y, Lo C Y 1998 Metastatic tumors of the thyroid gland: a study of 79 cases in Chinese patients. Arch Pathol Lab Med 122: 37–41
958. Satoh Y, Sakamoto A, Yamada K et al. 1990 Psammoma bodies in metastatic carcinoma to the thyroid. Mod Pathol 3: 267–270
959. Heffess C S, Wenig B M, Thompson L D 2002. Metastatic renal cell carcinoma to the thyroid gland. A clinicopathologic study of 36 cases. Cancer 95: 1869–1878
960. Matias-Guiu X, LaGuette J, Puras-Gil A M et al. 1997 Metastatic neuroendocrine tumors to the thyroid gland mimicking medullary carcinoma: a pathologic and immunohistochemical study of six cases. Am J Surg Pathol 21: 754–762
961. Hirokawa M, Carney J A, Goellner J R et al. 2002 Observer variation of encapsulated follicular lesions of the thyroid gland. Am J Surg Pathol 26: 1508–1514
962. Lloyd R V, Erickson L A, Casey M B et al. 2004 Observer variation in the diagnosis of follicular variant of papillary thyroid carcinoma. Am J Surg Pathol 28: 1336–1340
963. Elsheikh T M, Asa S L, Chan J K C et al. 2004 Inter-observer variation among experts in diagnosis of follicular variant of papillary thyroid carcinoma (Abstract). Mod Pathol 17(suppl 1): 102A–103A
964. Renshaw A A, Gould E W 2002 Why there is the tendency to "overdiagnose" the follicular variant of papillary thyroid carcinoma. Am J Clin Pathol 117: 19–21
965. Williams E D, Abrosimov A, Bogdanova T et al. 2000 Guest editorial: two proposals regarding the terminology of thyroid tumors. Int J Surg Pathol 8: 181–183
966. Ghossein R A, Rosai J, Heffess C 1998 Dyshormonogenetic goiter: a clinicopathologic study of 56 cases. Endocr Pathol 8: 283–292
967. Fadda G, Baloch Z W, LiVolsi V A 1999 Dyshormonogenetic goiter pathology, a review. Int J Surg Pathol 7: 125–131
968. Oertel Y C, Oertel J E 1998 Diagnosis of malignant epithelial thyroid lesions: fine needle aspiration and histopathologic correlation. Ann Diagn Pathol 2: 377–400
969. Oertel Y C 1996 Fine-needle aspiration and the diagnosis of thyroid cancer. Endocrinol Metab Clin North Am 25: 69–91
970. Baloch Z W, LiVolsi V A 2004 Fine-needle aspiration of thyroid nodules: past, present, and future. Endocr Pract 10: 234–241
971. Chang H Y, Lin J D, Chen J F et al. 1997 Correlation of fine needle aspiration cytology and frozen section biopsies in the diagnosis of thyroid nodules. J Clin Pathol 50: 1005–1009
972. Baloch Z W, Wu H, LiVolsi V A 1999 Post–fine-needle aspiration spindle cell nodules of the thyroid (PSCNT). Am J Clin Pathol 111: 70–74
973. Axiotis C A, Merino M J, Ain K et al. 1991 Papillary endothelial hyperplasia in the thyroid following fine-needle aspiration. Arch Pathol Lab Med 115: 240–242
974. Tsang K, Duggan M A 1992 Vascular proliferation of the thyroid. A complication of fine-needle aspiration. Arch Pathol Lab Med 116: 1040–1042
975. Ito Y, Tomoda C, Uruno T et al. 2005 Needle tract implantation of papillary thyroid carcinoma after fine-needle aspiration biopsy. World J Surg 29: 1544–1549
976. McHenry C R, Raeburn C, Strickland T et al. 1996 The utility of routine frozen section examination for intraoperative diagnosis of thyroid cancer. Am J Surg 172: 658–661
977. Gibb G K, Pasieka J L 1995 Assessing the need for frozen sections: still a valuable tool in thyroid surgery. Surgery 118: 1005–1009

978. Sabel M S, Staren E D, Gianakakis L M et al. 1997 Use of fine-needle aspiration biopsy and frozen section in the management of the solitary thyroid nodule. Surgery 122: 1021–1026
979. Mulcahy M M, Cohen J I, Anderson P E et al. 1998 Relative accuracy of fine-needle aspiration and frozen section in the diagnosis of well-differentiated thyroid cancer. Laryngoscope 108(4 part 1): 494–496
980. Anton R C, Wheeler T M 2005 Frozen section of thyroid and parathyroid specimens. Arch Pathol Lab Med 129: 1575–1584
981. Baloch Z W, LiVolsi V A 2002 Intraoperative assessment of thyroid and parathyroid lesions. Semin Diagn Pathol 19: 219–226
982. Paphavasit A, Thompson G B, Hay I D et al. 1997 Follicular and Hurthle cell thyroid neoplasms. Is frozen-section evaluation worthwhile? Arch Surg 132: 674–678
983. Udelsman R, Westra W H, Donovan P I et al. 2001 Randomized prospective evaluation of frozen-section analysis for follicular neoplasms of the thyroid. Ann Surg 233: 716–722
984. Chen H, Nicol T L, Udelsman R 1995 Follicular lesions of the thyroid. Does frozen section evaluation alter operative management? Ann Surg 222: 101–106
985. Crowe P J, Chetty R, Dent D M 1993 Thyroid frozen section: flawed but helpful. Aust N Z J Surg 63: 275–278
986. Kingston G W, Bugis S P, Davis N 1992 Role of frozen section and clinical parameters in distinguishing benign from malignant follicular neoplasms of the thyroid. Am J Surg 164: 603–605
987. Montone K T, LiVolsi V 1996 Frozen section analysis of thyroidectomy specimens: experience over a 12-year period. Pathol Case Rev 2: 241–245
988. Shirzad M, Larijani B, Hedayat A et al. 2003 Diagnostic value of frozen section examination in thyroid nodule – surgery at the Shariati Hospital (1997–2000). Endocr Pathol 14: 263–268

第二部分

甲状旁腺　The parathyroid gland

John K. C. Chan 著

李忠武　刘毅强　孙宇　薛卫成 译

甲状旁腺

正常甲状旁腺	1080	非典型性甲状旁腺腺瘤	1091
甲状旁腺功能亢进	1080	（不能确定恶性潜能的甲状旁腺肿瘤）	
甲状旁腺腺瘤	1081	其他肿瘤	1092
甲状旁腺癌	1087	甲状旁腺功能亢进的术中诊断	1092

正常甲状旁腺
The normal parathyroid glands

大多数人拥有两对甲状旁腺。胚胎学上，上面一对甲状旁腺来源于第四鳃囊，而下面一对来源于第三鳃囊。上甲状旁腺紧贴于甲状腺的后表面，甲状腺下动脉于此处进入甲状腺。下甲状旁腺通常紧靠甲状腺下极[1]，但是有时会位于纵隔内，这是因为它们与同样也起源于第三鳃囊的胸腺共同迁移的结果。

甲状旁腺分泌甲状旁腺激素，该激素可以通过直接作用于肾和骨以及间接作用于肠道而增加血清中钙的水平。熟悉正常甲状旁腺的颜色（深棕黄色）、大小以及重量对于识别异常的甲状旁腺来说非常重要（表18B.1）[2-6]。

组织学上，甲状旁腺呈分叶状。多角形、立方形的实质细胞呈巢状、条索状或片状分布，其间被纤细的血管以及数量不等的脂肪细胞所分隔（图18B.1A）。甲状旁腺由胞浆略嗜酸性或嗜双染性的主细胞以及水样透明细胞和嗜酸性细胞（oxyphil cell）组成（图18B.1B）。在老年人，单个或多个嗜酸性细胞结节并不少见（图18B.2）。

甲状旁腺功能亢进
Hyperparathyroidism

甲状旁腺功能亢进指的是血清中甲状旁腺激素升高的状态，也是甲状旁腺最常见的病理状态，可分为三

表18B.1　正常甲状旁腺的基本资料

参数	正常范围	提示甲状旁腺异常（增生或肿瘤）的一些改变
数目	通常为4个，有时会有5个（范围：1~12个）	
大小	长3~6mm 宽2~4mm 厚0.5~2.0mm	增大的腺体，大小＞6mm
重量	每个腺体重量≈30mg，下面的甲状旁腺通常重于上面的甲状旁腺 总重量 120±3.5mg(男性) 142±5.2mg(女性)	任一腺体重量＞60mg
脂肪所占百分比	平均17%，很少超过50%； 女性（20.5%）高于男性（15.6%）	腺体中完全缺乏或散在分布少量的脂肪细胞，可能存在的陷阱有： (1) 脂肪腺瘤，但是因腺体增大可被识别出。 (2) 正常儿童甲状旁腺的脂肪细胞可以稀少或者缺如
细胞浆内脂滴 （通过脂肪染色显示）	通常丰富	稀少或者缺如

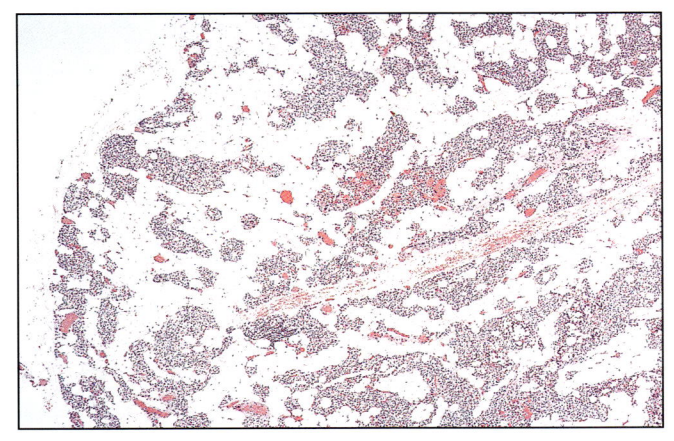

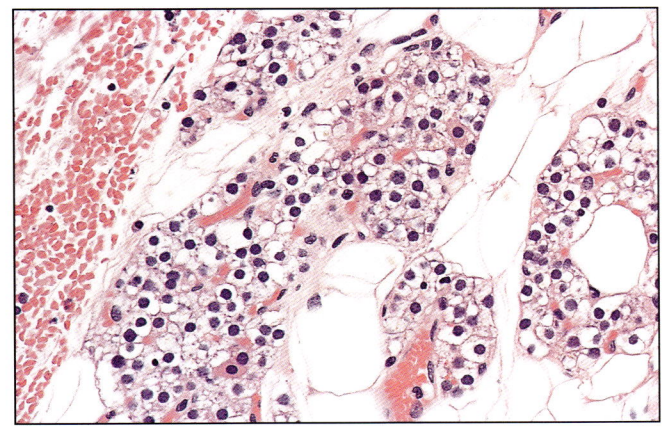

图18B.1　正常甲状旁腺。（A）正常甲状旁腺腺体通常被脂肪细胞所分隔。（B）甲状旁腺细胞主要是主细胞（含有细颗粒）或透明细胞。

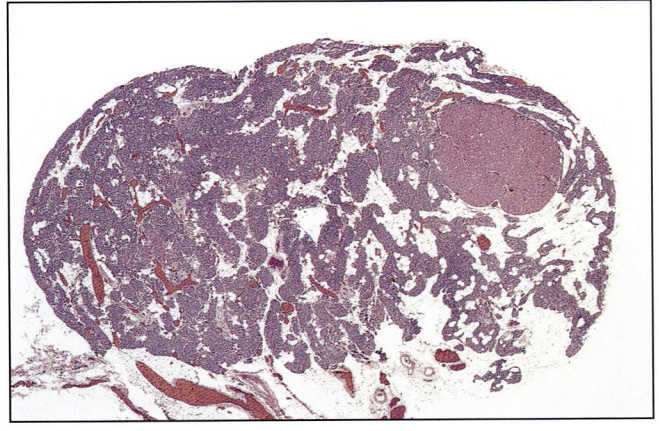

图18B.2　正常老年病例的甲状旁腺。右上方视野可见一个嗜酸（oxyphil）细胞结节。

种类型：原发性、继发性、三发性。只有原发性和三发性甲状旁腺功能亢进伴有高钙血症及其并发症，包括多尿、烦渴、肌无力、肾结石以及精神障碍。但是，三种类型均可以伴发甲状旁腺功能亢进性骨病，表现为骨痛或骨折（表 18B.2）[5,7-9]。最常见的原因包括甲状旁腺腺瘤（大约占85%）、甲状旁腺增生（大约占14%）和甲状旁腺癌（大约占1%）[10]。与甲状旁腺功能亢进相关的主要综合征见表 18B.3[11-20]。家族性孤立性甲状旁腺功能亢进具有多种临床表现形式，包括"顿挫型（forme fruste form）"多发内分泌肿瘤（MEN）Ⅰ型（最常见）、某些甲状旁腺功能亢进 - 颌骨肿瘤综合征病例、家族性低尿钙高钙血症以及一些未知的疾病[21-23]。

一些恶性肿瘤，特别是肺的鳞状细胞癌和肾细胞癌可以产生异位的甲状旁腺激素，引起高钙血症症状。然而这些激素性物质几乎均为甲状旁腺激素相关肽类，而非完整的甲状旁腺激素。

甲状旁腺腺瘤　Parathyroid adenoma

临床特征

甲状旁腺腺瘤是原发性甲状旁腺功能亢进的主要病因[24,25]，其主要的临床特征列于表 18B.4[25-30]。甲状旁腺腺瘤可以作为Ⅰ型或Ⅱ型多发内分泌肿瘤（MEN）以及甲状旁腺功能亢进 - 颌骨肿瘤综合征的组成部分（见表 18B.3）。头颈部辐射史可能是一些甲状旁腺腺瘤的病因[31,32]。

过去，多数患者表现出高钙血症并发症。如今，随着能检测包括血清钙在内的多通道临床化学分析仪的广泛使用，许多无症状的原发性甲状旁腺功能亢进患者通过此检测途径得以确诊[25,30]。那些表现为甲状旁腺功能亢进性骨病（如囊性纤维性骨炎和棕色瘤）的患者，其症状持续时间较短，但是肿瘤体积较大，甲状旁腺激素水平较高。表现为肾绞痛的患者症状持续时间相对较长[33]。

甲状旁腺功能亢进的诊断依赖于血清中甲状旁腺激素和血钙水平升高。多种成像技术可用来定位高功能甲状旁腺（甲状旁腺腺瘤），而锝-99m 标记的 sestamibi 扫描能够获得更高的诊断率[34-36]。

临床行为及治疗

单纯切除肿大腺体可以治愈甲状旁腺腺瘤，其结果是血清生化指标恢复正常，骨的无机盐密度增加[24,37,38]。然而，仍有大约 10% 的患者在术后或术后多年再发甲状旁腺功能亢进[39,40]。术中监测血浆甲状旁腺激素水平已被逐步用于判定甲状旁腺腺瘤是否被切除[41]。超声引导下将 96% 的乙醇注入甲状旁腺腺瘤引起肿瘤坏死的方法已经被应用于具有高手术风险的患者[42]。

对于无症状的原发性甲状旁腺功能亢进患者若不进行手术干预，随访 10 年发现他们的血清钙水平并没有进行性上升，但是大约 30% 的患者会出现并发症[38,43]。

甲状旁腺腺瘤

表18B.2 甲状旁腺功能亢进的不同类型

类型	定义	原因	病理表现
原发性	由于一个或多个甲状旁腺的内在异常而导致甲状旁腺激素生成过度,血清中钙升高而磷下降	甲状旁腺腺瘤（85%） 甲状旁腺癌（1%） 原发性甲状旁腺增生（14%） —散发性 —MEN1 —MEN2 —家族性孤立性甲状旁腺功能亢进 —家族性低尿钙高钙血症	腺瘤或癌（见正文）：通常累及单个腺体。 主细胞增生：尽管有时不对称，但是所有的甲状旁腺都增大。腺体表现为甲状旁腺细胞（主细胞、水样透明细胞以及嗜酸性细胞，其比例可以变化很大）的增生，以及实质脂肪组织显著减少。增生过程以弥漫方式开始，但是结节方式通常会占优势。 水样透明细胞增生：这种增生在过去几十年中已基本消失，没有家族性发生倾向或MEN相关性。甲状旁腺显著增大。组织学显示多数高度增生的甲状旁腺细胞有水样透明胞浆。
继发性	由于血清钙水平下降导致甲状旁腺代偿性增生，通常会使血清钙恢复正常	慢性肾功能衰竭（最常见的病因） 吸收不良 维生素D缺乏 肾小管性酸中毒	所有甲状旁腺都增生，与原发性甲状旁腺增生无法区分。下面甲状旁腺腺体通常比上面腺体大，多数病例会观察到多个结节（弥漫型增生通常为多克隆性，随着结节形成而出现占优势的单克隆群体）。
三发性	在继发性甲状旁腺功能亢进的基础上发生的自发性甲状旁腺功能亢进	病因同继发性甲状旁腺功能亢进	组织学特征类似继发性甲状旁腺功能亢进，但是腺体通常较大，伴有明显的结节。少数病例会伴发腺瘤或癌。

MEN1=多发内分泌肿瘤Ⅰ型；MEN2=多发内分泌肿瘤Ⅱ型

甲状旁腺异位(ectopic)的相关问题

甲状旁腺腺瘤可以发生于异位器官，如纵隔、甲状腺或食管。当患者在治疗原发性甲状旁腺功能亢进时，可能会导致徒劳的颈部探查[44-47]。尽管纵隔甲状旁腺肿瘤通常可以通过颈部通路手术切除，但有些病例需要开胸手术[45,47]。纵隔甲状旁腺肿瘤的形态学改变与正常部位甲状旁腺肿瘤相同[48]（见下文）。同样，完全包裹在甲状腺中的甲状旁腺肿瘤则可能在临床检查或手术探查时被漏查[44,46,49,50]。由于甲状旁腺腺瘤的组织学表现与甲状腺微滤泡型腺瘤和髓样癌相似，会引起组织学诊断方面的问题[44,51]。

双发性腺瘤 Double adenomas

以前对甲状旁腺双发腺瘤存在与否发生过争议，然而现在已被人们认可，尽管其发病率较低（仅占原发性甲状旁腺功能亢进的1.7%～12%）[30,52-56]。据Barsch等的研究报道[54]，与甲状旁腺单发腺瘤或甲状旁腺增生相比，双发腺瘤患者均有临床症状，而且肿瘤重量更重，甲状旁腺激素水平更高。73%的病例腺瘤位于双侧。由于与非对称性甲状旁腺增生难以鉴别，因此只有在手术切除两个增大腺体后进行临床随访，没有出现甲状旁腺功能亢进复发时该病才能确诊。同时应谨慎除外MEN，因为非对称性甲状旁腺增生也可以发生在这种综合征[53]。甲状旁腺双发腺瘤的诊断要点如下[52,53]：

1. 两个增大的甲状旁腺组织学表现为富于细胞。
2. 手术中证实其余的甲状旁腺正常（最好通过组织学活检证实）。
3. 没有MEN家族史或家族性甲状旁腺功能亢进的临床证据。
4. 单独切除两个增大腺体可以永久治愈高钙血症。

表18B.3 与甲状旁腺功能亢进有关的主要综合征

	MEN1	MEN2a	甲状旁腺功能亢进－颌骨肿瘤综合征
内分泌器官表现			
甲状旁腺	增生/肿瘤	增生/肿瘤	单发（或者偶尔双发）腺瘤/癌
甲状腺	结节 滤泡性腺瘤	髓样癌	－
肾上腺	无功能结节 功能性腺瘤	嗜铬细胞瘤	－
胰腺	胰岛细胞肿瘤	－	－
垂体前叶	垂体腺瘤	－	－
其他	胸腺类癌 支气管类癌	－	－
其他表现	面部血管纤维瘤 胶原瘤（collagenomas） 多发性脂肪瘤	苔藓样淀粉样变性（部分病例）	30%的病例有颌骨纤维骨化性病变，20%的病例有肾病变（如囊肿、错构瘤、癌）
遗传背景	常染色体显性遗传；染色体11q13的MEN1位点胚系突变	常染色体显性遗传；位于染色体10q11的RET原癌基因胚系突变，导致功能活化	常染色体显性遗传；基因位点与1q25-31连锁（HRPT2基因）
甲状旁腺功能亢进的自然病史	甲状旁腺功能亢进很常见，而且是该综合征的首要表现。累及肾和骨的几率与典型的原发性甲状旁腺功能亢进相似，但是血清钙的浓度偏低	出现在20%～30%的病例。一般症状轻微或无症状	大约80%的患者出现甲状旁腺功能亢进，一般在青春后期发生。高钙血症偏重。与MEN1和MEN2a相比，甲状旁腺癌的发生率较高（10%～15%）

基因表达谱研究证实甲状旁腺多发肿瘤（包括甲状旁腺双发腺瘤）是一种独特的分子疾病[57]。

大体表现

下甲状旁腺比上甲状旁腺更容易发生腺瘤[3]。腺瘤重量一般不超过1g（平均0.55g），但是曾有重达53g的报道[3,58]。通常，高钙血症越严重腺瘤越大[3]。大小从不足1厘米到几厘米。肿瘤界清、质软，呈橙黄色或橙红色孤立结节，可以发生出血或囊性变。嗜酸细胞腺瘤切面为红褐色。

只有腺瘤性甲状旁腺的体积增大，其余的甲状旁腺体积正常或较小。

组织学表现

甲状旁腺腺瘤界限清楚，一些呈分叶状或模糊结节状[59]。偶尔呈多结节状[1]。甲状旁腺腺瘤富于细胞而且通常缺乏脂肪细胞（脂肪腺瘤除外）。一些肿瘤周边可见一圈正常或者受压的甲状旁腺组织，较常见于甲状旁腺门部（图18B.3）。

肿瘤细胞排列成实性片状、条索状、腺泡状、滤泡状、微囊状（图18B.4至18B.7）。肿瘤中有纤细的窦状血管网穿过（图18B.8）。肿瘤细胞核通常朝向血管轴呈列兵样排列（图18B.9）。偶尔，滤泡内有淀粉样物沉积（图18B.7）[60,61]，更罕见的是会出现间质淀粉样物沉积[51]。肿瘤细胞呈多角形，有略嗜酸性或透明胞浆（图18B.10）。甲状旁腺腺瘤的细胞及细胞核通常大于正常甲状旁腺（图18B.11）。细胞核可以圆而规则，也可以显著增大、深染并具有多形性（图18B.10，18B.12）[3]。核分裂象稀少或缺如。伴有多形性或怪异细胞核的细胞通常散在分布于具有温和细胞核表现的细胞之间，在缺乏核分裂的情况下，不要误诊为恶性（图18B.12）。在甲状旁腺腺瘤中，散在分布着多个结节状病灶，这些细

表18B.4	甲状旁腺腺瘤与癌的临床特征比较	
	甲状旁腺腺瘤	甲状旁腺癌
发生率	显著高于甲状旁腺癌（≈85%的原发性甲状旁腺功能亢进）	少见（≈1%的原发性甲状旁腺功能亢进）
性别	女性>男性（3:1）	女性=男性
年龄	平均56~62岁	比甲状旁腺腺瘤发病年轻10岁；平均45~54岁
无症状	常见（12%~50%）	极少见（3%）
肾受累（肾结石）	4%~30%	常见（48%~56%）
骨受累	14%~20%	常见（63%~91%）
肾和骨同时受累	少见（<5%）	较常见（32%~53%）
颈部包块	少见（<2%）	较常见（38%~45%）
高钙血症	有（2.75~3mmol/l）	较严重（3.5~4mmol/l）
肿瘤重量	通常<1g	肿瘤较大，平均重量12g

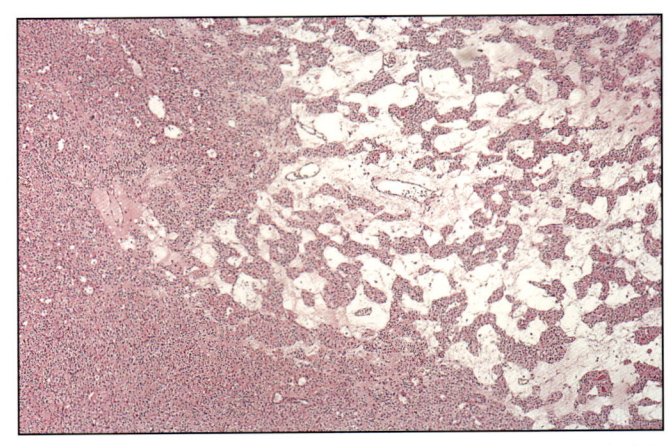

图18B.4 甲状旁腺腺瘤呈实性生长，伴有局灶间质水肿（右侧视野）。

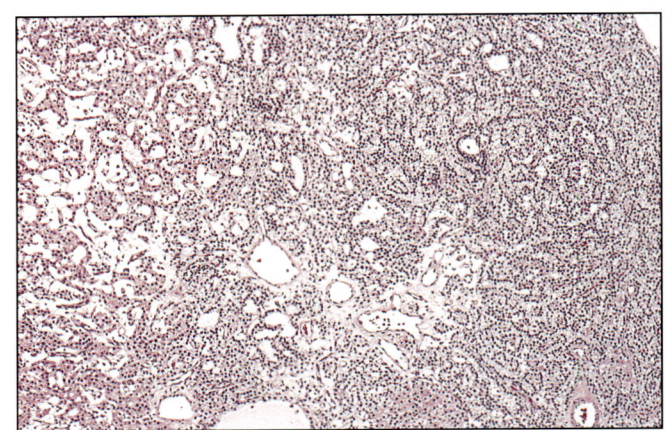

图18B.5 甲状旁腺腺瘤主要由相互连接的小管及相互吻合的条索构成。

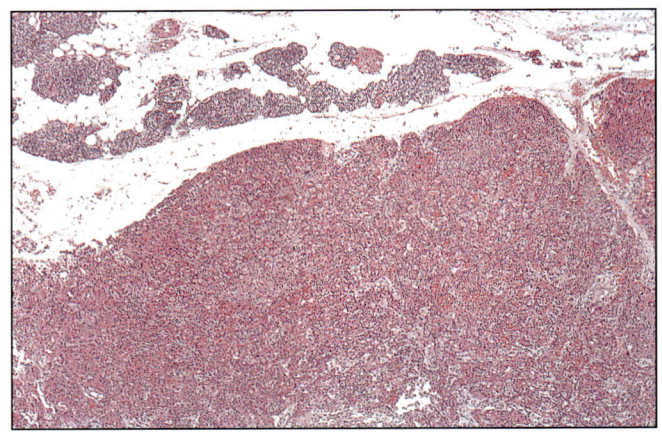

图18B.3 甲状旁腺腺瘤。注意肿瘤的界限及视野上方残余的甲状旁腺组织。

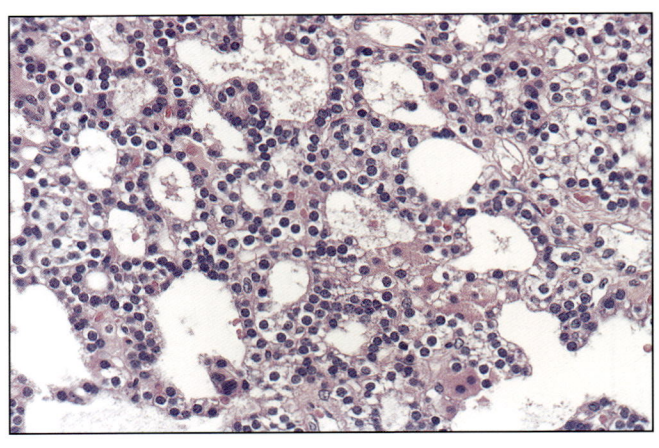

图18B.6 具有微腺性生长方式的甲状旁腺腺瘤，此种情况易被误诊为甲状腺滤泡性肿瘤。

胞比非结节区的细胞具有较高的增生指数（经Ki-67免疫组化染色证实）[62]。少数情况下，局灶会出现梭形肿瘤细胞[63]。

甲状旁腺腺瘤局灶会出现纤维化、出血、梗死及囊性变（图18B.13）。甲状旁腺腺瘤的囊性变在甲状旁腺功能亢进-颌骨肿瘤综合征患者中更为常见[20]。凝固性

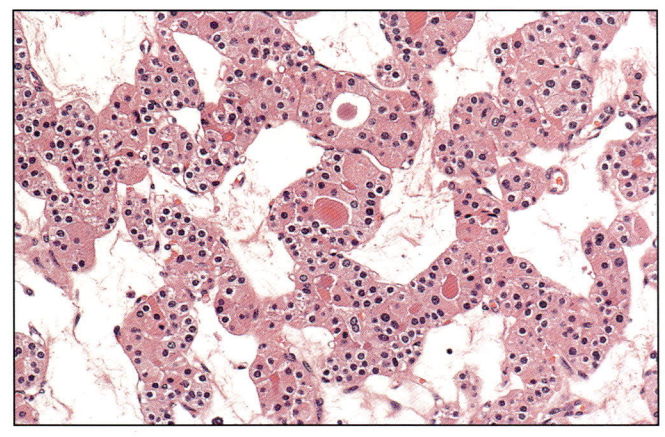

图18B.7 甲状旁腺腺瘤伴有滤泡状结构，类似甲状腺滤泡性肿瘤。本例管腔中的胶样物质实际是淀粉样物。

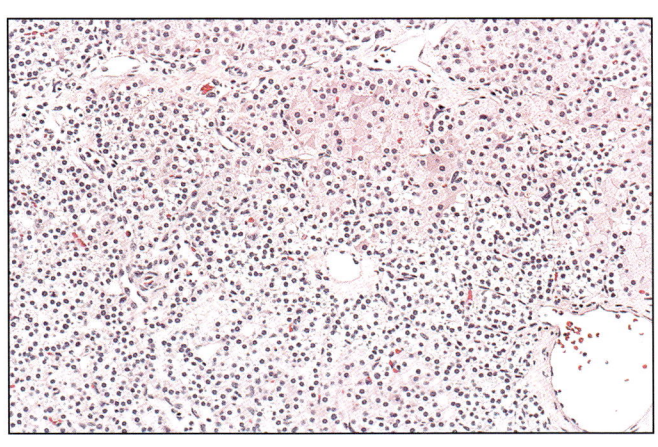

图18B.10 由主细胞、透明细胞和嗜酸性细胞混合形成的甲状旁腺腺瘤。在此例中，多角形细胞均匀一致，表现温和，缺少核分裂象。

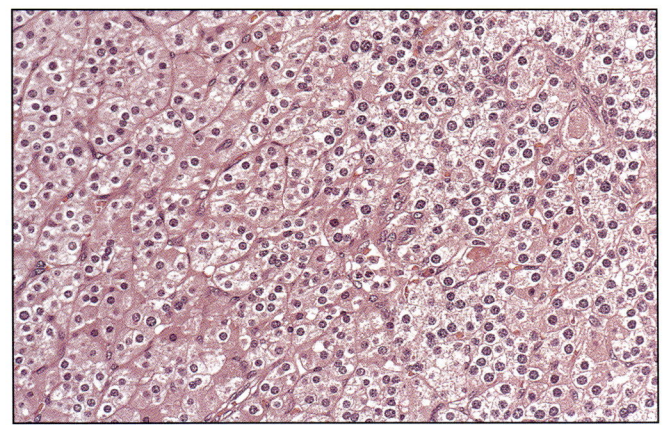

图18B.8 甲状旁腺腺瘤。呈弥漫性生长，其间有纤细的血管穿过，部分血管呈窦状。在视野左侧呈现条索状结构。

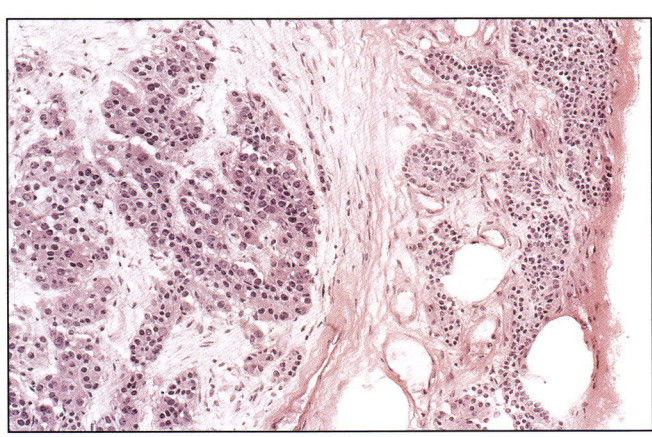

图18B.11 甲状旁腺腺瘤，冰冻切片。左侧多角形的肿瘤细胞无论是细胞体积还是细胞核体积均大于右侧残余的甲状旁腺细胞。

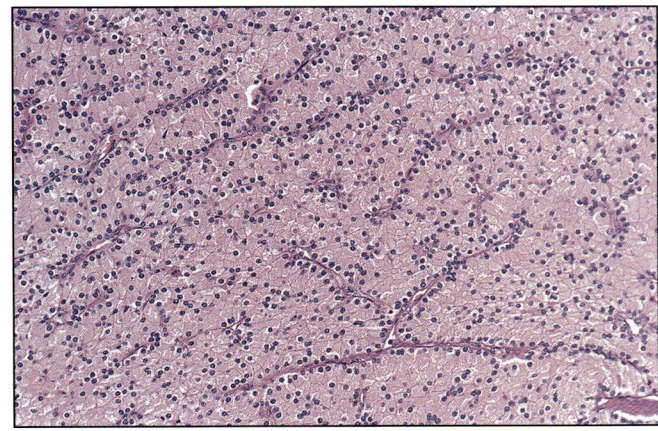

图18B.9 甲状旁腺腺瘤。其间有纤细的血管穿过，朝向血管间隙呈栅状排列的细胞核形成了列兵样结构——此结构为甲状旁腺病变（增生或肿瘤）的显著特征。

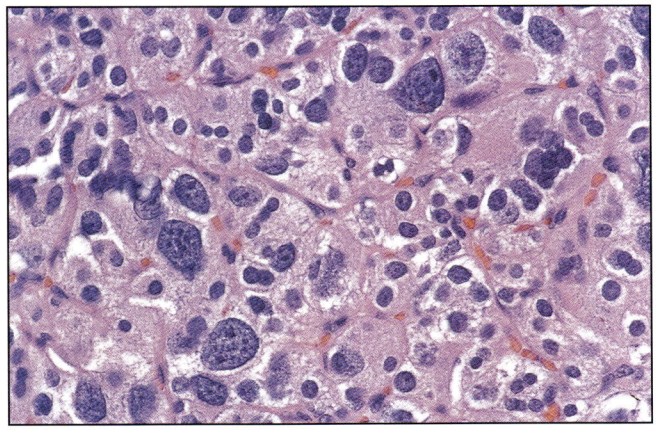

图18B.12 甲状旁腺腺瘤。即使出现散在的具有奇异、深染细胞核的大细胞，仍然属于甲状旁腺腺瘤的形态学范围之内。请注意其他的细胞具有温和均匀一致的细胞核，而且未见核分裂象。

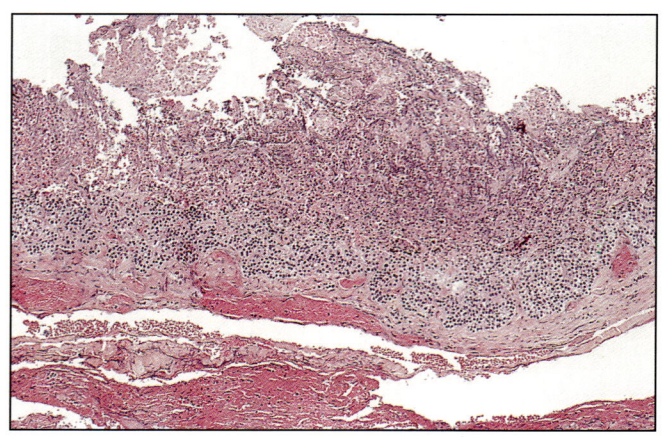

图18B.13 甲状旁腺腺瘤伴有梗死及囊性变。只看到一小圈存活的肿瘤细胞。视野上方为囊腔，囊壁腔面可见坏死组织。

肿瘤坏死不是良性甲状旁腺腺瘤的特征。少数情况下出现出血性梗死，能够导致甲状旁腺功能亢进自发性消退[64]。少数病例可以伴有淋巴细胞浸润，通常在肿瘤外围形成淋巴滤泡，但是淋巴细胞也可以与肿瘤细胞混杂在一起，导致肿瘤细胞变性和纤维化[65,66]。甲状旁腺腺瘤在酒精注射治疗后，可以出现梗死、纤维化以及血管形成增加，表现为肿瘤中心出现扩张的薄壁血管[67]。

甲状旁腺腺瘤的其他类型

脂肪腺瘤（甲状旁腺错构瘤）[Lipoadenoma (parathyroid hamartoma)][68-74] 脂肪腺瘤是甲状旁腺腺瘤中非常少见的一种类型，表现为主细胞/嗜酸性细胞与大量成熟的脂肪细胞混合在一起。脂肪细胞占肿瘤成分的20%～90%（图18B.14）。局灶可以出现黏液样间质。其腺瘤本质可以通过具有界限以及体积较大(1～15cm)而被识别，其余的甲状旁腺组织是正常的。至少一半病例伴有高钙血症。也有报道称一种极少见的甲状旁腺脂肪增生与甲状旁腺功能亢进有关[75]。

乳头状腺瘤(papillary variant) 少数病例表现为明显的乳头状结构，可能会被误诊为甲状腺乳头状癌[61,76]。

水样透明细胞腺瘤(water-clear variant) 少数甲状旁腺腺瘤完全由胞浆透明的多角形细胞构成，细胞膜清晰可见[77,78]。

滤泡型腺瘤(follicular variant) 明显的滤泡状（腺泡状）结构可能会导致误诊为甲状腺滤泡性肿瘤（见图18B.6和18B.7）。

嗜酸性（嗜酸细胞性）腺瘤 [oxyphil (oncocytic) adenoma] 偶尔肿瘤完全由具有大量线粒体的嗜酸性（嗜酸细胞性）细胞组成（图18B.15）。该肿瘤高钙血症通常较轻[79-81]。这些肿瘤（特别是位于甲状腺中的嗜酸性腺瘤）易被误诊为甲状腺 Hurthle 细胞肿瘤。与后者相比，甲状旁腺嗜酸性腺瘤的细胞膜通常更加清晰。

免疫组织化学

甲状旁腺腺瘤的诊断很少需要免疫组化研究。肿瘤细胞对于细胞角蛋白、广谱神经内分泌标志物以及甲状旁腺激素均为阳性[4,82,83]。当甲状旁腺腺瘤发生于其他部位或者形态学与甲状腺肿瘤（特别是滤泡型腺瘤）的鉴别有困难时，甲状旁腺激素免疫染色对于确认肿瘤的甲状旁腺本质是非常有帮助的。

细胞遗传学和分子学所见

X-连锁的限制性片段长度多态性的分子遗传学研究证实大多数甲状旁腺腺瘤具有单克隆性[84-86]。此外，还发现某些病例的甲状旁腺激素基因具有肿瘤特异的DNA改变[84]。

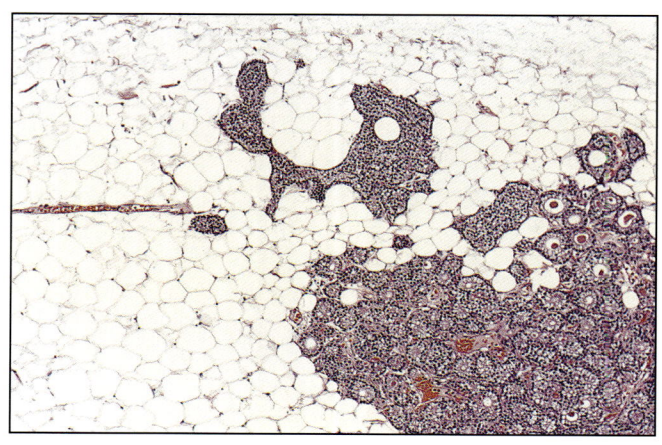

图18B.14 甲状旁腺脂肪腺瘤。肿瘤性甲状旁腺细胞呈滤泡状或岛状排列，与大量的脂肪细胞混合在一起。

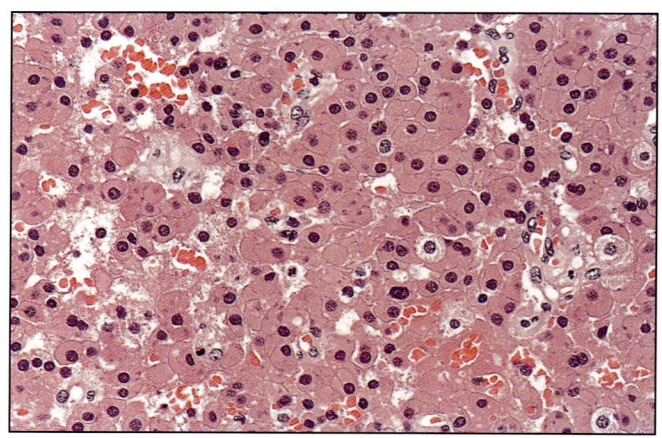

图18B.15 嗜酸细胞甲状旁腺腺瘤。细胞具有清晰的细胞膜和嗜酸性颗粒状胞浆。

少数甲状旁腺腺瘤存在11号染色体近着丝粒点倒置，从而使cyclin-D1基因（PRAD1）与甲状旁腺激素基因发生易位，导致cyclin-D1过表达[84,85,87-90]。Cyclin-D1在调控细胞周期中扮演重要角色，其过表达导致细胞增殖。使用免疫组化技术发现18%～39%的甲状旁腺腺瘤表达cyclin-D1，明显高于cyclin-D1基因重排率，提示cyclin-D1的表达失调存在其他分子机制[87,91]。正常甲状旁腺组织很少表达cyclin-D1，但是在甲状旁腺增生（61%）和甲状旁腺癌中cyclin-D1的表达较为常见[91]。

此外，位于11q13的 *MEN1* 位点（该基因胚系突变是MEN Ⅰ型的基本遗传学异常）与一些散发型甲状旁腺腺瘤有关，大约10%～23%的散发型甲状旁腺腺瘤患者存在该基因的体细胞突变[92,93]，而 *RET* 原癌基因（该基因胚系突变是MEN Ⅱ型的基本遗传学异常）似乎与散发型甲状旁腺腺瘤无关[94-98]。通过比较基因组杂交以及荧光原位杂交（FISH）技术，甲状旁腺腺瘤其他的一些染色体异常，如1p、1q、6q、11、13q以及15q缺失已被人们所认识[99,100]。

鉴别诊断

1. 原发性甲状旁腺增生：在原发性甲状旁腺增生中，所有的甲状旁腺均增大，尽管一些病例中各甲状旁腺增大程度不一致。这类患者应该检查可能存在的MEN[24]。对于甲状旁腺腺瘤而言，增大的只是单个腺体，而其他的甲状旁腺体积正常或变小。如果仅有一个甲状旁腺可供检查，而且该甲状旁腺体积增大并富于细胞，此时不能明确区分甲状旁腺腺瘤和甲状旁腺增生。这种情况下，必须检查其余的甲状旁腺（图18B.16；见后续章节术中诊断部分）。
2. 甲状旁腺癌（见后续章节及表18B.4和表18B.5）。
3. 继发性甲状旁腺增生：与甲状旁腺腺瘤的区别比较明显，因它与甲状旁腺腺瘤具有不同的临床表现，并且所有甲状旁腺呈多结节性增大（甲状旁腺腺瘤为单结节）（图18B.17）（见表18B.2）。
4. 甲状腺滤泡性腺瘤：当甲状旁腺肿瘤位于甲状腺内时，需要与甲状腺滤泡性腺瘤鉴别。
5. 嗜酸性细胞结节：与甲状旁腺腺瘤的不同点在于结节较小且通常多灶，不会导致高钙血症。

甲状旁腺癌　Parathyroid carcinoma

临床特征

甲状旁腺癌明显少于腺瘤，发病年龄也较甲状旁腺腺瘤年轻10岁（见表18B.4）。发病无性别倾向。多数

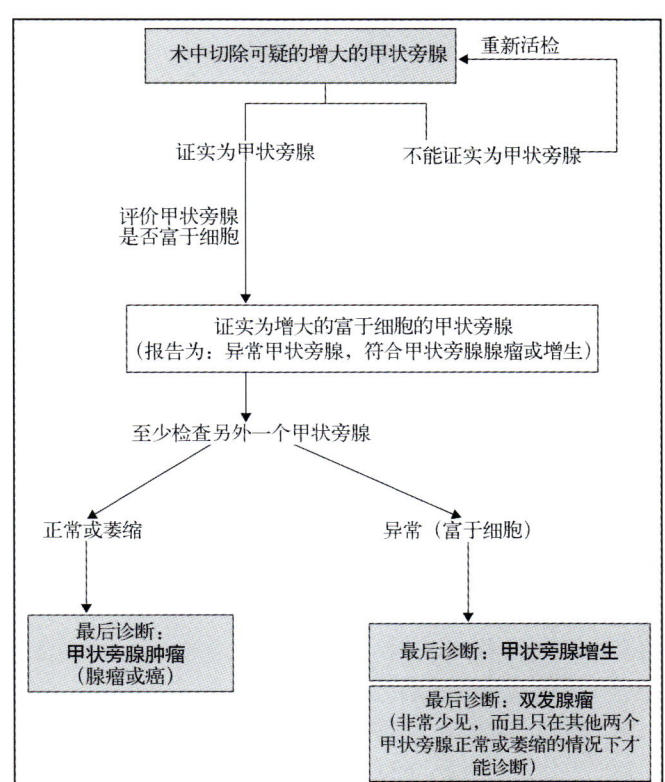

图18B.16　该流程图显示甲状旁腺功能亢进术中评价时的组织处理和诊断。

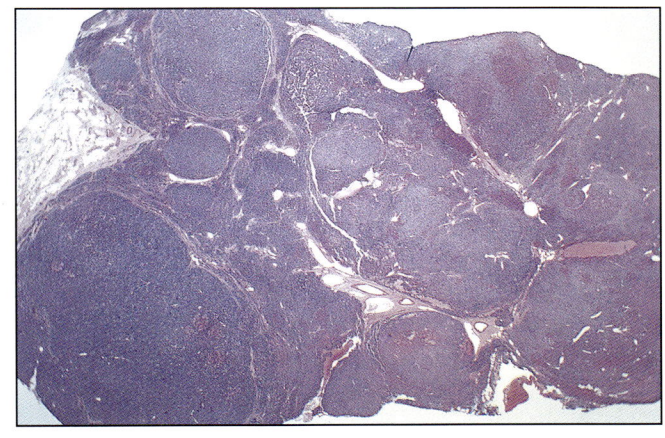

图18B.17　慢性肾功能衰竭患者的甲状旁腺结节状增生。该患者表现为三发性甲状旁腺功能亢进。请注意多结节结构及结节中丰富的细胞。

甲状旁腺癌是功能性的，可以引起严重的高钙血症和低磷血症，但也有一些是非功能性的[26-28,51,63,101-115]。多数患者表现为高钙血症或其并发症，如多尿、烦渴、虚弱、肾绞痛、骨痛、骨折以及复发性胰腺炎。下面一些特征无论单独或同时出现，对于诊断甲状旁腺癌而非甲状旁腺腺瘤具有提示作用：非常严重的高钙血症，同时出现

肾和骨疾病以及颈部可触及肿块。有些病例起初误诊为甲状旁腺腺瘤，但是在数年后由于复发或转移才显现出肿瘤的恶性本质[116,117]。

多数甲状旁腺癌是散发的，只有少数发生于多发内分泌肿瘤或甲状旁腺功能亢进-颌骨肿瘤综合征的基础上[17,20,103-118]。甲状旁腺癌偶尔可以发生在甲状旁腺腺瘤或甲状旁腺增生基础上[63]。

临床行为及治疗

甲状旁腺癌易于侵犯周围组织，特别是甲状腺，少数情况下还表现为甲状腺包块。大约30%的患者手术可以治愈[28,109,119]，如果在初次手术时进行充分的根治性(切除肿瘤、邻近的甲状腺叶、气管旁软组织、淋巴结和同侧胸腺)切除，治愈率还会提高[102,106,112,115,120,121]。就是说，治疗甲状旁腺癌的最佳时机是第一次手术时就认出病变的恶性本质，但这并非总是可能的[122]。

术后大约1/3的患者在三年内发生局部复发[112]。文献报道术后放疗可以降低局部复发率[105]。大约1/3的患者发生转移，通常发生在病程晚期，容易转移到颈部和纵隔区域淋巴结（30%）、肺、肝和骨。复发及转移通常表现为复发性高钙血症，因为肿瘤相对呈惰性，通过进一步（重复性）的手术可以治愈或很好地控制症状[27,28,101,107,109,117,120]。生存率以年计算，甲状旁腺癌的5年和10年生存率分别为60%～85%以及40%～70%[114,123]。复发病例平均生存期为7～8年。死亡通常是由于高钙血症引起的代谢性并发症，而非肿瘤对器官占位所致[26-28,123-125]。无功能甲状旁腺癌比功能性甲状旁腺癌更具有侵袭性[101]。

甲状旁腺癌的治疗主要依靠手术。术后放疗可以减少局部复发，特别是切缘被累及的情况下[123,126]。化疗的疗效尚未证实[103]。降低血钙的药物如二磷酸盐以及calcimimetic药物，可以控制高钙血症，但是长期使用常会降低其疗效[127,128]。有研究报道，新型免疫治疗可以有效控制严重的高钙血症[129-131]。

大体表现

甲状旁腺癌通常呈卵圆形，灰白、质硬，直径由1厘米至数厘米不等[26]。一般大于甲状旁腺腺瘤，平均重量12g[3]。可以界限清楚(通常有厚的纤维包膜)，也可以发生浸润。有时可出现坏死和钙化[124]。

组织学表现

甲状旁腺癌通常有厚的包膜。明显的浸润可有可无（图18B.18）[63]。细胞结构特征通常与甲状旁腺腺瘤相似，多角形细胞排列成实性片状、梁状和团块状（图

表18B.5	甲状旁腺恶性肿瘤(甲状旁腺癌)的组织学诊断标准
恶性的绝对标准	与恶性相关的特征

只要具备下述任何一条即可诊断恶性
1. 侵犯周围组织：
  —甲状腺
  —食管
  —神经
  —软组织
2. 组织学证明有局部或远处转移
	缺乏恶性绝对标准的情况下，具备以下至少2条、最好3条或3条以上的特征才可以确诊恶性
	1. 侵犯包膜
	2. 侵犯脉管
	3. 核分裂象易见（>5/10HPF）
	4. 肿瘤内宽大的纤维条索分割实质和膨胀性结节
	5. 肿瘤凝固性坏死（需要与梗死鉴别，梗死可见于甲状旁腺腺瘤）
	6. 弥漫成片的单一小细胞，核浆比很高。
	7. 弥漫的细胞非典型性
	8. 许多肿瘤细胞出现巨大核仁

注意：对于少数显示某些非决定性恶性特征的病例，可以采用"甲状旁腺非典型性腺瘤"的诊断术语。

18B.19）。基本不形成滤泡结构。细胞核可以均匀一致或者呈多形性（图18B.20至18B.22）。核多形性本身对于甲状旁腺癌的诊断没有意义，因为它也可以出现在甲状旁腺腺瘤或甲状旁腺增生中。大约一半的病例出现明显的核仁（大核仁）（见图18B.21和18B.22）[132]。细胞浆透明或嗜酸性[124]，偶尔可以完全由嗜酸细胞组成（图18B.23）[116,133,134]。一些病例可以见到小灶或大范围的凝固性坏死（见图18B.25A）[132]。

一些甲状旁腺癌具有欺骗性的温和表象（见图18B.20A和18B.23）[103]，而另一些病例的恶性特征却很直观，如浸润性生长、弥漫的细胞非典型性以及易于识别的核分裂象（见图18B.22）。对大多数病例，需要将所有特征综合考虑才能诊断恶性。组织学鉴别甲状旁腺癌和甲状旁腺腺瘤的可行性标准见表18B.5[135]。值得注意的是，少数病例完全缺乏恶性组织学特征，只有在以后复发或转移时，才出现明显的恶性特征（见图18B.23）[63]。包膜侵犯应该准确无误，肿瘤要超出纤维包膜的最外层或者浸润到周围脂肪组织（见图18B.18）。长期存在的甲状旁腺腺瘤会使部分肿瘤细胞陷入包膜内，不要误诊为包膜侵犯。脉管侵犯（大约有12%的病例）必须严格按照与诊断甲状腺滤泡癌相同的标准进行评估（图18B.24）。肿瘤中出现广泛而宽大的纤维间隔是有助于诊断恶性的特征（图18B.25），但是也必须与

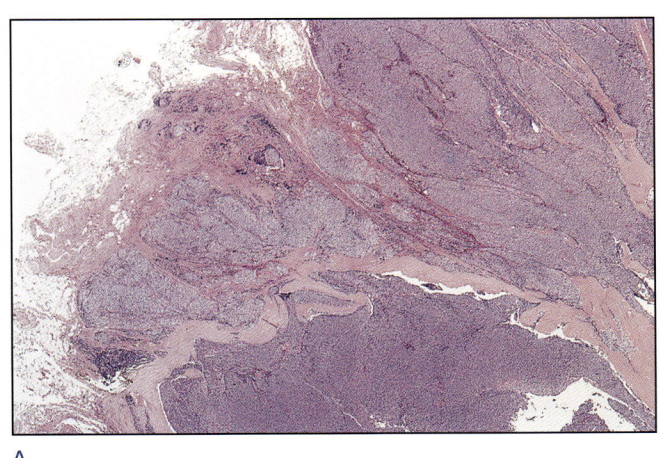 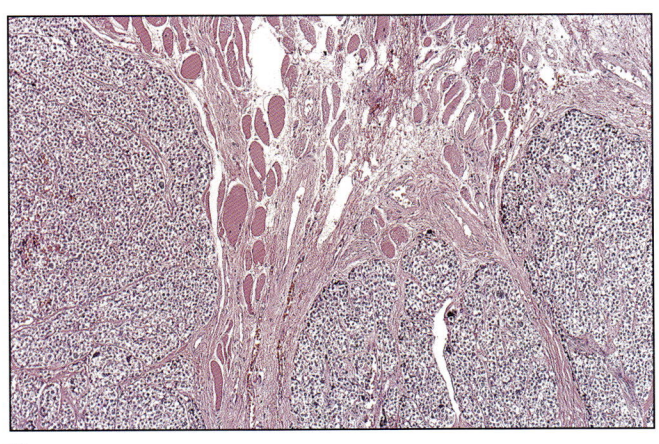

图18B.18 甲状旁腺癌。（A）肿瘤明显侵犯周围纤维脂肪组织（左上方）。（B）具有光滑轮廓的成片肿瘤细胞浸润到颈部的骨骼肌内。这些特征是诊断甲状旁腺恶性肿瘤的标准。

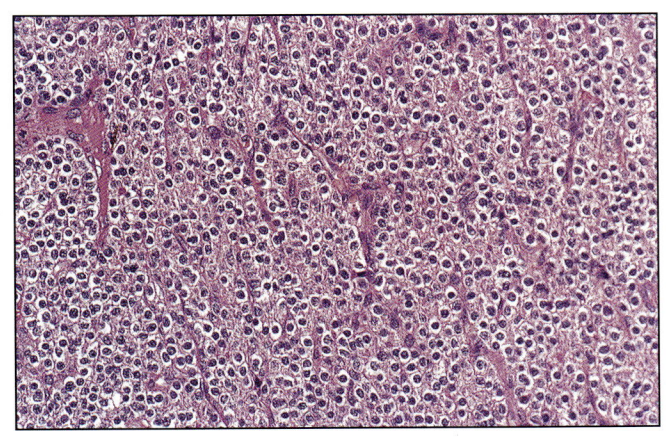

图18B.19 甲状旁腺癌。该例主要由温和的细胞构成，呈片状生长并穿插有纤细的血管。如果其他视野中没有确定的侵袭或恶性特征，就不能与甲状旁腺腺瘤相鉴别。

先前出血或手术形成局灶的瘢痕相鉴别[26]。这一特征只有与膨胀性结节同时出现时才有意义。当出现弥漫生长、形态单一、且核浆比例增加的小细胞时，提示甲状旁腺癌。广泛的细胞核非典型性和多形性，有别于偶尔出现的大而深染或怪异的细胞核，也提示甲状旁腺癌（见图18B.21和18B.22）。肿瘤细胞呈梁状排列，虽然有利于诊断甲状旁腺癌，但是不常出现而且不是甲状旁腺癌完全特异的表现[29]。

出现核分裂象是甲状旁腺癌最具争议性的特征。尽管Schantz & Castleman认为实质细胞（而非内皮细胞）出现核分裂象是诊断恶性最有价值的单一标准（见图

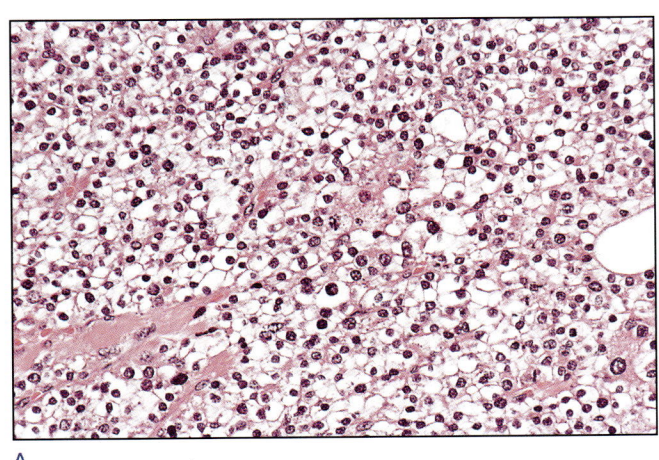 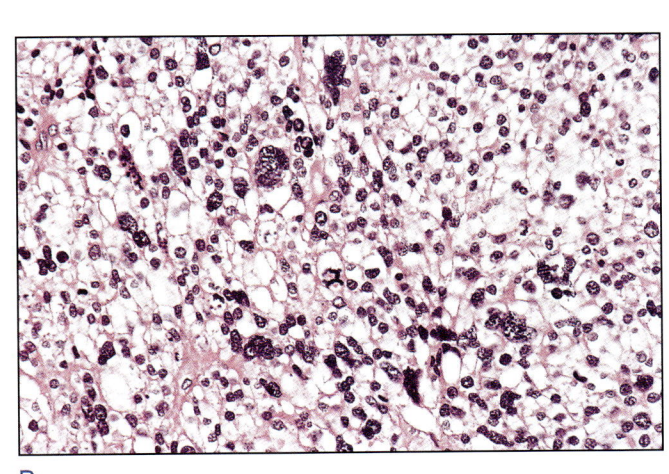

图18B.20 甲状旁腺癌。（A）该例主要展示温和表象的细胞，请注意中心部位有核分裂象。（B）该例主要展示多形性细胞与较温和的细胞混合。请注意中心部位异常的核分裂象。

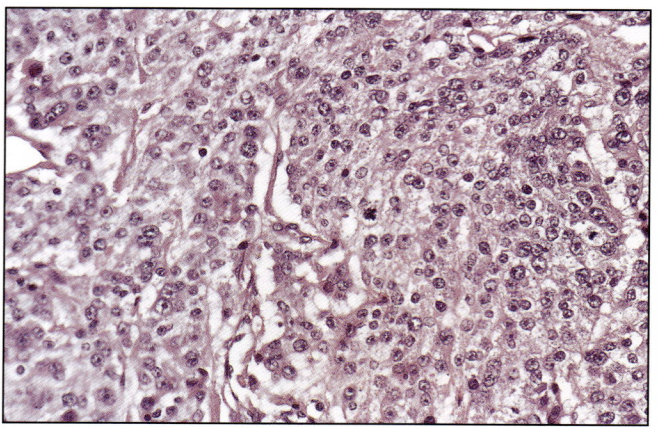

图18B.21 显示弥漫细胞非典型性的甲状旁腺癌。泡状细胞核具有大的核仁,可以看到数个核分裂象。

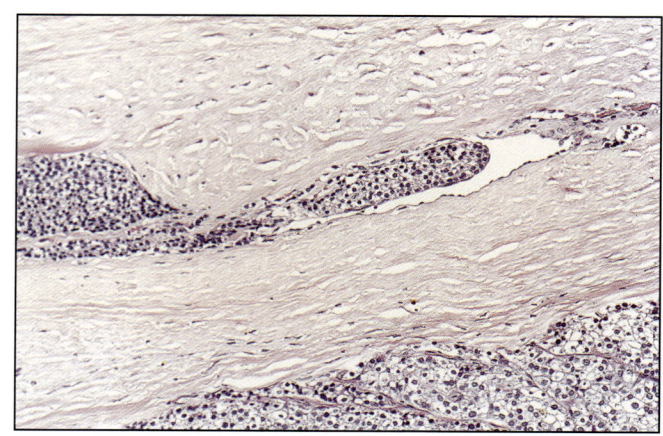

图18B.24 甲状旁腺癌。瘤栓进入衬覆内皮的脉管腔。该特征满足严格的脉管侵犯标准。

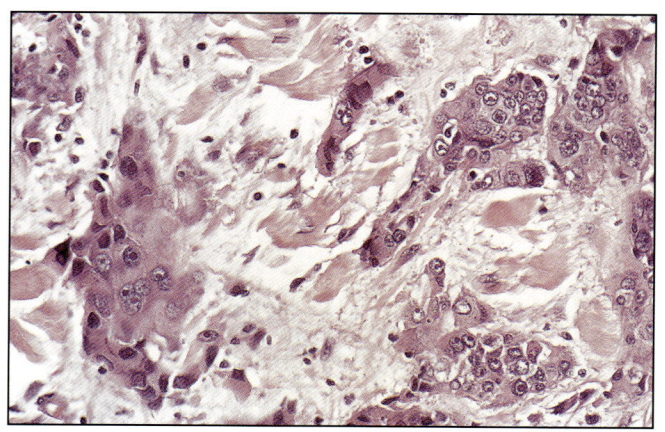

图18B.22 甲状旁腺癌。肿瘤呈现不规则的侵袭性岛状生长,细胞多形性很明显。该肿瘤的恶性本质易于识别,而甲状旁腺源性却难以识别。

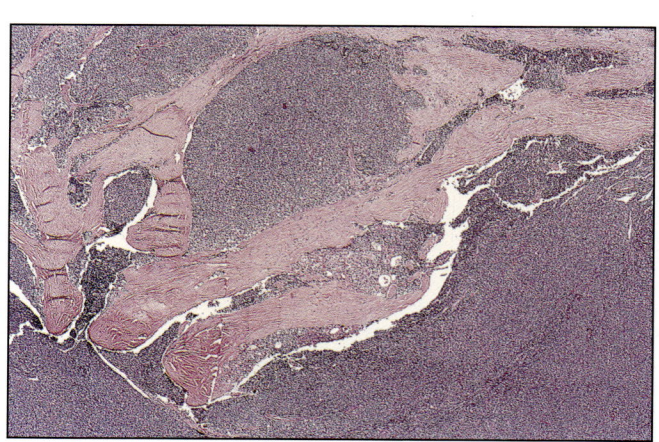

图18B.25 甲状旁腺癌。肿瘤被宽大的纤维条索分割,形成多个不规则的膨胀性、实性结节。

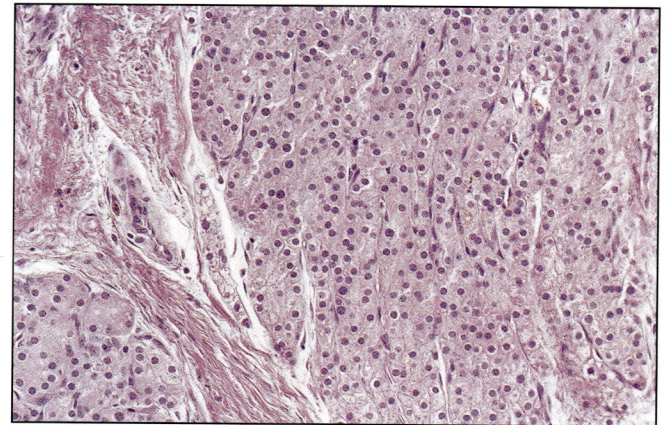

图18B.23 复发性甲状旁腺癌,嗜酸细胞型,发生于颈部软组织中。细胞表现温和而且核分裂不活跃。其恶性本质是根据局部复发来彰显的。

18B.20,18B.21)[26],但是核分裂象的重要性仍存在争议[135-137]。事实上核分裂象可以出现在甲状旁腺良性病变中(71%的甲状旁腺腺瘤以及80%的甲状旁腺增生,核分裂计数可以从几张切片中只有一个核分裂到每10个高倍视野5个核分裂)[63,137]。此外,在某些转移性甲状旁腺癌中可以完全没有核分裂象[26,132,135],有时形态学难以区分核分裂象与固缩细胞核。因此,甲状旁腺肿瘤出现核分裂象并不等同于恶性诊断,除非核分裂计数很高。

免疫组织化学

甲状旁腺激素的免疫染色对于确诊非功能性或异位甲状旁腺癌会有帮助(图18B.26)。

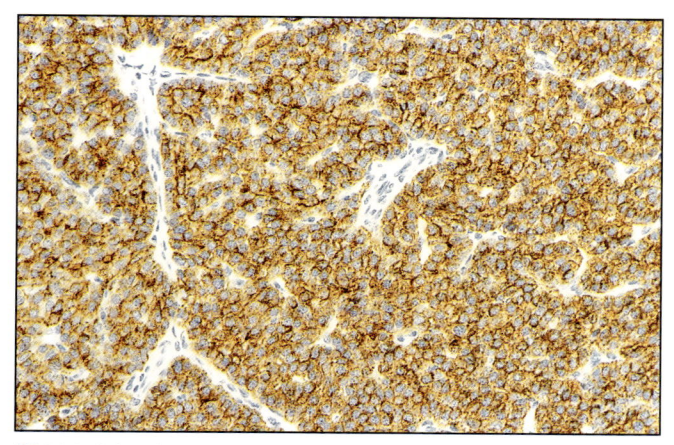

图18B.26　发生于纵隔的甲状旁腺癌。甲状旁腺激素免疫染色阳性证实肿瘤来源于甲状旁腺。

增殖指数标志物 Ki-67 有助于鉴别甲状旁腺癌（Ki-67 指数为 0.4%～26%，平均 6.05%～8.4%）和甲状旁腺腺瘤（Ki-67 指数为 0.5%～5.1%，平均 2.03%～3.28%）[138-141]。该项免疫染色也可以显示核分裂象，与模糊背景中的固缩细胞核相鉴别。然而，由于腺瘤与腺癌在核分裂计数上有一定的重叠，所以这项检查不能单独用于判断良恶性[142]。高增殖指数（>5%）提示恶性诊断，但是低增殖指数不能排除恶性的可能。

最近发现 Galectin-3 的表达对鉴别甲状旁腺癌（92.3%的病例阳性）和甲状旁腺腺瘤（3.3%的病例阳性）很有帮助[143]。其他有鉴别诊断价值的免疫组化标志物包括 parafibromin、Rb 蛋白和 p27（见下一章节）。

细胞遗传学和分子学所见

编码 parafibromin 蛋白的 *HRPT2* 基因失活性突变（该基因与甲状旁腺功能亢进-颌骨肿瘤综合征相关）在甲状旁腺癌的发病中发挥重要作用。这种突变至少出现在 2/3 的散发性甲状旁腺癌病例中，而基本不出现在甲状旁腺腺瘤中[144,145]。奇怪的是，某些病例中会发现 *HRPT2* 基因胚系突变，提示这一类病例可能是甲状旁腺功能亢进-颌骨肿瘤综合征中新的先证者或表型变异[144]。parafibromin 蛋白的一个已知功能是抑制 cyclinD1 的表达[146]。其免疫染色发现几乎所有的甲状旁腺癌都缺乏核染色，而甲状旁腺腺瘤则全部阳性（甲状旁腺功能亢进-颌骨肿瘤综合征相关性腺瘤除外）[147]。

视网膜母细胞瘤(*Rb*)抑癌基因的等位缺失在甲状旁腺癌中很常见[89,135,148,149]。曾有报道，20%～100%的甲状旁腺癌缺乏 Rb 蛋白免疫活性[138,148-150]。一些研究认为该项特征有助于甲状旁腺癌和甲状旁腺腺瘤的鉴别，另一些研究则认为该项特征并非可靠的鉴别指标[138,141,149]。总体上，甲状旁腺癌的 *Rb* 等位基因部分缺失较甲状旁腺腺瘤多见[151]。FISH 研究证实，与甲状旁腺腺瘤相比，甲状旁腺癌 11 号染色体的获得（gain）更为常见[152]。

甲状旁腺癌常见 cyclinD1 过表达（91%），提示细胞周期失调在肿瘤发生中扮演关键角色[87,91]。*p53* 等位基因的缺失与一些甲状旁腺癌的发生有关[150]。细胞周期依赖性激酶抑制蛋白 p27 的表达减少，对于鉴别甲状旁腺癌（平均标记指数为 13.9%）和甲状旁腺腺瘤（平均标记指数为 56.8%）很有帮助[140,153]。

非典型性甲状旁腺腺瘤（不能确定恶性潜能的甲状旁腺肿瘤）
Atypical parathyroid adenoma (parathyroid neoplasm of uncertain malignant potential)

非典型性腺瘤也称为不能确定恶性潜能的甲状旁腺肿瘤，并非一种临床病理学疾病，而是在甲状旁腺肿瘤存在一些令人担忧的特征但又没有充足的证据诊断恶性时所用的诊断术语。也就是说，肿瘤有一项或两项"恶性相关特征"，但是缺乏表 18B.5 中所列的"恶性的绝对标准"[154]。应用这一名称，就是承认了甲状旁腺肿瘤谱系中的灰区，并且说明准确预测临床结局有时存在困难。正如预期的那样，非典型性甲状旁腺腺瘤的免疫表达谱（如 Ki-67 和 p27 表达）介于甲状旁腺腺瘤和甲状旁腺癌之间[153]。一项研究表明，非整倍体的非典型性甲状旁腺腺瘤会发生术后复发，而整倍体的非典型性甲状旁腺腺瘤不会发生[155]。

例如，图 18B.27 显示一个界限清楚，重约 12g 的肿瘤。该肿瘤呈现局灶而非弥漫的细胞不典型性，局部有少数核分裂象以及数个高核浆比、形态单一的小细胞区。因此，只具备了一项"恶性相关特征"（片状单一小细胞），但是另外还有一些上述令人担忧的特征，可以使用"非典型性甲状旁腺腺瘤"术语来表明该病例有发生不良结局的少许可能性，这比应用甲状旁腺腺瘤和甲状旁腺癌都要好，前者可能会降低随访的警惕性；后者则会使患者思想上饱受恶性肿瘤的困扰。定期随访血清钙水平会有帮助。一例报告为"伴有非典型梭形细胞形态的甲状旁腺腺瘤"[156]，可能代表了这类肿瘤。该肿瘤界限清楚，但是存在多灶梭形细胞巢，且核分裂活跃（每 10 个高倍视野有 8 个核分裂象）。

我们预期少数非典型甲状旁腺腺瘤可以复发或转移，但是并未得到确切的数据来支持这一结论。同样，复发或转移风险可能会取决于存在何种令人担忧的特

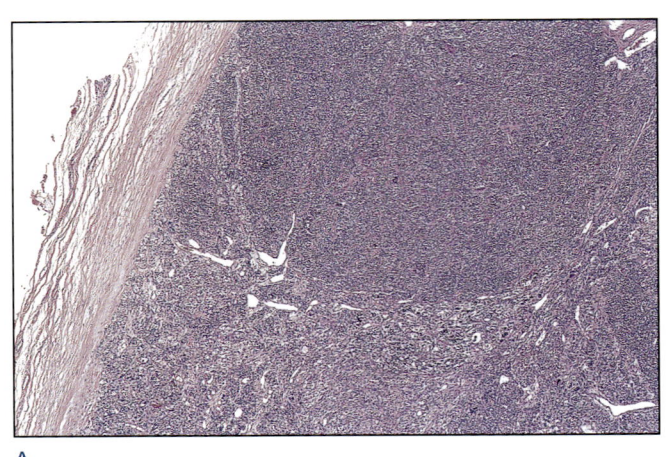
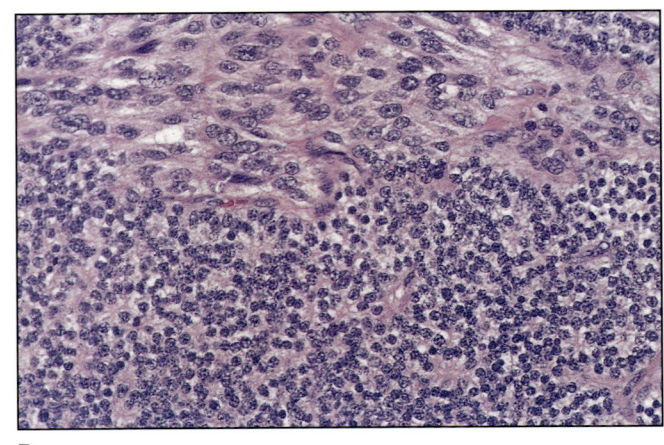

图18B.27 不能确定恶性潜能的甲状旁腺肿瘤。（A）该肿瘤较大（12g），但是包膜完整。视野上方显示形态单一的小细胞。（B）视野上方显示梭形肿瘤细胞，视野下方显示的是具有高核浆比的小细胞。该视野看不到核分裂象，其他视野可以见到少数核分裂象。

征，例如，显示脉管侵犯的肿瘤可能比只显示宽大纤维条索的肿瘤预后差。

其他肿瘤

除腺瘤和癌之外，甲状旁腺其他肿瘤均十分罕见。曾有报道，副神经节瘤可以发生于甲状旁腺[157]。甲状旁腺发生的肿瘤样病变还有甲状旁腺囊肿、鳃裂囊肿和淀粉样变性[158-160]。

甲状旁腺功能亢进的术中诊断

传统方法：手术探察和冰冻切片评估[161,162]

目的

在对甲状旁腺功能亢进患者进行术中冰冻切片评估时，病理医生的主要职责是指明病理改变，这对于治疗极为重要。对于甲状旁腺腺瘤，只切除受累的腺体即可治愈。对于甲状旁腺癌，识别其恶性本质使得初次手术就可以实施根治性切除，提供了最佳的治疗时机。如果诊断为甲状旁腺增生，则需甲状旁腺次全切除，即切除三个半腺体，只留下大约50mg的甲状旁腺组织。这是一种较激进的手术方式，可能会导致永久性甲状旁腺功能低下[24,37]。

首先，要确定送检组织确实是甲状旁腺而不是淋巴结、离散的甲状腺结节或异位胸腺组织。第二步，确定甲状旁腺组织是异常的（图18B.28）。此时，也只能诊

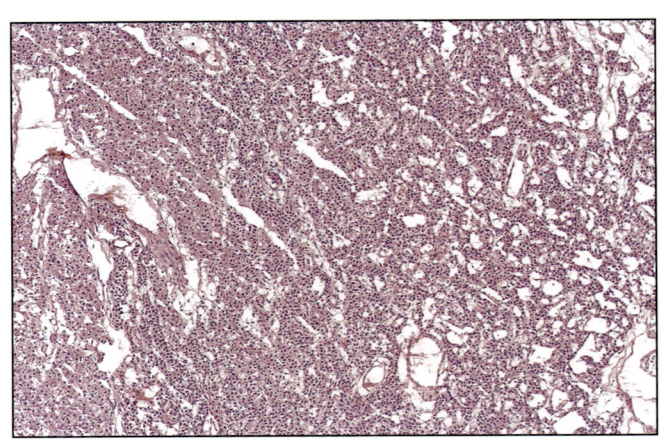

图18B.28 甲状旁腺腺瘤，冰冻切片。腺体富于细胞（异常），看不到散在的脂肪细胞。单凭这个标本，不能明确与甲状旁腺增生区分。

断异常甲状旁腺，符合腺瘤或增生。病理医师应该询问其他甲状旁腺的情况，并且要求从其他一个或多个甲状旁腺取活检（通常为切取活检），所遵循的步骤总结于图18B.16。尽管有人提倡用细胞刮片或者细胞印片作为术中冰冻诊断经济而快速的替代方法，但是其准确性不够高，尚未成为标准常规[10,163,164]。然而，细胞涂片确实是提高冰冻切片准确性的有益的辅助工作[165]。

少数情况下，切除的甲状旁腺中有提示恶性的表现（见表18B.5），病理医生要将这种印象或者诊断告知外科医生，进而使其考虑是否采用更为激进的手术方式。

正常或异常的甲状旁腺？

表18B.1列举了提示甲状旁腺异常（肿瘤或增生）的一些特征（见图18B.28）。如果整个甲状旁腺可供检查，就应该测量、称重并进行组织学检查。而当只有切取标本可供检查时，则很难做出评价。这种情况下，外科医

生所提供的腺体大小信息应该与组织学表现相结合。一个小且富于脂肪细胞的腺体应该考虑是正常或功能受抑制的甲状旁腺。一个增大且基本没有脂肪细胞的腺体应该是异常的甲状旁腺（富于细胞）。如果所见不足以得出结论，那么脂肪染色会有帮助（见后续章节）。

细胞及细胞核大小的绝对增加是甲状旁腺增生或肿瘤的特征，这一点很难判断，除非有正常的甲状旁腺细胞提供对照（见图18B.11）。

一些作者发现在冰冻切片或细胞印片中应用脂肪染色（苏丹Ⅱ或Ⅳ，油红O）有助于鉴别正常和异常甲状旁腺[86,166-169]。快速脂肪染色可用于切取活检标本或最初切除的甲状旁腺组织。值得注意的是脂肪染色用来评估细胞内的脂质而非间质中的脂肪细胞。

正常甲状旁腺细胞内含有大量的胞浆脂滴，而增生或腺瘤细胞中通常缺乏细胞内脂滴。这一现象不适用于嗜酸细胞，因为无论正常、增生或肿瘤性嗜酸细胞都缺少胞浆内脂滴[1]。某些作者对于脂肪染色的价值持保守态度，因为有时腺瘤或增生性腺体可以含有胞浆内脂滴，而正常甲状旁腺可以缺乏脂滴[170-172]。然而，如果微弱或局灶染色被认为是阴性，胞浆中脂肪染色的差异就非常少（1.1%）[173]。

甲状旁腺腺瘤（Parathyroid adenoma）抑或甲状旁腺增生（parathyroid hyperplasia）？

如果出现一薄圈受挤压的正常甲状旁腺腺体，建议诊断为甲状旁腺腺瘤（见图18B.3），但是如果不出现也不能排除腺瘤的可能性，因为可能是正常腺体完全被肿瘤取代或者是取材问题。然而，这个标准并非完全可靠，因为这种薄圈也可见于某些甲状旁腺增生病例，而且多结节性甲状旁腺增生中受压的甲状旁腺实质也会产生类似结构[174,175]。

甲状旁腺腺瘤和增生最可靠的鉴别点在于通过组织学检查另外一个或多个甲状旁腺（见图18B.16）[1]。光凭手术台上观察是不可靠的，因为一些增生病变对甲状旁腺的影响不均衡，因此腺体可能仅仅略微增大[176]。所以，最好进行切取活检的组织学评估。

术中冰冻切片对于判断甲状旁腺组织有多准确？

Johns Hopkins的Westra等人对1579例术中冰冻切片进行回顾后发现，对于甲状旁腺探察术中组织类型的鉴定，准确率高达99.2%[177]。有时在鉴别甲状旁腺、甲状腺结节或淋巴结时存在困难，需要延期诊断（延期率为0.4%）[177]。主要问题包括冰冻造成的假象、脂肪的存在造成切片不理想、冰冻切片中细胞学细节不理想，以及取材错误。

术中冰冻切片诊断中的一些潜在陷阱[177]

1. 冰冻假象会使人将淋巴结误认为甲状旁腺组织，因为冰晶造成的组织裂隙会给人以间质脂肪细胞分割小梁状主细胞的印象。反之亦然（图18B.29）。
2. 甲状旁腺腺瘤有时会被误诊为甲状腺滤泡性腺瘤，特别是出现微滤泡或以嗜酸细胞为主时，以及甲状旁腺腺瘤位于甲状腺内时。反之，甲状腺结节也会被误诊为甲状旁腺病变，原因是将间质水肿误认为间质脂肪细胞，或者确实有散在的脂肪细胞。
3. 尽管只检查两个甲状旁腺不足以排除双发腺瘤的可能性，但是这种情况非常少见，因此许多外科医生在确定一侧颈部存在一个富于细胞的腺瘤和一个正常甲状旁腺后，就不再进行对侧颈部探察[37,161]。然而，也有一些医生提倡常规探察所有的甲状旁腺腺体[175]。
4. 对于发生率较低的脂肪腺瘤，因为散在分布大量的脂肪细胞，故很难被辨认出是肿瘤。但是其体积增大和重量增加无疑表明这是一个异常腺体。

替代方法：甲状旁腺微创切除术及术中辅助性甲状旁腺激素水平测定
Alternative approach: minimally invasive parathyroidectomy with the aid of intraoperative parathyroid hormone assay

原理

由于血液循环中甲状旁腺激素的起始半衰期非常短，所以手术切除增大的甲状旁腺后血浆中甲状旁腺激

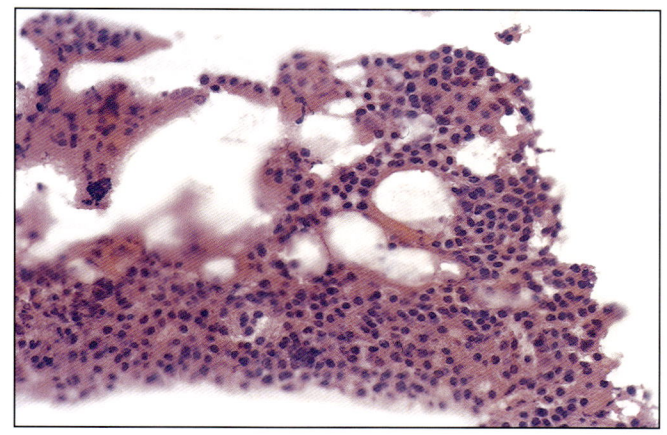

图18B.29　颈部淋巴结，冰冻切片。该活检标本来自甲状旁腺功能亢进患者的颈部探察，被误诊为甲状旁腺组织。冰晶造成的假象给人以散在脂肪细胞的错误印象，而淋巴细胞则被误认为甲状旁腺细胞。

素的迅速下降，证明确实切除了过度产生甲状旁腺激素的"元凶"。因此，术中快速检测甲状旁腺激素可用于指导甲状旁腺功能亢进的手术治疗[41,178]。通常不需要冰冻切片检查，除非是不能确定被切除组织的来源[41]。

过程和结果解释

甲状旁腺微创手术可以在门诊实施，探察过程创伤小且并发症发生几率低。该手术也适用于术前扫描发现单个腺体增大的甲状旁腺功能亢进患者。在对甲状旁腺进行任何操作前，采集一份参考血样（如在诱导麻醉后立即采血）。在手术切除增大腺体十分钟后，采集另一份血样（有时也采集系列血样）。与参考血样比较，如果血浆中甲状旁腺激素水平下降 50% 以上证明治疗成功。甲状旁腺激素水平未能显著下降可能由于：(1) 术前定位检查忽略了其他的高功能甲状旁腺，如双发腺瘤和甲状旁腺增生；(2) 切除的组织不是高功能甲状旁腺。这时需要进一步探察。

有效性

多项研究表明，术中检测甲状旁腺水平有利于提高原发性甲状旁腺功能亢进患者的手术疗效[179-183]。据 Boggs 等人的研究，治疗甲状旁腺功能亢进的手术失败率由 5%（传统的手术探察）降到 1.5%（术前定位以及术中甲状旁腺激素检测）[184]。在另一项 345 例连续的原发性甲状旁腺功能亢进病例研究中，均只有一个甲状旁腺增大而进行微创手术，第一组 157 例患者没有进行术中甲状旁腺激素水平检测，第二组 188 例患者进行了术中甲状旁腺激素水平检测。在第一组中，15 例（10%）因为没有发现其他高功能甲状旁腺而出现了术后高钙血症；在第二组中，170 名（90%）患者在手术切除单个甲状旁腺腺瘤后甲状旁腺激素水平下降超过 50%，从而得以治愈。其余 18 例（10%）由于甲状旁腺激素水平没有明显下降而实施了双侧颈部探察并且切除了另外的甲状旁腺组织（包括 9 例双发腺瘤和 9 例甲状旁腺增生）[180]。

参考文献

1. Grimelius L, Bondeson L 1995 Histopathological diagnosis of parathyroid diseases. Pathol Res Pract 191: 353–365
2. Dekker A, Dunsford H A, Geyer S J 1979 The normal parathyroid gland at autopsy: the significance of stromal fat in adult patients. J Pathol 128: 127–132
3. Castleman B, Roth S 1978 Tumors of the parathyroid glands. Atlas of tumor pathology, series 2, fascicle 14. Armed Forces Institute of Pathology, Washington, DC
4. Mendelsohn G 1988 Pathology of the parathyroid glands. In: Mendelsohn G (ed) Diagnosis and pathology of endocrine diseases. J B Lippincott, Philadelphia, p 139–177
5. DeLellis R A 1993 Tumors of the parathyroid gland. Atlas of tumor pathology, series 3, fascicle 6. Armed Forces Institute of Pathology, Washington, DC
6. Chryssochoos J T, Weber C J, Cohen C et al. 1995 DNA index and ploidy distinguish normal human parathyroids from parathyroid adenomas and primary hyperplastic parathyroids. Surgery 118: 1041–1049
7. Grimelius L, Akerstrom G, Johansson H. et al. 1998 The parathyroid glands. In: Kovacs K, Asa SL (eds) Functional endocrine pathology 2nd edn. Blackwell Science, Malden, p 381–414
8. Matsushita H 1997 Pathology of the parathyroid glands. In Lechago J, Gould V E (eds) Bloodworth's endocrine pathology 3rd edn. Williams & Wilkins, Baltimore, p 249–272
9. Tominaga Y, Kohara S, Namii Y et al. 1996 Clonal analysis of nodular parathyroid hyperplasia in renal hyperparathyroidism. World J Surg 20: 744–750
10. Roth S I, Faquin W C 2003 The pathologist's intraoperative role during parathyroid surgery. Arch Pathol Lab Med 127: 15
11. Barry M K, van Heerden J A, Grant C S et al. 1997 Is familial hyperparathyroidism a unique disease? Surgery 122: 1028–1033
12. Teh B T, Farnebo F, Twigg S et al. 1998 Familial isolated hyperparathyroidism maps to the hyperparathyroidism-jaw tumor locus in 1q21-q32 in a subset of families. J Clin Endocrinol Metab 83: 2114–2120
13. Huang S M, Duh Q Y, Shaver J et al. 1997 Familial hyperparathyroidism without multiple endocrine neoplasia. World J Surg 21: 22–28
14. Harach H R, Jasani B 1992 Parathyroid hyperplasia in tertiary hyperparathyroidism: a pathological and immunohistochemical reappraisal. Histopathology 21: 513–519
15. Dotzenrath C, Goretzki P E, Farnebo F et al. 1996 Molecular genetics of primary and secondary hyperparathyroidism. Exp Clin Endocrinol Diabetes 104: 105–107
16. Agarwal S K, Kester M B, Debelenko L V et al. 1997 Germline mutations of the MEN1 gene in familial multiple endocrine neoplasia type 1 and related states. Hum Mol Genet 6: 1169–1175
17. Yoshimoto K, Endo H, Tsuyuguchi M et al. 1998 Familial isolated primary hyperparathyroidism with parathyroid carcinomas: clinical and molecular features. Clin Endocrinol (Oxf) 48: 67–72
18. Kraimps J L, Denizot A, Carnaille B et al. 1996 Primary hyperparathyroidism in multiple endocrine neoplasia type IIa: retrospective French multicentric study. Groupe d'Etude des Tumeurs a Calcitonine (GETC, French Calcitonin Tumors Study Group), French Association of Endocrine Surgeons. World J Surg 20: 808–812
19. Fitzpatrick L A 1989 Hypercalcemia in the multiple endocrine neoplasia syndromes. Endocrinol Metab Clin North Am 18: 741–752
20. Teh B T, Sweet K M, Morrison C D 2004 Hyperparathyroidism-jaw tumour syndrome, In: DeLellis R A, Lloyd R V, Heitz P U et al. (eds) Pathology and genetics, tumours of endocrine organs, World Health Organization classification of tumours. IARC Press, Lyon, p 228–229
21. Cetani F, Pardi E, Ambrogini E et al. 2006 Genetic analyses in familial isolated hyperparathyroidism: implication for clinical assessment and surgical management. Clin Endocrinol (Oxf) 64: 146–152
22. Warner J, Epstein M, Sweet A et al. 2004 Genetic testing in familial isolated hyperparathyroidism: unexpected results and their implications. J Med Genet 41: 155–160
23. Simonds W F, Robbins C M, Agarwal S K et al. 2004 Familial isolated hyperparathyroidism is rarely caused by germline mutation in HRPT2, the gene for the hyperparathyroidism-jaw tumor syndrome. J Clin Endocrinol Metab 89: 96–102
24. Wang C A, Castleman B, Cope O. 1982 Surgical management of hyperparathyroidism due to primary hyperplasia. Ann Surg 195: 384–392
25. Dolgin C, Lo Gerfo P, LiVolsi V et al. 1979 Twenty-five year experience with primary hyperparathyroidism at Columbia Presbyterian Medical Center. Head Neck Surg 2: 92–98
26. Schantz A, Castleman B 1973 Parathyroid carcinoma. A study of 70 cases. Cancer 31: 600–605
27. Holmes E C, Morton D L, Ketcham A S 1969 Parathyroid carcinoma: a collective review. Ann Surg 169: 631–640
28. Shane E, Bilezikian J P 1982 Parathyroid carcinoma: a review of 62 patients. Endocr Rev 3: 218–226
29. Van Heerden J A, Weiland L H, ReMine W H et al. 1979 Cancer of the parathyroid glands. Arch Surg 114: 475–480
30. Heath H, Hodgson S F, Kennedy M A 1980 Primary hyperparathyroidism, incidence, morbidity and potential economic impact in a community. N Engl J Med 302: 189–193
31. Prinz RA, Barbato A L, Braithwaite S S et al. 1982 Prior irradiation and the development of coexistent differentiated thyroid cancer and hyperparathyroidism. Cancer 49: 874–877

32. Russ J E, Scanlon E F, Sener S F. 1979 Parathyroid adenomas following radiation. Cancer 43: 1078–1083
33. Mallette L E, Bilezikian J P, Heath D A et al. 1974 Primary hyperparathyroidism: clinical and biochemical features. Medicine (Baltimore) 53: 127–146
34. Royal R E, Delpassand E S, Shapiro S E et al. 2002 Improving the yield of preoperative parathyroid localization: technetium Tc 99m-sestamibi imaging after thyroid suppression. Surgery 132: 968–974
35. Calcutt V G, Franco-Saenz R, Morrow L B et al. 1998 Localization of abnormal parathyroid tissue with use of technetium-99m-sestamibi. Endocr Pract 4: 184–189
36. Moka D, Voth E, Dietlein M et al. 2000 Technetium 99m-MIBI-SPECT: a highly sensitive diagnostic tool for localization of parathyroid adenomas. Surgery 128: 29–35
37. Roth S I, Wang C A, Potts J T 1975 The team approach to primary hyperparathyroidism. Hum Pathol 6: 645–648
38. Silverberg S J, Shane E, Jacobs T P et al. 1999 A 10-year prospective study of primary hyperparathyroidism with or without parathyroid surgery. N Engl J Med 341: 1249–1255
39. Nordenstrom E, Westerdahl J, Bergenfelz A 2004 Long-term follow-up of patients with elevated PTH levels following successful exploration for primary hyperparathyroidism. World J Surg 28: 570–575
40. Hedback G, Oden A 2003 Recurrence of hyperparathyroidism; a long-term follow-up after surgery for primary hyperparathyroidism. Eur J Endocrinol 148: 413–421
41. Carter A B, Howanitz P J 2003 Intraoperative testing for parathyroid hormone: a comprehensive review of the use of the assay and the relevant literature. Arch Pathol Lab Med 127: 1424–1442
42. Khafif A, Halperin D, Marshak G 1998 Ethanol injection to parathyroid tissue: indications and limitations. Ear Nose Throat J 77: 538–540
43. Corlew D S, Bryda S L, Bradley E L et al. 1985 Observations on the course of untreated primary hyperparathyroidism. Surgery 98: 1064–1071
44. Sawady J, Mendelsohn G, Sirota R L et al. 1989 The intrathyroid hyperfunctioning parathyroid gland. Mod Pathol 2: 652–657
45. Russell C F, Edis A J, Scholz D A et al. 1981 Mediastinal parathyroid tumors: experience with 38 tumors requiring mediastinotomy for removal. Ann Surg 193: 805–809
46. Spiegel A M, Marx S J, Doppman J L et al. 1975 Intrathyroidal parathyroid adenoma or hyperplasia. An occasionally overlooked cause of surgical failure in primary hyperparathyroidism. J Am Med Assoc 234: 1029–1033
47. Nathaniels E K, Nathaniels A M, Wang C 1970 Mediastinal parathyroid tumours: a clinical and pathological study of 84 cases. Ann Surg 171: 165–170
48. Moran C A, Suster S 2005 Primary parathyroid tumors of the mediastinum. A clinicopathologic and immunohistochemical study of 17 cases. Am J Clin Pathol 124: 749–754
49. De la Cruz Vigo F, Ortega G, Gonzalez S et al. 1997 Pathologic intrathyroidal parathyroid glands. Int Surg 82: 87–90
50. Summers G W 1996 Parathyroid update: a review of 220 cases. Ear Nose Throat J 75: 434–439
51. Ordonez N G, Ibanez M L, Samaan N A et al 1983 Immunoperoxidase study of uncommon parathyroid tumors. Report of two cases of nonfunctioning parathyroid carcinoma and one intrathyroid parathyroid tumor-producing amyloid. Am J Surg Pathol 7: 535–542
52. Harness J K, Ramsburg S R, Nishiyama R H et al 1979 Multiple adenomas of the parathyroids: do they exist? Arch Surg 114: 468–474
53. Verdonk C C, Edias A J 1981 Parathyroid "double adenomas": fact or fiction? Surgery 90: 523–526
54. Bartsch D, Nies C, Hasse C et al. 1995 Clinical and surgical aspects of double adenoma in patients with primary hyperparathyroidism. Br J Surg 82: 926–929
55. Szabo E, Lundgren E, Juhlin C et al. 1998 Double parathyroid adenoma, a clinically nondistinct entity of primary hyperparathyroidism. World J Surg 22: 708–713
56. Abboud B, Sleilaty G, Helou E et al. 2005 Existence and anatomic distribution of double parathyroid adenoma. Laryngoscope 115: 1128–1131
57. Morrison C, Farrar W, Kneile J et al. 2004 Molecular classification of parathyroid neoplasia by gene expression profiling. Am J Pathol 165: 565–576
58. Yao K, Singer F R, Roth S I et al. 2004 Weight of normal parathyroid glands in patients with parathyroid adenomas. J Clin Endocrinol Metab 89: 3208–3213
59. Castleman B, Schantz A, Roth S 1976 Parathyroid hyperplasia in primary hyperparathyroidism: a review of 85 cases. Cancer 38: 1668–1675
60. Leedham P W, Pollock D J 1970 Intrafollicular amyloid in primary hyperparathyroidism. J Clin Pathol 23: 811–817
61. Sahin A, Robinson R A 1988 Papillae formation in parathyroid adenoma, a source of possible diagnostic error. Arch Pathol Lab Med 122: 99–100
62. Loda M, Lipman J, Cukor B et al. 1994 Nodular foci in parathyroid adenomas and hyperplasias: an immunohistochemical analysis of proliferative activity. Hum Pathol 25: 1050–1056
63. Evans H L 1991 Criteria for diagnosis of parathyroid carcinoma: a critical study. Surg Pathol 4: 244–265
64. Natsui K, Tanaka K, Suda M et al. 1996 Spontaneous remission of primary hyperparathyroidism due to hemorrhagic infarction in the parathyroid adenoma. Intern Med 35: 646–649
65. Lawton T J, Feldman M, LiVolsi V A 1998 Lymphocytic infiltrates in solitary parathyroid adenomas, a report of four cases with review of the literature. Int J Surg Pathol 6: 5–10
66. Veress B, Nordenstrom J 1994 Lymphocytic infiltration and destruction of parathyroid adenomas: a possible tumour-specific autoimmune reaction in two cases of primary hyperparathyroidism. Histopathology 25: 373–377
67. Chow L T, Metreweli C, King W W et al. 1997 Histological changes of parathyroid adenoma after percutaneous injection of ethanol. Histopathology 30: 87–89
68. Abdul-Haj S K, Conklin H, Hewitt W C 1962 Functioning lipoadenoma of the parathyroid gland, report of a unique case. N Engl J Med 266: 121–123
69. Daroca P J Jr, Landau R L, Reed R J et al. 1977 Functioning lipoadenoma of the parathyroid gland. Arch Pathol Lab Med 101: 28–29
70. Obara T, Fujimoto Y, Ito Y et al. 1989 Functioning parathyroid lipoadenoma – report of four cases: clinicopathological and ultrasonographic features. Endocrinol Jpn 36: 135–145
71. Perosio P, Brooks J J, LiVolsi V A 1988 Orbital brown tumor as initial manifestation of parathyroid lipoadenoma. Surg Pathol 1: 77–82
72. Chow L S, Erickson L A, Abu-Lebdeh H S, Wermers R A 2006 Parathyroid lipoadenomas: a rare cause of primary hyperparathyroidism. Endocr Pract 12: 131–136
73. Weiland L H, Garrison R C, ReMine W H et al. 1978 Lipoadenoma of the parathyroid gland. Am J Surg Pathol 2: 3–7
74. Wolff M, Goodman E N 1980 Functioning lipoadenoma of a supernumerary parathyroid gland in the mediastinum. Head Neck Surg 2: 302–307
75. Straus F H, Kaplan E L, Nishiyama R H et al. 1983 Five cases of parathyroid lipohyperplasia. Surgery 94: 901–905
76. Ho K J 1996 Papillary parathyroid adenoma. A rare occurrence and its importance in differentiation from papillary carcinoma of the thyroid. Arch Pathol Lab Med 120: 883–884
77. Roth S I 1995 Water-clear cell "adenoma". A new entity in the pathology of primary hyperparathyroidism (editorial; comment). Arch Pathol Lab Med 119: 996–997
78. Grenko R T, Anderson K M, Kauffman G et al. 1995 Water-clear cell adenoma of the parathyroid. A case report with immunohistochemistry and electron microscopy. Arch Pathol Lab Med 119: 1072-1074
79. Bedetti C D, Dekker A, Watson C G 1984 Functioning oxyphil cell adenoma of the parathyroid gland: a clinicopathologic study of ten patients with hyperparathyroidism. Hum Pathol 15: 1121–1126
80. Natsui K, Tanaka K, Suda M et al 1996 Oxyphil parathyroid adenoma associated with primary hyperparathyroidism and marked post-operative hungry bone syndrome. Intern Med 35: 545–549
81. Wolpert H R, Vickery A L Jr, Wang C A 1989 Functioning oxyphil cell adenomas of the parathyroid gland. A study of 15 cases. Am J Surg Pathol 13: 500–504
82. Weiler R, Fischer-Colbrie R, Schmid K W et al. 1988 Immunological studies on the occurrence and properties of chromogranin A and B and secretogranin II in endocrine tumors. Am J Surg Pathol 12: 877–884
83. Miettinen M, Clark R, Lehto V P et al. 1985 Intermediate-filament proteins in parathyroid glands and parathyroid adenomas. Arch Pathol Lab Med 109: 986–989
84. Arnold A, Staunton C E, Kim H G et al. 1988 Monoclonality and abnormal parathyroid hormone genes in parathyroid adenomas. N Engl J Med 318: 658–662
85. Marx S J 1988 Genetic defects in primary hyperparathyroidism [editorial]. N Engl J Med 318: 699–701
86. Grimelius L, Johansson H 1997 Pathology of parathyroid tumors. Semin Surg Oncol 13: 142–154
87. Hsi E D, Zukerberg L R, Yang W I et al. 1996 Cyclin D1/PRAD1 expression in parathyroid adenomas: an immunohistochemical study. J Clin Endocrinol Metab 81: 1736–1739
88. Abati A, Skarulis M C, Shawker T et al. 1995 Ultrasound-guided fine-needle aspiration of parathyroid lesions: a morphological and immunocytochemical approach. Hum Pathol 26: 338–343
89. Arnold A 1994 Molecular mechanisms of parathyroid neoplasia. Endocrinol Metab Clin North Am 23: 93–107
90. Arnold A, Motokura T, Bloom T et al. 1992 PRAD1 (cyclin D1): a parathyroid neoplasia gene on 11q13. Henry Ford Hosp Med J 40: 177–180
91. Vasef M A, Brynes R K, Sturm M et al. 1999 Expression of cyclin D1 in parathyroid carcinomas, adenomas, and hyperplasias: a paraffin immunohistochemical study. Mod Pathol 12: 412–416
92. Heppner C, Kester M B, Agarwal S K et al. 1997 Somatic mutation of the MEN1 gene in parathyroid tumours. Nat Genet 16: 375–378
93. Shan L, Nakamura Y, Nakamura M et al. 1998 Somatic mutations of multiple endocrine neoplasia type 1 gene in the sporadic endocrine tumors. Lab Invest 78: 471–475
94. Kimura T, Yoshimoto K, Tanaka C et al. 1996 Obvious mRNA and protein expression but absence of mutations of the RET proto-oncogene in parathyroid tumors. Eur J Endocrinol 134: 314–319
95. Komminoth P, Roth J, Muletta-Feurer S et al. 1996 RET proto-oncogene point mutations in sporadic neuroendocrine tumors. J Clin Endocrinol Metab 81: 2041–2046
96. Pausova Z, Soliman E, Amizuka N et al. 1996 Role of the RET proto-oncogene in sporadic hyperparathyroidism and in hyperparathyroidism of multiple endocrine neoplasia type 2. J Clin Endocrinol Metab 81: 2711–2718
97. Padberg B C, Schroder S, Jochum W et al. 1995 Absence of RET proto-oncogene point mutations in sporadic hyperplastic and neoplastic lesions of the parathyroid gland. Am J Pathol 147: 1600–1607

98. Williams G H, Rooney S, Carss A et al. 1996 Analysis of the RET proto-oncogene in sporadic parathyroid adenomas. J Pathol 180: 138–141
99. Palanisamy N, Imanishi Y, Rao P H et al. 1998 Novel chromosomal abnormalities identified by comparative genomic hybridization in parathyroid adenomas. J Clin Endocrinol Metab 83: 1766–770
100. Agarwal S K, Schrock E, Kester M B et al. 1998 Comparative genomic hybridization analysis of human parathyroid tumors. Cancer Genet Cytogenet 106: 30–36
101. Aldinger K A, Hickey R C, Ibanez M L et al. 1982 Parathyroid carcinoma: a clinical study of seven cases of functioning and two cases of nonfunctioning parathyroid cancer. Cancer 49: 388–397
102. Shortell C K, Andrus C H, Phillips C E Jr et al. 1991 Carcinoma of the parathyroid gland: a 30-year experience. Surgery 110: 704–708
103. Wynne A G, van Heerden J, Carney J A et al. 1992 Parathyroid carcinoma: clinical and pathologic features in 43 patients. Medicine (Baltimore) 71: 197–205
104. Park S T, Condemi G, Shakir K M et al. 1998 Parathyroid carcinoma: report of three cases and review of the literature. Mil Med 163: 246–249
105. Chow E, Tsang R W, Brierley J D et al. 1998 Parathyroid carcinoma – the Princess Margaret Hospital experience. Int J Radiat Oncol Biol Phys 41: 569–572
106. Cohn K, Silverman M, Corrado J et al. 1985 Parathyroid carcinoma: the Lahey Clinic experience. Surgery 98: 1095–1100
107. Cordeiro A C, Montenegro F L, Kulcsar M A et al. 1998 Parathyroid carcinoma. Am J Surg 175: 52–55
108. McPheeters G O, Bender C A 1985 Parathyroid carcinoma: a case report and review. Hawaii Med J 44: 104–108
109. Shane E 1997 Parathyroid carcinoma. Curr Ther Endocrinol Metab 6: 565–568
110. Vetto J T, Brennan M F, Woodruff J et al. 1993 Parathyroid carcinoma: diagnosis and clinical history. Surgery 114: 882–892
111. Vazquez-Quintana E 1997 Parathyroid carcinoma: diagnosis and management. Am Surg 63: 954–957
112. Wang C A, Gaz R D 1985 Natural history of parathyroid carcinoma. Diagnosis, treatment, and results. Am J Surg 149: 522–527
113. Robert J H, Trombetti A, Garcia A et al. 2005 Primary hyperparathyroidism: can parathyroid carcinoma be anticipated on clinical and biochemical grounds? Report of nine cases and review of the literature. Ann Surg Oncol 12: 526–532
114. Kleinpeter K P, Lovato J F, Clark P B et al. 2005 Is parathyroid carcinoma indeed a lethal disease? Ann Surg Oncol 12: 260–266
115. DeLellis R A 2005 Parathyroid carcinoma: an overview. Adv Anat Pathol 12: 53–61
116. Obara T, Fujimoto Y, Yamaguchi K et al. 1985 Parathyroid carcinoma of the oxyphil cell type. A report of two cases, light and electron microscopic study. Cancer 55: 1482–1489
117. Vainas I G, Tsilikas C, Grecu A et al. 1997 Metastatic parathyroid carcinoma (mPCa): natural history and treatment of a case. J Exp Clin Cancer Res 16: 429–432
118. Jenkins P J, Satta M A, Simmgen M et al. 1997 Metastatic parathyroid carcinoma in the MEN2A syndrome. Clin Endocrinol (Oxf) 47: 747–751
119. Fujimoto Y, Obara T, Ito Y et al. 1984 Surgical treatment of ten cases of parathyroid carcinoma: importance of an initial en bloc tumor resection. World J Surg 8: 392–400
120. Obara T, Okamoto T, Kanbe M et al. 1997 Functioning parathyroid carcinoma: clinicopathologic features and rational treatment. Semin Surg Oncol 13: 134–141
121. Wiseman S M, Rigual N R, Hicks W L Jr et al. 2004 Parathyroid carcinoma: a multicenter review of clinicopathologic features and treatment outcomes. Ear Nose Throat J 83: 491–494
122. Hundahl S A, Fleming I D, Fremgen A M et al. 1999 Two hundred eighty-six cases of parathyroid carcinoma treated in the US. between 1985–1995: a National Cancer Data Base Report. The American College of Surgeons Commission on Cancer and the American Cancer Society. Cancer 86: 538–544
123. Busaidy N L, Jimenez C, Habra M A et al. 2004 Parathyroid carcinoma: a 22-year experience. Head Neck 26: 716–726
124. Anderson B J, Samaan N A, Vassilopoulou-Sellin R et al. 1983 Parathyroid carcinoma: features and difficulties in diagnosis and management. Surgery 94: 906–915
125. Stevenson H U 1950 Malignant tumours of the parathyroid gland: a review of the literature with report of a case. Arch Surg 60: 247–266
126. Munson N D, Foote R L, Northcutt R C et al. 2003 Parathyroid carcinoma: is there a role for adjuvant radiation therapy? Cancer 98: 2378–2384
127. Collins M T, Skarulis M C, Bilezikian J P et al. 1998 Treatment of hypercalcemia secondary to parathyroid carcinoma with a novel calcimimetic agent. J Clin Endocrinol Metab 83: 1083–1088
128. Sandelin K, Thompson N W, Bondeson L 1991 Metastatic parathyroid carcinoma: dilemmas in management. Surgery 110: 978–986
129. Bradwell A R, Harvey T C 1999 Control of hypercalcaemia of parathyroid carcinoma by immunisation. Lancet 353: 370–373
130. Schott M, Feldkamp J, Schattenberg D et al. 1999 Dendritic cell immunotherapy in disseminated parathyroid carcinoma (letter). Lancet 353: 1188–1189
131. Betea D, Bradwell A R, Harvey T C et al. 2004 Hormonal and biochemical normalization and tumor shrinkage induced by anti-parathyroid hormone immunotherapy in a patient with metastatic parathyroid carcinoma. J Clin Endocrinol Metab 89: 3413–3420
132. Bondeson L, Sandelin K, Grimelius L 1993 Histopathological variables and DNA cytometry in parathyroid carcinoma. Am J Surg Pathol 17: 820–829
133. Nasser G, Loberant N, Salameh A et al. 1995 Oxyphil cell carcinoma of the parathyroid: a rare cause of hyperparathyroidism. Clin Oncol 7: 323–324
134. Erickson L A, Jin L, Papotti M et al. 2002 Oxyphil parathyroid carcinomas: a clinicopathologic and immunohistochemical study of 10 cases. Am J Surg Pathol 26: 344–349
135. Chan J K, Tsang W Y 1995 Endocrine malignancies that may mimic benign lesions. Semin Diagn Pathol 12: 45–63
136. Chaitin B A, Goldman R L 1981 Mitotic activity in benign parathyroid disease (letter). Am J Clin Pathol 76: 363–364
137. Snover D C, Foucar K 1981 Mitotic activity in benign parathyroid disease. Am J Clin Pathol 75: 345–347
138. Vargas M P, Vargas H I, Kleiner D E et al. 1997 The role of prognostic markers (MiB-1, RB, and bcl-2) in the diagnosis of parathyroid tumors. Mod Pathol 10: 12–17
139. Abbona G C, Papotti M, Gasparri G et al. 1995 Proliferative activity in parathyroid tumors as detected by Ki-67 immunostaining. Hum Pathol 26: 135–138
140. Erickson L A, Jin L, Wollan P et al. 1999 Parathyroid hyperplasia, adenomas, and carcinomas: differential expression of p27/KipI protein. Am J Surg Pathol 23: 288–295
141. Lloyd R V, Carney J A, Ferreiro J A et al. 1995 Immunohistochemical analysis of the cell cycle-associated antigens Ki-67 and retinoblastoma protein in parathyroid carcinomas and adenomas. Endocr Pathol 6: 279–287
142. DeLellis R A 1997 Proliferation markers in neuroendocrine tumors: useful or useless? A critical reappraisal. Verh Dtsch Ges Pathol 81: 53–61
143. Bergero N, De Pompa R, Sacerdote C et al. 2005 Galectin-3 expression in parathyroid carcinoma: immunohistochemical study of 26 cases. Hum Pathol 36: 908–914
144. Shattuck T M, Valimaki S, Obara T et al. 2003 Somatic and germ-line mutations of the HRPT2 gene in sporadic parathyroid carcinoma. N Engl J Med 349: 1722–1729
145. Howell V M, Haven C J, Kahnoski K et al. 2003 HRPT2 mutations are associated with malignancy in sporadic parathyroid tumours. J Med Genet 40: 657–663
146. Woodard G E, Lin L, Zhang J H et al. 2005 Parafibromin, product of the hyperparathyroidism-jaw tumor syndrome gene HRPT2, regulates cyclin D1/PRAD1 expression. Oncogene 24: 1272–1276
147. Tan M H, Morrison C, Wang P et al. 2004 Loss of parafibromin immunoreactivity is a distinguishing feature of parathyroid carcinoma. Clin Cancer Res 10: 6629–6637
148. Cryns V L, Thor A, Xu H J et al. 1994 Loss of the retinoblastoma tumor-suppressor gene in parathyroid carcinoma. N Engl J Med 330: 757–761
149. Cetani F, Pardi E, Viacava P et al. 2004 A reappraisal of the Rb1 gene abnormalities in the diagnosis of parathyroid cancer. Clin Endocrinol (Oxf) 60: 99–106
150. Cryns V L, Rubio M P, Thor A D et al. 1994 p53 abnormalities in human parathyroid carcinoma. J Clin Endocrinol Metab 78: 1320–1324
151. Hunt J L, Carty S E, Yim J H et al. 2005 Allelic loss in parathyroid neoplasia can help characterize malignancy. Am J Surg Pathol 29: 1049–1055
152. Erickson L A, Jalal S M, Harwood A et al. 2004 Analysis of parathyroid neoplasms by interphase fluorescence in situ hybridization. Am J Surg Pathol 28: 578–584
153. Stojadinovic A, Hoos A, Nissan A et al. 2003 Parathyroid neoplasms: clinical, histopathological, and tissue microarray-based molecular analysis. Hum Pathol 34: 54–64
154. Levin K E, Galante M, Clark O H 1987 Parathyroid carcinoma versus parathyroid adenoma in patients with profound hypercalcemia. Surgery 101: 649–660
155. Levin K E, Chew K L, Ljung B M et al. 1988 Deoxyribonucleic acid cytometry helps identify parathyroid carcinomas. J Clin Endocrinol Metab 67: 779–784
156. Alpers C E, Clark O H 1989 Atypical spindle cell pattern (? carcinoma) arising in a parathyroid adenoma. Surg Pathol 2: 157–161
157. McCluggage W G, Cameron C H, Brooker D et al. 1996 Paraganglioma: an unusual tumour of the parathyroid gland. J Laryngol Otol 110: 196–199
158. Chetty R 1995 Branchial cysts in thyroid and parathyroid glands (letter). Hum Pathol 26: 930
159. Rangnekar N, Bailer W J, Ghani A et al. 1996 Parathyroid cysts. Report of four cases and review of the literature. Int Surg 81: 412–414
160. Koelmeyer T D 1977 Generalised amyloidosis with involvement of the parathyroids: case report. NZ Med J 85: 372–373
161. LiVolsi V A, Hamilton R 1994 Intraoperative assessment of parathyroid gland pathology. A common view from the surgeon and the pathologist. Am J Clin Pathol 102: 365–373
162. Anton R C, Wheeler T M 2005 Frozen section of thyroid and parathyroid specimens. Arch Pathol Lab Med 129: 1575–1584
163. Wong N A, Mihai R, Sheffield E A et al. 2000 Imprint cytology of parathyroid tissue in relation to other tissues of the neck and mediastinum. Acta Cytol 44: 109–113
164. Yao D X, Hoda S A, Yin D Y et al. 2003 Interpretative problems and preparative technique influence reliability of intraoperative parathyroid touch imprints. Arch Pathol Lab Med 127: 64–67
165. Shidham V B, Rao R N, Chavan A et al. 2003 Reliability of intraoperative parathyroid touch imprints. Arch Pathol Lab Med 127: 1082–1083
166. Dekker A, Watson C G, Barnes E L 1979 The pathologic assessment of primary hyperparathyroidism and its impact on therapy, a prospective evaluation of 50 cases with oil-red-O stain. Ann Surg 190: 671–675

167. Ljungberg O, Tibblin S 1979 Perioperative fat staining of frozen sections in primary hyperparathyroidism. Am J Pathol 95: 633–641
168. Roth S I, Gallagher M J 1976 The rapid identification of "normal" parathyroid glands by the presence of intracellular fat. Am J Pathol 84: 521–528
169. Sasano H, Geelhoed G W, Silverberg S G 1988 Intraoperative cytologic evaluation of lipid in the diagnosis of parathyroid adenoma. Am J Surg Pathol 12: 282–286
170. Dufour D R, Durkowski C 1982 Sudan IV stain. Its limitations in evaluating parathyroid functional status. Arch Pathol Lab Med 106: 224–227
171. Kasdon E J, Rosen S, Cohen R B et al. 1981 Surgical pathology of hyperparathyroidism. Usefulness of fat stain and problems in interpretation. Am J Surg Pathol 5: 381–384
172. King D T, Hirose F M 1979 Chief cell intracytoplasmic fat used to evaluate parathyroid disease by frozen section. Arch Pathol Lab Med 103: 609–612
173. Clarke M R, Hoover W W, Carty S E et al 1996 Atypical fat staining patterns in hyperparathyroidism. Int J Surg Pathol 3: 163–168
174. Black W C, Utley J R 1968 The differential diagnosis of parathyroid adenoma and chief cell hyperplasia. Am J Pathol 49: 761–775
175. Kay S 1976 The abnormal parathyroid. Hum Pathol 7: 127–138
176. Black W C, Haff R C 1970 The surgical pathology of parathyroid chief cell hyperplasia. Am J Clin Pathol 53: 565–579
177. Westra W H, Pritchett D D, Udelsman R 1998 Intraoperative confirmation of parathyroid tissue during parathyroid exploration: a retrospective evaluation of the frozen section. Am J Surg Pathol 22: 538–544
178. Baloch Z W, LiVolsi V A 2002 Intraoperative assessment of thyroid and parathyroid lesions. Semin Diagn Pathol 19: 219–226
179. Boggs J E, Irvin G L 3rd, Molinari A S et al. 1996 Intraoperative parathyroid hormone monitoring as an adjunct to parathyroidectomy. Surgery 120: 954–958
180. Chen H, Pruhs Z, Starling J R et al. 2005 Intraoperative parathyroid hormone testing improves cure rates in patients undergoing minimally invasive parathyroidectomy. Surgery 138: 583–587; 587–590
181. Jortay A M, Verougstraete G, Wittersheim E et al. 2004 Intraoperative measurement of parathyroid hormone in minimally invasive surgery for parathyroid adenoma. Acta Otorhinolaryngol Belg 58: 125–128
182. Iacobone M, Scarpa M, Lumachi F et al. 2005 Are frozen sections useful and cost-effective in the era of intraoperative qPTH assays? Surgery 138: 1159–1164
183. Guarda L A 2004 Rapid intraoperative parathyroid hormone testing with surgical pathology correlations: the "chemical frozen section". Am J Clin Pathol 122: 704–712
184. Boggs J E, Irvin G L 3rd, Carneiro DM et al. 1999 The evolution of parathyroidectomy failures. Surgery 126: 998–1002

肾上腺肿瘤
Tumors of the adrenal gland

Ernest E. Lack 著

张晓波 译　回允中 校

正常肾上腺	1099	髓脂肪瘤	1117
结节性肾上腺	1099	恶性淋巴瘤和浆细胞瘤	1117
肾上腺皮质腺瘤	1100	恶性黑色素瘤	1117
伴有男性化或女性化的肾上腺皮质肿瘤	1103	其他少见的肾上腺原发性肿瘤	1118
肾上腺皮质癌	1105	肾上腺转移性肿瘤	1118
嗜铬细胞瘤	1109		

正常肾上腺　The normal adrenal gland

肾上腺是一种由皮质和髓质两部分组成的内分泌腺体，其中每一部分都有不同的胚胎发生、结构和功能。肾上腺皮质来源于一种与体腔上皮相关的细胞，这种细胞起源于中胚层。肾上腺皮质在调解水和电解质平衡中起着重要的作用，主要通过分泌盐皮质激素，并通过糖皮质激素发挥作用，它能调节中间代谢、伤口愈合、生长发育、炎症的变化，而且也能影响免疫系统的某些方面。肾上腺皮质还是性类固醇的来源。肾上腺髓质起源于神经嵴，分泌儿茶酚胺类，主要是肾上腺素，它能调节机体对于应激和环境变化的快速适应能力。在成人，右侧肾上腺大体上是锥形的，而左侧肾上腺则较长或为新月形。单侧或两侧肾上腺的重量取决于各种因素的变化，诸如年龄、各种疾病的存在和慢性程度，最重要的是在称重之前是否尽量仔细去除与其相连的结缔组织和脂肪[1]。在新生儿，由于胎儿肾上腺皮质（或暂时）退化，最初几周肾上腺重量明显减轻。一项研究显示，足月新生儿两侧肾上腺平均总的重量在6g到7g之间，而在9~14周之间已减轻到2g左右[1]。在成人，手术切除的单侧肾上腺的平均重量大约是4g（1 SD=0.8g），肾上腺髓质大约占整个肾上腺重量的10%[1]。

在成人，正常肾上腺皮质的厚度约为2 mm，组织学检查常常显示不同的带状分布。球状带较薄，通常在被膜下呈不连续性分布，在腺体的某些部位占皮质厚度的5%~10%。束状带约占皮质厚度的70%，正常情况下由放射状排列的细胞柱或细胞条索组成，细胞胞浆富于脂质、淡染。皮质其余部分是由内部的网状带组成的。肾上腺髓质主要集中在伴有嗜铬细胞的肾上腺的头部和体部，排列成散在的细胞巢或相互吻合的条索[1]。肾上腺脉管系统的解剖学也是很独特的，肾上腺中心静脉分支的中层具有畸形排列的平滑肌，有时造成皮质或嗜铬细胞与血管腔隙并列。

结节性肾上腺
The nodular adrenal gland

在没有皮质醇增多症（hypercortisolism）临床或实验室证据的病人，也可见到一个或多个的肾上腺皮质结节[1]（图19.1）。肾上腺皮质结节的发生率随年龄而增加，并与高血压和糖尿病有关[2-4]。肾上腺结节性增大可能是应用高分辨率CT扫描时的偶然发现，并被误认为是真正的肿瘤。这些"偶发瘤"（incidentalomas）大多数被认为是腺瘤[5,6]。在类固醇的生物合成中，某些结节吸收放射性核素的前体，因此，是非高功能性而不是非功能性。根据类固醇生成酶（steroidogenic enzymes）的免疫组化分析，大多数小的非功能性的肾上腺皮质腺瘤（在无症状的病人中偶然发现）能够产生具有生物活性的类固醇，包括皮质醇（cortisol）[8]。据报告，某些临床前或亚临床Cushing综合征病人，根据基础和动态内分泌试验显示有轻微的皮质醇增多症的证据；在某些病例，肾上腺切除的主要危险是肾上腺皮质功能不全。

在垂体依赖性Cushing综合征（Cushing病）以及异位促肾上腺皮质激素（ACTH）综合征，肾上腺可能

肾上腺皮质腺瘤

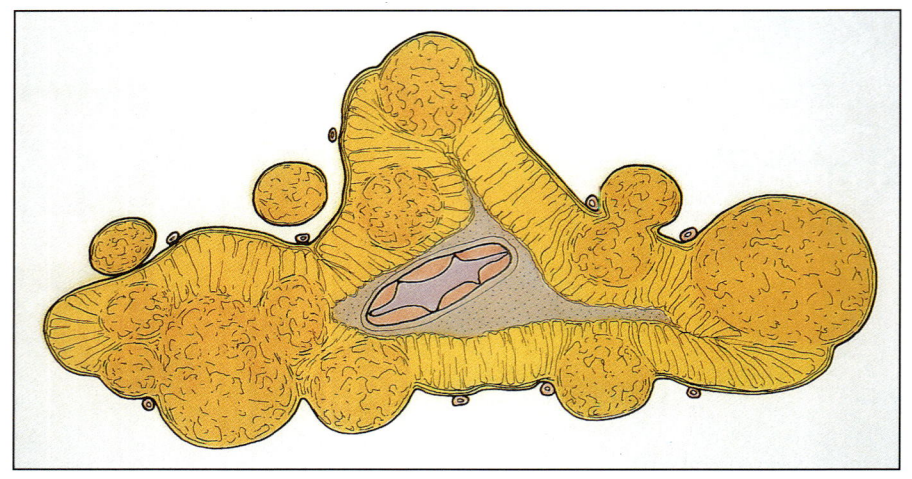

图19.1 横切面具有许多膨胀皮质结节的肾上腺的示意图；某些结节从被膜下突出形成皮质结节，与其下的皮质连续，而另外一些结节似乎与肾上腺被膜融合，或游离在邻近的结缔组织内。较大的皮质内结节可能类似于一个良性肿瘤。(Reproduced with permission from Lack E E, Travis W D, Oertel J E 1990 Adrenal cortical nodules, hyperplasia, and hyperfunction. In: Lack E E (ed) Pathology of the adrenal glands. Churchill Livingstone, New York, p75-113.)

显示有小的结节状区域，这些结节通常只有几个毫米大小。在某些Cushing病病例，肾上腺可有明显的增生，伴有巨大结节形成，这些巨大结节可能是弥漫性和微小结节状增生的后期，或者在少数情况下，表面上可能是自主性肾上腺皮质增生，它可能类似于肿瘤[1,5]。

肾上腺皮质腺瘤
Adrenal cortical adenomas

一般来说，大多数肾上腺皮质腺瘤发生在成人，女性发病率略高。儿童发生腺瘤的情况非常罕见，并且通常伴有男性化[9]。除了偶然发现的以外，这些腺瘤大部分伴有某一种类固醇激素分泌过多。

发生于Cushing综合征的腺瘤
Adenomas in Cushing's syndrome

这些肿瘤的重量通常小于50g[1,5]，横切面常有明显的界限清楚的包膜（图19.2）。肿瘤重量偶有超过100g。整个切面呈淡黄色或金黄色，或有不规则的花斑状深色色素沉着区。偶尔可见出血区，但是融合性肿瘤性坏死非常少见。仔细检查附着的肾上腺皮质或对侧面的肾上腺，可能发现皮质萎缩[10]。镜下，肿瘤常有一个相对光滑的推挤性边缘，伴有假包膜形成，这是由于压迫邻近组织或推挤肾上腺包膜引起的。肿瘤细胞胞浆淡染，富含脂质，类似于束状带的细胞（图19.3）。可以证实胞浆内有丰富的中性脂质（图19.4）。某些肿瘤细胞中可能混有具有较致密嗜酸性胞浆的细胞，类似于网状带的细胞（图19.5）；某些细胞可能含有明显的脂色素。常见的结构形态是小梁状（或短条索状）和伴有圆形细胞巢的腺泡状[1,11]。细胞核通常为空泡状，伴有小的点状核仁；偶尔细胞核小而固缩，而另外一些细胞核可能增大，并呈多形性。可能出现脂肪瘤或髓脂肪瘤改变的区域（图19.6）。超微结构检查示，细胞含有丰富的脂质和呈管状或囊泡状嵴结构的线粒体，并有明显的滑面内质网（图19.7）。

发生于原发性醛固酮增多症的腺瘤
Adenomas in primary hyperaldosteronism

这些肿瘤（"醛固酮瘤"，aldosteronomas）常小而单发，直径大多小于2～3cm[12]，1%～6%的病例肿瘤为双侧或多发性[1,11]。偶尔肿瘤非常大，重达75g或更重。在完整的腺体中，一些非常小的肿瘤可能难于发现，但横切面可见圆形或卵圆形的肿瘤，常呈亮黄色（或鲜黄色）（图19.8）。某些较大的肿瘤可见变性改变伴有出血。

组织学检查，肿瘤细胞具有腺泡状结构，或排列成短条索或小梁状（图19.9）。根据文献描述，肿瘤细胞具有四种形态学变异[13]。其中类似于束状带的淡染富含脂质的细胞最常见（图19.10）；其他细胞具有较高的核浆比例，胞浆淡染，类似于球状带细胞，或具有较致密的嗜酸性胞浆，类似于网状带细胞。介于球状带细胞和网状带细胞特征之间的"混合性"细胞也有描述。伴随

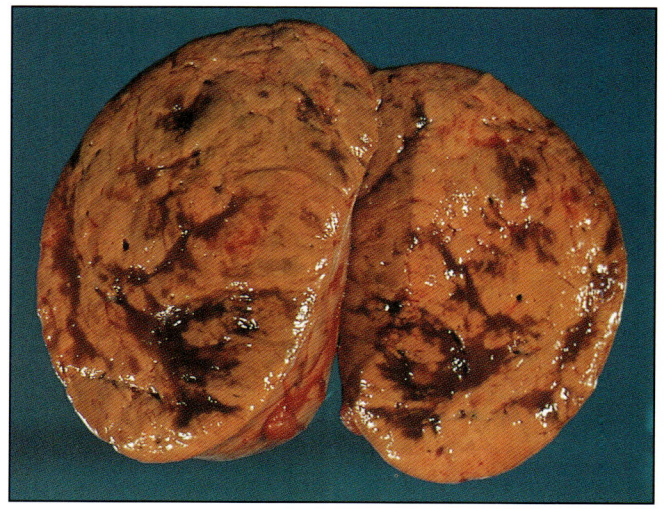

图19.2 肾上腺皮质腺瘤切面橙黄色，由于充血和出血，可见伴有色素沉着的不规则区域。

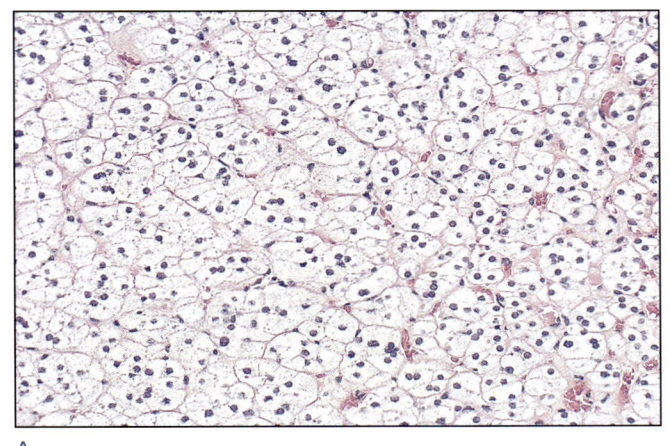
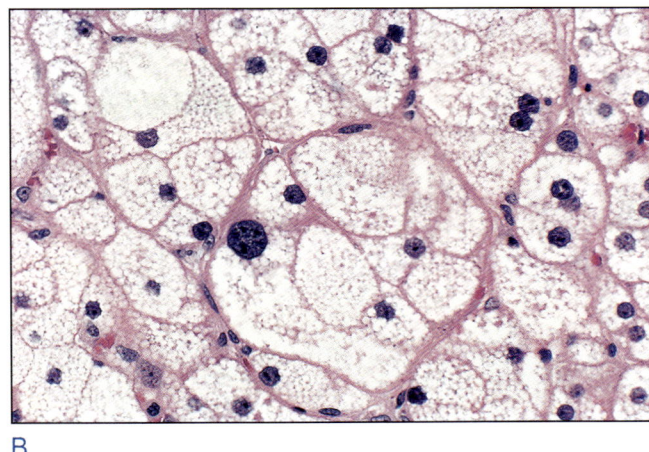

图19.3 （A）伴有Cushing综合征的肾上腺皮质腺瘤是由腺泡状成簇的富含脂质的细胞构成的，类似于束状带的细胞。大多数细胞核呈圆形，略呈空泡状，伴有小的点状核仁。（B）肾上腺皮质腺瘤含有丰富的淡染胞浆，呈细空泡状。虽然这种类型的细胞被称为"透明细胞"，但是胞浆内脂质使其呈细空泡状或网状结构。大多数细胞核含有一个小核仁。

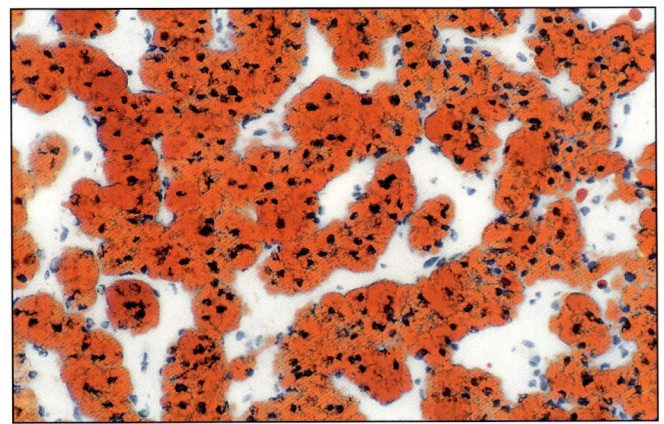

图19.4 来自Cushing综合征病人的肾上腺皮质腺瘤，具有丰富的细胞内中性脂质。油红O染色。

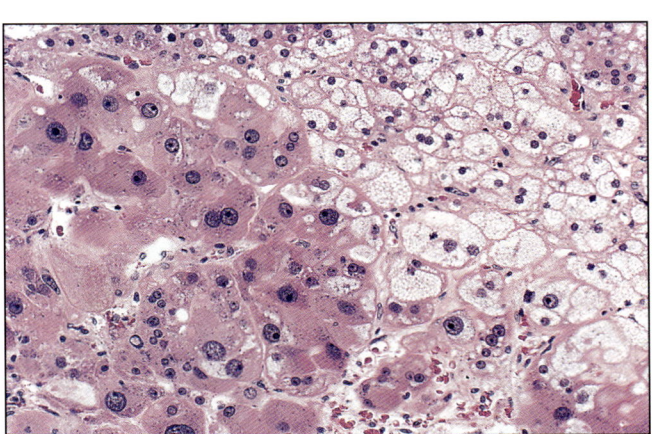

图19.5 由于脂质缺失，某些肿瘤细胞具有致密的嗜酸性胞浆，而另外一些胞浆淡染，呈空泡状。某些细胞内有稀疏的颗粒状色素沉着，可能是脂褐质。注意某些细胞核大伴有明显的核仁。

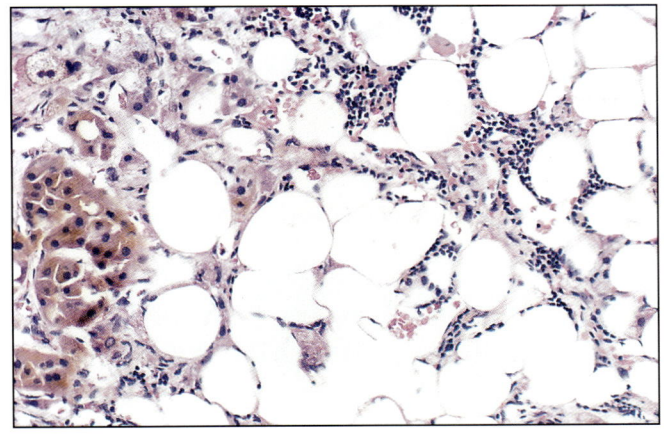

图19.6 显示髓脂肪瘤成分的肾上腺皮质腺瘤（可能是一种化生），某些肿瘤细胞有显著的脂色素沉着。

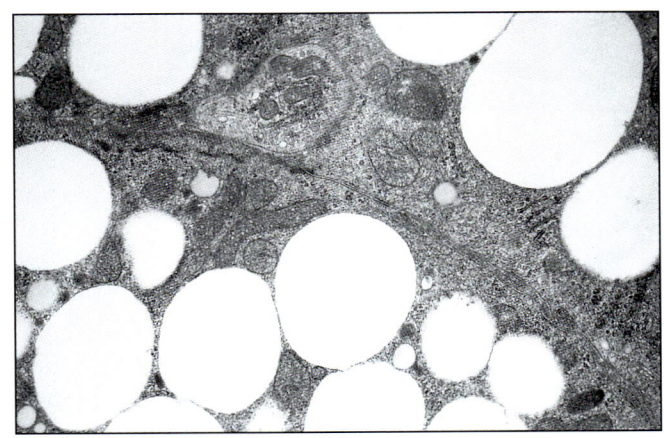

图19.7 肾上腺皮质腺瘤肿瘤细胞中有丰富的脂质，病人伴有Cushing综合征。线粒体呈卵圆形并变长，伴有明显的管泡状嵴。某些区域滑面内质网突出，伴有少量的粗面内质网。

肾上腺皮质腺瘤

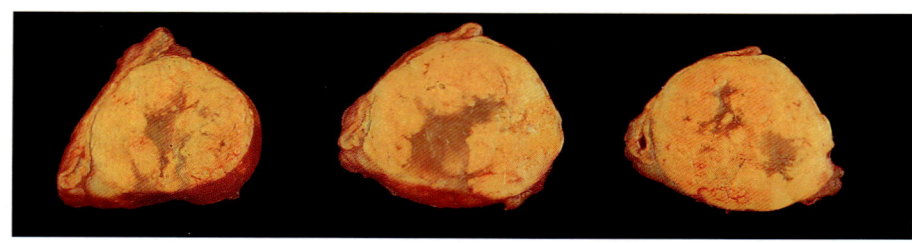

图19.8 分泌醛固酮的肾上腺皮质腺瘤（"醛固酮瘤"）切面呈橙黄色，伴有不规则的黑色区域。肿瘤的一侧边缘有明显的残余的肾上腺皮质。

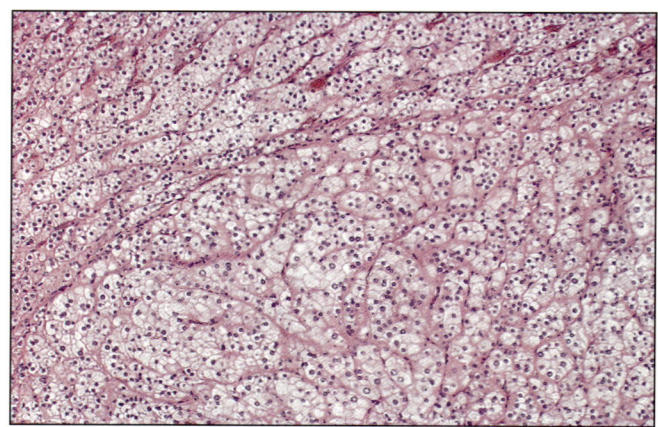

图19.9 分泌醛固酮的肾上腺皮质腺瘤的切面，视野的较下部分显示肿瘤的交界面，而肾上腺皮质轻微受压（视野的左上部分）。注意其缺乏真正的包膜。

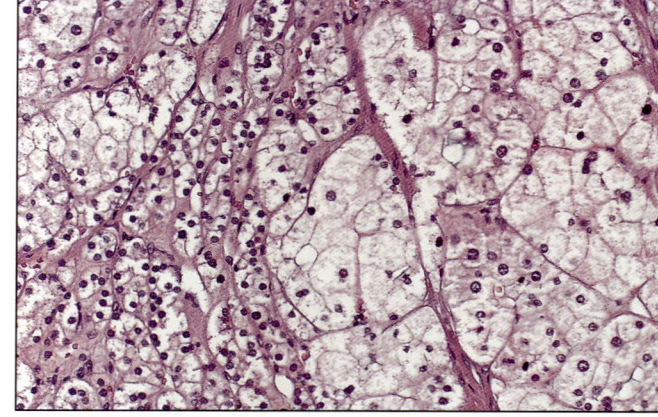

图19.10 在分泌醛固酮的肾上腺皮质腺瘤的视野内，显示其细胞类似于球状带细胞（左中）、束状带细胞（右半部分），以及介于这两种细胞之间的"混合性"细胞。细胞排列成短条索状或成簇的腺泡。

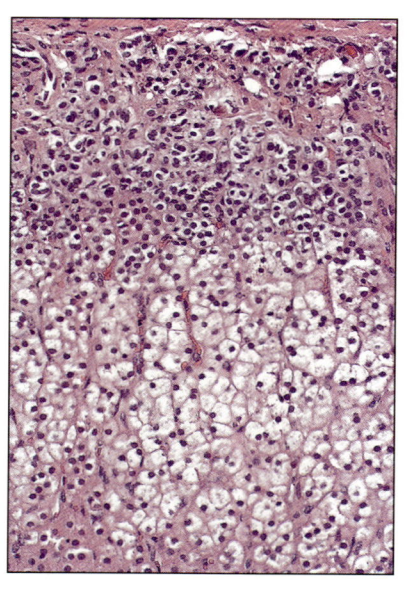

图19.11 附着于分泌醛固酮腺瘤的肾上腺皮质，显示球状带增生，其证据是被膜下球状带连续增厚。

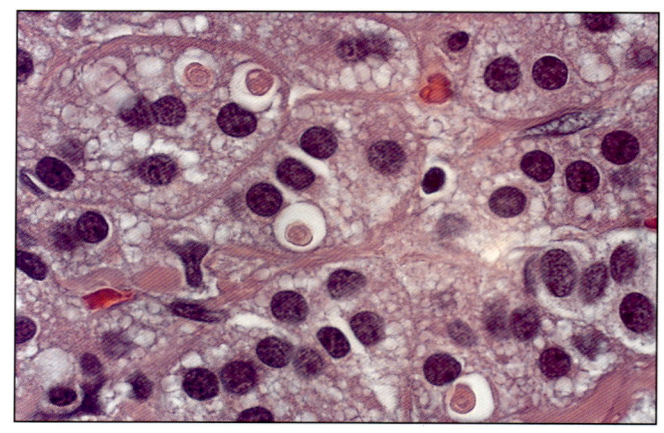

图19.12 分泌醛固酮的皮质腺瘤病人，同侧肾上腺皮质有小的嗜酸性"漩涡样"包涵体，位于某些球状带细胞的胞浆中。包涵体大小从2 mm到12 mm不等，常常类似于细胞核的大小。

的或对侧肾上腺皮质常常显示球状带的增生[1,10,14]（图19.11）。应用醛固酮拮抗剂治疗的病人可见"螺旋内酯小体"[1,15]；虽然这种包涵体在肿瘤细胞中已有描述，但在非肿瘤性球状带细胞中也是比较常见的，这种包涵体呈嗜酸性，"漩涡样（scroll-like）"，伴有周围透明空晕（图19.12）。

功能性色素沉着性（"黑色"）腺瘤
Functional pigmented ("black") adenomas

这种肿瘤非常少见，切面可见弥漫性色素沉着或呈黑色；这种肿瘤通常伴有Cushing综合征，但个别肿瘤引起原发性醛固酮增多症[1,11]。大多数肿瘤重量小于35 g，平均直径在2.5 cm左右。整个肿瘤通常有黑色素沉着（图19.13），但在某些病例色素沉着可能并不完全。

镜下，细胞具有致密的嗜酸性胞浆，伴有可与其他皮质腺瘤相比的结构特征。细胞内色素呈褐色至金褐

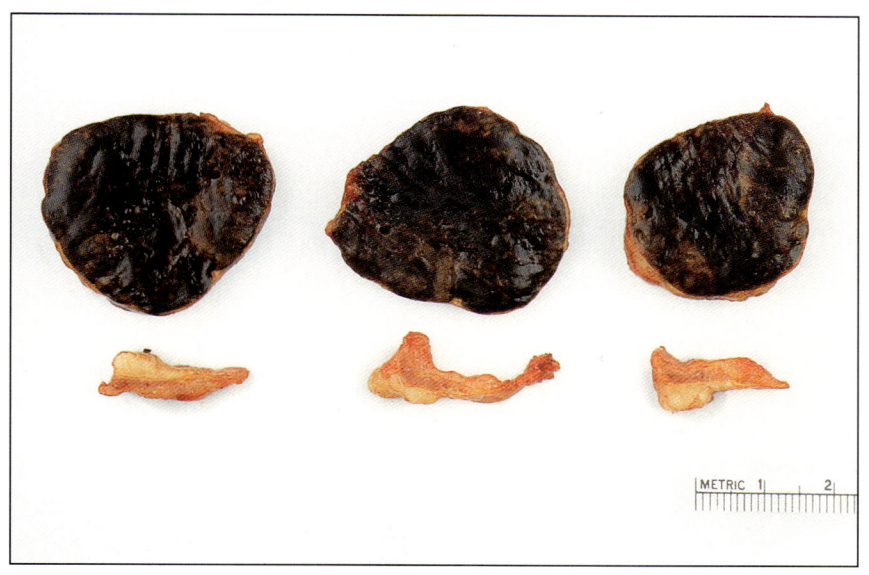

图19.13 色素沉着性("黑色")肾上腺皮质腺瘤,男性,58岁,伴有Cushing综合征。肿瘤重约30g,由于含有丰富的脂色素,整个切面呈黑色。

色,邻近核的胞浆常常没有色素沉着(图19.14)。这种色素具有脂褐质的染色特点,尽管一项研究根据色素漂白的不稳定性提示某些色素可能是神经黑色素[16]。电子显微镜检查,有数量不等的与脂褐质相关的电子致密颗粒;某些颗粒含有小的脂质包涵体(图19.15),某些颗粒可以出现界膜。没有黑色素小体或前黑色素小体。

伴有男性化或女性化的肾上腺皮质肿瘤
Adrenal cortical neoplasms associated with virilization or feminization

这些肿瘤中的某些肿瘤常常较大,其大体和显微镜下特征可能引起有关其潜在的生物学行为方面的担忧(见下文)[1,17]。女性化的肾上腺皮质肿瘤特别令人担忧,在一项52例的回顾分析中,肿瘤平均重量为1 000g(从175g到2 650g不等)[17]。肿瘤通常呈淡褐色至淡棕色,多数细胞具有致密的嗜酸性胞浆(图19.16)。然而,组织学表现是非特异性的,如果没有临床和(或)生物化学资料,人们不能可靠地预测其伴随发生的内分泌综合征。有报告肾上腺Leydig细胞腺瘤(含有Reinke类晶体)可以伴有男性化[18]以及含有Leydig细胞的分泌睾酮的肾上腺神经节瘤(ganglioneuroma)[19]。

嗜酸细胞性肾上腺皮质肿瘤
Oncocytic adrenal cortical neoplasms

这种肿瘤非常少见[20],切面通常为暗棕色至红褐色(图19.17A),由具有丰富的颗粒状嗜酸性胞浆的细胞组成(图19.17B)。在迄今为止报告的几个病例中,胞浆内脂质成分少或几乎没有,超微结构研究显示有丰富

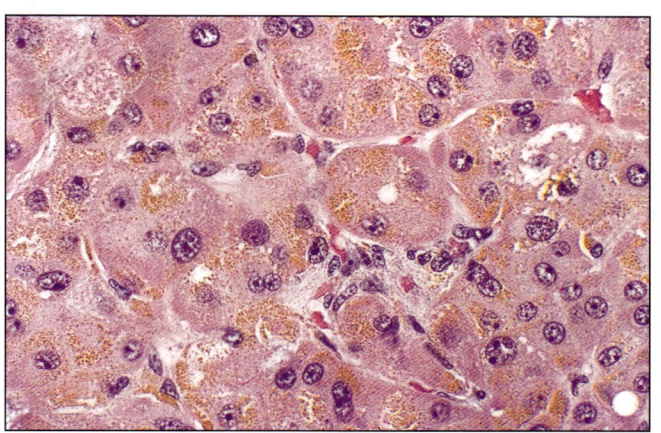

图19.14 这个"黑色"腺瘤具有腺泡状或巢状结构。单个细胞具有致密的嗜酸性胞浆,许多细胞的胞浆内有明显的颗粒状色素沉着。核呈空泡状,伴有位于中心或偏心的核仁。这个视野内个别核有"假包涵体"。

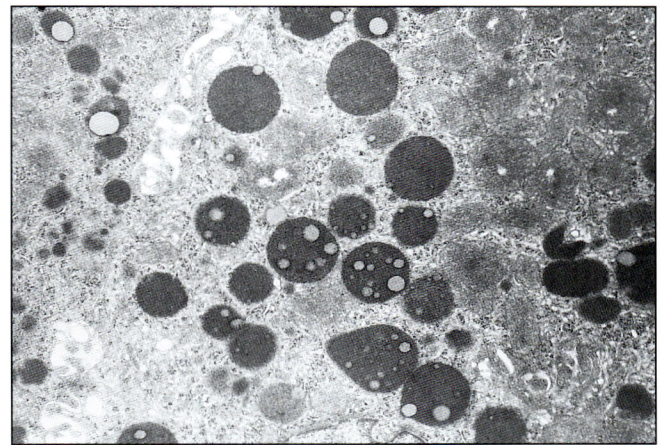

图19.15 这个"黑色"腺瘤中可见许多电子致密颗粒,某些颗粒有小的脂质包涵体。线粒体呈圆形或卵圆形,伴有不规则的管状嵴。

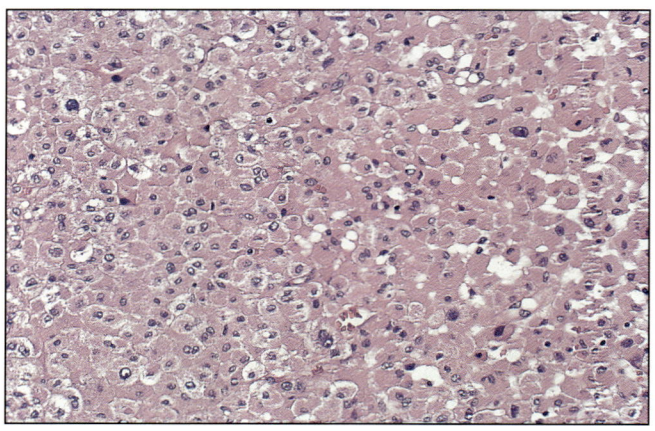

图19.16 这个男性化的肾上腺皮质肿瘤是由具有致密嗜酸性胞浆的细胞组成的，细胞弥漫排列或呈实性结构。没有诸如血管浸润或核分裂象等提示恶性的组织学特征。

表19.1	21-羟化酶缺乏：临床类型和发病率
经典型	
发病率：出生人口的1:5 000到1:15 000	
盐缺失：2/3的病例	
单纯性女性化疾病：1/3的病例	
非经典型	
发病率：占普通白色人群的0.3%	
病人在出生时表面上是正常的	
在儿童后期或青春期出现雄激素过多的征象	
隐蔽型	
无症状	

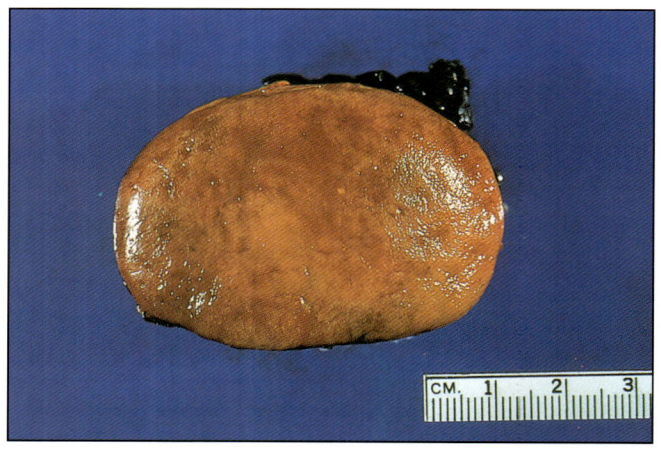

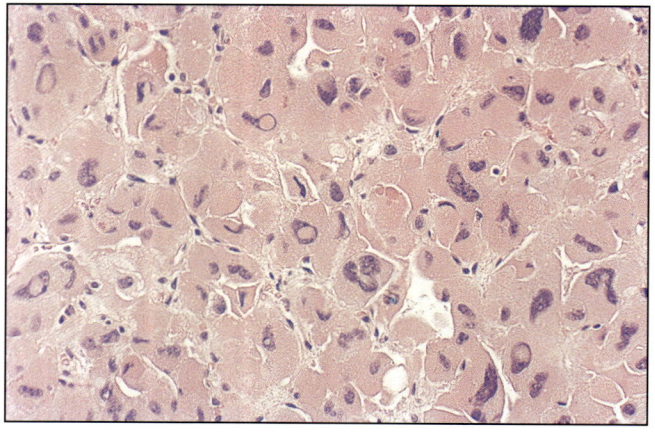

图19.17 嗜酸细胞性肾上腺皮质肿瘤。（A）肿瘤为非功能性，重70g，切面呈红褐色（Courtesy by Dr. Victor Reuter, New York City）。（B）肿瘤细胞具有丰富的颗粒状嗜酸性胞浆，核具有中度多形性，伴有"假包涵体"形成。

的线粒体[1]。某些研究认为，这些肿瘤是真正的非功能性肿瘤，因为缺乏参与类固醇生物合成的酶的表达[21]。而报告的大多数肿瘤是腺瘤（或"嗜酸细胞腺瘤"，oncocytoma），偶尔有嗜酸细胞性肾上腺皮质癌的报告[20,23]。

发生在先天性肾上腺增生的性腺肿瘤
Gonadal tumors in congenital adrenal hyperplasia

先天性肾上腺增生也称为肾上腺生殖器综合征（adrenogenital syndrome），是一种不常见的常染色体隐性遗传性疾病，它是由于缺乏参与类固醇生物合成的五种酶中的任何一种酶而引起的。90%～95%的病例是由于缺乏21-羟化酶引起的，并被分为三种类型[1,24]（表19.1）。在患有先天性肾上腺增生的儿童中，已有几例发生肾上腺皮质腺瘤和癌的报告[1,25]，虽然病因尚不清楚，但是有人提出肿瘤转化与持续性的ACTH营养刺激有关。已经注意到性腺肿瘤发生在睾丸，而最新有发生在卵巢的报告[26]；异位肾上腺皮质残余沿着女性的阔韧带分布，而在男性则沿着精索和睾丸附件分布，特别是在睾丸门[27]（图19.18）。很少报告在Nelson综合征发生肾上腺皮质型的睾丸"肿瘤"（见第17章）[28,29]。睾丸肿瘤通常为双侧性，切面常常为褐色至棕色，呈粗结节状（图19.19）。许多较小的肿瘤位于睾丸门[30]。肿瘤细胞呈结节状分布，被交织排列的结缔组织束分开（图19.20）；虽然肿瘤细胞非常类似于Leydig细胞，但是没有Reinke结晶（图19.21）。在某些记录完好的病例中，显示肿瘤是ACTH依赖性，并且具有类似于肾上腺皮质的功能[31]。迄今尚没有报告证实这些睾丸肿瘤在临床上是恶性的。

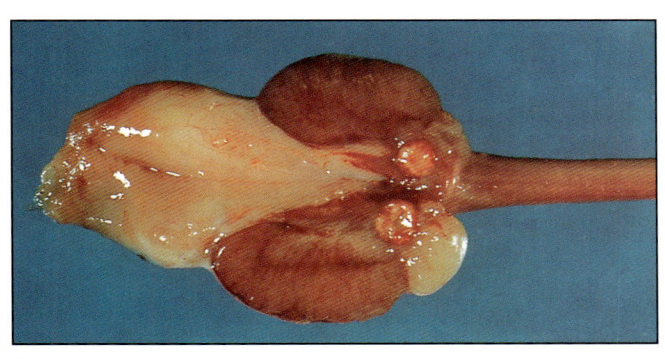
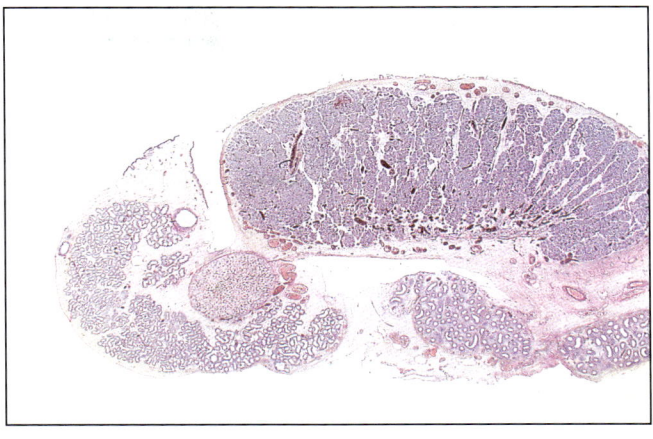

A

B

图19.18 （A）新生儿睾丸和附件剖面显示睾丸门处有界限清楚的肾上腺皮质细胞。这个儿童死于单纯疱疹，这个皮质残余和位置正常的肾上腺显示明显的坏死，含有典型的疱疹病毒核包涵体。（B）新生儿睾丸门处小的肾上腺皮质残余，邻近附睾头部，不同于图（A）所见。组织主要是由胎儿或暂定的皮质细胞组成。(Both illustrations reproduced with permission from Lack E E, Kozakewich H P W 1990 Embryology, developmental anatomy and selected aspects of non-neoplastic pathology. In: Lack E E (ed) Pathology of the adrenal glands. Churchill Livingstone, New York, p1-74.)

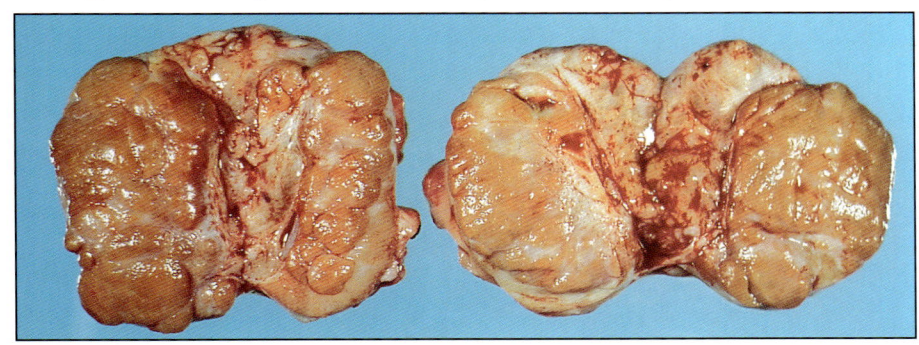

图19.19 双侧睾丸切除标本，来自21-羟化酶缺乏的25岁男性病人，十多岁时发展为双侧睾丸肿瘤。肿瘤剖面可见暗褐色隆起的结节，大部分睾丸实质被其取代。(Reproduced with permission from Lack E E, Kozakewich H P W 1990 Embryology, developmental anatomy and selected aspects of non-neoplastic pathology. In: Lack E E (ed) Pathology of the adrenal glands. Churchill Livingstone, New York, p1-74.)

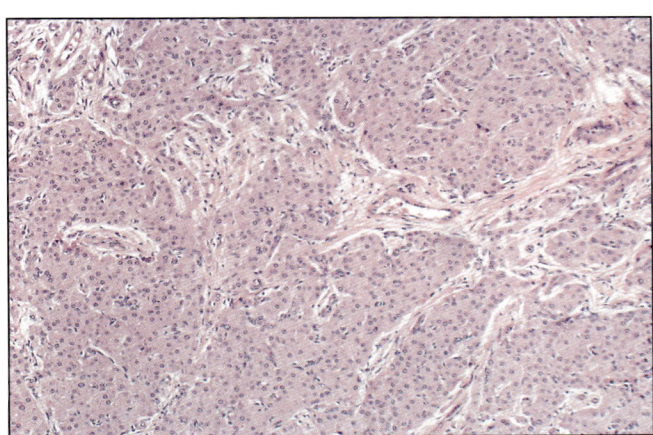
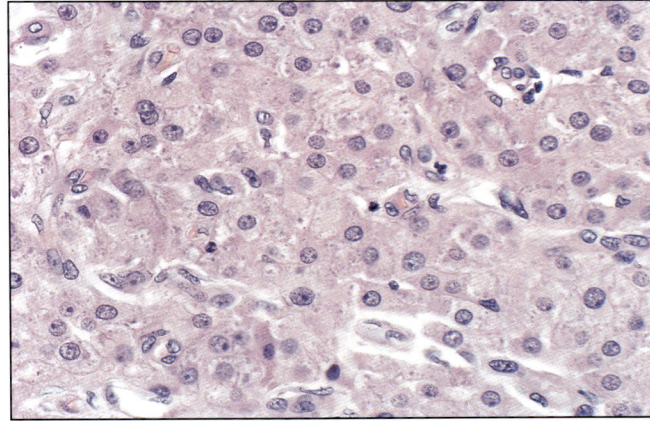

图19.20 睾丸"肿瘤"具有不规则的分叶，由交织排列的纤维血管结缔组织分开。网织纤维包绕单个或成簇的肿瘤细胞，呈现复杂的染色形态。

图19.21 睾丸"肿瘤"。肿瘤细胞具有致密的嗜酸性胞浆，核呈空泡状，核仁小点状。注意某些细胞含有少量颗粒状棕色色素，可能是脂褐素。没有发现Reinke晶体。

肾上腺皮质癌
Adrenal cortical carcinoma

肾上腺皮质癌是一种罕见的肿瘤（估计终生发病率为每百万人2例），通常累及40～70岁的年龄较大的个体，但也可以发生在儿科年龄组[1,9,11]。多数为非功能性肿瘤。与腺瘤相比，肾上腺皮质癌通常是较大的肿瘤[32,33]，但是在少数情况下，非常小的肾上腺皮质肿瘤（例如少于40g）可能发生转移，而某些非常大的肿瘤（1400g或更大）可能没有恶性行为[1,11]。几项研究显示肿瘤的平均重量从705g（96～2460g）到1210g（160～3000g）不等[34-36]。肾上腺皮质癌通常表现为粗结节巨大的肿块，

肾上腺皮质癌

伴有坏死、出血，偶尔有囊性退变的区域（图19.22）。存活的肿瘤可能表现为黄色、橘黄色、或褐色到棕色。

镜下，典型的结构特征一般可以分为小梁状、腺泡状（或巢状）或弥漫性（实性），在任何一个肿瘤中这几种形态均可混合存在。特征性的形态是小梁状结构，呈现宽的相互吻合的细胞条索或细胞柱，其间为纤细的血管间隙（图19.23）；个别切面的某些区域可能显示游离分布的肿瘤细胞"球"。还可能见到由圆钝的细胞条索或蜿蜒排列的细胞组成的比较纤细的小梁状结构（图19.24）。黏液样结构也有描述（图19.25）。大部分黏液样肾上腺皮质肿瘤是恶性的，但是某些仍可归入腺瘤。多数细胞不含脂质，具有致密的嗜酸性；个别情况下胞浆浓缩（图19.24），而且少数肿瘤胞浆内可见透明小体（图19.26）。在一项30例儿童肾上腺皮质肿瘤的研究中，仅有3例可见透明小体（一例为肾上腺皮质腺瘤，两例为肾上腺皮质癌）[37]。应该注意的是，在某些情况下，肾上腺皮质肿瘤与嗜铬细胞瘤的鉴别诊断是非常困难的[1,38,39]。这可能是因为核磁共振成像（MRI）检查具有意

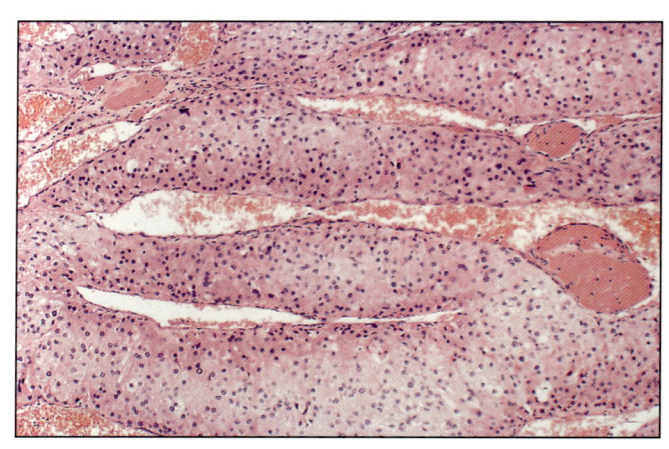

图19.23　肾上腺皮质癌。注意宽的相互吻合的小梁状结构，伴有纤细的裂隙样血管腔。单独根据这种形态要作出绝对良性的诊断，病理医师往往犹豫不定。

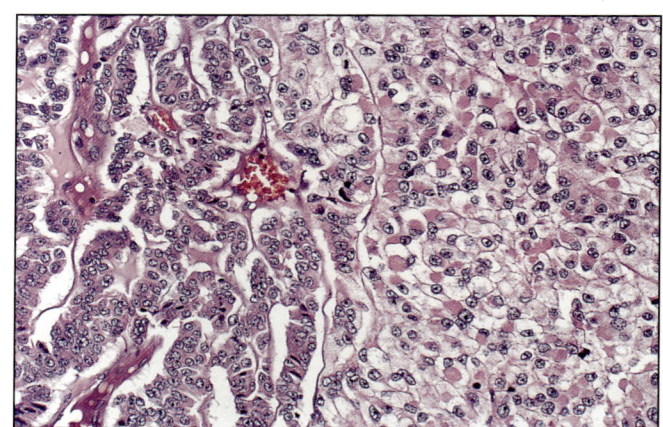

图19.24　肾上腺皮质癌。图的左侧显示蜿蜒的带状结构，细胞具有致密的嗜酸性胞浆；图的右侧具有比较弥漫或实性的结构，胞浆凝聚类似于透明小体。

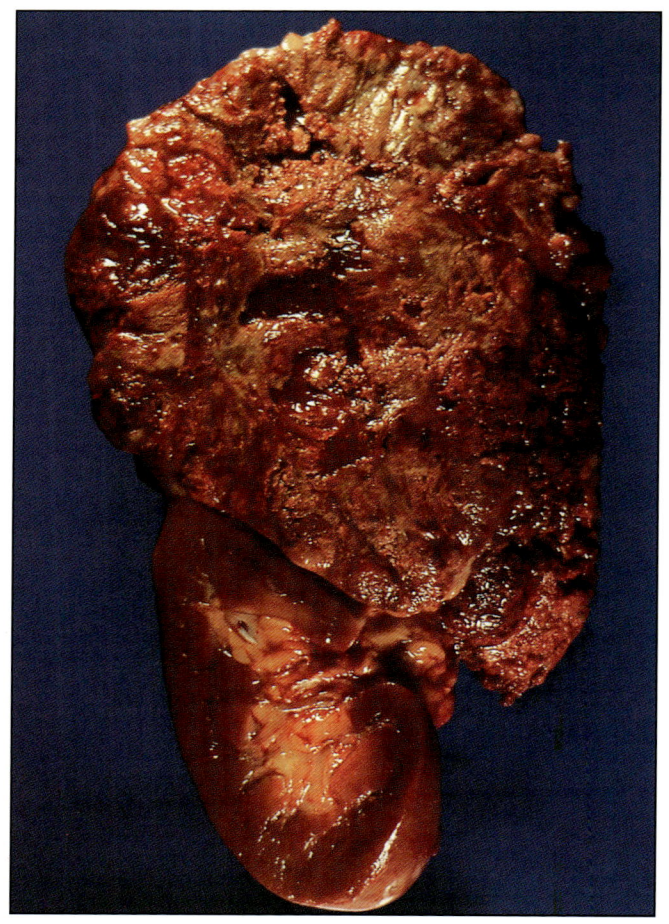

图19.22　肾上腺皮质癌。57岁女性病人的根治性肾切除标本。病人有巨大的肾上腺皮质癌，显示广泛坏死。没有皮质功能障碍的体征和症状。有广泛的肝转移，病人于9个月内死于广泛转移。

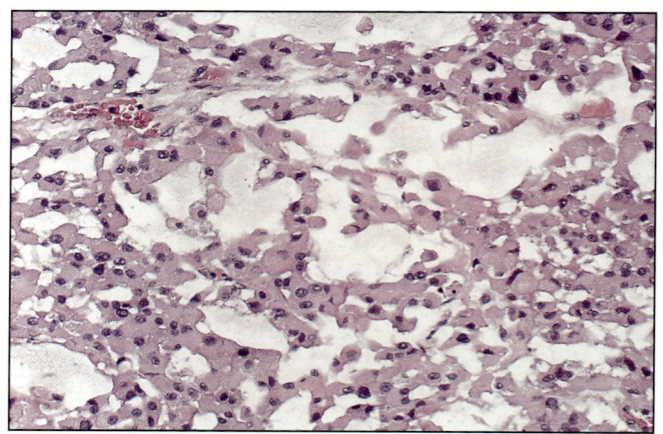

图19.25　肾上腺皮质癌。本例可见黏液样结构。不规则的条索状排列的肿瘤细胞被淡染的黏液样间质分开，这种形态有点类似于脊索瘤。

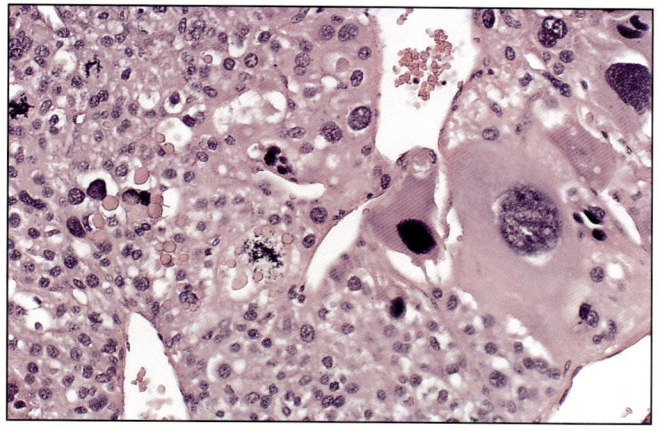

图19.26 肾上腺皮质癌显示明显的核多形性，核深染以及几个核分裂象，有些为非典型性核分裂象。注意这些肿瘤的少数部分还可见到胞浆内透明小体。

表19.2	应用统计学方法分析恶性肾上腺皮质肿瘤的组织学标准
组织学标准	出现转移的最大可能性
宽的纤维带	p<0.0001
弥漫性生长方式	p<0.001
血管浸润	p<0.001
广泛肿瘤坏死	p<0.0001
核分裂象>10个/100HPF	p<0.02
细胞多形性	p<0.001
包膜浸润	p<0.03

From Hough A J, Hallifield J W, Page D L et al. 1979 Prognostic factors in adrenal cortical tumors. A mathematical analysis of clinical and morphologic data. Am J Clin Pathol 72:390-399.
©1979 American Society of Clinical Pathologists. Reprinted with permission.

想不到的影像特征，呈器官样或巢状生长方式，致密的缺乏脂质的胞浆，胞浆内存在透明小体，以及对神经内分泌标记物呈阳性免疫染色，例如神经元特异性烯醇化酶（NSE）和突触素（Synaptophysin）（图19.27A）。在罕见的情况下，由于儿茶酚胺分泌增加，有报告肾上腺皮质肿瘤在临床上酷似嗜铬细胞瘤[40]。

明确诊断恶性肾上腺皮质肿瘤可能是困难的。已经建立的最好的标准列在表19.2和表19.3中。在某些肾上腺皮质癌中，核多形性可能是一种显著的特征（图19.26），但仅有这种表现并不能可靠地预示临床行为。核分裂象可能明显，包括非典型性核分裂象[41-43]。核分裂计数已被用于区分低级别（≤20/50 HPF）和高级别（>20/50 HPF）肾上腺皮质癌，后者中位生存率较短（图19.27B）[43]。肿瘤坏死可能是一种突出的特征，可以是大片融合性坏死，孤立的存活细胞分布在血管周围。可能有小灶状的钙化，或者在宽的纤维组织带中，或者在坏死区内[1,11,37]。与恶性相关的另外一个特征是血管浸润[1,37,41,42,44]，常常表现为血管腔内有显著的疏松的肿瘤细胞栓子（图19.28）。真正的包膜浸润是微妙的，显微镜下难以辨认，包膜浸润本身对于确定肿瘤是良性还是恶性的价值相对较小。肾上腺基底以外区域的局部浸润和（或）侵犯到邻近器官或组织是更加可靠的恶性指征。

肾上腺皮质肿瘤的特征是呈现Melan-A（MART-1）[45,46]以及抑制素（inhibin）（图19.29B）和钙视网膜蛋白（calretinin）[46]免疫反应，包括良性和恶性肿瘤。某些

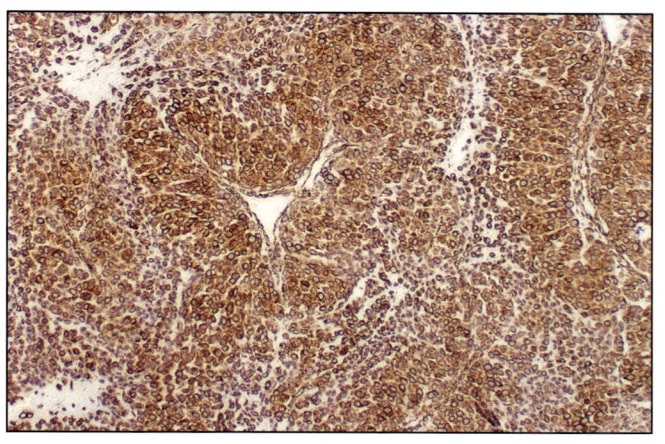

A

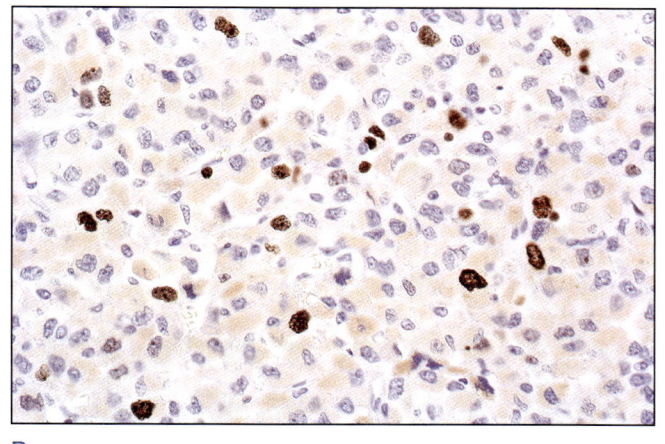

B

图19.27 （A）肾上腺皮质癌显示突触素强阳性免疫染色。肿瘤嗜铬素完全阴性（过氧化物酶-抗过氧化物酶染色）。（B）肾上腺皮质癌显示核Ki-67阳性反应。肿瘤其他部位标记指数更高。核分裂象每50个高倍视野少于20个（过氧化物酶-抗过氧化物酶染色）。

表19.3	转移性和复发性肾上腺皮质肿瘤的组织学特征
18例转移性或复发性肿瘤中见于50%以上病例的组织学特征	
高核分级（例如Ⅲ级或Ⅳ级）	14/18
核分裂象≥6/50 HPF	14/18
细胞成分显著（例如＞75%）	16/18
弥漫性结构	13/18
肿瘤坏死	17/18
窦样结构浸润	10/18
包膜浸润	10/18
仅见于转移性或复发性肾上腺皮质肿瘤的特征	
核分裂象≥6/50 HPF	
非典型性核分裂象	
静脉浸润	

From Weiss L M 1984 Comparative histologic study of 43 metastasizing and nonmetastasizing adrenocortical tumors. Am J Surg Pathol 8:163-169.

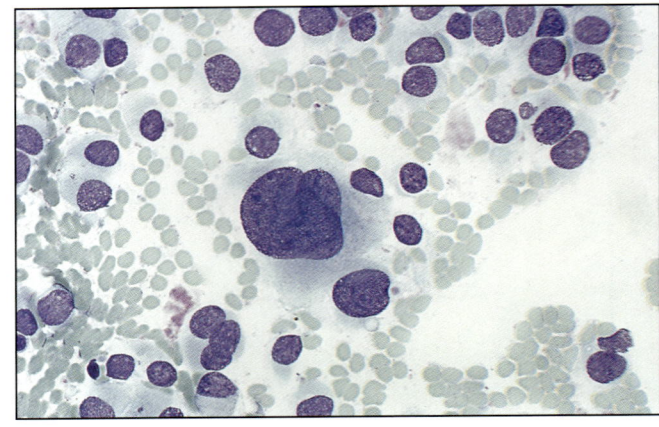

A

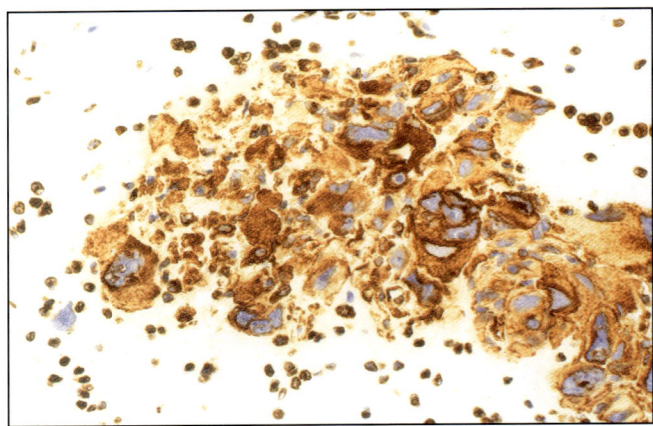

B

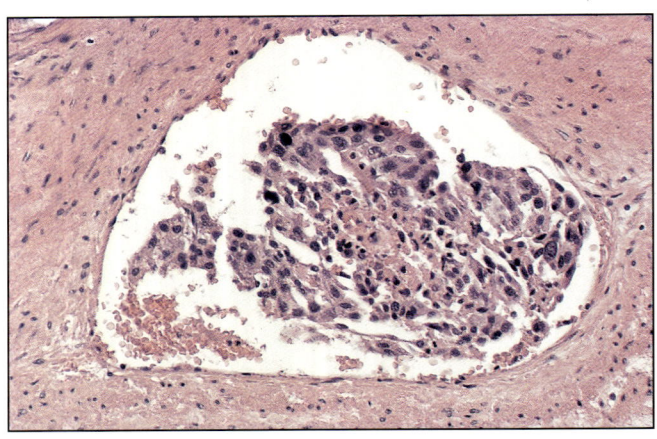

图19.28　肾上腺皮质癌。血管浸润表现为血管腔隙内疏松的肿瘤栓子。（Reproduced with permission from Lack E E, Travis W D, Oertel J E 1990 Adrenal cortical neoplasms. In: Lack E E (ed) Pathology of the adrenal glands. Churchill Livingstone, New York, p115-171.）

作者报告，常规固定的肾上腺皮质癌（和肾上腺皮质腺瘤）石蜡包埋组织波形蛋白（vimentin）阳性，而细胞角蛋白（cytokeratin）、EMA和血型组抗原（blood group antigens）阴性。应用蛋白酶消化或新鲜的冰冻组织细胞角蛋白可能阳性。[47] 另外一项研究指出，肾上腺皮质癌可能具有神经内分泌特征，表现为NSE、实触素和神经微丝蛋白（neurofilament protein）[48] 染色阳性（图19.27A）。应用mRNA原位杂交技术已经证实，肾上腺皮质癌有突触素的合成[49]。肾上腺皮质癌嗜铬素（Chromogranin）A免疫染色阴性，而嗜铬细胞瘤阳性，这可能有助于这两种肿瘤的鉴别诊断。已经显示单克隆抗体D11在鉴别肾上腺皮质肿瘤和其他肿瘤方面具有作用，但是不能鉴别良性和恶性肾上腺皮质肿瘤[50]；据报告，肾上腺皮质标记物D11核的免疫反应见于44%的

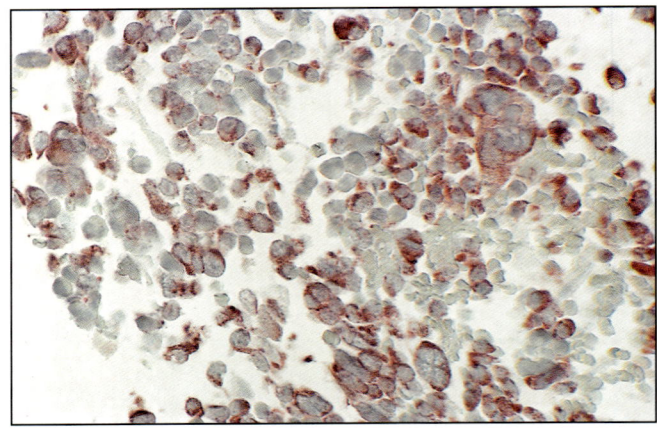

C

图19.29　肾上腺皮质癌。（A）成人巨大肾上腺肿块细针吸取，伴有多发性肺转移。注意核的显著多形性。病人有轻度高血压，可能与肿瘤产生的醛固酮有关。（B）巨大肾上腺肿块细针吸取活检，显示肿瘤细胞具有显著的核的多形性。制备的细胞块中的肿瘤细胞抑制素免疫反应强阳性。（C）制备的细胞块中肿瘤细胞波形蛋白明显阳性。上皮标记物、嗜铬素A和CEA阴性。

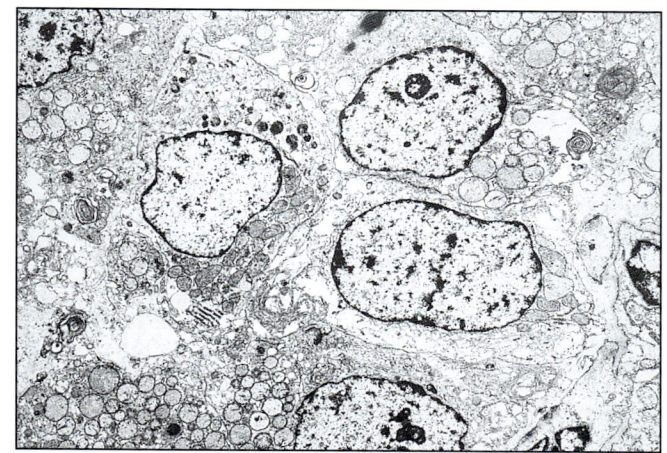

图19.30 肾上腺皮质癌。肿瘤细胞内几乎没有脂质；某些瘤细胞中线粒体丰富，伴有少数粗面内质网堆积。偶尔出现髓磷脂结构。

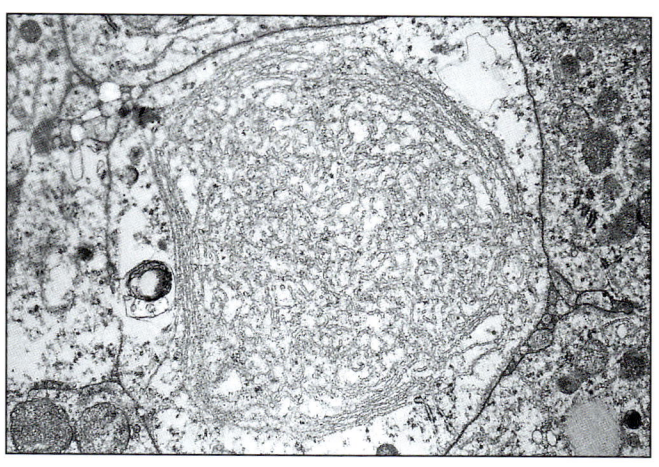

图19.31 肾上腺皮质癌。可见相互缠结的滑面内质网，伴有少数粗面内质网结构。（Reproduced with permission from Lack E E, Travis W D, Oertel J E 1990 Adrenal cortical neoplasms. In: Lack E E (ed) Pathology of the adrenal glands. Churchill Livingstone, New York, p115-171.）

肾上腺皮质癌，而且较常见于高分化肿瘤[51]。肾上腺4结合蛋白（adrenal 4 binding protein）核的免疫反应主要在参与类固醇合成的细胞有表达，可能有助于肾上腺皮质癌的鉴别诊断，因为其他类型的肿瘤（例如嗜铬细胞瘤、肾细胞癌）阴性[52]。免疫组化染色显示，核增殖相关抗原（Ki-67）肿瘤增殖指数增高（图19.27B）以及p53阳性与恶性行为密切相关[53,54]。

细针吸取可能有助于诊断，但是必须考虑其与临床和内分泌学资料的相关性以及肿瘤的大小和部位（图19.29）；因腹部CT扫描偶然发现肾上腺结节而诊断为肾上腺皮质癌的可能性极低[1]。

流式细胞技术已被用于分析DNA倍体和生物学行为的相互关系[1,55-58]。然而，已经发现临床上良性的肾上腺皮质肿瘤存在DNA非整倍体，而且一项研究没有证实DNA倍体是预示恶性的可靠指标[58]。测定DNA的价值似乎仅仅局限于那些外科可能治愈的病人，因为不管倍体如何，其预后都是不良的[56]。超微结构检查，肾上腺皮质癌胞浆内脂质非常稀少甚至缺乏（图19.30）。线粒体可能丰富，具有板样嵴或管状（空泡状）断面。可见粗面内质网和滑面内质网池（图19.31）。某些肾上腺皮质癌可见致密轴心颗粒；这些可能是原始的溶酶体[59]，但是几项研究将其解释内分泌型颗粒[40,48]。

成人肾上腺皮质癌的死亡率从70%到92%不等[1,33,34,60,61]，多数肿瘤相关性死亡发生在诊断之后的头12个月内。肝和肺是最常见的转移部位（表19.4）[1,11]。预后参数包括肿瘤分期，核分裂象率和邻近器官浸润[62]。在儿童，可能往往倾向于将肾上腺皮质肿瘤诊断为不能确定潜能或诊断为肾上腺皮质癌[63,64]。在这些较为年轻的病人中，根据年龄临床上分成两组：婴儿组和青少年组，后者的生存率明显较差[37,65]。

表19.4	美国国家卫生研究所50例肾上腺皮质癌尸检转移部位的分布				
部位	病例数	（%）	部位	病例数	（%）
肝	46	（92）	骨	9	（18）
肺	39	（78）	腹膜	8	（16）
腹膜后	24	（48）	肾	6	（12）
下腔静脉	14	（28）	横膈	6	（12）
肠浆膜	11	（22）	心	6	（12）
淋巴结			脾	4	（8）
腹部	16	（32）	胰	4	（8）
胸腔	13	（26）	甲状腺	3	（6）
			脑	2	（4）
			皮肤	1	（2）

嗜铬细胞瘤　Pheochromocytoma

嗜铬细胞瘤最常见于30～50岁的病人，而家族性病例倾向于发生在较早的年龄。多数研究指出，男女发病率大致相同[1,38,39]。大约10%的肿瘤发生在儿科年龄组[1]。超过2/3的嗜铬细胞瘤好像是功能性的，因而有症状，最常见的是引起高血压和与心动过速有关的症状。典型的散发性嗜铬细胞瘤为孤立性单中心性病变，切面可以出现包膜（图19.32），大多数肿瘤的大小从2～10cm不等；单个肿瘤重量差别很大，但是多数临床上良性的嗜铬细胞瘤重50～100g[1,39]，嗜铬细胞瘤通常为实性，质硬韧而有弹性，切面呈灰白色、淡褐色或暗红色。某些肿瘤可有出血或变性的区域（图19.33）；某些肿瘤可能有囊性变，在少数情况下仅仅可

嗜铬细胞瘤

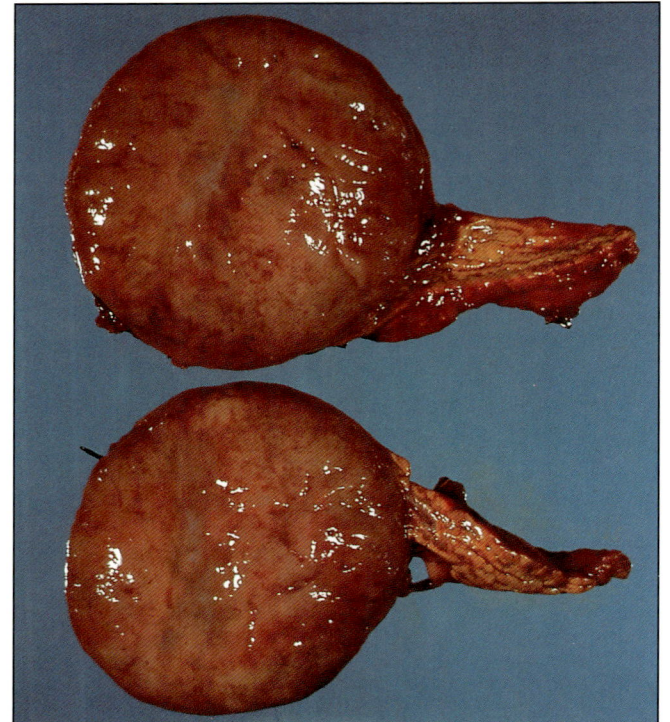

图19.32 肾上腺髓质副神经节瘤（嗜铬细胞瘤）。肿瘤界限清楚，切面褐色隆起，略呈分叶状。残余的肾上腺附着其上。(Reproduced with permission from Linnoila R I, Keiser H R, Steinberg S M, Lack E E. 1990 Histopathology of benign versus malignant sympathoadrenal paragangliomas. Clinicopathologic study of 120 cases including unusual histologic features. Hum Pathol 21: 1168-1180.)

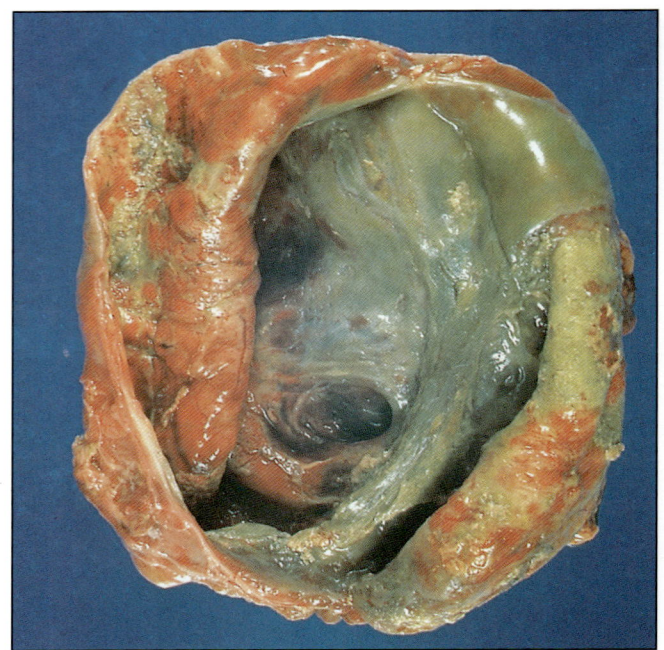

图19.34 囊性嗜铬细胞瘤。这个肾上腺肿瘤呈明显的囊性结构，囊壁取材显示残余的肿瘤和周围的棕色脂肪。(Reproduced with permission from Lack E E 1990 Adrenal medullary hyperplasia and pheochromocytoma. In: Lack E E (ed) Pathology of the adrenal glands. Churchill Linvingstone, New York, p 173-235.)

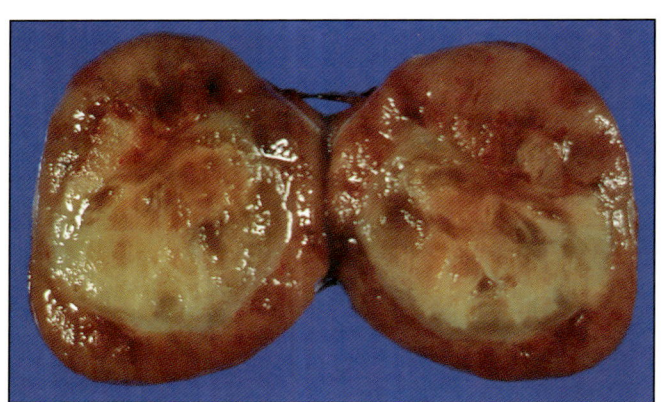

图19.33 来自儿童的嗜铬细胞瘤切除标本。肿瘤切面显示中心坏死和变性，而周围组织是存活的。临床上证实肿瘤是良性的。

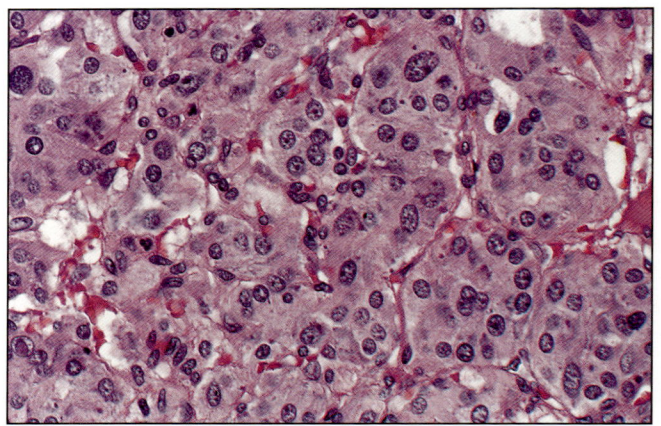

图19.35 嗜铬细胞瘤。注意器官样（腺泡状）细胞簇，这个视野的形态类似于头颈部的副神经节瘤，诸如颈动脉体肿瘤。

见薄薄的一圈肿瘤（图19.34）[1,39]。偶尔肿瘤可以钙化。

可见三种主要的组织学特征：腺泡状（或巢状）（图19.35），小梁状伴有相互吻合的细胞条索（图19.36）以及细胞呈实性排列。偶尔可见梭形细胞结构，但这很少是主要的特征[1,39]。可以出现假乳头或细胞排列在血管周围，但这通常与肿瘤处理的手工操作或血管充血有关。少数情况下，肿瘤突入肾上腺中心静脉分支腔内，可能导致明显的继发性充血和出血[1,39]。可能没有明显的包膜（除了肾上腺本身的包膜之外），肿瘤和非肿瘤性肾上腺之间仅有一个纤细的交界面（图19.36），甚至可以见到肿瘤和邻近的肾上腺皮质细胞混合[1,39]。

单个肿瘤细胞常呈多角形，伴有中等量的颗粒状嗜酸性（图19.35）或嗜双染（图19.37）的胞浆。在形态学上某些细胞可能类似于神经元或神经节细胞（图19.38）。核深染和多形性可能是突出的特征，但是对于预示恶性行为并不可靠；事实上某些作者主张，在正

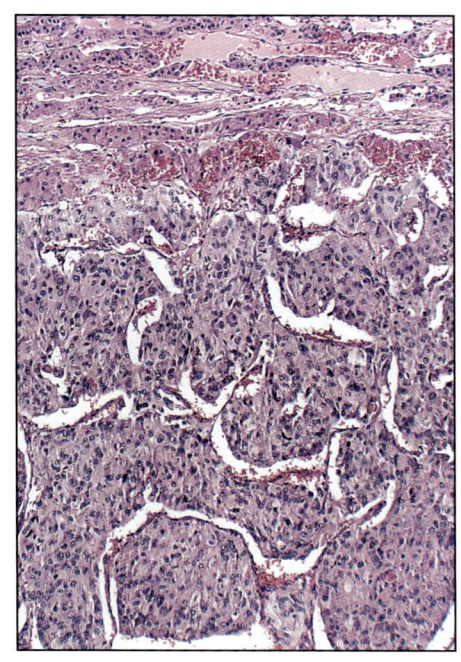

图19.36 嗜铬细胞瘤。相互吻合的小梁状结构，肿瘤细胞相互连接形成缠绕的条索。在肿瘤和邻近的肾上腺皮质交界处没有真正的包膜。

常情况下，没有嗜铬组织的部位出现转移性肿瘤是唯一绝对的恶性标准[66]。大约1/3的嗜铬细胞瘤可见核内"假包涵体"[67]，这是胞浆内折的结果（图19.37）。大约47%的嗜铬细胞瘤胞浆内有透明小体[68]，透明小体呈嗜酸性，PAS染色阳性，抗淀粉酶预消化[1,38,39]（图19.39）。出现透明小体可能有助于嗜铬细胞瘤和肾上腺皮质肿瘤的鉴别诊断，但在一小部分肾上腺皮质肿瘤中也会出现透明小体[1,11,37]。嗜铬细胞瘤还可能类似于肾上腺皮质肿瘤，因为产生ACTH[38,39]或肿瘤内的脂质变性（图19.40）[69]。某些病例肾上腺周围的棕色脂肪可能是一个显著特征[70]，但与嗜铬细胞瘤是否密切相关尚有争议[71]。据报道大约9%的肿瘤间质中有淀粉样物质沉积（图19.41）[72]。

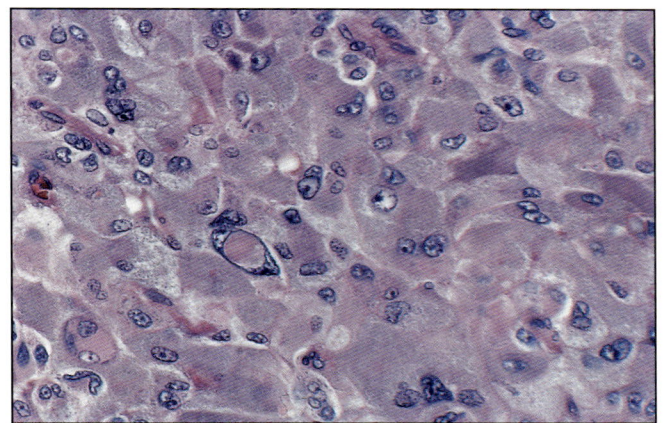

图19.37 嗜铬细胞瘤显示肿瘤细胞比较弥漫或实性的排列。光镜检查肿瘤细胞胞浆呈淡紫色，伴有显著可溶解的点状颗粒。接近视野中心的瘤细胞核内可见"假包涵体"。

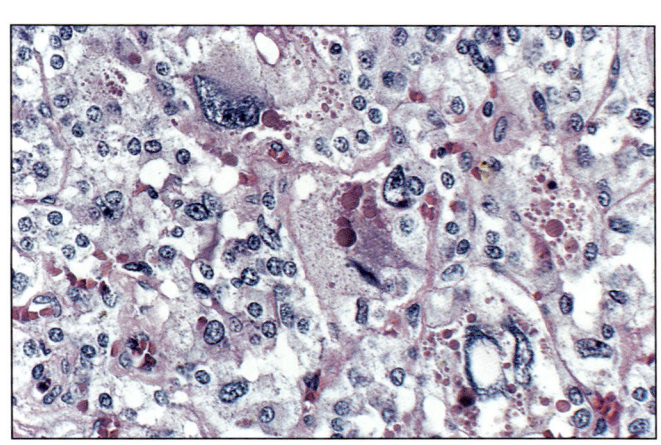

图19.39 嗜铬细胞瘤。注意核的多形性和胞浆内透明小体。视野右下角增大的细胞核内可见"假包涵体"。

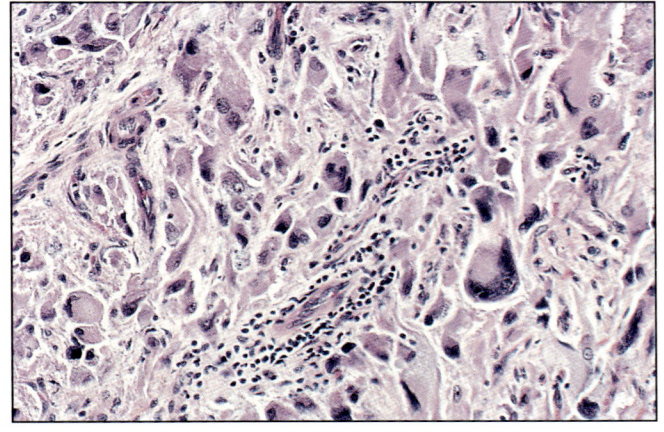

图19.38 嗜铬细胞瘤伴有奇异性多核细胞，某些可见变细的胞浆突起。某些病灶的形态学特征提示神经元或神经节细胞分化。

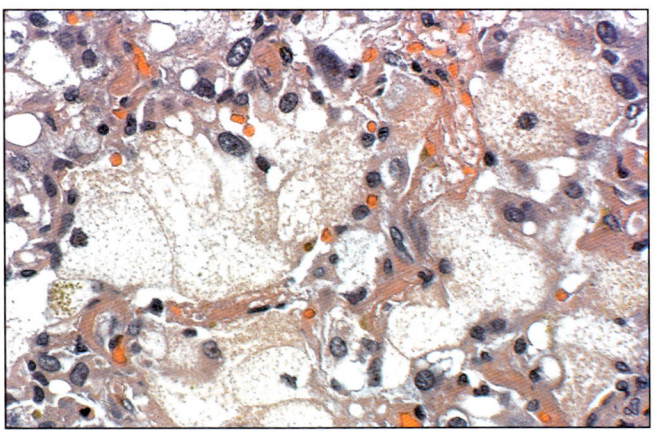

图19.40 嗜铬细胞瘤伴有增大的富含脂质细胞的区域，是为脂质变性。其他区域具有比较典型的组织学特征。

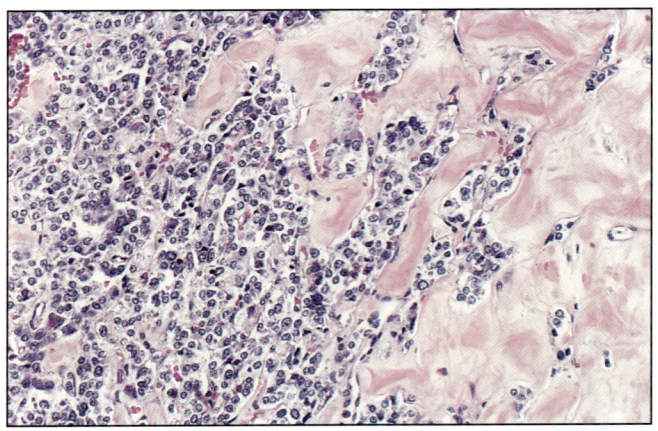

图19.41 嗜铬细胞瘤中的玻璃样变间质类似于淀粉样物。

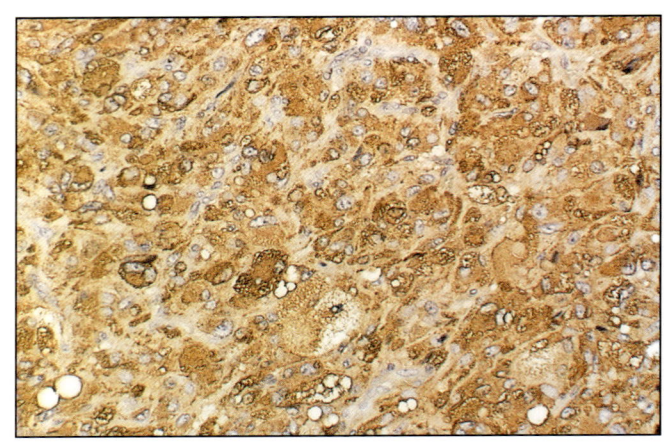

图19.43 嗜铬细胞瘤显示嗜铬粒蛋白阳性免疫染色。（过氧化物酶-抗过氧化物酶染色）。

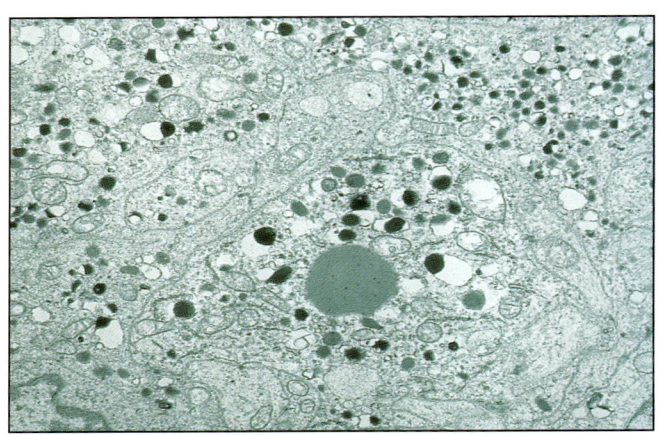

图19.42 嗜铬细胞瘤细胞含有许多致密轴心神经分泌型颗粒；某些颗粒是"去甲肾上腺素型"颗粒，在电子致密轴心与界膜之间有偏心的透明区，而其他颗粒则有狭窄而均一空晕（"肾上腺素型颗粒"）。某些颗粒的多形性可能相当明显，而且一般来说，不能将颗粒的形态学和任何特殊激素或神经肽的储存联系起来。注意复杂的相互交错的细胞突起。

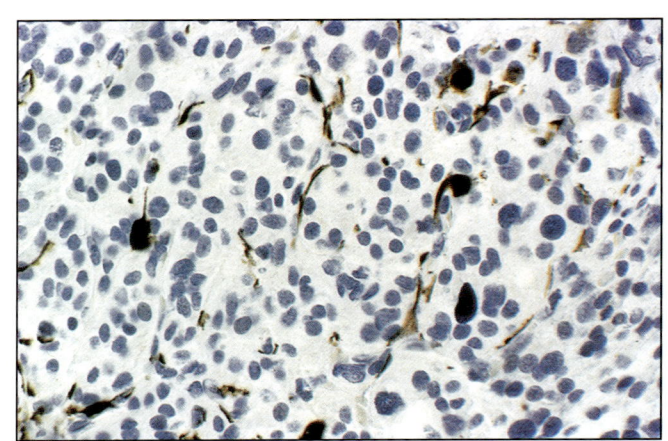

图19.44 嗜铬细胞瘤。S-100阳性细胞有角或呈星形，位于腺泡状肿瘤细胞簇的周围。注意细胞核染色阳性。这些细胞是支持细胞。（过氧化物酶-抗过氧化物酶染色）。

嗜铬细胞瘤的超微结构特点是出现具有结合膜（membrane-bound）的致密轴心颗粒，直径常为150～250 nm。据报道，去甲肾上腺素型颗粒具有宽而偏心的空晕，伴有界膜（limiting membrane），而与肾上腺素有关的颗粒则比较均匀一致（图19.42）[1]，但是颗粒的形态学差异可能很大，使之无法与任何特殊激素或神经肽的储存有机地联系起来[1,38,39]。嗜铬细胞瘤的免疫组化谱显著不同，它能产生多种神经肽[73]（图19.5）。NSE和诸如嗜铬粒蛋白和突触素等神经内分泌标记物免疫染色阳性具有特征性[1,38,39]（图19.43）。S-100蛋白核染色阳性可以证实支持细胞（sustentacular cells）[1,39]（图19.44）。重要的是，嗜铬细胞瘤角蛋白和EMA阴性。阳性的嗜铬反应可能有助于诊断，而且在适当的情况下，几乎所有嗜铬细胞瘤的胞浆均呈嗜银性（argyrophilia）[1,38,39]。许多嗜铬细胞瘤显示1号染色体短臂丢失，提示这个位点有推定的肿瘤抑制因子[74]。

表19.5	临床良性和恶性的副神经节瘤的免疫组化表达	
	阳性肿瘤的百分比	
	临床上良性 (n=55)	临床上恶性 (n=25)
[Leu-5]-脑啡肽	85	48
[Met-5]-脑啡肽	89	40
生长抑素	78	48
胰多肽	60	33
血管活性肠多肽	45	2
P物质	29	24
促肾上腺皮质激素	21	36
降钙素	24	8
蛙皮素	12	4
神经降压素	12	13

混合性嗜铬细胞瘤
Composite pheochromocytoma

这个术语是指具有类似于神经母细胞瘤（图 19.45A），神经节母细胞瘤（图 19.45B），神经节瘤[1,38,39,75,76]（图 19.45C～E），乃至恶性外周神经鞘肿瘤（恶性神经鞘瘤）成分的嗜铬细胞瘤。曾有一例报道，双侧嗜铬细胞瘤-恶性外周神经鞘肿瘤发生于 von Recklinghausen 病病人[77]。还有一例报道，混合性嗜铬细胞瘤-神经节瘤发生于 2A 型多发性内分泌肿瘤（MEN）的病人[78]。

肾上腺髓质的胚胎发生有助于解释这种歧异的分化[38,39]（图 19.46）。这些罕见的肿瘤通常伴有儿茶酚胺分泌过多引起的症状或体征；个别具有神经节型细胞的病例，由于血管活性肠多肽（VIP）而引起水泻综合征[75]。一例双侧混合性嗜铬细胞瘤-神经节瘤伴有神经纤维瘤病[79]。根据迄今为止相对少数的病例报告，出现类似于神经母细胞瘤或神经节母细胞瘤区域并不一定代表预后较差，而且这些肿瘤的生物学行为可能难以预测，如同比较传统的嗜铬细胞瘤一样[1]。新近报道一例混合性嗜铬细胞瘤-ACA，两种类型的细胞不规则

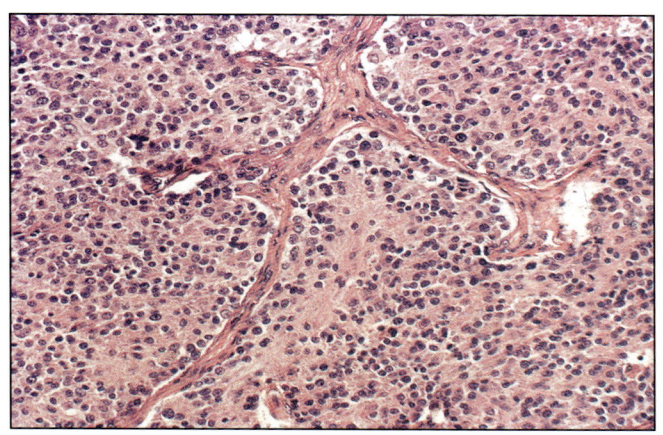

A

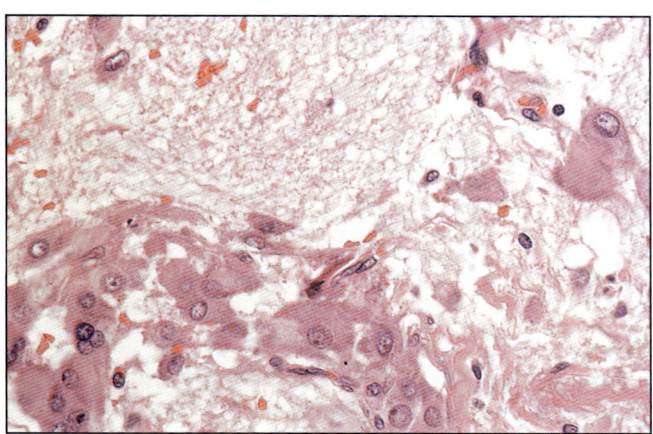

B

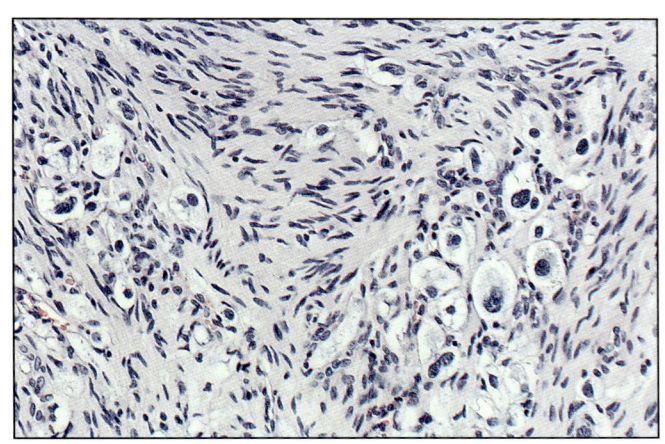

C

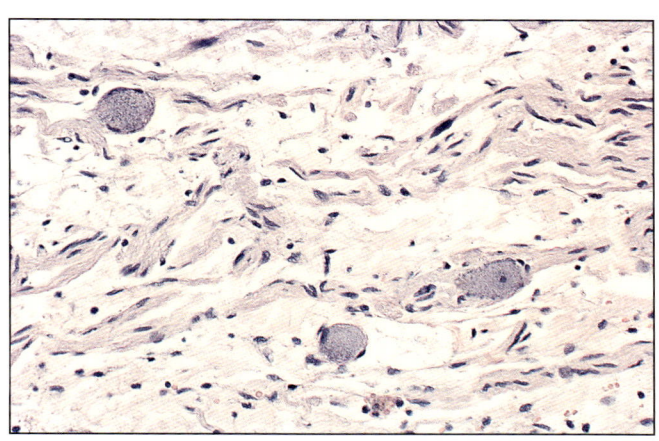

D

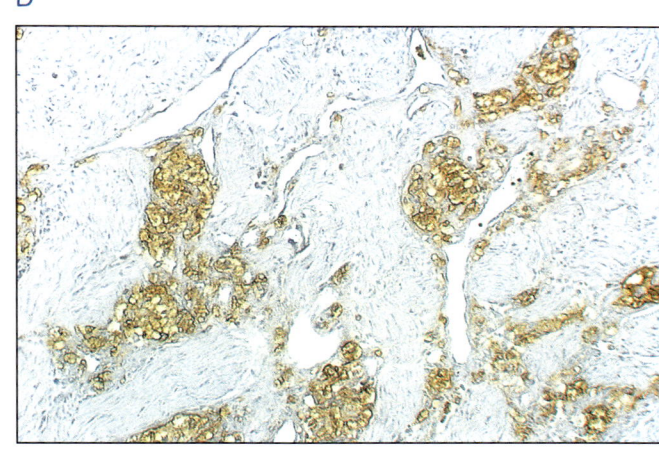

E

图19.45 （A）混合性嗜铬细胞瘤具有类似于神经母细胞瘤的区域。（B）不同的混合性嗜铬细胞瘤，视野中类似于神经节母细胞瘤的区域伴有缠结的神经原纤维基质，肿瘤细胞类似于神经元或神经节细胞。（C）混合性嗜铬细胞瘤显示梭形细胞神经鞘间质，混有嗜铬细胞瘤。（D）同一肿瘤的另外一个部位由神经节瘤组成。（E）嗜铬粒蛋白免疫染色突出了位于神经节瘤中的嗜铬细胞瘤的瘤细胞（过氧化物酶-抗过氧化物酶染色）。

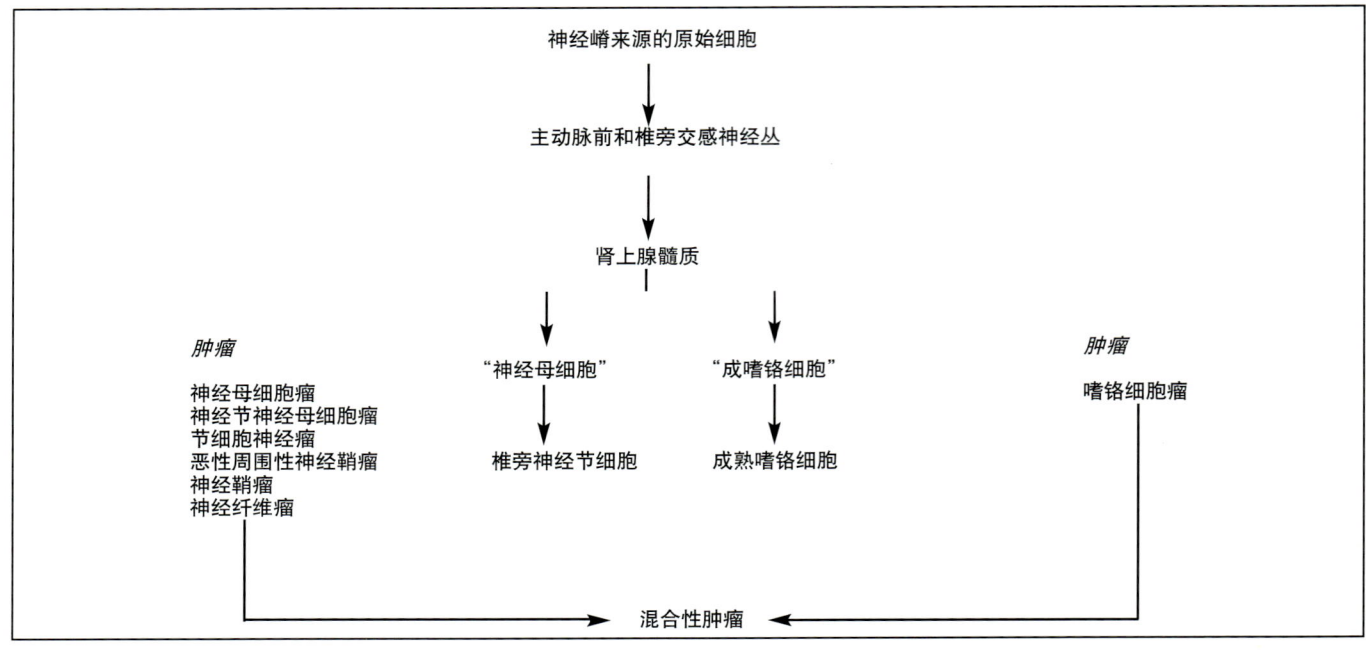

图19.46 神经嵴来源的原始细胞的胚胎发育过程，图示原始细胞发展成熟为嗜铬细胞和神经节细胞的过程，列出了理论上可能发生的肿瘤。混合性嗜铬细胞瘤可能沿着两个途径呈现歧异的分化。（Reproduced with permission from Lack E E 1990 Adrenal medullary hyperplasia and pheochromocytoma. In: Lack E E (ed) Pathology of the adrenal glands. Churchill Linvingstone, New York, p 173-235.）

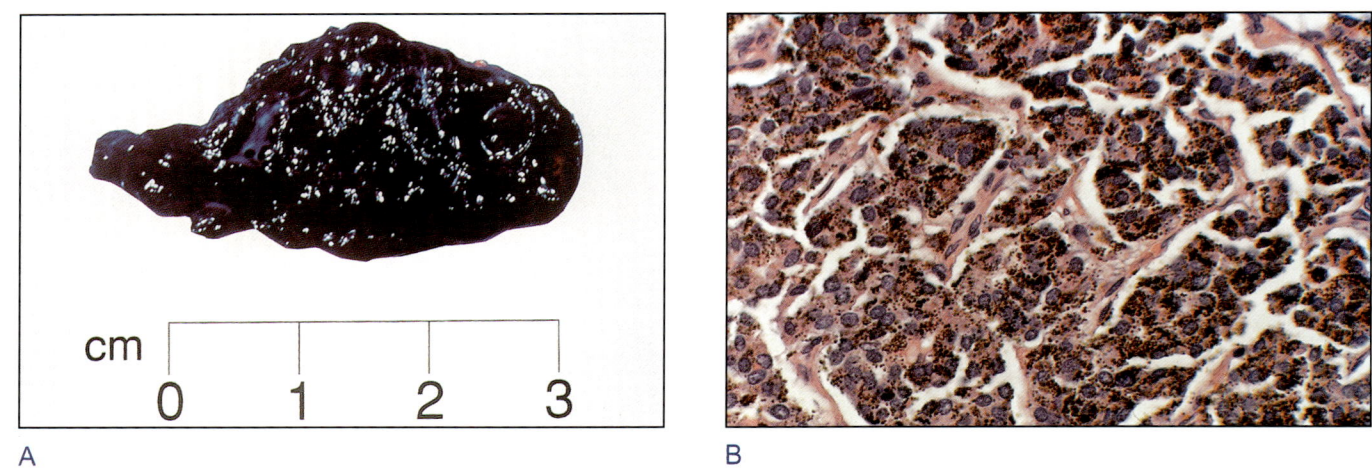

图19.47 色素性（"黑色"）副神经节瘤。（A）这个重225g的肿瘤完全呈深黑色，发生在接近右肾上极的腹膜后。（B）肿瘤细胞排列成巢和相互吻合的条索，含有大量粗糙的暗棕色至墨黑色的色素颗粒。

地混合在一起[80]。

色素性嗜铬细胞瘤
Pigmented pheochromocytoma

近年来，色素性嗜铬细胞瘤和肾上腺外副神经节瘤已有报道。根据组织化学染色或超微结构研究，推测这些包含的色素颗粒是真正的黑色素[1]。这种肿瘤可能呈深黑色（图19.47A），类似于恶性黑色素瘤。曾有一例报道，肿瘤中的色素具有神经黑色素的特点（图19.47B），神经黑色素（neuromelanin）是一种儿茶酚胺代谢过程中产生的不含酶或氧化物的废物[81]。

家族性嗜铬细胞瘤
Familial pheochromocytoma

2型多发性内分泌肿瘤（MEN）是由 RET 原癌基因突变引起的一组与常染色体显性遗传有关的癌症综合征[82-84]。嗜铬细胞瘤是2型多发性内分泌肿瘤综合征重要的组成部分（表19.6）；肾上腺髓质增生[弥漫性和（或）结节性]被认为是嗜铬细胞瘤的前体病变[85-87]。也有报道指肾上腺髓质增生发生于非家族性的情况下，病人具有类似于嗜铬细胞瘤的症状和体征[1,39,88]。结节性增生和嗜铬细胞瘤的区别是人为的，某些作者提出以1cm作为帮助诊断的切点[85]（图19.48）。在这种情况下，嗜

表19.6	2a型和2b型多发性内分泌肿瘤（MEN）临床和病理学特征比较
2a型MEN	**2b型MEN**
双侧MCT	双侧MCT
嗜铬细胞瘤	嗜铬细胞瘤
甲状旁腺增生	甲状旁腺疾病罕见
没有特异表型	常有Marfan综合征表型 黏膜神经瘤常见
家族性遗传，表现为Mendel常染色体显性特征	可以发生在Mendel常染色体显性遗传病人，但可能不是家族性
进展为MCT几率不同，常常为惰性	通常迅速进展为MCT

MCT，medullary carcinoma of the thyroid，甲状腺髓质癌

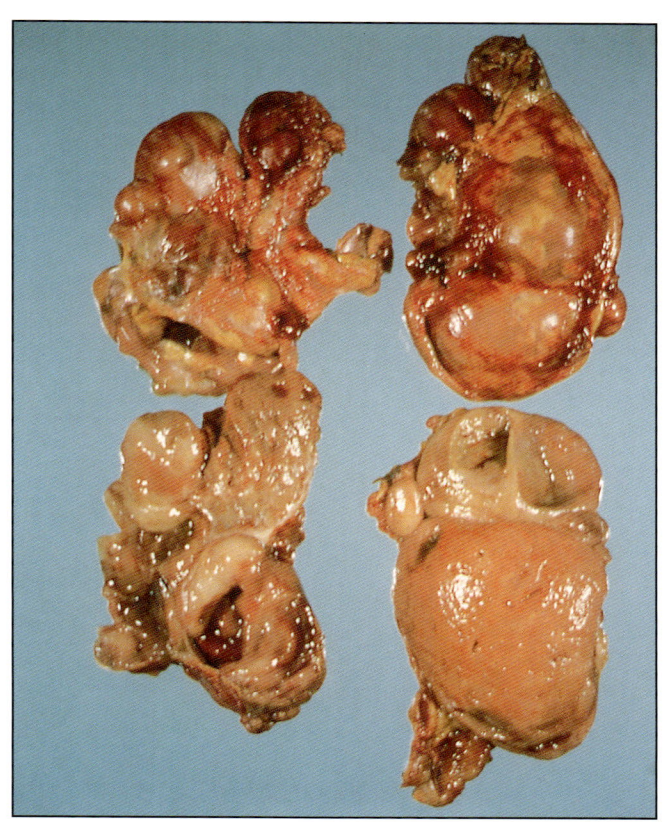

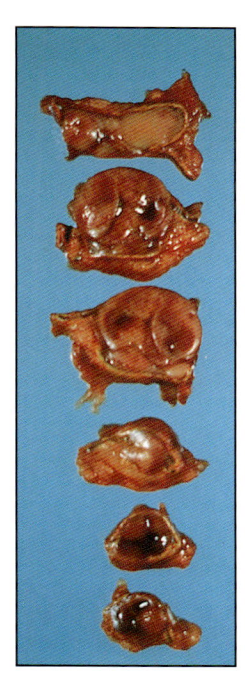

图19.48 来自2a型多发性内分泌肿瘤病人（Sipple综合征）的右肾上腺的横断面，显示结节状髓质增生；如果武断地应用"1cm的标准"作为切点，多数结节为早期的嗜铬细胞瘤。（Reproduced with permission from Lack E E 1990 Adrenal medullary hyperplasia and pheochromocytoma. In: Lack E E (ed) Pathology of the adrenal glands. Churchill Linvingstone, New York, p 173-235.）

图19.49 来自2a型多发性内分泌肿瘤病人的双侧多结节状嗜铬细胞瘤（Sipple综合征）。上方显示每个肿瘤的外貌，下方显示切面。这种表现与图19.32和19.33的单中心性孤立性嗜铬细胞瘤形成鲜明对比。（Reproduced with permission from Lack E E 1990 Adrenal medullary hyperplasia and pheochromocytoma. In: Lack E E (ed) Pathology of the adrenal glands. Churchill Linvingstone, New York, p 173-235.）

铬细胞瘤常常是多中心性和双侧性，仅仅根据大体形态就能提醒病理医师注意潜在的综合征[89]（图19.49）。2b型多发性内分泌肿瘤病人可能有明显的胃肠表现，而且胃肠症状可能先于内分泌疾病出现[90]。有一种特征性的"神经瘤性"增生，伴有唇、舌、颊黏膜和其他部位受累（图19.50）。神经节瘤病（ganglioneuromatosis）通常出现在整个消化道，伴有神经鞘细胞、轴突（neurites）和神经节细胞的错构瘤性增生（图19.51）。还可能出现角膜神经（corneal nerves）变粗。

其他的多内分泌综合征已有描述，如嗜铬细胞瘤伴有胰腺胰岛细胞瘤[91]，以及von Recklinghausen病、嗜铬细胞瘤和富于生长抑素的壶腹部类癌相伴发生[92]。

恶性嗜铬细胞瘤
Malignant pheochromocytoma

在报告的多数嗜铬细胞瘤的系列中，恶性嗜铬细胞瘤的发病率从2.4%到14%不等[39,93,94]；根据报告，腹部的肾上腺外副神经节瘤的发病率还要高些（见第28章）[1,39,95]。嗜铬细胞瘤的恶性行为较常见于伴有*SDHB*基因种系突变的病人[96]。出现转移是恶性唯一可靠的指征，虽然广泛局部浸润和融合的坏死区域是怀疑恶性的特征。近来报道了一种用来区分嗜铬细胞瘤良恶性的评分系统[97]，但这需要得到其他人员的重复。局部和远处转移最常见的部位是肝、淋巴结、肺和骨。DNA成分的定量分析已经得到应用[98]，但临床上良性的肿瘤也可见到非整倍体，因而限制了它在诊断恶性方面的应用[99]。其他资料提示，MIB-1免疫染色可能具有预后价值[100]。

髓脂肪瘤

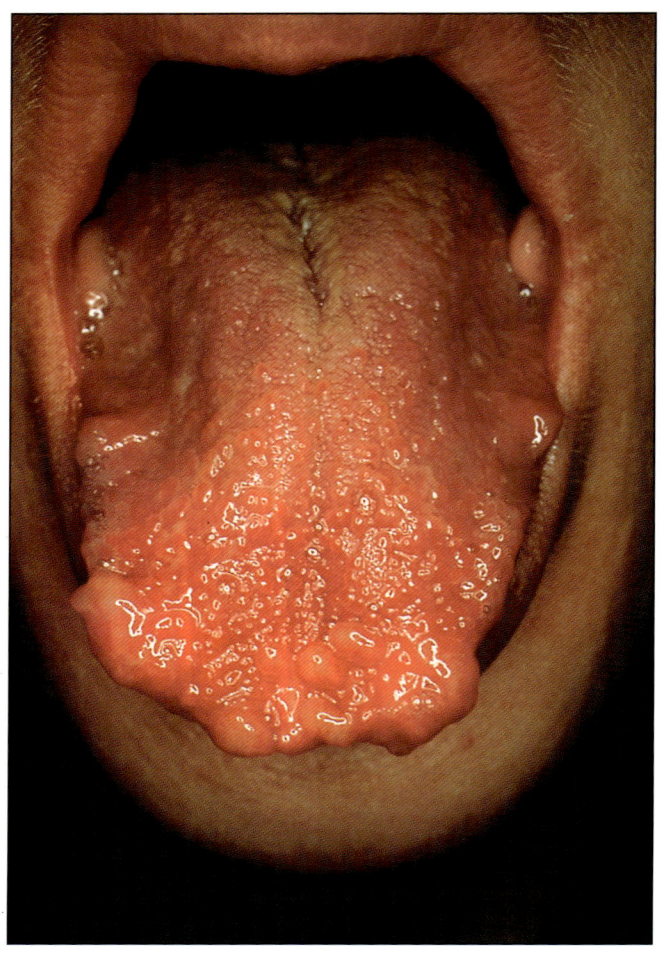

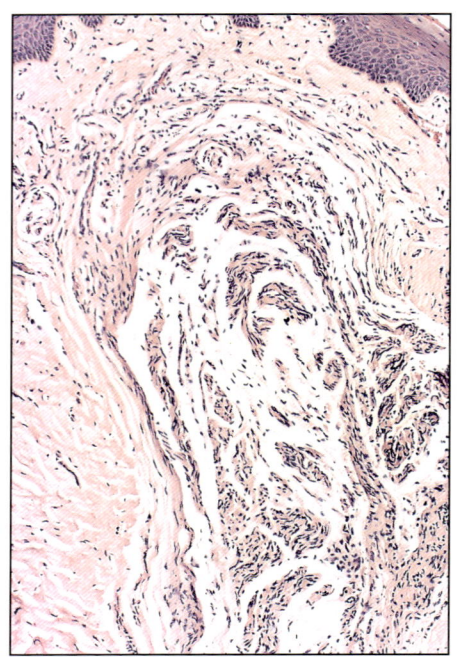

图19.50 （A）2b型多发性内分泌肿瘤病人舌表面散布黏膜神经瘤结节，特别是沿着侧缘和尖端。本病没有家族史。病人在一年以后死于甲状腺髓质癌广泛转移。(Reproduced with permission from Lack E E 1990 Adrenal medullary hyperplasia and pheochromocytoma. In: Lack E E (ed) Pathology of the adrenal glands. Churchill Linvingstone, New York, p 173-235.) （B）2b型多发性内分泌肿瘤。注意弯弯曲曲的神经增生，伴有间质水肿。病变类似于断肢（外伤性）神经瘤。未见神经节细胞。

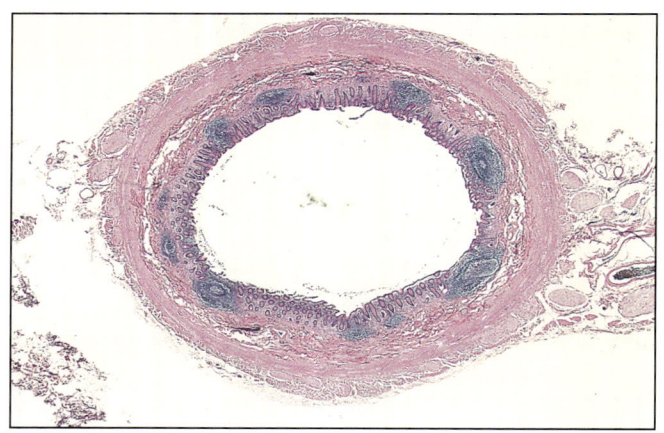

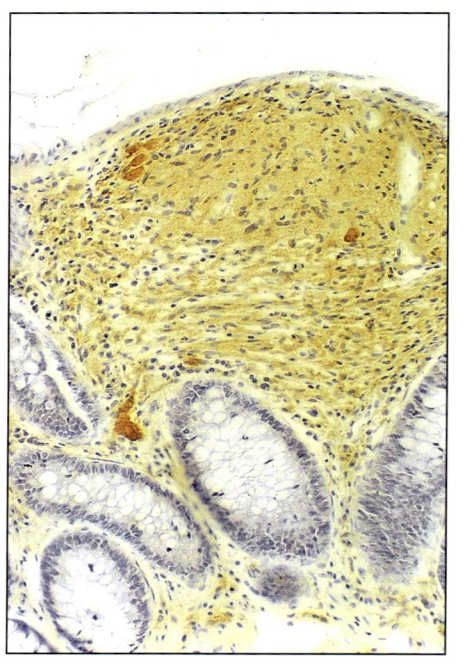

图19.51 （A）2b型多发性内分泌肿瘤病人的阑尾切除标本。在这个横切面上，浆膜面和阑尾系膜可见明显增大的神经束。（B）固有膜内可见明显的神经节瘤病，伴有少数NSE深染的神经节细胞。过氧化物酶-抗过氧化物酶染色。

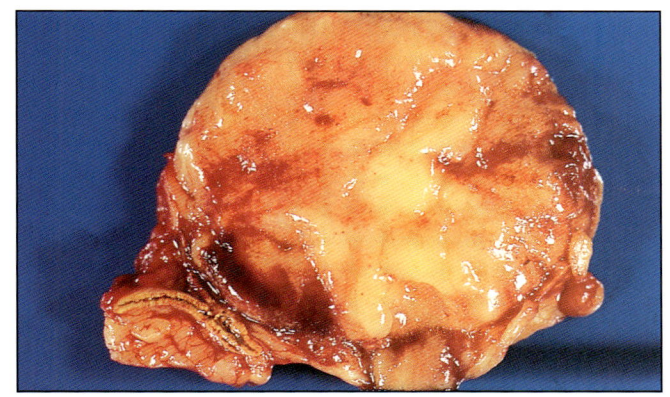

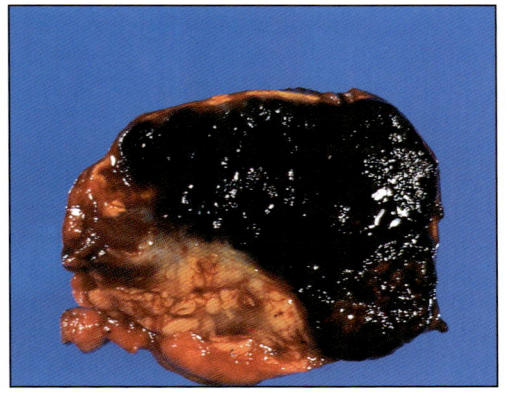

A

图19.52 肾上腺髓脂肪瘤的横切面，肿瘤呈叶状，黄色，伴有不规则的暗红色区域。图的左下方可见残余的肾上腺，伴有肾上腺周围脂肪组织。（Reproduced with permission from Travis W D, Oertel J E, Lack E E 1990 Miscellaneous tumors and tumefactive lesions of the adrenal gland. In: Lack E E (ed) Pathology of the adrenal glands. Churchill Livingstone, New York, p351-378）

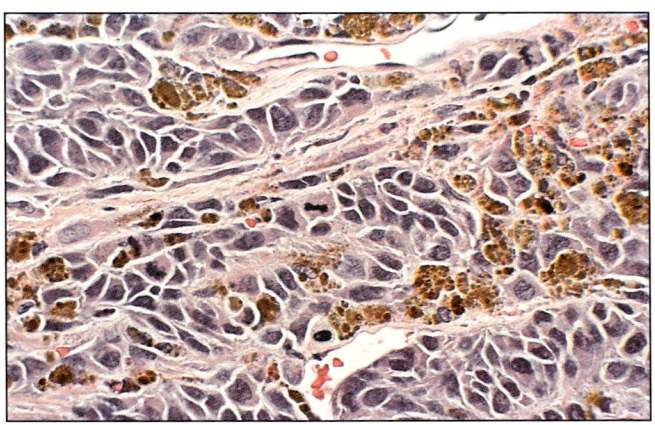

B

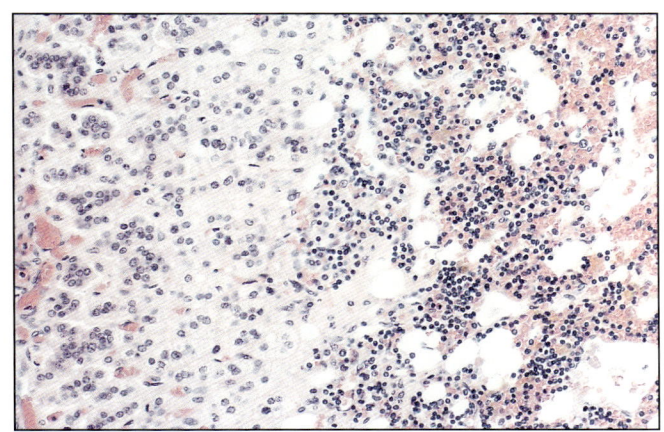

图19.53 肾上腺髓脂肪瘤由造血细胞和脂肪组织组成，前者主要是髓系和红系前体细胞。在其他区域可见巨核细胞。

图19.54 （A）年轻女性的肾上腺恶性黑色素瘤，表现为间断性胁腹痛。肿瘤是在腹部CT扫描时发现的，大小接近6cm。肿瘤切除之后仔细检查了病人的皮肤、黏膜和眼睛，没有发现原发性肿瘤。切面肿瘤呈黑色，几乎取代了整个肾上腺；肿瘤上部可见线样到点状残余的黄色肾上腺皮质。标本的下方可见肾上腺周围脂肪组织。（B）为肿瘤（A）有代表性的视野，显示恶性黑色素瘤伴有较多的黑色素沉着。

髓脂肪瘤 Myelolipoma

肾上腺髓脂肪瘤是一种良性肿瘤性病变，在肾上腺外部位也有报告（见第24章）。多数肿瘤发生于40～70岁的病人，男女发病率大致相等[1,101]。多数髓脂肪瘤为孤立性单侧性病变，但是双侧多灶性也可发生[102]。肿瘤大小差别很大，虽然多数病例为偶然发现，但其中某些为巨大肿瘤。大体表现从黄色到红棕色不等，取决于髓细胞和脂肪的相对比例（图19.52）。肿瘤界限清楚，但通常没有包膜。髓脂肪瘤由成熟的脂肪组织和髓细胞组成（图19.53）。偶尔可见梗死、出血或骨化生。还需提出的是，化生性髓脂肪瘤性病灶可以见于各种肾上腺皮质疾病，特别是与肾上腺皮质功能亢进有关的肾上腺皮质疾病。另据报告，髓脂肪瘤与先天性肾上腺增生有关[102]。

恶性淋巴瘤和浆细胞瘤
Malignant lymphoma and plasmacytoma

据报告，18%～25%的伴有播散性疾病的恶性淋巴瘤病人累及肾上腺[103,104]。得到公认的肾上腺原发性恶性淋巴瘤（以及浆细胞瘤）非常少见[1,105]，仔细检查可以发现肾上腺外受累。肾上腺原发性恶性淋巴瘤与EB病毒感染有关[106]。

恶性黑色素瘤 Malignant melanoma

肾上腺原发性恶性黑色素瘤已有报告，但是非常罕见，而且最后难以得到证实[1]。诊断标准包括单侧肾上腺受累，皮肤、黏膜或眼缺乏任何可疑的色素性病变，

其他少见的肾上腺原发性肿瘤
Other unusual primary adrenal tumors

良性间叶性肿瘤包括：肾上腺血管瘤（通常为海绵状，其次为毛细血管性）[1,107]，平滑肌瘤，神经鞘瘤[107a]和神经纤维瘤[1,108]（图19.55）。腺瘤样瘤也有报告，具有间皮本质[109,110]（图19.56），一例报告发生在获得性免疫缺陷综合征（AIDS）病人[111]。卵巢卵泡膜化生可能是一种性索间质来源的病变[112-114]（图19.57），可能与所谓的肾上腺肿瘤性梭形细胞病变（adrenal tumefactive spindle cell lesion）有关[115]。已有一例原发性肾上腺的颗粒卵泡膜细胞瘤的报告[116]。肾上腺孤立性纤维性肿瘤的病例也已描述[117,118]。作者遇到过两例肾上腺炎症性肌纤维母细胞肿瘤。

恶性间叶性肿瘤包括血管肉瘤[119]，通常为上皮样型（见第3章）（图19.58），以及平滑肌肉瘤[120]（图19.59）。据报告一例男性AIDS病人发生肾上腺原发性平滑肌肉瘤，在这种情况下，平滑肌肿瘤与EB病毒感染有关[121]。恶性外周神经鞘肿瘤（恶性神经鞘瘤）已有病例报告，有时是放射治疗的并发症[1]。唯一一例肾外Wilms瘤已经报告，发生在4岁男孩的肾上腺[122]。

肾上腺转移性肿瘤
Tumors metastatic to the adrenal gland

肾上腺转移性肿瘤的发生率不同，占癌症病人尸检病例的9%到27%，但是随着诸如CT扫描等影像

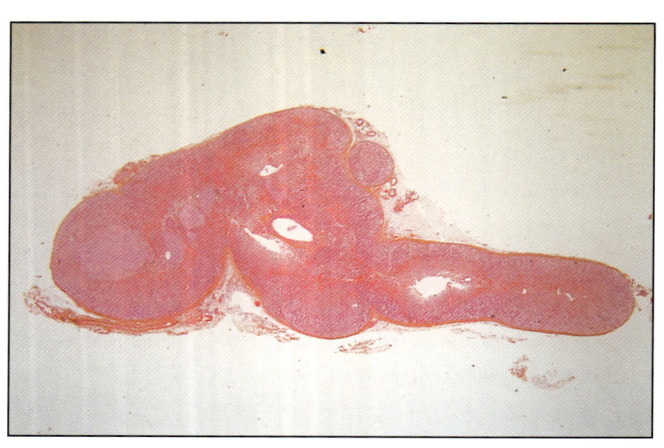

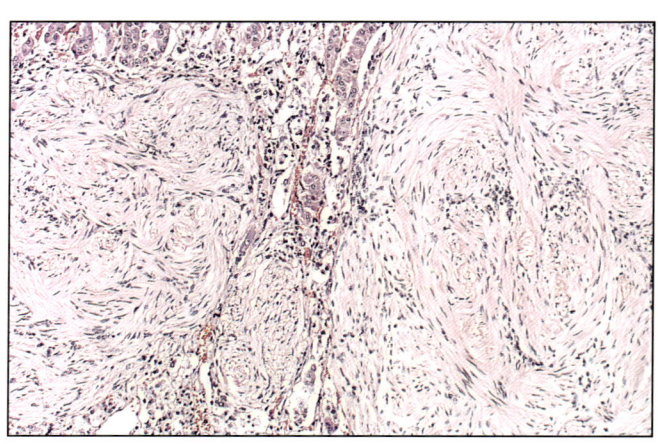

图19.55 （A）肾上腺神经纤维瘤。成人尸检肾上腺横切面，显示髓质中神经增生形成的结节状区域。病变是偶然发现的。（B）高倍放大显示梭形细胞交互排列成束。没有发现神经节细胞，认为这个病变是神经纤维瘤。（Reproduced with permission from Lack E E, Kozakewich H P W 1990 Adrenal neuroblastoma, ganglioneuroblastoma and related tumors. In: Lack E E (ed) Pathology of the adrenal glands. Churchill Linvingstone, New York, p 277-309.）

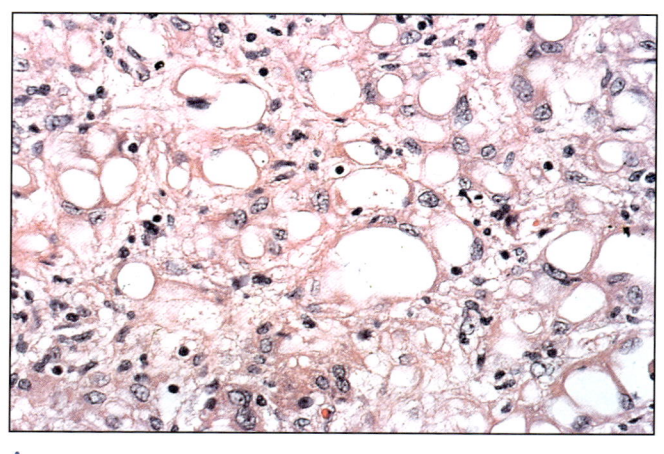

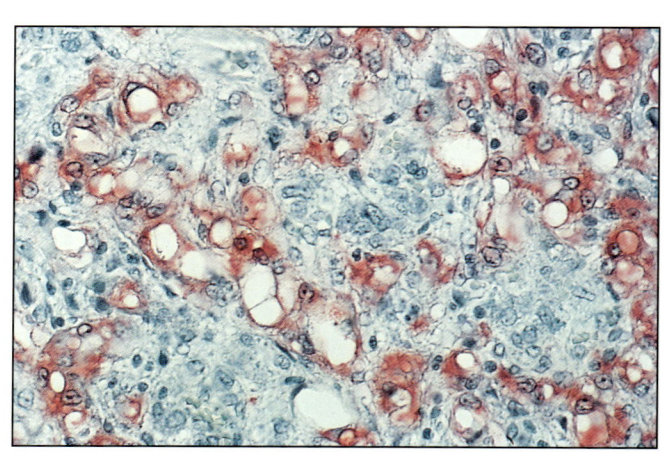

图19.56 （A）肾上腺原发性腺瘤样瘤，显示内衬扁平细胞的不规则的腺样间隙，胞浆淡颗粒状。在这个常规染色的切面上，难以辨认残余的皮质细胞。（B）细胞角蛋白免疫染色显著阳性，腺瘤样瘤细胞与残留的皮质形成鲜明对比。（链霉亲和素-碱性磷酸酶方法）

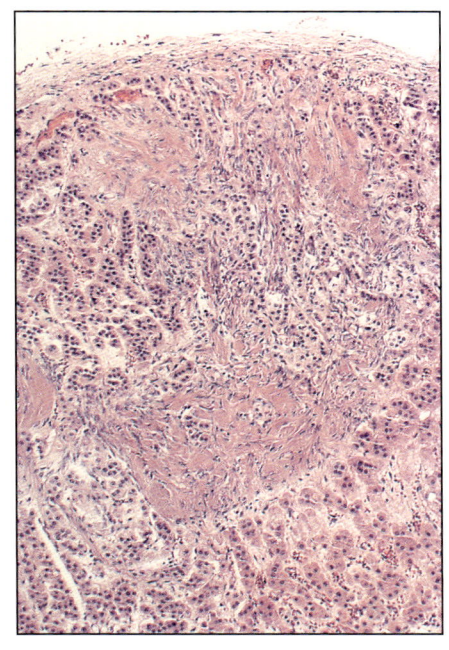

图19.57 肾上腺的卵巢卵泡膜化生。病变略呈楔形，图的上方附着于包膜，并有一些玻璃样变的区域。

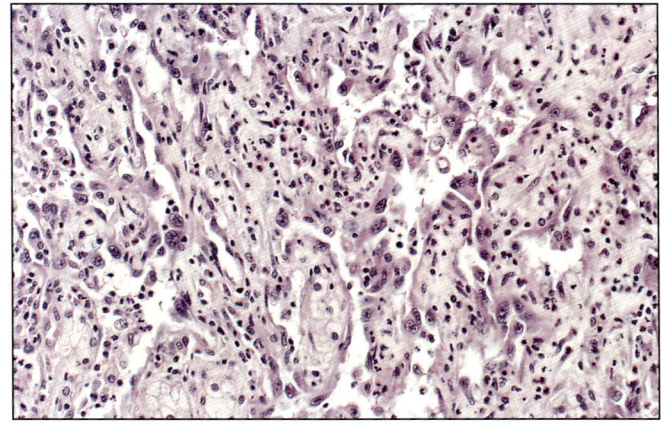

图19.58 肾上腺原发性血管肉瘤。可见血管增生形态，伴有恶性细胞形成的乳头状突起和裂隙样结构。间质中的某些淡染空泡状细胞是残余的肾上腺皮质细胞。

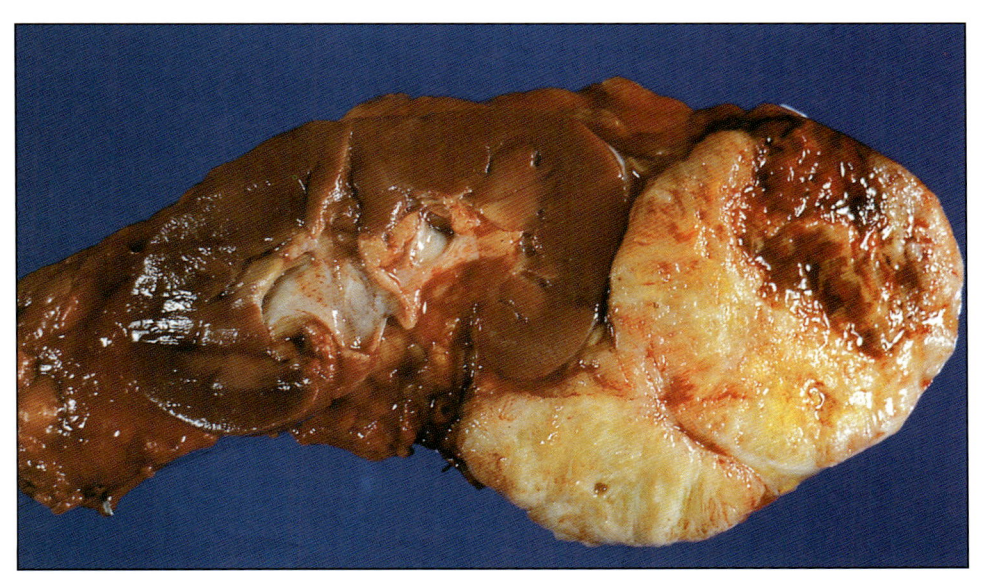

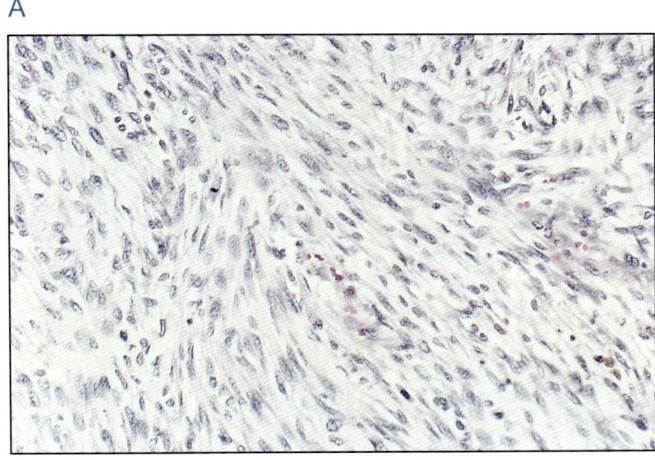

图19.59 （A）肾上腺平滑肌肉瘤。肿瘤取代了大部分肾上腺组织。注意局灶出血和坏死。肿瘤可能起源于肾上腺中心静脉的分支。(Reproduced with permission from Lack E E, Graham C W, Azumi N et al. 1991 Primary leiomyosarcoma of adrenal gland. Case report with immunohistochemical and ultrastructural study. Am J Surg Pathol 15:899-905.) （B）肾上腺平滑肌肉瘤。超微结构研究以及肌肉特异性和平滑肌特异性肌动蛋白免疫染色阳性证实有平滑肌分化。

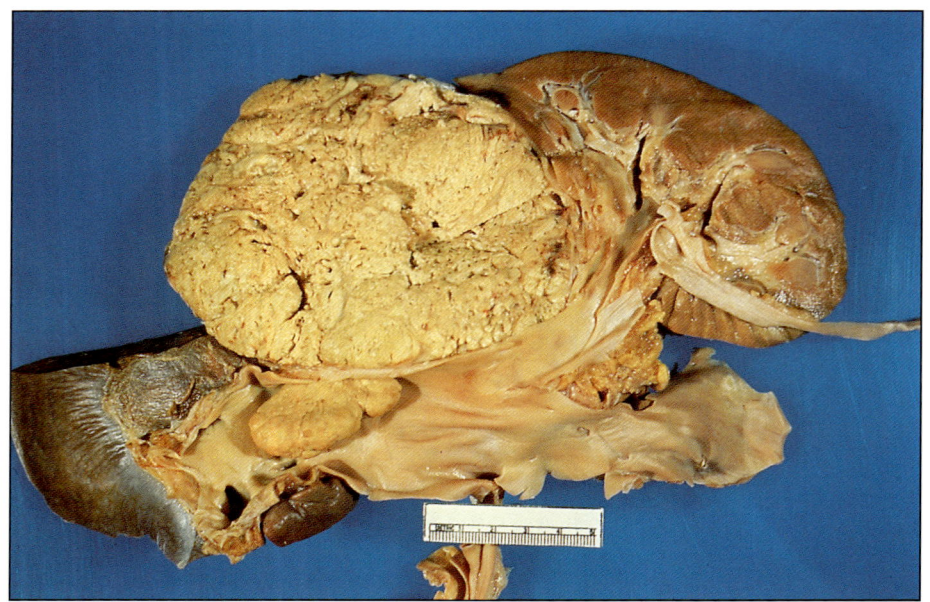

图19.60 肾上腺转移性肺癌。病人的肺有多发性肿瘤性结节。肾上腺肿块很大,大体检查侵犯下腔静脉,提出有肾上腺皮质癌的可能性。

技术的进步,死前常常能够诊断肾上腺受累[1,101]。某些肿瘤,例如转移性肺癌,可能与原发性肾上腺肿瘤混淆(图19.60)。肺和乳腺是最常见的原发部位,而其他转移常常来源于恶性黑色素瘤、胃和结肠腺癌以及肾细胞癌[1,101,123]。两侧肾上腺转移性肿瘤可能导致亚临床甚至明显的肾上腺皮质功能不全(Addison病)[1]。某些AIDS病人可见Kaposi肉瘤累及肾上腺(图19.61)。

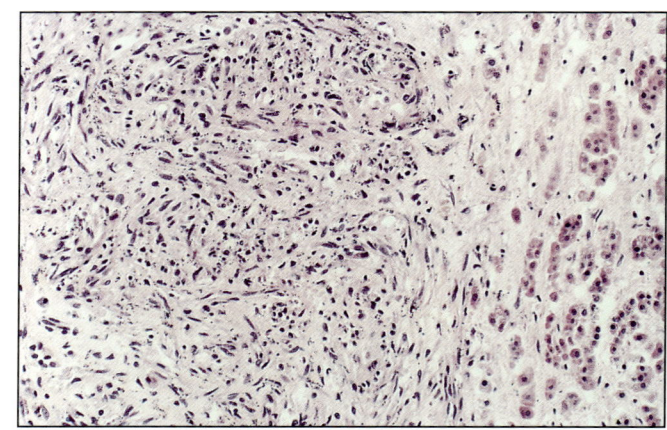

图19.61 Kaposi肉瘤累及肾上腺,病人死于获得性免疫缺陷综合征(AIDS)。病人有广泛的Kaposi肉瘤,肾上腺受累是偶然所见。

参考文献

1. Lack E E 1997 Tumors of the adrenal gland and extra-adrenal paraganglia. Atlas of tumor pathology, 3rd series, fascicle 19. Armed Forces Institute of Pathology, Washington, D C
2. Shamma A H, Goddard J W, Sommers S C 1958 A study of the adrenal status in hypertension. J Chronic Dis 8: 587–595
3. Hedeland H, Ostberg G, Hokfelt B 1968 On the prevalence of adrenocortical adenomas in an autopsy material in relation to hypertension and diabetes. Acta Med Scand 184: 211–214
4. Dobbie J W 1969 Adrenocortical nodular hyperplasia: the ageing adrenal. J Pathol 99: 1–18
5. Lack E E, Travis W D, Oertel J E 1990 Adrenal cortical nodules, hyperplasia, and hyperfunction. In: Lack E E (ed) Pathology of the adrenal glands. Churchill Livingstone, New York, p 75–113
6. Grumbach M M, Biller B M K, Braunstein G D et al. 2003 Management of the clinically inapparent adrenal mass ("incidentaloma"). Ann Intern Med 138: 424–429
7. Gross M D, Wilton G P, Shapiro B et al. 1987 Functional and scintigraphic evaluation of the silent adrenal mass. J Nucl Med 28: 1401–1407
8. Suzuki T, Sasano H, Sawai T et al. 1992 Small adrenocortical tumors without apparent clinical endocrine abnormalities. Immunolocalization of steroidogenic enzymes. Pathol Res Pract 188: 883–889
9. Wieneke J A, Thompson L D R, Heffess C S 2003 Adrenal cortical neoplasms in the pediatric population. A clinicopathologic and immunophenotypic analysis of 83 patients. Am J Surg Pathol 27: 867–881
10. Neville A M, O'Hare M J 1985 Histopathology of the human adrenal cortex. Clin Endocrinol Metab 14: 791–820
11. Lack E E, Travis W D, Oertel J E 1990 Adrenal cortical neoplasms. In: Lack E E (ed) Pathology of the adrenal glands. Churchill Livingstone, New York, p 115–171
12. Conn J W, Knopf R F, Nesbit R M 1964 Clinical characteristics of primary aldosteronism from an analysis of 145 cases. Am J Surg 107: 159–172
13. Neville A M, Symington T 1966 Pathology of primary aldosteronism. Cancer 19: 1854–1868
14. Conn J W 1955 Primary aldosteronism. J Lab Clin Med 45: 661–664
15. Janigan D T 1963 Cytoplasmic bodies in the adrenal cortex of patients treated with spironolactone. Lancet i: 850–852
16. Damron T A, Schelper R L, Sorensen L 1987 Cytochemical demonstration of neuromelanin in black pigmented adrenal nodules. Am J Clin Pathol 87: 334–341
17. Gabrilove J L, Sharma D C, Woftiz H H et al. 1965 Feminizing adrenocortical tumors in the male. A review of 52 cases including a case report. Medicine 44: 37–79

18. Pollock W J, McConnell C F, Hilton C et al. 1986 Virilizing Leydig cell adenoma of adrenal gland. Am J Surg Pathol 10: 816–822
19. Aquirre P, Scully R E 1983 Testosterone-secreting adrenal ganglioneuroma containing Leydig cells. Am J Surg Pathol 7: 699–705
20. Bisceglia M. Ludovico O, Di Mattia A et al. 2004 Adrenocortical oncocytic tumors: report of 10 cases and review of the literature. Int J Surg Pathol 12: 231–243
21. Sasano H, Suzuki T, Sano T et al. 1991 Adrenocortical oncocytoma. A true nonfunctioning adrenocortical tumor. Am J Surg Pathol 15: 949–956
22. Lin B T-Y, Bonsib S M, Mierau G W et al. 1998 Oncocytic adrenocortical neoplasms. A report of seven cases and review of the literature. Am J Surg Pathol 22: 603–614
23. Hoang M P, Ayala A G, Albores-Saavedra J 2002 Oncocytic adrenocortical carcinoma. A morphologic, immunohistochemical and ultrastructural study of four cases. Mod Pathol 15: 973–978
24. Lack E E, Kozakewich H P W 1990 Embryology, developmental anatomy and selected aspects of non-neoplastic pathology. In: Lack E E (ed) Pathology of the adrenal glands. Churchill Livingstone, New York, p 1–74
25. Hamwi G J, Serbin R A, Kruger F A 1957 Does adrenocortical hyperplasia result in adrenocortical carcinoma? N Engl J Med 257: 1153–1157
26. Al-Ahmadie H A, Stanek J, Liv J et al. 2001 Ovarian tumor of the adrenogenital syndrome. The first reported case. Am J Surg Pathol 25: 1443–1450
27. Dahl E V, Bahn R C 1962 Aberrant adrenal cortical tissue near the testis in human infants. Am J Pathol 40: 587–598
28. Verdonk C, Guerin C, Lufkin E 1982 Activation of virilizing adrenal rest tissues by excessive ACTH production. An unusual presentation of Nelson's syndrome. Am J Med 73: 455–459
29. Johnson R E, Scheithauer B 1982 Massive hyperplasia of testicular adrenal rests in a patient with Nelson's syndrome. Am J Clin Pathol 77: 501–507
30. Rutgers J L, Young R H, Scully R E 1988 The testicular "tumor" of the adrenogenital syndrome. A report of six cases and review of the literature on testicular masses in patients with adrenocortical disorders. Am J Surg Pathol 12: 503–513
31. Radfar N, Bartter F C, Easley R et al. 1977 Evidence for endogenous LH suppression in a man with bilateral testicular tumors and congenital adrenal hyperplasia. J Clin Endocrinol Metab 45: 1194–1204
32. Tang C K, Gray G F 1975 Adrenocortical neoplasms. Prognosis and morphology. Urology 5: 691–695
33. King D R, Lack E E 1979 Adrenal cortical carcinoma. A clinical and pathologic study of 49 cases. Cancer 44: 239–244
34. Van Slooten H, Schaberg A, Smeenk D et al. 1985 Morphologic characteristics of benign and malignant adrenocortical tumors. Cancer 55: 766–773
35. Cohn K, Gottesman L, Brennan M F 1986 Adrenocortical carcinoma. Surgery 100: 1170–1177
36. Brown F M, Gaffey T A, Wold L E et al. 2000. Myxoid neoplasms of the adrenal cortex. A rare histologic variant. Am J Surg Pathol 24: 396–401
37. Lack E E, Mulvihill J J, Travis W D et al. 1992 Adrenal cortical neoplasms in the pediatric and adolescent age group. Clinicopathologic study of 30 cases with emphasis on epidemiologic and prognostic factors. Pathol Annu 27: 1–53
38. Lack E E 1990 Adrenal medullary hyperplasia and pheochromocytoma. In: Lack E E (ed) Pathology of the adrenal glands. Churchill Livingstone, New York, p 173–235
39. Lack E E 1994 Pathology of adrenal and extra-adrenal paraganglia. Major problems in surgical pathology, vol 29. W B Saunders, Philadelphia
40. Alsabeh R, Mazoujian G, Goates J et al. 1995 Adrenal cortical tumors clinically mimicking pheochromocytoma. Am J Clin Pathol 104: 382–390
41. Hough A J, Hollifield J W, Page D L et al. 1979 Prognostic factors in adrenal cortical tumors. A mathematical analysis of clinical and morphological data. Am J Clin Pathol 72: 390–399
42. Weiss L M 1984 Comparative histologic study of 43 metastasizing and nonmetastasizing adrenocortical tumors. Am J Surg Pathol 8: 163–169
43. Weiss L M, Medeiros L J, Vickery A L Jr 1989 Pathologic features of prognostic significance in adrenal cortical carcinoma. Am J Surg Pathol 13: 202–206
44. Wieneke J A, Thomspon L D R, Heffess C S 2003 Adrenal cortical neoplasms in the pediatric population. A clinicopathologic and immunophenotypic analysis of 83 patients. Am J Surg Pathol 27: 867–881
45. Loy T S, Phillips R W, Linder C L 2002 A103 immunostaining in the diagnosis of adrenal cortical tumors. An immunohistochemical study of 316 cases. Arch Pathol Lab Med 126: 170–172
46. Zhang P J, Genega E M, Tomaszewski J E et al. 2003 The role of calretinin, inhibin, Melan-A, BCL-2 and C-kit in differentiating adrenal cortical and medullary tumors: an immunohistochemical study. Mod Pathol 16: 591–597
47. Gaffey M J, Traweek S J, Mills S E et al. 1992 Cytokeratin expression in adrenocortical neoplasia: an immunohistochemical and biochemical study with implications for the differential diagnosis of adrenocortical, hepatocellular, and renal cell carcinoma. Hum Pathol 23: 144–153
48. Miettinen M 1992 Neuroendocrine differentiation in adrenocortical carcinoma. New immunohistochemical findings supported by electron microscopy. Lab Invest 66: 169–174
49. Komminoth P, Roth J, Schröder S et al. 1995 Overlapping expression of immunohistochemical markers and synaptophysin mRNA in pheochromocytomas and adrenocortical carcinomas. Implications for the differential diagnosis of adrenal gland tumors. Lab Invest 72: 424–431
50. Schroder S, Niendorf A, Achilles E et al. 1990 Immunocytochemical differential diagnosis of adrenocortical neoplasms using the monoclonal antibody D11. Virchows Arch [A] 417: 89–96
51. Tartour E, Caillou B, Tenenbaum F et al. 1993 Immunohistochemical study of adrenocortical carcinoma. Predictive value of the D11 monoclonal antibody. Cancer 72: 3296–3303
52. Sasano H, Shizawa S, Suzuki T et al. 1995 Transcription factor adrenal 4 binding protein as a marker of adrenocortical malignancy. Hum Pathol 26: 1154–1156
53. Vargas M P, Vargas H I, Kleiner D E et al. 1997 Adrenocortical neoplasms: role of prognostic markers MIB-1, p53 and RB. Am J Surg Pathol 21: 556–562
54. Aubert S, Wacrenier A, Leroy X et al. 2002 Weiss system revisited. A clinicopathologic and immunohistochemical study of 49 adrenocortical tumors. Am J Surg Pathol 26: 1612–1619
55. Amberson J B, Vaughan E D Jr, Gray G F et al. 1987 Flow cytometric analysis of nuclear DNA from adrenocortical neoplasms. A retrospective study using paraffin-embedded tissue. Cancer 59: 2091–2095
56. Hosaka Y, Rainwater L M, Grant C S et al. 1987 Adrenocortical carcinoma: nuclear deoxyribonucleic acid ploidy studied by flow cytometry. Surgery 102: 1027–1034
57. Cibas E S, Medeiros L J, Weinberg D S et al. 1990 Cellular DNA profiles of benign and malignant adrenocortical tumors. Am J Surg Pathol 14: 948–955
58. Zerbini C, Kozakewich H A W, Weinberg D S et al. 1992 Adrenocortical neoplasms in childhood and adolescence. Analysis of prognostic factors including DNA content. Endocrine Pathol 3: 116–128
59. Silva E G, Mackay B, Samaan N A et al. 1982 Adrenocortical carcinomas: an ultrastructural study of 22 cases. Ultrastruct Pathol 3: 1–7
60. MacFarlane D A 1958 Cancer of the adrenal cortex. The natural history, prognosis and treatment in a study of fifty-five cases. Ann R Coll Surg Engl 23: 155–186
61. Henley D J, van Heerden J A, Grant C S et al. 1983 Adrenal cortical carcinoma – a continuing challenge. Surgery 94: 926–931
62. Stojadinovic A, Ghossein R A, Hoos A et al. 2002 Adrenocortical carcinoma: clinical, morphologic and molecular characterization. J Clin Oncol 20: 941–950
63. Cagle P T, Hough A J, Pysher T J et al. 1986 Comparison of adrenal cortical tumors in children and adults. Cancer 57: 2235–2237
64. Bugg M F, Ribeiro R C, Roberson P K et al. 1994 Correlation of pathologic features with clinical outcome in pediatric adrenocortical neoplasia. Am J Clin Pathol 101: 625–629
65. Humphrey G B, Pysher T, Holcombe J et al. 1983 Overview of the management of adrenocortical carcinoma (ACC). In: Humphrey G B, Brindey G B, Dehner L P et al. (eds) Adrenal and endocrine tumors in children. Martinus Nijhoff, Boston, p 349–358
66. Neville A M 1969 The adrenal medulla. In: Symington T (ed) Functional pathology of the human adrenal gland. Williams & Wilkins, Baltimore, MD, p 217–289
67. Medeiros L J, Wolf B C, Balogh K et al. 1985 Adrenal pheochromocytoma: a clinicopathologic review of 60 cases. Hum Pathol 16: 580–589
68. Linnoila R I, Keiser H R, Steinberg S M et al. 1990 Histopathology of benign versus malignant sympathoadrenal paragangliomas. Clinicopathologic study of 120 cases including unusual histologic features. Hum Pathol 21: 1168–1180
69. Unger P D, Cohen J M, Thung S N et al. 1990 Lipid degeneration in a pheochromocytoma histologically mimicking an adrenal cortical tumor. Arch Pathol Lab Med 114: 892–894
70. Melicow M M 1957 Hibernating fat and pheochromocytoma. Arch Pathol 63: 367–372
71. Medeiros L J, Katsas G G, Balogh K 1985 Brown fat and adrenal pheochromocytoma. Association or coincidence? Hum Pathol 16: 970–972
72. Miranda R N, Wu C D, Nayak R N et al. 1995 Amyloid in adrenal gland pheochromocytomas. Arch Pathol Lab Med 119: 827–830
73. Linnoila R I, Lack E E, Steinberg S M et al. 1988 Decreased expression of neuropeptides in malignant paragangliomas. An immunohistochemical study. Hum Pathol 19: 41–50
74. Benn D E, Dwight T, Richardson A L et al. 2000 Sporadic and familial pheochromocytomas are associated with loss of at least two discrete intervals on chromosome 1p. Cancer Res 60: 7048–7051
75. Trump D L, Livingstone J N, Baylin S B 1977 Watery diarrhea syndrome in an adult with ganglioneuroma–pheochromocytoma. Identification of vasoactive intestinal peptide, calcitonin, and catecholamines and assessment of their biologic activity. Cancer 40: 1526–1552
76. Tischler A S, Dayal Y, Balogh K et al. 1987 The distribution of immunoreactive chromogranins, S-100 protein, and vasoactive intestinal peptide in compound tumors of the adrenal medulla. Hum Pathol 18: 909–917
77. Sakaguchi N, Sano K, Ito M et al. 1996 A case of von Recklinghausen's disease with bilateral pheochromocytoma-malignant peripheral nerve sheath tumors of the adrenal and gastrointestinal autonomic nerve tumors. Am J Surg Pathol 20: 889–897
78. Brady S, Lechan R M, Schwaitzberg S D et al. 1997 Composite pheochromocytoma/ganglioneuroma of the adrenal gland associated with multiple endocrine neoplasia 2A. Case report with immunohistochemical analysis. Am J Surg Pathol 21: 102–108
79. Chetty R, Duhig J D 1993 Bilateral pheochromocytoma–ganglioneuroma of the adrenal in type I neurofibromatosis. Am J Surg Pathol 17: 837–841

80. Wieneke J A, Thompson L D R, Heffess C S 2001 Cortico-medullary mixed tumor of the adrenal gland. Ann Diagn Pathol 5: 304–308
81. Lack E E, Kim H, Reed K 1998 Pigmented ("black") extraadrenal paraganglioma. Am J Surg Pathol 22: 265–269
82. Brandi M L, Gagel R F, Angeli A et al. 2001 Guidelines for diagnosis and therapy of MEN type 1 and type 2. J Clin Endocrinol Metab 86: 5658–5671
83. Dannenberg H, Komminoth P, Dinjens W N M et al. 2003 Molecular genetic alterations in adrenal and extra-adrenal pheochromocytomas and paragangliomas. Endocr Pathol 2003; 4: 329–350
84. Powers J F, Brachold J M, Tischler A S 2003 Ret protein expression in adrenal medullary hyperplasia and pheochromocytoma. Endocr Pathol 4: 351–362
85. Carney J A, Sizemore G W, Tyce G M 1975 Bilateral adrenal medullary hyperplasia in multiple endocrine neoplasia, type 2. The precursor of bilateral pheochromocytoma. Mayo Clin Proc 50: 3–10
86. DeLellis R A, Wolfe H J, Gagel R F et al. 1976 Adrenal medullary hyperplasia. A morphometric analysis in patients with familial medullary thyroid carcinoma. Am J Pathol 83: 177–196
87. Carney J A, Sizemore G W, Sheps S G 1976 Adrenal medullary disease in multiple endocrine neoplasia, type 2. Pheochromocytoma and its precursors. Am J Clin Pathol 66: 279–290
88. Rudy F R, Bates R D, Cimorelli A J et al. 1980 Adrenal medullary hyperplasia: a clinicopathologic study of four cases. Hum Pathol 11: 50–657
89. Webb T A, Sheps S G, Carney J A 1980 Differences between sporadic pheochromocytoma and pheochromocytoma in multiple endocrine neoplasia, type 2. Am J Surg Pathol 4: 121–126
90. Carney J A, Go V L W, Sizemore G W et al. 1976 Alimentary-tract ganglioneuromatosis. A major component of the syndrome of multiple endocrine neoplasia, type 2b. N Engl J Med 295: 1287–1291
91. Carney J A, Go V L W, Gordon H et al. 1980 Familial pheochromocytoma and islet cell tumor of the pancreas. Am J Med 68: 515–521
92. Wheeler M H, Curley I R, Williams E D 1986 The association of neurofibromatosis, pheochromocytoma and somatostatin-rich duodenal carcinoid tumor. Surgery 100: 1163–1168
93. Melicow M M 1977 One hundred cases of pheochromocytoma (107 tumors) at the Columbia–Presbyterian Medical Center 1926–1976. A clinicopathological analysis. Cancer 40: 1987–2004
94. Van Heerden J A, Sheps S G, Hamberger B et al. 1982 Pheochromocytoma: current status and changing trends. Surgery 91: 367–373
95. Lack E E, Cubilla A L, Woodruff J M et al. 1980 Extra-adrenal paragangliomas of the retroperitoneum. A clinicopathologic study of 12 tumors. Am J Surg Pathol 4: 109–120
96. Gimenez-Roqueplo A, Favier J, Rustin P et al. 2003 Mutations in the SDHB gene are associated with extra-adrenal and/or malignant phaeochromocytomas. Cancer Res 63: 5615–5621
97. Thompson L D R 2002 Pheochromocytoma of the adrenal gland scaled score (PASS) to separate benign from malignant neoplasms. A clinicopathologic and immunophenotypic study of 100 cases. Am Surg Pathol 26: 551–566
98. Nativ O, Grant C S, Sheps S G et al. 1992 The clinical significance of nuclear DNA ploidy pattern in 184 patients with pheochromocytoma. Cancer 69: 2683–2687
99. Amberson J B, Vaughan E D Jr, Gray G F et al. 1987 Flow cytometric determination of nuclear DNA content in benign adrenal pheochromocytomas. Urology 30: 102–104
100. Clarke M R, Weyant R J, Watson C G et al. 1998 Prognostic markers in pheochromocytoma. Hum Pathol 28: 522–526
101. Travis W D, Oertel J E, Lack E E 1990 Miscellaneous tumors and tumefactive lesions of the adrenal gland. In: Lack E E (ed) Pathology of the adrenal glands. Churchill Livingstone, New York, p 351
102. Allison K H, Mann G N, Norwood T H et al. 2003 An unusual case of multiple giant myelolipomas: Clinical and pathogenetic features. Endocr Pathol 14: 93–100
103. Rosenberg S A, Diamond H D, Jaslowitz B et al. 1961 Lymphosarcoma: a review of 1269 cases. Medicine 40: 31–84
104. Richmond J, Sherman R S, Diamond H D et al. 1962 Renal lesions associated with malignant lymphomas. Am J Med 32: 184–207
105. Page D L, DeLellis R A, Hough A J 1986 Tumors of the adrenal. Atlas of tumor pathology, series 2, fascicle 23. Armed Forces Institute of Pathology, Washington, DC
106. Ohsawa M, Tomita Y, Hashimoto M et al. 1996 Malignant lymphoma of the adrenal gland: its possible correlation with the Epstein–Barr virus. Mod Pathol 9: 534–543
107. Plaut A 1962 Hemangiomas and related lesions of the adrenal gland. Virchows Arch [A] 335: 345–355
107a. Lau S K, Spagnolo D V, Weiss L M 2006 Schwannoma of the adrenal gland: report of two cases. Am J Surg Pathol 30: 630–634
108. Lack E E, Kozakewich H P W 1990 Adrenal neuroblastoma, ganglioneuroblastoma and related tumors. In: Lack E E (ed) Pathology of the adrenal gland. Churchill Livingstone, New York, p 277–309
109. Travis W D, Lack E E, Azumi N et al. 1990 Adenomatoid tumor of the adrenal gland with ultrastructure and immunohistochemical demonstration of a mesothelial origin. Arch Pathol Lab Med 114: 722–724
110. Isotalo P A, Keeney G L, Sebo T J et al. 2003 Adenomatoid tumor of the adrenal gland. A clinicopathologic study of five cases and review of the literature. Am J Surg Pathol 27: 969–977
111. Angeles-Angeles A, Reyes E, Muñoz-Fernandez K et al. 1997 Adenomatoid tumor of the right adrenal gland in a patient with AIDS. Endocrine Pathol 8: 59–64
112. Reed R J, Patrick J T 1967 Nodular hyperplasia of the adrenal cortical blastoma. Bull Tulane Univ Med Fac 26: 151–157
113. Wong T-W, Warner N E 1971 Ovarian thecal metaplasia in the adrenal gland. Arch Pathol 92: 319–328
114. Fidler W J 1977 Ovarian thecal metaplasia in adrenal glands. Am J Clin Pathol 67: 318–323
115. Carney J A 1987 Unusual tumefactive spindle cell lesions in the adrenal glands. Hum Pathol 18: 980–985
116. Orselli R C, Bassler T J 1973 Theca granulosa tumor arising in adrenal. Cancer 31: 474–477
117. Prévot S, Penna C, Imbert J-C et al. 1996 Solitary fibrous tumor of the adrenal gland. Mod Pathol 9: 1170–1174
118. Bongiovanni M, Viberti L, Giraudo G et al. 2000 Solitary fibrous tumour of the adrenal gland associated with pregnancy. Virchows Arch 437: 445–449
119. Wenig B M, Abbondanzo S L, Heffess C S 1994 Epithelioid angiosarcoma of the adrenal glands. A clinicopathologic study of nine cases with a discussion of the implications of finding epithelial-specific markers. Am J Surg Pathol 18: 62–73
120. Lack E E, Graham C W, Azumi N et al. 1991 Primary leiomyosarcoma of adrenal gland. Case report with immunohistochemical and ultrastructural study. Am J Surg Pathol 15: 899–905
121. Zetler P J, Filipenko J D, Bilbey J H et al. 1995 Primary adrenal leiomyosarcoma in a man with acquired immunodeficiency syndrome (AIDS). Further evidence for an increase in smooth muscle tumors related to Epstein–Barr infection in AIDS. Arch Pathol Lab Med 119: 1164–1167
122. Santonja C, Diaz M A, Dehner L P 1996 A unique dysembryonic neoplasm of the adrenal gland composed of nephrogenic rests in a child. Am J Surg Pathol 20: 118–124
123. Lau W K, Zincke H, Lohse C M et al. 2003 Contralateral adrenal metastasis of renal cell carcinoma: treatment, outcome and review. BJU Int 91: 775–779

胰腺内分泌肿瘤
Tumors of the endocrine pancreas

Gunter Klöppel 和 Philipp U. Heitz 著

回允中　李莹杰　译

命名和分类	1123	形态学特征	1125
病因和发病机制	1123	主要肿瘤类型	1128
流行病学	1124	鉴别诊断	1133
生物学行为	1125		

命名和分类

相对于较早的胰岛细胞瘤这一术语，本章更偏好于应用胰腺内分泌肿瘤这一术语。如果符合恶性标准，肿瘤应该称为恶性、转移性，或最好称为内分泌癌（表20.1）。新近公布的修订的 WHO 分类[1,2]，根据较早的建议[3,4]，考虑到了大多数的恶性指征（表20.2）。

由于分泌激素异常而伴有内分泌综合征的肿瘤被称为功能性或综合征性肿瘤，并且根据引起综合征的激素分类，例如，胰岛素瘤、胰高血糖素瘤、生长抑素瘤或血管活性肠多肽瘤（VIPoma）。这种分类也用于由异位到成人胰腺的激素而引起的伴有综合征的肿瘤，例如胃泌素、促肾上腺皮质激素（ACTH）、5-羟色胺或生长激素释放因子，即使根据免疫细胞化学检查证实这种肿瘤是由多种激素引起的。非功能性或非综合征性胰腺内分泌肿瘤包括不伴有特殊激素综合征的所有肿瘤，虽然多数细胞表达而且常常也分泌激素，例如胰多肽、神经紧张肽或降钙素[5]。

直径小于 0.5 cm 的肿瘤结节被称为微小腺瘤（microadenoma），这是肉眼发现肿瘤所需要的最低大小[6]。区分这种肿瘤与大的胰岛（300μm）可能有困难，但是通过免疫细胞化学检查可以区别开来，大的胰岛表现为不同类型内分泌细胞的不规则分布。微小腺瘤病（microadenomatosis）这一术语表示胰腺出现多发性微小腺瘤，可以见于 1 型多发性内分泌肿瘤形成（MEN 1；见下文 MEN 1 中的胰腺内分泌肿瘤）。

病因和发病机制

散发性胰腺内分泌肿瘤的病因尚不清楚。危险因素还未确定，但是可能有致癌剂参与，因为经过链佐星（streptozotocin）结合烟酰胺（nicotinamide）处理可以

表20.1　胰腺内分泌肿瘤分类[2]

高分化内分泌肿瘤

功能性
　胰岛素生成性（胰岛素瘤）
　胰高血糖素生成性（胰高血糖素瘤）
　生长抑素生成性（生长抑素瘤）
　胃泌素生成性（胃泌素瘤）
　VIP生成性（VIPoma瘤）
　其他
非功能性
　微小腺瘤（小于0.5 cm）
　其他

高分化内分泌癌

功能性
　胰岛素生成性（胰岛素瘤）
　胰高血糖素生成性（胰高血糖素瘤）
　生长抑素生成性（生长抑素瘤）
　胃泌素生成性（胃泌素瘤）
　VIP生成性（VIPoma）
　5-羟色胺生成性伴有类癌综合征
　ACTH生成性伴有Cushing综合征
非功能性

低分化内分泌癌-小细胞癌

混合性外分泌-内分泌癌

VIP，血管活性肠多肽；ACTH，促肾上腺皮质激素；
TNM分期系统没有用于胰腺内分泌肿瘤。

表20.2	胰腺内分泌肿瘤的临床病理学分类
高分化内分泌肿瘤	
良性行为：局限于胰腺，没有血管浸润，大小<2 cm，每10个高倍视野核分裂象≤2，每10个高倍视野Ki-67阳性细胞≤2%	
功能性：胰岛素瘤	
非功能性	
行为不能确定：局限于胰腺，大小≤2 cm，每10个高倍视野核分裂象>2，每10个高倍视野Ki-67阳性细胞>2%，或有血管浸润	
功能性：胃泌素瘤，胰岛素瘤，VIPoma，胰高血糖素瘤，生长抑素瘤或其他肿瘤[a]	
非功能性	
高分化内分泌癌	
低级别恶性肿瘤，伴有大体局部浸润和（或）转移	
功能性：胃泌素瘤，胰岛素瘤，胰高血糖素瘤，VIPoma，生长抑素瘤或其他肿瘤[a]	
非功能性	
低分化内分泌癌	
高级别恶性肿瘤（小到中等大小细胞）癌	

[a]Cushing（促肾上腺皮质激素），肢端肥大症，或巨人症（生长释放激素）等

诱导鼠发生胰腺内分泌肿瘤[7]。

有关散发性人类肿瘤的癌基因和分子基础知之甚少。在散发性胰腺内分泌肿瘤，癌基因的活性不是常见的事件。发生在胰腺外分泌或胃肠道癌的常见突变，例如p53，K-ras，p16，DPC4或DCC，在散发性胰腺内分泌肿瘤可能无法确定[8-13]。

每个肿瘤的基因组变化总数与肿瘤体积和疾病分期有关，说明在肿瘤进展期间，基因变化有积累[14]。这样，大的肿瘤和（或）恶性肿瘤，特别是转移性肿瘤，基因改变的数目比小的肿瘤和良性肿瘤多[14,15]。这些发现表明，肿瘤抑制通路和染色体不稳定性是与肿瘤进展有关的重要机制。发现基因组有扩增，特别是染色体4pq（17%的肿瘤），5q（25%），7pq（41%），9q（28%），12q（23%），14q（32%），17pq（31%）和20q（27%）；而基因组丢失发生在1p（21%），3p（19%），6q（28%），10pq（14%），11q（30%），Y（31%）和X（31%）[14-17]。1号染色体和11q丢失以及9q扩增似乎是早期事件[14]，而3p、6pq和10pq丢失以及5q、12q、18q和20q扩增与恶性行为有关[14,18,19]，4号和7号染色体扩增以及21q丢失与转移有关[15]。

胰岛素瘤的基因组改变数目比胰腺其他内分泌肿瘤少[15-17]，3p、6q和进一步的恶性相关性改变在胰岛素瘤罕见[18,19]。这些发现常常与胰岛素瘤的良性表型有关。在胃泌素瘤，发现只有少数染色体失衡，例如3p和18q21丢失，分别发生于33%和22%的胃泌素瘤病例[14,15,17]。有趣的是，18q丢失也常见于胃肠道内分泌肿瘤，说明这些肿瘤和胰腺胃泌素瘤可能有关。非功能性胰腺内分泌肿瘤一般具有比功能性肿瘤更多数量的染色体扩增和丢失。4号染色体扩增和6q丢失好像是早期事件，因为它们已经分别见于40%和50%的直径小于2 cm的非功能性肿瘤[14,15]。

散发性胰腺内分泌肿瘤还显示有MEN 1基因的体细胞突变[20]。这些突变和11q13杂合性丢失在不同类型的特发性胰腺内分泌肿瘤的发生频率不同，例如在胰岛素瘤分别是7.7%和39%，非功能性肿瘤（8%和75%），胃泌素瘤（37%和90%），胰高血糖素瘤（67%和75%）以及VIPoma（44%和80%）；对于所有类型肿瘤的平均值是MEN 1突变21%和11q13杂合性丢失68%。

伴有MEN 1、von Hippel-Lindau病（VHL）[21,22]和1型神经纤维瘤病（NF 1）的肿瘤的分子基础已经确立[23,24]。

遗传性胰腺内分泌肿瘤是MEN 1综合征最常见的组成部分。这是一个外显率非常高的具有遗传倾向的肿瘤（见下文MEN 1中胰腺内分泌肿瘤）。这种基因位点定位于染色体11q13（长约9 kb，包括10个外显子；转录物大约2 kb）[25]。MEN 1基因被确定为肿瘤抑制基因，它的蛋白被称为menin（660个氨基酸）[23]。一个等位基因遗传突变结合来源于正常父母的第二个等位基因体细胞缺失，能够导致它的灭活。到目前为止，已知在MEN 1基因的9个外显子（外显子2～10）中大约发生了300个突变。

流行病学

内分泌肿瘤大约占所有胰腺肿瘤的1%～2%[26]。然而，胰腺内分泌肿瘤的精确发病率仍不清楚。因为总的来说，它们的预后相当好，所以实际上其发病率可能低于流行病学发病率，据估计，后者低于1/100 000[27]。根据计算，胰岛素瘤的发病率大约为4例/百万人/年[28]。根据德国人长达10年的调查，在六千二百万居民中，每年大约有30例肿瘤被切除[29]。有人报告，尸检发现的没有症状的小肿瘤（直径通常小于1 cm）的发生率从0.5%到10%不等[30]。

胰腺内分泌综合征引起危及生命的代谢综合征。在手术切除肿瘤的大的系列研究中，功能性肿瘤一般占所有肿瘤的60%～85%，胰岛素瘤是最常见的类型（多达70%），其次为胃泌素瘤[26,31-33]。新近638例手术切除肿瘤的资料显示，功能性肿瘤只占60.3%[5]，或许是因为现代影像技术发现非功能性病变比较敏感所致。所有胰腺

内分泌肿瘤中，大约15%～25%可能伴有MEN 1。

对于整个胰腺内分泌肿瘤来说没有明显的性别差异，但是女性略占优势（女性大约55%，男性大约45%）。肿瘤可以出现在任何年龄，但是主要发生在30岁到60岁之间（见主要肿瘤类型）。

生物学行为

胰腺内分泌肿瘤是潜在的恶性肿瘤。然而，不同肿瘤类型之间的恶性率有所不同（表20.2）。在功能性肿瘤中，多数胰岛素瘤显示良性行为[27,34]。它们或许具有恶性潜能，但是由于早期表现出低血糖的症状，加之随后手术切除肿瘤中断了其自然病史，所以阻止了这种潜能的表达。相反，其他类型的功能性肿瘤或者属于不能确定行为的高分化肿瘤（大约占10%～15%），或者属于高分化癌（大约占85%～90%），但后者较为常见。绝大多数的非功能性肿瘤是高分化癌（约占90%～95%）。低分化内分泌癌不常见[5,30]。

一般来说，恶性转移性胰腺内分泌肿瘤是缓慢生长的肿瘤。从诊断时开始的生存期通常在2年到10年之间。在散发性转移性胃泌素瘤，来源于十二指肠的比来源于胰腺的生存期长[35,36]。

胰腺MEN 1相关性肿瘤很少发生转移，这不同于十二指肠[6,37,38]。尽管早期转移，总的来说十二指肠胃泌素瘤比胰腺胃泌素瘤的侵袭性低[35,39]。

许多神经内分泌肿瘤，包括胰腺肿瘤，表达生长抑素受体（SSTR1～5），可以通过放射自显影[40]，甚至是在经皮穿刺活检标本[41]，闪烁成像（octreoscan）[42]或免疫组织化学染色得以证实[43,44]。后一种方法有助于肿瘤定位和诊断，而且可能与治疗有关，因为出现生长抑素受体在某种程度上与生长抑素类似物奥曲肽（octreotide）抑制这些肿瘤释放激素和生长作用有关[42]。

形态学特征

大体

不同类型的胰腺肿瘤可能有不同的好发部位，胰头、胰体或胰尾（见下文）。某些类型的肿瘤（例如胃泌素瘤、生长抑素瘤，VIPoma）还可能发生在胰腺外（见主要类型肿瘤）。多数肿瘤境界清楚，但是缺乏明确的包膜，肿瘤质硬，或少数肿瘤质软（图20.1）。切面呈黄白色或棕粉色，或少数呈暗红色或囊性[45]。肿瘤直径在1 cm到5 cm之间。手术切除的胰岛素瘤和十二指肠

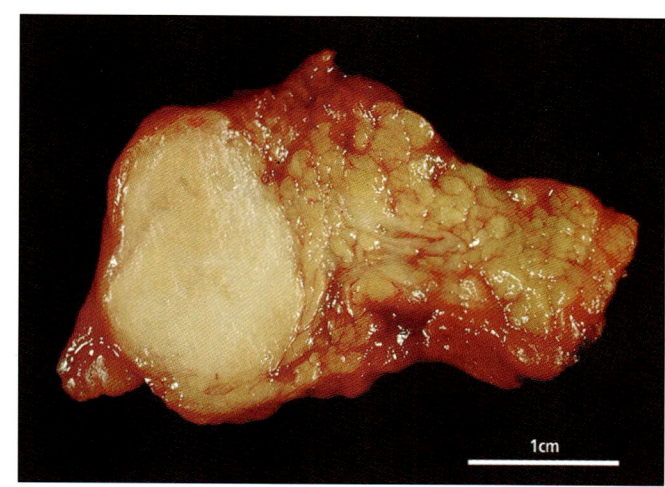

图20.1　胰腺内分泌肿瘤的大体表现。肿瘤与周围正常胰腺界限分明。

胃泌素瘤一般比其他功能性肿瘤小（小于2 cm），提示胰高血糖素瘤、VIPoma和其他功能活性的肿瘤需要达到相对大的体积才能产生临床症状。肿瘤大小与激素引起的症状的严重性无关。在少数病例，发现有一个以上的肿瘤。这种情况总是应该怀疑有无MEN 1的可能性，并及时进行分子遗传学分析。

较大或者位于胰腺大导管附近的胰腺内分泌肿瘤可能引起阻塞性慢性胰腺炎。在少数病例，还有伴有原发性慢性胰腺炎的报告[46]。

组织学

多数肿瘤为高分化。肿瘤由相对一致的立方细胞组成，胞浆嗜酸性，细颗粒状，核圆形或卵圆形，位于中心，常有显著的核仁。核分裂象通常罕见。偶尔，在大小相对一致的细胞群中可见细胞核大的细胞。少数病例可见黏液产物，PAS阳性小体，横纹肌样包涵体，透明细胞，富于脂质的空泡细胞，或有嗜酸细胞改变[47-52a]。可见两种主要的组织学类型：包括缎带样，脑回状和腺体结构在内的小梁状结构（图20.2），以及实性髓样结构（图20.3）。在同一个肿瘤内可以出现混合性形态。小梁状肿瘤核有极性，而伴有实性生长方式的肿瘤则没有。血管间质的数量和间质硬化程度不同，可以非常突出（图20.4）。玻璃样变的间质可以显示小灶状钙化。肿瘤边缘可见诸如胰岛和导管等正常胰腺成分陷入肿瘤组织[53]。

少数肿瘤细胞多形性显著，核深染，核分裂象常见，其组织学结构不定[53a]。这些低分化的肿瘤可能类似于胰腺腺癌或肺的小细胞癌，第一眼几乎辨认不出是内分泌肿瘤，需要进行免疫细胞化学检查以揭示其神经内分

形态学特征

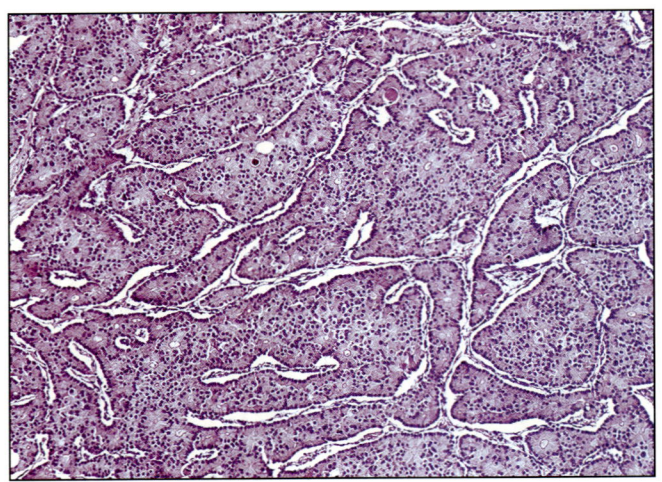

图20.2　胰腺内分泌肿瘤（胰岛素瘤）伴有小梁状核假腺样生长方式。

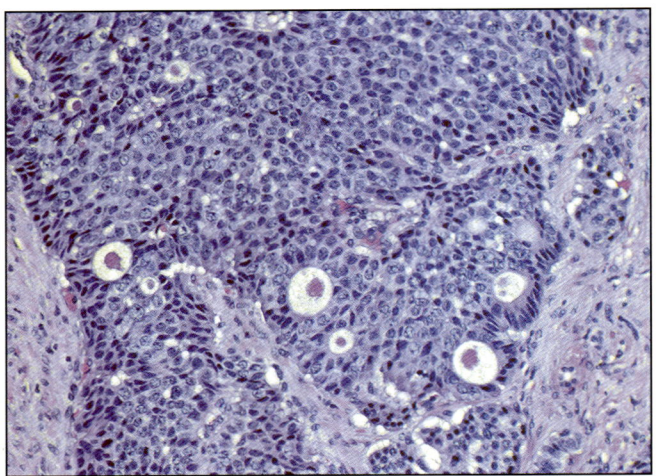

图20.3　胰腺内分泌肿瘤伴有实性生长方式和腺体结构。

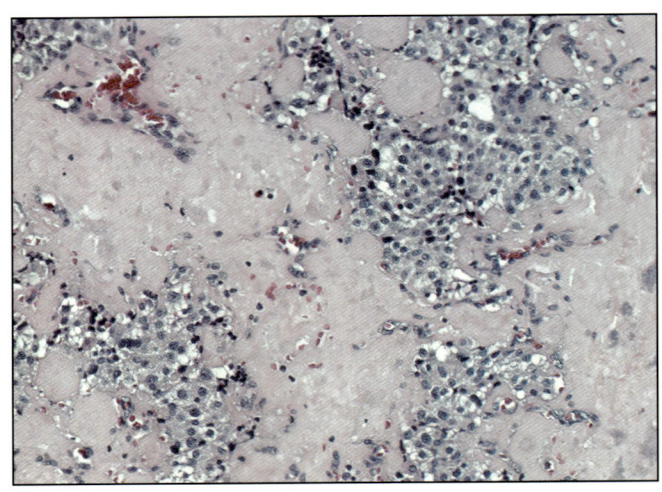

图20.4　胰腺内分泌肿瘤伴有实性生长方式和玻璃样变间质硬化。

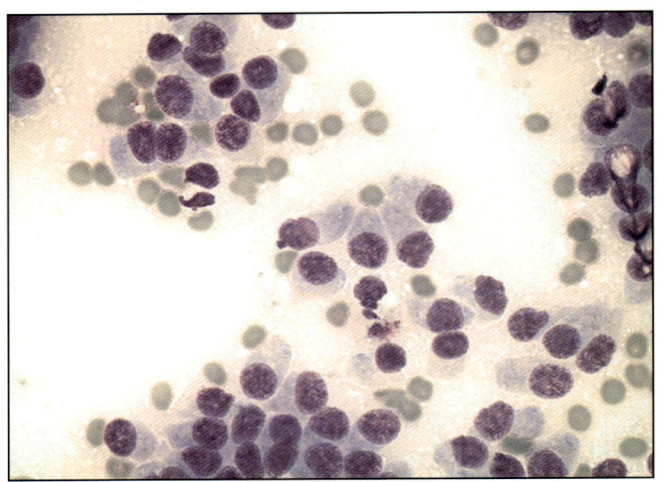

图20.5　胰腺内分泌肿瘤细针吸取细胞学，显示高分化的细胞伴有浆细胞样表现和颗粒状胞浆。

泌本质。它们常常显示核的p53免疫反应[26]。

从肿瘤的组织学表现不可能得出有关其功能状态或产生激素类型的结论。然而，存在3种例外情况：（1）含有沙粒体的腺体结构常常见于生长抑素瘤，通常发生在壶腹部[54,55]；（2）淀粉样物沉积提示胰岛素瘤（见下文，胰岛素瘤一节）；（3）透明细胞肿瘤提示von Hippel-Lindau综合征[56,57]。

细胞学

细针吸取（FNA）对于研究胰腺内分泌肿瘤是有用的。现在常常应用导向技术，包括CT以及经腹和内窥镜超声检查。从胰腺内分泌肿瘤吸出的标本非常富于细胞。低倍镜下，以疏松黏着的细胞为主。然而，在整个涂片中可见一些分散的细胞簇（由几个细胞到上百个细胞组成）[26,58]。细胞均匀一致，相对较小，核小圆形，通常偏心（图20.5）。胞浆常常稀少，呈灰粉色或颗粒状，从透明到致密不一。核的位置偏心以及胞浆的特征可能使得细胞呈浆细胞样表现。

免疫表型

神经内分泌表型标记物[59]，例如突触素（synaptophysin）[60]，嗜铬素（chromogranin）A、B和C[61,62]，HISL-19[63]，神经元特异性烯醇化酶（NSE）[64]，前蛋白转化酶（proprotein convertases）PC2和PC3[65]，网状淋巴细胞表位Leu-7[66]以及神经细胞黏连分子（NCAM或CD56）[67]显示胰腺内分泌肿瘤的神经内分泌分化，与激素产物无关。NSE是一种胞浆蛋白，而突触素属于小泡膜蛋白家族复合体，它还包括突触小泡蛋白（synaptobrevin），SV2和SNAP25[68]。这些标记物的染色强度与细胞内分泌颗粒含量或激素产物类型无关[69]（图20.6）。解释NSE的染色结果时应多加小心，因为这个标记物特异性低。相反，抗各种嗜铬素的抗体和抗血清，HISL-19，Leu-7，前白蛋白（pre-albumin），胰抑素（pancreastatin）[70]可以识别神经内分泌成分，它们的染色强度取决于细胞内分泌颗粒的含量（即分化程度）（图20.7）。嗜铬素A免疫反应与用于检测嗜银的银染色技术大致平行[62]。除了神经内分泌标记物以外，胰腺内分泌肿瘤角蛋白8、18和19染色阳性，少数情况下角蛋白7[71,72]和神经丝蛋白阳性[73]。

在光镜和电镜水平，多数功能性肿瘤的激素（细胞类型）特异性标记物染色有助于检测引起症状的激素[26,74]。然而，不管染色强度还是阳性细胞数目均与激素引起的症状的严重性无关。由于激素分泌异常和快速，或分泌不全，个别产生激素的胰腺肿瘤相应的肽的免疫细胞化学染色可能阴性，虽然原位杂交定位相关mRNA可能取得阳性结果[75,76]。如果应用一组抗胰腺和异位激素的抗血清染色，结果证明，许多肿瘤为多种激素性[26,74,77,78]。

PP是所有类型胰腺内分泌肿瘤的一种特别常见的成分[6,79,80]。一般来说，免疫染色阳性细胞的分布并不均匀，而且转移灶可能产生激素，而原发性肿瘤却没有发现激素。

电子显微镜检查

超微结构检查，可见许多胰腺内分泌肿瘤细胞以出现有界膜的电子致密分泌颗粒为特征[26]。分泌颗粒的数目，大小和形状取决于肿瘤细胞分化程度。在某些高分化的肿瘤，分泌颗粒的形态学可以提示包含的激素，因而有可能辨认细胞类型（图20.8）。多数肿瘤，特别是低分化的肿瘤[26]，肿瘤细胞的颗粒不具有诊断性，或者可能完全缺乏。

恶性标准

大体侵犯邻近器官以及淋巴结或肝转移是胰腺内分泌肿瘤肯定恶性的证据，而组织学分化差伴有高度细胞间变和具有小细胞癌的特征（图20.9）是诊断恶性很好的指征（表20.3）。然而，没有这些特征的胰腺内分泌肿瘤的生物学行为难以评估。此外，确定这样的肿瘤具有良性本质需要长期临床随访，因为直到手术切除原发性肿瘤之后多年才可能发生转移。近年来，为了确定几项指标的预后价值已经做了许多研究[81]。这些研究显示，在高分化肿瘤，肿瘤大小（＞2～3 cm），肿瘤坏死，淋巴管、血管或神经微小浸润（图20.10），高核分裂指数（即每10个高倍视野大于2个核分裂象）和高增生活性（即Ki-67/MIB-1指数＞2%和PCNA指数＞5%）（图20.11和图20.12），以及肿瘤生物学（胰岛素瘤还是非胰岛素瘤）与恶性行为密切相关（表20.2）[34,82-87]。新近发现角蛋白19与恶性有关[88]。DNA分析（倍体状态）[89]，

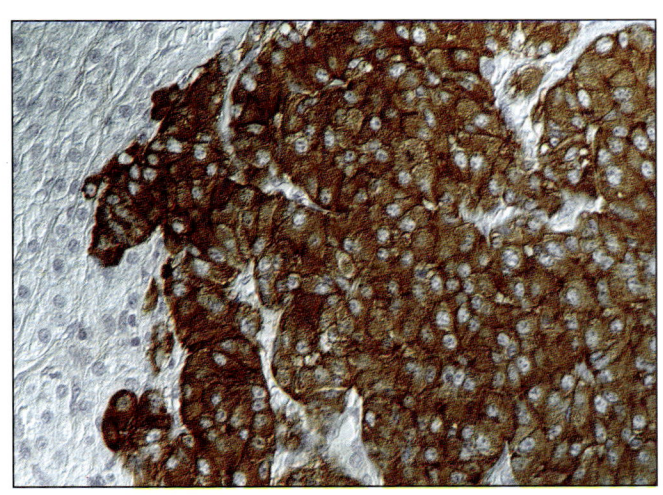

图20.6 胰腺内分泌肿瘤突触素免疫染色。实际上所有的肿瘤细胞均呈免疫反应。

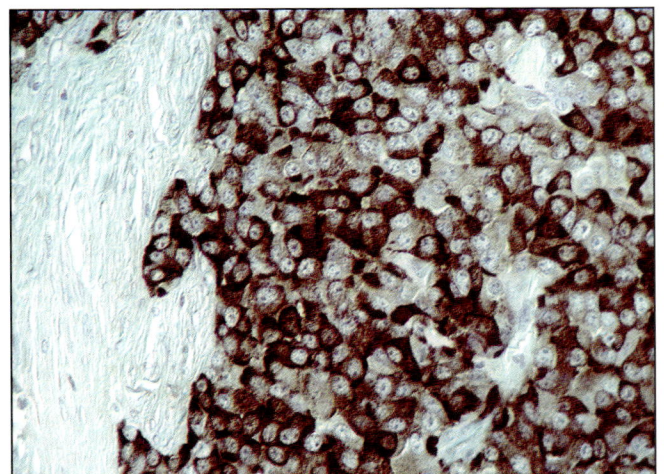

图20.7 与图20.6为同一肿瘤，嗜铬素A免疫染色。嗜铬素出现在多数但不是所有的肿瘤细胞。

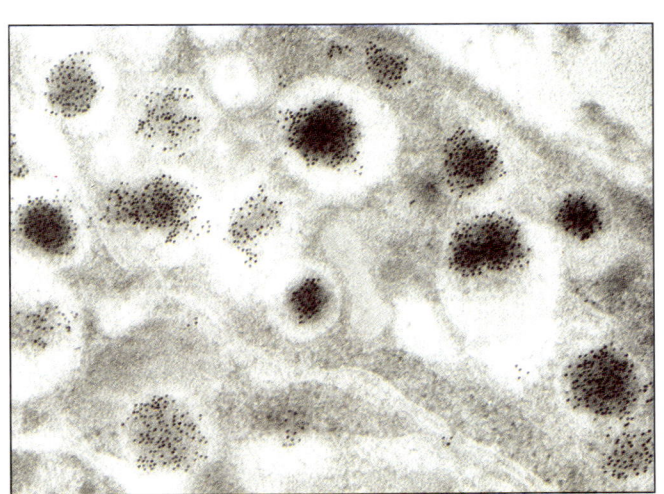

图20.8 胰岛素瘤的电子显微镜照片，显示有界膜的分泌颗粒。颗粒轴心圆形或呈结晶状，含有胰岛素。胰岛素免疫金反应。

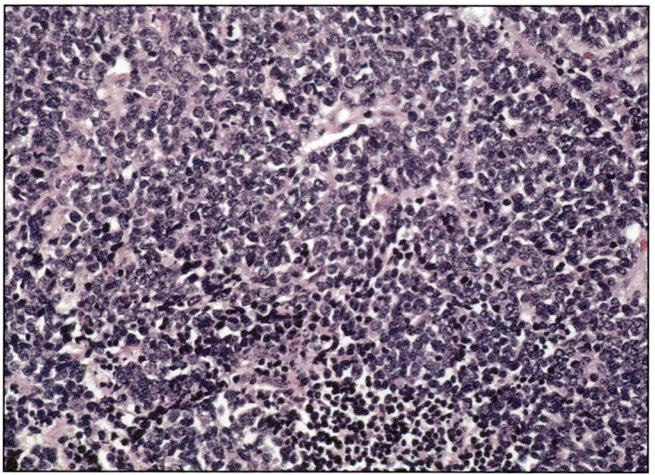

图20.9 低分化胰腺内分泌癌。

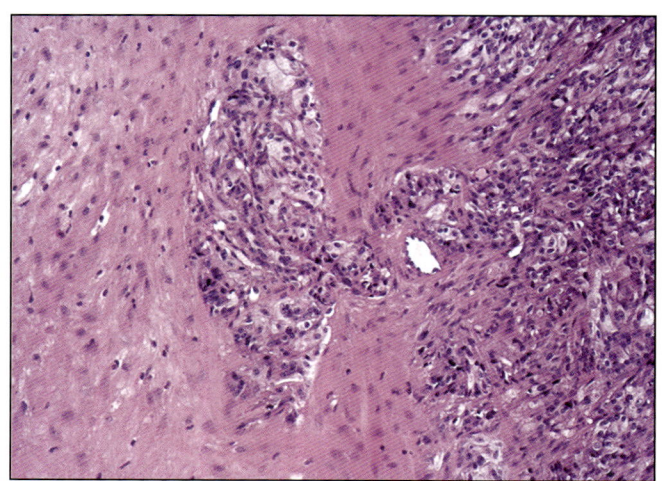

图20.10 胰腺内分泌癌侵犯淋巴管。

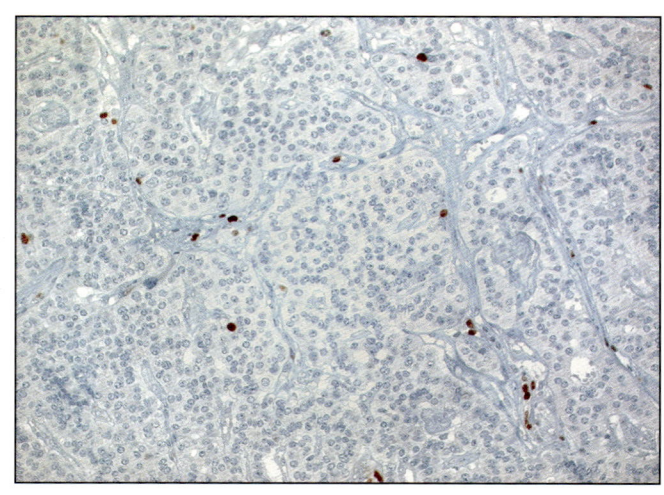

图20.11 胰岛素瘤伴有低增生活性（Ki-67/MIB-1＜2%）。

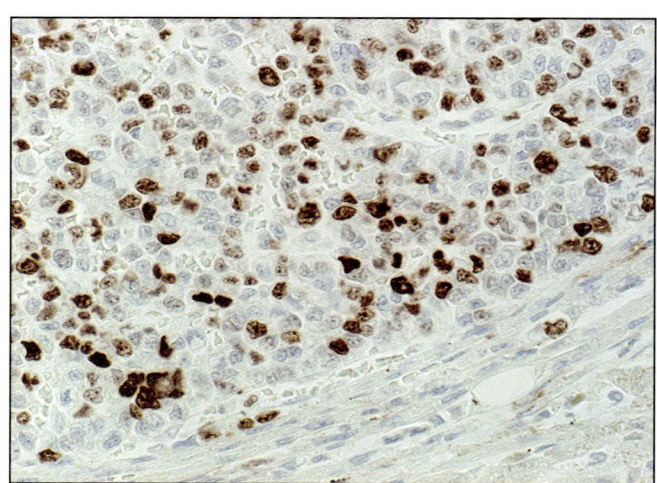

图20.12 胃泌素瘤伴有高增生活性（Ki-67/MIB-1＞2%）。

表20.3	高分化胰腺内分泌肿瘤预后不良（危险）因素[2]
转移	局部淋巴结，肝
大体浸润	邻近器官
肿瘤直径	2 cm 或 ＞2 cm
侵犯脉管	静脉，淋巴管
周围神经浸润	胰腺内神经
核分裂象	每10个高倍视野超过2个
增生指数（Ki-67）	超过2%
坏死	除了胰岛素瘤的功能性肿瘤

AgNORs 染色[90]以及癌基因产物表达[75]，孕激素受体（PR）[84,91]，层黏连蛋白受体（laminin receptor）[83]和α链人绒毛膜促性腺激素（hCG-α）[90,92]预后价值较小[81]。目前还没有可以预测肿瘤生物学行为的分子生物学资料[93]。

主要肿瘤类型 Special tumor types

胰岛素瘤 Insulinomas

胰岛素瘤病人表现为高胰岛素血症性低血糖症状，即 Whipple 三征，由精神错乱、虚弱疲乏和癫痫发作组成，不进食物时血糖水平低于 50 mg/dl，进食葡萄糖后症状立即缓解[94]。多数病人体重增加。对于占优势的血浆葡萄糖浓度来说，血清胰岛素水平不恰当的升高，而且前胰岛素通常比正常所见比率要高。胰岛素瘤还可以发生在非胰岛素依赖性糖尿病病人的胰腺，而且可能导致症状的改善[95]。

胰岛素瘤是最常见的功能性胰腺内分泌肿瘤，诊断时年龄范围广泛，但是 15 岁之前非常少见[96,97]。高峰发病年龄在 40 到 60 岁之间。

伴有持续性高胰岛素血症性低血糖症的新生儿和婴儿，最常患有由内分泌胰腺 β 细胞钾离子通道失效引起的胰岛素分泌异常，这是由于钾离子通道各种蛋白点突变引起的[98]。形态学上，可见弥漫性或局灶性胰岛母细胞增生症（nesidioblastosis）[99-102]。成人也可能发生弥漫性胰岛母细胞增生症，但非常罕见[103-107]。

实际上，所有的胰岛素瘤均发生于胰腺。它们几乎均匀地分布于整个胰腺，或附着于胰腺之上[108]。其令人信服的证据是胰岛素产物和低血糖症状的位于胰腺外的神经内分泌肿瘤的报告罕见。到目前为止，这样的肿瘤在十二指肠[109]、回肠[110,111]、肺[112]、宫颈[113]和卵巢[114]已有报告。

85%到99%的胰岛素瘤是良性孤立性肿瘤，发现时直径小于2.5 cm[34,108,115]（图20.13）。证明是恶性的胰岛素瘤直径通常大于3 cm，大约1/3的病例在诊断时已有转移[108]。2%～7%的病人同时或异时发生多发性胰岛素瘤，多发性神经内分泌肿瘤1型（multiple endocrine neoplasia type 1，MEN 1）相关性胰岛素瘤占6%[34]。

免疫组化检查显示，所有的胰岛素瘤均可发现产生胰岛素和前胰岛素的细胞。胰岛素（在细胞的基底）和前胰岛素（在核的周围区域）强阳性通常见于伴有小梁状生长方式的高分化胰岛素瘤[116]（图20.14和图20.15）。相反，伴有实性生长方式的胰岛素瘤，前胰岛素和胰岛素可能仅仅显示微弱反应和弥漫性胞浆分布[114]。胰岛素瘤还常常表达胰岛淀粉样多肽（islet amyloid polypeptide，IAPP）[117,118]，这些IAPP肿瘤大约5%间质中可能有淀粉样物沉积[119]。正常情况下胰腺β细胞释放IAPP连同胰岛素；IAPP又叫支链淀粉（amylin）。恶性胰腺肿瘤大量分泌IAPP已有报告[120]。胰岛素瘤还可能表达胰岛素以外的激素，不管是良性或恶性[34,74]。

电子显微镜检查显示，伴有典型β颗粒的颗粒形成完好的细胞（图20.8），伴有非典型性，有时是多形性的细胞，以及几乎没有颗粒的细胞均有描述。此外，可能见到伴有典型α颗粒和PP颗粒的细胞。根据肿瘤性β细胞不同的超微结构特征，提出了胰岛素瘤的三种工作分类[121-123]，在某种程度上可能与这些胰岛素瘤分泌的前胰岛素的比例有关（例如与前胰岛素与胰岛素不同程度的转化有关）。

在伴有胰岛素瘤的非肿瘤性内分泌胰腺的病人，胰岛成分胰岛素免疫反应可能降低。这可能是由于正常β细胞对于长期低血糖的适应性反应[124]。

胃泌素瘤 Gastrinomas

胃泌素瘤分泌异常的胃泌素引起Zollinger-Ellison综合征（ZES）。ZES以胃酸分泌过多、难治性消化性溃疡以及偶尔有严重的腹泻为特征[125,126]。60%到70%的ZES病人此综合征为孤立性疾病（散发性ZES）；其余的ZES病人是MEN 1综合征的一部分[6,26,127]。假Zollinger-Ellison综合征（pseudo-ZES）（也叫1型ZES，与由胃

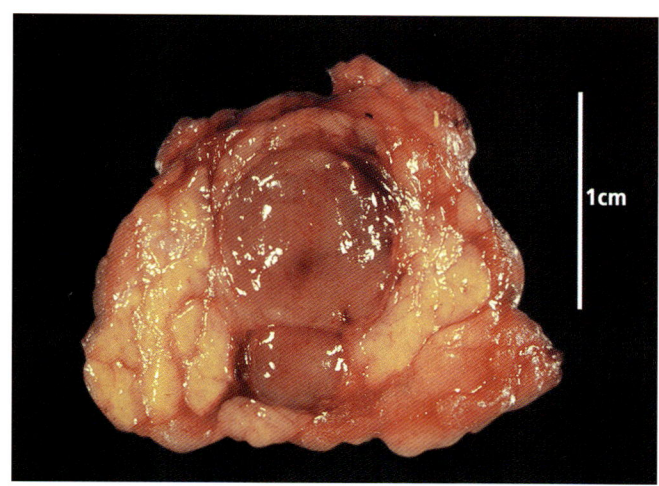

图20.13 小的胰岛素瘤的大体表现，切面呈红棕色。

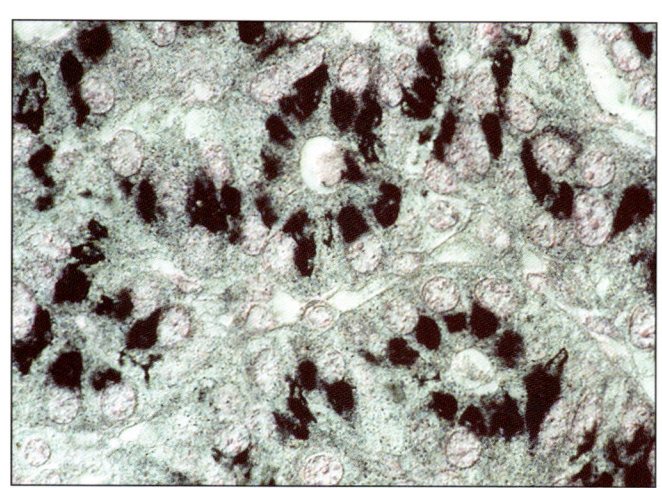

图20.14 小梁状胰岛素瘤，显示细胞核周围Golgi器区域前胰岛素免疫反应。

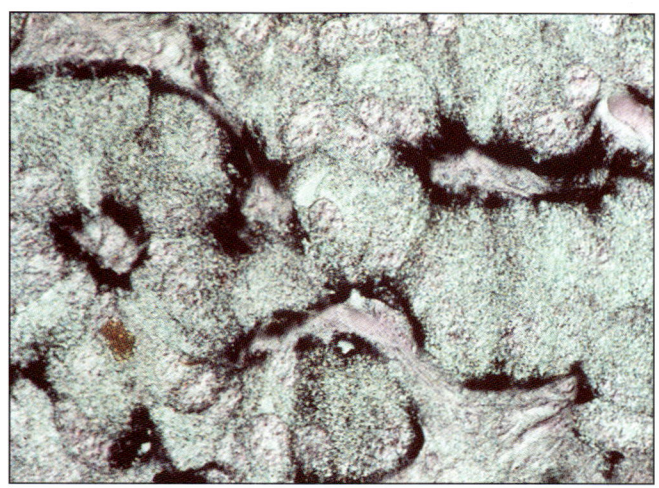

图20.15 小梁状胰岛素瘤，显示肿瘤细胞分泌部位的胰岛素免疫反应。

泌素瘤引起的2型ZES不同）这一术语用于伴有类似于ZES症状的综合征，可能是由胃窦G细胞功能亢进和G细胞增生引起的[128,129]。事实上，近些年来这个综合征已经不再描述，有人提出了它是否存在的疑问。在罕见的情况下，可能发现复发性和难治性消化性溃疡综合征与并不产生和分泌胃泌素的胰腺内分泌肿瘤有关[130]。引起这种病人消化性溃疡的因素尚未确定[131]。

胃泌素瘤的发病率仅次于胰岛素瘤，而且最常见的是恶性胃泌素瘤。胃泌素瘤的发病高峰年龄在40岁和50岁之间；儿童（5～15岁）很少受累[125]。

大约50%～70%的伴有散发性ZES的胃泌素瘤发生在胰腺，特别是胰头（图20.16），其余的主要见于十二指肠[35]。在解剖学部位上，胃泌素瘤主要位于胰头以及十二指肠的第一和第二部分，这个区域被称为胃泌素瘤三角（gastrinoma triangle）[132]。胃泌素瘤少见的部位是胃[133]、空肠[134,135]、胆道、肝[132]和肾[136]。含有足够数量的，伴有胃泌素产物的活性内分泌细胞的卵巢或胰腺黏液性囊性肿瘤，也可以引起ZES，但不常见[137,138]。

存在于十二指肠的胃泌素瘤大约90%伴有MEN 1综合征[38]。这些肿瘤通常小于1 cm，多中心性，发生于胃泌素细胞前体病变[139]。因为肿瘤较小，所以难以发现，如同散发性十二指肠胃泌素瘤一样（图20.17）。伴有MEN 1的胰腺胃泌素瘤罕见[6,140]，虽然这些病人的胰腺通常含有多发性内分泌肿瘤。然而，这些肿瘤实际上从不产生可以检测到的胃泌素[6,38]。

发生在胰腺或十二指肠的散发性胃泌素瘤主要是孤立性肿瘤。在胰腺，肿瘤直径通常为2 cm或大于2 cm（图20.16），而在十二指肠，肿瘤直径多数小于1 cm[35,141-143]（图20.18）。胰腺胃泌素瘤病人大约60%转移到局部淋巴结[144]，而在十二指肠胃泌素瘤则有更高的转移率[35]。十二指肠胃泌素瘤在非常小的时候即可转移，它们可以引起十二指肠周围淋巴结转移，转移性肿瘤大于原发性肿瘤。因此有人提出，所谓的胰腺周围和十二指肠周围淋巴结胃泌素瘤可能是来自十二指肠微小胃泌素瘤的转移，而不是真正的原发性肿瘤，十二指肠微小胃泌素瘤在手术时多被漏掉[39,145,146]。

与淋巴结转移的分布相比，十二指肠胃泌素瘤发生肝转移的比率似乎比胰腺胃泌素瘤小，不管是散发性还是MEN 1相关性肿瘤[39,144,145]。因而，十二指肠胃泌素瘤病人的10年生存率（84%）高于胰腺胃泌素瘤病人（57%）[36,147]。

组织学检查，胃泌素瘤最常显示小梁状或假腺体结构（图20.18）。免疫细胞化学检查，几乎所有的肿瘤均可以证实含有胃泌素（图20.19）[26,74]。大约50%的胃

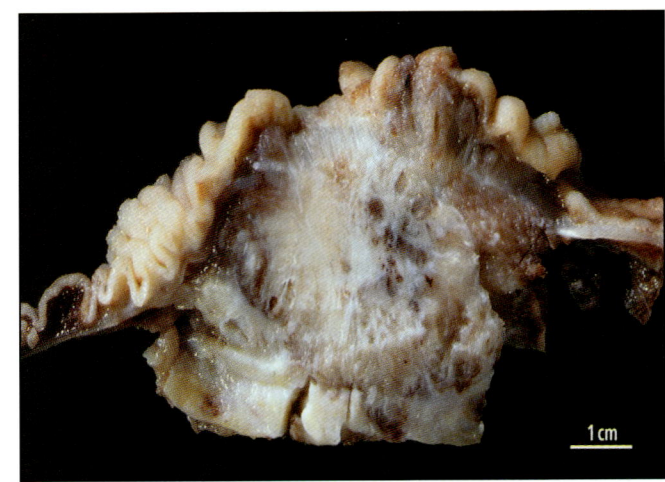

图20.16 胰头境界不清的恶性胃泌素瘤，侵犯十二指肠壁。病人患有Zollinger-Ellison综合征。

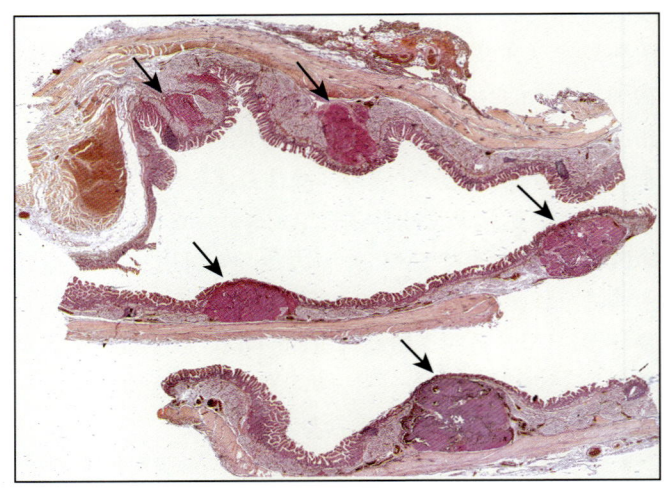

图20.17 十二指肠小的（<0.5 cm）黏膜下胃泌素瘤，来自一个患有多发性内分泌肿瘤1型相关性Zollinger-Ellison综合征的病人。

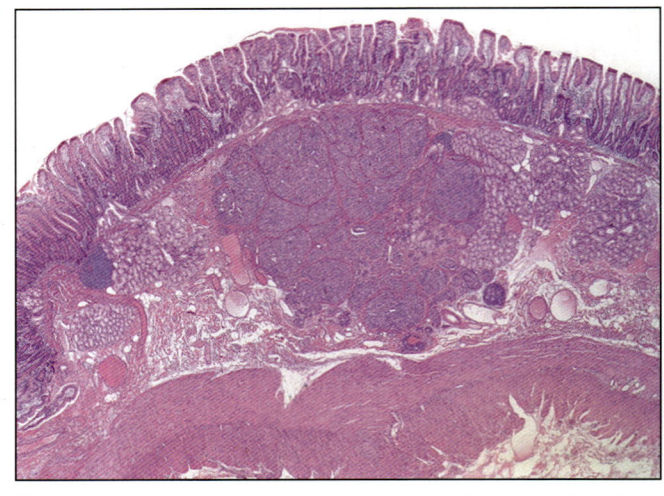

图20.18 多发性内分泌肿瘤1型：十二指肠胃泌素瘤位于十二指肠黏膜下。

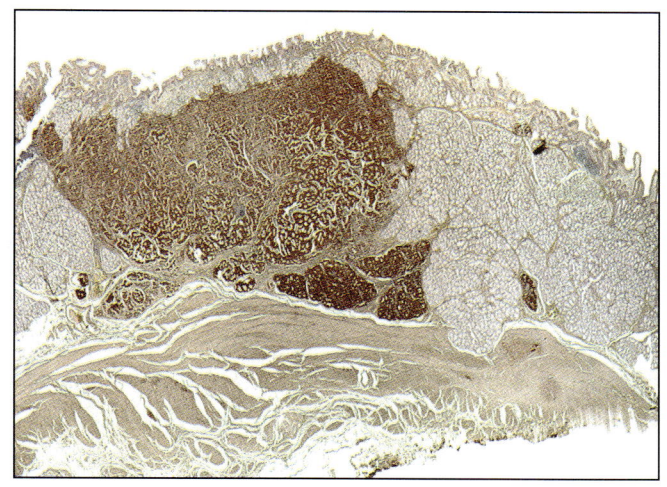

图20.19 多发性内分泌肿瘤1型：十二指肠黏膜下胃泌素瘤，胃泌素免疫反应。

泌素瘤为多种激素性，除了胃泌素外，还含有PP、胰高血糖素和（或）胰岛素。

反复描述胃泌素瘤病人的非肿瘤性胰腺有胰岛增生和胰岛母细胞增生症，但是这些所见并没有能够被形态学证实[148]。然而，新近形态测量显示胰头腹面派生部位PP细胞增生[149]。迄今尚未完全弄清高胃泌素血症对于这些变化具有什么样的影响。然而，在胃黏膜持续的高胃泌素血症可引起壁细胞增生伴有黏膜皱襞增厚和胃酸分泌亢进。此外，胃底黏膜肠嗜铬样（enterochromaffin-like，ECL）细胞数目增加[150-152]。众所周知，胃底ECL细胞瘤是患有恶性贫血伴有慢性A型胃炎病人的并发症，在散发性ZES病人好像非常少见[26]。然而，在ZES和MEN 1病人已有报告。在这些情况下，它们可能是MEN 1综合征的另外一种肿瘤性表现，而不仅仅是胃泌素营养作用的结果[150,153]。

胰高血糖素瘤　Glucagonomas

这个综合征包括称为松解坏死性游走性红斑（necrolytic migratory erythema）的皮疹，体重减轻，抑郁症和倾向于发生深静脉血栓形成[154]。认为这种症状是反映了胰高血糖素血清浓度明显升高的分解代谢作用[155]。在胰腺外产生胰高血糖素的肿瘤中，这种综合征尚无令人信服的病例描述。

功能活跃的胰高血糖素瘤相当大（直径从2 cm到35 cm），常常发生在胰腺的远端部分或附着于胰腺，多数为恶性[154]。含有产生胰高血糖素的细胞，但是不伴有胰高血糖素瘤综合征的肿瘤常常是良性的，通常为小的肿瘤，在尸检或在MEN 1病人的胰腺发现[6,156,157]。

免疫细胞化学染色，胰高血糖素瘤常常显示胰高血糖素染色呈弱阳性，对于由前胰高血糖素（proglucagon）衍化而来的肽类（肠高血糖素，glicentin；胰高血糖素样肽1和2，glucagons-like peptides 1 and 2）也有反应[158]。此外，常常可见许多PP细胞。电子显微镜检查，在功能上静止的产生胰高血糖素的肿瘤中，可能见到容易辨认的A细胞颗粒，而非典型性分泌颗粒主要见于伴有综合征的胰高血糖素瘤[26]。

血管活性肠多肽瘤　Vipomas

血管活性肠多肽瘤（vipomas）异常分泌血管活性肠多肽（vasoactive intestinal polypeptide，VIP）引起水样泻、低钾血症和胃酸缺乏（watery diarrhea, hypokalemia, and achlorhydria，WDHA）综合征，也叫Verner-Morrison综合征[159]。虽然WDHA综合征很可能是由VIP介导的，但是其他激素样物质也可能参与，例如甲硫氨基酸组胺酸肽（peptide histidine methionine）[26]。

在成人，绝大多数vipomas来源于胰腺。某些罕见的产生VIP的嗜铬细胞瘤[160,161]和肠内分泌肿瘤则是例外[162]。在儿童，据报告WDHA综合征还与分泌VIP的神经节细胞瘤和神经节母细胞瘤有关[163,164]。WDHA综合征还起因于胰岛增生[165,166]。这些报告难以解释，因为在正常成人胰腺VIP仅存在于自主神经，而不存在于胰岛细胞中。

胰腺vipomas通常为孤立性大肿瘤（平均4～5 cm），常常发生在胰尾（大约50%），至少80%的病例为恶性[26,162]。免疫细胞化学检查，在保存完好的常规福尔马林固定的组织中或在干冰和汽化固定（vapor-fixed）的标本中，可以见到VIP[74,162]。固定不满意的组织VIP反应性可能丧失。有时，应用原位杂交技术有助于寻找mRNA。产生VIP的肿瘤细胞还有PHM-27表达，PHM-27是一种与VIP共有大的前体肽的蛋白（prepro-VIP/PHM-27）[167]。此外，它们常常表达PP[74,167]，而且不常表达降钙素（calcitonin）和神经紧张素（neurotensin）[167]。

生长抑素瘤　Somatostatinomas

胰腺生长抑素瘤病人，可能患有被认为是由于生长抑素作用广泛受到抑制而引起的综合征。这种综合征由糖尿病、胆石症、脂肪痢、消化不良、胃酸过少、以及偶尔伴贫血所组成[168,169]。

胰腺生长抑素瘤非常罕见。这种肿瘤实际上总是恶性的[26,170]，偶尔可能含有沙粒体性钙化[169]。

胰腺外生长抑素瘤最常发生在十二指肠的第二部分，常常在Vater乳头的部位或非常接近Vater乳头，有时伴有NF 1（von Recklinghausen病）和嗜铬细胞瘤[142]。

产生异位激素或多种激素的功能性肿瘤
Functioning tumors producing ectopic hormones or multiple hormones

胰腺内分泌肿瘤不常见的和由异位激素引起的综合征是由 ACTH（Cushing 综合征）[171,172]、5-羟色胺（类癌综合征）[173]、生长激素释放因子（肢端肥大症，acromegaly）[174-176]、酷似副肿瘤性高钙血症（PTH）作用的副肿瘤性高钙血症相关蛋白（PTHrP）[177,178] 和降钙素（50% 的病例腹泻）[179] 等产物引起的。

由异位激素引起的伴有综合征的多数肿瘤是恶性肿瘤，而且是较大的肿瘤。它们的组织学结构通常与其他胰腺内分泌肿瘤相同。例外的是，某些肿瘤产生生长激素释放因子，引起肢端肥大症，这些肿瘤可能显示独特的副神经节瘤样微小分叶状结构[180] 和梭形细胞[174]。

不同的激素综合征共同存在或从一种综合征转变成另外一种综合征均有描述，但是似乎并不常见。已知的联合存在的综合征是 ZES 和高钙血症[181]，ZES 和 Cushing 综合征[182-184]，低血糖和 Cushing 综合征[185]，以及低血糖伴有 ZES[186]，或类癌综合征[187,188]。在某些罕见的情况下，胰高血糖素瘤综合征在细胞生长抑制（cytostatic）治疗后出现低血糖综合征[189]。应该强调的是，许多伴有联合临床综合征的病人显示患有 MEN 1，特别是 ZES 和 Cushing 综合征[26]。

非功能性肿瘤　Non-functioning tumors

非功能性肿瘤的临床症状（腹痛、黄疸、体重减轻）明显，或者是由于体积较大侵犯邻近器官，或者是由于发生转移。少数病人可以表现为胰腺炎[190]，或伴有血液学改变，例如全血细胞减少[191] 或皮肤嗜酸性粒细胞浸润[192]。缺乏激素引起的综合征有各种各样的解释，即使是在出现免疫细胞化学可以检测到激素的病人：（1）产生和释放激素的量可能太低以致不能引起综合征；（2）虽然肿瘤合成和分泌的主要激素过多，但不引起任何特殊的临床征象，例如胰多肽瘤（PPomas）和神经紧张素瘤（neurotensinomas）[79,193]；（3）肿瘤分泌没有功能活性的前体激素或激素样物质；或（4）肿瘤的激素产物尚未被认识。

手术切除的非功能性肿瘤直径多数 > 5 cm，并且显示恶性行为[26,194]。其症状或与转移的表现有关，或与肿瘤大小和部位有关。

免疫细胞化学检查，大约 10% 的肿瘤是无颗粒性，仅有稀疏的激素阳性细胞[74]。这些肿瘤的无颗粒性反映在嗜铬素蛋白（chromogranin）染色非常弱，而突触素（synaptophysin）保持阳性。在嗜铬素蛋白 A 反应阳性的非功能性肿瘤，PP 常常阳性。因为有时 PP 是主要的激素，所以这些肿瘤被称为 PPomas[79]，虽然它们不是一种临床上的疾病。在富于胰多肽（PP）细胞的胰腺外肿瘤中，主要是十二指肠的节细胞性副神经节瘤[195]（见第 28 章）和某些直肠神经内分泌肿瘤[196]。免疫细胞化学染色显示少数非功能性恶性肿瘤有 5-羟色胺（serotonin）产物[173,197,198]。被描述为神经紧张素瘤（neurotensinomas）[170,193]、降钙素瘤（calcitoninomas）[171] 或产生蛙皮素（bombesin）的肿瘤[199] 或者激素不活跃，或者伴有难以与这些激素作用联系起来的综合征。

发生在 MEN 1 的胰腺内分泌肿瘤
Pancreatic endocrine tumors in MEN 1

胰腺肿瘤是累及甲状旁腺（80%~98% 的病人），垂体前部（9%~40%）和十二指肠（40%~85%）肿瘤谱系的一部分[200,201]，偶尔也是胃、回肠、肺或胸腺肿瘤的一部分[153,202,203]。

发生在 MEN 1 的胰腺病变的显著特征是，与一个或几个大肿瘤（直径 > 0.5 cm）相伴的弥漫性微小腺瘤病（microadenomatosis）[6,200,204,204a]。组织学检查，多数小的肿瘤显示特征性的小梁状结构，而且许多肿瘤均有结缔组织包膜（图 20.20）。这些肿瘤共同的所见是多激素性（multihormonality），通常以一种激素为主[204a]。最常见的是胰高血糖素瘤和 PPomas，其次为胰岛素瘤[6]。因此，推荐在 MEN 1 病人中筛查血清胰多肽（PP）激素[205]，虽然随后的资料提示激素类型分布广泛[206]。在伴有低血糖的 MEN 1 病人中注意到，尽管存在多个肿瘤，但通常只有一个大的肿瘤产生胰岛素。切除这个肿瘤能够缓解病人的低血糖综合征[6,34]。大约 60% 的 MEN 1 病人伴有 ZES，这些病人的胰腺胃泌素瘤非常少见，尽管这些病人的胰腺可能布满产生其他激素的不同大小的

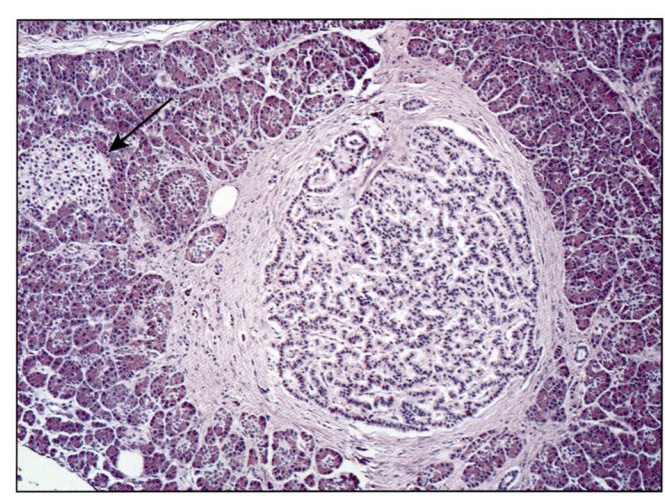

图 20.20　MEN 1 病人胰腺小的内分泌微小腺瘤。注意肿瘤的小梁状结构和结缔组织包膜。

肿瘤[38]。这些病人的胃泌素瘤主要位于十二指肠的近端，直径通常 < 1 cm，而且为多中心性（见上文胃泌素瘤一节）。在 MEN 1 的情况下，发生 WDHA 综合征[6,167]，胰高血糖素瘤综合征[207,208]，或由于肿瘤分泌生长激素释放因子而引起肢端肥大症[174,175]的非常罕见。

混合性内分泌-外分泌肿瘤
Mixed endocrine-exocrine tumors

胰腺真正的混合性内分泌-外分泌肿瘤（亦即导管内分泌或腺泡内分泌肿瘤，ductal endocrine or acinar-endocrine tumors）非常罕见，它的两种成分界限分明[26,209-211]。有证据支持肿瘤的内分泌-外分泌本质存在于原发性肿瘤及其转移性肿瘤，超微结构发现含有激素颗粒和含有酶原或黏液颗粒两种细胞。

内分泌肿瘤中含有正常导管（所谓的小管胰岛瘤，ductuloinsular tumors），或胰腺导管腺癌的肿瘤性腺体附着有内分泌细胞，均不能作为这种肿瘤在本质上是真正的内分泌-外分泌肿瘤的证据[53,211]。

鉴别诊断

大多数胰腺内分泌肿瘤通过常规组织学检查可能容易诊断。然而，有时候在与慢性胰腺炎的胰岛集聚、某些胰腺外分泌肿瘤、混合性内分泌-外分泌肿瘤、非上皮性肿瘤或继发性浸润胰腺的肿瘤进行鉴别时，可能出现问题（表 20.4）。

显著的分叶状胰岛集聚（lobular islet aggregation）可能见于慢性胰腺炎。它的特征是在纤维组织中有胰岛集聚。单个的胰岛可能增大，但是结构正常，包括分布间隙规律的 4 种类型的细胞。

可能与神经内分泌肿瘤混淆的外分泌肿瘤是实性假乳头状肿瘤、腺泡细胞癌、胰腺母细胞瘤、低分化导管腺癌、透明细胞癌和嗜酸细胞癌。这些病变已在第 11 章详细描述。简而言之，免疫细胞化学检查可以识别实性假乳头状肿瘤（solid pseudopapillary tumor），波形蛋白和 NSE 弥漫阳性，β-catenin 核阳性[212]，形成对比的是角蛋白，突触素和嗜铬素蛋白反应非常弱或为阴性[213]。腺泡细胞癌（acinar cell carcinomas）和胰腺母细胞瘤（pancreatoblastoma）胰腺酶染色阳性（例如胰蛋白酶，脂酶和其他），在某些情况下，甲胎蛋白阳性；低分化导管腺癌（poorly differentiated ductal adenocarcinomas）包括透明细胞癌（clear cell carcinoma）和嗜酸细胞癌（oncocytic carcinoma）显示黏液，癌胚抗原（CEA）和 CA19.9 局灶性表达[214]。腺泡细胞癌和胰腺母细胞瘤可以出现少数内分泌细胞，导致神经内分泌标记物有散在的表达。

真正的混合性腺泡-内分泌或导管-内分泌癌罕见[210,211]。内分泌细胞成分至少应该占整个细胞群的 30%[26]。不管内分泌细胞的量，混合性外分泌-内分泌肿瘤（mixed exocrine-endocrine tumors）的预后是由外分泌成分决定的。某些高分化导管腺癌可能伴有明显的散在的内分泌细胞或胰岛细胞集聚。然而，这样的肿瘤不应该认为是真正的混合性腺泡-内分泌癌，因为这种肿瘤转移仅见于肿瘤的外分泌成分[210]。

可能与内分泌肿瘤混淆的非上皮性肿瘤是上皮样胃肠道间质瘤（epithelioid gastrointestinal stromal tumors）和外周神经外胚层肿瘤（peripheral neuroectodermal tumors），特别是在小的活检标本中，两者均以独特的免疫表型为特征（见第 8 章和第 27 章）。

可能酷似内分泌肿瘤的胰腺转移性肿瘤包括来自肾细胞癌，小细胞肺癌和回肠内分泌肿瘤的转移性肿瘤。来自回肠内分泌肿瘤的胰腺转移可以通过其P物质（substance P）和 5-羟色胺（serotonin）的一致阳性进行分类（除了神经内分泌标记物的表达以外）。肾透明细胞癌缺乏神经内分泌标记物，但是显示嗜铬素蛋白强阳性染色，而且常常与波形蛋白和 MUC1 共存。小细胞肺癌转移在形态学上不能与胰腺原发性（神经内分泌）小细胞癌鉴别[26]，但与多数胰腺神经内分泌肿瘤不同，TTF-1 免疫染色阳性[216]。

表20.4	胰腺内分泌肿瘤的鉴别诊断					
	I-CP	AC	PB	SPT	DAC	MET
年龄	所有年龄	>50岁	<8岁	10~50岁	>50岁	所有年龄
性别	两性	男性>女性	两性	女性	两性	两性
组织学	分叶状胰岛集聚	腺泡-小梁状	腺泡状，鳞状巢	假乳头状，出血性-囊性	小管状，腺管状	实性
标记物	胰岛细胞激素，神经内分泌标记物，弥漫性	胰蛋白酶，脂酶，神经内分泌标记物，散在性	胰蛋白酶，脂酶，甲胎蛋白，神经内分泌标记物，散在性	波形蛋白，神经元特异性烯醇化酶，β连环蛋白	癌胚抗原，MUC1, p53	无神经内分泌标记物

I-CP，慢性胰腺炎胰岛集聚；AC，腺泡细胞癌；PB，胰母细胞瘤；SPT，实性假乳头状肿瘤；DAC，导管腺癌；MET，转移性肿瘤。

参考文献

1. Solcia E, Klöppel G, Sobin L H et al. 2000 Histological typing of endocrine tumours, 2nd edn. WHO international histological classification of tumours. Springer, Berlin
2. DeLellis R A, Lloyd R V, Heitz P U et al. 2004 Pathology and genetics: tumours of endocrine organs. WHO classification of tumors. IARC Press, Lyon
3. Capella C, Heitz P U, Höfler H et al. 1995 Revised classification of neuroendocrine tumours of the lung, pancreas and gut. Virchows Arch 425: 547–560
4. Klöppel G 1997 Classification of neuroendocrine tumors. Verh Dtsch Ges Pathol 81: 111–117
5. Heitz P U, Komminoth P, Perren A et al. 2004 Pancreatic endocrine tumours: introduction. In: DeLellis R A, Lloyd R V, Heitz P U et al. (ed) Pathology and genetics: tumours of endocrine organs. WHO classification of tumors. IARC Press, Lyon, p 177–182
6. Klöppel G, Willemer S, Stamm B et al. 1986 Pancreatic lesions and hormonal profile of pancreatic tumors in multiple endocrine neoplasia type I. An immunocytochemical study of nine patients. Cancer 57: 1824–1832
7. Rakieten N, Gordon B S, Beaty A et al. 1971 Pancreatic islet cell tumors produced by the combined action of streptozotocin and nicotinamide. Proc Soc Exp Biol Med 137: 280–283
8. Lohmann D R, Funk A, Niedermeyer H P et al. 1993 Identification of p53 gene mutations in gastrointestinal and pancreatic carcinoids by nonradioisotopic SSCA. Virchows Arch [B] Cell Pathol 64: 293–296
9. Komminoth P, Roth J, Muletta-Feurer S et al. 1996 RET proto-oncogene point mutations in sporadic neuroendocrine tumors. J Clin Endocrinol Metab 81: 2041–2046
10. Lollgen R M, Hessman O, Szabo E et al. 2001 Chromosome 18 deletions are common events in classical midgut carcinoid tumors. Int J Cancer 92: 812–815
11. Moore P S, Orlandini S, Zamboni G et al. 2001 Pancreatic tumours: molecular pathways implicated in ductal neoplasia and in ampullary but not in exocrine nonductal or endocrine tumorigenesis. Br J Cancer 84: 253–262
12. Hruban R H, Iacobuzio-Donahue C, Wilentz R E et al. 2001 Molecular pathology of pancreatic cancer. Cancer J 7: 251–258
13. Serrano J, Goebel S U, Peghini P L et al. 2000 Alterations in the p16INK4a/CDKN2A tumor suppressor gene in gastrinomas. J Clin Endocrinol Metab 85: 4146–4156
14. Speel E J, Scheidweiler A F, Zhao J et al. 2001 Genetic evidence for early divergence of small functioning and nonfunctioning endocrine pancreatic tumors: gain of 9Q34 is an early event in insulinomas. Cancer Res 61: 5186–5192
15. Zhao J, Moch H, Scheidweiler A F et al. 2001 Genomic imbalances in the progression of endocrine pancreatic tumors. Genes Chromos Cancer 32: 364–372
16. Speel E J, Richter J, Moch H et al. 1999 Genetic differences in endocrine pancreatic tumor subtypes detected by comparative genomic hybridization. Am J Pathol 155: 1787–1794
17. Stumpf E, Aalto Y, Hoog A et al. 2000 Chromosomal alterations in human pancreatic endocrine tumors. Genes Chromos Cancer 29: 83–87
18. Barghorn A, Komminoth P, Bachmann D et al. 2001 Deletion at 3p25.3-p23 is frequently encountered in endocrine pancreatic tumours and is associated with metastatic progression. J Pathol 194: 451–458
19. Barghorn A, Speel E J, Farspour B et al. 2001 Putative tumor suppressor loci at 6q22 and 6q23-q24 are involved in the malignant progression of sporadic endocrine pancreatic tumors. Am J Pathol 158: 1903–1911
20. Gortz B, Roth J, Krahenmann A et al. 1999 Mutations and allelic deletions of the MEN1 gene are associated with a subset of sporadic endocrine pancreatic and neuroendocrine tumors and not restricted to foregut neoplasms. Am J Pathol 154: 429–436
21. Probst A, Lotz M, Heitz P U 1978 Von Hippel–Lindau's disease, syringomyelia and multiple endocrine tumors: a complex neuroendocrinopathy. Virchows Arch [A] Pathol Anat 378: 265–272
22. Mount S L, Weaver D L, Taatjes D J et al. 1995 Von Hippel–Lindau disease presenting as pancreatic neuroendocrine tumour. Virchows Arch 426: 523–528
23. Chandrasekharappa S C, Guru S C, Manickam P et al. 1997 Positional cloning of the gene for multiple endocrine neoplasia type 1. Science 276: 404–407
24. Latif F, Tory K, Gnarra J et al. 1993 Identification of the von Hippel–Lindau disease tumor suppressor gene. Science 260: 1317–1320
25. Larsson C, Skogseid B, Öberg K et al. 1988 Multiple endocrine neoplasia type 1 gene maps to chromosome 11 and is lost in insulinoma. Nature 332: 85–87
26. Solcia E, Capella C, Klöppel G 1997 Tumors of the pancreas. AFIP atlas of tumor pathology, third series, fascicle 20. Armed Forces Institute of Pathology, Washington, D C
27. Moldow R E, Connelly R R 1968 Epidemiology of pancreatic cancer in Connecticut. Gastroenterology 55: 677–686
28. Service F J, McMahon M M, O'Brien P C et al. 1991 Functioning insulinoma – incidence, recurrence, and long-term survival of patients: a 60-year study. Mayo Clin Proc 66: 711–719
29. Kümmerle F, Rückert K 1978 Chirurgie des endokrinen Pankreas in der Bundesrepublik. Ergebnisse einer Umfrage [Surgery of pancreatic endocrine tumours in the German Federal Republic: results of a survey]. Dtsch Med Wochenschr 103: 729–732
30. Kimura W, Kuroda A, Morioka Y 1991 Clinical pathology of endocrine tumors of the pancreas. Analysis of autopsy cases. Dig Dis Sci 36: 933–942
31. Klöppel G, Heitz P U 1988 Pancreatic endocrine tumors. Pathol Res Pract 183: 155–168
32. Kent R B 3rd, van Heerden J A, Weiland L H 1981 Nonfunctioning islet cell tumours. Ann Surg 193: 185–190
33. Broughan T A, Leslie J D, Soto J M et al. 1986 Pancreatic islet cell tumors. Surgery 99: 671–678
34. Donow C, Pipeleers-Marichal M, Stamm B et al. 1990 Pathologie des Insulinoms und Gastrinoms. Lokalisation, Größe, Multizentrizität, Assoziation mit der multiplen endokrinen Neoplasie Typ I und Malignität. Dtsch Med Wochenschr 115: 1386–1391
35. Donow C, Pipeleers-Marichal M, Schröder S et al. 1991 Surgical pathology of gastrinoma. Site, size, multicentricity, association with multiple endocrine neoplasia type 1, and malignancy. Cancer 68: 1329–1334
36. Weber H C, Venzon D J, Lin J T et al. 1995 Determinants of metastatic rate and survival in patients with Zollinger–Ellison syndrome: A prospective long-term study. Gastroenterology 108: 1637–1649
37. Thompson N W, Lloyd R V, Nishiyama R H et al. 1984 MEN 1 pancreas: a histological and immunohistochemical study. World J Surg 8: 561–574
38. Pipeleers-Marichal M, Somers G, Willems G et al. 1990 Gastrinomas in the duodenums of patients with multiple endocrine neoplasia type 1 and the Zollinger–Ellison syndrome. N Engl J Med 322: 723–727
39. Pipeleers-Marichal M, Donow C, Heitz P U et al. 1993 Pathologic aspects of gastrinomas in patients with Zollinger–Ellison syndrome with and without multiple endocrine neoplasia type I. World J Surg 17: 481–488
40. Reubi J C, Häcki W H, Lamberts S W 1987 Hormone-producing gastrointestinal tumors contain a high density of somatostatin receptors. J Clin Endocrinol Metab 65: 1127–1134
41. Reubi J C, Kvols L K, Waser B et al. 1990 Detection of somatostatin receptors in surgical and percutaneous needle biopsy samples of carcinoids and islet cell carcinomas. Cancer Res 50: 5969–5977
42. Lamberts S W, Hofland L J, van Koetsveld P M et al. 1990 Parallel in vivo and in vitro detection of functional somatostatin receptors in human endocrine pancreatic tumors: consequences with regard to diagnosis, localization, and therapy. J Clin Endocrinol Metab 71: 566–574
43. Kulaksiz H, Eissele R, Rössler D et al. 2002 Identification of somatostatin receptor subtypes 1, 2A, 3 and 5 in neuroendocrine tumours with subtype specific antibodies. Gut 50: 52–60
44. Papotti M, Bongiovanni M, Volante M et al. 2002 Expression of somatostatin receptor types 1–5 in 81 cases of gastrointestinal and pancreatic endocrine tumors. A correlative immunohistochemical and reverse-transcriptase polymerase chain reaction analysis. Virchows Arch 440: 461–475
45. Davtyan H, Nieberg R, Reber H A 1990 Pancreatic cystic endocrine neoplasms. Pancreas 5: 230–233
46. Prescott R J, Manson J, Haboubi N Y 1993 Malignant islet cell tumour arising in chronic pancreatitis. Histopathology 22: 499–501
47. Tomita T, Bhatia P, Gourley W 1981 Mucin producing islet cell adenoma. Hum Pathol 12: 850–853
48. Perez-Montiel M D, Frankel W L, Suster S 2003 Neuroendocrine carcinomas of the pancreas with rhabdoid features. Am J Surg Pathol 27: 642–649
49. Guarda L A, Silva E G, Ordóñez N G et al. 1983 Clear cell islet cell tumor. Am J Clin Pathol 79: 512–517
50. Radi M J, Fenoglio-Preiser C M, Chiffelle T 1985 Functioning oncocytic islet-cell carcinoma. Report of a case with electron-microscopic and immunohistochemical confirmation. Am J Surg Pathol 9: 517–524
51. Gotchall J, Traweek S T, Stenzel P 1987 Benign oncocytic endocrine tumor of the pancreas in a patient with polyarteritis nodosa. Hum Pathol 18: 967–969
52. Ordóñez N G, Silva E G 1997 Islet cell tumour with vacuolated lipid-rich cytoplasm: a new histological variant of islet cell tumour. Histopathology 31: 157–160
52a. Singh R, Basturk O, Klimstra D S et al. 2006 Lipid-rich variant of pancreatic endocrine neoplasms. Am J Surg Pathol 30: 194–200
53. van Eeden S, de Leng W W J, Offerhaus G J A et al. 2004 Ductuloinsular tumors of the pancreas. Endocrine tumors with entrapped nonneoplastic ductules. Am J Surg Pathol 28: 813–820
53a. Zee S Y, Hochwald S N, Conlon K C et al. 2005 Pleomorphic pancreatic endocrine neoplasms: a variant commonly confused with adenocarcinoma. Am J Surg Pathol 29: 1194–1200
54. Dayal Y, Doos W G, O'Brien M J et al. 1983 Psammomatous somatostatinomas of the duodenum. Am J Surg Pathol 7: 653–665
55. Taccagni G L, Carlucci M, Sironi M et al. 1986 Duodenal somatostatinoma with psammoma bodies: an immunohistochemical and ultrastructural study. Am J Gastroenterol 81: 33–37
56. Lubensky I A, Pack S, Ault D et al. 1998 Multiple neuroendocrine tumors of the pancreas in von Hippel–Lindau disease patients: histopathological and molecular genetic analysis. Am J Pathol 153: 223–231

57. Hoang M P, Hruban R H, Albores-Saavedra J 2001 Clear cell endocrine pancreatic tumor mimicking renal cell carcinoma: a distinctive neoplasm of von Hippel–Lindau disease. Am J Surg Pathol 25: 602–609
58. Oertel J E, Heffess C S, Oertel Y C 1989 Pancreas. Diagn Surg Pathol 2: 1057–1093
59. Lloyd R V 2003 Practical markers used in the diagnosis of neuroendocrine tumors. Endocr Pathol 14: 293–301
60. Gould V E, Wiedenmann B, Lee I et al. 1987 Synaptophysin expression in neuroendocrine neoplasms as determined by immunocytochemistry. Am J Pathol 126: 243–257
61. Hagn C, Schmid K W, Fischer-Colbrie R et al. 1986 Chromogranin A, B and C in human adrenal medulla and endocrine tissues. Lab Invest 55: 405–411
62. Lloyd R V, Mervak T, Schmidt K et al. 1984 Immunohistochemical detection of chromogranin and neuron-specific enolase in pancreatic endocrine neoplasms. Am J Surg Pathol 8: 607–614
63. Krisch K, Horvat G, Krisch I et al. 1988 Immunochemical characterization of a novel secretory protein (defined by monoclonal antibody HISL-19) of peptide hormone producing cells which is distinct from chromogranin A, B, and C. Lab Invest 58: 411–420
64. Schmechel D, Marangos P J, Brightman M 1978 Neurone-specific enolase is a molecular marker for peripheral and central neuroendocrine cells. Nature 276: 834–836
65. Lloyd R V, Jin L, Qian X et al. 1995 Analysis of the chromogranin A post-translational cleavage product pancreastatin and the prohormone convertases PC2 and PC3 in normal and neoplastic human pituitaries. Am J Pathol 146: 1188–1198
66. Tischler A S, Mobtaker H, Mann K et al. 1986 Anti-lymphocyte antibody Leu-7 (HNK-1) recognizes a constituent of neuroendocrine granule matrix. J Histochem Cytochem 34: 1213–1216
67. Jin L, Hemperly J J, Lloyd R V 1991 Expression of neural cell adhesion molecule in normal and neoplastic human neuroendocrine tissues. Am J Pathol 138: 961–969
68. Schmitt-Gräff A, Müller H, Rancso C et al. 1997 Molecules of regulated secretion are differentiation markers of neuroendocrine tumors (in German). Verh Dtsch Ges Pathol 81: 157–161
69. Bordi C, Pilato F P, D'Adda T 1988 Comparative study of seven neuroendocrine markers in pancreatic endocrine tumours. Virchows Arch [A] Pathol Anat 413: 387–398
70. Schmidt W E, Siegel E G, Lamberts R et al. 1988 Pancreastatin: molecular and immunocytochemical characterization of a novel peptide in porcine and human tissues. Endocrinology 123: 1395–1404
71. Höfler H, Denk H, Lackinger E et al. 1986 Immunocytochemical demonstration of intermediate filament cytoskeleton proteins in human endocrine tissues and (neuro-) endocrine tumours. Virchows Arch [A] Pathol Anat 409: 609–626
72. Hoorens A, Prenzel K, Lemoine N R et al. 1998 Undifferentiated carcinoma of the pancreas: analysis of intermediate filament profile and Ki-ras mutations provides evidence of a ductal origin. J Pathol 185: 53–60
73. Perez M A, Saul S H, Trojanowski J Q 1990 Neurofilament and chromogranin expression in normal and neoplastic neuroendocrine cells of the human gastrointestinal tract and pancreas. Cancer 65: 1219–1227
74. Heitz P U, Kasper M, Polak J M et al. 1982 Pancreatic endocrine tumours. Immunohistochemical analysis of 125 tumours. Hum Pathol 13: 263–271
75. Höfler H, Ruhri C, Pütz B et al. 1988 Oncogene expression in endocrine pancreatic tumors. Virchows Arch [B] Cell Pathol 55: 355–361
76. McKenzie K J, Hind C, Farquharson M A et al. 1997 Demonstration of insulin production and storage in insulinomas by in situ hybridization and immunochemistry. J Pathol 181: 218–222
77. Larsson L I, Grimelius L, Håkanson R et al. 1975 Mixed endocrine pancreatic tumors producing several peptide hormones. Am J Pathol 79: 271–284
78. Mukai K, Grotting J C, Greider M H, Rosai J 1982 Retrospective study of 77 pancreatic endocrine tumors using the immunoperoxidase method. Am J Surg Pathol 6: 387–399
79. Tomita T, Friesen S R, Kimmel J R et al. 1983 Pancreatic polypeptide-secreting islet cell tumors. A study of three cases. Am J Pathol 113: 134–142
80. Heitz P, Polak J M, Bloom S R et al. 1976 Cellular origin of human pancreatic polypeptide (HPP) in endocrine tumours of the pancreas. Virchows Arch [B] Cell Pathol 21: 259–265
81. Capella C, La Rosa S, Solcia E 1997 Criteria for malignancy in pancreatic endocrine tumors. Endocr Pathol 8: 87–90
82. La Rosa S, Sessa F, Capella C et al. 1996 Prognostic criteria in nonfunctioning pancreatic endocrine tumours. Virchows Arch 429: 323–333
83. Pelosi G, Pasini F, Bresaola E et al. 1997 High-affinity monomeric 67-kD laminin receptors and prognosis in pancreatic endocrine tumours. J Pathol 183: 62–69
84. Pelosi G, Bresaola E, Bogina G et al. 1996 Endocrine tumors of the pancreas: Ki-67 immunoreactivity on paraffin sections is an independent predictor for malignancy: a comparative study with proliferating-cell nuclear antigen and progesterone receptor protein immunostaining, mitotic index, and other clinicopathologic variables. Hum Pathol 27: 1124–1134
85. Clarke M R, Baker E E, Weyant R J et al. 1997 Proliferative activity in pancreatic endocrine tumors: association with function, metastases, and survival. Endocr Pathol 8: 181–187
86. Pelosi G, Zamboni G, Doglioni C et al. 1992 Immunodetection of proliferating cell nuclear antigen assesses the growth fraction and predicts malignancy in endocrine tumors of the pancreas. Am J Surg Pathol 16: 1215–1225
87. Hochwald S N, Zee S, Conlon K C et al. 2002 Prognostic factors in pancreatic endocrine neoplasms: an analysis of 136 cases with a proposal for low grade and intermediate grade groups. J Clin Oncol 20: 2633–2642
88. Deshpande V, Fernandez-del Castillo C, Muzikansky A et al. 2004 Cytokeratin 19 is a powerful predictor of survival in pancreatic endocrine tumors. Am J Surg Pathol 28: 1145–1153
89. Klöppel G, Höfler H, Heitz P U 1993 Pancreatic endocrine tumours in man. In: Polak J M (ed) Diagnostic histopathology of neuroendocrine tumours. Churchill Livingstone, Edinburgh, p 91–121
90. Rüschoff J, Willemer S, Brunzel M et al. 1993 Nucleolar organizer regions and glycoprotein-hormone alpha-chain reaction as markers of malignancy in endocrine tumours of the pancreas. Histopathology 22: 51–57
91. Viale G, Doglioni C, Gambacorta M et al. 1992 Progesterone receptor immunoreactivity in pancreatic endocrine tumors. An immunocytochemical study of 156 neuroendocrine tumors of the pancreas, gastrointestinal and respiratory tracts, and skin. Cancer 70: 2268–2277
92. Heitz P U, Kasper M, Klöppel G et al. 1983 Glycoprotein-hormone alpha-chain production by pancreatic endocrine tumors: a specific marker for malignancy. Immunocytochemical analysis of tumors of 155 patients. Cancer 51: 277–282
93. Perren A, Komminoth P, Heitz P U 2004 Molecular genetics of gastroenteropancreatic endocrine tumors. Ann NY Acad Sci 1014: 199–208
94. Field J B 1993 Insulinoma. In: Mazzaferri E L, Samaan N A (ed) Endocrine tumors. Blackwell Scientific Publications, Boston, p 497–530
95. Heik S C W, Klöppel G, Krone W et al. 1988 Hypoglykämie durch Insulinom bei Diabetes mellitus. Dtsch Med Wochenschr 113: 1714–1717
96. Mann J R, Rayner P H, Gourevitch A 1969 Insulinoma in childhood. Arch Dis Child 44: 435–442
97. Lo C Y, Lam K Y, Kung A W et al. 1997 Pancreatic insulinomas. A 15-year experience. Arch Surg 132: 926–930
98. Fournet J C, Junien C 2004 Genetics of congenital hyperinsulinism. Endocr Pathol 15: 233–240
99. Sempoux C, Guiot Y, Dahan K et al. 2003 The focal form of persistent hyperinsulinemic hypoglycemia of infancy: morphological and molecular studies show structural and functional differences with insulinoma. Diabetes 52: 784–794
100. Goossens A, Gepts W, Saudubray J M et al. 1989 Diffuse and focal nesidioblastosis: a clinicopathological study of 24 patients with persistent neonatal hyperinsulinemic hypoglycemia. Am J Surg Pathol 13: 766–775
101. de Lonlay P, Fournet J C, Touati G et al. 2002 Heterogeneity of persistent hyperinsulinaemic hypoglycaemia. A series of 175 cases. Eur J Pediatr 161: 37–48
102. Reinecke-Lüthge A, Koschoreck F, Klöppel G 2000 The molecular basis of persistent hyperinsulinemic hypoglycemia of infancy and its pathologic substrates. Virchows Arch 436: 1–5
103. Keller A, Stone A M, Valderrama E et al. 1983 Pancreatic nesidioblastosis in adults. Report of a patient with hyperinsulinemic hypoglycemia. Am J Surg 145: 412–416
104. Gould V E, Chejfec G, Shah K et al. 1984 Adult nesidiodysplasia. Semin Diagn Pathol 1: 43–53
105. Weinstock G, Margulies P, Kahn E et al. 1986 Islet cell hyperplasia: an unusual cause of hypoglycemia in an adult. Metabolism 35: 110–117
106. Albers N, Löhr M, Bogner U et al. 1989 Nesidioblastosis of the pancreas in an adult with persistent hyperinsulinemic hypoglycemia. Am J Clin Pathol 91: 336–340
107. Anlauf M, Wieben D, Perren A et al. 2005 Persistent hyperinsulinemic hypoglycemia in 15 adults with diffuse nesidioblastosis: diagnostic criteria, incidence and characterization of β-cell changes. Am J Surg Pathol 29: 524–533
108. Stefanini P, Carboni M, Patrassi N et al. 1974 Beta-islet cell tumors of the pancreas: results of a study on 1067 cases. Surgery 75: 597–609
109. Miyazaki K, Funakoshi A, Nishihara S et al. 1986 Aberrant insulinoma in the duodenum. Gastroenterology 90: 1280–1285
110. Adamson A R, Grahame-Smith D G, Bogomoletz V et al. 1971 Malignant argentaffinoma with carcinoid syndrome and hypoglycaemia. Br Med J 3: 93–94
111. Pelletier G, Cortot A, Launay J M et al. 1984 Serotonin-secreting and insulin-secreting ileal carcinoid tumor and the use of in vitro culture of tumoral cells. Cancer 54: 319–322
112. Shames J M, Dhurandhar N R, Blackard W G 1968 Insulin-secreting bronchial carcinoid tumor with widespread metastases. Am J Med 44: 632–637
113. Kiang D T, Bauer G E, Kennedy B J 1973 Immunoassayable insulin in carcinoma of the cervix associated with hypoglycemia. Cancer 31: 801–805
114. Ashton M A 1995 Strumal carcinoid of the ovary associated with hyperinsulinaemic hypoglycaemia and cutaneous melanosis. Histopathology 27: 463–467
115. Liu T H, Tseng H C, Zhu Y et al. 1985 Insulinoma. An immunohistochemical and morphologic analysis of 95 cases. Cancer 56: 1420–1429
116. Roth J, Klöppel G, Madsen O D et al. 1992 Distribution patterns of proinsulin and insulin in human insulinomas: an immunohistochemical analysis in 76 tumors. Virchows Arch [B] Cell Pathol 63: 51–61
117. Westermark P, Engström U, Johnson K H et al. 1990 Islet amyloid polypeptide: pinpointing amino acid residues linked to amyloid fibril formation. Proc Natl Acad Sci USA 87: 5036–5040

118. Rindi G, Terenghi G, Westermark G et al. 1991 Islet amyloid polypeptide in proliferating pancreatic B cells during development, hyperplasia, and neoplasia in humans and mice. Am J Pathol 138: 1321–1334
119. Westermark P, Grimelius L, Polak J M et al. 1977 Amyloid in polypeptide hormone-producing tumors. Lab Invest 37: 212–215
120. Stridsberg M, Berne C, Sandler S et al. 1993 Inhibition of insulin secretion, but normal peripheral insulin sensitivity, in a patient with a malignant endocrine pancreatic tumour producing high amounts of an islet amyloid polypeptide-like molecule. Diabetologia 36: 843–849
121. Suzuki H, Matsuyama M 1971 Ultrastructure of functioning beta cell tumors of the pancreatic islets. Cancer 28: 1302–1313
122. Creutzfeldt W, Arnold R, Creutzfeldt C et al. 1973 Biochemical and morphological investigations of 30 human insulinomas. Correlation between the tumour content of insulin and proinsulin-like components and the histological and ultrastructural appearance. Diabetologia 9: 217–231
123. Berger M, Bordi C, Cüppers H J et al. 1983 Functional and morphologic characterization of human insulinomas. Diabetes 32: 921–931
124. Bani-Sacchi T, Bani D, Biliotti G 1989 The endocrine pancreas in patients with insulinomas. An immunocytochemical and ultrastructural study of the nontumoral tissue with morphometrical evaluations. Int J Pancreatol 5: 11–28
125. Jensen R T, Gardner J D 1993 Gastrinoma. In: Go V L W, DiMagno E P, Gardner J D et al. (eds) The pancreas: biology, pathobiology and disease. Raven Press, New York, p 931–978
126. Zollinger R M 1987 Gastrinoma: the Zollinger–Ellison syndrome. Semin Oncol 14: 247–252
127. Ruszniewski P, Podevin P, Cadiot G et al. 1993 Clinical, anatomical, and evolutive features of patients with the Zollinger–Ellison syndrome combined with type I multiple endocrine neoplasia. Pancreas 8: 295–304
128. Polak J M, Stagg B, Pearse A G 1972 Two types of Zollinger–Ellison syndrome: immunofluorescent, cytochemical and ultrastructural studies of the antral and pancreatic gastrin cells in different clinical states. Gut 13: 501–512
129. Friesen S R, Tomita T 1981 Pseudo-Zollinger–Ellison syndrome: hypergastrinemia, hyperchlorhydria without tumor. Ann Surg 194: 481–493
130. Mehring U M, Jäger H J, Klöppel G et al. 1997 Pankreatischer Polypeptid-sezernierender endokriner Pankreastumor assoziiert mit multiplen Ulcera ventriculi et duodeni. Langenbecks Arch Chir 382: 134–137
131. Chey W Y, Chang T M, Lee K Y et al. 1989 Ulcerogenic tumor syndrome of the pancreas associated with a nongastrin acid secretagogue. Ann Surg 210: 139–149
132. Stabile B E, Morrow D J, Passaro E Jr 1984 The gastrinoma triangle: operative implications. Am J Surg 147: 25–31
133. Klöppel G, Clemens A 1996 The biological relevance of gastric neuroendocrine tumors. Yale J Biol Med 69: 69–74
134. Solcia E, Capella C, Buffa R et al. 1980 Pathology of the Zollinger–Ellison syndrome. In: Fenoglio L M, Wolf M (ed) Progress in surgical pathology. Masson, New York, p 119–133
135. Antonioli D A, Dayal Y, Dvorak A M et al. 1987 Zollinger–Ellison syndrome. Cure by surgical resection of a jejunal gastrinoma containing growth hormone releasing factor. Gastroenterology 92: 814–823
136. Nord K S, Joshi V, Hanna M et al. 1986 Zollinger–Ellison syndrome associated with a renal gastrinoma in a child. J Pediatr Gastroenterol Nutr 5: 980–986
137. Margolis R M, Jang N 1984 Zollinger–Ellison syndrome associated with pancreatic cystadenocarcinoma. N Engl J Med 311: 1380–1381
138. Morgan D R, Wells M, MacDonald R C et al. 1985 Zollinger–Ellison syndrome due to a gastrin secreting ovarian mucinous cystadenoma. Case report. Br J Obstet Gynaecol 92: 867–869
139. Anlauf M, Perren A, Meyer C L et al. 2005 Precursor lesions in patients with multiple endocrine neoplasia type 1-associated duodenal gastrinomas. Gastroenterology 128: 1187–1198
140. Vella M A, Cowie A G, Gorsuch A N et al. 1988 Giant gastrinoma in a patient with multiple endocrine adenopathy (type 1). J R Soc Med 81: 359–360
141. Oberhelman H A Jr, Nelsen T S 1964 Surgical consideration in the management of ulcerogenic tumors of the pancreas and duodenum. Am J Surg 108: 132–141
142. Stamm B, Hedinger C E, Saremaslani P 1986 Duodenal and ampullary carcinoid tumors. A report of 12 cases with pathological characteristics, polypeptide content and relation to the MEN 1 syndrome and von Recklingshausen's disease (neurofibromatosis). Virchows Arch [A] Pathol Anat 408: 475–489
143. Thompson N W, Vinik A I, Eckhauser F E 1989 Microgastrinomas of the duodenum. A cause of failed operations for the Zollinger–Ellison syndrome. Ann Surg 209: 396–404
144. Stabile B E, Passaro E Jr 1985 Benign and malignant gastrinoma. Am J Surg 149: 144–150
145. Delcore R Jr, Cheung L Y, Friesen S R 1988 Outcome of lymph node involvement in patients with the Zollinger–Ellison syndrome. Ann Surg 208: 291–298
146. Wolfe M M, Alexander R W, McGuigan J E 1982 Extrapancreatic, extraintestinal gastrinoma: effective treatment by surgery. N Engl J Med 306: 1533–1536
147. Thompson J C, Lewis B G, Wiener I et al. 1983 The role of surgery in the Zollinger–Ellison syndrome. Ann Surg 197: 594–607
148. Schwarting H, Osse G, Sippel M et al. 1983 Morphometry of the pancreatic islets in patients with insulinomas and gastrinomas. In: Mutt V, Uvnäs-Moberg K (ed) Regulatory peptides. Abstracts of the 4th international symposium on gastrointestinal hormones. Elsevier, Amsterdam, p 129
149. Martella E M, Ferraro G, Azzoni C et al. 1997 Pancreatic-polypeptide cell hyperplasia associated with pancreatic or duodenal gastrinomas. Hum Pathol 28: 149–153
150. Bordi C, Costa A, Missale G 1975 ECL cell proliferation and gastrin levels. Gastroenterology 68: 205–206
151. Solcia E, Bordi C, Creutzfeldt W et al. 1988 Histopathological classification of nonantral gastric endocrine growths in man. Digestion 41: 185–200
152. D'Adda T, Corleto V, Pilato F P et al. 1990 Quantitative ultrastructure of endocrine cells of oxyntic mucosa in Zollinger–Ellison syndrome. Correspondence with light microscopic findings. Gastroenterology 99: 17–26
153. Solcia E, Capella C, Fiocca R et al. 1990 Gastric argyrophil carcinoidosis in patients with Zollinger–Ellison syndrome due to type 1 multiple endocrine neoplasia. A newly recognized association. Am J Surg Pathol 14: 503–513
154. Mallinson C N, Bloom S R, Warin A P et al. 1974 A glucagonoma syndrome. Lancet ii: 1–5
155. Fujita J, Seino Y, Ishida H et al. 1986 A functional study of a case of glucagonoma exhibiting typical glucagonoma syndrome. Cancer 57: 860–865
156. Ruttman E, Klöppel G, Bommer G et al. 1980 Pancreatic glucagonoma with and without syndrome. Immunocytochemical study of 5 tumour cases and review of the literature. Virchows Arch [A] Pathol Anat 388: 51–67
157. Bordi C, Ravazzola M, Baetens D et al. 1979 A study of glucagonomas by light and electron microscopy and immunofluorescence. Diabetes 28: 925–936
158. Hamid Q A, Bishop A E, Sikri K L et al. 1986 Immunocytochemical characterization of 10 pancreatic tumours, associated with the glucagonoma syndrome, using antibodies to separate regions of the pro-glucagon molecule and other neuroendocrine markers. Histopathology 10: 119–133
159. Bloom S R, Polak J M, Pearse A G E 1973 Vasoactive intestinal peptide and watery-diarrhoea syndrome. Lancet ii: 14–16
160. Trump D L, Livingston J N, Baylin S B 1977 Watery diarrhea syndrome in an adult with ganglioneuroma-pheochromocytoma: identification of vasoactive intestinal peptide, calcitonin, and catecholamines and assessment of their biologic activity. Cancer 40: 1526–1532
161. Mendelsohn G, Eggleston J C, Olson J L et al. 1979 Vasoactive intestinal peptide and its relationship to ganglion cell differentiation in neuroblastic tumors. Lab Invest 41: 144–149
162. Capella C, Polak J M, Buffa R et al. 1983 Morphologic patterns and diagnostic criteria of VIP-producing endocrine tumors. A histologic, histochemical, ultrastructural and biochemical study of 32 cases. Cancer 52: 1860–1874
163. Udall J N Jr 1989 Diarrhea due to hormone-secreting tumours. In: Lebenthal E (ed) Textbook of gastroenterology and nutrition in infancy, 2nd edn. Raven, New York, p 1193–1205
164. Long R G, Bryant M G, Mitchell S J et al. 1981 Clinicopathological study of pancreatic and ganglioneuroblastoma tumours secreting vasoactive intestinal polypeptide (vipomas). Br Med J (Clin Res Ed) 282: 1767–1771
165. Verner J V, Morrison A B 1974 Endocrine pancreatic islet disease with diarrhea. Report of a case due to diffuse hyperplasia of nonbeta islet tissue with a review of 54 additional cases. Arch Intern Med 133: 492–499
166. Tomita T, Kimmel P R, Friesen S R 1980 Pancreatic polypeptide cell hyperplasia with and without watery diarrhea syndrome. J Surg Oncol 14: 11–20
167. Ooi A, Kameya T, Tsumuraya M et al. 1985 Pancreatic endocrine tumours associated with WDHA syndrome. An immunohistochemical and electron microscopic study. Virchows Arch [A] Pathol Anat 405: 311–323
168. Krejs G J, Orci L, Conlon J M et al. 1979 Somatostatinoma syndrome. Biochemical, morphologic and clinical features. N Engl J Med 301: 285–292
169. Sessa F, Arcidiaco M, Valenti L et al. 1997 Metastatic psammomatous somatostatinoma of the pancreas causing severe ketoacedotic diabetes cured by surgery. Endocr Pathol 8: 327–333
170. Vinik A I, Strodel W E, Eckhauser F E et al. 1987 Somatostatinomas, PPomas, neurotensinomas. Semin Oncol 14: 263–281
171. Heitz P U, Klöppel G, Polak J M et al. 1981 Ectopic hormone production by endocrine tumors: localization of hormones at the cellular level by immunocytochemistry. Cancer 48: 2029–2037
172. Melmed S, Yamashita S, Kovacs K et al. 1987 Cushing's syndrome due to ectopic proopiomelanocortin gene expression by islet cell carcinoma of the pancreas. Cancer 59: 772–778
173. Wilander E, El-Salhy M, Willén T et al. 1981 Immunocytochemistry and electron microscopy of an argentaffin endocrine tumor of the pancreas. Virchows Arch [A] Pathol Anat 392: 263–269
174. Sano T, Asa S L, Kovacs K 1988 Growth hormone-releasing hormone-producing tumors: clinical, biochemical, and morphological manifestations. Endocr Rev 9: 357–373
175. Berger G, Trouillas J, Bloch B et al. 1984 Multihormonal carcinoid tumor of the pancreas. Secreting growth hormone-releasing factor as a cause of acromegaly. Cancer 54: 2097–2108
176. Bostwick D G, Quan R, Hoffman A R et al. 1984 Growth-hormone-releasing factor immunoreactivity in human endocrine tumors. Am J Pathol 117: 167–170
177. Rasbach D A, Hammond J M 1985 Pancreatic islet cell carcinoma with hypercalcemia. Primary hyperparathyroidism or humoral hypercalcemia of malignancy. Am J Med 78: 337–342

178. Broadus A E, Mangin M, Ikeda K et al. 1988 Humoral hypercalcemia of cancer. Identification of a novel parathyroid hormone-like peptide. N Engl J Med 319: 556–563
179. Fleury A, Fléjou J F, Sauvanet A et al. 1998 Calcitonin-secreting tumors of the pancreas: About six cases. Pancreas 16: 545–550
180. Saeger W, Schulte H M, Klöppel G 1986 Morphology of a GHRH producing pancreatic islet cell tumor causing acromegaly. Virchows Arch [A] Pathol Anat 409: 547–554
181. Cryer P E, Hill G J 2d 1976 Pancreatic islet cell carcinoma with hypercalcemia and hypergastrinemia: response to streptozotocin. Cancer 38: 2217–2221
182. Hammar S, Sale G 1975 Multiple hormone producing islet cell carcinomas of the pancreas. A morphological and biochemical investigation. Hum Pathol 6: 349–362
183. Asa S L, Kovacs K, Killinger D W et al. 1980 Pancreatic islet cell carcinoma producing gastrin, ACTH, alpha-endorphin, somatostatin and calcitonin. Am J Gastroenterol 74: 30–35
184. Maton P N, Gardner J D, Jensen R T 1986 Cushing's syndrome in patients with the Zollinger–Ellison syndrome. N Engl J Med 315: 1–5
185. Sadoff L, Gordon J, Goldman S 1975 Amelioration of hypoglycemia in a patient with malignant insulinoma during the development of the ectopic ACTH syndrome. Diabetes 24: 600–603
186. Wynick D, Williams S J, Bloom S R 1988 Symptomatic secondary hormone syndromes in patients with established malignant pancreatic endocrine tumors. N Engl J Med 319: 605–607
187. Gloor F, Pletscher A, Hardmeier T 1964 Metastasierendes Inselzelladenom des Pankreas mit 5-Hydroxytryptamin- und Insulin-Produktion. Schweiz Med Wochenschr 94: 1476–1480
188. Appleyard T N, Losowsky M S 1970 A pancreatic tumor with carcinoid syndrome and hypoglycemia. Postgrad Med J 46: 159–171
189. Ohneda A, Otsuki M, Fujiya H et al. 1979 A malignant insulinoma transformed into a glucagonoma syndrome. Diabetes 28: 962–969
190. Simpson W F, Adams D B, Metcalf J S et al. 1988 Nonfunctioning pancreatic neuroendocrine tumors presenting as pancreatitis: report of four cases. Pancreas 3: 223–231
191. Aabo K, Romond E, Dimitrov N V et al. 1983 Pancreatic islet cell carcinoma associated with multiple hormone secretion and pancytopenia. Evidence of a serum factor suppressing hematopoiesis. Cancer 51: 1691–1696
192. Kniffin W D Jr, Spencer S K, Memoli V A et al. 1988 Metastatic islet cell amphicrine carcinoma of the pancreas. Association with an eosinophilic infiltration of the skin. Cancer 62: 1999–2004
193. Feurle G E, Helmstaedter V, Tischbirek K et al. 1981 A multihormonal tumor of the pancreas producing neurotensin. Dig Dis Sci 26: 1125–1133
194. Eckhauser F E, Cheung P S, Vinik A I et al. 1986 Nonfunctioning malignant neuroendocrine tumors of the pancreas. Surgery 100: 978–988
195. Perrone T, Sibley R K, Rosai J 1985 Duodenal gangliocytic paraganglioma. An immunohistochemical and ultrastructural study and a hypothesis concerning its origin. Am J Surg Pathol 9: 31–41
196. Alumets J, Alm P, Falkmer S et al. 1981 Immunohistochemical evidence of peptide hormones in endocrine tumors of the rectum. Cancer 48: 2409–2415
197. Carstens P H, Cressman F K Jr 1989 Malignant oncocytic carcinoid of the pancreas. Ultrastruct Pathol 13: 69–75
198. Kanavaros P, Hoang C, Le Bodic M F et al. 1990 Serotonin-producing pancreatic endocrine tumour. Histological, ultrastructural and immunohistochemical study of a case. Histol Histopathol 5: 325–328
199. Bostwick D G, Bensch K G 1985 Gastrin releasing peptide in human neuroendocrine tumours. J Pathol 147: 237–244
200. Padberg B, Schröder S, Capella C et al. 1995 Multiple endocrine neoplasia type 1 (MEN 1) revisited. Virchows Arch 426: 541–548
201. Samaan N A, Ouais S, Ordóñez N G et al. 1989 Multiple endocrine syndrome type I. Clinical, laboratory findings, and management in five families. Cancer 64: 741–752
202. Rosai J, Higa E, Davie J 1972 Mediastinal endocrine neoplasm in patients with multiple endocrine adenomatosis. A previously unrecognized association. Cancer 29: 1075–1083
203. Duh Q Y, Hybarger C P, Geist R et al. 1987 Carcinoids associated with multiple endocrine neoplasia syndromes. Am J Surg 154: 142–148
204. Komminoth P, Heitz P U, Klöppel G 1998 Multiple endocrine disorders. In: Stefaneanu L, Sasano T, Kovacs K (ed) Molecular and cellular endocrine pathology. Chapman & Hall, Philadelphia, PA
204a. Anlauf M, Schlenger R, Perren A et al. 2006 Microadenomatosis of the endocrine pancreas in patients with and without the multiple endocrine neoplasia type 1 syndrome. Am J Surg Pathol 30: 560–574
205. Friesen S R 1982 Tumors of the endocrine pancreas. N Engl J Med 306: 580–590
206. Le Bodic M F, Heymann M F, Lecomte M et al. 1996 Immunohistochemical study of 100 pancreatic tumors in 28 patients with multiple endocrine neoplasia, type I. Am J Surg Pathol 20: 1378–1384
207. Warner T F, Block M, Hafez G R et al. 1983 Glucagonomas. Ultrastructure and immunohistochemistry. Cancer 51: 1091–1096
208. Stacpoole P W, Jaspan J, Kasselberg A G et al. 1981 A familial glucagonoma syndrome: genetic, clinical and biochemical features. Am J Med 70: 1017–1026
209. Eusebi V, Capella C, Bondi A et al. 1981 Endocrine-paracrine cells in pancreatic exocrine carcinomas. Histopathology 5: 599–613
210. Ohike N, Jürgensen A, Pipeleers-Marichal M et al. 2003 Mixed ductal-endocrine carcinomas of the pancreas and ductal adenocarcinomas with scattered endocrine cells: characterization of the endocrine cells. Virchows Arch 442: 258–265
211. Ohike N, Kosmahl M, Klöppel G 2004 Mixed acinar-endocrine carcinoma of the pancreas. A clinicopathological study and comparison with acinar-cell carcinoma. Virchows Arch 445: 231–235
212. Tanaka Y, Kato K, Notohara K et al. 2001 Frequent β-catenin mutation and cytoplasmic/nuclear accumulation in pancreatic solid-pseudopapillary neoplasm. Cancer Res 61: 8401–8404
213. Kosmahl M, Seada L S, Jänig U et al. 2000 Solid-pseudopapillary tumor of the pancreas: its origin revisited. Virchows Arch 436: 473–480
214. Klöppel G, Heitz P U, Capella C et al. 1996 Pathology and nomenclature of human gastrointestinal neuroendocrine (carcinoid) tumors and related lesions. World J Surg 20: 132–141
215. Lüttges J, Pierré E, Zamboni G et al. 1997 Maligne nicht-epitheliale Tumoren des Pankreas. Pathologe 18: 233–237
216. Du EZ, Goldstraw P, Zacharias J et al. 2004. TTF-1 expression is specific for lung primary in typical and atypical carcinoids: TTF-1 positive carcinoids are predominantly in peripheral location. Hum Pathol 35: 825–831

淋巴网状系统肿瘤
Tumors of the lymphoreticular system

21

第一部分

淋巴结　The lymph node

John K.C. Chan 著
陈定宝 译　薛卫成 校

淋巴结	
淋巴结和有结构的淋巴组织	1139
淋巴瘤的诊断	1142
Hodgkin淋巴瘤（HL）	1152
非Hodgkin淋巴瘤（NHL）	1168
前体淋巴母细胞淋巴瘤	1172
外周B细胞淋巴瘤	1176
外周T细胞肿瘤和有争议的NK细胞肿瘤	1213
免疫缺陷相关性淋巴组织增生异常	1234
组织细胞和树突状细胞肿瘤	1237
白血病及相关病变	1243
淋巴结转移性肿瘤	1244
淋巴结非淋巴造血系统肿瘤和瘤样病变	1245
淋巴组织增生性病变诊断的实践问题	1250

淋巴结和有结构的淋巴组织
Lymph node and organized lymphoid tissues

淋巴结的正常组织学和免疫结构
Normal histology and immunoarchitecture of lymph node

淋巴结的框架和淋巴窦
The framework and sinuses of the node

淋巴结包裹在一层薄的延续性纤维被膜内，后者的纤细的纤维梁伸入其实质内[1,2]。在皮质表面，输入淋巴管引流入被膜下淋巴窦，后者通过中间窦和髓窦连接进入输出淋巴管，输出淋巴管在门部离开淋巴结。淋巴窦被覆窦衬附细胞，含有数量不等的组织细胞和小淋巴细胞。肠系膜淋巴结窦隙常常扩张，含有淋巴液。淋巴结实质由纤维母细胞性树突状细胞网架支撑，后者可对细胞角蛋白显示不同程度的免疫反应。

皮质　The cortex

皮质是淋巴结的外凸部分，其中有散在B细胞性淋巴滤泡（图21A.1和21A.2）。初级滤泡是由圆形聚集的小淋巴细胞组成，核呈圆形或轻度不规则，染色质致密，胞浆稀少。这些淋巴细胞呈IgG$^+$IgD$^+$。次级滤泡主要由IgD$^-$的中心母细胞（大无裂细胞）和中心细胞（小裂细胞）构成的滤泡中心以及周围的小淋巴细胞套（IgM$^+$、IgD$^+$）组成。中心母细胞具有圆形泡状核和多层膜包绕的核仁，胞浆层薄，位于边缘，呈嗜双色性。中心细胞具有成角的折叠形核，染色质相当致密，核仁不明显，胞浆稀少（图21A.1B）。这些滤泡中心B细胞（CD10$^+$、bcl-6$^+$）混杂有内含可染小体的巨噬细胞、滤泡树突状细胞（FDC）和滤泡内的小T淋巴细胞（通常CD4$^+$、CD10$^+$、bcl-6$^+$，不同程度的CD57$^+$）。FDC的特点是核膜薄，呈紫罗兰色，核质空，核仁小而明显，细胞边界不清楚；有些细胞可能为双核。有时在套区的外周可见边缘区，由中等大小的细胞组成，胞浆量中等，淡染至透明。边缘区常常不明显，除非是腹腔内淋巴结。

在某些反应性淋巴结病，单核样B细胞在淋巴窦形成带状或弧形结构，围绕反应性滤泡。它们是中等大小的细胞，核呈锯齿状，胞浆丰富而透明。常常混合中性粒细胞。

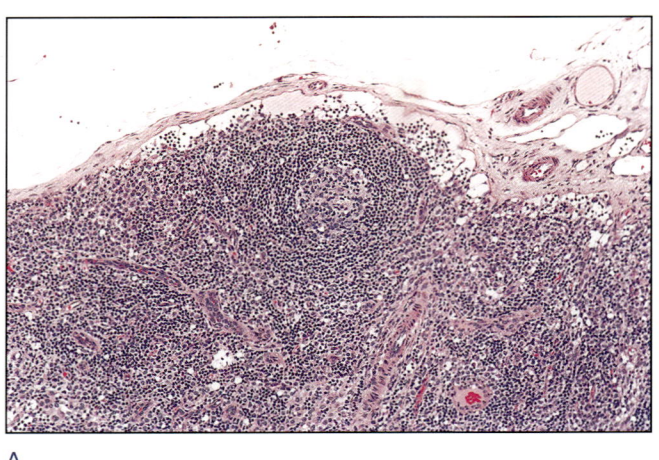 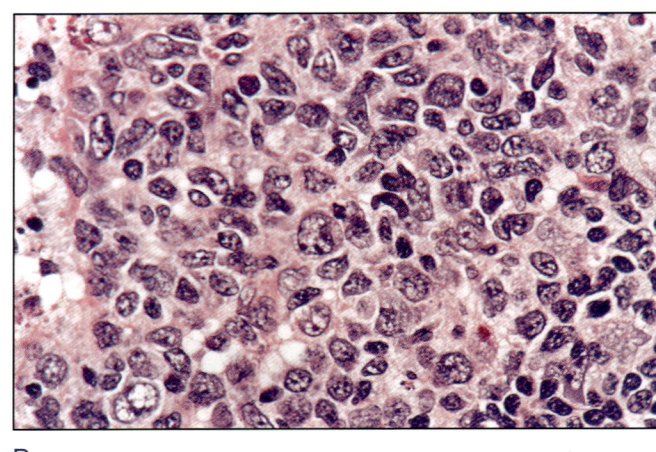

图21A.1 正常淋巴结。（A）被膜和被膜窦下方是皮质区，含有淋巴滤泡。在副皮质区可见明显的微静脉。（B）生发中心由中心母细胞（大无裂细胞）和中心细胞（小裂细胞）混合组成。后者的核呈三角形或长形，胞浆几乎见不到。

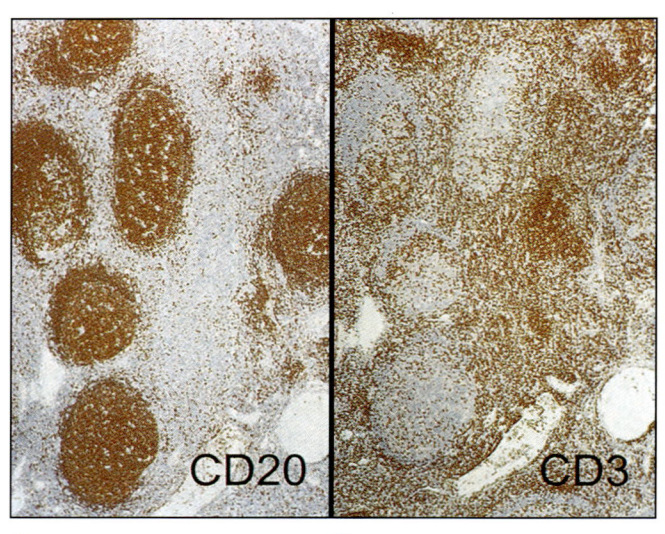

图21A.2 正常淋巴结的免疫结构。（A）CD20免疫染色显示结节状聚集的B细胞，代表滤泡。滤泡间区仅含有少数B细胞。（B）CD3免疫染色显示副皮质区的T细胞。有些T细胞也可见于淋巴滤泡内。

副皮质区 The paracortex

副皮质区包括滤泡间和紧贴滤泡下的部分。主要由T细胞（小淋巴细胞和较大的母细胞）组成，它们混合有一些组织细胞、B淋巴细胞（包括免疫母细胞）、指状树突状细胞和Langerhans细胞（图21A.2）。后两种细胞可通过其核沟和扭曲的核以及丰富的轻度嗜酸性胞浆而被识别，S100蛋白免疫染色可清楚地显示。有时副皮质区可形成模糊结节状，被称为T结节。由立方形内皮细胞衬覆的高内皮细胞微静脉是副皮质的典型特征；它们是淋巴细胞运输的门户。

副皮质区可包含浆细胞样单核细胞聚集（CD68$^+$、CD123$^+$），其细胞中等大小，具有偏心性圆形细胞核，染色质相当致密，胞浆呈偏心轮状，嗜双色性。通常有散在的凋亡小体，有时可见含有可染性小体的巨噬细胞。

髓质和门部 The medulla and the hilum

髓质是淋巴结的深在部分，由富于浆细胞的髓索散在于髓窦之间组成。髓窦汇入门部输出淋巴管，门部也是动脉和静脉出入淋巴结的部位。

结外淋巴组织，包括Waldeyer环 Extranodal lymphoid tissues, including Waldeyer's ring

人体含有大量没有包膜的淋巴组织，大多数位于黏膜部位，如Waldeyer环（监护咽部通道开口的环状淋巴组织）、肠道和呼吸道。它们提供针对感染性病原体和外来抗原的免疫防御。这些淋巴聚集体被称为"黏膜相关淋巴组织（MALT）"。与淋巴结不同，它们通常缺乏被膜和窦。在结构上它们有两种成分：B细胞滤泡和富于T细胞的分隔性滤泡间区。这两种成分的比例及其活性因部位和时间而异。通常可见淋巴细胞和被覆上皮细胞之间密切的相互作用。

淋巴细胞的发生 Lymphocyte development

淋巴细胞有三种谱系：B细胞、T细胞和自然杀伤细胞（NK）。B和T淋巴细胞的发生阶段以及伴随细胞分化的免疫表型改变见图21A.3和21A.4[1,3,4]。许多淋巴瘤类型可能与淋巴细胞成熟的某个阶段有关。

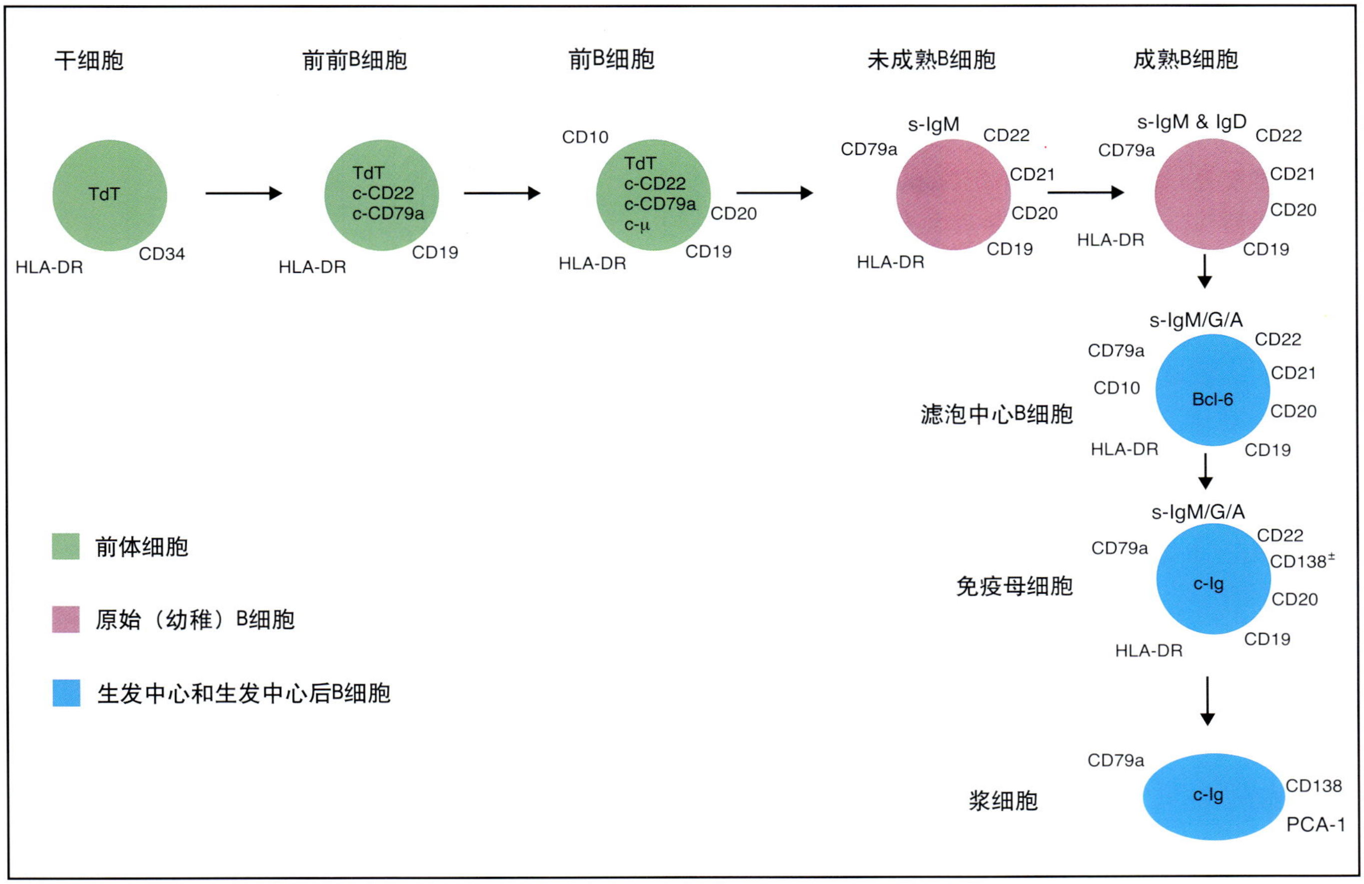

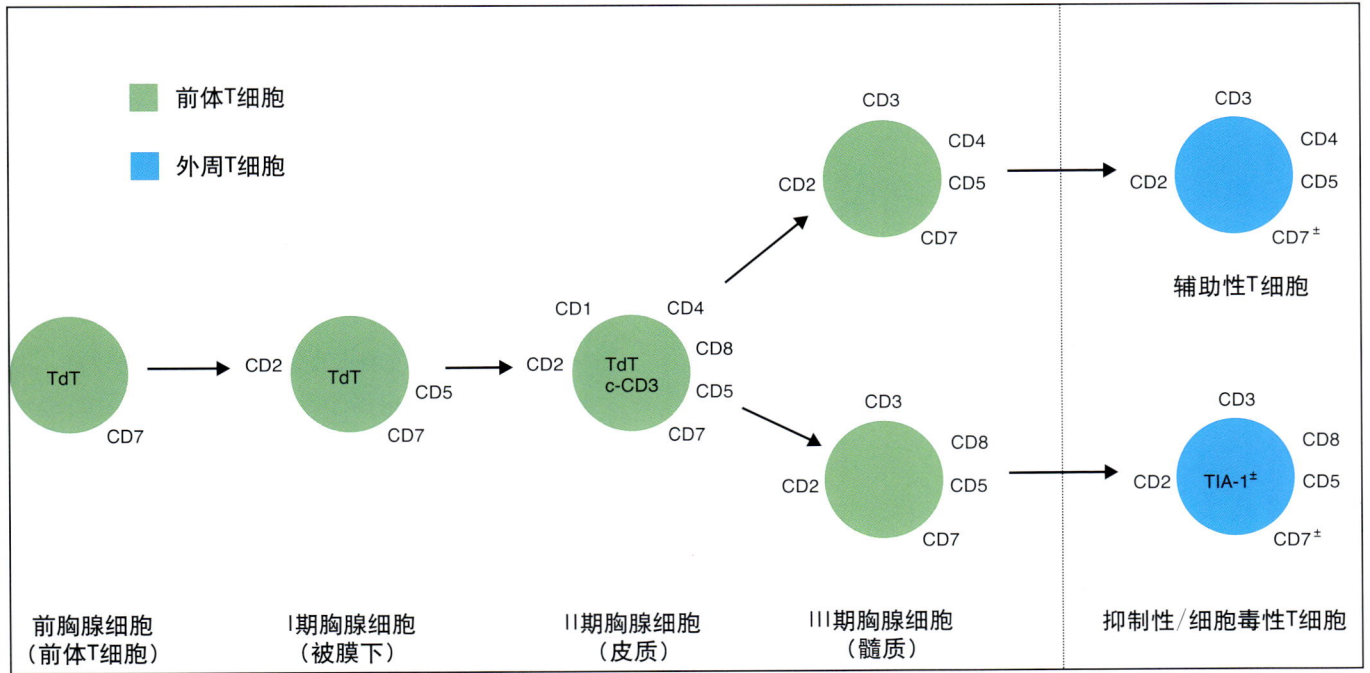

图21A.3 B淋巴细胞的发生及其不同分化阶段免疫表型特征的改变。圈内（细胞）显示的标记物在胞浆（c-）或核内表达，而圈外显示的标记物在细胞表面（s-）表达。注意常见的表面B细胞标记物随着向浆细胞分化的成熟而丢失。

图21A.4 T淋巴细胞的发生及其不同分化阶段免疫表型特征的改变。圈内（细胞）显示的标记物在胞浆（c-）或核表达，而圈外显示的标记物在细胞表面表达。

淋巴瘤的诊断
Diagnosis of lymphomas

淋巴瘤是一种淋巴网状系统肿瘤，可发生于淋巴结或结外部位。淋巴瘤包括Hodgkin淋巴瘤（Hodgkin lymphoma，HL）和非Hodgkin淋巴瘤（non Hodgkin lymphoma，NHL），后者较常见。

做出淋巴瘤诊断的必备条件：技术因素

对于可疑淋巴瘤，通过正确的处理方法从组织标本中获取最大信息量是非常重要的：（1）制作印片以进行详细的细胞学评估；（2）如果需要冰冻切片进行免疫组织化学或基因型分析，则进行快速冷冻组织保存；（3）如果需要，则进行细胞培养；（4）将组织用于其他必要的研究，例如细胞遗传学、流式细胞术。然而，最重要的是保留足够的组织用于石蜡包埋切片诊断。缓冲甲醛溶液是良好的"多用途"固定液，可以很好地提供细胞学细节，保护抗原以进行免疫组织化学检查，并可以相当好地保留mRNA和DNA用于分子学研究。由于细胞核细节易碎，有些实验室使用B5固定液，但B5固定液有含汞的缺点，不可预测抗原可否保留，并且由于有酸存在，不利于分子学研究。

高质量的HE染色切片是诊断的关键，但有些病理医生喜欢Giemsa染色。切片厚度最好是2～4μm，因为较厚的切片很难评估细胞学细节。

形态学评估

一般形态学评估

由于淋巴组织较脆，活检挤压或牵拉、干燥、固定过度、固定延迟等均易引起人工假象。淋巴结最外层常常发生固定过度或发生干燥，导致淋巴细胞显得小而黑。淋巴结的中心部分常常发生固定延迟，导致核增大和染色质透明。一般情况下，中间区最适于细胞学评估。许多误诊是由于组织切片质量欠佳而掩盖了真正的病变。

淋巴瘤病变的确定

恶性淋巴瘤可能类似或被误以为是转移癌或黑色素瘤。最重要的是不要将反应性淋巴组织增生误诊为淋巴瘤。有帮助的鉴别诊断特征将在各类淋巴瘤中以及本章末尾讨论。

淋巴瘤，尤其是弥漫的大B细胞淋巴瘤和滤泡性淋巴瘤，可以自发梗死，而难以或不可能从活检标本中做出淋巴瘤诊断。因此诊断为完全性淋巴结梗死的病例应该密切随访，以除外淋巴瘤，必要时应重复活检[5,6]。

淋巴瘤细胞大小和分类的判定

淋巴瘤诊断作出后，下一步是进行分类。按照细胞大小进行分类时，可将肿瘤细胞与其间散在的反应性组织细胞进行对比。小细胞、中等细胞和大细胞分别是指它们的细胞核小于、等于或大于反应性组织细胞的细胞核。如果找不到组织细胞，则可将内皮细胞核作为替代性"尺度"应用，虽然内皮细胞核呈卵圆形或长形而较不满意。淋巴瘤分类要考虑细胞的大小、细胞核形态、胞浆的特点、细胞的结构（如滤泡性和弥漫性）以及其他辅助特征。

免疫组织化学检查

免疫组织化学检查在评估淋巴组织增生中有多重要？

免疫组织化学在评估淋巴组织增生中具有重要作用，通过勾画常规显微镜下不明显的结构、细胞间隔、细胞类型和细微特征等，其可提供较为详细和准确的疾病评估。

对于形态学评估明显为良性的淋巴组织增生，如反应性滤泡增生或窦组织细胞增生，不需要进行免疫组织化学染色，虽然选择性抗体常常应用于某些特殊淋巴结病的诊断，如S100蛋白在Rosai-Dorfman病中呈阳性。对于不能确定是反应性还是恶性的淋巴组织增生，免疫组织化学检查对明确诊断十分重要。对于淋巴瘤，免疫组织化学检查对确定其谱系、分类和预测都是重要的。

使用冰冻切片或石蜡切片免疫组织化学还是流式细胞术？

冰冻组织免疫染色的优点是可以做出全面评估，因为几乎所有抗体均可应用于这种组织，其主要的缺点是：需要额外的处理程序，且有时染色结果和细胞成分难以对应。目前，由于抗原修复技术的提高和抗体应用范围的扩展，几乎所有的白细胞抗原在常规石蜡切片上都可以可靠地显示。由于操作方便（包括易于邮寄至其他中心进行染色操作）且能保持良好的细胞形态，目前石蜡切片免疫组织化学是首选的常规技术，冰冻切片免疫组织化学则用于显示石蜡包埋组织中不能可靠检测的抗原，如表面CD3、CD103和$\gamma\delta$-TCR。

流式细胞术是另一种在免疫表型方面应用较多的技术。流式细胞术需要使用新鲜组织，必须用物理方法将细胞分离以制备细胞悬液，后者与荧光染料标记的抗体一起孵育后，使用流式细胞仪进行分析。由此可形成一个分布图，显示每个细胞的大小和荧光浓度。通过分选可进行特殊细胞群的分析。流式细胞术免疫表型的优点包括：（1）可以迅速获得结果；（2）可以同时分析两种或多种标记物，易于识别伴有特殊或异常免疫表型的细胞群；（3）在检测表面 Ig 表达方面具有优越性，因为细胞已经脱离了间质血清——不同于在冰冻或石蜡切片中，由于间质染色重可导致解释 Ig 染色困难。流式细胞术免疫表型的主要缺点是：（1）需要新鲜组织；（2）缺乏与局部解剖学或细胞学的直接对应性，例如，由于肿瘤标本富于不成熟表型的 T 细胞，胸腺瘤可被误诊为 T 淋巴母细胞性淋巴瘤；（3）由于纤维化或存活的肿瘤细胞数量少，肿瘤细胞群在细胞悬液中可能不具有代表性。因此，当结果与组织学所见矛盾时，应将其忽略，建议在冰冻或石蜡包埋组织应用免疫组织化学染色进一步检查。

用于分析淋巴造血系统增生的抗体

有助于评估淋巴造血系统增生和淋巴瘤亚型分类的抗体在表 21A.1 和 21A.2 中列出。在有的情况下应尽可能使用 CD（cluster of differentiation）名称[7-11]。在国际白细胞分型工作会议上（International Leukocyte Typing Workshops），对相应的单克隆抗体已指定了特定的 CD 数。

免疫组织化学染色的解释

免疫组织化学染色必须在形态学检查的前提下解释并仔细与细胞群相对应。对于许多淋巴瘤类型，背景中可能有许多反应性细胞，在非典型（肿瘤性）细胞，检查者必须确定哪种标记物呈阳性。如果结果是阴性，必须通过寻找内部阳性对照判定染色的有效性，如果没有内部阳性对照，则使用外部阳性对照。而且，细胞中的信号部位必须与所用的抗体一致，否则结果不能被认为是阳性的，如 CD20 的核仁染色或 CD30 的弥漫性胞浆染色都应被忽略（图 21A.5）[12]。

细胞遗传学研究

一些类型的淋巴瘤具有特殊的染色体易位。它们已成为淋巴瘤分类的辅助因素，其检测有助于诊断（表 21A.3）[13-17]。这些易位常常（但不总是）累及并列的原癌基因与免疫球蛋白基因（14 号染色体的重链基因，或 2 号和 22 号染色体的轻链基因），导致结构正常的

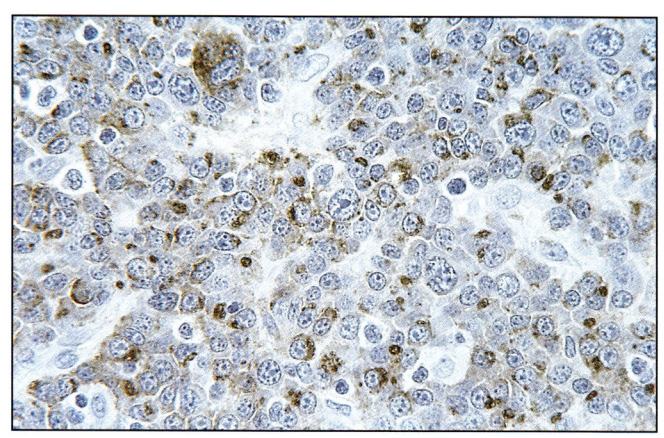

图21A.5　大B细胞淋巴瘤显示单形性 λ 轻链染色，表现为核旁小球。免疫球蛋白染色常常难以解释，因为免疫球蛋白能从间质中被动蔓延至胞浆。核旁小球染色（高尔基区），伴有或不伴有弥漫的胞浆染色，总是有意义的，因为它可提示细胞的免疫球蛋白合成。核周区染色也提示细胞免疫球蛋白合成（未显示）。

原癌基因过表达。其他染色体易位有时可导致嵌合体蛋白产物。

分子学研究

分子学分析的价值

分子学研究是很有用的研究手段，但在常规实践中，只有在形态学和免疫组织化学检查得不出结论时才使用。组织的 DNA 水平分析可提供如下信息[1,18-20]：

1. 淋巴组织增生的克隆性。分子学研究有助于鉴别淋巴瘤与反应性淋巴组织增生、检测治疗后微量残留病变以及早期复发。应用Southern印迹技术可检测到克隆细胞所占比例＞5%的细胞群。如果应用聚合酶链反应（PCR），则敏感性会更高。
2. 淋巴组织增生的谱系。实际上所有B细胞性淋巴瘤均显示免疫球蛋白（Ig）重链和Ig轻链基因的重排，而大多数T细胞性淋巴瘤显示T细胞受体（TCR）β 或 γ 链基因的重排。NK细胞淋巴瘤和组织细胞肿瘤通常缺乏Ig和TCR基因重排。

淋巴瘤的诊断

表21A.1　用于评估淋巴增生性病变的抗体

CD（抗体）	染色形式	正常淋巴造血细胞中的主要反应者	淋巴造血系统肿瘤中的主要反应者	染色结果判定及注意事项
普通白细胞标记物				
CD45RB/白细胞共同抗原	细胞膜，有时为高尔基区	所有白细胞，除了浆细胞（阴性或不同程度地阳性）	淋巴瘤和白血病。一些淋巴瘤病例可能是CD45RB−，特别是淋巴母细胞性淋巴瘤和间变大细胞淋巴瘤。浆细胞肿瘤的CD45RB染色结果不一致。	绝大多数非淋巴造血系统肿瘤CD45RB阴性。经典Hodgkin淋巴瘤中的Reed-Sternberg细胞阴性。
B细胞相关性				
CD19	细胞膜	B细胞，除了浆细胞	B细胞肿瘤，包括B淋巴母细胞性肿瘤	在B细胞发生中，CD19表达较早，因此与CD20相比是检查淋巴母细胞性肿瘤较敏感的B系标记物。浆细胞肿瘤阴性。
CD20（例L26）	细胞膜	B细胞，除了前前B细胞和浆细胞	B细胞肿瘤；B-CLL/SLL的染色较弱，B淋巴母细胞肿瘤可能为阴性。结节性淋巴细胞为主型Hodgkin淋巴瘤（L&H细胞）。一些经典型Hodgkin淋巴瘤病例（Reed-Sternberg细胞）	B细胞的良好标记物；极少数T细胞性肿瘤也呈CD20阳性。浆细胞肿瘤通常为CD20阴性。使用热诱导抗原修复的病例可出现非特异性核仁染色。一些胸腺瘤，特别是A型，CD20阳性。
CD22	高尔基区和（或）细胞膜	B细胞，除了浆细胞	B细胞肿瘤，包括B淋巴母细胞肿瘤	CD22胞浆表达见于B细胞发生的早期（同CD19一样早），之后是细胞表面CD22表达。浆细胞肿瘤阴性。
CD23	细胞膜	B细胞亚群；滤泡性树突状细胞亚群（淋巴滤泡顶端的亮区和套区）	B-CLL/SLL。一些滤泡中心细胞淋巴瘤，特别是在弥漫性区域。纵隔大B细胞淋巴瘤。滤泡性树突状细胞肿瘤。	CD23可显示滤泡性树突状细胞网，可见于各种类型的淋巴瘤，如滤泡性淋巴瘤、套细胞淋巴瘤；CD23有助于鉴别B-CLL/SLL（阳性）与套细胞淋巴瘤（阴性）和结外边缘区B细胞淋巴瘤（阴性）
CD79a/mb-1	弥漫性胞浆	B细胞，包括浆细胞	B细胞肿瘤，包括浆细胞肿瘤（50%）和B淋巴母细胞性肿瘤。结节性淋巴细胞为主型Hodgkin淋巴瘤（L&H细胞）。少数经典型Hodgkin淋巴瘤病例（Reed-Sternberg细胞）。	CD79a与B细胞表面的免疫球蛋白有关，类似于T细胞中CD3与TCR的关系。一些T淋巴母细胞性肿瘤可表达CD3和CD79a；因此用于谱系判定时要加以注意。平滑肌细胞可显示微弱的胞浆染色。

表21A.1 用于评估淋巴增生性病变的抗体（续）

CD（抗体）	染色形式	正常淋巴造血细胞中的主要反应者	淋巴造血系统肿瘤中的主要反应者	染色结果判定及注意事项
PAX-5（B细胞特异性活化蛋白）	细胞核	B细胞，除了浆细胞	B细胞肿瘤，包括B淋巴母细胞肿瘤。结节性淋巴细胞为主型Hodgkin淋巴瘤（L&H细胞）。经典型Hodgkin淋巴瘤（Reed-Sternberg细胞通常呈弱～中等染色）	浆细胞肿瘤阴性。证实B淋巴母细胞性肿瘤的应用价值高。Merkel细胞癌和小细胞癌PAX-5常常呈阳性。
Oct-2	细胞核	B细胞，包括浆细胞	B细胞肿瘤，包括浆细胞肿瘤	在经典型Hodgkin淋巴瘤，Reed-Sternberg细胞通常不表达Oct-2
Bob.1	细胞核+/−细胞浆	B细胞，包括浆细胞	B细胞肿瘤，包括浆细胞肿瘤	在经典型Hodgkin淋巴瘤，Reed-Sternberg细胞通常不表达Bob.1 一些T细胞淋巴瘤可能Bob.1阳性
免疫球蛋白（IgM、IgG、IgA、IgD、κ、λ）	胞浆高尔基区，细胞核周或细胞膜	B细胞，在浆细胞、浆母细胞、免疫母细胞和滤泡中心细胞亚型可见强阳性染色	B细胞肿瘤。浆细胞肿瘤。	轻链染色有助于确定B细胞增生的克隆性。IgD染色有助于鉴别B-CLL/SLL、套细胞淋巴瘤和脾边缘区B细胞淋巴瘤与结外边缘区B细胞淋巴瘤。从组织液中非特异性摄取免疫球蛋白常见于组织细胞、Reed-Sternberg细胞、大淋巴细胞和变性细胞；这可以通过缺乏核周或高尔基区染色以及同一细胞中既有κ又有λ轻链染色来鉴别。
T细胞相关性				
CD2	细胞膜+/−高尔基区	T细胞，除了很不成熟的T细胞；NK细胞	T细胞肿瘤。NK细胞肿瘤。	一种对T和NK细胞很敏感的标记物
CD3，表面*	细胞膜	T细胞，从晚期胸腺细胞开始	T细胞肿瘤	CD3分子在T细胞表面与TCR非共价结合。抗表面CD3抗体与完整CD3分子的抗原决定簇发生反应（由ε、γ和δ亚单位组成）。表面CD3在NK细胞肿瘤通常呈阴性。
CD3ε（胞浆CD3）	胞浆，伴有核周或高尔基区增强；少数细胞膜	T细胞；NK细胞	T细胞肿瘤。NK细胞肿瘤。	髓细胞阴性。组织细胞和浆细胞可显示微弱的非特异性弥漫性胞浆染色。

表21A.1 用于评估淋巴增生性病变的抗体（续）

CD（抗体）	染色形式	正常淋巴造血细胞中的主要反应者	淋巴造血系统肿瘤中的主要反应者	染色结果判定及注意事项
CD4	细胞膜	辅助性/诱导性T细胞；单核细胞/组织细胞；Langerhans细胞	许多T细胞肿瘤。组织细胞肿瘤。Langerhans细胞组织细胞增生症	—
CD5	细胞膜	T细胞；少数B细胞亚型	T细胞肿瘤。一些B细胞肿瘤，尤其是B-CLL/SLL和套细胞淋巴瘤；也见于少数大B细胞淋巴瘤亚型	NK细胞肿瘤通常呈阴性。CD5表达对小B细胞肿瘤的分类很有帮助。胸腺癌常常CD5阳性。
CD7	细胞膜	T细胞	T细胞肿瘤。少数髓细胞肉瘤病例。	CD7表达于T细胞发生早期，在一些T淋巴母细胞肿瘤，可能是仅有的T细胞表达标记物。
CD8	细胞膜	抑制性/细胞毒性T细胞；NK细胞亚群	一些T细胞肿瘤病例。一些NK细胞肿瘤病例。	脾窦内衬细胞CD8阳性。
CD43	细胞膜；少数高尔基区	T细胞；组织细胞；髓细胞；B细胞的少数亚型；浆细胞（不一致）；EVB感染的B细胞；巨核细胞	T细胞肿瘤。一些B细胞淋巴瘤（CD43与特异性B系标记物共表达）。组织细胞和单核细胞肿瘤。髓细胞肉瘤。浆细胞瘤（偶尔）	增生B细胞的CD43染色异常提示病变为肿瘤性。"仅仅CD43$^+$"表型的淋巴造血系统肿瘤应高度怀疑为髓细胞肉瘤。
CD45RO	细胞膜；少数高尔基区	T细胞；组织细胞；髓细胞	T细胞肿瘤。组织细胞肿瘤。髓细胞肉瘤。	弥漫胞浆染色应该考虑为非特异性染色
LAT	细胞膜	T细胞（包括不成熟性T细胞）；NK细胞	T细胞肿瘤 NK细胞肿瘤	巨核细胞和肥大细胞LAT阳性
αβ-TCR（即βF1）	细胞膜	T细胞（主要群体）；非NK细胞	大多数T细胞肿瘤	NK细胞淋巴瘤通常呈阴性
γδ-TCR*（即TCR-δ1）	细胞膜	T细胞（少数群体）；非NK细胞	极少数T细胞肿瘤，如肝脾T细胞淋巴瘤	NK细胞淋巴瘤通常呈阴性

NK细胞相关性

CD56	细胞膜	NK细胞；T细胞亚群（NK样T细胞）	NK细胞肿瘤。一些T细胞淋巴瘤，尤其是表达γδ-TCR的淋巴瘤。	CD56识别神经元细胞黏附分子（N-CAM）。神经组织、神经内分泌细胞和一些其他类型细胞CD56阳性。因此神经肿瘤，神经内分泌肿瘤和一些非淋巴造血系统肿瘤CD56可以阳性。

表21A.1　用于评估淋巴增生性病变的抗体（续）

CD（抗体）	染色形式	正常淋巴造血细胞中的主要反应者	淋巴造血系统肿瘤中的主要反应者	染色结果判定及注意事项
CD57	细胞膜	NK细胞；T细胞亚群（NK样T细胞）	T细胞大颗粒淋巴细胞白血病。极少数T淋巴母细胞淋巴瘤病例	NK细胞淋巴瘤通常CD57阴性。CD57有助于鉴别结节性淋巴细胞为主型Hodgkin淋巴瘤（许多小淋巴细胞阳性）与富于T细胞的大B细胞淋巴瘤（少数CD57⁺细胞）。CD57还可着染神经外胚层组织和前列腺。
细胞毒性标记物				
TIA-1	胞浆颗粒	活化和非活化性NK细胞；T细胞亚群（NK样T细胞）	NK细胞淋巴瘤。一些外周T细胞淋巴瘤，尤其是间变大细胞淋巴瘤和结外淋巴瘤。	–
粒酶B	胞浆颗粒	活化性NK细胞，T细胞亚群（NK样T细胞）	NK细胞淋巴瘤。一些外周T细胞淋巴瘤，尤其是间变大细胞淋巴瘤和结外淋巴瘤。	–
穿孔素	胞浆颗粒	活化性NK细胞；T细胞亚群（NK样T细胞）	NK细胞淋巴瘤。一些外周T细胞淋巴瘤，尤其是间变大细胞淋巴瘤和结外淋巴瘤。	–
活化和增生相关性				
CD25/白介素-2受体	细胞膜	活化性T细胞，B细胞或巨噬细胞	有些B或T细胞肿瘤，尤其是成人T细胞淋巴瘤/白血病、毛细胞白血病和间变大细胞淋巴瘤。经典型Hodgkin淋巴瘤。	–
CD30	细胞膜和（或）高尔基区	活化性T或B细胞	经典型Hodgkin淋巴瘤。间变大细胞淋巴瘤。个别外周T细胞和大B细胞淋巴瘤病例。浆细胞瘤（有些病例）	单纯胞浆染色应该忽略。胚胎性癌常常CD30阳性。
Ki-67	细胞核	增生性细胞（细胞周期中的细胞）	阳性细胞百分数因不同的淋巴瘤类型而不同。低度恶性者通常Ki-67指数低，而高度恶性者Ki-67指数高。	Ki-67染色对诊断Burkitt淋巴瘤尤其有帮助：实际上所有肿瘤细胞均阳性
分化阶段相关性				
TdT/末端脱氧核苷转移酶	细胞核	不成熟（前体细胞）B、T或NK淋巴细胞	B、T或NK淋巴母细胞肿瘤。母细胞性NK细胞淋巴瘤。	TdT是鉴别淋巴母细胞肿瘤与外周T细胞淋巴瘤和成熟B细胞淋巴瘤的唯一最有用的标记物。TdT偶尔可表达于非淋巴造血系统小圆细胞肿瘤。

表21A.1　用于评估淋巴增生性病变的抗体（续）

CD（抗体）	染色形式	正常淋巴造血细胞中的主要反应者	淋巴造血系统肿瘤中的主要反应者	染色结果判定及注意事项
CD10	细胞膜	滤泡中心B细胞；滤泡中心T细胞；前体淋巴细胞；粒细胞	滤泡性淋巴瘤和滤泡中心细胞来源的B细胞淋巴瘤（一些弥漫大B细胞淋巴瘤和弥漫小细胞淋巴瘤）。Burkitt淋巴瘤。B淋巴母细胞肿瘤。血管免疫母细胞性T细胞淋巴瘤。	CD10可识别常见的急性淋巴母细胞性白血病抗原（CALLA）。CD10表达还见于广泛多样的非淋巴造血系统组织。
CD99a/MIC2	细胞膜	不成熟T细胞（胸腺细胞）；NK细胞；单核细胞	淋巴母细胞肿瘤	CD99a在Ewing肉瘤/外周原始神经外胚瘤常为阳性
Bcl-2	核周间隙	大多数B细胞和T细胞，除了反应性滤泡中心B细胞	滤泡性淋巴瘤。许多其他类型的B或T细胞肿瘤。	Bcl-2蛋白具有较强的抗凋亡功能。Bcl-2免疫染色有助于鉴别滤泡性淋巴瘤与反应性滤泡增生，但对淋巴瘤的分类没有帮助。Burkitt淋巴瘤bcl-2通常呈阴性。
Bcl-6	细胞核	滤泡中心B细胞；滤泡中心T细胞；$CD30^+$的滤泡周细胞；少数T细胞亚群	滤泡性淋巴瘤。滤泡中心细胞来源的B细胞淋巴瘤（一些弥漫大B细胞淋巴瘤和弥漫小细胞淋巴瘤）。Burkitt淋巴瘤。间变大细胞淋巴瘤。血管免疫母细胞性T细胞淋巴瘤。结节性淋巴细胞为主型Hodgkin淋巴瘤（L&H细胞）。	—
CD103/黏膜淋巴细胞抗原*	细胞膜	肠上皮内淋巴细胞	肠病型T细胞淋巴瘤。毛细胞白血病。	在上皮细胞，CD103（整合素αE亚单位/αEβ7）结合至钙粘连蛋白
EMA/上皮膜抗原	细胞膜和（或）高尔基区	浆细胞	间变大细胞淋巴瘤。浆细胞肿瘤。结节性淋巴细胞为主型Hodgkin淋巴瘤（L&H细胞）。少数大细胞淋巴瘤。	EMA在许多上皮性肿瘤中呈阳性
CD138/多配体（蛋白）聚糖-1	细胞膜	浆细胞，浆母细胞；有些免疫母细胞	浆细胞肿瘤。一些大B细胞淋巴瘤。	CD138在正常上皮细胞和许多不同类型的上皮性肿瘤中呈阳性
MUM-1	细胞核和细胞浆	浆细胞；少部分生发中心B细胞（bcl-6阴性）；少部分活化性T细胞	浆细胞肿瘤。淋巴母细胞淋巴瘤。弥漫大B细胞淋巴瘤（75%）。其他B细胞淋巴瘤（比例不等）。有些T细胞淋巴瘤（比例不等）。Hodgkin淋巴瘤。	MUM-1对于淋巴造血系统并不特异，恶性黑色素瘤常呈阳性

表21A.1　用于评估淋巴增生性病变的抗体（续）

CD（抗体）	染色形式	正常淋巴造血细胞中的主要反应者	淋巴造血系统肿瘤中的主要反应者	染色结果判定及注意事项
淋巴瘤相关性				
Cyclin D1	细胞核	有些组织细胞 正常和反应性淋巴细胞全部呈阴性	套细胞淋巴瘤	极少数B-CLL/SLL病例cyclin D1呈阳性。部分毛细胞白血病和骨髓瘤表达cyclin D1。一些内皮细胞和上皮细胞cyclin D1阳性。
ALK/间变性淋巴瘤激酶	细胞核或胞浆	没有（正常和反应性淋巴细胞全部呈阴性）	间变性大细胞淋巴瘤，T/裸细胞性，原始系统型。ALK$^+$大B细胞淋巴瘤。ALK$^+$组织细胞增生症	除少数例外，ALK染色的出现与t(2;5)或累及2号染色体的易位密切相关
组织细胞、树突状细胞和髓细胞相关性				
CD68	胞浆颗粒	KP1着染组织细胞/单核细胞和粒细胞。PGM1只着染组织细胞/单核细胞。	组织细胞肿瘤和单核细胞白血病。KP1还着染髓细胞肉瘤。	许多非淋巴造血系统肿瘤可呈CD68阳性，如恶性黑色素瘤、颗粒细胞瘤
CD163	细胞膜$^{+/-}$胞浆	组织细胞（除了生发中心和脾白髓的组织细胞以及上皮样组织细胞和肉芽肿中的多核巨细胞），不着染树突状细胞	组织细胞肉瘤。急性单核细胞白血病。	树突状细胞肿瘤呈阴性。纤维组织细胞瘤亚型可显示CD163免疫反应。
S100蛋白	细胞核，伴有或不伴有弥漫胞浆染色	Langerhans细胞；指状树突状细胞；少数T细胞亚群	Langerhans细胞组织细胞增生症。指状树突状细胞肿瘤。个别组织细胞肉瘤病例。	许多非淋巴造血系统细胞类型S100蛋白呈阳性
CD1a	细胞膜	Langerhans细胞；未定类细胞；不成熟T细胞（胸腺皮质细胞）	Langerhans细胞组织细胞增生症。未定类细胞肿瘤。有些T淋巴母细胞肿瘤。	–
Langerin	细胞膜+胞浆（颗粒）	Langerhans细胞	Langerhans细胞组织细胞增生症	淋巴结和肝的窦内衬细胞常常Langerin阳性
CD15	高尔基区和（或）细胞膜	粒细胞；单核细胞/组织细胞（常常呈颗粒状结构）；CMV感染细胞	经典型Hodgkin淋巴瘤。少数T或B细胞淋巴瘤（大细胞）。组织细胞肿瘤，包括Langerhans细胞组织细胞增生症。粒细胞肉瘤（结果不一致）。	CD15抗体针对糖类X半抗原。敏感性可通过单价（抗IgM）连接抗体的使用而提高。有些腺癌CD15也呈阳性，可用于鉴别间皮瘤

表21A.1　用于评估淋巴增生性病变的抗体（续）

CD（抗体）	染色形式	正常淋巴造血细胞中的主要反应者	淋巴造血系统肿瘤中的主要反应者	染色结果判定及注意事项
CD21/C3d受体	细胞膜	滤泡树突状细胞；B细胞亚群	滤泡树突状细胞肿瘤。一些B细胞淋巴瘤，如地方性Burkitt淋巴瘤、滤泡性淋巴瘤。	最常用的滤泡树突状细胞标记物。CD21识别CD3d/EBV受体（CR2）。
CD35/C3b受体	细胞膜	滤泡树突状细胞；B细胞亚群；单核细胞；粒细胞	滤泡树突状细胞肿瘤。一些髓细胞白血病。	一种有用的滤泡树突状细胞的标记物，可与CD21抗体联合来增加敏感性
丛生蛋白（Clusterin）	细胞膜	滤泡树突状细胞	滤泡树突状细胞肿瘤。大多数间变大细胞淋巴瘤。	–
CD123（白介素-3受体，低亲和力）	细胞膜	浆细胞样单核细胞（浆细胞样树突状细胞）	母细胞性NK细胞淋巴瘤。浆细胞样单核细胞聚集的肿瘤。	
溶菌酶（Lysozyme）	胞浆颗粒	组织细胞；髓细胞	组织细胞肉瘤。髓细胞肉瘤。一些T细胞淋巴瘤。	许多非淋巴造血系统肿瘤Lysozyme也呈阳性
髓过氧化物酶（Myeloperoxidase）	胞浆颗粒	粒细胞（各分化阶段）	髓细胞肉瘤和髓性白血病	髓系最敏感和特异的标记物

*目前仅能在新鲜或冰冻组织中显示。TCR：T细胞受体；B-CLL/SLL：B细胞慢性淋巴细胞白血病/小淋巴细胞淋巴瘤。

3. 检测某种淋巴瘤类型的特征性癌基因或染色体易位，如滤泡性淋巴瘤的 *BCL-2* 重排。
4. 判定所发现的不同淋巴瘤成分的克隆性关系或在不同时点，或通过比较重排的Ig分子或TCR基因大小，或通过更准确地比较重排的Ig或TCR的DNA序列。

Southern印迹分析（参见第32章）
Southern blot analysis

Ig 和 TCR 基因重排分别是 B 和 T 细胞的标志，因此是淋巴组织增生谱系敏感而特异的标志物[20,21]。检测 Ig 基因重排的原则如下文所述。原本的 Ig 基因是由许多可变区片段、多样区片段、连接区片段和恒定区（原型）片段组成。当细胞定向为 B 细胞系时，Ig 基因重排，于是可变区的一条片段可与多样区的一条片断、连接区和恒定区的一条片段进行特异组合；Ig 的多样性由此产生。B 细胞淋巴瘤是一种克隆性增生，其所有的肿瘤细胞具有相同的 Ig 基因重排。当提取的 DNA（需要新鲜或冰冻组织）用限制性核酸内切酶消化时，可产生恒定大小的 DNA 片段。电泳之后它们与有放射活性的探针杂交，在 Ig 基因的恒定区出现清晰的重排带。另一方面，混合性细胞组成的多克隆性 B 细胞增生具有不同的 Ig 基因重排结构，可产生大小不同的 Ig DNA 片段，因此检测不到一条明确的条带。TCR 基因重排的原则也一样，因为 TCR 基因也是由可变区、多样区和连接区构成的。

聚合酶链反应（参见第32章）
Polymerase chain reaction (PCR)

PCR 为检测克隆性淋巴组织增生提供了高敏感性方法，可用于常规石蜡包埋的组织[18,20,22]。这种方法不需要限制性核酸内切酶消化，也不需要有放射活性的 DNA 探针以及耗时的自动放射自显影过程。

表21A.2　评估淋巴造血系统增生的最有用的抗体

面对的问题	推荐的一线抗体
B系？	CD20（或CD79a）
T系？	CD3
NK系？	CD56
髓细胞？	髓过氧化物酶（MPO）
滤泡中心细胞？	CD10（或bcl-6）
滤泡性淋巴瘤或滤泡增生？	Bcl-2
B细胞慢性淋巴细胞性白血病？	CD5、CD23
正常套区细胞？	IgD
套细胞淋巴瘤？	Cyclin D1
Burkitt淋巴瘤？	Ki-67、CD10/bcl-6、bcl-2
不成熟（前体淋巴母细胞）细胞？	TdT
间变大细胞淋巴瘤？	CD30、ALK1
浆细胞？	CD20（阴性） CD138（阳性）
组织细胞？	CD68（或CD163）
指状树突状细胞或Langerhans细胞？	S100（对后一种细胞类型，langerin也呈阳性）
滤泡树突状细胞？	CD21或CD35
Hodgkin淋巴瘤？	CD30、CD15

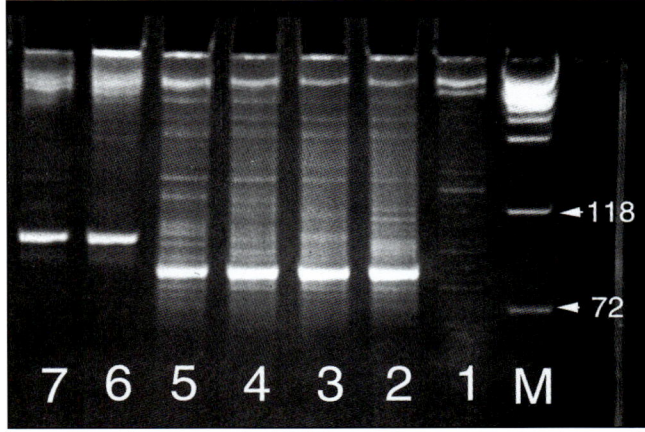

图21A.6　免疫球蛋白基因的聚合酶链反应（PCR）。PCR之后，凝胶用溴化乙啶进行染色并在紫外灯下观察扩增的DNA凝胶电泳结果。M泳道：分子大小标记物。泳道1：可见多条带（梯形结构），符合多克隆性结构。泳道2～4：在许多条弱带的背景下，可见明显分离的带，提示在反应性B细胞的背景中存在单个一条带的B细胞克隆；这个结果支持B细胞淋巴瘤的诊断。泳道6～7：已知的B细胞淋巴瘤阳性对照；单一条带提示存在克隆性免疫球蛋白基因重排。

如果一种淋巴瘤可显示某种特异性染色体易位（如滤泡性淋巴瘤中 *IGH* 基因的 JH 区与 *BCL-2* 并列），则通过 PCR 显示这种独特 DNA 序列可支持诊断。由于 PCR 反应使用与重组区互补的引物，所以正常细胞不出现阳性信号。

通过应用引物识别这些基因的保守序列，PCR 技术还可以用于检测 Ig 或 TCR 基因重排。如果存在克隆性淋巴细胞群，则可见到一条清晰的带（或者是 Ig 或 TCR 基因的等位基因产生的两条清晰带），因为扩增的 DNA 产物其分子大小是相同的（图 21A.6）。如果细胞群是多克隆性的，则可见到一条阶梯状（许多条带）或模糊形态的结构，因为来自不同细胞的 DNA 扩增产物的分子大小不同，因而电泳时迁移至不同的部位（图 21A.6）。肿瘤性克隆细胞群若占到标本的 1%，即可被检测到。然而，与 Southern 印迹分析相比，其有 10%～40% 的假阴性率。假阴性是由于部分重排或体细胞超突变，导致与重排的 Ig 或 TCR 基因杂交的"通用型"引物失效。假阴性率在生发中心和生发中心后 B 细胞肿瘤较高（如滤泡性淋巴瘤和结外边缘区 B 细胞淋巴瘤，MALT 型），原因是：重排的 Ig 基因显示体细胞超突变[22]。但是通过采用针对重排基因不同区域的多对引物，如 Biomed-2 多重 PCR 策略，假阴性率可以明显降低[23-26]。

荧光原位杂交
Fluorescence in situ hybridization (FISH)

FISH 可应用于新鲜、冰冻或石蜡包埋组织，由于其有高敏感性和特异性，正普遍用于检测特异性染色体易位。根据选择的探针，检测者可寻找共同迁移的两个信号（提示基因融合）或信号的分离（提示染色体断裂点），以提示存在染色体易位。FISH 也是一种检测染色体单体或三体的便利方法。

RNA/DNA微阵列分析
RNA/DNA microarray analysis

应用微阵列技术可将寡核苷酸或其他 DNA 序列有序地排列在固相支持物上，利用一小块组织标本就可同时分析成千上万的基因。其主要应用在于识别遗传学改变和评估基因表达谱[27]。这种技术已成功地应用于研究淋巴造血系统肿瘤，例如，应用基因表达谱来确定疾病实体并识别其正常的对应者，在已知的肿瘤实体内识别临床和生物学相关亚型并预测存活和对治疗的反应。

表21A.3　特殊类型的淋巴瘤的特征性遗传学表现

淋巴瘤类型	特异性染色体易位	涉及的癌基因或肿瘤抑制基因	淋巴瘤发生的机制
滤泡性淋巴瘤	t(14;18) (q32;q21)	BCL-2	由于与IGH基因并列引起bcl-2过表达
套细胞淋巴瘤	t(11;14) (q13;q32)	BCL-1 (CCND1)	由于与IGH基因并列引起bcl-1 (cyclin D1)过表达
结外边缘区B细胞淋巴瘤，MALT型	t(11;18) (q21;q21) t(1;14) (q22;q32) t(14;18) (q32;q21) t(3;14) (p141;q32)	API2、MALT1 BCL-10 MALT1 FOXP1	产生API2-MALT1嵌合体蛋白，激活NFκB 由于与IGH基因并列引起bcl-10过表达 由于与IGH基因并列引起MALT1过表达 由于与IGH基因并列引起FOXP1过表达
Burkitt淋巴瘤	t(8;14) (q24;q32) t(8;22) (q24;q11) t(2;8) (p12;q24)	C-MYC	由于与IGH、IGκ或IGλ基因并列引起c-myc表达失调
弥漫大B细胞淋巴瘤	累及3q27及许多染色体配体的易位	BCL-6	由于与IG或其他基因并列引起bcl-6过表达
前体T淋巴母细胞淋巴瘤/白血病	t(1;14) (p32-34;q11)	TAL1	由于与TCR基因并列引起tal-1过表达
间变大细胞淋巴瘤，原始系统型	t(2;5) (p23;q35)	NPM、ALK	产生嵌合体蛋白NPM-ALK，具有构成性酪氨酸激酶活性
	累及2p23的易位，如t(1;2)、t(2;3)和inv(2) (p23;q35)	ALK及其他配体基因	产生嵌合体ALK蛋白，具有构成性酪氨酸激酶活性

虽然DNA微阵列目前还没有应用于常规诊断工作中，但是相关研究的重要信息将来可用于诊断，例如，根据有限的基因表达来确定疾病类型或亚型，使用针对过表达基因蛋白的一组抗体可以起到鉴别作用。

Hodgkin淋巴瘤
Hodgkin lymphoma (HL)

定义

Hodgkin淋巴瘤（HL）的特点是：在一个适当的炎症细胞背景中可以见到Reed-Sternberg细胞及其变型。它包括两种不同的生物学和临床病变：结节性淋巴细胞为主型Hodgkin淋巴瘤（N-LPHL）和经典型Hodgkin淋巴瘤（C-HL）。N-LPHL是一种B细胞性肿瘤，而几乎所有的C-HL病例均为"残缺的"（crippled）B细胞肿瘤[28,29]。虽然HL最初只是依据形态学标准来定义的，用免疫组化染色证实是建议进行，事实上在不典型病例，用免疫组化染色证实是必需的[30]。

在高加索人，HL占所有淋巴瘤的25%～40%，一个发病高峰年龄为11～30岁，另一个发病高峰年龄为51～60岁。在东方人和来自不发达国家的人中，HL仅占所有淋巴瘤的5%～10%[31]。与散发病例相比，发生于AIDS患者的HL可表现许多少见的特征（表21A.4）[32-35a]。

分类

Rye分类已广泛应用了很多年。在修订的欧美淋巴瘤或世界卫生组织（REAL/WHO）分类中，为了保持淋巴细胞为主型HL（LPHL）种类的单纯性，加入了"富于淋巴细胞的C-HL"型（表21A.5）[36-42]。最常见的HL类型是结节硬化型HL（NSHL），占＞50%（高达80%）的病例。除了在不发达国家和免疫受损患者，淋巴细胞削减型HL极其罕见。未分类的病例过去常常归入混合细胞型[43]，但REAL/WHO分类推荐将这种病例称为"HL，未定类"[39]。大多数"间变性大细胞淋巴瘤，Hodgkin样"病例已证明是C-HL，通常是结节硬化型[40]。

过去，淋巴细胞为主型、结节硬化型（NS）、混合细胞型（MC）和淋巴细胞削减型（LD）HL被证明临床预后极为不同，但现在这些差异已经被现代治疗手段极大地降低了[44]。

表21A.4	与散发性HL相比，发生于HIV阳性患者的HL的特殊特征

- 出现症状时为进展期（90%为III/IV期）
- 全身症状常见
- 常常累及结外和少见部位
- 常常累及骨髓（40%~50%）
- 纵隔累及较少见
- 不连续的播散方式
- 更可能是侵袭性HL亚型：混合细胞型和淋巴细胞削减型较常见（占66%的病例，散发性HL只占29%）
- 背景T细胞大多数为$CD8^+$细胞，而不是$CD4^+$细胞
- 肿瘤细胞显示生发中心后B细胞分化，并且缺乏散发性HL病例的滤泡中心细胞分化的证据
- 临床过程呈侵袭性且通常对治疗反应差。但是早期疾病积极治疗后仍有可能治愈
- 与EBV具有较强的相关性（80%~100%）

表21A.6	Hodgkin淋巴瘤的Ann Arbor分期
I期	累及单一淋巴结区（I）或单一淋巴外器官（IE）
II期	累及横膈同侧的两个或多个淋巴结区（II），或局限累及横膈同侧的一个淋巴外器官以及一个或多个淋巴结区（IIE）
III期	累及横膈两侧淋巴结区（III），可能还伴有一个淋巴外器官（IIIE）或脾（IIIS）局限累及或二者皆有（IIISE）
IV期	弥漫性或播散性累及一个或多个淋巴外器官或组织或没有相关淋巴结肿大

亚分类：
A 没有下列症状
B 系统性症状：
— 无法解释的发热38℃
— 在前6个月中，无法解释的体重减轻10%
— 盗汗

*淋巴外器官被定义为淋巴结、脾、胸腺、Waldeyer环、阑尾和Peyer结以外的器官。

与非Hodgkin淋巴瘤的关系：复合性淋巴瘤、灰区淋巴瘤及转化
Relationship with non-Hodgkin lymphomas: composite lymphoma, gray zone lymphoma and transformation

虽然HL被认为是一种不同于NHL的肿瘤，但两者可以有重叠和灰区[45-52]。几乎任何类型的NHL（滤泡性淋巴瘤最常见）都可与HL同时发生，这种病例被称为"复合性淋巴瘤"（composite lymphoma）；至少在有些病例其克隆相关性可由于存在共同的B细胞前体而被证实[53,54]。HL患者发生NHL的风险增加。已观察到，有些B细胞慢性淋巴细胞白血病（B-CLL）病例可进展为HL。其他类型的淋巴瘤患者，如滤泡性淋巴瘤和蕈样霉菌病，少数情况下可继发HL。另一方面，有的病例尽管应用了各种技术进行了彻底分析，也难以明确区分HL和NHL（尤其是弥漫性大B细胞淋巴瘤），这种病例被称为"灰区淋巴瘤"（gray zone lymphoma）[55]。

分期

Ann Arbor分期系统已广泛用于HL和NHL的分期（表21A.6）[56,57]。临床分期依据病史、体检、影像学检查、同位素扫描和实验室检查进行，与病理学分期没有必然的对应关系。脾的组织学受累可发生于重量少于200g的脾，但增大的脾并不一定受累。1/3~1/4的临床分期为I/II期的患者出现膈下病变。

表21A.5	Hodgkin淋巴瘤的分类比较	
REAL/WHO	**Rye**	**Lukes & Butler**
结节性淋巴细胞为主型	淋巴细胞为主型	淋巴细胞和组织细胞型，结节和弥漫型
经典型　经典的富于淋巴细胞型		
混合细胞型	混合细胞型	混合细胞型
结节硬化型	结节硬化型	结节硬化型
淋巴细胞削减型	淋巴细胞削减型	网状型
		弥漫纤维化型

结节性淋巴细胞为主型Hodgkin淋巴瘤
Nodular lymphocyte-predominant Hodgkin lymphoma (N-LPHL)

临床特征

N-LPHL 也称为结节性副颗粒细胞瘤（nodular paragranuloma），仅占所有 HL 的 5%。其最常发生于儿童和中青年人（表 21A.7）。男性好发（男女比例为 3:1）。患者通常表现为外周淋巴结孤立性增大，最常见于颈部、腹股沟或腋窝。纵隔淋巴结很少累及。多数患者的病变是早期的（80% 为 I 期或 II 期），系统性症状不常见[58-66]。骨髓受累很少见，与预后差有关[67]。

表21A.7　不同亚型的Hodgkin淋巴瘤（HL）的突出的临床和病理学特征

	结节性淋巴细胞为主型HL	经典型HL			
		富于淋巴细胞性经典型HL	结节硬化型HL	混合细胞型HL	淋巴细胞削减型HL
临床特征					
发生率（%）	~5	~5	~60	~25	15~50
性别	男>女	男>女	女>男	男>女	男>女
年龄	通常中青年人（中位年龄35岁）	年龄较大（中位年龄43岁）	通常为青年（中位年龄28岁）	任何年龄（中位年龄35岁）	老年人（中位年龄51岁）
纵隔累及	少见（7%）	少见（15%）	常见（80%）常累及肺	有时（40%）	少见
病变部位和临床特征	通常伴有长期淋巴结肿大，通常发生于外周淋巴结。临床过程较好	淋巴结肿大	纵隔肿物伴锁骨上淋巴结累及是最常见的表现。病变巨大。25%的病例显示隐匿性脾病变。	病变可累及许多部位，但通常不特别大。常累及脾。	病变常常广泛。淋巴结可大可小。常见发热、消瘦、血细胞减少和肝功能失调。
B症状	少见，~10%	少见，~10%	42%	35%	>50%
I/II期	80%	70%~80%	60%	50%	仅仅20%
病理学					
诊断性RS细胞	少见或缺乏	少见	存在	通常易于找到	通常易于找到
主要RS细胞变型	L&H细胞；少数情况下细胞具有大核仁，类似单核或诊断性RS细胞	单核RS细胞	陷窝细胞	单核RS细胞	单核RS细胞；多形性RS细胞
相应的炎症背景	仅仅为淋巴细胞和（或）组织细胞	淋巴细胞、浆细胞、组织细胞、嗜酸性粒细胞和（或）中性粒细胞			
其他诊断特征	结节性结构	结节性比弥漫性常见	RS细胞及其变型细胞容易聚集，形成模糊结节。致密纤维带分割病变。	RS细胞及其变型细胞显示散在分布，没有结节	可显示弥漫纤维化

RS：Reed-Sternberg。

临床行为

结节性淋巴细胞为主型 Hodgkin 淋巴瘤（N-LDPL）的自然病史明显不同于经典型 Hodgkin 淋巴瘤（C-HL）[68]。常见同一部位或其他部位淋巴结复发（19%～32%），并且可间隔许多年（中位复发时间是 4 年，比 C-HL 时间长）（表 21A.7）。其中，25% 的患者表现为多处复发[60-62,65,66,69-71]。复发病变的组织学保持不变，预后仍然良好[61,72]。

Ⅰ期病变患者的预后良好，生存率与正常人群的相近[60,73]。Ⅰ期和Ⅱ期的 8 年 HL 特异性生存率和无病生存率分别为 95% 和 80%。另一方面，Ⅳ期的相应数值分别为 41% 和 24%[61,74-76]。对治疗没有反应的高分期疾病患者通常死于 1～2 年内[60]。

当像 C-HL 一样治疗时，N-LPHL 预后良好。但是，其他原因导致的死亡，尤其是第二种恶性肿瘤和心脏疾病，比死于该肿瘤者更常见[75]。而且，有些单独外科切除肿瘤的患者能健康地生存[60,69]。因此建议使用较轻的治疗，如仅对受累区域实施放疗，并使用较小的放射剂量，虽然这种肿瘤的首选治疗方案仍未出台[74,75]。对于Ⅰ期患者，甚至可以考虑只进行随访[61,62]。利妥昔单抗（rituximab）的治疗价值仍不清楚[77]。

病理学

淋巴结结构通常被破坏，虽然可见受压的淋巴组织边缘和反应性淋巴滤泡[43,58,78]。有拥挤的或分割的多发深染结节，主要由小细胞组成。当结节背靠背时，彼此可以嵌合（图 21A.7）。结节呈圆形、卵圆形或匐行性[79]。14% 的病例结节内可见小的生发中心[79]。由于混有粉染的组织细胞，结节呈斑驳状，有时组织细胞呈花环状围绕结节[80]。嗜酸性粒细胞和浆细胞通常稀少或缺乏。出现纤维化不否定诊断[58,79]。有些病例可见程度不同的弥漫区域（图 21A.8）[62,79]。

大多数肿瘤细胞（淋巴细胞和组织细胞；L&H 细胞）分布在结节内，然而也可见于结节之间（图 21A.9），可占细胞成分的 10%。肿瘤细胞通常具有扭曲的或分叶状核，核膜薄，染色质细腻，有多个嗜碱性或嗜酸性小核仁，因此被称为"爆米花细胞"（popcorn cell）。诊断性 Reed-Sternberg 细胞通常少见或缺乏，且并非诊断 N-LPHL 所必需。然而也有例外。在少数病例，许多 L&H 细胞具有大核仁，类似陷窝细胞（lacunar cell）或诊断性 Reed-Sternberg 细胞；只有结合免疫组织化学检查才能将这种病例与 C-HL 鉴别开（图 21A.10）。

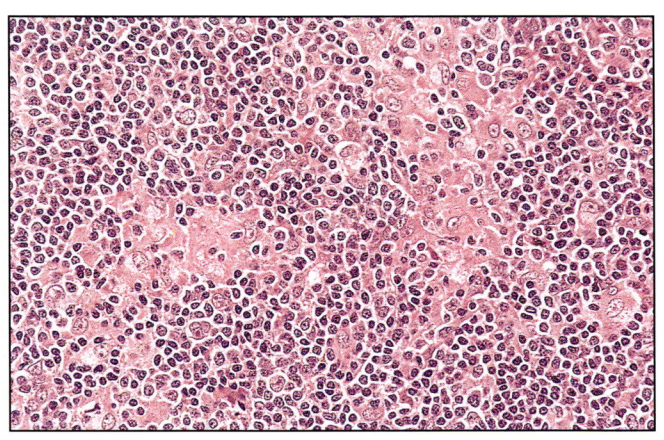

图 21A.8　结节性淋巴细胞为主型 Hodgkin 淋巴瘤。在这种弥漫成分中，大的 L&H 细胞散布在小淋巴细胞（当病变弥漫时，大多数细胞为 T 系）和组织细胞背景中。

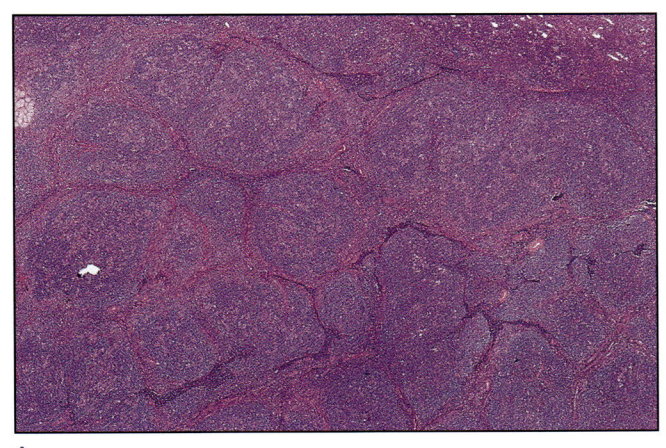

A

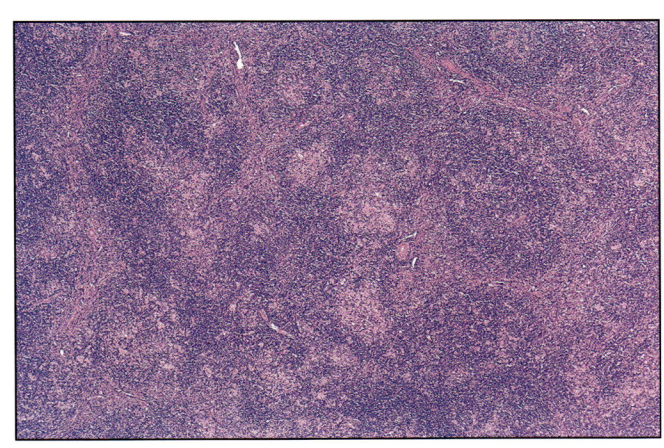

B

图 21A.7　结节性淋巴细胞为主型 Hodgkin 淋巴瘤。（A）典型病例的特点是呈明显的多发深染大结节，其中混杂有组织细胞组成的粉染灶。结节密集，局部彼此镶嵌。（B）另一个病例显示结节模糊且局部融合。

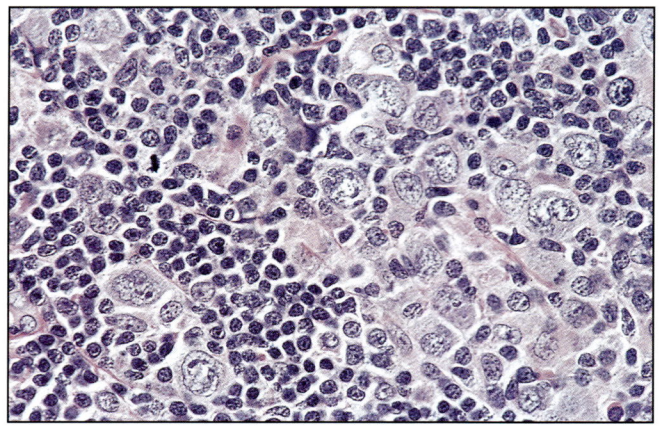

图21A.9 结节性淋巴细胞为主型Hodgkin淋巴瘤。肿瘤细胞（L&H细胞）由于核膜折叠或分叶而类似爆米花。核仁通常不明显。肿瘤细胞在结节内最容易见到。缺少浆细胞和嗜酸性粒细胞。

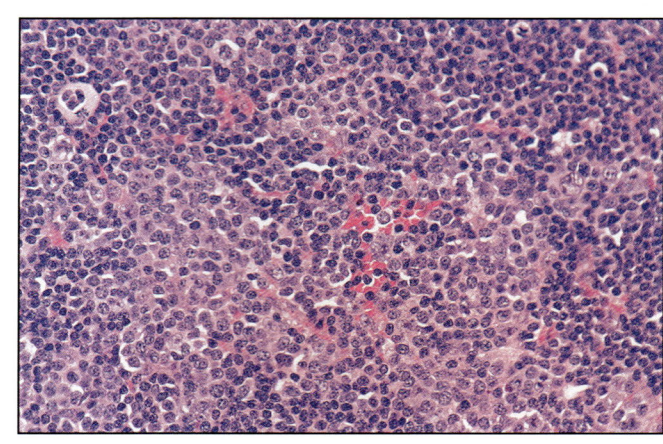

图21A.11 结节性淋巴细胞为主型Hodgkin淋巴瘤。在有些病例，结节内可见淡染的中等大小的淋巴细胞群，胞浆淡染；这些是T细胞。L&H细胞常常散在于这些细胞群中。

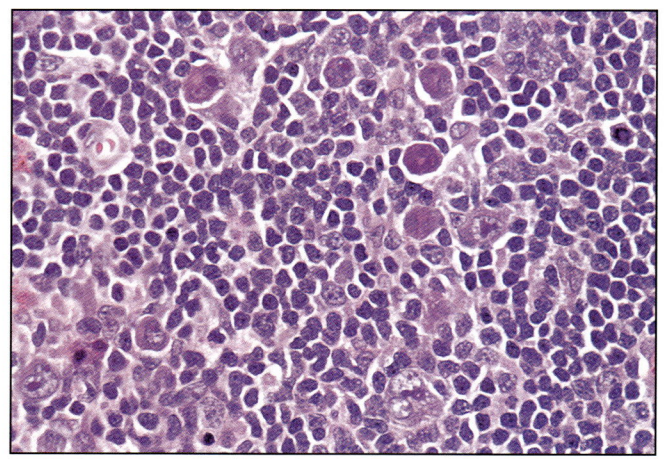

图21A.10 结节性淋巴细胞为主型Hodgkin淋巴瘤，类似于富于淋巴细胞的经典型Hodgkin淋巴瘤。在这个少见病例中，肿瘤细胞具有大的嗜酸性核仁，类似于诊断性或单核Reed-Sternberg细胞。需要通过免疫组织化学确诊。

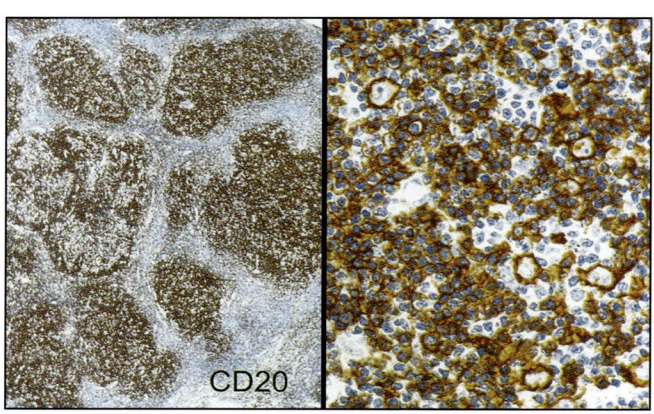

图21A.12 结节性淋巴细胞为主型Hodgkin淋巴瘤CD20免疫染色。左侧：结节结构因为富含B淋巴细胞而明显。右侧：高倍镜显示这种肿瘤的诊断性结构。阳性染色的大细胞见于小B细胞结节内，由于大细胞周围是一圈未染色的T淋巴细胞，因此格外明显。

虽然结节内或结节之间的淋巴细胞大多数是表现温和的小淋巴细胞，但在少数病例，染色质较分散的中等大小的淋巴细胞可形成淡染聚集区，围绕L&H细胞。这种细胞是反应性T淋巴细胞（图21A.11）。

在结外部位，其病理学和细胞学结构类似于淋巴结中所见[81,82]。当累及脾时，常常一致累及白髓（见本章第2部分）。

诊断N-LPHL需要进行免疫组化检查吗？

虽然以前认为单独通过形态学评估可以确诊N-LPHL，但现在认为其诊断需要免疫组化染色证实。在von Wasielewski等[83]的指导性研究中，根据形态学诊断的N-LPHL病例只有76%经免疫组化证实是真正的N-LPHL。反之，12%的诊断为C-HL的病例被证实是N-LPHL[83]。对于诊断N-LPHL，生存资料显示，免疫组化标准优于单独的形态学评估。显示N-LPHL免疫组化特征的淋巴瘤（即真正的N-LPHL）其生存率明显高于缺乏这种特征的淋巴瘤（即淋巴细胞为主型C-HL）。

免疫细胞化学

N-LPHL最典型的免疫表型特征是可见B细胞标记物CD20阳性大细胞（L&H细胞）出现在小B细胞结节中。大细胞与背景小B淋巴细胞反差明显，因为大细胞周围存在一圈未染色的细胞（T淋巴细胞）（图21A.12）。

表21A.8　结节性LPHL与经典型HL中肿瘤细胞的免疫表型比较

	结节性LPHL	经典型HL
CD45RB	阳性，但常常难以解释，因为L&H细胞周围紧紧围绕着小淋巴细胞	R-S细胞及其变型呈阴性，但常常难以解释，因为这些细胞混合在淋巴细胞中
CD20	阳性 许多L&H细胞（CD20⁺）细胞位于CD20⁺的小B细胞结节内 阳性染色的L&H细胞周围通常围绕着一圈CD20⁻细胞（T细胞）	阴性或阳性。如果阳性，通常不一致：有些细胞呈强阳性，有些细胞呈弱阳性，有些细胞呈阴性
CD79a	阳性	阴性或阳性；阳性率低于CD20⁺的阳性率
CD30	通常阴性（有些细胞可呈弱阳性）	阳性
CD15	阴性	通常阳性（～75%）
EMA	通常阳性	阴性
J链	阳性	阴性
Bcl-6	阳性（几乎所有的肿瘤细胞）	通常阴性。如果阳性，通常＜10%的肿瘤细胞
EBV LMP-1	阴性	阳性常见（30%～60%）

L&H细胞：L&H细胞一致表达各种B系标记物，如CD20和CD79a以及B细胞相关转录因子，如PAX-5、PU.1、Oct-2和Bob.1（图21A.12）。其免疫组化谱系不同于C-HL的Reed-Sternberg细胞，见表21A.8[68,84-88]。CD30阳性可见于高达7%～19%的病例，CD15阴性[79,88]。50%的病例EMA阳性。有些研究报道，L&H细胞存在Ig轻链限制性，几乎所有的病例表达κ轻链[89,90]。但是Ig轻链限制性可能难以显示。

L&H细胞bcl-6和CD40呈阳性，但CD10和fascin呈阴性[88,91,92]。MUM-1染色呈阴性或弱阳性[93,94]。

27%的病例L&H细胞表达IgD。这种亚型显示了某些不同于IgD阴性亚型的特征：中位年龄较年轻（21岁与44岁）；明显以男性为主（男女比例23:1与5:1）；更常累及颈部淋巴结（56%与18%）；L&H细胞主要位于滤泡外[95]。

背景细胞：在N-LPHL，结节富于多型性小B淋巴细胞（IgM⁺、IgD⁺），由密集的FDC网支持，常常显示虫蚀状结构[96,97]。在结节内，L&H细胞通常被CD3⁺的T淋巴细胞呈花环状包绕，其中有些共表达CD57和bcl-6（图21A.13）[87,88,98-100]。这种独特的bcl-6⁺CD57⁺T细胞群在结节性淋巴细胞为主型C-HL中少见或缺乏[100]。有些CD30⁺细胞可见于结节周围或结节之间[101]。

在27%的病例中组成结节的小淋巴细胞几乎全是T细胞而不是B细胞（图21A.14）[79]。结节之间和弥漫区域内的小淋巴细胞主要是T细胞（CD3⁺），很少有小B细胞。弥漫区域内很少有CD57⁺的小淋巴细胞。

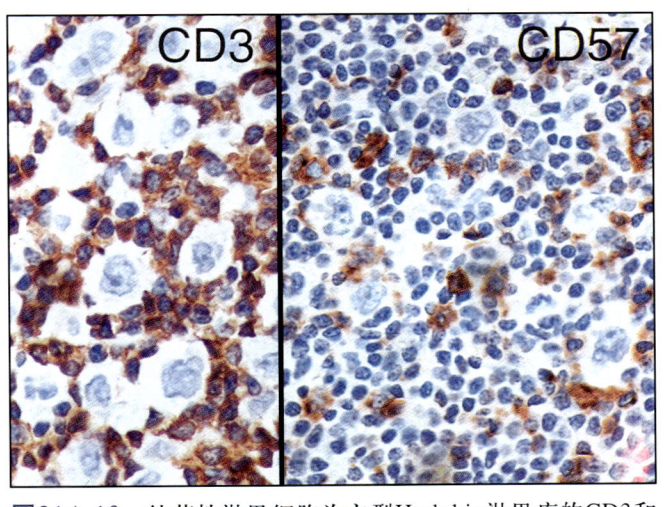

图21A.13　结节性淋巴细胞为主型Hodgkin淋巴瘤的CD3和CD57免疫染色。左侧：CD3染色显示花环状T细胞围绕L&H细胞。右侧：其中一些T细胞CD57呈阳性。

遗传学特征

无论是应用Southern印迹分析还是应用标准的PCR技术，在N-LPHL组织标本中通常检测不到克隆性Ig基因重排[101,102]。但是，通过PCR分析显微切割的L&H细胞可显示Ig基因的克隆性重排，证实肿瘤细胞为B细胞源性[28,103-107]。在L&H细胞中可检测到Ig mRNA转录。存在Ig基因体细胞超突变和克隆内部多样性、畸变的体细胞超突变（PIM1、PAX5、RhoH/TTF、C-MYC基因），48%的病例存在BCL-6基因重排，以及有组织学和免疫组化所见（存在特征改变的滤泡结节；存在

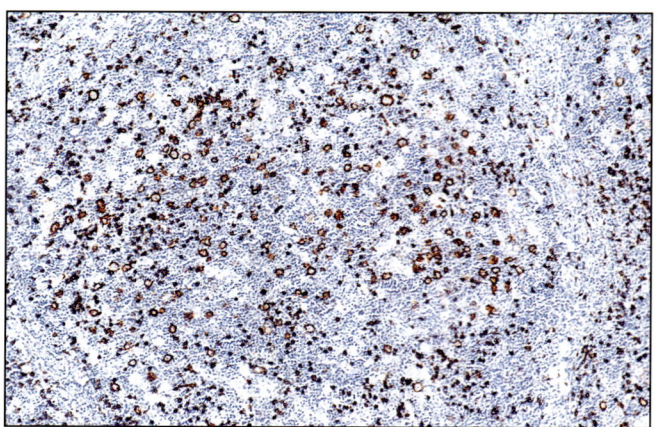

图21A.14 结节性淋巴细胞为主型Hodgkin淋巴瘤，富于T细胞的结节的CD20免疫染色。结节内CD20⁺的大肿瘤细胞分布于少数CD20⁺的小B细胞之间。

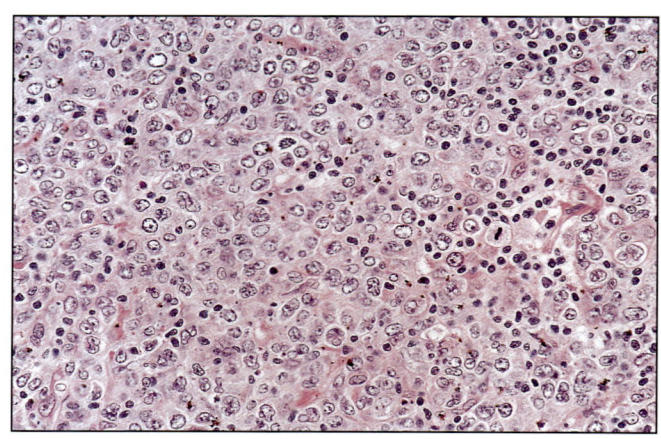

图21A.15 大B细胞淋巴瘤合并结节性淋巴细胞为主型Hodgkin淋巴瘤。可见单一形态增生的大细胞，其中一些类似L&H细胞。

分离的FDC网；表达B系标记物和bcl-6），强烈提示N-LPHL与生发中心B细胞的相关性[108,109]。然而由于缺乏 *BCL-2* 基因重排，它不是滤泡性淋巴瘤的一种亚型[110]。

尚未发现特异性细胞遗传学异常。比较性基因组杂交提示：有大量的基因组失衡（平均每例10.8种，包括多种染色体或染色体片段的获得和丢失）[111]。除了极少数例外，均与EBV无关[28,112]。

转化为非Hodgkin淋巴瘤

大约3%~4%的N-LPHL病例伴有弥漫大B细胞淋巴瘤，可在最初或之后发现（间隔0.5~24年，中位间隔期为1年）[45,69,113-118]。大B细胞淋巴瘤由融合成片的类似于中心母细胞（常为分叶状）或免疫母细胞的大细胞组成（图21A.15），表达B系标记物，常常表达单一型Ig。尚不清楚大细胞淋巴瘤是真正的NHL还是仅仅是L&H细胞的肿瘤性过度生长[119]。分子证据显示，有些（但非全部）大B细胞淋巴瘤和N-LPHL之间存在克隆关系[102,119-121]。EBV在转化中不起作用。虽然有些研究提示，来源于N-LPHL的大B细胞淋巴瘤预后良好，但其他研究显示其预后与原发性弥漫大B细胞淋巴瘤相似[79,114,118]。

已有报道，极少数外周T细胞淋巴瘤在N-LPHL同时或之后发生[122-124]。一些N-LPHL病例会伴发C-HL[125]。

鉴别诊断

- **生发中心的进行性转化**（progressive transformation of germinal centers, PTGC）：PTGC是一种反应性病变，其特点是滤泡大而深染，散在分布于普通型反应性滤泡的背景中（图21A.16）。这些大滤泡的大

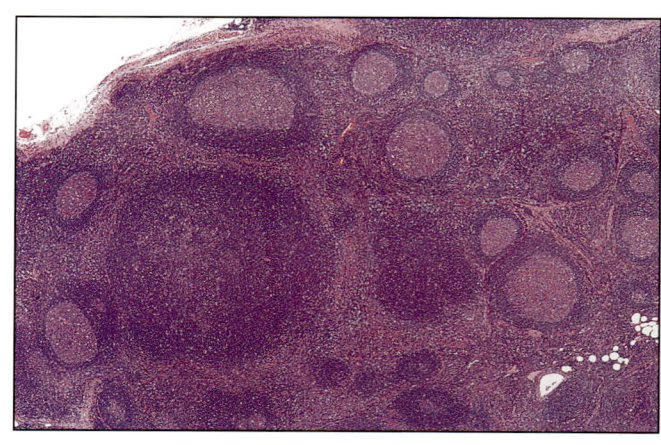

图21A.16 生发中心进行性转化。在反应性淋巴滤泡背景中出现深染大结节。根据定义，其直径是反应性滤泡的几倍。

小是周围反应性滤泡的几倍，主要由小淋巴细胞组成，散在分布有生发中心细胞。其中有些仍含有多个小的残留生发中心。PTGC和N-LPHL之间的发病机制关系已提出。它们可以共同存在于同一个淋巴结内；有些N-LPHL患者随访中发生PTGC；少部分PTGC患者后来发生了N-LPHL[59,80,126-131]。因此当N-LPHL患者发生复发的淋巴结肿大时，必须进行淋巴结活检以确定患者是否为肿瘤复发、PTGC或其他不相关的病变。在所有显著的PTGC病例，应通过寻找明确的膨胀性融合滤泡和L&H除外细胞早期的N-LPHL[80]。围绕CD20⁺大细胞的T细胞花环是N-LPHL的恒定特征，但在PTGC则极少见[97]。见"淋巴组织增生性病变的诊断实践问题"（第1250页）。

- **滤泡性淋巴瘤**（follicular lymphoma）：少数滤泡性淋巴瘤病例可显示类似于N-LPHL的结构特征。与

后者不同，其组成结节的淋巴细胞是滤泡中心细胞（中心细胞常常富于三角形或长形核，CD10和bcl-6阳性）而不是小淋巴细胞和L&H细胞[132]。见"淋巴组织增生性病变的诊断实践问题"（第1250页）。

- B细胞慢性淋巴细胞白血病/小淋巴细胞淋巴瘤（B-CLL/SLL）：N-LPHL以小淋巴细胞为主，可误诊为小淋巴细胞淋巴瘤。但是，小淋巴细胞淋巴瘤在40岁以下者极少见，且小B淋巴细胞共表达CD5并显示轻链限制性。
- 经典型Hodgkin淋巴瘤（classical HL）：见"淋巴组织增生性病变的诊断实践问题"（第1250页）。
- 结节性富于B细胞的滤泡树突状细胞肿瘤（nodular B cell-rich FDC tumor）：见"滤泡树突状细胞肉瘤"（第1240页）。

弥漫性淋巴细胞为主型Hodgkin淋巴瘤存在吗？

目前还不能识别或界定弥漫LPHL（图21A.17）。当网状纤维染色或B细胞标记物免疫染色发现弥漫LPHL肿瘤中具有较少结节时，应诊断为N-LPHL[86]。如果整个标本中未见结节成分，则诊断为"富于T细胞的大B细胞淋巴瘤"。

出现明显弥漫成分的N-LPHL与疾病高分期（III/IV期）和高复发率有关[62,66,73,79,133]。

经典型Hodgkin淋巴瘤
Classical Hodgkin lymphoma (C-HL)

临床特征

大多数C-HL患者表现为淋巴结肿大。淋巴结肿大常常是多发的，质硬韧、无触痛且无光泽。C-HL极少表现为单独的结外病变。临床上，结节硬化型HL（NSHL）不同于其他C-HL类型的特点是：前者好发于女性，常常累及纵隔。不同的HL亚型的主要临床特征见表21A.7[1,39,62,134-136]。

C-HL的播散

C-HL主要向邻近部位播散，经分期探查术所见和早期患者放疗成功例证已证实[137]。HL可以单病灶起病，以类似于癌转移的方式（包括逆流）通过淋巴管播散至下一组淋巴结。脾播散发生在主动脉旁淋巴结和脾门淋巴结受累之后。一旦累及脾，则可发生血行播散，如播散至肝和骨髓。但是这种理论不能解释某些病例，例如，"跳跃性转移"，双侧颈部/腋窝淋巴结受累而其间没有淋巴结受累，输入淋巴管未受累的脾转移[138]。这种理论也不能解释AIDS患者发生的HL。

临床行为和治疗

未经治疗的C-HL的5年生存率小于5%[139]。应用目前的治疗方法，大部分患者可以治愈[1,140]。在美国，1960—1992年间，HL患者的5年生存率已从40%上升至82%，体现了现代癌症治疗的巨大成功[141]。根据临床分期和不同的预后因素，治疗模式已经个体化，目的是减少治疗毒性而保持高的治愈率。对非大块肿物的IA或IIA期患者，选择ABVD（阿霉素、博来霉素、长春碱和氮烯唑胺）化疗4个疗程，对未达到完全缓解的患者，实施2个疗程化疗加受累部位放疗[142,143]。5年总体生存率可达95%。对进展期患者，行ABVD化疗至完全缓解后2个疗程，然后或者强化化疗，或者化疗加上肿块区域放疗。5年总体生存率>80%[142,144]。

绝大多数患者可以得到缓解[145]。大约30%的缓解患者会复发，尤其是分期较高的患者，通常在2～3年内。通过补救治疗常常可以再次缓解[145-147]。但是在HL的长期生存者中，与治疗有关的第二种肿瘤（如急性白血病和实体癌）应予以关注[148-150]。

肿瘤细胞：Reed-Sternberg细胞及其变型

HL的肿瘤细胞是Reed-Sternberg细胞及其变型[78]。诊断性Reed-Sternberg细胞是必需的但并不足以诊断C-HL，因为类似于Reed-Sternberg的细胞可见于NHL、反应性淋巴结病（包括传染性单核细胞增多症）及其他恶性肿瘤[151,152]。因此，要诊断HL，必须在相应亚型细胞背景中找到Reed-Sternberg细胞（表21A.7）。

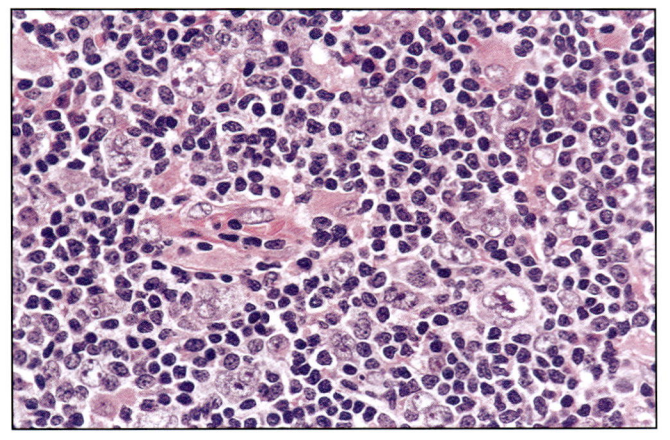

图21A.17 所谓的弥漫性淋巴细胞为主型Hodgkin淋巴瘤。L&H细胞具有分叶状核，位于小淋巴细胞背景中。没有见到局灶结节结构，无法与富于T细胞的大B细胞淋巴瘤鉴别。

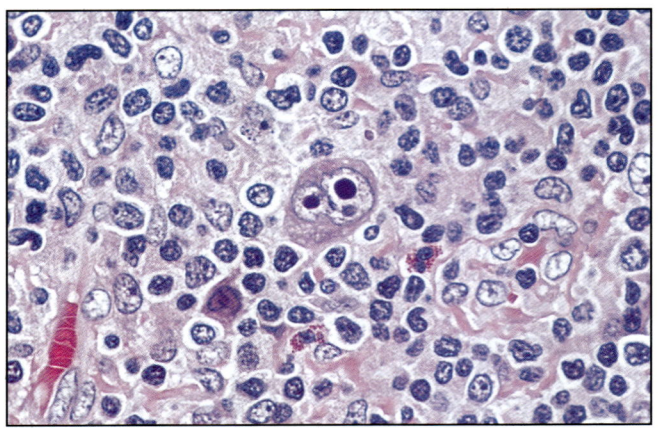

图21A.18 经典型Hodgkin淋巴瘤的诊断性Reed-Sternberg细胞（视野中央）。可见巨大嗜酸性包涵体样核仁。背景由非活化小淋巴细胞、浆细胞和嗜酸性粒细胞组成。

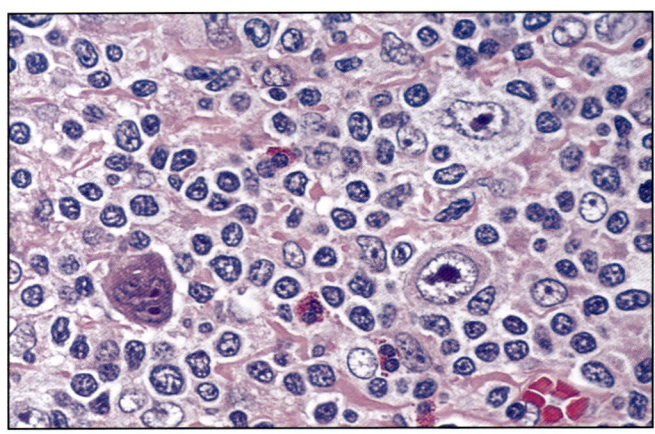

图21A.20 经典型Hodgkin淋巴瘤（混合细胞型）的单核Reed-Sternberg细胞。核仁位于中央。诊断性Reed-Sternberg细胞可见于视野左侧。

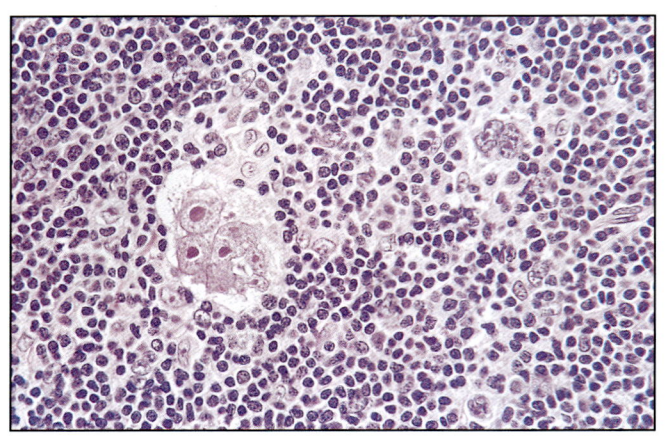

图21A.19 经典型Hodgkin淋巴瘤的诊断性Reed-Sternberg细胞。与普通细胞相比，肿瘤细胞含有较多的分叶。加之细胞显示多倍体特征、核仁足够大，就可以考虑为诊断性Reed-Sternberg细胞。

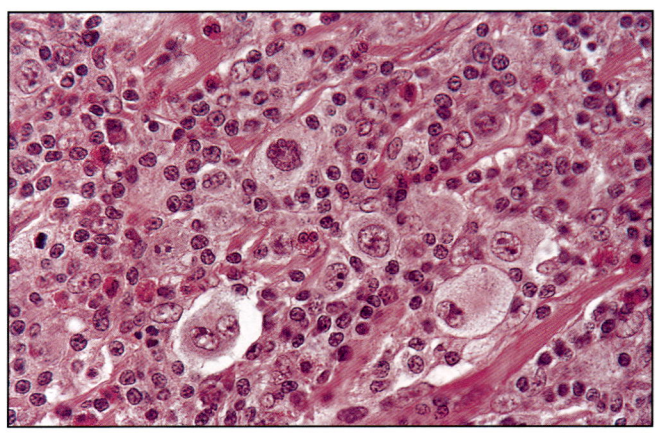

图21A.21 结节硬化型Hodgkin淋巴瘤的陷窝细胞。可见特征性淡染收缩的胞浆。核仁通常相对较小。

诊断性 Reed-Sternberg 细胞：是大细胞（20～30μm），形态学标志为多倍体（双核、多核或分叶核），并不需要教科书中所描述的镜影双核（图21A.18和21A.19）。核膜厚，有大的包涵体样嗜酸性核仁（大于红细胞），周围常常有空晕。胞浆轻度嗜酸性至嗜双色性。除了N-LPHL之外，诊断性Reed-Sternberg细胞可见于所有的HL亚型。

单核 Reed-Sternberg 细胞：除了具有单一圆形或卵圆形核以外，其他特征与诊断性 Reed-Sternberg 细胞相同（图21A.20）。其可见于不同亚型的 HL，但在 N-LPHL 中少见或缺乏。

陷窝细胞（lacunar cells）：是结节硬化型 HL（NSHL）的特点。核呈圆形或分叶状，染色质呈空泡状，具有多个明显的小到中等的核仁。胞浆量多，淡染收缩，因此肿瘤细胞明显位于陷窝内（图21A.21）。这种诊断特征是甲醛溶液固定的人工假象，因为在 Zenker 或 B5 固定的组织中见不到。

多形性 Reed-Sternberg 细胞：核大，呈奇异形、多倍体。其虽然是淋巴细胞削减型 HL（LDHL）的特点，但也可见于 NSHL 和混合细胞型 HL（MCHL）。

干尸细胞（mummified cells）：是渐进性坏死的大细胞，核的细节不清楚，胞浆深染嗜酸性（图 21A.22）。在 HL 中常见，但本身不具有诊断性。

Reed-Sternberg细胞识别的实际问题

虽然文献和教科书中强调诊断 HL 需要见到诊断性 Reed-Sternberg 细胞，但并不需要花费过多的精力寻找 Reed-Sternberg 细胞。在有些 C-HL 病例，诊断性 Reed-Sternberg 细胞稀少，大多数肿瘤细胞更类似于普通的大细胞淋巴瘤。实际上，如果具备了相应的细胞背景，只要出现一些大细胞（单核、双叶或多叶核），核仁大且显示典型的免疫表型，就可以诊断 C-HL（图21.23）。

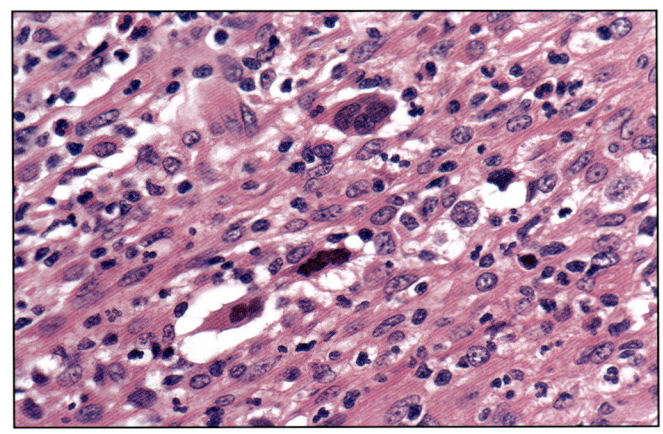

图21A.22 经典型Hodgkin淋巴瘤的干尸细胞。核大，污秽。

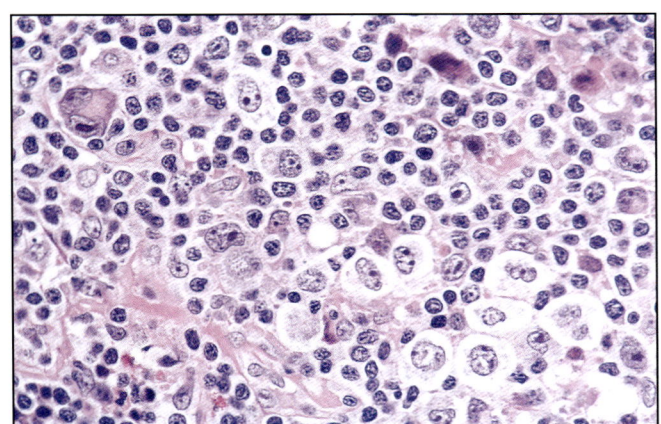

图21A.23 结节硬化型Hodgkin淋巴瘤，BNLI 1级。小淋巴细胞中可见陷窝细胞和干尸细胞。陷窝细胞与大细胞淋巴瘤难以鉴别。左边可见一个诊断性Reed-Sternberg细胞。

Reed-Sternberg细胞的性质

Reed-Sternberg细胞的组织学发生存在争议。组织细胞、指状树突状细胞、滤泡树突状细胞（FDC）、髓细胞和淋巴细胞均被提示可能为其细胞来源[28]。近期的研究显示，几乎所有C-HL病例的Reed-Sternberg细胞都是B细胞来源，证据是：表达B细胞特异性激活蛋白PAX-5，有时表达CD20，存在Ig基因重排，以及基因组表达方式符合B细胞[28,29,153-155]。这些细胞显示生发中心或生发中心后B淋巴细胞特征，但是处于"残缺"状态，因此尽管存在Ig基因重排，它们不能产生功能性Ig mRNA转录和Ig蛋白，而且常常缺乏B细胞特异性抗原表达。这种不一致性的原因可能是Ig基因的残缺突变（～25%的病例）或B细胞转录因子（Oct-2、Bob.1和PU.1）的下调和中断[28,84,155-161]。

少数C-HL病例的Reed-Sternberg细胞可显示T细胞或FDC分化的免疫组化或分子学证据[28,162,163]。

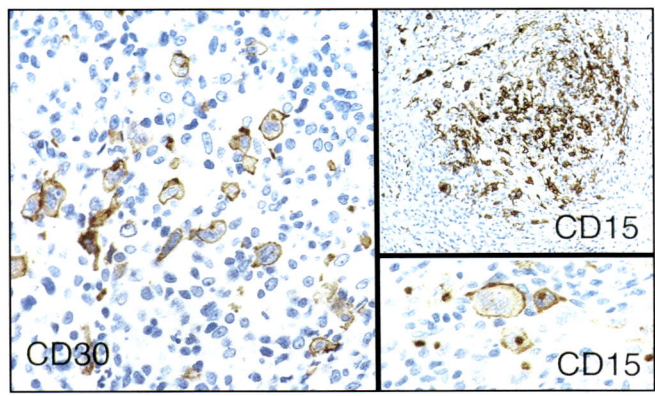

图21A.24 经典型Hodgkin淋巴瘤的免疫染色。左侧：Reed-Sternberg细胞显示细胞膜和高尔基区CD30阳性。右侧：在这个结节硬化型Hodgkin淋巴瘤中，CD15染色使肿瘤细胞的结节性聚集更加突出。右下：Reed-Sternberg细胞的CD15染色位于细胞膜或高尔基区。

免疫细胞化学

Reed-Sternberg细胞及其变型：在C-HL，Reed-Sternberg细胞及其变型常常是CD45RB$^-$、CD30$^+$、CD15$^+$（表21A.8）。在高达100%的病例，CD30阳性[164]。在高达75%的病例，CD15阳性。阳性表现应该呈核旁小球状，伴有或不伴细胞膜染色（图21A.24）[164,165]。缺乏CD15表达与以下因素有关：年龄较大，男性为主，疾病分期较高，混合细胞型比结节硬化型更常见[166]。CD15阳性还可见于B细胞淋巴瘤（5%）、T细胞淋巴瘤（20%）和非淋巴造血系统肿瘤[167,168]。Reed-Sternberg细胞常常表达HLA-DR、CD25、CD40、MUM-1和fascin[91-94,169-172]。只有30%的病例可见少数肿瘤细胞表达bcl-6[85]。

B细胞系标记物染色的可变率已有报道[173,174]。当CD20着染时，几乎总是异质性的，有些细胞呈强阳性，有些细胞呈弱阳性，有些细胞呈阴性（图21A.25）。Reed-Sternberg细胞常常显示Ig着染，但κ和λ轻链在同一细胞内均可显示，提示Ig是从周围组织中吸收而不是细胞自身合成的[175,176]。PAX-5通常呈阳性，强度弱至中等。B细胞相关转录因子PU.1、Oct-2和Bob.1通常都为阴性，或仅表达其中一种或两种。高达5%的病例可以显示T细胞系标记物着染，如CD2、CD3、CD4、CD5和CD8（通常在一部分肿瘤细胞中表达单一抗体）[163,177,178]。

虽然常可见p53蛋白表达，但*P53*基因突变少见[179,180]。

背景淋巴细胞成分：大多数背景小淋巴细胞是T细胞，CD4$^+$细胞远远多于CD8$^+$细胞（图21A.26）[181]。T细胞常常表达细胞毒性分子，但不表达CD57[182]。网络

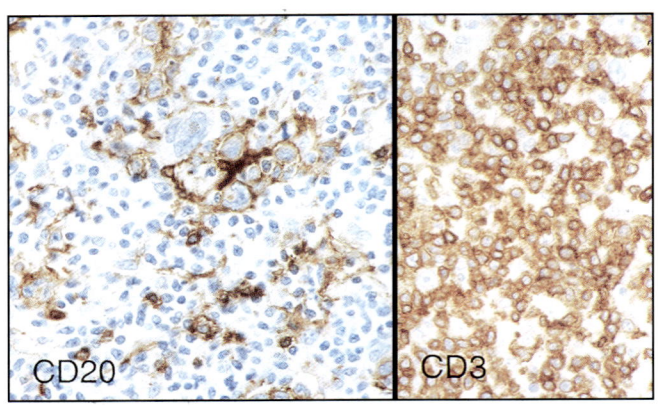

图21A.25 经典型Hodgkin淋巴瘤的免疫染色。左侧：在有些病例，有些大的肿瘤细胞显示CD20弱阳性或强阳性，而有些肿瘤细胞显示阴性。右侧：背景富含CD3⁺T细胞，但肿瘤细胞阴性。

Reed-Sternberg 细胞及其变型的 FDC 网可见于 50% 的结节硬化型 Hodgkin 淋巴瘤（NSHL）和 20% 的混合细胞型 Hodgkin 淋巴瘤（MCHL）[183]。

遗传学特征

在 Southern 印迹分析中，C-HL 通常缺乏 Ig 基因重排，除非是富含 Reed-Sternberg 细胞的病例[184-189]。当应用 PCR 检测整个组织的克隆性 Ig 基因重排时，23%～50% 的病例可获得阳性结果，显示 CD20 免疫反应的病例阳性率较高[155,190-192]。应用 Southern 印迹分析或 PCR 均检测不到 TCR 基因重排，只有以前的一个报道是个例外[28,193]。

组织显微切割获取单个肿瘤细胞的 PCR 分析表明，Ig 基因有重排且显示体细胞超突变。同一病例中不同细胞的 Ig 基因重排的 DNA 序列对比分析证实，肿瘤细胞具有克隆性本质[28,155,157,194-198]。生发中心细胞还常常有靶基因的异常体细胞超突变（*PIM1*、*PAX5*、*RhoH/TTF*、*C-MYC*）[109]。

C-HL 中可见多种染色体数量异常，但没有特定的染色体异常[155,199]。

基因表达谱研究表明，Reed-Sternberg 细胞表达的 B 细胞特异性基因 mRNA 较少，可影响 B 细胞信号激活途径的多种成分，包括 B 细胞受体信号[200]。可以识别具有不同临床预后的分子组：预后好的组别具有凋亡诱导和细胞信号基因过表达，而预后差的组别涉及纤维母细胞激活、血管生成、细胞外基质重建、细胞增殖的基因上调以及肿瘤抑制基因的下调[201]。

与EBV的关系

在西方国家，40%～50% 的 C-HL 病例与 Epstein-Barr 病毒（EBV）有关，提示 EBV 在 C-HL 发生中的作用。EBV 与混合型的相关性最强（>60%），与结节硬化型的相关性较弱（大约35%）[202-205]。发生在头颈部的 C-HL 以及发生在年龄较小或较大的 HL 与 EBV 具有较强的相关性[202,203,206,207]。在东方国家，这种相关比约为 60%[203,208]。在发展中国家的患者和 AIDS 患者，EBV 与 C-HL 的相关性接近 100%，提示当免疫活性水平低时，EBV 在 C-HL 的发生中可能具有较为重要的作用。

EBV 以克隆性游离体形式（clonal episomal form）存在，提示感染在肿瘤性克隆扩增之前。在 EBV 相关的肿瘤中，EBV 基因的表达形式是可变的，有三种主要的潜伏形式（表 21A.9）。C-HL 通常显示 II 型潜伏形式[209]。

许多不同的技术可用于显示 EBV 的存在。PCR 的缺点是：即使 EBV 仅仅存在于某些反应性淋巴细胞

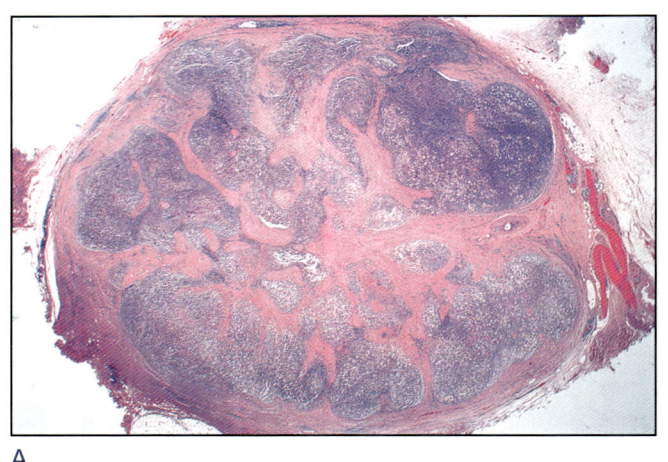

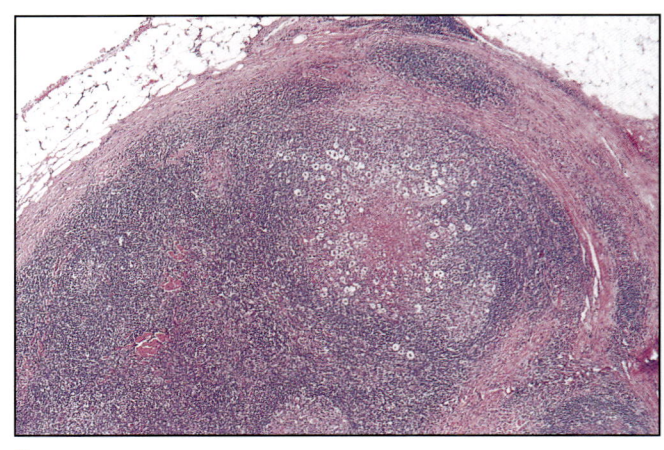

图21A.26 结节硬化型Hodgkin淋巴瘤。（A）典型病例显示广泛纤维化和结节形成。可见明显的纤维性被膜增厚。（B）宽厚的纤维带从增厚的被膜蔓延至实质。陷窝细胞结节内常出现明显的中心坏死。

表21A.9　EBV相关肿瘤中EBV基因的表达模式

	EBV潜伏		
	I型	II型	III型
EBNA1	+	+	+
EBNA2-6	–	–	+
LMP1	–	+	+
疾病类型	Burkitt淋巴瘤	Hodgkin淋巴瘤；鼻咽癌；非B细胞NHL（如NK/T细胞淋巴瘤，外周T细胞淋巴瘤）	移植后淋巴组织增生性病变

EBNA：EBV核抗原；LMP1：潜伏膜蛋白-1。

中，也可以获得阳性信号。检测EBV编码的早期RNA（EBER）的原位杂交技术具有高度敏感性，是在细胞水平可显示EBV的相对简单的方法。Reed-Sternberg细胞和个别小淋巴细胞显示阳性核标记[210-121]。EBV潜伏膜蛋白-1（LMP-1）免疫染色是另一种显示EBV的简单方法，因为这种蛋白在EBV相关的C-HL的Reed-Sternberg细胞中恒定表达[205,212,213]。染色应位于细胞膜和高尔基区。

虽然EBV阳性与C-HL的预后关系存在争议，但近期的研究表明，50岁以上的C-HL患者，如果EBV呈阳性，则预后差[214-217]。

结节硬化型Hodgkin淋巴瘤
Nodular sclerosis Hodgkin lymphoma (NSHL)

临床行为：应用现代治疗，5年生存率可达80%。可发生局部或远处复发，复发的HL保持结节硬化类型，即使肿瘤细胞的比例可以增加（表21A.7）。

病理学：即使HL中仅仅出现局灶性结节硬化，也要优先诊断NSHL[78,218]。淋巴结显示局灶性、部分性或全部受累。典型的病例被膜增厚，伴有多处宽的、双折射性血管化胶原带，蔓延至实质，导致多个结节形成（图21A.26）。但有些病例的纤维化较轻微；有人提出，诊断NSHL至少要出现一条有极向的纤维带[43]。即使没有硬化，也要有形成模糊的结节结构的肿瘤细胞松散聚集的趋势（图21A.26B）。结节中心可显示坏死和（或）化脓（图21A.26）。结节可随着时间的迁延形成闭塞性纤维化。

在结节内，陷窝细胞混合有数量不等的小淋巴细胞、浆细胞、嗜酸性粒细胞、中性粒细胞和组织细胞。有些病例的背景细胞几乎均由小淋巴细胞组成（图21A.21，21A.23）。陷窝细胞可呈单个，或成团、成片分布。可表现为单一形态，也可显示一定的多形性，核仁或大或小（图21A.21，21A.23，21A.27）。诊断性Reed-Sternberg细胞少见。

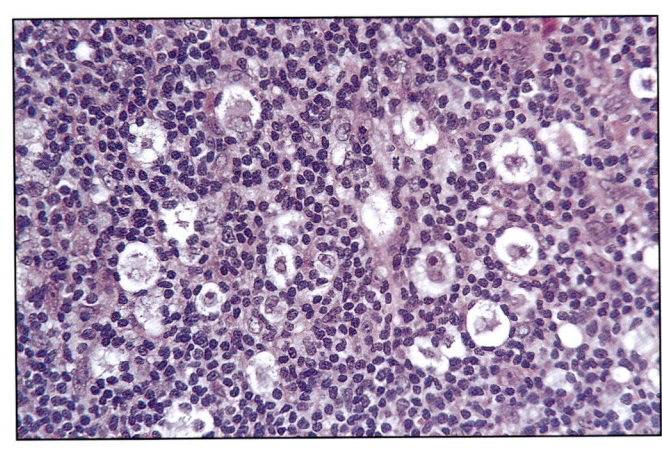
A

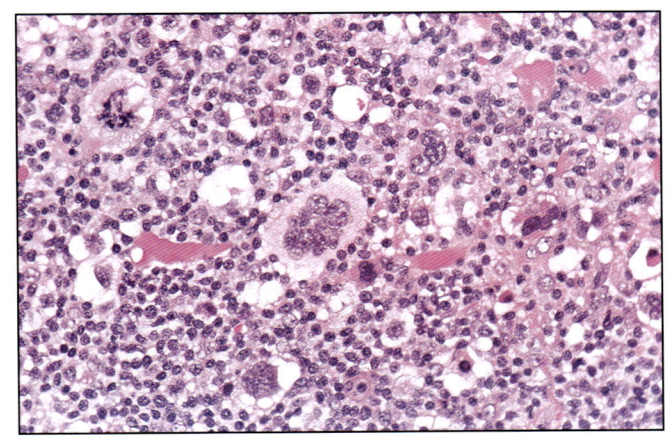
B

图21A.27　结节硬化型Hodgkin淋巴瘤。（A）陷窝细胞可见于富于小淋巴细胞的背景中，符合BNLI 1级。（B）在这个病例中，大多数结节内可见奇异形陷窝细胞，没有淋巴细胞削减，符合BNLI 2级。

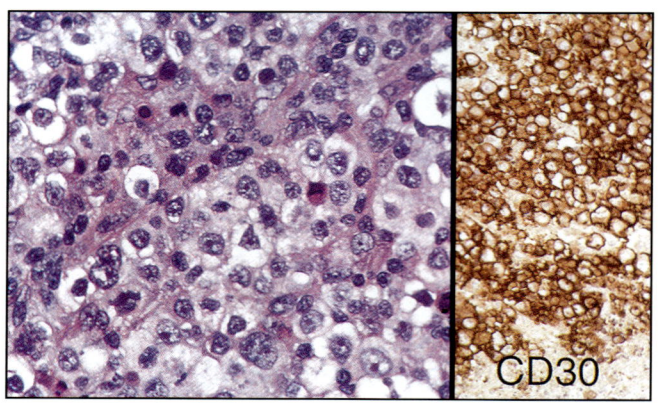

21A.28 结节硬化型Hodgkin淋巴瘤，合体细胞型或BNLI2级。左侧：肿瘤细胞成片，其间淋巴细胞少见或没有，符合BNLI2级。这种病变与大细胞淋巴瘤难以鉴别。右侧：CD30免疫染色显示成片的肿瘤细胞。

表21A.10	结节硬化型Hodgkin淋巴瘤：BNLI 1级和2级病变的行为差异	
	NSHD 1级 (NS1)（%）	NSHD 2级 (NS2)（%）
B症状的出现	29	51
5年生存率：		
I/II期	92	74
III/IV期	77	55
总体	83	66
完全缓解率	84	66
5年无病生存率	54	37

合体细胞型NSHL的特点是肿瘤细胞形成合性细胞团块（图21A.28）。肿瘤细胞可能不显示典型的陷窝细胞的细胞学特征，类似于普通的大细胞淋巴瘤[30,219]。坏死常见，有时呈地图形[220]。这种变型可被误诊为转移癌、转移性黑色素瘤或大细胞淋巴瘤。其表现为高分期疾病[220]。

富于细胞期NSHL是有争议的病变。它是指可见结节结构和明显陷窝细胞的病例，但缺乏纤维化条带。将这种病变归于NSHL而不是MCHL是正确的，因为进一步活检常常显示典型NSHL的特征[218]。

结节硬化型Hodgkin淋巴瘤的亚型/分级：根据淋巴细胞和肿瘤细胞的数量，NSHL有时可再分为淋巴细胞为主型、混合细胞型和淋巴细胞削减型（LP、MC和LD）三种亚型。虽然有些研究显示这种分类缺乏预后意义[134,221]，但有些研究表明这种分类是重要的[222]。不建议应用这些名称,因为容易与各种组织学类型的HL混淆。

英国国立淋巴瘤研究（British National Lymphoma Investigation，BNLI）发现，NSHL的分级具有重要的预后意义（表21A.10）[73,222-224]。NSHL分为1级（NS1）或2级（NS2）。对于NS2,局部病变有效放疗后可以复发，这种复发与晚期腹部复发对于补救治疗通常无效[225]。应用强化治疗可改善NS2的预后。一些研究证实这种分级是有用的[226-228]，然而也有不同观点[229-231]。这些矛盾结果的一个可能解释是：强化治疗可消除1级和2级NSHL之间预后的差异[39]。另一种解释是：仅仅观察了在进展期疾病分级之间的预后差异而不是在疾病早期和中期的预后差异，所以包括或主要包括早期疾病患者的研究可能不显示差异[228]。

当出现以下任何一种特征时，病变归属于2级（图21A.27B，21A.28，21A.29）：

1. 25%的细胞结节含有多量奇异性和高度间变的

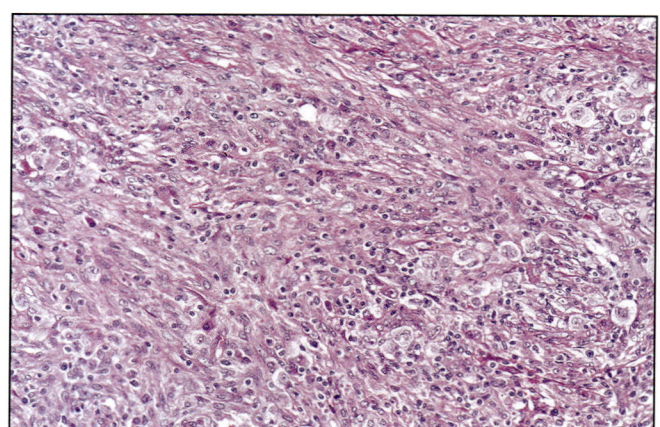

图21A.29 结节硬化型Hodgkin淋巴瘤，BNLI 2级。纤维组织细胞结构，右侧区域可见一些肿瘤细胞。

Hodgkin细胞，没有淋巴细胞削减。
2. 25%的细胞结节显示淋巴细胞削减，无论肿瘤细胞表现为一致性还是表现为间变性。
3. 80%的细胞结节显示纤维组织细胞形态（许多组织细胞和纤维母细胞，相对少量的陷窝细胞或Reed-Sternberg细胞）（图21A.29）。

总体上，80%的病例属于1级。可疑的或交界性病例也归类为1级。合体细胞型属于2级病变。"纤维母细胞型"在Stanford[134]以前的研究中与无复发生存期较短有关，相当于纤维组织细胞型的NS2。

von Wasielewski 等[228]提出的另一种分级系统,考虑以下三种因素：

1. 嗜酸性粒细胞（在所有细胞中所占比例＞5%，或在至少5个高倍视野中成群出现）。
2. 淋巴细胞削减（在整张切片所有细胞中所占比例＜33%）。

3. 非典型性（＞25%的Hodgkin细胞或Reed-Sternberg细胞呈奇异形和高度间变形，具有多形性核特征，深染，核轮廓高度不规则）。

不显示以上任何因素的病例被认为是"低危险性"，而显示一种或多种因素的病例被认为是"高危险性"。这两种危险类别的病例各占一半，总体和无进展生存率具有显著差异。

鉴别诊断

1. **坏死性淋巴结炎和猫抓病**（necrotizing lymphadenitis and cat-scratch disease）：有些NSHL病例可显示广泛的凝固性或化脓性坏死而掩盖肿瘤性质，导致误诊为坏死性淋巴结炎或猫抓病。对于纵隔或低位颈部淋巴结，要防止漏诊NSHL。由于核仁小，与组织细胞难以鉴别，寻找肿瘤细胞的最佳部位是坏死灶周围。CD30免疫染色对于显示这种细胞极有帮助。
2. **硬化性炎症或硬化性纵隔炎**（sclerosing inflammation or sclerosing mediastinitis）：显示明显闭塞性硬化的NSHL小活检可能被误诊为硬化性炎症。应当连续切片寻找陷窝细胞和Reed-Sternberg细胞。如果临床上怀疑HL但组织学检查不能诊断，则应重新活检。
3. **恶性纤维组织细胞瘤**（malignant fibrous histiocytoma）：纤维组织细胞-纤维母细胞型NSHL可被误诊为所谓的恶性纤维组织细胞瘤（多形性肉瘤）。然而，梭形细胞缺乏明确的异型性。更仔细地寻找偶尔可见陷窝细胞和Reed-Sternberg细胞。
4. **转移癌**（metastatic cancer）：合体细胞型NSHL可能与转移癌或黑色素瘤难以鉴别。出现梭形肿瘤细胞，明显的窦状隙结构，明显的核多形性和肿瘤细胞吞噬中性粒细胞强烈提示转移癌[232]。如果怀疑，则应进行免疫组化。
5. **大细胞淋巴瘤**（large cell lymphoma）：合体细胞型NSHL和大细胞淋巴瘤的鉴别可能很困难。出现典型的NSHL灶倾向于前者。见"淋巴组织增生性病变诊断的实践问题"（第1250页）。

混合细胞型Hodgkin淋巴瘤
Mixed cellularity Hodgkin's lymphoma（MCHL）

临床特征和行为：没有独特的临床特征（表21A.7）。除了颈部和锁骨上淋巴结，还容易累及腹腔内淋巴结。应用现代治疗，70%以上的病例可以达到完全缓解。这种HL可进展为淋巴细胞削减型HL（LDHL）。

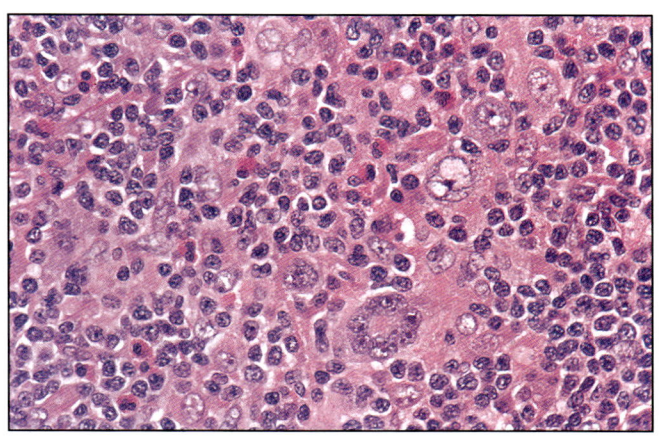

图21A.30 混合细胞型Hodgkin淋巴瘤。淋巴细胞、嗜酸性粒细胞和浆细胞背景中可见到Reed-Sternberg细胞。不显示结节硬化型Hodgkin淋巴瘤中的结节性结构。

病理学：淋巴结部分或弥漫受累。在小淋巴细胞、嗜酸性粒细胞、中性粒细胞和组织细胞背景中，易于见到单核细胞和诊断性Reed-Sternberg细胞（图21A.18，21A.20，21A.30）。肿瘤细胞均匀散在，不同于在NSHL中的结节性结构。并非所有的肿瘤细胞均显示Reed-Sternberg细胞及其变型的典型特征；有些可类似于免疫母细胞或显示界于免疫母细胞和单核Reed-Sternberg细胞之间的特征。有些病例富于上皮样组织细胞，类似于Lennert淋巴瘤。可见灶状坏死和继发性纤维化。后者缺乏在NSHL中见到的折光性带状纤维组织。

虽然HL背景中的淋巴细胞通常被描述为"小圆形淋巴细胞"、"非活化性"且"缺乏母细胞"，事实上，有些病例的淋巴细胞核轻度增大且不规则（图21A.20）。也可以出现少数活化的母细胞性大细胞。

鉴别诊断

1. **外周T细胞淋巴瘤**（peripheral T-cell lymphoma）：在外周T细胞淋巴瘤，小淋巴细胞通常可见异型性和不规则形的核皱折，常常连续出现小细胞、中等细胞和大细胞。出现透明细胞也倾向于诊断T细胞性淋巴瘤。需要免疫组化检查来证实诊断。
2. **富于T细胞的大B细胞淋巴瘤**（T cell-rich large B-cell lymphoma）：见"淋巴组织增生性病变诊断的实践问题"（第1250页）。
3. **反应性免疫母细胞增生，如传染性单核细胞增多症**（reactive immunoblastic proliferations, such as infectious mononucleosis）：反应性免疫母细胞增生与Reed-Sternberg细胞不容易鉴别[151]。但是，富于活化淋巴细胞和免疫母细胞的背景从未出现在HL中。见"淋巴组织增生性病变诊断的实践问题"（第1250页）。
4. **滤泡间Hodgkin样淋巴结炎**（interfollicular Hodgkinoid

lymphadenitis）：是一种以滤泡间淋巴细胞、浆细胞、嗜酸性粒细胞和上皮样组织细胞增生为特征的反应性病变，类似于HL[233]。但是，免疫母细胞小于单核Reed-Sternberg细胞，其核仁一般呈嗜碱性，而不是呈嗜酸性，胞浆呈嗜碱性/嗜双色性而不是呈嗜酸性。这些细胞与B细胞或T细胞抗体发生反应，但CD15呈阴性。

5. **转移癌或黑色素瘤**（metastatic carcinoma or melanoma）。

6. **Castleman病，浆细胞型**（castleman disease, plasma cell type）：极少数MCHL最初可表现为类似浆细胞型Castleman病的组织学特征，只有在复发时才能明确诊断HL。因此，在诊断浆细胞型Castleman病之前，必须仔细检查淋巴结寻找HL潜在的证据[234-236]。

富于淋巴细胞的经典型Hodgkin淋巴瘤 Lymphocyte-rich classical HL (LRCHL)

临床特征和行为：LRCHL少见，仅占所有HL的4%[237]。同N-LPHL一样，不同于NSHL或MCHL，LRCHL患者的病变常常为早期，B症状和纵隔受累少见[72,237]。但是，中位年龄比N-LPHL大（表21A.7）。根据一组研究，LRCHL的生存率比N-LPHL的差（5年生存率为80%与98%）[83]。但是，在其他研究中，LRCHL的生存率与N-LPHL的没有显著差异（8年HL特异性生存率为87%与95%；8年无病生存率为75%与74%）[62,72,238]。但是，与N-LPHL相比，多处复发较不常见（5%与27%），复发后的生存率较差[62,72]。

病理学：LRCHL的特点是单个Reed-Sternberg细胞及其变型散在于富于小淋巴细胞的背景中，粒细胞稀少

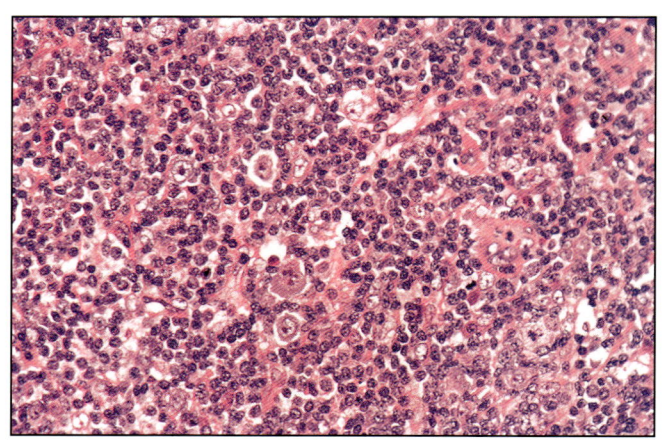

图21A.31 弥漫性富于淋巴细胞型Hodgkin淋巴瘤。单核Reed-Sternberg细胞散在于小淋巴细胞背景中。几乎没有浆细胞或嗜酸性粒细胞。

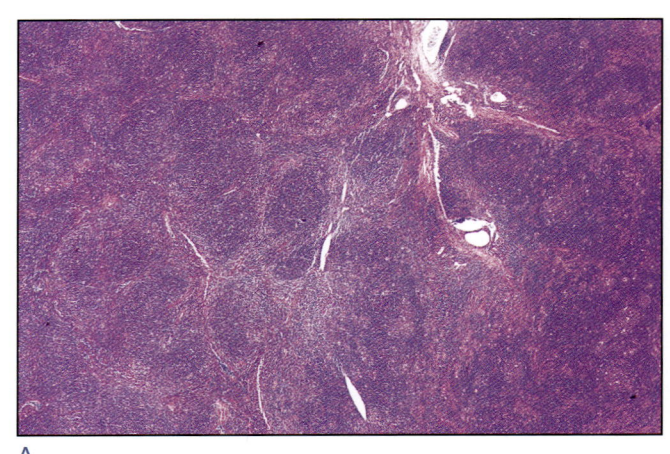

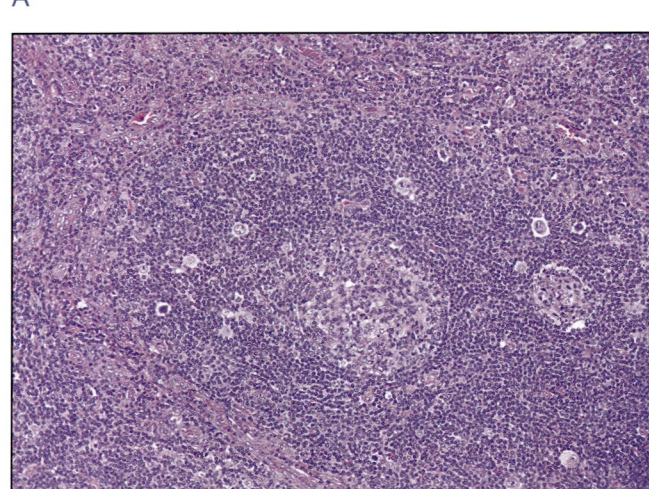

图21A.32 结节性富于淋巴细胞型经典型Hodgkin淋巴瘤。（A）淋巴细胞结节紧密排列、深染而大，是这种类型Hodgkin淋巴瘤的低倍镜特征。（B）有些结节由套区增厚的滤泡组成，其中散在Reed-Sternberg细胞。

或缺乏（图21A.31）。生长方式可呈结节状（较常见），也可呈弥漫性。

在结节型，低倍镜可见密集的大结节，结构非常类似于N-LPHL。结节主要由小淋巴细胞组成，但有些结节具有小的生发中心。Reed-Sternberg细胞及其变型可散在于淋巴细胞结节中，也可位于结节之间（图21A.32）[239]。在一些病例的淋巴细胞结节内，Reed-Sternberg细胞及其变型细胞周围聚集着淡染的中等大小的细胞（T细胞）。混合性浆细胞和多形核细胞少见。

免疫组化评估显示大细胞具有Reed-Sternberg细胞典型的免疫表型[39]。组成结节的小淋巴细胞大多数为CD20阳性的B细胞，表达IgD。常有CD3阳性的T细胞花环围绕肿瘤性大细胞，但CD57阳性细胞少见[100]。CD21阳性FDC网格通常显示为由大肿瘤细胞及其周围的T细胞形成的多个小"空洞"。滤泡间区富于T细胞。分子学分析显示突变性Ig基因重排，没有明显的克隆

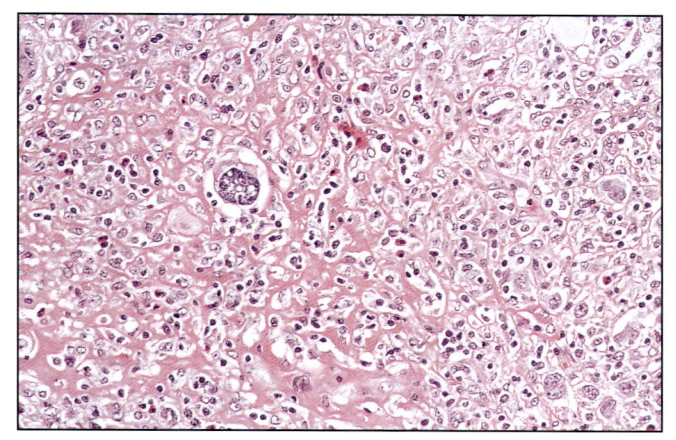

图21A.33 淋巴细胞削减型Hodgkin淋巴瘤,弥漫纤维化型。细胞成分减少,具有纤维组织背景。

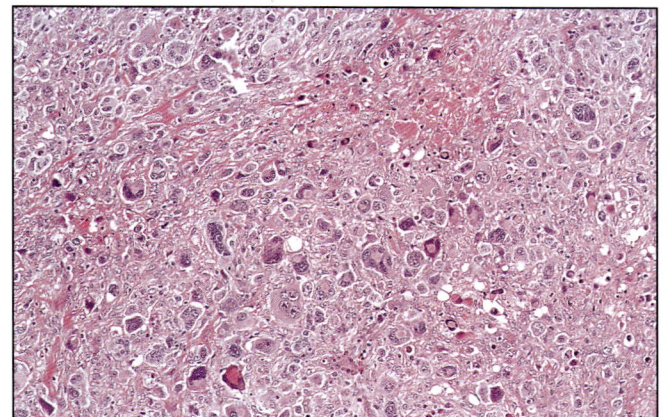

图21A.34 淋巴细胞削减型Hodgkin淋巴瘤,网状型。可见多量多形性Reed-Sternberg细胞。

内多样性,类似于其他经典型 HL 中所见[240]。

淋巴细胞削减型Hodgkin淋巴瘤
Lymphocyte-depleted Hodgkin lymphoma (LDHL)

病理学

已识别的 LDHL 类型有两种[43,241,242]:

1. **弥漫纤维化型** (diffuse fibrosis type):在网状纤维（非双折射性）和无定形蛋白物质不规则分布的背景中,所有细胞成分明显减少。诊断性Reed-Sternberg细胞少见（图21A.33）。坏死可能明显。
2. **网状型** (reticular type):病变高度富于细胞,伴有多量诊断性和多形性Reed-Sternberg细胞（图21A.34）。成熟淋巴细胞稀少,浆细胞、嗜酸性粒细胞、组织细胞和中性粒细胞也少见。可见不均匀无双折射性的纤维组织。常见坏死。

淋巴细胞削减型 Hodgkin 淋巴瘤的再评估:随着对各种类型的非 Hodgkin 淋巴瘤（NHL）的准确分类,目前已极少诊断 LDHL。过去诊断的多数 LDHL 病例经过评估后可重新归类[30,243,244]为伴淋巴细胞减少的结节硬化型 Hodgkin 淋巴瘤;大细胞 NHL,通常是间变大细胞、外周 T 细胞和富于 T 细胞的大 B 细胞淋巴瘤。极少数病例是真正的 LDHL 病例。不管 Reed-Sternberg 细胞的数目及其变型,如果以陷窝细胞为主且伴有纤维化,则将该病例归类为 NSHL[43,218]。没有免疫组化的支持就不能诊断 LDHL。

LDHL 患者的确切生存率差,几乎 80% 死于 3 个月以内[73,242]。但正确的化疗可挽救一些患者[136]。

经典型Hodgkin淋巴瘤的特殊形态学特征
Special morphologic features in C-HL

- 滤泡间Hodgkin淋巴瘤 (interfollicular HL):不同亚型的HL均可表现为以滤泡间生长为主。伴发的反应性滤泡增生可能非常明显,以致于病理医生忽视了不显眼的HL成分[245]。
- Hodgkin淋巴瘤中的泡沫状组织细胞 (foamy histiocytes in HL):有些HL病例中可见多量泡沫状组织细胞,导致其与黄色肉芽肿性炎或脂质贮积性疾病混淆[246]。
- Hodgkin淋巴瘤中的上皮样组织细胞 (epithelioid histiocytes in HL):有些HL病例可能伴有融合成团的上皮样组织细胞,形态类似Lennert淋巴瘤[247]。多数属于混合细胞型。
- 单核样B细胞团中发生的Hodgkin淋巴瘤 (HL occuring in monocytoid B-cell clusters):完全或主要局限于反应性单核样B细胞团中的HL非常少见,因此可能漏诊（图21A.35）[248,249]。
- 治疗改变的Hodgkin淋巴瘤 (treatment-altered HL):

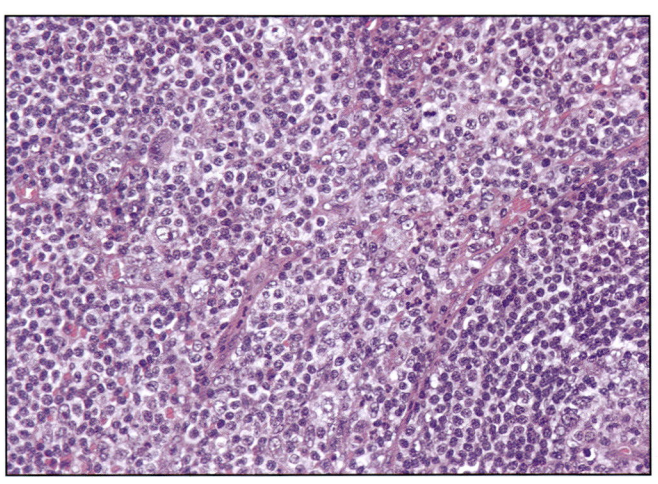

图21A.35 发生于单核样B细胞团的经典型Hodgkin淋巴瘤。在淋巴滤泡（右下视野）周围的单核样B细胞宽带中,散在大的Reed-Sternberg细胞。

治疗后复发的HL可显示非常不典型的组织细胞特征。细胞增生可呈单一形态，使之难以与NHL鉴别[250,251]。有时HL治疗后持续存在的肿物病变可仅仅由玻璃样变组织组成，没有残留病变的证据[252,253]。

其他组织受累和分期性剖腹术标本的评估
Involvement of other tissues and assessment of staging laparotomy materials

虽然分期性剖腹术一度盛行，但现在已极少使用。当C-HL的组织学诊断已经明确，诊断其他组织受累的标准可以不太严格。只要在适当的背景中见到具有典型免疫表型的非典型大细胞，就可以诊断HL累及，即使缺乏诊断性Reed-Sternberg细胞。

在脾，应该计数异常结节的数目，因为出现≥5个异常结节与较差的预后有关[44]。HL首先累及白髓，在小动脉周围或边缘区；肿瘤逐渐蚕食淋巴滤泡和红髓，形成融合性结节（见本章第2部分）。

在肝，累及门脉管道，逐渐侵入实质。在骨髓，即使缺乏非典型细胞，出现灶状或弥漫纤维化伴非特异性淋巴细胞、组织细胞、嗜酸性粒细胞和浆细胞浸润也提示受累。骨髓嗜酸性粒细胞增多是一种反应形式，有时见于经典型Hodgkin淋巴瘤患者；单独出现不应认为是C-HL累及骨髓。

经典型Hodgkin淋巴瘤的预后因素[254]

1. **临床**：高分期疾病是预后不良因素[44]。男性、进展期、B症状、肿物体积大以及没有得到完全缓解均与较差的预后有关[255]。
2. **病理学**：随着现代治疗的应用，组织学类型的预后意义实际上已消失[44]。但是，当使用严格的分类标准时，组织学类型仍对预后具有影响，只是影响力有所减少。预后最差的是淋巴细胞削减型[73]。血管侵犯与较差的预后有关[256,257]。结节硬化型Hodgkin淋巴瘤的组织学分级也具有预后意义（见"结节硬化型Hodgkin淋巴瘤"第1163页）。
3. **免疫表型**：缺乏CD15或CD20的表达与预后较差有关[166]。在肿瘤细胞中出现FDC网与较好的预后有关[258,259]。

非Hodgkin淋巴瘤
Non-Hodgkin lymphoma（NHL）

分类

在过去的许多年中已提出很多NHL分类。由于名称混乱，又制定了工作分类（Working Formulation）方法，试图用它来解释不同的淋巴瘤分类，在20世纪80～90年代这种方法得到了广泛应用[260]。1994年，国际淋巴瘤研究小组提出修订的欧美淋巴瘤（REAL）分类方法[36]。这种分类方法包括多种不同的临床病理学疾病，可以应用有效的技术进行区分，而不是建立在假定的正常对应者基础之上。它代表一种新的淋巴瘤分类范例，因为它强调生物学行为，而不是单纯依靠形态学分类。事实上，每一种类型的淋巴瘤均可显示广泛的形态学特征和一系列临床行为，但是统一的特征是具有独特的免疫表型和（或）基因型。一般情况下，保留了常用名称，但改进了有些病变的诊断标准。REAL分类方法自发表以来在全世界得到广泛应用，许多研究已经证明了其临床相关性（表21A.11）[261-264]。2001年发表的新版世界卫生组织（WHO）分类方法结合了REAL分类，并根据1994年后获得的新资料进行了一些修订（表21A.12）[36,40-42,265-267]。在确定疾病的性质时，着重强调疾病的部位。

REAL/WHO分类的有效性
Validation of the REAL/WHO classification

来自8个国家的9个研究所提供的1378例淋巴瘤的回顾性研究证实，REAL分类在可重复性和临床相关性方面有效[264]。总体上，组内和组间观察者的诊断可重复性很好（≥85%），优于大多数以往的分类。对于许多类型的淋巴瘤，免疫表型明显影响诊断的可重复性。只有三种类型的淋巴瘤具有很低的可重复性（53%～63%），包括Burkitt样淋巴瘤、淋巴浆细胞性淋巴瘤和淋巴结型边缘区B细胞淋巴瘤，但这些是淋巴瘤诊断中公认的有问题领域。

REAL分类中的淋巴瘤类型被证实具有不同的临床和行为特征（表21A.11，21A.13）[264,268,270]。这些研究还证实了国际预后指数（international prognostic index）的重要性，为每一种类型的淋巴瘤提供了进一步的预后信息。

非Hodgkin淋巴瘤概述

NHL的分类不仅是学术性活动，而且对患者的治疗和预后都是重要的，因为每种类型的淋巴瘤均显示不同的临床病理学特征。总体上根据生物学行为可将淋巴瘤分为三种主要类型：惰性、侵袭性和高度侵袭性，也就是所谓的"好、差和极差"（表21A.14）。侵袭性和高度侵袭性淋巴瘤的长期生存率有可能优于惰性淋巴瘤，这种看似矛盾的现象是因为：侵袭性淋巴瘤是可治愈的[271,272]。有两种类型的淋巴瘤具有不同于上述三种类型的特征：包括原发性皮肤间变性大细胞淋巴

表21A.11 NHL常见类型的临床特征和生存率（资料来自NHL分类方案）

NHL的组织学类型	发病率	中位年龄（岁）	男女比例	分期分布 I	II	III	IV	巨大病变≥10cm	骨髓累及	IPI评分差	5年总体生存率	5年无病生存率
淋巴母细胞性淋巴瘤（T或B系）	2%	28	1.8:1	0%	11%	14%	75%	32%	50%	26%	26%	24%
B-CLL/SLL	6%	65	1.1:1	4%	5%	8%	83%	13%	72%	13%	51%	25%
淋巴浆细胞性淋巴瘤	1%	63	1.1:1	7%	13%	7%	73%	25%	73%	15%	59%	25%
套细胞淋巴瘤	6%	63	2.8:1	13%	7%	9%	71%	25%	64%	23%	27%	11%
滤泡性淋巴瘤	22%	59	0.7:1	18%	15%	16%	51%	28%	42%	7%	72%	40%
弥漫大B细胞淋巴瘤	31%	64	1.2:1	25%	29%	13%	33%	30%	16%	19%	46%	41%
纵隔大B细胞淋巴瘤	2%	37	0.5:1	10%	56%	3%	31%	52%	3%	11%	50%	48%
Burkitt淋巴瘤	<1%	31	8.1:1	37%	25%	0%	38%	22%	33%	14%	44%	44%
Burkitt样淋巴瘤	2%	57	1.4:1	26%	26%	7%	41%	42%	21%	22%	47%	43%
结外边缘区B细胞淋巴瘤，MALT型	5%	60	0.92:1	39%	28%	2%	31%	8%	14%	8%	81%	65%
边缘区B细胞淋巴瘤，淋巴结型	1%	58	0.7:1	13%	13%	34%	40%	0%	32%	13%	56%	28%
外周T细胞淋巴瘤	6%	61	1.2:1	8%	12%	15%	65%	12%	36%	31%	25%	18%
间变大细胞淋巴瘤	2%	34	2.2:1	19%	32%	10%	39%	17%	13%	21%	77%	58%

IPI：国际预后指数。

瘤和MALT型结外边缘区B细胞淋巴瘤，两者均具有良好的预后，可自然消退或在根除病原后消退。这种简单的概况可作为概念性框架，有助于理解和学习各种类型的淋巴瘤。

成人和儿童最常见的非Hodgkin淋巴瘤类型

如表21A.11所示，成人最常见的两种NHL类型是弥漫大B细胞淋巴瘤和滤泡性淋巴瘤，共占所有病例的50%以上[264]。T细胞淋巴瘤相对少见。

在儿童，以侵袭性淋巴瘤为主，几乎所有的病例均分属于淋巴母细胞性淋巴瘤（～35%）、Burkitt淋巴瘤（～40%）和大细胞淋巴瘤（～20%）。大细胞淋巴瘤类型包括间变大细胞淋巴瘤、弥漫大B细胞淋巴瘤和其他一些外周T细胞淋巴瘤[273]。

国际预后指数
International Prognostic Index（IPI）

在治疗NHL患者时，必须考虑预后因素和组织学类型。国际预后指数(IPI)由几种参数组成，已得到广泛验证，对各种类型的淋巴瘤的预后分组极为有用（表21A.15）。适用于惰性和侵袭性淋巴瘤[264,274-277]。

非Hodgkin淋巴瘤的病因学

有关NHL的病因学知之甚少。淋巴瘤发病率有些种族差异提示遗传易感性和环境因素是起作用的。例如，滤泡性淋巴瘤、B细胞慢性淋巴细胞白血病/小淋巴细胞淋巴瘤和肠病型T细胞淋巴瘤在东方人和不发达国家人群中比在高加索人中少见，而NK细胞淋巴瘤在东方人中较常见。

免疫缺陷（先天性、获得性或医源性）和自身免疫性疾病患者易于发生恶性淋巴瘤。免疫监测缺陷导致具有增生优势的异常克隆出现，如EBV感染细胞。慢性刺激或化脓也可提供淋巴瘤发生的微环境[278]。

有些淋巴瘤类型与感染因素有关，包括细菌和病毒，详细描述见表21A.16[279-308]。识别这些相关因素的重要性有几方面：（1）证明有EBV或HHV-8可能有助于诊断某些淋巴瘤类型；（2）根治细菌能使胃的结外边缘区B细胞淋巴瘤和小肠免疫增生性疾病消退；（3）免疫能力的恢复可使某些EBV相关的淋巴增生性病变消退；（4）应用免疫调节剂可治疗有些病毒相关性淋巴瘤，如淋巴瘤样

表21A.12	WHO非Hodgkin淋巴瘤分类（2001）
B细胞肿瘤	**T细胞和NK细胞肿瘤**
前体B细胞肿瘤 • 前体B淋巴母细胞白血病/淋巴母细胞淋巴瘤	前体T细胞肿瘤 • 前体T淋巴母细胞白血病/淋巴母细胞淋巴瘤
成熟B细胞肿瘤 • 慢性淋巴细胞白血病/小淋巴细胞淋巴瘤 • B细胞幼稚淋巴细胞白血病 • 淋巴浆细胞性淋巴瘤 • 脾边缘区淋巴瘤 • 毛细胞白血病 • 浆细胞骨髓瘤/浆细胞瘤 • 结外边缘区B细胞淋巴瘤，黏膜相关淋巴组织（MALT淋巴瘤） • 淋巴结边缘区B细胞淋巴瘤 • 滤泡性淋巴瘤 • 套细胞淋巴瘤 • 弥漫大B细胞淋巴瘤 • 纵隔大B细胞淋巴瘤 • 血管内大B细胞淋巴瘤 • 原发渗出性淋巴瘤 • Burkitt淋巴瘤 • 淋巴瘤样肉芽肿	外周T细胞和NK细胞肿瘤 • T细胞幼稚淋巴细胞白血病 • T细胞大颗粒淋巴细胞白血病 • 侵袭性NK细胞白血病 • 成人T细胞淋巴瘤/白血病 • 结外NK/T细胞淋巴瘤，鼻型 • 肠病型T细胞淋巴瘤 • 肝脾T细胞淋巴瘤 • 皮下脂膜炎样T细胞淋巴瘤 • 母细胞性NK细胞淋巴瘤 • 蕈样霉菌病/Sezary综合征 • 原发性皮肤间变大细胞淋巴瘤 • 外周T细胞性淋巴瘤，非特指 • 血管免疫母细胞T细胞淋巴瘤 • 间变大细胞淋巴瘤

表21A.13	根据生存数据对非Hodgkin淋巴瘤进行分组*（数据来自NHL分类方案）
总体5年生存率	**病变**
生存率很好（~70%）	• 结外边缘区B细胞淋巴瘤，MALT型 • 间变大细胞淋巴瘤，T/裸细胞型 • 滤泡性淋巴瘤
生存率好（~55%）	• 淋巴浆细胞性淋巴瘤 • B细胞慢性淋巴细胞白血病/小淋巴细胞淋巴瘤 • 淋巴结边缘区B细胞淋巴瘤
生存率差（~45%）	• 弥漫大B细胞淋巴瘤 • Burkitt淋巴瘤
生存率很差（<30%）	• 套细胞淋巴瘤 • T淋巴母细胞淋巴瘤 • 外周T细胞淋巴瘤（除外间变大细胞淋巴瘤）

*此表的分组依据是基于接受现代治疗的患者生存率，不同于表21A.14所显示的分组，后者是基于淋巴瘤类型的自然病史。同组病变可能接受极为不同的治疗；例如，滤泡性淋巴瘤可采用观察或非强化治疗，而间变大细胞淋巴瘤则需要强化化疗。

肉芽肿、成人T细胞淋巴瘤/白血病；以及（5）预防性措施能极大地降低某些感染因素相关性淋巴瘤的发病率。

免疫细胞化学

虽然有一些淋巴瘤类型能够单独通过形态学诊断（如B细胞慢性淋巴细胞白血病/小淋巴细胞淋巴瘤，滤泡性淋巴瘤和结外边缘区B细胞淋巴瘤，MALT型）[264]，但目前免疫表型分析是淋巴瘤诊断的组成部分，因为其能提高分类的准确性。在描述各种淋巴瘤类型时，将常规列举下列标记物：

1. 提示淋巴瘤谱系的标记物。
2. 有助于明确或辅助诊断的标记物。
3. 证明免疫表型，但一般没有诊断意义的标记物。
4. 可能导致误诊的标记物。

淋巴瘤的免疫表达谱在治疗后可能改变；例如，应用抗CD20抗体（如美罗华）治疗可导致残留或复发病变中CD20表达的丢失。在这种情况中，需要使用其他B系标记物（如PAX-5）证明其细胞系。

表21A.14　非Hodgkin淋巴瘤主要类型的一般特征

	惰性淋巴瘤（"好"）	侵袭性淋巴瘤（"坏"）	高度侵袭性淋巴瘤（"极坏"）
典型病变	• 滤泡性淋巴瘤 • B细胞慢性淋巴细胞白血病/小淋巴细胞淋巴瘤 • 淋巴浆细胞性淋巴瘤 • 套细胞淋巴瘤 • 脾边缘区B细胞淋巴瘤	• 弥漫大B细胞淋巴瘤 • 各种外周T细胞和NK细胞淋巴瘤，除了蕈样霉菌病、T细胞大颗粒淋巴细胞白血病和原发性皮肤间变大细胞淋巴瘤	• Burkitt淋巴瘤 • 淋巴母细胞淋巴瘤
年龄组	老年人	任何年龄	儿童和年轻人
生长速度	慢；偶尔出现增大和回缩过程	快	很快（肿瘤突然出现）
首诊分期	通常为高分期（>80%为III/IV期）	各期分布均匀（I~IV期）	通常呈高分期，尤其是淋巴母细胞淋巴瘤
外周血和骨髓累及	很常见	少见；累及提示预后很差	常见
中枢神经系统累及	少见	少见	常见
未经治疗的自然病史	惰性过程，患者经多年死亡。一部分病例可能转化为大细胞淋巴瘤	1~2年内患者死亡	早期播散，几周至几个月内患者死亡
对治疗的反应和治愈性	生长分数低，使用化疗或放疗常常不能治愈，除了少数早期病变患者	生长分数高，因此使用化疗或放疗可能治愈	生长分数很高，对强化化疗反应高；普通化疗效果不满意，因为在化疗周期间可发生"逃逸"
治疗的临床后果	治疗可控制疾病，但是疾病会反复复发。由于治疗难以改变最终预后，无症状患者可采取观察，无需积极治疗	化疗可使70%~80%的患者达到完全缓解；其中2/3可以治愈	使用强化化疗可以治愈，尤其是早期患者。中枢神经系统预防也需要考虑
生存曲线	连续下降，意味着不可治愈	起初下降（没有缓解或部分缓解者死亡），随后稳定（患者治愈）	起初急剧下降（未达到缓解者迅速死亡），随后稳定（患者治愈）

* 以上分类例外的是：结外边缘区B细胞淋巴瘤和原发性皮肤间变大细胞淋巴瘤。
- 所有年龄组。
- 通常为早期；很少累及骨髓或中枢神经系统。
- 可治愈，预后良好。
- 不经过细胞毒性治疗即可消退，如自发性（原发性皮肤间变大细胞淋巴瘤）或应用抗幽门螺杆菌治疗（胃结外边缘区B细胞淋巴瘤，MALT型）。

表21A.15	非Hodgkin淋巴瘤的国际预后指数（IPI）
参数	
年龄	≥60岁
分期	进展期（III或IV期）
结外受累部位数目	>1
表现状况（performance status）	≥2
血清LDH水平	异常
国际预后指数（IPI）	
出现上述特征的总数	
根据指数进行的危险性分组	
0～1	低危
2	低-中等危险
3	高-中等危险
4～5	高危

未分类的或无法分类的淋巴瘤
The unclassified or unclassifiable lymphoma

有些淋巴瘤病例（百分之几）难以分类，甚至在所有的工作都做到的情况下亦如此。其可被称为"恶性淋巴瘤，未定型"。如果可能，提供谱系信息并推断肿瘤是低度恶性还是高度恶性的[40]。应该指出分类困难的原因，如不能归入现有的淋巴瘤类型，组织取材不充分，组织保存欠佳，不能进行特殊检查，或不能获得临床信息。如果原因是组织取材不充分，可通过进一步获取组织来解决。

前体淋巴母细胞淋巴瘤
Precursor lymphoblastic lymphoma

淋巴母细胞淋巴瘤
Lymphoblastic lymphoma

定义

淋巴母细胞淋巴瘤是一种高度侵袭性肿瘤，由T、B或NK细胞前体组成。淋巴母细胞淋巴瘤和急性淋巴母细胞白血病可能是同一病变谱系的两端。在大多数研究中，采用一种主观的标准"骨髓中淋巴母细胞<25%"来鉴别二者[309]。尽管明显类似，T细胞急性淋巴母细胞白血病和T淋巴母细胞淋巴瘤有明确的基因表达谱差异[310]。

总体上，80%～90%的淋巴母细胞淋巴瘤是T细胞来源。大多数B细胞淋巴母细胞肿瘤表现为急性淋巴母细胞白血病，很少表现为淋巴瘤。

临床特征

T细胞型（T-cell type）：T淋巴母细胞淋巴瘤最常发生于青少年和年轻成人，但任何年龄均可发病[272,311,312]。男女比例为2:1。大多数患者由于纵隔大肿物而表现为呼吸困难，常伴有上腔静脉阻塞症状、胸水和锁骨上淋巴结肿大。其他表现为淋巴结肿大或结外病变。85%以上的患者出现症状时即为进展期（III或IV期）。易于播散至骨髓和中枢神经系统。

迅速做出淋巴母细胞淋巴瘤诊断是重要的，以便及时进行治疗，阻止肿瘤迅速生长。虽然以往的预后不容乐观，但采用治疗急性淋巴母细胞白血病的强化化疗后治愈率高，儿童生存率可达80%～90%，成人生存率为60%[313-320]。

伴有组织和外周血嗜酸性粒细胞增多的少数T淋巴母细胞淋巴瘤，之后可发生急性髓性白血病、骨髓增生异常综合征或髓性增生[321]。这种少见而高度侵袭性的综合征（8p11髓性增生综合征，或干细胞白血病-淋巴瘤综合征）具有独特的易位t(8;13)(p11;q11)，导致*FGFR1/ZNF198*基因融合[320,322,323]。

已有个别T淋巴母细胞增生病例呈惰性表现的报告，单独手术切除可延长生存期[324,325]。组织学和免疫表型特征与T淋巴母细胞淋巴瘤不易区分。仅有的区别是缺乏克隆性TCR基因重排。

B细胞型（B-cell type）：至少有些文献报告的T淋巴母细胞淋巴瘤实际上是母细胞样套细胞淋巴瘤[326]。B淋巴母细胞淋巴瘤发病年龄范围广，从儿童到老人，平均年龄32岁。女性发病略高[326-331]。患者表现为明显的淋巴结肿大或结外病变，好发部位为皮肤和骨。皮肤病变最常发生于头颈部，骨病变呈溶骨性，累及单个或多个部位。很少累及纵隔[329,332,333]。总体生存率在最初2～3年内好于T淋巴母细胞淋巴瘤[330]。局部病变的预后很好。

NK细胞型（NK-cell type）：这种类型少见，有关的临床和行为特征知之甚少[334-336]。与所谓的母细胞性NK细胞淋巴瘤有重叠（见第1233页）。

病理学

组织学所见不能判断细胞来源。主要特征是淋巴细胞中等大小，呈弥漫、致密、单一形浸润，核仁不明显，核分裂计数高。核可呈圆形或脑回状；脑回状核显示多个深

表21A.16 非Hodgkin淋巴瘤发生中感染因素的作用

感染因素	与感染因素有关的NHL类型	说明
幽门螺杆菌（Hp）	胃结外边缘区B细胞淋巴瘤，MALT型	根治Hp可使>70%的淋巴瘤病例消退
空肠弯曲杆菌	小肠免疫增生性病变（地中海淋巴瘤），常常被认为是结外边缘区B细胞淋巴瘤的特殊类型	应用四环素治疗可消退
EB病毒（EBV）	• 移植后淋巴组织增生性病变 • 免疫缺陷相关性淋巴瘤，如原发性渗出性淋巴瘤，AIDS患者原发性中枢神经系统淋巴瘤，类风湿关节炎患者氨甲蝶呤相关性淋巴组织增生性病变 • Burkitt淋巴瘤（地方性：100%，非地方性：仅20%） • 淋巴瘤样肉芽肿病 • 伴有Reed-Sternberg样细胞的B细胞慢性淋巴细胞白血病 • 脓胸相关性大B细胞淋巴瘤 • 老年性EBV$^+$B细胞淋巴组织增生性病变 • 结外NK/T细胞淋巴瘤 • 各种组织学类型的淋巴瘤散发病例，较常见于黏膜部位	• 减少免疫抑制可使有些移植后淋巴组织增生性病变和氨甲蝶呤相关性淋巴组织增生性病变消退 • 淋巴瘤样肉芽肿可能对免疫调控有反应：例如干扰素-α
人类疱疹病毒8（HHV-8）	• 原发性渗出性淋巴瘤 • 来源于Castleman病的浆母细胞性淋巴瘤 • HHV8$^+$生发中心大B细胞淋巴瘤	HHV8编码一些人类细胞同源基因
人类T淋巴细胞病毒1	• 成人T细胞淋巴瘤/白血病	• 在日本、台湾北部、巴西和加勒比海流行 • 有时抗病毒治疗有效（zidovudine加干扰素-α）
丙型肝炎	• 脾边缘区B细胞淋巴瘤 • 淋巴浆细胞性淋巴瘤或单克隆γ球蛋白病伴冷球蛋白血症 • 结外边缘区B细胞淋巴瘤	• 丙型肝炎与B细胞淋巴瘤的相关性有地理差异，相关性在意大利和日本最高 • 病毒不整合入淋巴细胞，认为肿瘤克隆发生于丙型肝炎抗原引起的慢性B细胞刺激背景；丙型肝炎还可诱导B细胞突变 • 当应用抗病毒药物和（或）干扰素治疗时，高达75%的丙型肝炎相关性低级别B细胞淋巴瘤消退
鹦鹉热衣原体	眼眶结外边缘区B细胞淋巴瘤	鹦鹉热衣原体与眼眶结外边缘区B细胞淋巴瘤的相关性是有争议的。在意大利、德国和某些国家有强相关性，但有些研究没能证明这种相关性。报告显示应用抗生素治疗鹦鹉热衣原体之后，眼眶结外边缘区B细胞性淋巴瘤可消退。
博氏疏螺旋体（Borrelia burgdorferi）	原发性皮肤B细胞淋巴瘤	博氏疏螺旋体与皮肤B细胞淋巴瘤的相关性几乎全部来自英国，有些病例在根治博氏疏螺旋体之后消退

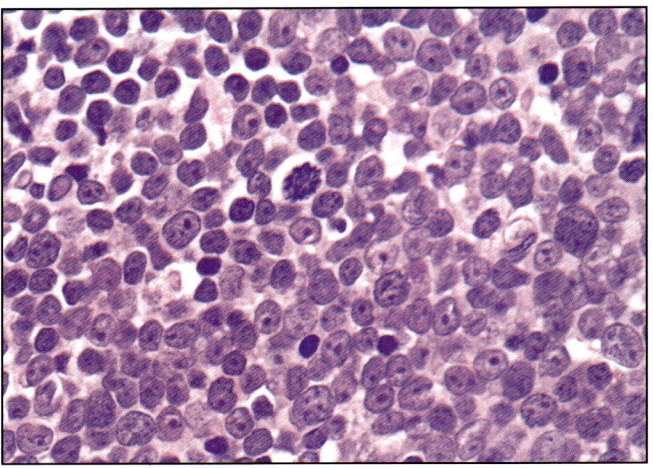

图21A.36 T淋巴母细胞淋巴瘤。细胞中等大小，形态单一，核圆形，核仁小，胞浆稀少。核分裂活跃。

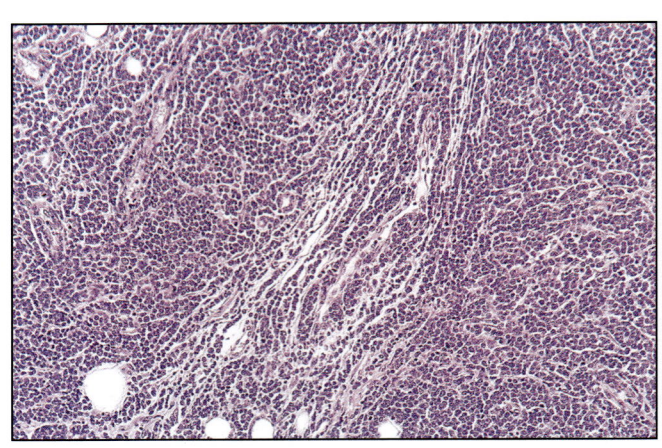

图21A.38 淋巴母细胞淋巴瘤。当这种淋巴瘤浸润淋巴结周围组织和纤维组织时，常常可见单排列结构（视野中央）。

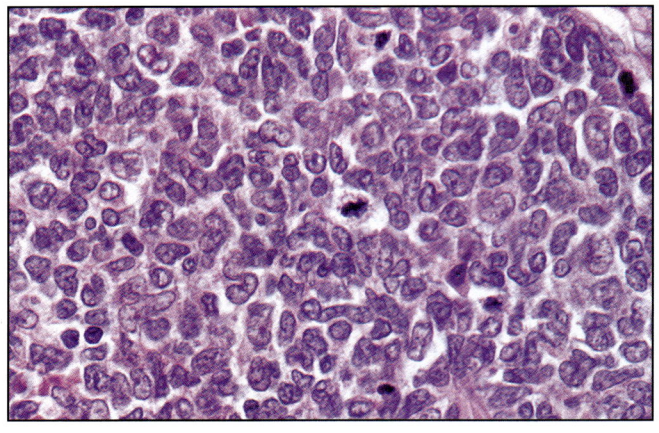

图21A.37 B淋巴母细胞淋巴瘤。大多数核可见明显的核沟回。染色质纤细。淋巴母细胞性淋巴瘤的核外形与细胞来源没有相关性。

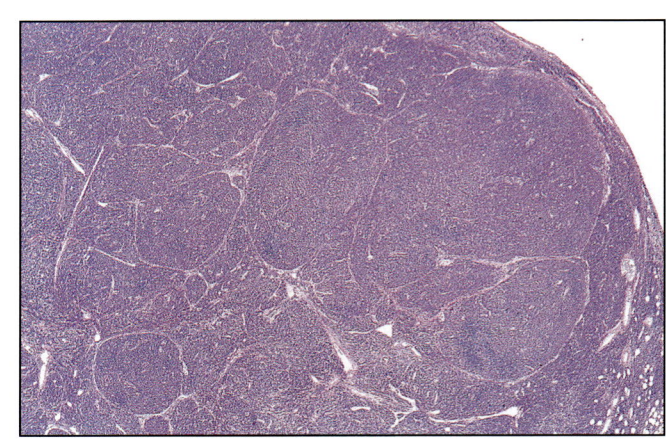

图21A.39 结节状T淋巴母细胞淋巴瘤。结节由纤维网状组织延伸组成，结节周围可见纤细粉染的纤维间隔和血管，不同于滤泡性淋巴瘤中所见到的结节。

的折叠，总体保持圆形轮廓（图21A.36和21A.37）。胞质稀少，细胞核密集。细胞大小略有差异，多核瘤细胞很少见。可见散在的含有可染小体的巨噬细胞，呈"星天"现象。

淋巴结结构可完全或部分消失，淋巴结周围组织的浸润常常呈单行排列（图21A.38）。当淋巴瘤细胞浸润纤维组织时，核可呈长形。偶尔伸展的网状纤维网或血管可形成多结节（假滤泡）结构，可误诊为滤泡性淋巴瘤（图21A.39）[337]。

免疫细胞化学

末端脱氧核苷转移酶（TdT）是淋巴母细胞淋巴瘤明确的标记物，有助于与T细胞淋巴瘤或成熟B细胞淋巴瘤鉴别。TdT免疫染色局限于核（图21A.40）[338]。CD99a是Ewing肉瘤/外周原始神经外胚叶肿瘤的典型抗原，是淋巴母细胞淋巴瘤的另一种标记物，但特异性较差。

淋巴母细胞淋巴瘤的细胞来源鉴定可能存在困难，因为CD20在B淋巴母细胞淋巴瘤中可能呈阴性，CD3在T淋巴母细胞淋巴瘤中可能呈阴性，CD79a在有些T淋巴母细胞淋巴瘤中可能呈阳性。少数病例具有双表型（表达T和B细胞标记物，或同时表达髓性标记物）或出现裸细胞免疫表型[339,340]。

T细胞型 T cell type

1. CD7在T细胞发生的极早期即开始表达，是最恒定的标记[341,342]。广谱T细胞标记物CD2、CD3（胞浆$CD3^+$，胞膜$CD3^{+/-}$）和CD5阳性程度不同（图21A.40）[340,343]。

2. TdT和CD99呈阳性（图21A.40）。CD1a和CD10表

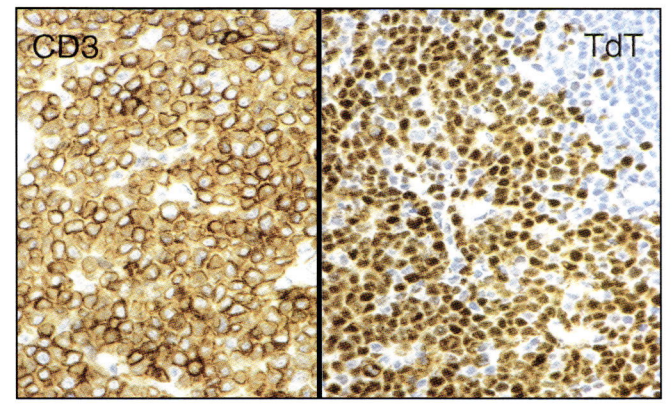

图21A.40 T淋巴母细胞淋巴瘤的免疫染色。左侧：肿瘤细胞CD3呈阳性。右侧：可见核TdT呈阳性。

达程度不同。CD43常常呈阳性，CD45RO常常呈阴性。TAL1表达于50%～75%的病例，不管是否有TAL1基因的结构改变[344,345]。

3. CD4和CD8的表达不恒定，表型可为CD4$^+$CD8$^+$，CD4$^-$CD8$^-$，CD4$^+$CD8$^-$或CD4$^-$CD8$^+$。TCR类型可能是αβ或γδ，或可能不表达。极少数病例表达NK细胞相关标记物，如CD16或CD57，提示侵袭性较强[312,346]。

4. 10%的T淋巴母细胞淋巴瘤CD79a与CD3共表达，可引起细胞系判定困难。这种病例是真正的T细胞源性，因为可见TCR基因重排[347,348]。

B细胞型　B-cell type

1. B细胞标记物阳性（如CD19、PAX-5和CD79a）：PAX-5和CD19的表达最恒定[349,350]。CD20常常呈阴性。某些病例可显示胞浆Igμ链，但胞膜Ig表达少见。
2. TdT呈阳性，CD10和CD99通常呈阳性。
3. HLA-DR$^+$，CD34$^{+/-}$。
4. 有些病例可见细胞角蛋白斑点状染色[328,351]。CD43常常呈阳性。

NK细胞型　NK-cell type

1. 胞膜CD3$^-$，胞浆CD3$^+$、CD5$^-$、CD56$^+$。
2. TdT$^+$。

遗传学特征

T细胞型（T cell type）：大约95%的T淋巴母细胞淋巴瘤显示TCR β和γ链基因重排，但20%可额外显示Ig重链基因重排，无Ig轻链基因重排[18,352]。细胞遗传学异常较多，大多显示14q11（TCR-α/δ）或7q35（TCR-β）TCR基因易位[1,352]。易位涉及许多参与基因，如TAL1（1p32-34）、TTG2/RHOM2（11p13）、HOX11（10q24）和MYC（8q24）。TAL1是最常见的受累基因，表现形式是t(1;14)(p32-34;q11)，或更为常见的是90kb间隙缺失。后者导致TAL1与上游位点SIL连接，导致TAL1过表达，因为TAL受到SIL的调控成分控制[345,353]。

基因表达谱研究识别出了几种信号，它们在正常胸腺细胞发生特殊阶段可抑制白血病：LYL1$^+$信号（前T）、HOX11$^+$（早期胸腺皮质细胞）和TAL1$^+$（晚期胸腺皮质细胞）。HOX11活化与预后良好有关，而TAL1或LYL1表达则与治疗反应较差有关[354]。

B细胞型（B-cell type）：近100%的B淋巴母细胞淋巴瘤病例显示Ig重链基因重排，只有20%～30%显示可重复性TCR β链基因克隆性重排[18,352]。在B细胞急性淋巴母细胞白血病，已识别出许多不同的细胞遗传学异常，t(9;22)(q34;q11)、t(1;19)(q23;p13)、t(4;11)(q21;q23)以及亚二倍体与预后较差有关，>50条染色体的超二倍体与预后良好有关[352]。有关淋巴瘤形式与细胞遗传学异常的关系和意义知之甚少。

鉴别诊断

1. **髓细胞肉瘤**（myeloid sarcoma）：髓细胞肉瘤可极其类似于淋巴母细胞淋巴瘤。应该慎重地排除这种可能性，尤其是出现以下任何"可疑"特征时：
   - (a) 核仁比正常时明显。
   - (b) 许多核具有肾形外观。
   - (c) 核仁清楚。
   - (d) 散在嗜酸性粒细胞
   - (e) 胞浆中可见细颗粒。

2. **B细胞慢性淋巴细胞白血病/小淋巴细胞淋巴瘤**（B-cell chronic lymphocytic leukemia/small lymphocytic lymphoma）：在固定欠佳的标本中，淋巴母细胞可皱缩而深染，类似小淋巴细胞。患者年轻以及核分裂活跃有可能是淋巴母细胞淋巴瘤。使用苏木素浅染（如PAS，或苏木素复染的免疫组化切片）组织切片检查，有助于识别淋巴母细胞纤细的染色质结构和核分裂象。

3. **胸腺瘤**（Thymoma）：见本章第3部分。

4. **套细胞淋巴瘤，母细胞样型**（mantle cell lymphoma, blastoid variant）：淋巴母细胞淋巴瘤TdT$^+$、cyclin D1$^-$，而套细胞淋巴瘤则显示相反的免疫反应表型。

5. **滤泡性淋巴瘤**（follicular lymphoma）：见"淋巴组织增生性病变诊断实践问题"（第1250页）。

6. **Burkitt淋巴瘤**（Burkitt lymphoma）见表21A.17和

表21A.17 有助于鉴别淋巴母细胞淋巴瘤和Burkitt淋巴瘤的特征

	淋巴母细胞淋巴瘤	Burkitt淋巴瘤
核	圆形或脑回状；通常无明显挤压变形	通常呈圆形，但偶尔可显示核突起；核挤压嵌合，核膜呈"方形"
染色质结构	纤细、尘状	粗糙、颗粒状
核仁	不明显	明显，核仁2～5个，常常没有膜包绕
胞浆	稀少，常规组织切片难以见到。在Giemsa染色印片中，部分核周可见明显的胞浆	有明确的嗜碱性圆环状或浆细胞样胞浆，胞浆轮廓呈"方形"。在Giemsa染色印片中，嗜碱性胞浆中可见小的脂质空泡
细胞谱系	通常为T细胞，有时为B或NK细胞	总是B细胞
Ki-67指数	高，但通常＜80%	～100%

"淋巴组织增生性病变诊断实践问题"（第1250页）。

外周B细胞淋巴瘤
Peripheral B-cell lymphomas

外周（成熟）B细胞淋巴瘤包括原始（virgin）/幼稚（naive）B细胞、滤泡/生发中心细胞和生发中心后细胞，以及经历了滤泡外T细胞非依赖性抗原反应的记忆性B细胞肿瘤。这些不同的B细胞分化阶段可以通过Ig基因重排的突变形式以及免疫组化标记物来界定。滤泡中心细胞通常显示Ig基因体细胞超突变，具有克隆内多样性（进行性突变）的证据。体细胞超突变是指以单核苷酸改变为主的突变，但有时也出现缺失或重复，主要发生在可变区基因[355]。这是产生Ig基因多样性从而生成高亲和性Ig分子的机制。

B细胞慢性淋巴细胞白血病/小淋巴细胞淋巴瘤
B-cell chronic lymphocytic leukemia/small lymphocytic lymphoma (B-CLL/SLL)

定义

B细胞慢性淋巴细胞白血病/小淋巴细胞淋巴瘤（B-CLL/SLL）是一种非活化的、成熟表现的小淋巴细胞肿瘤性增生。大多数病例具有白血病的表现（B-CLL），仅有少数病例为局限性疾病（B-SLL）；它们是同一生物学病变的不同表现[272,356]。以往文献所报道的许多局限性小淋巴细胞淋巴瘤可能是结外边缘区B细胞淋巴瘤而不是B-CLL/SLL。

如果在诊断时有明显的淋巴细胞增生，则可诊断为"B-CLL"。如果信息不明确，则通常诊断为"B-CLL/SLL"。

临床特征

B-CLL/SLL通常发生于老年患者（表21A.11）。大多数患者偶然发现淋巴细胞增生、淋巴结肿大或脾大。淋巴结肿大通常是全身性的。常见骨髓受累[272,356-358]。大约40%的患者具有B症状，预示生存期较短。副蛋白血症不常见。患者容易出现感染并发症，有些患者发生自身免疫性溶血性贫血。对于B-CLL，通常应用Rai或Binet分期系统来替代Ann Arbor系统[359,360]。

B-CLL/SLL呈惰性，可见未经特殊治疗的无症状患者[271]。对单一药物或多种药物化疗具有令人满意的反应，包括嘌呤类似物，但难以治愈[361,362]。病程特点是反复复发，多年后死亡。中位生存期大约为10年。然而，一些病例会呈现快速进展。预后差的相关因素包括：临床分期高、白细胞计数高（＞50×10^9/L）、血液中幼稚淋巴细胞百分比高（＞10%）、细胞遗传学异常del(11q)或del(17p)，表达CD38，表达ZAP-70，无Ig基因突变[363]。

病理学

淋巴结结构弥漫消失，极少数肿瘤可选择性地累及淋巴结滤泡间区或B区[364-366]。肿瘤常常侵犯淋巴结周围组织。在大多数病例，深染的淋巴组织中散布着淡染的圆形增生中心灶（"假滤泡"），这种结构本身是B-CLL/SLL的特异性病征（图21A.41）。然而，在有些病例见不到增生中心。

淋巴瘤细胞小，核圆形，染色质致密，核仁不明显，胞浆稀少。有时可见轻至中度的核不规则性，可导致误诊为套细胞淋巴瘤。浆细胞散在或缺乏。核分

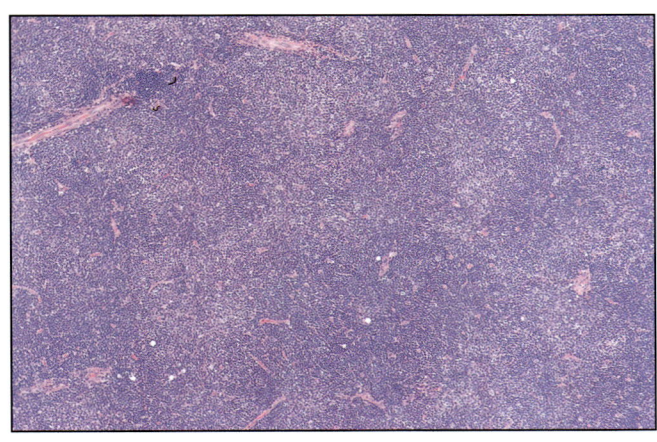

图21A.41 B细胞慢性淋巴细胞白血病/小淋巴细胞淋巴瘤。许多淡染"褪色的"病灶是诊断性增生中心,散在于深染的淋巴组织中。

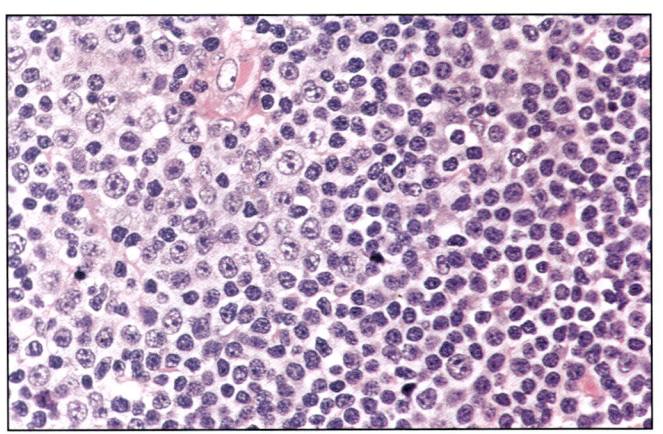

图21A.43 B细胞慢性淋巴细胞白血病/小淋巴细胞淋巴瘤。左上视野显示一个增生中心,由幼稚淋巴细胞和副免疫母细胞组成。

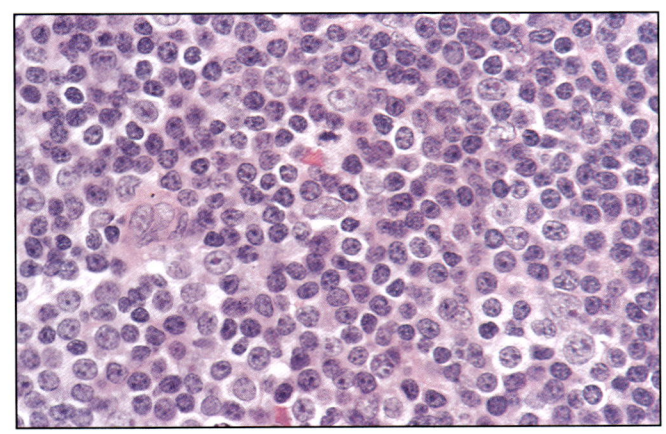

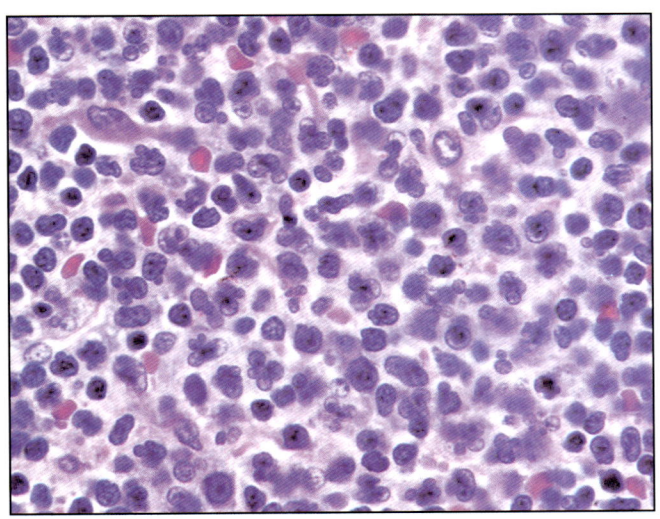

图21A.42 B细胞慢性淋巴细胞白血病/小淋巴细胞淋巴瘤。(A)副免疫母细胞和幼稚淋巴细胞与成群的小淋巴细胞密切混杂,可见圆形核轮廓,染色质致密,胞浆稀少。(B)少数病例可见明显的核分叶或折叠。

裂计数通常较低。增生中心通常呈非膨胀性,由幼稚淋巴细胞和副免疫母细胞混合组成(图 21A.42 和 21A.43)。幼稚淋巴细胞比小淋巴细胞略大,染色质较松散,核仁清楚,胞浆多而淡染。副免疫母细胞较大,伴有泡状染色质和明显的中央核仁;与免疫母细胞的区别是体积较小、胞浆染色较淡。小淋巴细胞之间也可见到散在的幼稚淋巴细胞和副免疫母细胞(图 21A.42A 和 21A.43)[367]。它们是 B-CLL/SLL 的标志,即使它们或小细胞的核不规则,也可作出这种诊断(图 21A.42B)。个别情况下可形成假玫瑰花结[368]。在非典型 B-CLL 患者(定义为幼稚淋巴细胞 > 10% 或核裂细胞或浆细胞样细胞 > 10%),淋巴结可显示较大的增生中心,淋巴细胞常常显示核的不规则性[369]。当出现成片或成群的副免疫母细胞时,称为"副免疫母细胞型";这种变型的预后较差(图 21A.44)[370,371]。

有些典型的 B-CLL/SLL 病例可出现淋巴浆细胞样细胞。这些细胞具有小淋巴细胞的核特征,但是具有中等量嗜双色性胞浆环,缺乏明显的高尔基区(图 21A.45)。浆细胞少见。胞浆 Ig 可显示,可有副蛋白血症。这种亚群相当于 Kiel 分类的淋巴浆细胞样免疫细胞瘤[272]。

免疫细胞化学

1. 广谱B细胞标记物(如CD20、CD79a)呈阳性。但CD20常常呈弱表达。单型性表面Ig(通常为IgD和IgM)常常呈弱表达。

2. 通常CD5$^+$、C10$^-$和CD23$^+$(图21A.46)[356,372]。除极少数例外,cyclin D1呈阴性[373]。

3. Ki-67(增生)指数较低,除非在增生中心。Ki-67

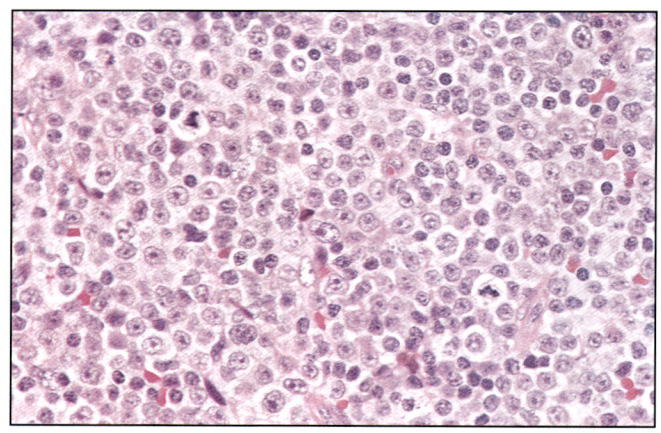

图21A.44 B细胞慢性淋巴细胞白血病/小淋巴细胞淋巴瘤，副免疫母细胞型。副免疫母细胞明显增生，这种病例可被误诊为大B细胞淋巴瘤。

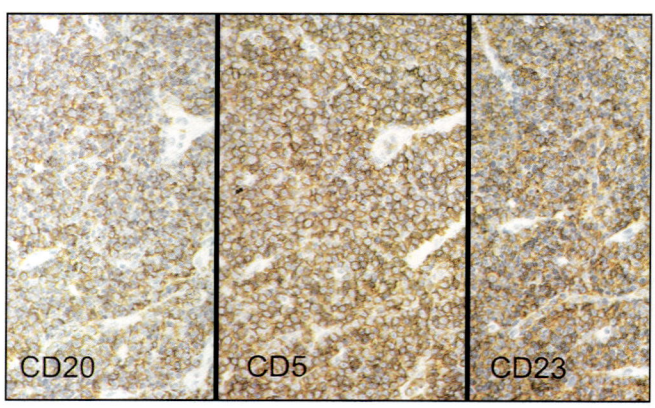

图21A.46 B细胞慢性淋巴细胞白血病/小淋巴细胞淋巴瘤的免疫染色。左侧：CD20呈弱阳性。中间：肿瘤细胞表达CD5。右侧：常常表达CD23。

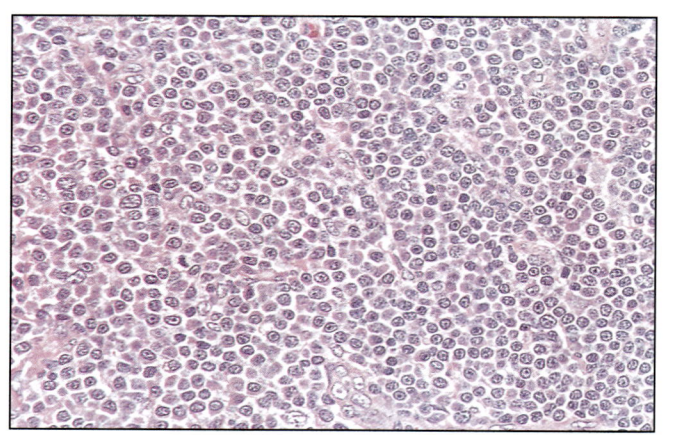

图21A.45 伴有浆细胞样特征的B细胞慢性淋巴细胞白血病/小淋巴细胞淋巴瘤。小淋巴样细胞显示小淋巴细胞的核特征和偏心性嗜双色性胞浆环。

增生指数＞25%提示预后较差[374]。界限不清的FDC网有时可见于增生中心[375,376]。背景中反应性T细胞通常稀少。常常表达TCL-1[377]。

4. 由于CD20表达较弱或缺乏，而CD43常常呈阳性，单独应用CD20和CD43可误诊为T细胞淋巴瘤[378]。

遗传学特征

Ig基因重排。虽然先前的研究提示B-CLL/SLL是幼稚的B细胞肿瘤，伴有非突变性Ig基因，但近期的研究明确显示，这种疾病来源于经过抗原刺激的B淋巴细胞，在Ig V基因突变水平上有差异[379,380]。也有人认为B-CLL/SLL可能来源于边缘区B细胞[379,381]。大约50%的病例显示非突变性Ig基因，大约50%的病例显示体细胞超突变[382-385]。非突变组的预后通常较差[386,387]。基因表达谱研究显示，B-CLL/SLL为同源性表型，与记忆性B细胞最相似，并且非突变组和突变组均显示数量有限的基因表达差异[380,388]，ZAP-70基因过表达能最好地区分非突变组和突变组[389]。免疫组化ZAP-70的表达可作为非突变组的代表性标记物[387,389-394]。

确诊时，B-CLL常常显示13q14缺失（50%的病例），可以是纯合子或半合子[395,396]。位于该染色体区域的两种小RNA基因在多数B-CLL病例中缺失或下调[379,397]。11q22-q23缺失可见于14%的B-CLL/SLL，这种特征与淋巴结广泛受累和预后较差有关[398]。受累基因是ATM（在共济失调性毛细管扩张症中突变），体细胞等位基因缺失或点突变引起的异常对于B-CLL/SLL具有致病作用[399-401]。10%的B-CLL可发生17p13缺失和P53基因突变/缺失，与疾病晚期和预后差有关[398,402]。

15%的B-CLL可见12号染色体三体，但仅见于部分肿瘤细胞，因此可能代表进展性而非原发性遗传学改变[395,403]。较高的临床分期、非典型CLL血象与预后较差有关[404-406]。

B-CLL/SLL合并大B细胞淋巴瘤
B-CLL/SLL complicated by large B-cell lymphoma

在一部分B-CLL（3%～10%），当疾病急剧恶化时，可并发大B细胞淋巴瘤（Richter综合征），导致1年内死亡。大B细胞淋巴瘤由大细胞组成，常常显示明显的细胞多形性和奇异性，包括Reed-Sternberg样细胞（图21A.47）。分子学研究表明，大细胞淋巴瘤或与B-CLL/SLL克隆相关（真性转化），或与B-CLL/SLL克隆不相关（易患病者的一种新的肿瘤事件）[18,54,407-411]。少数情

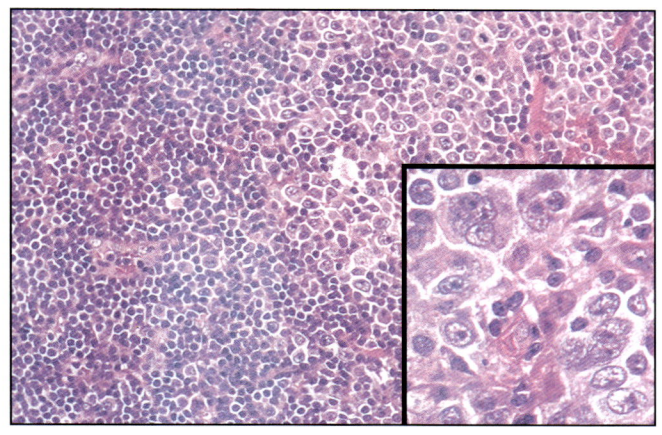

图21A.47　B细胞慢性淋巴细胞白血病合并弥漫大B细胞淋巴瘤（Richter综合征）。左侧视野可见慢性淋巴细胞白血病成分。右侧视野可见大细胞淋巴瘤成分。常见大的多形性和Reed-Sternberg样细胞（插图）。

况下，还可并发其他类型的侵袭性淋巴瘤[412-414]。

伴有Reed-Sternberg样细胞的B-CLL/SLL或并发Hodgkin淋巴瘤
B-CLL/SLL with Reed-Sternberg-like cells or superimposed Hodgkin lymphoma (HL)

极少数情况下，类似Reed-Sternberg细胞的孤立性大细胞散在于小淋巴瘤细胞之间，但缺乏典型的HL炎症背景（图21A.48）[415,416]。这些Reed-Sternberg样细胞显示活化的B细胞和典型Reed-Sternberg细胞免疫表型，或B细胞与Reed-Sternberg细胞混合性免疫表型[415,417,418]。EBV在这些大细胞的发生中起着关键作用，EBV在大细胞中恒定显示，但在B-CLL/SLL细胞中则见不到[48,416,419,420]。有时，在适当的炎症背景中可合并典型的HL组成性Reed-Sternberg细胞[48,418,421]。这种现象在近些年有较高的发生率，与应用氟达拉滨（fludarabine）治疗B-CLL/SLL的增加有关[422-424]。B-CLL/SLL和HL可以具有或不具有克隆相关性[54,424,425]。

鉴别诊断

1. **结节性淋巴细胞为主型Hodgkin淋巴瘤（N-LPHL）**：尤其是在年轻患者，在作出B-CLL/SLL诊断之前，必须除外N-LPHL。免疫组化检查，B-CLL/SLL的小淋巴细胞是单一类型，异常表达CD5和CD43，而N-LPHL的小淋巴细胞是多种类型，不显示异常免疫表型。
2. **其他小B细胞淋巴瘤**：见"淋巴组织增生性病变诊断的实践问题"（第1250页）。
3. **淋巴母细胞淋巴瘤**（lymphoblastic lymphoma）。
4. **反应性淋巴组织增生**（reactive lymphoid hyperplasia）：见"淋巴组织增生性病变诊断的实践问题"（第1250页）。
5. **滤泡性淋巴瘤**（follicular lymphoma）：出现明显增生中心的B-CLL/SLL可被误诊为滤泡性淋巴瘤。与肿瘤性滤泡不同，其增生中心是非膨胀性的，通常由具有圆形核和中央核仁的细胞组成（幼稚淋巴细胞和副免疫母细胞）。网状纤维染色会显示滤泡性淋巴瘤肿瘤性滤泡周围的致密纤维。B-CLL/SLL是$CD5^+CD10^-$，而滤泡性淋巴瘤常常$CD5^-CD10^+$。

B细胞幼稚淋巴细胞性白血病
B-cell prolymphocytic leukemia

见第22章（第1409页）。

淋巴浆细胞性淋巴瘤
Lymphoplasmacytic lymphoma

定义

淋巴浆细胞性淋巴瘤是少见的低级别B细胞淋巴瘤，由小淋巴细胞组成，伴有不同程度的浆细胞分化。它相当于Keil分类中的淋巴浆细胞性免疫细胞瘤[36]。这是一种排除性诊断。如果出现特殊淋巴瘤类型的特征，如滤泡性淋巴瘤或结外边缘区B细胞淋巴瘤，则不应该作出淋巴浆细胞性淋巴瘤的诊断。

临床特征

淋巴浆细胞性淋巴瘤发生于中老年人，发现时通常为播散性的（表21A.11）。患者表现为淋巴结肿大、脾大或高黏滞性综合征的症状（Waldenstrom巨球蛋白血

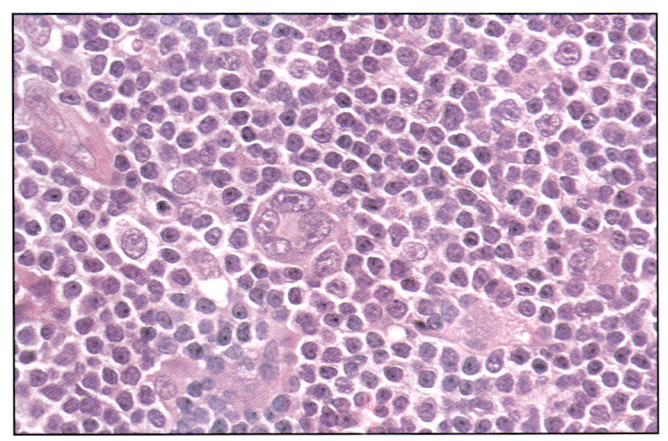

图21A.48　B细胞慢性淋巴细胞白血病伴有Reed-Sternberg样细胞。在小淋巴细胞（$CD20^+$的单一型）背景中，有散在的单个Reed-Sternberg细胞（显示$CD20^+$、$CD30^+$）。这不符合Hodgkin淋巴瘤的诊断，因为缺乏这种诊断所需要的炎症背景（比如T细胞）。

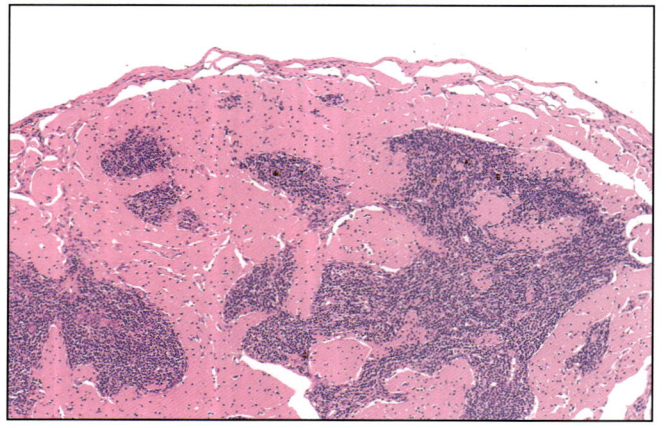

图21A.49 淋巴浆细胞性淋巴瘤。淋巴窦扩张伴有蛋白液体（免疫球蛋白）。

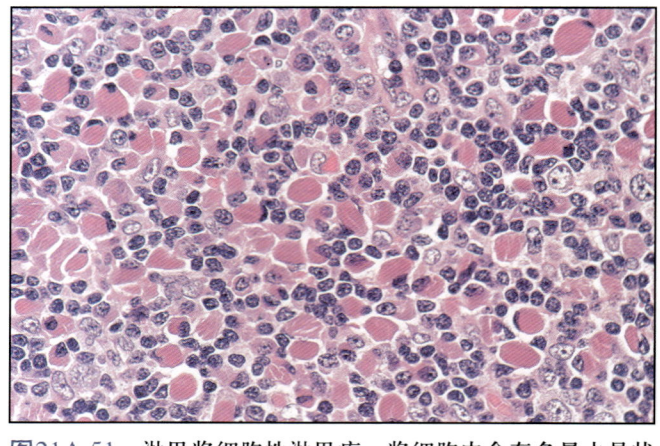

图21A.51 淋巴浆细胞性淋巴瘤。浆细胞内含有多量水晶状免疫球蛋白包涵体。淋巴浆细胞中也有许多相同的水晶状包涵体，强烈提示淋巴瘤，而不是反应性病变。

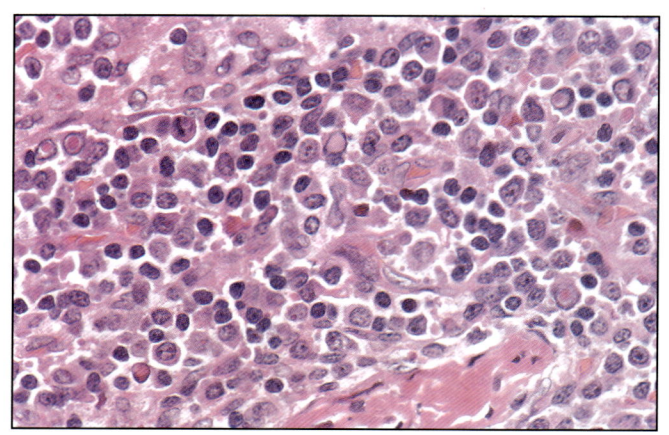

图21A.50 淋巴浆细胞性淋巴瘤。浆细胞散在于小淋巴细胞和淋巴浆样细胞之间。可见嗜酸性核内假包涵体（Dutcher小体）。

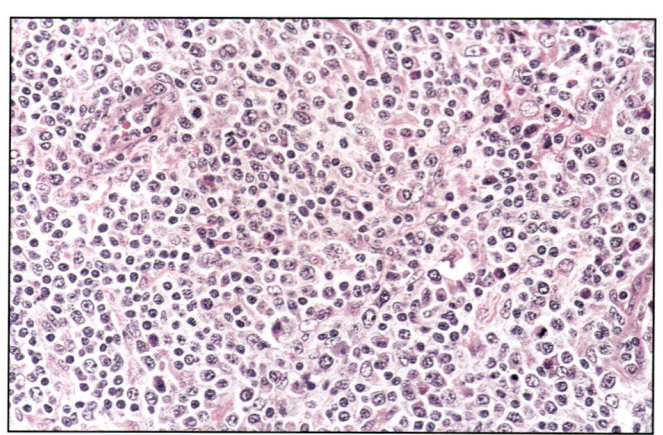

图21A.52 淋巴浆细胞性淋巴瘤伴大细胞增多。相当数量的活化大细胞混杂在淋巴浆样细胞和浆细胞之间。

症）、乏力、头痛和视觉障碍[356,426]。

有时淋巴细胞计数增多，骨髓常常受累。常见副蛋白血症：通常是IgM，有时是IgG或IgA。有些患者可患有Coombs阳性溶血性贫血。疾病呈惰性复发过程。中位生存期为6.5～9年[426,427]。当疾病迅速恶化时，有些病例可转化为大B细胞淋巴瘤（EBV通常阴性）[428]。

病理学

淋巴结结构通常全部被破坏，但淋巴窦可存在或扩张，内含蛋白性液体（图21A.49）[272]。病变常常弥漫分布，缺乏增殖中心。小淋巴细胞与淋巴浆细胞样细胞和浆细胞混合。常常可见鲜明嗜酸性、PAS阳性的核内Dutcher小体，是陷入核内的胞浆Ig（图21A.50）。在淋巴浆细胞样细胞和浆细胞胞浆中常见球形包涵体（Russell小体）或Ig水晶状包涵体（图21A.51）。可以混合一些大的活化淋巴细胞。肥大细胞常常增多。有些病例可有广泛的上皮样组织细胞反应[429]。细胞外可见无定形或结晶状Ig沉积，有时可见伴有异物巨细胞反应。少数病例伴有多量含有结晶的组织细胞，类似于成人横纹肌瘤[430]。

有些淋巴浆细胞性淋巴瘤病例具有相当多的混合性大细胞，曾被称为"伴母细胞增多的淋巴浆细胞性淋巴瘤"或"富于大细胞的免疫细胞瘤"（图21A.52）[272,431]。其预后稍差。

免疫细胞化学

1. B系标记物（如CD20，CD79a）呈阳性。单一型胞浆Ig，通常是IgM型。还常常显示表面Ig，通常呈IgM$^+$IgD$^-$，但有时呈IgM$^+$IgD$^+$（图21A.53）。
2. CD5、CD10和CD23常常呈阴性[356,427]。但是，流式细胞分析显示61%的病例CD23弱表达[432]。少数病例

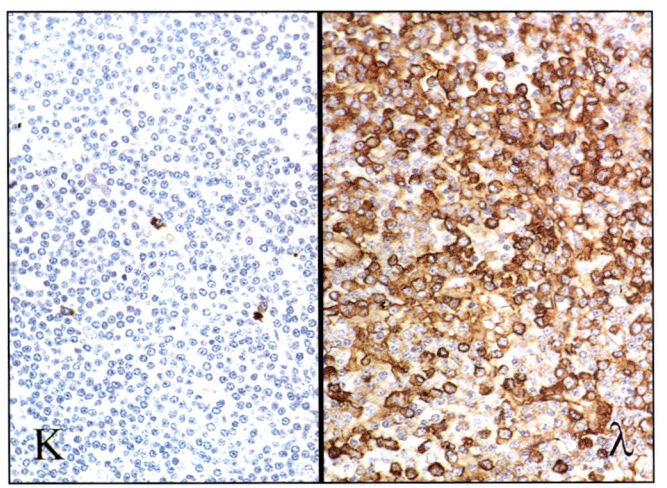

图21A.53 淋巴浆细胞性淋巴瘤的免疫染色。有特征性的轻链限制性。左侧：少数细胞κ轻链染色（残留的浆细胞）。右侧：多数细胞λ轻链染色。

（5%）CD5呈阳性[432]。

3. 55%的病例可见核表达bcl-10[433]。

遗传学特征

Ig基因重排。较早期的研究提示，染色体易位t(9;14)(p13;q32)，伴有 *PAX-5/IGH* 基因融合是淋巴浆细胞性淋巴瘤的独特特征[396,434,435]，近期研究发现，这种易位很少发生于这种淋巴瘤[436-438]。虽然不特异，但6q21缺失是最常见的遗传学改变[395,439]。蛋白质组学和基因表达谱系研究显示，淋巴浆细胞性淋巴瘤/Waldenstrom巨球蛋白血症与多发性骨髓瘤的表达模式不同，但有重叠[437,440]。

鉴别诊断

1. 其他小B细胞淋巴瘤：见"淋巴组织增生性病变诊断的实践问题"（第1250页）。
2. 外周T细胞淋巴瘤伴淋巴上皮样结构（Lennert淋巴瘤）[peripheral T-cell lymphoma with lymphoepithelioid pattern (Lennert lymphoma)]：淋巴浆细胞性淋巴瘤可显示明显的上皮样细胞反应，类似于Lennert淋巴瘤，不同之处在于：存在许多浆细胞和浆细胞样细胞。应用免疫组化检查较易做出鉴别。
3. 浆细胞瘤（plasmacytoma）：浆细胞瘤是由单一形浆细胞组成，而不是由混合性淋巴细胞、浆细胞和淋巴浆细胞样细胞组成。
4. Burkitt淋巴瘤（Burkitt lymphoma）：见"淋巴组织增生性病变诊断的实践问题"（第1250页）。

套细胞淋巴瘤　Mantle cell lymphoma

定义

套细胞淋巴瘤是由套区或原始滤泡淋巴细胞形成的B细胞淋巴瘤[36,441,442]。相当于Keil分类中的中心细胞淋巴瘤[272]。Cyclin D1过表达是这种肿瘤的标志。

临床特征

套细胞淋巴瘤通常发生于中老年人。好发于男性，男女比例7:1，是常见淋巴瘤类型中差别最大者[441-447]。患者常常表现为淋巴结肿大，但结外受累也常见，尤其是脾和胃肠道。胃肠道受累可以产生也可以不产生症状；有些患者表现为回盲部多发息肉（淋巴瘤性息肉病）。大多数患者的疾病分期较高，骨髓受累很常见（表21A.11）。

临床过程呈进展性，对目前可行的治疗反应差（缓解率仅为50%）；大多数有反应的患者在20个月内复发[444,448-451]。虽然美罗华联合化疗可使总体反应率提高（>90%），但并没有延长无进展生存期[452-454]。中位总生存年为3.5年，5年总生存率仅为30%[443,446-448]。因为预后如此差，所以必须考虑骨髓移植或新的治疗（如CDK4激酶抑制剂），尤其是在较年轻的患者[448,455]。另一方面，有少部分患者没有症状，疾病呈惰性[456-458]。

套细胞淋巴瘤可显示转化为母细胞样形式（见下文），但很少转化为弥漫大B细胞淋巴瘤[442]。

病理学

结构和一般特征：淋巴组织呈弥漫性、模糊结节状或结节状浸润。有时肿瘤细胞围绕残留的反应性生发中心增生，犹如套区增宽，融合并蔓延至滤泡间区（图21A.54）。不出现增生中心[441,459]。转化性大细胞缺乏或仅有少量，可能是残留的淋巴细胞。有典型散在的"裸露"淡染核，代表滤泡树突状细胞（图21A.55）。常常可见散在的孤立的上皮样组织细胞，这是有帮助的诊断线索（图21A.56）。常常显示血管玻璃样变和网状纤维增厚。

典型细胞学特征：淋巴瘤细胞常常呈单形性，比小淋巴细胞稍大。核有不同程度的凹陷和尖角，总体上保持球形。有时核非常圆（图21A.54A和21A.55A）。染色质致密，核仁不明显。核分裂计数多少不等，可高可低。胞浆稀少。在一些病例，部分肿瘤细胞胞浆丰富、淡染，类似于单核样B细胞[459,460]。少数病例可显示灶状分化成熟的浆细胞[461]。

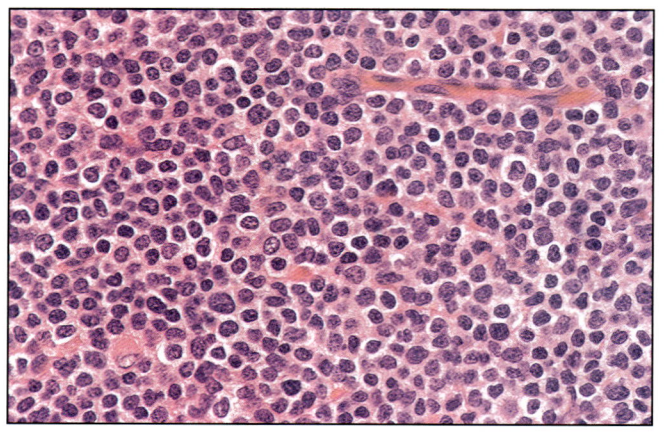

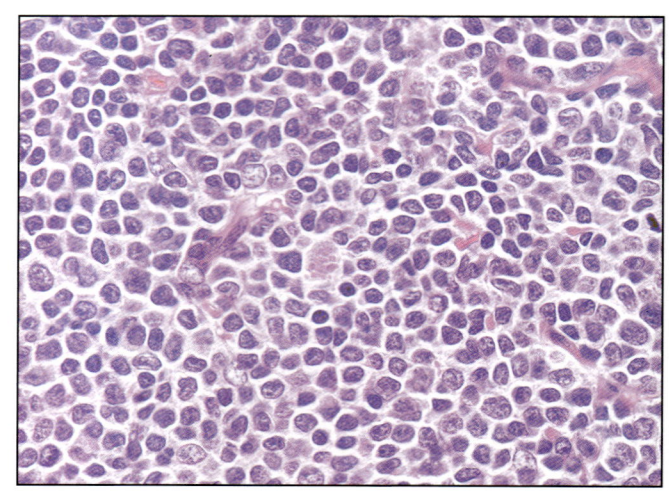

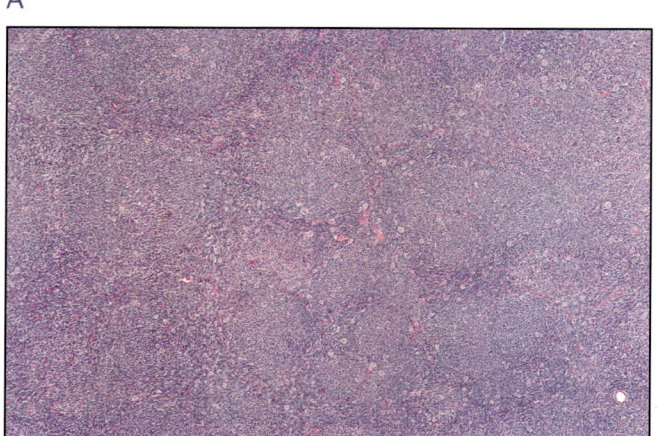

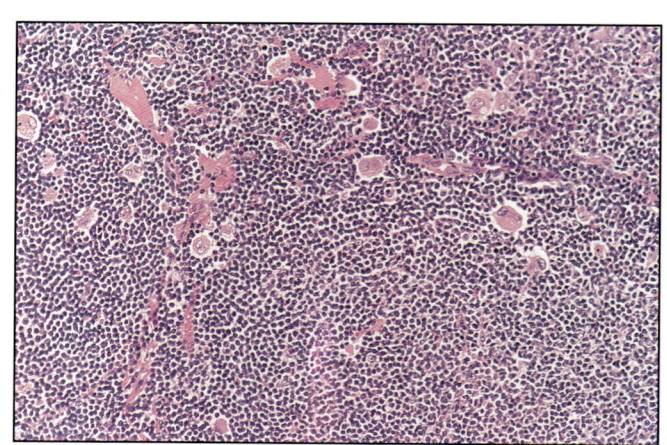

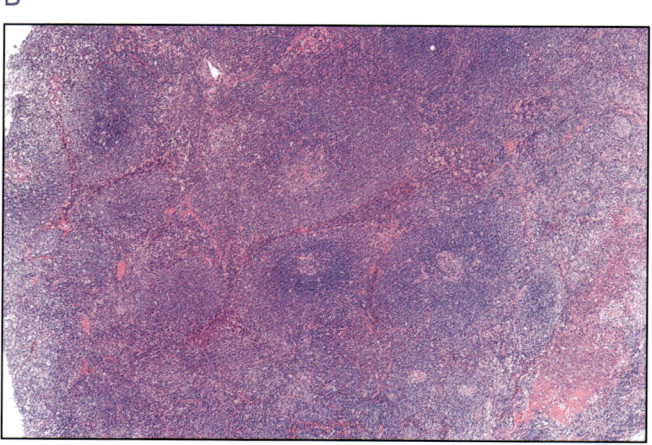

图21A.54 套细胞淋巴瘤，有不同的生长方式。（A）弥漫性生长。该病例显示套细胞淋巴瘤典型的细胞学特征，核不规则，染色质深染，胞浆稀少。（B）结节性生长，可误诊为滤泡性淋巴瘤。（C）套区生长，围绕残留的生发中心。

母细胞样变型（blastoid variant）：偶尔淋巴瘤细胞可呈"母细胞样"，类似淋巴母细胞[442,462-464]。细胞染色质细腻，易见核分裂象（图21A.55B）。同一活检中可显示形态学典型区域和母细胞样表现区域。母细胞样特征也可见于典型套细胞淋巴瘤患者的后续活检中，反之亦然。

图21A.55 套细胞淋巴瘤。（A）经典型。小淋巴样细胞显示核折叠，染色质相当致密。有散在的较大的"裸"核，是滤泡树突状细胞。（B）母细胞型。核染色质开放，类似淋巴母细胞淋巴瘤。常常可见核分裂象。该肿瘤TdT呈阴性。

图21A.56 套细胞淋巴瘤。淋巴瘤细胞之间散在孤立性组织细胞和玻璃样变微静脉，高度提示这种小细胞淋巴瘤是套细胞淋巴瘤。

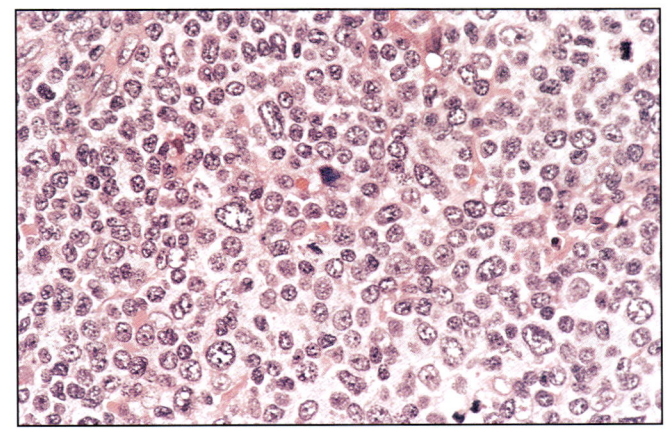

图21A.57 套细胞淋巴瘤,多形性变型。细胞中等大小,偶尔较大。染色质松散。与大B细胞淋巴瘤难以鉴别。诊断必须经免疫组化证实;该病例CD5+cyclin D1+。

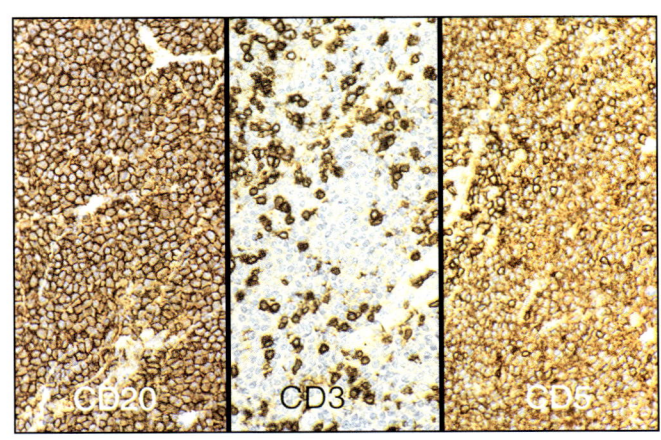

图21A.58 套细胞淋巴瘤的免疫表型特征。左侧:CD20呈阳性。中间:肿瘤细胞之间散在CD3阳性T淋巴细胞。右侧:B细胞(肿瘤细胞)表达CD5,与CD3(T细胞)染色相比,阳性细胞较多。

多形性(间变性、大细胞)变型 [pleomorphic (anaplastic, large cell) variant]:文献中,这种变型常常包括在"母细胞样变型"中。特点是出现不均一的肿瘤细胞群,核不规则,核仁明显[442]。与大B细胞淋巴瘤的不同之处在于:染色质结构中等致密,类似经典型,核仁常较小,胞浆稀少;免疫组化检查对于证实诊断是必要的(图21A.57)。可见散在的奇异形大细胞。

原位套细胞淋巴瘤(In-situ mantle cell lymphoma):在少数套细胞淋巴瘤病例,肿瘤细胞局限于反应性滤泡套区,没有融合或侵入滤泡间区。受累套区可见增厚或不增厚。不借助于免疫组化很难与反应性滤泡增生鉴别。

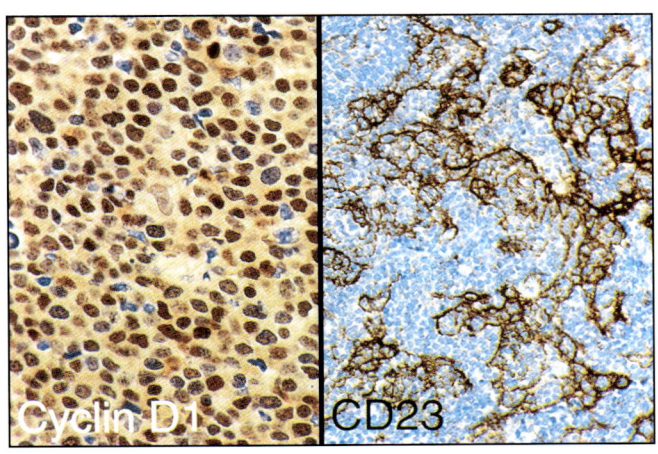

图21A.59 套细胞淋巴瘤的免疫表型。左侧:免疫组化标志是cyclin D1呈阳性。核着色。右侧:CD23染色显示滤泡树突状细胞网通常不规则,而淋巴瘤细胞是阴性的。

免疫细胞化学

1. B系标记物阳性。常见的表面Ig表型是IgM ± IgD,比在B-CLL/SLL中表达强。在B细胞淋巴瘤中,套细胞淋巴瘤不常见,其中λ轻链比κ的表达更常见。
2. CD5+、CD23-、CD10-、bcl-6-、cyclin D1+(图21A.58)。Cyclin D1表达是套细胞淋巴瘤的标志(阳性率>90%)(图21A.59);绝大多数其他类型的淋巴瘤Cyclin D1呈阴性[373,465-468]。然而,少数病例可偏离这种经典免疫表型:例如,高达11%的病例可能为CD5阴性,高达7%的病例可能为Cyclin D1阴性[458,469,470]。对于Cyclin D1呈阴性的病例,Cyclin D2或D3的上调可以替代Cyclin D1[470]。分散或偶尔呈结节状的网状FDC散布在整个病变中(图21A.59B)[471]。
3. CD43常常呈阳性。常常混合少数T细胞。
4. 极少数病例表达CD8[472]。

Cyclin D1表达对于诊断套细胞淋巴瘤是必要的或足够的吗?

高达7%的套细胞淋巴瘤病例免疫组化cyclin D1可能呈阴性;这种病例的确切诊断将依赖于典型的形态学、CD5表达和(或)其他类型的cyclin的表达[458]。在淋巴造血系统肿瘤中,Cyclin D1表达也不是套细胞淋巴瘤所特有的,也见于少数B-CLL/SLL、一部分毛细胞白血病和一部分多发性骨髓瘤或浆细胞瘤病例[373]。

遗传学特征

Ig基因发生重排。70%~80%的病例未突变,20%~30%的病例显示体细胞超突变[382,473-475]。与B-CLL/SLL不同,未突变和突变组之间的临床预后没有差异。最常应用的 V（H）基因是 V（H）3-21 和 V（H）4-34[476]。已有提示套细胞淋巴瘤可能不是先前认为的生发中心前（幼稚）B 细胞肿瘤，而是来源于边缘区或外周血的记忆性 B 细胞，即已经历了滤泡外 T 非依赖性抗原反应[477-479]。

大约 50%~65% 的病例显示 t(11;14)(q13;q32) 细胞遗传学异常，将 11q13 上的 *BCL-1* 癌基因与 *IGH* 基因连接起来[480,481]。前者编码一种细胞周期素，称为 *CYCLIN D1*、*PRAD1*（甲状旁腺腺瘤病）或 *CCND1*[482]。应用 Southern 印迹技术，50%~60% 的套细胞淋巴瘤可显示 *BCL-1* 基因重排[445]。应用 PCR，只有 25%~50% 的病例可显示 *BCL-1* 基因重排[483-485]。另一方面，应用 FISH 分析 11q13 易位，或应用 Northern 印迹分析 cyclin D1 过表达，几乎所有病例均得到阳性结果[477,486-488]。这些观察提示，对于缺乏 t(11;14) 的病例，其他机制或隐含的易位可能导致 *CYCLIN D1* 基因失调。

继发性细胞遗传学改变很常见。最常见的改变是：13 号和 Y 染色体丢失；1p、2p11、6q、8p、11q22-23、13q14、13q34 和 17p 缺失；3q26-29 和 11q 获得；以及 12 号染色体三体[489-494]。46% 的病例可见染色体 11q 缺失，累及 *ATM* 基因[495,496]。*P53* 基因突变，*P16* 基因缺失，P16 表达丢失，P21 表达丢失，以及 P13K/Akt 信号途径的组成性激活与母细胞样/多形性变型有关，常常显示四倍体、高水平 DNA 扩增和频发染色体失衡[497-502]。

基因表达谱研究表明，套细胞淋巴瘤具有独特的表达谱，不同于其他低级别 B 细胞淋巴瘤[458,503]。其标志基因涉及有关凋亡、细胞周期、信号转导和细胞结构的基因。肿瘤坏死因子(TNF)和 NFκB 途径也有改变[504]。有趣的是，在标志基因表达方面，cyclin D1 阴性病例与 cyclin D1 阳性病例相似；生存率也没有差异[458]。母细胞变型与经典型套细胞淋巴瘤之间存在一些基因表达差异，包括肿瘤抑制因子、转录因子、原癌基因以及细胞周期调控、增生、染色质组装、核分裂和纺锤体组装相关基因[505]。

预后因素

1. **临床**：年龄较大（>65~70 岁）与预后较差有关[444,446,447,451]。表现状态差、国际预后指数（IPI）高或滤泡性淋巴瘤 IPI（FLIPI）高是预后不良的因素[443,446,447,449,506,507]。诊断时外周血受累、脾大和乳酸脱氢酶水平高与预后较差有关[443,444,446,447,449,451,508]。
2. **形态学**：母细胞样/多形性变型比经典型套细胞淋巴瘤预后差[443,451,458,501]。类似于原始滤泡的结节性滤泡树突状细胞结构与预后较好有关[471]。
3. **增生**：核分裂计数高，>20/10HPF 或 Ki-67 指数 >10% 与预后较差有关[443,449,459,506]。增生基因高表达可用于识别 5 年生存期不同的患者亚群[458]。
4. **分子学**：V(H)3-21 与较长的中位生存期有关，确诊时患者常常较年轻[476,479,509]。*P53* 基因突变、P53 蛋白过表达或 *P16* 基因缺失与预后差有关[458,498,499]。

鉴别诊断

1. **其他小 B 细胞淋巴瘤**：少数套细胞淋巴瘤具有类似 MALT 型结外边缘区 B 细胞淋巴瘤的细胞结构特征[510,511]。见"淋巴组织增生性病变诊断的实践问题"（第 1250 页）。
2. **淋巴母细胞淋巴瘤** (lymphoblastic lymphoma)：由于核皱褶不规则，淋巴母细胞淋巴瘤可类似于套细胞淋巴瘤，鉴别点是前者的染色质较细腻，核分裂象较多，更可能是 T 细胞表型，患者年龄较小。母细胞型套细胞淋巴瘤不易与淋巴母细胞淋巴瘤鉴别，但 TdT 呈阴性。
3. **套区增生** (mantle zone hyperplasia)：套区增生有时发生于年轻患者的单个淋巴结[512]。与套细胞淋巴瘤的套区增生不同，滤泡局限于皮质，没有结构破坏，没有套区融合。
4. **玻璃样血管型 Castleman 病** (castleman disease of hyaline-vascular type)。

滤泡性淋巴瘤　Follicular lymphoma

定义

滤泡性淋巴瘤是由滤泡中心 B 淋巴细胞组成的肿瘤，显示滤泡结构形态[1]。

临床特征

在高加索人中，滤泡性淋巴瘤占所有 NHL 的 22%~40%，但在东方和不发达国家所占比例较低（5%~10%）[513]。滤泡性淋巴瘤主要发生于中老年人（表 21A.11）。患者通常表现为隐匿性、无痛性多发淋巴结肿大，可能有淋巴结肿大和衰退病史。常见脾大。有些患者具有全身症状，如发热和不适。

发病时疾病总是表现为 III/IV 期。骨髓受累常见（30%~50% 的病例，在小细胞为主的病例中较常见），但似乎不影响预后[260,514]。在一部分患者，循环血中可见淋巴瘤细胞，核有小凹（"臀细胞"，buttock cell），即所谓的淋巴肉瘤白血病。即使缺乏形态学累及证据，应用流式细胞术或基因型分析，在外周血中也常常能检测到克隆群[515,516]。此外，治疗后"完全缓解"的病例常常有克隆群持续存在[517,518]。

在大多数患者，疾病呈惰性迁延过程，并在多年后多次复发。尽管疾病对放疗和（或）化疗反应良好，但总会复发。也就是说，应用目前的治疗方法不能治愈滤泡性淋巴瘤，除非是I期疾病和滤泡性大细胞淋巴瘤。中位生存期是5～10年[519,520]。大多数患者最终死于疾病[521]。因此，对于无明显症状和生命危险的患者，可以不用治疗，直到有肿瘤进展证据时[522]。高达30%的患者会自发消退，但是最终还会复发[522]。少数患者疾病进展迅速，常常转化为侵袭性淋巴瘤并早期死亡。

滤泡性淋巴瘤有时表现为皮肤局部疾病[523,523a]。预后很好，但晚期可发生播散。原发性皮肤滤泡性淋巴瘤不同于普通型滤泡性淋巴瘤，其中只有少数具有bcl-2免疫反应和*BCL-2*基因重排[524,525]。滤泡性淋巴瘤有时也可发生于其他结外部位，尤其是胃肠道[525a]。

少数情况下，滤泡性淋巴瘤可发生于儿童[526-529]。与成人肿瘤不同，其显示以下特征：

1. 大多数患者的疾病为I/II期。
2. 头颈部常常受累。
3. 大多数病例是混合型或大细胞型（II级或III级）。
4. 疾病可治愈。
5. Bcl-2表达不常见（30%），*BCL-2*基因重排不常见（仅为12.5%）。

病理学

淋巴结结构被肿瘤性滤泡破坏，其中有些滤泡可蔓延至淋巴结周围组织。重要的是要在低倍镜下降低亮度检查组织学切片，这有助于识别滤泡结构。在大多数病例，滤泡呈背靠背排列，仅有少许滤泡间组织（图21A.60、21A.61和21A.62）[530]。如果细胞学评估证实滤泡是由滤泡中心细胞组成，则可确诊为滤泡性淋巴瘤。在其他病例，滤泡是离散、完全隔开的（图21A.63）。确诊滤泡性淋巴瘤较为困难，需要考虑其他特征（如细胞学组成，有无套区、含可染小体的巨噬细胞及极性）和（或）免疫组化评估。见"淋巴组织增生性病变诊断的实践问题"（第1250页）。

肿瘤性滤泡通常呈圆形，但也可以不规则。其大小不等，通常比反应性滤泡小[530]。滤泡界限不清，有时可见套区存在或均匀增厚（图21A.61、21A.63和21A.64）。肿瘤性滤泡缺乏反应性滤泡的细胞极性。大

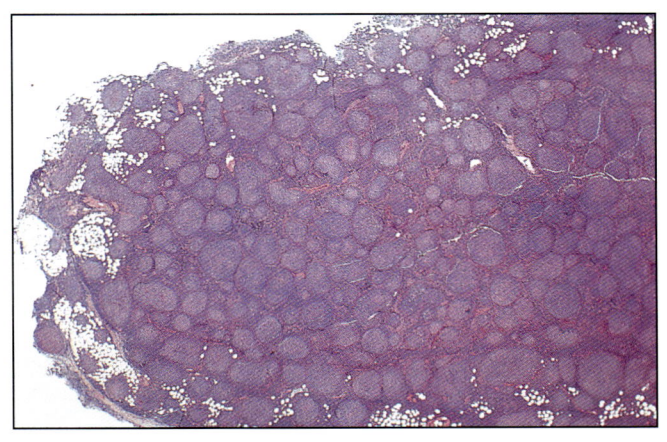

图21A.60　滤泡性淋巴瘤。显示滤泡性淋巴瘤的典型低倍镜下表现。淋巴结被密集排列的结节取代，仅有少量滤泡间组织。这种表现是滤泡性淋巴瘤的特异表现。此外，淋巴结周围脂肪中可见许多相似的滤泡。

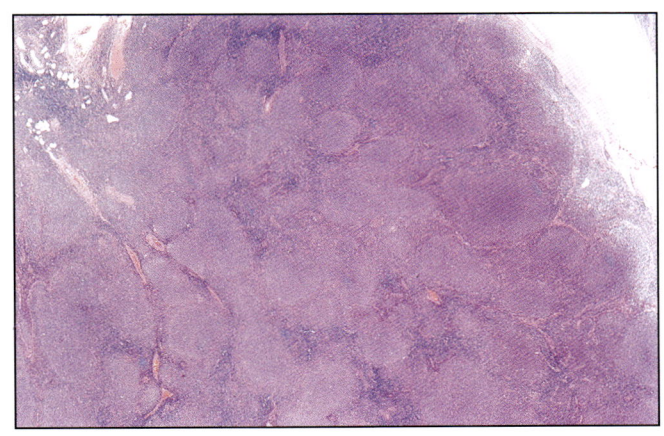

图21A.61　滤泡性淋巴瘤。与图21A.60相比，本例的滤泡界限不太清楚，并显示融合。

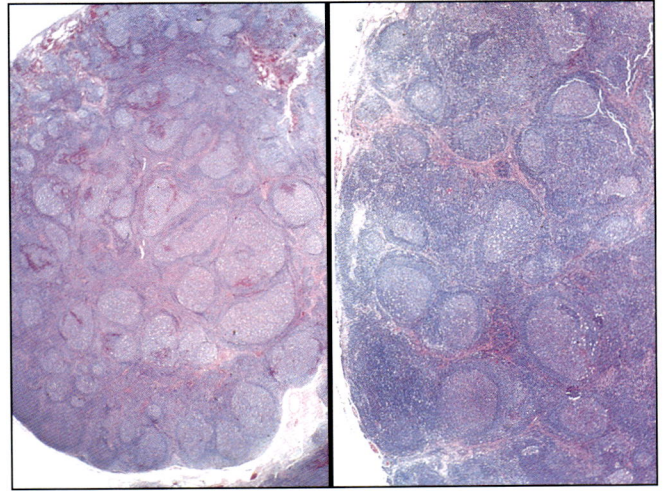

图21A.62　反应性滤泡增生。滤泡通常离散，周围是深染的套区。滤泡排列不太紧密，滤泡间组织明显。有些滤泡呈不规则形。

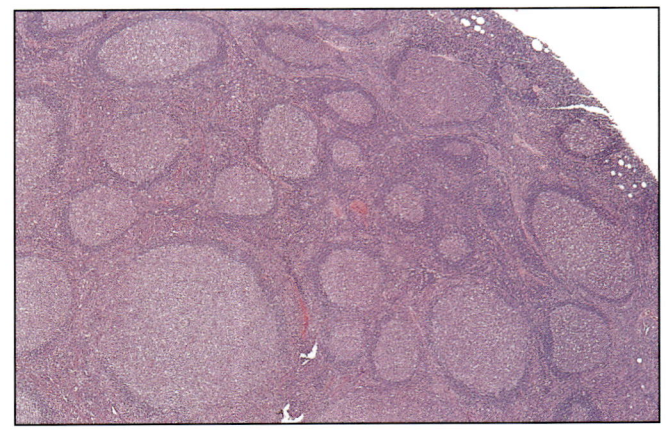

图21A.63 滤泡性淋巴瘤。本例类似于反应性滤泡增生，特点是滤泡间隙增宽，套区分离。诊断滤泡性淋巴瘤的依据是：（1）淋巴结外出现滤泡（右上方）；（2）滤泡中心形态单一（缺乏含可染小体的巨噬细胞和极性）；（3）高倍镜下显示滤泡以中心细胞为主。

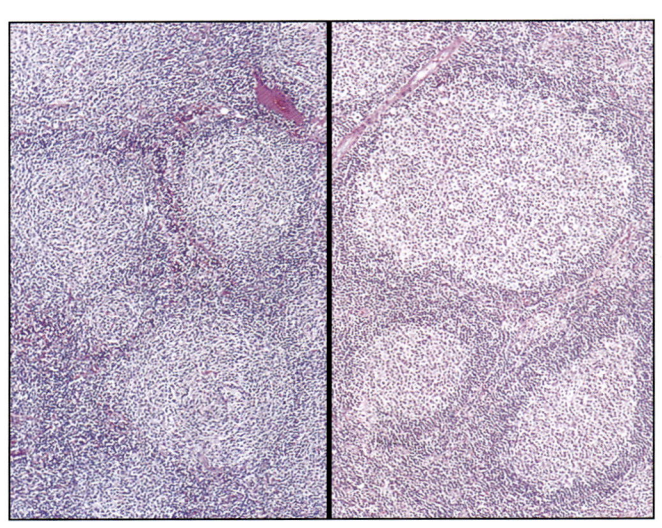

图21A.64 滤泡性淋巴瘤。滤泡由形态单一的细胞群组成，没有含可染小体的巨噬细胞。缺乏极性。左侧：滤泡排列紧密。右侧：滤泡排列不太紧密，可见薄的套区。

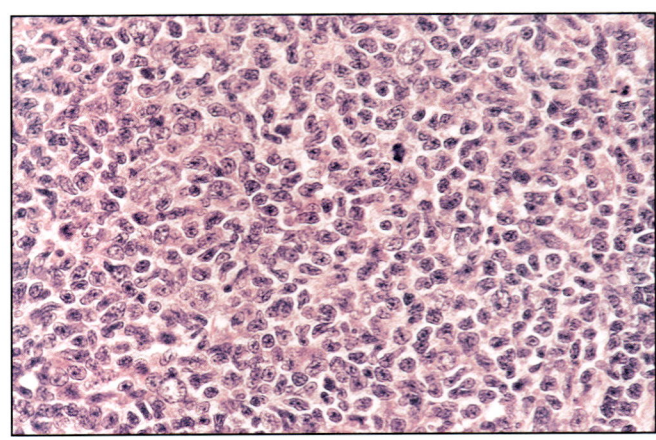

图21A.65 滤泡性淋巴瘤，显示细胞组成的谱系。（A）1级，由中心细胞（小裂细胞）组成。几乎总是可以见到少数大细胞，缺乏含可染小体的巨噬细胞。（B）2级，由大小不一的混合性细胞组成。有相当多的母细胞，核仁清楚，可见明显嗜双色性的胞浆环，混合有中心细胞（小裂细胞）。（C）3级，主要由大细胞组成。

多数病例缺乏或少见含可染小体的巨噬细胞，但也会有例外（图21A.64）。有趣的是，在淋巴结活检中可以出现残留的反应性淋巴滤泡，与早期（I/II）疾病有关[531]。

滤泡的细胞成分多样。主要由中心细胞（小裂细胞）组成的病例最容易诊断，因为反应性滤泡见不到这种形态单一的细胞成分。中心细胞通常具有折叠、成角和长形核，大小约为小淋巴细胞的2倍。染色质致密，但程度不及小淋巴细胞。胞浆稀少（图21A.65A）。较少见的是，中心细胞呈圆形，类似于小淋巴细胞。偶尔可见大的母细胞（中心母细胞或大无裂细胞）。肿瘤性滤泡内散在的FDC与母细胞不同，其核膜纤细呈蓝紫色，染色质"空"，核仁很小，细胞边界不清。

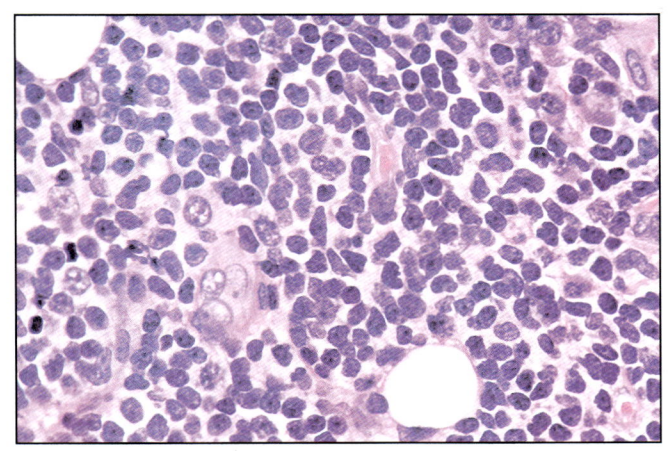

图21A.66 滤泡性淋巴瘤的滤泡间区。本例可见轻度增大的异常淋巴细胞，核形较不规则，染色质致密程度不及小淋巴细胞。其出现代表滤泡间区受侵，当其他特征模糊时，这一特征可用于支持滤泡性淋巴瘤的诊断。

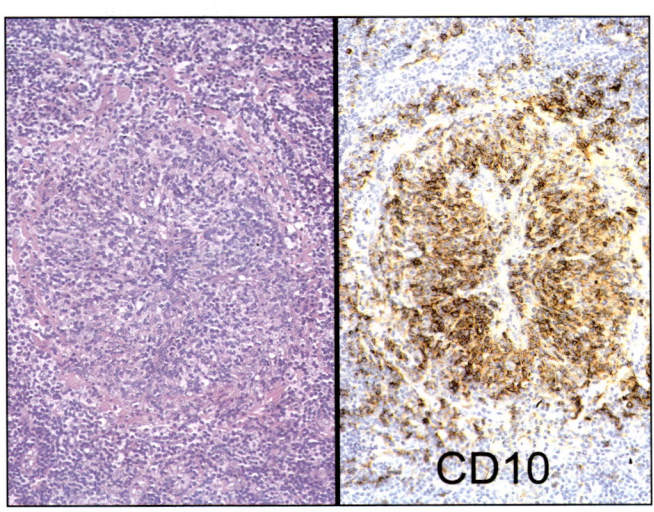

图21A.67 滤泡性淋巴瘤。左侧：滤泡性淋巴瘤的常见而具有高度特征性的特点是淋巴瘤细胞浸润静脉壁。与结外NK/T细胞淋巴瘤的血管侵犯不同，血管壁内或周围没有纤维素沉积，通常没有凝固性坏死。右侧：CD10免疫染色显示肿瘤细胞群，证实了滤泡中心细胞分化。

由混合性细胞组成或以大细胞为主的滤泡性淋巴瘤不易诊断，因为细胞成分类似于反应性滤泡（图21A.65B）。大细胞（中心母细胞或大无裂细胞）的核呈圆形，有时呈分叶状，染色质呈泡状，具有多个膜包被的核仁，胞浆嗜双色性或嗜碱性。少数细胞类似 Reed-Sternberg 细胞。

在宽窄不等的滤泡间区，可见形态温和的小淋巴细胞或成群的较大淋巴细胞，核不规则（图21A.66）。后者代表滤泡间区受累，是支持滤泡性淋巴瘤而非反应性滤泡的重要特征之一[532]。

常见某种程度的硬化，尤其是病变发生在腹膜后和腹股沟的病例[533]。淋巴结周围组织和弥漫生长区域的硬化最明显。可以形成宽胶原带，将肿瘤分隔成不规则的结节，或者形成纤细的淋巴细胞纤维分隔。静脉壁浸润是滤泡性淋巴瘤的另一个常见而高度具有特征性的特点（图21A.67）。

骨髓累及常发生于骨小梁旁，常伴有网状纤维增多（图21A.68）。附近骨髓组织可有不同程度受累。与淋巴结相比，大细胞数量通常较少，提示小细胞更容易进入血液循环[534,535]。

脾受累呈粟粒状，淋巴瘤选择性替代白髓。然而，红髓也可受累（见本章第2部分）。

滤泡性淋巴瘤的分级和亚分类
Grading or subclassification of follicular lymphoma

在滤泡性淋巴瘤的分级中，最重要的是要将富于

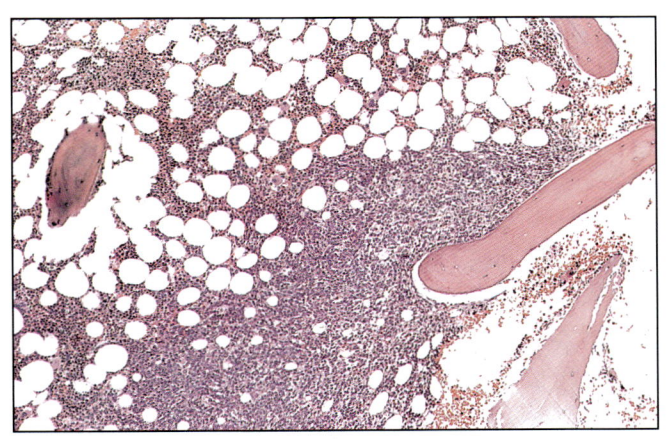

图21A.68 滤泡性淋巴瘤累及骨髓。可见典型的骨梁旁浸润形态。

大细胞的病例分开，因为其复发较早，有可能治愈，但这仍有争议[40,536-538]。已提出许多分级系统，推荐使用 Mann 和 Berard 提出的分类方法，因为其已得到广泛的使用和验证。应用10倍目镜和40倍物镜计数有核仁的大细胞。至少计数20个肿瘤性滤泡视野，取平均值，根据计数结果分为3个级别（表21A.18）[539,540]。计数结果要根据目镜和物镜视野大小进行校正。还应该注意，不要把FDC计数成大淋巴细胞。这种分级与生存期有关，

表21A.18　滤泡性淋巴瘤的分级或亚分类

分级		类似的名称	标准（每个高倍视野中有核仁的大细胞数目，基于视野大小为0.117mm²）
1		小裂细胞（中心母细胞-中心细胞）为主	≤5
2		小细胞和大细胞（中心母细胞-中心细胞）混合	5～15
3	3a	大细胞（中心母细胞-中心细胞）为主	>15，但仍有混合性中心细胞（小裂细胞）
	3b	大细胞（中心母细胞）	全部为有核仁的大细胞

伴有较多大细胞的病例预后较差，经过治疗可明显改善预后[541,542]。

3b级滤泡性淋巴瘤是特殊类型，其完全由中心母细胞（大无裂细胞）组成。不同于3a级滤泡性淋巴瘤，CD10表达较不常见（50%与100%），t(14;18)不常见（22%与73%），常见其他染色体异常，如3q27易位、+1/1q、del（6q）和+7/7p。也就是说似乎其生物学行为与弥漫大B细胞淋巴瘤更相似[543-546]。但是，3b和3a级滤泡性淋巴瘤的生存期没有差异[547]。

滤泡性淋巴瘤中的弥漫性成分
Diffuse component in follicular lymphoma

滤泡性淋巴瘤中可能有弥漫性成分，这被认为该区域完全被淋巴瘤浸润而缺乏肿瘤性滤泡。如果不确定，进行CD21免疫染色有助于证实病变区域没有FDC网。增宽的滤泡间区不符合弥漫性成分。建议用以下术语来量化弥漫性成分：滤泡为主型（滤泡成分＞75%）；滤泡和弥漫性混合型（滤泡成分占25%～75%），以及弥漫性为主型（滤泡成分＜25%）[40]。

在滤泡性淋巴瘤，弥漫性区域的出现被认为是进展现象，然而其对预后的影响并不确定[1]。对于1级和2级滤泡性淋巴瘤，只有弥漫性区域至少占肿瘤成分的25%～50%时，预后才较差。而对于3级滤泡性淋巴瘤，任何弥漫性成分均使预后变差；事实上，这种病例应该命名为"滤泡性淋巴瘤伴有弥漫大B细胞淋巴瘤"，而不是"滤泡性淋巴瘤，3级，滤泡和弥漫性混合型"[40]。

滤泡性淋巴瘤的形态学变型
Morphologic variants of follicular lymphoma

滤泡性淋巴瘤伴有边缘区分化（follicular lymphoma with marginal zone differentiation）：大约9%的滤泡性淋巴瘤伴有明显的肿瘤性边缘区成分，由类似于边缘区或单核样B细胞的细胞组成（图21A.69和21A.70）。与肿瘤性滤泡中心不同，边缘区细胞不表达CD10和bcl-6[548]。

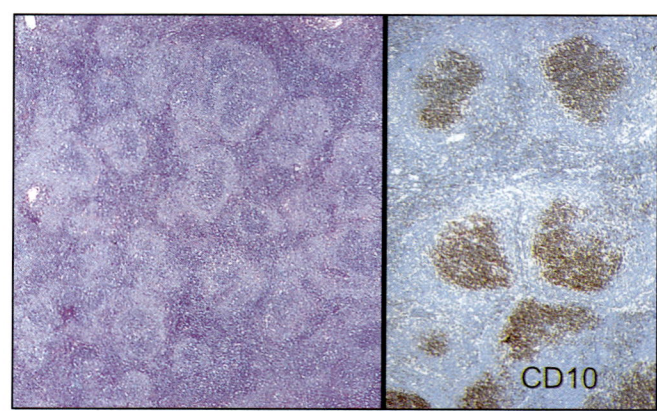

图21A.69　滤泡性淋巴瘤伴边缘区分化。左侧：肿瘤性滤泡中心周围是宽的、淡染的空晕，由单核样B细胞组成。右侧：CD10免疫染色选择性地显示肿瘤性滤泡中心，但不显示边缘区细胞。

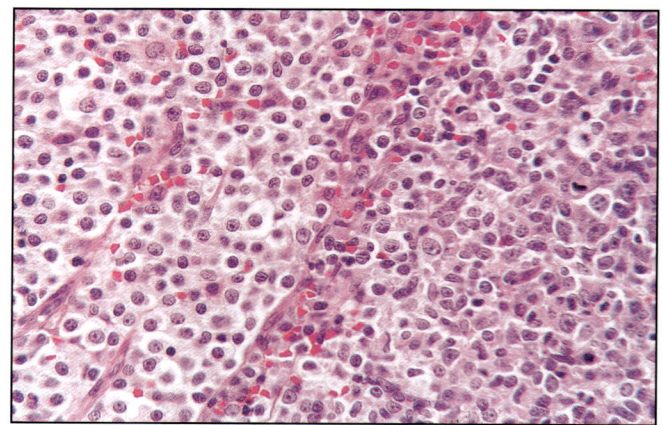

图21A.70　滤泡性淋巴瘤伴边缘区分化。右侧视野显示肿瘤性滤泡中心，而左侧显示宽带状排列的透明细胞，类似于单核样B细胞。

有些研究提示，边缘区B细胞成分＞5%的滤泡性淋巴瘤与进展期疾病（87%）、骨髓受累（69%）及5年无病生存期差有关[549-551]，但其他研究未显示这种特征具有预后意义[552]。

印戒细胞型（signet-ring cell type）：有些滤泡性淋

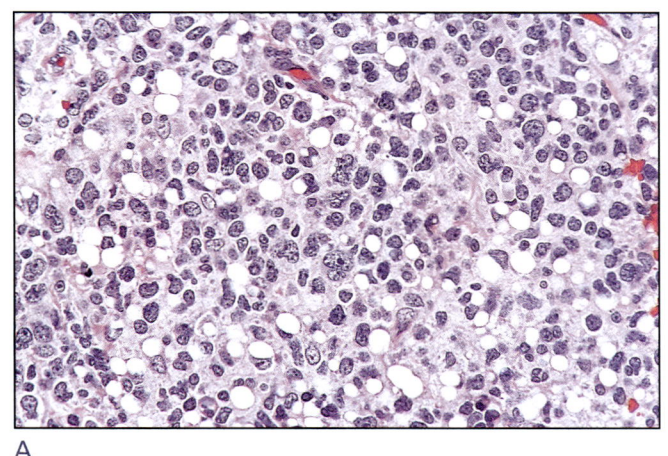
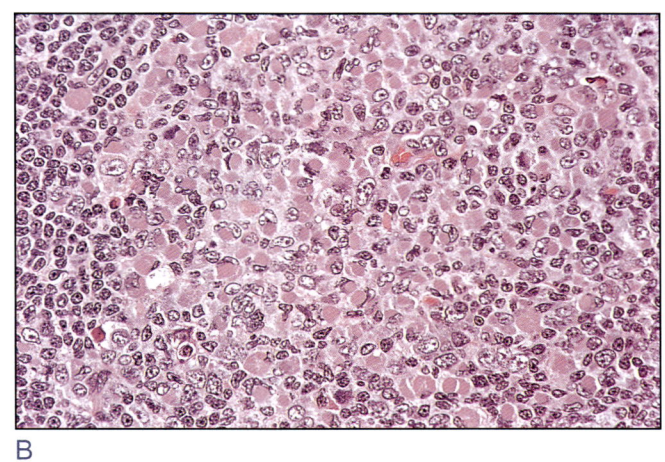

图21A.71 滤泡性淋巴瘤,印戒细胞型。(A)核偏位,可见胞浆内空泡。这种变型常常为IgG型。(B)在这种变型(通常为IgM型)中,是由嗜酸性胞浆小球引起核偏位。

巴瘤部分或全部由印戒细胞组成,核一侧由空泡或嗜酸性PAS阳性小球(Russell小体)代替(图21.A.71)[1,553]。透明空泡常常在边缘处呈Ig染色(通常为IgG),超微结构显示由大小均匀的小球或不规则的电子致密团块组成。嗜酸性小球通常呈IgM染色,超微结构显示在扩张的粗面内质网内可见无定形电子致密物质。

滤泡性淋巴瘤伴有丰富的嗜酸性沉积物(follicular lymphoma with abundant eosinophilic precipitate):有些滤泡性淋巴瘤含有丰富的细胞外PAS阳性无定形嗜酸性沉积物,超微结构显示其由膜包被的囊和电子致密小体组成[554,555]。因为这些是膜结构,可着染各种B细胞系表面标记物和Ig。

滤泡性淋巴瘤伴有玫瑰花结(follicular lymphoma with rosettes):玫瑰花结由肿瘤性淋巴细胞围绕嗜酸性原纤维物质组成[556]。因为原纤维物质是网状胞浆突起,对各种B细胞系标记物均着色。

花样变型(floral variant):当套区小淋巴细胞明显向肿瘤性生发中心延伸时,结构可类似于生发中心进行性转化(图21.72)[557,558]。背景中缺乏反应性滤泡,细胞成分和淋巴结周围组织受累倾向于诊断滤泡性淋巴瘤,但需要免疫组化证实诊断。

反转变型(reverse variant):少数滤泡性淋巴瘤显示"区域(zonation)"反转,滤泡中心多由深染的小细胞组成,而边缘由淡染的大细胞组成(图21A.73)[559]。这种变型不同于滤泡性淋巴瘤伴边缘区分化,因为两个区的细胞均呈CD10$^+$和bcl-6$^+$。

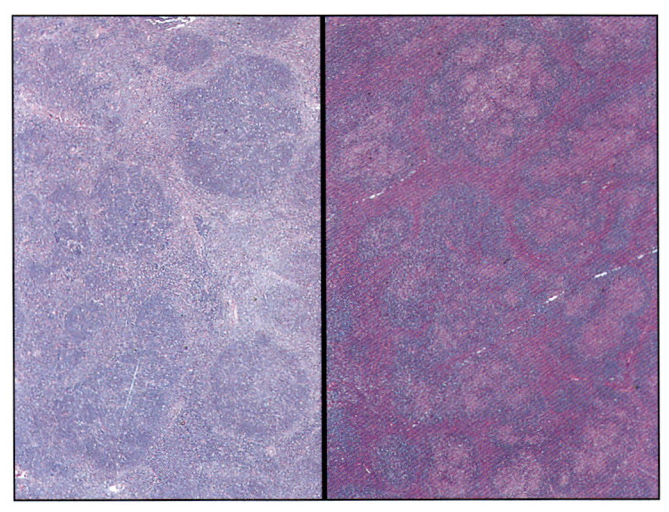

图21A.72 滤泡性淋巴瘤类似于结节性淋巴细胞为主型Hodgkin淋巴瘤或生发中心进行性转化。左侧:滤泡大且深染。右侧:淋巴细胞舌状蔓延入滤泡,形成花样外观。

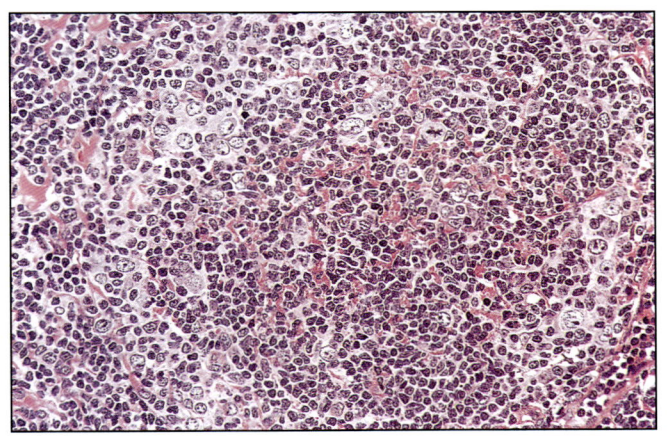

图21A.73 滤泡性淋巴瘤,反转型。滤泡的中心部分由中心细胞组成,周边以大细胞为主。

多形性/间变性变型 (pleomorphic/anaplastic variant)：有些滤泡性淋巴瘤由非常多形性和奇异形的细胞组成。

滤泡性淋巴瘤伴有脑回状核 (follicular lymphoma with cerebriform nuclei)：肿瘤细胞核具有极不规则的折叠，呈脑回状，类似于蕈样霉菌病的细胞核[560]。

滤泡性免疫母细胞-浆母细胞淋巴瘤 (follicular immunoblastic-plasmablastic lymphoma)：有些滤泡性淋巴瘤主要由免疫母细胞和浆母细胞组成。

滤泡性淋巴瘤伴有浆细胞分化 (follicular lymphoma with plasmacytic differentiation)：在有些滤泡性淋巴瘤，在其滤泡间区或滤泡内可见与肿瘤性滤泡相同的Ig轻链染色的浆细胞群（图21A.74）[563,564]。其中一些病例伴有副蛋白血症。在少数病例，肿瘤性滤泡全部由浆细胞组成（"滤泡性浆细胞瘤"）[565]。

Castleman病样变型 (Castleman disease-like variant)：少数肿瘤性滤泡可见穿插的玻璃样变血管，类似于玻璃样变血管型Castleman病。

富于T细胞变型 (T cell-rich variant)：这种类型的滤泡充满多量小的T细胞，掩盖了少数肿瘤性滤泡中心B细胞成分。经仔细观察，CD3+细胞是小淋巴细胞，CD20+细胞较大，还可见CD10+细胞侵入滤泡间区。

原位滤泡性淋巴瘤 (in-situ follicular lymphoma)：当淋巴结显示常见的反应性滤泡增生或非典型滤泡增生时，应用"原位滤泡性淋巴瘤"这个术语，但有些生发

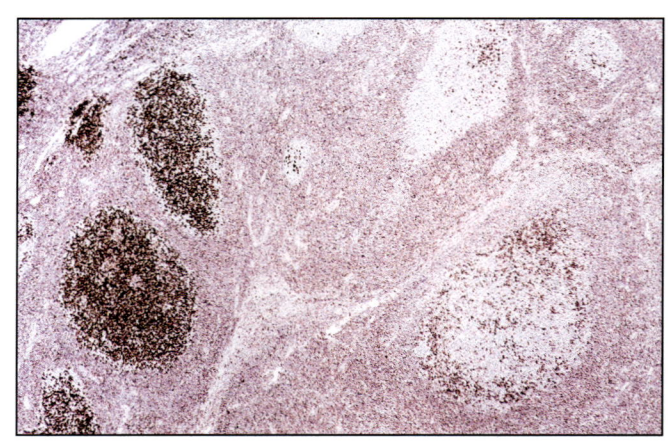

图21A.75 原位滤泡性淋巴瘤，BCL-2免疫染色。滤泡不拥挤，但有些滤泡充满了BCL-2强阳性细胞（肿瘤性细胞巢）。有些滤泡没有这种细胞或只有少数类似细胞（滤泡性淋巴瘤部分受累）。

中心可见bcl-2强阳性滤泡中心细胞聚集（图21A.75）[566]。分子学研究证实，bcl-2阳性滤泡是单克隆性的，常常显示*BCL-2*基因重排，而bcl-2阴性滤泡是多克隆性的。在有些患者，另一个部位同时出现滤泡性淋巴瘤。如果没有，至少23%的患者后来会发生滤泡性淋巴瘤。因此，原位滤泡性淋巴瘤可能是滤泡性淋巴瘤在反应性生发中心中的早期克隆化，或可能是最早期的滤泡性淋巴瘤或癌前病变[566-568]。

免疫细胞化学

1. B细胞系标记物呈阳性。常见的同型Ig是IgM，但也可表达第二种同型（IgG、IgD或IgA）。有些肿瘤Ig呈阴性，尤其是主要由大细胞组成的肿瘤[569-572]。
2. Bcl-2+、CD10+、bcl-6+、CD5−、cyclin D1−。正常滤泡中心B细胞bcl-2呈阴性（图21A.76），85%的

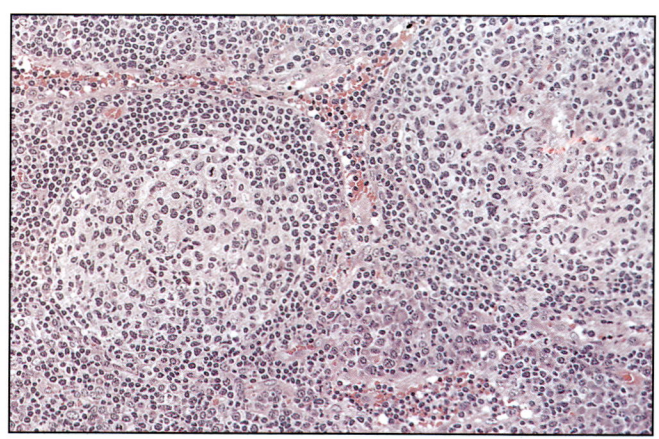

图21A.74 滤泡性淋巴瘤伴浆细胞分化。在肿瘤性滤泡之间，免疫组化显示浆细胞表达与淋巴瘤细胞相同的轻链。这种病例类似于反应性滤泡增生。诊断线索是滤泡内缺乏含可染小体的巨噬细胞。

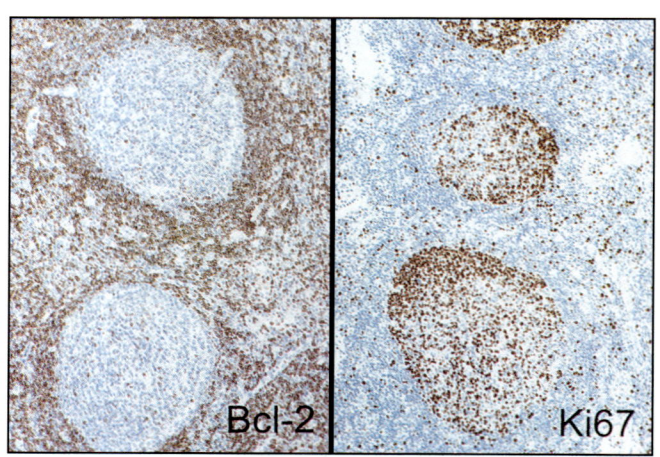

图21A.76 反应性滤泡增生的免疫染色。左侧：只有套区和滤泡间区细胞BCL-2呈阳性，滤泡中心呈阴性。右侧：Ki-67染色可显示滤泡的极性和很高的增生活性。

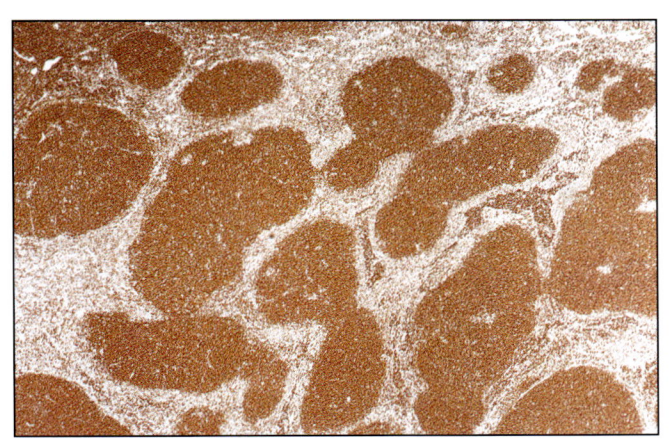

图21A.77 滤泡性淋巴瘤免疫染色。滤泡中心显示BCL-2强阳性。

肿瘤性滤泡表达bcl-2（图21A.77）。阳性率在以大细胞为主的病例中较低[573-576]。Bcl-2阴性染色可能是由于缺乏t(14;18)或BCL-2基因出现突变造成的[577]。极少数滤泡性淋巴瘤病例表达CD5，尤其是花样型[578-580]。组成致密网或变形网状结构的FDC可见于肿瘤性滤泡内[581]。滤泡间组织富于T细胞，若以B细胞为主时，提示滤泡间区被滤泡性淋巴瘤累及[1,532,582]。Ki-67（增殖）指数不恒定，常常比反应性滤泡增生低（平均15.6%与64.9%）[583]。

3. CD43常常呈阴性[10]。对CD23可能有不同的免疫反应。如果出现淋巴细胞套，可呈单一型（肿瘤病变的一部分）或多样型（反应性）[571,584]。T淋巴细胞通常CD4$^+$，散在分布于肿瘤性滤泡内[585,586]。反应性CD57$^+$细胞常常分散于肿瘤性滤泡中，有时出现在滤泡间区[581,587]。

遗传学特征

Ig基因重排显示体细胞超突变和进行性突变[383]。

滤泡性淋巴瘤通常显示t(14;18)(q32;q21)，造成18号染色体上的BCL-2基因与14号染色体上的IGH基因连接[18]。这种易位见于70%～90%的病例。虽然据说t(14;18)在东方人较少见[588,589]，但近期的研究表明其比率与西方人的相近[590-592]。易位导致肿瘤性滤泡中心细胞中结构正常的bcl-2蛋白过表达。由于bcl-2蛋白在阻断凋亡中具有重要作用，过表达有利于肿瘤细胞生存[593]。可应用Southern印迹分析或PCR进行检测t(14;18)，但这些技术可能得出假阴性结果[18]；荧光原位杂交可能是显示t(14;18)最敏感的技术[594]。有趣的是，大多数皮肤和其他结外滤泡性淋巴瘤似乎缺乏该易位[523a,525a]。t(14;18)还可见于一些弥漫大B细胞淋巴瘤；这种病例被认为是从隐匿性滤泡性淋巴瘤转化而来[595,596]。

BCL-6基因重排可见于5%～15%的滤泡性淋巴瘤[597,598]。伴有BCL-6重排的滤泡性淋巴瘤其临床和组织学类似于伴有BCL-2重排者[18]。这种肿瘤具有转化为大细胞淋巴瘤的高风险[599]。有些滤泡性淋巴瘤可显示BCL-2和BCL-6重排。47%的病例可发生BCL-6基因体细胞突变，来自滤泡中心细胞的普遍的非Ig基因超突变[600-602]。

微阵列研究显示，虽然滤泡性淋巴瘤具有正常生发中心B细胞的基因表达谱，但与后者相比，有些基因出现上调或下调[603]。

预后因素

1. **患者相关因素**：老年（＞70岁）、状态差和男性提示预后较差[604]。

2. **预后指数**（prognostic indices）：有些研究显示，滤泡性淋巴瘤国际预后指数（FLIPI）可将滤泡性淋巴瘤患者分成不同的预后组，比IPI的作用好。五种预后较差的因素包括：年龄（＞60岁与≤60岁）、Ann Arbor分期（III-IV与I-II）、血红蛋白水平（＜12g/dL与≥12g/dL）、受累淋巴结区域的数目（＞4与≤4）以及血清LDH水平（正常水平以上与正常水平以下）。已界定了三个危险组：低危组（0～1个不利因素），中等危险组（2个不利因素），以及高危组（≥3个不利因素）[605,606]。意大利淋巴瘤合作组（ILI）预后指数考虑：年龄、性别、B症状、结外部位的数目、ESR和乳酸脱氢酶水平，在判定患者生存期方面优于IPI[607]。

3. **肿瘤范围**：早期患者预后较好。肿瘤负荷表现为淋巴结大小、结外部位的数目、骨髓受累程度、肝脾肿大程度和循环血中淋巴瘤细胞的有无，与预后有关[604,608]。血红蛋白水平低、ESR增高、血清乳酸脱氢酶水平增高以及β$_2$-微球蛋白水平高是肿瘤负荷加重的实验室代表性标记物，与治疗反应较差和生存期较短有关[604]。

4. **组织学分级和增殖指数**（histologic grade and proliferative index）：与3级滤泡性淋巴瘤者相比，1级或2级滤泡性淋巴瘤患者的总体生存期明显长，虽然疾病特异性生存期不具有统计学差异[609]。在1级或2级滤泡性淋巴瘤中，有一组患者的增生指数不一致地增高（Ki-67指数≥30%），总体生存曲线显示最初几年迅速下降，然后达到平台水平，疾病特异性生存期明显比普通型1级或2级滤泡性淋巴瘤差。因此，这一组的临床表现与3级滤泡性淋巴瘤者较一致[609]。

5. **微环境**（microenvironment）：淋巴瘤相关性巨噬细胞含量高是独立的预后不良指标[610]。FOXP3阳性T调节细胞数量增多与预后较好有关[611]。

6. **其他遗传学改变** (additional genetic changes)：除了 t(14;18)之外的基因组畸变，尤其是6q和17p缺失，与生存期较短和弥漫大B细胞性淋巴瘤转化可能性较高具有相关性[612-614]。
7. **基因表达谱** (gene expression profiling)：根据一项研究，81个基因的基因表达谱可鉴别低级别和高级别滤泡性淋巴瘤。与目前应用的组织学分级和临床标准相比，这种分类谱能更可靠地预测临床表现[615]。根据另一项研究，滤泡性淋巴瘤患者的生存时间与肿瘤浸润免疫细胞的分子学特征有关，是独立的临床预后变量[616]。

鉴别诊断

1. **反应性滤泡增生** (reactive follicular hyperplasia)：见"淋巴组织增生性病变诊断的实践问题"（第1250页）。
2. **B细胞慢性淋巴细胞白血病/小淋巴细胞淋巴瘤** (B-CLL/SLL)：见"CLL/SLL"（第1176页）。
3. **淋巴母细胞性淋巴瘤**：见"淋巴母细胞性淋巴瘤"（第1172页）。
4. **结节性淋巴细胞为主型Hodgkin淋巴瘤** (N-LPHL)：见"淋巴组织增生性病变诊断的实践问题"（第1250页）。

滤泡性淋巴瘤的进展及遗传学基础
Progression of follicular lymphoma and genetic basis

滤泡性淋巴瘤是一种动态的和"不稳定的"肿瘤，表现为不同时间、不同部位的不同表现。其中一个淋巴结活检可显示为以小细胞为主，呈单纯的滤泡性生长，而同一患者的另一个活检可显示混合细胞成分，伴有滤泡性和弥漫性结构[617,618]。有些患者最初诊断为弥漫大B细胞淋巴瘤，治疗后发现具有残留的滤泡性淋巴瘤[619,620]。这些患者可能最初患有滤泡性淋巴瘤，经一段时间后转化为大细胞淋巴瘤。化疗后两种成分同样明显，对化疗更敏感的成分被根除了。同样，有些弥漫大B细胞淋巴瘤患者在分期时发现（如骨髓检查）具有潜在的滤泡性淋巴瘤。

由于bcl-2表达可抑制凋亡，淋巴瘤细胞存活期长，能够积累其他遗传学改变。这种变化可导致滤泡性淋巴瘤进展，出现弥漫性生长方式，转化为大细胞淋巴瘤和母细胞转化。

弥漫性生长方式 (diffuse growth pattern)：滤泡性淋巴瘤可进展为弥漫性生长期，而细胞学组成没有改变。这种现象不一定代表预后较差，尤其是当弥漫性成分较少时。但是，如果滤泡性淋巴瘤是大细胞型（3级），则预后较差。

转化为大B细胞淋巴瘤 (transformation to diffuse large B-cell lymphoma)：可转化为弥漫大B细胞淋巴瘤，长期随访发现几率>50%[54,621-623]。转化似乎是滤泡性淋巴瘤自然病史的一部分，而不是化疗或放疗所致遗传改变的结果。发生在滤泡性淋巴瘤诊断后7～300个月之间[624]。一般情况下，转化与侵袭性临床过程有关，但矛盾的是这种肿瘤可以治愈，大约1/3的经强化治疗的患者可以长期无病生存，治愈率类似于经强化化疗的原发性弥漫大B细胞淋巴瘤[625,626]。报告的中位生存期为4～22个月，预后良好的因素包括：病变局限，先前无化疗，以及治疗后完全缓解[623,624]。大细胞淋巴瘤通常表现为普通型大B细胞淋巴瘤，但可具有间变表现，呈窦隙分布，表达CD30[627]。一些遗传学改变能调节淋巴瘤转化，如*P53*基因突变，易位的*BCL-2*基因发生体细胞突变，*RAS*突变（少见），*C-MYC*重排，以及*P16*缺失或失活[628-640]。有趣的是，与原发性弥漫大B细胞淋巴瘤相比，转化性弥漫大B细胞淋巴瘤的基因表达谱更类似于先前的滤泡性淋巴瘤[638]。

母细胞转化 (blastic transformation)：少数病例可转化为类似Burkitt淋巴瘤或淋巴母细胞性淋巴瘤（图21A.78）[641-644]。这种转化的淋巴瘤称为"高级别B细胞淋巴瘤，未定型（具有类似Burkitt淋巴瘤或母细胞形态的特征）[645]"。具有淋巴母细胞性淋巴瘤特征者可以显示或不显示TdT免疫反应。由于t(8;14)，两种母细胞转化常常显示*C-MYC*易位，临床过程迅速进展[54,646-648]。

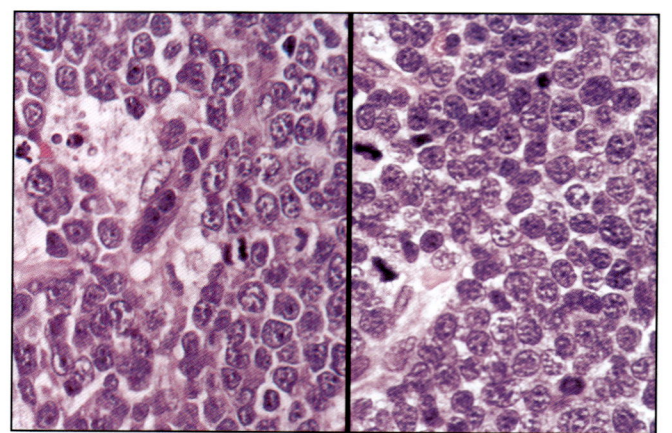

图21A.78 滤泡性淋巴瘤的母细胞转化。（A）转化的淋巴瘤类似于Burkitt淋巴瘤，具有星天结构，细胞中等大小，核仁小而清楚，胞浆嗜双色性，核分裂活性高。（B）转化的淋巴瘤类似于淋巴母细胞性淋巴瘤，细胞中等大小，核仁不清楚，胞浆稀少，核分裂活性高。本例是B细胞系，表达TdT（未显示）。

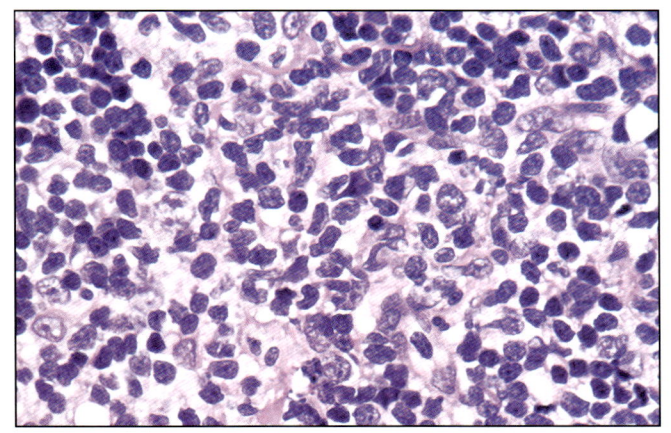

图21A.79 弥漫性滤泡中心淋巴瘤，I级。可见单纯的弥漫浸润性中心细胞，核有棱角，混合有少数大细胞。诊断必须得到免疫组化支持（CD5⁻、CD10⁺）。

弥漫性滤泡中心性淋巴瘤
Diffuse follicle center lymphoma

存在一种弥漫型的滤泡中心性淋巴瘤，主要由中心细胞（小裂细胞）组成，混杂一些中心母细胞（大无裂细胞），即1级或2级（图21A.79）。这种病变不常见，不借助于免疫组化或遗传学检查则难以确诊，表达CD10、bcl-6或*BCL-2*基因重排[40]。如果在随后活检发现患者有滤泡性淋巴瘤，或过去有滤泡性淋巴瘤病史，则应该认为肿瘤是滤泡性淋巴瘤的进展类型，不应该包括在这一类型中。

黏膜相关淋巴组织型结外边缘区B细胞淋巴瘤
Extranodal marginal zone B-cell lymphoma of MALT type

定义

黏膜相关淋巴组织型结外边缘区B细胞淋巴瘤也称为MALT淋巴瘤，是一种惰性淋巴瘤，结构和细胞学表现类似于各种黏膜和淋巴结外的正常淋巴组织[649,650]。在过去，这些淋巴瘤常被误诊为假性淋巴瘤、滤泡中心细胞淋巴瘤、淋巴浆细胞或浆细胞型淋巴瘤[651]。

临床特征

结外边缘区B细胞淋巴瘤可发生于多种不同的结外部位，尤其是胃肠道、甲状腺、涎腺和肺，较少发生在眼眶、胸腺、皮肤、软组织、乳腺、舌、扁桃体、胆囊、肝、泌尿生殖道和硬脑膜[652-655]。可发生于任何性别和任何年龄（表21A.11）。表现为肿物病变或非特异性症状；有些是偶然发现患有淋巴瘤。已知的易感因素是慢性炎症（例如螺杆菌相关性胃炎）、自身免疫性疾病（如桥本甲状腺炎和干燥综合征）[656]。

因为在发生播散之前，淋巴瘤常常局限于受累器官和（或）区域淋巴结很长一段时间，应用局部治疗可满意地医治很大一部分病例。然而，可能同时或异时累及多个黏膜部位，是由于黏膜淋巴细胞的归巢特性而产生的一种现象[657]。近期研究表明，局部或系统播散比最初预料的更为常见[658]。根据仔细分期，25%的胃结外边缘区B细胞淋巴瘤患者有多器官累及，40%的病例伴有胃肠道外播散[659]。胃以外的结外边缘区B细胞淋巴瘤更容易播散至另一个黏膜相关淋巴组织器官（46%）。据报道，骨髓受累发生于2%~15%的病例[658,659]。在胃淋巴瘤，多灶性与t(11;18)(q21;q21)明显相关，胃外淋巴瘤伴有18号染色体三体。然而在局部病变和播散性病变患者之间，生存期没有显著差异[658,659]。

虽然晚期可发生局部或远处复发，但预后很好。根据非Hodgkin淋巴瘤分类方案，5年总体生存率为74%[264]，胃淋巴瘤的5年生存率＞90%[660-662]。复发率为37%（胃肿瘤为22%，胃外肿瘤为48%），复发的中位时间为47个月[663]。

9%~30%的结外边缘区B细胞淋巴瘤病例可伴有大细胞淋巴瘤，使预后变差[269,431,660,664]。已有极少数复合性结外边缘区B细胞淋巴瘤和经典型Hodgkin淋巴瘤的病例报道[665]。

近年来，在治疗胃结外边缘区B细胞淋巴瘤的方法中，最引人注意的改变是应用抗生素。应用抗螺杆菌治疗，大约70%~80%的伴有螺杆菌胃炎的胃结外边缘区B细胞淋巴瘤显示完全缓解[655,666-673]。淋巴瘤消退通常发生在几周内，但也可能在1年内。抗生素治疗似乎主要在局限于黏膜和黏膜下层的单纯性低级别疾病中有效[672]。根治螺杆菌能抑制螺杆菌相关性黏膜的T细胞增生，通过CD40和CD40配体的相互作用为肿瘤性B细胞提供接触依赖，导致肿瘤消退[674]。基于PCR的研究显示，分子学反应比形态学反应滞后1~2年，肿瘤的分子学证据可持续存在于某些患者中[669,672,675,676]。尽管临床和组织学证实为缓解，可能有些残留肿瘤细胞仍维持休眠，再次刺激后能迅速生长，某些例证显示螺杆菌再感染可引起迅速复发[677]。有趣的是，螺杆菌阴性的早期胃结外边缘区B细胞淋巴瘤患者也能从单独的抗生素治疗中获益[678]。另一方面，螺杆菌根治对于胃以外的边缘区B细胞淋巴瘤无效[679]。

病理学

结外边缘区 B 细胞淋巴瘤显示结外组织单灶或多灶受累。反应性淋巴滤泡常常散布其间。肿瘤性淋巴组织浸润呈弥漫性，滤泡间或滤泡周分布（图 21A.80）。浸润常常呈异源性，由混合细胞类型组成，然而少数病例可显示单一形细胞群（图 21.81）[649,653,655,680]。最典型的细胞呈中心细胞样，小至中等大，核轻度折叠或长形成角，染色质中等致密，核仁不清楚，胞浆量少，淡染或透明（21A.81）。有些细胞稍大，胞浆丰富透明，类似于单核样 B 细胞（图 21A.81A）。有些细胞具有深染、圆形核，不易与正常淋巴细胞区分。常常有孤立的混合性大的母细胞，类似于中心母细胞或免疫母细胞。

淋巴瘤易于侵犯附近的上皮结构，形成"淋巴上皮病变"（图 21A.81A），定义为超过 3 个淋巴细胞的积聚使上皮扩张或变形[681]。随着时间进展，受损的上皮细胞可维持孤立或小巢状嗜酸性或印戒细胞（图 21A.82A）。有趣的是，上皮结构内和周围的淋巴瘤细胞常常呈中心细胞样或单核 B 细胞样表现，形成淡染的"环"围绕淋巴上皮病变，常见于涎腺中（图 21A.83）。虽然淋巴上皮病变是结外边缘区 B 细胞淋巴瘤的特征，但没有特异性，有时可见于其他淋巴瘤类型或反应性淋巴组织增生。

浆细胞常常混合在肿瘤中，或见于表面上皮细胞之下。大约 1/3 的病例浆细胞呈单一类型，因此是肿瘤性克隆的一部分。在有些病例，浆细胞很明显，与髓外浆细胞瘤难以鉴别。浆细胞可显示非典型特征，如核增大、核仁清楚、胞浆结晶和 Dutcher 小体。有时可见细胞外 Ig 或淀粉样沉积物。

滤泡克隆化是常见现象。肿瘤细胞侵犯并取代反应性滤泡，形成模糊或明确的结节，类似于滤泡性淋巴瘤[664,682,683]。滤泡克隆化的肿瘤细胞可显示浆细胞分化增多或有更多的母细胞表现。

30% 的病例累及局部淋巴结[653]。早期病变局限于反应性滤泡的边缘区。随着时间进展，出现边缘区增宽、融合，滤泡克隆化并侵犯滤泡间区，导致结构消失[680]。在少数脾受累的病例，边缘区常常受累，而白髓滤泡的反应性生发中心和套区并无受累[684]。

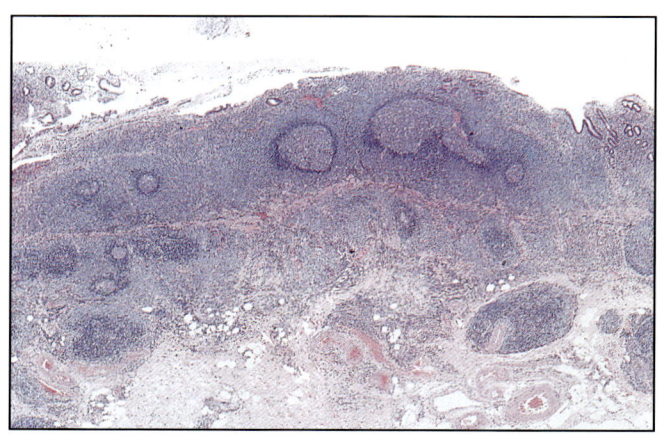

图 21A.80　胃结外边缘区 B 细胞淋巴瘤。围绕反应性淋巴滤泡的淋巴组织侵占黏膜。黏膜下层也受累。

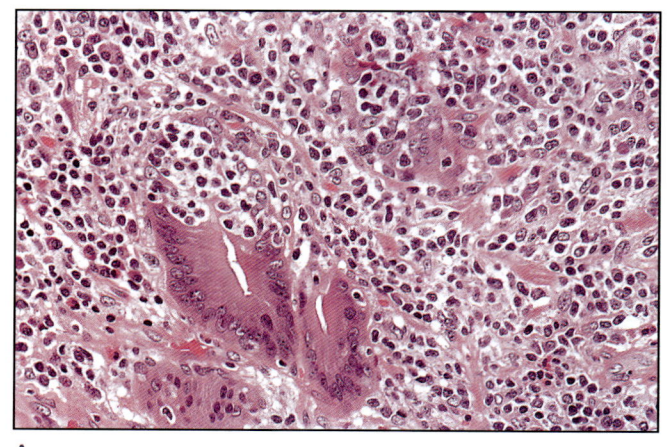

A

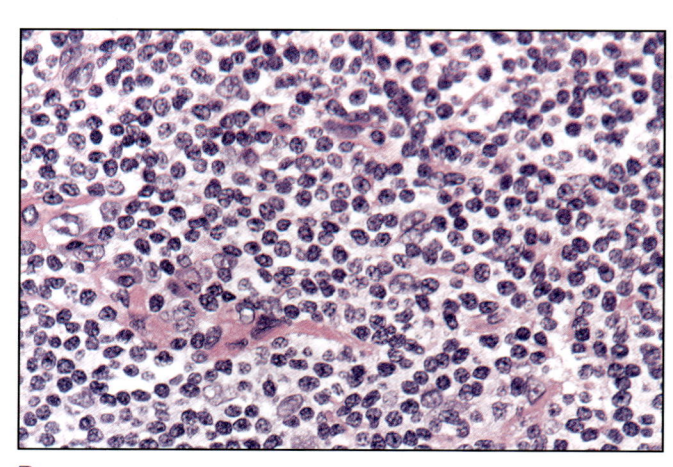

B

图 21A.81　胃结外边缘区 B 细胞淋巴瘤。（A）可见典型的淋巴上皮病变，淋巴瘤细胞使胃腺体扩张并破坏。淋巴瘤细胞呈中心细胞样，胞浆透明。可见混合的细胞类型，包括浆细胞。（B）在本例，有单一形态的小细胞巢。

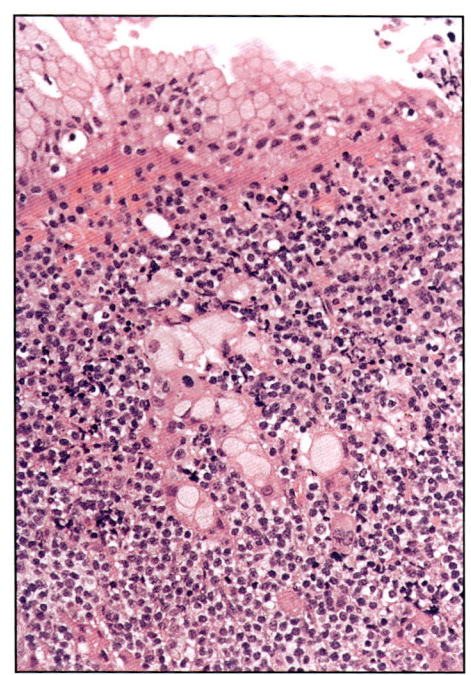

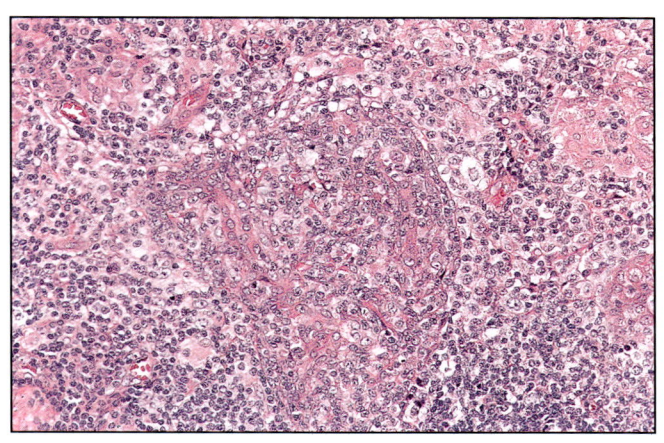

图21A.83 腮腺的结外边缘区B细胞淋巴瘤。中间的淋巴上皮病变表现为淋巴瘤细胞引起腺体明显扩张。围绕上皮岛的淋巴瘤细胞通常呈单核样B细胞表现,低倍镜下形成淡染环。

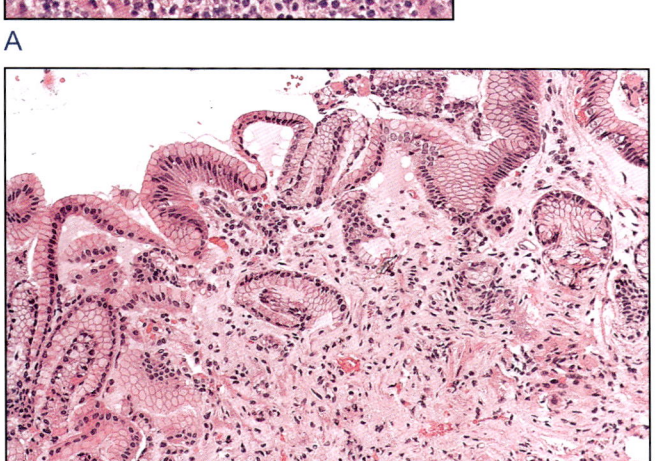

图21A.82 胃结外边缘区B细胞淋巴瘤。(A)有明显的腺体破坏,残留的上皮细胞具有嗜酸性或毛玻璃样外观。在活检标本,这种特征能导致误诊为弥漫型胃癌。(B)该活检显示抗螺杆菌治疗后,淋巴瘤消退的典型改变。有由于先前淋巴瘤破坏导致的腺体丢失。固有层由松散的纤维血管组织组成,伴有少数淋巴细胞,这些空间曾经被淋巴瘤细胞侵占,现在消失了。

与胃结外边缘区B细胞淋巴瘤抗螺杆菌治疗有关的诊断问题
Diagnostic problems related to anti-Helicobacter therapy in gastric extranodal marginal zone B-cell lymphoma

对抗螺杆菌的反应主要见于胃结外边缘区B细胞淋巴瘤,其他小细胞或大细胞淋巴瘤则没有反应,然而有些早期胃大B细胞淋巴瘤已证实有消退[685,686]。因此在进行抗螺杆菌治疗之前,必须证实组织学诊断和分类。

完成抗螺杆菌治疗后6周,通常要进行胃活检证实根除了螺杆菌,并要评估淋巴瘤的组织学反应[653,680]。之后,每隔3~6个月检测淋巴瘤的状态。目前,评估抗螺杆菌治疗反应的金标准仍然是组织学检查而不是分子学检查。淋巴瘤消退的特征性改变是:固有层细胞减少,由疏松结缔组织和散在的浆细胞组成,缺乏淋巴细胞有结构的聚集(图21A.82B)[669,680,687]。由于淋巴瘤细胞消失和先前的淋巴瘤破坏腺体,形成间质空区。

免疫细胞化学

1. B细胞系标记物。Ig通常为IgM,有时为IgG或IgA型,但不是IgD。
2. $CD5^-$、$CD10^-$、$CD23^-$、cyclin $D1^-$、bcl-6^-。少数病例可能为$CD5^+$;虽然已有提示,表达CD5的结外边缘区B细胞淋巴瘤易于累及骨髓,但并非总是如此[688,689]。具有t(11;18)或t(1;14)易位的病例会出现bcl-10异常核表达;在胃,这种特征与抗螺杆菌治疗无效有关。对于缺乏这些易位的病例,bcl-10免疫反应通常仅见于胞浆,如同在正常B淋巴细胞中一样[690-694]。
3. Bcl-2常常呈阳性[653],CD43表达见于大约50%的病例[695,696]。Ki-67(增生)指数低。

遗传学特征

表现为Ig基因重排,体细胞超突变[697]。也有Ig基因进行性突变证据,提示抗原刺激在克隆扩展方面起作用[698]。通常缺少 BCL-1、BCL-2 和 BCL-6 基因重排[653,683,699-701]。在这种淋巴瘤类型中有几种独特的互换性染色体易位，而在淋巴结或脾边缘区B细胞淋巴瘤中则见不到。易位的发生率随不同的结外部位而极为不同[702]。有趣的是，这些不同的易位都可导致NFκB的组成性激活（反式激活基因，如对细胞活化、增生和生存具有重要作用的细胞因子和生长因子的基因）[703]：

1. t(11;18)(q21;q21)导致11q21上的*API2*（凋亡基因的抑制子）与18q21上的*MALT1*融合，发生于18%～35%的病例[704-708]。染色体易位导致嵌合体蛋白的产生，可直接激活NFκB，绕过正常的信号序列途径[696]。通常作为单一的遗传学异常而发生。t(11;18)选择性地见于结外边缘区B细胞淋巴瘤，但不见于伴有大细胞成分或大B细胞性淋巴瘤者，提示易位具有对抗转化的"免疫力"[704,709]。染色体易位主要见于胃和肺的结外边缘区B细胞淋巴瘤，在其他结外部位则不常见。携带t(11;18)的肿瘤易于显示相对单一形态的淋巴瘤浸润；在胃，这种易位与抗螺杆菌治疗无效有关[710,711]。
2. t(1;14)(q22;q32)仅发生于1%～2%的病例，与较具播散性或侵袭性的肿瘤有关。易位连接*BCL-10*基因和*IGH*基因，引起野生型bcl-10蛋白过表达[712,713]。Bcl-10蛋白形成寡聚物，不需要通过表面抗原受体刺激途径的上游信号，连接MALT1并调节其寡聚合，接着触发引起NFκB激活的分子[696]。
3. t(14;18)(q32;q21)发生于大约15%的病例，连接*MALT1*和*IGH*基因，导致MALT1蛋白过表达[714]。肿瘤细胞显示胞浆MALT1和bcl-10高表达，可能是MALT1影响bcl-10并使其稳定[693]。寡聚合的MALT1导致NFκB激活[696]。这种染色体易位主要见于涎腺、眼、皮肤和肺的结外边缘区B细胞淋巴瘤[714,715]。常见其他遗传学畸变，如3号和（或）18号染色体三体。
4. t(3;14)(p14.1;q32)发生于大约10%的病例，导致*IGH*和*FOXP1*融合[716]。这种染色体易位主要见于甲状腺、眼和皮肤的结外边缘区B细胞淋巴瘤。

其他常见的遗传学改变是：3、12、18号染色体三体，杂合性丢失或*P53*突变，*P15*和*P16*启动子甲基化，以及*FAS*基因突变[696,717]。应用染色体原位杂交，3号染色体三体见于60%的病例[718,719]，但矛盾的是，常规细胞遗传学分析很难检测到[704]。遗传学不稳定性，表现为复制错误修复表型，见于50%的结外边缘区B细胞淋巴瘤[720]。

鉴别诊断

1. **反应性淋巴组织增生**：见"淋巴组织增生性病变诊断的实践问题"（第1250页）。
2. **其他小B细胞淋巴瘤**：见"淋巴组织增生性病变诊断的实践问题"（第1250页）。

结外边缘区B细胞淋巴瘤的大细胞转化
Large cell transformation of extranodal marginal zone B-cell lymphoma

弥漫大B细胞淋巴瘤常见于各种结外部位。目前，只有伴发低级别成分的病例（结外边缘区B细胞淋巴瘤）被认为与MALT淋巴瘤有关。即便如此，仍不鼓励使用"高级别MALT淋巴瘤"这个术语。

识别大细胞转化的重要性在于其预后较差（胃结外边缘区B细胞淋巴瘤的5年生存期从＞90%降至60%～70%）[660-662,721,722]。然而，有关大细胞转化的组成尚无一致意见。当有致密的细胞巢，融合成片的大细胞，位于克隆化滤泡边界以外时，可作出"弥漫大B细胞淋巴瘤，源于结外边缘区B细胞淋巴瘤"的诊断（图21A.84A）[40,664,680]。简而言之，大细胞成分＞5%时，最好诊断为"结外边缘区B细胞淋巴瘤伴有大细胞增多"，因为预后较差（图21A.84B）[40,269,272]。

大细胞转化的遗传学资料有限。在一部分病例，*P53*基因失活（一个等位基因突变，另一个等位基因丢失）可调节转化[717]。出现t(11;18)易位能保护结外边缘区B细胞淋巴瘤不转化为大细胞淋巴瘤[709]。

淋巴结边缘区B细胞淋巴瘤（所谓的单核样B细胞淋巴瘤）
Nodal marginal zone B-cell lymphoma (so-called monocytoid B-cell lymphoma)

定义

淋巴结边缘区B细胞淋巴瘤是一种不常见的原发性淋巴结B细胞肿瘤，形态学类似于累及淋巴结的结外或脾边缘区B细胞淋巴瘤，但没有结外或脾疾病证据[723]。根据定义，如果伴发滤泡性淋巴瘤成分，则应归类为滤泡性淋巴瘤伴有边缘区分化。

临床特征

淋巴结边缘区B细胞淋巴瘤主要发生于成人，女性发病率稍高（表21A.11）[268,724]。患者表现为淋巴结肿大。有些患者可有副蛋白血症[725]。高分期疾病

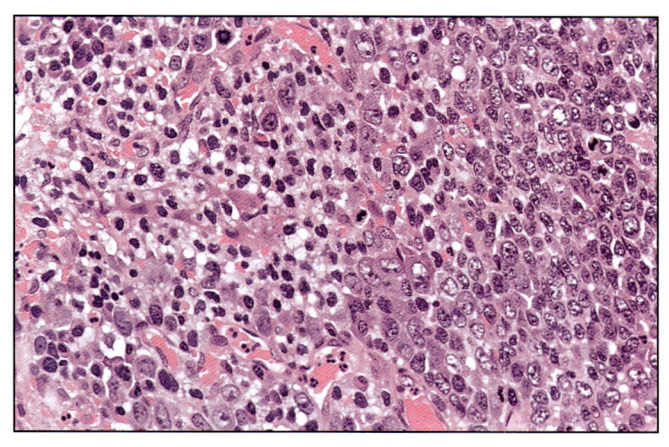
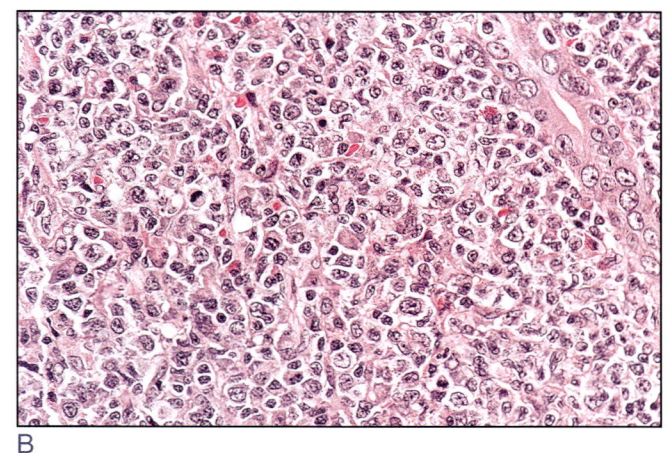

图21A.84　胃结外边缘区B细胞淋巴瘤。（A）低级别成分（左侧视野）与右侧视野的大细胞性淋巴瘤混合。（B）有数目增多的大的母细胞，与小细胞紧密混合，不形成片状细胞巢。可称为"结外边缘区B细胞淋巴瘤伴有大细胞增多"。

（Ⅲ期或Ⅳ期）发生于38%～76%的患者，但B症状不常见。与结外边缘区B细胞淋巴瘤相比，骨髓受累较常见（29%～62%与14%），预后较差（5年总体生存率为56%～65%与81%；5年无进展生存率为35%）[268,269,724-728]。常常复发。临床行为类似于低级别惰性淋巴瘤。20%的病例可转化为弥漫大B细胞淋巴瘤，预后较差[729-731]。与丙型肝炎感染没有明显相关性[724,725]。有趣的是，少数年轻患者发生的淋巴结边缘区B细胞淋巴瘤通常分期较低[731a]。

病理学

通常淋巴结结构破坏不完全。背景中常常散在反应性淋巴滤泡，伴有完好的或受侵犯的套区。淡染的肿瘤细胞形成巢状、带状和片状，分布在窦隙、边缘区和滤泡间区（图21A.85）[269,724,732-734]。它们也可能使反应性滤泡生发中心克隆化并呈现大细胞[725]。仅有少数病例可见完全的弥漫性结构消失。

细胞学成分常常为混合性的，包括小淋巴细胞、类似于单核样B细胞的细胞、浆细胞样细胞、浆细胞和大细胞[725]。单核细胞样细胞的核呈卵圆形，有切迹或呈锯齿状，染色质细腻，核仁不清楚，胞浆宽带状透明淡染（图21A.86）。浆细胞聚集可显示细胞学非典型性，可见于某些病例；常常被证实是肿瘤的一部分。可能有一些混合性中性粒细胞。有时，花环状上皮样组织细胞围绕淋巴瘤细胞巢（图21A.87）。混杂的大的母细胞甚至可以形成小的聚集。

免疫细胞化学

免疫表型与MALT型结外边缘区B细胞淋巴瘤相同。最常表达的Ig类型是IgM，但可能是IgM+IgD、IgG或IgA[725]。Bcl-2通常呈阳性，不同于反应性单核细胞样B细胞[724,732,735]。有些大细胞可表达bcl-6[725]。没有bcl-10核的表达[724]。

遗传学特征

重排的Ig基因通常显示体细胞超突变，与生发中心后B细胞一致[724,736]。最常见的遗传学改变包括：3、18和7号染色体三体，t(3;14)(q27;q32)，1号染色体结构异常，以及17号染色体遗传学物质丢失[725,737-739]。淋巴结边缘区B细胞淋巴瘤中见不到结外边缘区B细胞淋巴瘤的染色体易位特征，提示这两种肿瘤在生物学上是不同的[709,724,725]。

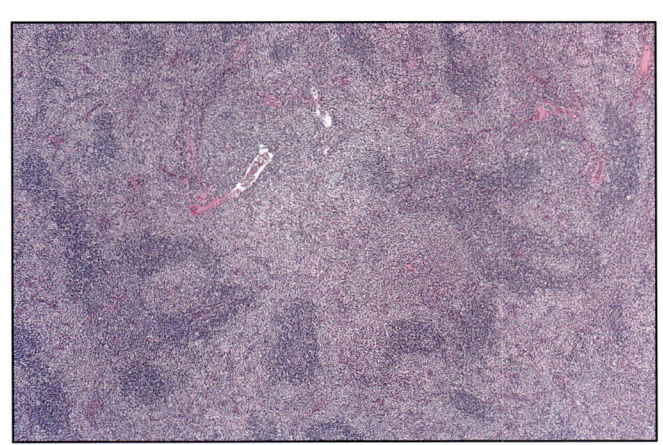

图21A.85　淋巴结边缘区B细胞淋巴瘤。这张图描绘了特征性斑片状受累的淋巴结，表现为淡染的斑块或片状。可见残留的反应性淋巴滤泡。

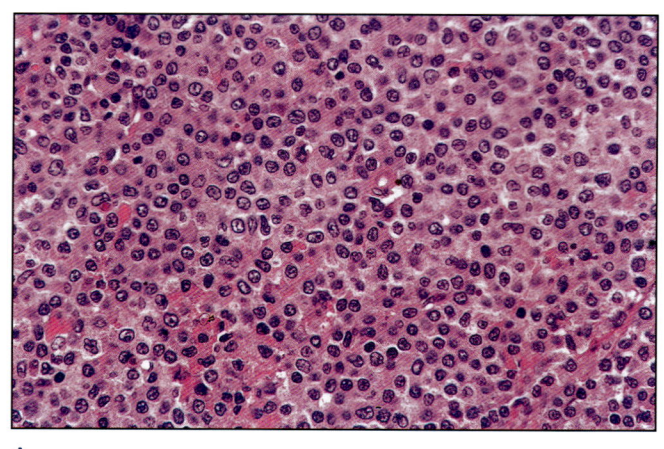
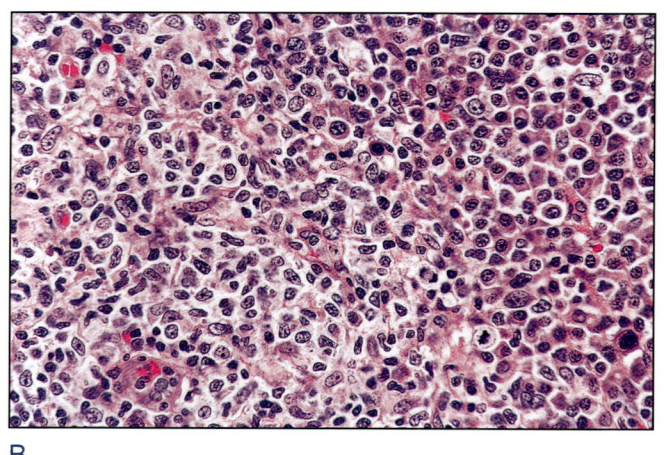

图21A.86 淋巴结边缘区B细胞淋巴瘤。(A)淋巴瘤细胞核圆形,核膜的表面有凹陷。有可识别的淡染胞浆,类似于单核细胞样B细胞。(B)淋巴瘤细胞极其类似于中心细胞样细胞(左侧视野),右侧视野可见许多浆细胞(肿瘤性)。

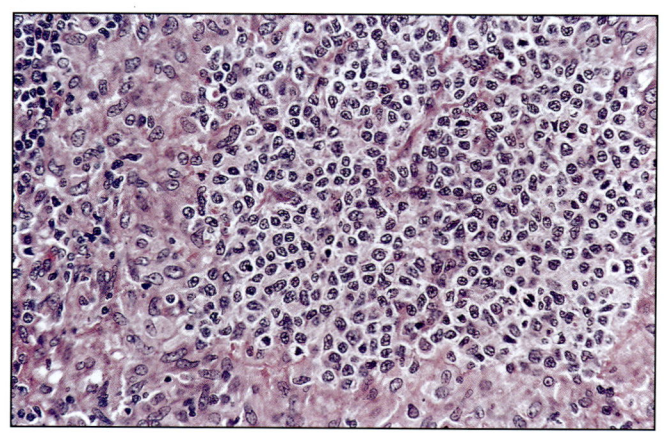

图21A.87 淋巴结边缘区B细胞淋巴瘤。病例中成片的肿瘤细胞,周围是花环状上皮样组织细胞。

变型:脾型淋巴结边缘区B细胞淋巴瘤
Variant: Nodal marginal zone B-cell lymphoma of splenic type

17%的淋巴结边缘区B细胞淋巴瘤病例其形态学和免疫表型特征极其类似于脾边缘区B细胞淋巴瘤,不同于结外边缘区B细胞淋巴瘤[732]。患者为成人,表现为淋巴结肿大,但无脾大。大多数疾病为Ⅰ期或Ⅱ期。临床行为信息有限,但短期生存率良好。

组织学上,淋巴结结构完全消失,被结节状或模糊结节状淋巴组织增生取代。有些结节的中心可见残留生发中心,常常缺乏套区结构。淋巴瘤细胞小至中等大,核不规则,核仁或小或无,胞浆淡染。偶尔混有大的母细胞,或集中在结节周边。免疫表型类似于普通的淋巴结边缘区B细胞淋巴瘤者,不同点是总会表达IgD。

鉴别诊断

1. **毛细胞白血病**(hairy cell leukemia):细胞学与毛细胞白血病有相似之处,但临床表现完全不同。
2. **单核细胞样B细胞增生**(monocytoid B-cell hyperplasia):许多反应性淋巴组织增生可见明显的单核细胞样B细胞。这些细胞局限于淋巴窦和滤泡周区域,不引起正常淋巴结结构消失。出现融合成大片的单核细胞样B细胞倾向于诊断淋巴瘤。肿瘤性单核细胞样B细胞更可能显示较大的核的不规则性、核分裂和核仁较多[740]。在困难的病例,可见轻链限制性,bcl-2免疫反应或基因型研究能证实淋巴瘤的诊断[735]。
3. **系统性肥大细胞增多症**(systemic mastocytosis):肥大细胞病可类似于结外边缘区B细胞淋巴瘤,胞浆透明,片状淋巴结受累。纤维化和嗜酸性粒细胞的出现应考虑肥大细胞增多症。
4. **外周T细胞淋巴瘤**(peripheral T-cell lymphoma):透明细胞常见于外周T细胞淋巴瘤,需要进行免疫组化检查来鉴别。

弥漫大B细胞淋巴瘤
Diffuse large B-cell lymphoma

定义

弥漫大B细胞淋巴瘤是一种侵袭性、生长迅速的肿瘤,由细胞核等于或大于反应性组织细胞核的淋巴细胞组成。细胞学可选择性地亚分类为中心母细胞(大无裂细胞)和免疫母细胞。这是一种异质性分类[36,41,42]。

临床特征

弥漫大B细胞淋巴瘤通常为原发性,但可由低级别淋巴瘤转化而来,如滤泡性淋巴瘤、B-CLL/SLL、结外边缘区 B 细胞淋巴瘤或淋巴浆细胞性淋巴瘤。关于弥漫大 B 细胞淋巴瘤的病因知之甚少。有些病例的发生有自身免疫性疾病或免疫缺陷背景。有些结外病例可发生于局部慢性炎症或刺激背景，如乳腺切除术后的淋巴水肿、骨与软组织慢性化脓性炎、金属植入以及长期脓胸[278,741-743]。

弥漫大 B 细胞淋巴瘤的发病年龄范围广泛，男性发病率略高（表 21A.11）。通常表现为淋巴结肿大，但结外症状也常见[268]。肿瘤常常生长迅速。可出现全身症状，尤其是在高分期疾病患者。大约一半的患者在发病时为 I 期或 II 期。

分期骨髓检查可提示淋巴瘤累及（IV 期）。重要的是要确定：是大细胞淋巴瘤累及，还是隐匿性滤泡性淋巴瘤累及（"形态学不一致"，占大约一半的病例），因为前者的预后较差，而后者不影响预后，除非疾病在完全缓解后更可能复发，常常表现为滤泡性淋巴瘤的形式[618,744-747]。

弥漫大 B 细胞淋巴瘤是一种侵袭性肿瘤，如果不治疗，通常能够致命。但是，采用现代治疗有可能治愈，大约 50% 的病例可以长期无病生存。标准治疗是 CHOP 方案联合化疗（环磷酰胺、阿霉素、长春新碱和泼尼松）或其他，通常联合美罗华（抗 CD20 嵌合性抗体）[748,749]。

病理学

弥漫大 B 细胞淋巴瘤的特点是淋巴结或结外部位弥漫破坏浸润[1]（图 21A.88）。常见淋巴结周围组织和血管浸润。有些病例伴有明显纤维化（图 21A.89）。常见坏死，偶尔发生完全性梗死，可掩盖诊断。有些病例可显示"星天"结构，由反应性组织细胞形成。有时背景中可见上皮样细胞、组织细胞、浆细胞和嗜酸性粒细胞[750]。

淋巴瘤细胞的大小在不同病例及同一病例内可存在极大的不同。核比反应性组织细胞的核大，或者两者相似。核呈圆形，或有凹陷或不规则折叠。染色质结构呈囊泡状或粗颗粒状。常见大小不等的嗜碱性或嗜酸性核仁。核仁单个或多个，与核膜连接或位于中心（图 21A.90）。胞浆量中等至多量，可呈嗜双色性、嗜碱性、淡染或透明。在有些病例，胞浆呈浆细胞样，具有淡染的核旁高尔基区。可见分离的嗜碱性胞浆片段，类似于炎症反应中见到的"浆细胞小体"。可见类似于 Reed-Sternberg 细胞的多核细胞或奇异细胞。易见核分裂象，常见非典型核分裂象。核碎可能明显（图 21A.91）。

仅仅根据形态学很难可靠地区分弥漫大 B 细胞淋巴瘤和外周 T 细胞淋巴瘤。

弥漫大B细胞淋巴瘤的不寻常的和少见的形态学变型
Unusual and uncommon morphologic variant of diffuse large B-cell lymphoma

黏液型（myxoid variant）：由于可见多量黏液性间质，大 B 细胞淋巴瘤可类似于各种肉瘤（如黏液纤维肉瘤或黏液性软骨肉瘤），其中散布着圆形、梭形或星形的淋巴瘤细胞（图 21A.92）[751,752]。

伴有原纤维基质或玫瑰花结的淋巴瘤（lymphoma with fibrillary matrix/rosettes）：出现多量原纤维基质，伴有或不伴有玫瑰花结形成，由此可类似于神经性肿瘤（图 21A.93）。因为基质由相互连接的细胞突起组成，故对 CD45 和 B 细胞系标记物染色[753]。

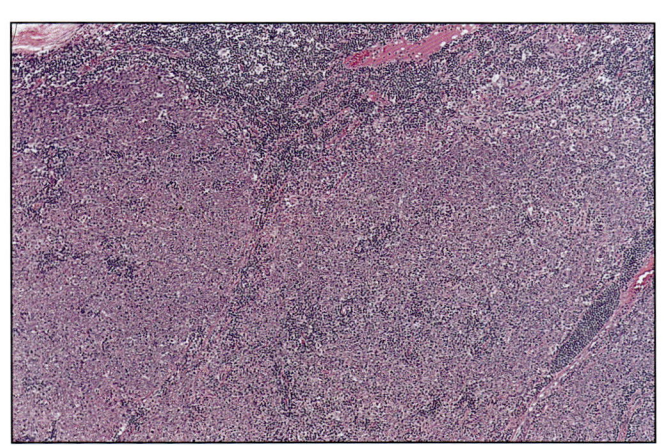

图21A.88 淋巴结弥漫大B细胞淋巴瘤。可见弥漫成片的淋巴瘤细胞。本例中，肿瘤与残留淋巴组织的交界非常明显，形成黏附性（癌样）质地。

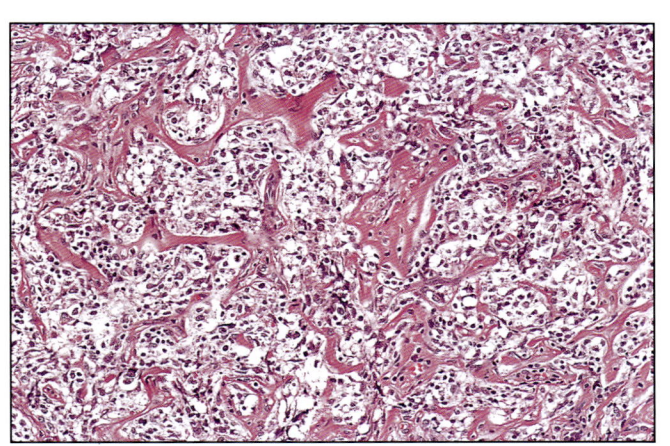

图21A.89 伴有纤维化的弥漫大B细胞淋巴瘤。纤维化导致巢状结构形成。由于收缩而产生的人工假象，纤维化区的淋巴瘤细胞显得比实际上小。

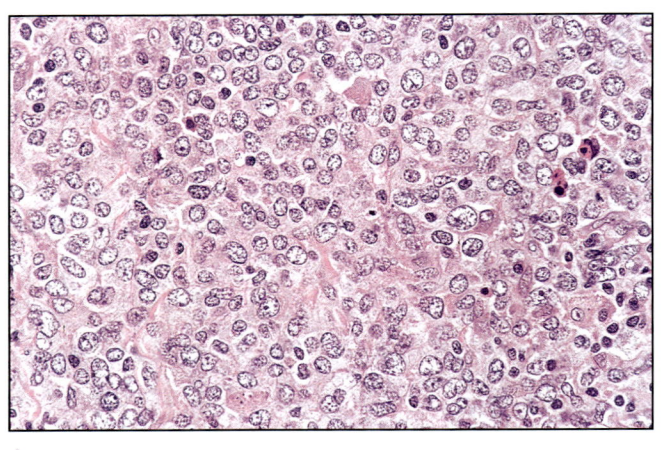 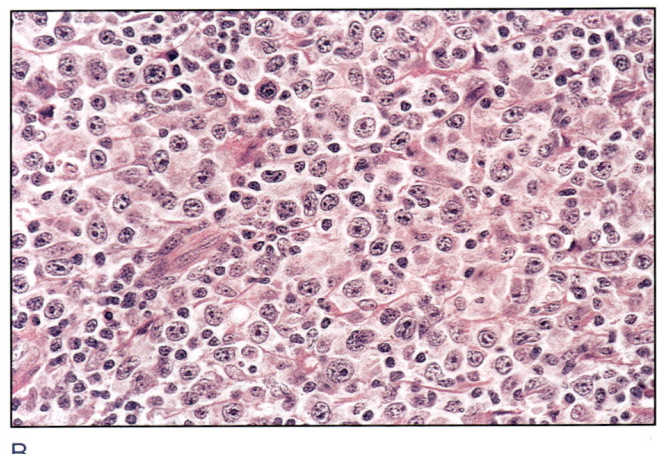

图21A.90 弥漫大B细胞淋巴瘤。(A) 大细胞具有临近核膜的小核仁。通常将其称为中心母细胞或大无裂细胞淋巴瘤。(B) 多数大细胞是免疫母细胞,核仁居中。然而也混杂具有中心母细胞特征的细胞(大无裂细胞)。

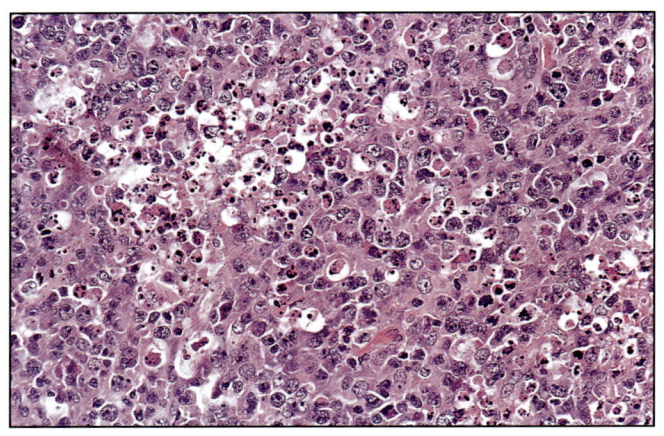 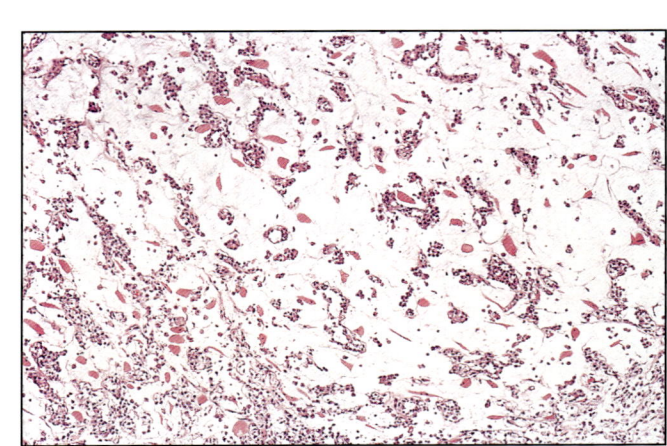

图21A.91 弥漫大B细胞淋巴瘤。淋巴瘤细胞核大,核仁明显。本例中核碎明显。

图21A.92 弥漫大B细胞淋巴瘤累及骨骼肌。有明显的黏液性间质。

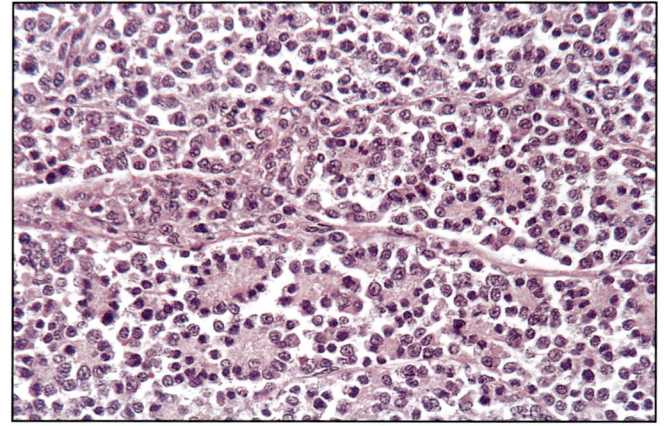

图21A.93 弥漫大B细胞淋巴瘤伴有玫瑰花结形成。(Courtesy of Dr Saul Suster, Ohio)

伴有梭形细胞的淋巴瘤 (lymphoma with spindle cells):淋巴瘤细胞可以由于陷入纤维化间质内而呈现一种梭形细胞结构或以梭形细胞束的形式自然生长[1](图21A.94)。尽管类似于各种肉瘤,但至少局部常常可见较易诊断的淋巴瘤区域。

印戒细胞淋巴瘤 (signet-ring cell lymphoma):印戒细胞大B细胞淋巴瘤的特点是透明空泡或嗜酸性小球使核呈偏心性移位,可能被误诊为印戒细胞癌[1,754]。

透明细胞变型 (clear cell variant):有些大B细胞淋巴瘤具有明显的透明胞浆,可类似于外周T细胞淋巴瘤、生殖细胞肿瘤或癌[755](图21A.95)。

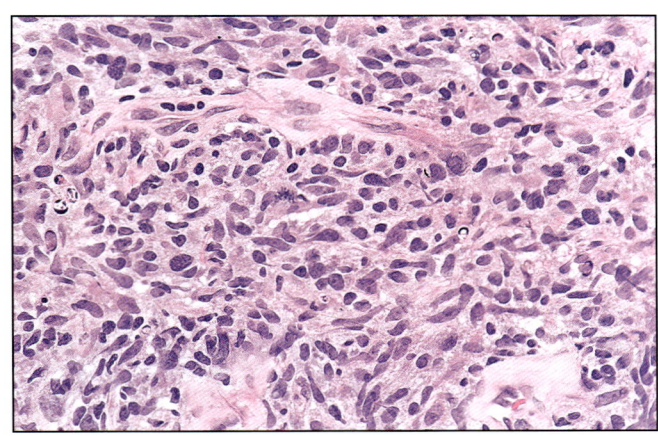

图21A.94 伴有明显梭形肿瘤细胞的弥漫大B细胞淋巴瘤。可被误诊为肉瘤。

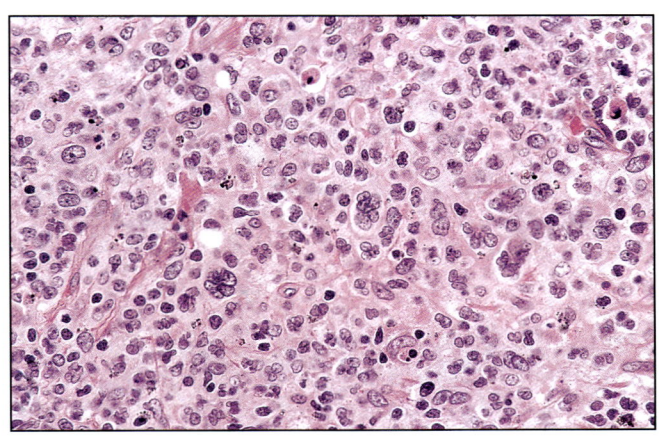

图21A.96 弥漫大B细胞淋巴瘤,核呈多个分叶型。核的分叶类似于花瓣。

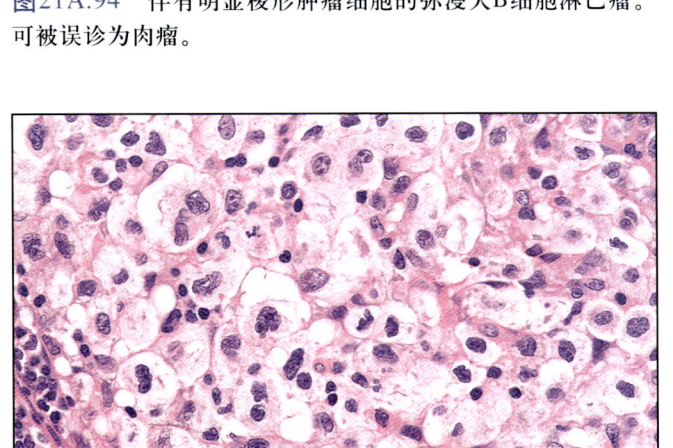

图21A.95 伴有透明胞浆的弥漫大B细胞淋巴瘤。透明细胞不是T细胞所特有的,也可见于有些B细胞淋巴瘤。

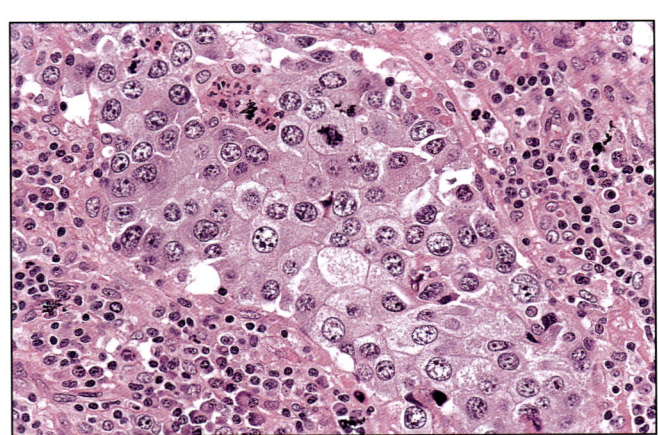

图21A.97 伴有间变大细胞的弥漫大B细胞淋巴瘤。多角形淋巴瘤细胞具有明显的细胞膜和淡染的胞浆。易于误诊为分化差的鳞状细胞癌。B细胞标记物能将这种肿瘤与间变大细胞淋巴瘤鉴别开。

海葵细胞/丝状/微绒毛大细胞淋巴瘤(anemone cell/filiform/microvillous large cell lymphoma):有些大细胞淋巴瘤的超微结构显示长的"丛状"细胞突起,类似于间皮细胞,只是没有张力丝和桥粒[756,757]。常规显微镜下,这些淋巴瘤通常没有明确特征,只是可见淋巴窦受累;大多数是B细胞[757]。CD30和EMA呈阴性。少见的特征是大约50%的病例表达CD56[758]。

淋巴窦大细胞淋巴瘤(sinusoidal large cell lymphoma):有些大B细胞淋巴瘤只累及淋巴结的窦隙,类似转移癌或黑色素瘤[759]。然而,典型的淋巴瘤细胞学特点以及免疫组化检查可用于证实诊断。与微绒毛大细胞淋巴瘤有相似的特点[757]。

滤泡间大B细胞淋巴瘤(interfollicular large B-cell lymphoma):大B细胞淋巴瘤有时可主要累及淋巴滤泡间区,生长方式类似于外周T细胞淋巴瘤[760,761]。

多分叶核大细胞淋巴瘤(multilobated large cell lymphoma):细胞核分叶状,特点是核膜折叠,类似于花瓣。事实上在大B细胞淋巴瘤并不少见(图21A.96)。当50%的肿瘤细胞显示这种特征时,则称为"多分叶核淋巴瘤"[762,763]。

间变大细胞型(anaplastic large cell type):有些大B细胞淋巴瘤由胞浆丰富的大的马蹄形或奇异核大细胞组成,形态学与T/裸细胞型间变大细胞淋巴瘤难以鉴别(图21A.97)。这种病例的行为与普通大B细胞淋巴瘤没有区别[764]。

伴浆细胞分化的大B细胞淋巴瘤(large B-cell lymphoma with plasma cell differentiation):有时肿瘤性大细胞混合有浆细胞,显示含有相同的Ig轻链。浆细胞可显示或不显示细胞学非典型性(图21A.98)。

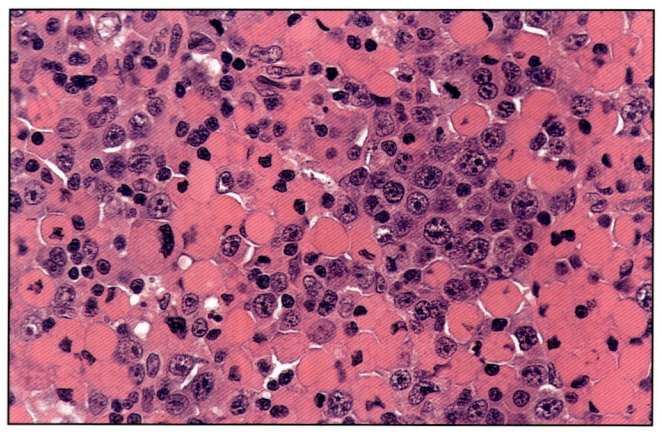

图21A.98 伴浆细胞分化的弥漫大B细胞淋巴瘤。在本例，浆细胞因含有免疫球蛋白包涵体而肿胀。

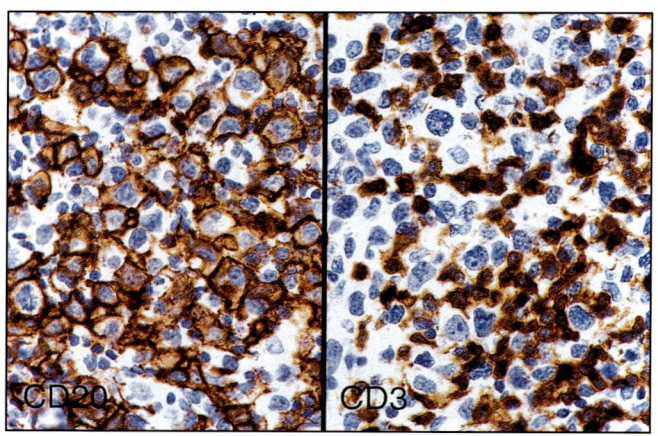

图21A.99 弥漫大B细胞淋巴瘤的免疫染色。左侧：大细胞显示膜CD20强阳性。右侧：CD3染色显示反应性小淋巴细胞。

免疫细胞化学

1. B细胞系标记物阳性（图21A.99）。免疫表型可发生异常，会出现一种或多种正常情况下表达的B细胞标记物丢失[765,766]。一项研究表明，缺乏CD20或CD22表达与预后较差有关[765]。淋巴瘤细胞常常表达表面和（或）胞浆Ig，但有些病例Ig阴性[767]。
2. 40%的病例CD10呈阳性，60%的病例bcl-6呈阳性；这些病例均为滤泡中心细胞起源，如果这两种标记物均呈阴性而MUM-1或CD138呈阳性，则起源于生发中心后细胞[768]。
3. 大约50%的病例bcl-2呈阳性，与化疗不敏感有关。活化标记物如CD25和CD30有时呈阳性。20%的病例可见CD43异常表达[9,10]。大约10%的病例表达CD5；有些研究提示这种亚组与预后较差有关[769,770]。Ki-67平均指数是55%，少数病例可高达100%。

遗传学特征

Ig基因重排，显示体细胞超突变。关于弥漫大B细胞淋巴瘤的发生，似乎至少有三种不同的分子途径：（1）原始途径，涉及 *BCL-6* 重排；（2）转化途径，涉及BCL-2激活，单独或伴有 *P53* 突变；（3）原始途径，但具有胚系 *BCL-2* 和 *BCL-6*，分子学机制尚未可知[771]。

20%～30%的弥漫大B细胞淋巴瘤病例 *BCL-2* 基因易位至 *IGH* 基因，提示这种病例与滤泡性淋巴瘤有关。与结外疾病相比，*BCL-2* 重排更常见于原发性淋巴结疾病[772]。患者大约比缺乏这种重排者大11岁[773,774]。伴有和不伴有 *BCL-2* 重排组之间的总体生存率没有差异，但前者复发的可能性增加，行为类似于滤泡性淋巴瘤[596,772,775]。

大约35%的弥漫大B细胞淋巴瘤具有 *BCL-6* 基因重排；与淋巴结淋巴瘤相比，这种特征更常见于结外淋巴瘤[597,598,772,776]。*BCL-6* 基因位于3q27，且可能相互易位至许多配体，包括（但不局限于）携带Ig基因位点者（14q32、2p12、22q11）。其编码锌指型（zinc finger-type）转录因子，正常情况下选择性表达于滤泡中心细胞，提示是生发中心发生和维持所必需的[16,777]。虽然有一项研究报告 *BCL-6* 重排的出现与预后较好有关，其他研究未证实其预后意义[598,772,776]。多发性（常常是双等位基因）突变见于73%的 *BCL-6* 基因5'非编码区，无论 *BCL-6* 基因有无重排。在B细胞迁移经由生发中心过程中，*BCL-6* 突变累积，因此也可见于各种生发中心细胞和生发中心后细胞的淋巴瘤中[600,777,778]。

C-MYC 基因重排发生于10%的弥漫大B细胞淋巴瘤病例，但主要见于结外病变[772,779,780]。通常发生于复杂遗传学改变背景上，与预后较差有关[780-782]。

REL 原癌基因位于2p14-15，在20%的弥漫大B细胞淋巴瘤中扩增；主要见于结外而非原发淋巴结病变[771]。基因扩增被认为是进展相关性事件。*P53* 基因突变见于20%的弥漫大B细胞淋巴瘤，对生存期具有负面影响[783,784]。

异常超突变可出现多个靶点，包括原癌基因 *PIM1*、*MYC*、*RhoH/TTF*（*ARHH*）和 *PAX5*，发生于50%以上的弥漫大B细胞淋巴瘤。突变分布于5'未翻译区或编码序列，是独立的染色体易位并具有Ig基因V区相关性体细胞超突变的典型特征，如同在正常滤泡中心细胞中见到的一样。它们可能通过DNA双链断裂的产生形成染色体易位而引发淋巴瘤[785]。

除了在下面讨论的特定变型，散发的弥漫大B细胞淋巴瘤很少有EBV感染（<10%）。

基于基因表达谱的组织发生分组
Histogenetic groups based on gene expression profiles

基因表达谱研究发现弥漫大B细胞淋巴瘤的组织发生分为三组[786-788]。

1. 生发中心B细胞样组（约占50%的病例）：显示生发中心B细胞标记基因高表达。CD10表达、BCL-2基因重排或C-REL扩增完全发生于这一组，为该组大B细胞淋巴瘤的生发中心细胞分化进一步提供了证据[787,789]。
2. 活化B细胞样组（约占30%的病例）：表达外周血B淋巴细胞体外激活时的正常诱导基因。NFκB信号途径的激活选择性地发生于这一组[790-792]。
3. 第3组：没有上述两组基因标记的高表达。

这三种组织发生组的预后有差异。5年总体生存率分别为60%、35%和39%[787]。根据另一项独立的研究，生发中心B细胞样和活化B细胞样组的5年生存率分别为51%和12%[782]。

预后因素

1. **临床**：国际预后指数（IPI）可准确地预测弥漫大B细胞淋巴瘤患者的生存期（表21A.15）[274]。肿瘤体积大以及血清β_2-微球蛋白水平高也是预后不良因素[793]。
2. **形态学**：虽然有些研究显示中心母细胞性淋巴瘤的预后比免疫母细胞性淋巴瘤好，但这种结论尚不确定，因为缺乏可重复性标准来鉴别这两种类型淋巴瘤[36,371,794-797]。而且，其他研究也不能重复出该结果[770,798-801]。
3. **免疫表型**：Bcl-2表达（不要与生发中心B细胞表型混淆）是弥漫大B细胞淋巴瘤最强的独立预后不良因素之一[792,802-806]。这种特征提示对化疗不敏感，化疗药物加美罗华（抗CD20抗体）可极大地使其逆转[807,808]。然而，近期研究提示，不表达bcl-6提示预后差，CHOP化疗加美罗华能使其逆转，而其中的bcl-2表达情况不影响预后，不管是使用CHOP方案还是使用R-CHOP方案[809]。CD5表达是预后不良的特征，与IPI评分高和分期高的疾病有关[810,811]。缺乏HLA-DR表达与预后差有关，提示肿瘤免疫监测丢失对于预后具有负面影响[812-814]。
4. **增殖指数**：增生比例高（如胸腺嘧啶核苷标记指数或Ki-67免疫染色指数>60%~80%）与弥漫大B细胞淋巴瘤的预后差和早期死亡有关[802,812,815]。
5. **生发中心细胞分化**：基因表达研究清楚地显示，弥漫大B细胞淋巴瘤的生发中心样B细胞组预后好[786,787]。应用其他参数的多数研究也发现，生发中心细胞分化的病例预后好，例如HGAL基因高表达（正常情况下在生发中心B细胞中高表达）、BCL-6 mRNA转录水平高以及对CD10和bcl-6的免疫反应[792,804-806,809,816-818]。
6. **微环境**：背景中反应性CD8$^+$细胞百分率低（<6%）与无复发生存期短有关[819,820]。活化粒酶B阳性细胞毒性T淋巴细胞≥15%的病例与无进展和总体生存期明显短强相关[821]。
7. **遗传学特征**：C-MYC重排与预后差有关（5年生存率仅为15%），不管分期和年龄如何[782]。染色体3p11-p12区的获得与预后差有关，不管基于基因表达生存模式如何[822]。P53基因突变与预后差有关[784,823]。
8. **基因表达谱**：四种基因表达标记和单基因BMP-6的表达与临床预后强相关：生发中心B细胞标记（预后好），MHC分类II标记（预后好），淋巴结标记（预后好），增生标记（预后差），以及BMP-6（预后差）[787,788]。由这些成分相加所得的预测评分与预后强相关，独立于弥漫大B细胞淋巴瘤的IPI评分或组织发生类型[787]。其他研究显示类似的基因表达谱（包括调节B细胞受体信号反应的基因，丝氨酸/苏氨酸磷酸化关键途径和凋亡）可推测预后[824]。氧化还原标记（抗氧化剂防御酶表达减少与硫氧还蛋白系统功能增加联合）与预后差有关[825]。一项研究显示，应用实时PCR单独对六种基因表达水平进行定量（LMO2、BCL-6、FN1、CCND2、SCYA3、BCL-2）能够预测弥漫大B细胞淋巴瘤患者的生存期[826]。

鉴别诊断

1. **转移癌或黑色素瘤**（metastatic carcinoma or melanoma）：见"淋巴组织增生性病变诊断的实践问题"（第1250页）。
2. **传染性单核细胞增多症**（infectious mononucleosis）：见"淋巴组织增生性病变诊断的实践问题"（第1250页）。
3. **Kikuchi淋巴结炎**（Kikuchi lymphadenitis）：见"淋巴组织增生性病变诊断的实践问题"（第1250页）。
4. **Burkitt淋巴瘤**（Burkitt lymphoma）。
5. **经典型Hodgkin淋巴瘤**（classic HL）：见"淋巴组织增生性病变诊断的实践问题"（第1250页）。

弥漫大B细胞淋巴瘤的特殊临床病理表现

有些类型的弥漫大B细胞淋巴瘤显示下列特殊的临床病理学特征，不包括本章第3部分讨论的纵隔大B细胞淋巴瘤。

血管内大B细胞淋巴瘤
Intravascular large B-cell lymphoma

疾病的本质：血管内大B细胞淋巴瘤是大B细胞淋巴瘤的一种特殊亚型，也称为血管内淋巴瘤病，嗜血管性淋巴瘤和（以前所认为的）肿瘤性血管内皮细胞瘤病，特点是：肿瘤细胞几乎都在血管内增生[827-834]。尽管肿瘤位于血管内，循环血中通常没有淋巴瘤细胞。虽然骨髓检查呈阴性，但分子学分析常常显示受累的证据[835]。

临床特征：大多数患者为中年人或老年人，表现出特殊的神经症状（由于血管阻塞引起多部位梗死）或皮肤病变，但任何器官（如肺、肾、肾上腺和肝）均可受累[1,832]。常有发热。疾病通常进展迅速而导致死亡，但是正确化疗能使一些病例完全缓解[832,834]。

病理学：淋巴瘤细胞大，没有黏附性，具有泡状核，核仁清楚。肿瘤细胞特征性地阻塞中、小血管腔（图21A.100）。肿瘤细胞常常陷在纤维素或血小板血栓中。血管阻塞常常导致广泛梗死。肿瘤细胞可沿着血管腔呈栅栏状排列，类似于被覆的内皮细胞。有时可见血管外的淋巴瘤成分。

免疫细胞化学和遗传学特征：绝大多数血管内淋巴瘤病例为B细胞来源，极少数病例显示T、NK或组织细胞来源[827,832,836-842]。一部分血管内大B细胞淋巴瘤病例表达CD5[843,844]。淋巴瘤细胞表达CD11a和CD49以及内皮细胞表达相应的配体CD54和CD106，可以解释为何淋巴瘤倾向于局限在血管腔内[844]。Ig基因重排[845]。一小部分病例可检测到EBV，主要是T或NK细胞来源患者[841,842,844,846]。

恶性组织细胞增生症样大B细胞淋巴瘤
Malignant histiocytosis-like large B-cell lymphoma

已有提示，恶性组织细胞增生症样大B细胞淋巴瘤是血管内大B细胞淋巴瘤的一种独特形式，好发于亚洲人[847,848]。患者表现为发热、肝脾大和噬血细胞综合征，没有淋巴结肿大或皮肤病变。疾病的临床过程呈侵袭性。骨髓活检显示肿瘤性大B细胞窦隙性浸润，伴有噬血性组织细胞。肝窦和肝门可见肿瘤细胞和噬血性组织细胞浸润。脾浸润发生于红髓，没有肿瘤性结节形成。

富于T细胞的大B细胞淋巴瘤
T cell-rich large B-cell lymphoma (TCRBCL)

定义和本质：TCRBCL是一种大B细胞淋巴瘤，具有明显的反应性T淋巴细胞成分，后者占细胞的90%以上[849]。尚不清楚TCRBCL是弥漫大B细胞淋巴瘤独特的临床病理亚型，还是仅仅为一种形态学变型。有些病例似乎是进展型滤泡中心细胞淋巴瘤或N-LPHL[850-852]。

临床特征和预后：所报告的病例包含的诊断标准差别很大，因此结果总是不容易解释或进行对比。有些研究报告，TCRBCL的行为与普通型大B细胞淋巴瘤没有区别[853,854]。但是，如果采用严格的诊断标准，超过90%的患者疾病为Ⅲ期或Ⅳ期，常见骨髓受累（>50%）。预后差，5年生存率仅为20%[855,856]，原因可能是高分期和高IPI病例所占比例较高[857]。

病理学：TCRBCL的特点是小淋巴细胞背景中散在孤立性或小灶状淋巴瘤大细胞，混有不同数量的组织细胞、上皮样细胞、嗜酸性粒细胞和浆细胞（图21A.101）。在有些病例，组织细胞丰富，以至于得名"富于T/组织细胞的大B细胞淋巴瘤"（图21A.101B）[857]。大细胞具有圆形、分叶状或不规则核皱褶，核仁清楚，类似于L&H细胞或Reed-Sternberg细胞。根据定义，肿瘤细胞不应该形成密集的巢状或片状。背景小淋巴细胞具有深染的小圆形核，具有轻度非典型性，核不规则或呈长形[760,849,852-854,858-860]。如果出现任何可识别的N-LPHL成分，则不属于这一类别，应该诊断为"伴有弥漫成分的

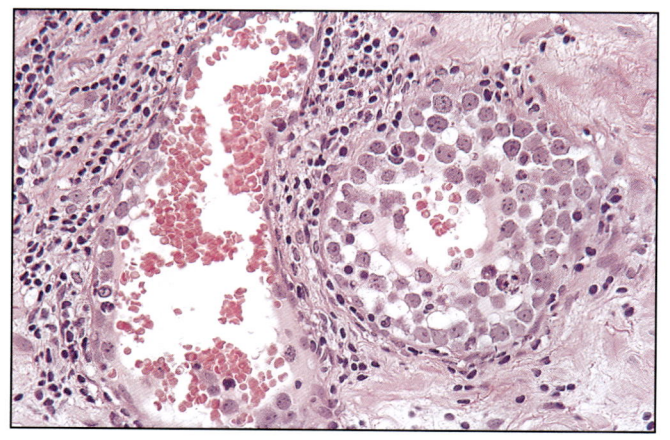

图21A.100 血管内大B细胞淋巴瘤。血管充满大的单核细胞。在左侧视野，有些淋巴瘤细胞似乎衬覆在血管腔面。

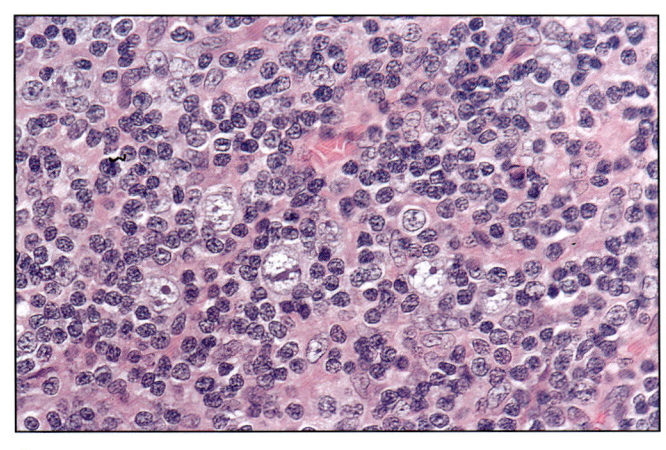
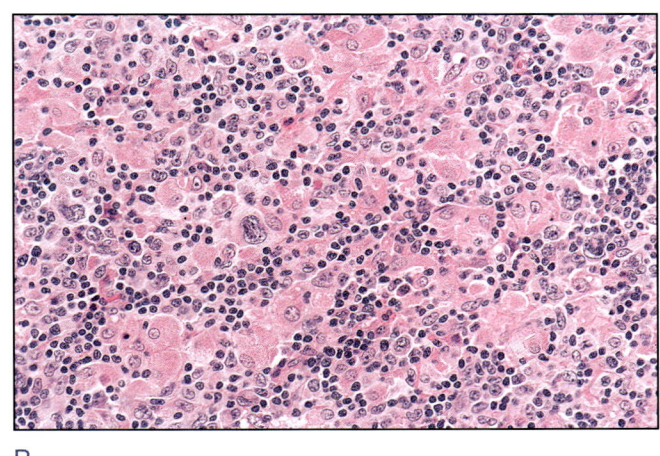

图21A.101 富于T细胞的大B细胞淋巴瘤。（A）非典型大细胞稀疏地散布于小淋巴细胞背景中。（B）在本例，大细胞显示不规则的核折叠。还混有许多组织细胞，成为所谓的富于T细胞/组织细胞的大B细胞淋巴瘤。与结节性淋巴细胞为主型Hodgkin淋巴瘤的鉴别很困难。

N-LPHL"。

免疫表型和基因型：散在的大细胞表达B细胞标记物，有时可显示轻链限制性（图21A.102）。背景中很少有小B细胞。Bcl-6常有表达[852]。有些病例恒定表达EMA，但并非所有的病例均如此[182,859,860]。偶尔表达CD30[852]。背景含有大量CD8和细胞毒性标记物阳性的小T淋巴细胞（图21A.102）[182]。背景中没有滤泡性树突状细胞（FDC）网。

分子学研究显示Ig基因克隆性重排[861]。除少数病例外，EBV呈阴性[852,862]。

鉴别诊断：需要考虑许多鉴别诊断，如反应性免疫母细胞增生、经典型Hodgkin淋巴瘤、伴明显弥漫成分的N-LPHL以及外周T细胞淋巴瘤。见"淋巴组织增生性病变诊断的实践问题"（第1250页）。

淋巴瘤样肉芽肿病
Lymphomatoid granulomatosis

淋巴瘤样肉芽肿病概念的演变：淋巴瘤样肉芽肿病最初由Liebow等[863]描述为肺的血管中心性、多形性、非典型淋巴网状浸润性病变，伴有明显坏死。尚未确定是肿瘤性或是炎症性病变。后来发现这种疾病也可累及皮肤、中枢神经系统和肾[864-866]。在20世纪70年代晚期和80年代早期，肺淋巴瘤样肉芽肿病与鼻腔多形性网状组织增生症的相似性受到关注[867]。Jaffe[868]使用"血管中心性免疫增生性病变"来统一涵盖这些病变。由于免疫组织化学分析显示大量的T细胞，它们被认为是特殊形式的T细胞淋巴瘤[868]。然而，重新评估这种病变显示其鼻腔的多形性网状组织增生症通常是NK/T细胞淋巴瘤，而肺的淋巴瘤样肉芽肿病通常是EBV⁺的克隆性B细胞增生，伴有明显的反应性T细胞成分[869-873]。

临床特征：中位发病年龄为40～60岁，好发于男性[874]。多数患者表现为肺病变，导致咳嗽、胸痛或呼吸困难。胸部X线检查通常显示双侧外周肺结节，孤立性肿物或弥漫性浸润。其他患者表现为肺外疾病，如皮肤病变（斑丘疹、皮肤结节或斑块）、中枢神经系统病变（肿块或皮质梗死，引起意识错乱、痴呆、共济失调或颅神经卒中）、肾和其他器官病变。骨髓通常不受累。肿瘤有时发生在免疫缺陷的背景下，包括AIDS和移植后。甚至在免疫缺陷不明显的患者，常常发现细胞介导免疫缺陷[875-879]。

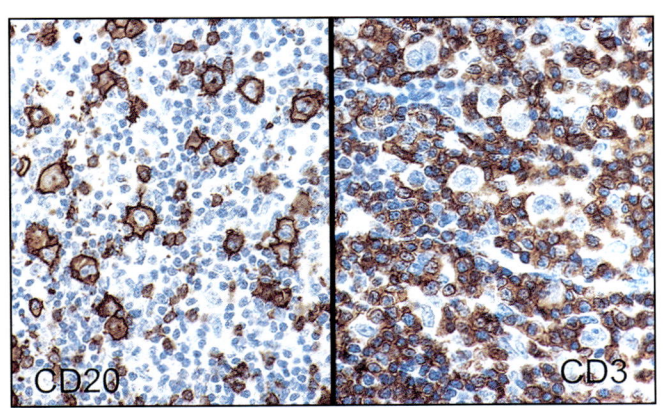

图21A.102 富于T细胞的大B细胞淋巴瘤的免疫染色。左侧：大的肿瘤细胞显示一致的CD20强阳性。不形成大的巢或片。右侧：背景中有许多小T细胞（CD3⁺）。

病理学：组织学三联征为：（1）非典型淋巴组织浸润，常常为混合性；（2）脉管侵犯（血管侵犯）；（3）明显的凝固性坏死，常常呈区域性（图21A.103）。浸润细胞

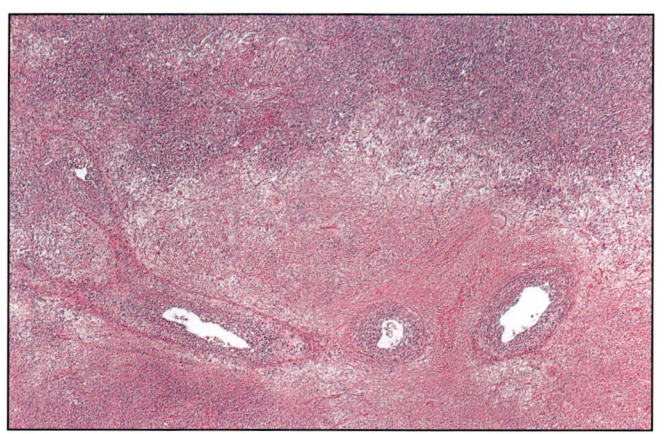

图21A.103 淋巴瘤样肉芽肿病。在这一肺病变中，有致密的淋巴浸润和中心区域性坏死。血管壁可见淋巴细胞侵犯（血管中心性侵犯）。

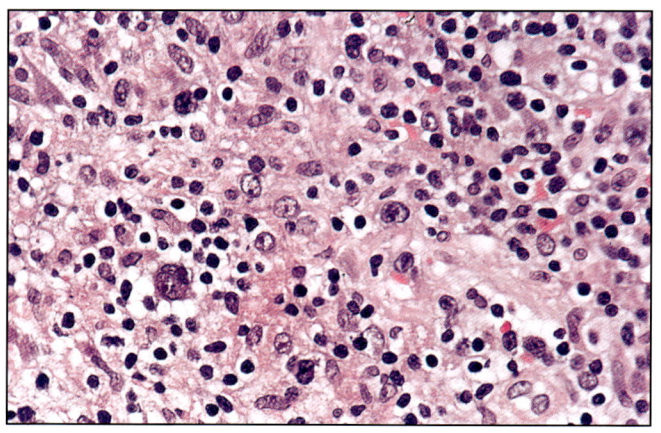

图21A.104 淋巴瘤样肉芽肿病，I级。混合性炎症背景中仅有少数非典型大细胞。

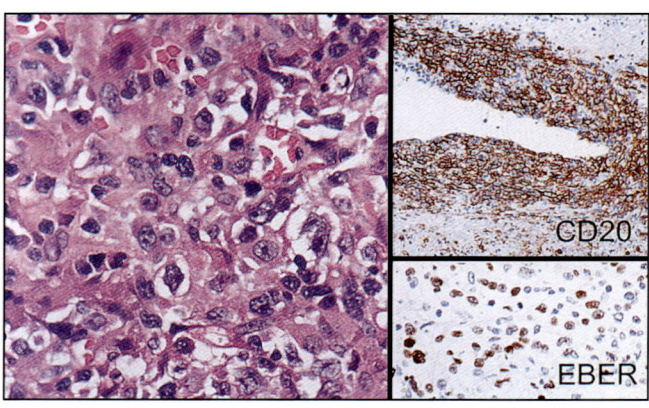

图21A.105 淋巴瘤样肉芽肿病，III级。左侧：可见许多非典型大细胞，类似于大细胞淋巴瘤的细胞。右上：CD20免疫染色显示大量肿瘤细胞（B细胞）浸润血管壁。右下：EBER原位杂交显示非典型大细胞。

常常包括小淋巴细胞、非典型大淋巴细胞和组织细胞，有时伴有肉芽肿形成。非典型大淋巴细胞类似于中心母细胞（大无裂细胞）、免疫母细胞或Reed-Sternberg细胞。常见奇异形细胞，核巨大，不规则形折叠，染色质粗大（图21A.104和21A.105）。非典型大细胞数量或者稀少（有时需要免疫组化染色来显示）或者较多。根据数量可进行组织学分级：I级（少数非典型大细胞），II级（明显的大、小细胞混合），III级（主要是非典型大细胞）。

免疫细胞化学和遗传学特征：CD20染色选择性地显示非典型大细胞，其中许多细胞为增生性，由Ki-67染色证实（图21A.105）[873]。CD20$^+$大细胞呈CD30和CD15阴性。背景富于反应性小T淋巴细胞，大多数为细胞毒性CD8$^+$细胞[880]。病变的B细胞本质由克隆性Ig基因重排进一步证实。EBV可见于非典型大细胞（图21A.105）[872,873]。

临床预后：自然病史相差很大。14%～27%的患者自发消退，但大多数疾病呈进展性，治疗失败则导致死亡。不利的预后因素有：组织学分级II～III级，年龄＞25岁，以及出现神经性疾病[873,874,881]。常见的治疗手段为类固醇和（或）化疗（如环磷酰胺），完全缓解率可达50%。其他治疗包括干扰素-α_{2b}或美罗华，加或不加化疗，两者均可获得良好的预期效果[876,882,883]。III级疾病通常像侵袭性淋巴瘤那样治疗[876]。

与富于T细胞的B细胞淋巴瘤（TCRBCL）鉴别：虽然淋巴瘤样肉芽肿病在概念上可认为是TCRBCL的一种形式，但是具有许多不同的特征：

1. 完全为淋巴结外病变（TCRBCL则为淋巴结或结外病变）。
2. 凝固性坏死是恒定特征（TCRBCL缺乏或仅有灶状坏死）。
3. 血管中心性-血管破坏性生长为明显的特征（TCRBCL通常缺乏）。
4. 总是与EBV有关（TCRBCL通常阴性）。

老年性EBV$^+$B细胞淋巴组织增生性疾病
Senile EBV$^+$ B-cell lymphoproliferative disorder

定义和临床特征：老年性EBV$^+$B细胞淋巴组织增生性疾病是EBV$^+$大B细胞淋巴瘤的一种形式，发生于没有免疫缺陷证据的老年患者（60岁以上）[884]。其被认为是随着衰老发生的细微免疫退化，EBV$^+$淋巴组织肿瘤易于发生。患者通常表现为淋巴结肿大或全身症状，如发热和体重减轻。常见结外受累。

病理学：组织病理学上，常常有凝固性坏死和血管中心性-血管破坏性生长。淋巴组织浸润可以是多形

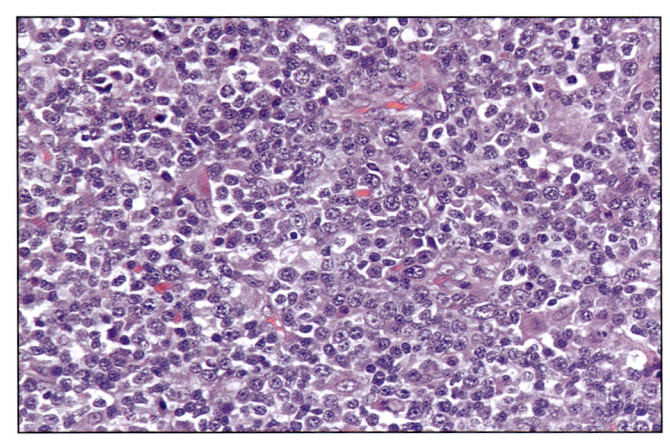

图21A.106 老年性EBV+B细胞淋巴组织增生性疾病,多形性亚型。可见混合性细胞浸润,包括免疫母细胞、浆母细胞和浆细胞,类似于传染性单核细胞增生症的组织学图像。

性(大淋巴细胞、小淋巴细胞和浆细胞混合,类似于移植后淋巴组织增生性病变)或单形性(类似普通型大B细胞淋巴瘤)(图21A.106)。有些大细胞常常巨大、奇异形,类似于Reed-Sternberg细胞。大细胞的免疫表型为:CD20+、CD79a+、CD30-/+、CD5-、CD10-、EBV-LMP1+。多形性组的预后明显好于单形性组(疾病相关死亡率分别为8%和78%)。

脓胸相关性大B细胞淋巴瘤
Pyothorax-associated large B-cell lymphoma

定义和临床特征:脓胸相关性大B细胞淋巴瘤是一种少见的淋巴瘤,合并因人工气胸治疗肺结核或结核性胸膜炎而引起的长期脓胸[743,885,886]。表现为形成胸膜肿块。慢性脓胸和淋巴瘤诊断的平均间隔为37年。已有提示,非自身免疫性慢性炎症刺激可能是病因[885,886]。这种淋巴瘤类型最初由日本人报告,也可见于其他亚洲人和高加索人[887-889]。

患者为成人,中位发病年龄为64岁,明显好发于男性(男女之比>10:1)[890]。最常见的表现是胸痛、痰咳、呼吸困难以及胸壁肿物。确诊时通常有胸壁、肺、心包和横膈侵犯,但很少远处播散[743]。这是一种侵袭性淋巴瘤,5年生存率仅为20%[890]。

病理学:组织学上,胸膜明显纤维性增厚,大细胞淋巴瘤密集浸润。绝大多数脓胸相关性淋巴瘤是大B细胞淋巴瘤,少数病例显示T细胞或双表型[886,891]。特征性免疫表型为CD20+、CD79a+、CD10-、bcl-6-、MUM1+、CD138+/-,符合生发中心晚期或生发中心后B细胞来源[892]。然而常见T细胞标记物异常表达,如CD2、CD3和CD4[892]。

遗传学特征:几乎总是与EBV(III型潜伏)有关,与人类疱疹病毒8无关[886,892-896]。在遗传学水平,P53基因突变很常见(70%)[886]。脓胸相关性大B细胞淋巴瘤显示基因表达谱不同于普通型弥漫大B细胞淋巴瘤;尤其是有干扰素诱导蛋白27明显过表达者[897]。

原发性渗出性淋巴瘤
Primary effusion lymphoma

临床特征:原发性渗出性淋巴瘤也称为体腔发生的淋巴瘤,是大B细胞淋巴瘤的一种特殊形式,几乎全部发生于AIDS患者。这种淋巴瘤明显好发于男性,同性恋是危险因素。患者表现为胸膜、心包或腹膜渗液,不形成独立的肿物。疾病常常局限于起源的体腔[898]。近年来,累及淋巴结或不同结外部位的一种不伴有渗出的体腔外实性淋巴瘤已被认识[899-903]。与经典型原发性渗出性淋巴瘤的主要差别在于:B细胞性抗原(25%)和免疫球蛋白(25%)的表达率稍高,生存期较长(中位生存期为11个月,而渗出性淋巴瘤为3个月)[900]。

肿瘤的侵袭性高[896,904-908]。中位生存期为6.2个月,1年总体生存率仅为39%[909]。

病理学:肿瘤细胞大,胞浆丰富、嗜碱性,高尔基区淡染。核常常呈高度多形性(图21A.107)。淋巴瘤在体腔外呈弥漫性浸润,常常伴有高核分裂活性和凋亡碎片[900]。

免疫细胞化学和遗传学特征:典型的免疫表型为CD45RB+、CD20-、CD22-、CD3-、MUM1+、CD138+、CD10-、bcl-6-,不同程度地表达活化标记物,如HLA-DR

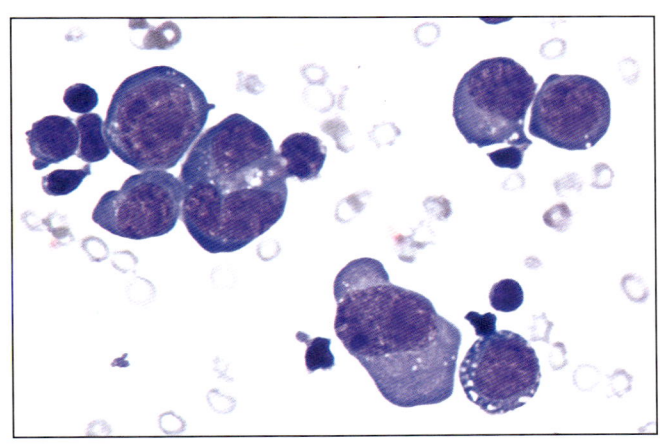

图21A.107 原发性渗出性淋巴瘤(胸腔积液涂片Giemsa染色)。可见大细胞核呈多形性,胞浆丰富,嗜碱性。

和 CD30[900,910]。支持这种肿瘤来源于 B 细胞的证据是出现 Ig 基因重排。这种淋巴瘤最明显的特征是几乎总是同时与两种病毒有关：人类疱疹病毒-8（HHV8）和 EBV[904,911]。C-MYC、BCL-2、BCL-6、RAS 和 P53 基因没有改变。

原发性渗出性淋巴瘤的基因表达谱与恶性浆细胞极其相似，提示为浆母细胞瘤的一种类型[912,913]。HHV8 在发病机制中具有重要作用，它的存在能选择特殊的细胞基因表达类型（如细胞周期和信号转导调节子的表达）[914]，HHV8 G 蛋白配对受体和周期素基因类似物也能调节恶性转化[900,906]。

HHV8⁺嗜生发中心大B细胞淋巴瘤
HHV8⁺ germinotropic large B-cell lymphoma

HHV8⁺ 嗜生发中心大 B 细胞淋巴瘤发生于具有免疫活性的宿主，表现为淋巴结肿大[915]。对化疗或放疗的反应良好。组织学上，先前存在的滤泡生发中心部分或完全被聚集的大细胞取代，核呈奇异形或多分叶状，胞浆嗜双色性。肿瘤性大细胞显示浆母细胞表型（CD20⁻、CD79a⁻、CD10⁻、bcl-6⁻），伴有免疫球蛋白轻链限制性。同时伴有 EBV 和 HHV8 感染。

ALK⁺大B细胞淋巴瘤
ALK⁺ large B-cell lymphoma

临床特征：ALK⁺ 大 B 细胞淋巴瘤是 B 细胞淋巴瘤的一种很少见类型，特点是表达 ALK 蛋白[916]。患者为成人，明显好发于男性。通常表现为淋巴结肿大，常常累及多个部位。多数患者疾病分期为 III 或 IV 期。临床过程呈高度侵袭性。

病理学：淋巴结结构破坏，常常累及淋巴窦。肿瘤细胞大，核圆形、空泡状，核仁明显，位于中央，胞浆丰富嗜双色性，有或没有核凹陷。可呈具有欺骗性的黏附性，类似于癌。

免疫细胞化学：不同标记物的阳性率如下：CD45RB 为 68%，CD20 为 5%，CD79a 为 10%，EMA 为 100%，CD30 为 24%，IgA 为 50%，CD138 为 100%，CD4 为 71%[645,917]。免疫表型提示浆母细胞分化阶段。ALK 染色通常为胞浆，常常具有颗粒状结构[918,919]。少数情况下，ALK 出现核和胞浆共同染色[920,921]。

遗传学特征：Ig 基因重排，支持肿瘤的 B 细胞本质，EBV 阴性。在大多数病例，t(2;17)(p23;q23) 引起 ALK 表达，伴有 CLTC-ALK 融合。少数病例显示 t(2;5)，伴有 NPM-ALK 融合[918-921]。因此这种类型淋巴瘤的 ALK 表达机制类似于间变大细胞淋巴瘤（见第 1223 页）。

浆母细胞性淋巴瘤 Plasmablastic lymphoma

定义和临床特征：浆母细胞性淋巴瘤目前缺乏统一的定义，是一种少见的高度侵袭性的大 B 细胞淋巴瘤，形态学和免疫表型特征提示终末 B 细胞分化[903]。这种异质性类型包括的病变不止一种[903]。

最初认为浆母细胞性淋巴瘤有两种表现形式：(1) 出现在 AIDS 患者的口腔和颌骨[922,923]；(2) 发生于多中心 Castleman 病的背景，患者常常为 HIV 阳性，累及淋巴结和脾[924,925]。现在认为其临床表现较广泛，可累及淋巴结或结外部位（如胃肠道、上呼吸道、骨和软组织）[926,927]。这种淋巴瘤不仅可发生于免疫相容的宿主（如 AIDS、移植后和类固醇治疗），也可发生于具有免疫活性的患者[903,928-930]。这种疾病通常呈局部侵犯，早期出现系统性播散，对治疗反应差，生存期短。

此外，有三种类型的弥漫大 B 细胞淋巴瘤也显示浆母细胞形态学和免疫表型特征：(1) 原发性渗出性淋巴瘤，(2) ALK⁺ 大 B 细胞淋巴瘤，以及 (3) HHV8⁺ 嗜生发中心的大 B 细胞淋巴瘤[903,915]。由 Simonitsch-Klupp 等[931] 报告的"弥漫大 B 细胞淋巴瘤伴有浆母细胞/浆细胞特征"的病例可能不是真性浆母细胞性淋巴瘤，因为其 CD20 呈阳性。

病理学：可见两种组织学亚型[903]。经典亚型的特点是母细胞停止分化。大淋巴瘤细胞显示单形性黏附性特征。核圆形至卵圆形，偏心位，空泡状，核仁或大而单一、位于中央，或几个核仁位于周边（图 21A.108）。胞浆丰富，嗜碱性至嗜双色性，伴有明显的核旁凹陷。凋亡明显，核分裂活跃[922]。浸润成分常含有巨噬细胞内可染小体，呈星天状。

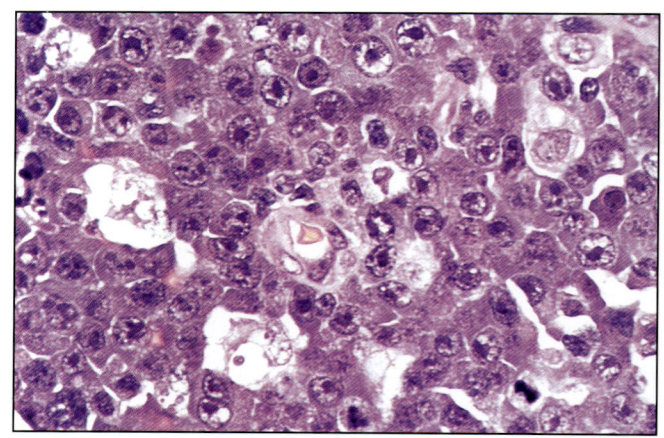

图21A.108　浆母细胞性淋巴瘤。大的淋巴瘤细胞呈单形性，核空泡状，核仁清楚。胞浆嗜双色性。

第二种亚型的特点是出现浆细胞分化。以免疫母细胞和浆母细胞为主，但这些细胞显示向浆细胞成熟分化。浆母细胞不同于免疫母细胞，可见稍小的核，染色质粗大，核仁较小。

免疫细胞化学特征：CD20 和 PAX-5 通常呈阴性，然而有些病例可见少部分肿瘤细胞表达 CD20。大约半数的病例表达 CD45RB、CD79a、Ig 或 EMA。CD38、CD138 和 MUM-1 呈阳性，但 bcl-6 通常呈阴性[903,932]。Ki-67 指数常常很高（>90%）[922,923,933]。

遗传学特征：Ig 基因重排。有些病例（40%）显示 Ig 基因的体细胞超突变[932]。50%～74% 的病例可见 EBV[922]。某项研究认为其与 HHV-8 具有强相关性[934]，但是没有被其他研究所证实[903,927,935]。对于发生于多中心性 Castleman 病的浆母细胞性淋巴瘤，HHV-8 呈阳性，但 EBV 呈阴性[924]。浆母细胞性淋巴瘤的散发病例也可能与 HHV-8 有关[936]。

鉴别诊断：浆母细胞性淋巴瘤与浆细胞瘤/骨髓瘤的浆母细胞型之间的鉴别可能很困难，因为它们的组织学和免疫表型相似。与骨髓瘤相比，前者在临床上更接近于淋巴瘤，与单克隆丙种球蛋白病无关。

浆细胞瘤　Plasmacytoma

临床特征

浆细胞瘤是肿瘤性浆细胞的肿瘤性聚集，可单独出现或发生于多发性骨髓瘤背景。孤立性浆细胞瘤患者一般比多发性骨髓瘤患者年轻[1]。孤立性浆细胞瘤可发生于任何部位，最常见于上呼吸消化道、骨和软组织。孤立性浆细胞瘤的预后比多发性骨髓瘤的好得多，中位生存期为 7～9 年。经随访，大约 40%～50% 的孤立性骨浆细胞瘤和 10%～20% 的孤立性髓外浆细胞瘤将进展为多发性骨髓瘤[1]。淋巴结浆细胞瘤很少见，预后很好[937,938]。有人认为，髓外浆细胞瘤和结外边缘区 B 细胞淋巴瘤具有共同特点，两种病变均主要显示为局限性疾病，预后良好[939]。

孤立性浆细胞瘤通常对放疗反应好。辅助化疗不影响转化为多发性骨髓瘤的发生率，但的确可延迟转化[940-942]。

病理学

浆细胞瘤取代部分或整个淋巴结。浆细胞常呈单一形态，可为成熟、不成熟或间变性。成熟浆细胞具有偏

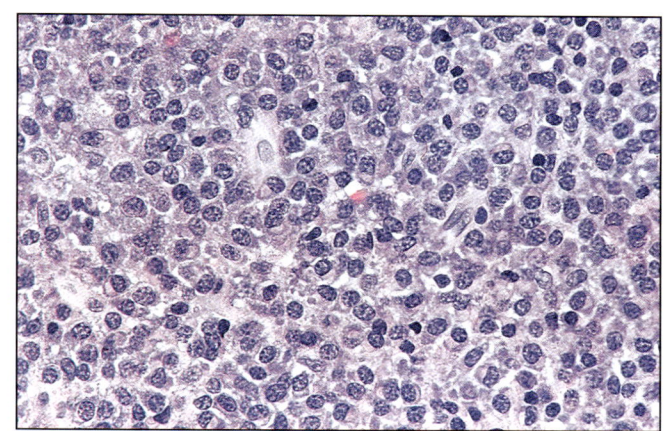

图 21A.109　淋巴结浆细胞瘤，主要由成熟或稍不成熟的浆细胞组成。通过显示轻链限制性来确诊。

心性、圆形核，染色质粗大、团块状（"钟盘状"），胞浆嗜碱性，核旁具有淡染的凹陷（图 21A.109）。不成熟浆细胞核较大且不规则，染色质不太致密，偶见核仁。间变性浆细胞（浆母细胞）核大小差异明显，染色质空泡状或粗大，核仁清楚（图 21A.110）。可见多核细胞。浆细胞可含有核内 Ig 包涵体（Dutcher 小体）或胞浆内结晶。

可形成血湖，导致假血管瘤表现[272]。有些病例可见 PAS 阳性蛋白沉积物（免疫球蛋白/轻链沉积病）、淀粉样沉积物或黏液样变。

免疫细胞化学

1. 胞浆 Ig 呈单一型染色，通常是 IgG 或 IgM（图 21A.111）。50% 的病例 CD79a 呈阳性。
2. CD45RB 常常但不总是呈阴性。CD20 和 PAX-5 呈阴性，而 CD138、MUM-1、Oct-2 和 Bob.1 呈阳性。
3. 上皮膜抗原不同程度呈阳性。虽然 CD56 和 cyclin D1 在多发性骨髓瘤病例中的表达率分别为 70% 和 25%，这些标记物在原发性髓外浆细胞瘤中较少表达[373,943-946]。
4. 有些病例表达细胞角蛋白[947]，连同 CD45RB 阴性和 EMA 阳性，可误诊为癌。有些病例 CD43 呈阳性连同 CD20 呈阴性一起可误诊为 T 细胞淋巴瘤。CD31 可以呈阳性，有可能误诊为血管肿瘤。

遗传学特征

关于孤立性浆细胞瘤的遗传学改变知之甚少。

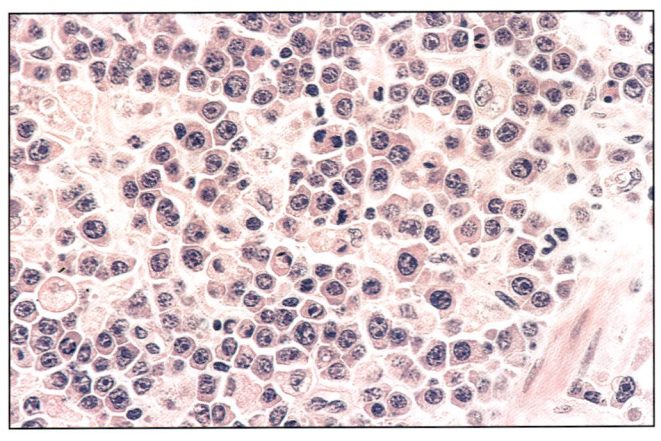
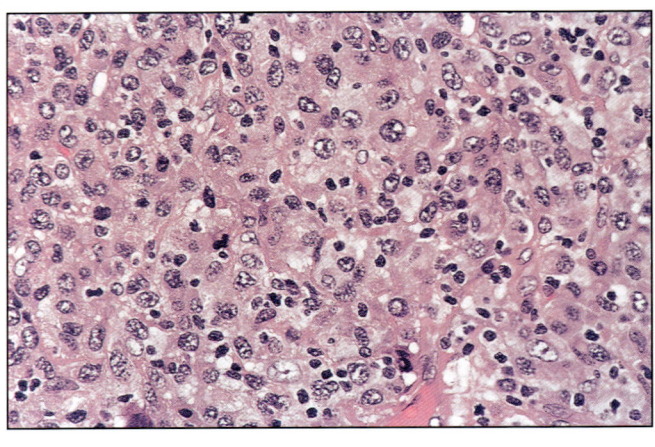

图21A.110 浆母细胞瘤和间变性浆细胞瘤。（A）本例由具有明显核仁的浆母细胞组成，浆细胞的特征性表盘状染色质仍然存在。（B）本例中肿瘤细胞与大细胞性淋巴瘤不易区分。个别细胞显示浆细胞染色质结构。

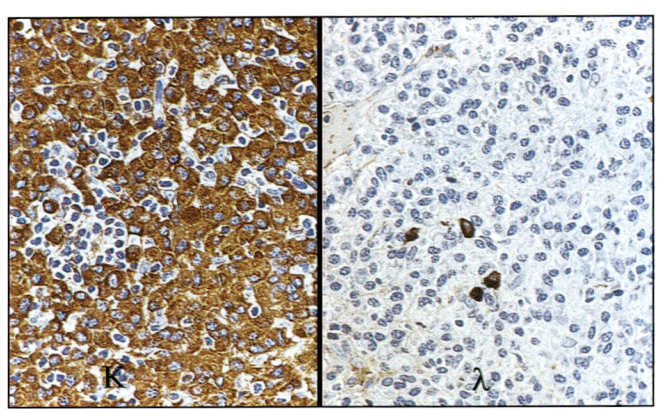

图21A.111 浆细胞瘤免疫染色。左侧：浆细胞κ轻链呈阳性。右侧：大多数细胞λ轻链呈阴性。少数阳性细胞是残留的浆细胞；比肿瘤性浆细胞小。

鉴别诊断

1. **反应性浆细胞增生症**（reactive plasmacytosis）：浆细胞在许多反应性和炎症性病变中可能很丰富（包括炎性假瘤），可显示某种程度的非典型性。但是，Dutcher小体的频繁出现仅见于肿瘤性浆细胞增生。Ig免疫染色对于判断有无轻链限制性在做出鉴别方面很有帮助。

2. **Castleman病**（Castleman disease）：浆细胞型Castleman病在淋巴结的髓质和滤泡间区常有丰富的成熟性浆细胞。背景中出现多个反应性滤泡和一些玻璃样血管滤泡，应该考虑这种诊断。但是，免疫组化并不一定能与浆细胞瘤相鉴别，因为浆细胞型Castleman病的浆细胞可显示轻链限制性[948]。

3. **弥漫大B细胞淋巴瘤**（diffuse large B-cell lymphoma）：间变性浆细胞瘤与弥漫大B细胞淋巴瘤的形态学鉴别可能很困难。前者一般可见较多粗大的块状染色质，类似于浆细胞核。肿瘤性浆细胞的免疫组化特征与正常浆细胞的相似，通常不表达CD45RB和表面B细胞标记物（如CD20）[949]。

4. **浆母细胞性淋巴瘤**（plasmablastic lymphoma）。

5. **淋巴浆细胞性淋巴瘤**（lymphoplasmacytic lymphoma）：小淋巴细胞和淋巴浆细胞样细胞的混合出现，倾向于诊断淋巴浆细胞性淋巴瘤而不是浆细胞瘤。

6. **癌**（carcinoma）。

毛细胞性白血病　Hairy cell leukemia

见本章第2部分和第22章。

Burkitt淋巴瘤（包括不典型Burkitt淋巴瘤）Burkitt lymphoma (including atypical Burkitt lymphoma)

定义

Burkitt淋巴瘤是一种侵袭性淋巴瘤，最初报道的为东非儿童一种颌骨的"圆形细胞肉瘤"。Burkitt淋巴瘤是生长最迅速的人类肿瘤之一，倍增时间为24~48小时[950]。

临床特征

有三种主要形式的Burkitt淋巴瘤[951,952]。

地方性Burkitt淋巴瘤（endemic Burkitt lymphoma）：地方性Burkitt淋巴瘤发生于非洲赤道附近，在那里，疟疾也是地方病。这种肿瘤通常发生于儿童，高峰年龄为7岁。最常见的受累部位是肾、肝、肠系膜、后腹膜、性腺和内分泌腺体。颌骨受累是典型特征，但较常见于幼儿[950]。淋巴结和骨髓受累不常见。这种肿瘤与EBV

有很强的相关性（95%）。如果不治疗，这种肿瘤致死性高。需要注意的是，有些发生于非洲的Burkitt淋巴瘤病例有AIDS相关性而非地方性。

散发性Burkitt淋巴瘤（sporadic Burkitt lymphoma）：对于散发于非洲国家以外的Burkitt淋巴瘤，与EBV的相关性是可变的，范围从高加索人群中的15%到发展中国家的60%~80%[280,950,953]。患者大多数为儿童和年轻成人，常常表现为腹部肿物或累及回盲部而引起肠套迭，或伴有Waldeyer环受累。其骨髓受累比地方性Burkitt淋巴瘤更常见。

AIDS相关性Burkitt淋巴瘤（AIDS-associated Burkitt lymphoma）：AIDS患者中，Burkitt淋巴瘤的发生率相当高（占所有非Hodgkin淋巴瘤的24%~40%，而其在普通人群中的比例<5%）[954,955]。患者大多数为年轻成人。易于累及淋巴结和结外部位，如脑、骨髓、肝和胃肠道。30%的病例伴有EBV感染[280,950,953]。

虽然非洲病例对环磷酰胺和氨甲蝶呤反应明显，但常见复发。应用强化化疗，I~III期疾病患者的5年生存率可达78%，但IV期病例的生存率较低（25%）[956]。

病理学

Burkitt淋巴瘤通常弥漫生长，但少数病例显示灶状滤泡结构[957,958]。尚不清楚后者是属于滤泡原发形成还是属于先前存在的滤泡归巢。由散在的含有可染小体的巨噬细胞形成的星天结构是其高度特征性表现，但不具有特异性（图21A.112）。

淋巴瘤以单一形中等细胞浸润为特征，核圆形，

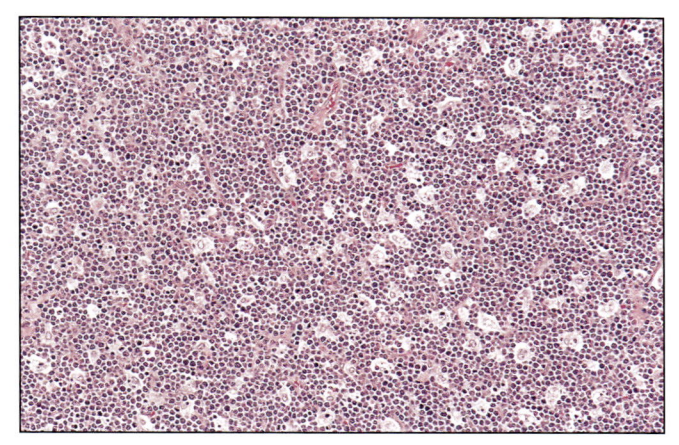

图21A.112 Burkitt淋巴瘤。病例的典型特征是单一形淋巴组织浸润，伴有星天表现。

染色质粗大，核仁为2~5个，嗜碱性，可见一圈嗜碱性胞浆（图21A.113）[959-961]。细胞和细胞核的大小变化很小。另一个特征是个别淋巴瘤细胞的核和细胞膜常常显示成形（molding）和"铺路石样外观（squaring off）"。有些病例显示小的细胞核突起（图21A.114）。胞浆明显呈浆细胞样[959]，间质中有时可见分离的嗜碱性胞浆碎片。有时可能有胞浆Ig包涵体[962]。在Giemsa染色印片中，强嗜碱性胞浆内常常可见小的脂质空泡，这种特征也可见于组织学薄切片中。核碎片和核分裂象常常是其特征。在有些病例，广泛坏死和（或）上皮样肉芽肿反应可混淆诊断[963-965]。有趣的是，Burkitt淋巴瘤的肉芽肿反应与EBV阳性、疾病早期和良好预后具有强相关性[965,966]。

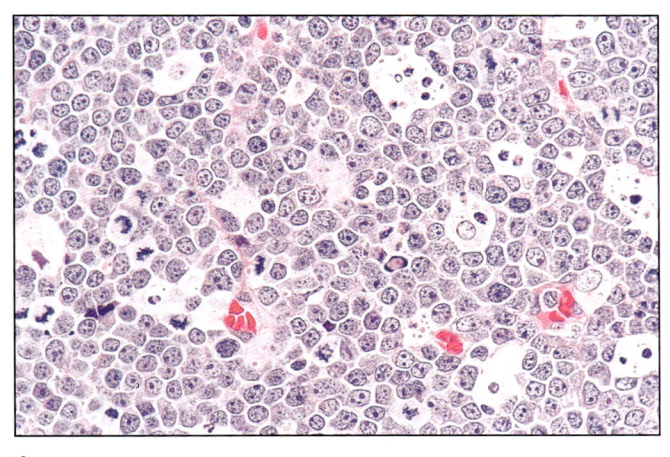

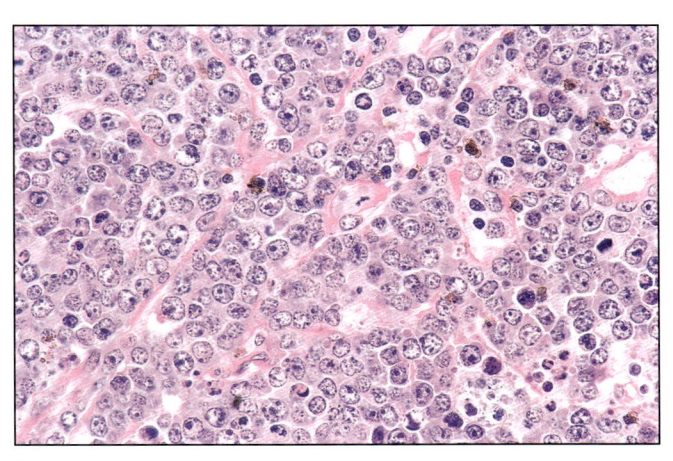

A

B

图21A.113 Burkitt淋巴瘤。（A）甲醛溶液固定的组织。肿瘤细胞中等大小，显示核膜和细胞膜"铺路石样外观"。可见典型的粗大染色质，具有多个明显的核仁，常见核分裂象。核仁通常没有膜包被。可见许多凋亡小体。（B）B5固定的组织。与甲醛溶液固定的组织比较，染色质团块更加粗大，细胞或细胞核成形通常较不明显。

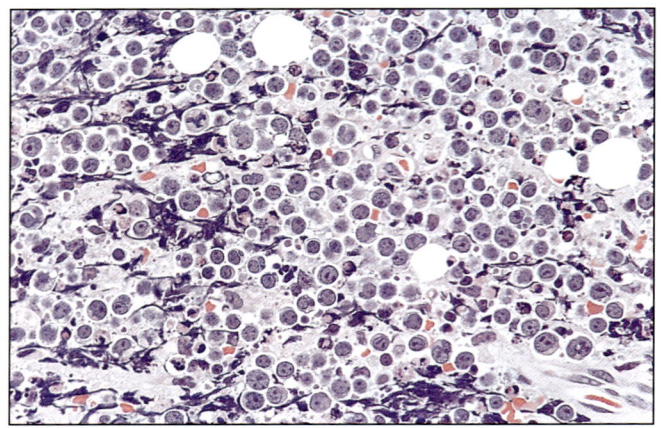

图21A.114 Burkitt淋巴瘤。在少数病例，可见细胞核突起，可能是一种变性现象。

非典型Burkitt淋巴瘤和诊断问题
Atypical Burkitt lymphoma and problems in diagnosis

非典型Burkitt淋巴瘤被认为是Burkitt淋巴瘤的一种变型，其特点是核的大小和形状变化较大，核仁更明显（有时孤立且位于中央），星天现象不太一致（图21A.115）。根据WHO的分类方法，这种名称用于生长分数接近100%以及推断有MYC易位的病例，然而对于如何"推断"，尚未进一步说明[967]。

"Burkitt样淋巴瘤"这个术语习惯上用于表示显示某些但并非全部Burkitt淋巴瘤典型特征的病例。这种分类显示的诊断可重复性低[264]。Burkitt样淋巴瘤是一种笼统性分类，包括真性Burkitt淋巴瘤（包括WHO分类中定义的非典型Burkitt淋巴瘤）、伴母细胞转化的滤泡性淋巴瘤以及增殖分数很高的弥漫大B细胞淋巴瘤。因此，部分病例可见BCL-2重排[968,969]。

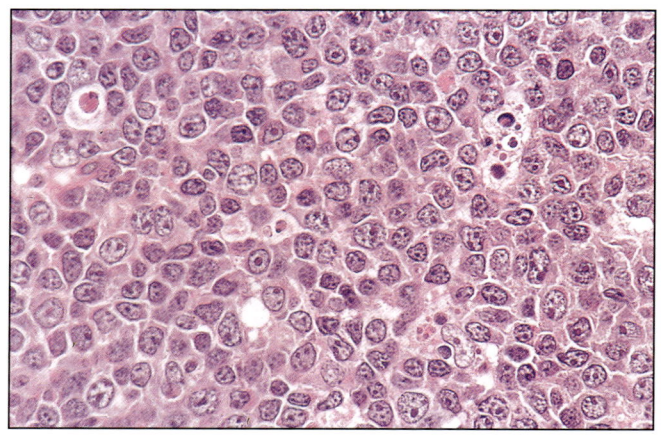

图21A.115 非典型Burkitt淋巴瘤。核大小有些差异。有些细胞具有明显的中心核仁。

免疫细胞化学

1. 全B细胞标记物呈阳性，例如CD19、CD20、CD22。表面Ig阳性（通常是IgM）[970]。
2. 滤泡中心细胞标记物CD10和bcl-6几乎总是呈阳性。CD5、bcl-2和TdT呈阴性[971,972]。增生分数（Ki-67指数）通常很高（接近100%）。
3. 不同程度地表达CD21（CD3d/EBV受体），但地方性病例常常呈阳性。常见CD43异常表达[10]。EBV阳性肿瘤不表达EBV LMP-1，提示为EBV潜伏I型（表21A.9）。

遗传学特征

Ig基因重排且显示体细胞超突变[973]。

Burkitt淋巴瘤特异的染色体易位包括t(8;14)(q24;q32)以及较少见的t(2;8)(p12;q24)和t(8;22)(q24;q11)。原癌基因C-MYC位于8q24，易位至14号、2号或22号染色体的Ig重链或轻链基因[18,952,974-976]。不同类型其Ig重链基因的断点也不同。在地方性Burkitt淋巴瘤，断点累及连接区，提示易位发生于早期B细胞，在完成Ig基因重排之前。在散发性Burkitt淋巴瘤，断点累及转换区（switch region），提示易位发生于B细胞发生的晚期。此外，C-MYC基因经常发生突变，造成基因失调[977]。因此Burkitt淋巴瘤发生的关键分子改变是C-MYC失调；肿瘤细胞永久地保留在细胞周期中而不分化，使肿瘤具有细胞学一致性[951]。

P53基因突变见于35%~50%的病例，这可能是进展性事件，导致对化疗和放疗不敏感[952]。

识别Burkitt淋巴瘤的基因表达谱
Gene expression profile for identification of Burkitt lymphoma

基于具有经典形态学和免疫表型的Burkitt淋巴瘤病例，能够建立一种基因表达谱（Burkitt淋巴瘤分子印迹）[782,978]。Burkitt淋巴瘤不同于弥漫大B细胞淋巴瘤之处在于：其C-MYC靶基因高表达，表达部分生发中心B细胞基因，以及主要组织相容性复合体I基因和NFκB靶基因低表达。对于形态学诊断为Burkitt淋巴瘤、非典型Burkitt淋巴瘤、弥漫大B细胞淋巴瘤或未分类高度恶性B细胞淋巴瘤的病例，根据表达Burkitt淋巴瘤的印迹可作出"分子学Burkitt淋巴瘤"的诊断。在"分子学Burkitt淋巴瘤"组中，95%的病例显示C-MYC重排，配对基因几乎总是IG基因；没有BCL-2或BCL-6重排，染色体复杂性低。"分子学Burkitt淋巴瘤"患者的预后明显好于缺乏Burkitt淋巴瘤印迹的高度恶性B细胞淋巴瘤患者（5年生存率分别为75%和39%），虽然多变量分析表明，前者的预后良好主要是由于患者的岁数小且疾病分期局限[782]。经强化药物治疗的患者明显好于经CHOP或CHOP样药物治疗者[978]。这些临床相关性提示，与目前的诊断标准相比，Burkitt淋巴瘤的分子学诊断可得出这种病变的较为准确的定义。弥漫大B细胞淋巴瘤可显示 C-MYC 重排，配对基因可能是免疫球蛋白或非免疫球蛋白基因。然而，染色体复杂性常常较高，同时伴有累及 BCL-2 或 BCL-6 的基因重排。

大量值得关注的观察显示，目前应用形态学和免疫组化方法诊断Burkitt淋巴瘤是不准确的[782,978]：

- 专业病理医生诊断为Burkitt淋巴瘤或非典型Burkitt淋巴瘤的少数病例不显示分子学Burkitt淋巴瘤印迹。
- 专业病理医生认为形态学肯定不是Burkitt淋巴瘤（或非典型Burkitt淋巴瘤）而符合弥漫大B细胞淋巴瘤的部分病例结果，却显示Burkitt淋巴瘤的分子学印迹。
- 高达21%的"分子学Burkitt淋巴瘤"病例表达bcl-2（虽然常常呈弱表达）。
- 高达34%的"分子学Burkitt淋巴瘤"病例显示Ki-67指数<95%。
- 但是，少数"分子学Burkitt淋巴瘤"病例可显示 IGH-BCL2 基因重排。

鉴别诊断

1. 淋巴母细胞性淋巴瘤（lymphoblastic lymphoma）：见第1176页，表21A.17。
2. 小B细胞淋巴瘤（small B-cell lymphoma）：在固定差的组织，Burkitt淋巴瘤细胞缩小，可被误诊为淋巴浆细胞性淋巴瘤或其他小细胞淋巴瘤。患者年轻是正确诊断的重要线索。
3. 弥漫大B细胞淋巴瘤（diffuse large B-cell lymphoma）：根据细胞中等大小和显示星天结构可能难以鉴别非典型Burkitt淋巴瘤与弥漫大B细胞淋巴瘤。以下特征倾向于诊断Burkitt淋巴瘤[40,971,979]：核分裂象和核碎裂小体很常见，细胞核与胞浆被挤压呈方形，免疫表型CD20+、CD10+、bcl-6+、bcl-2−、Ki-67指数>90%，以及FISH分析显示 MYC 易位，缺乏 BCL-2 和 BCL-6 易位。

外周T细胞肿瘤和有争议的NK细胞肿瘤
Peripheral T-and putative NK-cell neoplasms

外周T细胞和NK细胞淋巴瘤占所有非Hodgkin淋巴瘤的10%～30%，在高加索人群中所占百分率较低，在东方人群中较高，尤其是在日本和台湾北部等HTLV-1流行区[513]。

个别类型的外周T细胞和NK细胞淋巴瘤病例常显示细胞学的杂合性和免疫表型的广泛重叠性。与B淋巴瘤不同，相关的特异性细胞遗传学或分子学改变知之甚少。目前，临床综合征（尤其是在发病部位）在WHO的病变分类中被多种病变的定义引用。

从组织学特征能正确预测T细胞和NK细胞表型吗？

没有一种组织学特征是外周T细胞淋巴瘤（PTCL）或NK细胞淋巴瘤所特有的，然而当见到以下某些特征时应该考虑[980]：

1. 主要累及淋巴结副皮质区。
2. 小静脉内皮明显增高。
3. 细胞大小和形状多样，包括小、中和大细胞（图21A.116A）。
4. 核形状不规则，如多分叶和脑回状。
5. 许多细胞具有淡染至透明胞浆（图21A.116B），虽然有些B细胞淋巴瘤/白血病（毛细胞性白血病，淋巴结边缘区B细胞淋巴瘤，有些大B细胞淋巴瘤）也可见到透明细胞。
6. 可见许多上皮样组织细胞和（或）嗜酸性粒细胞。
7. 结外疾病具有明显的围血管生长和坏死。

外周T细胞和NK细胞淋巴瘤的诊断通常能经免疫组化染色证实。

识别淋巴瘤的T细胞系重要吗？

以往不能确定外周T细胞淋巴瘤是否比相应级别的B细胞淋巴瘤更具侵袭性，然而现在已证实，外周T细胞淋巴瘤（除了间变大细胞淋巴瘤）确实比弥漫大B细胞淋巴瘤预后差，甚至在应用国际预后指数分级时也是如此[262,264,981-986]。因此，确定淋巴瘤的细胞系非常重要，至少就预后而言[980]。

幼稚T淋巴细胞白血病
T-cell prolymphocytic leukemia

在WHO分类中，考虑到细胞遗传学畸变和预后的相似性，"慢性T淋巴细胞白血病"被认为是幼稚T淋巴细胞白血病的小细胞亚型，而不是一种独立的病变[987]。伴有毛细血管扩张的共济失调者发生幼稚T淋巴细胞白血病的危险性增加[40]。较详细的描述见第22章。

幼稚T淋巴细胞白血病的特点是：循环血中可见小

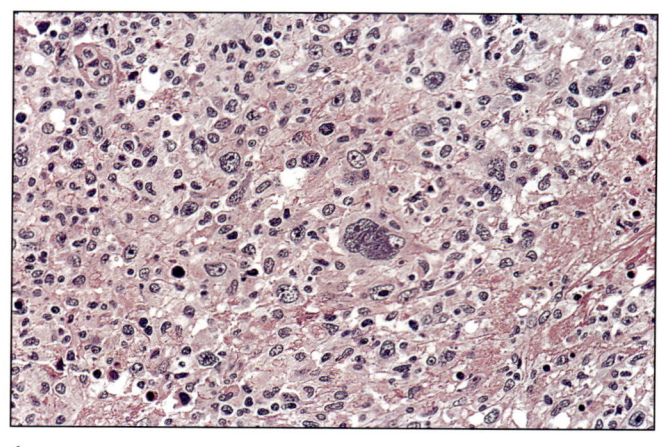 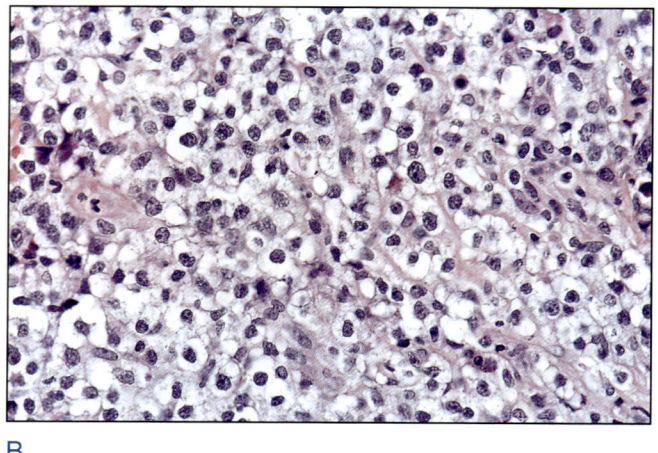

图21A.116 外周T细胞淋巴瘤，非特指。（A）细胞大小的变化以及较小淋巴细胞的非典型性很明显。中央的大细胞有些类似于Reed-Sternberg细胞。还可见典型的细条索状纤维化。（B）本例主要为透明细胞（所谓的"透明细胞免疫母细胞淋巴瘤"）。

到中等大的淋巴细胞，核圆形，染色质较致密，核仁清楚，胞浆嗜碱性，没有嗜苯胺蓝颗粒。小细胞亚型由小细胞组成，核有丘状突起，染色质致密，胞浆稀少。脑回状亚型的特点是核皱褶明显，类似于Sézary细胞。

最常见的免疫表型是CD2⁺、CD3⁺、CD4⁺、CD8⁻。少数病例可以是CD4⁺CD8⁺或CD4⁻CD8⁻。预后比B细胞慢性淋巴细胞白血病差，中位生存期为12个月或不足12个月[988]。组织学上，小淋巴细胞弥漫浸润，伴有不规则的核折叠（图21A.117）。与B-CLL不同，缺乏增生中心且有明显的高内皮细胞小静脉。可见少数散在较大的母细胞。脾脏红髓明显受累，伴有脾被膜和白髓浸润[989]。

T细胞颗粒性淋巴细胞白血病
T-cell granular lymphocytic leukemia

此病也称为"大颗粒性T淋巴细胞白血病"、"T淋巴细胞增生症"或"Tγ-淋巴组织增生性疾病"。更详细

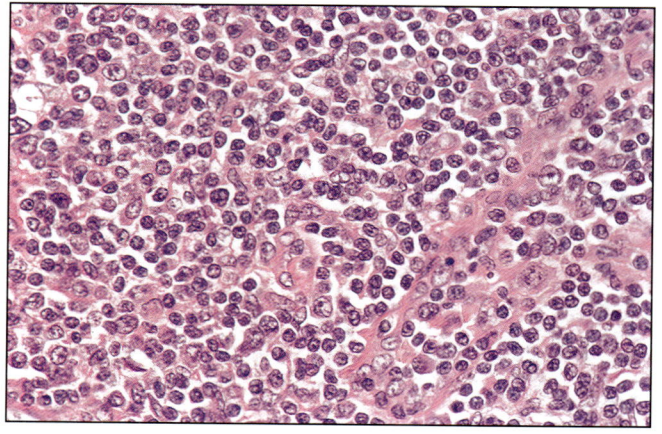

图21A.117 幼稚T淋巴细胞白血病（小细胞亚型）的淋巴结活检。小淋巴细胞显示轻度核凹陷，染色质致密。可见明显的高内皮细胞小静脉，该特征在B细胞慢性淋巴细胞白血病中见不到。没有增生中心。

的描述见第22章。

患者没有症状或表现为乏力、体重减轻和感染。有些患者具有类风湿性关节炎的血清学证据。常见脾大，但淋巴结肿大不常见。淋巴细胞增多通常不明显，常见中性粒细胞减少症。疾病通常呈稳定或慢性进展过程，常常由于感染并发症而死亡。循环血中淋巴细胞具有大颗粒淋巴细胞的特征，不同器官中的组织学改变已由Agnarsson和其他作者进行了总结[989,990]。多数病例显示免疫表型CD2⁺、CD3⁺、TCR-αβ⁺、CD4⁻和CD8⁻。NK细胞相关标记物的表达不一致，CD16和CD57常有不同程度表达，但很少表达CD56，其表达提示临床过程较具侵袭性[342,991]。TCRβ链基因重排。

蕈样霉菌病/Sézary综合征
Mycosis fungoides/Sézary syndrome

蕈样霉菌病是一种嗜表皮性皮肤T细胞淋巴瘤，由小到中等大的细胞组成，核呈脑回状。患者通常具有多发皮肤损害，由斑点进展成斑块或肿瘤[36,992-994]。Sézary综合征的特点是红皮病，淋巴结肿大和循环血中出现异常T淋巴细胞[995]。被认为是蕈样霉菌病的一种变型，但更具侵袭性。

典型的免疫表型为CD2⁺、CD3⁺、CD5⁺、CD7⁺/⁻、TCR-αβ⁺、CD4⁺、CD8⁻，在瘤块期常见异常的T细胞免疫表型。更详细的描述见第23章。

外周T细胞淋巴瘤，非特指
Peripheral T-cell lymphoma, unspecified

定义

外周T细胞淋巴瘤（PTCL）是一种成熟T细胞肿瘤，不同于T淋巴母细胞性淋巴瘤，后者由不成熟（前体）T

细胞组成。不显示其他明确类型的 PTCL 被诊断为外周 T 细胞性淋巴瘤，非特指（PTCL-U）。因此这是一个废纸篓和异质性类型，其中有意义的亚型将来可能会得到"拯救"。

临床特征

PTCL-U 的发病年龄范围广泛，高峰年龄为 50～70 岁[268,986,996-1001]。没有性别差异或仅仅男性略多。有些患者之前有免疫性疾病（如系统性红斑狼疮、类风湿性关节炎、桥本甲状腺炎）或淋巴组织增生性疾病（如滤泡性淋巴瘤）。常有全身症状。临床表现差异较大。虽然大多数患者表现为全身淋巴结肿大，但经常会同时或全部累及淋巴结外。常见皮肤、胸膜、肺、肝、脾和骨髓受累。大多数患者发病时表现为 III/IV 期（表 21A.11）。实验室检查提示多克隆高丙种球蛋白血症，Coombs 试验呈阳性或嗜酸性粒细胞增多。如果出现血钙升高，则应该考虑成人 T 细胞淋巴瘤/白血病。

PTCL-U 的行为常常不可预测。有些患者在短期内死亡，而少数病例则自然消退或呈惰性过程。总体上，PTCL-U 是侵袭性肿瘤。高分期疾病(III/IV 期)预后较差，IV 期疾病的生存率＜10%[1002,1003]。国际预后指数也具有预后意义[1004]。

伴噬血综合征的外周 T 细胞淋巴瘤 (peripheral T-cell lymphoma associated with hemophagocytic syndrome)：有些 PTCL-U 伴有噬血综合征、发热、全血细胞减少和肝脾肿大，可能是由于淋巴瘤细胞分泌的淋巴因子[1005-1007]。噬血综合征可以是淋巴瘤的首发症状，或在终末期发生。

病理学

PTCL-U 具有不同的组织学表现。淋巴组织浸润副皮质或呈弥漫性。常显示明显的高内皮细胞小静脉，淋巴细胞"拥堵"在小静脉中。常见反应性成分如嗜酸性粒细胞、浆细胞、组织细胞和上皮样组织细胞。细条索状胶原穿越病变，形成"分隔"现象。细胞成分因病例而异，可以是小、中和大细胞，或者这些细胞混合出现。细胞大小常常呈连续谱系，然而有时可见形态单一的细胞。核常常不规则性明显，表面有多个凹陷、脑回状、多分叶状或胶冻状[988]。染色质呈颗粒状或粗大（图 21A.118）。常见多核细胞和 Reed-Sternberg 样肿瘤细胞。胞浆可透明、淡染、嗜酸性、嗜双色性或嗜碱性。PTCL-U 的细胞学分级是非强制的，因为分级困难且未证明有预后意义[40,1004]。

形态学亚型

目前还没有明确的证据表明形态学亚型具有预后意义。

多分叶状 T 细胞淋巴瘤 (multilobated T-cell lymphoma)：特点是核呈明显分叶状，通常出现在淋巴结外部位[1008,1009]。虽然以前认为多分叶核是 T 细胞淋巴瘤的形态学标志，事实上这种核形在 B 细胞淋巴瘤中更常见（图 21A.118D）[1010]。

噬红细胞性 Tγ 淋巴瘤 (erythrophagocytic Tγ lymphoma)：累及器官的窦隙且淋巴瘤细胞吞噬红细胞，类似于"恶性组织细胞增生症"[1011]。这种病变与肝脾 T 细胞淋巴瘤有共同点。

Lennert（淋巴上皮样）淋巴瘤 [lennert (lymphoepithelioid) lymphoma]：特点是出现许多小灶状上皮样组织细胞，不形成独立的肉芽肿（图 21A.119）。其间淋巴细胞大多数是小淋巴细胞，核圆形或不规则形，染色质致密，胞浆稀少。其中混杂一些中等和大淋巴细胞，通常位于上皮样细胞附近。透明细胞不常见。很少出现 Reed-Sternberg 样细胞。高内皮细胞小静脉不明显。浆细胞较少，常见嗜酸性粒细胞。复发时，反应性上皮样细胞成分可以不明显。Lennert 淋巴瘤可转化为 T 细胞系大细胞淋巴瘤，缺少上皮样组织细胞反应[1012,1013]。

T 区淋巴瘤 (T-zone lymphoma)：是一种由 T 区的正常成分组成的淋巴瘤[272,988,1014]。淋巴瘤浸润特征为反应性淋巴滤泡之间的副皮质区扩大，然而在病变晚期，滤泡可以消失。淋巴细胞的大小及表现不一致，一般为小到中等大；一些细胞有丰富的透明胞浆。散布一些大的母细胞（图 21A.120）。可见巢状浆细胞样单核细胞、上皮样组织细胞、指状树突状细胞、浆细胞和嗜酸性粒细胞。高内皮细胞小静脉明显。随着疾病的进展，大细胞数目增加。在年轻患者，必须与自身免疫性淋巴组织增生综合征鉴别。

单形性中等大细胞的外周 T 细胞淋巴瘤 (monomorphous medium-sized cell PTCL)：特点是细胞形态单一、中等大小，核呈不规则折叠状，染色质相当致密，核仁不清楚，胞浆丰富透明或稀少（图 21A.121）[1016]。高内皮细胞小静脉常常丰富。主要鉴别诊断包括淋巴结边缘区 B 细胞淋巴瘤和系统性肥大细胞增生症。

印戒细胞 T 细胞淋巴瘤 (signet-ring T-cell lymphoma)：很少见，显示透明的胞浆空泡，类似于印戒细胞[1017,1021]。患者常常表现为皮肤病变。超微结构显示空泡含有微球体。细胞膜吞噬作用和异常膜循环被认为是空泡形成的可能机制。

伴有玫瑰花结的外周 T 细胞淋巴瘤 (peripheral T-cell lymphoma with rosettes)：很少见，可误诊为神经内分泌肿瘤[368]。

结节性 T 细胞淋巴瘤 (nodular T-cell lymphoma)：

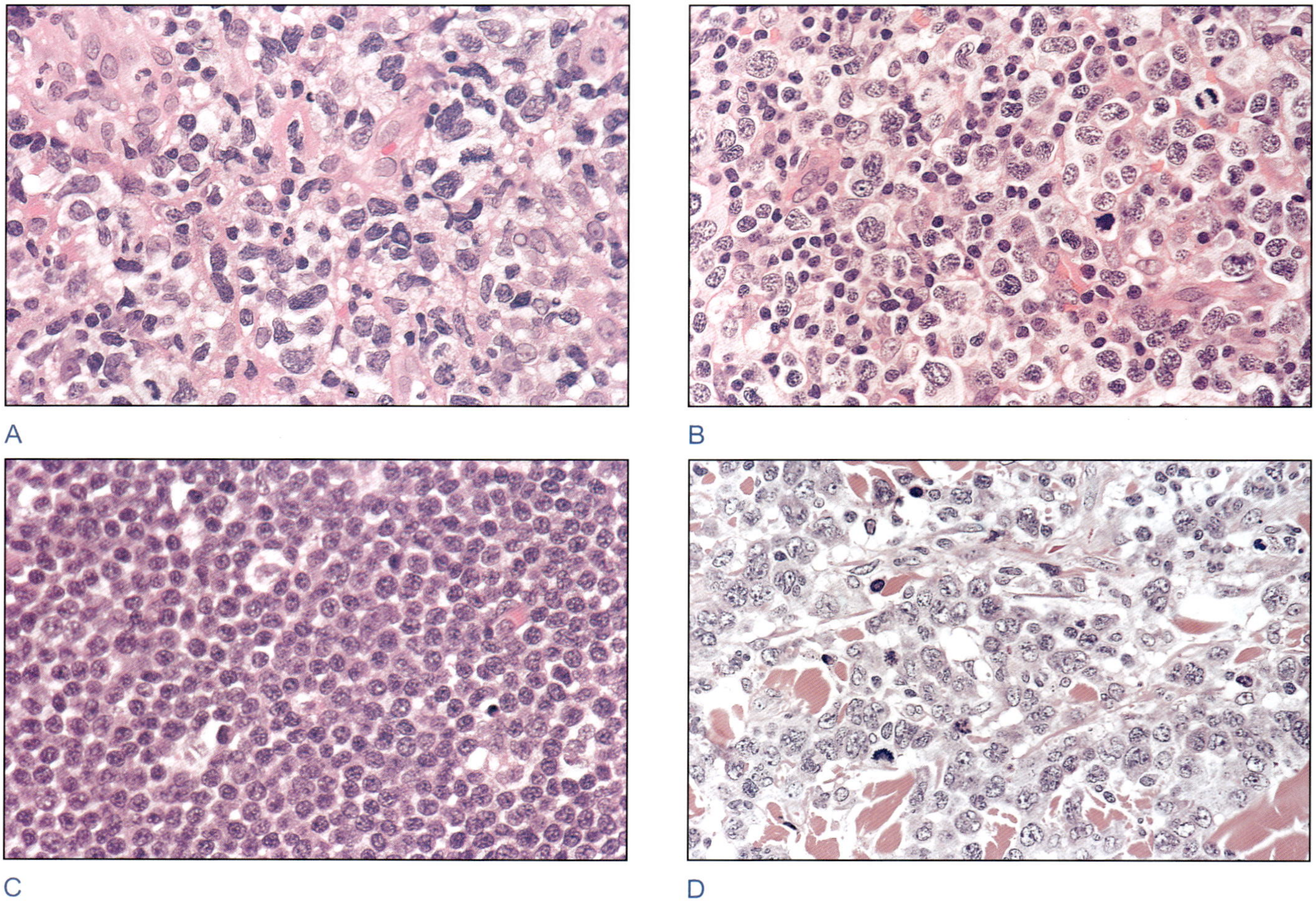

图21A.118 外周T细胞淋巴瘤，非特指。（A）本例主要由中等大小的细胞组成。常常可见核不规则折叠。（B）淋巴细胞核大小有变化。较小的细胞染色质较致密，而较大的细胞染色质呈粗糙、颗粒状。后者不符合正常活化的淋巴细胞（免疫母细胞）的表现。其中有些显示核折叠。（C）此例由单一形态的小细胞巢组成，核轻度不规则。（D）此例显示许多多分叶核细胞。

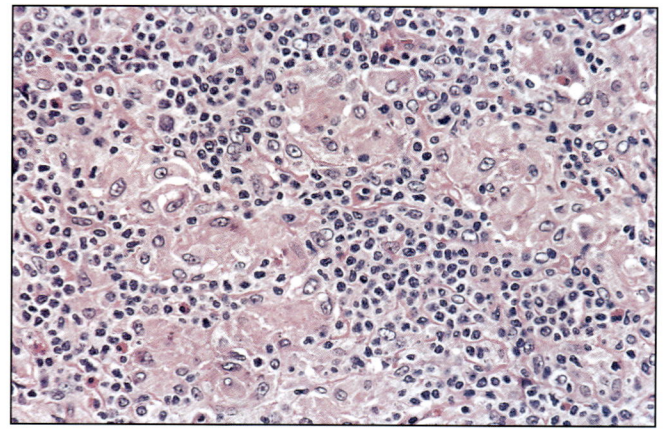

图21A.119 外周T细胞性淋巴瘤，非特指——所谓的Lennert淋巴瘤。淋巴细胞分布于上皮样组织细胞之间，大多数是小细胞，显示轻微的核异型性。偶尔有大淋巴细胞。

特点是副皮质区呈结节状生长。结节主要由小淋巴细胞组成，核不规则，混合散在大细胞。两种细胞类型均有透明胞浆。窦隙常常显著[1022]。

滤泡性T细胞淋巴瘤(follicular T-cell lymphoma)：是呈真性滤泡生长方式的外周T细胞淋巴瘤，极其类似滤泡性淋巴瘤。患者通常表现为全身淋巴结肿大。组织学上，滤泡界限明显或大而模糊，含有大量滤泡性树突状细胞，肿瘤性淋巴细胞小到中等大，核具有不规则裂隙或呈圆形，胞浆透明（图21A.122）。免疫表型谱系为$CD4^+CD8^-CD57^-bcl\text{-}6^+$和$CD10^{+/-}$ [1023,1024]。与血管免疫母细胞T细胞淋巴瘤（一种生发中心辅助T细胞肿瘤）的关系仍未阐明。

滤泡周T细胞淋巴瘤(perifollicular T-cell lymphoma)：特点是淋巴结结构部分破坏，边缘区被中等大小的淋巴

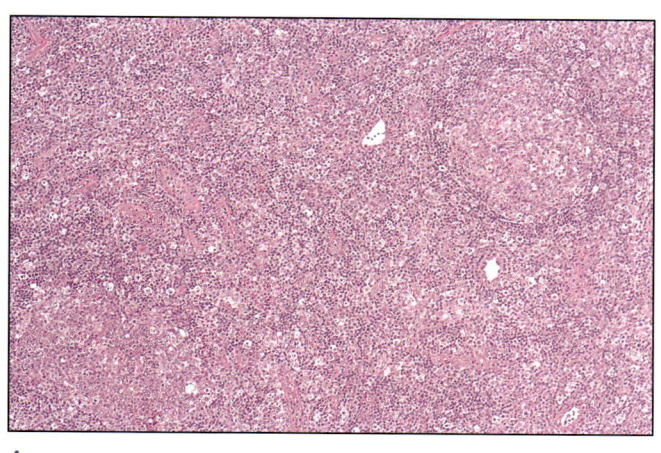
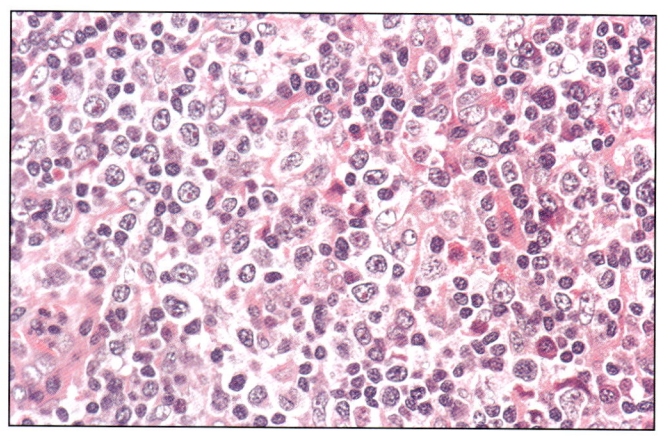

图21A.120 外周T细胞淋巴瘤,T区型。(A)淋巴瘤占据反应性滤泡之间的滤泡间区,间区扩大。(B)细胞学由混合细胞类型组成,包括有些透明细胞。许多淋巴细胞显示核折叠。还混合有些嗜酸性粒细胞。淋巴细胞的异型性(尤其是透明细胞)有助于与反应性副皮质区增生相鉴别。

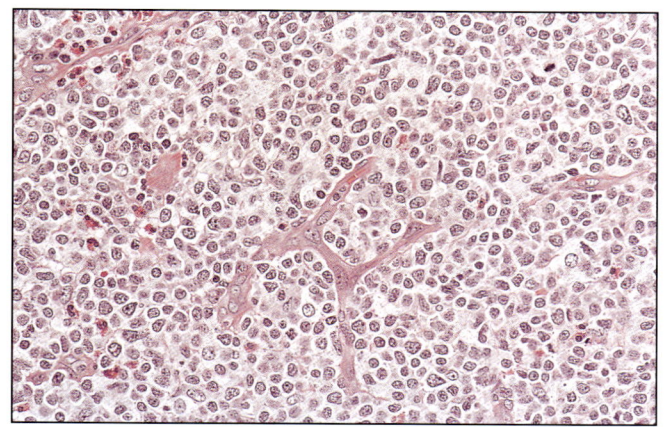

图21A.121 外周T细胞淋巴瘤显示单一形态的中等大小的细胞群。淋巴瘤细胞含有较丰富的透明胞浆。

细胞浸润,胞浆透明,核异型性明显。在副皮质T区有明显增生的高内皮细胞小静脉。其他明显的特征还包括浆细胞增生和被膜纤维化。淋巴瘤细胞显示T辅助细胞免疫表型（CD3$^+$、CD4$^+$、CD5$^{+/-}$、CD8$^-$、TIA1$^-$）[1025]。

S100蛋白阳性T细胞淋巴瘤（S100 protein-positive T-cell lymphoma）：是一种少见的淋巴瘤,通常发生于年轻患者,表现为发热、脾大明显和血细胞减少,但外周淋巴结肿大不明显[1026,1027]。疾病呈高度侵袭性过程。组织学上,中等到大的淋巴细胞浸润淋巴窦,实质有不同程度受累。在脾,可见红髓广泛受累。肝受累主要发生于肝窦。这些病例CD3$^+$,常常表达CD56[1026]。

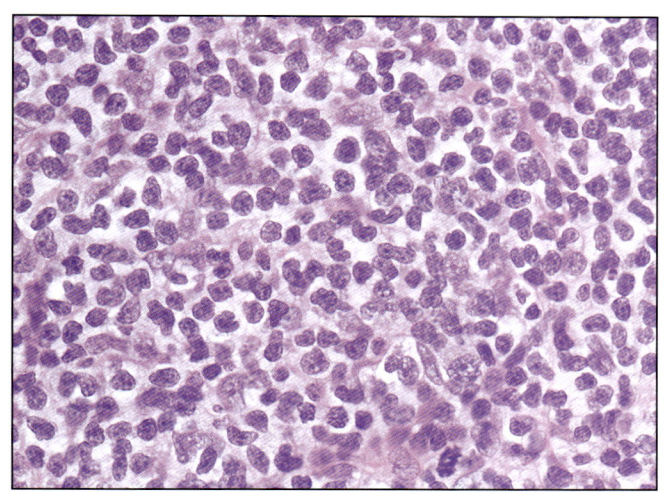
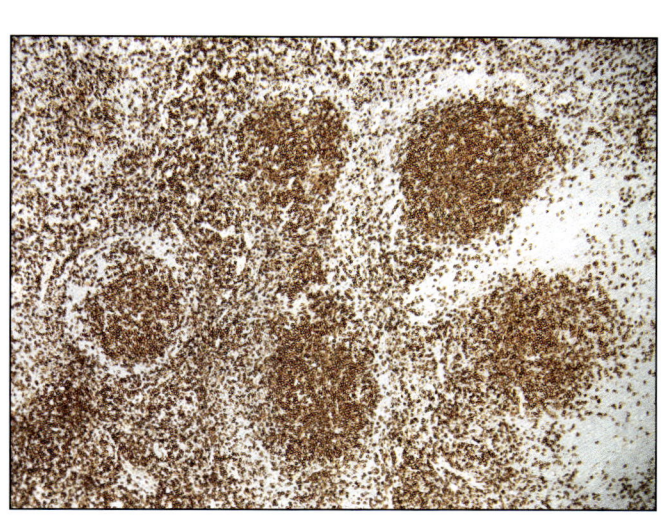

图21A.122 滤泡性T细胞淋巴瘤。(A)滤泡由小细胞组成,核不规则折叠,形态与普通滤泡性淋巴瘤I级难以区分。(B)然而CD3免疫染色显示增生的细胞是T细胞,而不是B细胞。

可能的临床病理学变型

黏膜皮肤γδT细胞淋巴瘤(mucocutaneous γδ T-cell lymphoma)：黏膜皮肤γδT细胞淋巴瘤组成非特指的外周T细胞淋巴瘤的一种独特亚型[1028]。大多数患者出现B症状，没有外周淋巴结肿大。好发部位是皮肤、鼻腔、胃肠道和呼吸道[1029]。常伴有慢性组织限制性抗原接触（如慢性鼻窦炎或慢性感染）和免疫缺陷，淋巴瘤一般呈侵袭性[1029,1030]。细胞组成大小不等。常见亲上皮性、血管中心性生长和坏死。淋巴瘤细胞显示CD2+、CD3+、TCR-γδ+以及cytotoxic（细胞毒性）阳性的免疫表型。大多数病例CD5⁻、CD4⁻、CD8⁻。大约半数病例具有EBV感染。

淋巴结细胞毒性T细胞淋巴瘤(nodal cytotoxic T-cell lymphoma)：与非细胞毒性组相比，淋巴结细胞毒性PTCL-U患者较年轻（中位年龄为55岁与64岁），状态较差，较常见B症状（68%与35%），血清乳酸脱氢酶水平较高，结外受累较常见，与EBV相关性较强（51%与2%）。完全缓解率（30%与63%）和总体生存率明显较低[1031]。细胞毒性组没有独特的形态学特征，只是多核肿瘤细胞相对常见，背景中浆细胞和嗜酸性粒细胞较少[1031]。

非特指外周T细胞淋巴瘤的进展
Progression of PTCL-U

PTCL-U的肿瘤复发可以伴有或不伴有组织学进展。组织学进展常常表现为大细胞的比例增加[1013,1032]。这可能与表型改变有关（表面抗原丢失）。

免疫细胞化学

1. T细胞系标记物阳性，例如CD2、CD3。在显示混合细胞群的肿瘤，较大的细胞呈CD3阴性或仅仅弱呈阳性，而较小的细胞则呈强阳性[1033]。
2. 多数PTCL（80%的病例）的典型特征是免疫表型异常，即一种或多种全T细胞抗原丢失[996,1016,1034,1035]。最常丢失的抗原是CD7和CD5（图21A.123），但CD7的丢失必须慎重评估，因为正常情况下CD7仅着染一部分T淋巴细胞[342,1034]。PTCL-U中的CD4表达比CD8更常见，但二者可同时缺失或共表达[767,998]。
3. 可不同程度地表达活化标记物，如HLA-DR、CD25、CD30和CD134。有趣的是，显示CD134表达的病例实际上从不表达CD30[1036]。有时可见较大细胞表达CD15[168,342,1037]。大多数病例表达αβ-TCR，有些病例表达γδ-TCR[1029]。可以表达细胞毒性分子，与淋巴结病例相比，这种特征较常见于结外病例[1038]。一部分表达细胞毒性标记物或γδ-TCR的PTCL-U还可表达CD56，即所谓的NK样T细胞淋巴瘤[1038-1040]。

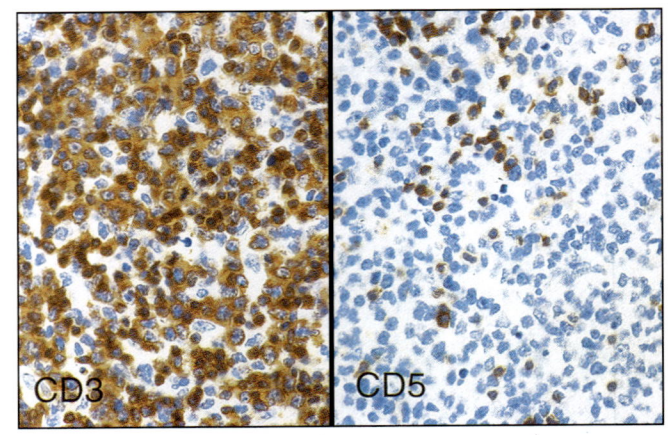

图21A.123 非特指外周T细胞淋巴瘤的免疫染色。左侧：非典型细胞显示CD3呈阳性。右侧：本例可见CD5表达异常缺失。

4. 有极少数表达CD20的外周T细胞淋巴瘤的报道，导致细胞系分类困难或混淆[1041-1045]。应用其他T细胞系标记物（CD2、CD5、CD7）和B细胞标记物（如PAX-5、CD79a）以及Ig和TCR基因重排等分子学研究可能有助于解决细胞系分类。

遗传学研究

TCRβ链基因重排是单克隆性和T细胞系淋巴组织增生的最好证据[18,342,1046]。TCRγ链基因也总是出现重排。只有极少数情况下同时有Ig重链基因重排。没有特异性的细胞遗传学或分子学改变[996]。

与类型明确的T细胞淋巴瘤不同，如血管免疫母细胞性T细胞淋巴瘤和间变大细胞淋巴瘤，基因表达谱研究显示，PTCL-U不具有单一的分子学谱系。至少可见三种分子亚型：U1印迹型包括已知与其他肿瘤预后差有关的基因，如*CCND2*；U2与T细胞活化和凋亡基因有关，包括*NFκB1*和*BCL-2*；U3主要涉及IFN/JAK/STAT通路基因的过表达[1047]。

有些基因可具有EBV感染，原位杂交可以观察到几种结构：（1）实际上几乎所有肿瘤细胞均呈阳性，提示肿瘤的EBV相关性；（2）少部分肿瘤细胞呈阳性，提示EBV感染发生于肿瘤转化之后，或EBV基因组在转化之后部分丢失；（3）孤立性大的阳性细胞主要是反应性B细胞而不是肿瘤细胞[1048,1049]。

血管免疫母细胞性T细胞淋巴瘤
Angioimmunoblastic T-cell lymphoma

定义

血管免疫母细胞性T细胞淋巴瘤是一种外周T细胞淋巴瘤,以系统性病变、淋巴结中多形性淋巴组织浸润以及高内皮细胞小静脉和滤泡树突状细胞增生为特征[1050]。近期的证据提示,这是一种生发中心T辅助细胞肿瘤[1051-1054]。

临床特征

血管免疫母细胞性T细胞淋巴瘤通常发生于老年人(中位年龄为64岁),男性发病稍多[1055-1057]。患者常常表现为全身淋巴结肿大、肝脾大、发热、全身症状、皮疹和渗出。淋巴结最大径通常<3cm,可自由活动。大约25%的患者有先前药物反应史或病毒感染史。常见多克隆丙种球蛋白病、自身免疫溶血性贫血、血循环中免疫复合物及自身抗体;90%的患者疾病为III期或IV期。患者易患各种感染,如分枝杆菌、巨细胞病毒、曲霉菌和卡氏肺囊虫感染,高达50%的死亡是由感染并发症引起的。

临床经过很不一致。在一些患者,疾病呈惰性过程,有时甚至自行消退。有些患者对化疗很敏感,可达到持久性缓解。另一些患者呈极具侵袭性过程,对治疗反应差[1056]。应用泼尼松伴或不伴加强化疗,60%的患者可达到完全缓解,但只有1/3的患者可以达到长期无病生存,因为56%的缓解患者会发生复发[1055,1057,1058]。

组织学特征

淋巴结结构破坏,但被膜下窦常常保持开放。分枝状高内皮细胞小静脉横穿淋巴结(图21A.124)。可见有些主要由滤泡树突状细胞组成的燃尽的生发中心。增生细胞主要为小到中等大的淋巴细胞,核圆形。其中有些细胞具有透明胞浆,聚集成团,在低到中倍放大时,形成高度特征性的花斑状结构(图21A.124)。常见胞浆嗜碱性的免疫母细胞灶,有时位于血管内。另外,常常可见混合性浆细胞、浆母细胞和嗜酸性粒细胞。在有些病例,上皮样细胞灶较明显[1059]。在少数病例,可见散在的单核或双核大细胞,类似Reed-Sternberg细胞(CD30+、CD15+、CD20+/-)且伴有EBV感染;这种病例可被误诊为Hodgkin淋巴瘤[1060]。随着疾病进展,中等的和大的淋巴细胞增加,形成弥漫片状。

一种独特的特征是常常出现不规则形的、细胞减少的淡染嗜酸性病灶,由成束和旋涡状的肥胖梭形细胞组成,胞浆丰富,细胞界限不清,核卵圆形,染色质纤细,是滤泡外增生的FDC(图21A.125)[980]。

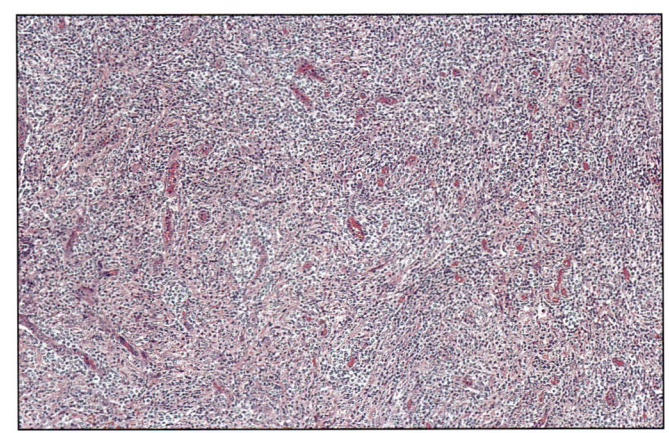

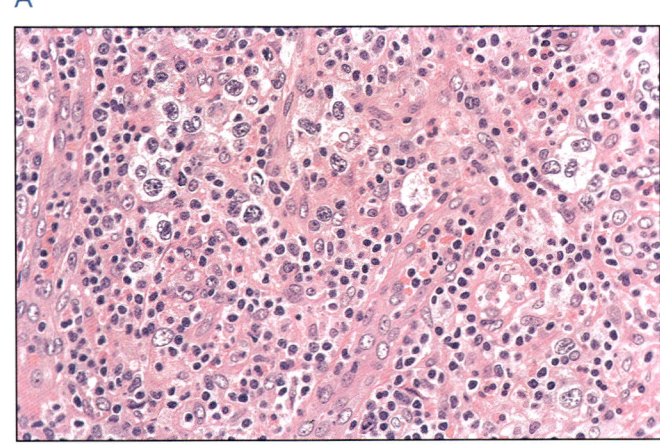

图21A.124 血管免疫母细胞性T细胞淋巴瘤。(A)可见分枝状高内皮细胞小静脉和特征性的巢状淡染细胞。(B)可见明显的小静脉。可见混合性淋巴细胞,包括一些透明细胞。背景中还可见有些嗜酸性粒细胞和浆细胞。

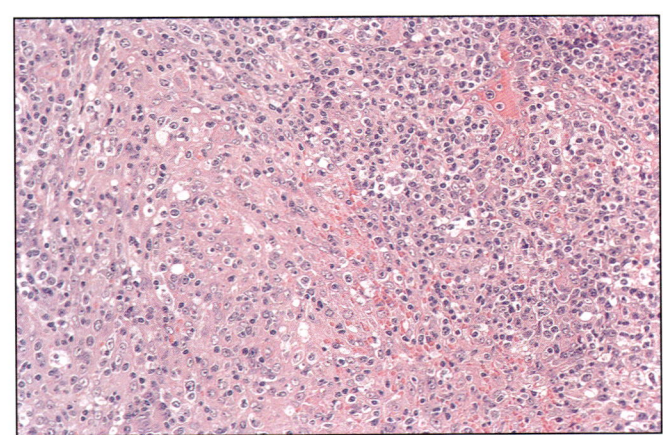

图21A.125 血管免疫母细胞性T细胞淋巴瘤。在左侧视野,可见粉染的细胞减少区,是滤泡外增生的滤泡树突状细胞。肥胖的梭形细胞没有明显的细胞轮廓。

血管免疫母细胞性T细胞淋巴瘤的早期病变

现在已认识到一种伴有增生性生发中心的早期血管免疫母细胞性T细胞淋巴瘤[1061-1063]。随着时间，其可进展为上述典型病例。

淋巴结结构部分保留。在皮质，可见增生的淋巴滤泡，套区形成较差。副皮质区扩张，充满多形性细胞，包括淋巴细胞、转化的淋巴细胞、浆细胞、组织细胞和嗜酸性粒细胞，伴有明显的高内皮细胞小静脉。在这一阶段，萌芽状CD21+的FDC蔓延至生发中心界限外，偶尔包绕小血管[1061]。

免疫细胞化学

1. T细胞系标记物阳性，通常为CD2+、CD3+、CD5+、CD7− （图21A.126）[1064]。
2. 通常可见大的不规则形滤泡外CD21+的FDC网，位于小静脉周围 （图21A.127）[272,1066]。肿瘤细胞常常表达CD10和bcl-6[1061,1066]。CXCL13是一种涉及B细胞迁移入生发中心的关键趋化因子，是生发中心T辅助细胞的特征，表达于89%～100%的血管免疫母细胞性T细胞淋巴瘤病例，其很少见于其他T细胞淋巴瘤[1051,1053]。PD-1（程序性死亡因子-1）是一种生发中心相关性T细胞标记物，实际上表达于所有病例[1052]。
3. 增生细胞几乎总是辅助（CD4+）类型[988,1064,1067-1070]。
4. 常常可见一定数量散在的大B细胞（CD20+），需要与B细胞淋巴瘤鉴别（图21A.126）。较具非典型细胞（包括透明细胞）——是T细胞来源，以及大B细胞具有多型性Ig，可做出正确诊断[980,1071]。

遗传学特征

大约90%的病例可见TCR重排。20%～30%的病

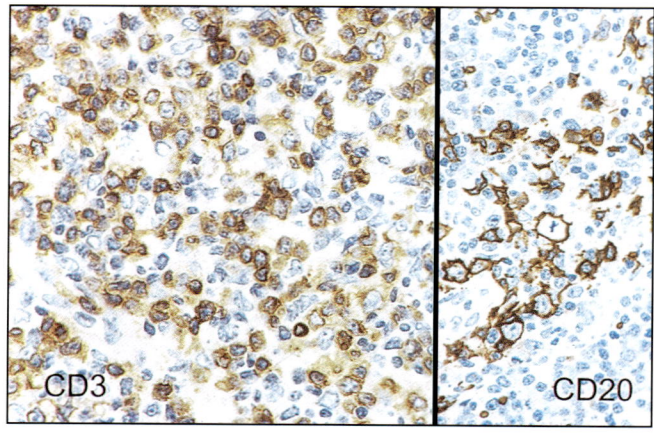

图21A.126　血管免疫母细胞性T细胞淋巴瘤的免疫染色。左侧：非典型细胞着染CD3。右侧：CD20染色常常显示相当数量的B细胞，其中有些是大细胞。

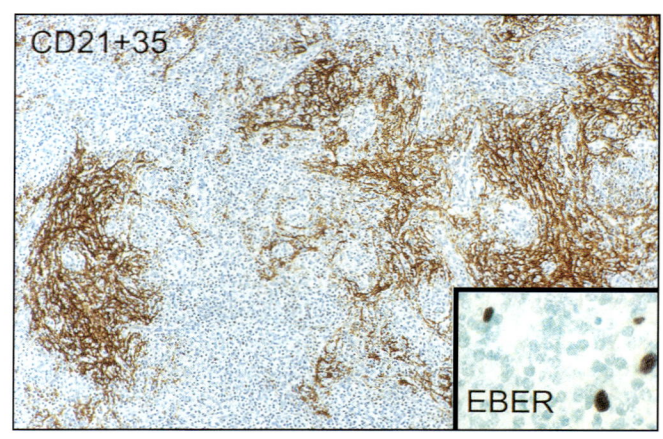

图21A.127　血管免疫母细胞性T细胞淋巴瘤的免疫染色。滤泡外的滤泡树突状细胞网，常常位于小静脉周围，是这种淋巴瘤类型的高度典型特征。常常散在有孤立的EBER阳性细胞（插图）。

例同时可检测到克隆性Ig重链基因重排。10%～20%的病例甚至可见Ig轻链基因重排[18,1072]。

没有特异性核型异常[1071]。3号、5号染色体三体和+X是最常见的染色体异常。这种淋巴瘤类型比较特殊，细胞遗传学不相关克隆的发生率较高（约50%）[1073]。

在大多数病例，可见散在的EBV感染的大淋巴细胞；它们主要是B细胞，但有时可以是T细胞（图21A.127）。EBV+ B细胞增多可能反映免疫系统的选择性缺陷[1074-1076]。极少数情况下，这些B细胞可进展为弥漫大B细胞淋巴瘤[1077]。

鉴别诊断

1. **外周T细胞淋巴瘤，非特指（PTCL-U）**：PTCL-U具有明显的小静脉和混合性淋巴细胞浸润，可能难以与血管免疫母细胞性T细胞淋巴瘤鉴别[980]。倾向于诊断后者的特征是出现上述独特的临床特征；有明显的分枝状小静脉；淋巴细胞具有圆形核轮廓，而非不规则形；常常可见透明细胞；背景富于浆细胞和嗜酸性粒细胞；CD10和CXCL13阳性；以及滤泡外出现不规则的FDC网[1065]。
2. **富于T细胞的大B细胞淋巴瘤** (T cell-rich large B-cell lymphoma)。
3. **伴异常蛋白血症的血管免疫母细胞性淋巴结病** (angioimmunoblastic lymphadenopathy with dysproteinemia)。

伴异常蛋白血症的血管免疫母细胞性淋巴结病（AILD）确实存在吗？
Does angioimmunoblastic lymphadenopathy with dysproteinemia (AILD) exist at all?

AILD的诊断以前很流行，现在却极少诊断[1078]。虽然有些"AILD"病例可能事实上是反应性或淋巴瘤前

期病变，但过去诊断的大多数病例可能是血管免疫母细胞性T细胞淋巴瘤，证据显示具有非随机染色体异常和TCR基因重排[1079-1081]。目前，根据淋巴组织增生伴有分枝状小静脉得出AILD诊断时必须应用严格的标准：

- 总体而言，细胞较少；
- 缺乏透明细胞；
- 缺乏明确的细胞学非典型性。

肠病型T细胞淋巴瘤
Enteropathy-type T-cell lymphoma

临床特征

这是一种肠上皮内的T细胞淋巴瘤。诊断时的中位年龄是60岁，男性发生率略高[654]。患者表现为小肠肿物或溃疡，常为多灶性[1082]。病变表现为急性肠穿孔、梗阻或出血。可以有短暂的成人乳糜泻病史、长期乳糜泻、疱疹样皮炎病史或根本没有乳糜泻病史。有些患者表现为重度乳糜泻，并丧失了谷胶敏感性。少数情况下，淋巴瘤首先出现在肠道之外，如肺和皮肤。预后很差，即使对治疗有反应也只是暂时的[654,1082-1084]。

相关病变是溃疡性空肠炎，表现为表浅的"良性"黏膜溃疡和绒毛萎缩。T细胞群的单克隆性证实这种病变是早期肠病型T细胞淋巴瘤[1085,1086]。

病理学

这种淋巴瘤最常累及空肠，表现为单个或多发溃疡性肿物[654]。多数肿瘤主要由多形性或间变性大细胞组成，虽然有些肿瘤可由小到中等大的细胞组成（图21A.128A和21A.129）。常见亲上皮性。有些病例伴有大量嗜酸性粒

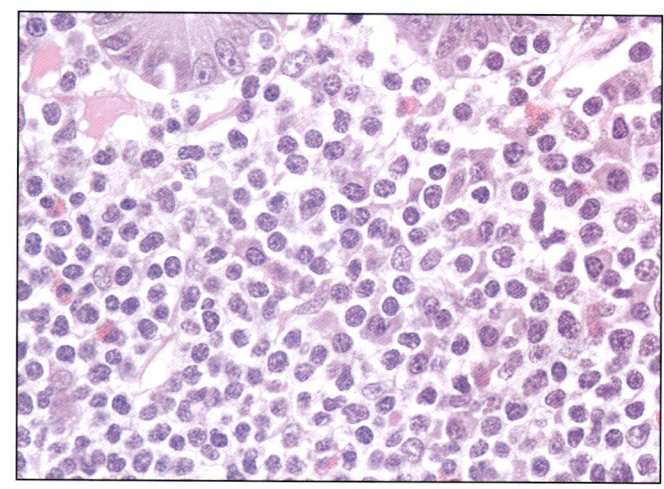

图21A.129　肠病型T细胞淋巴瘤。本例由单一形态的中等细胞组成，具有圆形或不规则折叠的细胞核。现有证据表明，这种形态学亚型显示免疫表型和基因型均不同于普通的肠病型T细胞淋巴瘤。

细胞或组织细胞浸润，可能迷惑诊断。周围的小肠黏膜通常显示绒毛萎缩、隐窝增生和上皮内淋巴细胞浸润，提示乳糜泻（可以是亚临床性）（图21A.128B）。

在溃疡性空肠炎，空肠溃疡显示重度混合性炎症细胞浸润，常常包括许多嗜酸性粒细胞。浸润灶内可见孤立和小巢状非典型大细胞。这种细胞由于CD30呈阳性而易于识别[1087]。

免疫细胞化学

1. T细胞系标记物阳性，如CD3、CD7和CD5通常呈阳性。
2. CD103（HML-A）常常呈阳性[1088]。细胞毒性分子常常呈阳性[1089]。

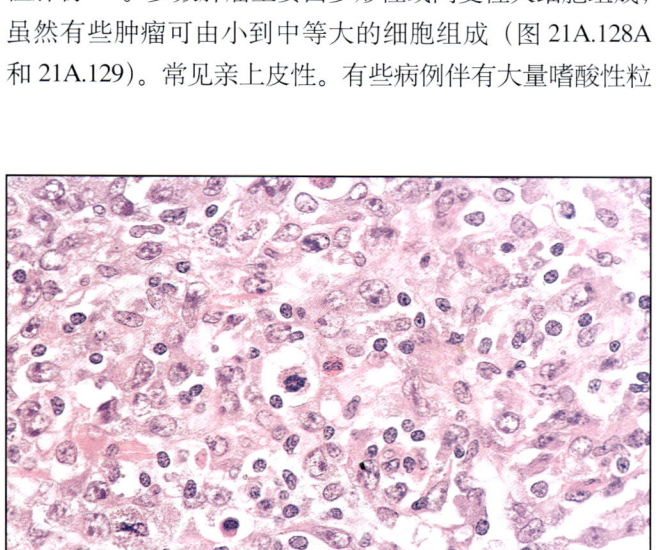

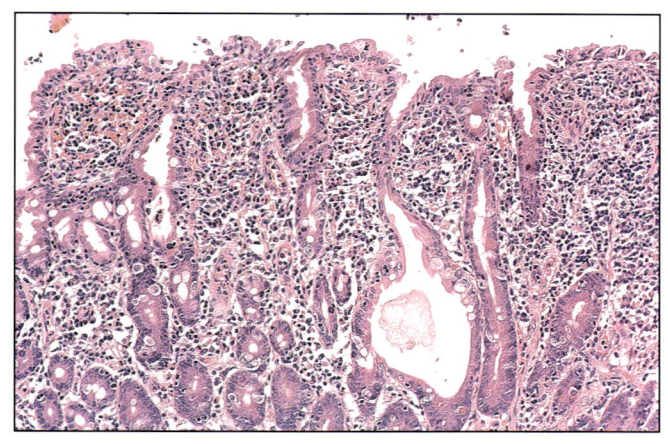

图21A.128　肠病型T细胞淋巴瘤。（A）此淋巴瘤由大细胞组成。（B）附近的小肠显示绒毛萎缩、隐窝增生和上皮内淋巴细胞增多，符合乳糜泻的特征。

3. CD30在富于大细胞的病例中呈阳性。CD4和CD8常常呈阴性。CD56在21%的病例中表达；这些病例主要常常由形态单一的中等细胞组成，显示CD4⁻CD5⁻CD8⁺的免疫表型[1082,1090]。

在已知为"难治性口炎性腹泻"的病变，上皮内淋巴细胞异常免疫表型的出现（CD8或TCR-β表达丢失）标志着肠病型T细胞淋巴瘤的早期表现。这还与TCR基因克隆性重排的出现有关[1091]。

遗传学特征

TCR基因重排。EBV通常呈阴性[654,1082]。大多数患者显示乳糜泻的特征性HLA DQA1*0501、DQB1*0201基因型[1091]。

常见的遗传学异常是9q扩增，提示为NOTCH1基因[1093,1094]。其他常见的异常包括+1q、+5q、+8q和-16q以及9p21杂合性缺失（尤其是具有大细胞形态学的肿瘤）[1093,1095,1096]。有两种不同形式的肠病型T细胞淋巴瘤：（1）较常见的是CD56⁻组，特点是+1q和+5q；（2）CD56⁺形态学组，特点是+8q。然而，二者均常常显示+9q和-16q。

肝脾T细胞淋巴瘤
Hepatosplenic T-cell lymphoma

见本章第2部分。

皮下脂膜炎样T细胞淋巴瘤
Subcutaneous panniculitis-like T-cell lymphoma

定义

这是一种细胞毒性T细胞淋巴瘤，倾向于累及皮下组织[1097,1098]。许多报告为"组织细胞吞噬性脂膜炎"的病例可能代表这种病变[1099]。

临床特征

这种淋巴瘤类型主要发生于成人，中位发病年龄为35岁[1100,1101]。没有性别差异。患者表现为孤立性或多发性皮下结节，最常见于四肢和躯干。结节大小0.5～12cm，可为坏死性。病变常常局限于皮下组织，很少播散至淋巴结或其他器官。发病时或疾病过程中，可能伴有噬血综合征，通常呈突发性临床过程。不伴噬血综合征的病例呈惰性过程，预后良好[1100-1105]。

病理学

淋巴组织浸润局限于皮下组织，不累及真皮。浸润的组织呈缎带样结构（图21A.130）。多数病例以小到中等大的淋巴瘤细胞为主，核不规则，有些病例可能以大细胞为主。淋巴瘤细胞常常呈环状围绕脂肪空隙。核碎常常明显，坏死广泛。常有散在的组织细胞，具有明显的吞噬活性。有些病例可见血管侵犯或肉芽肿。

有些病例由于细胞学非典型性轻微，难以作出明确诊断。随着时间的进展，细胞学非典型性增加，使诊断逐渐明确[1097]。

免疫细胞化学

1. T细胞系标记物呈阳性。
2. 细胞毒性标记物，如TIA-1、穿孔素和粒酶B阳性，但是粒酶M呈阴性（图21A.131）[1100,1106]。淋巴瘤细胞常常CD4⁻CD8⁺，CD56通常呈阴性。
3. 大多数病例表达αβ-TCR。表达γδ-TCR的病

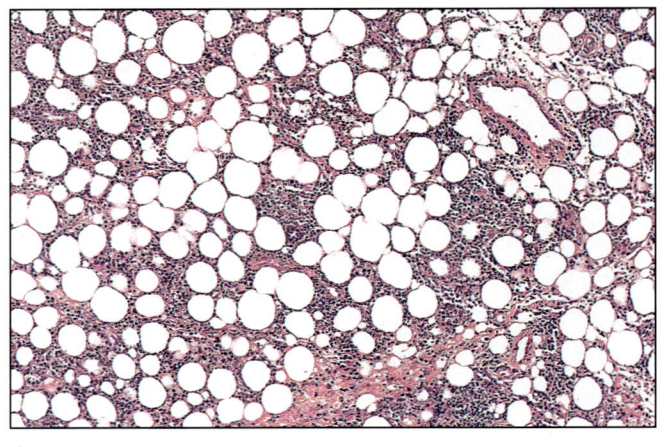

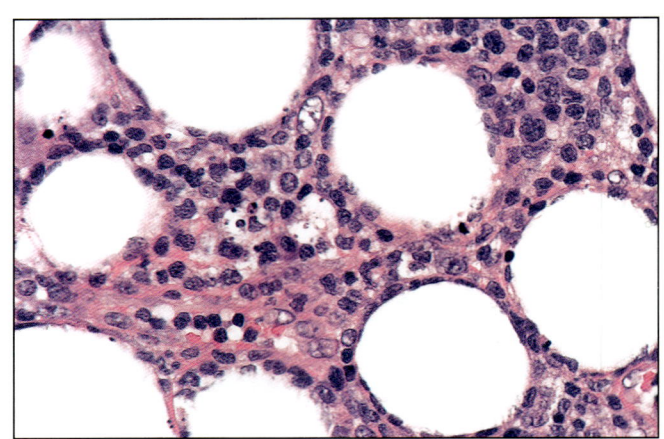

图21A.130 皮下脂膜炎样T细胞淋巴瘤。（A）在皮下脂肪小叶中可见缎带状淋巴细胞浸润，类似于小叶脂膜炎。（B）浸润性病变由非典型中等大小细胞组成，伴有明显的凋亡小体。可见围绕脂肪空泡的淋巴细胞环。

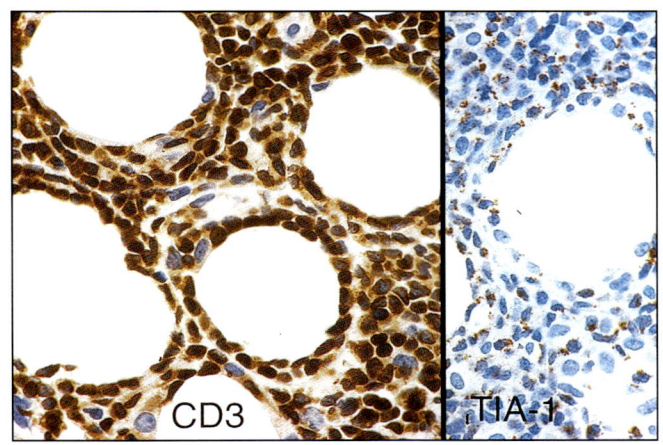

图21A.131 皮下脂膜炎样T细胞淋巴瘤免疫染色。左侧：CD3呈阳性。围绕脂肪空泡的淋巴瘤细胞环尤其明显。右侧：淋巴瘤细胞表达细胞毒性标记物，如TIA-1。

例（先前归类于皮下脂膜炎样T细胞淋巴瘤，常常表达CD56）现在分类为皮肤γδ-T细胞淋巴瘤[1098,1100,1101,1104]。

遗传学特征

TCR基因重排。不伴有EBV感染[1097,1100,1101]。关于这种淋巴瘤类型的遗传学异常知之甚少。

鉴别诊断

1. **小叶脂膜炎(lobular panniculitis)**：脂膜炎缺乏明确的细胞学非典型性和围绕脂肪空泡的淋巴细胞环。可见混合性CD4$^+$、CD8$^+$和CD20$^+$细胞，以及仅仅少量细胞毒性标记物染色细胞[1100]。
2. **累及皮肤的NK/T细胞淋巴瘤(NK/T cell lymphoma involving skin)**：这种淋巴瘤常常累及真皮和皮下组织，CD56呈阳性，EBV呈阳性，但没有TCR基因重排。
3. **皮肤γδ T细胞淋巴瘤(cutaneous γδ T-cell lymphoma)**：淋巴瘤皮下浸润灶可能不易与皮下脂膜炎样T细胞淋巴瘤鉴别，但在真皮中部和深层常常可见围血管和附属器累及。根据定义，表达γδ-TCR，CD56常常呈阳性[1098]。这种淋巴瘤呈高度侵袭性。
4. **外周T细胞淋巴瘤，非特指(peripheral T-cell lymphoma unspecified)**：以下特征倾向于诊断皮下脂膜炎样T细胞淋巴瘤而不是外周T细胞淋巴瘤（非特指）伴有皮肤累及：淋巴瘤浸润局限于皮下组织伴有轻微真皮受累，皮下组织中缎带样结构浸润不融合，部分脂肪空隙周围出现淋巴瘤细胞环，具有细胞毒性表型[980]。

间变大细胞淋巴瘤（ALCL），T或裸细胞型，原发系统性
Anaplastic large cell lymphoma (ALCL), T or null cell type, primary systemic form

定义

间变大细胞淋巴瘤(ALCL)是一种CD30$^+$的淋巴瘤，来源于T细胞或裸细胞，特点是细胞体积大，具有丰富的胞浆，也会出现小细胞组成的变型[1107-1111]。原发系统性的特点是原始发生且主要是播散性疾病，常累及淋巴结和结外部位。合并其他淋巴瘤的类型，如蕈样霉菌病和Lennert淋巴瘤（继发型），不包括在这种类别中。如果淋巴瘤由间变大细胞组成，但显示其他独特淋巴瘤类型的临床病理学特征（如肠病型T细胞淋巴瘤），也不包括在内。

裸细胞型是T细胞类型谱系的一部分，因为二者均表达细胞毒性标记物且通过敏感的PCR技术均常常能检测到TCR基因重排[1112-1114]。如果肿瘤表达B细胞系标记物，则将其归入弥漫大B细胞淋巴瘤[36,1115]。

CD30是一种活化标记物[1116]，可表达于滤泡旁淋巴细胞群、多种反应性病变中活化的淋巴细胞、Hodgkin淋巴瘤和某些非Hodgkin淋巴瘤。CD30呈阳性本身不足以将淋巴瘤归类为间变大细胞淋巴瘤，因为各种淋巴瘤类型中散在的肿瘤大细胞均可呈CD30阳性，有些普通的B或T细胞的大细胞淋巴瘤可显示广泛的CD30染色。

临床特征

原发性系统性ALCL的特点是发病年龄呈双峰分布，一个峰在青少年和年轻成人，另一个峰在老年人[1107-1110,1117-1124]。较常发生于男性。

临床表现非常不一致。除了淋巴结肿大，还常常出现结外部位如皮肤、骨、软组织和胃肠道发病。如果皮肤受累，还可见到皮肤外的额外部位受累。有些患者表现为淋巴网状系统弥漫受累，伴有或不伴有反应性噬血综合征，类似于恶性组织细胞增生症。

形态学评估发现，骨髓受累的发生率为10%~17%，但如果在骨髓活检中采用CD30免疫组化，则高达36%的病例能显示造血细胞之间散在的肿瘤细胞[1125,1126]。骨髓受累与预后较差有关[1126]。

肿瘤呈侵袭性，但应用多种药物化疗可达到完全缓解而获得良好的预后。根据非Hodgkin淋巴瘤分类方案，5年总体生存率为77%，在各种淋巴瘤生存率排位中列于生存率最好的结外边缘区B细胞淋巴瘤之后，居第二位[264]。生存率优于弥漫大B细胞淋巴瘤和其他外周T细胞淋巴瘤。

根据间变性淋巴瘤激酶（ALK）重新定义间变大细胞淋巴瘤
Redefining ALCL based on expression of anaplastic lymphoma kinase (ALK)

随着 ALCL 细胞遗传学标记物 t(2;5) 的发现以及对相关基因（*NPM* 和 *ALK*）的了解，有证据表明，表达间变性淋巴瘤激酶（ALK）蛋白的 ALCL 构成一个独特的种群[1115,1127-1137]，称为"间变大细胞淋巴瘤，T/裸细胞性，原发系统型，ALK$^+$"，或使用首字母缩略语"ALKoma"[1127]。它们属于同源性病变，具有以下特征[1114,1115,1128,1131,1138]：

- 年轻、单一年龄高峰在30岁以下。由双峰年龄分布组成的全部原发系统性间变大细胞淋巴瘤实际上是由发生在年轻患者（中位年龄17岁）的 ALK$^+$ 组和发生于老年患者（中位年龄60岁）的 ALK$^-$ 组混合组成。
- 患者有原发系统性疾病，但不是原发皮肤疾病。
- 常表达EMA，不伴有EBV感染。
- 预后很好。对于 ALK$^+$ 组，中位生存期为165个月，而对于 ALK$^-$ 组，则中位生存期为35个月。两组的5年生存率分别为72%和30%。累及 ALK 基因的各种染色体易位病例其行为与显示 t(2;5) 的病例一样[1130]。根据国际预后指数，可进一步将患者分为不同的预后组[1128]。白血病播散与预后差有关[1139]。

因此重要的是要识别 ALCL 中的 ALK$^+$ 组，因其预后非常好。在识别该组时，免疫组化优于分子学分析，因为方法简单且较敏感：ALK 免疫反应可见于累及 *ALK* 的各种易位，而配体不局限于 *NPM*。

ALK 免疫组化作为 ALK$^+$ 组 ALCL 的标记物其形态学谱系已被扩展。有些以前不被认识的例子（常常归类为非特指外周 T 细胞淋巴瘤）现在根据 ALK 免疫反应明确归为 ALCL。其良好的预后证实了这种重新分类的正确性，因为外周 T 细胞淋巴瘤预后很差。

事实上，对于非间变表现的淋巴组织肿瘤（如小细胞或混合细胞型），如果 ALK 阳性，应该诊断为 ALCL。对于形态学类似 ALCL 而缺乏 ALK 表达的病例，鉴别 ALCL 和非特指外周 T 细胞淋巴瘤是困难的，这也仅仅是个称谓问题，因为 ALK$^-$ 的 ALCL 和非特指外周 T 细胞淋巴瘤的行为极其相似[1140]。

病理学

ALCL 累及整个或部分淋巴结。相当一部分病例的

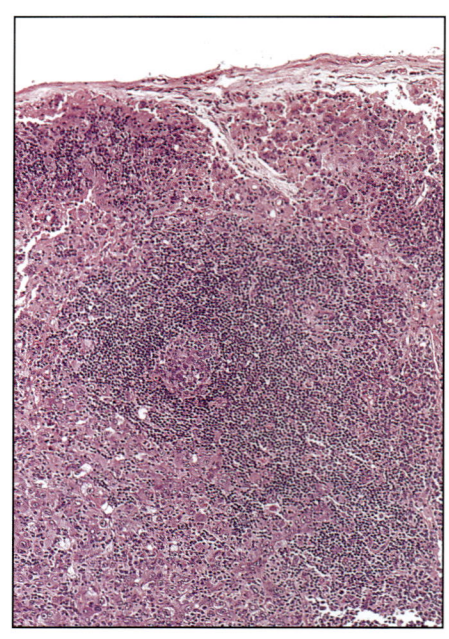

图21A.132　间变大细胞淋巴瘤，T细胞型，原发系统性。淋巴结典型地显示淋巴窦受累，也可见到副皮质区受累。

特征是明显累及或主要累及淋巴窦（图 21A.132）。淋巴结副皮质或滤泡周区域轻微受累的病例容易被漏诊。淋巴瘤细胞呈单个散在分布或形成灶状或片状，类似于癌的生长方式。**标志细胞**（hallmark cell）是特征性的，但不是 ALK$^+$ 病例所特有（图 21A.133）[1127]。下面列出的变型中标志细胞数量不等，表现为大细胞，核呈偏心胚芽状或肾形，丰富的胞浆中可见独特的嗜酸性高尔基区和多个小核仁。

常见被膜和实质纤维化[1108,1109,1114]。在有些病例，可见宽的纤维带，类似于结节硬化型 Hodgkin 淋巴瘤[1141]。

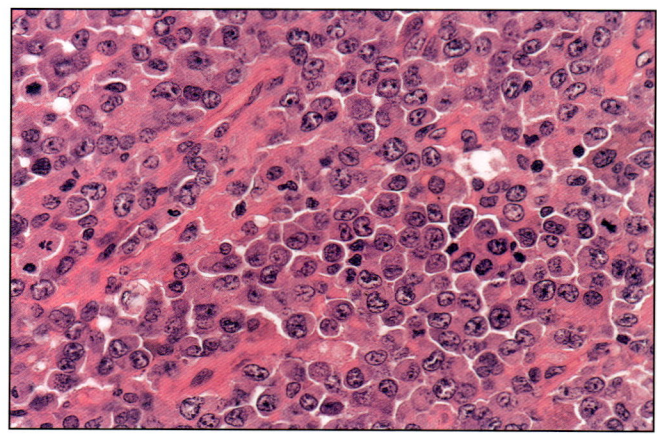

图21A.133　间变大细胞淋巴瘤，ALK呈阳性，普通型。该视野显示许多标志性细胞。

肿瘤细胞常与多种反应细胞混杂很常见，如小淋巴细胞、浆细胞、组织细胞、嗜酸性粒细胞和中性粒细胞[1142,1143]。

有些 ALCL 变型（ALK⁺ 或 ALK⁻）已被识别。某一病例在相同或不同淋巴结内可显示两种或多种变型特征，并且某种类型在反复活检时可进展为另一种类型。到目前为止，这些变型尚未显示有预后意义。

普通型（common type）：这种类型符合 ALCL 的经典描述。由大的（或很大的）细胞组成，核圆形或马蹄形。可见呈花环样排列的多核细胞或 Reed-Sternberg 样细胞。核仁通常为多个而不是单个，一般不是很大。胞浆呈嗜双色性至嗜碱性，常常可见淡染的核旁区域（图 21A.133、21A.134 和 21A.135）。

单一形态型（monomorphic variant）：这种变型的特点是中到大细胞，细胞形态、大小一致，呈单一性表现（图 21A.136）。通常可见一些标志性细胞。

淋巴组织细胞型（lymphohistiocytic variant）：在小淋巴细胞和奇异形组织细胞背景中，可见散在的中等至大的肿瘤细胞，染色质粗大或空泡状，核仁小而明显，胞浆嗜碱性，类似免疫母细胞。组织细胞呈卵圆形，核圆形、偏心，胞浆丰富嗜酸性，表面上类似浆细胞（图 21A.137）[1127,1129,1144-1146]。在常规组织学切片中，难以识别肿瘤细胞巢，因此这种变型常常被误诊为反应性淋巴结病。通过 CD30 或 ALK 免疫染色能很好地显示肿瘤细胞。

小细胞型（small cell variant）：这种变型的特点是具有许多 CD30 阴性的、核明显不规则的小 T 淋巴细胞以及少数 CD30⁺ 的较大细胞群[1127,1128,1147]。较大细胞易于形成血管周袖套；这种 ALK⁺ ALCL 的高度典型特征可为正确诊断提供重要的组织学线索（图 21A.138, 21A.139）。小细胞和大细胞均为肿瘤性，但仅仅后者表达 CD30。ALK 表

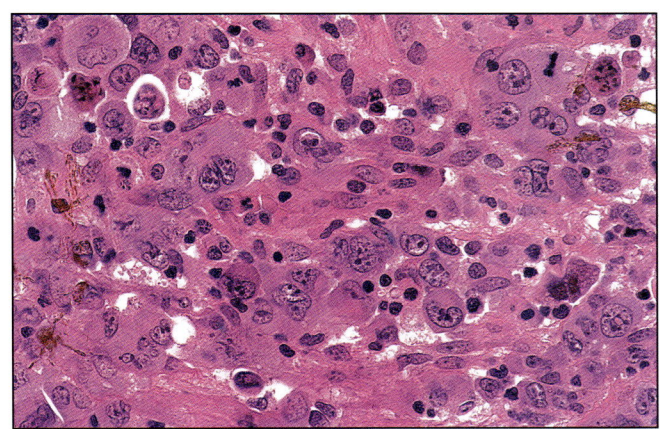

图 21A.134 间变大细胞淋巴瘤，ALK 阳性，普通型。肿瘤性大细胞具有丰富的嗜双色性胞浆和明显的高尔基区。有些核呈胚胎样。

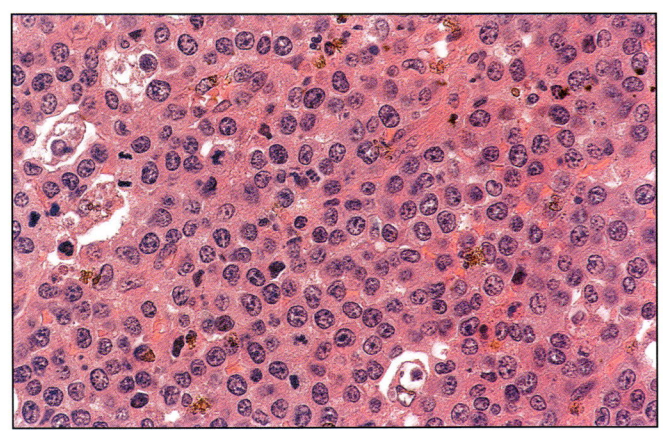

图 21A.136 间变大细胞淋巴瘤，ALK 阳性，单一形态型。细胞为中到大细胞，形态一致。与普通的大细胞淋巴瘤鉴别困难。偶尔可见标志性细胞。

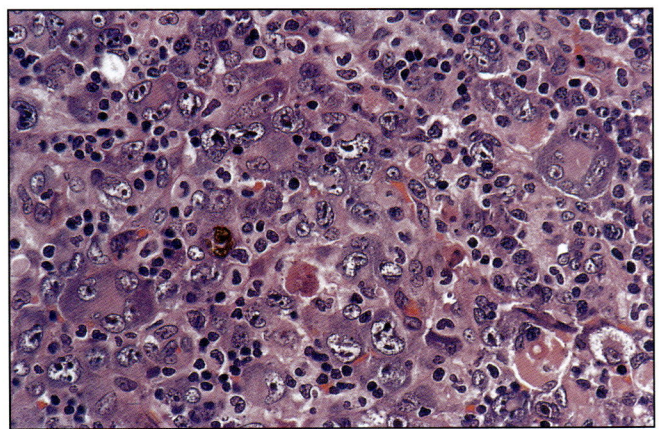

图 21A.135 间变大细胞淋巴瘤，ALK 阳性，普通型。肿瘤大细胞具有嗜双色性胞浆和明显的高尔基区，有些细胞显示花环样核。

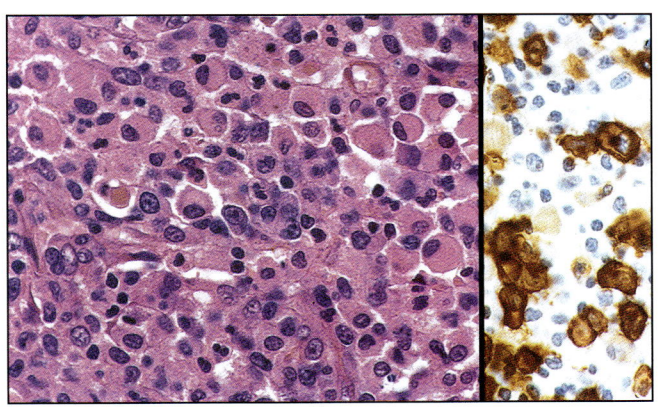

图 21A.137 间变大细胞淋巴瘤，ALK 阳性，淋巴组织细胞型。左侧：肿瘤细胞难以识别：中等到大的细胞，具有明显核仁。背景富于小淋巴细胞和奇异形组织细胞。右侧：CD30 免疫染色显示大量常规显微镜下看不清的肿瘤细胞。

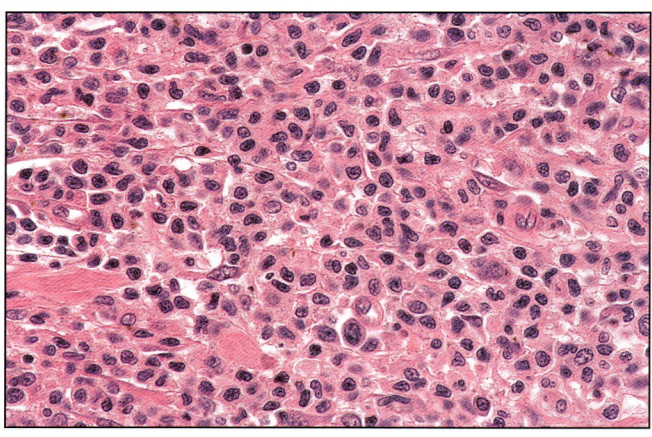

图21A.138　间变大细胞淋巴瘤，ALK阳性，小细胞型。小细胞具有不规则的核，偶尔混合有大的母细胞。根据形态学难以与非特指外周T细胞淋巴瘤鉴别。

达于大细胞，小细胞不表达或仅仅微弱表达。

24%的病例在1～146个月之后可转化为单一形态或普通型ALCL。转化的发生提示临床过程进展加速，75%的患者死于1年内。免疫表型没有变化，可能发生了其他遗传学改变[1148]。

混合细胞型（mixed cell variant）：混合细胞型有别于小细胞型之处仅仅在于可见数量较多的中等到大的细胞（图21A.140A）。不依靠ALK免疫染色很难与非特指外周T细胞淋巴瘤鉴别。

细胞减少型（hypocelluler variant）：淋巴结显示细胞成分减少，小到中等大小的淋巴细胞之间间隔增宽，由

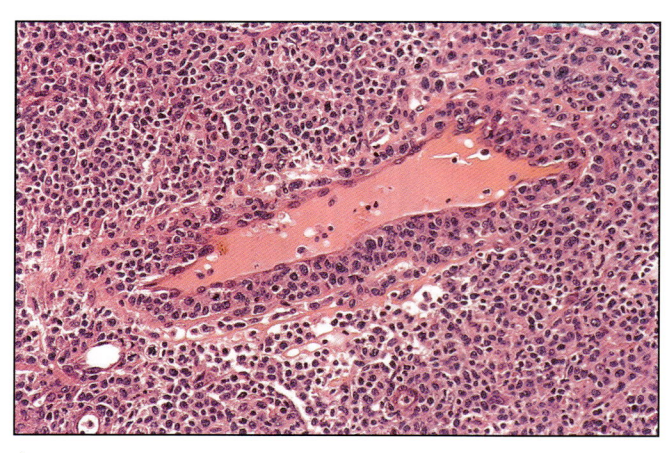
A

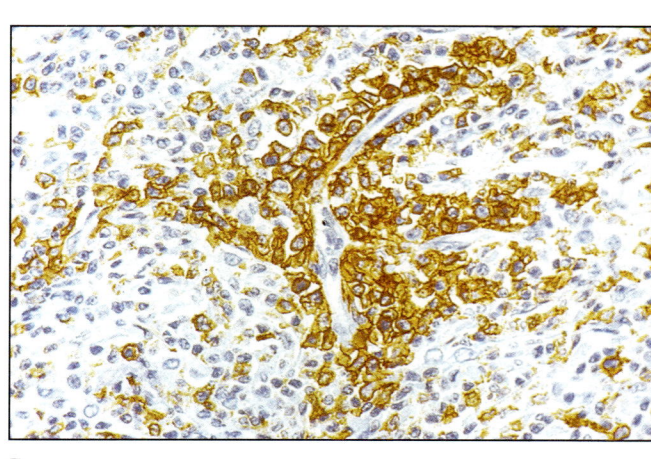
B

图21A.139　间变大细胞淋巴瘤，ALK阳性，小细胞型。（A）小静脉周围的大淋巴细胞袖套对于识别这种淋巴瘤类型、排除反应性淋巴组织增生是极其有用的指标。（B）CD30免疫染色显示血管周袖套中的较大细胞。

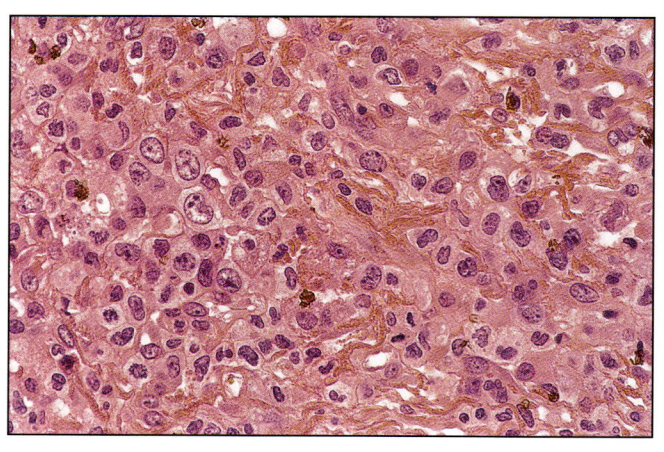
A

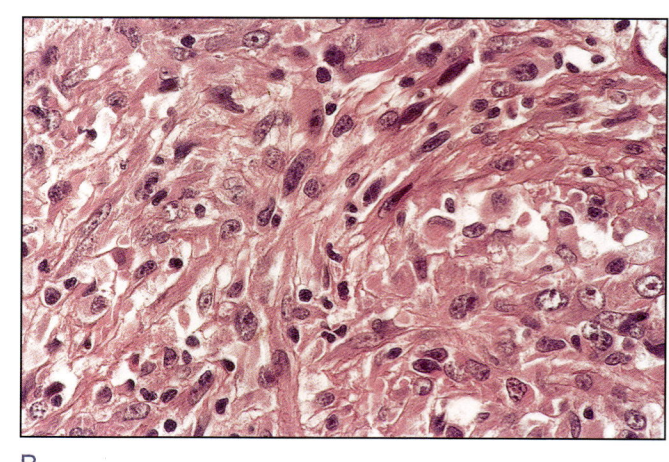
B

图21A.140　间变大细胞淋巴瘤。（A）混合细胞型。可见大小、形状不等的细胞。如果没有免疫组化支持，很难与非特指外周T细胞淋巴瘤鉴别。（B）肉瘤样型。丰满的梭形细胞可被误诊为肉瘤细胞。

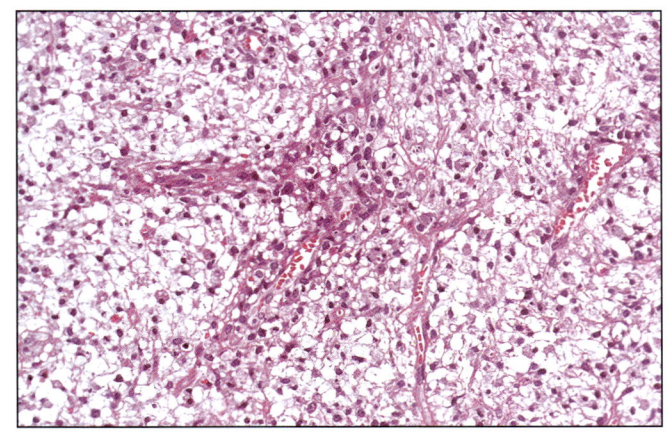

图21A.141 间变大细胞淋巴瘤，细胞减少型。淋巴瘤显示水肿、血管增加和组织细胞浸润，类似于肉芽组织，然而许多细胞实际上是淋巴瘤细胞。这种独特的组织学结构高度提示间变大细胞淋巴瘤。

丰富的水肿或纤维黏液样间质取代（图21A.141）。可见散在的组织细胞和肿瘤性梭形细胞，形成广泛的短束。具有非典型核的大细胞常常稀少，常常形成小静脉周围袖套。事实上，肉芽组织样间质如此明显，可为正确诊断ALCL提供首要线索，尤其是对于发生于儿童的各种特殊淋巴组织病变[1149]。

巨细胞型（giant cell varint）：这种少见变型的特点是出现许多多形性、奇异形的大细胞和多核肿瘤细胞。仅有1/3的病例表达ALK[1128]。

肉瘤样型（sarcomatoid variant）：少数由梭形细胞组成的病例可出现席纹状或黏液样生长结构（图21A.140B）[1150]。

免疫细胞化学

1. T细胞型表达T细胞系标记物。然而CD3常常呈阴性，可能需要使用多种T细胞标记物（如CD45RO、CD4、CD2、LAT、CD43）证实T细胞系。裸细胞型不表达T和B细胞系标记物。
2. 所有或大多数肿瘤细胞CD30呈阳性（图21A.142A），除非小细胞变型，其中仅有较大的细胞呈阳性（图21A.139）。EMA通常呈阳性（～80%）[1151]。大约50%～80%的病例表达ALK。ALK染色常常同时见于核和胞浆，但单纯胞浆染色见于15%的病例（图21A.142B）。因为正常或反应性淋巴细胞全部呈ALK阴性，出现任何ALK$^+$细胞均有意义[1127,1129,1130]。T细胞型和裸细胞型常常表达细胞毒性标记物（60%～80%），但这种特征不具有预后意义[1113,1131,1152-1154]。丛生蛋白（clusterin）免疫反应（着

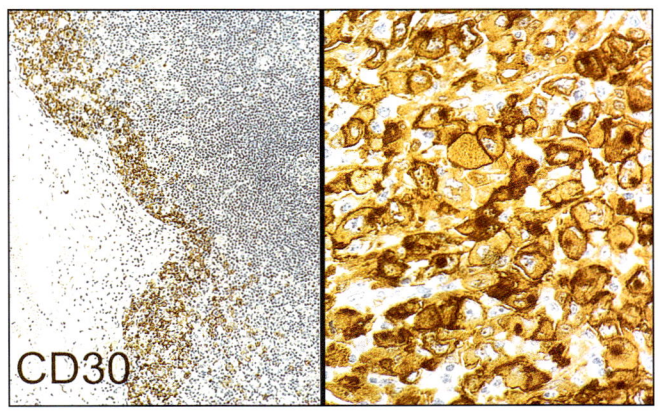

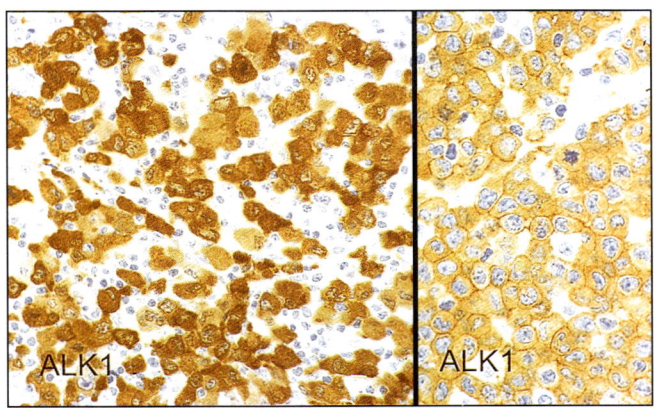

图21A.142 原发系统性间变大细胞淋巴瘤的免疫染色。（A）左侧：CD30染色常常显示肿瘤分布在淋巴窦。右侧：另一例显示弥漫性生长，肿瘤细胞显示细胞膜和高尔基区CD30染色。（B）左侧：ALK染色通常同时位于核和胞浆。右侧：少数病例的染色局限于胞浆。这种现象通常由ALK与NPM之外基因配体的多种易位引起。

染Golgi体）见于＞90%的病例，这种标记物很少表达于其他淋巴瘤类型[1155-1157]。

3. PAX-5总是呈阴性。活化标记物如HLA-DR和CD25常常呈阳性[1110,1151]。部分病例可表达CD15[1151,1158]。多数病例表达CD4，但有些病例表达CD8。TCR为γδ或αβ型[1152]。皮肤淋巴细胞抗原（HECA452）通常呈阴性。有些病例表达CD56，与预后较差有关[1159]。
4. 相当一部分病例（38%）缺乏CD45RB表达[1151,1160,1161]。更复杂的是少数病例细胞角蛋白阳性[1161]。因此这种大细胞肿瘤的淋巴组织本质可能被误解，即使是在免疫组化评估时。

遗传学特征

TCR基因克隆性重排仅见于60%～70%的病例，高达10%的病例同时显示Ig重链基因重排[18]。但是，应用敏感的PCR技术，近100%的病例可检测到TCR基

因克隆性重排[1112]。

有些 ALCL 显示特征性的染色体异常 t(2;5)(p23;q35)[1121,1162]。引起 5q35 上的 *NPM*（核磷蛋白）与 1p23 上的 *ALK*（间变性淋巴瘤激酶）连接[14,15,1114,1163,1164]。正常情况下淋巴细胞不表达 ALK，发生 t(2;5) 易位的 ALCL 可使 ALK 与 NPM 基因融合而促使其表达，产生嵌合型蛋白组成性激活 ALK 结构域，后者对这种淋巴瘤类型的发生起关键作用。

有些病例显示涉及 *ALK* 基因与其他配体基因融合的多种易位，这些基因广泛表达于淋巴细胞或许多细胞类型中[1165-1171]：

- t(1;2)(q25;p23)中的 *TPM3*（原肌球蛋白-III 基因）
- t(2;19)(p23;p13)中的 *TPM4*（原肌球蛋白-IV 基因）
- t(2;3)(p23;q21)中的 *TFG*（TRK 融合基因）
- inv (2)(p23;q35)中的 *ATIC*
- t(2;22)(p23;q11.2)中的 *CLTL*
- t(X;2)(q11-12;p23)中的 *MSN*（膜突蛋白）
- t(2;11;2)(p23;p15;q31)中的 *CARS*
- t(2;22)(p23;q11.2)中的 *MYH9*

但是最终结果是相似的，可见 ALK 蛋白表达和组成性激活。这些病例的 ALK 蛋白免疫染色通常显示单纯的胞浆或细胞膜染色（除了 *CLTL/ALK* 融合病例，其显示颗粒状染色），与携带 t(2;5) 者不同，后者显示核与胞浆染色[1130]。

基因表达谱研究显示，ALK⁺ ALCL 中具有编码信号转导分子（*SYK*、*LYN*、*CDC37*）的基因过表达和转录因子基因（包括 *HOXC6* 和 *HOXA3*）低表达，不同于 ALK⁻ ALCL。两组均有类似的激酶（*LCK*、蛋白激酶 C、vav2 和 *NKIAMRE*）和抗凋亡分子高表达[1172]。比较基因组杂交研究显示，虽然 ALK⁺ ALCL 显示少数可重复性染色体失衡，但 ALK⁻ ALCL 显示 1q41-qter 可重复性染色体获得（46%），以及 6q21（31%）和 13q21-q22（23%）的缺失[1173]。

虽然来自印度的一项研究报告，EBV 与原发系统性 ALCL 具有相关性[1174]，但其他研究尚未发现这种相关性[1131,1175]。

鉴别诊断

1. **转移癌或黑色素瘤**（metastatic carcinoma or melanoma）：ALCL 的窦隙生长方式可导致误诊为转移癌。若患者年轻，一定要考虑 ALCL，尤其是当肿瘤细胞显示丰富的嗜双色性胞浆并伴有明显的高尔基区时。
2. **Hodgkin 淋巴瘤**（Hodgkin's lymphoma）：见"淋巴组织增生性病变诊断的实践问题"（第 1250 页）。
3. **组织细胞肉瘤和恶性组织细胞增生症**（histiocytic sarcoma and malignant histiocytosis）。
4. **反应性淋巴组织增生**（reactive lymphoid hyperplasia）：有些 ALCL 患者由于缺乏大的淋巴瘤细胞，可被误诊为反应性淋巴结病。正确诊断的三个重要线索是患者年龄小、血管周袖套状大细胞以及可见肉芽组织样纤维黏液间质[1176]。

原发性皮肤间变大细胞淋巴瘤（ALCL），T 或裸细胞型
Primary cutaneous anaplastic large cell lymphoma (ALCL), T-or null-cell type

定义

原发性皮肤间变大细胞淋巴瘤（ALCL），T 或裸细胞型，其特点是在皮肤发病，诊断时没有先前存在的淋巴瘤或皮肤外播散的证据。属于原发性皮肤 T 细胞/裸细胞 CD30⁺ 淋巴组织增生性疾病范畴[980,1114,1177]。

临床特征

患者大多为成人，平均发病年龄为 49 岁，常常表现为孤立皮肤结节，少数病例可为多发皮肤结节[1177-1179]。较大的病变可为溃疡性。18%～44% 的病例可自发消退。疾病常常局限，皮肤复发率为 36%。预后很好，5 年累计生存率为 90%。预后良好的因素包括自发消退、年龄小于 60 岁以及缺乏皮肤外播散[1178-1180]。

病理学所见

真皮和（或）皮下组织可见片状淋巴瘤大细胞弥漫浸润，胞浆丰富。肿瘤细胞类似于普通型原发系统性 ALCL，虽然其常常显示程度较高的核多形性（图 21A.143）。但是，有些病例的细胞学特征与普通型大细胞淋巴瘤相同。被覆的表皮显示增生、溃疡或淋巴瘤细胞浸润。有些病例富于中性粒细胞[1142]。

免疫细胞化学

1. 在 T 细胞病例，T 细胞系标记物呈阳性，但在裸细胞病例则呈阴性。B 细胞系标记物呈阴性。
2. CD30 呈阳性，细胞毒性分子常常呈阳性。ALK 呈阴性。大约半数病例丛生蛋白呈阳性[1155]。
3. T 细胞病例常常 CD4⁺。约半数病例表达皮肤淋巴细胞抗原 HECA452。EMA 不常表达（0～28%）[1181]。

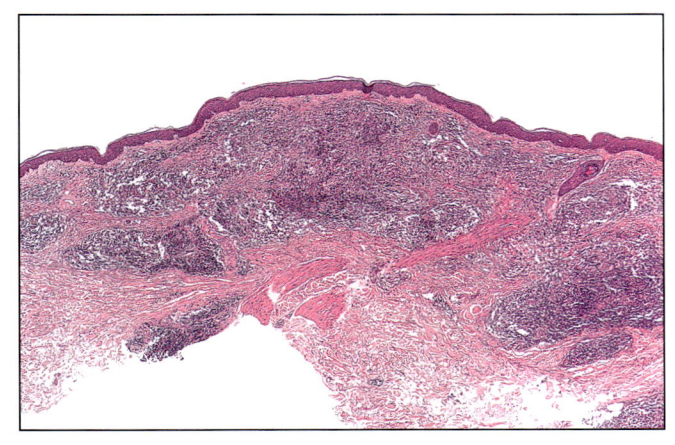
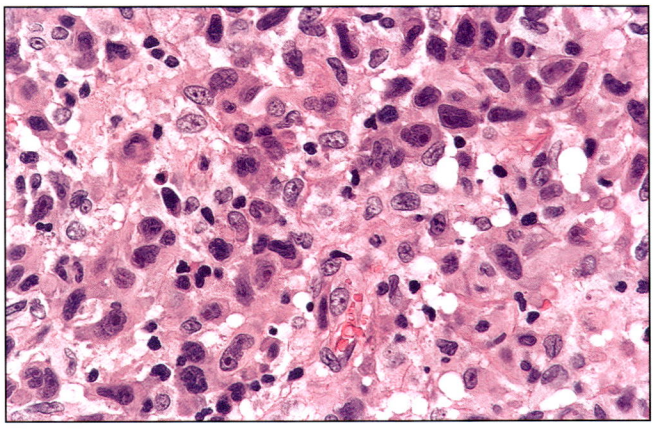

图21A.143 原发性皮肤间变大细胞淋巴瘤。（A）可见致密的真皮浸润。（B）浸润灶由间变淋巴细胞组成。

遗传学特征

TCR 基因重排。很少见到原发系统性 ALCL 典型的 t(2;5) 易位。EBV 呈阴性。

原发性皮肤T细胞/裸细胞CD30⁺的淋巴组织增生性病变谱系
The spectrum of primary cutaneous T-/null-cell CD30⁺ lymphoproliferative disorders

原发性皮肤 T 细胞 / 裸细胞 CD30⁺ 的淋巴组织增生性病变构成一个系列性病变，特点是病变完全局限于皮肤至少 6 个月，增生的淋巴组织富于 CD30⁺ 的大细胞，常常可自发消退[1177,1180,1182-1184]。已有提示，自发性消退可能是由同时表达 CD30 和 CD30 配基的淋巴细胞介导，CD30 配基对 CD30⁺ 细胞起到抗增生作用[1185]。淋巴瘤样丘疹病、原发性皮肤 ALCL 和交界性病变属于这种淋巴组织增生性病变谱系。这一概念也可应用于发生在口腔的类似病变[1186]。

淋巴瘤样丘疹病 (lymphomatoid papulosis)：是反复发作的自限性皮疹，可表现为片状，但 4% ～ 10% 的病例最终可发生播散性淋巴瘤[1180]。组织学上，可见真皮浅层楔形浸润或浅表和深部血管周浸润的 CD30⁺ 间变性大淋巴细胞，混合有许多炎细胞。有不同程度的亲表皮性。可见单克隆性 T 细胞群，但这种病变一般不被认为是淋巴瘤形式[1187]。

交界性病变 (borderline lesions)：介于淋巴瘤样丘疹病和原发性皮肤 ALCL 特征之间（如在病变中可见某些大片的 CD30⁺ 大细胞，其他特点与淋巴瘤样丘疹病相同），或临床和组织学特征不一致（如临床特征为淋巴瘤样丘疹病，但组织学检查有皮下受累证据）。自发消退比例高达 78%。5 年累计生存率为 100%[1178]。

鉴别诊断

1. **原发系统性ALCL** (primary systemic ALCL)：鉴别诊断必须考虑临床特征，如果肿瘤细胞对ALK有免疫反应，则必须慎重考虑以皮肤为首发的原发系统性ALCL。
2. **蕈样霉菌病大细胞转化** (large cell transformation of mycosis fungoides)。
3. **CD30阴性的原发皮肤外周T细胞淋巴瘤** (primary cutaneous peripheral T-cell lymphoma，CD30⁻ negtive)：对于原发皮肤T细胞或裸细胞大细胞淋巴瘤，重要的是确定CD30的状况。不考虑形态学，CD30表达与良好的预后有关，而缺乏CD30表达与差的预后有关[1183,1188]。

HTLV1⁺的成人T细胞淋巴瘤/白血病
Adult T-cell lymphoma/leukemia, HTLV1⁺

更详细的描述见第 22 章。有几种变型：急性、淋巴瘤性、慢性和冒烟型（smoldering）[1189]。后两者的预后比前两者的好。在有些冒烟型病例，淋巴结可显示 Hodgkin 样组织学表现：副皮质区因小到中等大淋巴细胞浸润而扩张，核轻度不规则，混杂有表达 CD30 和 CD15 的 Reed-Sternberg 样细胞[1190]。

根据形态学难以区分成人 T 细胞淋巴瘤/白血病和非特指外周 T 细胞淋巴瘤（图 21A.144A）。当出现以下某些特征时，应考虑前者：

- 患者来自日本、加勒比地区或巴西
- 出现皮肤病变
- 高钙血症
- 溶骨性病变
- 血循环中有"花形"细胞（图21A.144B）

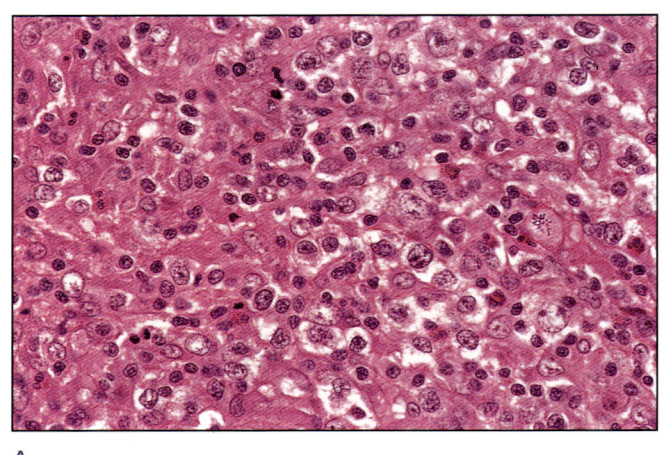
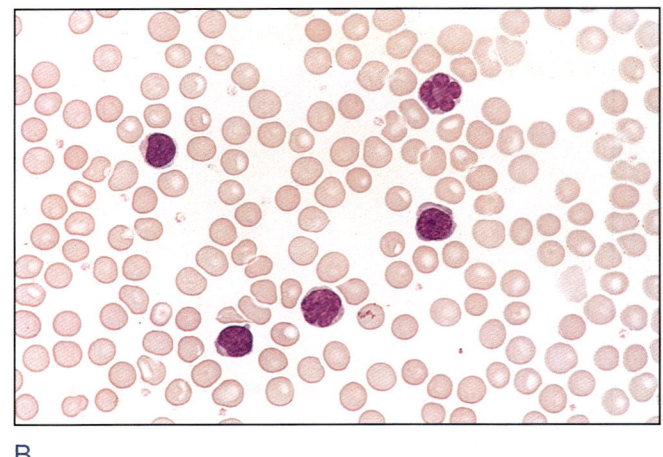

图21A.144 成人T细胞淋巴瘤/白血病。（A）淋巴结活检所见常常难以归类，类似非特指普通外周T细胞淋巴瘤。（B）血中可见循环性异常淋巴细胞，有些具有花形外观。

- CD25阳性。

最常见的免疫表型是 CD2⁺、CD3⁺、CD5⁺、CD7⁻、CD4⁺、CD8⁻、CD25⁺。大细胞可表达 CD30。成人T细胞淋巴瘤/白血病的诊断需要显示 HTLV-1 原病毒 DNA 单克隆性整合，如果病毒血清学呈阳性，则可作出假设诊断[980]。认识成人T细胞淋巴瘤/白血病的重要性在于：这是一种高度侵袭性肿瘤，并且有些病例可能对抗病毒加干扰素治疗有反应。

结外NK/T细胞淋巴瘤
Extranodal NK/T-cell lymphoma

定义

这是一种所谓的NK细胞淋巴瘤，几乎总是出现在淋巴结外部位。之所以称为"NK/T"是因为：一部分病例明显为细胞毒性T细胞而不是NK细胞来源。血管中心性和血管破坏性生长明显，因此在REAL分类中，这种病变被称为"血管中心性淋巴瘤"[1191-1196]。少数报告显示，NK/T细胞淋巴瘤可原发于淋巴结[1038,1197]。

临床特征和行为

NK/T细胞淋巴瘤多发生于成人，中位发病年龄为53岁，好发于男性。鼻型和鼻外型分别占病例的2/3和1/3[1191,1198-1202]。

NK/T细胞淋巴瘤在亚洲人、墨西哥人和南美洲人的发病率比在西方人高。与在成人不同，儿童和年轻人病例常发生在各种EBV相关疾病之后，如慢性活动性EBV感染，蚊子叮咬后过敏，病毒相关性噬血综合征，以及牛痘样水疱样皮疹[1203]。NK/T细胞淋巴瘤也可发生于实性器官移植受者，作为移植后淋巴组织增生性疾病的一种形式[1204-1206]。

鼻型NK/T细胞淋巴瘤 (nasal NK/T-cell lymphoma)：出现在鼻腔、鼻咽部或上呼吸消化道其他部位，不同程度地蔓延至鼻旁窦、眼眶、口腔、上颚和口咽。可见广泛破坏性/溃疡性病变（颜面中部破坏性疾病或所谓的"致死性中线肉芽肿"）或肿物性病变。大多数患者发病时处于早期。有些病例可并发噬血综合征[1207]。即使经过联合治疗，也常发生局部或系统性复发（好发部位为皮肤、肝、胃肠道和睾丸）。单独放疗或之前与化疗联合可以获得最好的效果[1208-1210]。常规联合化疗的治疗结果令人失望，可能与NK/T细胞淋巴瘤常常表达多耐药基因有关[1211]。最近，依托泊苷（etoposide）和L-门冬酰胺酶作为化疗药物已显示对这种淋巴瘤类型具有一定前景[1212,1213]。在回顾性研究中，完全缓解率为60%～80%，5年总体生存率通常为40%左右[1200,1214,1215]。有些近期研究显示，5年生存率为80%左右[1208,1216]。

鼻外型NK/T细胞淋巴瘤 (extranasal NK/T-cell lymphoma)：表现为淋巴结外疾病，常常累及多个解剖部位，通常没有浅表淋巴结肿大。好发于皮肤、胃肠道、

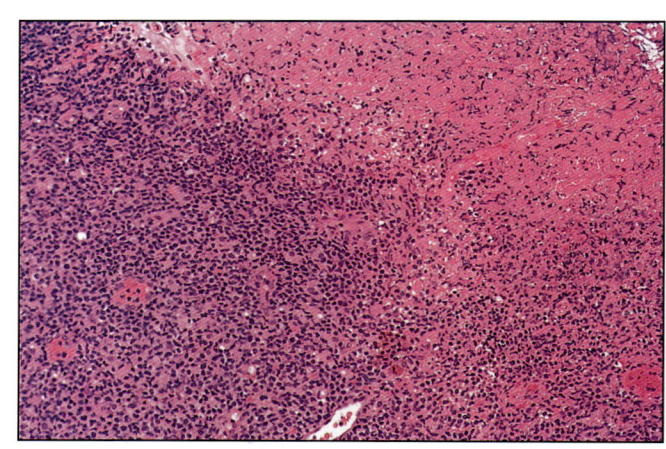

图21A.145 鼻型NK/T细胞淋巴瘤。淋巴瘤通常显示明显坏死。

睾丸和软组织。多数患者发病时疾病为Ⅲ期或Ⅳ期，常见系统性症状。有些患者在发病时或终末期，可并发噬血综合征[1207]。疾病呈高度侵袭性过程，对治疗反应差，复发早，死亡早。大多数患者6个月内死于疾病。2年总体生存率仅为20%[1199]。

病理学所见

最典型的特征是：溃疡组织伴有致密的异常淋巴细胞集聚，大片坏死累及肿瘤组织和未受累组织(图21A.145)[1191,1217]。

细胞学谱系广泛：(1) 小细胞，核不规则折叠，有角或呈卷曲状，染色质相当致密或呈颗粒状，核仁不清楚；(2) 中等大小的细胞，核圆形或折叠形，染色质颗粒状，核仁小；以及 (3) 大细胞，染色质呈空泡状或颗粒状，核仁清楚。肿瘤细胞常常具有中等量透明或淡染胞浆（图21A.146）。细胞组成可呈混合性。在Giemsa染色的细胞学涂片，胞浆可见嗜苯胺蓝颗粒。常常可见散在的凋亡小体和炎症细胞。

表面鳞状上皮可显示活跃的假上皮瘤样增生，类似于鳞状细胞癌（图21A.147）。鼻腔/鼻咽部黏膜内陷的黏膜腺体常常显示特殊的透明细胞变，可能是由于淋巴瘤细胞释放的细胞溶解分子引起细胞病变所造成。淋巴瘤细胞常常浸润表面上皮细胞和黏膜腺体。在皮肤，浸润常常围绕血管和皮肤附属器，但有些病例显示弥漫性真皮浸润；常累及皮下。

常见血管中心性和血管破坏性生长。血管中心性是指肿瘤细胞易于围绕血管或聚集于血管内，伴有血管壁浸润和破坏（图21A.148）。仅有血管周袖套或血管陷入成片的淋巴瘤浸润灶内表现者不足以使用这种名称。常常可见纤维素样坏死和血管弹力层断裂，伴有血管闭塞。

免疫细胞化学

1. NK/T细胞淋巴瘤最典型的免疫表型是：CD2[+]、

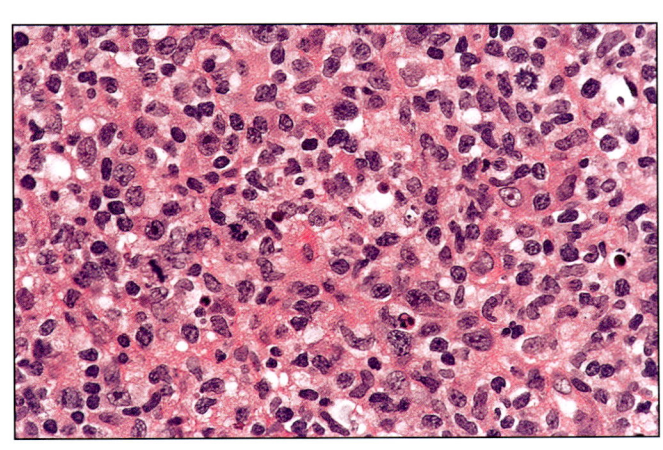

A

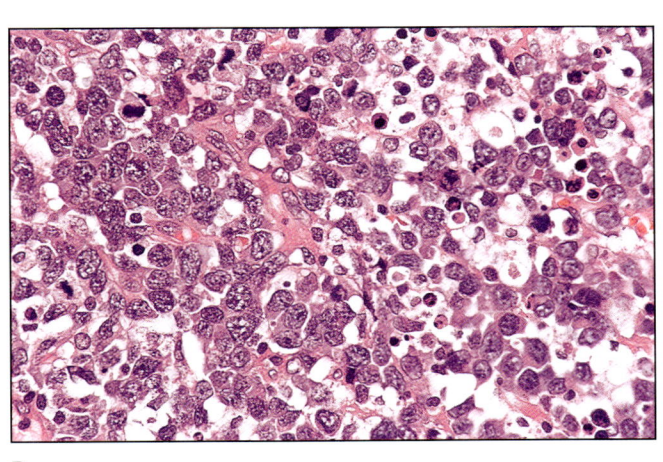

B

图21A.146　鼻型NK/T细胞淋巴瘤。这种淋巴瘤类型可显示宽广的形态学谱系。(A) 以中等细胞为主的病例，核常常拉长或不规则折叠，染色质颗粒状。混合一些核仁清楚的较大细胞。(B) 一例以大细胞为主的病例。可见明显的凋亡小体，常常是这种淋巴瘤的特点。

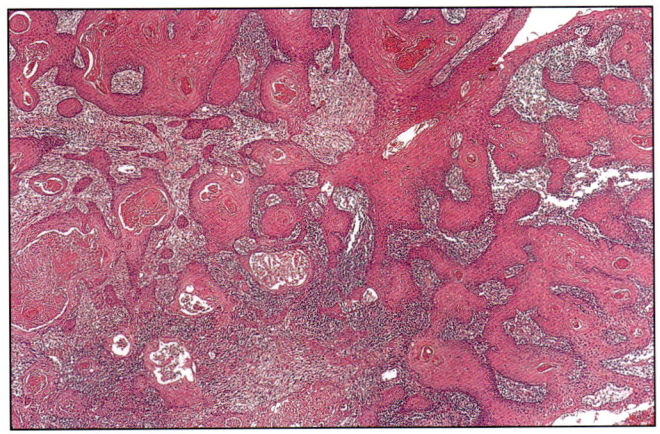

图21A.147　鼻型NK/T细胞淋巴瘤。此病例伴有增生活跃的鳞状上皮，类似于鳞状细胞癌。

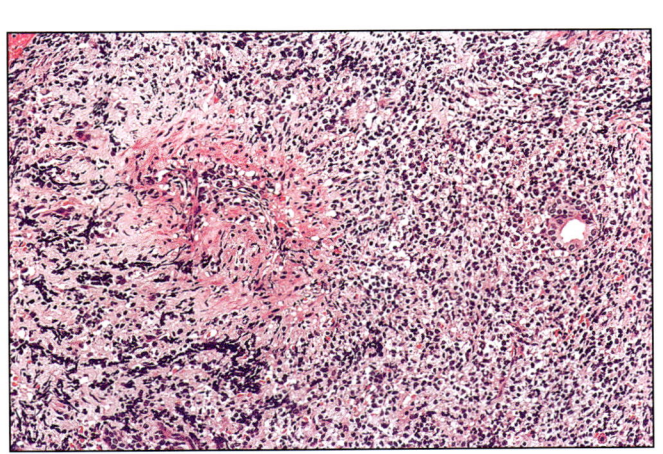

图21A.148　鼻型NK/T细胞淋巴瘤。左侧视野可见血管壁浸润。血管中心性-血管破坏性生长方式是其特征，但并非NK/T细胞淋巴瘤所特有。

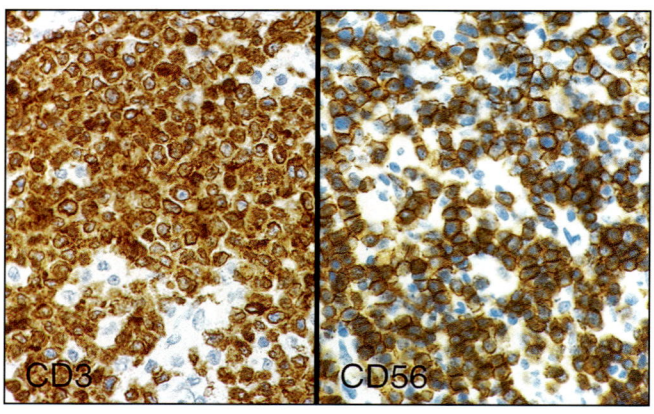

图21A.149 鼻型NK/T细胞淋巴瘤的免疫染色。左侧：在石蜡切片上，淋巴瘤细胞通常呈CD3阳性。右侧：细胞膜表达NK细胞标记物CD56。

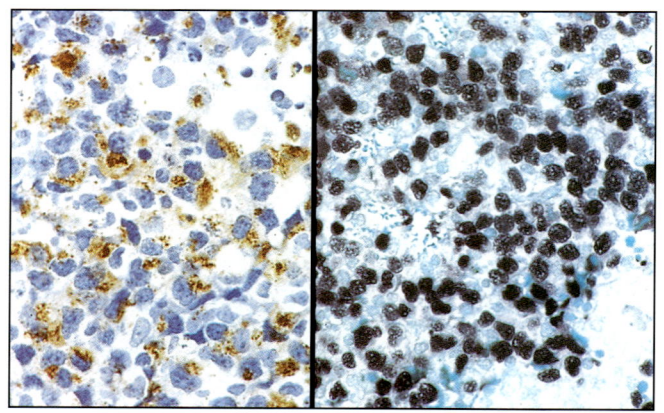

图21A.150 鼻型NK/T细胞淋巴瘤的免疫染色。左侧：淋巴瘤通常表达细胞毒性分子，如粒酶B。可见颗粒状胞浆染色。右侧：实际上所有淋巴瘤细胞都显示EBER原位杂交阳性。由于该技术高度敏感，可用于检测治疗后的残留病变或早期复发。

表面CD3/Leu4$^-$、胞浆CD3ε$^+$、CD5$^-$、CD56$^+$（图21A.149）[1191,1217-1221]。CD56$^-$的鼻腔淋巴瘤如果显示CD3ε$^+$、细胞毒性标记物$^+$、EBV$^+$表型，也包括在鼻型NK/T细胞淋巴瘤范围中[1196]。

2. TCR呈阴性。细胞毒性标记物，如TIA-1、粒酶B和穿孔素呈阳性（图21A.150）。NK细胞受体呈阳性[1222,1223]。

3. 有时表达CD7，但CD4、CD8、CD16和CD57通常呈阴性。CD43和CD45RO常常呈阳性。有些病例可表达CD25或CD30。Fas（CD95）和Fas配体常呈阳性[1223,1224]。在NK细胞受体中，CD94/NGK2常常表达，但KIR仅仅表达于少部分病例[1225-1228]。

遗传学研究

大多数病例TCR基因无重排[1191]。鼻型NK/T细胞淋巴瘤与EBV具有很强的相关性（>95%），而与患者的种族无关（图21A.150）。EBV可能起着病因学作用，而不仅仅是旁观者，因为鼻型CD56阴性的T细胞淋巴瘤和B细胞淋巴瘤显示与EBV具有弱相关性。因此鼻型NK/T细胞淋巴瘤是在所有人群中与EBV相关性最一致的淋巴瘤类型。EBV显示潜伏型Ⅱ型基因表达（表21A.9，第1163页）。在东方人群中，鼻外型NK/T细胞淋巴瘤也显示与EBV有很强的相关性（>90%），但在高加索人群中其相关性似乎较弱[1191,1202,1229,1230]。

导致NK/T细胞淋巴瘤的关键分子事件仍未可知。细胞遗传学、比较基因组杂交和核型谱系分析提示：位于以下染色体片段的基因可能对其发病机制具有重要作用：6q22-23、17p22-23、13q14-34、1p32-pter、Xp和8p23[1125,1191,1231-1234]。

诊断NK/T细胞肿瘤的金标准

确定某种淋巴瘤是NK细胞系的最可靠参数是：表达CD56，缺乏表面CD3而出现胞浆CD3，以及缺乏TCR基因重排（最好使用Southern印迹）。然而，常常只有甲醛溶液固定石蜡包埋组织可用于诊断，使其不能用于Southern印迹检测TCR基因重排，也不能用于表面CD3的研究。因此淋巴瘤表达胞浆CD3和CD56就暂且被认为是NK细胞来源，然而有些外周T细胞淋巴瘤，尤其是表达γδ-TCR者和累及皮肤或胃肠道者，可能具有这种胞浆CD3$^+$、CD56$^+$表型。

以下附加表现可进一步支持NK细胞来源，尽管不如利用新鲜/冰冻组织可靠：

- 不表达CD5
- αβ-TCR阴性（应用βF1）
- EBER原位杂交显示EBV阳性（因为表达CD56的外周T细胞淋巴瘤常常EBV阴性）
- PCR检测没有发现TCR基因重排

鉴别诊断

对于由中等或大的细胞组成的病例，NK/T细胞淋巴瘤的诊断常常很直观。然而，对于小淋巴细胞为主或显示混合细胞的病例，则很难与反应性淋巴组织增生区分，尤其是混合许多炎症细胞时。倾向于诊断肿瘤的特征包括（图21A.151）：

1. 致密的扩张性浸润，伴有黏膜腺体扭曲或破坏；
2. 出现透明胞浆；
3. 出现组织溃疡和坏死；
4. 出现明显的非典型细胞群：细胞中等大小，显著不规则性核或染色质呈颗粒状。这些非典型细胞常常位于活检组织深部，远离表面溃疡；

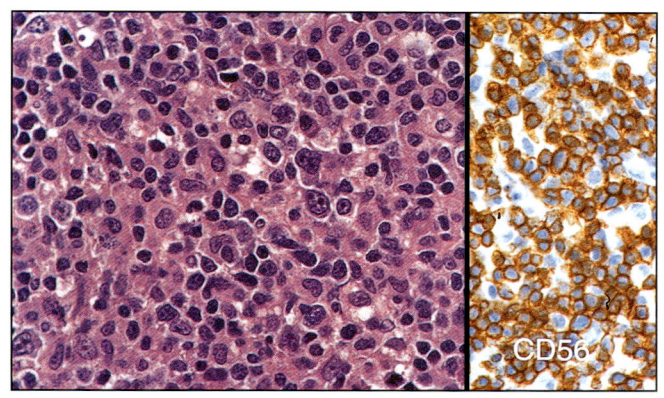

图21A.151　鼻型NK/T细胞淋巴瘤。左侧：本例难以鉴别淋巴瘤和反应性淋巴组织增生。细胞仅显示很轻微的非典型性，混杂有浆细胞。右侧：CD56广泛阳性染色支持淋巴瘤诊断，因为在反应性淋巴组织中，CD56⁺细胞通常稀少。

5. 在小淋巴细胞中容易见到核分裂象；
6. 出现血管侵犯性生长。

怀疑NK/T细胞淋巴瘤时，CD56免疫染色最有帮助。显示大的巢状和成片阳性细胞强烈支持诊断。但应该注意的是，CD56免疫染色阴性不能完全排除淋巴瘤（如CD56阴性的NK/T细胞淋巴瘤和非特指外周T细胞淋巴瘤）。另一种有帮助的手段是EBER原位杂交：出现大片阳性细胞支持淋巴瘤诊断。Ki-67免疫染色可能也有帮助，因为NK/T细胞淋巴瘤通常增殖分数很高（常常>80%），即使是小细胞为主的病变。

侵袭性NK细胞白血病
Aggressive NK-cell leukemia

临床特征和表现

侵袭性NK细胞白血病通常发生于10～40岁的患者，男女发病率相等或男性发病率稍高。患者表现为发热、系统性症状、肝脾大，有时伴有系统性淋巴结肿大，皮肤病变少见。通常病变很重，有些病例可伴有噬血综合征[1191,1199,1235-1242]。

疾病呈暴发性过程，治疗反应差或仅有短暂反应。多数患者死于数天或数周[1240]。发病时或终末期常见多器官衰竭和播散性血管内凝血[1243]。

病理学所见

血计数常提示贫血、中性粒细胞减少和血小板减少，伴有不同程度的淋巴细胞增多。大颗粒淋巴细胞占所有淋巴细胞的百分之几到>80%；核圆形，染色质致密，或核较大，伴有轻度不规则折叠。有些病例核仁明显。胞浆略呈嗜碱性，含有嗜苯胺蓝颗粒。骨髓受累轻微，斑片状或很广泛。

组织学显示肿瘤浸润呈弥漫性、破坏性和渗透性。常常形态单一。核圆形或不规则形，染色质相当致密。常见凋亡小体、凝固性坏死、血管侵犯和血管破坏。

免疫细胞化学、遗传学表现以及EBV相关性
Immunocytochemistry, genetic findings, and EBV association

除了CD16常常表达（40%～50%）外，免疫表型与鼻型NK/T细胞淋巴瘤相同。*TCR*基因无重排。EBV呈阳性[1191,1240]。可重复性染色体畸变包括1q获得以及6q22-23、7p15.1-p22.3和17p13.1丢失[1233,1234]。

鉴别诊断

1. **惰性NK淋巴组织增生性疾病**（indolent NK lymphoproliferative disease）：这是NK细胞增生的一种形式（尚未明确是反应性还是肿瘤性），伴有无进展病程，极少数病例可转化为侵袭性。以下特征不同于侵袭性NK/T细胞白血病：（a）通常没有症状，但有些病例可出现症状，如血管炎性皮肤病变、发热或复发性中性粒细胞减少性感染；（b）无肝脾大；（c）CD16和CD57常常呈阳性；（d）EBV呈阴性[1237,1238,1244]。

2. **T细胞颗粒性淋巴细胞白血病**（T-cell granular lymphocytic leukemia）：形态学上，侵袭性NK/T细胞白血病/淋巴瘤难以与T细胞颗粒性淋巴细胞白血病鉴别，虽然前者中细胞可显示某种程度的非典型性或不成熟性。以下特征可识别T细胞颗粒性淋巴细胞白血病：（a）临床过程呈惰性；（b）表达表面CD3；（c）*TCR*基因重排；以及（d）EBV阴性。

母细胞性NK细胞淋巴瘤
Blastic NK-cell lymphoma

疾病的定义和本质

母细胞性NK细胞淋巴瘤是一种由淋巴母细胞样细胞组成的肿瘤，免疫表型通常显示CD56⁺、sCD3⁻、cCD3⁻/⁺、CD4⁺[1245]，是一种异质性类别，至少由两种病变组成：CD4⁺CD56⁺的皮肤造血（hematodermic）肿瘤，是一种前体浆细胞样树突状细胞肿瘤，而不是NK细胞，由表达CD123（白介素3受体）而证实[1246-1249]；前体NK细胞淋巴母细胞淋巴瘤/白血病，是一种前体NK细胞或双潜能NK/T细胞[1250]，为定向NK细胞系；还包括一些无特征化的病变。

CD4⁺CD56⁺皮肤造血肿瘤
CD4⁺CD56⁺ hematodermic neoplasm

临床特征：CD4⁺CD56⁺皮肤造血肿瘤是最常见的"母细胞性NK细胞淋巴瘤"类型。其主要发生于成人，表现为皮肤结节或斑块。常常同时累及淋巴结和骨髓。有些病例可具有白血病症状。尽管最初的治疗反应良好，但几乎总会复发。平均生存期为14个月[1191,1194,1201,1247,1251-1256]。

病理学检查：皮肤显示真皮中致密、弥漫性浸润的单形性中等大母细胞，类似于淋巴母细胞性淋巴瘤或髓性白血病（图21A.152）。嗜苯胺蓝颗粒通常可见于Giemsa染色印片中。核分裂象易于见到。极少数情况下，可形成假玫瑰花结[1191,1257]。常呈单排浸润胶原。通常没有凝固性坏死或血管中心性。

免疫细胞化学和遗传学检查：典型的免疫表型是CD56⁺、表面CD3⁻、cCD3⁻/⁺、CD4⁺、CD123⁺，TdT在大约60%的病例中呈阳性。TCL1和CLA常常表达。与髓性/NK急性白血病不同，不表达髓性标记物[1247-1249,1255,1258-1261]。TCR基因位于胚系，EBV呈阴性[1191]。

前体NK细胞淋巴母细胞性淋巴瘤/白血病
Precursor NK-cell lymphoblastic lymphoma/leukemia

这是"母细胞性NK细胞淋巴瘤"的一种少见亚型，是NK细胞淋巴母细胞性淋巴瘤/白血病。患者通常表现为纵隔和淋巴结受累，而不是皮肤受累。组织学上，可见弥漫浸润性中等大小的母细胞。典型的免疫表型是CD56⁺，表面CD3⁻、CD4⁻、CD7⁺、CD123⁻、TdT⁺。TCR基因无重排，EBV呈阴性[334,1250]。

免疫缺陷相关性淋巴组织增生异常
Lymphoproliferative disorders associated with immunodeficiency

移植后淋巴组织增生异常
Post-transplant lymphoproliferative disorders (PTLD)

器官移植受者发生各种类型的淋巴组织增生异常的危险增加（<2%～10%），这是由抗移植排斥药物引起的医源性免疫抑制造成的。免疫抑制剂越强，如使用抗OKT3，危险性越高。移植后淋巴组织增生异常（PTLD）

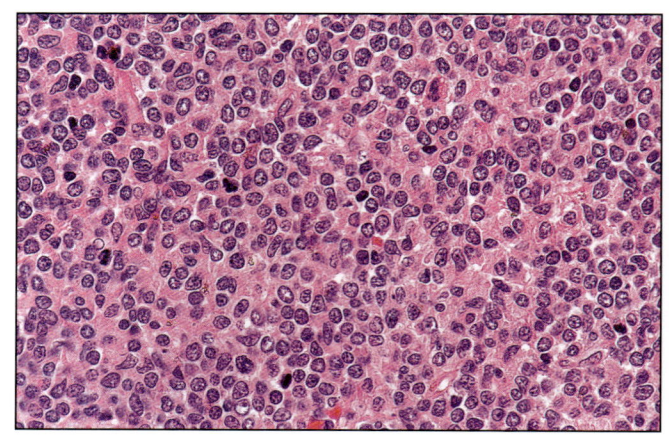

图21A.152 母细胞性NK/T细胞淋巴瘤。淋巴细胞中等大小，极其类似于淋巴母细胞性淋巴瘤。

常常出现在移植后数月至数年，中位间期为4.5～11个月。其表现为肿物性病变，常常累及淋巴结外部位和移植物。PTLD常常由EBV引起，有些病变随着免疫抑制的减少和停止，可显示明显消退。EBV基因组的表达方式常常相当于III型潜伏（表21A.9，第1163页）。评估循环血中EBV病毒含量可能有助于筛查和监测PTLD的发生，但结果有时可能具有争议[1262,1263]。

发生于实性器官移植后晚期的PTLD与EBV相关性较小（44%）。这种情况发生的淋巴瘤的临床病理学特征类似于散发性淋巴瘤，但临床预后差[1206]。

各种形式的PTLD的显著临床病理学特征见表21A.19（图21A.153和21A.154）[911,1265-1276]。PTLD包括一系列淋巴细胞异常增生，从良性多克隆性淋巴组织增生到侵袭性、常常是致死的单克隆非Hodgkin淋巴瘤。虽然就具体病例而言难以准确预测随着免疫移植减少PTLD是否会消退，但首选治疗方案是逐渐减少免疫抑制剂，加用或不加用干扰素和抗病毒治疗。对于局限性疾病可考虑手术。对于弥漫性或持续性疾病，必须给

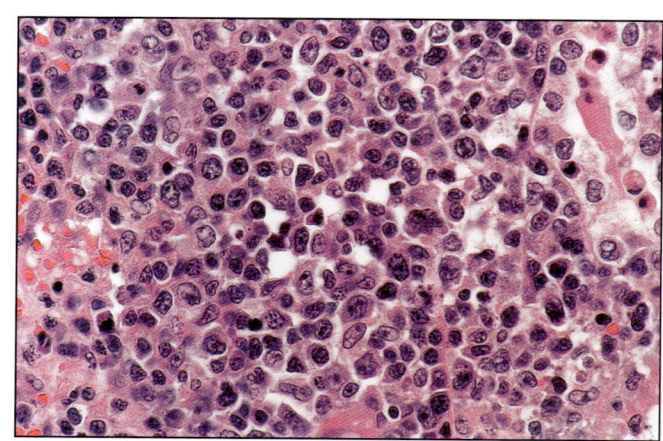

图21A.153 移植后的多形性淋巴组织增生异常。特点是细胞呈一个谱系，从免疫母细胞、浆母细胞至浆细胞。较大的细胞可显示非典型性。

表21A.19	移植后淋巴组织增生异常（PTLD）的主要类型的临床病理学特征*				
PTLD类型	临床特征和预后	常见受累部位	病理学特征	EBV状况	分子学特征
早期病变：反应性浆细胞增生和传染性单核细胞增多症样	通常发生于儿童和年轻患者，先前没有EBV感染，常常在移植后早期出现。病变通常自然消退或随着免疫抑制剂的最小化减少而消退。	扁桃体和淋巴结	结构保留或至少部分保留。增生的细胞没有非典型性。浆细胞增生：混合性浆细胞和淋巴浆样细胞；生发中心增生、退化或缺乏。传染性单核细胞增多症样：免疫母细胞增多，类似于免疫活性宿主的传染性单核细胞增多症	阳性（多克隆性或微弱单克隆方式）	多克隆Ig基因重排。癌基因或肿瘤抑制基因没有改变。
多形性PTLD	发生于所有年龄组。患者表现为I期、II期或III期疾病。随着免疫抑制剂的减少而消退。有些病例应用外科和放疗或化疗可消退。但是，尽管像淋巴瘤一样进行治疗，有些病例也可进展	淋巴结、肺、胃肠道和同种异体移植物	破坏性病变伴有结构消失。混合性小淋巴细胞、浆细胞、免疫母细胞和浆母细胞，重演了B淋巴细胞分化的全过程。大细胞可显示或不显示非典型性。坏死程度多样性。可进展为单形性PTLD。	阳性（克隆性）	克隆性Ig基因重排。癌基因或肿瘤抑制基因没有改变。通常缺乏BCL-6重排，但不一定有BCL-6突变。
单形性PTLD（根据淋巴瘤分类进行归类）	发生于各年龄组。发病时疾病常呈播散性。虽然少数病例随着免疫抑制剂减少可消退，但大多数病例进展迅速，即使进行了强化治疗。	淋巴结、骨髓和结外部位	弥漫性淋巴组织浸润导致结构消失，常见坏死。单形性细胞中等或偏大，但有些病例可显示细胞大小和形态明显不同。不要将这种细胞多形性误认为是多形性PTLD见到的细胞谱系。最常见的组织学类型是弥漫大B细胞淋巴瘤、Burkitt和Burkitt样淋巴瘤	通常呈阳性（克隆性）	克隆性Ig基因重排。常常显示癌基因突变，如BCL-6、RAS、C-MYC、P53
Hodgkin淋巴瘤和Hodgkin淋巴瘤样PTLD	发生Hodgkin淋巴瘤的时间平均在移植后49个月。Hodgkin淋巴瘤样PTLD似乎好发于男性和年轻组（儿童和青少年）。发病可早可晚（移植后4个月至12年）。	淋巴结或结外部位	根据经典的形态学和免疫组化特征（CD30$^+$CD15$^+$）得出Hodgkin淋巴瘤的诊断；最常见的亚型是混合细胞型。Hodgkin淋巴瘤样PTLD在形态学上类似于混合细胞型或淋巴细胞削减型Hodgkin淋巴瘤，但非典型大细胞表达CD45、CD20和CD79a；CD30的表达不一致，CD15呈阴性。因此是B细胞PTLD的一种形式，而不是真正的Hodgkin淋巴瘤	EBER呈阳性（原位杂交），主要见于Hodgkin淋巴瘤的大细胞，但还可见于Hodgkin淋巴瘤样PTLD中的小淋巴细胞	没有可用性

*极少数情况下，PTLD可能为浆细胞瘤或骨髓瘤的形式。T细胞型单形性PTLD出现需要的时间较长（中位发病时间为5年），极少累及同种异体移植物，显示EBV相关性的病例仅为50%左右。

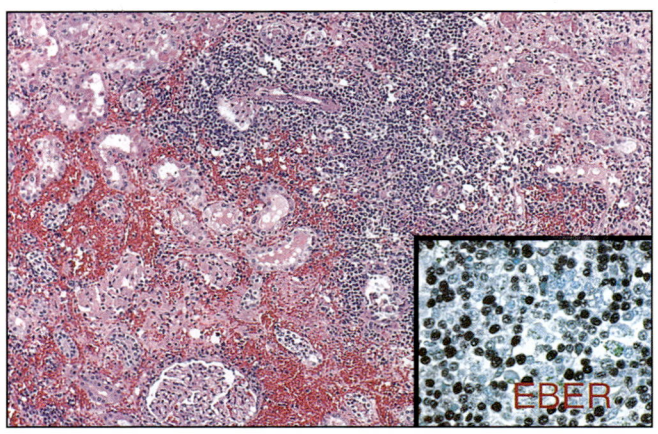

图21A.154 多形性形式的移植后淋巴组织增生异常。病变累及同种异体移植物（肾）。可见破坏性淋巴组织浸润。插图：淋巴细胞特征性显示EBV标记。

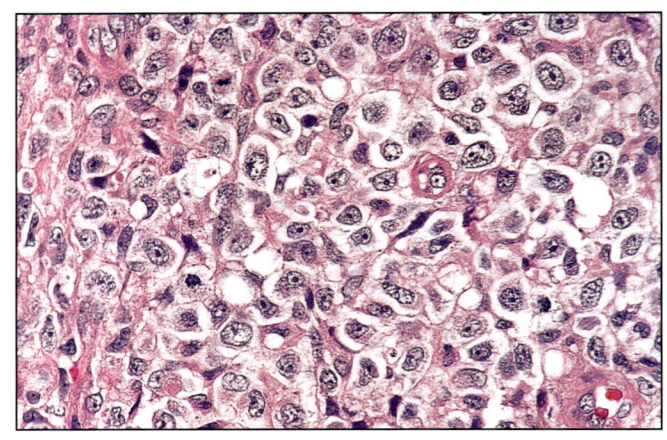

图21A.155 氨甲蝶呤相关性淋巴组织增生异常。本例的形态学特征与普通大B细胞淋巴瘤无法区分，但停用氨甲蝶呤后消退。

予美罗华和联合化疗[1277]。

获得性免疫缺陷综合征（AIDS）
Acquired immunodeficiency syndrome (AIDS)

各组（不考虑危险性）AIDS患者均易于发生恶性淋巴瘤，随着CD4+淋巴细胞计数的减少，其危险性增加。事实上，对于HIV阳性AIDS患者，非Hodgkin淋巴瘤是一种必然的疾病[32,911,955]。最常见的淋巴瘤类型是弥漫大B细胞淋巴瘤（伴有免疫母细胞形态者25%显示C-MYC重排，0%显示P53突变，100%显示EBV，19%显示BCL-6重排）和Burkitt淋巴瘤（100%显示C-MYC重排，63%显示P53突变，31%显示EBV，0%显示BCL-6重排）。发病时，淋巴瘤常广泛播散（Ⅲ/Ⅳ期）。好发于结外部位，如中枢神经系统、胃肠道、骨髓和肝。中枢神经系统淋巴瘤恒定与EBV有关，但总体上所有AIDS相关性NHL仅有40%与EBV有关。淋巴瘤细胞中检测不到HIV序列。虽然AIDS相关性淋巴瘤预后差，但近年来使用高活性抗反转录病毒治疗同时给予化疗后，生存率得以改善[1278,1279]。加用美罗华的价值仍不清楚[1280]。

发生于AIDS患者的两种特殊淋巴瘤类型是原发性渗出性淋巴瘤和浆母细胞淋巴瘤（见"弥漫大B细胞淋巴瘤"）。近期报道HIV阳性患者可以发生一种多形性淋巴组织增生性病变，类似于多形性移植后淋巴组织增生性病变[1281]。大多数病例的分子学分析显示克隆性B细胞群，但这可能仅仅代表多形性病变中的一种亚群。

在HIV阳性患者中，Hodgkin淋巴瘤的发生率略增加，尤其是中青年男性同性恋者，但不能将其认为是HIV感染AIDS患者的必然病变[32,34]。AIDS患者发生的HL其特征见第1153页的表21A.4。

与移植无关的医源性淋巴组织增生异常
Iatrogenic lymphoproliferative disorders in non-transplantation setting

使用氨甲蝶呤或其他免疫抑制药物治疗的类风湿性关节炎或皮肌炎患者，可发生淋巴结或结外淋巴组织增生异常，其特征类似非典型多形性淋巴组织增生异常、大B细胞淋巴瘤、HL或HL样淋巴组织增生（图21A.155）。大多数病例的非典型细胞有EBV感染。识别这种形式的淋巴组织增生异常的重要性在于：停用免疫抑制药物后大部分病例可以消退，避免了患者的毒性化疗[1282-1287]。但是，其中有些淋巴组织增生异常是进展性的、致死性的。顺便说一句，大多数发生于类风湿病患者的淋巴瘤，伴发自身免疫性疾病或与自身免疫性疾病有关，而不是与免疫抑制药物治疗有关，这种淋巴瘤通常EBV呈阴性[1285,1288]。

先天性免疫异常
Congenital immune disorders

先天性免疫缺陷（如Wiskott-Aldrich综合征，各种常见的免疫缺陷，共济失调-毛细血管扩张，重症联合免疫缺陷，X-连锁淋巴组织增生异常，以及高IgM综合征）常常伴发淋巴组织增生异常，患者发病年龄小，病变好发于淋巴结外部位，尤其是胃肠道和中枢神经系统。病变谱系包括反应性淋巴组织增生、非典型淋巴组织增生、B细胞或T细胞NHL、HL和白血病。仅有部分病例与EBV有关[911,1287,1289-1292]。淋巴瘤在临床上呈侵袭性。分子学研究的一些特殊发现是：临床与组织学呈良性的淋巴组织增生，有时显示克隆性Ig或TCR基因重排，以及某些可见于NHL代表明确恶性的寡克隆带[911]。

表21A.20　组织细胞和组织细胞增生的分类

	单核-吞噬细胞系统	树突状细胞系统（抗原呈递细胞）	
		非滤泡树突状细胞	滤泡树突状细胞
细胞类型	• 单核细胞（血和骨髓） • 组织巨噬细胞（各种部位） • 含可染小体的巨噬细胞（滤泡B细胞） • 窦组织细胞（淋巴结） • 上皮样组织细胞	• Langerhans细胞（皮肤） • 指状树突状细胞（T区） • 未定类细胞 • 面纱（veiled）细胞（淋巴管） • 浆细胞样树突状细胞（以前的"浆细胞样单核细胞"）	• 滤泡树突状细胞
酶谱系	• ATP酶阴性/弱 • 各种酶（溶菌酶、酸性磷酸酶、α1-抗胰蛋白酶）+	• ATP酶+ • 各种酶/弱	• ATP酶- • 各种酶-
免疫表型	• CD68+、CD163+（除了滤泡性巨噬细胞和上皮样组织细胞） • S100-（除了少数亚型） • CD1a- • CD4+ • HLA-DR不确定	• S100+ • CD68-（+活化时），CD163- • Langerhans和未定型细胞CD1a+，但指状树突状细胞和面纱细胞- • Langerhans细胞Langerin+ • CD4+/- • HLA-DR+	• CD21、CD23、CD35+ • CD68-、CD163- • S100-/+ • CD1a- • CD4-
反应性增生	• 窦组织细胞增生症 • Rosai-Dorfman病 • 噬血综合征 • 家族性噬红细胞性淋巴组织细胞增生症 • 对感染或异物的组织细胞反应 • 贮积性疾病	• 皮病性淋巴结病	• 滤泡树突状细胞过度生长
肿瘤性增生	• 急性单核细胞白血病和单核细胞肉瘤 • 组织细胞肉瘤 • 恶性组织细胞增生症 • ALK+的组织细胞增生症	• Langerhans细胞组织细胞增生症 • 指状树突状细胞肉瘤 • 其他树突状细胞肿瘤 • 浆细胞样单核细胞成瘤性聚集	• 滤泡树突状细胞肉瘤

组织细胞和树突状细胞肿瘤
Tumors of histiocytes and dendritic cells

过去曾经笼统地使用"网状细胞肉瘤"或"组织细胞淋巴瘤"来描述大细胞性淋巴造血系统肿瘤。重新评估显示：几乎所有肿瘤均属于B细胞或T细胞大细胞淋巴瘤[1293]。组织细胞肉瘤的诊断总是需要免疫组化或超微结构研究来支持。

组织细胞和树突状细胞肿瘤主要包括两种类型的组织细胞：单核/吞噬细胞和树突状细胞。相应的反应性或肿瘤性增生异常见表21A.20[1294-1300]。

组织细胞肉瘤　Histiocytic sarcoma

临床特征

肿瘤显示巨噬细胞分化，占所有非Hodgkin淋巴瘤的比例不足0.5%[1301,1302]。只有近十年来或基于大量免疫细胞化学和基因型研究的病例报告是可信的[1300-1307]。

肿瘤发病年龄范围广泛，平均为44岁，男性好发。患者表现为淋巴结肿大或结外肿物，最常累及皮肤、胃肠道和软组织[1307]。大多数患者表现为高分期疾病。少数情况下，急性淋巴母细胞性淋巴瘤治疗后可发生组织细胞肉瘤。有一例研究显示这两种疾病具有共同的克隆起源[1308,1309]。少数病例还可发生于纵隔生殖细胞肿瘤基础上[1310]。

多数患者2年内死于播散性疾病，虽然可能有幸存者（尤其是疾病局限者）[1307]。根据一项大的研究，7/12的患者死于疾病，2例带病生存[1300]。

病理学

受累淋巴结显示弥漫性、窦隙或副皮质区受累，但结外部位病变呈弥漫性。肿瘤细胞常常很大，类似于大细胞或间变大细胞淋巴瘤，只是胞浆通常丰富呈嗜酸性。胞浆还可呈小空泡状（图21.A156）。核偏心，圆形、卵圆形、不规则形或有核沟，染色质纤细或粗大。核仁常

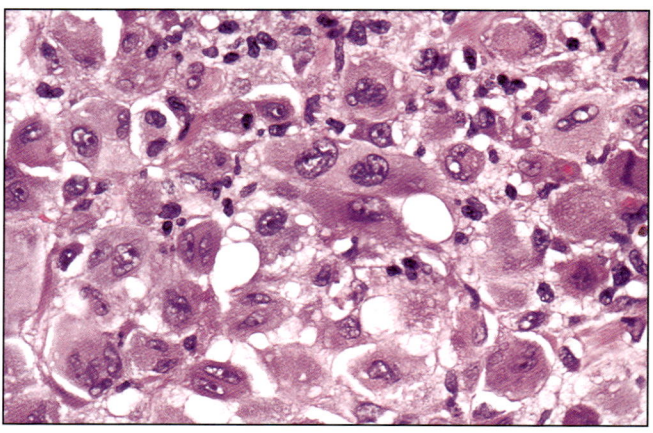

图21A.156 组织细胞肉瘤。这一肿瘤的特点是大细胞伴有多量嗜酸性胞浆，有时含有小空泡。核显示凹陷或核沟。

较小。细胞多形性程度不一。可见多核细胞。吞噬活性少见。可混杂不同数量的淋巴细胞、浆细胞、中性粒细胞和嗜酸性粒细胞。炎症成分明显者能掩盖肿瘤细胞，尤其是组织细胞肉瘤累及中枢神经系统时[1311]。在少数病例，可见黏液样或肉瘤样生长方式。

免疫细胞化学

1. CD68、CD163和溶菌酶呈阳性。
2. T细胞、B细胞、髓细胞和FDC标记物呈阴性。
3. 可表达多种组织细胞标记物，如CD4、CD11c、CD14和CD15。CD45RB染色不确定，但CD43和CD45RO通常呈阳性。有些病例S100蛋白阳性，但染色常呈斑片状，而不是弥漫一致。CD1a、langerin和CD30呈阴性[1300,1304,1305]。

遗传学特征

基因型研究显示Ig和TCR基因为胚系构型。组织细胞肉瘤缺少特异性遗传学或分子学异常。

鉴别诊断

1. 大细胞淋巴瘤(large cell lymphoma)：当"大细胞淋巴瘤"显示丰富的嗜酸性胞浆时，应该考虑组织细胞肉瘤。需要免疫组化确诊。
2. 单核细胞肉瘤（急性单核细胞白血病的局限性肿瘤）[monocytic sarcoma (localized tumor of acute monocytic leukemia)]：可识别的特征包括：肿瘤细胞较小，外观较单一。
3. 对于表达S100蛋白的病例，鉴别诊断还应该包括指状树突状细胞肉瘤。倾向后者的特征包括：S100免疫染色或超微结构检查显示长的树突状细胞突起，S100蛋白染色较强、较弥漫，CD68染色多样且常常较弱。

恶性组织细胞增生症
Malignant histiocytosis

Rappaport[1312]所定义的"恶性组织细胞增生症"是由形态学非典型性的组织细胞及其前体细胞构成的系统性、进展性和侵袭性增生。如同文献所述，患者通常表现发热、全身性症状、淋巴结肿大和肝脾肿大。常见全血减少。患者通常呈病态，疾病呈迅速致死性过程[1005,1312,1313]。传统的恶性组织细胞增生症被认为是组织细胞的恶性病变，但根据免疫表型和遗传学分析，几乎所有的病例均重新归类为大细胞淋巴瘤（通常是T细胞系，有时为B细胞系，常常表达CD30），伴有或不伴有反应性噬血综合征[1005,1006,1293,1314,1315]。

真正组织细胞来源的恶性组织细胞增生症极其少见[1316,1317]。其不同于组织细胞肉瘤之处在于其肿瘤细胞分散，不形成致密的肿块，常常不会造成受累组织正常结构的完全破坏。有些恶性组织细胞增生症病例与纵隔生殖细胞肿瘤一同发生[1318]。

ALK⁺的组织细胞增生症　ALK⁺ histiocytosis

ALK⁺的组织细胞增生症是发生于婴儿的一种罕见类型的系统性组织细胞增生，患者表现为苍白，块状肝脾大，生命衰竭。外周血通常显示明显贫血和血小板减少。肝活检显示，巨大组织细胞散在窦隙和（或）门脉通道中。组织细胞显示核不规则折叠，染色质纤细，核仁不明显，胞浆丰富呈弱嗜酸性，可呈小空泡状。细胞膜/胞浆显示ALK免疫反应，细胞也表达组织细胞标记物（CD68、CD163）和S100蛋白。有一项研究检测到TPM3/ALK融合基因。临床过程的特点是可缓慢消退，虽然疾病早期可危及生命。

Langerhans细胞组织细胞增生症（组织细胞增生症X；嗜酸性肉芽肿）
Langerhans' cell histiocytosis(histiocytosis X; eosinophilic granuloma)

临床特征

Langerhans细胞组织细胞增生症是Langerhans细胞的局限性或系统性克隆性增生[1319,1320]。主要发生于儿童和年轻人，但任何年龄均可累及。实际上任何器官均可受累，骨和皮肤为好发部位。患者分为单系统疾病（单部位或多部位）以及多系统疾病[1294]。总体死亡率大约为10%。单系统疾病对目前的治疗有效，预后很好。有些多系统疾病患者，尤其是年龄小的儿童，可死于疾病[1321]。基因表达谱研究显示，多系统Langerhans细胞

组织细胞增生症中 *MMP12* 表达增高，其可能在疾病进展中起作用[1322]。

淋巴结肿大是少数病例的最初或单一表现，与预后好有关，多数患者未经特殊治疗而痊愈[1323-1325]。少数情况下，Langerhans 细胞组织细胞增生症是患有淋巴瘤(HL 或 NHL) 淋巴结的偶然发现[1326]。

病理学

任何部位的病变其典型特征均表现为 Langerhans 细胞的簇状或片状增生[1327]。细胞核通常有核沟和不规则扭曲，核膜薄，染色质纤细，核仁不明显。胞浆丰富，略嗜酸性（图 21A.157）。常见多核巨细胞。虽然常见嗜酸性粒细胞，但不是诊断所必需。有时可见嗜酸性脓肿和大片坏死。在晚期，Langerhans 细胞稀疏，病变被混合有组织细胞的纤维组织取代，其中有些组织细胞呈泡沫状。出现轻度核异型性和较明显的核仁是可以接受的。但是，如果非典型性明显，伴有易于识别的核分裂象，则应该归为肉瘤型[1300]（见下文）。

在淋巴结，病变常常位于淋巴窦，伴有邻近实质不同程度受累（图 21.A158）[1323-1325,1328]。淋巴结周围组织常常受累，被膜常显示纤维化。少数情况下，Langerhans 细胞形成独立的结节，类似于上皮样肉芽肿；其本质只有通过免疫组化染色证实[1328]。

免疫细胞化学和组织化学

1. S100 蛋白呈阳性（多核巨细胞通常 S100 呈阴性）（图 21A.159）。
2. Langerin（CD207）是一种诱导 Birbeck 颗粒形成的细胞表面受体，是最重要的诊断标记物，在所有病例中呈阳性[1329]。CD1a 阳性还有助于鉴别 Langerhans 细

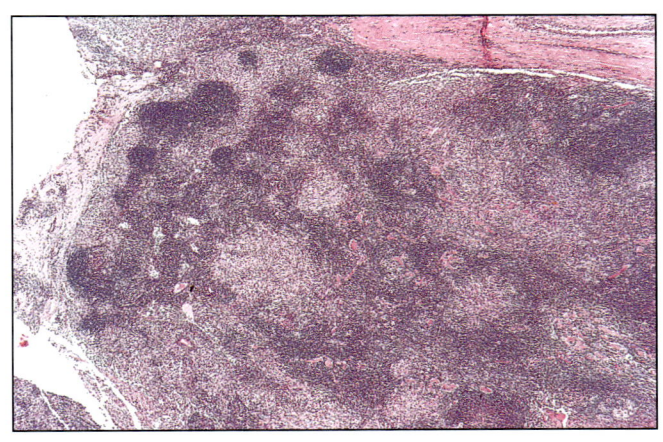

图21A.158 淋巴结Langerhans细胞组织细胞增生症。可见典型的窦隙受累（淡染区），被膜增厚，淋巴结周围受累。

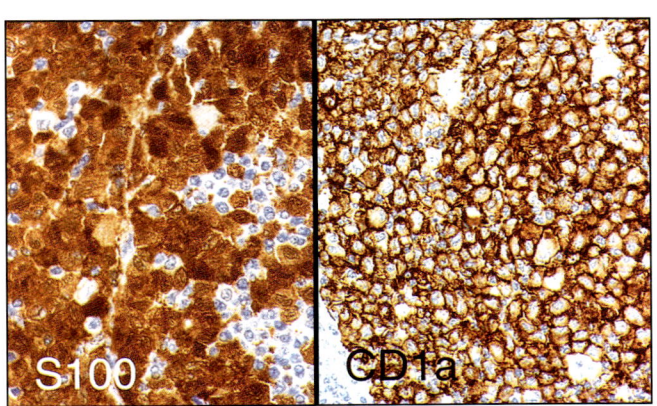

A

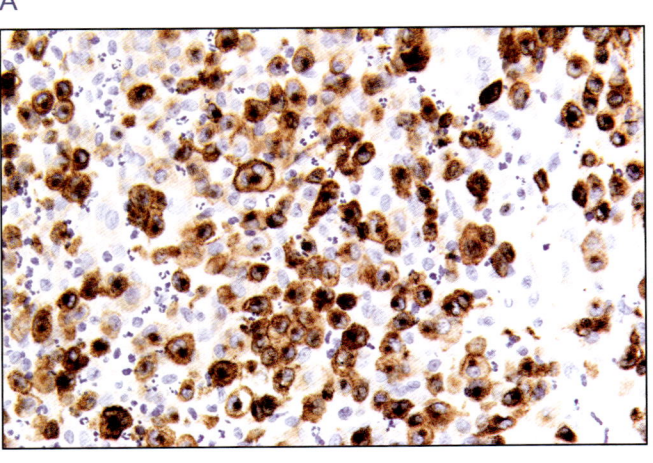

B

图21A.159 Langerhans细胞组织细胞增生症的免疫染色。（A）左侧：组织细胞显示核和胞浆S100蛋白染色。与正常的Langerhans细胞不同，树突状细胞的突起短或缺乏。右侧：CD1a免疫反应（细胞膜染色）是Langerhans细胞组织细胞增生症的重要标记物。（B）Langerin是近期发现的Langerhans细胞组织细胞增生症的限定性标记物，比CD1a更具特异性。染色呈颗粒状位于细胞膜和高尔基区。

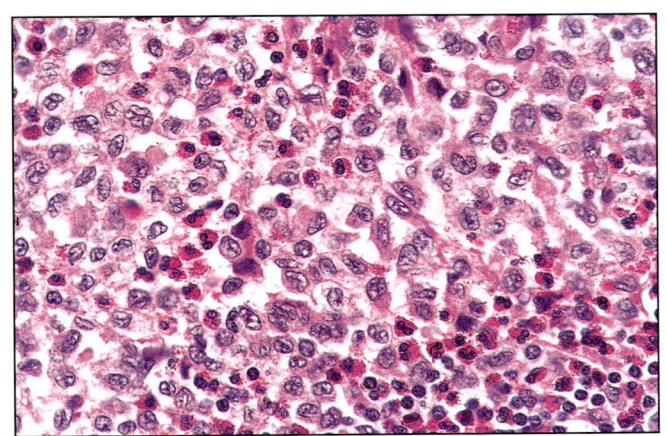

图21A.157 Langerhans细胞组织细胞增生症。细胞通常呈卵圆形，有核沟或扭曲。染色质纤细，胞浆丰富。可见混合性嗜酸性粒细胞。

细胞组织细胞增生症和其他树突状细胞及组织细胞增生（图21A.159）。ATP酶（三磷腺苷酶）通常呈阳性，常常可见花生凝集素标记[1330,1331]。

3. 表达普通组织细胞标记物，如溶菌酶、CD4、CD11c、CD15（经神经氨酸酶治疗后）和CD68[1299,1327]。HLA-DR和CD45RB常常呈阳性。

电子显微镜

超微结构特点是Birbeck颗粒，呈网球拍状或拉链形结构，宽33nm，具有中心条纹线[1299,1327]。

鉴别诊断

1. **皮病性淋巴结病**（dermatopathic lymphadenopathy）：在皮病性淋巴结病，可见大量的Langerhans细胞或指状树突状细胞，具有核沟。其与Langerhans细胞组织细胞增生症鉴别的特点有：主要为副皮质区而不是窦隙受累，混合的淋巴细胞较多，细胞边界较不明显，缺乏多核细胞，混杂有含黑色素的吞噬细胞，以及S100免疫染色显示的是树突状细胞而不是卵圆形细胞（图21A.160）。

2. **窦组织细胞增生症伴巨大淋巴结病**(sinus histiocytosis with massive lymphadenopathy)：这是另一种呈窦隙状分布且S100呈阳性的组织细胞增生。可识别的特征包括：组织细胞较大，核圆形，核仁清楚，胞浆丰富淡染。有些细胞可见吞噬现象（伸入运动）。这些组织细胞langerin和CD1a呈阴性。

肉瘤样Langerhans细胞组织细胞增生症
Sarcomatous Langerhans'cell histiocytosis

肉瘤样型的特点是具有明显恶性的细胞学特征，通常显示S100⁺CD1a⁺免疫表型（图21A.161）。核分裂象易见。嗜酸性粒细胞常常少见。这种变型发生于年龄较大的患者，平均年龄为40岁。疾病呈侵袭性，4/8的患者死于疾病，1例带病生存[1300]。"恶性组织细胞增生症X"这个术语也曾用于文献中，指代有明显细胞非典型性的Langerhans细胞组织细胞增生症病例；与侵袭性行为有关，但并不一定如此[1332]。

滤泡树突状细胞（FDC）肉瘤
Follicular dendritic cell (FDC) sarcoma

临床特征

FDC肉瘤（也称为树突网状细胞肿瘤）少见，也可能是认识不足。FDC肉瘤可发生于淋巴结或淋巴结外部位，尤其是扁桃体和腹腔内[1333-1345]。患者通常为成人，平均

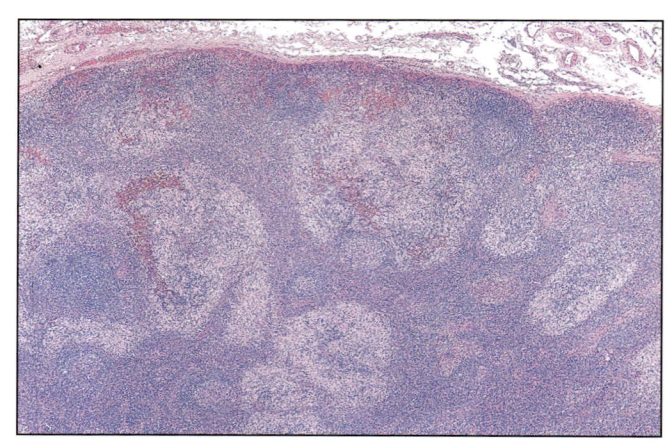

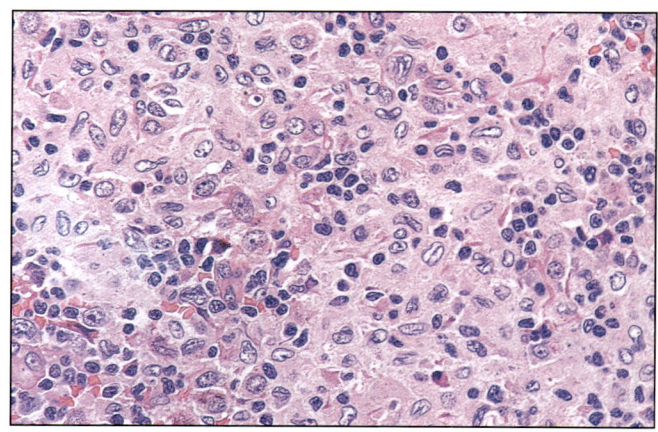

图21A.160 皮病性淋巴结病。（A）与Langerhans细胞组织细胞增生症不同，这种病变显示副皮质区受累，而不是窦隙受累，表现为淡染斑片状，有时呈结节状。（B）受累区域显示组织细胞具有核沟。这些细胞常常较细长，细胞界限不清楚。还可混杂许多淋巴细胞。

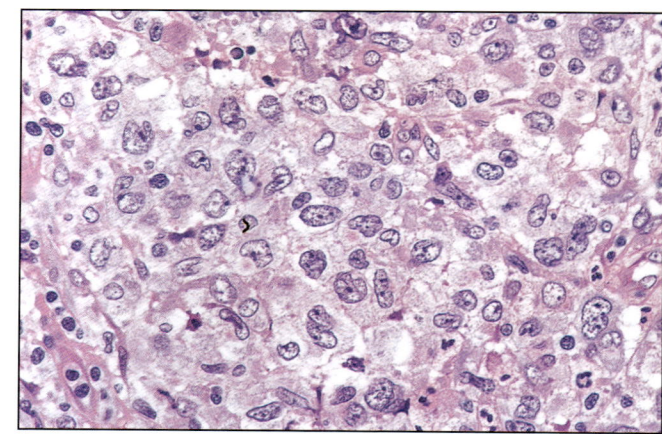

图21A.161 肉瘤样Langerhans细胞组织细胞增生症。细胞大，显示明显的核多形性。核沟仍可识别。在其他视野，易见核分裂象。

年龄为44岁。没有性别差异。有些病例明显发生于玻璃样变血管型Castleman病背景中,有时经历一个可识别的滤泡间FDC过度生长期[1346]。Castleman病病变可与FDC肉瘤同时发生或可发生于FDC肉瘤之前许多年[1336,1338,1347]。少数病例与精神分裂症有关[1348,1349],但极可能是巧合。

肿瘤常呈惰性进展,病程长,复发率＞40%,转移率＞25%(肺、淋巴结和肝最常见)[1339,1345]。这些可在最初诊断后10多年发生,复发仍可伴有长的生存期。但是在个别病例,尤其是在发生于腹腔内部位和显示凝固性坏死特征者(细胞非典型性明显,凝固性坏死和核分裂象常见),疾病可能呈迅速致死性过程。首选完整手术切除;辅助放疗或化疗的作用尚不清楚。

病理学

肿瘤平均大小为7cm,肿瘤界限清楚或显示推挤性边缘。肿瘤细胞呈梭形、较肥胖或呈卵圆形,形成旋涡状、束状或席纹状结构,弥漫成片或模糊结节状。肿瘤细胞通常边界不清,胞浆嗜酸性,通常呈纤维样(图21A.162)。核卵圆形或长形,核膜薄,染色质囊泡状,核仁小而明显。细胞常常分布不均匀,显示灶状集聚。常常可见散在的多核肿瘤细胞。有些病例可显示明显的核多形性、凝固性坏死和较多核分裂。肿瘤通常弥漫分布,伴有散在小淋巴细胞,常形成血管周袖套。

有些少见特征,包括:多角形细胞,具有玻璃样变胞浆、嗜酸性胞浆、透明胞浆,出现黏液样变,神经内分泌肿瘤样血管系统,假血管腔,血管周腔隙,胸腺瘤样分叶,以及混合性破骨巨细胞。

炎性假瘤样变型(inflammatory pseudotumor-like variant):这种变型全部发生于肝和脾。致密的淋巴浆细胞浸润掩盖了梭形或星形肿瘤细胞。有些肿瘤细胞类似于Reed-Sternberg细胞,貌似Hodgkin淋巴瘤[1350]。这种变型总是与EBV有关(见本章第2部分)。

结节性富于B细胞变型(nodular B cell-rich variant):这种少见的FDC肉瘤变型类似于结节性淋巴细胞为主型Hodgkin淋巴瘤(N-LPHL),因为肿瘤性FDC散在分布于小B淋巴细胞结节内。肿瘤细胞可识别的特征是:核大囊泡状,核仁呈包涵体样,位于中心,其本质可进一步由免疫染色所证实。肿瘤细胞还可见于结节间区[1351]。

免疫细胞化学和电子显微镜

1. FDC标记物阳性,如CD21、CD23、CD35、R4/23、KiM4p(图21A.163)。FDC相关标记物CAN.42敏感但特异性较差[1352]。Clusterin常常呈强阳性,但其

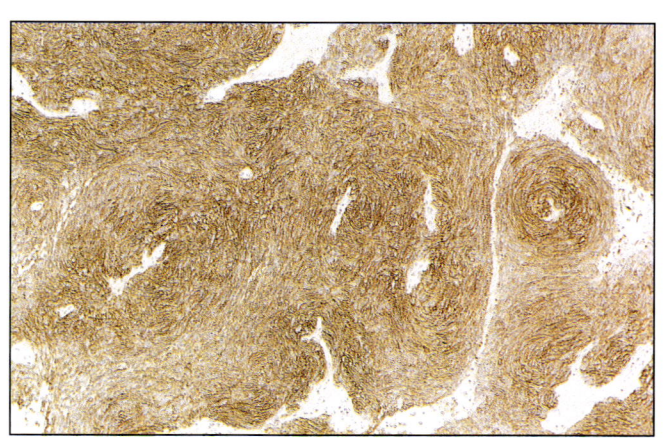

图21A.163 滤泡树突状细胞肉瘤的CD21免疫染色。可见细长的树突状细胞突起,是滤泡树突状细胞的特点。环形旋涡也明显,重现了细胞形成滤泡的能力。

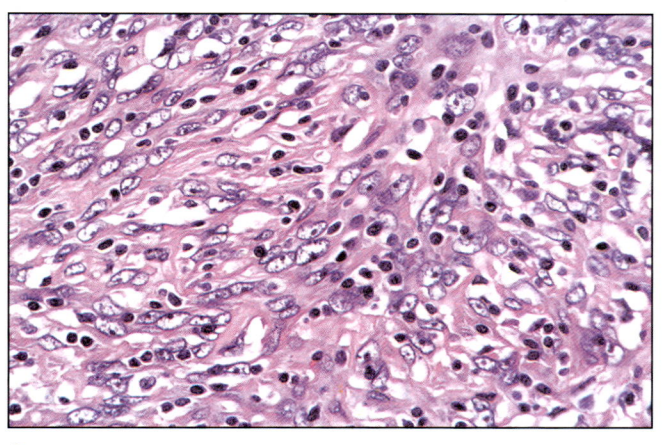

A

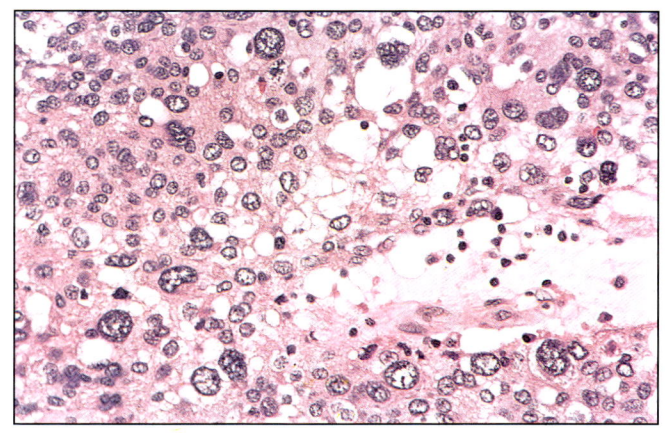

B

图21A.162 滤泡树突状细胞肉瘤。(A)梭形细胞边界不清、形成席纹状结构是该肿瘤的特点。可见特征性的囊泡状染色质结构,核仁小而明显,散在分布有小淋巴细胞。(B)本例显示细胞肥胖卵圆形,核大小不等。可见合体细胞样胞浆,是由于细胞突起交织而成。

他树突状细胞肿瘤常常呈阴性或弱阳性[1353,1354]。

2. 细胞角蛋白、CD45RB、B细胞系标记物、T细胞系标记物和CD1a均为阴性。
3. 桥粒蛋白和表皮生长因子受体常常呈阳性[1338,1355]。S100蛋白、CD68和actin的免疫反应不恒定。
4. 有些FDC肿瘤对上皮膜抗原呈阳性,因此可被误诊为癌。

超微结构可见长而复杂的指状胞浆突起,通过桥粒样连接相连。细胞器常常稀少。

遗传学特征

没有Ig和TCR基因重排。除发生于肝、脾的炎性假瘤样变型外,EBV均为阴性。FDC肉瘤的细胞遗传学或分子学改变知之甚少。

鉴别诊断

FDC肉瘤可类似于胸腺瘤、胸腺癌、脑膜瘤、多形性肉瘤、血管肉瘤、未分化癌、淋巴上皮瘤样癌或胃肠道间质瘤,反之亦然。

指状树突状细胞肉瘤
Interdigitating dendritic cell sarcoma

临床特征

指状树突状细胞肉瘤比FDC肉瘤更少见,更难以确定。这种肿瘤常发生于成人,表现为淋巴结肿大或结外疾病,尤其是在胃肠道。发病时疾病常常为高分期,系统性症状常见[1198,1300,1340,1356-1364]。少数病例可能与先前的低度恶性B细胞淋巴瘤有关[1365]。

这种肿瘤呈侵袭性。强化化疗常常仅有部分反应或短期缓解。至少1/3的患者在1周到3年死于广泛播散性疾病。总体中位生存期大约为15个月[1,1362,1366]。

病理学

肿瘤或局限于淋巴结副皮质区,或引起总体结构消失。组织学特征高度多变(图21A.164):

1. 肿瘤细胞可呈梭形,形态学酷似FDC肉瘤;与后者的严格区别只能依靠免疫组化染色。
2. 肿瘤细胞大,圆形或卵圆形,胞浆丰富,核具有多个深凹,类似肉瘤样Langerhans细胞组织细胞增生症。
3. 有些病例由多形性大细胞组成,类似于组织细胞肉瘤。

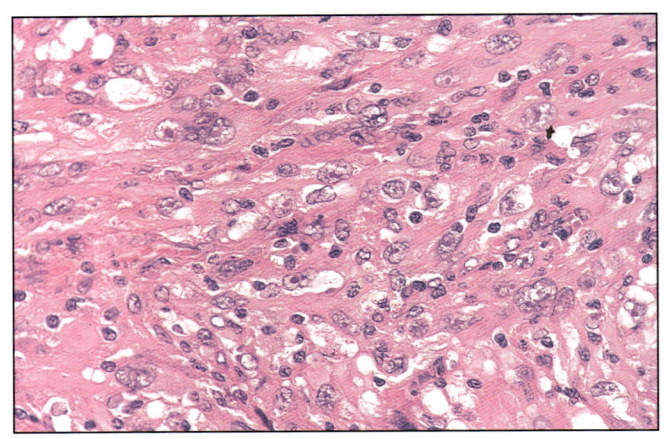

图21A.164　指状树突状细胞肉瘤。本例由肥胖的梭形和卵圆形细胞组成,核呈中等程度多形性。偶尔显示核沟。可见组织细胞样典型的嗜酸性胞浆。

免疫细胞化学、组织化学和电子显微镜

1. S100蛋白阳性。CD1a和langerin呈阴性。
2. CD68和ATP酶常常呈阳性。FDC标记物呈阴性。
3. CD45RB和CD4常常呈阳性。

超微结构可见长的胞浆突起,但没有桥粒或Birbeck颗粒。

鉴别诊断

淋巴结S100⁺梭形细胞恶性肿瘤的主要鉴别诊断包括:转移性恶性黑色素瘤和指状树突状细胞肉瘤,前者比后者更常见。为了得出指状树突状细胞肉瘤的诊断,必须注意S100染色的形态:应该出现细长的树状突,更可靠的是(有人认为绝对必要)显示其他淋巴造血系统标记物,如CD45RB、CD4和CD43。

纤维母细胞型树突状细胞肿瘤和非特指树突状细胞肿瘤
Fibroblastic dendritic cell tumors and dendritic cell tumor, not otherwise specified

有些淋巴结梭形细胞肿瘤显示类似于FDC肉瘤或指状树突状细胞肉瘤的组织学特征(只是常常出现细胞间胶原纤维),但缺乏FDC标记物和S100蛋白免疫反应。其中一些可能是纤维母细胞型树突状细胞肿瘤;可显示不同程度的细胞角蛋白、Actin、desmin和CD68免疫反应(图21A.165)[1360,1367-1369]。细胞角蛋白阳性染色并不奇怪,因为淋巴结的网状细胞可表达细胞角蛋白,但这种免疫表型可导致误诊为转移癌。其余完全不表达这些标记物的病例,可暂时归为"非特指树突状细胞肿瘤"。

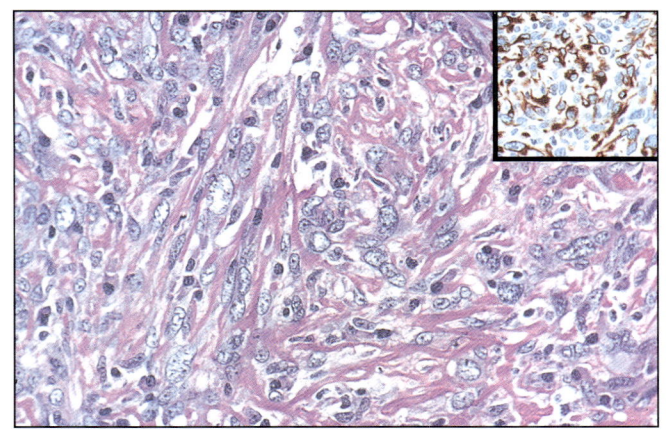

图21A.165 淋巴结纤维母细胞型树突状细胞肿瘤。梭形细胞与胶原纤维共存。本例显示desmin免疫反应，但对细胞角蛋白无反应（插图）。

浆细胞样单核细胞成瘤性聚集（所谓的浆细胞样单核细胞淋巴瘤）
Tumor-forming accumulation of plasmacytoid monocytes (so-called plasmacytoid monocytic lymphoma)

浆细胞样单核细胞（以前称为"浆细胞样 T 细胞"，最近称为"浆细胞样树突状细胞"），是正常时生成干扰素的细胞，是中等大小的单核细胞/组织细胞，形态学类似于浆细胞（核圆形或略不规则，染色质纤细，核仁小而不清楚，嗜双色性偏心性环状胞浆，没有高尔基区）[1370]。它们通常呈小簇状位于副皮质区，伴有许多核碎片。它们可发生于各种反应性淋巴组织增生中，尤其是 Kikuchi 淋巴结炎[1371-1375]。免疫表型谱系为 CD2⁻、CD3⁻、CD4⁺、CD68⁺、CD123⁺。

浆细胞样单核细胞成瘤性聚集已有报告（图

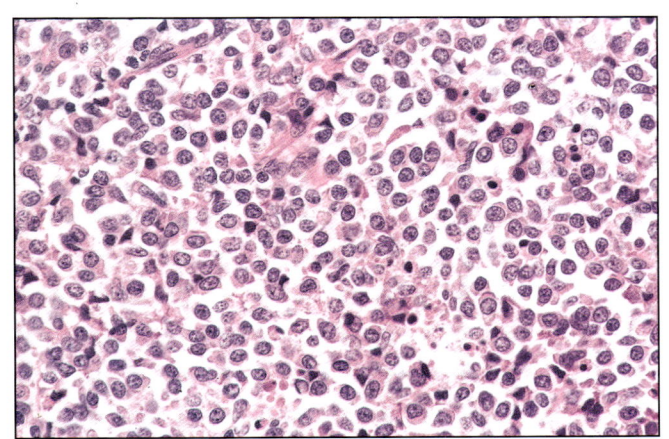

图21A.166 浆细胞样单核细胞成瘤性聚集（所谓的浆细胞样单核细胞淋巴瘤）。这些中等大小的细胞具有偏心性环状嗜双色性胞浆，类似于浆细胞。（Courtesy of Dr F. Facchetti, Brescia, Italy.）

21A.166）。几乎总是伴有髓性单核细胞性白血病、急性髓性白血病或髓性增生性病变，为浆细胞样单核细胞和单核细胞系列之间的联系提供了依据。在肿瘤性病变，除表达 CD4、CD68 和 CD123 以外，还可见 CD5 表达[1376-1383]。少数情况下，疾病表现为急性白血病[1384]。

Harris 和 Demirjian[1385] 提出，浆细胞样单核细胞仅仅是反应性的，因为与白血病浸润界限清楚，不显示髓细胞分化。类似的活跃性浆细胞样单核细胞反应也见于急性淋巴母细胞性白血病中[1379]。然而，至少有一例浆细胞样单核细胞显示与髓性白血病细胞相同的细胞遗传学异常，提示二者具有克隆相关性[1383]。

白血病及相关病变
Leukemia and related conditions

髓细胞肉瘤　Myeloid sarcoma

临床特征

髓细胞肉瘤（粒细胞性白血病）是一种原发于髓细胞的局部肿瘤[1,1386]。其可发生于不同部位，如皮肤、淋巴结、眼眶、心脏、骨、鼻咽、胃肠道、前列腺、睾丸、乳腺和女性生殖道[1386-1391]。肿瘤可出现于急性髓性白血病诊断之前、同时伴发或之后。对于彻底检查没有显示白血病证据的病例，如果没有给予系统性治疗，白血病几乎总是发生于间隔数周到数年之后。少数情况下，髓细胞肉瘤可以是骨髓增生异常综合征或慢性髓性增生性病变的首发体征。症状包括肿块、疼痛或与肿瘤部位有关的症状。

病理学

髓细胞肉瘤也称为"绿色瘤"（chloroma），因为新鲜标本略呈绿色。甲醛溶液固定时间过长，绿色可丢失，但将标本浸入过氧化氢中常常可恢复。

肿瘤特点是单形性中等到大细胞弥漫浸润，常伴有散在的嗜酸性粒细胞。肿瘤细胞核圆形或有折叠，染色质纤细，核仁清楚，胞浆量中等。有些细胞通常可见纤细的胞浆颗粒（图 A21A.167）。

鉴别诊断

髓细胞肉瘤常常被误诊为淋巴瘤，尤其是以前没有白血病病史的病例。正确诊断需要提高警觉性。组织学和免疫组化线索是[1]：

1. 任何少见的、不寻常表现或难以分类的"淋巴瘤"
2. 胞浆嗜酸性而不是嗜双色性或嗜碱性

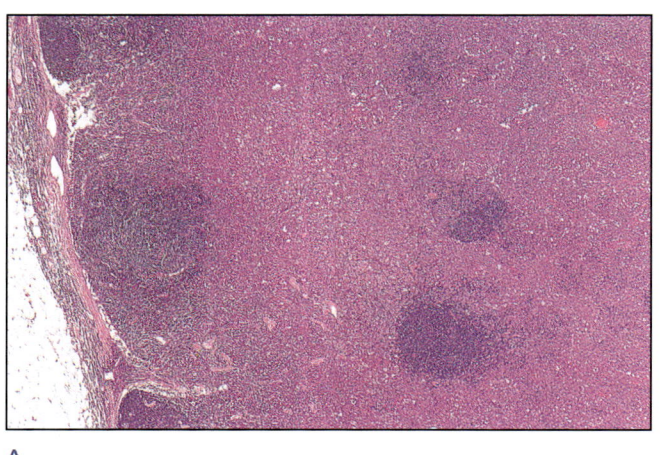
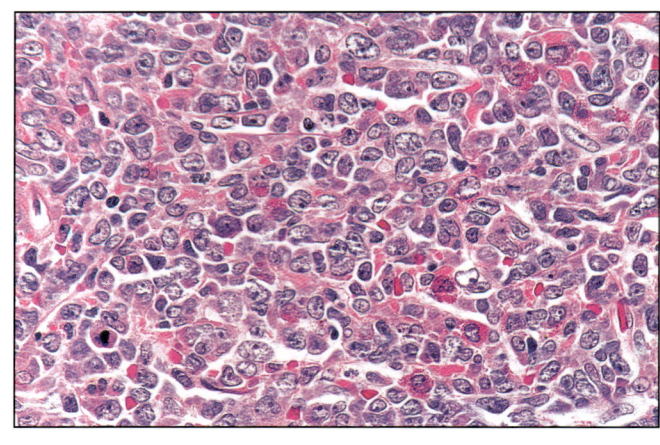

图21A.167 淋巴结髓细胞肉瘤。（A）常常呈部分受累，病变主要累及副皮质（淡染区）。（B）组织学图像类似于大细胞淋巴瘤。正确诊断的线索是可见散在的嗜酸性粒细胞。

3. 胞浆纤细颗粒状
4. 散在嗜酸性粒细胞
5. 斑片状或窦隙性累及淋巴结，伴有纤维间质中明显的"印第安纵队"结构浸润
6. 免疫表型"仅有CD43+"，即CD3⁻、CD20⁻、CD43+ [1392]。

Giemsa染色印片有利于观察嗜苯胺蓝胞浆颗粒，进一步为诊断提供支持。氯乙酸酯酶（Leder 染色）组织化学染色具有特异性（除了肥大细胞也着色之外），但对于证实髓细胞肉瘤的诊断不太敏感。目前最敏感和特异的免疫组化标记物是髓过氧化物酶 [1386,1393-1396]。在分化差的髓细胞肉瘤，髓过氧化物酶可呈阴性，诊断可由CD117和CD34阳性染色而支持 [1397]。在单核细胞型髓细胞肉瘤，髓过氧化物酶阴性，而CD68和CD163通常呈阳性。

毛细胞白血病 Hairy cell leukemia

见本章第2部分和第22章。

系统性肥大细胞增多症（系统性肥大细胞疾病） Systemic mastocytosis (systemic mast cell disease)

见本章B部分和第22章。

淋巴结转移性肿瘤 Metastatic tumor in lymph node

淋巴结常常被转移癌累及。淋巴结转移性肿瘤的病理学评估是重要的：（1）肿瘤的分期；（2）肿瘤复发的证实；（3）转移癌和恶性淋巴瘤的鉴别；以及（4）对于原发部位不明的转移癌，推测最可能的原发部位。

癌的分期或复发的证明

恶性黑色素瘤、多数癌和少数肉瘤容易转移至淋巴结。转移性肿瘤最初常常以孤立性细胞巢出现于被膜下窦，逐渐取代淋巴结实质。可伴有纤维组织增生性反应或炎症反应，包括肉芽肿形成。免疫组化检查有利于发现隐匿灶，如癌表达细胞角蛋白，黑色素瘤表达S100蛋白或HMB-45（图21A.168）。对于单个或小灶状细胞组成显微镜下转移灶，如果只有免疫组化染色能发现而形态学评估见不到，其临床意义仍有争议 [1398,1399]。

对于各种类型的癌，淋巴结受累的数目和水平，淋巴结转移灶的大小，以及有无结外蔓延，通常是最

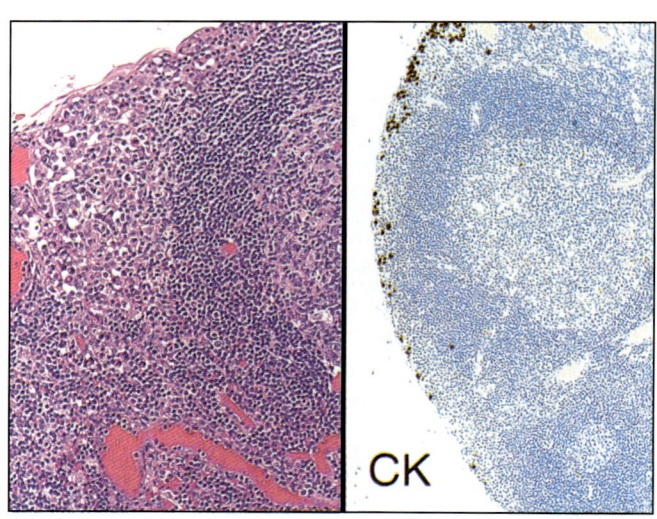

图21A.168 淋巴结转移性乳腺癌。左侧：可见被膜下窦隐匿受累。右侧：细胞角蛋白免疫染色有助于显示肿瘤细胞。在本例，病灶位于被膜下窦。

有意义的预后信息，这些可从切除检查的淋巴结标本中获得。近些年来前哨（第一站）淋巴结活检已受到越来越多的关注，可用其来预测下游区域淋巴结受累的可能性，免除某些患者不必要的淋巴结切除，这也有利于预后，如在乳腺癌和皮肤黑色素瘤[1400-1408]。

不要把淋巴结中的良性上皮或痣细胞包涵体误诊为转移癌。反之，转移癌可以呈欺骗性的良性表现而被误认为是发生性病变；例如，头颈部的鳞状细胞癌或甲状腺乳头状癌的囊性转移可被误诊为鳃裂囊肿。

转移癌与淋巴瘤的比较

有些转移癌（来源于鼻咽、乳腺或肺等部位）、黑色素瘤和生殖细胞肿瘤与恶性淋巴瘤难以鉴别（见"淋巴组织增生性病变诊断的实践问题"，第1250页）。儿童常见的问题是小圆细胞肿瘤，主要的鉴别诊断包括淋巴瘤/白血病、神经母细胞瘤、横纹肌肉瘤和Ewing肉瘤/原始外周神经外胚层肿瘤。

免疫组化研究很有帮助。应该使用一组抗体，至少包括细胞角蛋白、CD45RB（LCA）和S100抗体。免疫组化检查必须根据组织学和临床表现进行解释，要记住可能出现的陷阱，如淋巴结中树突状细胞会出现细胞角蛋白阳性，淋巴瘤偶尔会缺乏CD45RB表达[1409]。随着抗体可利用范围的扩展，电子显微镜的作用大大削弱了。

预测转移癌的原发部位
Prediction of the primary site for metastatic carcinoma

大约3%～4%的癌表现为隐匿性原发肿瘤转移[1410]。如果病理医生能提示可能的原发部位，尤其是对于可治愈或可有效缓解的肿瘤，在深入检查和治疗患者方面就极有帮助，如乳腺、前列腺、甲状腺和卵巢癌[1411]。患者性别、年龄和受累淋巴结的确切部位是至关重要的信息。例如，对于腋窝淋巴结转移，要考虑原发于乳腺或肺；对于锁骨上淋巴结转移要考虑乳腺、肺或生殖器官原发。

形态学评估可提供重要的诊断线索，有助于选择特殊检查。肿瘤细胞中出现胆汁可诊断肝细胞癌。成片界限不清的细胞，具有密集的泡状核和明显的核仁，要考虑鼻咽部未分化癌（图21A.169）。在有选择的情况下，免疫组化检查尤其有帮助，见表21A.21。一般情况下，腺癌会比鳞状细胞癌获得更多信息。虽然免疫组化所见并非总有定论，但常常有助于缩窄原发肿瘤的可能部位，例如"转移性腺癌；原发部位不可能在胃肠道"。

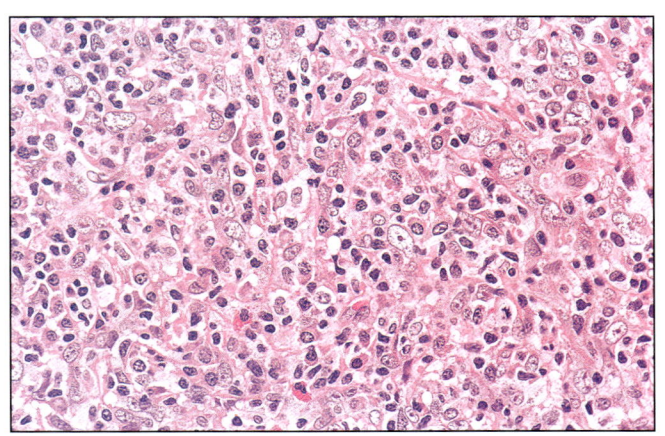

图21A.169　颈淋巴结转移性未分化鼻咽癌。滤泡间存在肿瘤细胞和淋巴细胞混合浸润，可被误诊为淋巴瘤。右侧视野出现模糊的细胞巢结构提示肿瘤的上皮性本质。在鼻咽癌，细胞边界通常不清楚，核呈空泡状。

淋巴结非淋巴造血系统肿瘤和瘤样病变
Non-hematolymphoid tumors and tumor-like lesions of lymph nodes

淋巴结各种非淋巴造血系统肿瘤和瘤样病变见表21A.22。

伴石棉样纤维的出血性梭形细胞肿瘤（栅栏状或淋巴结内肌纤维母细胞瘤）
Hemorrhagic spindle cell tumor with amianthoid fibers (palisaded or intranodal myofibroblastoma)

这是一种罕见的肿瘤，可发生于各年龄段[1412-1417]。患者表现为淋巴结肿大，最常见于腹股沟区。肿瘤界限非常清楚，周边可见受压的淋巴结组织。由表现良性、actin阳性的交叉的束状梭形细胞组成，核呈梭形，代表肌纤维母细胞。独特的特征是形成星形胶原结节（石棉样纤维）（图21A.170），并常常出现灶性栅栏状核排列。有些病例可见胞浆内线状包涵体。间质出血常常很明显，周边可见出血区。与Kaposi肉瘤不同，HHV8免疫染色呈阴性。

淋巴结非淋巴造血系统肿瘤和瘤样病变

表21A.21　有助于预测转移癌的可能的原发部位的抗体或探针组合

癌的组织学类型	预测可能的原发部位的抗体或探针	解释
腺癌结构	CK7和CK20	CK7⁺CK20⁻：非特异性表型，见于许多部位的腺癌 CK7⁻CK20⁺：肠癌 CK⁺CK20⁺：有些胃和胰腺胆管腺癌；女性生殖道黏液腺癌 CK7⁻CK20⁻：考虑肾和前列腺腺癌
	表面活性物质	肺腺癌
	甲状腺转录因子1	甲状腺癌或肺腺癌
	BRST-2（GCDFP-15）	乳腺癌；唾液腺癌；汗腺癌
	甲状腺球蛋白	甲状腺滤泡细胞肿瘤
	降钙素	甲状腺髓样癌
	前列腺特异性抗原	前列腺癌
	CDX-2	肠癌；肠类癌；一部分胰腺胆管癌病例，胃癌，食管癌和卵巢癌
	CA-125	女性生殖道癌，但少部分胰腺胆管癌、乳腺癌、肺癌、甲状腺癌、胃癌和肝腺癌也可呈阳性
	WT1	卵巢浆液性腺癌；间皮瘤
	HEP-PAR1	肝细胞癌；某些胃癌
	钙网素（calretinin）	间皮瘤；某些中到低分化结直肠腺癌
	CK5/6（高分子量角蛋白）	间皮瘤
	CD30	胚胎性癌
	胎盘碱性磷酸酶	可能为生殖细胞肿瘤
	Oct-3/4	胚胎性癌（或生殖细胞瘤/精原细胞瘤）
鳞状细胞，移行细胞或未分化癌	CD5	胸腺癌
	CK20	尿路上皮癌
	凝血调节蛋白	尿路上皮癌
	EBER原位杂交	鼻咽癌；原始咽和前肠来源部位的淋巴上皮瘤样癌
小细胞癌	CK20	Merkel细胞癌（皮肤、涎腺或少数淋巴结来源）

淋巴结中平滑肌增生
Smooth muscle proliferations in lymph nodes

淋巴结门部平滑肌增生
Smooth muscle proliferation in the nodal hilum

这是一种偶尔的发现，以淋巴结门部杂乱的平滑肌细胞增生为特点，伴有纤维化和明显的血管成分[1418]。

淋巴管肌瘤病和血管肌脂肪瘤
Lymphangiomyomatosis and angiomyolipoma

淋巴管肌瘤病是一种淋巴管和肥胖的胞浆淡染的平滑肌细胞增生（图21A.171），多发生于育龄女性[1,1419]。虽然肺最先受累，也可累及纵隔和腹腔内淋巴结。有时病变为盆腔淋巴结（淋巴结的淋巴管肌瘤）的偶然发现。除了对各种肌样标记物染色以外，淋巴管肌瘤/淋巴管肌瘤病还通常可着染黑色素瘤抗体 HMB45 或 Melan-A。因此，这些病变属于血管周上皮样细胞肿瘤家族（见第24章）。

淋巴结也可极为罕见地被血管肌脂肪瘤累及。与淋巴管肌瘤病有很多共同的形态学特征[1,1420]。

表21A.22	淋巴结原发非淋巴造血系统肿瘤和瘤样病变

A	间质，包括平滑肌和肌纤维母细胞
	  1. 伴石棉样纤维的出血性梭形细胞肿瘤（栅栏状肌纤维母细胞瘤）
	  2. 平滑肌增生
	    a. 淋巴结门部平滑肌增生
	    b. 血管肌脂肪瘤
	    c. 淋巴管肌瘤病/淋巴管肌瘤
	    d. 平滑肌瘤病
	    e. 血管肌瘤性错构瘤
	    f. 淋巴结内平滑肌瘤
	  3. 炎性假瘤
	  4. 蜕膜病

B	血管
	  1. Kaposi肉瘤
	  2. 血管瘤，血管内皮细胞瘤和血管肉瘤
	  3. 淋巴管瘤
	  4. Castleman病中的血管肌样增生性病变
	  5. Castleman病中的血管肿瘤
	  6. 淋巴窦血管转化
	  7. 杆菌性血管瘤病

C	上皮细胞和痣包涵体
	  1. 腺体包涵体
	  2. 痣细胞聚集和蓝痣

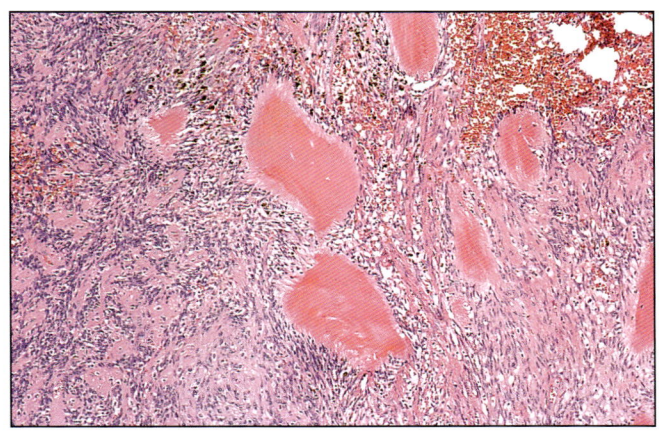

图21A.170　伴石棉样纤维的腹股沟淋巴结的出血性梭形细胞肿瘤（栅栏状肌纤维母细胞瘤）。短束状梭形细胞伴有散在的星形胶原结节。可见间质出血。（Courtesy of Dr Saul Suster, Columbus, Ohio.）

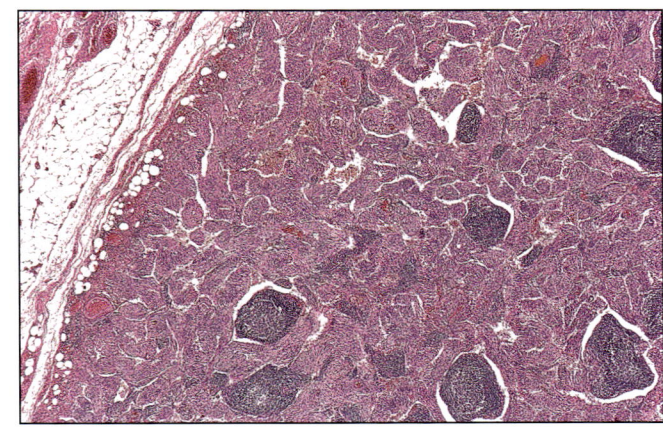

图21A.171　淋巴管肌瘤病累及淋巴结。短束状梭形细胞与细分枝状血管空隙交错排列。

血管肌瘤性错构瘤
Angiomyomatous hamartoma

这种病变几乎全部发生于腹股沟淋巴结，可能伴有同侧淋巴水肿。淋巴结门部厚壁血管增生延伸入淋巴结实质，表现为硬化性间质中杂乱排列的平滑肌细胞（图21A.172）[1421]。

淋巴结平滑肌瘤病和平滑肌瘤
Nodal leiomyomatosis and leiomyoma

少数情况下，淋巴结可被平滑肌瘤病或平滑肌瘤累及[1]。

淋巴结炎性假瘤
Inflammatory pseudotumor of lymph node

这是一种少见的、发生于年轻成人的良性淋巴结肿大，患者常有发热[2,1422-1426]。常见血沉加快、贫血和高丙种球蛋白血症。淋巴结常常肿大、缠结。病变主要累及淋巴结结缔组织网，特点是梭形细胞增生（主要为活化的组织细胞和纤维母细胞）、薄壁血管和单核细胞[1427]。淋巴结周边组织常可见静脉炎。

淋巴结炎性假瘤在临床和形态学上不同于肺及其他部位所谓的炎性假瘤（炎性肌纤维母细胞瘤），至少有些病例可能与特发性纤维硬化病有关[1426,1428]。分枝杆菌梭形细胞假瘤必须应用Ziehl-Neelsen染色予以排除。

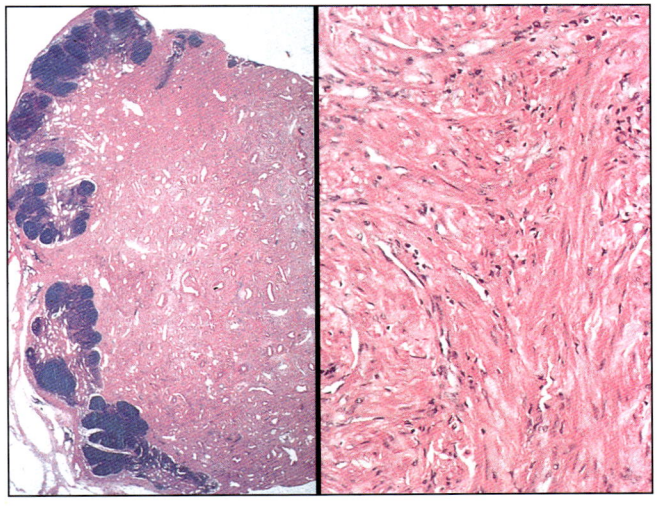

图21A.172　淋巴结血管肌瘤性错构瘤。左图：淋巴结组织被病变广泛替代。在门部（右侧视野）可见增生的厚壁血管。右图：在实质，平滑肌细胞杂乱排列在硬化性间质中。血管腔明显。

淋巴结蜕膜病　Deciduosis of lymph nodes

在妊娠女性，成片的蜕膜细胞可见于腹腔内淋巴结[1]。蜕膜细胞为多角形，细胞膜清楚，胞浆丰富，嗜双色性（有时呈空泡状），核略呈多形性。缺少纤维组织增生性反应、核分裂象和角化，不同于转移性鳞状细胞癌。

淋巴结Kaposi肉瘤
Kaposi sarcoma of lymph node

临床特征

Kaposi 肉瘤是一种独特的血管肿瘤，可能来源于淋巴管，常常显示多中心性生长。已显示其为一种克隆性（肿瘤性）病变，至少某些病例如此[1429,1430]（更详细的内容见第 3 章）。淋巴结受累可见于流行性 HIV 感染、其他免疫抑制患者，或者是非洲儿童迅速进展的淋巴肿大。

Kaposi 肉瘤与人类疱疹病毒 8 型（HHV-8）恒定相关，与临床背景无关[1440,1441]。

病理学

淋巴结中成型的 Kaposi 肉瘤表现为单一或多发结节，有时完全取代淋巴结实质（图 21A.173）[1442,1443]。早期病变常局限于被膜区（图 21A.174），但许多病变显示沿着纤维条索蔓延至淋巴结[1432,1444]。窦隙受累极少见。

成型的 Kaposi 肉瘤的特点是弯曲交错的梭形细胞束，导致纵切面显示为并排的束状结构，而横切面显示滤网状结构。小血管腔和裂隙含有外渗的红细胞，后者常常更明显。梭形细胞通常（但不一定）呈良性外观，核分裂不活跃（图 21A.175A）。还可见肥胖的卵圆形细胞，常常与某些隧道样的血管腔融合（图

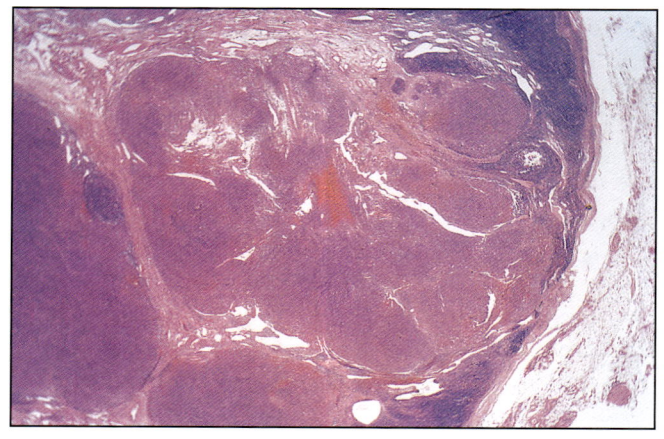

图 21A.173　Kaposi肉瘤累及淋巴结。肿瘤呈多结节形生长。可见淋巴管扩张围绕肿瘤结节。

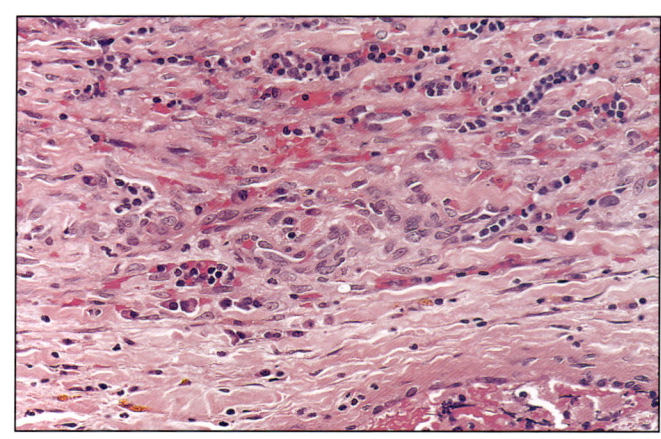

图 21A.174　累及淋巴结被膜的早期的、轻微的Kaposi肉瘤。梭形细胞、薄壁血管和浆细胞轻度增多提示诊断，中心细胞可见玻璃样变小体，有助于明确诊断。

21A.175B）。非常独特的表现是梭形或卵圆形细胞胞浆内出现大小不等的 PAS 阳性嗜酸性玻璃样变小体（图 21A.175B）[1431,1432]。这种肿瘤的血管本质可以通过 CD31 或 CD34 免疫染色进一步证实。

淋巴结被膜的早期 Kaposi 肉瘤很难诊断，仅有不明显的不规则血管腔增多，混有浆细胞和少数梭形细胞（图 21A.174）。玻璃样变小体的出现强烈支持这种诊断，可由 HHV-8 免疫染色阳性证实[1441]。

Kaposi 肉瘤必须与以下病变鉴别：淋巴窦血管转化、伴石棉样纤维的出血性梭形细胞肿瘤、杆菌性血管瘤病、炎性假瘤以及其他淋巴结血管肿瘤。与良性血管瘤不同，Kaposi 肉瘤中没有或少有 actin 阳性的周细胞。

淋巴结原发性血管肿瘤
Primary vascular tumors of lymph node

除 Kaposi 肉瘤外，其他淋巴结原发血管肿瘤很少见[1,1421,1445,1446]，包括血管瘤、血管内皮细胞瘤、上皮样血管瘤和淋巴管瘤（图 21A.176）。绝大多数为良性。诊断淋巴结上皮样血管内皮细胞瘤应仔细排除其他原发部位的可能性。

合并玻璃样变血管型Castleman病的血管增生性病变
Vasoproliferative lesions complicating hyaline-vascular Castleman disease

多种血管增生性病变可与玻璃样变血管型 Castleman 病并存。从良性到恶性的各种血管肿瘤均有报道[1446,1447]。滤泡间区可以发生明显的间质过度增生，由小静脉（CD34[+]）和梭形细胞（actin[+]）组成，不形成明确的肿瘤（图 21A.177）：这种血管肌样增生性病变预后良好[1347]。要与滤泡间 FDC 增生性病变鉴别，后者具

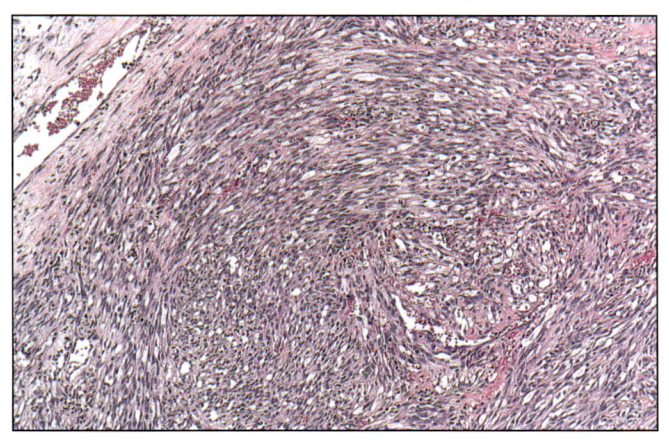
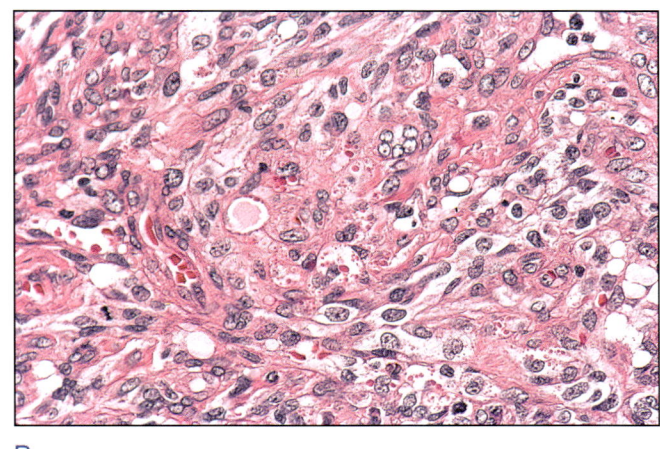

图21A.175　淋巴结Kaposi肉瘤。（A）交错弯曲的梭形细胞束，纵切面细胞与横切面细胞并行。裂隙中可见红细胞。（B）这一视野的许多细胞显示Kaposi肉瘤特征性的嗜酸性玻璃样小体。

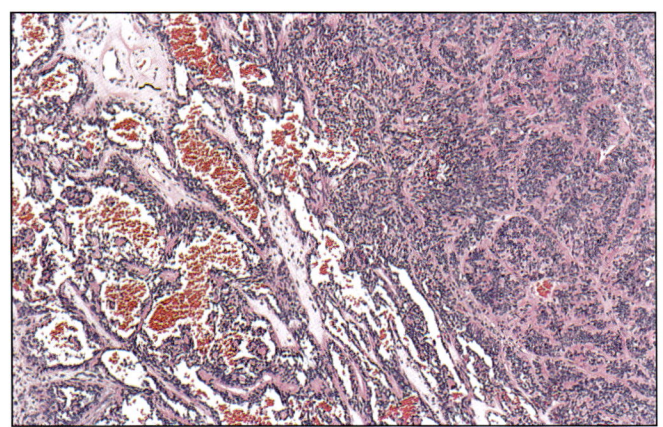

图21A.176　淋巴结原发性多形性血管内皮细胞瘤。这种少见肿瘤的特点是外观良性的细胞呈实性"器官样"生长（右侧视野），与不规则的血管裂隙（视野上方）混合，并在海绵状血管腔内生长（左侧视野）。

有复发和转移潜能[1347]。

淋巴窦血管转化
Vascular transformation of lymph node sinuses

这是一种反应性疾病，常常伴有淋巴管阻塞[1445,1448]。它可能是手术切除淋巴结时的偶然发现，或可表现为淋巴结肿大。复杂吻合的内衬扁平内皮细胞的血管腔使淋巴窦扩张，常伴有间质硬化。可出现富于梭形或肥胖细胞的区域，也可见朝向被膜的成熟的结构良好的血管腔（图21A.178）。常见红细胞外渗。少数情况下血管腔形成丛状，或形成模糊的或明显的结节[1446,1449]。淋巴窦血管转化不同于Kaposi肉瘤之处在于：仅累及淋巴窦，不累及淋巴结被膜，"成熟"方向朝向被膜下窦，缺乏PAS阳性玻璃样变小体，HHV-8染色呈阴性。

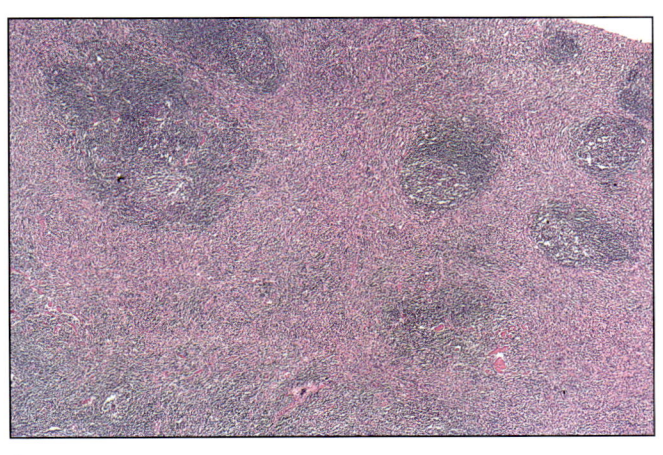
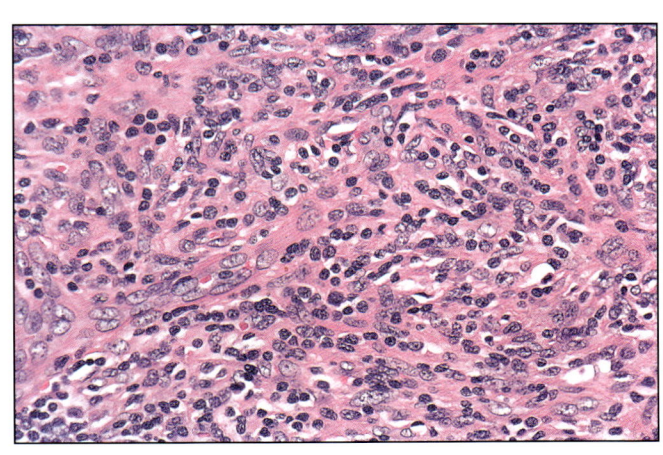

图21A.177　玻璃样变血管型Castleman病中的血管肌样增生性病变。（A）滤泡间区明显增宽。（B）病变由梭形细胞组成，核淡染，伴有血管，混合有小淋巴细胞。需要通过免疫染色将其与滤泡树突状细胞增生性病变相鉴别。

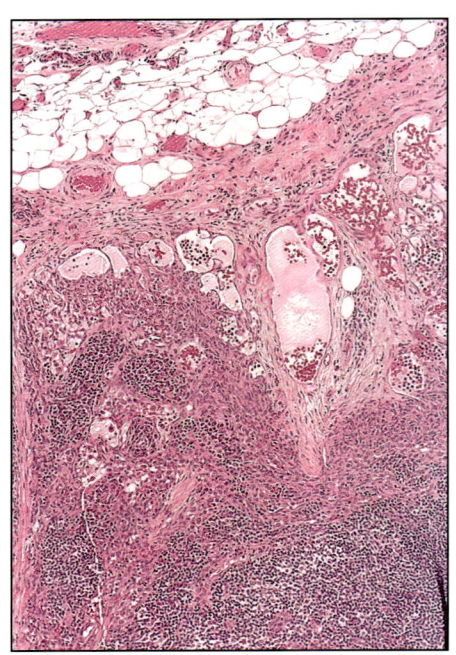

图21A.178 淋巴窦血管转化。窦隙转化成血管腔，位于纤维间质中。富于细胞的区域由梭形细胞组成，散在分布一些分枝状血管裂隙。合并成形成完好的血管，朝向被膜下窦（顶部）。

杆菌性血管瘤病　Bacillary angiomatosis

杆菌性血管瘤病是一种瘤样血管增生性病变，由巴尔通体属的 *henselae* 或 *quintana* 引起[1430-1460]。前一种微生物也是猫抓病的病原体。杆菌性血管瘤病几乎全部发生于免疫抑制患者，尤其是 AIDS 患者，在抗结核预防情况下已极其少见。皮肤是最常见的受累部位（表现为多发性皮肤结节），但淋巴结和脾也可受累。疾病可为致死性的，但对抗生素（红霉素）反应良好。

淋巴结杆菌性血管瘤病的特点是多发融合性结节，结节由内衬肥胖内皮细胞的管状或扩张血管组成，可显示某种程度的核多形性[1461]。典型特征是可见细胞外嗜双色性物质，Wharthin-Starry 染色或免疫组化染色可显示密集的巴尔通体属 *henselae* 杆菌[1462]。虽然间质中通常富于中性粒细胞，但有时可稀少或缺乏。

淋巴结中的上皮细胞或间皮细胞包涵体　Epithelial or mesothelial inclusions in lymph node

上皮成分有时可见于淋巴结内，类似于转移癌。良性 müller 包涵体偶尔可见于女性腹腔内淋巴结[1]。腺体可呈囊性，常常被覆纤毛或分泌性上皮。缺乏核非典型性、核分裂象和纤维组织增生性反应。子宫内膜异位症有时可引起淋巴结增大。

涎腺包涵体常常可见于腮腺内淋巴结和颈部淋巴结[1]。许多肿瘤，如 Warthin 瘤、多形性腺瘤和黏液表皮样癌，可来源于这些包涵体[1]。少数情况下，乳腺包涵体可见于腋窝淋巴结。

颈部淋巴结内甲状腺滤泡包涵体很少见，必须应用严格的标准诊断，包括显微镜下大小、缺乏细胞学非典型性及没有间质反应，因为淋巴结中见到甲状腺滤泡更可能代表隐匿性甲状腺乳头状癌转移[1]。

良性间皮细胞有时可见于纵隔或腹腔内淋巴结，几乎总是伴有浆膜腔渗出或炎症。间皮细胞主要见于淋巴窦内，呈孤立的细胞或簇状，可被误诊为转移癌。细胞呈多角形，核呈良性，胞浆丰富，嗜酸性，伴有细胞间"窗"。有时常规组织学切片难以识别间皮细胞，只有通过细胞角蛋白或钙网素免疫染色来显示。其被认为是通过淋巴管栓塞到达淋巴结的[1463-1470]。

淋巴结内痣细胞　Nevus cells in lymph node

淋巴结内痣细胞聚集很少见，最常位于颈腋部，表现为被膜内形态良性的细胞结节或条索，不同程度地蔓延到淋巴结周围组织和实质。更少见的是痣细胞完全聚集在实质内[1470a]。常常缺乏黑色素。蓝痣也可少见地发生于淋巴结被膜，有时伴有相似的皮肤病变[1,1471]。

淋巴组织增生性病变诊断的实践问题

以下内容中以星号（*）标记的病变是鉴别诊断中最重要的考虑。

中等大小的滤泡：诊断思路

主要的鉴别诊断

- 反应性滤泡增生*
- 滤泡性淋巴瘤*
- 结节性套细胞淋巴瘤*
- 边缘区B细胞淋巴瘤伴有滤泡克隆化*
- Castleman病
- 滤泡性T细胞淋巴瘤

淋巴母细胞性淋巴瘤显示多结节性生长结构，可误诊为滤泡性淋巴瘤。结节不是真性滤泡，而是大量聚集性肿瘤细胞，周围有纤维网或血管包绕（图21A.39）。细胞成分也与滤泡中心细胞淋巴瘤的不一致。其他线索包括单形性细胞群和高核分裂计数。

怎样鉴别反应性滤泡增生和滤泡性淋巴瘤？

反应性滤泡增生的滤泡是独立的，至少由一些滤泡间淋巴组织分隔；滤泡大小和形状常常不一，常见哑铃状或扭曲结构（图21A.62和21A.179）。具有界限清楚的套区，然而有些反应性病变中缺少套区，尤其是在HIV相关性淋巴结肿大和儿童淋巴结（图21.A.180）。滤泡显示异源性滤泡中心细胞，大细胞数量常常超过小细胞。通常散在含可染小体的巨噬细胞，细胞极向分亮区和暗区（图21A.179B）。

滤泡性淋巴瘤最重要的诊断标准是看低倍镜下的滤泡排列。滤泡背靠背遍布整个淋巴结实质，只有少量的滤泡间组织，是滤泡性淋巴瘤的诊断标准（图21A.60和21A.61）。这种结构可见于80%的滤泡性淋巴瘤病例[530]。余下的病例诊断较困难。在这种情况下，当见到下列两种或多种特征时，应该考虑滤泡性淋巴瘤[1,2]：

- 总是没有含可染小体的巨噬细胞（图21A.61、21A.53和21A.64）
- 滤泡中以中心细胞为主（图21A.65A）
- 总是套区缺乏或不完整（图21A.61和21A.64）
- 滤泡中总是缺乏细胞的极向（图21A.64）
- 淋巴结周围组织中可见滤泡（图21A.60）
- 侵犯血管壁（图21A.67）
- 异常增生的滤泡中心细胞（细胞核很长，奇异形细胞，印戒细胞，许多多核细胞）
- 在滤泡间区可见非典型细胞（细胞比小淋巴细胞大，具有不规则核折叠），提示出现滤泡外侵犯（图21A.66）。

年龄也是重要的考虑因素。在儿童和年轻人，作出滤泡性淋巴瘤诊断应极其慎重。骨髓活检也很有帮助，因为出现小梁旁淋巴组织浸润可为诊断滤泡性淋巴瘤提供有力的支持。如果有任何可疑之处，则应该进行特殊

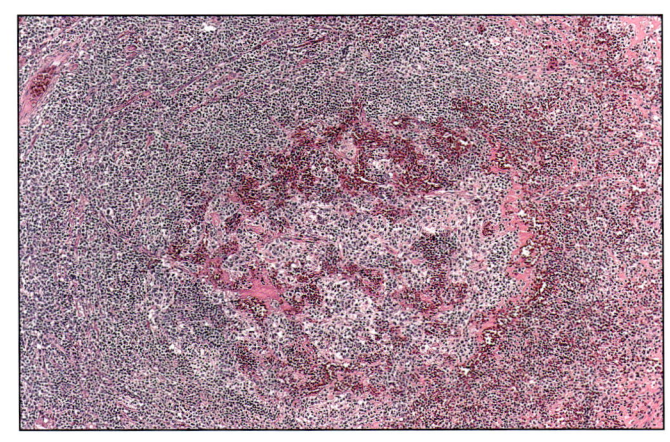

图21A.180 一例HIV阳性患者的爆发性反应性滤泡增生。淋巴滤泡缺乏明确的套区，显示滤泡裂解，出血和分散的细胞斑片是其证据。

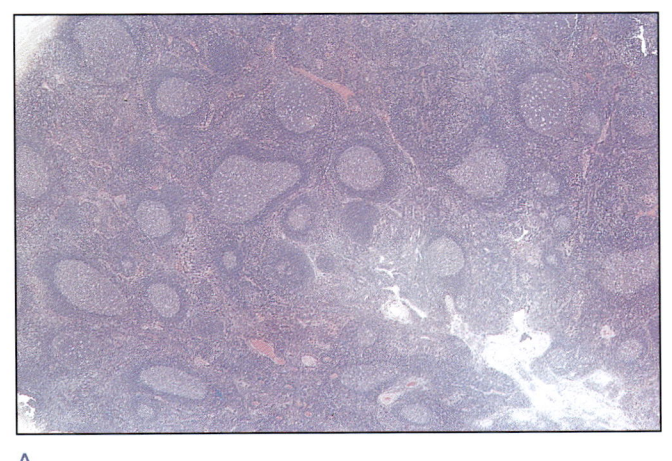

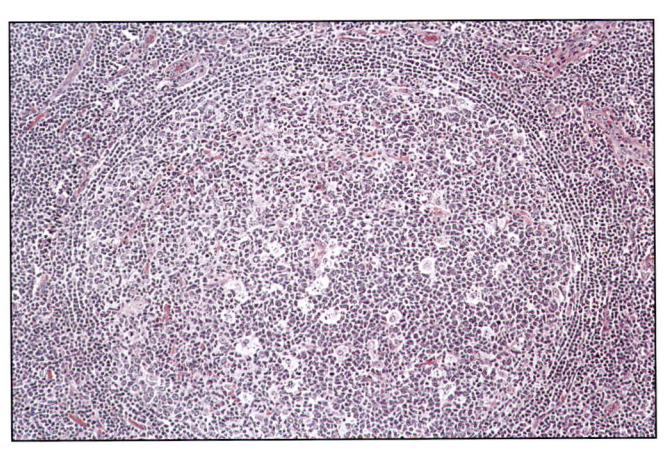

图21A.179 作为对照的反应性滤泡增生。（A）滤泡间隔宽，中心通常呈斑点状。有些滤泡显示极向（存在暗区和亮区）（B）有界限清楚的套区。由于具有含可染小体的巨噬细胞，生发中心部分生发中心浅染（亮区），部分深染，富于含可染小体的巨噬细胞。

形态学评估注意事项

对于上面列出的标准，可能有许多例外。含可染小体的巨噬细胞可见于一些滤泡性淋巴瘤病例。反应性滤泡中心浸润的众多反应性T淋巴细胞会给人小细胞为主或细胞单一的印象。在有些反应性滤泡增生病例，套区菲薄或缺乏，尤其是在儿童和HIV感染者。有些滤泡性淋巴瘤病例可显示某种程度的细胞极向，尤其是2级病例。当原本的反应性滤泡被滤泡性淋巴瘤部分累及时，组织学表现具有高度迷惑性。

免疫组化检查帮助诊断滤泡性淋巴瘤

1. 滤泡中心bcl-2阳性（图21A.77）。总体上，85%的滤泡性淋巴瘤bcl-2呈阳性，因此这是对鉴别滤泡性淋巴瘤和滤泡性增生唯一最有用的免疫染色[573,574]。但是，反应性滤泡可能偶尔具有一定数量的T淋巴细胞（bcl-2呈阳性）而被误认为阳性；与对应切片的T细胞染色结果进行对比可以解决这个问题[583]。Bcl-2染色呈阴性不能排除滤泡性淋巴瘤。在这种情况下，需要进行其他免疫染色提供支持性证据。

2. 滤泡间区密集排列CD20$^+$或CD79a$^+$B细胞，提示淋巴瘤侵犯滤泡间区[532]。在反应性滤泡增生，滤泡间区应该富于T细胞，仅有孤立或小灶状B细胞（图21A.2）。

3. 在滤泡间区出现数量较多的CD10$^+$细胞提示滤泡间侵犯（因此支持诊断滤泡性淋巴瘤），因为正常情况下该区域很少或没有CD10$^+$的淋巴细胞（图21A.181）[532]。滤泡间肿瘤细胞的CD10表达常常比滤泡内肿瘤细胞的弱。

4. 滤泡中心细胞可见轻链限制性[583]。在反应性滤泡增生，Ig轻链有多型性染色，常呈网状，而非不连续的滤泡中心细胞膜或胞浆染色。

5. Ki-67染色。在反应性滤泡，Ki-67免疫染色常显示极向，因为相当多的暗区滤泡中心细胞着染（图21A.76）。滤泡Ki-67（增生）指数低支持滤泡性淋巴瘤诊断，而不支持反应性滤泡增生（Ki-67平均指数分别为15.6%和64.9%），然而Ki-67指数高也不是决定性的[583]。

分子学研究支持诊断滤泡性淋巴瘤而不是反应性滤泡增生的依据如下：

1. Ig mRNA原位杂交显示单型性。

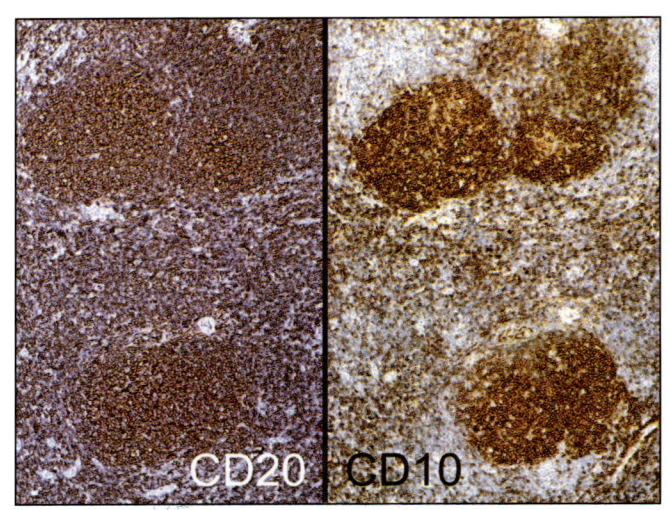

图21A.181　滤泡性淋巴瘤，疑难病例（滤泡孤立、分散）。诊断可通过免疫染色证实。左侧：CD20染色显示的不仅是滤泡，而且还显示滤泡之间的片状阳性细胞。右侧：CD10染色勾画出滤泡，但许多阳性细胞也见于滤泡间区，提示滤泡中心细胞侵犯这一区域。

2. 基因型研究：
   (a) 可见Ig基因重排
   (b) 可见*BCL-2*基因重排。

其他考虑

结节型套细胞淋巴瘤可极其类似于滤泡性淋巴瘤（图21A.54）。如果细胞成分单一或不规则折叠的核总体上呈圆形，则必须慎重考虑。一旦有任何疑问，免疫组化检查通常可澄清诊断（滤泡性淋巴瘤CD5$^-$、CD10$^+$、bcl-6$^+$、cyclin D1$^-$；套细胞淋巴瘤CD5$^+$、CD10$^-$、bcl-6$^-$、cyclin D1$^+$）。Bcl-2免疫染色在鉴别诊断方面没有价值，因为它不是滤泡中心细胞标记物，套细胞淋巴瘤几乎总是呈阳性。

边缘区B细胞淋巴瘤伴有明显的滤泡克隆化可能难以与滤泡性淋巴瘤鉴别。前者至少在有些区域通常具有明显的滤泡周围和滤泡间淋巴瘤浸润，有些淋巴瘤细胞通常显示单核样B细胞形态。免疫组化显示除少量残留的滤泡中心细胞外，滤泡内细胞不表达滤泡中心细胞标记物，如CD10、bcl-6。

滤泡性T细胞淋巴瘤极其罕见。在接受这种诊断之前，必须排除富于T细胞的滤泡性淋巴瘤（B细胞系）（见"滤泡性淋巴瘤"，第1184页）。

大淋巴结节：诊断思路

主要鉴别诊断

- 结节性淋巴细胞为主型 Hodgkin 淋巴瘤（N-LPHL）*
- 结节性富于淋巴细胞的经典型 Hodgkin 淋巴瘤（N-LRCHL）*
- 生发中心进行性转化（PTGC）*
- 结节硬化型 Hodgkin 淋巴瘤（NSHL）*
- 滤泡性淋巴瘤，花样亚型（floral variant）或类似于 N-LPHL 的亚型
- 结节性富于 B 细胞型滤泡树突状细胞瘤
- （伴假小叶生长结构的淋巴母细胞性淋巴瘤）。

诊断上的问题

一般情况下，N-LPHL、N-LRCHL 和 PTGC 的淋巴结节比滤泡性淋巴瘤的大（图 21A.7、21A.16、21A.182）。结节可密集或分散。虽然 N-LPHL 的肿瘤细胞（L&H 细胞）和 N-LRCHL 的肿瘤细胞（经典型 Reed-Sternberg 细胞及其变型）在典型病例中是不同的，但有些病例显示形态重合。因此慎重的做法是对所有的病例进行免疫组化检查来证实诊断。

PTGC 的特点是滤泡大而深染，散在分布于普通形态的反应滤泡之间。大滤泡的直径是反应性滤泡的 3～4 倍，并且富于小淋巴细胞，但可能含有孤立性或小灶状残留的滤泡中心细胞（图 21A.16）。滤泡不十分拥挤。缺乏 L&H 细胞，在大滤泡中，可见少数或没有围绕大淋巴细胞的 T 细胞花环[97]。PTGC 的诊断标准常常被误解，例如认为带状套区淋巴细胞"侵犯"滤泡中心足以作出诊断。

形态学评估

首先，大淋巴结节的分布和结构要在低倍镜下评估。

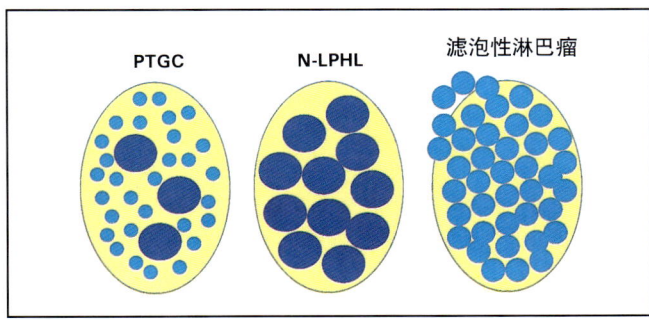

图21A.182 通过示意图显示生发中心进行性转化（PTGC）、N-LPHL和滤泡性淋巴瘤的结构差异。N-LPHL中的结节通常较大。在滤泡性淋巴瘤，结节常常紧密排列且侵犯淋巴结周围组织。

伴假小叶结构的淋巴母细胞性淋巴瘤可容易排除，因为结节是由纤细的粉染纤维间隔或血管勾画出来的，不是真正的滤泡。如果所有的大淋巴结节都是异常的，最不可能是 PTGC。如果偶尔有异常的大滤泡散在分布于普通反应性滤泡之间，则可能是 PTGC，尽管这种结构也能见于少数 N-LPHL 和 N-LRCHL 中。结节硬化型 HL 的结节通常易于识别，因为伴有硬化和出现结节性聚集中的陷窝细胞（图 21A.26）。

其次，评估大淋巴结节的细胞成分。N-LPHL、N-LRCHL 和 PTGC 的结节以小淋巴细胞为主。在 N-LPHL 的结节内通常见不到残留的生发中心。不规则形小生发中心常见于大结节 PTGC，萎缩的生发中心常见于 N-LRCHL 结节内。如果结节内大多数细胞显示生发中心细胞的形态学特征，则必须考虑滤泡性淋巴瘤。有些 N-LPHL 和 N-LRCHL 病例中存在令人迷惑的特征，在淋巴结节内可见大量聚集的中等细胞，胞浆淡染；这些是 T 淋巴细胞，通常围绕肿瘤性大细胞。

肿瘤性大细胞见于 Hodgkin 淋巴瘤和结节性富于 B 细胞的滤泡树突状细胞瘤内，但不应出现于 PTGC 内。在 Hodgkin 淋巴瘤，肿瘤细胞胞浆通常界限清楚，虽然在结节硬化型可见胞浆回缩（陷窝细胞）。在结节性富于 B 细胞的滤泡树突状细胞瘤，肿瘤细胞常呈大的"裸"核，因为胞浆边界不清。

免疫组化评估

CD20 免疫染色最有价值，能显示淋巴结节及其结构。在 PTGC，普通型反应性滤泡和散在的大滤泡均得以显示；使用 CD20 免疫染色可见后者具有单个或多个不规则形小生发中心。而且，这些 CD20+ 滤泡不形成虫蚀状。在 N-LPHL 和 N-LRCHL，结节富于 CD20+ 的小淋巴细胞，但明显的是肿瘤细胞及其周围的 T 细胞花环形成的多个无色区（图 21A.12）。生发中心在 N-LPHL 的结节中最少见，但可见于 N-LRCHL 的结节。在 NSHL，结节内淋巴细胞可以是 CD20+ 的 B 细胞或主要为 CD3+ 的 T 细胞。N-LPHL 的肿瘤细胞 CD20+，而 N-LRCHL 或 NSHL 的肿瘤细胞则呈阴性或染色呈不一致性。

在 N-LPHL、N-LRCHL 和一些 NSHL，CD3 显示肿瘤细胞周围的 T 细胞花环。N-LPHL 的 T 细胞花环常常共表达 bcl-6 和 CD57（图 21A.13），而 N-LRCHL 的 T 细胞花环极少表达这些标记物。在 PTGC，T 细胞花环很少见或缺乏。

在经典型 Hodgkin 淋巴瘤（N-LRCHL 和 NSHL），CD30 和 CD15 有助于显示肿瘤细胞，CD21 着染结节性富于 B 细胞的滤泡树突状细胞瘤的肿瘤细胞。

弥漫性小细胞或混合性淋巴细胞浸润是反应性的还是肿瘤性的？

形态学评估

当见到主要由小细胞或密切混合性小细胞和较大细胞组成的密集淋巴组织浸润时，无论是弥漫性浸润还是在滤泡间区形成分隔，主要的鉴别诊断包括淋巴瘤和淋巴组织增生。除少数病例外，反应性病变通常表现为[2]：

1. 结构保存（有时出现扭曲），具有完整的淋巴窦、反应性滤泡和可识别的副皮质成分；
2. 不形成分散的膨胀性肿物；
3. 不侵犯散在的反应性滤泡套区（图21A.183）；
4. 显示混合类型的淋巴细胞；
5. 缺乏细胞异型性，即没有偏离正常细胞和反应性细胞形态。如果出现一个明显的细胞群，表现为核中等大小，核膜明显折叠，染色质异常颗粒状，或胞浆透明，通常提示淋巴瘤（图21A.116，21A.124）。具有中等大小的核和透明胞浆的单核样B细胞是一种例外，可通过位于反应性滤泡周围而识别。浆细胞内出现易于见到的Dutcher小体或结晶状包涵体，也提示是肿瘤性病变（图21A.51）。

一个重要的例外是自身免疫性淋巴组织增生综合征（是一种遗传性疾病，特点是缺乏淋巴细胞凋亡），其中可见许多中等大小的淋巴细胞和透明细胞[1015]。在儿童和年轻人，总是应该考虑小细胞或淋巴组织细胞型间变大细胞淋巴瘤的可能性，尤其是当淋巴组织增生富于T细胞时。

怎样用免疫组化解决问题

当形态学特征不具有决定性意义或模棱两可时，免疫组化检查通过下列一种或多种特征非常有助于鉴别淋巴瘤与淋巴组织增生：（1）异常免疫结构；（2）异常免疫表型；或（3）单型性Ig（图21A.184）。

异常免疫结构（abnormal immunoarchitecture）：淋巴结和结外部位的反应性淋巴组织由B细胞结节组成（原发性或继发性滤泡），被富于T细胞的区域分隔开，T区中仅含有孤立性或小灶状B细胞（图21A.2）。因此，如果免疫染色显示广泛（至少半个低倍视野，应用4倍的目镜）、弥漫性、致密的B细胞（CD20$^+$或CD79a$^+$）浸润，伴有有限的散在T细胞（CD3$^+$），就代表异常的免疫结构，支持B细胞淋巴瘤的诊断（图21A.185）。另一方面，仅仅可见弥漫性致密浸润的T细胞（CD3$^+$），不足以诊断T细胞淋巴瘤，因为反应性淋巴组织增生可以主要由T细胞组成。

如果淋巴组织浸润由混合性CD20$^+$B细胞和CD3$^+$T细胞组成，但较大的或非典型性细胞选择性地着染CD20或CD3时，分别提示B细胞或T细胞淋巴瘤。

异常免疫表型（aberrant immunophenotype）：如果淋巴组织病变富于B细胞，若出现异常标记物表达（正常B细胞不表达或仅仅表达少数），如CD5、CD43、cyclin D1，支持淋巴瘤的诊断。但是，缺乏异常免疫表型不能排除淋巴瘤的可能性。在解释共表达时，重要的是要对比全B标记物（如CD20或CD79a）和全T标记物（如CD3）的显微镜下视野。如果CD43或CD5染色形态或阳性细胞数目与全B更加对应而不是与全T对应（除外由B细胞组成的淋巴滤泡，意外地共表达CD43或CD5），认为存在共表达（图21A.46，21A.58，21A.186）。淋巴细胞表达cyclin D1总是有意义的，因为所有正常和反应性淋巴细胞均为阴性（图21A.59）。

如果病变富于T细胞，不利的是没有满意的克隆性标记物来辅助诊断T细胞淋巴瘤。单纯以CD4$^+$或CD8$^+$细胞为主，不能作为单克隆的证据[2]。然而，在成熟T细胞增生中，出现异常的双阳性CD4$^+$CD8$^+$或双阴性CD4$^-$CD8$^-$表型，提示为肿瘤性病变，除了自身免疫性淋巴增生综合征患者。后者由淋巴细胞凋亡缺陷引起，最常见的原因是*FAS*（CD95）、*Fas*配体、*Caspase-8*或*Caspase-10*基因的胚系突变。淋巴结活检显示副皮质区

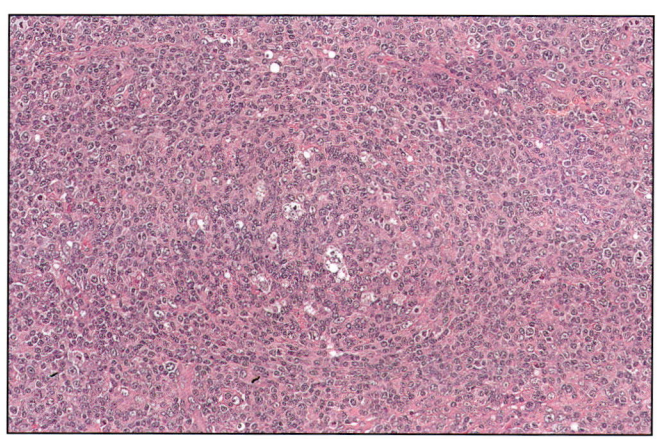

图21A.183 非特指外周T细胞淋巴瘤。视野中心显示反应性生发中心。套区消失，被淋巴组织增生所侵蚀。生发中心周边部分也被淋巴组织增生所替代。

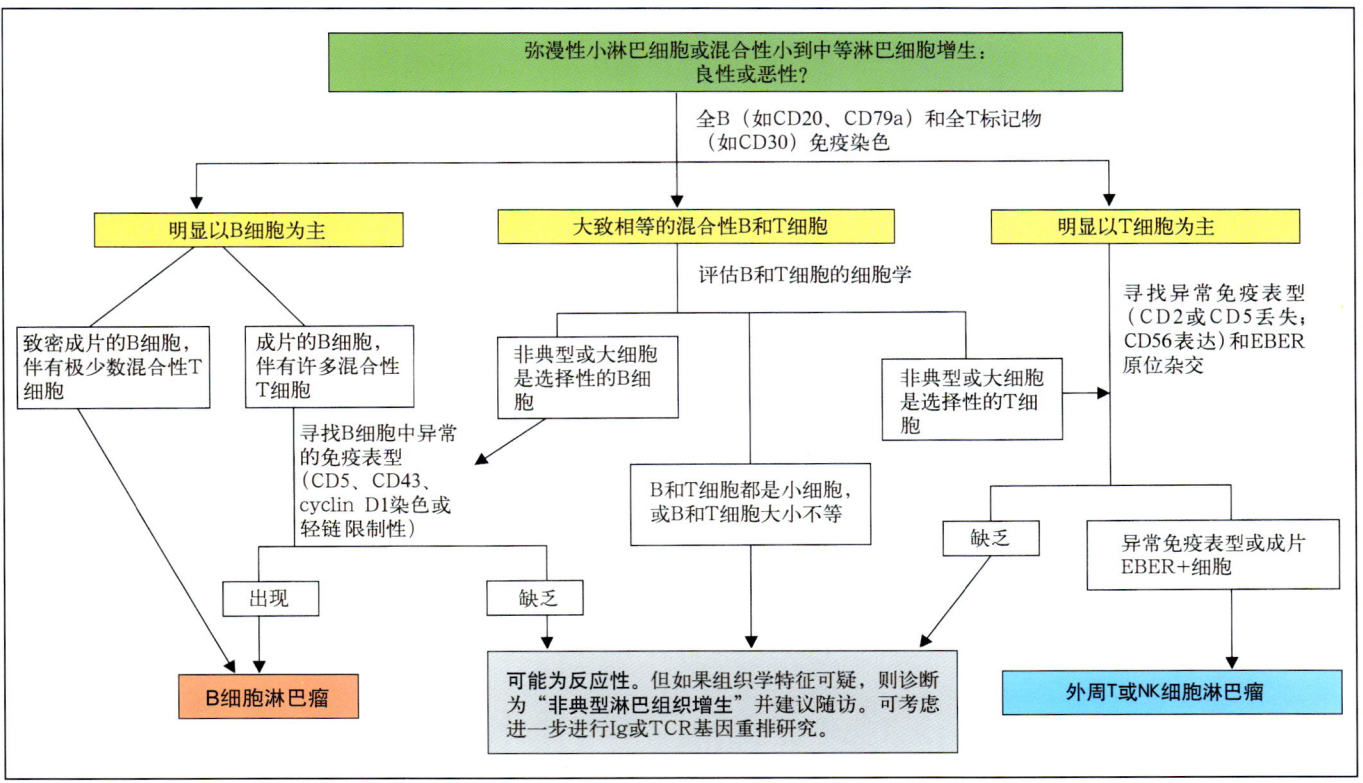

图21A.184 弥漫性小淋巴细胞或混合性淋巴细胞增生的诊断流程图。

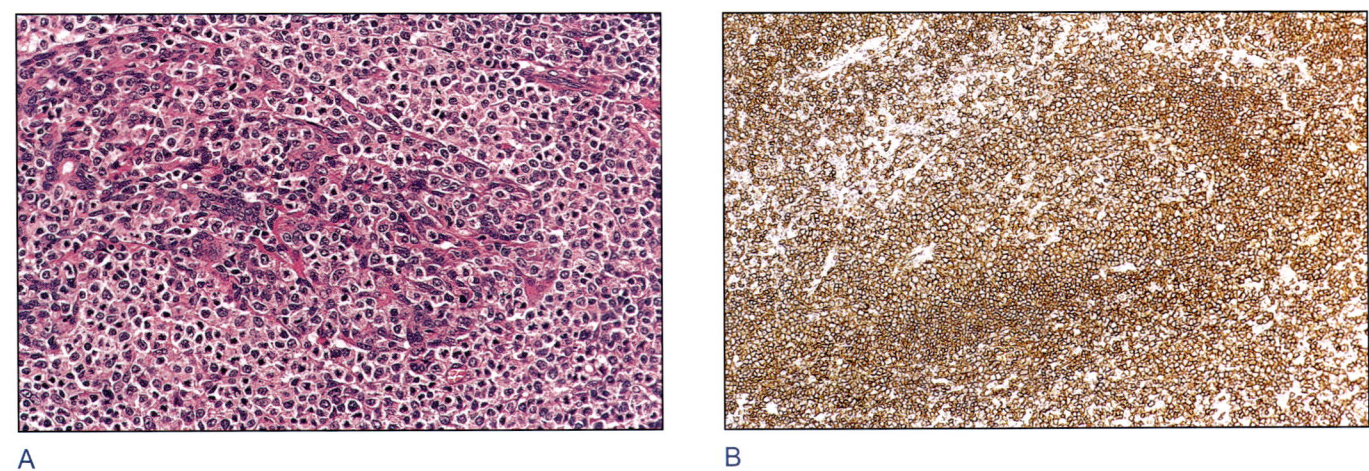

图21A.185 涎腺的结外边缘区B细胞淋巴瘤。（A）可见淋巴细胞浸润、充满导管引起的淋巴上皮病变。病变及周围细胞具有一定量的淡染胞浆，类似于单核样B细胞。（B）CD20免疫染色显示致密成片的B细胞，支持淋巴瘤诊断。

增大，可见淋巴细胞、浆细胞和免疫母细胞；淋巴细胞胞浆量中等，透明或嗜酸性，主要为T细胞，表型为$CD3^+CD4^-CD8^-CD45RO^-CD57^+$（图21A.187）[1015,1472-1476]。在评估T细胞增生时，全T标记物表达的丢失，如CD2、CD3、CD5、CD7，对于诊断淋巴瘤极其有价值（图21A.123）[2,1034]。出现成片表达CD10、CD56或γδ-TCR的细胞也强烈支持淋巴瘤诊断，因为这些标记物在正常情况下仅有极少数T淋巴细胞表达（图21A.149和21A.151）。出现任何ALK染色的淋巴细胞，均提示间变大细胞淋巴瘤的诊断（图21A.142B）。

单型性Ig (monotypic Ig)：对于B淋巴细胞增生，显示明显的Ig轻链限制性（κ：λ 比值＞10:1或＞1:10）可诊断淋巴瘤（图21A.53和21A.111）。在冰冻或石蜡

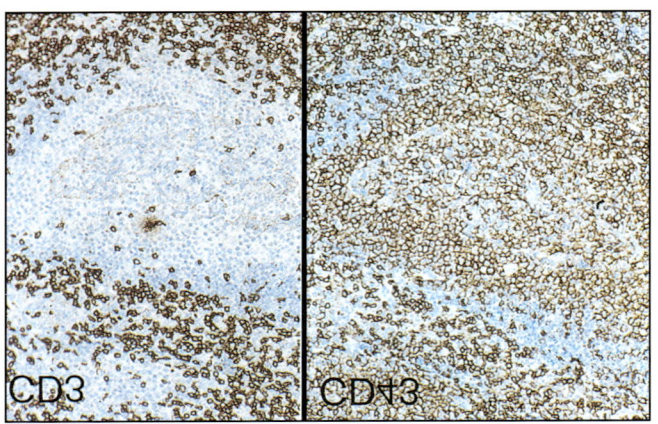

图21A.186 涎腺的结外边缘区B细胞淋巴瘤（与图21A.185为同一病例）。左侧：CD3免疫染色显示存在孤立性（斑片状）T细胞。右侧：CD43免疫染色显示大片阳性细胞，远远超过CD3$^+$细胞。因此得出淋巴细胞具有CD43的异常共表达。支持淋巴瘤的诊断。

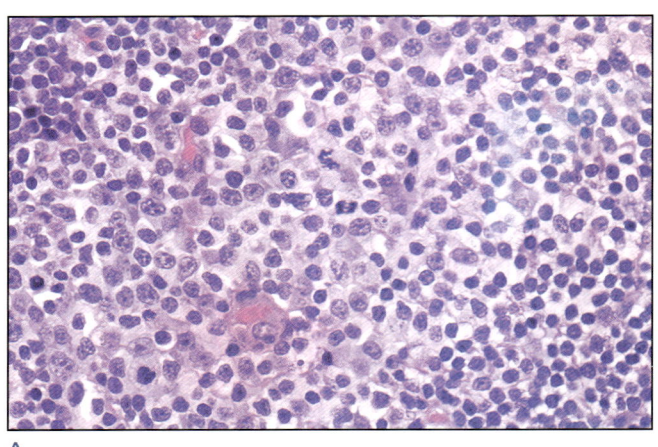

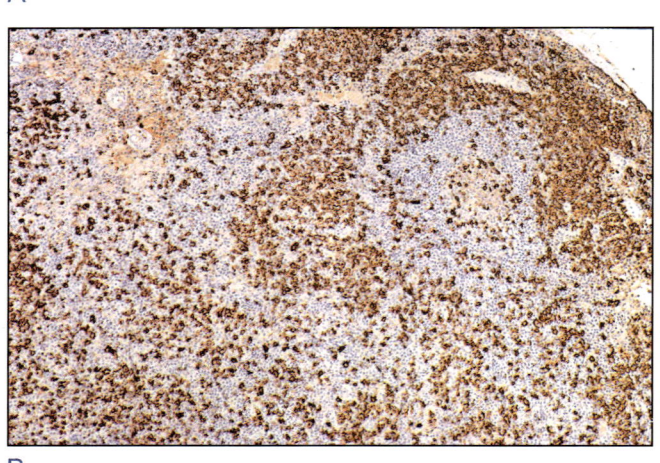

图21A.187 自身免疫淋巴组织增生综合征，淋巴结活检。
(A) 可见明显的活化淋巴细胞增生，不伴有凋亡小体。许多淋巴细胞中等或偏大，胞浆淡染或透明，形态学类似T区淋巴瘤。其中相当一部分细胞呈CD4$^-$、CD8$^-$（未显示）。
(B) 另一种显示免疫表型异常的便捷方式是使用CD57免疫染色：大量滤泡间T细胞着色。

包埋切片，应用流式细胞术或免疫组化染色可显示Ig。一般情况下，冰冻切片能更可靠地显示表面Ig。如果免疫组化未能显示轻链限制性，不能完全排除淋巴瘤，尤其是当小淋巴细胞染色结果不能令人信服时。Ig免疫染色的另一个问题是背景染色太强而难以判断。

分子学分析有帮助吗？

如果免疫组化检查没有得出结论，则Ig和TCR基因重排分子学分析可能有帮助，记住基于PCR的方法具有较高的假阴性率。

如果特殊检查没有得出结论该怎么办？

对于有些组织学特征怀疑为淋巴瘤但特殊检查没有得出明确的支持恶性的证据的病例，可以给出"意义不明的非典型淋巴组织浸润"诊断，建议随访，必要时重新活检。在重新活检时，要保存一些冰冻组织以显示表面Ig和各种T细胞系标记物，或行Southern印迹分析Ig和TCR基因重排。

弥漫性小B细胞淋巴瘤：分类方法
Diffuse small B-cell lymphomas: approach to classification

主要的鉴别诊断

- B细胞慢性淋巴细胞白血病/小淋巴细胞淋巴瘤（B-CLL/SLL）*
- 淋巴浆细胞性淋巴瘤
- 套细胞淋巴瘤*
- 结外边缘区B细胞淋巴瘤*
- 弥漫性滤泡中心淋巴瘤
- 脾边缘区B细胞淋巴瘤

诊断上的问题

对于由免疫组化证实为B细胞来源的弥漫性小细胞淋巴瘤，准确的分类很重要，因为不同类型的小B细胞淋巴瘤具有不同的临床进展。结外边缘区B细胞淋巴瘤常常局限、惰性，而套细胞淋巴瘤常常呈播散性，预后很差。

弥漫性小细胞淋巴瘤的分类可能很困难，尤其是小活检，其中的结构形态难以充分展示，挤压和人工假象使细胞学特征难以评估。更复杂的问题是：在小B细胞淋巴瘤中，可见明显的细胞形态重叠。多种淋巴瘤类型的细胞核均呈圆形或不规则折叠：例如，套细胞淋巴瘤的细胞核可以非常圆，而有些B-CLL/SLL病例可具有不规则折叠的核（图21A.42B）。

形态学线索

没有单一的组织学特征是某种弥漫性小细胞淋巴瘤所特异的。必须将特征综合考虑。

- 增生中心是 B-CLL/SLL 的诊断特征（图 21A.41）。
- 出现明显的淋巴上皮病变倾向于诊断结外边缘区B细胞淋巴瘤；破碎腺体可表现为淋巴细胞之间的嗜酸细胞碎片或印戒细胞（图21A.81、21A.82和21A.83）。然而，缺乏淋巴上皮病变不能完全除外这种淋巴瘤类型。
- 支持诊断套细胞淋巴瘤的特征：
  - 套区生长方式支持诊断套细胞淋巴瘤（图21A.54），虽然这种生长结构也可见于其他淋巴瘤类型。
  - 可见散在的孤立性上皮样组织细胞，尤其是当伴有玻璃样变小静脉时，高度提示为套细胞淋巴瘤（图21A.56）。
  - 单形性淋巴组织聚集支持诊断套细胞淋巴瘤，尤其是见到散在的"裸"核（FDC）时（图21A.55和21A.56）。少数情况下，结外边缘区B细胞淋巴瘤也可显示单形性肿瘤聚集（图21A.81B）。
- 当出现混有大淋巴细胞时，更可能是结外边缘区B细胞淋巴瘤或B-CLL/SLL。前者细胞组成杂乱，具有小淋巴细胞、中心细胞样细胞、单核样细胞、浆细胞和大淋巴细胞（图21A.81）。后者常显示混杂的幼稚淋巴细胞和副免疫母细胞（图21A.43和21A.44）。
- 出现许多Dutcher小体（核内Ig包涵体）是淋巴浆细胞性淋巴瘤的特征（图21A.50），但有时也可见于结外边缘区B细胞淋巴瘤。

淋巴浆细胞性淋巴瘤是排除性诊断：如果见到其他淋巴瘤类型特征，就不诊断淋巴浆细胞性淋巴瘤。在固定差或组织处理不理想时，Burkitt淋巴瘤或淋巴浆细胞性淋巴瘤可酷似小细胞淋巴瘤。将这些高度侵袭性的肿瘤误诊为低度恶性淋巴瘤的后果是严重的，对于年轻患者的"小B细胞淋巴瘤"，必须慎重考虑。

免疫组化评估

免疫组化研究在小B细胞淋巴瘤的鉴别诊断中极其重要，虽然结果偶尔不是结论性的，因为个别病例可能偏离经典的免疫表型（表21A.23）（图21A.46和21A.58）。注意：bcl-2免疫染色对分类没有帮助，因为

表21A.23　弥漫性小B细胞淋巴瘤诊断的抗体组合

淋巴瘤类型	CD5	CD23	IgD	Cyclin D1	Bcl-6 或 CD10
B-CLL/SLL	+	+	+	−	−
套细胞淋巴瘤	+	−*	+	+	−
淋巴浆细胞性淋巴瘤	−	−/+		−	−
结外边缘区B细胞淋巴瘤，MALT型	−	−*		−	−
脾边缘区B细胞淋巴瘤	−		+	−	−
滤泡中心淋巴瘤，弥漫性，小细胞为主型	−	+/−*	−	−	+

*滤泡树突状细胞网常常由CD23抗体显示。

其几乎在所有不同类型的小B细胞淋巴瘤中均呈阳性。免疫组化诊断结外边缘区B细胞淋巴瘤（MALT型）和淋巴浆细胞性淋巴瘤也基本上是排除性诊断，因为缺少特异性阳性标记物。

免疫组化显示cyclin D1曾经存在问题，但这个问题通过新近获得的兔单克隆抗体已得以解决[373]。如果肿瘤细胞cyclin D1呈阴性，重要的是要确定免疫染色的可靠性，要寻找内在的阳性对照，如散在的组织细胞、内皮细胞或可能的上皮细胞（复层鳞状上皮的副基底细胞和某些腺上皮的隐窝细胞cyclin D1常常呈阳性）。

基因型研究

基因型分析在有选择的条件下可能有帮助。采用Southern印迹技术、PCR或FISH显示 BCL-1（cyclin D1）基因重排，强烈支持诊断套细胞淋巴瘤。出现 BCL-2 基因重排支持诊断滤泡中心细胞淋巴瘤，但是如果显示特征性易位，如t(11;18)，支持诊断结外边缘区B细胞淋巴瘤。

未解决的问题

结外边缘区B细胞淋巴瘤和淋巴浆细胞性淋巴瘤之间的鉴别可能很困难，尤其是在结外部位[437]。根据定义，后者是排除性诊断。但是，即使见不到前者的典型特征（如淋巴上皮病变和类似于单核样B细胞的

细胞），结外边缘区 B 细胞淋巴瘤的可能性仍不能排除。在这种情况下，我们通常将病例报告为"小 B 细胞淋巴瘤，符合结外边缘区 B 细胞淋巴瘤或淋巴浆细胞性淋巴瘤；建议结合临床"。如果检查提示没有其他部位疾病，则可能诊断前者。否则，如果检查提示系统性受累和出现 Waldenström 巨球蛋白血症的特征，则更可能诊断后者。

对于有些即使经过全面检查仍然不能明确分类的病例，可合理地称为"小 B 细胞淋巴瘤，不能进一步分类"。如果分类困难是由于标本较小或技术因素，如挤压变形或固定差，则如有可能应该进一步活检。

小淋巴细胞背景中散在的大细胞：诊断方法
Large cells scattered in a background of small lymphocytes: approach to diagnosis

主要鉴别诊断

- 经典型Hodgkin淋巴瘤（C-HL），如富于淋巴细胞型、混合细胞型、结节硬化型*
- 结节性淋巴细胞为主型Hodgkin淋巴瘤（N-LPHL），主要呈弥漫性生长
- 富于T细胞的大B细胞淋巴瘤*
- 淋巴瘤样肉芽肿病
- 非特指外周T细胞淋巴瘤（很少显示这种细胞学结构）
- 伴Reed-Sternberg样细胞的B细胞慢性淋巴细胞白血病/小淋巴细胞淋巴瘤（B-CLL/SLL）（少见）
- 反应性淋巴组织增生*。

形态学评估

淋巴瘤样肉芽肿病最容易识别，因为其发生于结外部位且显示明显的凝固性坏死和血管侵犯性生长（图21A.103）。鉴别经典型 HL、弥漫为主型 N-LPHL 和富于 T 细胞的大 B 细胞淋巴瘤是最困难的，因为存在明显的组织学共性；有时甚至与反应性淋巴组织增生也难以鉴别（图 21A.10、21A.17、21A.19、21A.31 和 21A.101）。这三种病变中的大细胞均可表现为诊断性 Reed-Sternberg 细胞、L&H 细胞、多分叶核细胞或无法形容的大细胞；但富于 T 细胞的大 B 细胞淋巴瘤中的大细胞有时不易与反应性免疫母细胞区分（图 21A.188）。小淋巴细胞结节中出现大肿瘤细胞，即使很局限，也强烈提示诊断 N-LPHL。背景中反应性小淋巴细胞通常呈正常表现，但在富于 T 细胞的大 B 细胞淋巴瘤和有些 N-LPHL 病例可能表现轻度增大（图 21A.11 和 21A.101）。

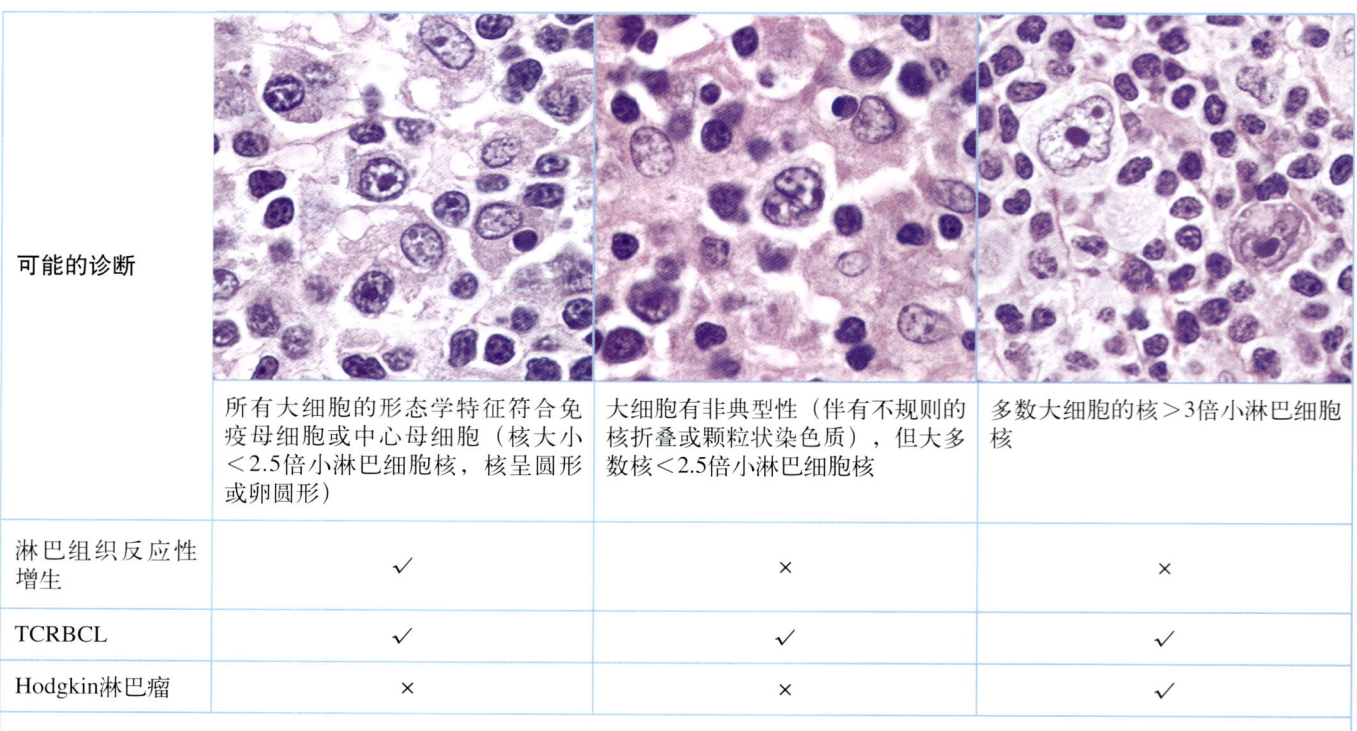

可能的诊断	所有大细胞的形态学特征符合免疫母细胞或中心母细胞（核大小<2.5倍小淋巴细胞核，核呈圆形或卵圆形）	大细胞有非典型性（伴有不规则的核折叠或颗粒状染色质），但大多数核<2.5倍小淋巴细胞核	多数大细胞的核>3倍小淋巴细胞核
淋巴组织反应性增生	✓	×	×
TCRBCL	✓	✓	✓
Hodgkin淋巴瘤	×	×	✓

TCRBCL：富于T细胞的大B细胞淋巴瘤。
✓：可能的诊断。
×：最不可能的诊断。

图21A.188　小淋巴细胞背景中散在大细胞的诊断思路。分析大细胞的形态学特征能缩小鉴别诊断范围。

表21A.24 经典型Hodgkin淋巴瘤、弥漫为主型结节性淋巴细胞为主型Hodgkin淋巴瘤、富于T细胞的大B细胞淋巴瘤和淋巴瘤样肉芽肿病的免疫表型比较

	经典型Hodgkin淋巴瘤	结节性淋巴细胞为主型Hodgkin淋巴瘤，主要为弥漫性	富于T细胞的大B细胞性淋巴瘤	淋巴瘤样肉芽肿病
大细胞 CD30	+	通常-	通常-	通常-
CD15	通常+	-	-	-
CD20	阴性或阳性；如果呈阳性，染色形态常常不均匀	+	+	+
CD79a	通常-，但偶尔阳性	+	+	+
PU1、Oct-2、Bob1	通常均为-，但偶尔其中一、两个标记物可能呈阳性	+	+	+
Ig轻链限制性	-（同一细胞常常既表达κ又表达λ轻链，原因是从周围组织摄取的）	有时具有Ig轻链限制性，但常常难以显示	有些病例易于显示轻链限制性	常常难以显示
EBV	30%~60%的病例呈阳性	-	通常-	+
背景小淋巴细胞CD20	少数	出现一些局灶结节，混合有CD20⁺大细胞	少数	少数
CD3	多量；CD3⁺细胞可形成花环围绕Reed-Sternberg细胞	弥漫区域较多；CD3⁺细胞常形成花环围绕CD20⁺大细胞	多量	多量
CD57	少数	常常很多，但在弥漫区域数量减少	少数	少数
TIA-1	许多	少数	许多	许多

免疫组化评估

细胞形态学与标记物表达相对应是避免误诊所必需的（表21A.24）[182]。N-LPHL、淋巴瘤样肉芽肿病和富于T细胞的大B细胞淋巴瘤中的大细胞CD20均呈一致强阳性，而经典型Hodgkin淋巴瘤中的大细胞CD20呈阴性或显示CD20染色结构异质性（图21A.12、21A.25、21A.102和21A.105）。CD20⁺小B细胞结节内出现CD20⁺大细胞，即使很局限，也可诊断N-LPHL，并且排除了富于T细胞的大B细胞淋巴瘤（图21A.12）。应该注意的是，在N-LPHL的弥漫区域，背景小淋巴细胞主要为T细胞而不是B细胞，这种区域常常难以与富于T细胞的大B细胞淋巴瘤鉴别。大细胞Ig轻链限制性支持诊断富于T细胞的大B细胞淋巴瘤而不是其他诊断。虽然T细胞花环围绕大细胞是N-LPHL的典型特征，但不具有特异性，还可见于经典型Hodgkin淋巴瘤，甚至偶尔可见于富于T细胞的大B细胞淋巴瘤（图21A.13）。然而，如果T细胞花环表达bcl-6和（或）CD57，则支持诊断N-LPHL[100]。

其他研究

EBV（EBER）原位杂交可能有帮助，因为淋巴瘤样肉芽肿病和伴Reed-Sternberg样细胞的B-CLL/SLL（信号局限于Reed-Sternberg样细胞）几乎总是为阳性，30%~60%的经典型Hodgkin淋巴瘤呈阳性，但在需

要鉴别的其他病变中一般呈阴性。

在极少数情况下，免疫组化检查得不到结论，Ig 和 TCR 基因重排分子学分析可能有助于确定细胞系。

弥漫性中等大小淋巴细胞增生：诊断方法
Diffuse medium-sized lymphoid cell proliferations: approach to diagnosis

主要的鉴别诊断

- Burkitt 淋巴瘤*
- 淋巴母细胞淋巴瘤*
- 母细胞样型套细胞淋巴瘤*
- 髓细胞肉瘤*
- 母细胞性 NK 细胞淋巴瘤
- 滤泡性淋巴瘤的母细胞转化
- 外周 T 细胞淋巴瘤或 NK/T 细胞淋巴瘤（以中等大细胞为主的病例）
- 弥漫大 B 细胞淋巴瘤（以中等大细胞为主的病例）
- 淋巴结边缘区 B 细胞淋巴瘤（有些病例）
- 系统性肥大细胞增生症

做出鉴别

有助于鉴别 Burkitt 淋巴瘤与淋巴母细胞淋巴瘤的特征见第 1176 页表 21A.17，鉴别 Burkitt 淋巴瘤和弥漫大 B 细胞淋巴瘤的特征在"Burkitt 淋巴瘤"部分讨论（见第 1210 页；图 21A.36、21A.37 和 21A.113）。

主要由中等大细胞组成的外周 T 细胞淋巴瘤和 NK/T 细胞淋巴瘤可与母细胞肿瘤组鉴别（见下一部分），前者核膜较厚，染色质颗粒状、粗大，缺乏 TdT 免疫反应。

具有母细胞形态学的肿瘤评估
Evaluation of tumors with blastic morphology

具有母细胞形态学的中等大细胞肿瘤包括：淋巴母细胞淋巴瘤、母细胞性 NK 细胞淋巴瘤、母细胞样型套细胞淋巴瘤、滤泡性淋巴瘤的母细胞转化和髓细胞肉瘤。根据形态学很难相互鉴别，除非是见到套细胞淋巴瘤或滤泡性淋巴瘤的典型区域。后两种病变在老年患者总是应该认真考虑（图 21A.55）。髓细胞肉瘤通常可见染色质较松散，核仁较明显，出现散在的嗜酸性粒细胞是强有力的诊断线索。

为了明确鉴别诊断，需要进行免疫组化研究。淋巴母细胞淋巴瘤、一些母细胞性 NK 细胞淋巴瘤和一些母细胞性滤泡性淋巴瘤 TdT 呈阳性，而母细胞样型套细胞淋巴瘤 TdT 总是呈阴性（图 21A.40）。诊断母细胞样型套细胞淋巴瘤可通过 cyclin D1 免疫反应进一步证实[464]。CD56 在母细胞性 NK 细胞淋巴瘤呈阳性，CD4 常常也呈阳性。髓过氧化物酶、CD117 和 CD34 免疫阳性可支持髓细胞肉瘤的诊断。

弥漫性大淋巴细胞增生：诊断方法
Diffuse large lymphoid cell proliferations: approach to diagnosis

淋巴瘤与非淋巴恶性肿瘤的鉴别
Distinction of lymphoma from non-lymphoid malignancies

大细胞为主的病变其恶性本质容易识别。而大细胞性淋巴瘤与癌、黑色素瘤和肉瘤的鉴别较困难。应该注意细胞排列和细胞学细节。癌的黏附性特征在中倍放大时最容易识别：与间质的界限通常清楚。核变形和水流状核在癌中也比在淋巴瘤中更常见。但是，淋巴瘤偶尔可呈黏附性，形成分离的结节或与周围组织界限清楚（图 21A.88）。黑色素瘤常被描述为"似黏非黏"，在细胞团内，各肿瘤细胞常常相互"分离"。淋巴瘤细胞常常呈非黏附性，显示弥散特性，其胞浆常常呈嗜碱性或嗜双色性。如果出现核膜明显不规则折叠，更可能是淋巴瘤而不是癌或黑色素瘤。由于淋巴瘤可显示多种欺骗性组织学特征，如淋巴窦浸润、印戒样形态、梭形细胞形态、黏液样间质、纤维性基质和花环结构，在大细胞肿瘤的鉴别诊断中总是应该考虑。CD45RB、细胞角蛋白和 S100 蛋白（加之 HMB45、Melan-A，如果可行）免疫染色通常可解决问题。但是，如果怀疑淋巴瘤但 CD45RB 呈阴性，应该进一步加做 B 细胞和 T 细胞标记物以及 CD30 以探讨这种可能性。

淋巴瘤与反应性淋巴结病的鉴别
Distinction of lymphoma from reactive lymphadenopathies

在传染性单核细胞增多症（infectious mononucleosis），显著的免疫母细胞增生常导致误诊为大细胞淋巴瘤。类似的显著的淋巴组织反应也可见于其他病毒感染和过敏反应（例如对苯妥英）。当形态学特征第一印象是大细胞淋巴瘤时，以下线索提示可能是传染性单核细胞增多症：

1. 患者年轻：在儿童和青少年中诊断大细胞淋巴瘤要非常慎重。
2. 结构破坏不彻底，保留一些完整的淋巴窦和反应性淋巴滤泡（常常显示生发中心部分坏死）（图 21A.189）。
3. 活化大淋巴细胞常缺乏明确的非典型性，如明显的核不规则性或粗大的染色质形态。
4. 大淋巴细胞不形成单形性细胞群，而显示向浆母细胞和浆细胞过渡（图 21A.189B）。

12. Cheuk W, Chan J K 2004 Subcellular localization of immunohistochemical signals: knowledge of the ultrastructural or biologic features of the antigens helps predict the signal localization and proper interpretation of immunostains. Int J Surg Pathol 12: 185–206
13. Whang-Peng J, Knutsen T 1997 Cytogenetics of non-Hodgkin's lymphomas. In: Magrath I (ed) The non-Hodgkin's lymphomas, 2nd edn. Arnold, London, 277–307
14. Chan J K C 1995 CD30+ (Ki-1) lymphoma: t(2; 5) translocation, the implicated genes, and more... Adv Anat Pathol 2: 99–104
15. Chan W C 1996 The t(2; 5) or NPM-ALK translocation in lymphomas: diagnostic considerations. Adv Anat Pathol 3: 396–399
16. Chan J K 1995 bcl-6 gene aberrations: the culprit of diffuse large B-cell lymphoma? Adv Anat Pathol 2: 153–158
17. Mrozek K, Bloomfield C D 1998 Major cytogenetic findings in non-Hodgkin's lymphoma. In: Cannelos G P, Lister T A, Sklar J L (eds) The lymphomas. WB Saunders, Philadelphia, 107–128
18. Medeiros L J 1996 Molecular hematopathology. In: Weiss L M (ed) Pathology of lymph nodes. Contemporary issues in surgical pathology, Vol. 21. Churchill Livingstone, New York, 1–80
19. Cossman J, Zehnbauer B, Garrett C T et al. 1991 Gene rearrangements in the diagnosis of lymphoma/leukemia. Guidelines for use based on a multiinstitutional study. Am J Clin Pathol 95: 347–354
20. Sklar J L 1998 The molecular diagnosis of lymphoma and related disorders. In: Cannelos G P, Lister T A, Sklar J L (eds) The lymphomas. WB Saunders, Philadelphia, 129–150
21. Cossman J, Uppenkamp M, Sundeen J 1988 Molecular genetics and the diagnosis of lymphoma. Arch Pathol Lab Med 112: 117–127
22. Segal G H 1996 Assessment of B-cell clonality by the polymerase chain reaction: a pragmatic overview. Adv Anat Pathol 3: 195–203
23. Gong J Z, Zheng S, Chiarle R et al. 1999 Detection of immunoglobulin kappa light chain rearrangements by polymerase chain reaction. An improved method for detecting clonal B-cell lymphoproliferative disorders. Am J Pathol 155: 355–363
24. van Dongen J J, Langerak A W, Bruggemann M et al. 2003 Design and standardization of PCR primers and protocols for detection of clonal immunoglobulin and T-cell receptor gene recombinations in suspect lymphoproliferations: report of the BIOMED-2 Concerted Action BMH4-CT98-3936. Leukemia 17: 2257–2317
25. Sandberg Y, van Gastel-Mol E J, Verhaaf B et al. 2005 BIOMED-2 multiplex immunoglobulin/T-cell receptor polymerase chain reaction protocols can reliably replace Southern blot analysis in routine clonality diagnostics. J Mol Diagn 7: 495–503
26. Droese J, Langerak A W, Groenen P J et al. 2004 Validation of BIOMED-2 multiplex PCR tubes for detection of TCRB gene rearrangements in T-cell malignancies. Leukemia 18: 1531–1538
27. Dunphy C H 2006 Gene expression profiling data in lymphoma and leukemia: review of the literature and extrapolation of pertinent clinical applications. Arch Pathol Lab Med 130: 483–520
28. Stein H, Diehl V, Marafioti T et al. 1999 The nature of Reed–Sternberg cells, lymphocytic and histiocytic cells and their molecular biology in Hodgkin's disease. In: Mauch P M, Armitage J O, Diehl V et al. (eds) Hodgkin's disease. Lippincott Williams & Wilkins, Philadelphia, 121–137
29. Stein H S, Hummel M 1999 Hodgkin's disease: biology and origin of Hodgkin's and Reed–Sternberg cells. Cancer Treat Rev 25: 161–168
30. Butler J J 1992 The histologic diagnosis of Hodgkin's disease. Semin Diagn Pathol 9: 252–256
31. Liang R, Choi P, Todd D et al. 1989 Hodgkin's disease in Hong Kong Chinese. Hematol Oncol 7: 395–403
32. Said J W 1997 Human immunodeficiency virus-related lymphoid proliferations. Semin Diagn Pathol 14: 48–53
33. Audouin J, Diebold J, Pallesen G 1992 Frequent expression of Epstein–Barr virus latent membrane protein-1 in tumor cells of Hodgkin's disease in HIV-positive patients. J Pathol 167: 381–384
34. Tirelli U, Carbone A, Straus D J 1999 HIV-related Hodgkin's disease. In: Mauch P M, Armitage J O, Diehl V et al. (eds) Hodgkin's disease. Lippincott Williams & Wilkins, Philadelphia, 701–711
35. Carbone A, Gloghini A, Larocca L M et al. 1999 Human immunodeficiency virus-associated Hodgkin's disease derives from post-germinal center B cells. Blood 93: 2319–2326
35a. Thompson L D R, Fisher S I, Chu W S et al. 2004 HIV-associated Hodgkin's lymphoma. A clinicopathologic and immunophenotypic study of 45 cases. Am J Clin Pathol 121: 727–738
36. Harris N L, Jaffe E S, Stein H et al. 1994 A revised European–American classification of lymphoid neoplasms: a proposal from the International Lymphoma Study Group. Blood 84: 1361–1392
37. Harris N L 1998 The many faces of Hodgkin's disease around the world: what have we learned from its pathology? Ann Oncol 9: S45–56
38. Harris N L 1999 Hodgkin's lymphomas: classification, diagnosis, and grading. Semin Hematol 36: 220–232
39. Harris N L 1999 Hodgkin's disease: classification and differential diagnosis. Mod Pathol 12: 159–175
40. Harris N L, Jaffe E S, Diebold J et al. 1999 World Health Organization classification of neoplastic diseases of the hematopoietic and lymphoid tissues: report of the Clinical Advisory Committee meeting, Airlie House, Virginia, November 1997. J Clin Oncol 17: 3835–3849
41. Chan J K, Banks P M, Cleary M L et al. 1995 A revised European–American classification of lymphoid neoplasms proposed by the International Lymphoma Study Group. A summary version. Am J Clin Pathol 103: 543–560
42. Chan J K, Banks P M, Cleary M L et al. 1994 A proposal for classification of lymphoid neoplasms (by the International Lymphoma Study Group). Histopathology 25: 517–536
43. Lukes R J 1971 Criteria for involvement of lymph node, bone marrow, spleen, and liver in Hodgkin's disease. Cancer Res 31: 1755–1767
44. Dorfman R F, Colby T V 1982 The pathologist's role in management of patients with Hodgkin's disease. Cancer Treat Rep 66: 675–680
45. Jaffe E S, Zarate-Osorno A, Medeiros L J 1992 The interrelationship of Hodgkin's disease and non-Hodgkin's lymphomas – lessons learned from composite and sequential malignancies. Semin Diagn Pathol 9: 297–303
46. Harris N L 1992 The relationship between Hodgkin's disease and non-Hodgkin's lymphoma. Semin Diagn Pathol 9: 304–310
47. Gonzalez C L, Medeiros L J, Jaffe E S 1991 Composite lymphoma. A clinicopathologic analysis of nine patients with Hodgkin's disease and B-cell non-Hodgkin's lymphoma. Am J Clin Pathol 96: 81–89
48. Momose H, Jaffe E S, Shin S S et al. 1992 Chronic lymphocytic leukemia/small lymphocytic lymphoma with Reed–Sternberg-like cells and possible transformation to Hodgkin's disease. Mediation by Epstein–Barr virus. Am J Surg Pathol 16: 859–867
49. Travis L B, Gonzalez C L, Hankey B F et al. 1992 Hodgkin's disease following non-Hodgkin's lymphoma. Cancer 69: 2337–2342
50. Zarate-Osorno A, Medeiros L J, Longo D L et al. 1992 Non-Hodgkin's lymphomas arising in patients successfully treated for Hodgkin's disease. A clinical, histologic, and immunophenotypic study of 14 cases. Am J Surg Pathol 16: 885–895
51. Marafioti T, Hummel M, Anagnostopoulos I et al. 1999 Classical Hodgkin's disease and follicular lymphoma originating from the same germinal center B cell. J Clin Oncol 17: 3804–3809
52. Jaffe E S, Muller-Hermelink H K 1999 Relationship between Hodgkin's disease and non-Hodgkin's lymphomas. In: Mauch P M, Armitage J O, Diehl V et al. (eds) Hodgkin's disease. Lipincott Williams & Wilkins, Philadelphia, 181–193
53. Brauninger A, Hansmann M L, Strickler J G et al. 1999 Identification of common germinal-center B-cell precursors in two patients with both Hodgkin's disease and non-Hodgkin's lymphoma. N Engl J Med 340: 1239–1247
54. Muller-Hermelink H K, Zettl A, Pfeifer W et al. 2001 Pathology of lymphoma progression. Histopathology 38: 285–306
55. Traverse-Glehen A, Pittaluga S, Gaulard P et al. 2005 Mediastinal gray zone lymphoma: the missing link between classic Hodgkin's lymphoma and mediastinal large B-cell lymphoma. Am J Surg Pathol 29: 1411–1421
56. Carbone P, Kaplan H S, Musshoff K 1971 Report of the Committee on Hodgkin's disease staging classification. Cancer Res 31: 1860–1861
57. Lister T A, Crowther D, Sutcliffe S B et al. 1989 Report of a committee convened to discuss the evaluation and staging of patients with Hodgkin's disease: Cotswolds meeting. J Clin Oncol 7: 1630–1636
58. Poppema S 1996 Nodular lymphocyte predominance type of Hodgkin's disease. In: Weiss L M (ed) Pathology of lymph nodes. Contemporary issues in surgical pathology, Vol. 21. Churchill Livingstone, New York, 215–228
59. Poppema S, Kaiserling E, Lennert K 1979 Hodgkin's disease with lymphocytic predominance, nodular type (nodular paragranuloma) and progressively transformed germinal centres – a cytohistological study. Histopathology 3: 295–308
60. Hansmann M L, Zwingers T, Boske A et al. 1984 Clinical features of nodular paragranuloma (Hodgkin's disease, lymphocyte predominance type, nodular). J Cancer Res Clin Oncol 108: 321–330
61. Diehl V, Franklin J, Sextro M et al. 1999 Clinical presentation and treatment of lymphocyte predominance Hodgkin's disease. In: Mauch P M, Armitage J O, Diehl V et al. (eds) Hodgkin's disease. Lippincott Williams & Wilkins, Philadelphia, 563–582
62. Diehl V, Sextro M, Franklin J et al. 1999 Clinical presentation, course, and prognostic factors in lymphocyte-predominant Hodgkin's disease and lymphocyte-rich classical Hodgkin's disease: report from the European Task Force on Lymphoma Project on Lymphocyte-Predominant Hodgkin's Disease. J Clin Oncol 17: 776–783
63. Crennan E, D'Costa I, Liew K H et al. 1995 Lymphocyte predominant Hodgkin's disease: a clinicopathologic comparative study of histologic and immunophenotypic subtypes. Int J Radiat Oncol Biol Phys 31: 333–337
64. Pappa V I, Norton A J, Gupta R K et al. 1995 Nodular type of lymphocyte predominant Hodgkin's disease. A clinical study of 50 cases. Ann Oncol 6: 559–565
65. Bodis S, Kraus M D, Pinkus G et al. 1997 Clinical presentation and outcome in lymphocyte-predominant Hodgkin's disease. J Clin Oncol 15: 3060–3066
66. Tefferi A, Zellers R A, Banks P M et al. 1990 Clinical correlates of distinct immunophenotypic and histologic subcategories of lymphocyte-predominance Hodgkin's disease. J Clin Oncol 8: 1959–1965
67. Khoury J D, Jones D, Yared M A et al. 2004 Bone marrow involvement in patients with nodular lymphocyte predominant Hodgkin's lymphoma. Am J Surg Pathol 28: 489–495
68. Mason D Y, Banks P M, Chan J et al. 1994 Nodular lymphocyte predominance Hodgkin's disease. A distinct clinicopathological entity. Am J Surg Pathol 18: 526–530

69. Miettinen M, Franssila K O, Saxen E 1983 Hodgkin's disease, lymphocyte predominance nodular, increased risk for subsequent non-Hodgkin's lymphomas. Cancer 51: 2293–2300
70. Regula D P Jr, Weiss L M, Warnke R A et al. 1987 Lymphocyte predominance Hodgkin's disease: a reappraisal based upon histological and immunophenotypical findings in relapsing cases. Histopathology 11: 1107–1120
71. Regula D P Jr, Hoppe R T, Weiss L M 1988 Nodular and diffuse types of lymphocyte predominance Hodgkin's disease. N Engl J Med 318: 214–219
72. Anagnostopoulos I, Hansmann M L, Franssila K et al. 2000 European Task Force on Lymphoma project on lymphocyte predominance Hodgkin's disease: histologic and immunohistologic analysis of submitted cases reveals 2 types of Hodgkin's disease with a nodular growth pattern and abundant lymphocytes. Blood 96: 1889–1899
73. Bennett M H, MacLennan K A, Vaughan Hudson B 1989 The clinical and prognostic relevance of histopathologic classification in Hodgkin's disease. In: Fenoglio-Preiser C M, Wolff M, Rilke F (eds) Progress in surgical pathology, Vol. 10. Field & Wood, New York, 127–151
74. Horning S 1999 Should lymphocyte predominance Hodgkin's disease be treated as a low grade lymphoma? In: Mason D Y, Harris N L (eds) Human lymphoma: clinical implications of the REAL classification. Springer, London, 48.41–48.44
75. Mauch P M 1999 Should lymphocyte predominance Hodgkin's disease be treated like classical Hodgkin's disease? In: Mason D Y, Harris N L (eds) Human lymphoma: clinical implications of the REAL classification. Springer, London, 47.41–47.45
76. Feugier P, Labouyrie E, Djeridane M et al. 2004 Comparison of initial characteristics and long-term outcome of patients with lymphocyte-predominant Hodgkin's lymphoma and classical Hodgkin's lymphoma at clinical stages IA and IIA prospectively treated by brief anthracycline-based chemotherapies plus extended high-dose irradiation. Blood 104: 2675–2681
77. Ekstrand B C, Lucas J B, Horwitz S M et al. 2003 Rituximab in lymphocyte-predominant Hodgkin's disease: results of a phase 2 trial. Blood 101: 4285–4289
78. Neiman R S 1978 Current problems in the histopathologic diagnosis and classification of Hodgkin's disease. Pathol Annu 13: 2289–2329
79. Fan Z, Natkunam Y, Bair E et al. 2003 Characterization of variant patterns of nodular lymphocyte predominant Hodgkin's lymphoma with immunohistologic and clinical correlation. Am J Surg Pathol 27: 1346–1356
80. Burns B F, Colby T V, Dorfman R F 1984 Differential diagnostic features of nodular L & H Hodgkin's disease, including progressive transformation of germinal centers. Am J Surg Pathol 8: 253–261
81. Chang K L, Kamel O W, Arber D A et al. 1995 Pathologic features of nodular lymphocyte predominance Hodgkin's disease in extranodal sites. Am J Surg Pathol 19: 1313–1324
82. Siebert J D, Stuckey J H, Kurtin P J et al. 1995 Extranodal lymphocyte predominance Hodgkin's disease. Clinical and pathologic features. Am J Clin Pathol 103: 485–491
83. von Wasielewski R, Werner M, Fischer R et al. 1997 Lymphocyte-predominant Hodgkin's disease. An immunohistochemical analysis of 208 reviewed Hodgkin's disease cases from the German Hodgkin's Study Group. Am J Pathol 150: 793–803
84. Carbone A, Gloghini A, Gaidano G et al. 1998 Expression status of BCL-6 and syndecan-1 identifies distinct histogenetic subtypes of Hodgkin's disease. Blood 92: 2220–2228
85. Falini B, Bigerna B, Pasqualucci L et al. 1996 Distinctive expression pattern of the BCL-6 protein in nodular lymphocyte predominance Hodgkin's disease. Blood 87: 465–471
86. Nicholas D S, Harris S, Wright D H 1990 Lymphocyte predominance Hodgkin's disease – an immunohistochemical study. Histopathology 16: 157–165
87. Pinkus G S, Said J W 1985 Hodgkin's disease, lymphocyte predominance type, nodular – a distinct entity? Unique staining profile for L&H variants of Reed–Sternberg cells defined by monoclonal antibodies to leukocyte common antigen, granulocyte-specific antigen, and B-cell-specific antigen. Am J Pathol 118: 1–6
88. Uherova P, Valdez R, Ross C W et al. 2003 Nodular lymphocyte predominant Hodgkin's lymphoma. An immunophenotypic reappraisal based on a single-institution experience. Am J Clin Pathol 119: 192–198
89. Schmid C, Sargent C, Isaacson P G 1991 L and H cells of nodular lymphocyte predominant Hodgkin's disease show immunoglobulin light-chain restriction. Am J Pathol 139: 1281–1289
90. Stoler M H, Nichols G E, Symbula M et al. 1995 Lymphocyte predominance Hodgkin's disease. Evidence for a kappa light chain-restricted monotypic B-cell neoplasm. Am J Pathol 146: 812–818
91. Carbone A, Gloghini A, Gattei V et al. 1995 Expression of functional CD40 antigen on Reed–Sternberg cells and Hodgkin's disease cell lines. Blood 85: 780–789
92. Pinkus G S, Pinkus J L, Langhoff E et al. 1997 Fascin, a sensitive new marker for Reed–Sternberg cells of Hodgkin's disease. Evidence for a dendritic or B cell derivation? Am J Pathol 150: 543–562
93. Falini B, Fizzotti M, Pucciarini A et al. 2000 A monoclonal antibody (MUM1p) detects expression of the MUM1/IRF4 protein in a subset of germinal center B cells, plasma cells, and activated T cells. Blood 95: 2084–2092
94. Carbone A, Gloghini A, Aldinucci D et al. 2002 Expression pattern of MUM1/IRF4 in the spectrum of pathology of Hodgkin's disease. Br J Haematol 117: 366–372
95. Prakash S, Fountaine T, Raffeld M, Jaffe E S, Pittaluga S 2006 IgD positive L&H cells identify a unique subset of nodular lymphocyte predominant Hodgkin's lymphoma. Am J Surg Pathol 30: 585–592
96. Hansmann M L, Wacker H H, Radzun H J 1986 Paragranuloma is a variant of Hodgkin's disease with predominance of B-cells. Virchows Arch A Pathol Anat Histopathol 409: 171–181
97. Nguyen P L, Ferry J A, Harris N L 1999 Progressive transformation of germinal centers and nodular lymphocyte predominance Hodgkin's disease: a comparative immunohistochemical study. Am J Surg Pathol 23: 27–33
98. Poppema S 1989 The nature of the lymphocytes surrounding Reed–Sternberg cells in nodular lymphocyte predominance and in other types of Hodgkin's disease. Am J Pathol 135: 351–357
99. Kamel O W, Gelb A B, Shibuya R B et al. 1993 Leu 7 (CD57) reactivity distinguishes nodular lymphocyte predominance Hodgkin's disease from nodular sclerosing Hodgkin's disease, T-cell-rich B-cell lymphoma and follicular lymphoma. Am J Pathol 142: 541–546
100. Kraus M D, Haley J 2000 Lymphocyte predominance Hodgkin's disease: the use of BCL-6 and CD57 in diagnosis and differential diagnosis. Am J Surg Pathol 24: 1068–1078
101. Hansmann M L, Weiss L M, Stein H et al. 1999 Pathology of lymphocyte predominance Hodgkin's disease. In: Mauch P M, Armitage J O, Diehl V et al. (eds) Hodgkin's disease. Lippincott Williams & Wilkins, Philadelphia, 169–180
102. Pan L X, Diss T C, Peng H Z et al. 1996 Nodular lymphocyte predominance Hodgkin's disease: a monoclonal or polyclonal B-cell disorder? Blood 87: 2428–2434
103. Ohno T, Stribley J A, Wu G et al. 1997 Clonality in nodular lymphocyte-predominant Hodgkin's disease. N Engl J Med 337: 459–465
104. Braeuninger A, Kuppers R, Strickler J G et al. 1997 Hodgkin's and Reed–Sternberg cells in lymphocyte predominant Hodgkin's disease represent clonal populations of germinal center-derived tumor B cells. Proc Natl Acad Sci USA 94: 9337–9342
105. Marafioti T, Hummel M, Anagnostopoulos I et al. 1997 Origin of nodular lymphocyte-predominant Hodgkin's disease from a clonal expansion of highly mutated germinal-center B cells. N Engl J Med 337: 453–458
106. Irsch J, Nitsch S, Hansmann M L et al. 1998 Isolation of viable Hodgkin's and Reed–Sternberg cells from Hodgkin's disease tissues. Proc Natl Acad Sci USA 95: 10117–10122
107. Vockerodt M, Soares M, Kanzler H et al. 1998 Detection of clonal Hodgkin's and Reed–Sternberg cells with identical somatically mutated and rearranged VH genes in different biopsies in relapsed Hodgkin's disease. Blood 92: 2899–2907
108. Wlodarska I, Nooyen P, Maes B et al. 2003 Frequent occurrence of BCL6 rearrangements in nodular lymphocyte predominance Hodgkin's lymphoma but not in classical Hodgkin's lymphoma. Blood 101: 706–710
109. Liso A, Capello D, Marafioti T et al. 2006 Aberrant somatic hypermutation in tumor cells of nodular-lymphocyte-predominant and classic Hodgkin's lymphoma. Blood 108: 1013–1020
110. Said J W, Sassoon A F, Shintaku I P et al. 1991 Absence of BCL-2 major breakpoint region and JH gene rearrangement in lymphocyte predominance Hodgkin's disease. Results of Southern blot analysis and polymerase chain reaction. Am J Pathol 138: 261–264
111. Franke S, Wlodarska I, Maes B et al. 2001 Lymphocyte predominance Hodgkin's disease is characterized by recurrent genomic imbalances. Blood 97: 1845–1853
112. Chang K C, Khen N T, Jones D et al. 2005 Epstein–Barr virus is associated with all histological subtypes of Hodgkin's lymphoma in Vietnamese children with special emphasis on the entity of lymphocyte predominance subtype. Hum Pathol 36: 747–755
113. Bennett M H, MacLennan K A, Vaughan Hudson G et al. 1991 Non-Hodgkin's lymphoma arising in patients treated for Hodgkin's disease in the BNLI: a 20-year experience. British National Lymphoma Investigation. Ann Oncol 2(Suppl 2): 83–92
114. Hansmann M L, Stein H, Fellbaum C et al. 1989 Nodular paragranuloma can transform into high-grade malignant lymphoma of B type. Hum Pathol 20: 1169–1175
115. Sundeen J T, Cossman J, Jaffe E S 1988 Lymphocyte predominant Hodgkin's disease nodular subtype with coexistent 'large cell lymphoma.' Histological progression or composite malignancy? Am J Surg Pathol 12: 599–606
116. Chittal S M, Alard C, Rossi J F et al. 1990 Further phenotypic evidence that nodular, lymphocyte-predominant Hodgkin's disease is a large B-cell lymphoma in evolution. Am J Surg Pathol 14: 1024–1035
117. Grossman D M, Hanson C A, Schnitzer B 1991 Simultaneous lymphocyte predominant Hodgkin's disease and large-cell lymphoma. Am J Surg Pathol 15: 668–676
118. Huang J Z, Weisenburger D D, Vose J M et al. 2003 Diffuse large B-cell lymphoma arising in nodular lymphocyte predominant Hodgkin's lymphoma. A report of 21 cases from the Nebraska Lymphoma Study Group. Leuk Lymphoma 44: 1903–1910
119. Greiner T C, Gascoyne R D, Anderson M E et al. 1996 Nodular lymphocyte-predominant Hodgkin's disease associated with large-cell lymphoma: analysis of Ig gene rearrangements by V–J polymerase chain reaction. Blood 88: 657–666

120. Wickert R S, Weisenburger D D, Tierens A et al. 1995 Clonal relationship between lymphocytic predominance Hodgkin's disease and concurrent or subsequent large-cell lymphoma of B lineage. Blood 86: 2312–2320
121. Ohno T, Huang J Z, Wu G et al. 2001 The tumor cells in nodular lymphocyte-predominant Hodgkin's disease are clonally related to the large cell lymphoma occurring in the same individual. Direct demonstration by single cell analysis. Am J Clin Pathol 116: 506–511
122. Delabie J, Greiner T C, Chan W C et al. 1996 Concurrent lymphocyte predominance Hodgkin's disease and T-cell lymphoma. A report of three cases. Am J Surg Pathol 20: 355–362
123. Tefferi A, Wiltsie J C, Kurtin P J 1992 Secondary T-cell lymphoma in the setting of nodular lymphocyte predominance Hodgkin's disease. Am J Hematol 40: 232–233
124. Rysenga E, Linden M D, Carey J L et al. 1995 Peripheral T-cell non-Hodgkin's lymphoma following treatment of nodular lymphocyte predominance Hodgkin's disease. Arch Pathol Lab Med 119: 88–91
125. Gelb A B, Dorfman R F, Warnke R A 1993 Coexistence of nodular lymphocyte predominance Hodgkin's disease and Hodgkin's disease of the usual type. Am J Surg Pathol 17: 364–374
126. Poppema S, Kaiserling E, Lennert K 1979 Nodular paragranuloma and progressively transformed germinal centers. Ultrastructural and immunohistologic findings. Virchows Arch B Cell Pathol Incl Mol Pathol 31: 211–225
127. Crossley B, Heryet A, Gatter K C 1987 Does nodular lymphocyte predominant Hodgkin's disease arise from progressively transformed germinal centres? A case report with an unusually prolonged history. Histopathology 11: 621–630
128. Hansmann M L, Fellbaum C, Hui P K, Moubayed P 1990 Progressive transformation of germinal centers with and without association to Hodgkin's disease. Am J Clin Pathol 93: 219–226
129. Osborne B M, Butler J J 1984 Clinical implications of progressive transformation of germinal centers. Am J Surg Pathol 8: 725–733
130. Osborne B M, Butler J J, Gresik M V 1992 Progressive transformation of germinal centers: comparison of 23 pediatric patients to the adult population. Mod Pathol 5: 135–140
131. Ferry J A, Zukerberg L R, Harris N L 1992 Florid progressive transformation of germinal centers. A syndrome affecting young men, without early progression to nodular lymphocyte predominance Hodgkin's disease. Am J Surg Pathol 16: 252–258
132. Algara P, Martinez P, Sanchez L et al. 1991 Lymphocyte predominance Hodgkin's disease (nodular paragranuloma) – a BCL-2 negative germinal centre lymphoma. Histopathology 19: 69–75
133. Hansmann M L, Stein H, Dallenbach F et al. 1991 Diffuse lymphocyte-predominant Hodgkin's disease (diffuse paragranuloma). A variant of the B-cell-derived nodular type. Am J Pathol 138: 29–36
134. Colby T V, Hoppe R T, Warnke R A 1982 Hodgkin's disease: a clinicopathologic study of 659 cases. Cancer 49: 1848–1858
135. Lukes R J, Butler J J, Hicks E B 1966 Natural history of Hodgkin's disease is related to its pathologic picture. Cancer 19: 317–344
136. Rosen P J 1986 Should we bother subclassifying Hodgkin's disease? J Clin Oncol 4: 275–277
137. Kaplan H S 1980 Hodgkin's disease: unfolding concepts concerning its nature, management and prognosis. Cacner 45: 2439–2474
138. DeVita V T, Hubbard S M, Longo D L 1990 Treatment of Hodgkin's disease. J Natl Cancer Inst Monogr 10: 19–28
139. Weinshel E L, Peterson B A 1993 Hodgkin's disease. CA Cancer J Clin 43: 327–346
140. Coleman C N 1999 Treatment of early-stage Hodgkin's lymphoma. In: Mason D Y, Harris N L (eds) Human lymphoma: clinical implications of the REAL classification. Springer, London, 50.51–50.56
141. Parker S L, Tong T, Bolden S et al. 1997 Cancer statistics. CA 47: 5–27
142. Connors J M 2005 Evolving approaches to primary treatment of Hodgkin's lymphoma. Hematology (Am Soc Hematol Educ Program): 239–244
143. Meyer R M, Gospodarowicz M K, Connors J M et al. 2005 Randomized comparison of ABVD chemotherapy with a strategy that includes radiation therapy in patients with limited-stage Hodgkin's lymphoma: National Cancer Institute of Canada Clinical Trials Group and the Eastern Cooperative Oncology Group. J Clin Oncol 23: 4634–4642
144. Diehl V, Behringer K 2006 Could BEACOPP be the new standard for the treatment of advanced Hodgkin's lymphoma? Cancer Invest 24: 461–465
145. Oza A M, Ganesan T S, Leahy M et al. 1993 Patterns of survival in patients with Hodgkin's disease: long follow up in a single centre. Ann Oncol 4: 385–392
146. Canellos G P, Horwich A 1999 Management of recurrent Hodgkin's disease. In: Mauch P M, Armitage J O, Diehl V et al. (eds) Hodgkin's disease. Lippincott Williams & Wilkins, Philadelphia, 507–519
147. Bartlett N L 2005 Therapies for relapsed Hodgkin's lymphoma: transplant and non-transplant approaches including immunotherapy. Hematology (Am Soc Hematol Educ Program): 245–251
148. Boivin J F, Hutchison G B, Zauber A G et al. 1995 Incidence of second cancers in patients treated for Hodgkin's disease. J Natl Cancer Inst 87: 732–741
149. Kaldor J M, Day N E, Band P et al. 1987 Second malignancies following testicular cancer, ovarian cancer and Hodgkin's disease: an international collaborative study among cancer registries. Int J Cancer 39: 571–585
150. Ng A K, Bernardo M V, Weller E et al. 2002 Second malignancy after Hodgkin's disease treated with radiation therapy with or without chemotherapy: long-term risks and risk factors. Blood 100: 1989–1996
151. Tindle B H, Parker J W, Lukes R J 1972 'Reed–Sternberg cells' in infectious mononucleosis? Am J Clin Pathol 58: 607–617
152. Symmers W S Sr 1968 Survey of the eventual diagnosis in 600 cases referred for a second histological opinion after an initial biopsy diagnosis of Hodgkin's disease. J Clin Pathol 21: 650–653
153. Cossman J, Annuziata C M, Barash S et al. 1999 Reed–Sternberg cell genome expression supports a B-cell lineage. Blood 94: 411–416
154. Foss H D, Reusch R, Demel G et al. 1999 Frequent expression of the B-cell-specific activator protein in Reed–Sternberg cells of classical Hodgkin's disease provides further evidence for its B-cell origin. Blood 94: 3108–3113
155. Stevenson F K, Wright D H 1998 Hodgkin's disease and immunoglobulin genetics. In: Kirkham N, Lemoine N R (eds) Progress in pathology, Vol. 4. Churchill Livingstone, Edinburgh, 99–111
156. Jox A, Zander T, Kuppers R et al. 1999 Somatic mutations within the untranslated regions of rearranged Ig genes in a case of classical Hodgkin's disease as a potential cause for the absence of Ig in the lymphoma cells. Blood 93: 3964–3972
157. Kanzler H, Kuppers R, Hansmann M L et al. 1996 Hodgkin's and Reed–Sternberg cells in Hodgkin's disease represent the outgrowth of a dominant tumor clone derived from (crippled) germinal center B cells. J Exp Med 184: 1495–1505
158. Yatabe Y, Mori N, Hirabayashi N, Asai J 1994 Natural killer cell leukemia. An autopsy case. Arch Pathol Lab Med 118: 1201–1204
159. Theil J, Laumen H, Marafioti T et al. 2001 Defective octamer-dependent transcription is responsible for silenced immunoglobulin transcription in Reed–Sternberg cells. Blood 97: 3191–3196
160. Stein H, Marafioti T, Foss H D et al. 2001 Down-regulation of BOB.1/OBF.1 and Oct2 in classical Hodgkin's disease but not in lymphocyte predominant Hodgkin's disease correlates with immunoglobulin transcription. Blood 97: 496–501
161. Re D, Muschen M, Ahmadi T et al. 2001 Oct-2 and BoB-1 deficiency in Hodgkin's and Reed Sternberg cells. Cancer Res 61: 2080–2084
162. Nakamura S, Nagahama M, Kagami Y et al. 1999 Hodgkin's disease expressing follicular dendritic cell marker CD21 without any other B-cell marker: a clinicopathologic study of nine cases. Am J Surg Pathol 23: 363–376
163. Tzankov A, Bourgau C, Kaiser A et al. 2005 Rare expression of T-cell markers in classical Hodgkin's lymphoma. Mod Pathol 18: 1542–1549
164. Charalambous C, Singh N, Isaacson P G 1993 Immunohistochemical analysis of Hodgkin's disease using microwave heating. J Clin Pathol 46: 1085–1088
165. Pinkus G S, Thomas P, Said J W 1985 Leu-M1 – a marker for Reed–Sternberg cells in Hodgkin's disease. An immunoperoxidase study of paraffin-embedded tissues. Am J Pathol 119: 244–252
166. von Wasielewski R, Mengel M, Fischer R et al. 1997 Classical Hodgkin's disease. Clinical impact of the immunophenotype. Am J Pathol 151: 1123–1130
167. Sheibani K, Battifora H, Burke J S et al. 1986 Leu-M1 antigen in human neoplasms. An immunohistologic study of 400 cases. Am J Surg Pathol 10: 227–236
168. Barry T S, Jaffe E S, Sorbara L et al. 2003 Peripheral T-cell lymphomas expressing CD30 and CD15. Am J Surg Pathol 27: 1513–1522
169. Ree H J, Neiman R S, Martin A W et al. 1989 Paraffin section markers for Reed–Sternberg cells. A comparative study of peanut agglutinin, Leu-M1, LN-2, and Ber-H2. Cancer 63: 2030–2036
170. Hsu S M, Jaffe E S 1984 Leu M1 and peanut agglutinin stain the neoplastic cells of Hodgkin's disease. Am J Clin Pathol 82: 29–32
171. Moller P 1982 Peanut lectin: a useful tool for detecting Hodgkin's cells in paraffin sections. Virchows Arch [Pathol Anat] 396: 313–317
172. O'Grady J T, Stewart S, Lowrey J et al. 1994 CD40 expression in Hodgkin's disease. Am J Pathol 144: 21–26
173. Schmid C, Pan L, Diss T et al. 1991 Expression of B-cell antigens by Hodgkin's and Reed–Sternberg cells. Am J Pathol 139: 701–707
174. Zukerberg L R, Collins A B, Ferry J A et al. 1991 Coexpression of CD15 and CD20 by Reed–Sternberg cells in Hodgkin's disease. Am J Pathol 139: 475–483
175. Landaas T O, Godal T, Halvorsen T B 1977 Characterization of immunoglobulins in Hodgkin's cells. Int J Cancer 20: 717–722
176. Kadin M E, Stites D P, Levy R et al. 1978 Exogenous immunoglobulin and the macrophage origin of Reed–Sternberg cells in Hodgkin's disease. N Engl J Med 299: 1208–1214
177. Kadin M E, Muramoto L, Said J 1988 Expression of T-cell antigens on Reed–Sternberg cells in a subset of patients with nodular sclerosing and mixed cellularity Hodgkin's disease. Am J Pathol 130: 345–353
178. Falini B, Stein H, Pileri S et al. 1987 Expression of lymphoid-associated antigens on Hodgkin's and Reed–Sternberg cells of Hodgkin's disease. An immunocytochemical study on lymph node cytospins using monoclonal antibodies. Histopathology 11: 1229–1242
179. Montesinos-Rongen M, Roers A, Kuppers R et al. 1999 Mutation of the p53 gene is not a typical feature of Hodgkin's and Reed-Sternberg cells in Hodgkin's disease. Blood 94: 1755–1760
180. Gupta R K, Norton A J, Thompson I W et al. 1992 p53 expression in Reed–Sternberg cells of Hodgkin's disease. Br J Cancer 66: 649–652

181. Abdulaziz Z, Mason D Y, Stein H et al. 1984 An immunohistological study of the cellular constituents of Hodgkin's disease using a monoclonal antibody panel. Histopathology 8: 1–25
182. Rudiger T, Ott G, Ott M M et al. 1998 Differential diagnosis between classic Hodgkin's lymphoma, T-cell-rich B-cell lymphoma, and paragranuloma by paraffin immunohistochemistry. Am J Surg Pathol 22: 1184–1191
183. Alavaikko M J, Hansmann M L, Nebendahl C et al. 1991 Follicular dendritic cells in Hodgkin's disease. Am J Clin Pathol 95: 194–200
184. Weiss L M, Strickler J G, Hu E et al. 1986 Immunoglobulin gene rearrangements in Hodgkin's disease. Hum Pathol 17: 1009–1014
185. Knowles D M, Neri A, Pelicci P G et al. 1986 Immunoglobulin and T-cell receptor beta-chain gene rearrangement analysis of Hodgkin's disease: implications for lineage determination and differential diagnosis. Proc Natl Acad Sci USA 83: 7942–7946
186. Hu E H, Ellison D, Zovich D et al. 1990 Molecular analysis of Hodgkin's disease with abundant Reed–Sternberg cells. Hematol Pathol 4: 27–35
187. Sundeen J, Lipford E, Uppenkamp M et al. 1987 Rearranged antigen receptor genes in Hodgkin's disease. Blood 70: 96–103
188. Cossman J, Sundeen J, Uppenkamp M et al. 1988 Rearranging antigen-receptor genes in enriched Reed–Sternberg cell fractions of Hodgkin's disease. Hematol Oncol 6: 205–211
189. Roth M S, Schnitzer B, Bingham E L et al. 1988 Rearrangement of immunoglobulin and T-cell receptor genes in Hodgkin's disease. Am J Pathol 131: 331–338
190. Tamaru J, Hummel M, Zemlin M et al. 1994 Hodgkin's disease with a B-cell phenotype often shows a VDJ rearrangement and somatic mutations in the VH genes. Blood 84: 708–715
191. Kamel O W, Chang P P, Hsu F J et al. 1995 Clonal VDJ recombination of the immunoglobulin heavy chain gene by PCR in classical Hodgkin's disease. Am J Clin Pathol 104: 419–423
192. Orazi A, Jiang B, Lee C H et al. 1995 Correlation between presence of clonal rearrangements of immunoglobulin heavy chain genes and B-cell antigen expression in Hodgkin's disease. Am J Clin Pathol 104: 413–418
193. Griesser H, Feller A C, Mak T W et al. 1987 Clonal rearrangements of T-cell receptor and immunoglobulin genes and immunophenotypic antigen expression in different subclasses of Hodgkin's disease. Int J Cancer 40: 157–160
194. Hummel M, Marafioti T, Stein H 1999 Clonality of Reed–Sternberg cells in Hodgkin's disease. N Engl J Med 340: 394–395
195. Hummel M, Ziemann K, Lammert H et al. 1995 Hodgkin's disease with monoclonal and polyclonal populations of Reed–Sternberg cells. N Engl J Med 333: 901–906
196. Hummel M, Marafioti T, Ziemann K et al. 1996 Ig rearrangements in isolated Reed–Sternberg cells: conclusions from four different studies. Ann Oncol 7: 31–33
197. Kuppers R, Rajewsky K, Zhao M et al. 1995 Hodgkin's disease: clonal Ig gene rearrangements in Hodgkin's and Reed–Sternberg cells picked from histological sections. Ann NY Acad Sci 764: 523–524
198. Kuppers R, Rajewsky K, Zhao M et al. 1994 Hodgkin's disease: Hodgkin's and Reed–Sternberg cells picked from histological sections show clonal immunoglobulin gene rearrangements and appear to be derived from B cells at various stages of development. Proc Natl Acad Sci USA 91: 10962–10966
199. Tilly H, Bastard C, Delastre T et al. 1991 Cytogenetic studies in untreated Hodgkin's disease. Blood 77: 1298–1304
200. Schwering I, Brauninger A, Klein U et al. 2003 Loss of the B-lineage-specific gene expression program in Hodgkin's and Reed–Sternberg cells of Hodgkin's lymphoma. Blood 101: 1505–1512
201. Devilard E, Bertucci F, Trempat P et al. 2002 Gene expression profiling defines molecular subtypes of classical Hodgkin's disease. Oncogene 21: 3095–3102
202. Glaser S L, Lin R J, Stewart S L et al. 1997 Epstein–Barr virus-associated Hodgkin's disease: epidemiologic characteristics in international data. Int J Cancer 70: 375–382
203. Chan J K, Yip T T, Tsang W Y et al. 1995 Detection of Epstein–Barr virus in Hodgkin's disease occurring in an Oriental population. Hum Pathol 26: 314–318
204. Herbst H, Niedobitek G, Kneba M et al. 1990 High incidence of Epstein–Barr virus genomes in Hodgkin's disease. Am J Pathol 137: 13–18
205. Pallesen G, Hamilton-Dutoit S J, Rowe M et al. 1991 Expression of Epstein–Barr virus latent gene products in tumour cells of Hodgkin's disease. Lancet 337: 320–322
206. O'Grady J, Stewart S, Elton R A et al. 1994 Epstein–Barr virus in Hodgkin's disease and site of origin of tumour. Lancet 343: 265–266
207. Jarrett R F, Gallagher A, Jones D B 1991 Detection of Epstein–Barr virus genomes in Hodgkin's disease: relation to age. J Clin Pathol 44: 844–848
208. Zhou X G, Hamilton-Dutoit S J, Yan Q H et al. 1993 The association between Epstein–Barr virus and Chinese Hodgkin's disease. Int J Cancer 55: 359–363
209. Ambinder R F, Weiss L M 1999 Association of Epstein–Barr virus with Hodgkin's disease. In: Mauch P M, Armitage J O, Diehl V et al. (eds) Hodgkin's disease. Lippincott Williams & Wilkins, Philadelphia, 79–98
210. Jiwa N M, Kanavaros P, De Bruin P C et al. 1993 Presence of Epstein–Barr virus harbouring small and intermediate-sized cells in Hodgkin's disease. Is there a relationship with Reed–Sternberg cells? J Pathol 170: 129–136
211. Herbst H, Pallesen G, Weiss L M et al. 1992 Hodgkin's disease and Epstein–Barr virus. Ann Oncol 3 Suppl 4: 27–30
212. Herbst H, Steinbrecher E, Niedobitek G et al. 1992 Distribution and phenotype of Epstein–Barr virus-harboring cells in Hodgkin's disease. Blood 80: 484–491
213. Herbst H, Dallenbach F, Hummel M et al. 1991 Epstein–Barr virus latent membrane protein expression in Hodgkin's and Reed–Sternberg cells. Proc Natl Acad Sci USA 88: 4766–4770
214. Murray P G, Billingham L J, Hassan H T et al. 1999 Effect of Epstein–Barr virus infection on response to chemotherapy and survival in Hodgkin's disease. Blood 94: 442–447
215. Fellbaum C, Hansmann M L, Niedermeyer H et al. 1992 Influence of Epstein–Barr virus genomes on patient survival in Hodgkin's disease. Am J Clin Pathol 98: 319–323
216. Jarrett R F, Stark G L, White J et al. 2005 Impact of tumor Epstein–Barr virus status on presenting features and outcome in age-defined subgroups of patients with classic Hodgkin's lymphoma: a population-based study. Blood 106: 2444–2451
217. Clarke C A, Glaser S L, Dorfman R F et al. 2001 Epstein–Barr virus and survival after Hodgkin's disease in a population-based series of women. Cancer 91: 1579–1587
218. Rappaport H, Berard C W, Butler J J et al. 1971 Report of the Committee on Histopathological Criteria Contributing to Staging of Hodgkin's Disease. Cancer Res 31: 1864–1865
219. Strickler J G, Michie S A, Warnke R A et al. 1986 The 'syncytial variant' of nodular sclerosing Hodgkin's disease. Am J Surg Pathol 10: 470–477
220. Ben-Yehuda-Salz D, Ben-Yehuda A, Polliack A et al. 1990 Syncytial variant of nodular sclerosis Hodgkin's disease. A new clinicopathologic entity. Cancer 65: 1167–1172
221. Keller A R, Kaplan H S, Lukes R J et al. 1968 Correlation of histopathology with other prognostic indicators in Hodgkin's disease. Cancer 22: 487–499
222. MacLennan K A, Bennett M H, Tu A 1985 Prognostic significance of cytologic subdivison in nodular sclerosing Hodgkin's disease: an analysis of 1156 patients. In: Cavalli F, Bonadonna G, Rosencweig M (eds) Malignant lymphomas and Hodgkin's disease, experimental and therapeutic advances. Martinus Nijhoff, Boston, 187–200
223. MacLennan K A, Bennett M H, Tu A et al. 1989 Relationship of histopathologic features to survival and relapse in nodular sclerosing Hodgkin's disease. A study of 1659 patients. Cancer 64: 1686–1693
224. MacLennan K A, Bennett M H, Vaughan Hudson B et al. 1992 Diagnosis and grading of nodular sclerosing Hodgkin's disease: a study of 2190 patients. Int Rev Exp Pathol 33: 27–51
225. Haybittle J L, Hayhoe F G, Easterling M J et al. 1985 Review of British National Lymphoma Investigation studies of Hodgkin's disease and development of prognostic index. Lancet 1: 967–972
226. Ferry J A, Linggood R M, Convery K M et al. 1993 Hodgkin's disease, nodular sclerosis type. Implications of histologic subclassification. Cancer 71: 457–463
227. Wijlhuizen T J, Vrints L W, Jairam R et al. 1989 Grades of nodular sclerosis (NSI–NSII) in Hodgkin's disease. Are they of independent prognostic value? Cancer 63: 1150–1153
228. von Wasielewski S, Franklin J, Fischer R et al. 2003 Nodular sclerosing Hodgkin's disease: new grading predicts prognosis in intermediate and advanced stages. Blood 101: 4063–4069
229. d'Amore E S, Lee C K, Aeppli D M et al. 1992 Lack of prognostic value of histopathologic parameters in Hodgkin's disease, nodular sclerosis type. A study of 123 patients with limited stage disease who had undergone laparotomy and were treated with radiation therapy. Arch Pathol Lab Med 116: 856–861
230. Masih A S, Weisenburger D D, Vose J M et al. 1992 Histologic grade does not predict prognosis in optimally treated, advanced-stage nodular sclerosing Hodgkin's disease. Cancer 69: 228–232
231. Hess J L, Bodis S, Pinkus G et al. 1994 Histopathologic grading of nodular sclerosis Hodgkin's disease. Lack of prognostic significance in 254 surgically staged patients. Cancer 74: 708–714
232. Bacchi C E, Dorfman R F, Hoppe R T et al. 1991 Metastatic carcinoma in lymph nodes simulating 'syncytial variant' of nodular sclerosing Hodgkin's disease. Am J Clin Pathol 96: 589–593
233. Fellbaum C, Hansmann M L, Lennert K 1988 Lymphadenitis mimicking Hodgkin's disease. Histopathology 12: 253–262
234. Zarate-Osorno A, Medeiros L J, Danon A D et al. 1994 Hodgkin's disease with coexistent Castleman-like histologic features. A report of three cases. Arch Pathol Lab Med 118: 270–274
235. Maheswaran P R, Ramsay A D, Norton A J et al. 1991 Hodgkin's disease presenting with the histological features of Castleman's disease. Histopathology 18: 249–253
236. Molinie V, Diebold J, Perie G 1995 Hodgkin's disease associated with localized or multicentric Castleman's disease. Arch Pathol Lab Med 119: 201
237. Shimabukuro-Vornhagen A, Haverkamp H, Engert A et al. 2005 Lymphocyte-rich classical Hodgkin's lymphoma: clinical presentation and treatment outcome in 100 patients treated within German Hodgkin's Study Group trials. J Clin Oncol 23: 5739–5745
238. de Jong D, Bosq J, MacLennan K A et al. 2006 Lymphocyte-rich classical Hodgkin's lymphoma (LRCHL): clinicopathological characteristics and outcome of a rare entity. Ann Oncol 17: 141–145

239. Ashton-Key M, Thorpe P A, Allen J P, Isaacson P G 1995 Follicular Hodgkin's disease. Am J Surg Pathol 19: 1294–1299
240. Braüninger A, Wacker H H, Rajewsky K et al. 2003 Typing the histogenetic origin of the tumor cells of lymphocyte-rich classical Hodgkin's lymphoma in relation to tumor cells of classical and lymphocyte-predominance Hodgkin's lymphoma. Cancer Res 63: 1644–1651
241. Anastasi J, Bitter M A, Vardiman J W 1989 The histopathologic diagnosis and subclassification of Hodgkin's disease. Hematol Oncol Clin North Am 3: 187–204
242. Neiman R S, Rosen P J, Lukes R J 1973 Lymphocyte-depletion Hodgkin's disease. A clinicopathological entity. N Engl J Med 288: 751–755
243. Tajima K, Suchi T, Hirose K et al. 1984 Re-evaluation of high incidence of Hodgkin's disease in Kyushu, Japan. Hematol Oncol 2: 373–380
244. Kant J A, Hubbard S M, Longo D L et al. 1986 The pathologic and clinical heterogeneity of lymphocyte-depleted Hodgkin's disease. J Clin Oncol 4: 284–294
245. Doggett R S, Colby T V, Dorfman R F 1983 Interfollicular Hodgkin's disease. Am J Surg Pathol 7: 145–149
246. Variakojis D, Strum S B, Rappaport H 1972 The foamy macrophages in Hodgkin's disease. Arch Pathol 93: 453–456
247. Patsouris E, Noel H, Lennert K 1989 Cytohistologic and immunohistochemical findings in Hodgkin's disease, mixed cellularity type, with a high content of epithelioid cells. Am J Surg Pathol 13: 1014–1022
248. Mohrmann R L, Nathwani B N, Brynes R K et al. 1991 Hodgkin's disease occurring in monocytoid B-cell clusters. Am J Clin Pathol 95: 802–808
249. Kojima M, Nakamura S, Shimizu K et al. 2003 Classical Hodgkin's lymphoma occurring in clusters of nodal marginal zone B-lymphocytes in association with progressive transformation of germinal center. A case report. Pathol Res Pract 199: 547–550
250. Grogan T M, Berard C W, Steinhorn S C et al. 1982 Changing patterns of Hodgkin's disease at autopsy: a 25-year experience at the National Cancer Institute, 1953–1978. Cancer Treat Rep 66: 653–665
251. Colby T V, Hoppe R T, Warnke R A 1981 Hodgkin's disease at autopsy: 1972–1977. Cancer 47: 1852–1862
252. Radford J A, Cowan R A, Flanagan M et al. 1988 The significance of residual mediastinal abnormality on the chest radiograph following treatment for Hodgkin's disease. J Clin Oncol 6: 940–946
253. Chen J L, Osborne B M, Butler J J 1987 Residual fibrous masses in treated Hodgkin's disease. Cancer 60: 407–413
254. Specht L K, Hasenclever D 1999 Prognostic factors of Hodgkin's disease. In: Mauch P M, Armitage J O, Diehl V et al. (eds) Hodgkin's disease. Lippincott Williams & Wilkins, Philadelphia, 295–325
255. Specht L, Lauritzen A F, Nordentoft A M et al. 1990 Tumor cell concentration and tumor burden in relation to histopathologic subtype and other prognostic factors in early stage Hodgkin's disease. The Danish National Hodgkin's Study Group. Cancer 65: 2594–2601
256. Rappaport H, Strum S B, Hutchison G, Allen L W 1971 Clinical and biological significance of vascular invasion in Hodgkin's disease. Cancer Res 31: 1794–1798
257. Strum S B, Hutchison G B, Park J K et al. 1971 Further observations on the biologic significance of vascular invasion in Hodgkin's disease. Cancer 27: 1–6
258. Baur A S, Meuge-Moraw C, Michel G et al. 1998 Prognostic value of follicular dendritic cells in nodular sclerosing Hodgkin's disease. Histopathology 32: 512–520
259. Alavaikko M J, Blanco G, Aine R et al. 1994 Follicular dendritic cells have prognostic relevance in Hodgkin's disease. Am J Clin Pathol 101: 761–767
260. The non-Hodgkin's Lymphoma Pathologic Classification Project Writing Committee 1982 National Cancer Institute sponsored study of classifications of non-Hodgkin's lymphomas: summary and description of a working formulation for clinical usage. Cancer 49: 2112–2135
261. Pittaluga S, Bijnens L, Teodorovic I et al. 1996 Clinical analysis of 670 cases in two trials of the European Organization for the Research and Treatment of Cancer Lymphoma Cooperative Group subtyped according to the Revised European–American Classification of Lymphoid Neoplasms: a comparison with the Working Formulation. Blood 87: 4358–4367
262. Melnyk A, Rodriguez A, Pugh W C et al. 1997 Evaluation of the Revised European–American Lymphoma classification confirms the clinical relevance of immunophenotype in 560 cases of aggressive non-Hodgkin's lymphoma. Blood 89: 4514–4520
263. Fisher R I, Dahlberg S, Nathwani B N et al. 1995 A clinical analysis of two indolent lymphoma entities: mantle cell lymphoma and marginal zone lymphoma (including the mucosa-associated lymphoid tissue and monocytoid B-cell subcategories): a Southwest Oncology Group study. Blood 85: 1075–1082
264. The Non-Hodgkin's Lymphoma Classification Project 1997 A clinical evaluation of the International Lymphoma Study Group classification of non-Hodgkin's lymphoma. Blood 89: 3909–3918
265. Jaffe E S, Harris N L, Diebold J et al. 1998 World Health Organization Classification of lymphomas: a work in progress. Ann Oncol 9: S25–30
266. Jaffe E S, Harris N L, Diebold J et al. 1999 World Health Organization classification of neoplastic diseases of the hematopoietic and lymphoid tissues. A progress report. Am J Clin Pathol 111: S8–12
267. Harris N L, Jaffe E S, Vardiman J W et al. 2001 WHO Classification of tumours of haematopoietic and lymphoid tissues: Introduction. In: Jaffe E S, Harris N L, Stein H et al. (eds) Pathology and genetics, tumours of haematopoietic and lymphoid tissues. IARC Press, Lyon, 12–13
268. Armitage J O, Weisenburger D D 1998 New approach to classifying non-Hodgkin's lymphomas: clinical features of the major histologic subtypes. Non-Hodgkin's Lymphoma Classification Project. J Clin Oncol 16: 2780–2795
269. Nathwani B N, Anderson J R, Armitage J O et al. 1999 Marginal zone B-cell lymphoma: A clinical comparison of nodal and mucosa-associated lymphoid tissue types. J Clin Oncol 17: 2486
270. Chan J K C 1997 Is the REAL classification for real? Do we need a separate classification for cutaneous lymphomas? Adv Anat Pathol 4: 359–369
271. Horning S J 1993 Natural history of and therapy for the indolent non-Hodgkin's lymphomas. Semin Oncol 20: 75–88
272. Lennert K, Feller A C 1992 Histopathology of non-Hodgkin's lymphomas (based on the updated Kiel classification), 2nd edn. Springer-Verlag, Berlin
273. Perkins S L, Segal G H, Kjeldsberg C R 1995 Classification of non-Hodgkin's lymphomas in children. Semin Diagn Pathol 12: 303–313
274. The International Non-Hodgkin's Lymphoma Prognostic Factors Project 1993 A predictive model for aggressive non-Hodgkin's lymphoma. N Engl J Med 329: 987–994
275. Hermans J, Krol A D, van Groningen K et al. 1995 International Prognostic Index for aggressive non-Hodgkin's lymphoma is valid for all malignancy grades. Blood 86: 1460–1463
276. Blay J, Gomez F, Sebban C et al. 1998 The International Prognostic Index correlates to survival in patients with aggressive lymphoma in relapse: analysis of the PARMA trial. Parma Group. Blood 92: 3562–3568
277. Bastion Y, Coiffier B 1994 Is the International Prognostic Index for Aggressive Lymphoma Patients useful for follicular lymphoma patients? J Clin Oncol 12: 1340–1342
278. Cheuk W, Chan A C, Chan J K et al. 2005 Metallic implant-associated lymphoma: a distinct subgroup of large B-cell lymphoma related to pyothorax-associated lymphoma? Am J Surg Pathol 29: 832–836
279. De Vita S, Sansonno D, Dolcetti R et al. 1995 Hepatitis C virus within a malignant lymphoma lesion in the course of type II mixed cryoglobulinemia. Blood 86: 1887–1892
280. Chan J K, Tsang W Y, Ng C S et al. 1995 A study of the association of Epstein–Barr virus with Burkitt's lymphoma occurring in a Chinese population. Histopathology 26: 239–245
281. Zuckerman E, Zuckerman T, Levine A M et al. 1997 Hepatitis C virus infection in patients with B-cell non-Hodgkin's lymphoma. Ann Intern Med 127: 423–428
282. Lai R, Weiss L M 1998 Hepatitis C virus and non-Hodgkin's lymphoma. Am J Clin Pathol 109: 508–510
283. Collier J D, Zanke B, Moore M et al. 1999 No association between hepatitis C and B-cell lymphoma. Hepatology 29: 1259–1261
284. Dammacco F, Gatti P, Sansonno D 1998 Hepatitis C virus infection, mixed cryoglobulinemia, and non-Hodgkin's lymphoma: an emerging picture. Leuk Lymphoma 31: 463–476
285. Gisbert J P, Garcia-Buey L, Pajares J M et al. 2003 Prevalence of hepatitis C virus infection in B-cell non-Hodgkin's lymphoma: systematic review and meta-analysis. Gastroenterology 125: 1723–1732
286. Libra M, Gasparotto D, Gloghini A et al. 2005 Hepatitis C virus (HCV) I hepatitis C virus (HCV) infection and lymphoproliferative disorders. Front Biosci 10: 2460–2471
287. Hermine O, Lefrere F, Bronowicki J P et al. 2002 Regression of splenic lymphoma with villous lymphocytes after treatment of hepatitis C virus infection. N Engl J Med 347: 89–94
288. Morgensztern D, Rosado A, Silva O et al. 2004 Prevalence of hepatitis C infection in patients with non-Hodgkin's lymphoma in South Florida and review of the literature. Leuk Lymphoma 45: 2459–2464
289. Giannoulis E, Economopoulos T, Mandraveli K et al. 2004 The prevalence of hepatitis C and hepatitis G virus infection in patients with B cell non-Hodgkin's lymphomas in Greece: a Hellenic Cooperative Oncology Group Study. Acta Haematol 112: 189–193
290. Engels E A, Chatterjee N, Cerhan J R et al. 2004 Hepatitis C virus infection and non-Hodgkin's lymphoma: results of the NCI-SEER multicenter case–control study. Int J Cancer 111: 76–80
291. Weng W K, Levy S 2003 Hepatitis C virus (HCV) and lymphomagenesis. Leuk Lymphoma 44: 1113–1120
292. Mele A, Pulsoni A, Bianco E et al. 2003 Hepatitis C virus and B-cell non-Hodgkin's lymphomas: an Italian multicenter case–control study. Blood 102: 996–999
293. Machida K, Cheng K T, Sung V M et al. 2004 Hepatitis C virus induces a mutator phenotype: enhanced mutations of immunoglobulin and protooncogenes. Proc Natl Acad Sci USA 101: 4262–4267
294. Gisbert J P, Garcia-Buey L, Pajares J M et al. 2005 Systematic review: regression of lymphoproliferative disorders after treatment for hepatitis C infection. Aliment Pharmacol Ther 21: 653–662
295. Chanudet E, Zhou Y, Bacon C M et al. 2006 *Chlamydia psittaci* is variably associated with ocular adnexal MALT lymphoma in different geographical regions. J Pathol 209: 344–351
296. Ferreri A J, Ponzoni M, Guidoboni M et al. 2005 Regression of ocular adnexal lymphoma after *Chlamydia psittaci*-eradicating antibiotic therapy. J Clin Oncol 23: 5067–5073
297. Rosado M F, Byrne G E Jr, Ding F et al. 2006 Ocular adnexal lymphoma: a clinicopathologic study of a large cohort of patients with no evidence for an association with *Chlamydia psittaci*. Blood 107: 467–472

298. Vargas R L, Fallone E, Felgar R E et al. 2006 Is there an association between ocular adnexal lymphoma and infection with *Chlamydia psittaci*? The University of Rochester experience. Leuk Res 30: 547–551
299. Mulder M M, Heddema E R, Pannekoek Y et al. 2006 No evidence for an association of ocular adnexal lymphoma with *Chlamydia psittaci* in a cohort of patients from the Netherlands. Leuk Res 30: 1305–1307
300. Daibata M, Nemoto Y, Togitani K et al. 2006 Absence of *Chlamydia psittaci* in ocular adnexal lymphoma from Japanese patients. Br J Haematol 132: 651–652
301. Liu Y C, Ohyashiki J H, Ito Y et al. 2006 *Chlamydia psittaci* in ocular adnexal lymphoma: Japanese experience. Leuk Res 30:1587–1589
302. Grunberger B, Hauff W, Lukas J et al. 2006 'Blind' antibiotic treatment targeting *Chlamydia* is not effective in patients with MALT lymphoma of the ocular adnexa. Ann Oncol 17: 484–487
303. Cerroni L, Zochling N, Putz B, Kerl H 1997 Infection by *Borrelia burgdorferi* and cutaneous B-cell lymphoma. J Cutan Pathol 24: 457–461
304. Roggero E, Zucca E, Mainetti C et al. 2000 Eradication of *Borrelia burgdorferi* infection in primary marginal zone B-cell lymphoma of the skin. Hum Pathol 31: 263–268
305. Goodlad J R, Davidson M M, Hollowood K et al. 2000 Primary cutaneous B-cell lymphoma and *Borrelia burgdorferi* infection in patients from the Highlands of Scotland. Am J Surg Pathol 24: 1279–1285
306. Wood G S, Kamath N V, Guitart J et al. 2001 Absence of *Borrelia burgdorferi* DNA in cutaneous B-cell lymphomas from the United States. J Cutan Pathol 28: 502–507
307. Li C, Inagaki H, Kuo T T et al. 2003 Primary cutaneous marginal zone B-cell lymphoma: a molecular and clinicopathologic study of 24 Asian cases. Am J Surg Pathol 27: 1061–1069
308. Lecuit M, Abachin E, Martin A et al. 2004 Immunoproliferative small intestinal disease associated with *Campylobacter jejuni*. N Engl J Med 350: 239–248
309. Bernard A, Boumsell L, Patte C 1986 Leukemia versus lymphoma in children: a worthless question? Med Pediatr Oncol 14: 148–157
310. Raetz E A, Perkins S L, Bhojwani D et al. 2006 Gene expression profiling reveals intrinsic differences between T-cell acute lymphoblastic leukemia and T-cell lymphoblastic lymphoma. Pediatr Blood Cancer 47: 130–140
311. Nathwani B N, Diamond L W, Winberg C D et al. 1981 Lymphoblastic lymphoma: a clinicopathologic study of 95 patients. Cancer 48: 2347–2357
312. Sheibani K, Nathwani B N, Winberg C D et al. 1987 Antigenically defined subgroups of lymphoblastic lymphoma. Relationship to clinical presentation and biologic behavior. Cancer 60: 183–190
313. Hvizdala E V, Berard C, Callihan T et al. 1988 Lymphoblastic lymphoma in children – a randomized trial comparing LSA2-L2 with the A-COP+ therapeutic regimen: a Pediatric Oncology Group Study. J Clin Oncol 6: 26–33
314. Morel P, Lepage E, Brice P et al. 1992 Prognosis and treatment of lymphoblastic lymphoma in adults: a report on 80 patients. J Clin Oncol 10: 1078–1085
315. van den Berg H, Zsiros J, Veneberg A et al. 1998 Favorable outcome after 1-year treatment of childhood T-cell lymphoma/T-cell acute lymphoblastic leukemia. Med Pediatr Oncol 30: 46–51
316. Crist W M, Shuster J J, Falletta J et al. 1988 Clinical features and outcome in childhood T-cell leukemia–lymphoma according to stage of thymocyte differentiation: a Pediatric Oncology Group Study. Blood 72: 1891–1897
317. Grenzebach J, Schrappe M, Ludwig W D et al. 2001 Favorable outcome for children and adolescents with T-cell lymphoblastic lymphoma with an intensive ALL-type therapy without local radiotherapy. Ann Hematol 80 Suppl 3: B73–76
318. Hoelzer D, Gokbuget N, Digel W et al. 2002 Outcome of adult patients with T-lymphoblastic lymphoma treated according to protocols for acute lymphoblastic leukemia. Blood 99: 4379–4385
319. Thomas D A, O'Brien S, Cortes J et al. 2004 Outcome with the hyper-CVAD regimens in lymphoblastic lymphoma. Blood 104: 1624–1630
320. Mora J, Filippa D A, Qin J, Wollner N 2003 Lymphoblastic lymphoma of childhood and the LSA2-L2 protocol: the 30-year experience at Memorial Sloan–Kettering Cancer Center. Cancer 98: 1283–1291
321. Abruzzo L V, Jaffe E S, Cotelingam J D et al. 1992 T-cell lymphoblastic lymphoma with eosinophilia associated with subsequent myeloid malignancy. Am J Surg Pathol 16: 236–245
322. Inhorn R C, Aster J C, Roach S A et al. 1995 A syndrome of lymphoblastic lymphoma, eosinophilia, and myeloid hyperplasia/malignancy associated with t(8; 13)(p11; q11): description of a distinctive clinicopathologic entity. Blood 85: 1881–1887
323. Somers G R, Slater H, Rockman S et al. 1997 Coexistent T-cell lymphoblastic lymphoma and an atypical myeloproliferative disorder associated with t(8; 13)(p21; q14). Pediatr Pathol Lab Med 17: 141–158
324. Velankar M M, Nathwani B N, Schlutz M J et al. 1999 Indolent T-lymphoblastic proliferation: report of a case with a 16-year course without cytotoxic therapy. Am J Surg Pathol 23: 977–981
325. Strauchen J A 2001 Indolent T-lymphoblastic proliferation: report of a case with an 11-year history and association with myasthenia gravis. Am J Surg Pathol 25: 411–415
326. Cheng A L, Su I J, Tien H F et al. 1994 Characteristic clinicopathologic features of adult B-cell lymphoblastic lymphoma with special emphasis on differential diagnosis with an atypical form probably of blastic lymphocytic lymphoma of intermediate differentiation origin. Cancer 73: 706–710
327. Sander C A, Medeiros L J, Abruzzo L V et al.1991 Lymphoblastic lymphoma presenting in cutaneous sites. A clinicopathologic analysis of six cases. J Am Acad Dermatol 25: 1023–1031
328. Ozdemirli M, Fanburg-Smith J C, Hartmann D P et al. 1998 Precursor B-lymphoblastic lymphoma presenting as a solitary bone tumor and mimicking Ewing's sarcoma: a report of four cases and review of the literature. Am J Surg Pathol 22: 795–804
329. Soslow R A, Baergen R N, Warnke R A 1999 B-lineage lymphoblastic lymphoma is a clinicopathologic entity distinct from other histologically similar aggressive lymphomas with blastic morphology. Cancer 85: 2648–2654
330. Yeh K H, Cheng A L, Su I J et al. 1997 Prognostic significance of immunophenotypes in adult lymphoblastic lymphomas. Anticancer Res 17: 2269–2272
331. Iravani S, Singleton T P, Ross C W et al. 1999 Precursor B lymphoblastic lymphoma presenting as lytic bone lesions. Am J Clin Pathol 112: 836–843
332. Sander C A, Jaffe E S, Gebhardt F C et al. 1992 Mediastinal lymphoblastic lymphoma with an immature B-cell immunophenotype. Am J Surg Pathol 16: 300–305
333. Kahwash S B, Qualman S J 2002 Cutaneous lymphoblastic lymphoma in children: report of six cases with precursor B-cell lineage. Pediatr Dev Pathol 5: 45–53
334. Ichinohasama R, Endoh K, Ishizawa K et al. 1996 Thymic lymphoblastic lymphoma of committed natural killer cell precursor origin: a case report. Cancer 77: 2592–2603
335. Nakamura F, Tatsumi E, Kawano S et al. 1997 Acute lymphoblastic leukemia/lymphoblastic lymphoma of natural killer (NK) lineage: quest for another NK-lineage neoplasm. Blood 89: 4665–4666
336. Tamura H, Ogata K, Mori S et al. 1998 Lymphoblastic lymphoma of natural killer cell origin, presenting as pancreatic tumour. Histopathology 32: 508–511
337. Ioachim H L, Finbeiner J A 1980 Pseudonodular pattern of T-cell lymphoma. Cancer 45: 1370–1378
338. Suzumiya J, Ohshima K, Kikuchi M et al. 1997 Terminal deoxynucleotidyl transferase staining of malignant lymphomas in paraffin sections: a useful method for the diagnosis of lymphoblastic lymphoma. J Pathol 182: 86–91
339. Childs C C, Chrystal G S, Strauchen J A 1986 Biphenotypic lymphoblastic lymphoma. An unusual tumor with lymphocytic and granulocytic differentiation. Cancer 57: 1019–1023
340. Weiss L M, Bindl J M, Picozzi V J et al. 1986 Lymphoblastic lymphoma: an immunophenotype study of 26 cases with comparison to T cell acute lymphoblastic leukemia. Blood 67: 474–478
341. Pittaluga S, Raffeld M, Lipford E H et al. 1986 3A1 (CD7) expression precedes T beta gene rearrangements in precursor T (lymphoblastic) neoplasms. Blood 68: 134–139
342. Knowles D M 1989 Immunophenotypic and antigen receptor gene rearrangement analysis in T cell neoplasia. Am J Pathol 134: 761–785
343. Feller A C, Parwaresch M R, Stein H et al. 1986 Immunophenotyping of T-lymphoblastic lymphoma/leukemia: correlation with normal T-cell maturation. Leuk Res 10: 1025–1031
344. Chetty R, Pulford K, Jones M et al. 1995 SCL/Tal-1 expression in T-acute lymphoblastic leukemia: an immunohistochemical and genotypic study. Hum Pathol 26: 994–998
345. Chetty R 1996 TAL1 gene and protein: an important gene and transcription factor involved in tumorigenesis. Adv Anat Pathol 3: 400–404
346. Sheibani K, Winberg C D, Burke J S et al. 1987 Lymphoblastic lymphoma expressing natural killer cell-associated antigens: a clinicopathologic study of six cases. Leuk Res 11: 371–377
347. Pilozzi E, Pulford K, Jones M et al. 1998 Co-expression of CD79a (JCB117) and CD3 by lymphoblastic lymphoma. J Pathol 186: 140–143
348. Pilozzi E, Muller-Hermelink H K, Falini B et al. 1999 Gene rearrangements in T-cell lymphoblastic lymphoma. J Pathol 188: 267–270
349. Tiacci E, Pileri S, Orleth A et al. 2004 PAX5 expression in acute leukemias: higher B-lineage specificity than CD79a and selective association with t(8; 21)-acute myelogenous leukemia. Cancer Res 64: 7399–7404
350. Torlakovic E, Torlakovic G, Nguyen P L et al. 2002 The value of anti-pax-5 immunostaining in routinely fixed and paraffin-embedded sections: a novel pan pre-B and B-cell marker. Am J Surg Pathol 26: 1343–1350
351. Menestrina F, Lestani M, Scarpa A et al. 1994 Common acute lymphoblastic leukaemia–lymphoma expressing cytokeratin: a case report. Virchows Arch 425: 83–87
352. Knowles D M 1999 Morphologic, immunologic and genetic features of precursor T and B cell neoplasms. In: Mason D Y, Harris N L (eds) Human lymphoma: clinical implications of the REAL classification. Springer, London, 43.41–43.45
353. Schichman S A, Aplan P D, Neri A et al. 1997 Pathogenesis of T-cell lymphomas. In: Magrath I (ed): The non-Hodgkin's lymphomas. Arnold, London, 411–442
354. Ferrando A A, Neuberg D S, Staunton J et al. 2002 Gene expression signatures define novel oncogenic pathways in T cell acute lymphoblastic leukemia. Cancer Cell 1: 75–87
355. Kuppers R, Klein U, Hansmann M L et al. 1999 Cellular origin of human B-cell lymphomas. N Engl J Med 341: 1520–1529
356. Pangalis G A, Angelopoulou M K, Vassilakopoulos T P et al. 1999 B-chronic lymphocytic leukemia, small lymphocytic lymphoma, and lymphoplasmacytic lymphoma, including Waldenström's macroglobulinemia: a clinical, morphologic, and biologic spectrum of similar disorders. Semin Hematol 36: 104–114

357. Pangalis G A, Boussiotis V A, Kittas C 1993 Malignant disorders of small lymphocytes. Small lymphocytic lymphoma, lymphoplasmacytic lymphoma, and chronic lymphocytic leukemia: their clinical and laboratory relationship. Am J Clin Pathol 99: 402–408
358. Morrison W H, Hoppe R T, Weiss L M et al. 1989 Small lymphocytic lymphoma. J Clin Oncol 7: 598–606
359. Rai K R, Sawitsky A, Cronkite E P 1975 Clinical staging of chronic lymphocytic leukemia. Blood 46: 219–234
360. Binet J L, Auquier A, Dighiero G et al. 1981 A new prognostic classification of chronic lymphocytic leukemia derived from a multivariate survival analysis. Cancer 48: 198–206
361. Ben-Ezra J, Burke J S, Swartz W G et al. 1989 Small lymphocytic lymphoma: a clinicopathologic analysis of 268 cases. Blood 73: 579–587
362. Cheson B D 1998 New prospects in the treatment of indolent lymphomas with purine analogues. Cancer J Sci Am 4(Suppl 2): S27–36
363. Montserrat E, Campo E 2006 Small lymphocytic lymphoma/chronic lymphocytic leukemia. In: Canellos G P, Lister T A, Young B D (eds) The lymphomas, 2nd edn. Saunders Elsevier, Philadelphia, 406–414
364. Ellison D J, Nathwani B N, Cho S Y et al. 1989 Interfollicular small lymphocytic lymphoma: the diagnostic significance of pseudofollicles. Hum Pathol 20: 1108–1118
365. Carbone A, Pinto A, Gloghini A et al. 1992 B-zone small lymphocytic lymphoma: a morphologic, immunophenotypic, and clinical study with comparison to 'well-differentiated' lymphocytic disorders. Hum Pathol 23: 438–448
366. Carbone A, Pinto A, Gloghini A et al. 1990 Report of an unusual small lymphocytic B-cell lymphoma selectively involving the B-zone of lymph node. Cancer 66: 302–312
367. Dick F R, Maca R D 1978 The lymph node in chronic lymphocytic leukemia. Cancer 41: 283–292
368. Koo C H, Shin S S, Bracho F et al. 1996 Rosette-forming non-Hodgkin's lymphomas. Histopathology 29: 557–563
369. Bonato M, Pittaluga S, Tierens A et al. 1998 Lymph node histology in typical and atypical chronic lymphocytic leukemia. Am J Surg Pathol 22: 49–56
370. Pugh W C, Manning J T, Butler J J 1988 Paraimmunoblastic variant of small lymphocytic lymphoma/leukemia. Am J Surg Pathol 12: 907–917
371. Brittinger G, Bartels H, Common H et al. 1984 Clinical and prognostic relevance of the Kiel classification of non-Hodgkin's lymphomas results of a prospective multicenter study by the Kiel Lymphoma Study Group. Hematol Oncol 2: 269–306
372. Medeiros L J, Strickler J G, Picker L J et al. 1987 'Well-differentiated' lymphocytic neoplasms. Immunologic findings correlated with clinical presentation and morphologic features. Am J Pathol 129: 523–535
373. Cheuk W, Wong K O, Wong C S et al. 2004 Consistent immunostaining for cyclin D1 can be achieved on a routine basis using a newly available rabbit monoclonal antibody. Am J Surg Pathol 28: 801–807
374. Medeiros L J, Picker L J, Gelb A B et al. 1989 Numbers of host 'helper' T cells and proliferating cells predict survival in diffuse small-cell lymphomas. J Clin Oncol 7: 1009–1017
375. Ratech H, Sheibani K, Nathwani B N et al. 1988 Immunoarchitecture of the 'pseudofollicles' of well-differentiated (small) lymphocytic lymphoma: a comparison with true follicles. Hum Pathol 19: 89–94
376. Schmid C, Isaacson P G 1994 Proliferation centres in B-cell malignant lymphoma, lymphocytic (B-CLL): an immunophenotypic study. Histopathology 24: 445–451
377. Narducci M G, Pescarmona E, Lazzeri C et al. 2000 Regulation of TCL1 expression in B- and T-cell lymphomas and reactive lymphoid tissues. Cancer Res 60: 2095–2100
378. Gelb A B, Rouse R V, Dorfman R F et al.1994 Detection of immunophenotypic abnormalities in paraffin-embedded B-lineage non-Hodgkin's lymphomas. Am J Clin Pathol 102: 825–834
379. Chiorazzi N, Rai K R, Ferrarini M 2005 Chronic lymphocytic leukemia. N Engl J Med 352: 804–815
380. Klein U, Tu Y, Stolovitzky G A et al. 2001 Gene expression profiling of B cell chronic lymphocytic leukemia reveals a homogeneous phenotype related to memory B cells. J Exp Med 194: 1625–1638
381. Klein U, Dalla-Favera R 2005 New insights into the phenotype and cell derivation of B cell chronic lymphocytic leukemia. Curr Top Microbiol Immunol 294: 31–49
382. Hummel M, Tamaru J, Kalvelage B et al. 1994 Mantle cell (previously centrocytic) lymphomas express VH genes with no or very little somatic mutations like the physiologic cells of the follicle mantle. Blood 84: 403–407
383. Nakamura N, Kuze T, Hashimoto Y et al. 1999 Analysis of the immunoglobulin heavy chain gene variable region of 101 cases with peripheral B cell neoplasms and B cell chronic lymphocytic leukemia in the Japanese population. Pathol Int 49: 595–600
384. Oscier D G, Thompsett A, Zhu D et al. 1997 Differential rates of somatic hypermutation in V(H) genes among subsets of chronic lymphocytic leukemia defined by chromosomal abnormalities. Blood 89: 4153–4160
385. Bahler D W, Aguilera N S, Chen C C et al. 2000 Histological and immunoglobulin VH gene analysis of interfollicular small lymphocytic lymphoma provides evidence for two types. Am J Pathol 157: 1063–1070
386. Oscier D G, Gardiner A C, Mould S J et al. 2002 Multivariate analysis of prognostic factors in CLL: clinical stage, IGVH gene mutational status, and loss or mutation of the p53 gene are independent prognostic factors. Blood 100: 1177–1184
387. Hamblin T J, Davis Z, Gardiner A et al. 1999 Unmutated Ig V(H) genes are associated with a more aggressive form of chronic lymphocytic leukemia. Blood 94: 1848–1854
388. Rosenwald A, Alizadeh A A, Widhopf G et al. 2001 Relation of gene expression phenotype to immunoglobulin mutation genotype in B cell chronic lymphocytic leukemia. J Exp Med 194: 1639–1647
389. Wiestner A, Rosenwald A, Barry T S et al. 2003 ZAP-70 expression identifies a chronic lymphocytic leukemia subtype with unmutated immunoglobulin genes, inferior clinical outcome, and distinct gene expression profile. Blood 101: 4944–4951
390. Del Principe M I, Del Poeta G, Buccisano F et al. 2006 Clinical significance of ZAP-70 protein expression in B-cell chronic lymphocytic leukemia. Blood 108: 853–861
391. Crespo M, Bosch F, Villamor N et al. 2003 ZAP-70 expression as a surrogate for immunoglobulin-variable-region mutations in chronic lymphocytic leukemia. N Engl J Med 348: 1764–1775
392. Rassenti L Z, Huynh L, Toy T L et al. 2004 ZAP-70 compared with immunoglobulin heavy-chain gene mutation status as a predictor of disease progression in chronic lymphocytic leukemia. N Engl J Med 351: 893–901
393. Durig J, Nuckel H, Cremer M et al. 2003 ZAP-70 expression is a prognostic factor in chronic lymphocytic leukemia. Leukemia 17: 2426–2434
394. Orchard J A, Ibbotson R E, Davis Z et al. 2004 ZAP-70 expression and prognosis in chronic lymphocytic leukaemia. Lancet 363: 105–111
395. Panayiotidis P, Kotsi P 1999 Genetics of small lymphocyte disorders. Semin Hematol 36: 171–177
396. Gaidano G, Pastore C, Capello D et al. 1997 Molecular pathways in low grade B-cell lymphoma. Leuk Lymphoma 26 Suppl 1: 107–113
397. Calin G A, Ferracin M, Cimmino A et al. 2005 A MicroRNA signature associated with prognosis and progression in chronic lymphocytic leukemia. N Engl J Med 353: 1793–1801
398. Dohner H, Stilgenbauer S, James M R 1997 11q deletions identify a new subset of B-CLL characeratized by extensive nodal involvement and inferior prognosis. Blood 89: 2516–2522
399. Schaffner C, Stilgenbauer S, Rappold G A et al. 1999 Somatic ATM mutations indicate a pathogenic role of ATM in B-cell chronic lymphocytic leukemia. Blood 94: 748–753
400. Bullrich F, Rasio D, Kitada S et al. 1999 ATM mutations in B-cell chronic lymphocytic leukemia. Cancer Res 59: 24–27
401. Stankovic T, Weber P, Stewart G et al. 1999 Inactivation of ataxia telangiectasia mutated gene in B-cell chronic lymphocytic leukaemia. Lancet 353: 26–29
402. Gaidano G, Ballerini P, Gong J Z et al. 1991 p53 mutations in human lymphoid malignancies: association with Burkitt lymphoma and chronic lymphocytic leukemia. Proc Natl Acad Sci USA 88: 5413–5417
403. Navarro B, Garcia-Marco J A, Jones D et al. 1998 Association and clonal distribution of trisomy 12 and 13q14 deletions in chronic lymphocytic leukaemia. Br J Haematol 102: 1330–1334
404. Oscier D G, Matutes E, Copplestone A et al. 1997 Atypical lymphocyte morphology: an adverse prognostic factor for disease progression in stage A CLL independent of trisomy 12. Br J Haematol 98: 934–939
405. Criel A, Verhoef G, Vlietinck R et al. 1997 Further characterization of morphologically defined typical and atypical CLL: a clinical, immunophenotypic, cytogenetic and prognostic study on 390 cases. Br J Haematol 97: 383–391
406. Matutes E, Oscier D, Garcia-Marco J et al. 1996 Trisomy 12 defines a group of CLL with atypical morphology: correlation between cytogenetic, clinical and laboratory features in 544 patients. Br J Haematol 92: 382–388
407. Jelic T, Jovanovic V, Milanovic N et al. 1997 Richter syndrome with emphasis on large-cell non-Hodgkin's lymphoma in previously unrecognized subclinical chronic lymphocytic leukemia. Neoplasma 44: 63–68
408. Matolcsy A, Casali P, Knowles D M 1995 Different clonal origin of B-cell populations of chronic lymphocytic leukemia and large-cell lymphoma in Richter's syndrome. Ann NY Acad Sci 764: 496–503
409. Traweek S T, Liu J, Johnson R M et al. 1993 High-grade transformation of chronic lymphocytic leukemia and low-grade non-Hodgkin's lymphoma. Genotypic confirmation of clonal identity. Am J Clin Pathol 100: 519–526
410. Brynes R K, McCourty A, Sun N C et al. 1995 Trisomy 12 in Richter's transformation of chronic lymphocytic leukemia. Am J Clin Pathol 104: 199–203
411. Bea S, Lopez-Guillermo A, Ribas M et al. 2002 Genetic imbalances in progressed B-cell chronic lymphocytic leukemia and transformed large-cell lymphoma (Richter's syndrome). Am J Pathol 161: 957–968
412. Lee A, Skelly M E, Kingma D W et al. 1995 B-cell chronic lymphocytic leukemia followed by high grade T-cell lymphoma. An unusual variant of Richter's syndrome. Am J Clin Pathol 103: 348–352
413. Pistoia V, Roncella S, Di Celle P F et al. 1991 Emergence of a B-cell lymphoblastic lymphoma in a patient with B-cell chronic lymphocytic leukemia: evidence for the single-cell origin of the two tumors. Blood 78: 797–804
414. Wetzler M, Kurzrock R, Goodacre A M et al. 1995 Transformation of chronic lymphocytic leukemia to lymphoma of true histiocytic type. Cancer 76: 609–617
415. Tsang W Y, Chan J K, Sing C 1993 The nature of Reed–Sternberg-like cells in chronic lymphocytic leukemia. Am J Clin Pathol 99: 317–323

416. Tsang W Y, Chan J K, Ng C S 1993 Epstein–Barr virus and Reed–Sternberg-like cells in chronic lymphocytic leukemia. Am J Surg Pathol 17: 853–854
417. Shin S S, Ben-Ezra J, Burke J S et al. 1993 Reed–Sternberg-like cells in low-grade lymphomas are transformed neoplastic cells of B-cell lineage. Am J Clin Pathol 99: 658–662
418. Williams J, Schned A, Cotelingam J D et al. 1991 Chronic lymphocytic leukemia with coexistent Hodgkin's disease. Implications for the origin of the Reed–Sternberg cell. Am J Surg Pathol 15: 33–42
419. Rubin D, Hudnall S D, Aisenberg A et al. 1994 Richter's transformation of chronic lymphocytic leukemia with Hodgkin's-like cells is associated with Epstein–Barr virus infection. Mod Pathol 7: 91–98
420. Pescarmona E, Pignoloni P, Mauro F R et al. 2000 Hodgkin's/Reed–Sternberg cells and Hodgkin's disease in patients with B-cell chronic lymphocytic leukaemia: an immunohistological, molecular and clinical study of four cases suggesting a heterogeneous pathogenetic background. Virchows Arch 437: 129–132
421. Weisenberg E, Anastasi J, Adeyanju M, Variakojis D, Vardiman J W 1995 Hodgkin's disease associated with chronic lymphocytic leukemia. Eight additional cases, including two of the nodular lymphocyte predominant type. Am J Clin Pathol 103: 479–484
422. Nemets A, Ben Dor D, Barry T et al. 2003 Variant Richter's syndrome: a rare case of classical Hodgkin's lymphoma developing in a patient with chronic lymphocytic leukemia treated with fludarabine. Leuk Lymphoma 44: 2151–2154
423. Thornton P D, Bellas C, Santon A et al. 2005 Richter's transformation of chronic lymphocytic leukemia. The possible role of fludarabine and the Epstein–Barr virus in its pathogenesis. Leuk Res 29: 389–395
424. de Leval L, Vivario M, De Prijck B et al. 2004 Distinct clonal origin in two cases of Hodgkin's lymphoma variant of Richter's syndrome associated with EBV infection. Am J Surg Pathol 28: 679–686
425. Tzankov A, Fong D 2006 Hodgkin's disease variant of Richter's syndrome clonally related to chronic lymphocytic leukemia arises in ZAP-70 negative mutated CLL. Med Hypotheses 66: 577–579
426. Kyrtsonis M C, Vassilakopoulos T P, Angelopoulou M K et al. 2001 Waldenström's macroglobulinemia: clinical course and prognostic factors in 60 patients. Experience from a single hematology unit. Ann Hematol 80: 722–727
427. Papamichael D, Norton A J, Foran J M et al. 1999 Immunocytoma: a retrospective analysis from St Bartholomew's Hospital, 1972 to 1996. J Clin Oncol 17: 2847–2853
428. Lin P, Mansoor A, Bueso-Ramos C et al. 2003 Diffuse large B-cell lymphoma occurring in patients with lymphoplasmacytic lymphoma/Waldenström macroglobulinemia. Clinicopathologic features of 12 cases. Am J Clin Pathol 120: 246–253
429. Patsouris E, Noel H, Lennert K 1990 Lymphoplasmacytic/lymphoplasmacytoid immunocytoma with a high content of epithelioid cells. Histologic and immunohistochemical findings. Am J Surg Pathol 14: 660–670
430. Kapadia S B, Enzinger F M, Heffner D K et al. 1993 Crystal-storing histiocytosis associated with lymphoplasmacytic neoplasms. Report of three cases mimicking adult rhabdomyoma. Am J Surg Pathol 17: 461–467
431. Berger F, Felman P, Sonet A et al. 1994 Nonfollicular small B-cell lymphomas: a heterogeneous group of patients with distinct clinical features and outcome. Blood 83: 2829–2835
432. Konoplev S, Medeiros L J, Bueso-Ramos C E et al. 2005 Immunophenotypic profile of lymphoplasmacytic lymphoma/Waldenström macroglobulinemia. Am J Clin Pathol 124: 414–420
433. Merzianu M, Jiang L, Lin P et al. 2006 Nuclear BCL-10 expression is common in lymphoplasmacytic lymphoma/Waldenström macroglobulinemia and does not correlate with p65 NF-kappaB activation. Mod Pathol 19: 891–898
434. Iida S, Rao P H, Nallasivam P et al. 1996 The t(9; 14)(p13; q32) chromosomal translocation associated with lymphoplasmacytoid lymphoma involves the PAX-5 gene. Blood 88: 4110–4117
435. Iida S, Rao P H, Ueda R et al. 1999 Chromosomal rearrangement of the PAX-5 locus in lymphoplasmacytic lymphoma with t(9; 14)(p13; q32). Leuk Lymphoma 34: 25–33
436. Cook J R, Aguilera N I, Reshmi-Skarja S et al. 2004 Lack of PAX5 rearrangements in lymphoplasmacytic lymphomas: reassessing the reported association with t(9; 14). Hum Pathol 35: 447–454
437. Lin P, Medeiros L J 2005 Lymphoplasmacytic lymphoma/Waldenström macroglobulinemia: an evolving concept. Adv Anat Pathol 12: 246–255
438. Andrieux J, Fert-Ferrer S, Copin M C et al. 2003 Three new cases of non-Hodgkin's lymphoma with t(9; 14)(p13; q32). Cancer Genet Cytogenet 145: 65–69
439. Mansoor A, Medeiros L J, Weber D M et al. 2001 Cytogenetic findings in lymphoplasmacytic lymphoma/Waldenström macroglobulinemia. Chromosomal abnormalities are associated with the polymorphous subtype and an aggressive clinical course. Am J Clin Pathol 116: 543–549
440. Mitsiades C S, Mitsiades N, Treon S P et al. 2003 Proteomic analyses in Waldenström's macroglobulinemia and other plasma cell dyscrasias. Semin Oncol 30: 156–160
441. Banks P M, Chan J, Cleary M L et al. 1992 Mantle cell lymphoma. A proposal for unification of morphologic, immunologic, and molecular data. Am J Surg Pathol 16: 637–640
442. Campo E, Raffeld M, Jaffe E S 1999 Mantle-cell lymphoma. Semin Hematol 36: 115–127
443. Argatoff L H, Connors J M, Klasa R J et al. 1997 Mantle cell lymphoma: a clinicopathologic study of 80 cases. Blood 89: 2067–2078
444. Oinonen R, Franssila K, Teerenhovi L et al. 1998 Mantle cell lymphoma: clinical features, treatment and prognosis of 94 patients. Eur J Cancer 34: 329–336
445. Pittaluga S, Wlodarska I, Stul M S et al. 1995 Mantle cell lymphoma: a clinicopathological study of 55 cases. Histopathology 26: 17–24
446. Samaha H, Dumontet C, Ketterer N et al. 1998 Mantle cell lymphoma: a retrospective study of 121 cases. Leukemia 12: 1281–1287
447. Zucca E, Roggero E, Pinotti G et al. 1995 Patterns of survival in mantle cell lymphoma. Ann Oncol 6: 257–262
448. Bertini M, Rus C, Freilone R et al. 1998 Mantle cell lymphoma: a retrospective study on 27 patients. Clinical features and natural history. Haematologica 83: 312–316
449. Bosch F, Lopez-Guillermo A, Campo E et al. 1998 Mantle cell lymphoma: presenting features, response to therapy, and prognostic factors. Cancer 82: 567–575
450. Meusers P, Hense J, Brittinger G 1997 Mantle cell lymphoma: diagnostic criteria, clinical aspects and therapeutic problems. Leukemia 11 Suppl 2: S60–64
451. Norton A J, Matthews J, Pappa V et al. 1995 Mantle cell lymphoma: natural history defined in a serially biopsied population over a 20-year period. Ann Oncol 6: 249–256
452. Howard O M, Gribben J G, Neuberg D S et al. 2002 Rituximab and CHOP induction therapy for newly diagnosed mantle-cell lymphoma: molecular complete responses are not predictive of progression-free survival. J Clin Oncol 20: 1288–1294
453. Lenz G, Dreyling M, Hoster E et al. 2005 Immunochemotherapy with rituximab and cyclophosphamide, doxorubicin, vincristine, and prednisone significantly improves response and time to treatment failure, but not long-term outcome in patients with previously untreated mantle cell lymphoma: results of a prospective randomized trial of the German Low Grade Lymphoma Study Group (GLSG). J Clin Oncol 23: 1984–1992
454. Forstpointner R, Dreyling M, Repp R et al. 2004 The addition of rituximab to a combination of fludarabine, cyclophosphamide, mitoxantrone (FCM) significantly increases the response rate and prolongs survival as compared with FCM alone in patients with relapsed and refractory follicular and mantle cell lymphomas: results of a prospective randomized study of the German Low-grade Lymphoma Study Group. Blood 104: 3064–3071
455. Marzec M, Kasprzycka M, Lai R et al. 2006 Mantle cell lymphoma cells express predominantly cyclin D1a isoform and are highly sensitive to selective inhibition of CDK4 kinase activity. Blood 108: 1744–1750
456. Vandenberghe E, De Wolf-Peeters C, Vaughan Hudson G et al. 1997 The clinical outcome of 65 cases of mantle cell lymphoma initially treated with non-intensive therapy by the British National Lymphoma Investigation Group. Br J Haematol 99: 842–847
457. Espinet B, Sole F, Pedro C et al. 2005 Clonal proliferation of cyclin D1-positive mantle lymphocytes in an asymptomatic patient: an early-stage event in the development or an indolent form of a mantle cell lymphoma? Hum Pathol 36: 1232–1237
458. Rosenwald A, Wright G, Wiestner A et al. 2003 The proliferation gene expression signature is a quantitative integrator of oncogenic events that predicts survival in mantle cell lymphoma. Cancer Cell 3: 185–197
459. Kurtin P J 1998 Mantle cell lymphoma. Adv Anat Pathol 5: 376–398
460. Swerdlow S H, Zukerberg L R, Yang W I et al. 1996 The morphologic spectrum of non-Hodgkin's lymphomas with BCL1/cyclin D1 gene rearrangements. Am J Surg Pathol 20: 627–640
461. Young K H, Chan W C, Fu K et al. 2006 Mantle cell lymphoma with plasma cell differentiation. Am J Surg Pathol 30: 954–961
462. Lardelli P, Bookman M A, Sundeen J et al. 1990 Lymphocytic lymphoma of intermediate differentiation. Morphologic and immunophenotypic spectrum and clinical correlations. Am J Surg Pathol 14: 752–763
463. Zucca E, Stein H, Coiffier B 1994 European Lymphoma Task Force (ELTF): Report of the Workshop on Mantle Cell Lymphoma (MCL). Ann Oncol 5: 507–511
464. Soslow R A, Zukerberg L R, Harris N L et al. 1997 BCL-1 (PRAD-1/cyclin D-1) overexpression distinguishes the blastoid variant of mantle cell lymphoma from B-lineage lymphoblastic lymphoma. Mod Pathol 10: 810–817
465. Chan J K, Miller K D, Munson P et al. 1999 Immunostaining for cyclin D1 and the diagnosis of mantle cell lymphoma: is there a reliable method? Histopathology 34: 266–270
466. Yang W I, Zukerberg L R, Motokura T et al. 1994 Cyclin D1 (BCL-1, PRAD1) protein expression in low-grade B-cell lymphomas and reactive hyperplasia. Am J Pathol 145: 86–96
467. Swerdlow S H, Yang W I, Zukerberg L R et al. 1995 Expression of cyclin D1 protein in centrocytic/mantle cell lymphomas with and without rearrangement of the BCL1/cyclin D1 gene. Hum Pathol 26: 999–1004
468. de Boer C J, Schuuring E, Dreef E et al. 1995 Cyclin D1 protein analysis in the diagnosis of mantle cell lymphoma. Blood 86: 2715–2723
469. Liu Z, Dong H Y, Gorczyca W et al. 2002 CD5– mantle cell lymphoma. Am J Clin Pathol 118: 216–224

470. Fu K, Weisenburger D D, Greiner T C et al. 2005 Cyclin D1-negative mantle cell lymphoma: a clinicopathologic study based on gene expression profiling. Blood 106: 4315–4321
471. Schrader C, Meusers P, Brittinger G et al. 2006 Growth pattern and distribution of follicular dendritic cells in mantle cell lymphoma: a clinicopathological study of 96 patients. Virchows Arch 448: 151–159
472. Hoffman D G, Tucker SJ, Emmanoulides C et al. 1998 CD8-positive mantle cell lymphoma: a report of two cases. Am J Clin Pathol 109: 689–694
473. Du M Q, Diss T C, Xu C F et al. 1997 Ongoing immunoglobulin gene mutations in mantle cell lymphomas. Br J Haematol 96: 124–131
474. Pittaluga S, Tierens A, Pinyol M et al. 1998 Blastic variant of mantle cell lymphoma shows a heterogenous pattern of somatic mutations of the rearranged immunoglobulin heavy chain variable genes. Br J Haematol 102: 1301–1306
475. Kienle D, Krober A, Katzenberger T et al. 2003 VH mutation status and VDJ rearrangement structure in mantle cell lymphoma: correlation with genomic aberrations, clinical characteristics, and outcome. Blood 102: 3003–3009
476. Walsh S H, Thorselius M, Johnson A et al. 2003 Mutated VH genes and preferential VH3-21 use define new subsets of mantle cell lymphoma. Blood 101: 4047–4054
477. Bertoni F, Rinaldi A, Zucca E et al. 2006 Update on the molecular biology of mantle cell lymphoma. Hematol Oncol 24: 22–27
478. Walsh S H, Rosenquist R 2005 Immunoglobulin gene analysis of mature B-cell malignancies: reconsideration of cellular origin and potential antigen involvement in pathogenesis. Med Oncol 22: 327–341
479. Bertoni F, Conconi A, Cogliatti S B et al. 2004 Immunoglobulin heavy chain genes somatic hypermutations and chromosome 11q22-23 deletion in classic mantle cell lymphoma: a study of the Swiss Group for Clinical Cancer Research. Br J Haematol 124: 289–298
480. Medeiros L J, Van Krieken J H, Jaffe E S et al. 1990 Association of BCL-1 rearrangements with lymphocytic lymphoma of intermediate differentiation. Blood 76: 2086–2090
481. De Wolf-Peeters C, Pittaluga S 1994 Mantle-cell lymphoma. Ann Oncol 5: 35–37
482. Swerdlow S H, Williams M E 1993 Centrocytic lymphoma: a distinct clinicopathologic, immunophenotypic, and genotypic entity. Pathol Annu 28: 171–197
483. Chibbar R, Leung K, McCormick S et al. 1998 BCL-1 gene rearrangements in mantle cell lymphoma: a comprehensive analysis of 118 cases, including B-5-fixed tissue, by polymerase chain reaction and Southern transfer analysis. Mod Pathol 11: 1089–1097
484. Luthra R, Hai S, Pugh W C 1995 Polymerase chain reaction detection of the t(11; 14) translocation involving the BCL-1 major translocation cluster in mantle cell lymphoma. Diagn Mol Pathol 4: 4–7
485. Rimokh R, Berger F, Delsol G et al. 1994 Detection of the chromosomal translocation t(11; 14) by polymerase chain reaction in mantle cell lymphomas. Blood 83: 1871–1875
486. Vaandrager J W, Schuuring E, Zwikstra E et al. 1996 Direct visualization of dispersed 11q13 chromosomal translocations in mantle cell lymphoma by multicolor DNA fiber fluorescence in situ hybridization. Blood 88: 1177–1182
487. Bigoni R, Negrini M, Veronese M L et al. 1996 Characterization of t(11; 14) translocation in mantle cell lymphoma by fluorescent in situ hybridization. Oncogene 13: 797–802
488. Bosch F, Jares P, Campo E et al. 1994 PRAD-1/cyclin D1 gene overexpression in chronic lymphoproliferative disorders: a highly specific marker of mantle cell lymphoma. Blood 84: 2726–2732
489. Cuneo A, Bigoni R, Rigolin G M et al. 1999 Cytogenetic profile of lymphoma of follicle mantle lineage: correlation with clinicobiologic features. Blood 93: 1372–1380
490. Wlodarska I, Pittaluga S, Hagemeijer A et al. 1999 Secondary chromosome changes in mantle cell lymphoma. Haematologica 84: 594–599
491. Bentz M, Plesch A, Bullinger L et al. 2000 t(11; 14)-positive mantle cell lymphomas exhibit complex karyotypes and share similarities with B-cell chronic lymphocytic leukemia. Genes Chromos Cancer 27: 285–294
492. Cuneo A, Bigoni R, Rigolin G M et al. 1999 13q14 deletion in non-Hodgkin's lymphoma: correlation with clinicopathologic features. Haematologica 84: 589–593
493. Kohlhammer H, Schwaenen C, Wessendorf S et al. 2004 Genomic DNA-chip hybridization in t(11; 14)-positive mantle cell lymphomas shows a high frequency of aberrations and allows a refined characterization of consensus regions. Blood 104: 795–801
494. Tagawa H, Karnan S, Suzuki R et al. 2005 Genome-wide array-based CGH for mantle cell lymphoma: identification of homozygous deletions of the proapoptotic gene BIM. Oncogene 24: 1348–1358
495. Stilgenbauer S, Winkler D, Ott G et al. 1999 Molecular characterization of 11q deletions points to a pathogenic role of the ATM gene in mantle cell lymphoma. Blood 94: 3262–3264
496. Greiner T C, Dasgupta C, Ho V V et al. 2006 Mutation and genomic deletion status of ataxia telangiectasia mutated (ATM) and p53 confer specific gene expression profiles in mantle cell lymphoma. Proc Natl Acad Sci USA 103: 2352–2357
497. Hernandez L, Fest T, Cazorla M et al. 1996 p53 gene mutations and protein overexpression are associated with aggressive variants of mantle cell lymphomas. Blood 87: 3351–3359
498. Greiner T C, Moynihan M J, Chan W C et al. 1996 p53 mutations in mantle cell lymphoma are associated with variant cytology and predict a poor prognosis. Blood 87: 4302–4310
499. Pinyol M, Hernandez L, Cazorla M et al. 1997 Deletions and loss of expression of p16INK4a and p21Waf1 genes are associated with aggressive variants of mantle cell lymphomas. Blood 89: 272–280
500. Ott G, Kalla J, Ott M M et al. 1997 Blastoid variants of mantle cell lymphoma: frequent BCL-1 rearrangements at the major translocation cluster region and tetraploid chromosome clones. Blood 89: 1421–1429
501. Parrens M, Belaud-Rotureau M A, Fitoussi O et al. 2006 Blastoid and common variants of mantle cell lymphoma exhibit distinct immunophenotypic and interphase FISH features. Histopathology 48: 353–362
502. Rudelius M, Pittaluga S, Nishizuka S et al. 2006 Constitutive activation of Akt contributes to the pathogenesis and survival of mantle cell lymphoma. Blood 108: 1668–1676
503. Thieblemont C, Nasser V, Felman P et al. 2004 Small lymphocytic lymphoma, marginal zone B-cell lymphoma, and mantle cell lymphoma exhibit distinct gene-expression profiles allowing molecular diagnosis. Blood 103: 2727–2737
504. Martinez N, Camacho F I, Algara P et al. 2003 The molecular signature of mantle cell lymphoma reveals multiple signals favoring cell survival. Cancer Res 63: 8226–8232
505. de Vos S, Krug U, Hofmann W K et al. 2003 Cell cycle alterations in the blastoid variant of mantle cell lymphoma (MCL-BV) as detected by gene expression profiling of mantle cell lymphoma (MCL) and MCL-BV. Diagn Mol Pathol 12: 35–43
506. Hui D, Reiman T, Hanson J et al. 2005 Immunohistochemical detection of cdc2 is useful in predicting survival in patients with mantle cell lymphoma. Mod Pathol 18: 1223–1231
507. Moller M B, Pedersen N T, Christensen B E 2006 Mantle cell lymphoma: prognostic capacity of the Follicular Lymphoma International Prognostic Index. Br J Haematol 133: 43–49
508. Wong K F, Chan J K, So JC et al. 1999 Mantle cell lymphoma in leukemic phase: characterization of its broad cytologic spectrum with emphasis on the importance of distinction from other chronic lymphoproliferative disorders. Cancer 86: 850–857
509. Thelander E F, Walsh S H, Thorselius M et al. 2005 Mantle cell lymphomas with clonal immunoglobulin V(H)3-21 gene rearrangements exhibit fewer genomic imbalances than mantle cell lymphomas utilizing other immunoglobulin V(H) genes. Mod Pathol 18: 331–339
510. Anagnostopoulos I, Foss H D, Hummel M et al. 2001 Extranodal mantle cell lymphoma mimicking marginal zone cell lymphoma. Histopathology 39: 561–565
511. Jacobson E, Burke P, Tindle B H 2005 Mantle cell lymphoma disguised as marginal zone lymphoma. Arch Pathol Lab Med 129: 929–932
512. Weisenburger D D, Duggan D J, Perry D A 1991 Non-Hodgkin's lymphomas of mantle zone origin. Pathol Annu 26: 139–158
513. Ng C S, Chan J K, Lo S T et al. 1986 Immunophenotypic analysis of non-Hodgkin's lymphomas in Chinese. A study of 75 cases in Hong Kong. Pathology 18: 419–425
514. Stein R S, Cousar J, Flexner J M et al. 1979 Malignant lymphomas of follicular center cell origin in man. III. Prognostic features. Cancer 44: 2236–2243
515. Smith B R, Weinberg D S, Robert N J et al. 1984 Circulating monoclonal B lymphocytes in non-Hodgkin's lymphoma. N Engl J Med 311: 1476–1481
516. Berliner N, Ault K A, Martin P et al. 1986 Detection of clonal excess in lymphoproliferative disease by kappa/lambda analysis: correlation with immunoglobulin gene DNA rearrangement. Blood 67: 80–85
517. Stetler-Stevenson M, Raffeld M, Cohen P et al. 1988 Detection of occult follicular lymphoma by specific DNA amplification. Blood 72: 1822–1825
518. Lambrechts A C, Hupkes P E, Dorssers L C et al. 1994 Clinical significance of t(14; 18)-positive cells in the circulation of patients with stage III or IV follicular non-Hodgkin's lymphoma during first remission. J Clin Oncol 12: 1541–1546
519. Gallagher C J, Lister T A 1987 Follicular non-Hodgkin's lymphoma. Baillières Clin Haematol 1: 141–155
520. de Jong D 2005 Molecular pathogenesis of follicular lymphoma: a cross talk of genetic and immunologic factors. J Clin Oncol 23: 6358–6363
521. Rohatiner A, Lister T A 1997 Follicular lymphoma. In: Magrath I (ed) The non-Hodgkin's lymphomas, 2nd edn. Arnold, London, 867–895
522. Horning S J, Rosenberg S A 1984 The natural history of initially untreated low-grade non-Hodgkin's lymphomas. N Engl J Med 311: 1471–1475
523. Garcia C F, Weiss L M, Warnke R A et al. 1986 Cutaneous follicular lymphoma. Am J Surg Pathol 10: 454–463
523a. Goodlad J R, Krajewski A S, Batstone P J et al 2002 Primary cutaneous follicular lymphoma: a clinicopathologic and molecular study of 16 cases in support of a distinct entity. Am J Surg Pathol 26: 733–741
524. Cerroni L, Volkenandt M, Rieger E et al. 1994 BCL-2 protein expression and correlation with the interchromosomal 14; 18 translocation in cutaneous lymphomas and pseudolymphomas. J Invest Dermatol 102: 231–235
525. Goodlad J R, Batstone P J, Hamilton D A et al. 2006 BCL2 gene abnormalities define distinct clinical subsets of follicular lymphoma. Histopathology 49: 229–241

525a. Goodlad J R, MacPherson S, Jackson R et al 2004 Extranodal follicular lymphoma: a clinicopathological and genetic analysis of 15 cases arising at non-cutaneous extranodal sites. Histopathology 44: 268–276
526. Pinto A, Hutchison R E, Grant L H et al. 1990 Follicular lymphomas in pediatric patients. Mod Pathol 3: 308–313
527. Winberg C D, Nathwani B N, Bearman R M et al. 1981 Follicular (nodular) lymphoma during the first two decades of life: a clinicopathologic study of 12 patients. Cancer 48: 2223–2235
528. Frizzera G, Murphy S B 1979 Follicular (nodular) lymphoma in childhood: a rare clinical–pathological entity. Report of eight cases from four cancer centers. Cancer 44: 2218–2235
529. Lorsbach R B, Shay-Seymore D, Moore J et al. 2002 Clinicopathologic analysis of follicular lymphoma occurring in children. Blood 99: 1959–1964
530. Nathwani B N, Winberg C D, Diamond L W et al. 1981 Morphologic criteria for the differentiation of follicular lymphoma from florid reactive follicular hyperplasia: a study of 80 cases. Cancer 48: 1794–1806
531. Adam P, Katzenberger T, Eifert M et al. 2005 Presence of preserved reactive germinal centers in follicular lymphoma is a strong histopathologic indicator of limited disease stage. Am J Surg Pathol 29: 1661–1664
532. Dogan A, Du M Q, Aiello A et al. 1998 Follicular lymphomas contain a clonally linked but phenotypically distinct neoplastic B-cell population in the interfollicular zone. Blood 91: 4708–4714
533. Waldron J A, Newcomer L N, Katz M E 1983 Sclerosing variants of follicular center cell lymphomas presenting in the retroperitoneum. Cancer 52: 712–720
534. Kluin P M, van Krieken J H, Kleiverda K et al. 1990 Discordant morphologic characteristics of B-cell lymphomas in bone marrow and lymph node biopsies. Am J Clin Pathol 94: 59–66
535. Bognar A, Csernus B, Bodor C et al. 2005 Clonal selection in the bone marrow involvement of follicular lymphoma. Leukemia 19: 1656–1662
536. Rodriguez J, McLaughlin P, Hagemeister F B et al. 1999 Follicular large cell lymphoma: an aggressive lymphoma that often presents with favorable prognostic features. Blood 93: 2202–2207
537. Horning S J, Weiss L M, Nevitt J B et al. 1987 Clinical and pathologic features of follicular large cell (nodular histiocytic) lymphoma. Cancer 59: 1470–1474
538. Armitage J O 1999 Clinical aspects of follicular lymphoma and the relevance of grading. In: Mason D Y, Harris N L (eds) Human lymphoma: clinical implications of the REAL classification. Springer, London, 13.11–13.14
539. Mann R B, Berard C W 1983 Criteria for the cytologic subclassification of follicular lymphomas: a proposed alternative method. Hematol Oncol 1: 187–192
540. Metter G E, Nathwani B N, Burke J S et al. 1985 Morphological subclassification of follicular lymphoma: variability of diagnoses among hematopathologists, a collaborative study between the Repository Center and Pathology Panel for Lymphoma Clinical Studies. J Clin Oncol 3: 25–38
541. Nathwani B N, Metter G E, Miller T P et al. 1986 What should be the morphologic criteria for the subdivision of follicular lymphomas? Blood 68: 837–845
542. Weisenburger D D, Chan W C 1993 Lymphomas of follicles. Mantle cell and follicle center cell lymphomas. Am J Clin Pathol 99: 409–420
543. Ott G, Katzenberger T, Lohr A et al. 2002 Cytomorphologic, immunohistochemical, and cytogenetic profiles of follicular lymphoma: 2 types of follicular lymphoma grade 3. Blood 99: 3806–3812
544. Bosga-Bouwer A G, van Imhoff G W, Boonstra R et al. 2003 Follicular lymphoma grade 3B includes 3 cytogenetically defined subgroups with primary t(14; 18), 3q27, or other translocations: t(14; 18) and 3q27 are mutually exclusive. Blood 101: 1149–1154
545. Bosga-Bouwer A G, van den Berg A, Haralambieva E et al. 2006 Molecular, cytogenetic, and immunophenotypic characterization of follicular lymphoma grade 3B; a separate entity or part of the spectrum of diffuse large B-cell lymphoma or follicular lymphoma? Hum Pathol 37: 528–533
546. Katzenberger T, Ott G, Klein T et al. 2004 Cytogenetic alterations affecting BCL6 are predominantly found in follicular lymphomas grade 3B with a diffuse large B-cell component. Am J Pathol 165: 481–490
547. Hsi E D, Mirza I, Lozanski G et al. 2004 A clinicopathologic evaluation of follicular lymphoma grade 3A versus grade 3B reveals no survival differences. Arch Pathol Lab Med 128: 863–868
548. Yegappan S, Schnitzer B, Hsi E D 2001 Follicular lymphoma with marginal zone differentiation: microdissection demonstrates the t(14; 18) in both the follicular and marginal zone components. Mod Pathol 14: 191–196
549. Nathwani B N, Anderson J R, Armitage J O et al. 1999 Clinical significance of follicular lymphoma with monocytoid B cells. Non-Hodgkin's Lymphoma Classification Project. Hum Pathol 30: 263–268
550. Cossman J 1999 A new, lethal form of follicular lymphoma? [editorial]. Hum Pathol 30: 249–250
551. Goodlad J R, Batstone P J, Hamilton D et al. 2003 Follicular lymphoma with marginal zone differentiation: cytogenetic findings in support of a high-risk variant of follicular lymphoma. Histopathology 42: 292–298
552. Avivi I, Bacon C M, Obsermann E C et al. 2002 Histological and clinical prognostic factors in follicular lymphoma: proposal for a prognostic model. [Abstract] Blood 100: Abstract 131
553. Kim H, Dorfman R F, Rappaport H 1978 Signet ring cell lymphoma. A rare morphologic and functional expression of nodular (follicular) lymphoma. Am J Surg Pathol 2: 119–132
554. Rosas-Uribe A, Variakojis D, Rappaport H 1973 Proteinaceous precipitate in nodular (follicular) lymphoma. Cancer 31: 532–542
555. Chittal S M, Caveriviere P, Voigt J A et al. 1987 Follicular lymphoma with abundant PAS-positive extracellular material. Immunohistochemical and ultrastructural observations. Am J Surg Pathol 11: 618–624
556. Frizzera G, Gajl-Peczalska K, Sibley R K et al. 1985 Rosette formation in malignant lymphoma. Am J Pathol 119: 351–356
557. Osborne B M, Butler J J 1987 Follicular lymphoma mimicking progressive transformation of germinal centers. Am J Clin Pathol 88: 264–269
558. Goates J J, Kamel O W, LeBrun D P et al. 1994 Floral variant of follicular lymphoma. Immunological and molecular studies support a neoplastic process. Am J Surg Pathol 18: 37–47
559. Chan J K, Ng C S, Hui P K 1988 An unusual morphological variant of follicular lymphoma. Report of two cases. Histopathology 12: 649–658
560. Nathwani B N, Sheibani K, Winberg C D et al. 1985 Neoplastic B cells with cerebriform nuclei in follicular lymphomas. Hum Pathol 16: 173–180
561. Chan J K, Ng C S, Hui P K 1990 Follicular immunoblastic lymphoma: neoplastic counterpart of the intrafollicular immunoblast? Pathology 22: 103–105
562. Brown R W, Pugh W C, Butler J J 1991 Follicular lymphoma of immunoblastic/plasmablastic type. [Abstract] Mod Pathol 4: 68A
563. Frizzera G, Anaya J S, Banks P M 1986 Neoplastic plasma cells in follicular lymphomas. Clinical and pathologic findings in six cases. Virchows Arch A Pathol Anat Histopathol 409: 149–162
564. Keith T A, Cousar J B, Glick A D 1985 Plasmacytic differentiation in follicular center cell lymphomas. Am J Clin Pathol 84: 283–290
565. Schmid U, Karow J, Lennert K 1985 Follicular malignant non-Hodgkin's lymphoma with pronounced plasmacytic differentiation: a plasmacytoma-like lymphoma. Virchows Arch A Pathol Anat Histopathol 405: 473–481
566. Cong P, Raffeld M, Teruya-Feldstein J et al. 2002 In situ localization of follicular lymphoma: description and analysis by laser capture microdissection. Blood 99: 3376–3382
567. Torlakovic E, Torlakovic G 2002 Follicular colonization by follicular lymphoma. Arch Pathol Lab Med 126: 1136–1137
568. Su W, Spencer J, Wotherspoon A C 2001 Relative distribution of tumour cells and reactive cells in follicular lymphoma. J Pathol 193: 498–504
569. Ngan B, Warnke A, Cleary M L 1989 Variability of immunoglobulin expression in follicular lymphoma. An immunohistologic and molecular genetic study. Am J Pathol 135: 1139–1144
570. Garcia C F, Warnke R A, Weiss L M 1986 Follicular large cell lymphoma. An immunophenotype study. Am J Pathol 123: 425–431
571. Warnke R A, Levy R 1978 Immunopathology of follicular lymphomas, a model of B-lymphocyte homing. N Engl J Med 298: 481–486
572. Hollema H, Poppema S 1988 Immunophenotypes of malignant lymphoma centroblastic–centrocytic and malignant lymphoma centrocytic: an immunohistologic study indicating a derivation from different stages of B cell differentiation. Hum Pathol 19: 1053–1059
573. Gaulard P, d'Agay M F, Peuchmaur M et al. 1992 Expression of the BCL-2 gene product in follicular lymphoma. Am J Pathol 140: 1089–1095
574. Pezzella F, Tse A G, Cordell J L et al. 1990 Expression of the BCL-2 oncogene protein is not specific for the 14;18 chromosomal translocation. Am J Pathol 137: 225–232
575. Pezzella F, Mason D Y 1990 The BCL-2 gene and 14;18 translocation in lymphoproliferative disorders. Nouv Rev Fr Hematol 32: 397–399
576. Utz G L, Swerdlow S H 1993 Distinction of follicular hyperplasia from follicular lymphoma in B5-fixed tissues: comparison of MT2 and BCL-2 antibodies. Hum Pathol 24: 1155–1158
577. Schraders M, de Jong D, Kluin P et al. 2005 Lack of BCL-2 expression in follicular lymphoma may be caused by mutations in the BCL2 gene or by absence of the t(14; 18) translocation. J Pathol 205: 329–335
578. Tiesinga J J, Wu C D, Inghirami G 2000 CD5+ follicle center lymphoma. Immunophenotyping detects a unique subset of 'floral' follicular lymphoma. Am J Clin Pathol 114: 912–921
579. Barry T S, Jaffe E S, Kingma D W et al. 2002 CD5+ follicular lymphoma: a clinicopathologic study of three cases. Am J Clin Pathol 118: 589–598
580. Manazza A D, Bonello L, Pagano M et al. 2005 Follicular origin of a subset of CD5+ diffuse large B-cell lymphomas. Am J Clin Pathol 124: 182–190
581. Stein H, Mason D Y 1985 Immunological analysis of tissue sections in diagnosis of lymphoma. Recent Adv Hematol 4: 127–169
582. Swerdlow S H, Murray L J, Habeshaw J A et al. 1985 B- and T-cell subsets in follicular centroblastic/centrocytic (cleaved follicular center cell) lymphoma: an immunohistologic analysis of 26 lymph nodes and three spleens. Hum Pathol 16: 339–352
583. Ashton-Key M, Diss T C, Isaacson P G, Smith M E 1995 A comparative study of the value of immunohistochemistry and the polymerase chain reaction in the diagnosis of follicular lymphoma. Histopathology 27: 501–508
584. Harris N L, Data R E 1982 The distribution of neoplastic and normal B-lymphoid cells in nodular lymphomas: use of an immunoperoxidase technique on frozen sections. Hum Pathol 13: 610–617

585. Harris N L, Nadler L M, Bhan A K 1984 Immunohistologic characterization of two malignant lymphomas of germinal center type (centroblastic/centrocytic and centrocytic) with monoclonal antibodies. Follicular and diffuse lymphomas of small cleaved-cell type are related but distinct entities. Am J Pathol 117: 262–272
586. Harris N L, Bhan A K 1983 Distribution of T-cell subsets in follicular and diffuse lymphomas of B-cell type. Am J Pathol 113: 172–180
587. Swerdlow S H, Murray L J 1984 Natural killer (Leu 7+) cells in reactive lymphoid tissues and malignant lymphomas. Am J Clin Pathol 81: 459–463
588. Amakawa R, Fukuhara S, Ohno H et al. 1989 Involvement of BCL-2 gene in Japanese follicular lymphoma. Blood 73: 787–791
589. Liang R, Chan V, Chan T K et al. 1990 Rearrangement of immunoglobulin, T-cell receptor, and BCL-2 genes in malignant lymphomas in Hong Kong. Cancer 66: 1743–1747
590. Au W Y, Fung A, Liang R 2005 Molecular epidemiology of follicular lymphoma in Chinese: relationship with BCL-2/IgH translocation and BCL-6 397G/C polymorphism. Ann Hematol 84: 506–509
591. Chuang S S, Hsieh P P, Lu C L et al. 2006 A clinicopathologic and molecular study of follicular lymphoma in Taiwan. Clin Lymphoma Myeloma 6: 314–318
592. Peh S C, Shaminie J, Tai Y C et al. 2004 The pattern and frequency of t(14; 18) translocation and immunophenotype in Asian follicular lymphoma. Histopathology 45: 501–510
593. Korsmeyer S J 1992 BCL-2 initiates a new category of oncogenes: regulators of cell death. Blood 80: 879–886
594. Hirose Y, Masaki Y, Ozaki M 2003 Fluorescence in situ hybridization detection of chromosome IGH/BCL2 translocations from paraffin-embedded tissue: evaluation in follicular lymphoma. Int J Hematol 78: 154–159
595. Aisenberg A C, Wilkes B M, Jacobson J O 1988 The BCL-2 gene is rearranged in many diffuse B-cell lymphomas. Blood 71: 969–972
596. Offit K, Koduru P R, Hollis R et al. 1989 18q21 rearrangement in diffuse large cell lymphoma: incidence and clinical significance. Br J Haematol 72: 178–183
597. Lo Coco F, Ye B H, Lista F et al. 1994 Rearrangements of the BCL6 gene in diffuse large cell non-Hodgkin's lymphoma. Blood 83: 1757–1759
598. Bastard C, Deweindt C, Kerckaert J P et al. 1994 LAZ3 rearrangements in non-Hodgkin's lymphoma: correlation with histology, immunophenotype, karyotype, and clinical outcome in 217 patients. Blood 83: 2423–2427
599. Akasaka T, Lossos I S, Levy R 2003 BCL6 gene translocation in follicular lymphoma: a harbinger of eventual transformation to diffuse aggressive lymphoma. Blood 102: 1443–1448
600. Migliazza A, Martinotti S, Chen W et al. 1995 Frequent somatic hypermutation of the 5′ noncoding region of the BCL6 gene in B-cell lymphoma. Proc Natl Acad Sci USA 92: 12520–12524
601. Peng H Z, Du M Q, Koulis A et al. 1999 Nonimmunoglobulin gene hypermutation in germinal center B cells. Blood 93: 2167–2172
602. Pasqualucci L, Migliazza A, Fracchiolla N et al. 1998 BCL-6 mutations in normal germinal center B cells: evidence of somatic hypermutation acting outside Ig loci. Proc Natl Acad Sci USA 95: 11816–11821
603. Husson H, Carideo E G, Neuberg D et al. 2002 Gene expression profiling of follicular lymphoma and normal germinal center B cells using cDNA arrays. Blood 99: 282–289
604. Luminari S, Federico M 2006 Prognosis of follicular lymphomas. Hematol Oncol 24: 64–72
605. Solal-Celigny P, Roy P, Colombat P et al. 2004 Follicular lymphoma international prognostic index. Blood 104: 1258–1265
606. Buske C, Hoster E, Dreyling M et al. 2006 The Follicular Lymphoma International Prognostic Index (FLIPI) separates high risk from intermediate or low risk patients with advanced stage follicular lymphoma treated front-line with rituximab and the combination of cyclophosphamide, doxorubicin, vincristine and prednisone (R–CHOP) with respect to treatment outcome. Blood 108: 1504–1508
607. Federico M, Vitolo U, Zinzani P L et al. 2000 Prognosis of follicular lymphoma: a predictive model based on a retrospective analysis of 987 cases. Intergruppo Italiano Linfomi. Blood 95: 783–789
608. Romaguera J E, McLaughlin P, North L et al. 1991 Multivariate analysis of prognostic factors in stage IV follicular low-grade lymphoma: a risk model. J Clin Oncol 9: 762–769
609. Wang S A, Wang L, Hochberg E P et al. 2005 Low histologic grade follicular lymphoma with high proliferation index: morphologic and clinical features. Am J Surg Pathol 29: 1490–1496
610. Farinha P, Masoudi H, Skinnider B F et al. 2005 Analysis of multiple biomarkers shows that lymphoma-associated macrophage (LAM) content is an independent predictor of survival in follicular lymphoma (FL). Blood 106: 2169–2174
611. Carreras J, Lopez-Guillermo A, Fox B C et al. 2006 High numbers of tumor infiltrating FOXP3-positive regulatory T-cells are associated with improved overall survival in follicular lymphoma. Blood 108:2957–2964
612. Viardot A, Barth T F, Moller P et al. 2003 Cytogenetic evolution of follicular lymphoma. Semin Cancer Biol 13: 183–190
613. Tilly H, Rossi A, Stamatoullas A et al. 1994 Prognostic value of chromosomal abnormalities in follicular lymphoma. Blood 84: 1043–1049
614. Hoglund M, Sehn L, Connors J M et al. 2004 Identification of cytogenetic subgroups and karyotypic pathways of clonal evolution in follicular lymphomas. Genes Chromos Cancer 39: 195–204
615. Glas A M, Kersten M J, Delahaye L J et al. 2005 Gene expression profiling in follicular lymphoma to assess clinical aggressiveness and to guide the choice of treatment. Blood 105: 301–307
616. Dave S S, Wright G, Tan B et al. 2004 Prediction of survival in follicular lymphoma based on molecular features of tumor-infiltrating immune cells. N Engl J Med 351: 2159–2169
617. Goffinet D R, Warnke R, Dunnick N R et al. 1977 Clinical and surgical (laparotomy) evaluation of patients with non-Hodgkin's lymphomas. Cancer Treat Rep 61: 981–992
618. Fisher R I, Jones R B, DeVita V T Jr et al. 1981 Natural history of malignant lymphomas with divergent histologies at staging evaluation. Cancer 47: 2022–2025
619. Marazuela M, Yebra M, Giron J A et al. 1991 Late relapse with nodular lymphoma after treatment for diffuse non-Hodgkin's lymphoma. Cancer 67: 1950–1953
620. Head D R, Avakian J, Kjeldsberg C R et al. 1988 Relapse of intermediate or high-grade (unfavorable) non-Hodgkin's lymphoma as a low-grade (favorable) non-Hodgkin's lymphoma. Report of four cases. Am J Clin Pathol 89: 106–108
621. Hubbard S M, Chabner B A, DeVita V T Jr et al. 1982 Histologic progression in non-Hodgkin's lymphoma. Blood 59: 258–264
622. Acker B, Hoppe R T, Colby T V et al. 1983 Histologic conversion in the non-Hodgkin's lymphomas. J Clin Oncol 1: 11–16
623. Horning S J 1999 Transformed follicular lymphoma. In: Mason D Y, Harris N L (eds) Human lymphoma: clinical implications of the REAL classification. Springer, London, 15.11–15.14
624. Yuen A R, Kamel O W, Halpern J et al. 1995 Long-term survival after histologic transformation of low-grade follicular lymphoma. J Clin Oncol 13: 1726–1733
625. Longo D L, Wilson W 1990 Follicular lymphomas. In: Magrath I T (ed) The non-Hodgkin's lymphomas. Williams & Wilkins, Baltimore, 293–308
626. Rohatiner A, Lister T A 1998 Follicular lymphoma. In: Canellos G P, Lister T A, Sklar J L (eds) The lymphomas. WB Saunders, Philadelphia, 371–387
627. Alsabeh R, Medeiros L J, Glackin C et al. 1997 Transformation of follicular lymphoma into CD30– large cell lymphoma with anaplastic cytologic features. Am J Surg Pathol 21: 528–536
628. Chang K L 1994 p53 invades pathology. Adv Anat Pathol 1: 38–43
629. Lo Coco F, Gaidano G, Louie D C et al. 1993 p53 mutations are associated with histologic transformation of follicular lymphoma. Blood 82: 2289–2295
630. Sander C A, Yano T, Clark H M et al. 1993 p53 mutation is associated with progression in follicular lymphomas. Blood 82: 1994–2004
631. Matolcsy A, Casali P, Warnke R A et al. 1996 Morphologic transformation of follicular lymphoma is associated with somatic mutation of the translocated BCL-2 gene. Blood 88: 3937–3944
632. Clark H M, Yano T, Sander C, Jaffe E S, Raffeld M 1996 Mutation of the ras genes is a rare genetic event in the histologic transformation of follicular lymphoma. Leukemia 10: 844–847
633. Yano T, Jaffe E S, Longo D L, Raffeld M 1992 MYC rearrangements in histologically progressed follicular lymphomas. Blood 80: 758–767
634. Elenitoba-Johnson K S, Gascoyne R D, Lim M S et al. 1998 Homozygous deletions at chromosome 9p21 involving p16 and p15 are associated with histologic progression in follicle center lymphoma. Blood 91: 4677–4685
635. Takimoto Y, Takafuta T, Imanaka F et al. 1996 Histological progression of follicular lymphoma associated with p53 mutation and rearrangement of the C-MYC gene. Hiroshima J Med Sci 45: 69–73
636. Davies A J, Lee A M, Taylor C et al. 2005 A limited role for TP53 mutation in the transformation of follicular lymphoma to diffuse large B-cell lymphoma. Leukemia 19: 1459–1465
637. Martinez-Climent J A, Alizadeh A A, Segraves R et al. 2003 Transformation of follicular lymphoma to diffuse large cell lymphoma is associated with a heterogeneous set of DNA copy number and gene expression alterations. Blood 101: 3109–3117
638. Lossos I S, Alizadeh A A, Diehn M et al. 2002 Transformation of follicular lymphoma to diffuse large-cell lymphoma: alternative patterns with increased or decreased expression of c-myc and its regulated genes. Proc Natl Acad Sci USA 99: 8886–8891
639. Boonstra R, Bosga-Bouwer A, Mastik M et al. 2003 Identification of chromosomal copy number changes associated with transformation of follicular lymphoma to diffuse large B-cell lymphoma. Hum Pathol 34: 915–923
640. Natkunam Y, Soslow R, Matolcsy A et al. 2004 Immunophenotypic and genotypic characterization of progression in follicular lymphomas. Appl Immunohistochem Mol Morphol 12: 97–104
641. Sham R L, Phatak P, Carignan J et al. 1989 Progression of follicular large cell lymphoma to Burkitt's lymphoma. Cancer 63: 700–702
642. Weiss L M, Warnke R A 1985 Follicular lymphoma with blastic conversion: a report of two cases with confirmation by immunoperoxidase studies on bone marrow sections. Am J Clin Pathol 83: 681–686
643. Nomdedeu J F, Baiget M, Gaidano G et al. 1998 p53 mutation in a case of blastic transformation of follicular lymphoma with double BCL-2 rearrangement (MBR and VCR). Leuk Lymphoma 29: 595–605
644. Natkunam Y, Warnke R A, Zehnder J L et al. 2000 Blastic/blastoid transformation of follicular lymphoma: immunohistologic and molecular analyses of five cases. Am J Surg Pathol 24: 525–534

645. Leoncini L, Delsol G, Gascoyne R D et al. 2005 Aggressive B-cell lymphomas: a review based on the workshop of the XI Meeting of the European Association for Haematopathology. Histopathology 46: 241–255
646. Karsan A, Gascoyne R D, Coupland R W et al. 1993 Combination of t(14; 18) and a Burkitt's type translocation in B-cell malignancies. Leuk Lymphoma 10: 433–441
647. Macpherson N, Lesack D, Klasa R et al. 1999 Small noncleaved, non-Burkitt's (Burkitt-like) lymphoma: cytogenetics predict outcome and reflect clinical presentation. J Clin Oncol 17: 1558–1567
648. Tomita N, Nakamura N, Kanamori H et al. 2005 Atypical Burkitt lymphoma arising from follicular lymphoma: demonstration by polymerase chain reaction following laser capture microdissection and by fluorescence in situ hybridization on paraffin-embedded tissue sections. Am J Surg Pathol 29: 121–124
649. Isaacson P G, Spencer J 1987 Malignant lymphoma of mucosa-associated lymphoid tissue. Histopathology 11: 445–462
650. Isaacson P G 1990 Lymphomas of mucosa-associated lymphoid tissue (MALT). Histopathology 16: 617–619
651. Spencer J, Diss T C, Isaacson P G 1989 Primary B cell gastric lymphoma. A genotypic analysis. Am J Pathol 135: 557–564
652. Isaacson P G, MacLennan K A, Subbuswamy S G 1984 Multiple lymphomatous polyposis of the gastrointestinal tract. Histopathology 8: 641–656
653. Isaacson P G 1999 Mucosa-associated lymphoid tissue lymphoma. Semin Hematol 36: 139–147
654. Isaacson P G 1999 Gastrointestinal lymphomas of T- and B-cell types. Mod Pathol 12: 151–158
655. Chan J K C 1994 Antibiotic-responsive gastric lymphoma? Adv Anat Pathol 1: 33–37
656. Wotherspoon A C, Ortiz-Hidalgo C, Falzon M R et al. 1991 Helicobacter pylori-associated gastritis and primary B-cell gastric lymphoma. Lancet 338: 1175–1176
657. Kerrigan D P, Irons J, Chen I M 1990 BCL-2 gene rearrangement in salivary gland lymphoma. Am J Surg Pathol 14: 1133–1138
658. Thieblemont C, Berger F, Dumontet C et al. 2000 Mucosa-associated lymphoid tissue lymphoma is a disseminated disease in one third of 158 patients analyzed. Blood 95: 802–806
659. Raderer M, Wohrer S, Streubel B et al. 2006 Assessment of disease dissemination in gastric compared with extragastric mucosa-associated lymphoid tissue lymphoma using extensive staging: a single-center experience. J Clin Oncol 24: 3136–3141
660. Cogliatti S B, Schmid U, Schumacher U et al. 1991 Primary B-cell gastric lymphoma: a clinicopathological study of 145 patients. Gastroenterology 101: 1159–1170
661. Akaza K, Motoori T, Nakamura S et al. 1995 Clinicopathologic study of primary gastric lymphoma of B cell phenotype with special reference to low-grade B cell lymphoma of mucosa-associated lymphoid tissue among the Japanese. Pathol Int 45: 832–845
662. Nakamura S, Akazawa K, Yao T et al. 1995 Primary gastric lymphoma, a clinicopathologic study of 233 cases with special reference to evaluation with the MIB-1 index. Cancer 76: 1313–1324
663. Raderer M, Streubel B, Woehrer S et al. 2005 High relapse rate in patients with MALT lymphoma warrants lifelong follow-up. Clin Cancer Res 11: 3349–3352
664. Chan J K, Ng C S, Isaacson P G 1990 Relationship between high-grade lymphoma and low-grade B-cell mucosa-associated lymphoid tissue lymphoma (MALToma) of the stomach. Am J Pathol 136: 1153–1164
665. Zettl A, Rudiger T, Marx A et al. 2005 Composite marginal zone B-cell lymphoma and classical Hodgkin's lymphoma: a clinicopathological study of 12 cases. Histopathology 46: 217–228
666. Wotherspoon A C, Doglioni C, Diss T C et al. 1993 Regression of primary low-grade B-cell gastric lymphoma of mucosa-associated lymphoid tissue type after eradication of Helicobacter pylori. Lancet 342: 575–577
667. Wotherspoon A C, Doglioni C, de Boni M et al. 1994 Antibiotic treatment for low-grade gastric MALT lymphoma. Lancet 343: 1503
668. Hussell T, Isaacson P G, Crabtree J E et al. 1993 The response of cells from low-grade B-cell gastric lymphomas of mucosal lymphoid tissue to Helicobacter pylori. Lancet 342: 571–574
669. Savio A, Franzin G, Wotherspoon A C et al. 1996 Diagnosis and post-treatment follow-up of Helicobacter pylori-positive gastric lymphoma of mucosa-associated lymphoid tissue: histology, polymerase chain reaction, or both? Blood 87: 1255–1260
670. Weber D M, Dimopoulos M A, Anandu D P et al. 1994 Regression of gastric lymphoma of mucosa-associated lymphoid tissue with antibiotic therapy for Helicobacter pylori. Gastroenterology 107: 1835–1838
671. Roggero E, Zucca E, Pinotti G et al. 1995 Eradication of Helicobacter pylori infection in primary low-grade gastric lymphoma of mucosa-associated lymphoid tissue. Ann Intern Med 122: 767–769
672. Bayerdorffer E, Neubauer A, Rudolph B et al. 1995 Regression of primary gastric lymphoma of mucosa-associated lymphoid tissue type after cure of Helicobacter pylori infection. MALT Lymphoma Study Group. Lancet 345: 1591–1594
673. Wundisch T, Thiede C, Morgner A et al. 2005 Long-term follow-up of gastric MALT lymphoma after Helicobacter pylori eradication. J Clin Oncol 23: 8018–8024
674. Hussell T, Isaacson P G, Crabtree J E et al. 1996 Helicobacter pylori-specific tumour-infiltrating T cells provide contact dependent help for the growth of malignant B cells in low-grade gastric lymphoma of mucosa-associated lymphoid tissue. J Pathol 178: 122–127
675. Montalban C, Manzanal A, Boixeda D et al. 1997 Helicobacter pylori eradication for the treatment of low-grade gastric MALT lymphoma: follow-up together with sequential molecular studies. Ann Oncol 8: 37–39
676. Fischbach W, Goebeler-Kolve M, Starostik P et al. 2002 Minimal residual low-grade gastric MALT-type lymphoma after eradication of Helicobacter pylori. Lancet 360: 547–548
677. Horstmann M, Erttmann R, Winkler K 1994 Relapse of MALT lymphoma associated with Helicobacter pylori after antibiotic treatment. Lancet 343: 1098–1099
678. Raderer M, Streubel B, Wohrer S et al. 2006 Successful antibiotic treatment of Helicobacter pylori negative gastric mucosa associated lymphoid tissue lymphomas. Gut 55: 616–618
679. Grunberger B, Wohrer S, Streubel B et al. 2006 Antibiotic treatment is not effective in patients infected with Helicobacter pylori suffering from extragastric MALT lymphoma. J Clin Oncol 24: 1370–1375
680. Chan J K 1996 Gastrointestinal lymphomas: an overview with emphasis on new findings and diagnostic problems. Semin Diagn Pathol 13: 260–296
681. Papadaki L, Wotherspoon A C, Isaacson P G 1992 The lymphoepithelial lesion of gastric low-grade B-cell lymphoma of mucosa-associated lymphoid tissue (MALT): an ultrastructural study. Histopathology 21: 415–421
682. Isaacson P G, Wotherspoon A C, Diss T et al. 1991 Follicular colonization in B-cell lymphoma of mucosa-associated lymphoid tissue. Am J Surg Pathol 15: 819–828
683. Isaacson P G, Androulakis-Papachristou A, Diss TC et al. 1992 Follicular colonization in thyroid lymphoma. Am J Pathol 141: 43–52
684. Du M Q, Peng H Z, Dogan A et al. 1997 Preferential dissemination of B-cell gastric mucosa-associated lymphoid tissue (MALT) lymphoma to the splenic marginal zone. Blood 90: 4071–4077
685. Morgner A, Miehlke S, Fischbach W et al. 2001 Complete remission of primary high-grade B-cell gastric lymphoma after cure of Helicobacter pylori infection. J Clin Oncol 19: 2041–2048
686. Chen L T, Lin J T, Tai J J et al. 2005 Long-term results of anti-Helicobacter pylori therapy in early-stage gastric high-grade transformed MALT lymphoma. J Natl Cancer Inst 97: 1345–1353
687. Copie-Bergman C, Gaulard P, Lavergne-Slove A et al. 2003 Proposal for a new histological grading system for post-treatment evaluation of gastric MALT lymphoma. Gut 52: 1656
688. Ferry J A, Yang W I, Zukerberg L R et al. 1996 CD5+ extranodal marginal zone B-cell (MALT) lymphoma. A low grade neoplasm with a propensity for bone marrow involvement and relapse. Am J Clin Pathol 105: 31–37
689. Ballesteros E, Osborne B M, Matsushima A Y 1998 CD5+ low-grade marginal zone B-cell lymphomas with localized presentation. Am J Surg Pathol 22: 201–207
690. Ohshima K, Muta H, Kawasaki C et al. 2001 Bcl10 expression, rearrangement and mutation in MALT lymphoma: correlation with expression of nuclear factor-kappaB. Int J Oncol 19: 283–289
691. Sagaert X, Laurent M, Baens M et al. 2006 MALT1 and BCL10 aberrations in MALT lymphomas and their effect on the expression of BCL10 in the tumour cells. Mod Pathol 19: 225–232
692. Ye H, Dogan A, Karran L et al. 2000 BCL10 expression in normal and neoplastic lymphoid tissue. Nuclear localization in MALT lymphoma. Am J Pathol 157: 1147–1154
693. Ye H, Gong L, Liu H et al. 2005 MALT lymphoma with t(14; 18)(q32; q21)/IGH-MALT1 is characterized by strong cytoplasmic MALT1 and BCL10 expression. J Pathol 205: 293–301
694. Ye H, Gong L, Liu H et al. 2006 Strong BCL10 nuclear expression identifies gastric MALT lymphomas that do not respond to H. pylori eradication. Gut 55: 137–138
695. Dorfman D M, Pinkus G S 1995 Utility of immunophenotypic studies in the diagnosis of low-grade lymphoma of mucosa-associated lymphoid tisuse (MALT) and other low-grade non-Hodgkin's lymphomas of extranodal sites. Appl Immunohistochem 3: 160–167
696. Isaacson P G, Du M Q 2005 Gastrointestinal lymphoma: where morphology meets molecular biology. J Pathol 205: 255–274
697. Qin Y, Greiner A, Trunk M J et al. 1995 Somatic hypermutation in low-grade mucosa-associated lymphoid tissue-type B-cell lymphoma. Blood 86: 3528–3534
698. Du M, Diss T C, Xu C et al. 1996 Ongoing mutation in MALT lymphoma immunoglobulin gene suggests that antigen stimulation plays a role in the clonal expansion. Leukemia 10: 1190–1197
699. Pan L, Diss T C, Cunningham D et al. 1989 The BCL-2 gene in primary B cell lymphoma of mucosa-associated lymphoid tissue (MALT). Am J Pathol 135: 7–11
700. Gaidano G, Volpe G, Pastore C et al. 1997 Detection of BCL-6 rearrangements and p53 mutations in MALT lymphomas. Am J Hematol 56: 206–213
701. Gaidano G, Capello D, Gloghini A et al. 1999 Frequent mutation of BCL-6 proto-oncogene in high grade, but not low grade, MALT lymphomas of the gastrointestinal tract. Haematologica 84: 582–588
702. Streubel B, Simonitsch-Klupp I, Mullauer L et al. 2004 Variable frequencies of MALT lymphoma-associated genetic aberrations in MALT lymphomas of different sites. Leukemia 18: 1722–1726

703. Farinha P, Gascoyne R D 2005 Molecular pathogenesis of mucosa-associated lymphoid tissue lymphoma. J Clin Oncol 23: 6370–6378
704. Ott G, Katzenberger T, Greiner A et al. 1997 The t(11; 18)(q21; q21) chromosome translocation is a frequent and specific aberration in low-grade but not high-grade malignant non-Hodgkin's lymphomas of the mucosa-associated lymphoid tissue (MALT) type. Cancer Res 57: 3944–3948
705. Auer I A, Gascoyne R D, Connors J M et al. 1997 t(11; 18)(q21; q21) is the most common translocation in MALT lymphomas. Ann Oncol 8: 979–985
706. Dierlamm J, Baens M, Wlodarska I et al. 1999 The apoptosis inhibitor gene API2 and a novel 18q gene, MLT, are recurrently rearranged in the t(11; 18)(q21; q21) associated with mucosa-associated lymphoid tissue lymphomas. Blood 93: 3601–3609
707. Akagi T, Motegi M, Tamura R et al. 1999 A novel gene, MALT1 at 18q21, is involved in t(11; 18) (q21; q21) found in low-grade B-cell lymphoma of mucosa-associated lymphoid tissue. Oncogene 18: 5785–5794
708. Morgan J A, Yin Y, Borowsky A D et al. 1999 Breakpoints of the t(11; 18)(q21; q21) in mucosa-associated lymphoid tissue (MALT) lymphoma lie within or near the previously undescribed gene MALT1 in chromosome 18. Cancer Res 59: 6205–6213
709. Rosenwald A, Ott G, Stilgenbauer S et al. 1999 Exclusive detection of the t(11; 18)(q21; q21) in extranodal marginal zone B cell lymphomas (MZBL) of MALT type in contrast to other MZBL and extranodal large B cell lymphomas. Am J Pathol 155: 1817–1821
710. Liu H, Ruskon-Fourmestraux A, Lavergne-Slove A et al. 2001 Resistance of t(11; 18) positive gastric mucosa-associated lymphoid tissue lymphoma to *Helicobacter pylori* eradication therapy. Lancet 357: 39–40
711. Liu H, Ye H, Ruskone-Fourmestraux A et al. 2002 T(11; 18) is a marker for all stage gastric MALT lymphomas that will not respond to H. pylori eradication. Gastroenterology 122: 1286–1294
712. Zhang Q, Siebert R, Yan M et al. 1999 Inactivating mutations and overexpression of BCL10, a caspase recruitment domain-containing gene. In: MALT lymphoma with t(1; 14)(p22; q32). Nat Genet 22: 63–68
713. Willis T G, Jadayel D M, Du M Q et al. 1999 Bcl10 is involved in t(1; 14) (p22; q32) of MALT B cell lymphoma and mutated in multiple tumor types. Cell 96: 35–45
714. Streubel B, Lamprecht A, Dierlamm J et al. 2003 T(14; 18)(q32; q21) involving IGH and MALT1 is a frequent chromosomal aberration in MALT lymphoma. Blood 101: 2335–2339
715. Streubel B, Scheucher B, Valencak J et al. 2006 Molecular cytogenetic evidence of t(14; 18)(IGH; BCL2) in a substantial proportion of primary cutaneous follicle center lymphomas. Am J Surg Pathol 30: 529–536
716. Streubel B, Vinatzer U, Lamprecht A et al. 2005 T(3; 14)(p14.1; q32) involving IGH and FOXP1 is a novel recurrent chromosomal aberration in MALT lymphoma. Leukemia 19: 652–658
717. Du M, Peng H, Singh N et al. 1995 The accumulation of p53 abnormalities is associated with progression of mucosa-associated lymphoid tissue lymphoma. Blood 86: 4587–4593
718. Wotherspoon A C, Finn T M, Isaacson P G 1995 Trisomy 3 in low-grade B-cell lymphomas of mucosa-associated lymphoid tissue. Blood 85: 2000–2004
719. Zhang Y, Cheung A N, Chan A C et al. 1998 Detection of trisomy 3 in primary gastric B-cell lymphoma by using chromosome in situ hybridization on paraffin sections. Am J Clin Pathol 110: 347–353
720. Peng H, Chen G, Du M et al. 1996 Replication error phenotype and p53 gene mutation in lymphomas of mucosa-associated lymphoid tissue. Am J Pathol 148: 643–648
721. Montalban C, Castrillo J M, Abraira V et al. 1995 Gastric B-cell mucosa-associated lymphoid tissue (MALT) lymphoma. Clinicopathological study and evaluation of the prognostic factors in 143 patients. Ann Oncol 6: 355–362
722. de Jong D, Boot H, van Heerde P et al. 1997 Histological grading in gastric lymphoma: pretreatment criteria and clinical relevance. Gastroenterology 112: 1466–1474
723. Isaacson P G, Nathwani B N, Piris M A et al. 2001 Nodal marginal zone B-cell lymphoma. In: Jaffe E S, Harris N L, Stein H et al. (eds) Pathology and genetics: tumours of haematopoietic and lymphoid tissues. World Health Organization Classification of Tumours. IARC Press, Lyon, 161
724. Camacho F I, Algara P, Mollejo M et al. 2003 Nodal marginal zone lymphoma: a heterogeneous tumor: a comprehensive analysis of a series of 27 cases. Am J Surg Pathol 27: 762–771
725. Traverse-Glehen A, Felman P, Callet-Bauchu E et al. 2006 A clinicopathological study of nodal marginal zone B-cell lymphoma. A report on 21 cases. Histopathology 48: 162–173
726. Berger F, Felman P, Thieblemont C et al. 2000 Non-MALT marginal zone B-cell lymphomas: a description of clinical presentation and outcome in 124 patients. Blood 95: 1950–1956
727. Arcaini L, Paulli M, Boveri E et al. 2004 Splenic and nodal marginal zone lymphomas are indolent disorders at high hepatitis C virus seroprevalence with distinct presenting features but similar morphologic and phenotypic profiles. Cancer 100: 107–115
728. Oh S Y, Ryoo B Y, Kim W S et al. 2006 Nodal marginal zone B-cell lymphoma: analysis of 36 cases. Clinical presentation and treatment outcomes of nodal marginal zone B-cell lymphoma. Ann Hematol 85: 781–786
729. Cogliatti S B, Lennert K, Hansmann M L et al. 1990 Monocytoid B cell lymphoma: clinical and prognostic features of 21 patients. J Clin Pathol 43: 619–625
730. Ngan B Y, Warnke R A, Wilson M et al. 1991 Monocytoid B-cell lymphoma: a study of 36 cases. Hum Pathol 22: 409–421
731. Traweek S T, Sheibani K, Winberg C D et al. 1989 Monocytoid B-cell lymphoma: its evolution and relationship to other low-grade B-cell neoplasms. Blood 73: 573–578
731a. Taddesse-Heath L, Pittaluga S, Sorbara L et al 2003 Marginal zone B-cell lymphoma in children and young adults. Am J Surg Pathol 27: 522–531
732. Campo E, Miquel R, Krenacs L et al. 1999 Primary nodal marginal zone lymphomas of splenic and MALT type. Am J Surg Pathol 23: 59–68
733. Nathwani B N, Kim H, Rappaport H 1976 Malignant lymphoma, lymphoblastic. Cancer 38: 964–983
734. Nathwani B N, Drachenberg M R, Hernandez A M et al. 1999 Nodal monocytoid B-cell lymphoma (nodal marginal-zone B-cell lymphoma). Semin Hematol 36: 128–138
735. Hernandez A M, Nathwani B N, Nguyen D et al. 1995 Nodal benign and malignant monocytoid B cells with and without follicular lymphomas: a comparative study of follicular colonization, light chain restriction, BCL-2, and t(14; 18) in 39 cases. Hum Pathol 26: 625–632
736. Miranda R N, Cousar J B, Hammer R D et al. 1999 Somatic mutation analysis of IgH variable regions reveals that tumor cells of most parafollicular (monocytoid) B-cell lymphoma, splenic marginal zone B-cell lymphoma, and some hairy cell leukemia are composed of memory B lymphocytes. Hum Pathol 30: 306–312
737. Dierlamm J, Rosenberg C, Stul M et al. 1997 Characteristic pattern of chromosomal gains and losses in marginal zone B cell lymphoma detected by comparative genomic hybridization. Leukemia 11: 747–758
738. Dierlamm J, Michaux L, Wlodarska I et al. 1996 Trisomy 3 in marginal zone B-cell lymphoma: a study based on cytogenetic analysis and fluorescence in situ hybridization. Br J Haematol 93: 242–249
739. Dierlamm J, Pittaluga S, Wlodarska I et al. 1996 Marginal zone B-cell lymphomas of different sites share similar cytogenetic and morphologic features. Blood 87: 299–307
740. Nathwani B N, Mohrmann R L, Brynes R K et al. 1992 Monocytoid B-cell lymphomas: an assessment of diagnostic criteria and a perspective on histogenesis. Hum Pathol 23: 1061–1071
741. d'Amore E S, Wick M R, Geisinger K R et al. 1990 Primary malignant lymphoma arising in postmastectomy lymphedema. Another facet of the Stewart–Treves syndrome. Am J Surg Pathol 14: 456–463
742. Copie-Bergman C, Niedobitek G, Mangham D C et al. 1997 Epstein–Barr virus in B-cell lymphomas associated with chronic suppurative inflammation. J Pathol 183: 287–292
743. Aozasa K, Takakuwa T, Nakatsuka S 2005 Pyothorax-associated lymphoma: a lymphoma developing in chronic inflammation. Adv Anat Pathol 12: 324–331
744. Cabanillas F, Velasquez W S, Hagemeister F B et al. 1992 Clinical, biologic, and histologic features of late relapses in diffuse large cell lymphoma. Blood 79: 1024–1028
745. Hodges G F, Lenhardt T M, Cotelingam J D 1994 Bone marrow involvement in large-cell lymphoma. Prognostic implications of discordant disease. Am J Clin Pathol 101: 305–311
746. Robertson L E, Redman J R, Butler J J et al. 1991 Discordant bone marrow involvement in diffuse large-cell lymphoma: a distinct clinical–pathologic entity associated with a continuous risk of relapse. J Clin Oncol 9: 236–242
747. Conlan M G, Bast M, Armitage J O et al. 1990 Bone marrow involvement by non-Hodgkin's lymphoma: the clinical significance of morphologic discordance between the lymph node and bone marrow. Nebraska Lymphoma Study Group. J Clin Oncol 8: 1163–1172
748. Fisher R I, Gaynor E R, Dahlberg S et al. 1993 Comparison of a standard regimen (CHOP) with three intensive chemotherapy regimens for advanced non-Hodgkin's lymphoma. N Engl J Med 328: 1002–1006
749. Sehn L H, Donaldson J, Chhanabhai M et al. 2005 Introduction of combined CHOP plus rituximab therapy dramatically improved outcome of diffuse large B-cell lymphoma in British Columbia. J Clin Oncol 23: 5027–5033
750. Navarro-Roman L, Medeiros L J, Kingma D W et al. 1994 Malignant lymphomas of B-cell lineage with marked tissue eosinophilia. A report of five cases. Am J Surg Pathol 18: 347–356
751. Tse C C, Chan J K, Yuen R W et al. 1991 Malignant lymphoma with myxoid stroma: a new pattern in need of recognition. Histopathology 18: 31–35
752. Fung D T, Chan J K, Tse C C et al. 1992 Myxoid change in malignant lymphoma. Pathogenetic considerations. Arch Pathol Lab Med 116: 103–105
753. Tsang W Y, Chan J K, Tang S K et al. 1992 Large cell lymphoma with fibrillary matrix. Histopathology 20: 80–82
754. Eyden B P, Cross P A, Harris M 1990 The ultrastructure of signet-ring cell non-Hodgkin's lymphoma. Virchows Arch A Pathol Anat Histopathol 417: 395–404
755. Nakamine H, Masih A S, Strobach R S et al. 1991 Immunoblastic lymphoma with abundant clear cytoplasm. A comparative study of B- and T-cell types. Am J Clin Pathol 96: 177–183
756. Osborne B M, Mackay B, Butler J J et al. 1983 Large cell lymphoma with microvillus-like projections: an ultrastructural study. Am J Clin Pathol 79: 443–450

757. Kinney M C, Glick A D, Stein H et al. 1990 Comparison of anaplastic large cell Ki-1 lymphomas and microvillous lymphomas in their immunologic and ultrastructural features. Am J Surg Pathol 14: 1047–1060
758. Hammer R D, Vnencak-Jones C L, Manning S S et al. 1998 Microvillous lymphomas are B-cell neoplasms that frequently express CD56. Mod Pathol 11: 239–246
759. Osborne B M, Butler J J, Mackay B 1980 Sinusoidal large cell ('histiocytic') lymphoma. Cancer 46: 2484–2491
760. Ng C S, Chan J K, Hui P K et al. 1989 Large B-cell lymphomas with a high content of reactive T cells. Hum Pathol 20: 1145–1154
761. Ng C S, Chan J K C, Hui P K 1991 Heterogeneity of interfollicular lymphomas [Abstract]. Surg Pathol 4: 372
762. Chan J K, Ng C S, Tung S 1986 Multilobated B-cell lymphoma, a variant of centroblastic lymphoma. Report of four cases. Histopathology 10: 601–612
763. van Baarlen J, Schuurman H J, van Unnik J A 1988 Multilobated non-Hodgkin's lymphoma. A clinicopathologic entity. Cancer 61: 1371–1376
764. MacLennan K A, Anderson J R, Armitage J O et al. 1998 Anaplastic large cell lymphoma (ALCL) of T/null-cell types is a distinctive clinicopathologic entity. (Abstr). Mod Pathol 11: 135A
765. Spier C M, Grogan T M, Lippman S M et al. 1988 The aberrancy of immunophenotype and immunoglobulin status as indicators of prognosis in B cell diffuse large cell lymphoma. Am J Pathol 133: 118–126
766. Borowitz M J, Bousvaros A, Brynes R K et al. 1985 Monoclonal antibody phenotyping of B-cell non-Hodgkin's lymphomas. The Southeastern Cancer Study Group experience. Am J Pathol 121: 514–521
767. Stein H, Lennert K, Feller A C et al. 1984 Immunohistological analysis of human lymphoma: correlation of histological and immunological categories. Adv Cancer Res 42: 67–147
768. de Leval L, Harris N L 2003 Variability in immunophenotype in diffuse large B-cell lymphoma and its clinical relevance. Histopathology 43: 509–528
769. Matolcsy A, Chadburn A, Knowles D M 1995 De novo CD5-positive and Richter's syndrome-associated diffuse large B cell lymphomas are genotypically distinct. Am J Pathol 147: 207–216
770. Harada S, Suzuki R, Uehira K et al. 1999 Molecular and immunological dissection of diffuse large B cell lymphoma: CD5+, and CD5− with CD10+ groups may constitute clinically relevant subtypes. Leukemia 13: 1441–1447
771. Houldsworth J, Mathew S, Rao P H et al. 1996 REL proto-oncogene is frequently amplified in extranodal diffuse large cell lymphoma. Blood 87: 25–29
772. Kramer M H, Hermans J, Wijburg E et al. 1998 Clinical relevance of BCL2, BCL6, and MYC rearrangements in diffuse large B-cell lymphoma. Blood 92: 3152–3162
773. Offit K, Chaganti R S 1991 Chromosomal aberrations in non-Hodgkin's lymphoma. Biologic and clinical correlations. Hematol Oncol Clin North Am 5: 853–869
774. Offit K, Wong G, Filippa D A et al. 1991 Cytogenetic analysis of 434 consecutively ascertained specimens of non-Hodgkin's lymphoma: clinical correlations. Blood 77: 1508–1515
775. Jacobson J O, Wilkes B M, Kwaiatkowski D J et al. 1993 BCL-2 rearrangements in de novo diffuse large cell lymphoma. Association with distinctive clinical features. Cancer 72: 231–236
776. Offit K, Lo Coco F, Louie D C et al. 1994 Rearrangement of the BCL-6 gene as a prognostic marker in diffuse large-cell lymphoma. N Engl J Med 331: 74–80
777. Gaidano G, Dalla-Favera R 1998 The biology of high-grade non-Hodgkin's lymphoma. In: Canellos G P, Lister T A, Sklar J L (eds) The lymphomas. WB Saunders, Philadelphia, 353–367
778. Capello D, Vitolo U, Pasqualucci L et al. 2000 Distribution and pattern of BCL-6 mutations throughout the spectrum of B-cell neoplasia. Blood 95: 651–659
779. van Krieken J H, Raffeld M, Raghoebier S et al. 1990 Molecular genetics of gastrointestinal non-Hodgkin's lymphomas: unusual prevalence and pattern of c-myc rearrangements in aggressive lymphomas. Blood 76: 797–800
780. Kawasaki C, Ohshim K, Suzumiya J et al. 2001 Rearrangements of BCL-1, BCL-2, BCL-6, and c-myc in diffuse large B cell lymphomas. Leuk Lymphoma 42: 1099–1106
781. Akasaka T, Akasaka H, Ueda C et al. 2000 Molecular and clinical features of non-Burkitt's, diffuse large-cell lymphoma of B-cell type associated with the c-MYC/immunoglobulin heavy-chain fusion gene. J Clin Oncol 18: 510–518
782. Hummel M, Bentink S, Berger H et al. 2006 A biologic definition of Burkitt's lymphoma from transcriptional and genomic profiling. N Engl J Med 354: 2419–2430
783. Koduru P R, Raju K, Vadmal V et al. 1997 Correlation between mutation in P53, p53 expression, cytogenetics, histologic type, and survival in patients with B-cell non-Hodgkin's lymphoma. Blood 90: 4078–4091
784. Ichikawa A, Kinoshita T, Watanabe T et al. 1997 Mutations of the p53 gene as a prognostic factor in aggressive B-cell lymphoma. N Engl J Med 337: 529–534
785. Pasqualucci L, Neumeister P, Goossens T et al. 2001 Hypermutation of multiple proto-oncogenes in B-cell diffuse large-cell lymphomas. Nature 412: 341–346
786. Alizadeh A A, Eisen M B, Davis R E et al. 2000 Distinct types of diffuse large B-cell lymphoma identified by gene expression profiling. Nature 403: 503–511
787. Rosenwald A, Wright G, Chan W C et al. 2002 The use of molecular profiling to predict survival after chemotherapy for diffuse large-B-cell lymphoma. N Engl J Med 346: 1937–1947
788. Staudt L M 2003 Molecular diagnosis of the hematologic cancers. N Engl J Med 348: 1777–1785
789. Huang J Z, Sanger W G, Greiner T C et al. 2002 The t(14; 18) defines a unique subset of diffuse large B-cell lymphoma with a germinal center B-cell gene expression profile. Blood 99: 2285–2290
790. Hill M E, MacLennan K A, Cunningham D C et al. 1996 Prognostic significance of BCL-2 expression and BCL-2 major breakpoint region rearrangement in diffuse large cell non-Hodgkin's lymphoma: a British National Lymphoma Investigation Study. Blood 88: 1046–1051
791. Gascoyne R D, Adomat S A, Krajewski S et al. 1997 Prognostic significance of BCL-2 protein expression and BCL-2 gene rearrangement in diffuse aggressive non-Hodgkin's lymphoma. Blood 90: 244–251
792. Colomo L, Lopez-Guillermo A, Perales M et al. 2003 Clinical impact of the differentiation profile assessed by immunophenotyping in patients with diffuse large B-cell lymphoma. Blood 101: 78–84
793. Swan F Jr, Velasquez W S, Tucker S et al. 1989 A new serologic staging system for large-cell lymphomas based on initial beta 2-microglobulin and lactate dehydrogenase levels. J Clin Oncol 7: 1518–1527
794. Engelhard M, Brittinger G, Huhn D et al. 1997 Subclassification of diffuse large B-cell lymphomas according to the Kiel classification: distinction of centroblastic and immunoblastic lymphomas is a significant prognostic risk factor. Blood 89: 2291–2297
795. Warnke R A, Strauchen J A, Burke J S et al. 1982 Morphologic types of diffuse large-cell lymphoma. Cancer 50: 690–695
796. Nathwani B N, Dixon D O, Jones S E et al. 1982 The clinical significance of the morphological subdivision of diffuse 'histiocytic' lymphoma: a study of 162 patients treated by the Southwest Oncology Group. Blood 60: 1068–1074
797. Diebold J, Anderson J R, Armitage J O et al. 2002 Diffuse large B-cell lymphoma: a clinicopathologic analysis of 444 cases classified according to the updated Kiel classification. Leuk Lymphoma 43: 97–104
798. Cossman J, Jaffe E S, Fisher R I 1984 Immunologic phenotypes of diffuse, aggressive, non-Hodgkin's lymphomas. Correlation with clinical features. Cancer 54: 1310–1317
799. Kwak L W, Wilson M, Weiss L M et al. 1991 Clinical significance of morphologic subdivision in diffuse large cell lymphoma. Cancer 68: 1988–1993
800. Simon R, Durrleman S, Hoppe R T et al. 1988 The Non-Hodgkin's Lymphoma Pathologic Classification Project. Long-term follow-up of 1153 patients with non-Hodgkin's lymphomas. Ann Intern Med 109: 939–945
801. Nakamine H, Bagin R G, Vose J M et al. 1993 Prognostic significance of clinical and pathologic features in diffuse large B-cell lymphoma. Cancer 71: 3130–3137
802. Sanchez E, Chacon I, Plaza M M et al. 1998 Clinical outcome in diffuse large B-cell lymphoma is dependent on the relationship between different cell-cycle regulator proteins. J Clin Oncol 16: 1931–1939
803. Kramer M H, Hermans J, Parker J et al. 1996 Clinical significance of bcl2 and p53 protein expression in diffuse large B-cell lymphoma: a population-based study. J Clin Oncol 14: 2131–2138
804. Barrans S L, Carter I, Owen R G et al. 2002 Germinal center phenotype and BCL-2 expression combined with the International Prognostic Index improves patient risk stratification in diffuse large B-cell lymphoma. Blood 99: 1136–1143
805. Muris J J, Meijer C J, Vos W et al. 2006 Immunohistochemical profiling based on BCL-2, CD10 and MUM1 expression improves risk stratification in patients with primary nodal diffuse large B cell lymphoma. J Pathol 208: 714–723
806. van Imhoff G W, Boerma E J, van der Holt B et al. 2006 Prognostic impact of germinal center-associated proteins and chromosomal breakpoints in poor-risk diffuse large B-cell lymphoma. J Clin Oncol 24: 4135–4142
807. Shivakumar L, Armitage J O 2006 BCL-2 gene expression as a predictor of outcome in diffuse large B-cell lymphoma. Clin Lymphoma Myeloma 6: 455–457
808. Mounier N, Briere J, Gisselbrecht C et al. 2003 Rituximab plus CHOP (R–CHOP) overcomes BCL-2-associated resistance to chemotherapy in elderly patients with diffuse large B-cell lymphoma (DLBCL). Blood 101: 4279–4284
809. Winter J N, Weller E A, Horning S J et al. 2006 Prognostic significance of BCL-6 protein expression in DLBCL treated with CHOP or R-CHOP: a prospective correlative study. Blood 107: 4207–4213
810. Yamaguchi M, Ohno T, Oka K et al. 1999 De novo CD5-positive diffuse large B-cell lymphoma: clinical characteristics and therapeutic outcome. Br J Haematol 105: 1133–1139
811. Yamaguchi M, Seto M, Okamoto M et al. 2002 De novo CD5+ diffuse large B-cell lymphoma: a clinicopathologic study of 109 patients. Blood 99: 815–821
812. Slymen D J, Miller T P, Lippman S M et al. 1990 Immunobiologic factors predictive of clinical outcome in diffuse large-cell lymphoma. J Clin Oncol 8: 986–993
813. Miller T P, Lippman S M, Spier C M et al. 1988 HLA–DR (Ia) immune phenotype predicts outcome for patients with diffuse large cell lymphoma. J Clin Invest 82: 370–372

814. Rimsza L M, Roberts R A, Miller T P et al. 2004 Loss of MHC class II gene and protein expression in diffuse large B-cell lymphoma is related to decreased tumor immunosurveillance and poor patient survival regardless of other prognostic factors: a follow-up study from the Leukemia and Lymphoma Molecular Profiling Project. Blood 103: 4251–4258
815. Miller T P, Grogan T M, Dahlberg S et al. 1994 Prognostic significance of the Ki-67-associated proliferative antigen in aggressive non-Hodgkin's lymphomas: a prospective Southwest Oncology Group trial. Blood 83: 1460–1466
816. Hans C P, Weisenburger D D, Greiner T C et al. 2004 Confirmation of the molecular classification of diffuse large B-cell lymphoma by immunohistochemistry using a tissue microarray. Blood 103: 275–282
817. Lossos I S, Jones C D, Warnke R et al. 2001 Expression of a single gene, BCL-6, strongly predicts survival in patients with diffuse large B-cell lymphoma. Blood 98: 945–951
818. Lossos I S, Alizadeh A A, Rajapaksa R et al. 2003 HGAL is a novel interleukin-4-inducible gene that strongly predicts survival in diffuse large B-cell lymphoma. Blood 101: 433–440
819. Lippman S M, Spier C M, Miller T P et al. 1990 Tumor-infiltrating T-lymphocytes in B-cell diffuse large cell lymphoma related to disease course. Mod Pathol 3: 361–367
820. Xu Y, Kroft S H, McKenna R W et al. 2001 Prognostic significance of tumour-infiltrating T lymphocytes and T-cell subsets in de novo diffuse large B-cell lymphoma: a multiparameter flow cytometry study. Br J Haematol 112: 945–949
821. Muris J J, Meijer C J, Cillessen S A et al. 2004 Prognostic significance of activated cytotoxic T-lymphocytes in primary nodal diffuse large B-cell lymphomas. Leukemia 18: 589–596
822. Bea S, Zettl A, Wright G et al. 2005 Diffuse large B-cell lymphoma subgroups have distinct genetic profiles that influence tumor biology and improve gene-expression-based survival prediction. Blood 106: 3183–3190
823. Leroy K, Haioun C, Lepage E et al. 2002 p53 gene mutations are associated with poor survival in low and low–intermediate risk diffuse large B-cell lymphomas. Ann Oncol 13: 1108–1115
824. Shipp M A, Ross K N, Tamayo P et al. 2002 Diffuse large B-cell lymphoma outcome prediction by gene-expression profiling and supervised machine learning. Nat Med 8: 68–74
825. Tome M E, Johnson D B, Rimsza L M et al. 2005 A redox signature score identifies diffuse large B-cell lymphoma patients with a poor prognosis. Blood 106: 3594–3601
826. Lossos I S, Czerwinski D K, Alizadeh A A et al. 2004 Prediction of survival in diffuse large B-cell lymphoma based on the expression of six genes. N Engl J Med 350: 1828–1837
827. Ferry J A, Harris N L, Picker L J et al. 1988 Intravascular lymphomatosis (malignant angioendotheliomatosis). A B-cell neoplasm expressing surface homing receptors. Mod Pathol 1: 444–452
828. Mori S, Itoyama S, Mohri N et al. 1985 Cellular characteristics of neoplastic angioendotheliosis. An immunohistological marker study of 6 cases. Virchows Arch A Pathol Anat Histopathol 407: 167–175
829. Sheibani K, Battifora H, Winberg C D et al. 1986 Further evidence that 'malignant angioendotheliomatosis' is an angiotropic large-cell lymphoma. N Engl J Med 314: 943–948
830. Wick M R, Mills S E, Scheithauer B W et al. 1986 Reassessment of malignant 'angioendotheliomatosis.' Evidence in favor of its reclassification as 'intravascular lymphomatosis.' Am J Surg Pathol 10: 112–123
831. Bhawan J 1987 Angioendotheliomatosis proliferans systemisata: an angiotropic neoplasm of lymphoid origin. Semin Diagn Pathol 4: 18–27
832. Stroup R M, Sheibani K, Moncada A et al. 1990 Angiotropic (intravascular) large cell lymphoma. A clinicopathologic study of seven cases with unique clinical presentations. Cancer 66: 1781–1788
833. Jalkanen S, Aho R, Kallajoki M et al. 1989 Lymphocyte homing receptors and adhesion molecules in intravascular malignant lymphomatosis. Int J Cancer 44: 777–782
834. DiGiuseppe J A, Nelson W G, Seifter E J et al. 1994 Intravascular lymphomatosis: a clinicopathologic study of 10 cases and assessment of response to chemotherapy. J Clin Oncol 12: 2573–2579
835. DiGiuseppe J A, Hartmann D P, Freter C et al. 1997 Molecular detection of bone marrow involvement in intravascular lymphomatosis. Mod Pathol 10: 33–37
836. Domizio P, Hall P A, Cotter F et al. 1989 Angiotropic large cell lymphoma (ALCL): morphological, immunohistochemical and genotypic studies with analysis of previous reports. Hematol Oncol 7: 195–206
837. Sepp N, Schuler G, Romani N et al. 1990 'Intravascular lymphomatosis' (angioendotheliomatosis): evidence for a T-cell origin in two cases. Hum Pathol 21: 1051–1058
838. O'Grady J T, Shahidullah H, Doherty V R et al. 1994 Intravascular histiocytosis. Histopathology 24: 265–268
839. Snowden J A, Angel C A, Winfield D A et al. 1997 Angiotropic lymphoma: report of a case with histiocytic features. J Clin Pathol 50: 67–70
840. Wu H, Said J W, Ames E D et al. 2005 First reported cases of intravascular large cell lymphoma of the NK cell type: clinical, histologic, immunophenotypic, and molecular features. Am J Clin Pathol 123: 603–611
841. Au W Y, Shek W H, Nicholls J et al. 1997 T-cell intravascular lymphomatosis (angiotropic large cell lymphoma): association with Epstein–Barr viral infection. Histopathology 31: 563–567
842. Kuo T T, Chen M J, Kuo M C 2006 Cutaneous intravascular NK-cell lymphoma: Report of a rare variant associated with Epstein–Barr virus. Am J Surg Pathol 30: 1197–1201
843. Khalidi H S, Brynes R K, Browne P et al. 1998 Intravascular large B-cell lymphoma: the CD5 antigen is expressed by a subset of cases. Mod Pathol 11: 983–988
844. Kanda M, Suzumiya J, Ohshima K et al. 1999 Intravascular large cell lymphoma: clinicopathological, immunohistochemical and molecular genetic studies. Leuk Lymphoma 34: 569–580
845. Otrakji C L, Voigt W, Amador A et al. 1988 Malignant angioendotheliomatosis – a true lymphoma: a case of intravascular malignant lymphomatosis studied by southern blot hybridization analysis. Hum Pathol 19: 475–478
846. Hsiao C H, Su I J, Hsieh S W et al. 1999 Epstein–Barr virus-associated intravascular lymphomatosis within Kaposi's sarcoma in an AIDS patient. Am J Surg Pathol 23: 482–487
847. Murase T, Nakamura S, Tashiro K et al. 1997 Malignant histiocytosis-like B-cell lymphoma, a distinct pathologic variant of intravascular lymphomatosis: a report of five cases and review of the literature. Br J Haematol 99: 656–664
848. Murase T, Nakamura S 1999 An Asian variant of intravascular lymphomatosis: an updated review of malignant histiocytosis-like B-cell lymphoma. Leuk Lymphoma 33: 459–473
849. Ramsay A D, Smith W J, Earl H M et al. 1987 T-cell lymphomas in adults: a clinicopathological study of eighteen cases. J Pathol 152: 63–76
850. De Jong D, Van Gorp J, Sie-Go D et al. 1996 T-cell rich B-cell non-Hodgkin's lymphoma: a progressed form of follicle centre cell lymphoma and lymphocyte predominance Hodgkin's disease. Histopathology 28: 15–24
851. Brauninger A, Kuppers R, Spieker T et al. 1999 Molecular analysis of single B cells from T-cell-rich B-cell lymphoma shows the derivation of the tumor cells from mutating germinal center B cells and exemplifies means by which immunoglobulin genes are modified in germinal center B cells. Blood 93: 2679–2687
852. Lim M S, Beaty M, Sorbara L et al. 2002 T-cell/histiocyte-rich large B-cell lymphoma: a heterogeneous entity with derivation from germinal center B cells. Am J Surg Pathol 26: 1458–1466
853. Rodriguez J, Pugh W C, Cabanillas F 1993 T-cell-rich B-cell lymphoma. Blood 82: 1586–1589
854. Krishnan J, Wallberg K, Frizzera G 1994 T-cell-rich large B-cell lymphoma. A study of 30 cases, supporting its histologic heterogeneity and lack of clinical distinctiveness. Am J Surg Pathol 18: 455–465
855. Gascoyne R D, Delabie J, de Wolfe-Peters C et al. 1999 'Paragranuloma-type' T-cell rich B-cell lymphoma (TCRBCL): a report of 50 cases. [Abstract] Mod Pathol 12: 137A
856. Delabie J, Vandenberghe E, Kennes C et al. 1992 Histiocyte-rich B-cell lymphoma. A distinct clinicopathologic entity possibly related to lymphocyte predominant Hodgkin's disease, paragranuloma subtype. Am J Surg Pathol 16: 37–48
857. Bouabdallah R, Mounier N, Guettier C et al. 2003 T-cell/histiocyte-rich large B-cell lymphomas and classical diffuse large B-cell lymphomas have similar outcome after chemotherapy: a matched-control analysis. J Clin Oncol 21: 1271–1277
858. Baddoura F K, Chan W C, Masih A S et al. 1995 T-cell-rich B-cell lymphoma. A clinicopathologic study of eight cases. Am J Clin Pathol 103: 65–75
859. Macon W R, Williams M E, Greer J P et al. 1992 T-cell-rich B-cell lymphomas. A clinicopathologic study of 19 cases. Am J Surg Pathol 16: 351–363
860. Chittal S M, Brousset P, Voigt J J et al. 1991 Large B-cell lymphoma rich in T-cells and simulating Hodgkin's disease. Histopathology 19: 211–220
861. Osborne B M, Butler J J, Pugh W C 1990 The value of immunophenotyping on paraffin sections in the identification of T-cell rich B-cell large-cell lymphomas: lineage confirmed by JH rearrangement. Am J Surg Pathol 14: 933–938
862. Loke S L, Ho F, Srivastava G et al. 1992 Clonal Epstein–Barr virus genome in T-cell-rich lymphomas of B or probable B lineage. Am J Pathol 140: 981–989
863. Liebow A A, Carrington C B, Friedman P J 1972 Lymphomatoid granulomatosis. Hum Pathol 3: 457–558
864. Katzenstein A L, Carrington C B, Liebow A A 1979 Lymphomatoid granulomatosis: a clinicopathologic study of 152 cases. Cancer 43: 360–373
865. James W D, Odom R B, Katzenstein A L 1981 Cutaneous manifestations of lymphomatoid granulomatosis. Report of 44 cases and a review of the literature. Arch Dermatol 117: 196–202
866. Beaty M W, Toro J, Sorbara L et al. 2001 Cutaneous lymphomatoid granulomatosis: correlation of clinical and biologic features. Am J Surg Pathol 25: 1111–1120
867. DeRemee R A, Weiland L H, McDonald T J 1978 Polymorphic reticulosis, lymphomatoid granulomatosis. Two diseases or one? Mayo Clin Proc 53: 634–640
868. Lipford E H Jr, Margolick J B, Longo D L et al. 1988 Angiocentric immunoproliferative lesions: a clinicopathologic spectrum of post-thymic T-cell proliferations. Blood 72: 1674–1681
869. Nicholson A G, Wotherspoon A C, Diss T C et al. 1996 Lymphomatoid granulomatosis: evidence that some cases represent Epstein–Barr virus-associated B-cell lymphoma. Histopathology 29: 317–324

870. Myers J L, Kurtin P J, Katzenstein A L et al. 1995 Lymphomatoid granulomatosis. Evidence of immunophenotypic diversity and relationship to Epstein–Barr virus infection. Am J Surg Pathol 19: 1300–1312
871. Jaffe E S, Wilson W H 1997 Lymphomatoid granulomatosis: pathogenesis, pathology and clinical implications. Cancer Surv 30: 233–248
872. Guinee D J Jr, Jaffe E, Kingma D et al. 1994 Pulmonary lymphomatoid granulomatosis. Evidence for a proliferation of Epstein–Barr virus infected B-lymphocytes with a prominent T-cell component and vasculitis. Am J Surg Pathol 18: 753–764
873. Guinee D G Jr, Perkins S L, Travis W D et al. 1998 Proliferation and cellular phenotype in lymphomatoid granulomatosis: implications of a higher proliferation index in B cells. Am J Surg Pathol 22: 1093–1100
874. Koss M N, Hochholzer L, Langloss J M et al. 1986 Lymphomatoid granulomatosis: a clinicopathologic study of 42 patients. Pathology 18: 283–288
875. Jaffe E S 1999 Nasal/nasal type NK/T cell lymphoma (angiocentric lymphoma) and Lymphomatoid granulomatosis. In: Mason D Y, Harris N L (eds) Human lymphoma: clinical implications of the REAL classification. Springer, London, 32.31–32.36
876. Wilson W H 1999 Clinical aspects and treatment options in nasal/nasal type lymphoma (angiocentric) and lymphomatoid granulomatosis. In: Mason D Y, Harris N L (eds) Human lymphoma: clinical implications of the REAL classification. Springer, London, 33.31–33.34
877. Saxena A, Dyker K M, Angel S et al. 2002 Post-transplant diffuse large B-cell lymphoma of 'lymphomatoid granulomatosis' type. Virchows Arch 441: 622–628
878. Kwon E J, Katz K A, Draft K S et al. 2006 Post-transplantation lymphoproliferative disease with features of lymphomatoid granulomatosis in a lung transplant patient. J Am Acad Dermatol 54: 657–663
879. Cachat F, Meagher-Villemure K, Guignard JP 2003 Lymphomatoid granulomatosis in a renal transplant patient. Pediatr Nephrol 18: 838–842
880. Morice W G, Kurtin P J, Myers J L 2002 Expression of cytolytic lymphocyte-associated antigens in pulmonary lymphomatoid granulomatosis. Am J Clin Pathol 118: 391–398
881. Fauci A S, Haynes B F, Costa J et al. 1982 Lymphomatoid granulomatosis: prospective clinical and therapeutic experience over 10 years. N Engl J Med 306: 68–74
882. Wilson W H, Kingma D W, Raffeld M et al. 1996 Association of lymphomatoid granulomatosis with Epstein–Barr viral infection of B lymphocytes and response to interferon-alpha 2b. Blood 87: 4531–4537
883. Rao R, Vugman G, Leslie W T et al. 2003 Lymphomatoid granulomatosis treated with rituximab and chemotherapy. Clin Adv Hematol Oncol 1: 658–660
884. Oyama T, Ichimura K, Suzuki R et al. 2003 Senile EBV+ B-cell lymphoproliferative disorders: a clinicopathologic study of 22 patients. Am J Surg Pathol 27: 16–26
885. Aozasa K 1996 Pyothorax-associated lymphoma. Int J Hematol 65: 9–16
886. Aozasa K, Ohsawa M, Kanno H 1997 Pyothorax-associated lymphoma: a distinctive type of lymphoma strongly associated with Epstein–Barr virus. Adv Anat Pathol 4: 58–63
887. Martin A, Capron F, Liguory-Brunaud M D et al. 1994 Epstein–Barr virus-associated primary malignant lymphomas of the pleural cavity occurring in longstanding pleural chronic inflammation. Hum Pathol 25: 1314–1318
888. Molinie V, Pouchot J, Navratil E et al. 1996 Epstein–Barr virus-related non-Hodgkin's lymphoma of the pleural cavity following long-standing tuberculous empyema. Arch Pathol Lab Med 120: 288–291
889. Androulaki A, Drakos E, Hatzianastassiou D et al. 2004 Pyothorax-associated lymphoma (PAL): a western case with marked angiocentricity and review of the literature. Histopathology 44: 69–76
890. Nakatsuka S, Yao M, Hoshida Y et al. 2002 Pyothorax-associated lymphoma: a review of 106 cases. J Clin Oncol 20: 4255–4260
891. Mori N, Yatabe Y, Narita M et al. 1996 Pyothorax-associated lymphoma. An unusual case with biphenotypic character of T and B cells. Am J Surg Pathol 20: 760–766
892. Petitjean B, Jardin F, Joly B et al. 2002 Pyothorax-associated lymphoma: a peculiar clinicopathologic entity derived from B cells at late stage of differentiation and with occasional aberrant dual B- and T-cell phenotype. Am J Surg Pathol 26: 724–732
893. Fukayama M, Ibuka T, Hayashi Y et al. 1993 Epstein–Barr virus in pyothorax-associated pleural lymphoma. Am J Pathol 143: 1044–1049
894. Fukayama M, Hayashi Y, Ooba T et al. 1995 Pyothorax-associated lymphoma: development of Epstein–Barr virus-associated lymphoma within the inflammatory cavity. Pathol Int 45: 825–831
895. Sasajima Y, Yamabe H, Kobashi Y et al. 1993 High expression of the Epstein–Barr virus latent protein EB nuclear antigen-2 on pyothorax-associated lymphoma. Am J Pathol 143:1280–1285
896. Cesarman E, Nador R G, Aozasa K et al. 1996 Kaposi's sarcoma-associated herpesvirus in non-AIDS related lymphomas occurring in body cavities. Am J Pathol 149: 53–57
897. Nishiu M, Tomita Y, Nakatsuka S et al. 2004 Distinct pattern of gene expression in pyothorax-associated lymphoma (PAL), a lymphoma developing in long-standing inflammation. Cancer Sci 95: 828–834
898. Banks P M, Warnke R 2001 Primary effusion lymphoma. In: Jaffe E S, Harris N L, Stein H et al. (eds) Pathology and genetics: tumours of haematopoietic and lymphoid tissues. World Health Organization Classification of Tumours. IARC Press, Lyon, 179–180
899. Carbone A, Gloghini A, Vaccher E et al. 2005 Kaposi's sarcoma-associated herpesvirus/human herpesvirus type 8-positive solid lymphomas: a tissue-based variant of primary effusion lymphoma. J Mol Diagn 7: 17–27
900. Chadburn A, Hyjek E, Mathew S et al. 2004 KSHV-positive solid lymphomas represent an extracavitary variant of primary effusion lymphoma. Am J Surg Pathol 28: 1401–1416
901. Deloose S T, Smit L A, Pals F T et al. 2005 High incidence of Kaposi sarcoma-associated herpesvirus infection in HIV-related solid immunoblastic/plasmablastic diffuse large B-cell lymphoma. Leukemia 19: 851–855
902. Mate J L, Navarro J T, Ariza A et al. 2004 Oral solid form of primary effusion lymphoma mimicking plasmablastic lymphoma. Hum Pathol 35: 632–635
903. Colomo L, Loong F, Rives S et al. 2004 Diffuse large B-cell lymphomas with plasmablastic differentiation represent a heterogeneous group of disease entities. Am J Surg Pathol 28: 736–747
904. Said J W 1996 Body cavity-based (primary effusion) lymphoma: a new lymphoma subtype associated with Kaposi's sarcoma herpesvirus (human herpesvirus 8). Adv Anat Pathol 3: 254–258
905. Cesarman E, Knowles D M 1997 Kaposi's sarcoma-associated herpesvirus: a lymphotropic human herpesvirus associated with Kaposi's sarcoma, primary effusion lymphoma, and multicentric Castleman's disease. Semin Diagn Pathol 14: 54–66
906. Cesarman E, Nador R G, Bai F et al. 1996 Kaposi's sarcoma-associated herpesvirus contains G protein-coupled receptor and cyclin D homologs which are expressed in Kaposi's sarcoma and malignant lymphoma. J Virol 70: 8218–8223
907. Cesarman E, Chang Y, Moore P S et al. 1995 Kaposi's sarcoma-associated herpesvirus-like DNA sequences in AIDS-related body cavity-based lymphomas. N Engl J Med 332: 1186–1191
908. Simonelli C, Spina M, Cinelli R et al. 2003 Clinical features and outcome of primary effusion lymphoma in HIV-infected patients: a single-institution study. J Clin Oncol 21: 3948–3954
909. Boulanger E, Gerard L, Gabarre J et al. 2005 Prognostic factors and outcome of human herpesvirus 8-associated primary effusion lymphoma in patients with AIDS. J Clin Oncol 23: 4372–4380
910. Carbone A, Gloghini A, Cozzi M R et al. 2000 Expression of MUM1/IRF4 selectively clusters with primary effusion lymphoma among lymphomatous effusions: implications for disease histogenesis and pathogenesis. Br J Haematol 111: 247–257
911. Knowles D M 1999 Immunodeficiency-associated lymphoproliferative disorders. Mod Pathol 12: 200–217
912. Jenner R G, Maillard K, Cattini N et al. 2003 Kaposi's sarcoma-associated herpesvirus-infected primary effusion lymphoma has a plasma cell gene expression profile. Proc Natl Acad Sci USA 100: 10399–10404
913. Klein U, Gloghini A, Gaidano G et al. 2003 Gene expression profile analysis of AIDS-related primary effusion lymphoma (PEL) suggests a plasmablastic derivation and identifies PEL-specific transcripts. Blood 101: 4115–4121
914. Fan W, Bubman D, Chadburn A et al. 2005 Distinct subsets of primary effusion lymphoma can be identified based on their cellular gene expression profile and viral association. J Virol 79: 1244–1251
915. Du M Q, Diss T C, Liu H et al. 2002 KSHV- and EBV-associated germinotropic lymphoproliferative disorder. Blood 100: 3415–3418
916. Delsol G, Lamant L, Mariame B et al. 1997 A new subtype of large B-cell lymphoma expressing the ALK kinase and lacking the 2;5 translocation. Blood 89: 1483–1490
917. Delsol G 2002 Present state of diffuse large B-cell lymphomas, including morphological variants [Abstract]. J Clin Pathol 55: A10
918. Gascoyne R D, Lamant L, Martin-Subero J I et al. 2003 ALK-positive diffuse large B-cell lymphoma is associated with Clathrin–ALK rearrangements: report of 6 cases. Blood 102: 2568–2573
919. De Paepe P, Baens M, van Krieken H et al. 2003 ALK activation by the CLTC–ALK fusion is a recurrent event in large B-cell lymphoma. Blood 102: 2638–2641
920. Adam P, Katzenberger T, Seeberger H et al. 2003 A case of a diffuse large B-cell lymphoma of plasmablastic type associated with the t(2; 5)(p23; q35) chromosome translocation. Am J Surg Pathol 27: 1473–1476
921. Onciu M, Behm F G, Downing J R et al. 2003 ALK-positive plasmablastic B-cell lymphoma with expression of the NPM–ALK fusion transcript: report of 2 cases. Blood 102: 2642–2644
922. Delecluse H J, Anagnostopoulos I, Dallenbach F et al. 1997 Plasmablastic lymphomas of the oral cavity: a new entity associated with the human immunodeficiency virus infection. Blood 89: 1413–1420
923. Carbone A, Gaidano G, Gloghini A et al. 1999 AIDS-related plasmablastic lymphomas of the oral cavity and jaws: a diagnostic dilemma. Ann Otol Rhinol Laryngol 108: 95–99
924. Dupin N, Diss T L, Kellam P et al. 2000 HHV-8 is associated with a plasmablastic variant of Castleman disease that is linked to HHV-8-positive plasmablastic lymphoma. Blood 95: 1406–1412
925. Oksenhendler E, Boulanger E, Galicier L et al. 2002 High incidence of Kaposi sarcoma-associated herpesvirus-related non-Hodgkin's lymphoma in patients with HIV infection and multicentric Castleman disease. Blood 99: 2331–2336
926. Chetty R, Hlatswayo N, Muc R et al. 2003 Plasmablastic lymphoma in HIV+ patients: an expanding spectrum. Histopathology 42: 605–609

927. Dong H Y, Scadden D T, de Leval L et al. 2005 Plasmablastic lymphoma in HIV-positive patients: an aggressive Epstein–Barr virus-associated extramedullary plasmacytic neoplasm. Am J Surg Pathol 29: 1633–1641
928. Teruya-Feldstein J, Chiao E, Filippa D A et al. 2004 CD20-negative large-cell lymphoma with plasmablastic features: a clinically heterogenous spectrum in both HIV-positive and -negative patients. Ann Oncol 15: 1673–1679
929. Verma S, Nuovo G J, Porcu P et al. 2005 Epstein–Barr virus- and human herpesvirus 8-associated primary cutaneous plasmablastic lymphoma in the setting of renal transplantation. J Cutan Pathol 32: 35–39
930. Scheper M A, Nikitakis N G, Fernandes R et al. 2005 Oral plasmablastic lymphoma in an HIV-negative patient: a case report and review of the literature. Oral Surg Oral Med Oral Pathol Oral Radiol Endod 100: 198–206
931. Simonitsch-Klupp I, Hauser I, Ott G et al. 2004 Diffuse large B-cell lymphomas with plasmablastic/plasmacytoid features are associated with TP53 deletions and poor clinical outcome. Leukemia 18: 146–155
932. Gaidano G, Cerri M, Capello D et al. 2002 Molecular histogenesis of plasmablastic lymphoma of the oral cavity. Br J Haematol 119: 622–628
933. Folk G S, Abbondanzo S L, Childers E L et al. 2006 Plasmablastic lymphoma: a clinicopathologic correlation. Ann Diagn Pathol 10: 8–12
934. Cioc A M, Allen C, Kalmar J R et al. 2004 Oral plasmablastic lymphomas in AIDS patients are associated with human herpesvirus 8. Am J Surg Pathol 28: 41–46
935. Carbone A, Gloghini A, Gaidano G 2004 Is plasmablastic lymphoma of the oral cavity an HHV-8-associated disease? Am J Surg Pathol 28: 1538–1540
936. Carbone A, Gloghini A, Vaccher E et al. 2005 KSHV/HHV-8 associated lymph node based lymphomas in HIV seronegative subjects. Report of two cases with anaplastic large cell morphology and plasmablastic immunophenotype. J Clin Pathol 58: 1039–1045
937. Lin B T, Weiss L M 1997 Primary plasmacytoma of lymph nodes. Hum Pathol 28: 1083–1090
938. Menke D M, Kyle R A, Horny H P 1993 Primary lymph node plasmacytomas (plasmacytic lymphomas). [Abstract] Mod Pathol 6: 96A
939. Hussong J W, Perkins S L, Schnitzer B et al. 1999 Extramedullary plasmacytoma. A form of marginal zone cell lymphoma? Am J Clin Pathol 111: 111–116
940. Holland J, Trenkner D A, Wasserman T H et al. 1992 Plasmacytoma. Treatment results and conversion to myeloma. Cancer 69: 1513–1517
941. Jyothirmayi R, Gangadharan V P, Nair M K et al. 1997 Radiotherapy in the treatment of solitary plasmacytoma. Br J Radiol 70: 511–516
942. Soesan M, Paccagnella A, Chiarion-Sileni V et al. 1992 Extramedullary plasmacytoma: clinical behaviour and response to treatment. Ann Oncol 3: 51–57
943. Martin P, Santon A, Bellas C 2004 Neural cell adhesion molecule expression in plasma cells in bone marrow biopsies and aspirates allows discrimination between multiple myeloma, monoclonal gammopathy of uncertain significance and polyclonal plasmacytosis. Histopathology 44: 375–380
944. Chang H, Samiee S, Yi Q L 2006 Prognostic relevance of CD56 expression in multiple myeloma: a study including 107 cases treated with high-dose melphalan-based chemotherapy and autologous stem cell transplant. Leuk Lymphoma 47: 43–47
945. Vasef M A, Medeiros L J, Yospur L S et al. 1997 Cyclin D1 protein in multiple myeloma and plasmacytoma: an immunohistochemical study using fixed, paraffin-embedded tissue sections. Mod Pathol 10: 927–932
946. Kremer M, Ott G, Nathrath M et al. 2005 Primary extramedullary plasmacytoma and multiple myeloma: phenotypic differences revealed by immunohistochemical analysis. J Pathol 205: 92–101
947. Wotherspoon A C, Norton A J, Isaacson P G 1989 Immunoreactive cytokeratins in plasmacytomas. Histopathology 14: 141–150
948. Radaszkiewicz T, Hansmann M L, Lennert K 1989 Monoclonality and polyclonality of plasma cells in Castleman's disease of the plasma cell variant. Histopathology 14: 11–24
949. Strickler J G, Audeh M W, Copenhaver C M et al. 1988 Immunophenotypic differences between plasmacytoma/multiple myeloma and immunoblastic lymphoma. Cancer 61: 1782–1786
950. Ziegler J L 1981 Burkitt's lymphoma. N Engl J Med 305: 735–743
951. Wright D H 1999 What is Burkitt's lymphoma and when is it endemic? [letter]. Blood 93: 758
952. Magrath I T, Bhatia K 1997 Pathogenesis of small noncleaved cell lymphomas (Burkitt's lymphoma). In: Magrath I (ed) The non-Hodgkin's lymphomas. Arnold, London, 385–409
953. Rowe M, Rooney C M, Rickinson A B et al. 1985 Distinctions between endemic and sporadic forms of Epstein–Barr virus-positive Burkitt's lymphoma. Int J Cancer 35: 435–441
954. Knowles D M 1996 Etiology and pathogenesis of AIDS-related non-Hodgkin's lymphoma. Hematol Oncol Clin North Am 10: 1081–1109
955. Knowles D M 1997 Molecular pathology of acquired immunodeficiency syndrome-related non-Hodgkin's lymphoma. Semin Diagn Pathol 14: 67–82
956. Lopez T M, Hagemeister F B, McLaughlin P et al. 1990 Small noncleaved cell lymphoma in adults: superior results for stages I–III disease. J Clin Oncol 8: 615–622
957. Pavlova Z, Parker J W, Taylor C R et al. 1987 Small noncleaved follicular center cell lymphoma: Burkitt's and non-Burkitt's variants in the US. II. Pathologic and immunologic features. Cancer 59: 1892–1902
958. Mann R B, Jaffe E S, Bryalan R C 1976 Non-endemic Burkitt lymphoma: a B-cell tumor related to germinal centers. N Engl J Med 295: 685–691
959. Hui P K, Feller A C, Lennert K 1988 High-grade non-Hodgkin's lymphoma of B-cell type. I. Histopathology. Histopathology 12: 127–143
960. Berard C W, O'Connor G T, Thomas L B 1969 Histopathological definition of Burkitt's tumour. Bull WHO 40: 601–607
961. Kelly D R, Nathwani B N, Griffith R C et al. 1987 A morphologic study of childhood lymphoma of the undifferentiated type. The Pediatric Oncology Group experience. Cancer 59: 1132–1137
962. Lee M H, Oliver J M, Gillooley J F 1988 Immunoglobulin inclusions in Burkitt's-like malignant lymphoma: a case report. Hum Pathol 19: 745–748
963. Hall P A, Kingston J, Stansfeld A G 1988 Extensive necrosis in malignant lymphoma with granulomatous reaction mimicking tuberculosis. Histopathology 13: 339–346
964. Hollingsworth H C, Longo D L, Jaffe E S 1993 Small noncleaved cell lymphoma associated with florid epithelioid granulomatous response. A clinicopathologic study of seven patients. Am J Surg Pathol 17: 51–59
965. Schrager J A, Pittaluga S, Raffeld M et al. 2005 Granulomatous reaction in Burkitt lymphoma: correlation with EBV positivity and clinical outcome. Am J Surg Pathol 29: 1115–1116
966. Haralambieva E, Rosati S, van Noesel C et al. 2004 Florid granulomatous reaction in Epstein–Barr virus-positive nonendemic Burkitt lymphomas: report of four cases. Am J Surg Pathol 28: 379–383
967. Diebold J, Jaffe E S, Raphael M et al. 2001 Burkitt lymphoma. In: Jaffe E S, Harris N L, Stein H et al. (eds) Pathology and genetics: tumours of haematopoietic and lymphoid tissues. World Health Organization Classification of Tumours. IARC Press, Lyon, 181–184
968. Yano T, van Krieken J H, Magrath I T et al. 1992 Histogenetic correlations between subcategories of small noncleaved cell lymphomas. Blood 79: 1282–1290
969. McClure R F, Remstein E D, Macon W R et al. 2005 Adult B-cell lymphomas with Burkitt-like morphology are phenotypically and genotypically heterogeneous with aggressive clinical behavior. Am J Surg Pathol 29: 1652–1660
970. Payne C M, Grogan T M, Cromey D W 1987 An ultrastructural, morphometric and immunophenotypic evaluation of Burkitt's and Burkitt's-like lymphomas. Lab Invest 57: 200–218
971. Garcia C F, Weiss L M, Warnke R A 1986 Small noncleaved cell lymphoma: an immunophenotypic study of 18 cases and comparison with large cell lymphoma. Hum Pathol 17: 454–461
972. Falini B, Fizzotti M, Pileri S et al. 1997 BCL-6 protein expression in normal and neoplastic lymphoid tissues. Ann Oncol 8: 101–104
973. Chapman C J, Wright D, Stevenson F K 1998 Insight into Burkitt's lymphoma from immunoglobulin variable region gene analysis. Leuk Lymphoma 30: 257–267
974. Grogan T M 1999 Morphologic, immunologic and genetic features of Burkitt's and Burkitt-like lymphomas. In: Mason D Y, Harris N L (eds) Human lymphoma: clinical implications of the REAL classification. Springer, London, 41.41–41.47
975. Taub R, Kirsch I, Morton C et al. 1982 Translocation of the c-myc gene into the immunoglobulin heavy chain locus in human Burkitt lymphoma and murine plasmacytoma cells. Proc Natl Acad Sci USA 79: 7837–7841
976. Berger R, Bernheim A 1982 Cytogenetic studies on Burkitt's lymphoma–leukemia. Cancer Genet Cytogenet 7: 231–244
977. Magrath I T, Shiramizu B 1989 Biology and treatment of small non-cleaved cell lymphoma. Oncology (Huntingt) 3: 41–53
978. Dave S S, Fu K, Wright G W et al. 2006 Molecular diagnosis of Burkitt's lymphoma. N Engl J Med 354: 2431–2442
979. Haralambieva E, Boerma E J, van Imhoff G W et al. 2005 Clinical, immunophenotypic, and genetic analysis of adult lymphomas with morphologic features of Burkitt lymphoma. Am J Surg Pathol 29: 1086–1094
980. Chan J K 1999 Peripheral T-cell and NK-cell neoplasms: an integrated approach to diagnosis. Mod Pathol 12: 177–199
981. Ascani S, Zinzani P L, Gherlinzoni F et al. 1997 Peripheral T-cell lymphomas. Clinicopathologic study of 168 cases diagnosed according to the REAL classification. Ann Oncol 8: 583–592
982. Brown D C, Heryet A, Gatter K C et al. 1989 The prognostic significance of immunophenotype in high-grade non-Hodgkin's lymphoma. Histopathology 14: 621–627
983. Lippman S M, Miller T P, Spier C M et al. 1988 The prognostic significance of the immunotype in diffuse large-cell lymphoma: a comparative study of the T-cell and B-cell phenotype. Blood 72: 436–441
984. Armitage J O, Vose J M, Linder J et al. 1989 Clinical significance of immunophenotype in diffuse aggressive non-Hodgkin's lymphoma. J Clin Oncol 7: 1783–1790
985. Coiffier B, Brousse N, Peuchmaur M et al. 1990 Peripheral T-cell lymphomas have a worse prognosis than B-cell lymphomas: a prospective study of 361 immunophenotyped patients treated with the LNH-84 regimen. The GELA (Groupe d'Etudes des Lymphomes Agressives). Ann Oncol 1: 45–50
986. Gisselbrecht C, Gaulard P, Lepage E et al. 1998 Prognostic significance of T-cell phenotype in aggressive non-Hodgkin's lymphomas. Groupe d'Etudes des Lymphomes de l'Adulte (GELA). Blood 92: 76–82
987. Catovsky D, Ralfkiaer E, Muller-Hermelink H K 2001 T-cell prolymphocytic leukaemia. In: Jaffe E S, Harris N L, Stein H et al. (eds)

988. Suchi T, Lennert K, Tu L Y et al. 1987 Histopathology and immunohistochemistry of peripheral T cell lymphomas: a proposal for their classification. J Clin Pathol 40: 995–1015
989. Osuji N, Matutes E, Catovsky D et al. 2005 Histopathology of the spleen in T-cell large granular lymphocyte leukemia and T-cell prolymphocytic leukemia: a comparative review. Am J Surg Pathol 29: 935–941
990. Agnarsson B A, Loughran T P Jr, Starkebaum G et al. 1989 The pathology of large granular lymphocyte leukemia. Hum Pathol 20: 643–651
991. Chan W C, Catovsky D, Foucar K et al. 2001 T-cell large granular lymphocyte leukaemia. In: Jaffe E S, Harris N L, Stein H et al. (eds) Pathology and genetics: tumours of haematopoietic and lymphoid tissues. World Health Organization Classification of Tumours. IARC Press, Lyon, 197–198
992. LeBoit P E 1991 Variants of mycosis fungoides and related cutaneous T-cell lymphomas. Semin Diagn Pathol 8: 73–81
993. Kim Y H, Hoppe R T 1997 Cutaneous T cell lymphomas. In: Magrath I (ed) The non-Hodgkin's lymphomas. Arnold, London, 907–926
994. Burg G, Kempf W, Smoller B et al. 2006 Mycosis fungoides. In: LeBoit P E, Burg G, Weedon D et al. (eds) Pathology and genetics. Skin tumours. World Health Organization Classification of Tumours. IARC Press, Lyon, 169–174
995. Russell-Jones R, Bernengo M, Burg G et al. 2006 Sézary syndrome. In: LeBoit P E, Burg G, Weedon D, Sarasin A (eds) Pathology and genetics. Skin tumours. World Health Organization Classification of Tumours. IARC Press, Lyon, 175–177
996. Jaffe E S 1999 Morphologic, immunologic and genetic features of peripheral T cell lymphomas (unspecified category). In: Mason D Y, Harris N L (eds) Human lymphoma: clinical implications of the REAL classification. Springer, London, 27.21–27.28
997. Armitage J O, Greer J P, Levine A M et al. 1989 Peripheral T-cell lymphoma. Cancer 63: 158–163
998. Pinkus G S, O'Hara C J, Said J W 1990 Peripheral/post-thymic T-cell lymphomas: a spectrum of disease. Clinical, pathologic, and immunologic features of 78 cases. Cancer 65: 971–998
999. Horning S J, Weiss L M, Crabtree G S et al. 1986 Clinical and phenotypic diversity of T cell lymphomas. Blood 67: 1578–1582
1000. Liang R, Todd D, Chan T K et al. 1987 Peripheral T cell lymphoma. J Clin Oncol 5: 750–755
1001. Coiffier B, Berger F, Bryon P A et al. 1988 T-cell lymphomas: immunologic, histologic, clinical, and therapeutic analysis of 63 cases. J Clin Oncol 6: 1584–1589
1002. Noorduyn L A, van der Valk P, van Heerde P et al. 1990 Stage is a better prognostic indicator than morphologic subtype in primary noncutaneous T-cell lymphoma. Am J Clin Pathol 93: 49–57
1003. Armitage J O, Carde P, Wolf M 1994 Non-Hodgkin's lymphoma: treatment of large cell lymphomas. Rev Invest Clin Suppl: 83–88
1004. Rudiger T, Weisenburger D D, Anderson J R et al. 2002 Peripheral T-cell lymphoma (excluding anaplastic large-cell lymphoma): results from the Non-Hodgkin's Lymphoma Classification Project. Ann Oncol 13: 140–149
1005. Wong K F, Chan J K 1991 Hemophagocytic disorders – a review. Hematol Rev 5: 5–37
1006. Falini B, Pileri S, De Solas I et al. 1990 Peripheral T-cell lymphoma associated with hemophagocytic syndrome. Blood 75: 434–444
1007. Jaffe E S, Costa J, Fauci AS et al. 1983 Malignant lymphoma and erythrophagocytosis simulating malignant histiocytosis. Am J Med 75: 741–749
1008. Van der Putte S C, Toonstra J, De Weger R A et al. 1982 Cutaneous T-cell lymphoma, multilobated type. Histopathology 6: 35–54
1009. Pinkus G S, Said J W, Hargreaves H 1979 Malignant lymphoma, T-cell type. A distinct morphologic variant with large multilobated nuclei, with a report of four cases. Am J Clin Pathol 72: 540–550
1010. O'Hara C J, Said J W, Pinkus G S 1986 Non-Hodgkin's lymphoma, multilobated B-cell type: report of nine cases with immunohistochemical and immunoultrastructural evidence for a follicular center cell derivation. Hum Pathol 17: 593–599
1011. Kadin M E, Kamoun M, Lamberg J 1981 Erythrophagocytic T gamma lymphoma: a clinicopathologic entity resembling malignant histiocytosis. N Engl J Med 304: 648–653
1012. Patsouris E, Engelhard M, Zwingers T et al. 1993 Lymphoepithelioid cell lymphoma (Lennert's lymphoma): clinical features derived from analysis of 108 cases. Br J Haematol 84: 346–348
1013. Patsouris E, Noel H, Lennert K 1988 Histological and immunohistological findings in lymphoepithelioid cell lymphoma (Lennert's lymphoma). Am J Surg Pathol 12: 341–350
1014. Nakamura S, Suchi T 1991 A clinicopathologic study of node-based, low-grade, peripheral T-cell lymphoma. Angioimmunoblastic lymphoma, T-zone lymphoma, and lymphoepithelioid lymphoma. Cancer 67: 2566–2578
1015. Lim M S, Straus S E, Dale J K et al. 1998 Pathological findings in human autoimmune lymphoproliferative syndrome. Am J Pathol 153: 1541–1550
1016. Weiss L M, Crabtree G S, Rouse R V et al. 1985 Morphologic and immunologic characterization of 50 peripheral T-cell lymphomas. Am J Pathol 118: 316–324
1017. Weiss L M, Wood G S, Dorfman R F 1985 T-cell signet-ring cell lymphoma. A histologic, ultrastructural, and immunohistochemical study of two cases. Am J Surg Pathol 9: 273–280
1018. Grogan T M, Richter L C, Payne C M et al. 1985 Signet-ring cell lymphoma of T-cell origin. An immunocytochemical and ultrastructural study relating giant vacuole formation to cytoplasmic sequestration of surface membrane. Am J Surg Pathol 9: 684–692
1019. Cross P A, Eyden B P, Harris M 1989 Signet ring lymphoma of T cell type. J Clin Pathol 42: 239–245
1020. Bellas C, Molina A, Montalban C et al. 1993 Signet-ring cell lymphoma of T-cell type with CD30 expression. Histopathology 22: 188–189
1021. Falini B, Liso A, Pasqualucci L et al. 1997 CD30+ anaplastic large-cell lymphoma, null type, with signet-ring appearance. Histopathology 30: 90–92
1022. Macon W R, Williams M E, Greer J P et al. 1995 Paracortical nodular T-cell lymphoma. Identification of an unusual variant of peripheral T-cell lymphoma. Am J Surg Pathol 19: 297–303
1023. de Leval L, Savilo E, Longtine J et al. 2001 Peripheral T-cell lymphoma with follicular involvement and a CD4+/BCL-6+ phenotype. Am J Surg Pathol 25: 395–400
1024. Starkey C R, Corn A I, Porensky R S et al. 2006 Peripheral T-cell lymphoma with extensive dendritic cell network mimicking follicular dendritic cell tumor: a case report with pathologic, immunophenotypic, and molecular findings. Am J Clin Pathol 126: 1–5
1025. Rudiger T, Ichinohasama R, Ott M M et al. 2000 Peripheral T-cell lymphoma with distinct perifollicular growth pattern: a distinct subtype of T-cell lymphoma? Am J Surg Pathol 24: 117–122
1026. Hanson C A, Bockenstedt P L, Schnitzer B et al. 1991 S100-positive, T-cell chronic lymphoproliferative disease: an aggressive disorder of an uncommon T-cell subset. Blood 78: 1803–1813
1027. Chan J K, Ng C S, Chu Y C et al. 1987 S100 protein-positive sinusoidal large cell lymphoma. Hum Pathol 18: 756–759
1028. Feldman A L, Pittaluga S, Jaffe E S 2006 Classification and histopathology of the lymphomas. In: Canellos G P, Lister T A, Young B (eds) The lymphomas, 2nd edn. Saunders Elsevier, Philadelphia, 2–38
1029. Arnulf B, Copie-Bergman C, Delfau-Larue M H et al. 1998 Nonhepatosplenic gammadelta T-cell lymphoma: a subset of cytotoxic lymphomas with mucosal or skin localization. Blood 91: 1723–1731
1030. Toro J R, Liewehr D J, Pabby N et al. 2003 Gamma-delta T-cell phenotype is associated with significantly decreased survival in cutaneous T-cell lymphoma. Blood 101: 3407–3412
1031. Asano N, Suzuki R, Kagami Y et al. 2005 Clinicopathologic and prognostic significance of cytotoxic molecule expression in nodal peripheral T-cell lymphoma, unspecified. Am J Surg Pathol 29: 1284–1293
1032. Jones D, Weissmann D J, Kraus M D et al. 2000 Recurrences in nodal T-cell lymphoma. Changes in histologic appearance and immunophenotype over the course of disease. Am J Clin Pathol 114: 438–447
1033. Wood K M, Pallesen G, Ralfkiaer E et al. 1993 Heterogeneity of CD3 antigen expression in T-cell lymphoma. Histopathology 22: 311–317
1034. Picker L J, Weiss L M, Medeiros L J et al. 1987 Immunophenotypic criteria for the diagnosis of non-Hodgkin's lymphoma. Am J Pathol 128: 181–201
1035. Hastrup N, Ralfkiaer E, Pallesen G 1989 Aberrant phenotypes in peripheral T cell lymphomas. J Clin Pathol 42: 398–402
1036. Jones D, Fletcher C D, Pulford K et al. 1999 The T-cell activation markers CD30 and OX40/CD134 are expressed in nonoverlapping subsets of peripheral T-cell lymphoma. Blood 93: 3487–3493
1037. Wieczorek R, Burke J S, Knowles D M D 1985 Leu-M1 antigen expression in T-cell neoplasia. Am J Pathol 121: 374–380
1038. Kagami Y, Suzuki R, Taji H et al. 1999 Nodal cytotoxic lymphoma spectrum: a clinicopathologic study of 66 patients. Am J Surg Pathol 23: 1184–1200
1039. Takeshita M, Yoshida K, Suzumiya J et al. 1999 Cases of cutaneous and nasal CD56 (NCAM)-positive lymphoma in Japan have differences in immunohistology, genotype, and etiology. Hum Pathol 30: 1024–1034
1040. Macon W R, Williams M E, Greer J P et al. 1996 Natural killer-like T-cell lymphomas: aggressive lymphomas of T-large granular lymphocytes. Blood 87: 1474–1483
1041. Quintanilla-Martinez L, Preffer F, Rubin D et al. 1994 CD20+ T-cell lymphoma. Neoplastic transformation of a normal T-cell subset. Am J Clin Pathol 102: 483–489
1042. Mohrmann R L, Arber D A 2000 CD20-positive peripheral T-cell lymphoma: report of a case after nodular sclerosis Hodgkin's disease and review of the literature. Mod Pathol 13: 1244–1252
1043. Yao X, Teruya-Feldstein J, Raffeld M et al. 2001 Peripheral T-cell lymphoma with aberrant expression of CD79a and CD20: a diagnostic pitfall. Mod Pathol 14: 105–110
1044. Yokose N, Ogata K, Sugisaki Y et al. 2001 CD20-positive T cell leukemia/lymphoma: case report and review of the literature. Ann Hematol 80: 372–375
1045. Sun T, Akalin A, Rodacker M et al. 2004 CD20 positive T cell lymphoma: is it a real entity? J Clin Pathol 57: 442–444
1046. Weiss L M, Picker L J, Grogan T M et al. 1988 Absence of clonal beta and gamma T-cell receptor gene rearrangements in a subset of peripheral T-cell lymphomas. Am J Pathol 130: 436–442
1047. Ballester B, Ramuz O, Gisselbrecht C et al. 2006 Gene expression profiling identifies molecular subgroups among nodal peripheral T-cell lymphomas. Oncogene 25: 1560–1570

1048. Anagnostopoulos I, Hummel M, Stein H 1995 Frequent presence of latent Epstein–Barr virus infection in peripheral T cell lymphomas. A review. Leuk Lymphoma 19: 1–12
1049. Ho J W, Ho F C, Chan A C et al. 1998 Frequent detection of Epstein–Barr virus-infected B cells in peripheral T-cell lymphomas. J Pathol 185: 79–85
1050. Jaffe E S, Ralfkiaer E 2001 Angioimmunoblastic T-cell lymphoma. In: Jaffe E S, Harris N L, Stein H et al. (eds) Pathology and genetics: tumours of haemaopoietic and lymphoid tissues. World Health Organization Classification of Tumours. IARC Press, Lyon, 225–226
1051. Dupuis J, Boye K, Martin N et al. 2006 Expression of CXCL13 by neoplastic cells in angioimmunoblastic T-cell lymphoma (AITL): a new diagnostic marker providing evidence that AITL derives from follicular helper T cells. Am J Surg Pathol 30: 490–494
1052. Dorfman D M, Brown J A, Shahsafaei A et al. 2006 Programmed death-1 (PD-1) is a marker of germinal center-associated T cells and angioimmunoblastic T-cell lymphoma. Am J Surg Pathol 30: 802–810
1053. Grogg K L, Attygale A D, Macon W R et al. 2006 Expression of CXCL13, a chemokine highly upregulated in germinal center T-helper cells, distinguishes angioimmunoblastic T-cell lymphoma from peripheral T-cell lymphoma, unspecified. Mod Pathol 19: 1101–1107
1054. Krenacs L, Schaerli P, Kis G et al. 2006 Phenotype of neoplastic cells in angioimmunoblastic T-cell lymphoma is consistent with activated follicular B helper T cells. Blood 108: 1110–1111
1055. Siegert W, Nerl C, Agthe A et al. 1995 Angioimmunoblastic lymphadenopathy (AILD)-type T-cell lymphoma: prognostic impact of clinical observations and laboratory findings at presentation. The Kiel Lymphoma Study Group. Ann Oncol 6: 659–664
1056. Wilson W H 1999 Clinical aspects and tratment of angioimmunoblastic T cell lymphoma (AILD). In: Mason D Y, Harris N L (eds) Human lymphoma: clinical implications of the REAL classification. Springer, London, 31.31–31.34
1057. Pautier P, Devidas A, Delmer A et al. 1999 Angioimmunoblastic-like T-cell non Hodgkin's lymphoma: outcome after chemotherapy in 33 patients and review of the literature. Leuk Lymphoma 32: 545–552
1058. Siegert W, Agthe A, Griesser H et al. 1992 Treatment of angioimmunoblastic lymphadenopathy (AILD)-type T-cell lymphoma using prednisone with or without the COPBLAM/IMVP-16 regimen. A multicenter study. Kiel Lymphoma Study Group. Ann Intern Med 117: 364–370
1059. Patsouris E, Noel H, Lennert K 1989 Angioimmunoblastic lymphadenopathy – type of T-cell lymphoma with a high content of epithelioid cells. Histopathology and comparison with lymphoepithelioid cell lymphoma. Am J Surg Pathol 13: 262–275
1060. Quintanilla-Martinez L, Fend F, Moguel L R et al. 1999 Peripheral T-cell lymphoma with Reed–Sternberg-like cells of B-cell phenotype and genotype associated with Epstein–Barr virus infection. Am J Surg Pathol 23: 1233–1240
1061. Attygalle A, Al-Jehani R, Diss T C et al. 2002 Neoplastic T cells in angioimmunoblastic T-cell lymphoma express CD10. Blood 99: 627–633
1062. Kojima M, Nakamura S, Itoh H et al. 2001 Angioimmunoblastic T-cell lymphoma with hyperplastic germinal centers: a clinicopathological and immunohistochemical study of 10 cases. Apmis 109: 699–706
1063. Ree H J, Kadin M E, Kikuchi M et al. 1998 Angioimmunoblastic lymphoma (AILD-type T-cell lymphoma) with hyperplastic germinal centers. Am J Surg Pathol 22: 643–655
1064. Lee S S, Rudiger T, Odenwald T et al. 2003 Angioimmunoblastic T cell lymphoma is derived from mature T-helper cells with varying expression and loss of detectable CD4. Int J Cancer 103: 12–20
1065. Leung C Y, Ho F C, Srivastava G et al. 1993 Usefulness of follicular dendritic cell pattern in classification of peripheral T-cell lymphomas. Histopathology 23: 433–437
1066. Yuan C M, Vergilio J A, Zhao X F et al. 2005 CD10 and BCL6 expression in the diagnosis of angioimmunoblastic T-cell lymphoma: utility of detecting CD10+ T cells by flow cytometry. Hum Pathol 36: 784–791
1067. Namikawa R, Suchi T, Ueda R et al. 1987 Phenotyping of proliferating lymphocytes in angioimmunoblastic lymphadenopathy and related lesions by the double immunoenzymatic staining technique. Am J Pathol 127: 279–287
1068. Watanabe S, Sato Y, Shimoyama M et al. 1986 Immunoblastic lymphadenopathy, angioimmunoblastic lymphadenopathy, and IBL-like T-cell lymphoma. A spectrum of T-cell neoplasia. Cancer 58: 2224–2232
1069. Tobinai K, Minato K, Ohtsu T 1988 Clinicopathologic, immunophenotypic and immunogenotypic analyses of immunoblastic lymphoadenopathy-like T-cell lymphoma. Blood 72: 1000–1006
1070. Willenbrock K, Roers A, Seidl C et al. 2001 Analysis of T-cell subpopulations in T-cell non-Hodgkin's lymphoma of angioimmunoblastic lymphadenopathy with dysproteinemia type by single target gene amplification of T cell receptor-beta gene rearrangements. Am J Pathol 158: 1851–1857
1071. Warnke R A 1999 Morphologic, immunologic and genetic features of angioimmunoblastic T cell lymphoma (AILD). In: Mason D Y, Harris N L (eds) Human lymphoma: clinical implications of the REAL classification. Springer, London, 30.31–30.35
1072. Tan B T, Warnke R A, Arber D A 2006 The frequency of B- and T-cell gene rearrangements and Epstein–Barr virus in T-cell lymphomas: a comparison between angioimmunoblastic T-cell lymphoma and peripheral T-cell lymphoma, unspecified with and without associated B-cell proliferations. J Mol Diagn 8: 466–475
1073. Schlegelberger B, Zhang Y, Weber-Matthiesen K et al. 1994 Detection of aberrant clones in nearly all cases of angioimmunoblastic lymphadenopathy with dysproteinemia-type T-cell lymphoma by combined interphase and metaphase cytogenetics. Blood 84: 2640–2648
1074. Anagnostopoulos I, Hummel M, Finn T et al. 1992 Heterogeneous Epstein–Barr virus infection patterns in peripheral T-cell lymphoma of angioimmunoblastic lymphadenopathy type. Blood 80: 1804–1812
1075. Ohshima K, Takeo H, Kikuchi M et al. 1994 Heterogeneity of Epstein–Barr virus infection in angioimmunoblastic lymphadenopathy type T-cell lymphoma. Histopathology 25: 569–579
1076. Weiss L M, Jaffe E S, Liu X F et al. 1992 Detection and localization of Epstein–Barr viral genomes in angioimmunoblastic lymphadenopathy and angioimmunoblastic lymphadenopathy-like lymphoma. Blood 79: 1789–1795
1077. Abruzzo L V, Schmidt K, Weiss L M et al. 1993 B-cell lymphoma after angioimmunoblastic lymphadenopathy: a case with oligoclonal gene rearrangements associated with Epstein–Barr virus. Blood 82: 241–246
1078. Frizzera G, Kaneko Y, Sakurai M 1989 Angioimmunoblastic lymphadenopathy and related disorders: a retrospective look in search of definitions. Leukemia 3: 1–5
1079. Weiss L M, Strickler J G, Dorfman R F et al. 1986 Clonal T-cell populations in angioimmunoblastic lymphadenopathy and angioimmunoblastic lymphadenopathy-like lymphoma. Am J Pathol 122: 392–397
1080. Feller A C, Griesser H, Schilling C V et al. 1988 Clonal gene rearrangement patterns correlate with immunophenotype and clinical parameters in patients with angioimmunoblastic lymphadenopathy. Am J Pathol 133: 549–556
1081. Lipford E H, Smith H R, Pittaluga S et al. 1987 Clonality of angioimmunoblastic lymphadenopathy and implications for its evolution to malignant lymphoma. J Clin Invest 79: 637–642
1082. Isaacson P G 1999 Intestinal (enteropathy-associated) T cell lymphoma. In: Mason D Y, Harris N L (eds) Human lymphoma: clinical implications of the REAL classification. Springer, London, 36.31–36.34
1083. Wohrer S, Chott A, Drach J et al. 2004 Chemotherapy with cyclophosphamide, doxorubicin, etoposide, vincristine and prednisone (CHOEP) is not effective in patients with enteropathy-type intestinal T-cell lymphoma. Ann Oncol 15: 1680–1683
1084. Gale J, Simmonds P D, Mead G M et al. 2000 Enteropathy-type intestinal T-cell lymphoma: clinical features and treatment of 31 patients in a single center. J Clin Oncol 18: 795–803
1085. Ashton-Key M, Diss T C, Pan L et al. 1997 Molecular analysis of T-cell clonality in ulcerative jejunitis and enteropathy-associated T-cell lymphoma. Am J Pathol 151: 493–498
1086. Bagdi E, Diss T C, Munson P et al. 1999 Mucosal intraepithelial lymphocytes in enteropathy-associated T-cell lymphoma, ulcerative jejunitis, and refractory celiac disease constitute a neoplastic population. Blood 94: 260–264
1087. Isaacson P G 1994 Gastrointestinal lymphoma. Hum Pathol 25: 1020–1029
1088. Spencer J, Cerf-Bensussan N, Jarry A et al. 1988 Enteropathy-associated T cell lymphoma (malignant histiocytosis of the intestine) is recognized by a monoclonal antibody (HML-1) that defines a membrane molecule on human mucosal lymphocytes. Am J Pathol 132: 1–5
1089. Daum S, Foss H D, Anagnostopoulos I et al. 1997 Expression of cytotoxic molecules in intestinal T-cell lymphomas. The German Study Group on Intestinal Non-Hodgkin's Lymphoma. J Pathol 182: 311–317
1090. Chott A, Haedicke W, Mosberger I et al. 1998 Most CD56+ intestinal lymphomas are CD8+CD5- T-cell lymphomas of monomorphic small to medium size histology. Am J Pathol 153: 1483–1490
1091. Daum S, Weiss D, Hummel M et al. 2001 Frequency of clonal intraepithelial T lymphocyte proliferations in enteropathy-type intestinal T cell lymphoma, coeliac disease, and refractory sprue. Gut 49: 804–812
1092. Howell W M, Leung S T, Jones D B et al. 1995 HLA-DRB, -DQA, and -DQB polymorphism in celiac disease and enteropathy-associated T-cell lymphoma. Common features and additional risk factors for malignancy. Hum Immunol 43: 29–37
1093. Zettl A, Ott G, Makulik A et al. 2002 Chromosomal gains at 9q characterize enteropathy-type T-cell lymphoma. Am J Pathol 161: 1635–1645
1094. Cejkova P, Zettl A, Baumgartner AK et al. 2005 Amplification of NOTCH1 and ABL1 gene loci is a frequent aberration in enteropathy-type T-cell lymphoma. Virchows Arch 446: 416–420
1095. Baumgartner A K, Zettl A, Chott A et al. 2003 High frequency of genetic aberrations in enteropathy-type T-cell lymphoma. Lab Invest 83: 1509–1516
1096. Obermann E C, Diss T C, Hamoudi R A et al. 2004 Loss of heterozygosity at chromosome 9p21 is a frequent finding in enteropathy-type T-cell lymphoma. J Pathol 202: 252–262
1097. Jaffe E S 1999 Subcutaneous panniculitis-like T cell lymphoma. In: Mason D Y, Harris N L (eds) Human lymphoma: clinical implications of the REAL classification. Springer, London, 34.31–34.34
1098. Jaffe E S, Burg G 2006 Subcutaneous panniculitis-like T-cell lymphoma. In: LeBoit P E, Burg G, Weedon D et al. (eds) Pathology and genetics. Skin tumours. World Health Organization Classification of Tumours. IARC Press, Lyon, 182–183

1099. Marzano A V, Berti E, Paulli M et al. 2000 Cytophagic histiocytic panniculitis and subcutaneous panniculitis-like T-cell lymphoma: report of 7 cases. Arch Dermatol 136: 889–896
1100. Kumar S, Krenacs L, Medeiros J et al. 1998 Subcutaneous panniculitic T-cell lymphoma is a tumor of cytotoxic T lymphocytes. Hum Pathol 29: 397–403
1101. Salhany K E, Macon W R, Choi J K et al. 1998 Subcutaneous panniculitis-like T-cell lymphoma: clinicopathologic, immunophenotypic, and genotypic analysis of alpha/beta and gamma/delta subtypes. Am J Surg Pathol 22: 881–893
1102. Gonzalez C L, Medeiros L J, Braziel R M et al. 1991 T-cell lymphoma involving subcutaneous tissue. A clinicopathologic entity commonly associated with hemophagocytic syndrome. Am J Surg Pathol 15: 17–27
1103. Perniciaro C, Zalla M J, White J W et al. 1993 Subcutaneous T-cell lymphoma: report of two additional cases and further observations. Arch Dermatol 129: 1171–1176
1104. Hoque S R, Child F J, Whittaker S J et al. 2003 Subcutaneous panniculitis-like T-cell lymphoma: a clinicopathological, immunophenotypic and molecular analysis of six patients. Br J Dermatol 148: 516–525
1105. Weenig R H, Ng C S, Perniciaro C 2001 Subcutaneous panniculitis-like T-cell lymphoma: an elusive case presenting as lipomembranous panniculitis and a review of 72 cases in the literature. Am J Dermatopathol 23: 206–215
1106. Krenacs L, Smyth M J, Bagdi E et al. 2003 The serine protease granzyme M is preferentially expressed in NK-cell, gamma delta T-cell, and intestinal T-cell lymphomas: evidence of origin from lymphocytes involved in innate immunity. Blood 101: 3590–3593
1107. Stein H, Mason D Y, Gerdes J et al. 1985 The expression of the Hodgkin's disease associated antigen Ki-1 in reactive and neoplastic lymphoid tissue: evidence that Reed–Sternberg cells and histiocytic malignancies are derived from activated lymphoid cells. Blood 66: 848–858
1108. Chan J K, Ng C S, Hui P K et al. 1989 Anaplastic large cell Ki-1 lymphoma. Delineation of two morphological types. Histopathology 15: 11–34
1109. Agnarsson B A, Kadin M E 1988 Ki-1 positive large cell lymphoma. A morphologic and immunologic study of 19 cases. Am J Surg Pathol 12: 264–274
1110. Chott A, Kaserer K, Augustin I et al. 1990 Ki-1-positive large cell lymphoma. A clinicopathologic study of 41 cases. Am J Surg Pathol 14: 439–448
1111. Stein H, Foss H D, Durkop H et al. 2000 CD30(+) anaplastic large cell lymphoma: a review of its histopathologic, genetic, and clinical features. Blood 96: 3681–3695
1112. Foss H D, Anagnostopoulos I, Araujo I et al. 1996 Anaplastic large-cell lymphomas of T-cell and null-cell phenotype express cytotoxic molecules. Blood 88: 4005–4011
1113. Krenacs L, Wellmann A, Sorbara L et al. 1997 Cytotoxic cell antigen expression in anaplastic large cell lymphomas of T- and null-cell type and Hodgkin's disease: evidence for distinct cellular origin. Blood 89: 980–989
1114. Chan J K 1998 Anaplastic large cell lymphoma: redefining its morphologic spectrum and importance of recognition of the ALK-positive subset. Adv Anat Pathol 5: 281–313
1115. Weisenburger D D, Anderson J R, Diebold J et al. 2001 Systemic anaplastic large-cell lymphoma: results from the non-Hodgkin's lymphoma classification project. Am J Hematol 67: 172–178
1116. Schwarting R, Gerdes J, Durkop H et al. 1989 Ber-H2: a new anti-Ki-1 (CD30) monoclonal antibody directed at a formol-resistant epitope. Blood 74: 1678–1689
1117. Schnitzer B, Roth M S, Hyder D M et al. 1988 Ki-1 lymphomas in children. Cancer 61: 1213–1221
1118. Nakamura S, Takagi N, Kojima M et al. 1991 Clinicopathologic study of large cell anaplastic lymphoma (Ki-1-positive large cell lymphoma) among the Japanese. Cancer 68: 118–129
1119. Kadin M E, Sako D, Berliner N et al. 1986 Childhood Ki-1 lymphoma presenting with skin lesions and peripheral lymphadenopathy. Blood 68: 1042–1049
1120. Salhany K E, Collins R D, Greer J P et al. 1991 Long-term survival in Ki-1 lymphoma. Cancer 67: 516–522
1121. Bitter M A, Franklin W A, Larson R A et al. 1990 Morphology in Ki-1(CD30)-positive non-Hodgkin's lymphoma is correlated with clinical features and the presence of a unique chromosomal abnormality, t(2; 5)(p23; q35). Am J Surg Pathol 14: 305–316
1122. Penny R J, Blaustein J C, Longtine J A et al. 1991 Ki-1-positive large cell lymphomas, a heterogenous group of neoplasms. Morphologic, immunophenotypic, genotypic, and clinical features of 24 cases. Cancer 68: 362–373
1123. Kinney M C, Greer J P, Glick A D et al. 1991 Anaplastic large-cell Ki-1 malignant lymphomas. Recognition, biological and clinical implications. Pathol Annu 26: 1–24
1124. Williams D M, Hobson R, Imeson J et al. 2002 Anaplastic large cell lymphoma in childhood: analysis of 72 patients treated on The United Kingdom Children's Cancer Study Group chemotherapy regimens. Br J Haematol 117: 812–820
1125. Wong K F, Chan J K, Ng C S et al. 1991 Anaplastic large cell Ki-1 lymphoma involving bone marrow: marrow findings and association with reactive hemophagocytosis. Am J Hematol 37: 112–119
1126. Fraga M, Brousset P, Schlaifer D et al. 1995 Bone marrow involvement in anaplastic large cell lymphoma. Immunohistochemical detection of minimal disease and its prognostic significance. Am J Clin Pathol 103: 82–89
1127. Benharroch D, Meguerian-Bedoyan Z, Lamant L et al. 1998 ALK-positive lymphoma: a single disease with a broad spectrum of morphology. Blood 91: 2076–2084
1128. Falini B, Pileri S, Zinzani P L et al. 1999 ALK+ lymphoma: clinicopathological findings and outcome. Blood 93: 2697–2706
1129. Falini B, Bigerna B, Fizzotti M et al. 1998 ALK expression defines a distinct group of T/null lymphomas ('ALK lymphomas') with a wide morphological spectrum. Am J Pathol 153: 875–886
1130. Falini B, Pulford K, Pucciarini A et al. 1999 Lymphomas expressing ALK fusion protein(s) other than NPM–ALK. Blood 94: 3509–3515
1131. Nakamura S, Shiota M, Nakagawa A et al. 1997 Anaplastic large cell lymphoma: a distinct molecular pathologic entity: a reappraisal with special reference to p80(NPM/ALK) expression. Am J Surg Pathol 21: 1420–1432
1132. Shiota M, Nakamura S, Ichinohasama R et al. 1995 Anaplastic large cell lymphoma expressing the novel chimeric protein p80NPM/ALK: a distinct clinicopathologic entity. Blood 86: 1954–1960
1133. Shiota M, Mori S 1996 The clinicopathological features of anaplastic large cell lymphomas expressing p80NPM/ALK. Leuk Lymphoma 23: 25–32
1134. Shiota M, Mori S 1997 Anaplastic large cell lymphomas expressing the novel chimeric protein p80NPM/ALK: a distinct clinicopathologic entity. Leukemia 11 Suppl 3: 538–540
1135. Aoun P, Greiner T, Vose J et al. 1998 Anaplastic lymphoma kinase (ALK): an important predictor of survival in peripheral T-cell lymphoma. [Abstract]. Mod Pathol 11: 125A
1136. Gascoyne R D, Aoun P, Wu D et al. 1999 Prognostic significance of anaplastic lymphoma kinase (ALK) protein expression in adults with anaplastic large cell lymphoma. Blood 93: 3913–3921
1137. Brugieres L, Deley M C, Pacquement H et al. 1998 CD30(+) anaplastic large-cell lymphoma in children: analysis of 82 patients enrolled in two consecutive studies of the French Society of Pediatric Oncology. Blood 92: 3591–3598
1138. Jaffe E S 2001 Anaplastic large cell lymphoma: the shifting sands of diagnostic hematopathology. Mod Pathol 14: 219–228
1139. Onciu M, Behm F G, Raimondi S C et al. 2003 ALK-positive anaplastic large cell lymphoma with leukemic peripheral blood involvement is a clinicopathologic entity with an unfavorable prognosis. Report of three cases and review of the literature. Am J Clin Pathol 120: 617–625
1140. ten Berge R L, de Bruin P C, Oudejans J J et al. 2003 ALK-negative anaplastic large-cell lymphoma demonstrates similar poor prognosis to peripheral T-cell lymphoma, unspecified. Histopathology 43: 462–469
1141. Vassallo J, Lamant L, Brugieres L et al. 2006 ALK-positive anaplastic large cell lymphoma mimicking nodular sclerosis Hodgkin's lymphoma: report of 10 cases. Am J Surg Pathol 30: 223–229
1142. Mann K P, Hall B, Kamino H et al. 1995 Neutrophil-rich, Ki-1-positive anaplastic large-cell malignant lymphoma. Am J Surg Pathol 19: 407–416
1143. McCluggage W G, Walsh M Y, Bharucha H 1998 Anaplastic large cell malignant lymphoma with extensive eosinophilic or neutrophilic infiltration. Histopathology 32: 110–115
1144. Pileri S, Falini B, Delsol G et al. 1990 Lymphohistiocytic T-cell lymphoma (anaplastic large cell lymphoma CD30+/Ki-1 + with a high content of reactive histiocytes). Histopathology 16: 383–391
1145. Pileri S A, Falini B, Mori S et al. 1997 Frequent expression of the NPM–ALK chimeric fusion protein in anaplastic large-cell lymphoma, lymphohistiocytic type. Am J Pathol 150: 1207–1211
1146. Ott G, Bastian B C, Katzenberger T et al. 1998 A lymphohistiocytic variant of anaplastic large cell lymphoma with demonstration of the t(2; 5)(p23; q35) chromosome translocation. Br J Haematol 100: 187–190
1147. Kinney M C, Collins R D, Greer J P et al. 1993 A small-cell-predominant variant of primary Ki-1 (CD30)+ T-cell lymphoma. Am J Surg Pathol 17: 859–868
1148. Hodges K B, Collins R D, Greer J P et al. 1999 Transformation of the small cell variant Ki-1+ lymphoma to anaplastic large cell lymphoma: pathologic and clinical features. Am J Surg Pathol 23: 49–58
1149. Cheuk W, Hill R W, Bacchi C et al. 2000 Hypocellular anaplastic large cell lymphoma mimicking inflammatory lesions of lymph nodes. Am J Surg Pathol 24: 1537–1543
1150. Chan J K, Buchanan R, Fletcher C D 1990 Sarcomatoid variant of anaplastic large-cell Ki-1 lymphoma. Am J Surg Pathol 14: 983–988
1151. Delsol G, Al Saati T, Gatter K C et al. 1988 Coexpression of epithelial membrane antigen (EMA), Ki-1, and interleukin-2 receptor by anaplastic large cell lymphomas. Diagnostic value in so-called malignant histiocytosis. Am J Pathol 130: 59–70
1152. Felgar R E, Salhany K E, Macon W R et al. 1999 The expression of TIA-1+ cytolytic-type granules and other cytolytic lymphocyte-associated markers in CD30+ anaplastic large cell lymphomas (ALCL): correlation with morphology, immunophenotype, ultrastructure, and clinical features. Hum Pathol 30: 228–236
1153. Foss H D, Demel G, Anagnostopoulos I et al. 1997 Uniform expression of cytotoxic molecules in anaplastic large cell lymphoma of null/T cell phenotype and in cell lines derived from anaplastic large cell lymphoma. Pathobiology 65: 83–90

1154. Dukers D F, ten Berge R L, Oudejans J J et al. 1999 A cytotoxic phenotype does not predict clinical outcome in anaplastic large cell lymphomas. J Clin Pathol 52: 129–136
1155. Lae M E, Ahmed I, Macon W R 2002 Clusterin is widely expressed in systemic anaplastic large cell lymphoma but fails to differentiate primary from secondary cutaneous anaplastic large cell lymphoma. Am J Clin Pathol 118: 773–779
1156. Nascimento A F, Pinkus J L, Pinkus G S 2004 Clusterin, a marker for anaplastic large cell lymphoma: immunohistochemical profile in hematopoietic and nonhematopoietic malignant neoplasms. Am J Clin Pathol 121: 709–717
1157. Wellmann A, Thieblemont C, Pittaluga S et al. 2000 Detection of differentially expressed genes in lymphomas using cDNA arrays: identification of clusterin as a new diagnostic marker for anaplastic large-cell lymphomas. Blood 96: 398–404
1158. Hall P A, d'Ardenne A J, Stansfeld A G 1988 Paraffin section immunohistochemistry. II. Hodgkin's disease and large cell anaplastic (Ki-1) lymphoma. Histopathology 13: 161–169
1159. Suzuki R, Kagami Y, Takeuchi K et al. 2000 Prognostic significance of CD56 expression for ALK-positive and ALK-negative anaplastic large-cell lymphoma of T/null cell phenotype. Blood 96: 2993–3000
1160. Falini B, Pileri S, Stein H et al. 1990 Variable expression of leucocyte common (CD45) antigen in CD30 (Ki-1)-positive anaplastic large-cell lymphoma: implications for the differential diagnosis between lymphoid and nonlymphoid malignancies. Hum Pathol 21: 624–629
1161. Gustmann C, Altmannsberger M, Osborn M et al. 1991 Cytokeratin expression and vimentin content in large cell anaplastic lymphomas and other non-Hodgkin's lymphomas. Am J Pathol 138: 1413–1422
1162. Mason D Y, Bastard C, Rimokh R et al. 1990 CD30-positive large cell lymphomas ('Ki-1 lymphoma') are associated with a chromosomal translocation involving 5q35. Br J Haematol 74: 161–168
1163. Morris S W, Kirstein M N, Valentine M B et al. 1994 Fusion of a kinase gene, ALK, to a nucleolar protein gene, NPM, in non-Hodgkin's lymphoma. Science 263: 1281–1284
1164. Morris S W, Naeve C, Mathew P et al. 1997 ALK, the chromosome 2 gene locus altered by the t(2; 5) in non-Hodgkin's lymphoma, encodes a novel neural receptor tyrosine kinase that is highly related to leukocyte tyrosine kinase (LTK). Oncogene 14: 2175–2188
1165. Ladanyi M, Cavalchire G 1996 Molecular variant of the NPM–ALK rearrangement of Ki-1 lymphoma involving a cryptic ALK splice site. Genes Chromos Cancer 15: 173–177
1166. Wlodarska I, De Wolf-Peeters C, Michaux L et al. 1995 A new t(2; 5) translocation in a null cell type CD30 positive anaplastic large cell lymphoma case. Leukemia 9: 1685–1688
1167. Wlodarska I, De Wolf-Peeters C, Falini B et al. 1998 The cryptic inv(2)(p23q35) defines a new molecular genetic subtype of ALK-positive anaplastic large-cell lymphoma. Blood 92: 2688–2695
1168. Hernandez L, Pinyol M, Hernandez S et al. 1999 TRK-fused gene (TFG) is a new partner of ALK in anaplastic large cell lymphoma producing two structurally different TFG–ALK translocations. Blood 94: 3265–3268
1169. Lamant L, Dastugue N, Pulford K et al. 1999 A new fusion gene TPM3–ALK in anaplastic large cell lymphoma created by a (1; 2)(q25; p23) translocation. Blood 93: 3088–3095
1170. Pittaluga S, Wiodarska I, Pulford K et al. 1997 The monoclonal antibody ALK1 identifies a distinct morphological subtype of anaplastic large cell lymphoma associated with 2p23/ALK rearrangements. Am J Pathol 151: 343–351
1171. Tort F, Pinyol M, Pulford K et al. 2001 Molecular characterization of a new ALK translocation involving moesin (MSN–ALK) in anaplastic large cell lymphoma. Lab Invest 81: 419–426
1172. Thompson M A, Stumph J, Henrickson S E et al. 2005 Differential gene expression in anaplastic lymphoma kinase-positive and anaplastic lymphoma kinase-negative anaplastic large cell lymphomas. Hum Pathol 36: 494–504
1173. Zettl A, Rudiger T, Konrad M A et al. 2004 Genomic profiling of peripheral T-cell lymphoma, unspecified, and anaplastic large T-cell lymphoma delineates novel recurrent chromosomal alterations. Am J Pathol 164: 1837–1848
1174. Agarwal S, Ramanathan U, Naresh K N 2002 Epstein–Barr virus association and ALK gene expression in anaplastic large-cell lymphoma. Hum Pathol 33: 146–152
1175. Herling M, Rassidakis G Z, Jones D et al. 2004 Absence of Epstein–Barr virus in anaplastic large cell lymphoma: a study of 64 cases classified according to World Health Organization criteria. Hum Pathol 35: 455–459
1176. Chan J K 2000 The perivascular cuff of large lymphoid cells: a clue to diagnosis of anaplastic large cell lymphoma. Int J Surg Pathol 8: 153–156
1177. Willemze R, Jaffe E S, Burg G et al. 2005 WHO–EORTC classification for cutaneous lymphomas. Blood 105: 3768–3785
1178. Paulli M, Berti E, Rosso R et al. 1995 CD30/Ki-1-positive lymphoproliferative disorders of the skin – clinicopathologic correlation and statistical analysis of 86 cases: a multicentric study from the European Organization for Research and Treatment of Cancer Cutaneous Lymphoma Project Group. J Clin Oncol 13: 1343–1354
1179. Vergier B, Beylot-Barry M, Pulford K et al. 1998 Statistical evaluation of diagnostic and prognostic features of CD30+ cutaneous lymphoproliferative disorders: a clinicopathologic study of 65 cases. Am J Surg Pathol 22: 1192–1202
1180. Bekkenk M W, Geelen F A, van Voorst Vader P C et al. 2000 Primary and secondary cutaneous CD30(+) lymphoproliferative disorders: a report from the Dutch Cutaneous Lymphoma Group on the long-term follow-up data of 219 patients and guidelines for diagnosis and treatment. Blood 95: 3653–3661
1181. de Bruin P C, Beljaards R C, van Heerde P et al. 1993 Differences in clinical behaviour and immunophenotype between primary cutaneous and primary nodal anaplastic large cell lymphoma of T-cell or null cell phenotype. Histopathology 23: 127–135
1182. Willemze R, Meijer C J 1999 EORTC classification for primary cutaneous lymphomas: the best guide to good clinical management. European Organization for Research and Treatment of Cancer. Am J Dermatopathol 21: 265–273
1183. Willemze R, Kerl H, Sterry W et al. 1997 EORTC classification for primary cutaneous lymphomas: a proposal from the Cutaneous Lymphoma Study Group of the European Organization for Research and Treatment of Cancer. Blood 90: 354–371
1184. Willemze R, Beljaards R C 1993 Spectrum of primary cutaneous CD30 (Ki-1)-positive lymphoproliferative disorders. J Am Acad Dermatol 28: 973–980
1185. Mori M, Manuelli C, Pimpinelli N et al. 1999 CD30–CD30 ligand interaction in primary cutaneous CD30(+) T-cell lymphomas: A clue to the pathophysiology of clinical regression. Blood 94: 3077–3083
1186. Alobeid B, Pan L X, Milligan L et al. 2004 Eosinophil-rich CD30+ lymphoproliferative disorder of the oral mucosa. A form of 'traumatic eosinophilic granuloma.' Am J Clin Pathol 121: 43–50
1187. Weiss L M, Wood G S, Trela M et al. 1986 Clonal T-cell populations in lymphomatoid papulosis. Evidence of a lymphoproliferative origin for a clinically benign disease. N Engl J Med 315: 475–479
1188. Willemze R, Beljaards R C, Meijer C J 1994 Classification of primary cutaneous T-cell lymphomas. Histopathology 24: 405–415
1189. Kikuchi M, Jaffe E S, Ralfkiaer E 2001 Adult T-cell leukaemia/lymphoma. In: Jaffe E S, Harris N L, Stein H et al. (eds) Pathology and genetics: tumours of haematopoietic and lymphoid tissues. World Health Organization Classification of Tumours. IARC Press, Lyon, 200–203
1190. Ohshima K, Kikuchi M, Yoshida T et al. 1991 Lymph nodes in incipient adult T-cell leukaemia–lymphoma with Hodgkin's disease-like histologic features. Cancer 67: 1622–1628
1191. Chan J K 1998 Natural killer cell neoplasms. Adv Anat Pathol 3: 77–145
1192. Jaffe E S, Berard C W 1978 Lymphoblastic lymphoma, a term rekindled with new precision. Ann Intern Med 89: 415–417
1193. Jaffe E S 1995 Nasal and nasal-type T/NK cell lymphoma: a unique form of lymphoma associated with the Epstein–Barr virus. Histopathology 27: 581–583
1194. Jaffe E S, Chan J K, Su I J et al. 1996 Report of the Workshop on Nasal and Related Extranodal Angiocentric T/Natural Killer Cell Lymphomas. Definitions, differential diagnosis, and epidemiology. Am J Surg Pathol 20: 103–111
1195. Jaffe E S 1996 Classification of natural killer (NK) cell and NK-like T-cell malignancies. Blood 87: 1207–1210
1196. Chan J K, Jaffe E S, Ralfkiaer E 2001 Extranodal NK/T-cell lymphoma, nasal type. In: Jaffe E S, Harris N L, Stein H et al. (eds) Pathology and genetics: tumours of haematopoietic and lymphoid tissues. World Health Organization Classification of Tumours. IARC Press, Lyon, 204–207
1197. Chim C S, Ma E S, Loong F et al. 2005 Diagnostic cues for natural killer cell lymphoma: primary nodal presentation and the role of in situ hybridisation for Epstein–Barr virus encoded early small RNA in detecting occult bone marrow involvement. J Clin Pathol 58: 443–445
1198. Chan W C, Zaatari G 1986 Lymph node interdigitating reticulum cell sarcoma. Am J Clin Pathol 85: 739–744
1199. Chan J K, Sin V C, Wong K F et al. 1997 Nonnasal lymphoma expressing the natural killer cell marker CD56: a clinicopathologic study of 49 cases of an uncommon aggressive neoplasm. Blood 89: 4501–4513
1200. Cheung M M, Chan J K, Lau W H et al. 1998 Primary non-Hodgkin's lymphoma of the nose and nasopharynx: clinical features, tumor immunophenotype, and treatment outcome in 113 patients. J Clin Oncol 16: 70–77
1201. Nakamura S, Suchi T, Koshikawa T et al. 1995 Clinicopathologic study of CD56 (NCAM)-positive angiocentric lymphoma occurring in sites other than the upper and lower respiratory tract. Am J Surg Pathol 19: 284–296
1202. Wong K F, Chan J K, Ng C S et al. 1992 CD56 (NKH1)-positive hematolymphoid malignancies: an aggressive neoplasm featuring frequent cutaneous/mucosal involvement, cytoplasmic azurophilic granules, and angiocentricity. Hum Pathol 23: 798–804
1203. Nitta Y, Iwatsuki K, Kimura H et al. 2005 Fatal natural killer cell lymphoma arising in a patient with a crop of Epstein–Barr virus-associated disorders. Eur J Dermatol 15: 503–506
1204. Hoshida Y, Li T, Dong Z et al. 2001 Lymphoproliferative disorders in renal transplant patients in Japan. Int J Cancer 91: 869–875
1205. Hoshida Y, Hongyo T, Nakatsuka S et al. 2002 Gene mutations in lymphoproliferative disorders of T and NK/T cell phenotypes developing in renal transplant patients. Lab Invest 82: 257–264
1206. Kwong Y L, Lam C C, Chan T M 2000 Post-transplantation lymphoproliferative disease of natural killer cell lineage: a clinicopathological and molecular analysis. Br J Haematol 110: 197–202

1207. Takahashi N, Miura I, Chubachi A et al. 2001 A clinicopathological study of 20 patients with T/natural killer (NK)-cell lymphoma-associated hemophagocytic syndrome with special reference to nasal and nasal-type NK/T-cell lymphoma. Int J Hematol 74: 303–308

1208. You J Y, Chi K H, Yang M H et al. 2004 Radiation therapy versus chemotherapy as initial treatment for localized nasal natural killer (NK)/T-cell lymphoma: a single institute survey in Taiwan. Ann Oncol 15: 618–625

1209. Cheung M M, Chan J K, Wong K F 2003 Natural killer cell neoplasms: a distinctive group of highly aggressive lymphomas/leukemias. Semin Hematol 40: 221–232

1210. Ribrag V, Ell Hajj M, Janot F et al. 2001 Early locoregional high-dose radiotherapy is associated with long-term disease control in localized primary angiocentric lymphoma of the nose and nasopharynx. Leukemia 15: 1123–1126

1211. Egashira M, Kawamata N, Sugimoto K et al. 1999 P-glycoprotein expression on normal and abnormally expanded natural killer cells and inhibition of P-glycoprotein function by ciclosporin A and its analogue, PSC833. Blood 93: 599–606

1212. Nagafuji K, Fujisaki T, Arima F et al. 2001 L-Asparaginase induced durable remission of relapsed nasal NK/T-cell lymphoma after autologous peripheral blood stem cell transplantation. Int J Hematol 74: 447–450

1213. Kwong Y L 2005 Natural killer-cell malignancies: diagnosis and treatment. Leukemia 19: 2186–2194

1214. Liang R, Todd D, Chan T K et al. 1995 Treatment outcome and prognostic factors for primary nasal lymphoma. J Clin Oncol 13: 666–670

1215. Chim C S, Ma S Y, Au W Y et al. 2004 Primary nasal natural killer cell lymphoma: long-term treatment outcome and relationship with the International Prognostic Index. Blood 103: 216–221

1216. Li Y X, Yao B, Jin J et al. 2006 Radiotherapy as primary treatment for stage IE and IIE nasal natural killer/T-cell lymphoma. J Clin Oncol 24: 181–189

1217. Chan J K, Ng C S, Lau W H, Lo S T 1987 Most nasal/nasopharyngeal lymphomas are peripheral T-cell neoplasms. Am J Surg Pathol 11: 418–429

1218. Chan J K, Tsang W Y, Pau M Y 1995 Discordant CD3 expression in lymphomas when studied on frozen and paraffin sections. Hum Pathol 26: 1139–1143

1219. Tsang W Y, Chan J K, Ng C S et al. 1996 Utility of a paraffin section-reactive CD56 antibody (123C3) for characterization and diagnosis of lymphomas. Am J Surg Pathol 20: 202–210

1220. Emile J F, Boulland M L, Haioun C et al. 1996 CD5−CD56+ T-cell receptor silent peripheral T-cell lymphomas are natural killer cell lymphomas. Blood 87: 1466–1473

1221. Kanavaros P, Lescs M C, Briere J et al. 1993 Nasal T-cell lymphoma: a clinicopathologic entity associated with peculiar phenotype and with Epstein–Barr virus. Blood 81: 2688–2695

1222. Ng C S, Lo S T, Chan J K et al. 1997 CD56+ putative natural killer cell lymphomas: production of cytolytic effectors and related proteins mediating tumor cell apoptosis? Hum Pathol 28: 1276–1282

1223. Ohshima K, Suzumiya J, Shimazaki K et al. 1997 Nasal T/NK cell lymphomas commonly express perforin and Fas ligand: important mediators of tissue damage. Histopathology 31: 444–450

1224. Ng C S, Lo S T, Chan J K 1999 Peripheral T and putative natural killer cell lymphomas commonly coexpress CD95 and CD95 ligand. Hum Pathol 30: 48–53

1225. Sawada A, Sato E, Koyama M et al. 2006 NK-cell repertoire is feasible for diagnosing Epstein–Barr virus-infected NK-cell lymphoproliferative disease and evaluating the treatment effect. Am J Hematol 81: 576–581

1226. Mori K L, Egashira M, Oshimi K 2001 Differentiation stage of natural killer cell-lineage lymphoproliferative disorders based on phenotypic analysis. Br J Haematol 115: 225–228

1227. Haedicke W, Ho F C, Chott A et al. 2000 Expression of CD94/NKG2A and killer immunoglobulin-like receptors in NK cells and a subset of extranodal cytotoxic T-cell lymphomas. Blood 95: 3628–3630

1228. Dukers D F, Vermeer M H, Jaspars L H et al. 2001 Expression of killer cell inhibitory receptors is restricted to true NK cell lymphomas and a subset of intestinal enteropathy-type T cell lymphomas with a cytotoxic phenotype. J Clin Pathol 54: 224–228

1229. Tsang W Y, Chan J K, Yip T T et al. 1994 In situ localization of Epstein–Barr virus encoded RNA in non-nasal/nasopharyngeal CD56-positive and CD56-negative T-cell lymphomas. Hum Pathol 25: 758–765

1230. Chan J K, Yip T T, Tsang W Y et al. 1994 Detection of Epstein–Barr viral RNA in malignant lymphomas of the upper aerodigestive tract. Am J Surg Pathol 18: 938–946

1231. Siu L L, Wong K F, Chan J K et al. 1999 Comparative genomic hybridization analysis of natural killer cell lymphoma/leukemia. Recognition of consistent patterns of genetic alterations. Am J Pathol 155: 1419–1425

1232. Wong K F, Chan J K, Kwong Y L 1997 Identification of del(6)(q21q25) as a recurring chromosomal abnormality in putative NK cell lymphoma/leukaemia. Br J Haematol 98: 922–926

1233. Wong K F, Zhang Y M, Chan J K 1999 Cytogenetic abnormalities in natural killer cell lymphoma/leukaemia – is there a consistent pattern? Leuk Lymphoma 34: 241–250

1234. Nakashima Y, Tagawa H, Suzuki R et al. 2005 Genome-wide array-based comparative genomic hybridization of natural killer cell lymphoma/leukemia: different genomic alteration patterns of aggressive NK-cell leukemia and extranodal Nk/T-cell lymphoma, nasal type. Genes Chromos Cancer 44: 247–255

1235. Kwong Y L, Chan A C, Liang R H 1997 Natural killer cell lymphoma/leukemia: pathology and treatment. Hematol Oncol 15: 71–79

1236. Imamura N, Kusunoki Y, Kawa-Ha K et al. 1990 Aggressive natural killer cell leukaemia/lymphoma: report of four cases and review of the literature. Possible existence of a new clinical entity originating from the third lineage of lymphoid cells. Br J Haematol 75: 49–59

1237. Oshimi K 1996 Lymphoproliferative disorders of natural killer cells. Int J Hematol 63: 279–290

1238. Oshimi K, Yamada O, Kaneko T et al. 1993 Laboratory findings and clinical courses of 33 patients with granular lymphocyte-proliferative disorders. Leukemia 7: 782–788

1239. Hamaguchi H, Yamaguchi M, Nagata K et al. 2001 Aggressive NK cell lymphoma/leukemia with clonal der(3)t(1; 3) (q12; p25), del(6)(q13) and del(13)(q12q14). Cancer Genet Cytogenet 130: 150–154

1240. Suzuki R, Suzumiya J, Nakamura S et al. 2004 Aggressive natural killer-cell leukemia revisited: large granular lymphocyte leukemia of cytotoxic NK cells. Leukemia 18: 763–770

1241. Chan J K, Wong K F, Jaffe E S et al. 2001 Aggressive NK-cell leukaemia. In: Jaffe E S, Harris N L, Stein H et al. (eds) Pathology and genetics: tumours of haematopoietic and lymphoid tissues. World Health Organization Classification of Tumours. IARC Press, Lyon, 198–200

1242. Murdock J, Jaffe E S, Wilson W H et al. 2004 Aggressive natural killer cell leukemia/lymphoma: case report, use of telesynergy and review of the literature. Leuk Lymphoma 45: 1269–1273

1243. Song S Y, Kim W S, Ko Y H et al. 2002 Aggressive natural killer cell leukemia: clinical features and treatment outcome. Haematologica 87: 1343–1345

1244. Rabbani G R, Phyliky R L, Tefferi A 1999 A long-term study of patients with chronic natural killer cell lymphocytosis. Br J Haematol 106: 960–966

1245. Chan J K, Jaffe E S, Ralfkiaer E 2001 Blastic NK-cell lymphoma. In: Jaffe E S, Harris N L, Stein H et al. (eds) Pathology and genetics: tumours of haematopoietic and lymphoid tissues. World Health Organization Classification of Tumours. IARC Press, Lyon, 214–215

1246. Petrella T, Dalac S, Maynadie M et al. 1999 CD4+ CD56+ cutaneous neoplasms: a distinct hematological entity? Groupe Francais d'Etude des Lymphomes Cutanes (GFELC). Am J Surg Pathol 23: 137–146

1247. Petrella T, Bagot M, Willemze R et al. 2005 Blastic NK-cell lymphomas (agranular CD4+CD56+ hematodermic neoplasms): a review. Am J Clin Pathol 123: 662–675

1248. Reichard K K, Burks E J, Foucar M K et al. 2005 CD4(+) CD56(+) lineage-negative malignancies are rare tumors of plasmacytoid dendritic cells. Am J Surg Pathol 29: 1274–1283

1249. Jacob M C, Chaperot L, Mossuz P et al. 2003 CD4+ CD56+ lineage negative malignancies: a new entity developed from malignant early plasmacytoid dendritic cells. Haematologica 88: 941–955

1250. Karube K, Ohshima K, Tsuchiya T et al. 2003 Non-B, non-T neoplasms with lymphoblast morphology: further clarification and classification. Am J Surg Pathol 27: 1366–1374

1251. Kobashi Y, Nakamura S, Sasajima Y et al. 1996 Inconsistent association of Epstein–Barr virus with CD56 (NCAM)-positive angiocentric lymphoma occuring in sites other than the upper and lower respiratory tract. Histopathology 28: 111–120

1252. DiGiuseppe J A, Louie D C, Williams J E et al. 1997 Blastic natural killer cell leukemia/lymphoma: a clinicopathologic study. Am J Surg Pathol 21: 1223–1230

1253. Nakamura S, Katoh E, Koshikawa T et al. 1997 Clinicopathologic study of nasal T/NK-cell lymphoma among the Japanese. Pathol Int 47: 38–53

1254. Bayerl M G, Rakozy C K, Mohamed A N et al. 2002 Blastic natural killer cell lymphoma/leukemia: a report of seven cases. Am J Clin Pathol 117: 41–50

1255. Suzuki R, Nakamura S, Suzumiya J et al. 2005 Blastic natural killer cell lymphoma/leukemia (CD56-positive blastic tumor): prognostication and categorization according to anatomic sites of involvement. Cancer 104: 1022–1031

1256. Ng A P, Lade S, Rutherford T et al. 2006 Primary cutaneous CD4+/CD56+ hematodermic neoplasm (blastic NK-cell lymphoma): a report of five cases. Haematologica 91: 143–144

1257. Ko Y H, Kim S H, Ree H J 1998 Blastic NK-cell lymphoma expressing terminal deoxynucleotidyl transferase with Homer–Wright type pseudorosettes formation. Histopathology 33: 547–553

1258. Nakamura S, Koshikawa T, Yatabe Y et al. 1998 Lymphoblastic lymphoma expressing CD56 and TdT. Am J Surg Pathol 22: 135–137

1259. Suzuki R, Yamamoto K, Seto M et al. 1997 CD7+ and CD56+ myeloid/natural killer cell precursor acute leukemia: a distinct hematolymphoid disease entity. Blood 90: 2417–2428

1260. Scott A A, Head D R, Kopecky K J et al. 1994 HLA-DR−, CD33+, CD56+, CD16− myeloid/natural killer cell acute leukemia: a previously unrecognized form of acute leukemia potentially misdiagnosed as French–American–British acute myeloid leukemia-M3. Blood 84: 244–255

1261. Petrella T, Meijer C J, Dalac S et al. 2004 TCL1 and CLA expression in agranular CD4/CD56 hematodermic neoplasms (blastic NK-cell lymphomas) and leukemia cutis. Am J Clin Pathol 122: 307–313

1262. Wagner H J, Cheng Y C, Huls M H et al. 2004 Prompt versus preemptive intervention for EBV lymphoproliferative disease. Blood 103: 3979–3981
1263. Oertel S, Trappe R U, Zeidler K et al. 2006 Epstein–Barr viral load in whole blood of adults with post-transplant lymphoproliferative disorder after solid organ transplantation does not correlate with clinical course. Ann Hematol 85: 478–484
1264. Dotti G, Fiocchi R, Motta T et al. 2000 Epstein–Barr virus-negative lymphoproliferate disorders in long-term survivors after heart, kidney, and liver transplant. Transplantation 69: 827–833
1265. Harris N L, Ferry J A, Swerdlow S H 1997 Post-transplant lymphoproliferative disorders: summary of Society for Hematopathology Workshop. Semin Diagn Pathol 14: 8–14
1266. Chadburn A, Cesarman E, Knowles D M 1997 Molecular pathology of post-transplantation lymphoproliferative disorders. Semin Diagn Pathol 14: 15–26
1267. Swerdlow S H 1997 Classification of the post-transplant lymphoproliferative disorders: from the past to the present. Semin Diagn Pathol 14: 2–7
1268. Swerdlow S H 1997 Post-transplant lymphoproliferative disorders: a working classification. Curr Diagn Pathol 2: 28–35
1269. Chadburn A, Chen J M, Hsu D T et al. 1998 The morphologic and molecular genetic categories of post-transplantation lymphoproliferative disorders are clinically relevant. Cancer 82: 1978–1987
1270. van Gorp J 1995 Post-transplant T-cell lymphoma: a review. Adv Anat Pathol 2: 132–134
1271. Knowles D M, Cesarman E, Chadburn A et al. 1995 Correlative morphologic and molecular genetic analysis demonstrates three distinct categories of post-transplantation lymphoproliferative disorders. Blood 85: 552–565
1272. Cesarman E, Chadburn A, Liu Y F et al. 1998 BCL-6 gene mutations in post-transplantation lymphoproliferative disorders predict response to therapy and clinical outcome. Blood 92: 2294–2302
1273. Harris N L, Swerdlow S H, Frizzera G et al. 2001 Post-transplant lymphoproliferative disorders. In: Jaffe E S, Harris N L, Stein H et al. (eds) Pathology and genetics, tumors of haematopoietic and lymphoid tissues. World Health Organization Classification of Tumours. IARC Press, Lyon, 264–269
1274. Ranganathan S, Webber S, Ahuja S et al. 2004 Hodgkin's-like post-transplant lymphoproliferative disorder in children: does it differ from post-transplant Hodgkin's lymphoma? Pediatr Dev Pathol 7: 348–360
1275. Pitman S D, Huang Q, Zuppan C W et al. 2006 Hodgkin's lymphoma-like post-transplant lymphoproliferative disorder (HL-like PTLD) simulates monomorphic B-cell PTLD both clinically and pathologically. Am J Surg Pathol 30: 470–476
1276. Garnier J L, Lebranchu Y, Dantal J et al. 1996 Hodgkin's disease after transplantation. Transplantation 61: 71–76
1277. Friedberg J W, Swinnen L J 2006 Post-transplant lymphoproliferative disease. In: Canellos G P, Lister A T, Young B (eds) The lymphomas, 2nd edn. Saunders Elsevier, Philadelphia, 555–565
1278. Diamond C, Taylor T H, Im T et al. 2006 Improved survival and chemotherapy response among patients with AIDS-related non-Hodgkin's lymphoma receiving highly active antiretroviral therapy. Hematol Oncol 24: 139–145
1279. Mounier N, Spina M, Gabarre J et al. 2006 AIDS-related non-Hodgkin's lymphoma: final analysis of 485 patients treated with risk-adapted intensive chemotherapy. Blood 107: 3832–3840
1280. Kaplan L D, Lee J Y, Ambinder R F et al. 2005 Rituximab does not improve clinical outcome in a randomized phase 3 trial of CHOP with or without rituximab in patients with HIV-associated non-Hodgkin's lymphoma: AIDS Malignancies Consortium Trial 010. Blood 106: 1538–1543
1281. Nador R G, Chadburn A, Gundappa G et al. 2003 Human immunodeficiency virus (HIV)-associated polymorphic lymphoproliferative disorders. Am J Surg Pathol 27: 293–302
1282. Kamel O W, Weiss L M, van de Rijn M et al. 1996 Hodgkin's disease and lymphoproliferations resembling Hodgkin's disease in patients receiving long-term low-dose methotrexate therapy. Am J Surg Pathol 20: 1279–1287
1283. Kamel O W 1997 Iatrogenic lymphoproliferative disorders in nontransplantation settings. Semin Diagn Pathol 14: 27–34
1284. Kamel O W, van de Rijn M, Hanasono M M et al. 1995 Immunosuppression-associated lymphoproliferative disorders in rheumatic patients. Leuk Lymphoma 16: 363–368
1285. Kamel O W, van de Rijn M, LeBrun D P et al. 1994 Lymphoid neoplasms in patients with rheumatoid arthritis and dermatomyositis: frequency of Epstein–Barr virus and other features associated with immunosuppression. Hum Pathol 25: 638–643
1286. Salloum E, Cooper D L, Howe G et al. 1996 Spontaneous regression of lymphoproliferative disorders in patients treated with methotrexate for rheumatoid arthritis and other rheumatic diseases. J Clin Oncol 14: 1943–1949
1287. Facchetti F, Blanzuoli L, Ungari M et al. 1998 Lymph node pathology in primary combined immunodeficiency diseases. Springer Semin Immunopathol 19: 459–478
1288. Kojima M, Itoh H, Shimizu K et al. 2006 Malignant lymphoma in patients with systemic rheumatic disease (rheumatoid arthritis, systemic lupus erythematosus, systemic sclerosis, and dermatomyositis): a clinicopathologic study of 24 Japanese cases. Int J Surg Pathol 14: 43–48
1289. Elenitoba-Johnson K S, Jaffe E S 1997 Lymphoproliferative disorders associated with congenital immunodeficiencies. Semin Diagn Pathol 14: 35–47
1290. Sander C A, Medeiros L J, Weiss L M et al. 1992 Lymphoproliferative lesions in patients with common variable immunodeficiency syndrome. Am J Surg Pathol 16: 1170–1182
1291. Harrington D S, Weisenburger D D, Purtilo D T 1987 Malignant lymphoma in the X-linked lymphoproliferative syndrome. Cancer 59: 1419–1429
1292. Borisch B, Raphael M, Swerdlow S H et al. 2001 Lymphoproliferative diseases associated with primary immune disorders. In: Jaffe E S, Harris N L, Stein H et al. (eds) Pathology and genetics, tumors of haematopoietic and lymphoid tissues. World Health Organization Classification of Tumours. IARC Press, Lyon, 257–259
1293. Weiss L M, Trela M J, Cleary M L et al. 1985 Frequent immunoglobulin and T-cell receptor gene rearrangements in 'histiocytic' neoplasms. Am J Pathol 121: 369–373
1294. Jaffe R 1999 The histiocytoses. Diagn Pediatr Hematol 19: 135–155
1295. Jaffe E S 1995 Malignant histiocytosis and true histiocytic lymphomas. In: Jaffe E S (ed) Surgical pathology of lymph nodes and related organs. Major problems in pathology, Vol. 16, 2nd edn. WB Saunders, Philadelphia, 560–593
1296. Jaffe E S 1988 Histiocytoses of lymph nodes: biology and differential diagnosis. Semin Diagn Pathol 5: 376–390
1297. Jaffe R 1987 Pathology of histiocytosis X. Perspect Pediatr Pathol 9: 4–47
1298. Foucar K, Foucar E 1990 The mononuclear phagocyte and immunoregulatory effector (M-PIRE) system: evolving concepts. Semin Diagn Pathol 7: 4–18
1299. Favara B E, Feller A C, Pauli M et al. 1997 Contemporary classification of histiocytic disorders. The WHO Committee on Histiocytic/Reticulum Cell Proliferations. Reclassification Working Group of the Histiocyte Society. Med Pediatr Oncol 29: 157–166
1300. Pileri S A, Grogan T M, Harris N L et al. 2002 Tumours of histiocytes and accessory dendritic cells: an immunohistochemical approach to classification from the International Lymphoma Study Group based on 61 cases. Histopathology 41: 1–29
1301. Hanson C A, Jaszcz W, Kersey J H et al. 1989 True histiocytic lymphoma: histopathologic, immunophenotypic and genotypic analysis. Br J Haematol 73: 187–198
1302. Ralfkiaer E, Delsol G, O'Connor N T et al. 1990 Malignant lymphomas of true histiocytic origin. A clinical, histological, immunophenotypic and genotypic study. J Pathol 160: 9–17
1303. Milchgrub S, Kamel O W, Wiley E et al. 1992 Malignant histiocytic neoplasms of the small intestine. Am J Surg Pathol 16: 11–20
1304. Copie-Bergman C, Wotherspoon A C, Norton A J et al. 1998 True histiocytic lymphoma: a morphologic, immunohistochemical, and molecular genetic study of 13 cases. Am J Surg Pathol 22: 1386–1392
1305. Kamel O W, Gocke C D, Kell D L et al. 1995 True histiocytic lymphoma: a study of 12 cases based on current definition. Leuk Lymphoma 18: 81–86
1306. Vos J A, Abbondanzo S L, Barekman C L et al. 2005 Histiocytic sarcoma: a study of five cases including the histiocyte marker CD163. Mod Pathol 18: 693–704
1307. Hornick J L, Jaffe E S, Fletcher C D 2004 Extranodal histiocytic sarcoma: clinicopathologic analysis of 14 cases of a rare epithelioid malignancy. Am J Surg Pathol 28: 1133–1144
1308. Soslow R A, Davis R E, Warnke R A et al. 1996 True histiocytic lymphoma following therapy for lymphoblastic neoplasms. Blood 87: 5207–5212
1309. Feldman A L, Minniti C, Santi M et al. 2004 Histiocytic sarcoma after acute lymphoblastic leukaemia: a common clonal origin. Lancet Oncol 5: 248–250
1310. Nichols C R, Roth B J, Heerema N et al. 1990 Hematologic neoplasia associated with primary mediastinal germ-cell tumors. N Engl J Med 322: 1425–1429
1311. Cheuk W, Walford N, Lou J et al. 2001 Primary histiocytic lymphoma of the central nervous system: a neoplasm frequently overshadowed by a prominent inflammatory component. Am J Surg Pathol 25: 1372–1379
1312. Rappaport H 1966 Tumors of the hematopoietic system. Atlas of tumor pathology, Series 1, Section 3. Armed Forces Institute of Pathology, Washington DC
1313. Warnke R A, Kim H, Dorfman R F 1975 Malignant histiocytosis (histiocytic medullary reticulosis). I. Clinicopatholigic study of 29 cases. Cancer 35: 215–230
1314. Cattoretti G, Villa A, Vezzoni P et al. 1990 Malignant histiocytosis. A phenotypic and genotypic investigation. Am J Pathol 136: 1009–1019
1315. Wilson M S, Weiss L M, Gatter K C et al. 1990 Malignant histiocytosis. A reassessment of cases previously reported in 1975 based on paraffin section immunophenotyping studies. Cancer 66: 530–536
1316. Mongkonsritragoon W, Li C Y, Phyliky R L 1998 True malignant histiocytosis. Mayo Clin Proc 73: 520–528
1317. Sato T, Terui T, Kogawa K et al. 2002 A case of true malignant histiocytosis: identification of histiocytic origin with use of immunohistochemical and immunocytogenetic methods. Ann Hematol 81: 285–288
1318. Suenaga M, Matsushita K, Kawamata N et al. 2006 True malignant histiocytosis with trisomy 9 following primary mediastinal germ cell tumor. Acta Haematol 116: 62–66

1319. Willman C L, Busque L, Griffith B B et al. 1994 Langerhans'-cell histiocytosis (histiocytosis X) – a clonal proliferative disease. N Engl J Med 331: 154–160
1320. Yu R C, Chu C, Buluwela L et al. 1994 Clonal proliferation of Langerhans' cells in Langerhans' cell histiocytosis. Lancet 343: 767–768
1321. Bernstrand C, Sandstedt B, Ahstrom L et al. 2005 Long-term follow-up of Langerhans' cell histiocytosis: 39 years' experience at a single centre. Acta Paediatr 94: 1073–1084
1322. Rust R, Kluiver J, Visser L et al. 2006 Gene expression analysis of dendritic/Langerhans' cells and Langerhans' cell histiocytosis. J Pathol 209: 474–483
1323. Motoi M, Helbron D, Kaiserling E et al. 1980 Eosinophilic granuloma of lymph nodes – a variant of histiocytosis X. Histopathology 4: 585–606
1324. Williams J W, Dorfman R F 1979 Lymphadenopathy as the initial manifestation of histiocytosis X. Am J Surg Pathol 3: 405–421
1325. Reid H, Fox H, Whittaker J S 1977 Eosinophilic granuloma of lymph nodes. Histopathology 1: 31–37
1326. Burns B F, Colby T V, Dorfman R F 1983 Langerhans' cell granulomatosis (histiocytosis X) associated with malignant lymphomas. Am J Surg Pathol 7: 529–533
1327. Favara B E, Jaffe R 1987 Pathology of Langerhans' cell histiocytosis. Hematol Oncol Clin North Am 1: 75–97
1328. Favara B E, Steele A 1997 Langerhans' cell histiocytosis of lymph nodes: a morphologic assessment of 43 biopsies. Pediatr Pathol Lab Med 17: 769–787
1329. Chikwava K, Jaffe R 2004 Langerin (CD207) staining in normal pediatric tissues, reactive lymph nodes, and childhood histiocytic disorders. Pediatr Dev Pathol 7: 607–614
1330. Ruco L P, Pulford K A, Mason D Y et al. 1989 Expression of macrophage-associated antigens in tissues involved by Langerhans' cell histiocytosis (histiocytosis X). Am J Clin Pathol 92: 273–279
1331. Ornvold K, Ralfkiaer E, Carstensen H 1990 Immunohistochemical study of the abnormal cells in Langerhans' cell histiocytosis (histiocytosis X). Virchows Arch A Pathol Anat Histopathol 416: 403–410
1332. Ben-Ezra J, Bailey A, Azumi N et al. 1991 Malignant histiocytosis X. A distinct clinicopathologic entity. Cancer 68: 1050–1060
1333. Monda L, Warnke R, Rosai J 1986 A primary lymph node malignancy with features suggestive of dendritic reticulum cell differentiation. A report of 4 cases. Am J Pathol 122: 562–572
1334. Hollowood K, Pease C, Mackay A M et al. 1991 Sarcomatoid tumours of lymph nodes showing follicular dendritic cell differentiation. J Pathol 163: 205–216
1335. Hollowood K, Stamp G, Zouvani I et al. 1995 Extranodal follicular dendritic cell sarcoma of the gastrointestinal tract. Morphologic, immunohistochemical and ultrastructural analysis of two cases. Am J Clin Pathol 103: 90–97
1336. Chan J K, Tsang W Y, Ng C S 1994 Follicular dendritic cell tumor and vascular neoplasm complicating hyaline–vascular Castleman's disease. Am J Surg Pathol 18: 517–525
1337. Chan J K, Tsang W Y, Ng C S et al. 1994 Follicular dendritic cell tumors of the oral cavity. Am J Surg Pathol 18: 148–157
1338. Chan J K, Fletcher C D, Nayler S J et al. 1997 Follicular dendritic cell sarcoma. Clinicopathologic analysis of 17 cases suggesting a malignant potential higher than currently recognized. Cancer 79: 294–313
1339. Chan J K 1997 Proliferative lesions of follicular dendritic cells: an overview, including a detailed account of follicular dendritic cell sarcoma, a neoplasm with many faces and uncommon etiologic associations. Adv Anat Pathol 4: 387–411
1340. Weiss L M, Berry G J, Dorfman R F et al. 1990 Spindle cell neoplasms of lymph nodes of probable reticulum cell lineage. True reticulum cell sarcoma? Am J Surg Pathol 14: 405–414
1341. Perez-Ordóñez B, Erlandson R A, Rosai J 1996 Follicular dendritic cell tumor: report of 13 additional cases of a distinctive entity. Am J Surg Pathol 20: 944–955
1342. Perez-Ordóñez B, Rosai J 1998 Follicular dendritic cell tumor: review of the entity. Semin Diagn Pathol 15: 144–154
1343. Biddle D A, Ro J Y, Yoon G S et al. 2002 Extranodal follicular dendritic cell sarcoma of the head and neck region: three new cases, with a review of the literature. Mod Pathol 15: 50–58
1344. Choi P C, To K F, Lai F M et al. 2000 Follicular dendritic cell sarcoma of the neck: report of two cases complicated by pulmonary metastases. Cancer 89: 664–672
1345. Shia J, Chen W, Tang L H et al. 2006 Extranodal follicular dendritic cell sarcoma: clinical, pathologic, and histogenetic characteristics of an underrecognized disease entity. Virchows Arch 449: 148–158
1346. Chan A C, Chan K W, Chan J K et al. 2001 Development of follicular dendritic cell sarcoma in hyaline–vascular Castleman's disease of the nasopharynx: tracing its evolution by sequential biopsies. Histopathology 38: 510–518
1347. Lin O, Frizzera G 1997 Angiomyoid and follicular dendritic cell proliferative lesions in Castleman's disease of hyaline–vascular type: a study of 10 cases. Am J Surg Pathol 21: 1295–1306
1348. Katano H, Kaneko K, Shimizu S et al. 1997 Follicular dendritic cell sarcoma complicated by hyaline–vascular type Castleman's disease in a schizophrenic patient. Pathol Int 47: 703–706
1349. Masunaga A, Nakamura H, Katata T et al. 1997 Follicular dendritic cell tumor with histiocytic characteristics and fibroblastic antigen. Pathol Int 47: 707–712
1350. Cheuk W, Chan J K, Shek T W et al. 2001 Inflammatory pseudotumor-like follicular dendritic cell tumor: a distinctive low-grade malignant intra-abdominal neoplasm with consistent Epstein–Barr virus association. Am J Surg Pathol 25: 721–731
1351. Chan J K C, Facchetti F, Chetty R et al. 1999 B-cell-rich nodular variant of follicular dendritic cell (FDC) tumor: a neoplasm with intriguing histologic features. [Abstract] Mod Pathol 12: 134A
1352. Raymond I, Al Saati T, Tkaczuk J et al. 1997 CNA.42, a new monoclonal antibody directed against a fixative-resistant antigen of follicular dendritic reticulum cells. Am J Pathol 151: 1577–1585
1353. Grogg K L, Lae M E, Kurtin P J et al. 2004 Clusterin expression distinguishes follicular dendritic cell tumors from other dendritic cell neoplasms: report of a novel follicular dendritic cell marker and clinicopathologic data on 12 additional follicular dendritic cell tumors and 6 additional interdigitating dendritic cell tumors. Am J Surg Pathol 28: 988–998
1354. Grogg K L, Macon W R, Kurtin PJ et al. 2005 A survey of clusterin and fascin expression in sarcomas and spindle cell neoplasms: strong clusterin immunostaining is highly specific for follicular dendritic cell tumor. Mod Pathol 18: 260–266
1355. Sun X, Chang K C, Abruzzo L V et al. 2003 Epidermal growth factor receptor expression in follicular dendritic cells: a shared feature of follicular dendritic cell sarcoma and Castleman's disease. Hum Pathol 34: 835–840
1356. Miettinen M, Fletcher C D, Lasota J 1993 True histiocytic lymphoma of small intestine. Analysis of two S-100 protein-positive cases with features of interdigitating reticulum cell sarcoma. Am J Clin Pathol 100: 285–292
1357. Nakamura S, Koshikawa T, Kitoh K et al. 1994 Interdigitating cell sarcoma: a morphologic and immunologic study of lymph node lesions in four cases. Pathol Int 44: 374–386
1358. Nakamura S, Hara K, Suchi T et al. 1988 Interdigitating cell sarcoma. A morphologic, immunohistologic, and enzyme-histochemical study. Cancer 61: 562–568
1359. Rousselet M C, Francois S, Croue A et al. 1994 A lymph node interdigitating reticulum cell sarcoma. Arch Pathol Lab Med 118: 183–188
1360. Andriko J W, Kaldjian E P, Tsokos M et al. 1998 Reticulum cell neoplasms of lymph nodes: a clinicopathologic study of 11 cases with recognition of a new subtype derived from fibroblastic reticular cells. Am J Surg Pathol 22: 1048–1058
1361. Luk I S, Shek T W, Tang V W et al. 1999 Interdigitating dendritic cell tumor of the testis: a novel testicular spindle cell neoplasm. Am J Surg Pathol 23: 1141–1148
1362. Gaertner E M, Tsokos M, Derringer G A et al. 2001 Interdigitating dendritic cell sarcoma. A report of four cases and review of the literature. Am J Clin Pathol 115: 589–597
1363. Kawachi K, Nakatani Y, Inayama Y et al. 2002 Interdigitating dendritic cell sarcoma of the spleen: report of a case with a review of the literature. Am J Surg Pathol 26: 530–537
1364. Pillay K, Solomon R, Daubenton J D et al. 2004 Interdigitating dendritic cell sarcoma: a report of four paediatric cases and review of the literature. Histopathology 44: 283–291
1365. Vasef M A, Zaatari G S, Chan W C et al. 1995 Dendritic cell tumors associated with low-grade B-cell malignancies. Report of three cases. Am J Clin Pathol 104: 696–701
1366. Fonseca R, Yamakawa M, Nakamura S et al. 1998 Follicular dendritic cell sarcoma and interdigitating reticulum cell sarcoma: a review. Am J Hematol 59: 161–167
1367. Gould V E, Warren W H, Faber L P et al. 1990 Malignant cells of epithelial phenotype limited to thoracic lymph nodes. Eur J Cancer 26: 1121–1126
1368. Chan A C, Serrano-Olmo J, Erlandson R A et al. 2000 Cytokeratin-positive malignant tumors with reticulum cell morphology: a subtype of fibroblastic reticulum cell neoplasm? Am J Surg Pathol 24: 107–116
1369. Jones D, Amin M, Ordóñez N G et al. 2001 Reticulum cell sarcoma of lymph node with mixed dendritic and fibroblastic features. Mod Pathol 14: 1059–1067
1370. Facchetti F, Vermi W, Mason D et al. 2003 The plasmacytoid monocyte/interferon producing cells. Virchows Arch 443: 703–717
1371. Horny H P, Feller A C, Horst H A et al. 1987 Immunocytology of plasmacytoid T cells: marker analysis indicates a unique phenotype of this enigmatic cell. Hum Pathol 18: 28–32
1372. Harris N L, Bhan A K 1987 'Plasmacytoid T cells' in Castleman's disease. Immunohistologic phenotype. Am J Surg Pathol 11: 109–113
1373. Vollenweider R, Lennert K 1983 Plasmacytoid T-cell clusters in non-specific lymphadenitis. Virchows Arch B Cell Pathol Incl Mol Pathol 44: 1–14
1374. Facchetti F, De Wolf-Peeters C, van den Oord J J et al. 1988 Plasmacytoid T cells: a cell population normally present in the reactive lymph node. An immunohistochemical and electronmicroscopic study. Hum Pathol 19: 1085–1092
1375. Facchetti F, de Wolf-Peeters C, Mason D Y et al. 1988 Plasmacytoid T cells. Immunohistochemical evidence for their monocyte/macrophage origin. Am J Pathol 133: 15–21
1376. Prasthofer E F, Prchal J T, Grizzle W E et al. 1985 Plasmacytoid T-cell lymphoma associated with chronic myeloproliferative disorder. Am J Surg Pathol 9: 380–387

1377. Beiske K, Langholm R, Godal T et al. 1986 T-zone lymphoma with predominance of 'plasmacytoid T-cells' associated with myelomonocytic leukaemia – a distinct clinicopathological entity. J Pathol 150: 247–255
1378. Muller-Hermelink H K, Stein H, Steinmann G et al. 1983 Malignant lymphoma of plasmacytoid T-cells. Morphologic and immunologic studies characterizing a special type of T-cell. Am J Surg Pathol 7: 849–862
1379. Facchetti F, De Wolf-Peeters C, Kennes C et al. 1990 Leukemia-associated lymph node infiltrates of plasmacytoid monocytes (so-called plasmacytoid T-cells). Evidence for two distinct histological and immunophenotypical patterns. Am J Surg Pathol 14: 101–112
1380. Koo C H, Mason D Y, Miller R et al. 1990 Additional evidence that 'plasmacytoid T-cell lymphoma' associated with chronic myeloproliferative disorders is of macrophage/monocyte origin. Am J Clin Pathol 93: 822–827
1381. Baddoura F K, Hanson C, Chan W C 1992 Plasmacytoid monocyte proliferation associated with myeloproliferative disorders. Cancer 69: 1457–1467
1382. Fontana P, Facchetti F, Fiaccavento S 1997 Fine-needle aspiration cytologic findings in a case of lymph node tumor of plasmacytoid monocytes. Diagn Cytopathol 17: 57–60
1383. Vermi W, Facchetti F, Rosati S et al. 2004 Nodal and extranodal tumor-forming accumulation of plasmacytoid monocytes/interferon-producing cells associated with myeloid disorders. Am J Surg Pathol 28: 585–595
1384. Caldwell C W, Yesus Y W, Loy T S et al. 1990 Acute leukemia/lymphoma of plasmacytoid T-cell type. Am J Clin Pathol 94: 778–786
1385. Harris N L, Demirjian Z 1991 Plasmacytoid T-zone cell proliferation in a patient with chronic myelomonocytic leukemia. Histologic and immunohistologic characterization. Am J Surg Pathol 15: 87–95
1386. Neiman R S, Barcos M, Berard C et al. 1981 Granulocytic sarcoma: a clinicopathologic study of 61 biopsied cases. Cancer 48: 1426–1437
1387. Long J C, Mihm M C 1977 Multiple granulocytic tumors of the skin: report of six cases of myelogenous leukemia with initial manifestations in the skin. Cancer 39: 2004–2016
1388. Furebring-Freden M, Martinsson U, Sundstrom C 1990 Myelosarcoma without acute leukaemia: immunohistochemical and clinicopathologic characterization of eight cases. Histopathology 16: 243–250
1389. Meis J M, Butler J J, Osborne B M et al. 1986 Granulocytic sarcoma in nonleukemic patients. Cancer 58: 2697–2709
1390. Krause J R 1979 Granulocytic sarcoma preceding acute leukemia: a report of six cases. Cancer 44: 1017–1021
1391. Hutchison R E, Kurec A S, Davey F R 1990 Granulocytic sarcoma. Clin Lab Med 10: 889–901
1392. Segal G H, Stoler M H, Tubbs R R 1992 The 'CD43 only' phenotype. An aberrant, nonspecific immunophenotype requiring comprehensive analysis for lineage resolution. Am J Clin Pathol 97: 861–865
1393. Menasce L P, Banerjee S S, Beckett E et al. 1999 Extra-medullary myeloid tumour (granulocytic sarcoma) is often misdiagnosed: a study of 26 cases. Histopathology 34: 391–398
1394. Pinkus G S, Pinkus J L 1991 Myeloperoxidase: a specific marker for myeloid cells in paraffin sections. Mod Pathol 4: 733–741
1395. Wong K F, Chan J K C 1995 Antimyeloperoxidase: antibody of choice for labeling of myeloid cells including diagnosis of granulocytic sarcoma. Adv Anat Pathol 2: 65–68
1396. Traweek S T, Arber D A, Rappaport H et al. 1993 Extramedullary myeloid cell tumors. An immunohistochemical and morphologic study of 28 cases. Am J Surg Pathol 17: 1011–1019
1397. Chen J, Yanuck R R 3rd, Abbondanzo S L et al. 2001 c-Kit (CD117) reactivity in extramedullary myeloid tumor/granulocytic sarcoma. Arch Pathol Lab Med 125: 1448–1452
1398. Hermanek P, Hutter R V, Sobin L H et al. 1999 International Union Against Cancer Classification of isolated tumor cells and micrometastasis. Cancer 86: 2668–2673
1399. Page D L, Anderson T J, Carter B A 1999 Minimal solid tumor involvement of regional and distant sites: when is a metastasis not a metastasis? Cancer 86: 2589–2592
1400. Pfeifer J D 1999 Sentinel lymph node biopsy. Am J Clin Pathol 112: 599–602
1401. Lukowsky A, Bellmann B, Ringk A et al. 1999 Detection of melanoma micrometastases in the sentinel lymph node and in nonsentinel nodes by tyrosinase polymerase chain reaction. J Invest Dermatol 113: 554–559
1402. Reintgen D, Shivers S 1999 Sentinel lymph node micrometastasis from melanoma. Proven methodology and evolving significance. Cancer 86: 551–552
1403. Cibull M L 1999 Handling sentinel lymph node biopsy specimens. A work in progress. Arch Pathol Lab Med 123: 620–621
1404. Tsang W Y 1999 Sentinel lymph node biopsy: not the state of art in the management of breast cancer yet. Adv Anat Pathol 6: 92–96
1405. Czerniecki B J, Scheff A M, Callans L S et al. 1999 Immunohistochemistry with pancytokeratins improves the sensitivity of sentinel lymph node biopsy in patients with breast carcinoma. Cancer 85: 1098–1103
1406. Cox C, White L, Allred N et al. 2006 Survival outcomes in node-negative breast cancer patients evaluated with complete axillary node dissection versus sentinel lymph node biopsy. Ann Surg Oncol 13: 708–711
1407. Essner R 2006 Sentinel lymph node biopsy and melanoma biology. Clin Cancer Res 12: 2320s–2325s
1408. Thompson J F, Scolyer R A, Uren R F 2006 Surgical management of primary cutaneous melanoma: excision margins and the role of sentinel lymph node examination. Surg Oncol Clin North Am 15: 301–318
1409. Doglioni C, Dell'Orto P, Zanetti G et al. 1990 Cytokeratin-immunoreactive cells of human lymph nodes and spleen in normal and pathological conditions. An immunocytochemical study. Virchows Arch A Pathol Anat Histopathol 416: 479–490
1410. Batsakis J G 1981 The pathology of head and neck tumors: the occult primary and metastases to the head and neck, Part 10. Head Neck Surg 3: 409–423
1411. Robert N J, Garnick M B, Frei E D 1982 Cancers of unknown origin: current approaches and future perspectives. Semin Oncol 9: 526–531
1412. Suster S, Rosai J 1989 Intranodal hemorrhagic spindle-cell tumor with 'amianthoid' fibers. Report of six cases of a distinctive mesenchymal neoplasm of the inguinal region that simulates Kaposi's sarcoma. Am J Surg Pathol 13: 347–357
1413. Bigotti G, Coli A, Mottolese M et al. 1991 Selective location of palisaded myofibroblastoma with amianthoid fibres. J Clin Pathol 44: 761–764
1414. Hisaoka M, Hashimoto H, Daimaru Y 1998 Intranodal palisaded myofibroblastoma with so-called amianthoid fibers: a report of two cases with a review of the literature. Pathol Int 48: 307–312
1415. Weiss S W, Gnepp D R, Bratthauer G L 1989 Palisaded myofibroblastoma. A benign mesenchymal tumor of lymph node. Am J Surg Pathol 13: 341–346
1416. Fletcher C D, Stirling R W 1990 Intranodal myofibroblastoma presenting in the submandibular region: evidence of a broader clinical and histological spectrum. Histopathology 16: 287–293
1417. Kleist B, Poetsch M, Schmoll J 2003 Intranodal palisaded myofibroblastoma with overexpression of cyclin D1. Arch Pathol Lab Med 127: 1040–1043
1418. Channer J L, Davies J D 1985 Smooth muscle proliferation in the hilum of superficial lymph nodes. Virchows Arch A Pathol Anat Histopathol 406: 261–270
1419. Chan J K, Tsang W Y, Pau M Y et al. 1993 Lymphangiomyomatosis and angiomyolipoma: closely related entities characterized by hamartomatous proliferation of HMB-45-positive smooth muscle. Histopathology 22: 445–455
1420. Ro J Y, Ayala A G, el-Naggar A et al. 1990 Angiomyolipoma of kidney with lymph node involvement. DNA flow cytometric analysis. Arch Pathol Lab Med 114: 65–67
1421. Chan J K, Frizzera G, Fletcher C D et al. 1992 Primary vascular tumors of lymph nodes other than Kaposi's sarcoma. Analysis of 39 cases and delineation of two new entities. Am J Surg Pathol 16: 335–350
1422. Perrone T, De Wolf-Peeters C, Frizzera G 1988 Inflammatory pseudotumor of lymph nodes. A distinctive pattern of nodal reaction. Am J Surg Pathol 12: 351–361
1423. Chan J K, Tsang W Y 1993 Uncommon syndromes of reactive lymphadenopathy. Semin Oncol 20: 648–657
1424. Moran C A, Suster S, Abbondanzo S L 1997 Inflammatory pseudotumor of lymph nodes: a study of 25 cases with emphasis on morphological heterogeneity. Hum Pathol 28: 332–338
1425. Davis R E, Warnke R A, Dorfman R F 1991 Inflammatory pseudotumor of lymph nodes. Additional observations and evidence for an inflammatory etiology. Am J Surg Pathol 15: 744–756
1426. Kutok J L, Pinkus G S, Dorfman D M et al. 2001 Inflammatory pseudotumor of lymph node and spleen: an entity biologically distinct from inflammatory myofibroblastic tumor. Hum Pathol 32: 1382–1387
1427. Facchetti F, De Wolf Peeters C, De Wever I et al. 1990 Inflammatory pseudotumor of lymph nodes. Immunohistochemical evidence for its fibrohistiocytic nature. Am J Pathol 137: 281–289
1428. Chan J K 1996 Inflammatory pseudotumor: a family of lesions of diverse nature and etiologies. Adv Anat Pathol 3: 156–171
1429. Rabkin C S, Bedi G, Musaba E et al. 1995 AIDS-related Kaposi's sarcoma is a clonal neoplasm. Clin Cancer Res 1: 257–260
1430. Rabkin C S, Janz S, Lash A et al. 1997 Monoclonal origin of multicentric Kaposi's sarcoma lesions. N Engl J Med 336: 988–993
1431. Dorfman R F 1984 Kaposi's sarcoma revisited. Hum Pathol 15: 1013–1017
1432. Dorfman R F 1986 Kaposi's sarcoma. With special reference to its manifestations in infants and children and to the concepts of Arthur Purdy Stout. Am J Surg Pathol 10: 68–77
1433. Krigel R L, Friedman-Kien A E 1990 Epidemic Kaposi's sarcoma. Semin Oncol 17: 350–360
1434. Penn I 1997 Kaposi's sarcoma in transplant recipients. Transplantation 64: 669–673
1435. Penn I 1979 Kaposi's sarcoma in organ transplant recipients: report of 20 cases. Transplantation 27: 8–11
1436. Slavin G, Cameron H M, Forbes C et al. 1970 Kaposi's sarcoma in East African children: a report of 51 cases. J Pathol 100: 187–199
1437. Ziegler J L, Templeton A C, Vogel C L 1984 Kaposi's sarcoma: a comparison of classical, endemic, and epidemic forms. Semin Oncol 11: 47–52
1438. Templeton A C 1981 Kaposi's sarcoma. Pathol Annu 16: 315–336
1439. Taylor J F, Templeton A C, Vogel C L et al. 1971 Kaposi's sarcoma in Uganda: a clinico-pathological study. Int J Cancer 8: 122–135
1440. Huang Y Q, Li J J, Kaplan M H 1995 Human herpesvirus-like nucleic acid in various forms of Kaposi's sarcoma. Lancet 345: 759–761
1441. Cheuk W, Wong K O, Wong C S et al. 2004 Immunostaining for human herpesvirus 8 latent nuclear antigen-1 helps distinguish Kaposi sarcoma from its mimickers. Am J Clin Pathol 121: 335–342

1442. Chan J K C 1997 Vascular tumours with a prominent spindle cell component. Curr Diagn Pathol 4: 76–90
1443. O'Connell K M 1977 Kaposi's sarcoma in lymph nodes: histological study of lesions from 16 cases in Malawi. J Clin Pathol 30: 696–703
1444. Finkbeiner W E, Egbert B M, Groundwater J R et al. 1982 Kaposi's sarcoma in young homosexual men: a histopathologic study with particular reference to lymph node involvement. Arch Pathol Lab Med 106: 261–264
1445. Chan J K, Warnke R A, Dorfman R 1991 Vascular transformation of sinuses in lymph nodes. A study of its morphological spectrum and distinction from Kaposi's sarcoma. Am J Surg Pathol 15: 732–743
1446. Tsang W Y, Chan J K, Dorfman RF et al. 1994 Vasoproliferative lesions of the lymph node. Pathol Annu 29: 63–133
1447. Gerald W, Kostianovsky M, Rosai J 1990 Development of vascular neoplasia in Castleman's disease. Report of seven cases. Am J Surg Pathol 14: 603–614
1448. Haferkamp O, Rosenau W, Lennert K 1971 Vascular transformation of lymph node sinuses due to venous congestion. Arch Pathol 92: 81–83
1449. Cook P D, Czerniak B, Chan J K et al. 1995 Nodular spindle-cell vascular transformation of lymph nodes. A benign process occurring predominantly in retroperitoneal lymph nodes draining carcinomas that can simulate Kaposi's sarcoma or metastatic tumor. Am J Surg Pathol 19: 1010–1020
1450. Adal K A, Cockerell C J, Petri W A Jr 1994 Cat scratch disease, bacillary angiomatosis, and other infections due to *Rochalimaea*. N Engl J Med 330: 1509–1515
1451. Cockerell C J 1992 The causative agent of bacillary angiomatosis. Int J Dermatol 31: 615–617
1452. Webster G F, Cockerell C J, Friedman-Kien A E 1992 The clinical spectrum of bacillary angiomatosis. Br J Dermatol 126: 535–541
1453. Cockerell C J, Tierno P M, Friedman-Kien A E et al. 1991 Clinical, histologic, microbiologic, and biochemical characterization of the causative agent of bacillary (epithelioid) angiomatosis: a rickettsial illness with features of bartonellosis. J Invest Dermatol 97: 812–817
1454. Koehler J E, Sanchez M A, Garrido C S et al. 1997 Molecular epidemiology of *Bartonella* infections in patients with bacillary angiomatosis–peliosis. N Engl J Med 337: 1876–1883
1455. Relman D A, Falkow S, LeBoit P E et al. 1991 The organism causing bacillary angiomatosis, peliosis hepatis, and fever and bacteremia in immunocompromised patients. N Engl J Med 324: 1514
1456. LeBoit P E, Berger T G, Egbert B M et al. 1989 Bacillary angiomatosis. The histopathology and differential diagnosis of a pseudoneoplastic infection in patients with human immunodeficiency virus disease. Am J Surg Pathol 13: 909–920
1457. Berger T G, Tappero JW, Kaymen A et al. 1989 Bacillary (epithelioid) angiomatosis and concurrent Kaposi's sarcoma in acquired immunodeficiency syndrome. Arch Dermatol 125: 1543–1547
1458. LeBoit P E 1990 The expanding spectrum of a new disease, bacillary angiomatosis. Arch Dermatol 126: 808–811
1459. Relman D A, Loutit J S, Schmidt T M et al. 1990 The agent of bacillary angiomatosis. An approach to the identification of uncultured pathogens. N Engl J Med 323: 1573–1580
1460. Tsang W Y, Chan J K 1992 Bacillary angiomatosis. A 'new' disease with a broadening clinicopathologic spectrum. Histol Histopathol 7: 143–152
1461. Chan J K, Lewin K J, Lombard C M et al. 1991 Histopathology of bacillary angiomatosis of lymph node. Am J Surg Pathol 15: 430–437
1462. Cheuk W, Chan A K, Wong M C et al. 2006 Confirmation of diagnosis of cat scratch disease by immunohistochemistry. Am J Surg Pathol 30: 274–275
1463. Parkash V, Vidwans M, Carter D 1999 Benign mesothelial cells in mediastinal lymph nodes. Am J Surg Pathol 23: 1264–1269
1464. Suarez Vilela D, Izquierdo Garcia F M 1998 Embolization of mesothelial cells in lymphatics: the route to mesothelial inclusions in lymph nodes? Histopathology 33: 570–575
1465. Argani P, Rosai J 1998 Hyperplastic mesothelial cells in lymph nodes: report of six cases of a benign process that can stimulate metastatic involvement by mesothelioma or carcinoma. Hum Pathol 29: 339–346
1466. Clement P B, Young R H, Oliva E et al. 1996 Hyperplastic mesothelial cells within abdominal lymph nodes: mimic of metastatic ovarian carcinoma and serous borderline tumor – a report of two cases associated with ovarian neoplasms. Mod Pathol 9: 879–886
1467. Brooks J S, LiVolsi V A, Pietra G G 1990 Mesothelial cell inclusions in mediastinal lymph nodes mimicking metastatic carcinoma. Am J Clin Pathol 93: 741–748
1468. Rutty G N, Lauder I 1994 Mesothelial cell inclusions within mediastinal lymph nodes. Histopathology 25: 483–487
1469. Colby T V 1999 Benign mesothelial cells in lymph node. Adv Anat Pathol 6: 41–48
1470. Kir G, Eren S, Kir M 2004 Hyperplastic mesothelial cells in pelvic and abdominal lymph node sinuses mimicking metastatic ovarian microinvasive serous borderline tumor. Eur J Gynaecol Oncol 25: 236–238
1470a. Biddle D A, Evans H L, Kemp B L et al 2003 Intraparenchymal nevus cell aggregates in lymph nodes. A possible diagnostic pitfall with malignant melanoma and carcinoma. Am J Surg Pathol 27: 673–681
1471. Mihic-Probst D, Saremaslani P, Komminoth P et al. 2003 Immunostaining for the tumour suppressor gene p16 product is a useful marker to differentiate melanoma metastasis from lymph-node nevus. Virchows Arch 443: 745–751
1472. Sneller M C, Straus S E, Jaffe E S et al. 1992 A novel lymphoproliferative/autoimmune syndrome resembling murine lpr/gld disease. J Clin Invest 90: 334–341
1473. Sneller M C, Wang J, Dale J K et al. 1997 Clinical, immunologic, and genetic features of an autoimmune lymphoproliferative syndrome associated with abnormal lymphocyte apoptosis. Blood 89: 1341–1348
1474. van den Berg A, Tamminga R, de Jong D et al. 2003 FAS gene mutation in a case of autoimmune lymphoproliferative syndrome type IA with accumulation of gammadelta+ T cells. Am J Surg Pathol 27: 546–553
1475. Worth A, Thrasher A J, Gaspar H B 2006 Autoimmune lymphoproliferative syndrome: molecular basis of disease and clinical phenotype. Br J Haematol 133: 124–140
1476. Holzelova E, Vonarbourg C, Stolzenberg M C et al. 2004 Autoimmune lymphoproliferative syndrome with somatic Fas mutations. N Engl J Med 351: 1409–1418
1477. Tsang W Y, Chan J K, Ng C S 1994 Kikuchi's lymphadenitis. A morphologic analysis of 75 cases with special reference to unusual features. Am J Surg Pathol 18: 219–231

第二部分

脾 The spleen

Wah Cheuk 和 John K.C. Chan 著

孙 雷 译

脾

正常脾	1289	脾的组织细胞和树突状细胞增生	1303
淋巴瘤和白血病累及脾的方式：诊断方法	1289	脾的间叶性肿瘤和瘤样病变	1304
脾的原发性淋巴瘤	1295	脾的罕见病变	1309
以脾受累为主要特征的淋巴瘤和白血病	1297	脾的转移性肿瘤	1310

正常脾 The normal spleen

脾有两个主要功能：免疫防御和过滤[1]。正常成人脾重 50～250g，由纤维性被膜包裹，并有细的纤维性小梁伸入脾实质内。结构上，脾由白髓和红髓组成，前者为明显的 1～2 mm 的白色小结节，均匀分布于实质内。

白髓是脾的淋巴组织部分，以中央动脉为中心，而中央动脉由小梁动脉分支而来（图 21B.1A）。T 细胞围绕中央动脉形成淋巴鞘，并有偏心性的 B 细胞结节状聚集（脾淋巴小体，malpighian corpuscle）。在脾淋巴小体内，生发中心细胞（IgD⁻、bcl2⁻）由外套小淋巴细胞（IgD⁺、bcl2⁺）围绕，其外是由 B 淋巴细胞（IgD⁻、bcl2⁺）构成的边缘区。边缘区淋巴细胞中等大小，伴有中等量的透明胞浆，类似于淋巴结内的单核细胞样 B 细胞（图 21B.1B）。

红髓是脾的过滤部分，由静脉窦构成，静脉窦由髓索和动脉系统的终末分支分开（图 21B.1）[1,2]。脾血窦是血管中的一种特殊结构，呈环状而不形成完整的网状纤维鞘，并且内衬细胞（衬细胞，littoral cell）表达 CD8、CD31 和 Ⅷ 因子相关抗原，而不表达 CD34。髓索是由巨噬细胞胞浆突起相互连接构成的网状结构（CD8⁺）。一些淋巴细胞单个或小灶状弥散分布于红髓内，其中 T 细胞远多于 B 细胞。

淋巴瘤和白血病累及脾的方式：诊断方法

一般情况下，淋巴瘤主要累及脾的白髓（除几种类型的淋巴瘤以外），而白血病倾向于累及红髓（除 B-CLL/

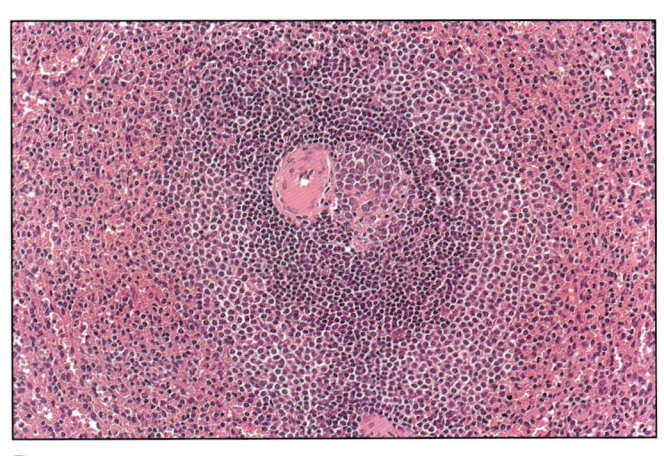

图21B.1　正常脾。（A）白髓由伴有滤泡结构的淋巴细胞小结构成。其间为静脉窦和髓索。（B）白髓滤泡有生发中心，周围绕以由小淋巴细胞组成的外套层。其外有边缘区，由含有较多浅染胞浆的细胞组成。

SLL以外）[1,3-6]。评估脾的淋巴组织增生性病变时，以下几个步骤有助于明确诊断：

1. 脾的重量。脾的重量超过500g实际上意味着存在病变。
2. 将脾每隔2～3mm做一切面，并仔细检查每一切面。病变可能小而局限，尤其是Hodgkin淋巴瘤累及脾的早期，如果脾的切面不够薄的话，病变容易被漏掉。
3. 大体检查脾切面能够提供非常重要的诊断线索（表21B.1）（图 21B.2至21B.4）[6]。应该分别从异常和明显正常的脾实质适当取材。
4. 必须对脾门淋巴结取材进行组织学检查。根据淋巴结受累的情况有时容易区分出淋巴瘤的种类。
5. 组织学评估包括确定受累部位（主要累及白髓，主要累及红髓，还是白髓红髓均受累）、细胞排列方式、细胞组成以及其他组织学特征。各种非Hodgkin淋巴瘤累及脾的模式见表21B.2[7-12]。
6. 免疫组织化学染色对于明确组织结构和淋巴细胞种类非常重要。
7. 在诸如自身免疫性疾病、感染、Castleman病以及自身免疫性淋巴细胞增生综合征等反应性病变，白髓滤泡可能增生，伴有明显的生发中心和（或）边缘区增宽[1,13]。此时可能很难与肿瘤性病变区分。支持淋巴瘤诊断的特征包括：
   - 白髓滤泡融合（图21B.5）。
   - 即使在低倍镜下也能看到红髓内小淋巴细胞呈小结节状聚集（图21B.5A）。

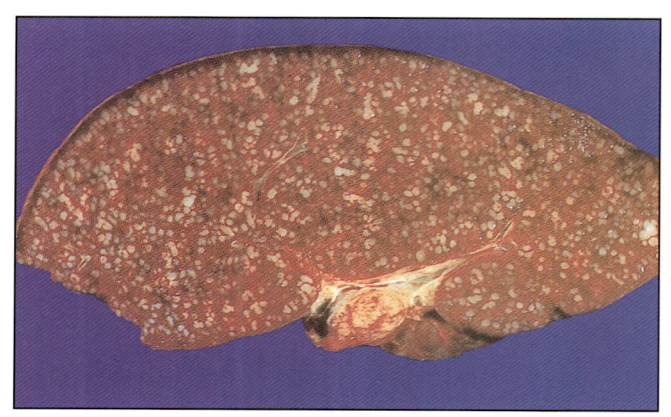

图21B.2 滤泡性淋巴瘤累及脾的切面。显示典型的粟粒状小结节状外观。

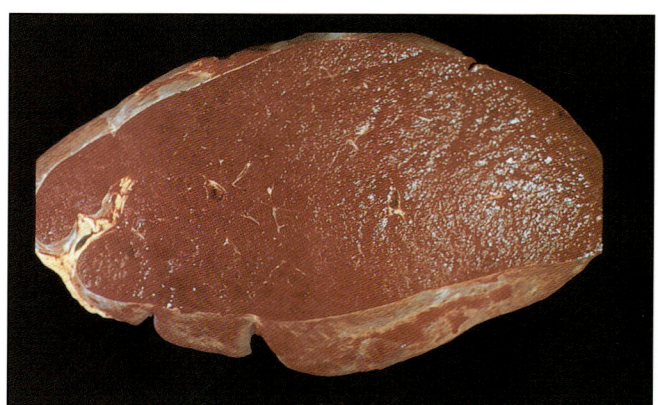

图21B.4 毛细胞淋巴瘤累及脾的切面。显示弥漫性牛肉红样外观，这是红髓广泛受累的特征。

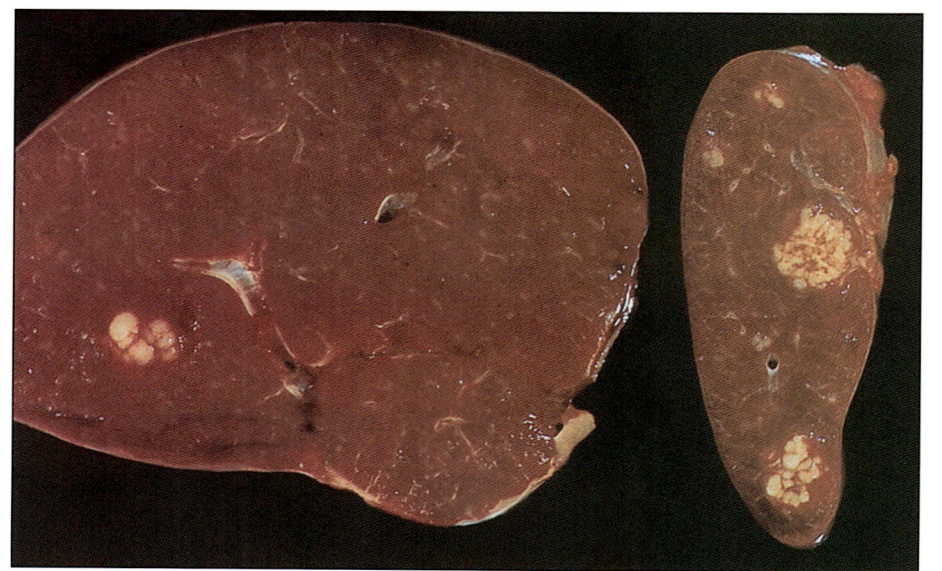

图21B.3 经典性Hodgkin淋巴瘤累及脾的切面。左侧：单个受累病灶由几个相邻的小的褐色结节组成。右侧：显示脾较广泛受累，伴有一些杂乱分布的小结节以及两个较大的结节。后者是由小结节融合而成。

表21B.1　淋巴血液系统肿瘤和其他疾病中脾累及的大体形态

脾切面的大体表现	鉴别诊断需要考虑的淋巴血液系统肿瘤	可能产生类似大体表现的其他疾病
分布于整个脾内的粟粒状白色小结节	滤泡性淋巴瘤 B-CLL/SLL 淋巴浆细胞性淋巴瘤 套细胞淋巴瘤（淋巴结、结外和脾） 边缘区B细胞淋巴瘤 Hodgkin淋巴瘤（罕见）	粟粒性结核病 分枝杆菌梭形细胞假瘤 淀粉样变（主要是白髓受累）
孤立性或几个簇状小结节	Hodgkin淋巴瘤	局限性淋巴组织增生
孤立性或多发性大的鱼肉样结节，伴有或不伴有散在的小结节	弥漫性大B细胞淋巴瘤 滤泡性淋巴瘤，3级 一些外周T细胞淋巴瘤 各种高级别淋巴瘤 Hodgkin淋巴瘤	各种非淋巴液系统肿瘤和瘤样病变，如炎性假瘤、脾错构瘤、转移癌和杆菌性血管瘤病
红髓扩大呈牛肉红样外观，而白髓病变不显著	各种类型的白血病，除了B-CLL/SLL以外 肝脾T细胞淋巴瘤 一些弥漫性大B细胞淋巴瘤和外周T细胞淋巴瘤（"恶性组织细胞增多症"的形态） 原因不明的骨髓化生（特发性骨髓纤维化） 系统性肥大细胞增生症（常有明显的纤维条纹和边界不清的小结节） Langerhans细胞组织细胞增生症	传染性单核细胞增多症和其他免疫反应 噬血细胞综合征 淤血性脾大 溶血性贫血 贮积病 淀粉样变（主要是红髓受累）

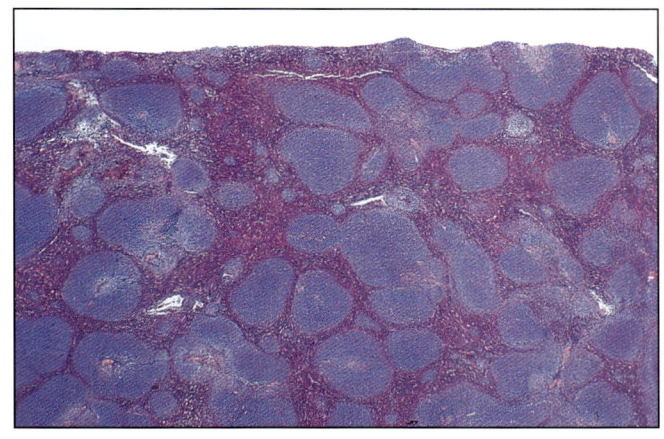
A

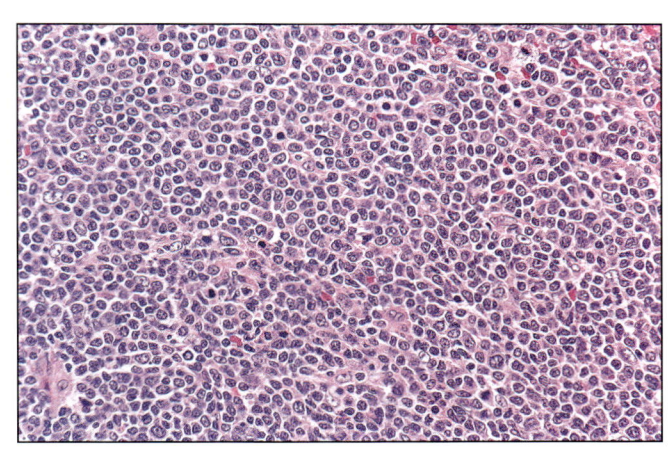
B

图21B.5　滤泡性淋巴瘤累及脾。（A）除白髓明显的膨胀和局灶性融合以外，红髓内也有显著的较小的淋巴瘤结节。（B）膨胀的白髓结节由滤泡中心细胞组成，不伴有散在的可染小体巨噬细胞。

- 浸润脾的纤维性小梁和血管内膜下（常见于白血病，而淋巴瘤少见）（图21B.6）。
- 免疫染色显示红髓内有致密成簇和片块状集聚的B淋巴细胞。

8. 扩大的红髓内出现大量大淋巴细胞，可出现在大细胞性淋巴瘤或传染性单核细胞增多症中。后者甚至可以浸润脾的纤维性小梁和血管内膜，更加类似于肿瘤性病变（图21B.7）不过，对于年轻患者，应该考虑传染性单核细胞增多症。此外，传染性单核细胞增多症的大淋巴细胞常常具有一系列的表现，有些细胞明显显示经由浆母细胞阶段向浆细胞的成熟过程。

9. 每当脾实质出现不能解释的硬化时，必须考虑系统性肥大细胞增生症的可能性（图21B.8）。

表21B.2	各种类型的非Hodgkin淋巴瘤累及脾的主要形态
淋巴瘤类型	脾受累的主要形态
B细胞淋巴瘤	
B-CLL/SLL	白髓明显膨胀，伴有红髓轻度受累
淋巴浆细胞性淋巴瘤	白髓明显膨胀，伴有红髓轻度受累
套细胞淋巴瘤	白髓明显膨胀，伴有红髓轻度受累；少数病例可能显示边缘区细胞分化
滤泡性淋巴瘤	白髓明显膨胀，伴有红髓轻度受累；少数病例可能显示边缘区细胞分化 3级滤泡性淋巴瘤可以形成大的结节状聚集，伴有脾结构的消失
结外和淋巴结边缘区B细胞淋巴瘤	白髓边缘区和（或）生发中心集聚，伴有红髓轻度受累
脾边缘区B细胞淋巴瘤	白髓明显膨胀，伴有红髓轻度受累
毛细胞淋巴瘤	红髓弥漫性受累，常见血池
弥漫性大B细胞淋巴瘤	淋巴瘤细胞呈大结节状聚集，伴有脾结构的消失（最为常见） 微小结节状结构（主要是富于T细胞/组织细胞的大B细胞淋巴瘤） 红髓弥漫性受累，窦状隙和脾索结构常常保留
Burkitt淋巴瘤	白髓和红髓常同时受累，虽然有些病例主要是白髓受累
T细胞淋巴瘤	
T细胞大颗粒状淋巴细胞白血病	红髓弥漫性受累（脾索更加明显），但是脾窦及脾索结构保留；白髓反应性滤泡增生（不受白血病性病变累及）
T细胞前淋巴细胞性白血病	红髓广泛受累（窦状隙和脾索），但是窦状隙和脾索结构常常保留；白髓破坏和萎缩
侵袭性NK细胞白血病	主要累及红髓；脾的纤维性小梁和血管壁常有浸润；常见坏死
成人T细胞白血病/淋巴瘤	主要累及红髓，但是白髓也可受到侵袭
蕈样霉菌病	红髓和白髓内不规则的结节 红髓弥漫性受累 选择性的聚集于小动脉周围淋巴鞘
结外NK/T细胞淋巴瘤	片块状或弥漫性浸润红髓；可局限于小动脉周围淋巴鞘；常浸润血管壁
肝脾T细胞淋巴瘤	红髓弥漫性受累，窦状隙和脾索结构常常保留
外周T细胞淋巴瘤，非特异性	淋巴瘤细胞呈大结节状聚集，伴有脾结构消失（最为常见） 红髓弥漫性受累 选择性地聚集于小动脉周围淋巴鞘
血管免疫母细胞性T细胞淋巴瘤	白髓扩张伴有红髓浸润
原发性系统性间变性大细胞淋巴瘤	淋巴瘤细胞呈大结节状聚集，伴有脾结构消失（最为常见）

由单一白髓受累形成的粟粒状小结节
Miliary small nodules produced by uniform white pulp involvement

主要累及白髓，切面形成粟粒状白色小结节，大小通常为几个毫米（图 21B.2）。有时结节可能较大，或大小明显不同。这是滤泡性淋巴瘤、各种小B细胞淋巴瘤和B-CLL/SLL累及脾的最具有特征性的表现。在少数情况下，Hodgkin淋巴瘤也可以形成这种大体表现。

组织学上，浸润引起白髓淋巴小体增大，而且可能表现为融合。然而，红髓也常受累，表现为整个实质内

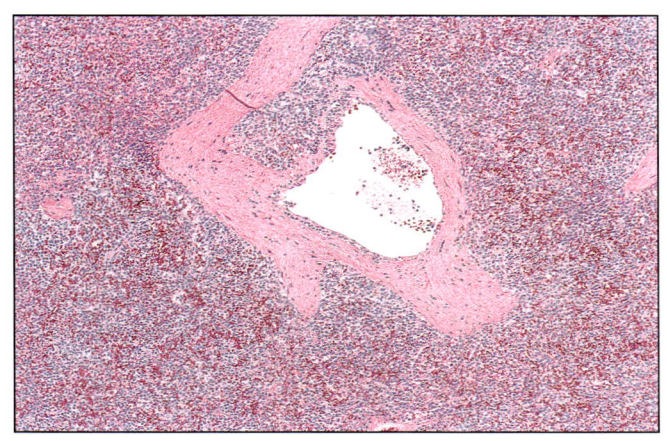

图21B.6　毛细胞性白血病累及的脾。小梁血管壁和内膜下有浸润。

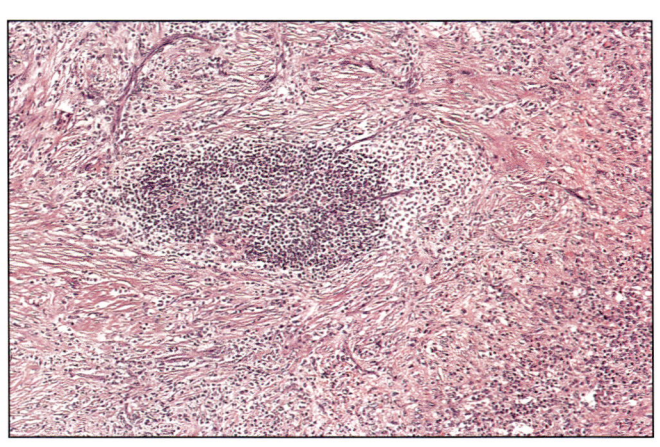

图21B.8　系统性肥大细胞增生症累及脾。肥大细胞簇常聚集于白髓的边缘区，伴有明显的硬化。

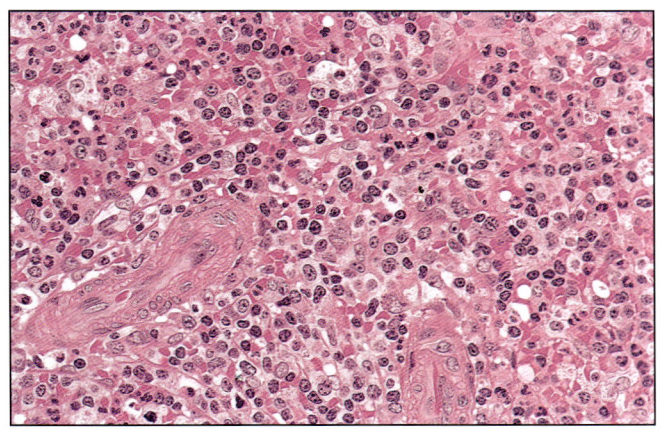

图21B.7　传染性单核细胞增多症累及脾。由于大细胞明显增加，可能被误诊为淋巴瘤。

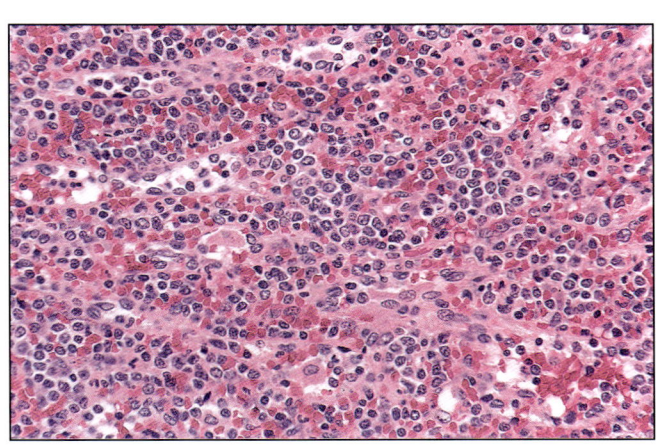

图21B.9　滤泡性淋巴瘤累及的脾。红髓有异常淋巴细胞（淋巴瘤细胞）浸润。

有散在分布的淋巴细胞微小结节（图21B.5和21B.9）。罕见的是，红髓受累非常广泛，以至于难以评估集中在白髓内的肿瘤性结节（图21B.10）。

仔细的形态学分析可以发现淋巴瘤分类的重要线索。受累的白髓结节周围是由胞浆透明的中等大小的细胞组成的边缘区，后者对于边缘区B细胞淋巴瘤并不特异，在各种类型的淋巴瘤中均可见到，尤其是滤泡性和套细胞淋巴瘤[14]。在套细胞淋巴瘤中，淋巴细胞浸润倾向于单形性。在滤泡性淋巴瘤中，结节是由具有滤泡中心细胞形态的细胞组成的，通常以中心细胞（小核裂细胞）为主（图21B.5B）。脾的边缘区B细胞淋巴瘤的典型表现为双相性细胞群，而前淋巴细胞和独特的具有中心核仁的拟免疫母细胞（paraimmunoblast）混合存在却是B-CLL/SLL的特征（图21B.10）。免疫组织化学染色对于这些小淋巴细胞肿瘤的分类具有重要作用（见第21章第1部分）。

系统性肥大细胞增生症也可选择性地累及白髓，类似于淋巴瘤（图21B.11）。倾向于在边缘区形成带状浸润，根据胞浆颗粒以及伴随的嗜酸性粒细胞和硬化可以鉴别诊断。

孤立性或几个小簇状结节
Solitary or several small clustered nodules

出现单个的由成簇的小而融合的结节构成的病变，或有几个这样的病变杂乱地分布在实质内，是Hodgkin淋巴瘤的显著特征，虽然较晚期的病例可以见到大块状多结节的受累（图21B.3）[6]。

在经典的Hodgkin淋巴瘤，小结节是由于混合性细胞浸润造成的淋巴小结膨大，包括Reed-Sternberg细胞及其亚型，伴有或不伴有硬化性的间质（图21B.12和21B.13）。这种浸润好像是从小动脉周围淋巴鞘和白髓边缘区开始。在Hodgkin淋巴瘤患者中，即使缺乏诊断性Reed-Sternberg细胞，也可做出脾受累的诊断，其条件是

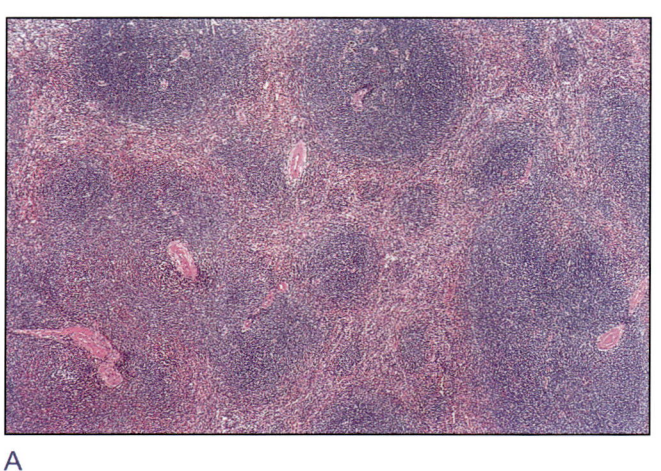
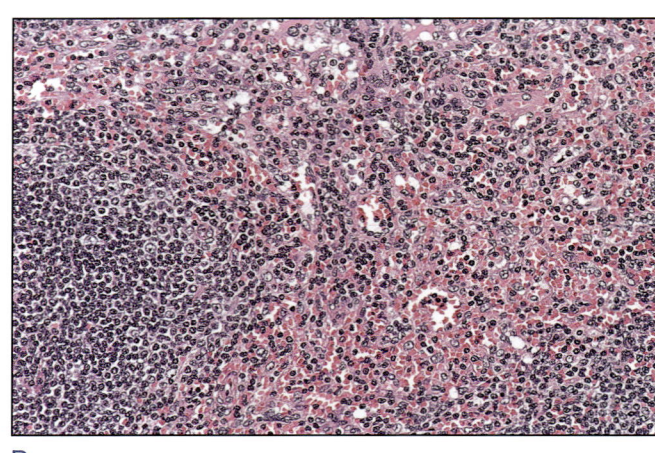

图21B.10　B细胞慢性淋巴细胞性白血病累及脾。（A）白髓膨胀，形成大小不等的结节，并且累及红髓，表现为弥漫性浸润或小结节状聚集。（B）白髓小结（左）由于单一淋巴细胞浸润而膨胀。红髓（右）同样也有明显的小淋巴细胞增加。

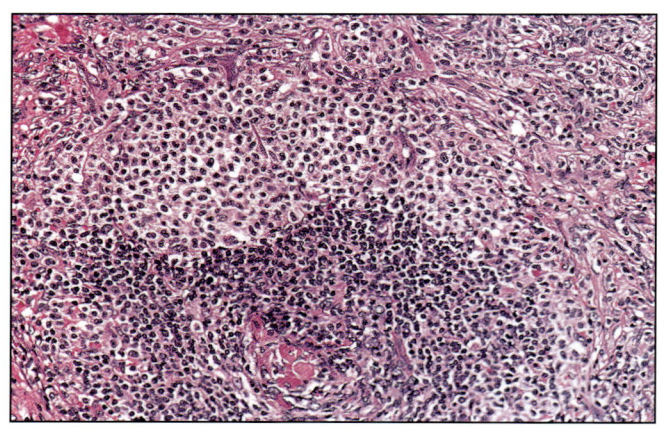

图21B.11　系统性肥大细胞增生症累及脾。白髓边缘区有带状肥大细胞聚集。肥大细胞有明显的淡染胞浆，可能被误认为淋巴瘤细胞。

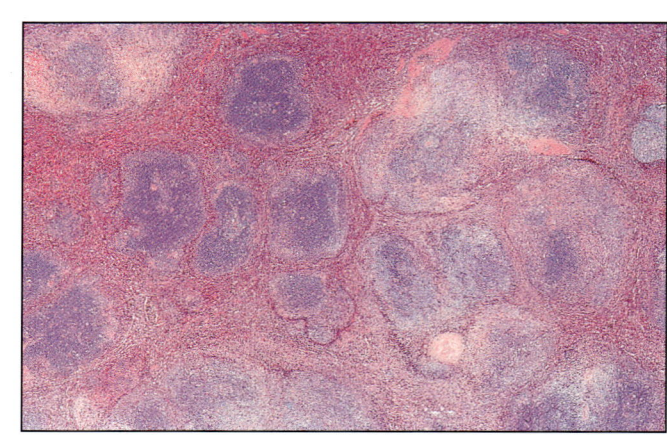

图21B.13　经典的Hodgkin淋巴瘤累及脾。本例显示受累范围比较广泛，伴有许多白髓淋巴小体增大和融合。

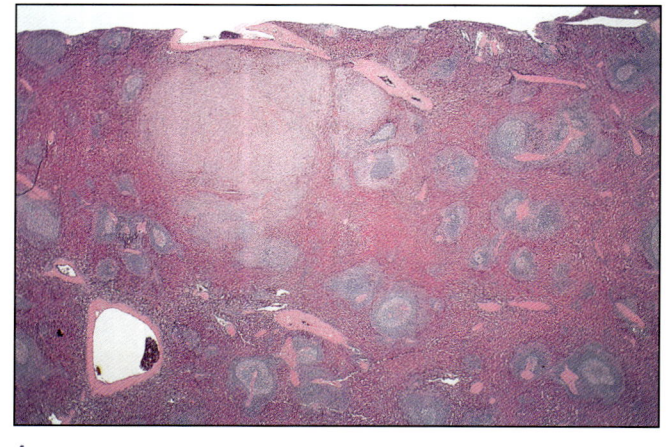
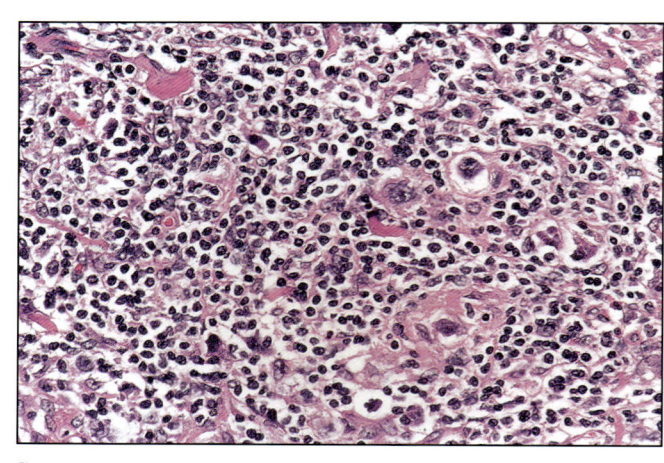

图21B.12　经典的Hodgkin淋巴瘤累及脾。（A）注意白髓淋巴小体的局灶性膨胀和融合，形成大的浅染的结节。（B）大结节内，在淋巴细胞和浆细胞的背景中可见Reed-Sternberg细胞的亚型。

在适当的背景中出现 Reed-Sternberg 细胞的亚型或具有突出核仁的大的非典型性细胞。如果怀疑，可以进行 CD30 和 CD15 免疫染色以证实这些大的非典型性细胞的本质。

当结节性淋巴细胞为主性 Hodgkin 淋巴瘤累及脾时，整个脾的淋巴小结常常均匀一致受累，并且病变不仅局限于肉眼可见的结节。实际上，脾的大体表现甚至可以是正常的[15]。与经典的 Hodgkin 淋巴瘤不同，后者的显微镜下受累程度一般与大体所见密切相关[16]。孤立性 L & H 细胞出现在小淋巴细胞（主要为 B 细胞）和组织细胞的背景中[15]。上皮样肉芽肿可能出现在肿瘤性病灶内或其周边。偶尔，肿瘤细胞可以延伸到红髓[17]。

脾的局限性反应性淋巴细胞增生可能类似于 Hodgkin 淋巴瘤累及脾[18]。在这种情况下，有局灶性集聚和融合的反应性大淋巴滤泡，伴有突出的生发中心。然而，在诊断前，必须对组织进行多方面的检查，以除外局灶性 Hodgkin 淋巴瘤和巨细胞病毒感染[19,20]。

孤立性或多发性大的鱼肉样结节
Solitary or multiple large fleshy nodules

B 细胞或 T 细胞系的大细胞淋巴瘤倾向于形成大而散在的瘤块，这些瘤块或为孤立性或为多发性（图 21B.14），一般呈鱼肉状、融合，常常出现坏死。有时，3 级滤泡性淋巴瘤和 Hodgkin 淋巴瘤累及脾也可有这种表现（图 21B.15）。组织学上，肿瘤细胞形成密集的片块，引起受累部位的正常脾实质结构完全破坏。

由弥漫性红髓膨胀引起的"牛肉红"脾
'Beefy-red' spleen caused by diffuse red pulp expansion

急性和慢性白血病，不论是淋巴细胞性还是髓细胞性，均倾向于主要累及红髓，导致切面呈均质性牛肉红外观，白髓受累不明显（图 21B.4）。组织学上，红髓显著弥漫性膨胀，伴有白髓消失或萎缩（图 21B.16）。B-CLL/SLL 是个例外，它主要累及白髓，虽然也有红髓浸润（图 21B.10）。

慢性髓细胞性白血病累及脾与原因不明的骨髓化生可能难以鉴别，因为这两种病变均有红髓内造血细胞浸润。支持前一种疾病诊断的特征是髓细胞明显，而不是混合性的造血细胞，并且浸润纤维小梁或血管壁（图 21B.16 和 21B.17）。

有几种类型的淋巴瘤选择性地累及红髓，伴有窦状隙和红髓框架保留。其中包括肝脾 T 细胞淋巴瘤、一些外周 T 细胞淋巴瘤病例（可能伴有噬血细胞综合征）以及少数大 B 细胞淋巴瘤病例[8]。在后两种病变，淋巴瘤

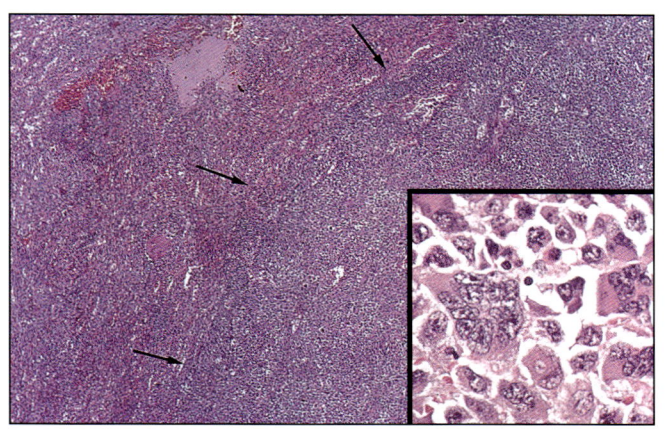

图21B.14　弥漫性大B细胞淋巴瘤累及脾。箭头所示为大的肿瘤结节。肿瘤累及区域结构完全消失。插图：肿瘤由大的多形性淋巴瘤细胞组成。

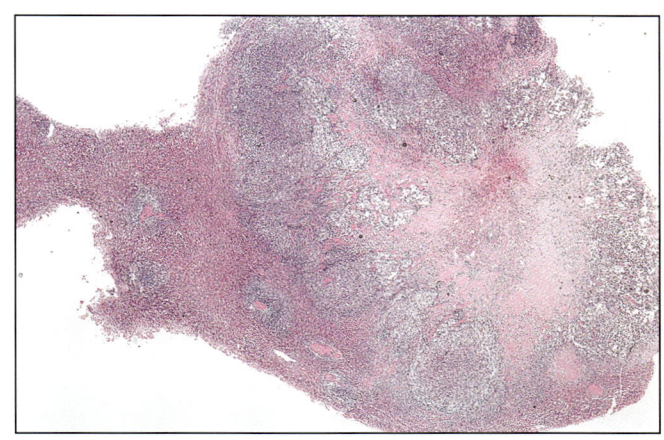

图21B.15　滤泡性大细胞淋巴瘤（3a级）累及脾。与 1 级和 2 级滤泡性淋巴瘤不同，3 级滤泡性淋巴瘤累及脾常常表现为形成大的肿瘤结节，而不是弥漫性粟粒状结构。

细胞散在分布于红髓内，不形成肿块性病变[21,22]。除非有明显的细胞学非典型性，否则在鉴别诊断时需要考虑传染性单核细胞增多症。

脾的原发性淋巴瘤
Primary lymphoma of the spleen

虽然脾常受到播散性淋巴瘤的累及，但脾的原发性淋巴瘤罕见。确定脾是原发部位的证据是：淋巴瘤应该局限于脾和（或）脾门淋巴结内，虽然有些作者也承认存在骨髓受累的病例[23]。由于不同研究应用不同的标准来选择病例，很难获得临床病理学特征性的同一标准[6]。

患者表现为脾大（腹痛或肿块）、伴有或不伴有发热、全身不适或血小板减少症[23-26]。不管组织学类型如何，总的生存率大约为 50%[6]。最近的研究提示，脾切除术后辅以化疗可以提高生存率[27]。

脾的原发性淋巴瘤

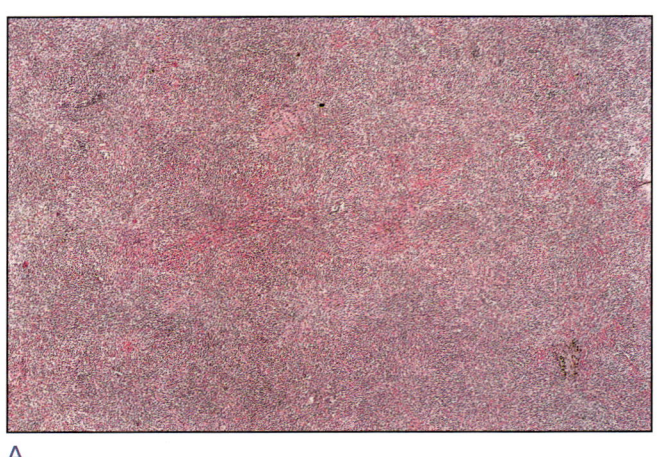

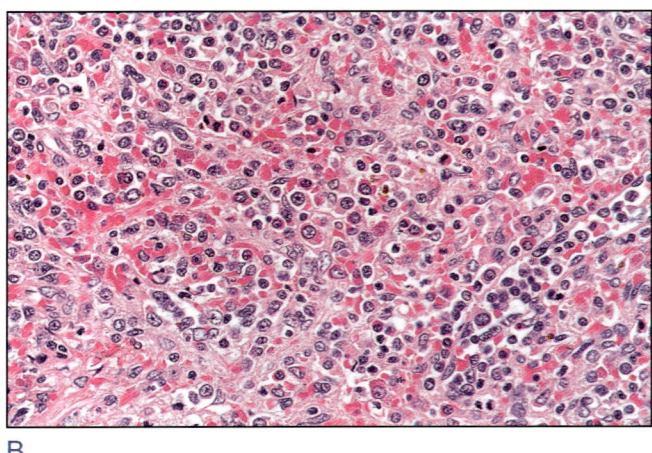

图21B.16 慢性髓细胞性白血病累及脾。（A）弥漫性浸润红髓，白髓结构消失。（B）浸润细胞为处于不同成熟阶段的粒细胞。

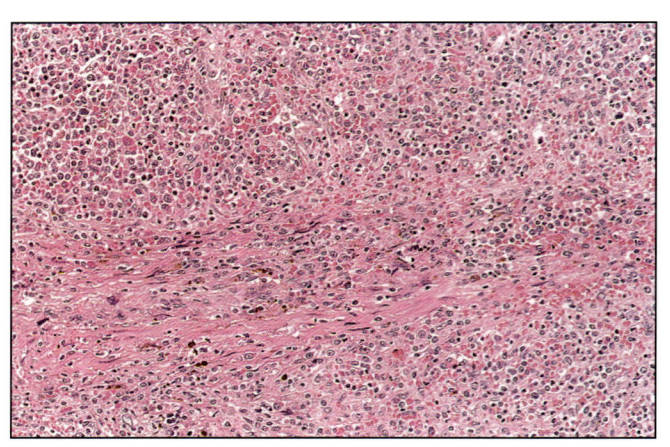

图21B.17 慢性髓细胞性白血病累及脾。显示纤维性小梁（水平切面，穿过视野中心）有异常细胞浸润。这种特征强烈提示：病变为肿瘤性而不是反应性的。

各种组织学类型的非Hodgkin淋巴瘤均可作为原发性淋巴瘤发生于脾。绝大多数病例为B细胞系来源，弥漫性大B细胞淋巴瘤最为常见[6,27,28]。罕见的是，淋巴瘤被显著的上皮样肉芽肿性反应所掩盖，以致难以辨认疾病过程的肿瘤性本质[29,30]。例外的是，组织细胞肉瘤和Hodgkin淋巴瘤也可以原发于脾[31,32]。

弥漫性大B细胞淋巴瘤累及脾有三种方式[22]：

- 巨大结节状肿块，以Ⅰ期疾病为主，bcl-6呈阳性，临床预后较好。
- 微小结节状结构，以晚期疾病为主，bcl-6呈阳性，预后不良。这种结构通常是由富于T细胞和（或）组织细胞的大B细胞淋巴瘤引起的（图21B.18）[33]。微小结节由大量CD3⁺的T细胞、CD68⁺的组织细胞以

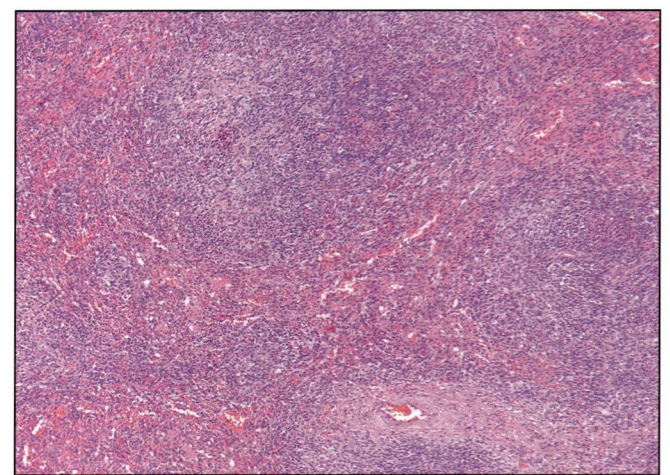

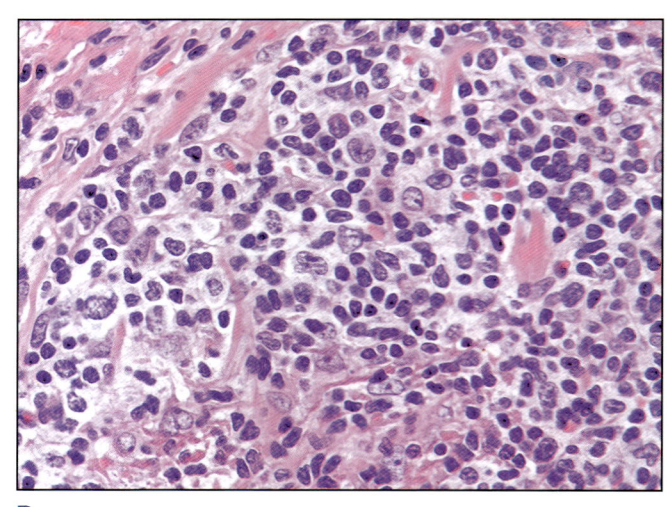

图21B.18 富于T细胞的大B细胞淋巴瘤累及脾。（A）低倍镜下可见明显的微小结节结构。（B）每个结节均由具有不规则折叠核的非典型性大细胞（CD20⁺淋巴瘤细胞）组成，散在分布于小淋巴细胞中。

1296

及具有免疫球蛋白轻链限制性的散在的CD20⁺的大B细胞组成。大B细胞bcl-6呈阳性，而CD10呈阴性。微小结节内没有滤泡树突状细胞。
- 弥漫性累及红髓，以晚期疾病为主，预后差。

以脾受累为主要特征的淋巴瘤和白血病
Lymphomas and leukemias with splenic involvement as a dominant feature

许多类型的淋巴瘤和白血病均可明显累及脾，虽然其他部位也常常受累。其中包括脾的边缘区B细胞淋巴瘤、肝脾T细胞淋巴瘤和毛细胞性白血病。罕见的是，滤泡性淋巴瘤或淋巴浆细胞性淋巴瘤最初可以表现为脾大[34]。系统性肥大细胞增生症也常常表现为脾受累。

脾边缘区B细胞淋巴瘤
Splenic marginal zone B-cell lymphoma

定义

脾边缘区B细胞淋巴瘤是一种少见的原发于脾的低级别B细胞淋巴瘤类型[35,36]。实际上，所有"伴有循环血液内绒毛状淋巴细胞（villous lymphocytes）的脾淋巴瘤"患者均表现出与脾边缘区B细胞淋巴瘤相同的脾的变化，但是并非所有脾边缘区B细胞淋巴瘤患者的外周血内都有绒毛状淋巴细胞（图21B.19）[37,38]。

临床特征

患者为老年人，平均发病年龄为68岁[39]。男性稍多见[35,36,40-45]。患者表现为脾大，外周淋巴结不大。外周血、骨髓和肝常常受累。某些病例可能有自身免疫性溶血性贫血或血小板减少症[46]。

部分脾边缘区B细胞淋巴瘤病例与丙型肝炎感染相关[47]，丙型肝炎抗体阳性病例在抗病毒治疗（干扰素-α₂ᵦ，合用或不用利巴韦林，ribavirin）之后，淋巴瘤可能消退[48,49]。

临床经过平稳，总的5年生存率为65%～78%[39,45]。病程进展中位数时间在5年以上[50]。治疗选择脾切除。某些患者可以只观察而不进行积极的治疗，对化疗的反应不确定。少数情况下可以合并大细胞淋巴瘤，这与侵袭性的临床经过相关。

病理学

脾通常明显增大，重量常超过1千克。切面可见粟粒大小的结节（图21B.20）。组织学上，白髓结节性膨大，伴有显著的边缘区结构，并有不同程度的融合（图21B.19）[36-38,40]。某些结节有残留的小的反应性生发中心（图21B.21）。组成结节的细胞显示特征性的双向结构，中心区为染色质致密的小淋巴细胞，外周区为伴有淡染至透明胞浆的中等大小的细胞（类似于正常脾的边缘区细胞）（图21B.22）。外周区偶尔可见转化的大细胞。然而，红髓也总是受累。红髓显示小淋巴细胞弥漫性浸润，伴有中等大小细胞的微小结节状集聚。常有明显的脾窦浸润。当红髓受累严重时，可能掩盖白髓的微小结节状结构。不常见的表现是浆细胞分化和上皮样肉芽肿。

受累的淋巴结有明显的结节状结构，常常伴有淋巴窦的扩张。结节是在先前存在的滤泡基础上形成的，可见小的残留的生发中心。结节是由小淋巴细胞组成的，伴有少数散在的转化性大细胞。与脾不同，通常缺乏伴

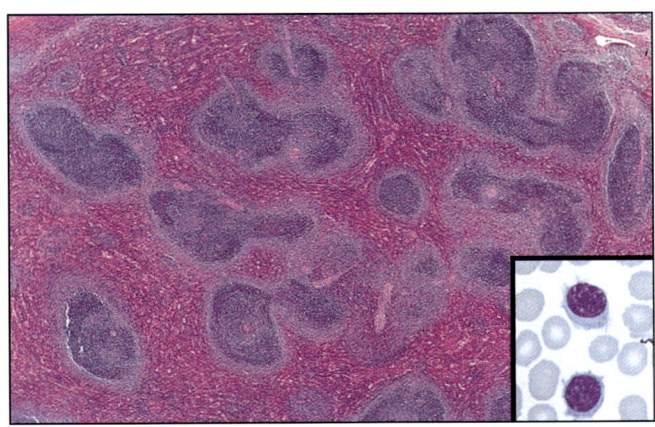

图21B.19　脾边缘区B细胞淋巴瘤。白髓淋巴小体显著膨大并融合。注意淋巴小体周围可见明显淡染的"边缘区"细胞套。插图：血液循环中的淋巴样细胞具有绒毛状突起。

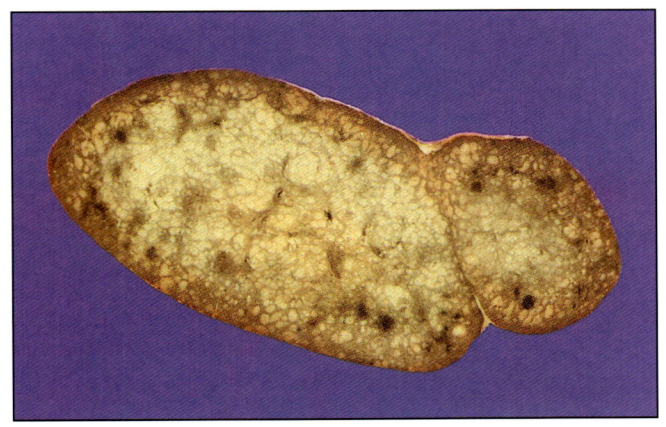

图21B.20　脾边缘区B细胞淋巴瘤累及的脾的切面。呈粟粒状受累的结构，但本例粟粒状结节相对较大并比较密集。

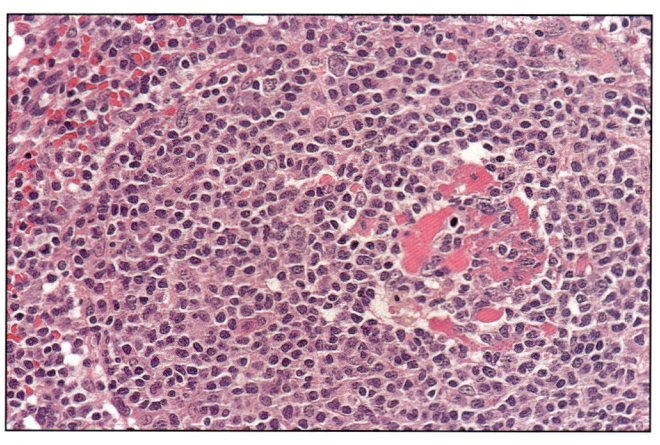

图21B.21 脾边缘区B细胞淋巴瘤。这个增大的白髓结节仍旧保留了残留的生发中心。生发中心由小淋巴样细胞环绕，融合到周围胞浆淡染的稍大细胞中。小淋巴细胞和较大的细胞都是肿瘤细胞。

免疫细胞化学

- B细胞系标记物阳性，即CD20、CD22、Ig（IgM，常常还有IgD）呈阳性。
- CD5、CD10、CD23、CD43、CD103、bcl-6 和 cyclin D1呈阴性[39,53,54]。
- Bcl-2呈阳性。CD21和CD35表达不定。Ki67免疫染色显示边缘区增生指数高，但是在深染小细胞区，增生指数则较低。许多反应性T淋巴细胞分布在所有的肿瘤间隔内。

遗传学特征

重排的Ig基因或者是非突变的，或者显示正在进行的体细胞超突变（somatic hypermutation），提示某些脾边缘区B细胞淋巴瘤起源于原始的B细胞，而其他病例来源于滤泡后B细胞[36,53,55-58]。具有没有重排的 *BCL1* 和 *BCL2* 基因[43,53,59]。

最常见的遗传学改变包括1、3、7和8号染色体的改变，尤其是表现为del（3）和del(7q21-32)[59-62]。某些病例显示有通过7q21位点的染色体易位的 *CDK6* 基因失调[63]。*p53* 基因通常不发生突变，除非是在伴有大细胞增加的侵袭性亚型[52,53,64]。

基因表达谱研究显示主要是单一的标记，伴有B细胞受体信号基因的下调、肿瘤坏死因子信号和核因子-κB（nuclear factor-κB，NFκB）的激活[65]。其他过表达的基因包括 *SELL* 和 *LPXN*（在脾内高表达）、淋巴瘤癌基因 *ARHH* 和 *TCL1*、AP-1转录因子和 *NOTCH2*[65,66]。位于缺失区7q31的 *CAV1*、*CAV2* 和 *GNG11* 基因下调。*ILF1*、*SENATAXIN* 和 *CD40* 的表达可将脾边缘区B细胞淋巴瘤与其他小B细胞淋巴瘤鉴别开来[65]。

有边缘区细胞表现的淋巴瘤细胞[51]。骨髓受累是在间质内，伴有小淋巴细胞结节状聚集及转化的母细胞。此外，常有窦状隙内的浸润，但是如果不借助于免疫染色，可能并不明显[45]。

侵袭性变型

侵袭性变型以大细胞数量增加为特征。伴有明显侵袭性的临床经过，6例死亡患者中5例（80%以上）死于4年之内[52]。组织学上，具有显著的伴有突出核仁的大淋巴细胞成分，位于受累白髓的外带，偶尔可超过外带。这种变型可能是脾边缘区B细胞淋巴瘤偶尔伴发的大细胞淋巴瘤的前兆。

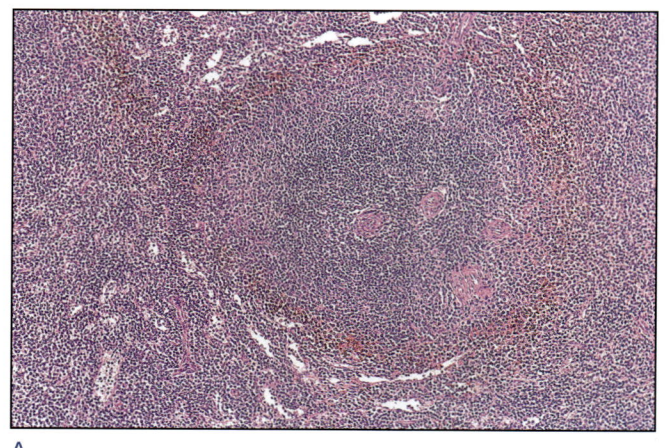

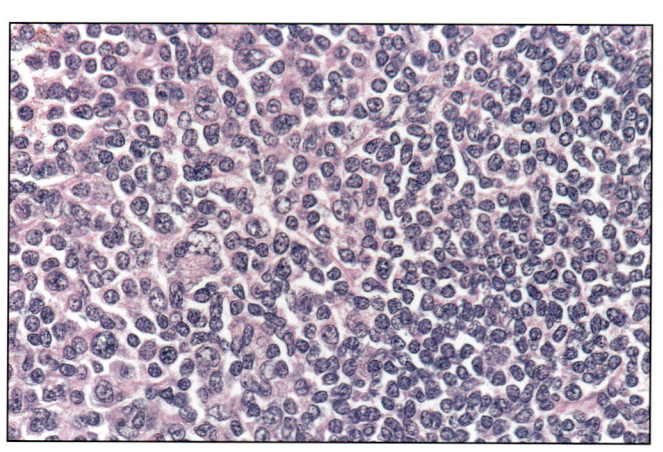

图21B.22 脾边缘区B细胞淋巴瘤。（A）这个增大的白髓结节不再有可辨认的残留的生发中心。注意中心的细胞较小且染色较深，而周围的细胞略大。（B）高倍镜下显示双相性细胞群。右侧为小淋巴细胞。左侧为胞浆淡染的略大一些的细胞。

与其他边缘区B细胞淋巴瘤的关系和命名问题

尽管形态学和免疫表型类似，但是脾边缘区B细胞淋巴瘤缺乏真正的边缘区生长方式，而且常常表达IgD，不同于淋巴结和结外边缘区B细胞淋巴瘤。脾边缘区B细胞淋巴瘤不显示结外边缘区B细胞淋巴瘤特有的染色体易位[67]。

淋巴瘤细胞与正常边缘区B细胞虽然相似，但是"边缘区"这一术语可能是一个误称，其理由如下[36,38,40,68]：

- 脾内受累的淋巴小结缺乏完整的外套区，严格地讲不在边缘区的间隔内。
- 肿瘤细胞不局限于边缘区。
- 双相性细胞学：有相当数量的小肿瘤细胞，这些细胞缺乏脾边缘区细胞的形态学特征。
- 组织学、免疫表型和细胞遗传学特征与其他边缘区B细胞淋巴瘤不同。
- 累及脾的其他低级别淋巴瘤可以表现出边缘区的形态[14,69,70]。

鉴别诊断

- 滤泡性淋巴瘤（follicular lymphoma）：滤泡性淋巴瘤累及脾时，滤泡可能被边缘区包绕，但是常常表现出明显的肿瘤性特征。
- 套细胞淋巴瘤（mantle cell lymphoma）：细胞比较单一，虽然可以出现由具有比较丰富透明胞浆的细胞组成的边缘区样区域，但几乎不存在混合的有核仁的转化细胞。Cyclin D1的免疫反应强烈支持套细胞淋巴瘤的诊断[38,40]。
- MALT型结外边缘区B细胞淋巴瘤（extranodal marginal zone B-cell lymphoma of MALT type）：在少数情况下可以累及脾。与脾边缘区B细胞淋巴瘤不同，白髓受累的形态真正位于边缘区，残留的生发中心周围保留套层细胞[70]。

肝脾T细胞淋巴瘤
Hepatosplenic T-cell lymphoma

定义

肝脾T细胞淋巴瘤，曾被命名为肝脾γδT细胞淋巴瘤，是一种不常见的独特类型的T细胞淋巴瘤，以肝和脾的窦状隙明显受累为特征，常常表达γδ型T细胞受体[71]。

临床特征

肝脾T细胞淋巴瘤的最大特征是发生于年轻人，年龄中位数为34岁，明显多见于男性[71,72]。患者表现为肝脾大，常常伴有全身症状，但是无淋巴结肿大。血小板减少症常见，而且即使脾切除后仍可持续存在。骨髓常常受累，而且循环血中也可出现少量淋巴瘤细胞。肝脾T细胞淋巴瘤可以发生于免疫抑制情况下，如器官移植受者[73-78]。

本病具有侵袭性的临床经过，生存时间中位数为16个月。虽然化疗最初有效，但是几乎总是复发。骨髓移植为长期生存提供了最大的希望[71,72,79-85]。

病理学

脾明显增大，重量通常超过1kg。切面显示均匀一致的牛肉红外观。组织学上，脾红髓明显膨大，内有中等大小的淋巴细胞浸润，而白髓淋巴小体消失或萎缩[80-83,86,87]。然而，红髓脾窦和白髓脾索结构依然保留。淋巴细胞表现单一，核呈圆形、椭圆形或偶尔呈不规则形，核染色质相当致密，具有中等量的淡染至透明的胞浆（图21B.23A）。核分裂象非常少见。一般没有坏死。

在肝，淋巴瘤细胞一般分布于肝窦，不同于普通淋巴瘤累及汇管区（图21B.23）。在骨髓，由于淋巴瘤细胞通常局限于窦状隙，所以在常规检查时可能被遗漏，但是通过应用T细胞系标记物进行免疫染色容易辨认。

免疫细胞化学

- T细胞系标记物阳性，如CD2、CD3和CD7。
- 多数病例γδT细胞受体呈阳性，少数病例表达αβT细胞受体[88]。TIA-1常常呈阳性，而穿孔素（perforin）常常呈阴性，表明肝脾T细胞淋巴瘤是一种非活化的细胞毒素T细胞肿瘤[87]。
- CD5、CD4和CD8通常呈阴性，虽然个别病例可能表达CD8[72]。
- CD56表达常见[72,87]。

遗传学特征

肿瘤显示γ链T细胞受体基因重排。β链受体基因可能是种系重排或部分重排。EB病毒呈阴性[72,78]，这一特征可能有助于与结外NK/T细胞淋巴瘤鉴别，后者同样表达细胞毒标记物和CD56，但EB病毒常阳性。

遗传分析表明，等臂染色体7q出现率高，而环状染色体7罕见。三倍体8和染色体Y缺失也常常出现[81-83,87,89-93]。

鉴别诊断和诊断中的问题

肝脾T细胞淋巴瘤的脾的组织学表现与毛细胞性白血病无法区分，除了血肿不常见以外，两者很难区别。免疫组化染色对于区分两者非常重要。

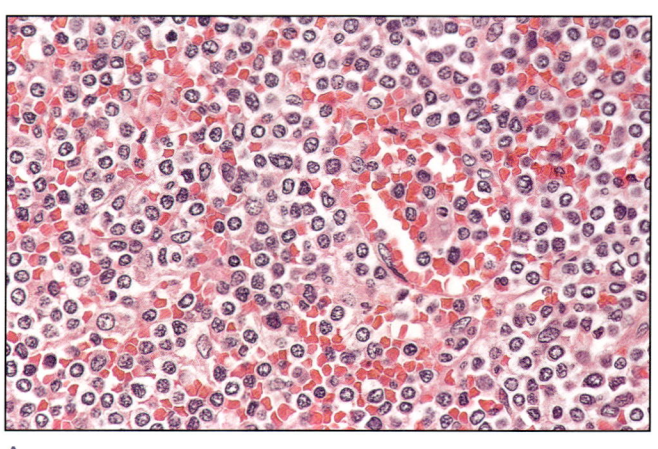 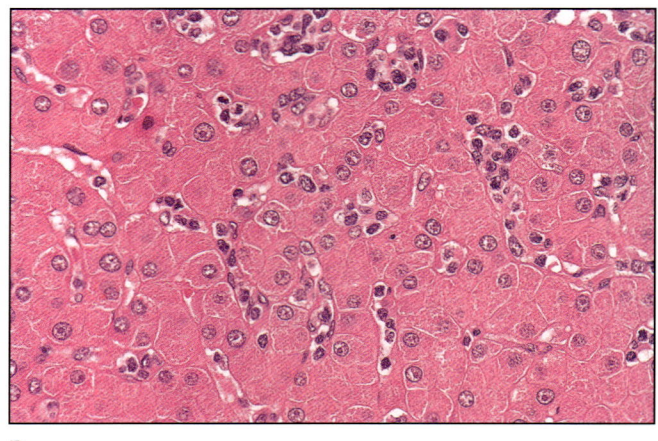

图21B.23 肝脾T细胞淋巴瘤。（A）单形性细胞群累及脾的红髓，细胞中等大小，胞浆淡染。核为圆形，或略有凹陷。注意在形态学上明显类似于毛细胞性白血病。（B）肝典型表现为肝窦受累。

一个普遍错误的概念是：存在 γ 链 T 细胞受体基因重排的证据则支持 γδT 细胞淋巴瘤的诊断。事实上，表达 αβT 细胞受体的普通 T 细胞淋巴瘤也总是显示 γ 链 T 细胞受体基因的重排。γδT 细胞淋巴瘤的确诊依赖于免疫细胞化学检查证实有 γδT 细胞受体表达，只有应用新鲜或冰冻组织才能可靠地进行此检查。免疫染色没有得到证实时，如果有 T 细胞标记物表达且缺乏 αβT 细胞受体表达（如通过应用 βF1 抗体），可以推测有 γδT 细胞受体表达。

毛细胞性白血病　Hairy cell leukemia

定义

毛细胞性白血病是一种经过缓慢的 B 细胞性白血病，以循环血内出现多个长的胞浆突起的白血病细胞为特征[6]。

临床特征

本章只讨论显著的特征和组织学所见（其他细节见第22章的详细讨论）[6,94]。毛细胞性白血病好发于中年人，临床表现为疲劳、劳累时呼吸困难、腹胀或感染。脾大常见，但淋巴结肿大少见。有些病例可能伴有坏死性血管炎。

本病临床经过缓慢，中位生存时间为 4～5 年。可能合并感染，导致死亡。治疗方式包括观察、脾切除术、α-干扰素治疗以及应用诸如 2'-脱氧柯福霉素（2'-deoxycoformycin）、2-氯脱氧腺苷（2-chlorodeoxyadenosine）和一磷酸氟达拉滨（fludarabine monophosphate）等药物[94-96]。

病理学

为了诊断或治疗的目的，常常需对毛细胞性白血病患者进行脾切除术。脾的重量通常大于 1 kg，均匀一致，呈红色，质硬（图 21B.4）[97,98]。组织学上，红髓内有弥漫性的形态单一的浸润细胞，并不形成结节，伴有白髓萎缩和消失（图 21B.24）。肿瘤细胞核中等大小，呈椭圆形、肾形，有时呈分叶状[97,99]，染色质细腻，核仁不显著，核分裂象罕见。细胞核的间隙一般较宽，因为有丰富的弱嗜酸性至透明的胞浆（图 21B.25）。有时可见交错的细胞界限。在肿瘤细胞"浸润"浆液内的区域，可以清楚地见到一圈宽的胞浆和纤细的胞浆突起（图 21B.26）。小梁血管常常有内膜下和管壁浸润（图 21B.6）。存在内衬白血病细胞的大小不同的血池（假窦）是毛细胞性白血病的特征（图 21B.24），这种结构可能非常突出，以至于类似海绵状血管瘤[97]。在受累不太广泛的脾，白血病浸润主要局限于脾小梁静脉内皮下区域，并在纤维性小梁周围也有浸润[98]。

淋巴结通常轻微肿大或不肿大。淋巴细胞浸润极少导致脾结构的完全消失，而是主要局限于副皮质区，

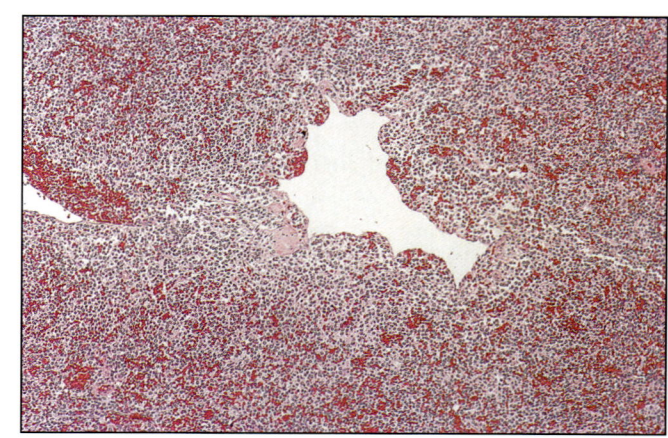

图21B.24 毛细胞性白血病累及脾。红髓弥漫性受累，伴有白髓消失。视野中央，肿瘤细胞浸润血管壁。整个红髓内散在分布多发性小血池。

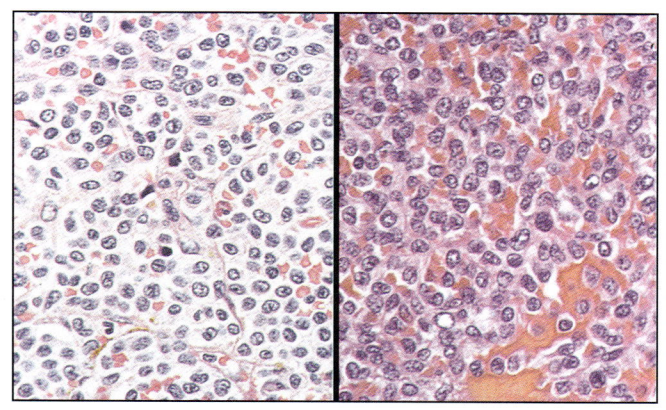

图21B.25 毛细胞性白血病累及脾。注意单一的单核细胞浸润，由于胞浆丰富造成核的间隔加宽。核呈卵圆形或有凹陷，具有细腻的染色质。左：胞浆透明。右：胞浆弱嗜酸性。由于组织切片较厚，细胞比较密集。有小而不规则的血池。

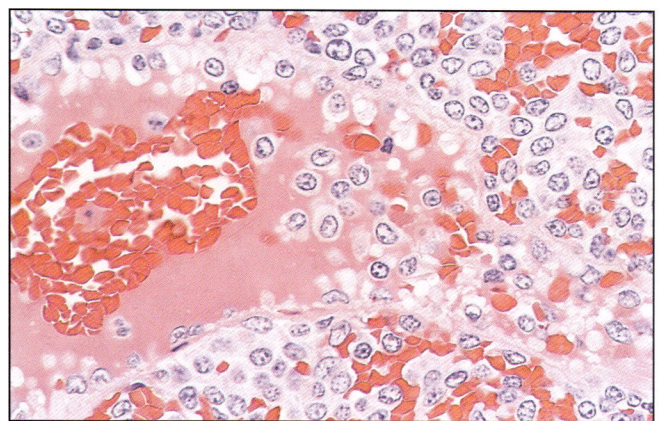

图21B.26 毛细胞性白血病累及脾。浸在血管浆液中的细胞能够最好地显示毛细胞的肿胀性胞浆和绒毛状的细胞轮廓。

表现为具有透明胞浆的均匀一致的细胞呈簇状或片状浸润。

组织化学和免疫细胞化学

- B细胞系标记物呈阳性，如CD19、CD20、CD22CD79a和表面免疫球蛋白。
- 抗酒石酸酸性磷酸酶反应呈阳性，这种酶现在可通过免疫组化方法检查[100]。常常阳性的有CD25、毛细胞性白血病相关抗原（HC1、HC2、B-ly7/CD103）、浆细胞相关性抗原（PCA-1）以及一些组织细胞标记物（CD11c和CD68）[94,101-103]。
- CD5、CD10和CD23通常为阴性。某些病例表达cyclin D1，但是没有 *BCL1* 基因的重排[104]。关于S100蛋白免疫反应的报告结果不一[105,106]。

遗传学特征

存在Ig基因重排。Ig基因中体细胞突变率常常较高，表明毛细胞性白血病是生发中心后B细胞肿瘤[55]。尚无一致性的细胞遗传学变化。毛细胞性白血病表现为同质性结构的基因表达谱，不同于其他B细胞淋巴瘤[107]。与记忆性B细胞密切相关，但是显示控制细胞粘附基因的表达和对趋化因子的反应发生改变[107]。

鉴别诊断

- 系统性肥大细胞增生症也以透明细胞为特征，但是为片块状分布，而且伴有硬化和嗜酸性细胞浸润。
- 低级别B细胞淋巴瘤常常伴有白髓内结节形成，而且肿瘤细胞核的间隔没有那么宽。应该注意的是，其他疾病偶尔也可出现血池结构，如B-CLL和骨髓瘤[97]。
- 肝脾T细胞淋巴瘤。

系统性肥大细胞增生症（系统性肥大细胞病）
Systemic mastocytosis (systemic mast cell disease)

临床特征

系统性肥大细胞增生症（见22章）以脾、淋巴结、骨髓和肝内肥大细胞异常浸润为特征，伴有或不伴有皮肤受累[108]。主要发生于男性，平均年龄为60岁[109]。患者表现为皮肤疾病、过敏反应、骨痛或骨折（骨质疏松、溶骨性病变、骨硬化，或以上病变混合出现）、胃肠道症状（腹痛、腹泻及消化性溃疡）、呼吸系统症状（哮喘、呼吸困难）、血液表现（血细胞减少症、嗜酸性细胞增多症、单核细胞增多症或血循环中出现肥大细胞）或肝脾大。这些症状多数都是由肥大细胞释放组胺（histamine）引起的。还可能伴有血液疾病和实体恶性肿瘤[109-113]。常常与髓细胞的肿瘤性疾病并存，提示系统性肥大细胞增生症本身可能是一种髓细胞疾病，而且肥大细胞也可能是髓细胞来源[112,114,115]。罕见的伴有纵隔生殖细胞肿瘤的病例也有报道[116]。

临床经过不定，总的5年存活率为52%[109]。死亡通常发生在最初3年之内。缺乏皮肤病变，出现细胞非典型性以及伴有血液疾病是预后不好的特征[112,115,117]。基本上采取对症治疗[109]。

肥大细胞增生症的分类 [108,109,112,115,118-122]

- 皮肤肥大细胞增生症(cutaneous mastocytosis)（色素性荨麻疹，urticaria pigmentosa）：仅有皮肤受累，预后良好。在青春期常常可自发性消退。
- 系统性肥大细胞增生症：以无自发性缓解的多器官受累为特征。有以下几型：
  - 惰性（indolent）系统性肥大细胞增生症：通常表现为色素性荨麻疹样皮肤病变，伴有内脏器官相对成熟的肥大细胞浸润，缺乏血液异常和进行性器官损害的征象。这种类型的预期寿命几乎正常。
- 系统性肥大细胞增生症伴有克隆性非肥大细胞系血液疾病：如骨髓异常增生综合征、慢性骨髓增生性疾病、急性髓细胞性白血病和淋巴瘤。
- 侵袭性（aggressive）系统性肥大细胞增生症：以肥大细胞进行性浸润各种器官为特征，肥大细胞常常表现为细胞学非典型性，但是缺乏伴随的克隆性血液疾病。存在下述一项或几项特征：骨髓功能障碍，表现为一种或一种以上血细胞减少；可以触及的肝大，伴有肝功能损伤、腹水和（或）门脉高压；骨骼受累；可以触及的脾大，伴有脾功能亢进；胃肠肥大细胞浸润导致吸收障碍，伴有体重下降。预后不良。
- 肥大细胞白血病（mast cell leukemia）：特征是血循环内非典型性肥大细胞大于10%，骨髓内肥大细胞大于20%。本病具有迅速致死的临床经过。

病理学

肥大细胞具有卵圆形、有切迹或二分叶的细胞核，核染色质细腻，核仁不明显。但是有些细胞可能呈梭形[114,115,117,125]。肥大细胞具有明显的淡染或透明的胞浆，胞浆内含有数量不等的细颗粒（图21B.27）。胞浆颗粒可能稀少，尤其是在侵袭性肥大细胞增生症。肥大细胞可呈簇状或岛屿状，或散在分布，但几乎总是伴有不同数量的嗜酸性细胞和纤细的硬化带。

脾一般显著增大，伴有被膜增厚。切面常常可见突出的纤维性条纹（图21B.28）。组织学上，最先累及白髓的边缘区和纤维性小梁，但是脾的其他区域也可受累（图21B.11）。随着病程的加长，肥大细胞可能变得不明显，代之以致密的硬化带（图21B.8）。

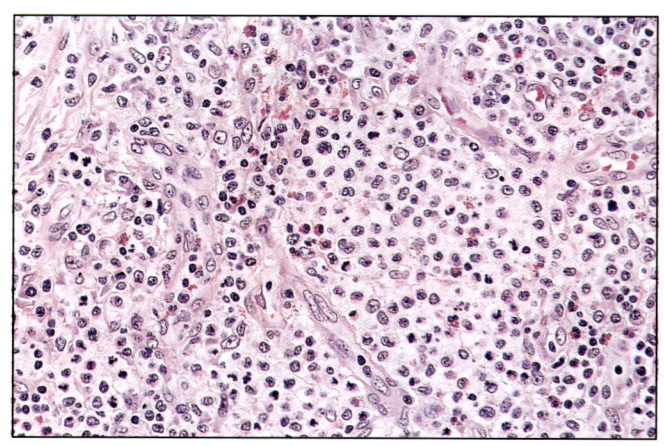

图21B.27 系统性肥大细胞增生症。本例主要是二分叶核。胞浆一般透明，或有时呈细颗粒状。混合存在的丰富的嗜酸性细胞提示为肥大细胞疾病，而不是淋巴瘤。

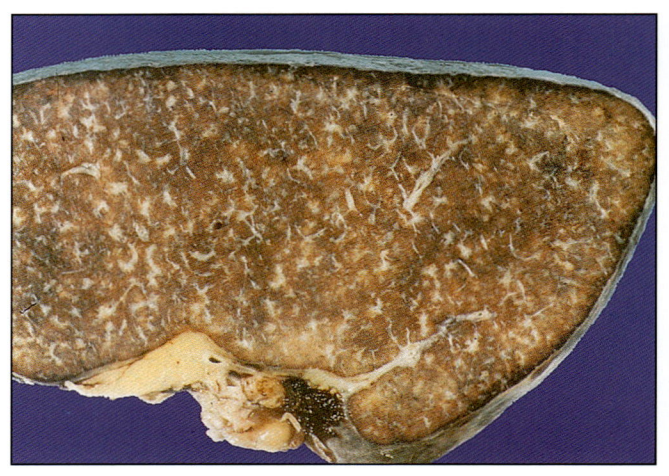

图21B.28 系统性肥大细胞增生症累及脾。明显增大的脾的切面显示明显的白色条纹，这是本病的特征。白色条纹相当于组织学上的硬化区域。

淋巴结的肥大细胞浸润发生在窦状隙、副皮质区、滤泡周围或在少数情况下形成假滤泡结构[114,115,117,123,124]。某些病例可能伴有明显的毛细血管或小静脉增生。在肝，肥大细胞主要见于汇管区，但是也可以散在分布于肝窦内[125]。骨髓受累可以是轻微的，伴有梭形肥大细胞的集聚，混有嗜酸性细胞和数量不等的淋巴细胞，即所谓的"嗜酸细胞性纤维组织细胞病变"（eosinophilic fibrohistiocytic lesion），或者可能是广泛的小梁旁和血管周围受累。有时，伴随的纤维化非常广泛，以至于类似于病因不明的骨髓外化生[110,117,126,127]。在皮肤，肥大细胞主要出现在血管周围或分布于真皮上部的皮肤附属器周围[115]。

遗传学特征

毫无疑问，现在认为系统性肥大细胞增生症是一种肿瘤性疾病[120,128,129]。在肥大细胞形成过程中具有重要作用的 *C-KIT* 基因与系统性肥大细胞增生症的发生有关。*C-KIT* 基因的酪氨酸激酶结构域的具有功能的体细胞突变（最常见的是 Asp816 → Val），几乎见于所有的侵袭性系统性肥大细胞增生症以及少数惰性系统性肥大细胞增生症患者[118,130-134]。然而，伴有 Asp816 → Val 突变的患者对酪氨酸激酶抑制剂伊玛替尼（imatinib）的治疗反应常常较差[135-138]，因为突变的位置导致了构象变化，会妨碍与伊玛替尼的结合，但并不一定发生。另一方面，系统性肥大细胞增生症-高嗜酸性粒细胞性综合征患者以及有 *FIP1L1-PDGFR-α* 融合、野生型 *C-KIT* 和一些 *C-KIT* 突变（如F522C）的患者对伊玛替尼的治疗反应良好[135-137]。具有遗传性 *C-KIT* 种系突变者常常发生多发性胃肠道间质瘤和系统性肥大细胞增生症[139]。

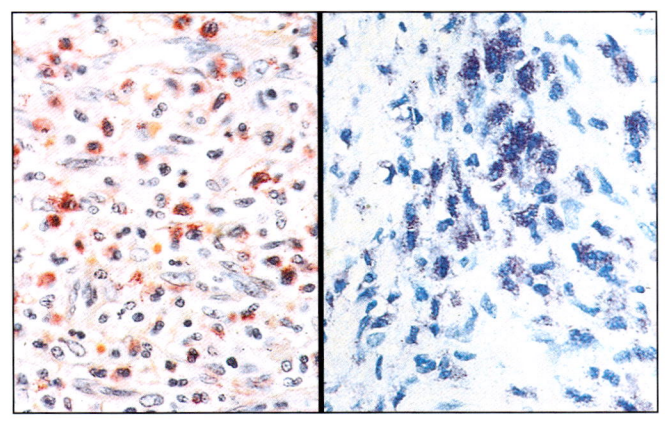

图21B.29 用于确诊系统性肥大细胞增生症的特殊染色。左侧：氯乙酸酯酶染色颗粒呈亮红色。细胞与细胞之间染色强度不同。右侧：甲苯胺蓝染色肥大细胞呈异染性。

鉴别诊断

由于在常规组织切片中不易辨认肥大细胞的颗粒，所以系统性肥大细胞增生症常被误诊为其他淋巴网状系统疾病，如淋巴瘤、毛细胞性白血病和反应性组织细胞增生。辨认肥大细胞的主要线索是出现成簇浅染的"单核细胞样"细胞，伴有嗜酸性细胞和硬化。通过 Giemsa（紫色颗粒）、甲苯胺蓝（异染性颗粒）或氯乙酸脂酶染色（亮红色颗粒，但是颗粒性白细胞也可阳性）可能容易确诊（图21B.29）[6]。在确定肥大细胞分化方面，肥大细胞类胰蛋白酶或 CD117/c-kit 免疫染色比组织化学染色敏感[122,140]。几乎所有的系统性肥大细胞增生症均有 CD25 表达，CD25 表达对于区分正常和反应性肥大细胞具有价值[141]。

脾的组织细胞和树突状细胞增生
Histiocytic and dendritic cell proliferations in the spleen

伴有组织细胞增生的各种脾的病变常常选择性地累及红髓。贮积性疾病（storage diseases），如脑苷脂沉积症（Gaucher 病）、类脂组织细胞增多症（Niemann-Pick 病）和神经节苷脂沉积症（gangliosidosis），特征为组织细胞积聚，其内充满由于酶的缺陷而未能代谢的物质[1]。尽管这些组织细胞看起来比较温和，但是有时可见局灶性核的非典型性。

某些感染性病变，如利什曼病、组织胞浆菌病、疟疾和伤寒沙门菌感染，均以脾内组织细胞增多为特征，通过在组织切片上辨认病原微生物或通过培养不难做出诊断。对感染的一种特殊类型的组织细胞反应是形成分枝杆菌梭形细胞假瘤（见下文）。

组织细胞肉瘤和恶性组织细胞增多症累及脾可能形成散在的肿块，或表现为弥散的红髓受累[6,32]。Langerhans 细胞组织细胞增生症可以累及脾，但是并不常见，表现为弥漫性红髓受累[3,142]。少数情况下，滤泡性树突状细胞和指状突树突状细胞肿瘤也可以发生于脾[143-145]。

噬血细胞综合征 Hemophagocytic syndrome

噬血细胞综合征是一种反应性但可致命的疾病，以全身性组织细胞增生为特征，伴有活跃的吞噬造血细胞现象。患者常常出现发热、全身症状、肝脾大和全血细胞减少[146-151]。肿大的脾因有良性的组织细胞增生而造成红髓扩张，伴有吞噬红细胞及其他造血成分的表现。因为吞噬血细胞的组织细胞可以见于正常的脾，所以只有当这些组织细胞明显增生并伴有相应的临床症状时，才能诊断噬血细胞综合征。淋巴瘤是最常见的伴随疾病，应仔细查找是否混有异常淋巴细胞以除外淋巴瘤的可能性[8]。

脾的上皮样肉芽肿
Epithelioid granulomas in the spleen

在许多情况下都可发生脾的上皮样肉芽肿，如感染、结节病、慢性尿毒症和淋巴瘤[1,152]。

大约 10% 的 Hodgkin 淋巴瘤患者脾内可以发现非干酪性上皮样肉芽肿[153]。这种肉芽肿可伴有淋巴瘤性浸润，也可以是单独的出现，因此肉芽肿本身并不代表 Hodgkin 淋巴瘤累及脾。没有发现 Hodgkin 淋巴瘤出现上皮样肉芽肿具有预后意义[154]。

累及脾的某些淋巴瘤伴有非常明显的上皮样肉芽肿，以至于淋巴瘤成分可能被掩盖[30,155]。B 细胞或 T 细胞淋巴瘤均可见到这种结构。在主要由小淋巴细胞组成的病例，仅仅根据形态学很难做出诊断。为了明确诊断，可能需要免疫组织化学和基因型检查。

因此，在脾内见到上皮样肉芽肿时，必须仔细查找微生物和恶性淋巴瘤。还有一些脾广泛性上皮样肉芽肿形成的病例，虽经广泛检查仍然不能发现明确的病因，这样的病例可以诊断为"上皮样肉芽肿病"（epithelioid granulomatosis）[156,157]。患者常常表现为发热、体重减轻、肝脾大和脾功能亢进，因此临床上往往怀疑为淋巴瘤。脾切除后症状消退，随访没有发现有进展为淋巴瘤的病例[156,157]。

分枝杆菌梭形细胞假瘤
Mycobacterial spindle cell pseudotumor

鸟胞内分枝杆菌（mycobacterium avium intracellulare）感染可能与梭形细胞假瘤形成有关，类似于炎性假瘤或平滑肌肿瘤。这一现象最常见于 AIDS 患者。受累的脾可见多发性梭形细胞结节，混有组织细胞、淋巴细胞和

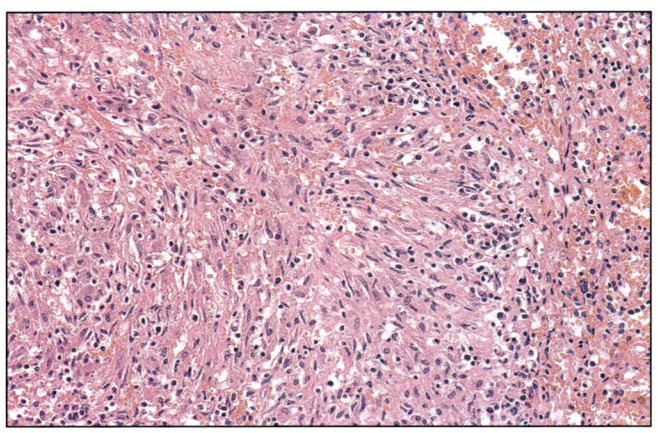

图21B.30 分枝杆菌梭形细胞假瘤累及脾。梭形组织细胞混有淋巴细胞和浆细胞。Ziehl-Neelsen染色显示组织细胞内有许多杆菌（没有显示）。

浆细胞（图21B.30）[158,159]。这种梭形细胞肥胖，含有显示蓝色条纹的颗粒状胞浆。如Ziehl-Neelsen染色显示梭形细胞胞浆内有大量抗酸杆菌，容易确定诊断。梭形细胞实际上是组织细胞（CD68阳性），但是可能显示结蛋白免疫反应阳性，具有误导性[158]。

炎性假瘤样滤泡性树突状细胞肿瘤
Inflammatory pseudotumor-like follicular dendritic cell tumor

临床特征

炎性假瘤样滤泡性树突状细胞肿瘤是滤泡性树突状细胞肿瘤的一种独特亚型，组织学上类似于炎性假瘤，可以发生于脾或肝[144,160,161]。好发于年轻到中年的妇女，表现为腹部不适或疼痛。全身性症状并不少见，如明显的体重减轻、发热或不适。本病的一些患者可出现复发。

炎性假瘤样滤泡性树突状细胞肿瘤在下列几个方面不同于普通的滤泡性树突状细胞肿瘤（在脾内极其少见）：女性明显常见；选择性地局限于腹腔内部位；常常出现全身症状；尽管位于腹腔，但呈惰性临床经过；肿瘤细胞散在分布，并有明显的淋巴浆细胞浸润；均与EBV相关。

病理学

肿瘤通常是孤立性的，呈鱼肉样，伴有大片出血和坏死。组织学上，背景富于淋巴细胞和浆细胞。有散在的梭形或卵圆形细胞，伴有空泡状核和明显的核仁，核的非典型性程度由轻微到显著，有些细胞核可能为奇形怪状（图21B.31A）。同普通的滤泡性树突状细胞肿瘤一样，一些病例可出现梭形细胞束。有些血管壁可见纤维蛋白样物沉积，具有特征性。少数病例可见丰富的嗜酸性细胞或上皮样肉芽肿。

滤泡性树突状细胞标记物免疫染色呈阳性，如CD21和CD35，虽然常呈局灶性。原位杂交检测EBV编码的RNA发现，梭形细胞核显著呈阳性。有些梭形细胞呈良性表现，而有些梭形细胞则明显增大且具有非典型性（图21B.31B）[144,162]。极少数病例的梭形细胞不表达滤泡性树突状细胞标记物，但存在EBV。这些病例与炎性假瘤和炎性假瘤样滤泡性树突状细胞肿瘤的相互关系尚不清楚[161,163]。

脾的间叶性肿瘤和瘤样病变
Mesenchymal tumors and tumor-like lesions of the spleen

脾的主要非淋巴血液系统肿瘤和瘤样病变见表21B.3。

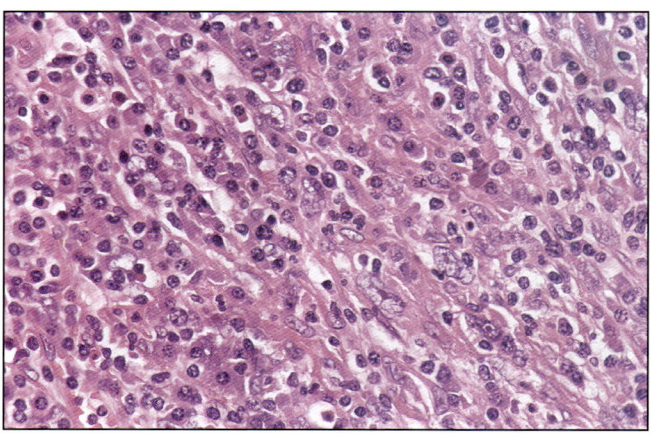

A

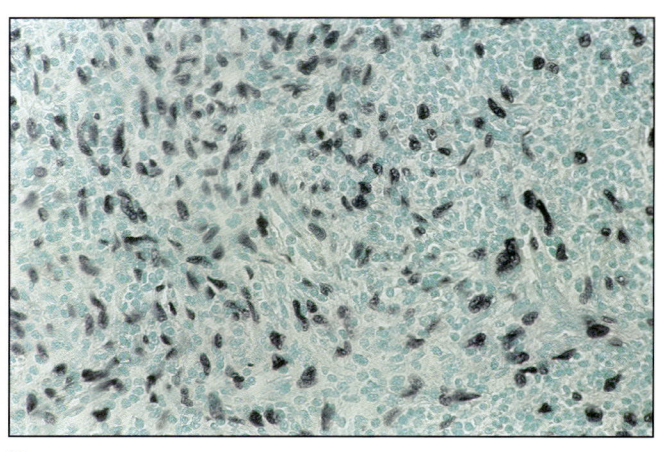

B

图21B.31 脾的炎性假瘤样滤泡性树突状细胞肿瘤。（A）伴有空泡状细胞核和界限不清的肥胖梭形细胞被大量淋巴浆细胞浸润所掩盖。免疫组织化学染色显示细胞为滤泡性树突状细胞。（B）EBER原位杂交能够最好地显示这些细胞。注意至少有一些细胞核大而奇异。

表21B.3	脾的非淋巴血液系统肿瘤和瘤样病变

A. 血管性
 1. 血管瘤（包括衬细胞血管瘤）和弥漫性血管瘤病
 2. 淋巴管瘤和淋巴管瘤病
 3. 脾紫癜
 4. 血管内皮细胞瘤
 5. 血管肉瘤（包括衬细胞血管肉瘤）
 6. Kaposi肉瘤
 7. 杆菌性血管瘤病
 8. 硬化性血管瘤样结节性转化

B. 其他
 1. 其他类型肉瘤
 2. 炎性假瘤
 3. 脾错构瘤
 4. 囊肿
  a. 上皮性囊肿
  b. 间皮性囊肿
  c. 寄生虫性囊肿
  d. 假囊肿

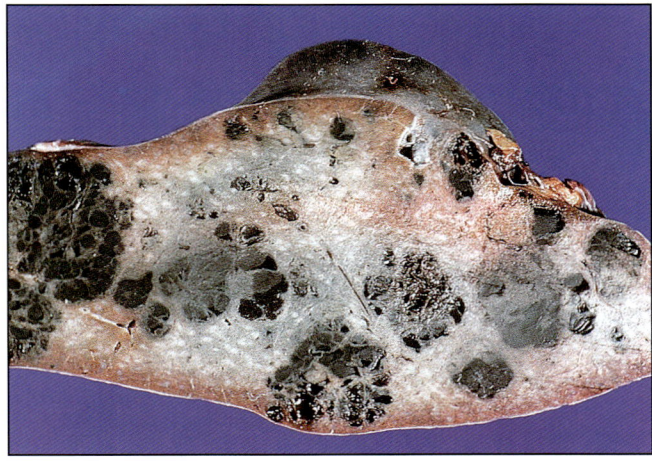

图21B.32 脾的衬细胞血管瘤。切面显示多灶性病变，由大的血管腔隙聚集而成。

脾的血管瘤和血管瘤病
Splenic hemangioma and hemangiomatosis

血管瘤是最常见的脾的原发性肿瘤[6,164-168]。脾血管瘤可为偶然发现，表现为脾大或出现脾大的并发症（如脾破裂、消耗性凝血障碍和血小板减少症）。多数病例为海绵状血管瘤，形成孤立性或多发性蓝红色结节。血管瘤免疫染色显示VIII因子相关抗原、CD31和CD34阳性，而CD8呈阴性[169]。

弥漫性血管瘤病以血管瘤弥漫广泛累及脾为特征。可伴有或不伴有其他器官受累[169-174]。本病常常合并消耗性凝血障碍。增生的血管可呈海绵状或为毛细血管型。

脾紫癜可与血管瘤鉴别，表现为杂乱分布的不规则的或圆形的充满血液的腔隙，并不形成散在的肿块，而且容易累及滤泡旁区域[1,6]。目前认为与应用合成代谢类固醇和消耗性疾病有关。

衬细胞血管瘤 Littoral cell angioma

临床特征

衬细胞血管瘤是脾窦内衬细胞中唯一的良性肿瘤，因此在软组织没有相应的肿瘤[175]。受累患者年龄范围广，无性别差异。多数患者表现为脾大，有时伴有脾功能亢进，但是有些患者可不出现症状[169]。部分病例可能伴有内脏肿瘤[176,177]。

病理学

肿瘤形成孤立性或多发性的散在结节，常常表现为海绵状并充满血液（图21B.32）。组织学上，相互吻合的狭窄血管腔隙中散在分布有扩张的血管腔和灶状假毛细血管。血管腔隙内衬肥胖的表现温和的细胞，有些细胞可脱落到管腔内（图21B.33）。有些肿瘤细胞胞浆内常常可见嗜酸性小体。肿瘤细胞免疫染色显示内皮标记物（VIII因子相关抗原和CD31，而不是CD34）、组织细胞标记物（CD68、CD163和溶菌酶）以及CD21阳性。另一方面，脾窦内衬细胞标记物CD8却呈阴性反应[169,175]。

脾的淋巴管瘤和淋巴管瘤病
Splenic lymphangioma and lymphangiomatosis

曾有报道，脾的淋巴管瘤或为孤立性或为多发性，常累及被膜和纤维性小梁[6,164,165,178]。衬于腔隙的细胞常常变薄。然而，重新评价本病表明，诊断为淋巴管瘤的绝大多数病例事实上是间皮囊肿（细胞角蛋白阳性）[179]。真正的脾淋巴管瘤的确存在，但极为少见，为境界清楚的孤立性肿瘤，由内衬扁平到局部肥胖的内皮细胞的血管间隙组成，有些病例伴有血管内乳头状丛形成（图21B.34）。血管腔内充满蛋白性物质[168,180,181]。当同时累及诸如肝等其他部位时，可以应用"淋巴管瘤病"这一术语[178,182,183]。

血管肉瘤，包括衬细胞血管肉瘤
Angiosarcoma, including littoral cell angiosarcoma

临床特征

脾的原发性血管肉瘤罕见，是一种高度侵袭性的肿瘤[6,168,184-189]。常发生于老年患者，表现为腹痛、腹部

脾的间叶性肿瘤和瘤样病变

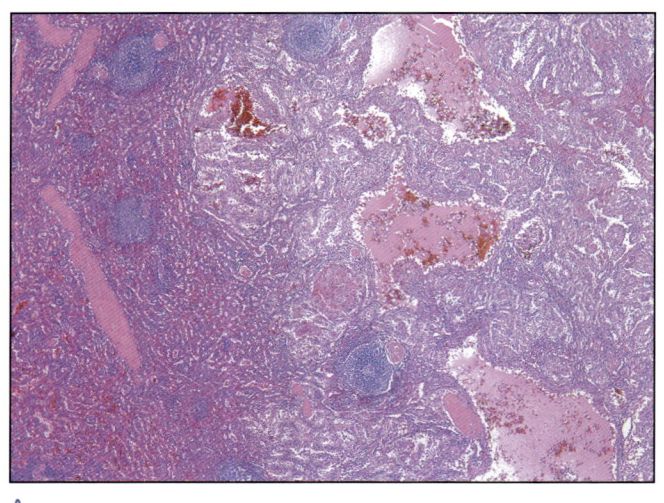
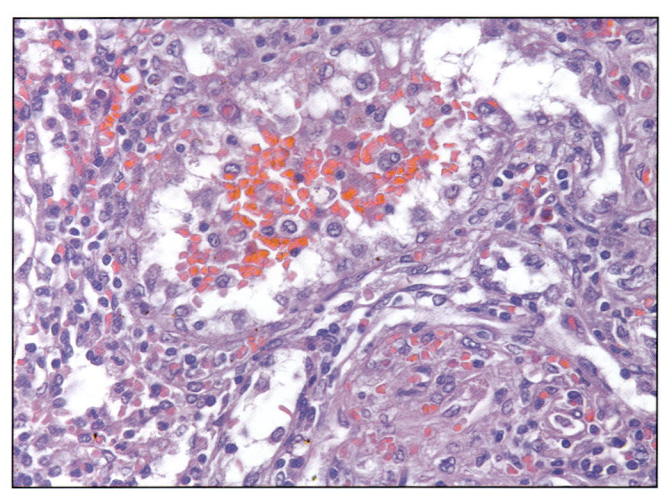

图21B.33　脾的衬细胞血管瘤。（A）与正常红髓血窦比较（左侧视野），构成衬细胞血管瘤的血管腔大而扩张，而且比较扭曲（右侧视野）。局部形成假乳头状结构。还可见到海绵状血管腔隙。（B）血管腔内衬肥胖细胞，伴有卵圆形到有切迹的细胞核，管腔内可见脱落细胞。少数细胞含有胞浆内透明小体。

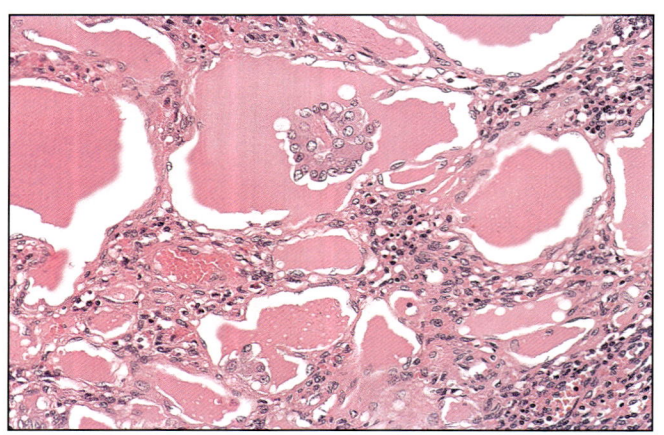

图21B.34　脾的淋巴管瘤。不同大小的内衬内皮的腔隙内含有蛋白性液体。有些内皮细胞形成乳头状突起突入血管腔内。

肿块或腹腔积血。在少数情况下，儿童也可受累[190,191]。有些病例同时显示广泛的肝受累。远处转移常见。尽管最近一项研究报告指出，生存年龄中位数为36个月，但多数患者于1年内死亡[191]。

病理学

脾被多发性边界不清的结节取代，或为弥漫性生长，伴有明显的出血和坏死。组织学上，有吻合的血管腔梭形细胞束、乳头状结构和实性区。细胞学非典型性通常明显，虽然某些病例可以出现具有迷惑性的、类似于血管瘤的良性区域（图21B.35）。梭形细胞血管肉瘤显示不同程度的内皮细胞标记物免疫染色阳性，如VIII因子

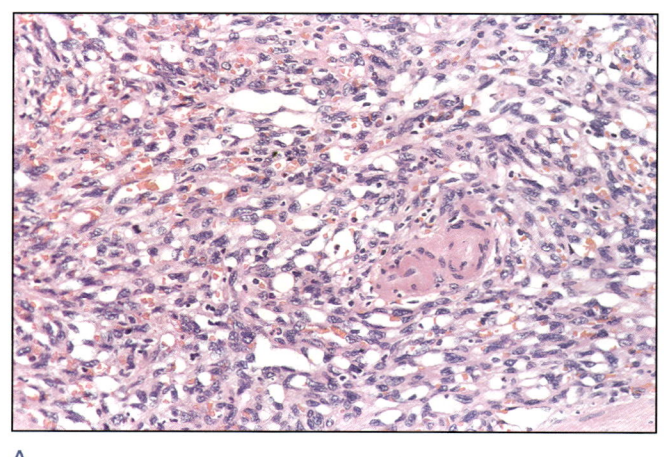
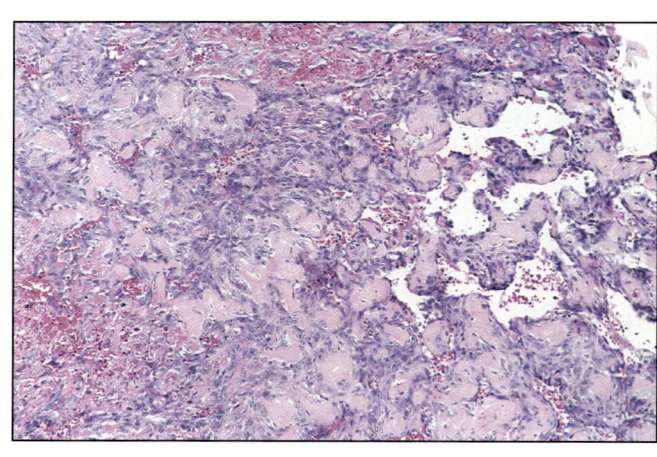

图21B.35　脾的血管肉瘤。（A）肿瘤由密集排列的血管腔隙构成，内衬细胞具有轻到中度的核非典型性。（B）肿瘤具有实性灶（左侧视野）和不规则相互吻合的血管腔，伴有乳头状突起（右侧视野）。

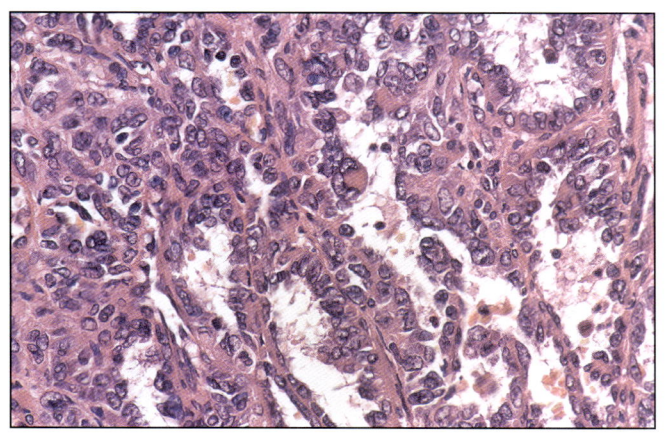

图21B.36 脾的衬细胞血管肉瘤。血管腔隙内衬肥胖细胞,伴有轻到中度非典型性。其结构和细胞学与衬细胞血管瘤相似,内衬细胞CD8免疫染色呈阳性(没有显示)。

相关抗原、CD31 和 CD34[169]。极少数病例还表达脾窦内衬细胞标记物 CD8,因此可能是衬细胞血管肉瘤(图21B.36)[192-195]。

鉴别诊断

- 脾的血管瘤。血管肉瘤具有核的多形性、核分裂象,而且常常出现实性结构,可与血管瘤区分。
- 杆菌性血管瘤病。
- 所谓的恶性纤维组织细胞瘤。低分化血管肉瘤可有实性区域,组织学上不能与高级别多形性肉瘤区分。在诊断之前,应该通过充分取材和免疫组织化学染色寻找血管分化的证据(如胞浆空泡和原始的血管腔隙)。

脾的血管内皮细胞瘤
Hemangioendothelioma of the spleen

累及脾的少数血管瘤显示介于血管瘤和血管肉瘤之间的形态学特征,生物学行为如同低级别恶性肿瘤[196-198]。

脾的杆菌性血管瘤病
Bacillary angiomatosis of the spleen

杆菌性血管瘤病累及脾时(见第21A章)形成多发性结节[199-203]。组织学上,内衬胞浆淡染的肥胖内皮细胞的小的毛细血管呈小叶状增生。内皮细胞可能表现出不同程度的核非典型性。有时,局部可能出现不规则的分枝状血管腔。间质内杆菌集聚形成嗜双色性物质,为杆菌性血管瘤病的组织学标志,通过 Warthin-Starry 等银染色或巴尔通杆菌(*Bartonella henselae*)免疫染色可以更好显示[204]。血管腔隙之间可以发现数量不等的中性粒细胞。

与血管肉瘤不同,杆菌性血管瘤病是由鱼肉样结节组成的,而不是出血性和坏死性结节,而且缺乏明显的核非典型性。间质内大量的嗜双色性物质和中性粒细胞是正确诊断本病的线索。

杆菌性血管瘤病可能被误诊为上皮样血管瘤或血管内皮细胞瘤,但是后者内皮细胞缺乏胞浆内透明物质。

硬化性血管瘤样结节性转化
Sclerosing angiomatoid nodular transformation (SANT)

临床特征

硬化性血管瘤样结节性转化是脾的一种独特的非肿瘤性血管病变[205],曾经称为"条索状毛细血管瘤"(cord capillary hemangioma)[206]。其主要发生于成人,发病年龄中位数为 56 岁,女性多见。最常见的表现是偶然发现的脾肿块、腹痛或腹部不适以及脾大。脾切除后无复发病例。

病理学

病变为孤立性的,大小为 3 ~ 17 cm,与周围脾实质界限分明。融合的红棕色结节位于致密的纤维性间质内。组织学上,单个结节呈血管瘤样外观,由内衬肥胖内皮细胞的裂隙样、圆形或不规则形状的血管腔隙组成,其间散在分布有成群的梭形或卵圆形细胞(图 21B.37)。某些结节(尤其是小的)被同心圆性排列的胶原纤维环绕,有外渗的红细胞和散在的炎症细胞。细胞核的非典型性轻微,核分裂象非常少见。结节之间的间质由不同程度的黏液样到密集的纤维组织构成,其内散在有肥胖的肌纤维母细胞、浆细胞、淋巴细胞和单核细胞。免疫染色显示血管瘤样结节内有三种不同类型的血管:$CD34^+/CD8^-/CD31^+$ 的毛细血管、$CD34^-/CD8^+/CD31^+$ 的窦状隙以及 $CD34^-/CD8^-/CD31^+$ 的小静脉,重现了正常脾红髓的组成成分。血管瘤样结节表现为变化了的红髓组织,其中包含非肿瘤性间质增生性病变。

炎性假瘤 Inflammatory pseudotumor

临床特征

类似于发生在肺和肺外的炎性假瘤可以发生于脾。可以是偶然发现,可表现为发热和腹痛[6,206-219]。脾切除一般可以治愈。

病理学

大体上病变通常为孤立性的,大小为小于 1 ~ 12 cm 不等(图 21B.38A)。为局限性或部分有浸润的质硬

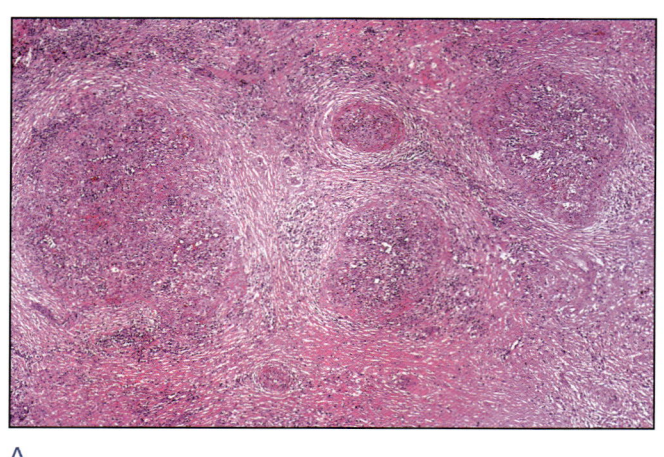 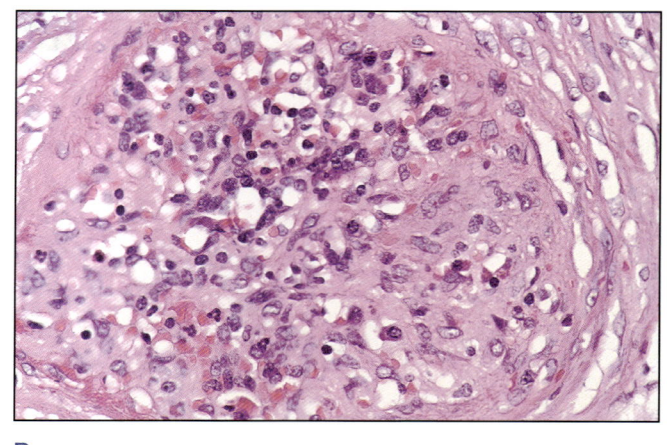

图21B.37 脾的硬化性血管瘤样结节性转化。（A）血管瘤样结节，常常被纤维蛋白样物质和同心圆性胶原纤维环绕，位于炎性硬化的间质中。（B）血管瘤样结节由内衬肥胖细胞的不同大小的血管腔隙构成，被一些卵圆形的细胞分隔。

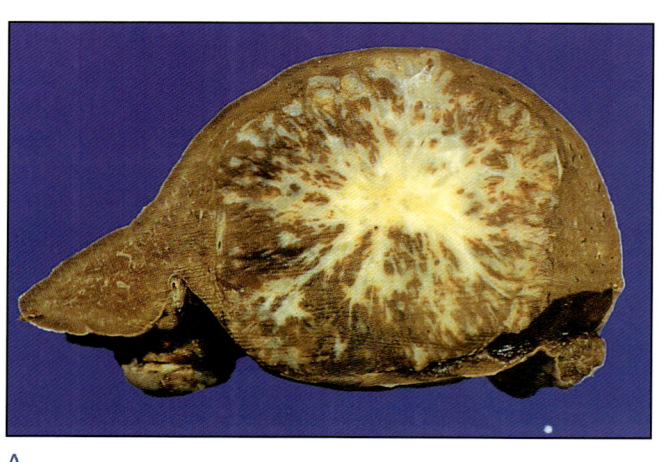 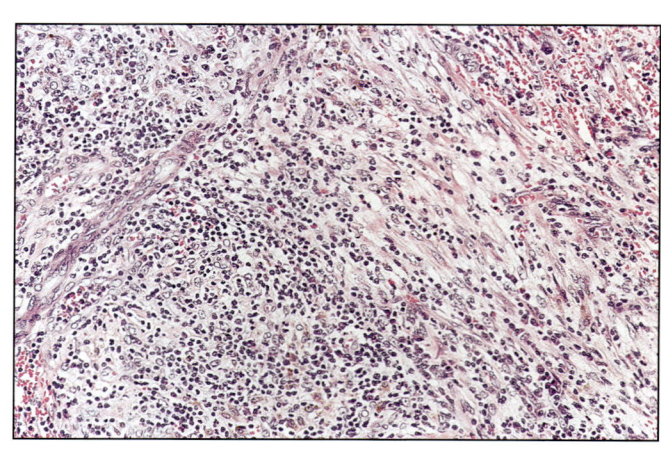

图21B.38 脾的炎性假瘤。（A）大而散在的肿瘤，切面质硬，呈褐色到白色。多发性散在的棕色病灶是陷入的红髓组织。（B）组织学上，病变由梭形细胞和血管组成，间质硬化，有淋巴细胞和浆细胞浸润。

白色肿块，可伴有突出的出血或坏死区域。组织学上，病变的特征是梭形肌纤维母细胞、淋巴细胞和浆细胞混合存在（图21B.38B）。可出现中性粒细胞，而且有些病例显示先前存在脓肿的证据。硬化比起其他部位的炎性假瘤更为突出。陷入的红髓组织有时可能导致交界性或恶性血管性肿瘤的错误诊断。目前，很难区分病变的本质是反应性还是肿瘤性（炎性肌纤维母细胞瘤）。不过，需要谨慎排除分枝杆菌假瘤（需要抗生素治疗）和炎性假瘤样滤泡性树突状细胞肿瘤。

脾的错构瘤 Splenic hamartoma

临床特征

脾的错构瘤是瘤样畸形，常为偶然发现。然而，部分患者可出现与肿块病变相关的症状或血液学的并发症[6,165,178,206,220-227]。少数病例发生在结节性硬化症患者[225]。脾的错构瘤发生年龄范围较广，无性别差异[206]。

病理学

脾的错构瘤通常为孤立性的，境界清楚，也可为多发性的（图21B.39）。肿瘤由内衬脾窦内皮细胞的不规则排列的扭曲的血管腔隙组成，由髓索样成分分开，即基本上是"混杂"的红髓（图21B.40）。网状纤维结构紊乱，不同于周围正常的脾实质。错构瘤内无脾淋巴小体（白髓的成分），如果出现淋巴细胞，也呈杂乱分布。时间较长的错构瘤可出现硬化。少数病例存在散在的类似于Reed-Sternberg细胞的大而奇异的间质细胞，可能被误诊为Hodgkin淋巴瘤[228,229]。

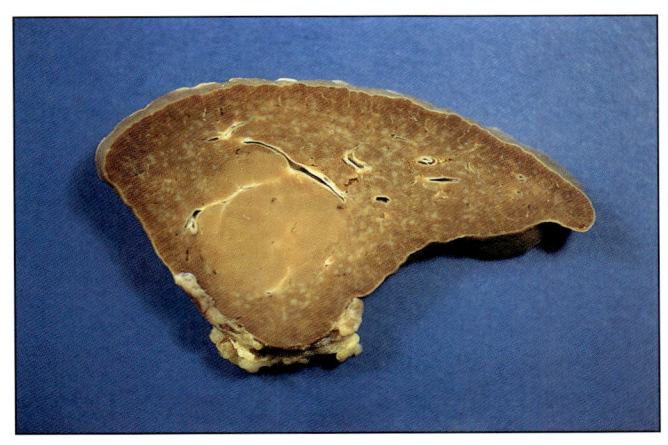

图21B.39 脾的错构瘤。形成同质性表现的散在结节，缺乏纤细的条纹和正常脾实质的细小白髓结节。

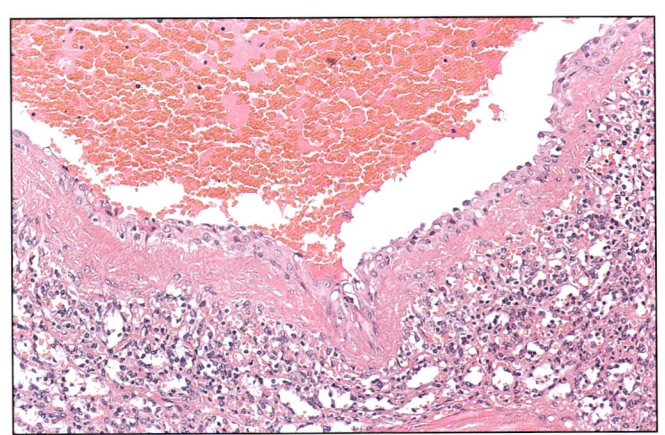

图21B.41 脾的上皮性囊肿。囊肿有纤维性囊壁，内衬局灶复层的上皮细胞。

CD8和CD31免疫组化染色可以突出窦状隙成分。Ⅳ型胶原明显增加[169]。

关于"肌样血管内皮细胞瘤"（myoid angioendothelioma）是一种独特的疾病还是仅仅是脾错构瘤的一个亚型（伴有奇异间质细胞的脾错构瘤，splenic hamartoma with bizarre stromal cells），目前尚不清楚[206,228,230-232]。病变界限清楚，有内衬扁平内皮细胞（CD34+）的小或中等大小的血管腔，偶尔为大血管腔，其间为大量卵圆形细胞，胞浆嗜酸性，细胞核呈卵圆形、扭曲或深染，常常伴有明显的核仁。少数细胞存在有核的假包涵体。椭圆形细胞表达肌肉标记物，如平滑肌肌动蛋白和肌肉特异性肌动蛋白。

脾囊肿　Splenic cysts

脾内可见几种类型的囊肿（表21B.3）[6,164,233-236]。除了寄生虫性囊肿以外，假囊肿占所有病例的4/5。假囊肿（false cysts，pseudocyst）可能发生于创伤后血肿的液化、错构瘤变性、梗死或上皮性囊肿上皮剥脱。腔面光滑或粗糙。无上皮内衬的纤维性囊壁可能出现钙化。

上皮性囊肿（epithelial cyst）通常为孤立性的，大体检查时腔面呈粗小梁状。内衬复层鳞状上皮，可有角化或黏液化生（图21B.41）。有时可见鞋钉样细胞。

间皮性囊肿（mesothelial cyst）位于脾被膜下。内衬表达间皮免疫表型的扁平细胞，细胞角蛋白、钙视网膜蛋白（calretinin）和HBME1呈阳性，而血管标记物呈阴性（图21B.42）。间皮性囊肿曾经常被误诊为淋巴管瘤[179,236]。

脾的罕见病变　Rare lesions of the spleen

已报道的脾的罕见病变包括淀粉样瘤[237]、脂肪瘤[238]、纤维瘤（可能仅仅是硬化性血管瘤或错构瘤）[239]、

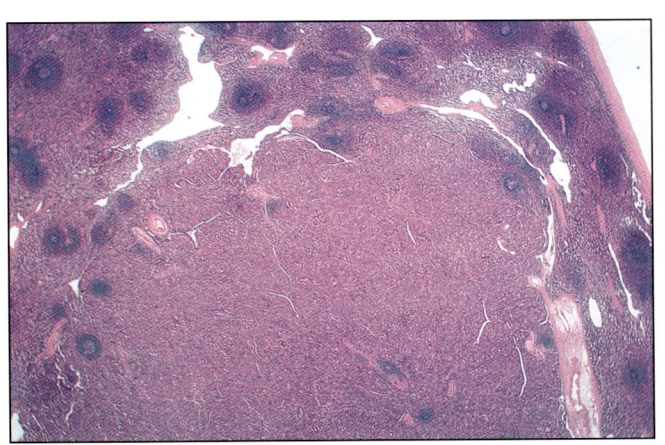

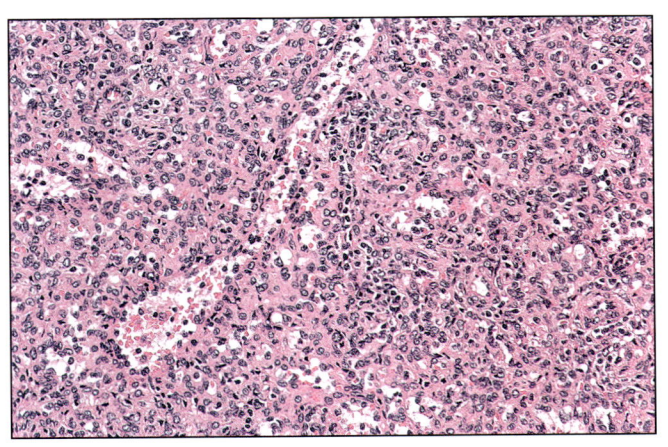

图21B.40 脾的错构瘤。（A）结节与周围脾实质界限非常清楚。注意缺乏白髓结节。（B）与正常红髓相比，髓索和窦状隙结构紊乱。

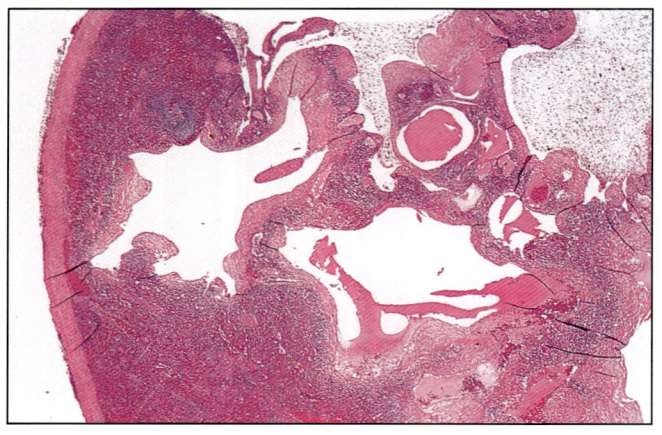

图21B.42 脾的间皮性囊肿。这个病变曾被误诊为淋巴管瘤。特征是发生于脾的被膜下区域,由内衬扁平细胞的囊腔组成。

血管肌脂肪瘤[240]、所谓的恶性纤维组织细胞瘤[241-243]、纤维肉瘤[164]、平滑肌肉瘤[164,165]、EB病毒相关性移植后平滑肌肿瘤[244,245]、横纹肌肉瘤[246,247]、血管外皮细胞瘤[248-250]、Dabska血管内乳头状血管内皮细胞瘤[251]、Kaposi肉瘤[252]、恶性畸胎瘤[253]、显著的囊性输卵管内膜异位[254]、癌肉瘤[255]以及原发性黏液性囊腺癌(可能与腹膜假黏液瘤有关)[256-258]。

脾的转移性肿瘤
Metastatic tumor in spleen

脾的转移性肿瘤发生于播散性肿瘤的晚期,最常见的来自于肺和乳腺,而且只在尸检时才被发现[1,5,259,260]。少数情况下,脾大是实体癌复发的首发体征,尤其是女性生殖道的肿瘤[261-266]。转移性肿瘤可以是大体所见(结节状或弥漫性取代),也可以是显微镜下所见(常为窦状隙)[6,267]。癌症累及脾的一种特殊类型是可能导致红髓的结节状转化,伴有少数癌细胞散在分布于红髓结节之间的纤维性条带中[268]。

参考文献

1. Neiman R S, Orazi A 1999 Disorders of the spleen. WB Saunders, Philadelphia
2. Kraus M D 2003 Splenic histology and histopathology: an update. Semin Diagn Pathol 20: 84–93
3. Burke J S 1981 Surgical pathology of the spleen: an approach to the differential diagnosis of splenic lymphomas and leukemias. Part II. Diseases of the red pulp. Am J Surg Pathol 5: 681–694
4. Burke J S 1981 Surgical pathology of the spleen: an approach to the differential diagnosis of splenic lymphomas and leukemias. Part I. Diseases of the white pulp. Am J Surg Pathol 5: 551–563
5. Butler J J 1983 Pathology of the spleen in benign and malignant conditions. Histopathology 7: 453–474
6. Warnke R A, Weiss L M, Chan J K, et al. 1995 Tumors of the lymph nodes and spleen. Atlas of tumor pathology, series 3, fascicle 14. Armed Forces Institute of Pathology, Washington DC, 411–526
7. Neiman R S, Orazi A 1999 Disorders of the spleen, 2nd edn. In: LiVolsi V A (ed) Major problems in pathology, Vol. 38. WB Saunders, Philadelphia, 65–285
8. Chan J K 2003 Splenic involvement by peripheral T-cell and NK-cell neoplasms. Semin Diagn Pathol 20: 105–120
9. Osuji N, Matutes E, Catovsky D, et al. 2005 Histopathology of the spleen in T-cell large granular lymphocyte leukemia and T-cell prolymphocytic leukemia: a comparative review. Am J Surg Pathol 29: 935–941
10. Arber D A, Rappaport H, Weiss L M 1997 Non-Hodgkin's lymphoproliferative disorders involving the spleen. Mod Pathol 10: 18–32
11. Burke J S 2004 The spleen. In: Mills S E, Carter D, Greenson J K, et al (eds) Sternberg's diagnostic surgical pathology, 4th edn. Lippincott Williams & Wilkins, Philadelphia, 849–875
12. Agnarsson B A, Loughran T P, Jr, Starkebaum G, et al. 1989 The pathology of large granular lymphocyte leukemia. Hum Pathol 20: 643–651
13. Lim M S, Straus S E, Dale J K, et al. 1998 Pathological findings in human autoimmune lymphoproliferative syndrome. Am J Pathol 153: 1541–1550
14. Piris M A, Mollejo M, Campo E, et al. 1998 A marginal zone pattern may be found in different varieties of non-Hodgkin's lymphoma: the morphology and immunohistology of splenic involvement by B-cell lymphomas simulating splenic marginal zone lymphoma. Histopathology 33: 230–239
15. Chang K L, Kamel O W, Arber D A, et al. 1995 Pathologic features of nodular lymphocyte predominance Hodgkin's disease in extranodal sites. Am J Surg Pathol 19: 1313–1324
16. Lukes R J 1971 Criteria for involvement of lymph node, bone marrow, spleen and liver in Hodgkin's disease. Cancer Res 31: 1755–1767
17. Siebert J D, Stuckey J H, Kurtin P J, et al. 1995 Extranodal lymphocyte predominance Hodgkin's disease. Clinical and pathologic features. Am J Clin Pathol 103: 485–491
18. Burke J S, Osborne B M 1983 Localized reactive lymphoid hyperplasia of the spleen simulating malignant lymphoma. A report of seven cases. Am J Surg Pathol 7: 373–380
19. Harris N L 1984 Localized lymphoid hyperplasia of the spleen [letter]. Am J Surg Pathol 8: 557–558
20. Isaacson P G, Norton A J 1994 Extranodal lymphomas. Churchill Livingstone, Edinburgh
21. Stroup R M, Burke J S, Sheibani K, et al. 1992 Splenic involvement by aggressive malignant lymphomas of B-cell and T-cell types. A morphologic and immunophenotypic study. Cancer 69: 413–420
22. Mollejo M, Algara P, Mateo M S, et al. 2003 Large B-cell lymphoma presenting in the spleen: identification of different clinicopathologic conditions. Am J Surg Pathol 27: 895–902
23. Falk S, Stutte H J 1990 Primary malignant lymphomas of the spleen. A morphologic and immunohistochemical analysis of 17 cases. Cancer 66: 2612–2619
24. Harris N L, Aisenberg A C, Meyer J E, et al. 1984 Diffuse large cell (histiocytic) lymphoma of the spleen. Clinical and pathologic characteristics of ten cases. Cancer 54: 2460–2467
25. Ahmann D L, Kiely J M, Harrison E G 1966 Malignant lymphoma of the spleen, a review of 49 cases in which the diagnosis was made at splenectomy. Cancer 19: 461–469
26. Kehoe J, Straus D J 1988 Primary lymphoma of the spleen. Clinical features and outcome after splenectomy. Cancer 62: 1433–1438
27. Grosskreutz C, Troy K, Cuttner J 2002 Primary splenic lymphoma: report of 10 cases using the REAL classification. Cancer Invest 20: 749–753
28. Ambulkar I, Kulkarni B, Borges A, et al. 2006 Primary non-Hodgkin's lymphoma of the spleen presenting as space occupying lesion: a case report and review of literature. Leuk Lymphoma 47: 135–139
29. Brox A, Bishinsky J I, Berry G 1991 Primary non-Hodgkin's lymphoma of the spleen. Am J Hematol 38: 95–100
30. Braylan R C, Long J C, Jaffe E S, et al. 1977 Malignant lymphoma obscured by concomitant extensive epithelioid granulomas: report of three cases with similar clinicopathologic features. Cancer 39: 1146–1155
31. Zellers R A, Thibodeau S N, Banks P M 1990 Primary splenic lymphocyte-depletion Hodgkin's disease. Am J Clin Pathol 94: 453–457
32. Franchino C, Reich C, Distenfeld A et al. 1988 A clinicopathologically distinctive primary splenic histiocytic neoplasm. Demonstration of its histiocyte derivation by immunophenotypic and molecular genetic analysis. Am J Surg Pathol 12: 398–404
33. Dogan A, Burke J S, Goteri G, et al. 2003 Micronodular T-cell/histiocyte-rich large B-cell lymphoma of the spleen: histology, immunophenotype, and differential diagnosis. Am J Surg Pathol 27: 903–911
34. Audouin J, Le Tourneau A, Diebold J, et al. 1989 Primary intestinal lymphoma of Ki-1 large cell anaplastic type with mesenteric lymph node and spleen involvement in a renal transplant recipient. Hematol Oncol 7: 441–449
35. Schmid C, Kirkham N, Diss T, et al. 1992 Splenic marginal zone cell lymphoma. Am J Surg Pathol 16: 455–466
36. Dogan A, Isaacson PG 2003 Splenic marginal zone lymphoma. Semin Diagn Pathol 20: 121–127

37. Isaacson P G, Matutes E, Burke M, et al. 1994 The histopathology of splenic lymphoma with villous lymphocytes. Blood 84: 3828–3834
38. Isaacson P G, Piris M A 1997 Splenic marginal zone lymphoma. Adv Anat Pathol 4: 191–201
39. Franco V, Florena A M, Iannitto E 2003 Splenic marginal zone lymphoma. Blood 101: 2464–2472
40. Isaacson P G 1999 Splenic marginal zone B cell lymphoma. In: Mason D Y, Harris N L (eds) Human lymphoma: clinical implications of the REAL classification. Springer Verlag, London, 7.1–7.6
41. Pittaluga S, Verhoef G, Criel A, et al. 1996 'Small' B-cell non-Hodgkin's lymphomas with splenomegaly at presentation are either mantle cell lymphoma or marginal zone cell lymphoma. A study based on histology, cytology, immunohistochemistry, and cytogenetic analysis. Am J Surg Pathol 20: 211–223
42. Palutke M, Eisenberg L, Narang S, et al. 1988 B lymphocytic lymphoma (large cell) of possible splenic marginal zone origin presenting with prominent splenomegaly and unusual cordal red pulp distribution. Cancer 62: 593–600
43. Mollejo M, Menarguez J, Lloret E, et al. 1995 Splenic marginal zone lymphoma: a distinctive type of low-grade B-cell lymphoma. A clinicopathological study of 13 cases. Am J Surg Pathol 19: 1146–1157
44. Hammer R D, Glick A D, Greer J P, et al. 1996 Splenic marginal zone lymphoma. A distinct B-cell neoplasm. Am J Surg Pathol 20: 613–626
45. Iannitto E, Ambrosetti A, Ammatuna E, et al. 2004 Splenic marginal zone lymphoma with or without villous lymphocytes. Hematologic findings and outcomes in a series of 57 patients. Cancer 101: 2050–2057
46. Van Huyen J-P D, Molina T, Delmer A, et al. 2000 Splenic marginal zone lymphoma with our without plasmacytic differentiation. Am J Surg Pathol 24: 1581–1592
47. Arcaini L, Paulli M, Boveri E, et al. 2004 Splenic and nodal marginal zone lymphomas are indolent disorders at high hepatitis C virus seroprevalence with distinct presenting features but similar morphologic and phenotypic profiles. Cancer 100: 107–115
48. Hermine O, Lefrere F, Bronowicki J P, et al. 2002 Regression of splenic lymphoma with villous lymphocytes after treatment of hepatitis C virus infection. N Engl J Med 347: 89–94
49. Weng W K, Levy S 2003 Hepatitis C virus (HCV) and lymphomagenesis. Leuk Lymphoma 44: 1113–1120
50. Berger F, Felman P, Thieblemont C, et al. 2000 Non-MALT marginal zone B-cell lymphomas: a description of clinical presentation and outcome in 124 patients. Blood 95: 1950–1956
51. Mollejo M, Lloret E, Menarguez J, et al. 1997 Lymph node involvement by splenic marginal zone lymphoma: morphological and immunohistochemical features. Am J Surg Pathol 21: 772–780
52. Lloret E, Mollejo M, Mateo M S, et al. 1999 Splenic marginal zone lymphoma with increased number of blasts: an aggressive variant? Hum Pathol 30: 1153–1160
53. Wu C D, Jackson C L, Medeiros L J 1996 Splenic marginal zone cell lymphoma. An immunophenotypic and molecular study of five cases. Am J Clin Pathol 105: 277–285
54. Savilo E, Campo E, Mollejo M, et al. 1998 Absence of cyclin D1 protein expression in splenic marginal zone lymphoma. Mod Pathol 11: 601–606
55. Miranda R N, Cousar J B, Hammer R D, et al. 1999 Somatic mutation analysis of IgH variable regions reveals that tumor cells of most parafollicular (monocytoid) B-cell lymphoma, splenic marginal zone B-cell lymphoma, and some hairy cell leukemia are composed of memory B lymphocytes. Hum Pathol 30: 306–312
56. Dunn-Walters D K, Boursier L, Spencer J, et al. 1998 Analysis of immunoglobulin genes in splenic marginal zone lymphoma suggests ongoing mutation. Hum Pathol 29: 585–593
57. Stamatopoulos K, Belessi C, Papadaki T, et al. 2004 Immunoglobulin heavy- and light-chain repertoire in splenic marginal zone lymphoma. Mol Med 10: 89–95
58. Traverse-Glehen A, Davi F, Ben Simon E, et al. 2005 Analysis of VH genes in marginal zone lymphoma reveals marked heterogeneity between splenic and nodal tumors and suggests the existence of clonal selection. Haematologica 90: 470–478
59. Sole F, Woessner S, Florensa L, et al. 1997 Frequent involvement of chromosomes 1, 3, 7 and 8 in splenic marginal zone B-cell lymphoma. Br J Haematol 98: 446–449
60. Mateo M, Mollejo M, Villuendas R, et al. 1999 7q31-32 allelic loss is a frequent finding in splenic marginal zone lymphoma. Am J Pathol 154: 1583–1589
61. Mollejo M, Camacho F I, Algara P, et al. 2005 Nodal and splenic marginal zone B cell lymphomas. Hematol Oncol 23: 108–118
62. Ibbotson R E, Parker A E, Oscier D G 2005 Splenic marginal zone lymphoma: 7q abnormalities. Methods Mol Med 115: 241–250
63. Corcoran M M, Mould S J, Orchard J A, et al. 1999 Dysregulation of cyclin dependent kinase 6 expression in splenic marginal zone lymphoma through chromosome 7q translocations. Oncogene 18: 6271–6277
64. Baldini L, Guffanti A, Cro L, et al. 1997 Poor prognosis in non-villous splenic marginal zone cell lymphoma is associated with p53 mutations. Br J Haematol 99: 375–378
65. Ruiz-Ballesteros E, Mollejo M, Rodriguez A, et al. 2005 Splenic marginal zone lymphoma: proposal of new diagnostic and prognostic markers identified after tissue and cDNA microarray analysis. Blood 106: 1831–1838
66. Troen G, Nygaard V, Jenssen T K, et al. 2004 Constitutive expression of the AP-1 transcription factors c-jun, junD, junB, and c-fos and the marginal zone B cell transcription factor Notch2 in splenic marginal zone lymphoma. J Mol Diagn 6: 297–307
67. Rosenwald A, Ott G, Stilgenbauer S, et al. 1999 Exclusive detection of the t(11; 18)(q21; q21) in extranodal marginal zone B cell lymphomas (MZBL) of MALT type in contrast to other MZBL and extranodal large B cell lymphomas. Am J Pathol 155: 1817–1821
68. Dierlamm J, Baens M, Wlodarska I, et al. 1999 The apoptosis inhibitor gene API2 and a novel 18q gene, MLT, are recurrently rearranged in the t(11; 18)(q21; q21) associated with mucosa-associated lymphoid tissue lymphomas. Blood 93: 3601–3609
69. Alkan S, Ross C W, Hanson C A, Schnitzer B 1996 Follicular lymphoma with involvement of the splenic marginal zone: a pitfall in the differential diagnosis of splenic marginal zone cell lymphoma. Hum Pathol 27: 503–506
70. Du M Q, Peng H Z, Dogan A, et al. 1997 Preferential dissemination of B cell gastric mucosa-associated lymphoid tissue (MALT) lymphoma to the splenic marginal zone. Blood 90: 4071–4077
71. Jaffe E S 1999 Hepatosplenic gamma delta T cell lymphoma. In: Mason D Y, Harris N L (eds) Human lymphoma: clinical implications of the REAL classification. Springer Verlag, London, 35.1–35.4
72. Belhadj K, Reyes F, Farcet J P, et al. 2003 Hepatosplenic gammadelta T-cell lymphoma is a rare clinicopathologic entity with poor outcome: report on a series of 21 patients. Blood 102: 4261–4269
73. Ross C W, Schnitzer B, Sheldon S, et al. 1994 Gamma/delta T-cell posttransplantation lymphoproliferative disorder primarily in the spleen. Am J Clin Pathol 102: 310–315
74. Salhany K E, Feldman M, Peritt D, et al. 1997 Cytotoxic T-lymphocyte differentiation and cytogenetic alterations in gammadelta hepatosplenic T-cell lymphoma and posttransplant lymphoproliferative disorders. Blood 89: 3490–3491
75. Kraus M D, Crawford D F, Kaleem Z, et al. 1998 T gamma/delta hepatosplenic lymphoma in a heart transplant patient after an Epstein–Barr virus positive lymphoproliferative disorder: a case report. Cancer 82: 983–992
76. Francois A, Lesesve J F, Stamatoullas A, et al. 1997 Hepatosplenic gamma/delta T-cell lymphoma: a report of two cases in immunocompromised patients, associated with isochromosome 7q. Am J Surg Pathol 21: 781–790
77. Steurer M, Stauder R, Grunewald K, et al. 2002 Hepatosplenic gammadelta-T-cell lymphoma with leukemic course after renal transplantation. Hum Pathol 33: 253–258
78. Khan W A, Yu L, Eisenbrey A B, et al. 2001 Hepatosplenic gamma/delta T-cell lymphoma in immunocompromised patients. Report of two cases and review of literature. Am J Clin Pathol 116: 41–50
79. Yao M, Tien H F, Lin M T, et al. 1996 Clinical and hematological characteristics of hepatosplenic T gamma/delta lymphoma with isochromosome for long arm of chromosome 7. Leuk Lymphoma 22: 495–500
80. Farcet J P, Gaulard P, Marolleau J P, et al. 1990 Hepatosplenic T-cell lymphoma: sinusal/sinusoidal localization of malignant cells expressing the T-cell receptor gamma delta. Blood 75: 2213–2219
81. Wong K F, Chan J K, Matutes E, et al. 1995 Hepatosplenic gamma delta T-cell lymphoma. A distinctive aggressive lymphoma type. Am J Surg Pathol 19: 718–726
82. Cooke C B, Krenacs L, Stetler-Stevenson M, et al. 1996 Hepatosplenic T-cell lymphoma: a distinct clinicopathologic entity of cytotoxic gamma delta T-cell origin. Blood 88: 4265–4274
83. Chang K L, Arber D A 1998 Hepatosplenic gamma delta T-cell lymphoma – not just alphabet soup. Adv Anat Pathol 5: 21–29
84. Moleti M L, Testi A M, Giona F, et al. 2006 Gamma-delta hepatosplenic T-cell lymphoma. Description of a case with immunophenotypic and molecular follow-up successfully treated with chemotherapy alone. Leuk Lymphoma 47: 333–336
85. Domm J A, Thompson M, Kuttesch J F, et al. 2005 Allogeneic bone marrow transplantation for chemotherapy-refractory hepatosplenic gammadelta T-cell lymphoma: case report and review of the literature. J Pediatr Hematol Oncol 27: 607–610
86. Sallah S, Smith S V, Lony L C, et al. 1997 Gamma/delta T-cell hepatosplenic lymphoma: review of the literature, diagnosis by flow cytometry and concomitant autoimmune hemolytic anemia. Ann Hematol 74: 139–142
87. Salhany K E, Feldman M, Kahn M J, et al. 1997 Hepatosplenic gammadelta T-cell lymphoma: ultrastructural, immunophenotypic, and functional evidence for cytotoxic T lymphocyte differentiation. Hum Pathol 28: 674–685
88. Macon W R, Williams M E, Greer J P, et al. 1996 Natural killer-like T-cell lymphomas: aggressive lymphomas of T-large granular lymphocytes. Blood 87: 1474–1483
89. Coventry S, Punnett H H, Tomczak E Z, et al. 1999 Consistency of isochromosome 7q and trisomy 8 in hepatosplenic gammadelta T-cell lymphoma: detection by fluorescence In situ hybridization of a splenic touch-preparation from a pediatric patient. Pediatr Dev Pathol 2: 478–483
90. Wang C C, Tien H F, Lin M T, et al. 1995 Consistent presence of isochromosome 7q in hepatosplenic T gamma/delta lymphoma: a new cytogenetic–clinicopathologic entity. Genes Chromos Cancer 12: 161–164

91. Jonveaux P, Daniel M T, Martel V, et al. 1996 Isochromosome 7q and trisomy 8 are consistent primary, non-random chromosomal abnormalities associated with hepatosplenic T gamma/delta lymphoma. Leukemia 10: 1453–1455
92. Alonsozana E L, Stamberg J, Kumar D, et al. 1997 Isochromosome 7q: the primary cytogenetic abnormality in hepatosplenic gammadelta T cell lymphoma. Leukemia 11: 1367–1372
93. Shetty S, Mansoor A, Roland B 2006 Ring chromosome 7 with amplification of 7q sequences in a pediatric case of hepatosplenic T-cell lymphoma. Cancer Genet Cytogenet 167: 161–163
94. Troussard X, Maloisel F, Flandrin G 1998 Hairy cell leukemia. What is new forty years after the first description? Hematol Cell Ther 40: 139–148
95. Kraut E H, Grever M R, Bouroncle B A 1994 Long-term follow-up of patients with hairy cell leukemia after treatment with 2′-deoxycoformycin. Blood 84: 4061–4063
96. Jehn U, Bartl R, Dietzfelbinger H, et al. 1999 Long-term outcome of hairy cell leukemia treated with 2-chlorodeoxyadenosine. Ann Hematol 78: 139–144
97. Burke J S, Rappaport H 1984 The diagnosis and differential diagnosis of hairy cell leukemia in bone marrow and spleen. Semin Oncol 11: 334–346
98. Burke J S, Sheibani K, Winberg C D, et al. 1987 Recognition of hairy cell leukemia in a spleen of normal weight. The contribution of immunohistologic studies. Am J Clin Pathol 87: 276–281
99. Hanson C A, Ward P C, Schnitzer B 1989 A multilobular variant of hairy cell leukemia with morphologic similarities to T-cell lymphoma. Am J Surg Pathol 13: 671–679
100. Hoyer J D, Li C Y, Yam L T, et al. 1997 Immunohistochemical demonstration of acid phosphatase isoenzyme 5 (tartrate-resistant) in paraffin sections of hairy cell leukemia and other hematologic disorders. Am J Clin Pathol 108: 308–315
101. Catovsky D, Foa R 1990 The lymphoid leukemias. Butterworths, London
102. Matutes E, Morilla R, Owusu-Ankomah K, et al. 1994 The immunophenotype of hairy cell leukemia (HCL). Proposal for a scoring system to distinguish HCL from B cell disorders with hairy or villous lymphocytes. Leuk Lymphoma 14: 57–61
103. Moller P, Mielke B, Moldenhauer G 1990 Monoclonal antibody HML-1, a marker for intraepithelial T cells and lymphomas derived thereof, also recognizes hairy cell leukemia and some B cell lymphomas. Am J Pathol 136: 509–512
104. Cheuk W, Wong K O, Wong C S, et al. 2004 Consistent immunostaining for cyclin D1 can be achieved on a routine basis using a newly available rabbit monoclonal antibody. Am J Surg Pathol 28: 801–807
105. Sansoni P, Rowden G, Manara G C, et al. 1988 Immunoelectronmicroscopic demonstration of S-100 protein in hairy cell leukemia cells. Am J Clin Pathol 89: 374–377
106. Strickler J G, Schmidt C M, Wick M R 1990 Methods in pathology. Immunophenotype of hairy cell leukemia in paraffin sections. Mod Pathol 3: 518–523
107. Basso K, Liso A, Tiacci E, et al. 2004 Gene expression profiling of hairy cell leukemia reveals a phenotype related to memory B cells with altered expression of chemokine and adhesion receptors. J Exp Med 199: 59–68
108. Valent P, Horny H P, Li C Y, et al. 2001 Mastocytosis. In: Jaffe E S, Harris N L, Stein H, et al. (eds) Pathology and genetics, tumours of haematopoietic and lymphoid tissues. World Health Organization classification of tumours. IARC Press, Lyon, 293–302
109. Travis W D, Li C Y, Bergstralh E J, et al. 1988 Systemic mast cell disease. Analysis of 58 cases and literature review. Medicine (Baltimore) 67: 345–368
110. Horny H P, Kaiserling E 1988 Lymphoid cells and tissue mast cells of bone marrow lesions in systemic mastocytosis: a histological and immunohistological study. Br J Haematol 69: 449–455
111. Travis W D, Li C Y, Bergstralh E J 1989 Solid and hematologic malignancies in 60 patients with systemic mast cell disease. Arch Pathol Lab Med 113: 365–368
112. Travis W D, Li C Y, Yam L T, et al. 1988 Significance of systemic mast cell disease with associated hematologic disorders. Cancer 62: 965–972
113. Horny H P, Ruck M, Wehrmann M, et al. 1990 Blood findings in generalized mastocytosis: evidence of frequent simultaneous occurrence of myeloproliferative disorders. Br J Haematol 76: 186–193
114. Lennert K, Parwaresch M R 1979 Mast cells and mast cell neoplasia: a review. Histopathology 3: 349–365
115. Parwaresch M R, Horny H P, Lennert K 1985 Tissue mast cells in health and disease. Pathol Res Pract 179: 439–467
116. Chariot P, Monnet I, Gaulard P, et al. 1993 Systemic mastocytosis following mediastinal germ cell tumor: an association confirmed. Hum Pathol 24: 111–112
117. Brunning R D, McKenna R W, Rosai J, et al. 1983 Systemic mastocytosis. Extracutaneous manifestations. Am J Surg Pathol 7: 425–438
118. Valent P, Escribano L, Parwaresch R M, et al. 1999 Recent advances in mastocytosis research. summary of the Vienna mastocytosis meeting 1998. Int Arch Allergy Immunol 120: 1–7
119. Valent P 1996 Biology, classification and treatment of human mastocytosis. Wien Klin Wochenschr 108: 385–397
120. Horny H P, Ruck P, Krober S, et al. 1997 Systemic mast cell disease (mastocytosis). General aspects and histopathological diagnosis. Histol Histopathol 12: 1081–1089
121. Kors J W, Van Doormaal J J, Breukelman H, et al. 1996 Long-term follow-up of indolent mastocytosis in adults. J Intern Med 239: 157–164
122. Horny H P, Sillaber C, Menke D, et al. 1998 Diagnostic value of immunostaining for tryptase in patients with mastocytosis. Am J Surg Pathol 22: 1132–1140
123. Travis W D, Li C Y 1988 Pathology of the lymph node and spleen in systemic mast cell disease. Mod Pathol 1: 4–14
124. Horny H P, Kaiserling E, Parwaresch M R, et al. 1992 Lymph node findings in generalized mastocytosis. Histopathology 21: 439–446
125. Horny H P, Kaiserling E, Campbell M, et al. 1989 Liver findings in generalized mastocytosis. A clinicopathologic study. Cancer 63: 532–538
126. Horny H P, Parwaresch M R, Lennert K 1985 Bone marrow findings in systemic mastocytosis. Hum Pathol 16: 808–814
127. Rywlin A M 1982 Mastocytic eosinophilic fibrohistiocytic lesion of the bone marrow. Haematology 2: 1–4
128. Krober S M, Horny H P, Ruck P, et al. 1997 Mastocytosis: reactive or neoplastic? J Clin Pathol 50: 525–527
129. Akin C 2005 Clonality and molecular pathogenesis of mastocytosis. Acta Haematol 114: 61–69
130. Nagata H, Okada T, Worobec A S, et al. 1997 c-kit mutation in a population of patients with mastocytosis. Int Arch Allergy Immunol 113: 184–186
131. Long J C, Aisenberg A C, Zamecnik P C 1974 An antigen in Hodgkin's disease tissue cultures: fluorescent antibody studies. Proc Natl Acad Sci USA 71: 2285–2289
132. Longley B J Jr, Metcalfe D D, Tharp M, et al. 1999 Activating and dominant inactivating c-KIT catalytic domain mutations in distinct clinical forms of human mastocytosis. Proc Natl Acad Sci USA 96: 1609–1614
133. Longley B J, Tyrrell L, Lu S Z, et al. 1996 Somatic c-KIT activating mutation in urticaria pigmentosa and aggressive mastocytosis: establishment of clonality in a human mast cell neoplasm. Nat Genet 12: 312–314
134. Worobec A S, Semere T, Nagata H, Metcalfe D D 1998 Clinical correlates of the presence of the Asp816Val c-kit mutation in the peripheral blood mononuclear cells of patients with mastocytosis. Cancer 83: 2120–2129
135. Metcalfe D D 2005 Mastocytosis. Novartis Found Symp 271: 232–242
136. Droogendijk H J, Kluin-Nelemans H J, van Doormaal J J, et al. 2006 Imatinib mesylate in the treatment of systemic mastocytosis: a phase II trial. Cancer 107: 345–351
137. Pardanani A, Akin C, Valent P 2006 Pathogenesis, clinical features, and treatment advances in mastocytosis. Best Pract Res Clin Haematol 19: 595–615
138. Ma Y, Zeng S, Metcalfe D D, et al. 2002 The c-KIT mutation causing human mastocytosis is resistant to STI571 and other KIT kinase inhibitors; kinases with enzymatic site mutations show different inhibitor sensitivity profiles than wild-type kinases and those with regulatory-type mutations. Blood 99: 1741–1744
139. Nishida T, Hirota S, Taniguchi M, et al. 1998 Familial gastrointestinal stromal tumours with germline mutation of the KIT gene [letter]. Nat Genet 19: 323–324
140. Arber D A, Tamayo R, Weiss L M 1998 Paraffin section detection of the c-kit gene product (CD117) in human tissues: value in the diagnosis of mast cell disorders. Hum Pathol 29: 498–504
141. Sotlar K, Horny H P, Simonitsch I, et al. 2004 CD25 indicates the neoplastic phenotype of mast cells: a novel immunohistochemical marker for the diagnosis of systemic mastocytosis (SM) in routinely processed bone marrow biopsy specimens. Am J Surg Pathol 28: 1319–1325
142. Yagita H, Iwai M, Yagita-Toguri M, et al. 2001 Langerhans cell histiocytosis of an adult with tumors in liver and spleen. Hepatogastroenterology 48: 581–584
143. Perez-Ordonez B, Erlandson R A, Rosai J 1996 Follicular dendritic cell tumor: report of 13 additional cases of a distinctive entity. Am J Surg Pathol 20: 944–955
144. Cheuk W, Chan J K, Shek T W, et al. 2001 Inflammatory pseudotumor-like follicular dendritic cell tumor: a distinctive low-grade malignant intra-abdominal neoplasm with consistent Epstein–Barr virus association. Am J Surg Pathol 25: 721–731
145. Kawachi K, Nakatani Y, Inayama Y, et al. 2002 Interdigitating dendritic cell sarcoma of the spleen: report of a case with a review of the literature. Am J Surg Pathol 26: 530–537
146. McKenna R W, Risdall R J, Brunning R D 1981 Virus associated hemophagocytic syndrome. Hum Pathol 12: 395–398
147. Risdall R J 1980 Pathologic anatomy: virus-associated hemophagocytic syndrome. Minn Med 63: 879–880
148. Risdall R J, McKenna R W, Nesbit M E, et al. 1979 Virus-associated hemophagocytic syndrome: a benign histiocytic proliferation distinct from malignant histiocytosis. Cancer 44: 993–1002
149. Wong K F, Chan J K 1992 Reactive hemophagocytic syndrome – a clinicopathologic study of 40 patients in an Oriental population. Am J Med 93: 177–180
150. Chan J K, Ng C S, Law C K, et al. 1987 Reactive hemophagocytic syndrome: a study of 7 fatal cases. Pathology 19: 43–50
151. Wong K F, Chan J K C 1991 Hemophagocytic disorders – a review. Hematol Rev 5: 5–37
152. Neiman R S 1977 Incidence and importance of splenic sarcoid-like granulomas. Arch Pathol Lab Med 101: 518–521
153. Sacks E L, Donaldson S S, Gordon J, et al. 1978 Epithelioid granulomas associated with Hodgkin's disease: clinical correlation in 55 previously untreated patients. Cancer 41: 562–567
154. Abrams J, Pearl P, Moody M, et al. 1988 Epithelioid granulomas revisited: long-term follow-up in Hodgkin's disease. Am J Clin Oncol 11: 456–460

155. Narang S, Wolf B C, Neiman R S 1985 Malignant lymphoma presenting with prominent splenomegaly: a clinicopathologic study with special reference to intermediate cell lymphoma. Cancer 55: 1948–1957
156. Kuo T, Rosai J 1974 Granulomatous inflammation in splenectomy specimens. Clinicopathologic study of 20 cases. Arch Pathol 98: 261–268
157. Falk S, Takeshita M, Stutte H J 1988 Epithelioid granulomatosis with initial and predominant manifestation in spleen. Morphological and immunohistochemical analysis of six cases. Virchows Arch A Pathol Anat Histopathol 414: 69–76
158. Suster S, Moran C A, Blanco M 1994 Mycobacterial spindle-cell pseudotumor of the spleen. Am J Clin Pathol 101: 539–542
159. Kumar S, Kumar D, Cowan D F, Alperin J B: Mycobacterial spindle cell pseudotumor of the spleen [letter]. Am J Clin Pathol 102: 863, 1994
160. Arber D A, Kamel O W, van de Rijn M, et al. 1995 Frequent presence of the Epstein–Barr virus in inflammatory pseudotumor. Hum Pathol 26: 1093–1098
161. Delsol G, Diebold J, Isaacson P G, et al. 1998 Pathology of the spleen: report on the workshop of the VIIIth meeting of the European Association for Haematopathology, Paris 1996. Histopathology 32: 172–179
162. Horiguchi H, Matsui-Horiguchi M, Sakata H, et al. 2004 Inflammatory pseudotumor-like follicular dendritic cell tumor of the spleen. Pathol Int 54: 124–131
163. Lewis J T, Gaffney R L, Casey M B, et al. 2003 Inflammatory pseudotumor of the spleen associated with a clonal Epstein–Barr virus genome. Case report and review of the literature. Am J Clin Pathol 120: 56–61
164. Garvin D F, King F M 1981 Cysts and nonlymphomatous tumors of the spleen. Pathol Annu 16: 61–80
165. Morgenstern L, Rosenberg J, Geller S A 1985 Tumors of the spleen. World J Surg 9: 468–476
166. Husni E A 1961 The clinical course of splenic hemangioma, with emphasis on spontaneous rupture. Arch Surg 83: 681–688
167. Chen L W, Chien R N, Yen C L, et al. 2004 Splenic tumour: a clinicopathological study. Int J Clin Pract 58: 924–927
168. Kutok J L, Fletcher C D 2003 Splenic vascular tumors. Semin Diagn Pathol 20: 128–139
169. Arber D A, Strickler J G, Chen Y Y, et al. 1997 Splenic vascular tumors: a histologic, immunophenotypic, and virologic study. Am J Surg Pathol 21: 827–835
170. Dufau J P, Le Tourneau A, Audouin J, et al. 1999 Isolated diffuse hemangiomatosis of the spleen with Kasbach–Merritt-like syndrome. Histopathology 35: 337–3s44
171. Ruck P, Horny H P, Xiao J C, et al. 1994 Diffuse sinusoidal hemangiomatosis of the spleen. A case report with enzyme-histochemical, immunohistochemical, and electron-microscopic findings. Pathol Res Pract 190: 708–714; discussion 715–717
172. Tarazov P G, Polysalov V N, Ryzhkov VK 1990 Hemangiomatosis of the liver and spleen: successful treatment with embolization and splenectomy. AJR Am J Roentgenol 155: 1235–1236
173. Shiran A, Naschitz J E, Yeshurun D, et al. 1990 Diffuse hemangiomatosis of the spleen: splenic hemangiomatosis presenting with giant splenomegaly, anemia, and thrombocytopenia. Am J Gastroenterol 85: 1515–1517
174. Tada S, Shin M, Takashima T, et al. Diffuse capillary hemangiomatosis of the spleen as a cause of portal hypertension. Radiology 104: 63–4, 1972
175. Falk S, Stutte H J, Frizzera G 1991 Littoral cell angioma. A novel splenic vascular lesion demonstrating histiocytic differentiation. Am J Surg Pathol 15: 1023–1033
176. Bisceglia M, Sickel J Z, Giangaspero F, et al. 1998 Littoral cell angioma of the spleen: an additional report of four cases with emphasis on the association with visceral organ cancers. Tumori 84: 595–599
177. Mohan V, Jones R C, Drake A J 3rd, et al. 2005 Littoral cell angioma presenting as metastatic thyroid carcinoma to the spleen. Thyroid 15: 170–175
178. Morgenstern L, Bello J M, Fisher B L, et al. 1992 The clinical spectrum of lymphangiomas and lymphangiomatosis of the spleen. Am Surg 58: 599–604
179. Arber D A, Strickler J G, Weiss L M 1997 Splenic mesothelial cysts mimicking lymphangiomas. Am J Surg Pathol 21: 334–338
180. Chan K W, Saw D 1980 Distinctive, multiple lymphangiomas of spleen. J Pathol 131: 75–81
181. Takayama A, Nakashima O, Kobayashi K, et al. 2003 Splenic lymphangioma with papillary endothelial proliferation: a case report and review of the literature. Pathol Int 53: 483–488
182. Schmid C, Beham A, Uranus S, et al. 1991 Non-systemic diffuse lymphangiomatosis of spleen and liver. Histopathology 18: 478–480
183. McQuown D S, Fishbein M C, Moran E T, et al. 1975 Abdominal cystic lymphangiomatosis: report of a case involving the liver and spleen and illustration of two cases with origin in the greater omentum and root of the mesentery. J Clin Ultrasound 3: 291–296
184. Falk S, Krishnan J, Meis J M 1993 Primary angiosarcoma of the spleen. A clinicopathologic study of 40 cases. Am J Surg Pathol 17: 959–970
185. Miyata T, Fujimoto Y, Fukushima M, et al. 1993 Spontaneous rupture of splenic angiosarcoma: a case report of chemotherapeutic approach and review of the literature. Surg Today 23: 370–374
186. Buckner J W, Porterfield G, Williams GR 1990 Spontaneous splenic rupture secondary to angiosarcoma. J Okla State Med Assoc 83: 211–213
187. De Vriese L, De Coster M, Noyez D 1989 Angiosarcoma of the spleen. Case report and review of literature. Acta Chir Belg 89: 46–48
188. Chen K T, Bolles J C, Gilbert E F 1979 Angiosarcoma of the spleen: a report of two cases and review of the literature. Arch Pathol Lab Med 103: 122–124
189. Neuhauser T S, Derringer G A, Thompson L D, et al. 2000 Splenic angiosarcoma: a clinicopathologic and immunophenotypic study of 28 cases. Mod Pathol 13: 978–987
190. Kren L, Kaur P, Goncharuk V N, et al. 2003 Primary angiosarcoma of the spleen in a child. Med Pediatr Oncol 40: 411–412
191. Hsu J T, Chen H M, Lin C Y, et al. 2005 Primary angiosarcoma of the spleen. J Surg Oncol 92: 312–316
192. Rosso R, Paulli M, Gianelli U, et al. 1995 Littoral cell angiosarcoma of the spleen. Case report with immunohistochemical and ultrastructural analysis. Am J Clin Pathol 102: 1203–1208
193. Rosso R, Gianelli U, Chan J K 1996 Further evidence supporting the sinus lining cell nature of splenic littoral cell angiosarcoma [letter]. Am J Surg Pathol 20: 1531
194. Meybehm M, Fischer H P 1997 Littoral cell angiosarcoma of the spleen. Morphologic, immunohistochemical findings and consideration of histogenesis of a rare splenic tumor. Pathologe 18: 401–405
195. Takato H, Iwamoto H, Ikezu M, et al. 1993 Splenic hemangiosarcoma with sinus endothelial differentiation. Acta Pathol Jpn 43: 702–708
196. Kaw Y T, Duwaji M S, Knisley R E, et al. 1992 Hemangioendothelioma of the spleen. Arch Pathol Lab Med 116: 1079–1082
197. Suster S 1992 Epithelioid and spindle-cell hemangioendothelioma of the spleen. Report of a distinctive splenic vascular neoplasm of childhood. Am J Surg Pathol 16: 785–792
198. Budke H L, Breitfeld P P, Neiman R S 1995 Functional hyposplenism due to a primary epithelioid hemangioendothelioma of the spleen. Arch Pathol Lab Med 119: 755–757
199. Cotell S L, Noskin G A 1994 Bacillary angiomatosis. Clinical and histologic features, diagnosis, and treatment. Arch Intern Med 154: 524–528
200. Slater L N, Welch D F, Min K W 1992 *Rochalimaea henselae* causes bacillary angiomatosis and peliosis hepatis. Arch Intern Med 152: 602–606
201. Slater L N, Pitha J V, Herrera L, et al. 1994 *Rochalimaea henselae* infection in acquired immunodeficiency syndrome causing inflammatory disease without angiomatosis or peliosis. Demonstration by immunocytochemistry and corroboration by DNA amplification. Arch Pathol Lab Med 118: 33–38
202. Tsang W Y, Chan J K 1992 Bacillary angiomatosis. A 'new' disease with a broadening clinicopathologic spectrum. Histol Histopathol 7: 143–152
203. Kemper C A, Lombard C M, Deresinski S C, et al. 1990 Visceral bacillary epithelioid angiomatosis: possible manifestations of disseminated cat scratch disease in the immunocompromised host: a report of two cases. Am J Med 89: 216–222
204. Cheuk W, Chan A K, Wong M C, et al. 2006 Confirmation of diagnosis of cat scratch disease by immunohistochemistry. Am J Surg Pathol 30: 274–275
205. Martel M, Cheuk W, Lombardi L, et al. 2004 Sclerosing angiomatoid nodular transformation (SANT): report of 25 cases of a distinctive benign splenic lesion. Am J Surg Pathol 28: 1268–1279
206. Krishnan J, Frizzera G 2003 Two splenic lesions in need of clarification: hamartoma and inflammatory pseudotumor. Semin Diagn Pathol 20: 94–104
207. Galindo Gallego M, Ortega Serrano M P, Ortega Lopez M, et al. 1997 Inflammatory pseudotumor of spleen. Report of two cases and literature review. Minerva Chir 52: 1379–1388
208. McHenry C R, Perzy-Gall H B, Mardini G, et al. 1995 Inflammatory pseudotumor of the spleen: a rare entity that may mimic hematopoietic malignancy. Am Surg 61: 1067–1071
209. Thomas R M, Jaffe E S, Zarate-Osorno A, et al. 1993 Inflammatory pseudotumor of the spleen. A clinicopathologic and immunophenotypic study of eight cases. Arch Pathol Lab Med 117: 921–926
210. Iwafuchi M, Watanabe H, Maejima T, et al. 1992 Inflammatory pseudotumor of the spleen. Report of a case with an immunohistochemical study. Acta Pathol Jpn 42: 376–381
211. Dalal B I, Greenberg H, Quinonez G E, et al. 1991 Inflammatory pseudotumor of the spleen. Morphological, radiological, immunophenotypic, and ultrastructural features. Arch Pathol Lab Med 115: 1062–1064
212. Monforte-Munoz H, Ro J Y, Manning J T Jr, et al. 1991 Inflammatory pseudotumor of the spleen. Report of two cases with a review of the literature. Am J Clin Pathol 96: 491–495
213. Wiernik P H, Rader M, Becker N H, et al. 1990 Inflammatory pseudotumor of spleen. Cancer 66: 597–600
214. Chang J L, Tzeng H H, Tu Y C, et al. 1989 Inflammatory pseudotumor of the spleen – case report and literature review. Chung Hua I Hsueh Tsa Chih 44: 139–144
215. Sheahan K, Wolf B C, Neiman R S 1988 Inflammatory pseudotumor of the spleen: a clinicopathology study of three cases. Hum Pathol 19: 1024–1029
216. Alpern H D, Olson J E, Kozak A J 1986 Inflammatory pseudotumor of the spleen. J Surg Oncol 33: 46–49
217. Cotelingam J D, Jaffe E S 1984 Inflammatory pseudotumor of the spleen. Am J Surg Pathol 8: 375–380
218. Seijo L, Unger P D, Strauchen J A 1996 Inflammatory pseudotumor of the spleen, a case report and review of the literature. Int J Surg Pathol 3: 289–298
219. Braun B, Cazorla A, Rivas C, et al. 2003 Inflammatory pseudotumor of the spleen in a patient with human immunodeficiency virus infection: a case report and review of the literature. Ann Hematol 82: 511–514

220. Falk S, Stutte H J 1989 Hamartomas of the spleen: a study of 20 biopsy cases. Histopathology 14: 603–612
221. Zukerberg L R, Kaynor B L, Silverman M L, et al. 1991 Splenic hamartoma and capillary hemangioma are distinct entities: immunohistochemical analysis of CD8 expression by endothelial cells. Hum Pathol 22: 1258–1261
222. Hayes T C, Britton H A, Mewborne E B, et al. 1998 Symptomatic splenic hamartoma: case report and literature review. Pediatrics 101: E10
223. Ferguson E R, Sardi A, Beckman E N 1993 Spontaneous rupture of splenic hamartoma. J LA State Med Soc 145: 48–52
224. Silverman M L, LiVolsi V A 1978 Splenic hamartoma. Am J Clin Pathol 70: 224–229
225. Darden J W, Teeslink R, Parrish A 1975 Hamartoma of the spleen: a manifestation of tuberous sclerosis. Am Surg 41: 564–566
226. Ross C F, Schiller K F 1971 Hamartoma of spleen associated with thrombocytopenia. J Pathol 105: 62–64
227. Morgenstern L, McCafferty L, Rosenberg J, et al. 1984 Hamartomas of the spleen. Arch Surg 119: 1291–1293
228. Cheuk W, Lee A K, Arora N, et al. 2005 Splenic hamartoma with bizarre stromal cells. Am J Surg Pathol 29: 109–114
229. Laskin W B, Alasadi R, Variakojis D 2005 Splenic hamartoma. Am J Surg Pathol 29: 1114–1115
230. Kraus M D, Dehner L P 1999 Benign vascular neoplasms of the spleen with myoid and angioendotheliomatous features. Histopathology 35: 328–336
231. Chan Y F, Kumar B, Auldist A, et al. 2005 Myoid angioendothelioma of the spleen in a child after successful treatment of a Wilms' tumour. Pathology 37: 181–184
232. Karim R Z, Ma-Wyatt J, Cox M, et al. 2004 Myoid angioendothelioma of the spleen. Int J Surg Pathol 12: 51–56
233. Burrig K F 1988 Epithelial (true) splenic cysts. Pathogenesis of the mesothelial and so-called epidermoid cyst of the spleen. Am J Surg Pathol 12: 275–281
234. Shousha S 1978 Splenic cysts: a report of six cases and a brief review. Postgrad Med J 54: 265–269
235. Tsakraklides V, Hadley T W 1973 Epidermoid cysts of the spleen. A report of five cases. Arch Pathol 96: 251–254
236. Palmieri I, Natale E, Crafa F, et al. 2005 Epithelial splenic cysts. Anticancer Res 25: 515–521
237. Chen K T K, Flam M S, Workman R D 1987 Amyloid tumor of the spleen. Am J Surg Pathol 11: 723–725
238. Easler R E, Dowlin W M 1969 Primary lipoma of the spleen, report of a case. Arch Pathol 88: 557–559
239. Bostick W L 1945 Primary splenic neoplasms. Am J Pathol 21: 1143–1165
240. Hulbert J C, Graf R 1983 Involvement of the spleen by renal angiomyolipoma: metastasis or multicentricity? J Urol 130: 328–329
241. Mallipudi B V, Chawdhery M Z, Jeffery P J 1998 Primary malignant fibrous histiocytoma of spleen. Eur J Surg Oncol 24: 448–449
242. Govoni E, Bazzocchi F, Pileri S, et al. 1982 Primary malignant fibrous histiocytoma of the spleen: an ultrastructural study. Histopathology 6: 351–366
243. Sieber S C, Lopez V, Rosai J, et al. 1990 Primary tumor of spleen with morphologic features of malignant fibrous histiocytoma. Immunohistochemical evidence for a macrophage origin. Am J Surg Pathol 14: 1061–1070
244. Le Bail B, Morel D, Merel P, et al. 1996 Cystic smooth-muscle tumor of the liver and spleen associated with Epstein–Barr virus after renal transplantation. Am J Surg Pathol 20: 1418–1425
245. Morel D, Merville P, Le Bail B, et al. 1996 Epstein–Barr virus (EBV)-associated hepatic and splenic smooth muscle tumours after kidney transplantation. Nephrol Dial Transplant 11: 1864–1866
246. Feakins R M, Norton A J 1996 Rhabdomyosarcoma of the spleen. Histopathology 29: 577–579
247. Gong J Z, Sullivan J D, Teichberg S, et al. 1999 Pleomorphic large cell sarcoma of the spleen with rhabdomyosarcomatous differentiation. Ann Clin Lab Sci 29: 303–307
248. Guadalajara Jurado J, Turegano Fuentes F, Garcia Menendez C, et al. 1989 Hemangiopericytoma of the spleen. Surgery 106: 575–577
249. Neill J S, Park H K 1991 Hemangiopericytoma of the spleen. Am J Clin Pathol 95: 680–683
250. Yilmazlar T, Kirdak T, Yerci O, et al. 2005 Splenic hemangiopericytoma and serosal cavernous hemangiomatosis of the adjacent colon. World J Gastroenterol 11: 4111–4113
251. Katz J A, Mahoney D H, Shukla L W, et al. 1988 Endovascular papillary angioendothelioma in the spleen. Pediatr Pathol 8: 185–193
252. Sarode V R, Datta B N, Savitri K, et al. 1991 Kaposi's sarcoma of spleen with unusual clinical and histologic features. Arch Pathol Lab Med 115: 1042–1044
253. Daftary M, Barnett R N 1971 Malignant teratoma of the spleen. Yale J Biol Med 43: 283–287
254. Tanahashi J, Kashima K, Daa T, et al. 2006 Florid cystic endosalpingiosis of the spleen. APMIS 114: 393–398
255. Westra W H, Anderson B O, Klimstra D S 1994 Carcinosarcoma of the spleen. An extragenital malignant mixed mullerian tumor? Am J Surg Pathol 18: 309–315
256. Hirota M, Hayashi N, Tomioka T, et al. 1999 Mucinous cystadenocarcinoma of the spleen presenting a point mutation of the Kirsten-ras oncogene at codon 12. Dig Dis Sci 44: 768–774
257. Morinaga S, Ohyama R, Koizumi J 1992 Low-grade mucinous cystadenocarcinoma in the spleen. Am J Surg Pathol 16: 903–908
258. Du Plessis D G, Louw J A, Warnz P A B 1999 Mucinous epithelial cysts of the spleen assoicated with psuedomyxoma peritonei. Histopathology 35: 551–557
259. Berge T 1974 Splenic metastases, frequencies and patterns. Acta Pathol Microbiol Scand Sect A 82: 499–506
260. Lam K Y, Tang V 2000 Metastatic tumors to the spleen. A 25-year clinicopathologic study. Arch Pathol Lab Med 124: 526–530
261. Giuliani A, Caporale A, Di Bari M, et al. 1999 Isolated splenic metastasis from endometrial carcinoma. J Exp Clin Cancer Res 18: 93–96
262. Jorgensen L N, Chrintz H 1988 Solitary metastatic endometrial carcinoma of the spleen. Acta Obstet Gynecol Scand 67: 91–92
263. Gilks C B, Acker B D, Clement P B 1989 Recurrent endometrial adenocarcinoma: presentation as a splenic mass mimicking malignant lymphoma. Gynecol Oncol 33: 209–211
264. Abrams H L, Spiro R, Goldstein N: Metastases in carcinoma, analysis of 1000 autopsied cases. Cancer 3: 74–85, 1950
265. Hadjileontis C, Amplianitis I, Valsamides C, et al. 2004 Solitary splenic metastasis of endometrial carcinoma ten years after hysterectomy. Case report and review of the literature. Eur J Gynaecol Oncol 25: 233–235
266. Goktolga U, Dede M, Deveci G, et al. 2004 Solitary splenic metastasis of squamous cell carcinoma of the uterine cervix: a case report and review of the literature. Eur J Gynaecol Oncol 25: 742–744
267. Marymount J H J, Gross S 1963 Patterns of metastatic cancer in the spleen. Am J Clin Pathol 40: 58–60
268. Fakan F, Michal M 1994 Nodular transformation of splenic red pulp due to carcinomatous infiltration. A diagnostic pitfall. Histopathology 25: 175–178

第三部分

胸腺　The thymus

Wah Cheuk 和 John K.C. Chan 著

关宏伟 译

胸腺

正常胸腺	1315
胸腺肿瘤	1317
胸腺上皮性肿瘤	1317
胸腺的神经内分泌肿瘤	1337
胸腺和纵隔的生殖细胞肿瘤	1340
淋巴细胞、组织细胞和树突状细胞肿瘤	1343
胸腺和前纵隔间叶性肿瘤	1349
发生于胸腺的异位肿瘤	1350
胸腺和前纵隔的罕见的肿瘤和瘤样病变	1350
胸腺或前纵隔转移性肿瘤	1351
纵隔肿瘤：诊断方法和误区	1351

正常胸腺　The normal thymus

解剖学

胸腺位于前纵隔，从胚胎学上讲是由第三咽囊衍生而来的，在少数情况下，第四咽囊也参与了其发育。在胸腺下降迁移至前纵隔的过程中，部分胸腺可能残留于颈部，形成异位胸腺组织、异位胸腺囊肿和异位胸腺肿瘤[1]。胸腺是锥体形的两叶器官，包埋在菲薄的纤维性包膜中。胎儿末期胸腺达到其相对最大重量，而在青春期达到其绝对最大重量30～40g。此后，胸腺随着年龄增长缓慢退化，并逐渐由脂肪组织取代[2,3]。

组织学和超微结构特征

胸腺是一种对T淋巴细胞的成熟、选择细胞组成成熟T细胞的所有成分以及清除与自身肽抗原具有高亲和力的细胞必不可少的淋巴上皮性器官。胸腺由以深染的皮质和淡染的髓质为特征的分枝状小叶构成（图21C.1）。在结构上，相互连接的上皮细胞形成网状支架结构，淋巴细胞位于其中。有些散在分布的血管周围间隙不经免疫组化染色很难辨认（图21C.2）。

皮质由于淋巴细胞密集而深染。上皮细胞被密集的淋巴细胞所掩盖，表现为散在的卵圆形"裸"核，染色质呈空泡状，核仁不明显（图21C.3）。在胸腺被膜下排列成行的上皮细胞比较容易辨认。超微结构上胸腺上皮细胞显示有多数纤细的细胞突起，相邻细胞之间的细胞突起通过桥粒相互连接，胞浆内含有张力丝。

髓质淋巴细胞不如皮质淋巴细胞排列紧密（图21C.3B）。除了形成支架的上皮细胞网外，可见特征性的胸腺小体（Hassall小体），伴有同心圆性角化或中心

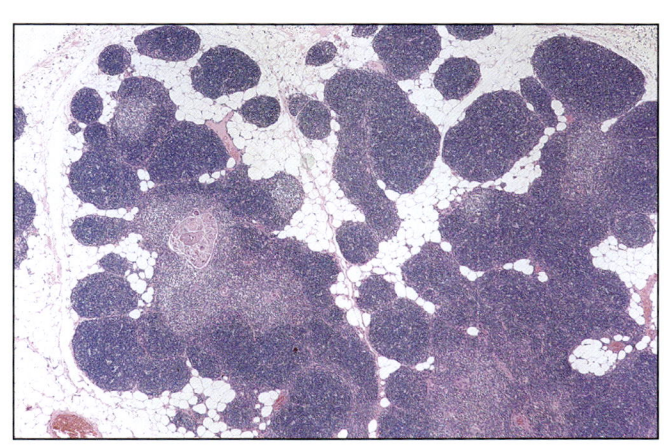

图21C.1　正常胸腺。胸腺小叶由深染的皮质和淡染的髓质构成。与胸腺瘤不同，其间的间质是由脂肪组织而不是由纤维组织构成的。

腔形成。偶尔可见淋巴滤泡或肌样细胞。

正常胸腺的免疫细胞化学

上皮成分：细胞角蛋白免疫染色可以很好地显示胸腺上皮细胞，特别是这些细胞的大量纤细、相互连接的胞浆突起（图21C.4）。根据解剖学部位不同，上皮细胞可有许多亚群，这些亚群的免疫组化染色和超微结构表现具有微细的差别[3-5]。

淋巴成分：皮质含有皮质胸腺细胞（不成熟的T细胞），这些细胞表达末端脱氧核苷酸转移酶（TdT）、胞浆CD3、CD1a和CD99a，但不表达表面CD3（surface CD3）（图21C.5和21C.6）[6]。这些淋巴细胞增殖率高，胸腺皮质内发育成熟时迁移到髓质，成为髓质胸腺细胞。髓质胸腺细胞通常表面CD3和胞浆CD3均呈阳性反应，

正常胸腺

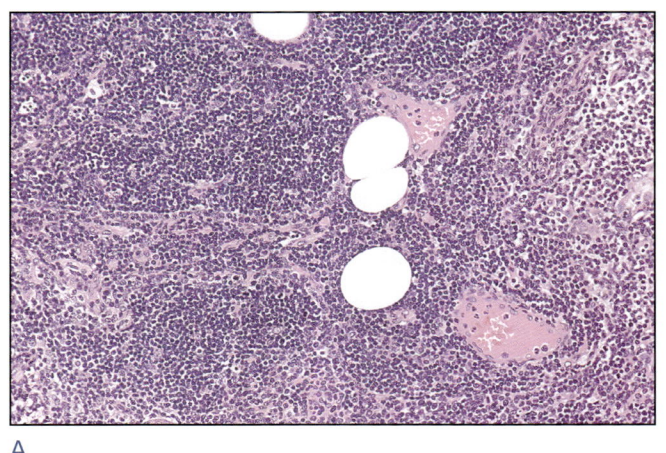
A

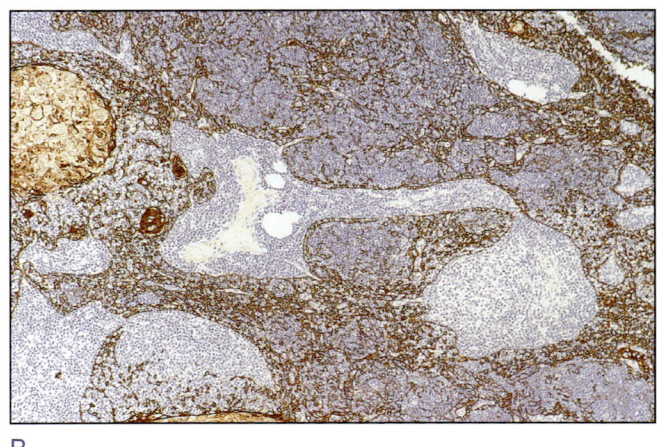
B

图21C.2 正常胸腺的血管周围间隙。（A）由于血管周围间隙常常充满小淋巴细胞，所以光镜下很难识别它的边界。（B）细胞角蛋白免疫组化染色可以非常容易辨认血管周围间隙，因为它完全不含细胞角蛋白阳性的胸腺上皮细胞。

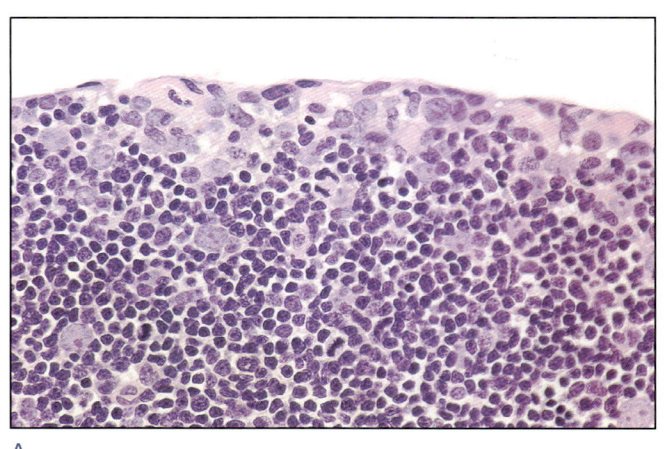
A

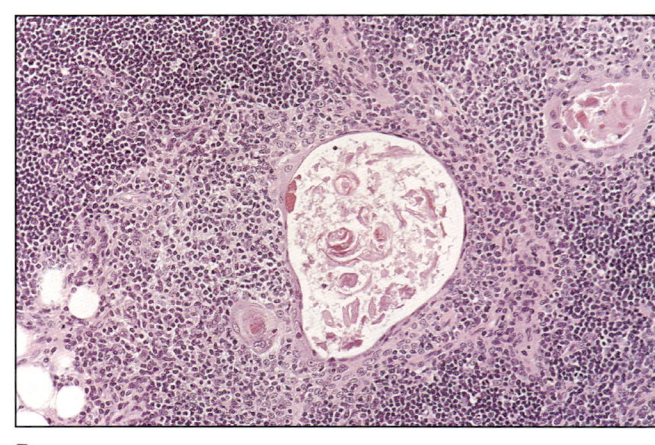
B

图21C.3 正常胸腺。（A）皮质富于淋巴细胞，胸腺上皮细胞核大而淡染容易识别。上皮细胞在被膜下方排列成行。（B）髓质的特征是细胞密度较小，可见胸腺小体，某些胸腺小体可出现囊性变。

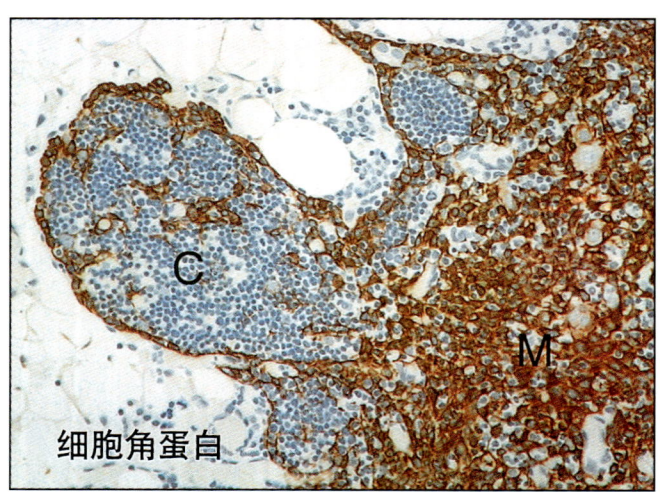
细胞角蛋白

图21C.4 正常胸腺的细胞角蛋白的免疫组化染色，显示复杂的胸腺上皮网。在皮质（C）、皮质的外部有成排的细胞，而皮质的内部却为疏松的网状结构所替代。在髓质（M），上皮细胞呈较密集的编织状排列。

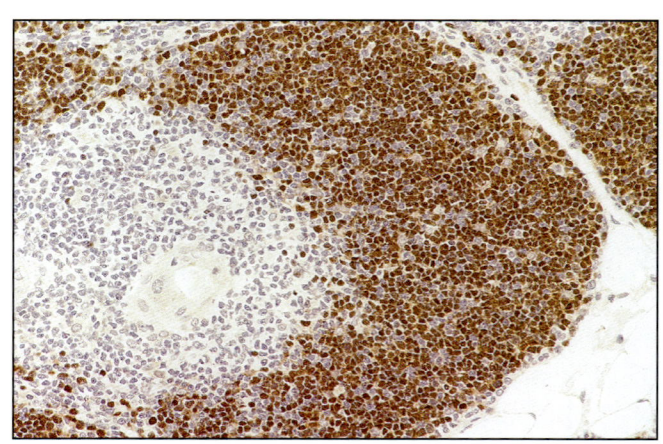

图21C.5 正常胸腺的TdT免疫组化染色。皮质的淋巴细胞（右侧）呈强阳性，而髓质的淋巴细胞（左侧）呈阴性。

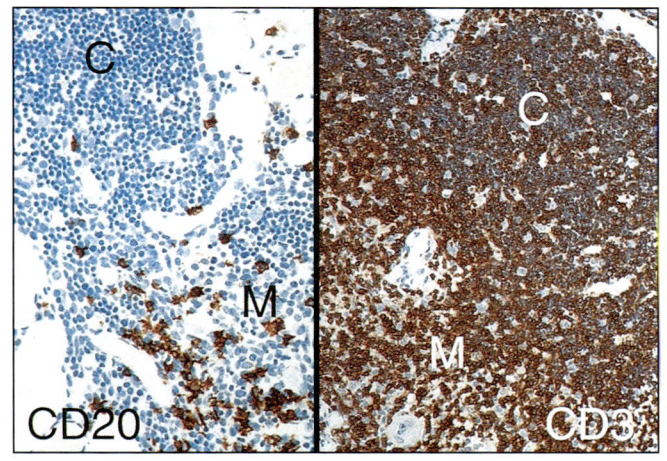

图21C.6 正常胸腺的免疫染色。左：CD20免疫染色显示，髓质（M）有一些B细胞，但后者在皮质（C）非常少见。右：CD3免疫染色显示，皮质（C）和髓质（M）均有大量T细胞，皮质胸腺细胞CD3染色阳性强度略弱于髓质胸腺细胞。

但是TdT、CD1a和CD99a呈阴性（图21C.5）。髓质胸腺细胞最终离开胸腺并定居于周围淋巴组织。

在胸腺髓质内还有相当数量的免疫表型独特的B细胞，这些细胞被认为是纵隔大B细胞淋巴瘤的前体细胞（图21C.6A）。由于T细胞插入，造成其中某些B细胞具有星状或星样形态表现。特征性的免疫表型是CD5[-]、CD19[+]、CD20[+]、CD21[-]、CD22[+]、CD23[+]、CD32[-]、CD35[-]，伴胞浆内IgD、IgM和IgG合成[7-9]。

胸腺肿瘤 Tumors of the thymus

胸腺原发性肿瘤少见。表21C.1所列的分类是根据2004版世界卫生组织（WHO）分类的修订版而来的[10-13]。在胸腺原发性肿瘤中，最常见的是胸腺瘤和淋巴瘤。胸腺生殖细胞肿瘤虽然少见，但是在鉴别诊断中总是应该予以考虑，因为采用现代疗法其治愈的可能性很高。

胸腺上皮性肿瘤 Thymic epithelial tumors

胸腺上皮性肿瘤是一个谱系，包括有包膜的胸腺瘤、浸润性胸腺瘤和胸腺癌。胸腺瘤（包括有包膜或浸润性的）的临床表现、组织学形态和生物学行为不同于胸腺癌（表21C.2）[13-22]。只有获得整个肿瘤进行组织学检查时才能明确区分有包膜的胸腺瘤和浸润性胸腺瘤。应用这种分类方法多数胸腺上皮性肿瘤易于分类，虽然有少数病例具有介于胸腺瘤和胸腺癌之间的交界性特征[6,23,24]。

胸腺瘤 Thymoma

定义

胸腺瘤是一种具有某些器官样特征并伴有不同数量反应性淋巴细胞的胸腺上皮性肿瘤[1,25]。器官样特征包括小叶状、髓质分化、血管周围间隙和不成熟的T淋巴细胞出现。

临床特征

胸腺瘤可以发生在任何年龄组，特别是41～50岁和51～60岁年龄组，平均年龄为49.5岁[1,26-29]。男女发病相等或女性略占优势。大约1/3～1/2的患者表现为胸部X线检查时发现无症状的前纵隔肿物。1/3的患者具有前纵隔肿物引起的症状，如咳嗽、呼吸困难、胸痛、咽下困难、声音嘶哑以及反复发生的胸部感染。1/3的患者出现瘤外表现（paraneoplastic manifestations），如重症肌无力、红细胞发育不全、获得性低丙种球蛋白血症、甲状腺炎和系统性红斑狼疮（表21C.3）[1,30-35]。组织学类型与临床表现相关，但不是绝对的。无论是A型还是B型，胸腺瘤均可伴有重症肌无力（A型或AB型胸腺瘤约15%，B1型胸腺瘤约40%，而B2型和B3型胸腺瘤约50%），但单纯红细胞发育不全和低丙种球蛋白血症却较常见于A型胸腺瘤的患者[5,31,36]。

极少数胸腺瘤病例伴有外周血T细胞淋巴细胞增多症，胸腺原发性肿瘤切除后通常可以恢复正常。这种胸腺瘤常常是浸润性胸腺瘤，富含淋巴细胞。外周血T淋巴细胞显示髓质胸腺细胞或外周T淋巴细胞的免疫表型，分子学分析发现，这些细胞是多克隆的。推测的发病机制可能包括：胸腺瘤免疫调节紊乱引起的反应性病变，以及来自胸腺瘤的较成熟的T淋巴细胞的溢出[37-44]。

人类胸腺瘤发生的病因学尚不明确。罕见的病例可以发生在胸腺囊肿内。与EB病毒无关，尽管过去曾这样认为[45-50]。

儿童胸腺瘤非常罕见。儿童胸腺瘤很少伴有重症肌无力[51]，并且预后良好。某些儿童胸腺瘤表现独特的间质改变，如小叶内和小叶周围有富于细胞的纤维性间质，伴嗜酸性细胞、组织细胞和肥大细胞浸润[52]。

临床行为和治疗

胸腺瘤最重要的单一预后因素是肿瘤分期[53-57]。表21C.4列出的Masaoka或修订的Masaoka分期方法已被广泛应用[58-60]。在一项有307例的病例研究中，分期分布如下：Ⅰ期44%、Ⅱ期23%、Ⅲ期27%和Ⅳ期6%[35]。这些分期的5年实际生存率分别为90%、88%、67%和50%，而10年实际生存率分别为80%、78%、47%和30%[35]。

表21C.1 胸腺肿瘤分类（根据2004 WHO分类方法修订）

上皮性肿瘤
1. 胸腺瘤
   - A型
   - AB型
   - B1型
   - B2型
   - B3型
   - 微小结节性胸腺瘤
   - 化生性胸腺瘤
2. 胸腺癌
   - 鳞状细胞癌
   - 淋巴上皮瘤样癌
   - 肉瘤样癌、梭形细胞癌和癌肉瘤
   - 透明细胞癌
   - 基底细胞样癌
   - 黏液表皮样癌
   - 乳头状腺癌
   - 腺癌
   - 未分化癌
   - 横纹肌样癌
   - 肝样癌
3. 胸腺上皮性肿瘤伴有介于胸腺瘤与胸腺癌之间的交界性特征

神经内分泌肿瘤
1. 类癌（典型和不典型）
   - 典型
   - 梭形细胞
   - 色素性
   - 伴有淀粉样物
   - 不典型
   - 黏液性
2. 小细胞癌，神经内分泌型
3. 大细胞神经内分泌癌

生殖细胞肿瘤
1. 精原细胞瘤
2. 胚胎性癌
3. 卵黄囊瘤
4. 绒毛膜癌
5. 畸胎瘤
   - 成熟畸胎瘤
   - 不成熟畸胎瘤
6. 混合性生殖细胞肿瘤
7. 伴有体细胞型恶性成分的生殖细胞肿瘤
8. 伴有造血恶性成分的生殖细胞肿瘤

淋巴细胞、组织细胞和树突状细胞肿瘤
1. Hodgkin淋巴瘤（尤其是结节硬化型）
2. 纵隔大B细胞淋巴瘤
3. T淋巴母细胞淋巴瘤的前体
4. 黏膜相关淋巴组织型结外边缘区B细胞淋巴瘤
5. Langerhans细胞组织细胞增生症
6. 组织细胞肉瘤（可以合并生殖细胞肿瘤）
7. 滤泡性树突状细胞肉瘤
8. 其他淋巴细胞，组织细胞或树突状细胞肿瘤

间叶性肿瘤
1. 脂肪瘤
2. 胸腺脂肪瘤
3. 胸腺脂肪肉瘤
4. 孤立性纤维性肿瘤
5. 恶性横纹肌样肿瘤
6. 滑膜肉瘤
7. 其他间叶性肿瘤

瘤样病变
1. 真性胸腺增生
2. 淋巴组织增生（淋巴滤泡性胸腺炎）
3. 多房性胸腺囊肿

发生于颈部的胸腺或相关鳃囊肿瘤
1. 异位错构瘤性胸腺瘤
2. 异位颈部胸腺瘤
3. 具有胸腺样分化的梭形细胞上皮性肿瘤（SETTLE）
4. 显示胸腺样分化的癌（CASTLE）

转移性肿瘤

未分类肿瘤

对于有包膜的（Ⅰ期）胸腺瘤，建议完全切除，包括胸腺及其周围的脂肪[2,26,30,61-63]。据报道，复发的危险为0%～12%不等，平均复发率为2%[15,17,19,26,28,35,64-68]。有些报告的复发率较高，可能由于肿瘤取材不完全，以致未能发现镜下浸润[15,66]。复发表现为纵隔局部肿块或多发性胸膜种植。远处转移非常罕见。

浸润性胸腺瘤的特征为穿透纤维性包膜的显微镜下浸润，或者明显浸润相邻结构（如心包、大血管或肺）（图21C.7）。有些病例还显示多发性胸膜和心包表面种植。约30%的病例复发，平均发生在最初切除之后5.5年，但是10年以后仍可复发[35,67]。术后3年之内的复发被定义为早期复发，早期复发常常导致死亡[59]。不到5%的浸润性胸腺瘤出现胸腔外转移，常见的转移部位是肝、肾、胸腔外淋巴结、骨和中枢神经系统[14,15,19,26,28,30,64,66,69-74]。完全切除肿瘤患者的生存率高于不完全切除肿瘤的生存率和仅做活检患者的生存率[15,35,56,75]。一般建议术后放射治疗，几组研究显示，术后放射治疗能使复发率从50%降到20%[2,30,66,68,76,77,77a]。对于Ⅲ期或Ⅳ期患者，常常给予顺铂为基础的化疗，有时疗效较好[2,30,66,77a,78-82]。对于复发病例，进一步完全切除复发的肿瘤或进行多学科的治疗偶尔有治愈的可能[30,67,83]。

尽管从前的研究发现重症肌无力是预后不好的因素，但最近的研究显示，重症肌无力并不具有预后意义，可能是因为重症肌无力的治疗得到改进的

表21C.2	胸腺瘤与胸腺癌的比较		
	有包膜的胸腺瘤	浸润性胸腺瘤	胸腺癌
包膜或周围组织浸润	无	有	常有，但少数病例可有包膜
自身免疫现象	常见		无
器官型组织学特征	有，如显著的小叶状、血管周围间隙、髓质分化和不成熟的T细胞出现 即使有浸润，小叶状生长方式依然保留		无 尽管有些肿瘤可出现小叶状结构，但是浸润灶呈片块状、岛状、条索状或单个细胞排列
上皮细胞的细胞学特征	细胞形态温和，轻度细胞非典型性，或偶尔可以出现大的非典型性核		恶性的
上皮成分的独特免疫反应	有些胸腺瘤表达CD20，尤其是A型胸腺瘤 有些胸腺瘤可能显示CD57免疫反应 CD5和CD117呈阴性		大约70%的胸腺癌CD5或CD117呈阳性
肿瘤内淋巴细胞	主要是不成熟的T细胞（TdT阳性）		成熟T细胞（TdT阴性）混有一些B细胞
临床行为	手术切除通常可以治愈；局部复发（0~3%）或转移非常罕见	局部复发常见（20%~41%）；转移罕见	迅速生长和早期局部复发；淋巴结转移；远处转移

表21C.3	与胸腺瘤相关的瘤外表现	
	胸腺瘤伴有这种表现（%）	与胸腺瘤相关的这种疾病的发生率（%）
重症肌无力	30~50	10~15
红细胞发育不全	5	30~50
低丙种球蛋白血症	5~12	10

表21C.4	胸腺瘤的临床分期
分期	修订的Masaoka系统*（1981、1994）
I	大体上和镜下均有完整的包膜；肿瘤侵入但未突破包膜，也归入I期
II	1. 镜下包膜穿透性浸润，或 2. 大体侵犯胸腺或周围脂肪组织，或与纵隔胸膜或心包粘连，但是并未突破
III	大体侵犯邻近器官，如心包、大血管或肺
IV	（IVa）胸膜或心包播散 （IVb）淋巴或血行转移

*在最初的Masaoka系统中，肿瘤侵犯纤维包膜被认为是II期，但是改良的分期要求肿瘤完全穿透纤维性包膜才能归为II期。

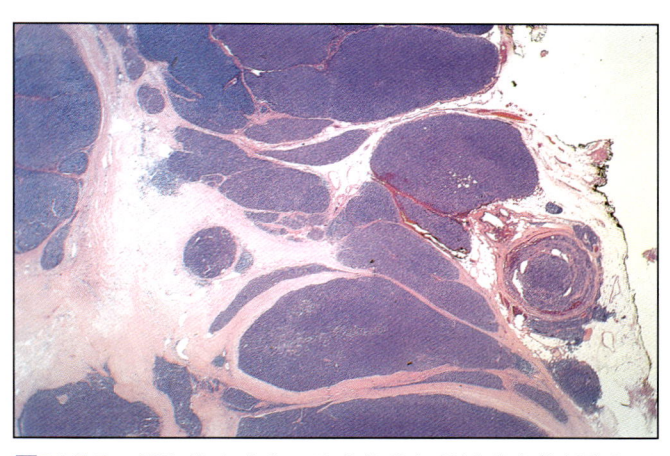

图21C.7 浸润性胸腺瘤。肿瘤的特征是被致密的纤维间隔分开的拼图样小叶结构。浸润性小叶（视野右侧）以"裸露"于脂肪组织中为特征，缺少纤维组织包裹。黑色墨水标记的切缘未被肿瘤累及。

结果[15,28,35,53,64]。

胸腺瘤的传统分类

传统上，根据形态学背景将胸腺瘤分为如下几种类型：淋巴细胞为主型、上皮细胞为主型、淋巴上皮混合型和梭形细胞型[26,65,84-86]。然而，这种分类不具预后意义[26,65,69,87-90]。

胸腺瘤的Muller-Hermelink分类

在20世纪80年代中期，根据胸腺瘤与胸腺皮质

表21C.5　胸腺上皮性肿瘤的各种分类的比较

WHO分类		Muller-Hermelink分类	Suster-Moran分类
A型胸腺瘤	良性胸腺瘤	髓质胸腺瘤	胸腺瘤
AB型胸腺瘤		混合性胸腺瘤	
B1型胸腺瘤	恶性胸腺瘤，I型	主要为皮质胸腺瘤	
B2型胸腺瘤		皮质胸腺瘤	
B3型胸腺瘤		高分化胸腺癌	非典型性胸腺瘤*
胸腺癌	恶性胸腺瘤，II型	恶性胸腺瘤，II型（低级或高级）	胸腺癌

*这种类型还包括显示胸腺瘤和胸腺癌重叠特征的交界性病例。

区和髓质区组织学和免疫表型的相似之处，Muller-Hermelink 提出了胸腺瘤的"功能性"分类（表21C.5）[5,91-97]。这种分类评估了胸腺瘤形态学的重要性。尽管许多研究证实组织学类型与肿瘤分期和临床结果相关（表21C.6）[53,87,92,97-104]，但一些研究根据多因素分析未能发现这种分类具有任何预后意义，而显示有无浸润是唯一最重要的预后因素[19,105,106]。应用"高分化胸腺癌"这一术语命名胸腺瘤的一种亚型也会造成命名上的混淆；例如，为了研究胸腺癌，一般来说有些临床研究会将这一组肿瘤与真正的胸腺癌放在一起[107]。

胸腺上皮性肿瘤的Suster-Moran分类

Suster-Moran 分类方法简单地将胸腺上皮性肿瘤分为三类：胸腺瘤（高分化胸腺癌）、非典型性胸腺瘤（中分化胸腺癌）和胸腺癌（低分化胸腺癌），因为作者认为，对于进一步分型来说，胸腺瘤的形态学表现过于多样，具有异质性，其他分类方法在不同观察者之间的可重复性太差，各种组织学起源的假说也尚未被证实（表21C.5）[22,24,108-111]。

胸腺瘤的WHO分类

1999版和2004版的胸腺瘤WHO分类方法基本采用了公认的Muller-Hermelink胸腺瘤分类方法，只是用字母数字代替了诊断术语（表21C.1和21C.5）[10,13,112]。这种命名方法避免了引起争议的组织学发生的含义（皮质还是髓质）和令人误解的"高分化胸腺癌"这一术语。组织学亚型与肿瘤分期有关，多数A型和AB型胸腺瘤为I期或II期（91%~94%），而III期或IV期病例所占比例从B1型到B2型以至B3型胸腺瘤有所增加（表21C.6）[13,36,97-99,112]。不同的研究一致显示，B3型胸腺瘤侵袭性最强，疾病10年特异性生存率为62%（其他类型胸腺瘤生存率大于80%）[36]。

大体表现

胸腺瘤大小不同，从显微镜下可见到很大的（重达几千克）[113]。肿瘤呈圆形或卵圆形，被覆厚薄不等的纤维性包膜（图21C.8）。切面一般呈褐色鱼肉样分叶状结构，有纤维性间隔，虽然少数胸腺瘤可能缺少分叶状结构（图21C.9）[4]。囊肿、出血灶和钙化常见。浸润性胸腺瘤可见明显的纤维性包膜破坏或侵犯邻近结构和器

表21C.6　根据WHO/Muller-Hermelink分类方法分类的胸腺瘤的临床特征，以及与临床分期的相互关系
(data compiled from two series, including a total of 277 cases)[97-99]

组织学类型	平均或中位年龄（岁）	性别（男:女）	平均大小（cm）	Masaoka分期（占肿瘤的%）			
				I	II	III	IV
A型	64~65	1:1.7	6.8	65	35	0	0
AB型	57~62	1:1.25	7.2	70	30	0	0
B1型	45~50	1:2.2	10.1	53	34	13	0
B2型	49~50	1:1.2	6.4	28	33	34	6
B3型	50~57	1:1	8.3	0	19	62	19
胸腺癌	53	2.5:1	—	0	7	64	29

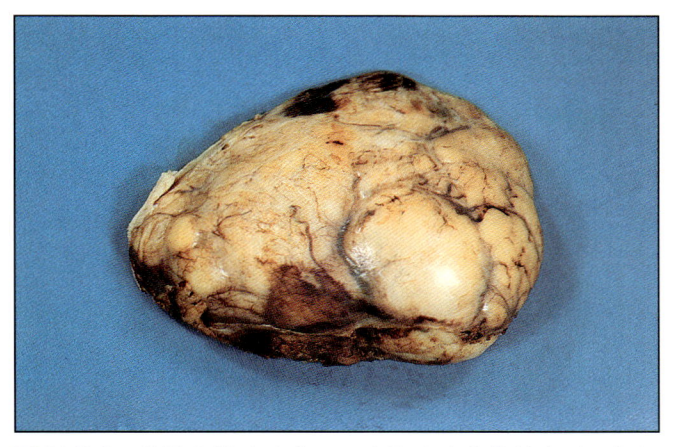

图21C.8 非浸润性胸腺瘤。切除的胸腺瘤的外表面一般呈现光滑的圆凸样外观。

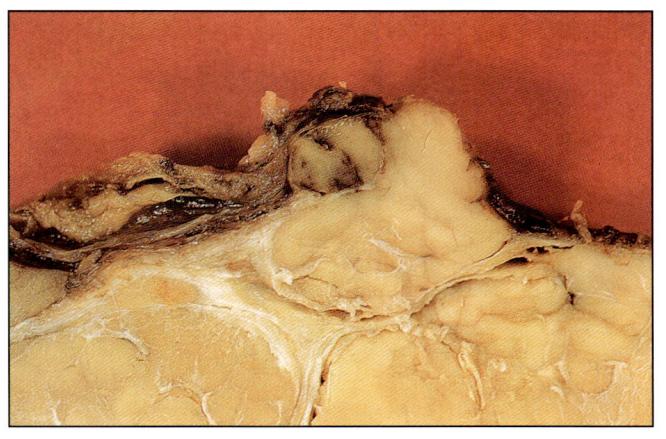

图21C.10 浸润性胸腺瘤。肿瘤主体由纤维性包膜围绕。浸润性肿瘤出芽穿破包膜,而且缺乏纤维性包裹。

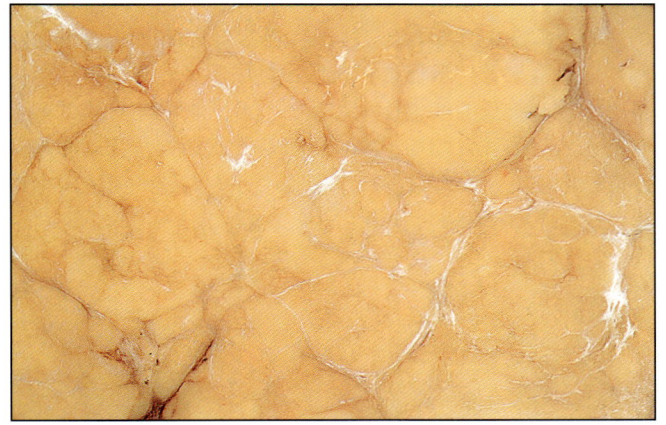

图21C.9 胸腺瘤。胸腺瘤的切面具有诊断性。大小不等的拼图样褐色肿瘤结节由白色纤维性间隔分开。

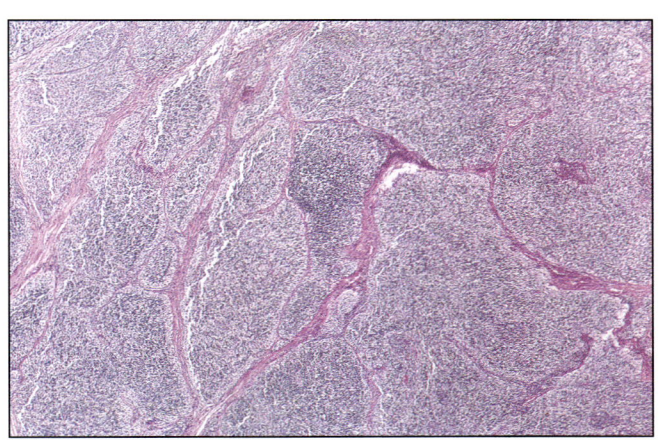

图21C.11 B2型胸腺瘤。拼图样小叶是胸腺瘤的特征性表现。在这个病例中,纤维性间隔相对较薄。许多小叶明显成角。

官(图21C.10)。

显微镜下表现

胸腺瘤低倍显微镜下最具特征性的表现是出现拼图样小叶(jigsaw puzzle-like lobules),被厚薄不均的无细胞纤维性条带所分隔(图21C.7和21C.11)。小叶大小不一,呈地图样,有一些经常明显成角。纤维性间隔可以发生局灶钙化。不同病例之间细胞组成和生长方式差异可能很大,甚至在同一肿瘤内不同小叶之间也有不同。本质上,增生的上皮成分是必需的。虽然常常含大量淋巴细胞,但是淋巴细胞也可以稀疏甚至缺失。

肿瘤性上皮成分:上皮细胞通常较大,表现为"合体状",呈卵圆形或多角形(图21C.12、21C.13和21C.14)。在深染的淋巴细胞中,上皮常常表现为浅染。其上皮本质可能难以辨认,除非在小叶边缘和血管周围间隙的周边出现上皮细胞团(图21C.15)。上皮细胞具有规则的圆形或卵圆形空泡状细胞核,核仁不明显或仅有小的核仁。个别细胞可以出现核的非典型性或多形性,但是核分裂象稀少。上皮细胞也可以呈梭形、细胞核变长、染色质致密、核仁不明显。

上皮细胞排列成片块状、簇状、假玫瑰花结样、相互吻合的网状或带状。梭形细胞常常排列呈束状、席纹状或呈血管外皮细胞瘤样生长。有时可见微囊性间隙、小圆形腺体、窄裂隙样腺腔、黏液腺、假乳头状结构以及发育不全的胸腺小体。在非常少见的情况下,肿瘤细胞间可见淀粉样物沉积[114]。

有助于诊断的特征是:出现大小不等的类似于正常胸腺内出现的血管周围间隙,其周围为肿瘤性上皮细胞,间隙内充满蛋白性液体,其中常常飘浮有小淋巴细胞和红细胞(图21C.15)。这些间隙可以发生玻璃样变纤维化。少数情况下,出现较多大的充满红细胞的囊性间隙,即所谓的胸腺紫癜(peliosis thymomis)[115]。

当胸腺瘤复发时,可以保留原来的组织学形态,或者

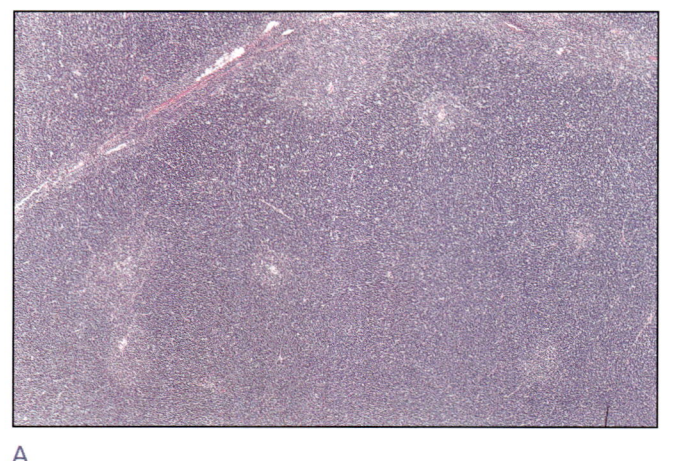

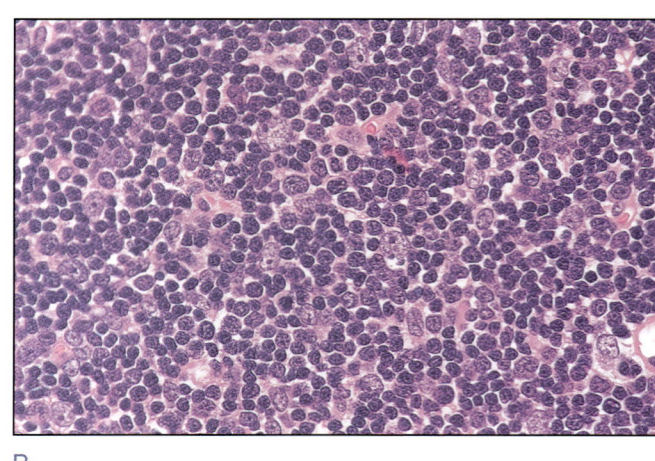

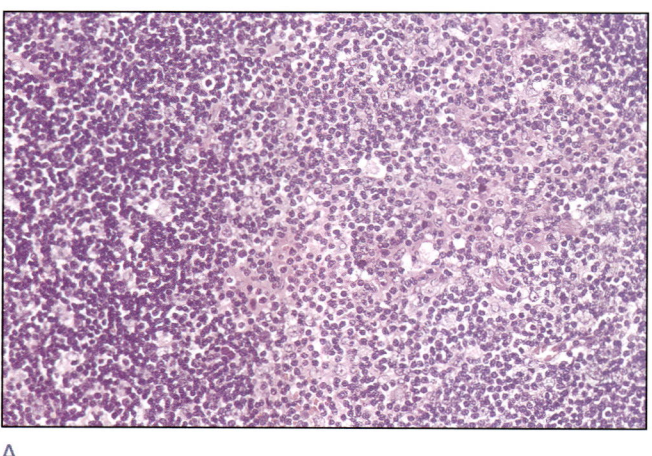

图21C.12　B1型胸腺瘤。在各种类型的胸腺瘤中，此类型具有最致密的淋巴细胞。（A）非常特征性的改变是出现散在的代表髓质分化的淡染灶。注意表面类似于B细胞慢性淋巴细胞性白血病累及的淋巴结，其特征是在深染的小淋巴细胞背景中散在有淡染的增生性中心区。（B）根据伴有淡染染色质和小核仁的较大的细胞核可以辨认上皮细胞。背景有大量小淋巴细胞。（C）血管周围间隙中心为血管，间隙内充满蛋白性液体和一些淋巴细胞。

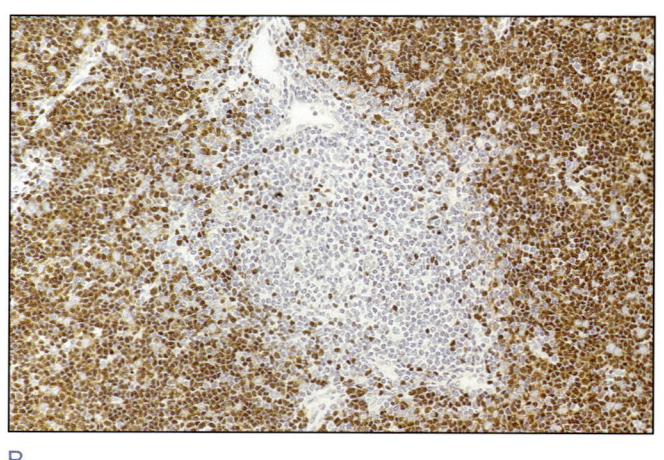

图21C.13　B1型胸腺瘤。显示髓质分化的细节。（A）髓质分化灶（视野右侧）淋巴细胞排列比较稀疏。（B）免疫组化染色显示灶内TdT阴性，与周围强阳性的淋巴细胞形成对比。注意非常类似于正常胸腺的结构。

可以从 B1 型进展为 B2 或 B3 型，或从 B2 型进展为 B3 型[116]。

反应性淋巴细胞成分：淋巴细胞通常较小、核圆形、染色质致密（图 21C.13A）。然而某些细胞可能有较大的细胞核，而且表现活跃。常常可见核分裂象。淋巴细胞通常与上皮细胞混合存在，但是可以彼此分开（图 21C.12 和 21C.14）。整个肿瘤中可见散在分布的可染小体巨噬细胞，呈现星空样外观。有时可见生发中心。在 B1 型胸腺瘤以及有时在 B2 型胸腺瘤，可见多发性界限清楚的非膨胀性淡染"髓质分化"区域，其中淋巴细胞排列比较松散，可能可见胸腺小体样结构，类似于正常胸腺的髓质部分（图 21C.12 和 21C.113）。

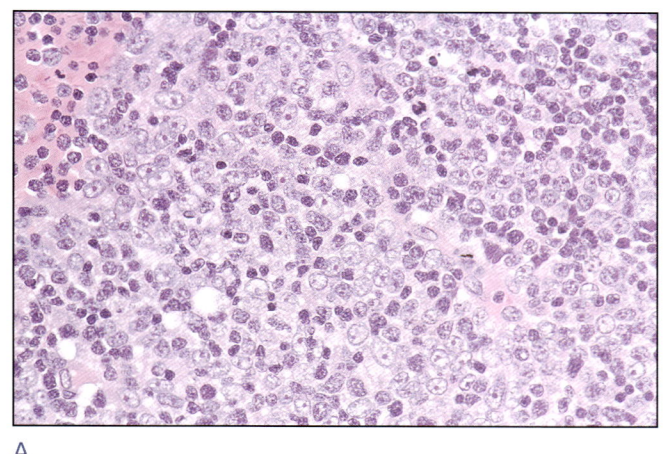
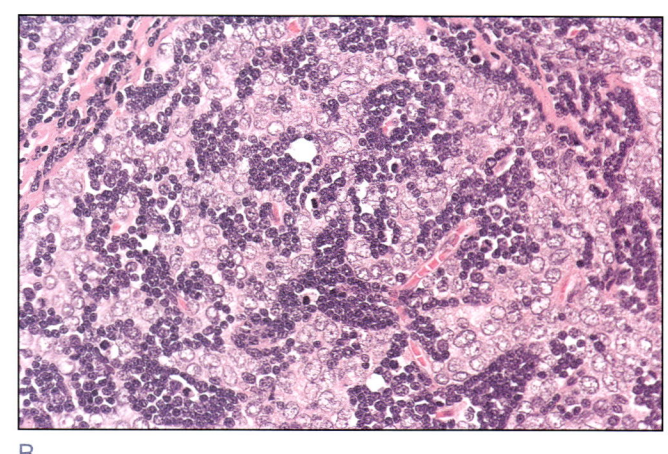

图21C.14 B2型胸腺瘤。(A)与B1型胸腺瘤相比,上皮细胞较为明显,伴有空泡状细胞核和清楚的核仁。淋巴细胞不丰富。(B)上皮细胞可形成散在的细胞巢,因此相对比较容易辨认这种肿瘤的上皮样性质。

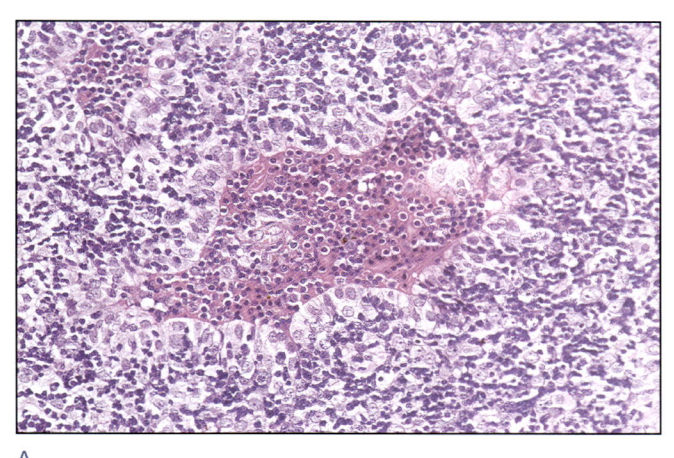
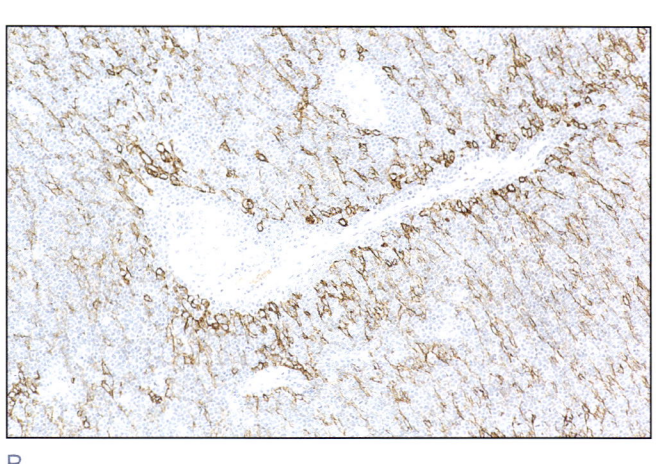

图21C.15 B2型胸腺瘤。(A)围绕血管周围间隙有栅栏状排列的上皮细胞,间隙内充满淋巴细胞。(B)免疫染色显示,血管周围间隙被细胞角蛋白阳性的上皮细胞围绕。注意非常类似于正常血管周围间隙,如图21C.2所示。

根据WHO分类的胸腺瘤类型

各种类型的胸腺瘤的发生率大致如下:A型10%、AB型28%、B1型15%、B2型28%以及B3型18%[36,112]。如出现两种不同类型的胸腺瘤特征的病例,则应分别估计每种成分所占的比例。

A型胸腺瘤:小叶常常较大,因此通过一张组织学切片检查可能很难辨认。上皮细胞常常呈梭形,排列成束状、席纹状或血管外皮细胞瘤样结构(图21C.16)。具有表现温和的细胞核,染色质致密,核仁不明显(图21C.16)。核分裂象缺乏或非常稀少。几乎所有的病例至少都有局灶性腺体分化,表现为分化好的腺体、发育不良的腺体或微囊,特别是在小叶的周围(图21C.17)。偶尔可见印戒细胞(图21C.18)[117]。有时形成假玫瑰花结结构(图21C.19)。血管周围间隙少见或发育不良。从未发现有胸腺小体或表皮样分化灶。在一些病例,肿瘤细胞为立方形而不是梭形,但是其细胞核仍然保留温和的外观(图21C.20)。淋巴细胞一般稀疏,其中多数为TdT染色阴性,即髓质胸腺细胞或成熟阶段的T细胞。

AB型胸腺瘤:小叶形态通常清楚。缺乏淋巴细胞成分的A型胸腺瘤与富含淋巴细胞成分的B型胸腺瘤混合存在,两种成分比例变化很大,在某些区域可能以一种类型为主,或表现为唯一的成分。两种成分可形成散在的独立小叶,或混合存在(图21C.21和21C.22)。

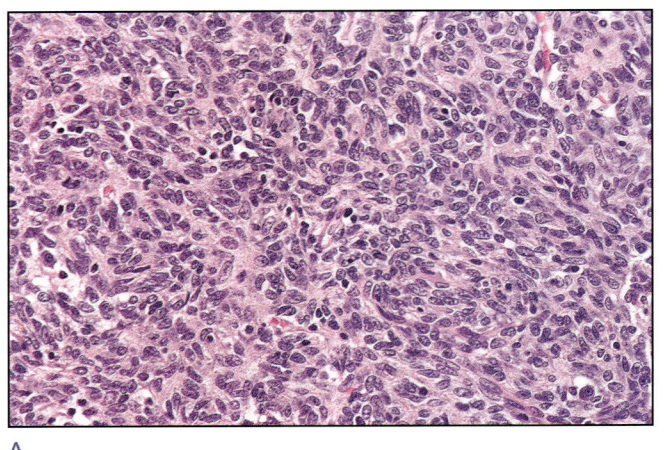
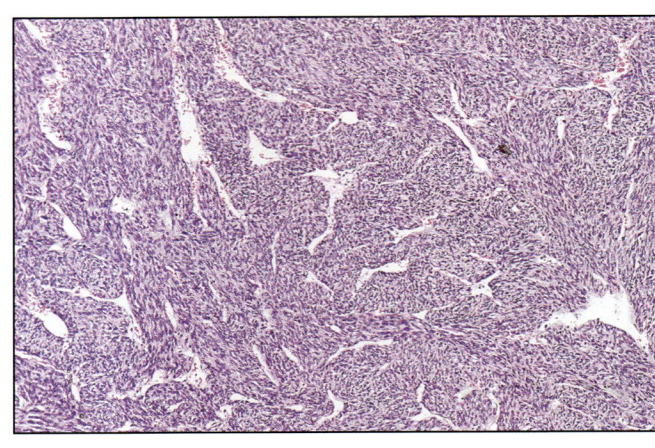

图21C.16 A型胸腺瘤。(A)梭形肿瘤细胞形成短束状或杂乱分布。这些细胞具有均匀一致的细长细胞核和致密的染色质。特征性表现是混有少量淋巴细胞。(B)梭形肿瘤细胞常常显示血管外皮细胞瘤的血管结构。

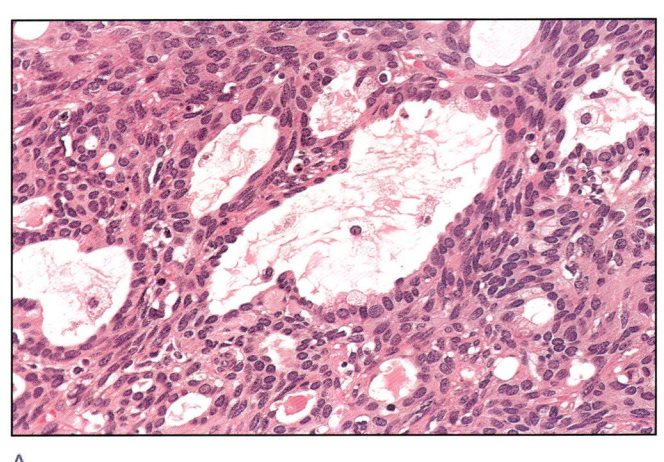
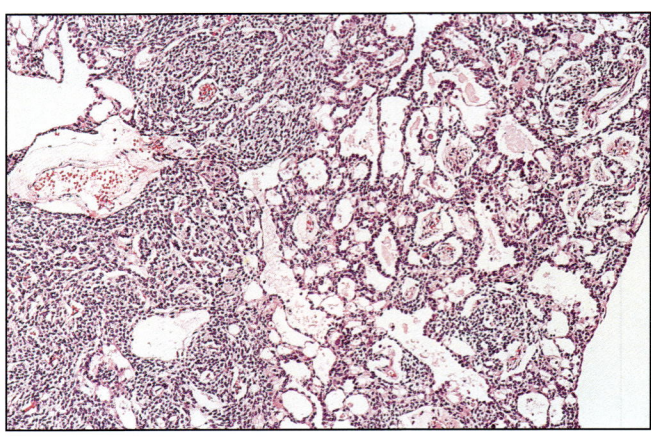

图21C.17 A型胸腺瘤。(A)散在于梭形细胞中的真正的腺体间隙,其中有些腺腔含有分泌物。注意腺体细胞染色质致密,核仁不明显,这正是A型胸腺瘤肿瘤细胞的特征。(B)本例显示微囊性和实性生长方式。那些腔隙并非真正的腺体结构,而是由间质水肿形成的。淋巴细胞稀少。

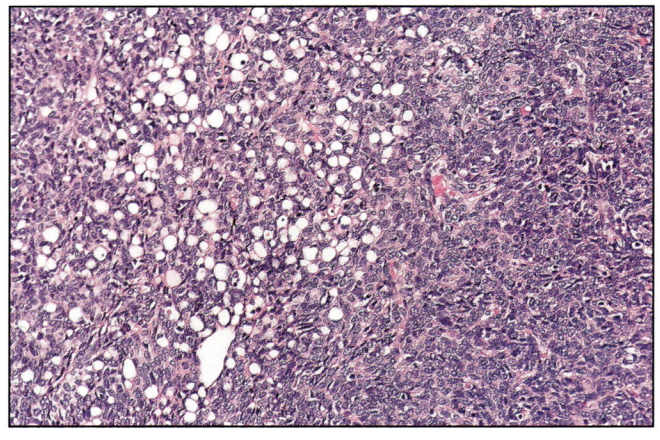
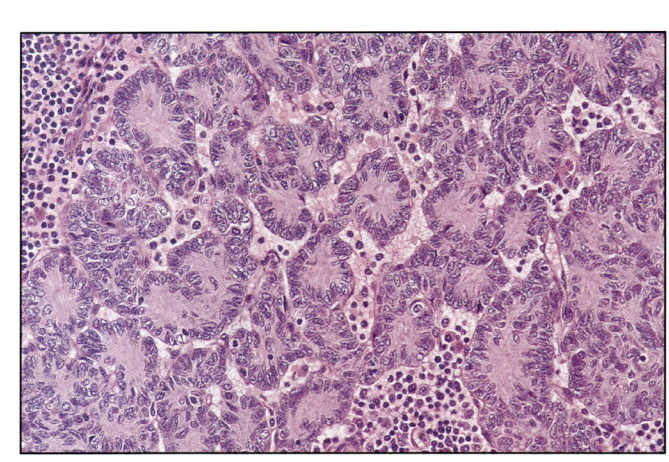

图21C.18 A型胸腺瘤。本例的梭形肿瘤细胞中散在许多印戒细胞,为腺体分化不良的表现(胞浆内腔)。

图21C.19 A型胸腺瘤。上皮细胞形成明显的假玫瑰花结结构。

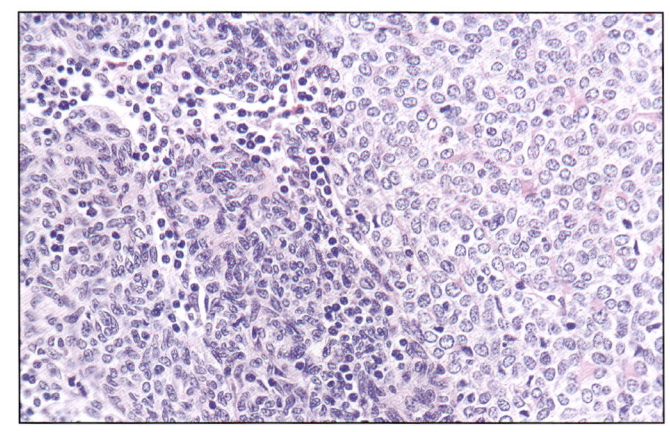

图21C.20 A型胸腺瘤。在一些病例中，肿瘤由均匀一致的具有淡染胞浆的立方形细胞构成（视野右侧）。注意其染色质形态类似于梭形细胞（视野左侧）。核仁不明显。

有时A型成分形成明显的"细胞间隔"，穿插于B型小叶之间（图21C.21B）。与B1型或B2型胸腺瘤相比，AB型胸腺瘤B型成分的肿瘤性上皮细胞常常具有较小的细胞核和不清楚的核仁。B型成分的淋巴细胞多为不成熟的T细胞（TdT阳性），而A型成分的淋巴细胞多为成熟的T细胞（TdT阴性）（图21C.23）。偶尔可以见到血管周围间隙。

B1型胸腺瘤：B1型胸腺瘤的细胞结构非常类似正常胸腺，因此也被称为"器官样胸腺瘤"（organoid thymoma）[118]。具有被硬化性间隔分开的发育良好的特征性小叶。上皮性成分相对不明显，表现为散在的卵圆形细胞，细胞核圆而淡染，伴有小的核仁，但是有些细胞可能为大而明显的核仁（图21C.12和21C.13）。上

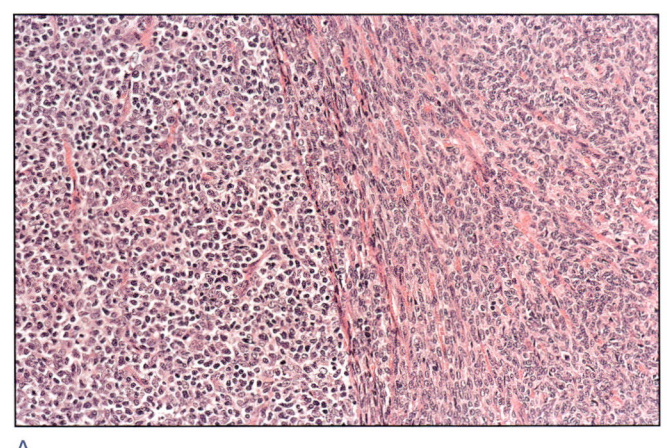

A

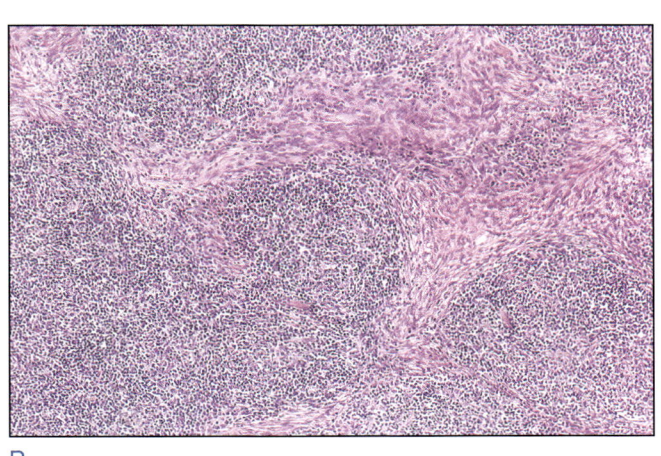

B

图21C.21 AB型胸腺瘤。（A）在本例中，两种成分是分开的，A型胸腺瘤小叶（右）与B型胸腺瘤小叶（左）明显并列存在。前者由梭形细胞构成，几乎无淋巴细胞，而后者由肥胖的卵圆形细胞构成，混合有大量淋巴细胞。（B）在本例中，富含淋巴细胞的B型胸腺瘤小叶与A型胸腺瘤紧密混合，后者形成富于细胞的间隔样结构。

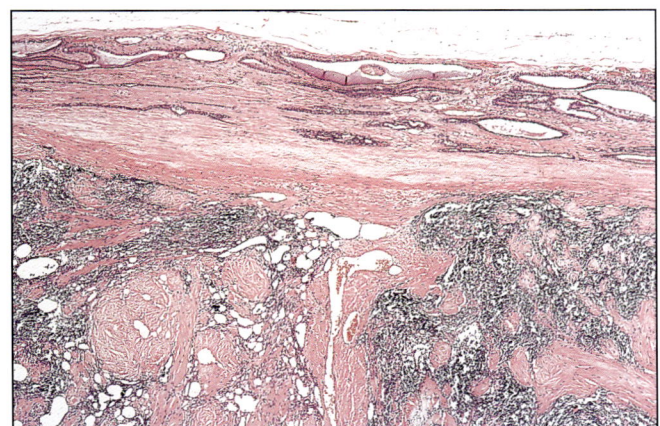

图21C.22 AB型胸腺瘤。深蓝色的成分是B型胸腺瘤。在肿瘤的外周部分和纤维性间隔内有内衬相对扁平细胞的狭窄管状腺体。腺体结构是A型胸腺瘤的特征，在单纯性B型胸腺瘤中没有腺体结构。

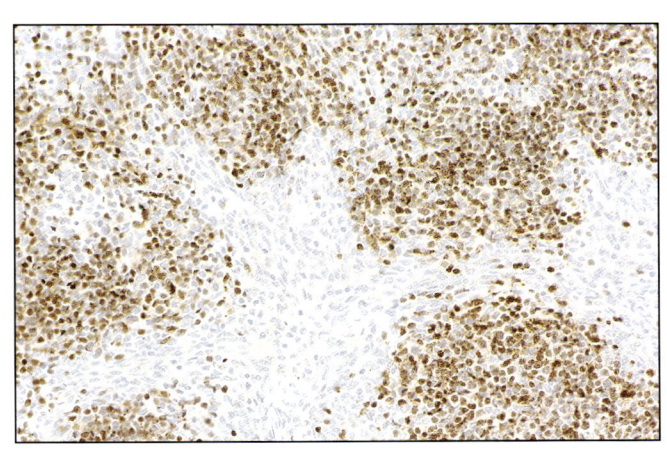

图21C.23 AB型胸腺瘤。TdT免疫染色显示，与B型成分相关的多数淋巴细胞呈阳性，而与A型成分相关的淋巴细胞则为阴性。

皮细胞并不形成细胞集聚或片块。在各种类型的胸腺瘤中，B1 型胸腺瘤具有最丰富的淋巴细胞成分。这些淋巴细胞主要是不成熟的 T 细胞（TdT 呈阳性）。通常有代表髓质分化的散在的淡染圆形灶，由较松散排列的具有较成熟表型的 T 淋巴细胞（TdT 呈阴性）组成（图21C.13）。可以见到散在的发育不好或发育良好的胸腺小体。常常出现血管周围间隙（图 21C.12C），但是比 B2 型或 B3 型胸腺瘤少见。这些间隙可扩张并充满淋巴细胞。

B2 型胸腺瘤：小叶结构常常明显。肿瘤细胞表现为单个或成簇排列的大卵圆形细胞，伴有空泡状核和明显的位于中心的核仁（图 21C.14）。这些细胞常常在血管周围间隙和纤维性间隔附近呈栅栏状排列（图 21C.15）。血管周围间隙常见且往往狭窄（图 21C.15）。淋巴细胞丰富，但是不如 B1 型胸腺瘤丰富。多数淋巴细胞为不成熟 T 细胞。髓质分化灶不明显或缺如。可以出现伴有生发中心的淋巴滤泡。约 20% 的病例有与 B3 型胸腺瘤相似的灶状富于上皮的区域，这样的病例被称为混合性 B2/B3 胸腺瘤（combined B2/B3 thymoma）（图21C.24）。

B3 型胸腺瘤：肿瘤是由多角形上皮细胞小叶构成的，小叶被增厚的硬化性间隔分开。上皮细胞常常显示鳞状上皮的特征，但是没有细胞间桥。细胞常常围绕血管周围间隙或沿着纤维性间隔呈显著的栅栏状排列（图21C.25 和 21C.26）。多数病例中，细胞具有"葡萄干样"细胞核，核仁不明显，胞浆嗜酸性或透明，类似于挖空细胞（图 21C.25A）。然而，在另外一些病例，细胞具有大的空泡状核和明显的核仁，类似于 B2 型胸腺瘤。

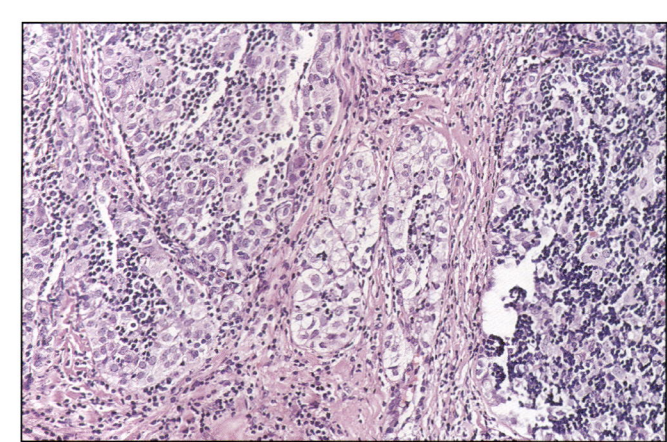

图21C.24　B2/B3 型胸腺瘤。本图显示从 B2 型胸腺瘤（视野右侧）向 B3 型胸腺瘤的过渡（视野左侧）。

核具有轻到中度非典型性，核分裂象常见。可出现局灶性角化。一些病例肿瘤细胞呈梭形，排列成束，与 A 型胸腺瘤的不同在于核具有非典型性（图 21C.27）。只有少量淋巴细胞，为不成熟的 T 细胞。血管周围间隙常常狭窄（图 21C.26）。含 B2 型胸腺瘤成分的病例并不少见。

微结节性胸腺瘤：在这种亚型的胸腺瘤中，有多发性小而分散的或融合性的表现温和的梭形上皮细胞结节，这些结节被伴有或不伴有明显生发中心的淋巴细胞所分隔（图 21C.28）[119-122]。常有多发散在的内衬上皮的囊性间腔。

淋巴成分的免疫组化分析显示：上皮结节周围或上皮结节内存在一些不成熟的 T 细胞（TdT⁺）。上皮结节之间的淋巴细胞主要是 B 细胞，混有一些成熟 T 细胞。细胞角蛋白染色可以明显将上皮与淋巴成分分开，淋巴细胞间质中没有细胞角蛋白阳性细胞出现（图 21A.29）。

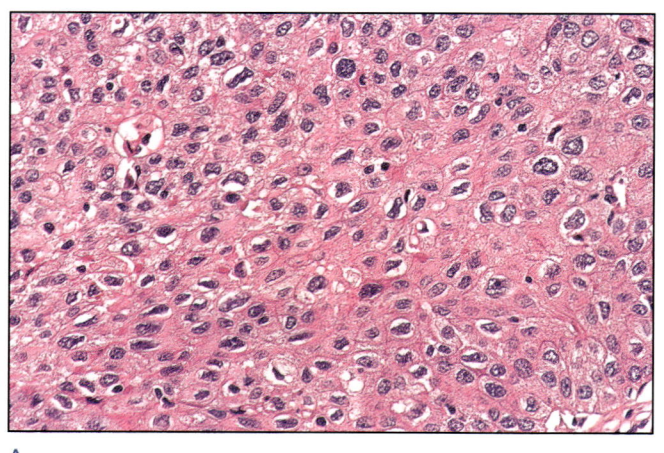

A

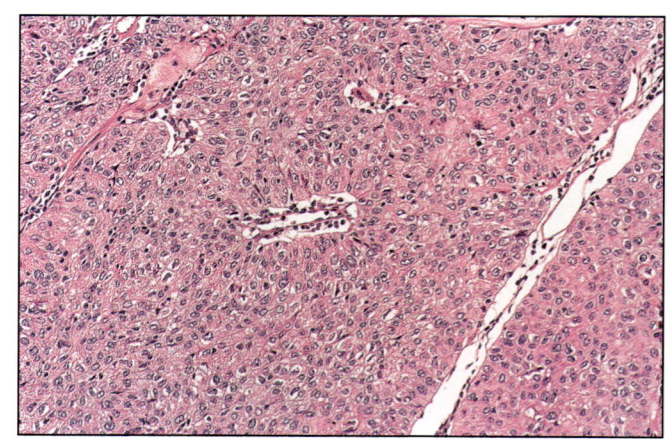

B

图21C.25　B3 型胸腺瘤。（A）多角形细胞具有卵圆形及不规则的细胞核和嗜酸性胞浆。注意由于出现核皱缩和核周胞浆透明，有些细胞类似于挖空细胞。（B）肿瘤由多角形上皮细胞小叶构成，并混有少量淋巴细胞。注意在视野中心的狭窄的血管周围间隙周围，有细胞呈栅栏状排列。

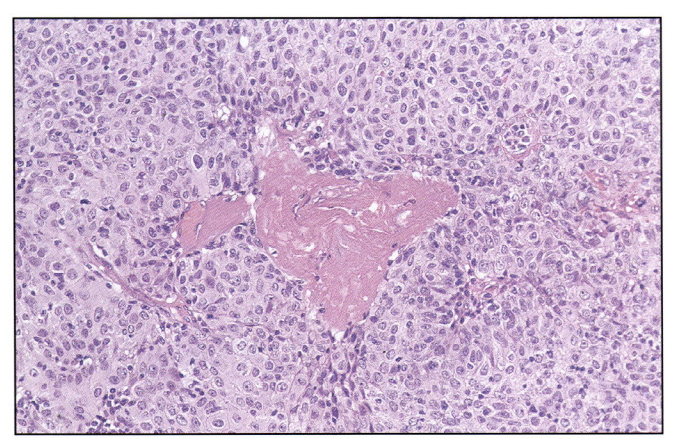

图21C.26 B3型胸腺瘤。胸腺瘤显示出鳞状特征。视野中心的血管周围间隙玻璃样变性。

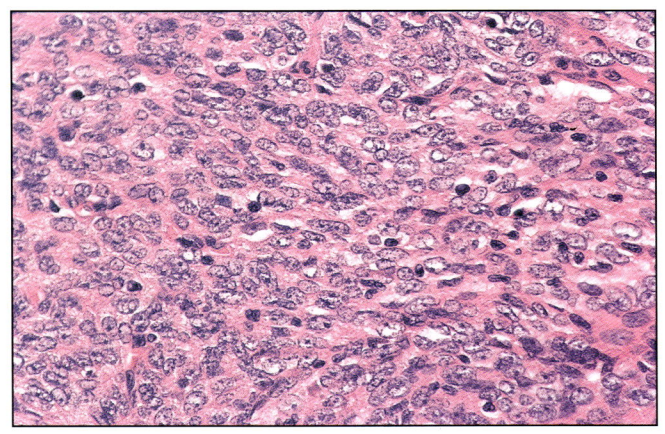

图21C.27 B3型胸腺瘤,梭形细胞型。这种类型不同于A型胸腺瘤,具有空泡状染色质和非典型性,并且缺乏均匀一致的细胞核。

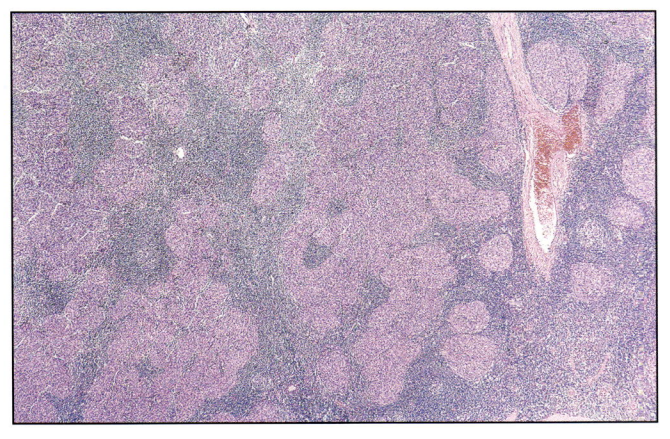

A

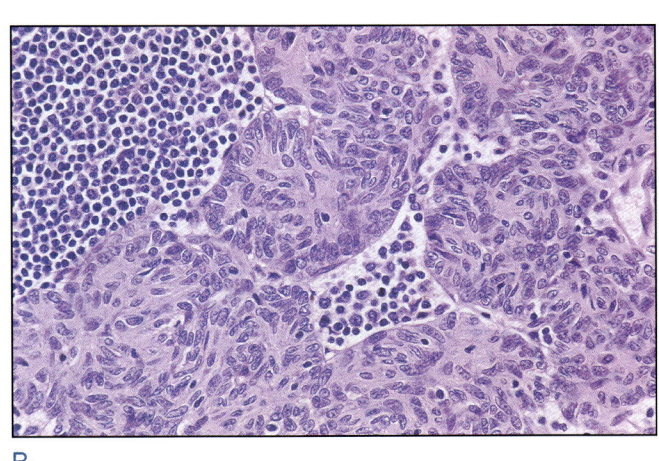

B

图21C.28 微结节性胸腺瘤。(A)多发性大小不一的融合性上皮细胞结节散布于成片的淋巴细胞中。(B)结节由表现温和的梭形细胞组成,并且与淋巴细胞间质分界清晰。

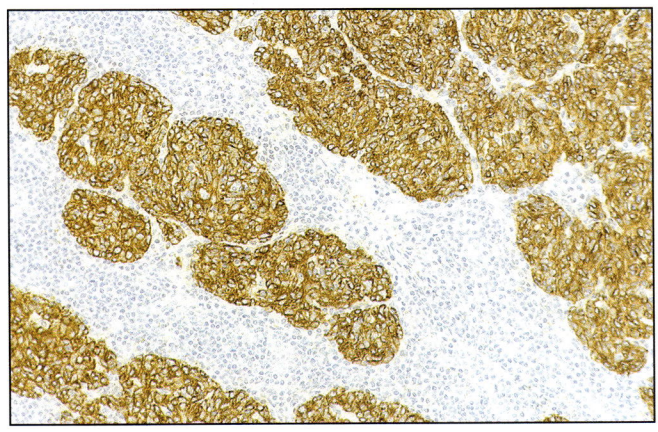

图21C.29 微结节性胸腺瘤。细胞角蛋白免疫染色显示上皮细胞结节。在淋巴细胞间质中没有发现上皮细胞,不同于B型和AB型胸腺瘤。

这种类型可能是A型胸腺瘤的少见形式,在一些病例中,微结节性胸腺瘤的特征可以见于普通胸腺瘤(最常见的是A型或AB型胸腺瘤)的一些小叶中。不伴有重症肌无力。约1/3的病例可能发现单克隆的B细胞群,其中半数显示有黏膜相关淋巴组织型肿瘤内结外边缘区B细胞淋巴瘤[120]。

化生性胸腺瘤:这种罕见类型的胸腺瘤在文献中已有报道,被称为"伴有假肉瘤性间质的胸腺瘤"(thymoma with pseudosarcomatous stroma)和"低级别化生性癌"(low-grade metaplastic carcinoma)[95,123]。患者多为成人,以男性为主。多数患者无症状,且常处于早期阶段(I期75%,II期17%)。患者均无重症肌无力表现[124]。随访的11名患者中,10名患者生存良好,1名患者在14个月时局部复发,6年时死亡[124]。

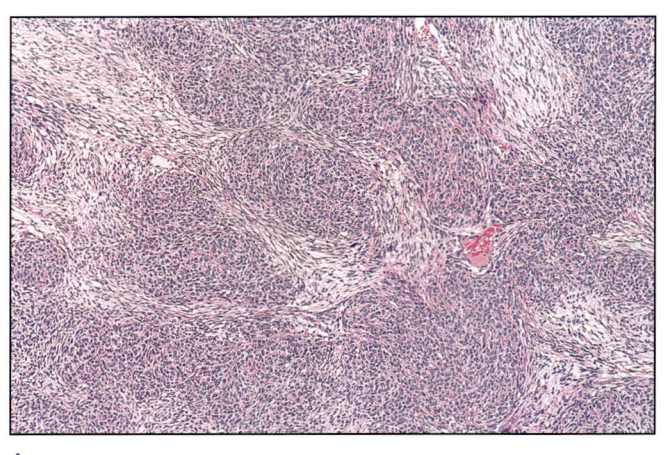 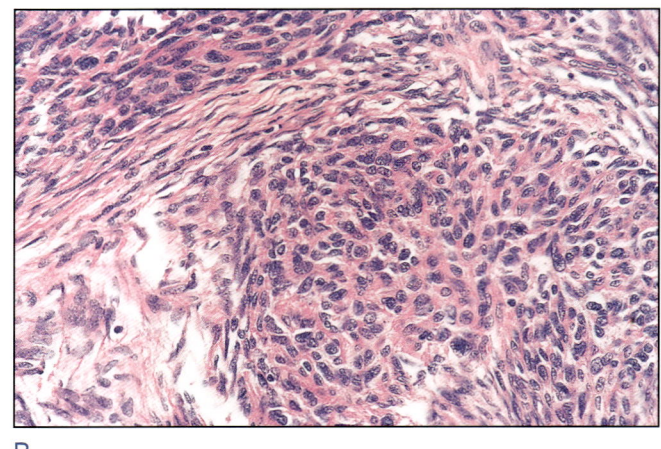

图21C.30　化生性胸腺瘤。（A）肿瘤具有双相性生长方式，由梭形细胞将卵圆形或多角形细胞分隔成细胞岛。（B）卵圆形细胞具有轻度核非典型性，可能含有散在的多形性细胞核，但是梭形细胞总是呈温和表现。

肿瘤有包膜，但是缺少普通胸腺瘤的特征性小叶结构。组织学上，相互吻合的卵圆形或多角形上皮细胞岛和小梁与相互缠绕的纤细的梭形细胞束形成双相性结构（图21C.30A）。上皮细胞常常显示鳞状特征，具有卵圆形空泡状细胞核、小而明显的核仁以及中等量的嗜酸性胞浆。尽管可能显示局灶性核的多形性，但是核分裂活性非常低（图21C.30B）。这些上皮细胞岛可以被胶原纤维细支分隔。上皮细胞细胞角蛋白和上皮膜抗原免疫反应呈阳性。梭形细胞呈温和表现，显示短束状或席纹状生长方式。从局部来看，梭形细胞可与上皮细胞逐渐融合或以梭形细胞为主。梭形细胞的细胞角蛋白和上皮膜抗原免疫染色呈局灶弱阳性或阴性反应，而vimentin呈阳性反应。Actin表达不一致。淋巴细胞稀少。分子生物学研究显示几乎不存在遗传学改变，提示这种肿瘤与A型或AB型胸腺瘤的关系比与胸腺癌或B3型胸腺瘤的关系更密切[124]。

梭形细胞成分很可能是肿瘤性成分（化生性改变）而不是活跃的间质反应。最重要的是要避免把化生性胸腺瘤误诊为侵袭性强的癌肉瘤（见1332页）。

形态学变异或少见的改变

继发性改变：有些胸腺瘤显示继发性改变，如累及单个肿瘤小叶或整个肿瘤的出血或梗死[125]。这种改变并不具有预后意义[125]。在罕见情况下，胸腺瘤可以发生退行性变，仅在显微镜下可见被硬化带包绕的残留的肿瘤灶（所谓的硬化性或陈旧性胸腺瘤，sclerosing or ancient thymoma）[126,127]。

囊性胸腺瘤：囊性改变有时可能非常明显，以至于胸腺瘤被误诊为胸腺囊肿[128]。大体上，病变由多发性大囊腔构成，其内充满透明、血性或黏稠的物质。组织学上，囊壁内可见残留的具有胸腺瘤组织学特征的实性细胞巢。与非肿瘤性胸腺囊肿不同，囊壁一般没有内衬上皮；多数囊腔显然是来自高度扩张和相互融合的血管周围间隙。在某些情况下，非肿瘤性胸腺组织周边发生炎症性的囊性改变，以致粘连并明显浸润邻近的纵隔结构。

类固醇治疗的影响：切除肿瘤之前接受过皮质类固醇治疗的患者，胸腺瘤可能显示未成熟淋巴细胞数量显著减少，导致上皮成分相对为主，因此B1型或B2型胸腺瘤有可能被误诊为B3型胸腺瘤。辨认类固醇影响的线索是：在上皮细胞中间出现小的空"晕"，这些空晕是淋巴细胞消失后留下的间隙；残留的淋巴细胞常常固缩，而且可能伴有组织细胞和泡沫细胞数量增加（图21C.31）[92,129]。

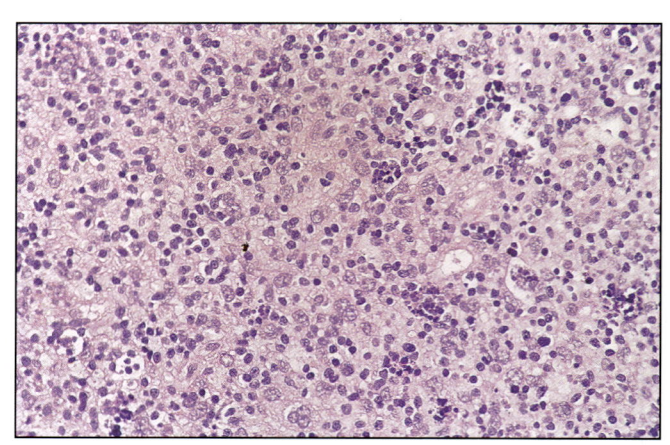

图21C.31　B1型胸腺瘤伴类固醇效应。经过皮质类固醇激素治疗后切除的胸腺瘤，典型地表现为淋巴细胞减少，导致上皮成分相对明显，类似于B2型或B3型胸腺瘤。存在典型的小空泡状空隙和残存的凋亡淋巴细胞。

富于浆细胞型胸腺瘤：少数胸腺瘤具有明显的浆细胞成分[130]。

透明细胞胸腺瘤：少数胸腺瘤（通常为B3或B2型胸腺瘤）可能显示为含大量糖原的透明细胞。因此，在胸腺上皮性肿瘤中出现透明细胞并不说明可以诊断为透明细胞癌（图21C.32）[109]。

横纹肌瘤性亚型：有时可以发现骨骼肌细胞[131]，偶尔可能非常多，以致有理由应用"横纹肌瘤性胸腺瘤"（rhabdomyomatous thymoma）这一术语[132]。

微小胸腺瘤、显微镜下胸腺瘤和结节性增生："显微镜下胸腺瘤"（microscopic thymoma）用来指在胸腺中偶然发现的散在的细小上皮岛[1]，其发生率在重症肌无力患者为15%，而在尸检标本为4%[113,133,134]。这种病变可以是孤立性的也可以是多发性，位于皮质或髓质，大小从0.2~0.4 mm不等。组织学上，病变是由界限清楚但无包膜的上皮细胞岛构成，形成实性细胞巢、玫瑰花结或小管状结构，典型者几乎不混有淋巴细胞。这种类型已被收入最新一版的WHO胸腺肿瘤分类中，而且后者还规定肿瘤大小上限为1mm[135]。然而，显微镜下胸腺瘤缺少器官型结构和膨胀性生长，在形态学上明显不同于普通胸腺瘤。它是否为早期胸腺瘤或胸腺瘤的前体病变尚未得到证实，类似的病变可能见于胸腺的各种生理性、非肿瘤性病变，如退化的胸腺和涉及T细胞的各种先天性免疫缺陷性疾病。因此，最好将所谓的显微镜下胸腺瘤重新命名为胸腺上皮结节性增生（nodular hyperplasia of thymic epithelium）[136,137]。

另一方面，微小胸腺瘤（microthymoma）是一种小型的胸腺瘤，除了大小小于1cm以外，它与普通胸腺瘤的组织学特征完全相同[137]。尽管肿瘤较小，也可出现瘤外综合征。微小胸腺瘤可累及没有纤维包膜的胸腺单个小叶，提示可能是胸腺瘤形态演变中最早可辨认的改变。

胸腺瘤浸润的组织学评估

评估胸腺瘤是否存在浸润非常重要。一项研究发现，在有显微镜下浸润并仅仅接受手术治疗的9例胸腺瘤患者中，4例出现术后复发[19]。在处理切除标本时，切缘应用墨水标记，并且充分取材非常重要。我们建议按肿瘤最大径至少每个厘米取一块，最好取两块组织，并应包括肿瘤包膜部位。

明显的浸润应该容易辨认，因为肿瘤可侵犯周围的解剖学结构（图21C.7）。显微镜下浸润的标准是肿瘤完全穿透包膜（图21C.33）[19,59]。如果肿瘤穿透包膜形成蘑菇状结构，则容易辨认（图21C.33A）。然而，当肿瘤以推进的方式浸润时，评估就比较困难。如果肿瘤周

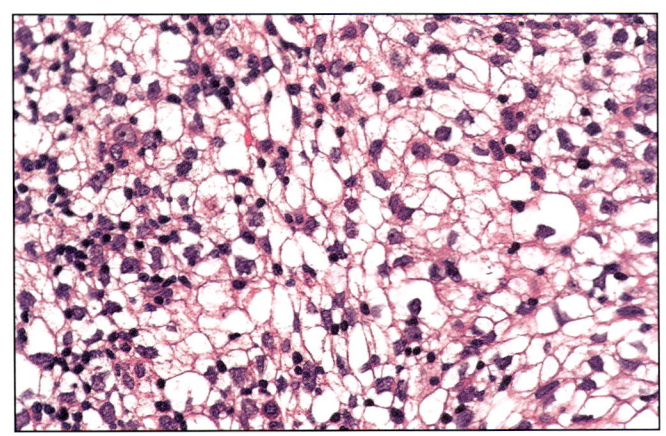

图21C.32 伴有透明细胞的B2型胸腺瘤。透明细胞有时可能出现在胸腺瘤中，并不一定是诊断透明细胞癌的证件。这些细胞富含糖原。

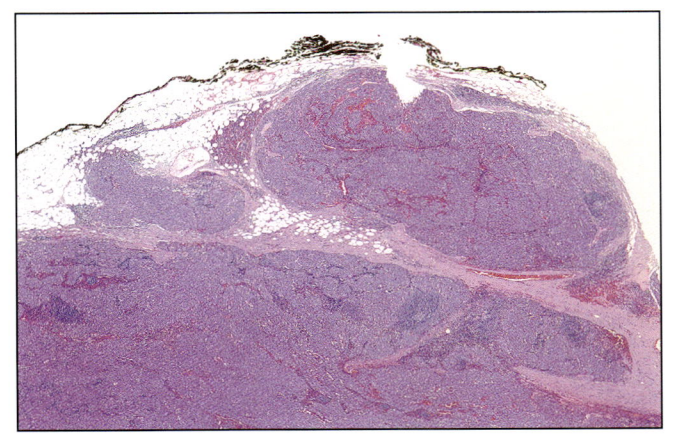

A

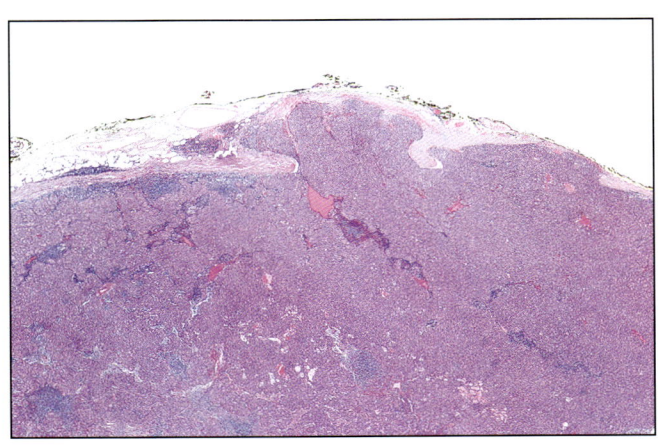

B

图21C.33 胸腺瘤：评估浸润。（A）蘑菇形出芽推挤穿过纤维性厚包膜进入周围脂肪组织，虽然芽外部仍然被覆一层纤维组织，但是显然已经扩展到肿瘤外面。（B）肿瘤周围部分的两个小叶没有纤维性间质，裸露于脂肪组织中，因此为浸润性生芽。

围部分的肿瘤小叶没有纤维性包膜包裹，与邻近的解剖学结构直接相连而无插入的纤维性包膜，或裸露于脂肪组织，可以推测有浸润（图21C.33B）。有时胸腺瘤与纵隔周围的结构粘连而没有真正的浸润；胸腺瘤与邻近的解剖学结构之间存在无细胞性纤维性间质支持这种表现。

免疫细胞化学

上皮成分：胸腺瘤的上皮成分表达细胞角蛋白和上皮膜抗原，并不同程度地表达CD57[19,89,138-140]。当细胞角蛋白免疫染色显示上皮细胞时，表现为伴有指突状细胞突起的复杂网状结构（B1型胸腺瘤、B2型胸腺瘤以及AB型胸腺瘤中的B型成分），或者表现为散在的多角形细胞（B3型胸腺瘤）及梭形细胞（A型胸腺瘤）（图21C.34）。在A型胸腺瘤中，散在的腺体结构细胞角蛋白染色阳性程度明显比梭形肿瘤细胞的强。不同的细胞角蛋白亚型在不同类型的胸腺瘤中表达具有差异[141]。

令人惊奇的发现是，某些胸腺瘤的肿瘤性上皮细胞可以表达B细胞标记物CD20，这种现象几乎都发生在A型胸腺瘤或AB型胸腺瘤（图21C.35）[142]。与胸腺癌不同，胸腺瘤的上皮细胞不表达CD5和CD117。

淋巴成分：淋巴成分主要是由不成熟T淋巴细胞构成，基因型研究显示：这些细胞是非克隆性的[143]。T淋巴细胞通常显示皮质胸腺细胞表型：TdT+、CD1a+和CD99a+（图21C.13B、21C.23和21C.35）[6,89,144-147]。在"髓质分化"区域，血管周围间隙或与A型胸腺瘤相关的淋巴细胞通常比较成熟，显示晚期（髓质）胸腺细胞表型：TdT−、表面CD3+、CD1−和CD99a−（图21C.13B）[6,148,149]。Ki67染色呈阳性说明淋巴细胞增殖指数高。通常出现少量B细胞，主要见于髓质分化区域和淋巴滤泡内[92,140,150,151]。

即使在转移性胸腺瘤或异位胸腺瘤，伴随的淋巴细胞也显示为不成熟的T细胞表型[149,152-154]，提示肿瘤性胸腺上皮与胸腺细胞之间有密切的关系和相互作用。

电子显微镜检查

胸腺瘤的肿瘤细胞具有较多长的指状细胞突起，突起间通过桥粒连接。细胞浆内常有突出的张力丝。

遗传学特征

A型胸腺瘤几乎无遗传学改变，经常发生的改变是6号染色体短臂缺失[112,156-159]。B3型胸腺瘤常常显示染色体失衡，最常见的改变是+1q、−6和−13q[156,158,159]。B2型胸腺瘤遗传学改变与B3型胸腺瘤相关[159]。

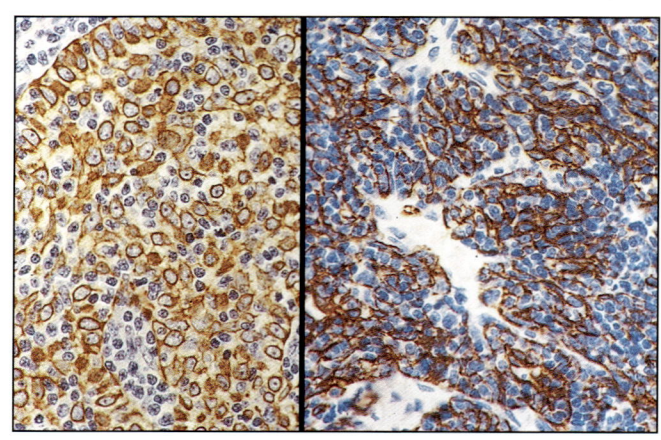

图21C.34 胸腺瘤的细胞角蛋白免疫组化染色。左：某些病例上皮细胞呈卵圆形，伴有少量纤细的胞浆突起。右：某些病例，尤其是B1型胸腺瘤，可见显著的树突状染色结构。核周几乎没有胞浆，但有明显的相互吻合的胞浆突起。

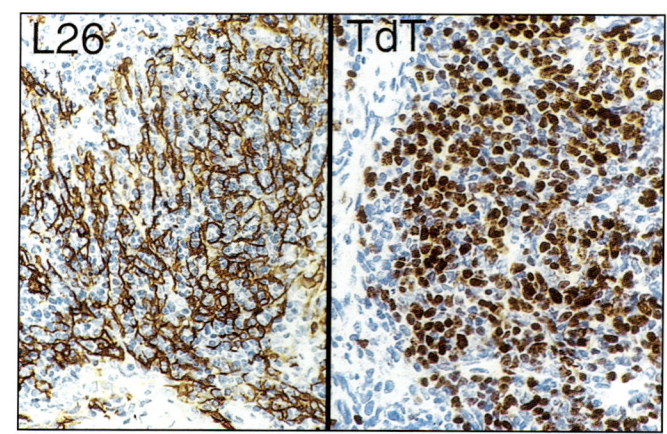

图21C.35 胸腺瘤免疫组化染色。左：某些A型胸腺瘤病例的梭形上皮细胞显示CD20阳性。右：伴随胸腺瘤的淋巴细胞一般为不成熟T细胞，TdT免疫染色可以证实。

预后因素

- 肿瘤分期是最有意义的预后因素[35,55-57,64,75,76,104-106,160,161]。10年生存率从非浸润性肿瘤的80%下降到浸润性肿瘤的35%。
- 完整切除[28,30,35,55,56,75,104]。完整切除与不完全切除或活检病例的10年实际生存率分别为76%和28%。Regnard等[35]发现，在多变量分析中这是唯一的预后因素。
- 组织学类型。许多研究显示WHO/Muller-Hermelink分类具有预后意义[36,55,56,75,97,99,101,104,160-162]。
- 大小。多变量分析显示肿瘤大于11cm是预后不好的因素[28,75]。

- 体力状态。多变量分析显示对于总的生存率来说，体力状态不好是不利的预后因素[76]。

鉴别诊断

主要鉴别诊断包括类癌、Hodgkin 淋巴瘤、淋巴母细胞性淋巴瘤和胸腺癌（见表21C.2）。如果胸腺上皮性肿瘤显示任何明显程度的鳞状分化，则应高度怀疑鳞状细胞癌。另一方面，在各种非上皮性胸腺肿瘤中发现残留的胸腺上皮细胞，可能与胸腺瘤混淆，但是通过其片块状分布可以进行鉴别。A 型胸腺瘤还应与各种间叶性肿瘤鉴别。

胸腺癌　Thymic carcinoma

定义

胸腺癌（曾被称为"C 型胸腺瘤"）是胸腺原发性上皮性肿瘤，具有明显恶性的细胞学特征并缺少器官型特征[10,13,20,25,112]。形态学上类似于其他器官发生的普通癌。

临床特征

胸腺癌大约占所有原发性胸腺上皮性肿瘤的15%[36]。大部分发生于成人，平均发病年龄为50岁，男性略多于女性[4,20,21,163-167]。虽然有些患者无症状，但多数患者表现为与纵隔肿块相关的症状[164,168]。肿瘤通常发生明显浸润（图 21C.36），相当一部分病例不能切除。除了少数由先前存在的胸腺瘤发展而来的病例外，胸腺癌不伴有重症肌无力或其他瘤外综合征。在非常罕见的情况下，鳞状细胞癌可能伴有瘤外高钙血症[169,170]。

临床行为和治疗

胸腺癌是浸润性肿瘤并常常发生局部淋巴结和远处转移，尤其是骨、肺和肝[20,21,164,165,168,171]。局部复发常见（>50%）[107,165,171]。需要多种方法联合治疗，包括手术切除、术后放疗和（或）化疗[2,77a,172-174]。低级别胸腺癌（高分化鳞状细胞癌、高分化黏液表皮样癌和基底细胞样癌）的 5 年和 10 年生存率分别为83%和67%。高级别胸腺癌（除上述三种胸腺癌之外）的 5 年和 10 年生存率分别为18%和15%[165]。然而，回顾性研究发现，许多包括在低级别组中的肿瘤现在可被重新归为 B3 型胸腺瘤或非典型性胸腺瘤。因此，按照目前的诊断标准确定为胸腺癌的多数肿瘤很可能是高级别的肿瘤[21]。

显微显微镜下表现

胸腺癌经常表现为广泛的周围组织浸润（图 21C.36）。细胞学非典型性明显，常见坏死区域。

鳞状细胞癌（表皮样癌，角化性或非角化性）：鳞状细胞癌是胸腺癌中最常见的类型，可能与肺鳞状细胞癌侵犯或转移到纵隔难以鉴别[5,10,20,21,164,165,168,175-179]。鉴别两者非常重要，因为胸腺鳞状细胞癌预后较好（生

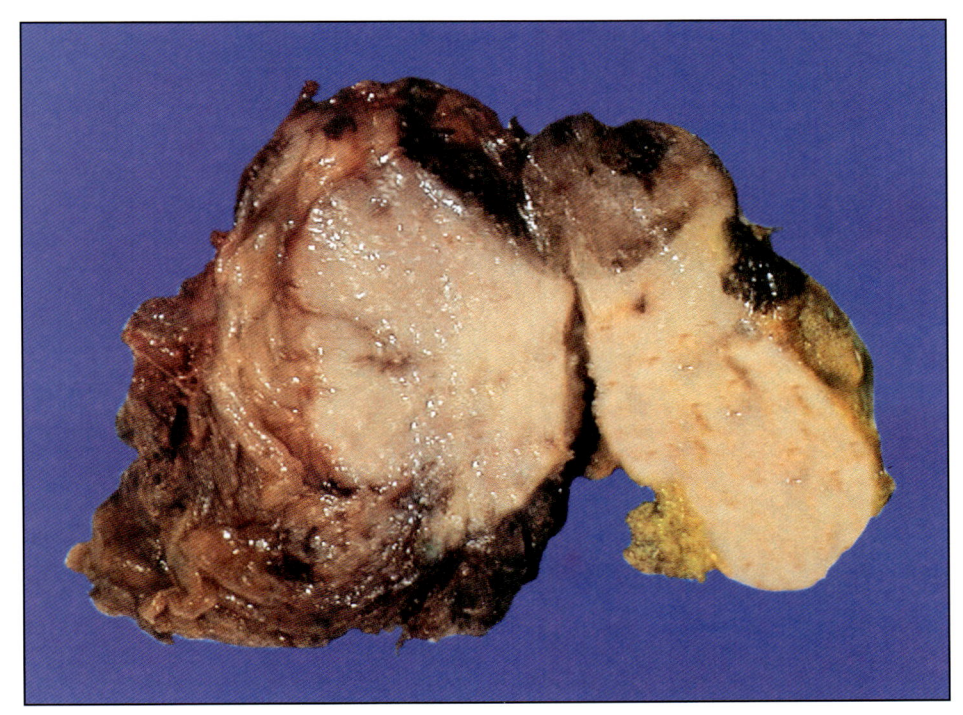

图21C.36　胸腺癌。肿瘤切面呈褐色鱼肉样。具有浸润性且缺少胸腺瘤的小叶状结构，右下方黄色是染料染色的切缘。

存率＞50%）[176]。支持胸腺鳞状细胞癌诊断的组织学特征是小叶状生长方式、玻璃样变的间质和空泡状核（图21C.37A）[180]。肿瘤小叶或肿瘤岛被有不同程度炎细胞浸润的纤维胶原性间质明显分隔（图21C.37B）。肿瘤岛常常有纤细的血管穿过。分化程度从好到差不等。在分化较好的肿瘤常有明显的角化和细胞间桥（图21C.38）。曾报道一例伴有显著的囊性改变，与胸腺囊肿相似[181]。

淋巴上皮瘤样癌：淋巴上皮瘤样癌在组织学上与鼻咽癌相同。肿瘤细胞岛和肿瘤细胞片块混有小淋巴细胞和浆细胞[20,46,50,168,175,182-184]。肿瘤细胞界限不清楚，核呈空泡状，核仁明显（图21C.39）。可有局灶性鳞状分化。

淋巴上皮瘤样癌最常发生于男性，年龄呈双峰分布，高峰在14岁和48岁。不管种族背景如何，约50%的病例与EB病毒感染有关（儿童和年轻人EB病毒常常呈阳性，而年龄超过30岁的患者不常呈阳性）[46,48,182,183,185,186]。

肉瘤样癌、癌肉瘤和梭形细胞胸腺癌：肉瘤样癌或癌肉瘤被定义为部分或全部肿瘤类似于软组织肉瘤的胸腺癌[10,165,175,177,187-189]。肿瘤可以完全是肉瘤样，也可能有明显的癌灶（癌肉瘤）。肉瘤样成分细胞角蛋白阴性或不同程度阳性[167,190]。有时可见骨骼肌或软骨分化[177,187,191]。

梭形细胞胸腺癌的特征是不同程度非典型性的梭形细胞排列成束或片状，某些区域出现大而深染的细胞核和明显的核仁，核分裂象常见[192]。梭形细胞细胞角蛋白染色弥漫强阳性。75%的病例与梭形细胞胸腺瘤有交叉，12%的病例混有癌的成分。肿瘤具有侵袭性，50%

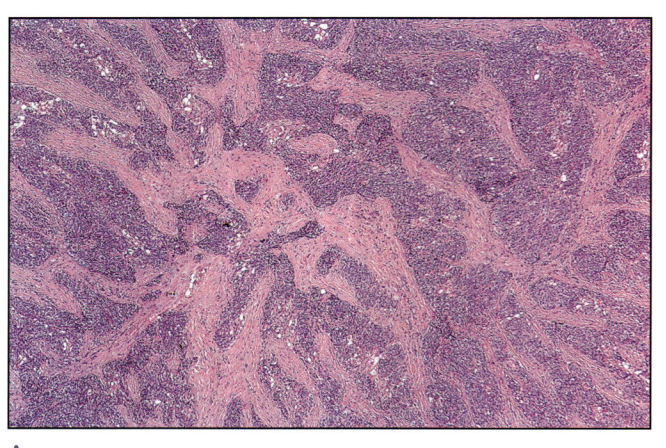

A

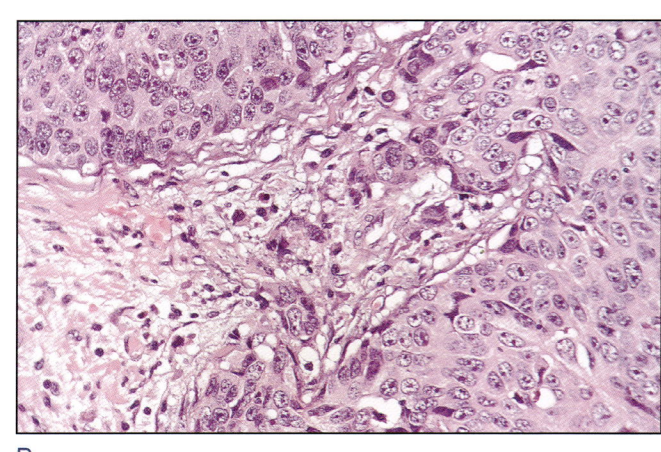

B

图21C.37 胸腺鳞状细胞癌，低分化。（A）不规则的肿瘤细胞岛浸润纤维组织增生性间质，但仍然具有一些模糊的类似于胸腺瘤的小叶结构。（B）肿瘤细胞岛由具有多形性细胞核的细胞构成。间质为纤维组织增生，并常有浆细胞浸润。

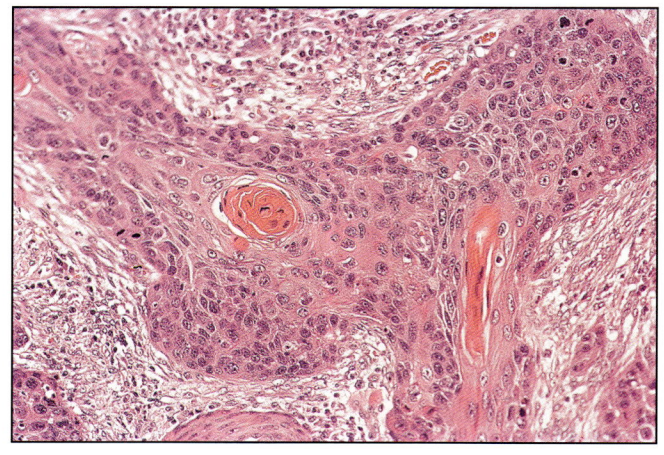

图21C.38 胸腺鳞状细胞癌，高分化。本例显示角化。注意纤维组织增生性间质伴有淋巴细胞和浆细胞浸润。

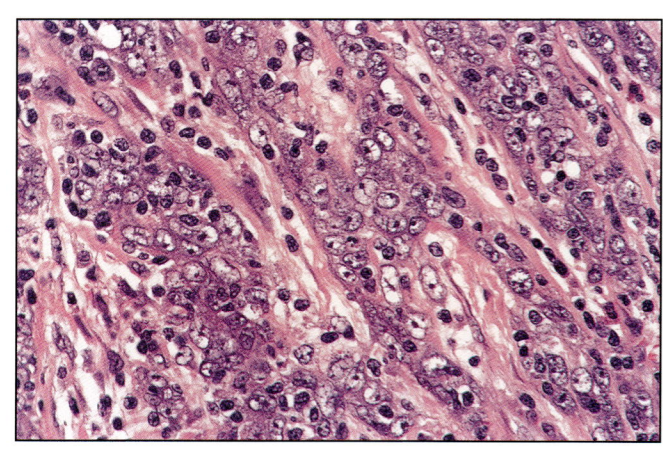

图21C.39 胸腺淋巴上皮样癌。不规则的合体细胞表现的肿瘤细胞岛具有空泡状细胞核和清楚的核仁。混有淋巴细胞。本例EB病毒阳性。

的患者在诊断之后 2～5 年间死亡。

黏液表皮样癌：胸腺黏液表皮样癌类似于涎腺黏液表皮样癌[164,165,168,177,193-195]。大体上，肿瘤为实性，伴有灶状黏液样改变，伴有或不伴有多发性散在的囊肿[193]。肿瘤由表皮样细胞岛构成，含散在分泌黏液的细胞和含有黏液的腔隙。可见局灶性单个细胞角化和细胞间桥。常有被炎症细胞浸润的硬化性间质。在某些病例中，肿瘤的发生似乎与多房性囊肿内衬上皮密切相关。低级别肿瘤比高级别肿瘤常见[194]。在前者，细胞多形性不明显、核分裂象罕见、预后好；在后者，核的非典型性明显、核分裂象常见，并且有坏死；多数患者死于后者（图21C.40）[194]。总之，预后不好与肿瘤级别高或肿瘤分期高有关[194]。

基底细胞样癌：基底细胞样癌的特征是小的基底样细胞排列成片块状、巢状和小梁状，周围呈栅栏状排列，常见核分裂象。常见囊性退变，囊壁内衬肿瘤细胞（图21C.41）。在罕见的情况下，细胞巢的中心可以出现灶状角化[5,20,165,167,196,197]。

透明细胞癌：透明细胞癌由排列成条索状、巢状和片块状的胞浆透明丰富的多角形细胞构成[164,165,167,168,171,198-201]。胞浆含糖原而不是黏液。核呈圆形或卵圆形，核染色质细而散在，单个核仁。核的非典型性一般不明显。常有硬化性间质，将肿瘤分隔成小叶状。在某些病例中可见与普通的鳞状细胞癌有移行。主要的鉴别诊断包括精原细胞瘤（细胞角蛋白常常阴性）、转移性肾细胞癌（具有富于血管的间质）、甲状旁腺癌（伴有富于血管的间

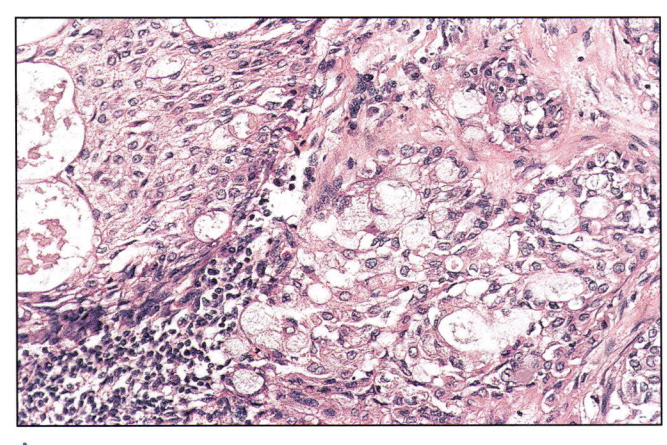

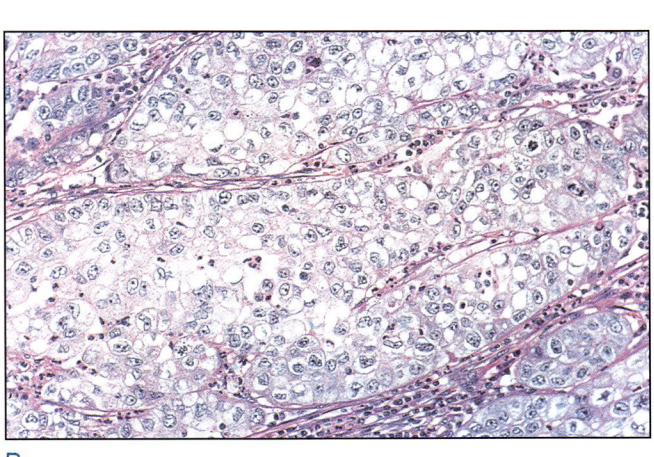

图21C.40 胸腺黏液表皮样癌。（A）本例为低级别肿瘤，类似于发生在涎腺的相应肿瘤。鳞状细胞岛内散在有分泌黏液的细胞和含有黏液的囊腔。肿瘤细胞核形态相对温和。（B）本例为高级别肿瘤，由胞浆淡染的实性细胞岛组成，类似于透明细胞癌。然而，黏液卡红染色说明肿瘤细胞内有大量黏液。

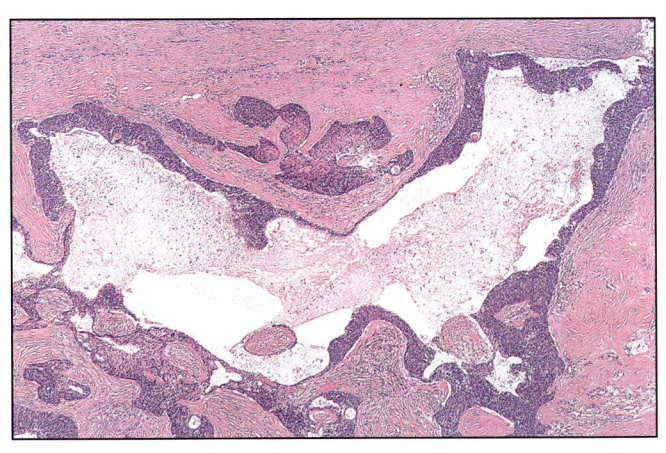

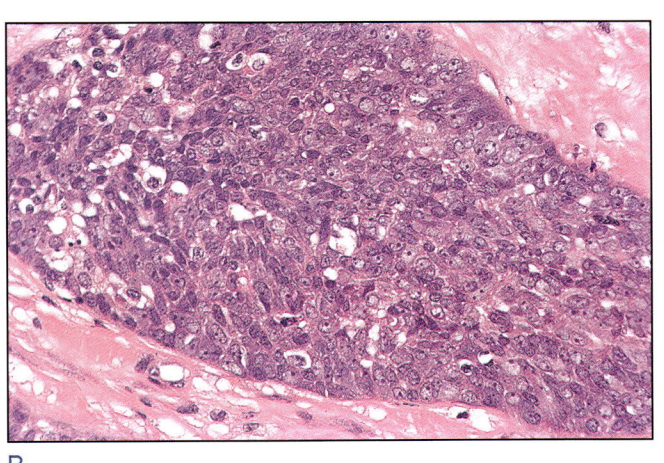

图21C.41 胸腺基底细胞样癌。（A）这种肿瘤通常含有内衬肿瘤细胞的大的囊性间隙。（B）肿瘤细胞岛具有基底细胞样细胞特征，胞浆稀少。

未分化（间变性）癌：这一名称用于不容易按上述分类方法进行分类的肿瘤，它们具有显著的细胞多形性并缺少特异的细胞分化谱系[165]。

乳头状腺癌：是胸腺癌中非常罕见的类型，可能被误诊为间皮瘤、转移性甲状腺乳头状腺癌或转移性肺腺癌[21,202,203]。肿瘤形成纤细的乳头或管状乳头，被覆立方及柱状细胞，伴有低级别或高级别核的非典型性。可以出现沙粒体（图 21C.42）。多数病例起源于先前存在的 A 型胸腺瘤。肿瘤癌胚抗原、CD15/LeuM1 和 BerEP4 呈阳性，CD5 不同程度呈阳性，但甲状球蛋白和表面活性物质（surfactant）呈阴性。

腺癌：在罕见的情况下，胸腺可以发生类似于肠和胆道腺癌的原发性胸腺癌[21,167,203-206]。可以表现为胶样（黏液）癌、囊腺癌或非特异性腺癌（图 21C.43）。其中有些病例似乎起源于先前存在的胸腺囊肿。重要的鉴别诊断是转移性腺癌、间皮瘤和生殖细胞肿瘤。

伴有 Castleman 病样反应的未分化大细胞癌：这是未分化大细胞癌中一种少见而又独特的类型，肿瘤周围区域伴有类似于透明血管性 Castleman 病的炎症性反应[207]。肿瘤成分由具有合体细胞样表现的大的多形性细胞结节构成。在某些区域，癌细胞位于淋巴滤泡的中心部分。多达 60% 的患者可以无症状。许多病例呈现惰性临床经过，令人奇怪的是，肿瘤却具有高级别的形态学改变。

罕见类型的癌：原发性胸腺肝样癌（hepatoid

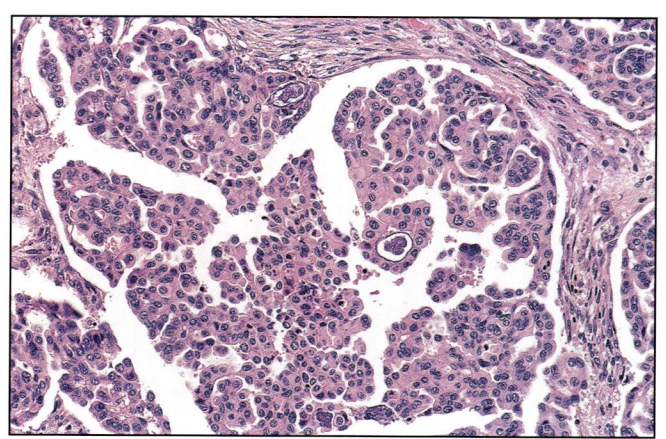

图21C.42 胸腺乳头状癌。纤细的乳头主要由细胞簇构成，可见沙粒体。这个肿瘤起源于A型胸腺瘤。

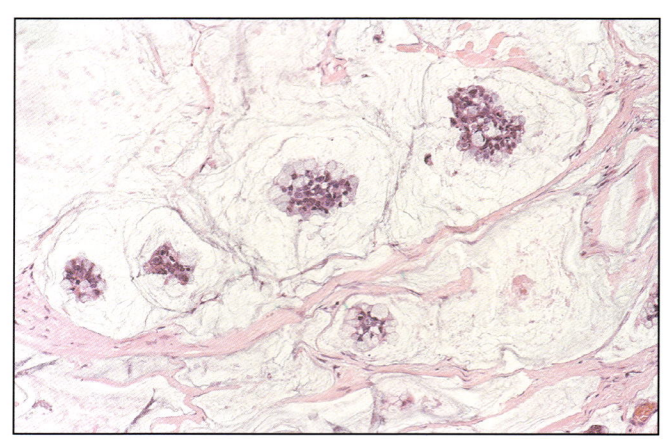

图21C.43 胸腺腺癌。这种黏液（胶样）腺癌是由漂浮于细胞外黏液湖内的肿瘤性腺样结构组成的。

carcinoma）、横纹肌样癌（rhabdoid carcinoma）、横纹肌瘤性癌（rhabdomyomatous carcinoma）、腺鳞癌和腺样囊性癌有少数报道[21,177 208-211]。

伴有 t(15;19) 易位的胸腺癌：发生在年轻人纵隔或胸腺的伴有 t(15;19) 易位的胸腺癌已有几篇报道[211a]。本病可迅速致死，伴有广泛的局部浸润和全身播散。组织学上，癌由成片排列的未分化细胞构成，虽然可有局灶性鳞状分化[212-215]。这种特征性的易位导致 *NUT* 基因的重排[211a]。

起源于胸腺瘤或胸腺囊肿的胸腺癌
Thymic carcinoma arising in thymoma or thymic cyst

多数胸腺癌是直接发生的，但是有些胸腺癌是由胸腺瘤恶变而来。这两种成分或分散存在，或在交界性特征的间插区域逐渐移行[216,217]。由于坏死常见于癌的成分，所以在胸腺瘤中发现肿瘤坏死时，病理医生应该警惕出现癌变的可能（图 21C.44）。有证据显示，未切除的胸腺瘤长期存在其恶变的危险性可能增加[216]。

胸腺瘤可以是任何组织学类型，而胸腺癌成分最常见的是低分化或高分化鳞状细胞癌[216,217]。肿瘤恶变可能伴有上皮膜抗原和 CK 7、8、18 和 19 表达上调，以及 p53 蛋白染色呈弥漫强阳性[217]。

某些胸腺癌可以发生于先前存在的单房性或多房性胸腺囊肿，如鳞状细胞癌或黏液表皮样癌[20,193,194,218-221]。

免疫细胞化学和特殊研究

胸腺癌表达广谱细胞角蛋白。此外，常常表达 CD5 和 CD117，这些标记物在其他部位的癌常不表达。

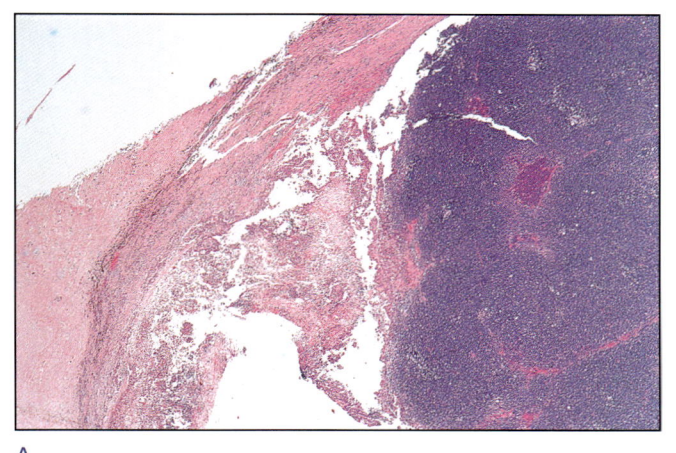
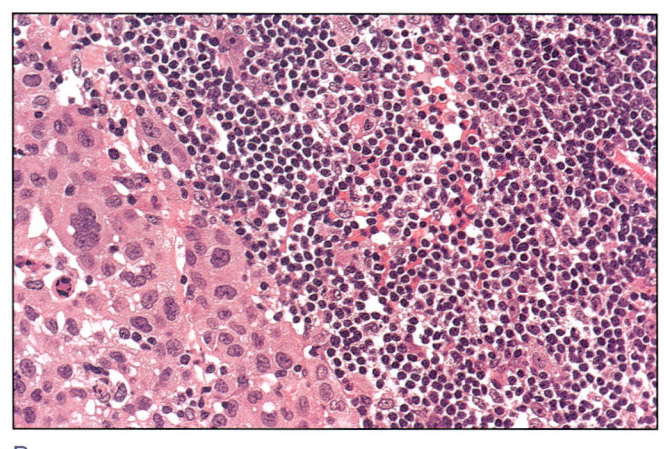

图21C.44 发生在B1型胸腺瘤的胸腺癌。（A）胸腺瘤成分深染（视野右侧）。包膜下方有坏死，此处可见并发的胸腺癌。（B）视野右侧显示胸腺瘤成分，左侧显示胸腺癌成分。后者可见明显的核多形性，核分裂活跃（没有显示）。

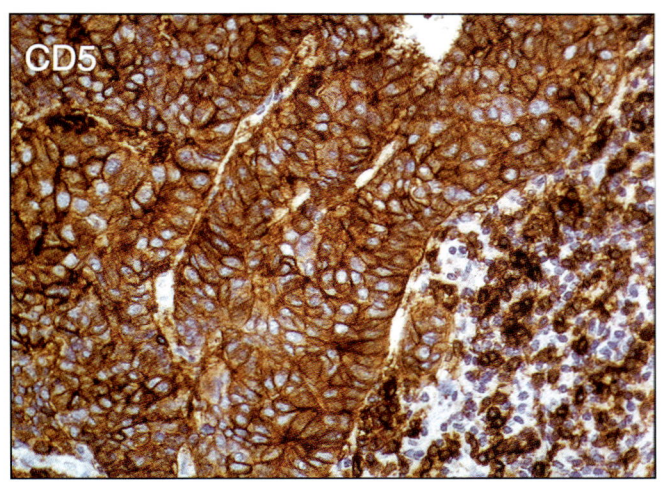

图21C.45 胸腺癌CD5免疫组化染色。癌细胞（视野左侧）显示细胞膜和胞浆CD5呈强阳性。肿瘤内的T淋巴细胞（视野右侧）为CD5染色提供了最好的内部阳性对照。

胸腺癌62%～80%表达CD5（图21C.45）[222-227]，而胸腺瘤CD5几乎总是呈阴性。80%～86%的胸腺癌表达CD117，而胸腺瘤仅有0～4%CD117呈阳性[228,229]。

散在的或成团的表达神经内分泌标记物的肿瘤细胞可见于约60%的胸腺癌和部分交界性胸腺上皮性肿瘤。另一方面，这些细胞在胸腺瘤中非常罕见[227,230,231]。这种现象可能与不同部位普通癌中出现神经内分泌细胞相似，反映了肿瘤内的多方向分化性。

与胸腺瘤不同，胸腺癌中的浸润淋巴细胞为成熟的T细胞和B细胞，缺乏TdT⁺的不成熟T淋巴细胞。

除了淋巴上皮瘤样癌（见上"显微显微镜下表现"）外，各种类型胸腺癌EB病毒呈阴性。

虽然有些研究显示在胸腺癌中，p53蛋白免疫反应常常呈阳性（74%），但其在胸腺瘤中则很少表达（6%）[232]，另外一些研究发现，胸腺瘤也常表达p53蛋白[233-236]。11%～22%的胸腺癌可见 *P53* 基因突变[232,237]。胸腺癌常常为非整倍体并显示高DNA指数[238,239]。

胸腺鳞状细胞癌常常显示多数染色体失衡：+1q、+17q、+18、−3p、−6、−13q、−16q 和 −17p[112,156,158,159]。与B3型胸腺瘤共有 +1q、−6 和 −13q，提示这两种类型的肿瘤密切相关。

胸腺癌的预后因素

- 组织学类型和分级见上文"临床行为和治疗"一节。
- 核分裂活性：每10个高倍视野核分裂象超过10个与预后不好相关，其死亡率为84%；而核分裂象计数低者死亡率为21%[165]。
- 大体浸润：浸润性、界线不清的肿瘤侵袭性行为比界限清楚的肿瘤的强（死亡率分别为88%和16.6%）[165]。肿瘤浸润大血管者预后不好[107,240]。
- 胸腺癌的Masaoka分期缺乏预后意义，而暂行的TNM分期系统分别考虑了局部浸润、淋巴结状况和远处转移，能够将患者分组，各组具有不同的预后[4,13,60]。

鉴别诊断

- 转移癌：因为除非有胸腺瘤成分存在，否则根据形态学检查不能准确地将胸腺癌和转移癌区分开来，所以为了确定原发性胸腺癌的诊断，必须进行充分的临床和放射学评估[167]。如果CD5和

CD117免疫反应呈阳性，则支持胸腺癌的诊断。
- 胸腺瘤（见表21C.2）。
- 大细胞淋巴瘤。
- 化生性胸腺瘤（可能被误诊为胸腺癌）。
- 生殖细胞肿瘤。

介于胸腺瘤和胸腺癌之间的交界性胸腺上皮性肿瘤（非典型性胸腺瘤）
Thymic epithelial tumor borderline between thymoma and thymic carcinoma (atypical thymoma)

组织学特征介于胸腺瘤和胸腺癌之间的胸腺上皮性肿瘤罕见[6]。也就是说，这类胸腺肿瘤细胞和结构的非典型性比普通胸腺瘤的明显，但是尚未充分发展为胸腺癌的特征（图21C.46）。这些交界性胸腺瘤有时被称为1.5型恶性胸腺瘤或非典型性胸腺瘤[6,23,227]。我们并不像Suster和Moran那样将B3型胸腺瘤包括在这种类型的胸腺瘤中[109]。

交界性胸腺上皮性肿瘤不是一种独立的疾病，而是反映了在胸腺瘤和胸腺癌之间的一个灰色地带。多数病例可能是B3型胸腺瘤（具有胸腺瘤的典型结构特征），这些病例的细胞非典型性超过了典型的胸腺瘤（所谓的"伴有间变的B3型胸腺瘤"，B3 thymoma with anaplasia）（图21C.47）。尚不清楚这种肿瘤是生物学意义上的B3型胸腺瘤，还是进展性B3型胸腺瘤伴异型增生或原位癌的改变。在其他一些病例中，肿瘤缺乏胸腺瘤的小叶结构和血管周围间隙的特征，但是细胞非典型性并不明显。

免疫组化研究有时可以进一步提供肿瘤在生物学上是接近于胸腺瘤还是接近于胸腺癌的信息。如果有较多

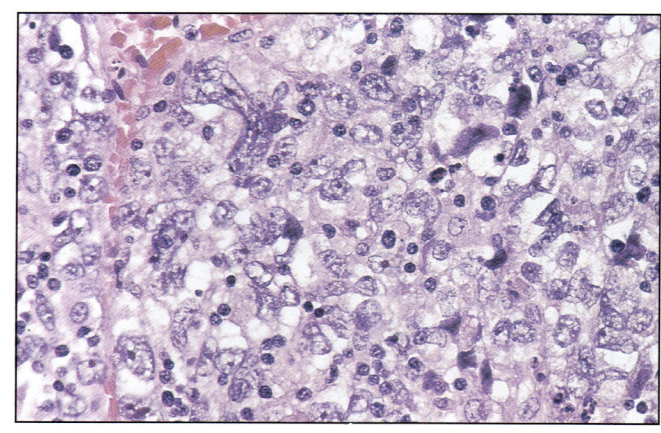

图21C.47　介于胸腺瘤和胸腺癌之间的交界性胸腺上皮性肿瘤（非典型性胸腺瘤）。这个肿瘤显示小叶结构和血管周围间隙，但肿瘤细胞显示高度的核深染和多形性。

TdT+淋巴细胞，在生物学特征上可能更接近于胸腺瘤。另一方面，如果上皮细胞显示CD5或CD117免疫反应阳性，肿瘤或许更接近于胸腺癌。

异位胸腺和相关的鳃肿瘤
Ectopic thymic and related branchial tumors

异位胸腺瘤　Ectopic thymoma

胸腺瘤可发生在前纵隔以外的部位，如颈部、甲状腺、肺和胸膜[152,241-245]。

这种现象可以解释为胚胎发育过程中胸腺下降不完全[241]。异位胸腺瘤容易被误诊为癌或淋巴瘤，因为可能根本没有考虑胸腺瘤的可能性。偶尔，有报告胸腺瘤发生在心脏黏液瘤内的报道[246]。

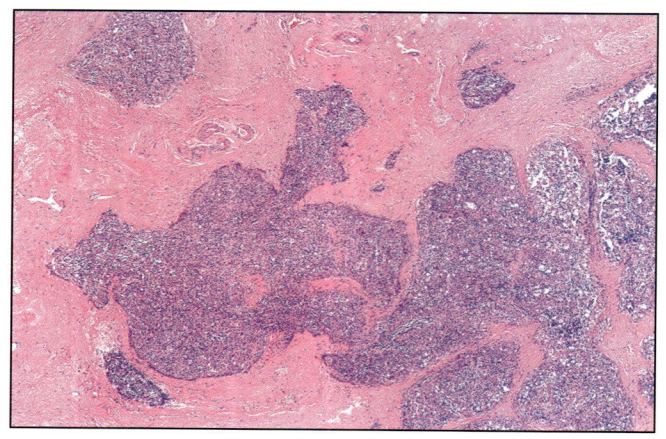

A

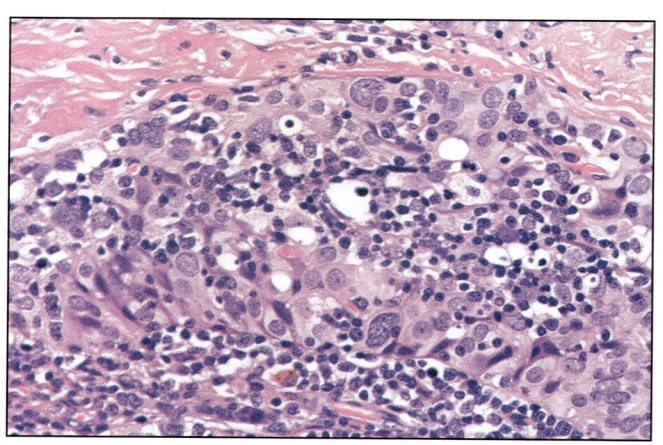

B

图21C.46　介于胸腺瘤和胸腺癌之间的交界性胸腺上皮性肿瘤（非典型性胸腺瘤）。（A）这个肿瘤显示胸腺瘤的结构特征，在致密的纤维性间质内可见有棱角的肿瘤小叶。（B）然而，核的非典型性超过典型的B3型胸腺瘤。

异位错构瘤性胸腺瘤
Ectopic hamartomatous thymoma

这是一种发生于下颈部软组织的独特的界限清楚的良性肿瘤，由错综复杂的上皮性成分、梭形细胞和脂肪细胞混合而成[241,247]。尽管某些肿瘤与正常胸腺结构相似，但目前还没有证据表明具有胸腺的本质。在形态学上不同于胸腺瘤，缺乏拼图样的分叶状结构。

伴有胸腺样成分的梭形上皮性肿瘤
Spindle epithelial tumor with thymus-like element (SETTLE)

见第18章第一部分。这种特殊而罕见的肿瘤可能是"胸腺母细胞瘤"（thymoblastoma）的一种形式，但是到目前为止还没有向胸腺方向分化的可靠证据。

显示胸腺样成分的癌
Carcinoma showing thymus-like element (CASTLE)

见第18章第一部分。现在有令人信服的证据表明，这种肿瘤是发生于甲状腺内的胸腺癌，因为CD5和CD117呈阳性，且在肿瘤附近偶尔可见残留的异位胸腺组织。

胸腺的神经内分泌肿瘤
Neuroendocrine tumors of the thymus

存在一系列胸腺原发性神经内分泌肿瘤，它们被认为是起源于正常存在于胸腺的Kultschizky型神经内分泌细胞。这个谱系中比较良性的一类是类癌，而较恶性的一类是小细胞和大细胞神经内分泌癌。有些病例不可避免地显示中间性或混合性的特征。命名法和诊断标准与发生在肺的神经内分泌肿瘤相同[248,249]。有些学者喜欢把类癌、非典型类癌以及小细胞/大细胞神经内分泌癌分别称为高分化、中分化和低分化神经内分泌癌，以便较清楚地表明其恶性性质[250-252]。然而，2004版WHO分类将典型类癌和非典型性类癌归为"高分化神经内分泌癌"，而将小细胞癌和大细胞神经内分泌癌归为"低分化神经内分泌癌"[253]。

类癌（典型和非典型性）
Carcinoid tumor (typical and atypical)

临床特征

胸腺类癌少见。发病年龄广泛，平均发病年龄为50岁[250,254-258]。男性多见，男女发病比例为3:1，患者或无症状，或出现与纵隔肿块有关的症状，或出现内分泌症状。约1/3的患者由于分泌ACTH而发生Cushing综合征[250,254,255,259]。偶尔可以发生其他瘤外综合征，如不适量的抗利尿激素产物、肥大性骨关节病和Eaton-Lambert综合征[256,260,261]。然而，相关的类癌综合征尚无报道[20]。

多达25%的胸腺类癌为1型多发性内分泌肿瘤（MEN1）的成分[254-256,262,263]，这样的肿瘤更具侵袭性[261]。MEN1相关性胸腺类癌通常发生于男性，平均发病年龄为37～44岁，许多患者为重度吸烟者[262-266]。与类癌综合征和Cushing综合征无关。预后一般不好，可能是由于肿瘤发现晚，且缺乏有效的治疗[264]。有人提出，所有的胸腺类癌患者均应检查以除外MEN1[264]。少见情况下，胸腺类癌的发生可作为MEN2的一部分[267]。

罕见的典型胸腺类癌呈相对惰性的经过，偶尔有局部复发和转移播散[250,251]。非典型类癌侵袭性较强，伴有复发和广泛转移的倾向[250,251]。包膜完整的肿瘤不常见，经手术切除可治愈。常见的浸润性肿瘤通常在纵隔、肺和胸壁反复复发，局部淋巴结转移常见[260]。约30%的病例将发生远处转移，尤其是肺、骨和肝转移[268]。骨转移经常是成骨性的。肿瘤放疗或化疗效果一般不好。尽管5年生存率为30%～60%，长期预后仍然较差，多数患者最终死于肿瘤[2,252,253,256,258,261,269]。

大体表现

胸腺类癌或包膜完整，或有明显浸润。肿瘤通常较大、实性鱼肉状、伴有坏死和出血区。由于钙化，切面可呈砂砾样。缺乏见于胸腺瘤的典型小叶结构。

显微镜下表现

类癌的特征是多角形细胞呈器官样簇状、片块状和缎带样排列，被纤细的纤维血管间质分隔（图21C.48）。可以出现真玫瑰花结、假玫瑰花结、血管周围玫瑰花结和球形肿块（常伴有粉刺样坏死）（图21C.49）。肿瘤细胞具有圆形或卵圆形细胞核，染色质细腻散在，核仁不明显。可见不同程度的核多形性。胞浆呈颗粒状（图21C.50）。偶尔可见鳞状分化灶。可以出现营养不良性钙化。血管浸润常见，见于多达50%以上的非典型性类癌患者。在罕见情况下，胸腺类癌可与胸腺瘤共存[20,270]。

大多数胸腺类癌的形态学和生物学与肺的非典型类癌相似而不是典型类癌。典型类癌（typical carcinoid）被定义为每10个高倍视野（2mm^2）核分裂象小于2个，并且没有坏死。非典型类癌（atypical carcinoid）被定义为每10个高倍视野（2mm^2）核分裂象2～10个，或

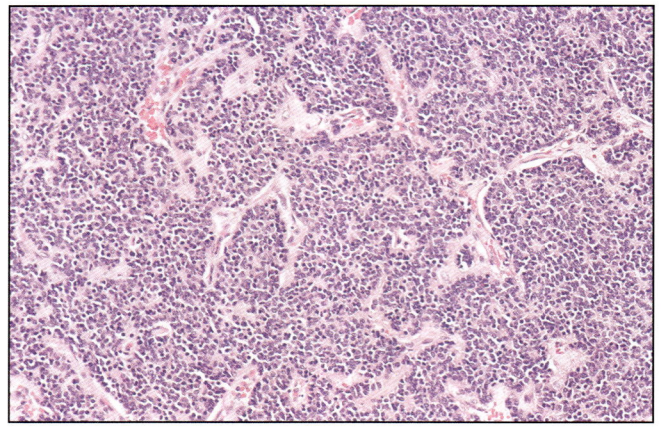

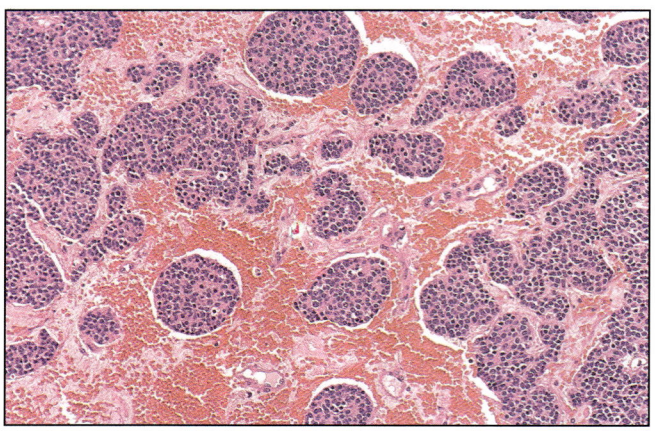

A

B

图21C.48 胸腺非典型类癌。（A）成片的多角形细胞被纤细的纤维血管间隔分割，具有内分泌肿瘤的特征。（B）肿瘤细胞团被血液或富于血管的间质分隔。

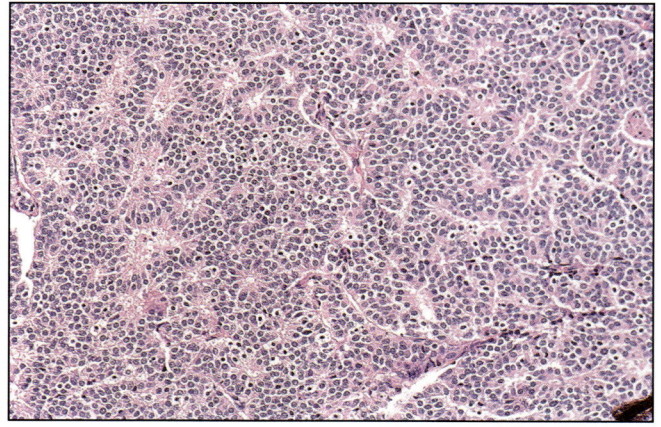

图21C.49 胸腺非典型类癌。肿瘤含有纤细的纤维血管间隔，并形成一些玫瑰花结结构。

出现凝固性坏死，后者常呈点灶状，每10个高倍视野核分裂计数多达10个（图21C.50）。

形态学亚型

胸腺类癌的许多形态学亚型已有描述，但并无预后

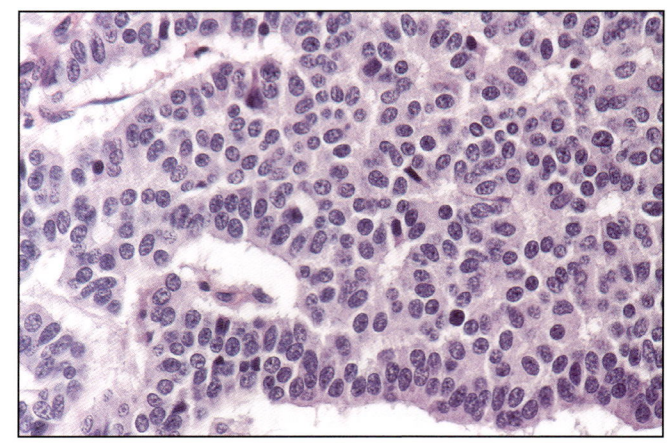

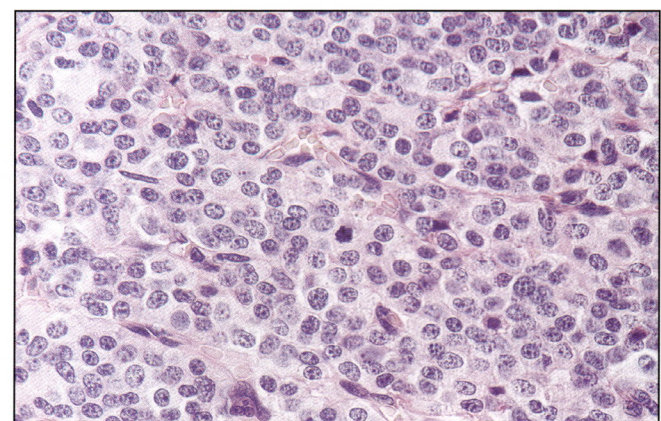

A

B

图21C.50 胸腺类癌。（A）典型类癌的肿瘤细胞均匀一致，核分裂象少见。（B）非典型类癌具有轻度的核非典型性和核分裂活性。

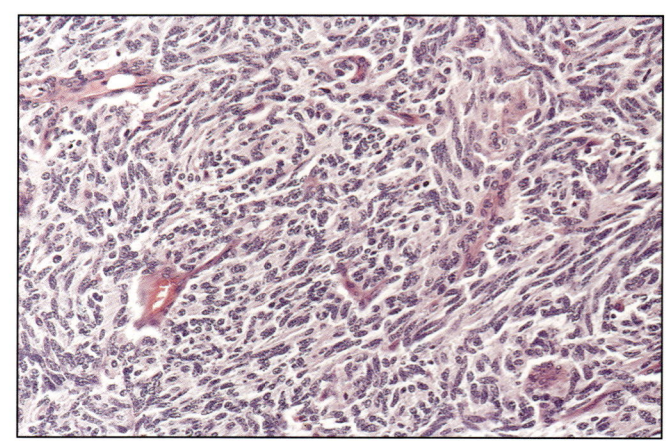

图21C.51 胸腺类癌，梭形细胞型。这种类型可能类似于梭形细胞胸腺瘤，但是颗粒状染色质、颗粒状胞浆和纤细的纤维血管间隔提示肿瘤具有神经内分泌本质。

意义。对于单个病例来说，进一步鉴别是典型类癌还是非典型类癌仍然十分重要。

- **梭形细胞亚型**（spindle cell variant）：由交织排列的梭形细胞束构成[271,272]。通过发现穿过肿瘤的纤细纤维

血管间隔和局灶性普通类癌的区域，可以与梭形细胞胸腺瘤鉴别。

- **色素性亚型** (pigmented variant)：有些肿瘤细胞中可出现蜡样色素（ceroid pigmemt）或黑色素[273-275]。
- **嗜酸细胞型亚型** (oncocytic variant)：其特征是明显的细胞嗜酸性改变[276,277]。肿瘤细胞排列成巢状、条索状和片块状，可能被误诊为转移癌、副神经节瘤和恶性黑色素瘤[278]。
- **硬化型亚型** (sclerotic variant)：伴有丰富的硬化性间质和局灶性印第安纵队排列的细胞[256]。
- **弥漫性亚型** (diffuse subtype)：片块样排列的肿瘤，几乎不能辨认器官样结构[256]。
- **甲状腺髓样癌样亚型** (medullary thyroid carcinoma-like variant)：其中的肿瘤细胞散在分布于丰富的淀粉样物质中[254,261]。
- **伴有明显黏液性间质的胸腺类癌** (thymic carcinoid with prominent mucinous stroma)：其特征是肿瘤细胞条带和肿瘤细胞岛被丰富的黏液性间质包绕，类似于黏液（胶样）腺癌（图21C.52）。然而，这种黏液性物质是透明质酸，因此是对肿瘤的一种间质反应而不是肿瘤细胞的分泌产物[279]。
- **血管瘤样亚型** (angiomatoid variant)：伴有多数充满血液的囊性间隙，容易误诊为血管瘤[280]。这些血液池由肿瘤细胞而不是由内皮细胞围绕。
- **伴有歧异肉瘤样分化的胸腺类癌** (thymic carcinoid with divergent sarcomatoid differentiation)：类癌和肉瘤成分混合存在，甚至可能出现骨和软骨分化（图21C.53）[281,282]。

免疫细胞化学

胸腺类癌细胞角蛋白阳性。绝大多数肿瘤细胞广谱神经内分泌标记物阳性，如嗜铬素和突触素，不同于胸腺癌中常见的局灶性染色。胸腺类癌各种激素染色也常常阳性，如ACTH、生长抑素、5-羟色胺和β-内啡肽（β-endorphin）[260]，并且多种激素表达并不少见[283]。

电子显微镜检查

超微结构显示，细胞膜光滑或有短而钝圆的指状突起。存在桥粒。胞浆含有线粒体、发育良好的粗面内质网和有致密轴心的神经内分泌颗粒[256]。

鉴别诊断

- 胸腺瘤：鉴别特征见表21C.7。
- 胸腺癌。
- 从其他部位转移而来的神经内分泌癌：鉴别诊断需

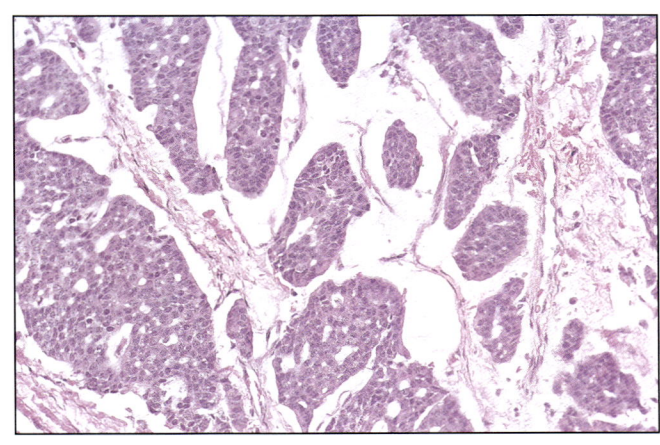

图21C.52 伴有黏液性间质的胸腺非典型类癌。注意与胶样癌相似。

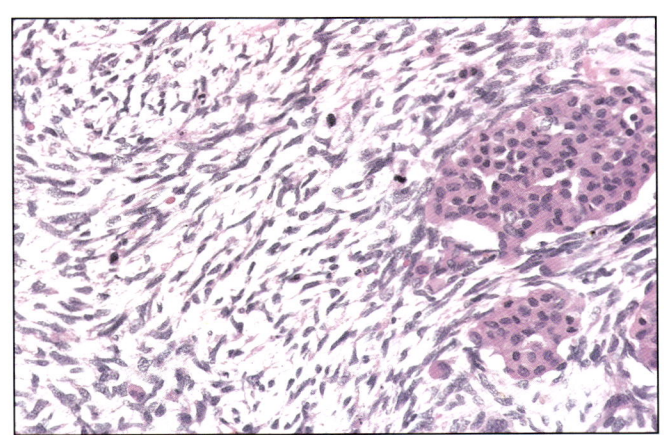

图21C.53 伴有歧异肉瘤样分化的胸腺类癌。视野右侧显示非典型类癌成分，具有嗜酸性颗粒状胞浆。视野左侧显示梭形细胞肉瘤，核分裂活跃。

要结合临床。

- 大细胞淋巴瘤：大细胞淋巴瘤可能类似于类癌，因为具有硬化性间质间隔。一般来说，大细胞淋巴瘤至少有些区域肿瘤细胞比较弥散，并且常常出现不规则的核折叠。
- 精原细胞瘤：弥漫性亚型的胸腺类癌可能类似于精原细胞瘤，但是后者经常出现突出的核仁、散在的淋巴细胞且缺乏细胞角蛋白染色或仅有局灶点状表达。
- 副神经节瘤：副神经节瘤显示特征性的细胞球形态而不形成小梁状结构。细胞角蛋白呈阴性，肿瘤细胞巢周围的支持细胞S-100呈阳性有助于与类癌的鉴别诊断。

小细胞癌
Small cell carcinoma

临床特征

只有通过临床、放射学、内镜和细胞学检查排除隐

表21C.7 胸腺类癌和胸腺瘤的鉴别特征

	胸腺类癌	胸腺瘤
性别	男性为主	没有性别差异或女性略占优势
瘤外或内分泌表现	Cushing综合征	重症肌无力、红细胞发育不全、低丙种球蛋白血症
伴随	MEN 1，而MEN 2罕见	不伴有综合征
局部或远处转移	非常常见	罕见
大体表现	通常均匀一致，但可有坏死区域	明显的纤维间隔穿过肿瘤，形成分叶状结构
显著的组织学特征	缺乏明显的分叶；有纤细的纤维血管间隔穿过；没有血管周围间隙；几乎无淋巴细胞；胞浆颗粒状	拼图样小叶被宽的硬化带分隔；缺乏内分泌型纤细的纤维血管间隔；血管周围间隙；常常出现大量淋巴细胞；胞浆无颗粒
免疫细胞化学	嗜铬素、突触素和其他内分泌产物阳性	神经内分泌标记物阴性
电子显微镜检查	短的指突状细胞突起；电子致密颗粒	长的指突状细胞突起；无电子致密颗粒

匿性支气管原发性小细胞癌的转移后，才能确诊胸腺小细胞癌[260,284]。与胸腺类癌不同，小细胞癌两性发病率相等。患者为年轻人或中年成人（平均年龄44.6岁），表现为与迅速生长的胸腺肿块相关的症状，上腔静脉阻塞并不少见。有些病例可出现转移[261]。到目前为止还没有出现Cushing综合征[164,168,175]。多数患者在诊断后3年内死亡，但平均生存期（25～36个月）比肺小细胞癌长[253,261]。

病理学

小细胞癌由成片块状或成簇的小细胞组成，其直径一般不到静止淋巴细胞（resting lymphocytes）的3倍[248,253]。细胞核圆形、卵圆形或梭形，染色质细颗粒状，核仁不明显[164,168,175]。胞浆一般稀少（图21C.54）。核碎裂、坏死和核分裂象常见。少数病例出现局灶鳞癌和腺鳞分化[167,168,177]。血管浸润常见（大于75%）[258]。有些病例可能显示向类癌转化[284]。

免疫细胞化学

肿瘤细胞角蛋白阳性，尤其是低分子量细胞角蛋白，

以及广谱神经内分泌标记物阳性。与Merkel细胞癌不同，细胞角蛋白20呈阴性反应[285]。

大细胞神经内分泌癌
Large cell neuroendocrine carcinoma

大细胞神经内分泌癌的定义是伴有神经内分泌形态学改变（器官样细胞巢、栅栏状、玫瑰花结和小梁状结构）、非小细胞癌细胞学特征（细胞大、核浆比例低）、神经内分泌标记物免疫染色阳性、凝固性坏死和高核分裂率（每10高倍视野核分裂象>11个）的肿瘤[10,248]。这种肿瘤在胸腺非常罕见，具有高度侵袭性[253,286]。

胸腺和纵隔的生殖细胞肿瘤
Germ cell tumors of the thymus and mediastinum

生殖细胞肿瘤　Germ cell tumors
临床特征

原发性生殖细胞肿瘤占所有纵隔肿瘤的10%～15%[287]。尽管在没有腹膜后淋巴结肿大的情况下，转移而来的可能性不大，然而，在检查时应该排除有隐匿性睾丸原发性生殖细胞肿瘤的可能[288]。畸胎瘤最常见，占所有病例的44%，在儿童所占比例甚至更高（70%）[12,289]。精原细胞瘤（生殖细胞瘤）占病例的37%，其他生殖细胞肿瘤占病例的19%[12,290-296]。Klinefelter综合征容易发生纵隔生殖细胞肿瘤[297,298]。

除了畸胎瘤外，纵隔生殖细胞肿瘤几乎全部发生于男性，女性畸胎瘤与男性畸胎瘤同样常见[12,291,293-295,299,300]。生殖细胞肿瘤发生年龄广泛，虽然多数患者年龄在15～35岁。在青春期前年龄组，实际上几乎所有的病例均为畸胎瘤和卵黄囊瘤，而在青春期后年龄组，所有各

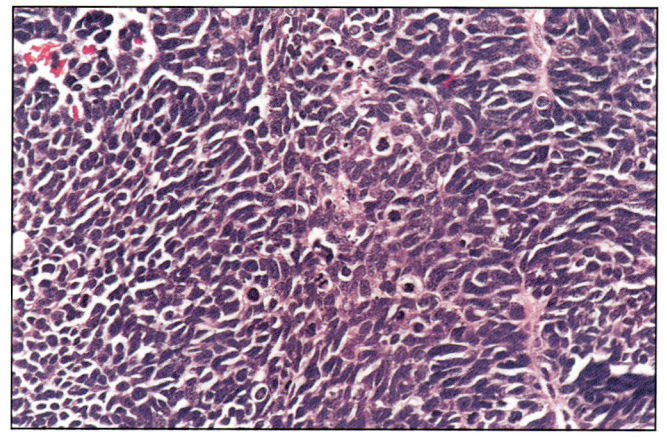

图21C.54　胸腺小细胞神经内分泌癌。组织学特征与肺小细胞癌无法区分。有显著的核变形。

种类型的生殖细胞肿瘤均可发生[301]。

一些患者表现为由纵隔肿块引起的非特异性症状，一些患者伴有上腔静脉阻塞，而另一些患者无症状。畸胎瘤罕见，具有诊断意义的表现是咳出毛发。非精原细胞瘤性恶性生殖细胞肿瘤常常伴有血清人绒毛膜促性腺激素和（或）甲胎蛋白升高。

并发或伴随的继发性肿瘤
Supervening or associated second neoplasms

有些纵隔生殖细胞肿瘤与血液系统肿瘤的发生有关[289,302-308]。这种并发症只发生在非精原细胞瘤性生殖细胞肿瘤，尤其是伴有卵黄囊瘤成分的肿瘤。血液系统恶性肿瘤同时或随后（通常在 1 年之内）发生，包括巨核细胞疾病、急性髓细胞性白血病、骨髓发育不良综合征、"恶性组织细胞增生症"、组织细胞肿瘤和系统性肥大细胞增生症。已经证实，一些这样的病例具有与纵隔肿瘤相同的染色体畸变（12p 等臂染色体），提示两种肿瘤有共同的起源[302,309]。有人提出，血液系统的恶性肿瘤起源于卵黄囊瘤成分内的血液前体细胞[307]。

少数情况下，体细胞型恶性肿瘤（癌或肉瘤）可以发生在生殖细胞肿瘤内，如畸胎瘤、精原细胞瘤、卵黄囊瘤或混合性生殖细胞肿瘤[12,310,311]。这种成分对常常用于治疗生殖细胞肿瘤的化疗药物没有反应。预后一般不良，平均生存时间仅为 9 个月[311]。

临床行为

成熟性畸胎瘤是良性肿瘤，在没有并发症的情况下，手术可以完全治愈[12,293,296]。罕见的纯粹不成熟性畸胎瘤常常在 I 期疾病时发现，预后通常较好[12]。伴有其他恶性生殖细胞肿瘤成分或体细胞型癌的畸胎瘤，生存率大约为 50%。伴有体细胞肉瘤成分的畸胎瘤，80% 的患者在 2 年内死亡[11,12]。

生殖细胞瘤（germinoma），也称为精原细胞瘤（seminoma），对放疗高度敏感，预后良好[290,312,313]。最近的研究表明，在治疗方案中加入化疗，85% 的病例可以长期生存[314]。分期是判断预后的最重要的单一因素，随访发现，实际上所有的一期患者均无病生存[12]。

非精原细胞瘤性恶性生殖细胞肿瘤的预后比发生在性腺的相应肿瘤要差[11,12,292,315-317]。诊断时大部分患者已经发生转移，如转移至肺、胸膜、淋巴结、肝和骨[314]。应用现代疗法，包括以顺铂为基础的化疗和（或）手术治疗，大约 50% 的患者可以获得长期生存[318,319]。儿童患者的预后似乎较好。然而，绒毛膜癌患者几乎全部死亡[12,316]。

其他预后因素包括年龄（小于 30 岁预后好）、存在远处转移（预后不好）、临床分期以及是否完全切除。

显微镜下表现

纵隔生殖细胞肿瘤的少见形态学特征：各种类型的生殖细胞肿瘤均可出现多发性囊腔，后者是残留的胸腺上皮化生的结果（图 21C.55）。残留的胸腺上皮对肿瘤组织可以产生明显的反应性增生，可能误诊为胸腺瘤（图 21C.56）。

生殖细胞瘤（精原细胞瘤）：生殖细胞瘤的形态学表现与性腺发生的生殖细胞瘤相同（见 14 章）。肿瘤可以被广泛的上皮样肉芽肿性反应、囊肿、反应性淋巴滤泡增生或纤维化所掩盖（图 21C.55、图 21C.56 和 21C.57）[12,312,313,322,323]。因此，胸腺囊肿出现上皮样肉芽肿或生发中心时应彻底检查并查找生殖细胞瘤（和 Hodgkin 淋巴瘤）[25]。

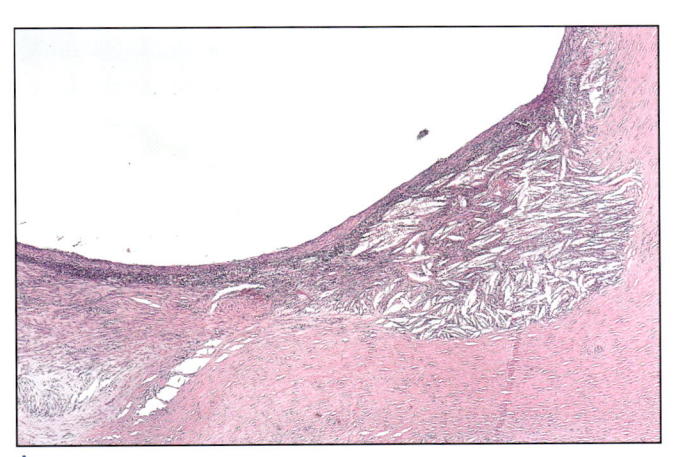
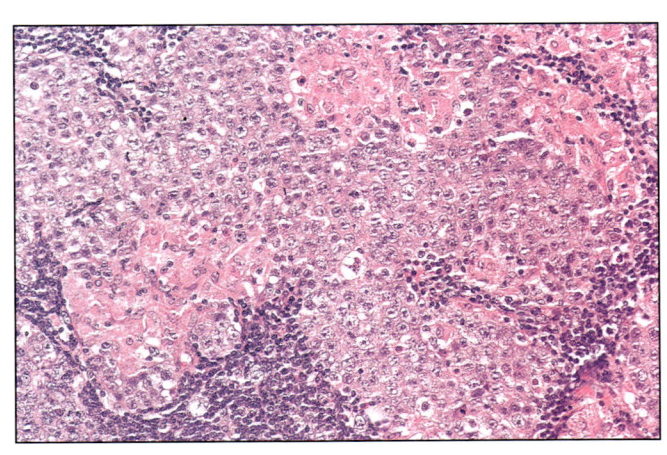

图 21C.55　酷似胸腺囊肿的精原细胞瘤。（A）这个囊性病变含有胆固醇结晶的纤维性囊壁。（B）囊壁内可见灶状精原细胞瘤成分，肿瘤细胞具有明显的核仁和淡染的胞浆。

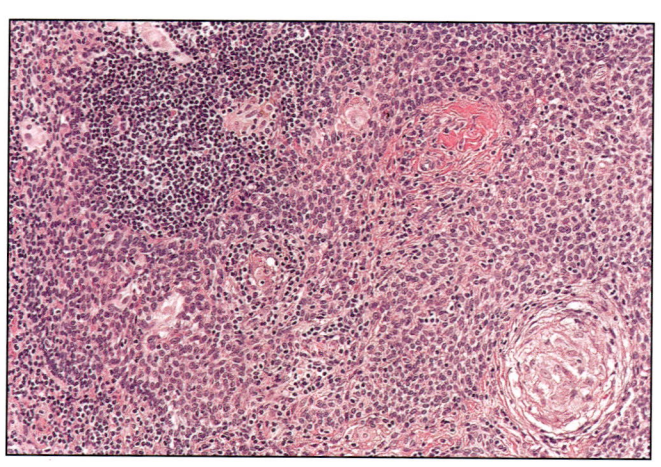

图21C.56 精原细胞瘤伴有胸腺上皮显著增生。这个视野没有显示精原细胞瘤的成分。图中可见伴随肿瘤的明显增生的胸腺上皮，可能误诊为胸腺瘤。

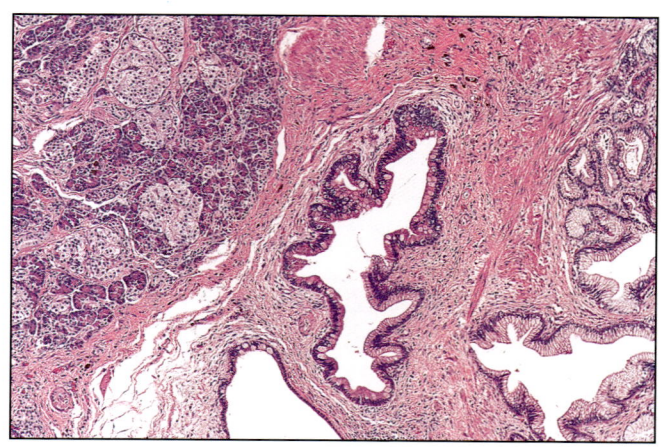

图21C.58 胸腺成熟畸胎瘤。所有的成分都是成熟的。注意出现胰腺组织（视野左侧）。

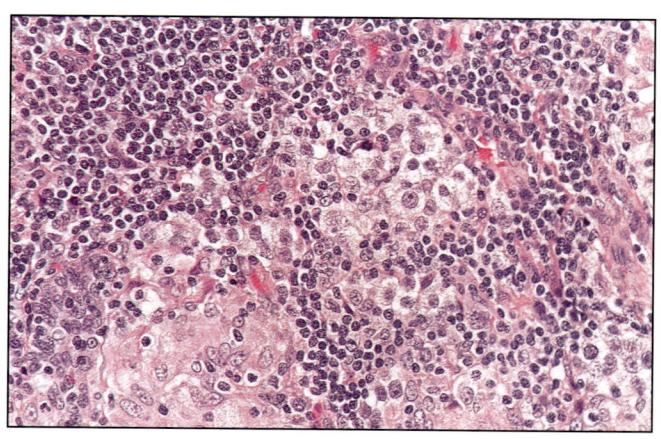

图21C.57 被肉芽肿性反应掩盖了的精原细胞瘤。小巢状的精原细胞瘤（具有明显的核仁和淡染的胞浆）隐藏于淋巴细胞和上皮样肉芽肿中。

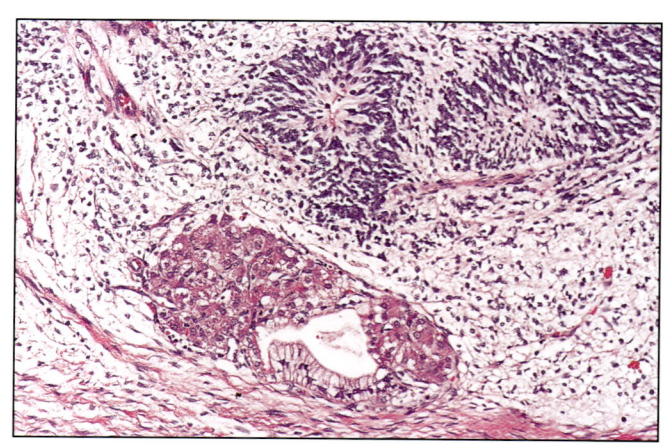

图21C.59 胸腺不成熟畸胎瘤。视野上方可见原始神经外胚层组织。视野下方显示腺体结构和胚胎性/胎儿性肝细胞。

纵隔畸胎瘤：多数纵隔畸胎瘤为成熟性畸胎瘤。胰腺组织在性腺畸胎瘤中极其罕见，其原因尚不清楚，而在纵隔畸胎瘤中却相当常见（图21C.58）[4,324,325]。推测这种胰腺成分可以产生蛋白分解酶而与周围组织紧密粘连。胰腺组织胰岛过度活跃可能导致低血糖[326]。纵隔单纯不成熟性畸胎瘤罕见，常常与其他类型的生殖细胞肿瘤混合存在（图21C.59）。

与性腺畸胎瘤相比，纵隔畸胎瘤较常伴有其他恶性成分，这些恶性成分可以是另外一种生殖细胞肿瘤，也可以是体细胞恶性肿瘤[11,12,327,328]。体细胞恶性肿瘤可为肉瘤，最常见的是横纹肌肉瘤和血管肉瘤；体细胞恶性肿瘤也可为癌，如腺癌、鳞状细胞癌甚至杯状细胞类癌（图21C.60）。与成熟性畸胎瘤有关的胎盘部位滋养叶细胞肿瘤非常罕见，仅有一例报告[329]。恶性成分或与畸胎瘤成分紧密混合，或形成散在独立的肿瘤包块。

纵隔卵黄囊瘤：与性腺卵黄囊瘤一样，纵隔卵黄囊瘤可有一系列形态学表现，如微囊性、内胚窦性、黏液瘤性、腺体-腺泡性、乳头、多囊状-卵黄性、附壁性、子宫内膜样和肝样性（图21C.61）[12,294,315,330,331]。最少见的肉瘤样结构在性腺部位以前没有描述过，其特征是非典型性的梭形细胞形成模糊的席纹状结构[332]。

纵隔胚胎癌和绒毛膜癌：形态学上这些肿瘤与性腺相应的肿瘤相同（见第14章）。

特殊诊断思考：当纵隔出现未分化癌或低分化腺癌而又不符合规定类型的胸腺癌诊断标准时，应该认真考虑性腺外生殖细胞恶性肿瘤综合征（extragonadal germ cell cancer syngrome）的可能性，即使组织学特征不是典型的生殖细胞肿瘤。人绒毛膜促性腺激素（HCG）和（或）甲胎蛋白免疫反应将支持这种诊断。不应该错过这种诊断的可能，因为有些患者对用于治疗生殖细胞肿瘤的化疗有非常明显的反应。

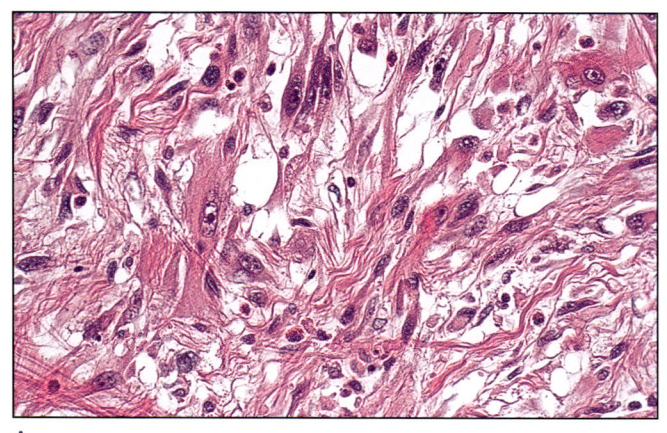
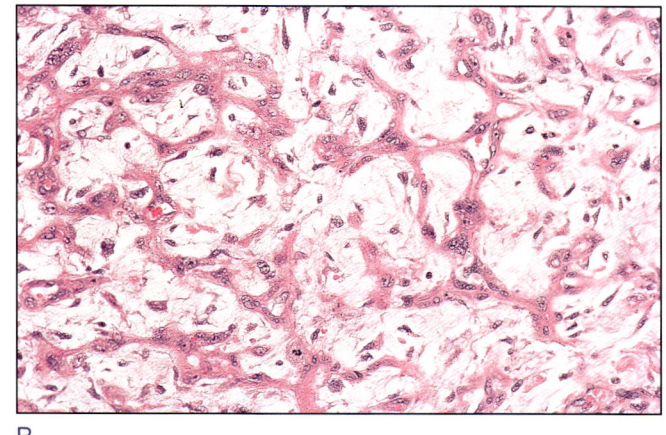

图21C.60 并发肉瘤的胸腺畸胎瘤。（A）这里显示发生于畸胎瘤的横纹肌肉瘤成分。（B）这种肉瘤是血管肉瘤，由狭窄而复杂的血管间隙构成，内衬核分裂活跃的非典型性细胞。

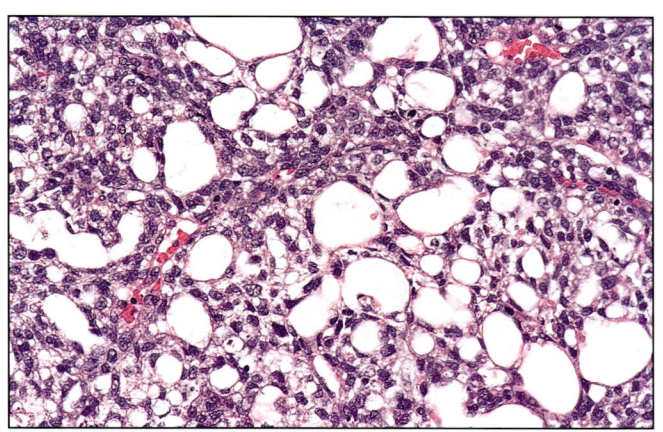

图21C.61 胸腺卵黄囊瘤。典型的卵黄囊瘤伴有微囊性结构。

鉴别诊断

- **胸腺癌**：胸腺癌与生殖细胞肿瘤相比倾向于发生在老年人。肿瘤细胞排列成片块状、小管状和乳头状，其中细胞核非常密集，呈空泡状者多半是胚胎性癌。出现微囊性结构、Schiller-Duval小体和丰富的细胞外基底膜样物质时，支持卵黄囊瘤的诊断。
- **大细胞淋巴瘤**：精原细胞瘤和大细胞淋巴瘤有时可能难以鉴别，尤其是当淋巴瘤主要是由成簇的透明细胞组成时。丰富的糖原支持精原细胞瘤的诊断，而核呈分叶状支持淋巴瘤的诊断。如果患者是女性，诊断纵隔精原细胞瘤时应慎重。

免疫细胞化学

各种类型的生殖细胞肿瘤细胞角蛋白均呈阳性反应，除精原细胞瘤细胞角蛋白染色为阴性或仅呈局灶性或片块状阳性反应（常常伴有点状结构）[12,20,294,334]。与胸腺癌不同，除了绒毛膜癌和畸胎瘤外，上皮膜抗原极少表达。

精原细胞瘤胎盘碱性磷酸酶免疫染色阳性，但是胚胎癌、卵黄囊瘤和绒毛膜癌也可以阳性。精原细胞瘤的另外一个标记物是c-kit（CD117），表达于细胞膜和（或）Golgi结构[335]。大部分胚胎性癌CD30呈阳性，尽管卵黄囊瘤也有不同程度的阳性表达。Oct-3/4是一个转录因子，仅在精原细胞瘤和胚胎性癌表达，而在卵黄囊瘤和畸胎瘤不表达[336]。HCG染色见于绒毛膜癌、胚胎性癌和伴有合体滋养细胞的精原细胞瘤。甲胎蛋白染色见于卵黄囊瘤、一些胚胎性癌和少数畸胎瘤[12,20,294,301,334]。

淋巴细胞、组织细胞和树突状细胞肿瘤
Lymphoid, histiocytic and dendritic cell tumors

尽管任何组织学类型的淋巴瘤均可发生于胸腺，但绝大部分病例为以下几个类型：

- 结节硬化性Hodgkin淋巴瘤
- 纵隔大B细胞淋巴瘤
- T淋巴母细胞淋巴瘤。

间变性大细胞淋巴瘤、结外边缘带黏膜相关淋巴组织型B细胞淋巴瘤以及罕见的外周T细胞淋巴瘤也可以发生于胸腺[337-339]。

由于各种类型的淋巴瘤在本章淋巴结一节中已有详细描述，所以本节仅讨论纵隔大B细胞淋巴瘤和发生于纵隔部位的淋巴瘤的特殊表现。

Hodgkin淋巴瘤 Hodgkin lymphoma (HL)

临床特征和病理学

发生于胸腺的Hodgkin淋巴瘤几乎完全是结节硬化型。多数患者为年轻人，女性多见。表现为与纵隔肿物相关的症状，或在胸部X线检查时偶然发现纵隔肿物。可能伴有锁骨上淋巴结肿大。

组织学特征与发生在其他部位的典型的结节硬化性Hodgkin淋巴瘤相同。然而，由纵隔部位引起的许多组织学变化可能造成诊断困难：

- 常有散在的内衬胸腺上皮的囊肿，而在囊壁上发现有Hodgkin淋巴瘤结节。这种现象可能是由于胸腺髓质导管阻塞扩张引起的（图21C.62）。因此，在做出胸腺多房性囊肿诊断前，必须仔细检查囊壁和间隔，看是否存在Hodgkin淋巴瘤或其他肿瘤。
- Hodgkin淋巴瘤可能伴有胸腺上皮的显著反应性增生，注意与胸腺瘤的鉴别诊断（图21C.63）。
- 在成功的放疗之后，可能形成大的内衬上皮的胸腺囊腔，临床上类似于复发的Hodgkin淋巴瘤[340]。
- 有些病例有突出的肉芽肿，可能被误诊为"肉芽肿性炎症"。
- 在一些病例，Hodgkin淋巴瘤可以与纵隔大B细胞淋巴瘤共存[341,342]。

鉴别诊断

由于存在厚的包膜，结节被纤维性间隔分开，而且明显混有大细胞和小淋巴细胞，因此结节硬化性Hodgkin淋巴瘤可能被误诊为胸腺瘤。然而，Hodgkin淋巴瘤的结节通常是圆形的不成角，且与纤维组织的分界不像胸腺瘤中见到的那样明显。细胞组成也不相同：

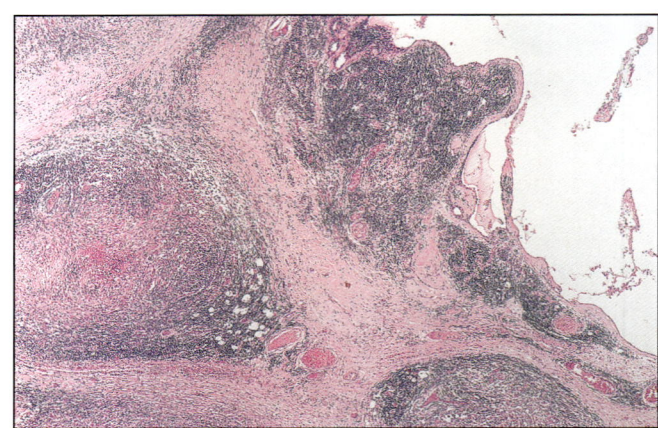

图21C.62 结节硬化性Hodgkin淋巴瘤累及胸腺。注意淋巴瘤结节由宽大的硬化带分隔。淋巴瘤常常伴有胸腺上皮囊肿形成（视野右侧）。

Hodgkin淋巴瘤混有组织细胞和嗜酸性粒细胞，而肿瘤细胞显示陷窝细胞和Reed-Sternberg细胞的特征。

对于富于陷窝细胞和Reed-Sternberg细胞的病例，可能难以与纵隔大B细胞淋巴瘤鉴别。以下特征支持Hodgkin淋巴瘤的诊断：

- 较明显的炎症性背景，常常伴有明显的嗜酸性粒细胞成分
- 在肿瘤细胞形成大的结节，或成片的区域中可见地图样坏死
- 缺乏CD45/LCA表达
- CD20呈阴性或染色不均匀
- Oct-2和Bob.1呈阴性，或两种标记物中至多一种呈阳性
- 缺乏MAL表达
- EB病毒呈阳性。

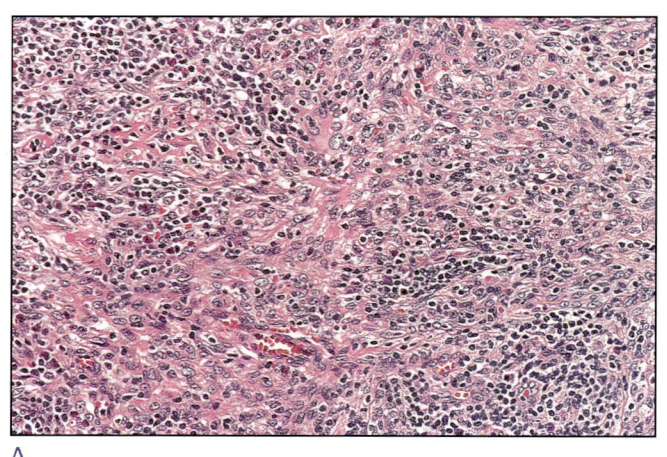

A

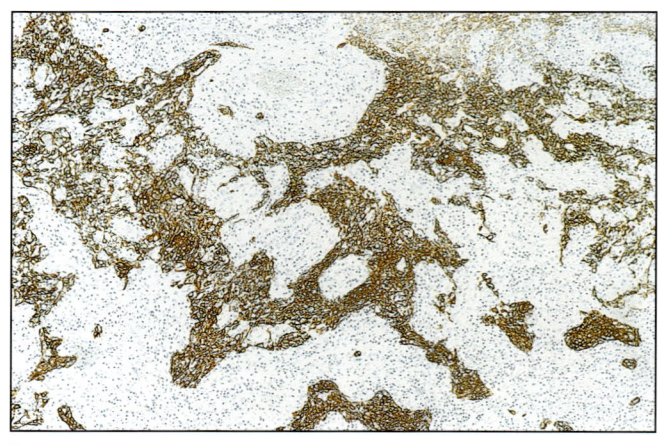

B

图21C.63 结节硬化性Hodgkin淋巴瘤伴有明显的胸腺上皮增生。（A）显著的梭形上皮细胞增生见于Hodgkin淋巴瘤累及的许多区域。（B）细胞角蛋白免疫染色显示增生的胸腺上皮呈强阳性。

纵隔大B细胞淋巴瘤
Mediastinal large B-cell lymphoma

定义

纵隔大B细胞淋巴瘤是发生在前纵隔的一种独特类型的淋巴瘤，常常起源于胸腺。可能是来源于胸腺髓质的固有B细胞群，与滤泡中心或外套区B细胞无明显关系[7,337,343-348]。

临床特征

纵隔大B细胞淋巴瘤占所有非Hodgkin淋巴瘤的2.4%[349]。最常见于年轻女性，平均发病年龄为37岁，男女比例为1:2。患者出现上腔静脉阻塞或与纵隔肿块相关的症状，如咳嗽和呼吸困难，少数患者没有症状[343,344,347,350-359]。肿瘤通常巨大（大于10 cm）。胸膜和心包渗出常见。多数患者（66%）发现时为I期或II期，骨髓受累非常罕见（纵隔为3%，而普通大B细胞淋巴瘤为17%）[349,360]。血清乳酸脱氢酶水平常常升高（约75%），但是 β_2-微球蛋白水平往往正常，原因是淋巴瘤细胞I型HLA表达不足[355]。

临床行为和治疗

淋巴瘤可以局灶侵犯心包、胸膜、肺、胸骨和胸壁。它可以播散到外周淋巴结和诸如卵巢、肾、肾上腺和肠等少见部位[347,356,361,362]，虽然在一些研究中并未观察到具有播散到少见部位的倾向[360,363]。26%的患者在发现时或在复发时出现脑实质和软脑膜受累。

对CHOP等标准化疗方案的反应一般并不令人满意（只有约50%的完全缓解率），但是当大剂量联合应用多种药物时，疗效一般可以得到改善。应用辅助放疗后这两种类型化疗的治疗效果进一步改善（大剂量化疗加上放疗的完全缓解率达到80%左右）[352,354,355,360,365,366]。经过最佳的治疗，10年病情无进展的生存率可以高达78%[349,354,360,363,366,367]。

预后不好的因素包括：肿瘤巨大（>10 cm）、血清乳酸脱氢酶水平高、心包积液、身体状态差以及国际预后指数（International Progaostic Index）高（指数为4或5，没有出现衰竭的患者5年生存率为0；而指数为0或1的患者则为69%）以及未能达到完全缓解[349,355,358,360,363,368]。治疗后通过放射线评估或镓扫描发现纵隔肿块持续存在时，伴有较高的复发危险率[358,360,367]。

病理学

淋巴瘤细胞从中等大小到很大，伴有圆形、肾形或多叶状细胞核，染色质空泡状，并有多个清楚的核仁（图21C.64）[343,344,347,350,351,369]。细胞具有中等量到丰富的淡染、透明或嗜双色性胞浆。虽然透明细胞具有特征性[344,370-372]，但仅出现在约40%的病例中[360,369,373]。肿瘤内可能混合有Reed-Sternberg样细胞、高度多形性的肿瘤细胞和小淋巴细胞[350,374]。在单个病例中，肿瘤细胞的形态学表现通常比较一致，但在不同病例之间，细胞形态学差别非常显著[369]。

肿瘤呈弥散性生长方式，但常常出现纤细的硬化带或宽的玻璃样变性带，常常导致"分隔"结构，类似于癌或精原细胞瘤（图21C.65和21C.66）。不过，硬化并不是诊断的必备条件[360,373]。淋巴瘤细胞可能表现为梭形，因为硬化性间质可以使之变形[350]。经常出现坏死。血管内膜下或透壁浸润常见，有助于诊断。残留的胸腺上皮岛可见淋巴瘤细胞浸润，也可显示反应性增生或出现囊性变，伴有多发性囊肿形成。罕见情况下，肿瘤细胞可显示残留反应性生发中心的趋向性[375]。

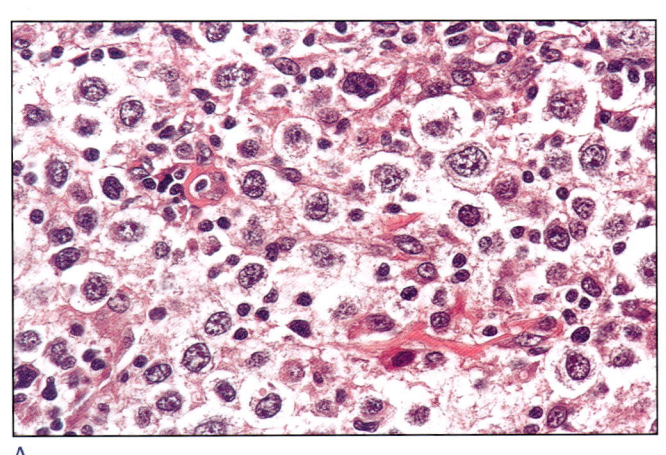

A

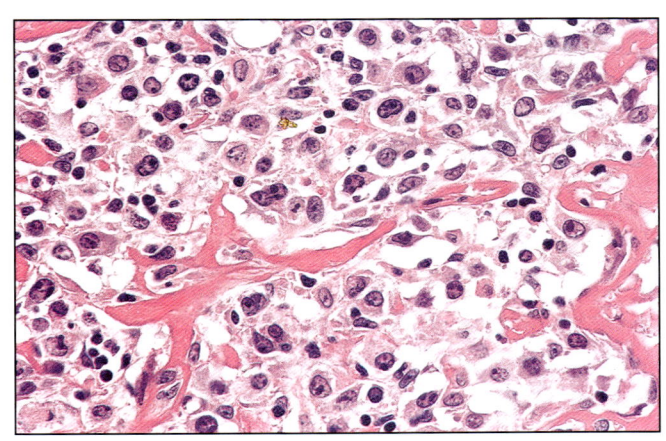

B

图21C.64 纵隔大B细胞淋巴瘤。（A）淋巴瘤细胞大，具有圆形细胞核和透明的胞浆。这种细胞容易被误认为是精原细胞瘤的细胞。（B）本例的特征是核有折叠，胞浆丰富呈淡嗜酸性。肿瘤内可见纤细的硬化带穿过。

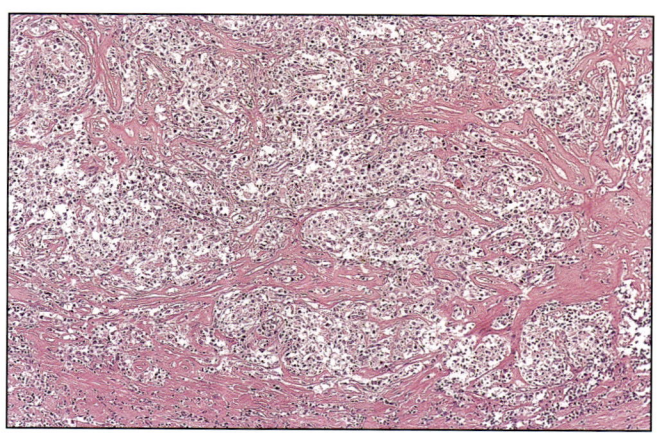

图21C.65 纵隔大B细胞淋巴瘤。肿瘤通常显示突出的硬化，形成巢状结构。

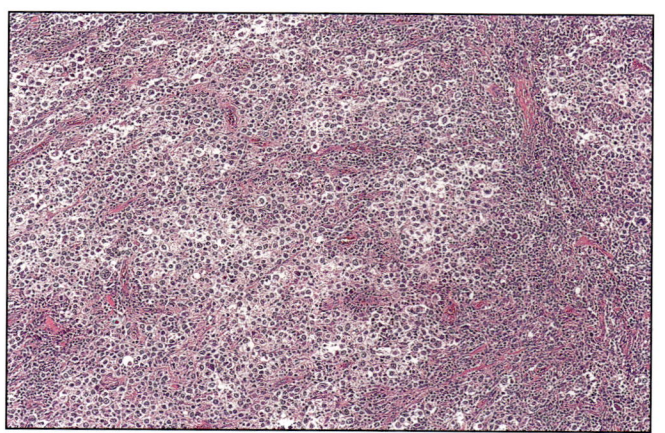

图21C.66 纵隔大B细胞淋巴瘤。出现间隔、透明细胞并混有淋巴细胞，形成一种非常类似于精原细胞瘤的结构。

免疫细胞化学

- 广谱B细胞标记物如CD20、CD79a、PAX5、Oct-2和Bob.1呈阳性[345,371,373,376,377]。
- CD5、CD10和CD21通常呈阴性。与普通的弥漫性大B细胞淋巴瘤不同，纵隔大B细胞淋巴瘤常常缺乏表面免疫球蛋白表达，尽管常常表达免疫球蛋白相关的CD79a分子[337,343,344,347,353,376-379]。CD23可能具有诊断意义，因为70%的纵隔大B细胞淋巴瘤表达CD23，而非纵隔大B细胞淋巴瘤只有约10%表达[9]。70%的病例表达一种T细胞限制性标记物MAL，而只有少数非纵隔大B细胞淋巴瘤表达MAL。
- CD30表达发生在约70%的病例，但是染色通常呈斑片状弱表达。CD15表达非常罕见[373,377]。通常缺乏主要组织相容性复合体（major histocompatibility complex, MHC）分子表达[370]，而且MHC II表达缺失与预后不良有关[381]。
- 14%~35%的病例可能缺乏CD45RB的表达[360,373]。人绒毛膜促性腺激素免疫反应已有少数报道[382]。

遗传学特征

我们对纵隔大B细胞淋巴瘤分子生物学的理解已经有了较大的突破。这种类型的淋巴瘤具有不同于普通弥漫性大B细胞淋巴瘤的特征性遗传学改变，包括染色体9p（JAK2基因所在位置）和Xq扩增[383,384]，以及BCL2和BCL6基因缺失或罕有的重排[360,385-387]。EB病毒呈阴性。纵隔大B细胞淋巴瘤常有MAL基因过表达，胸腺髓质的少数B细胞亚群也有MAL基因表达，纵隔大B细胞淋巴瘤可能起源于这种细胞[380,388]。基因表达谱显然不同于活化的B细胞或弥漫性大B细胞淋巴瘤生发中心的B细胞，但却与结节硬化性Hodgkin淋巴瘤的基因表达谱非常相似，包括B细胞受体成分和信号级联系统低表达、细胞因子通路成分、肿瘤坏死因子（TNF）家族成员和细胞外基质以及κ基因结合核因子（NF-κB）通路结构激活高表达[389,390]。因此，有人提出，纵隔大B细胞淋巴瘤和结节硬化性Hodgkin淋巴瘤可能起源于共同的前体细胞，或者这两种疾病可能是生物学谱系相对的两极，并且伴有表现为纵隔灰区淋巴瘤的中间体形式[391]。然而，纵隔大B细胞淋巴瘤和Hodgkin淋巴瘤的基因表达谱仍有明显差别，部分纵隔大B细胞淋巴瘤的特征基因和诸如CD19、CD20、CD22、CD79a和Oct-2等成熟B细胞基因在Hodgkin淋巴瘤中没有表达。

纵隔大B细胞淋巴瘤的界定问题

前纵隔大B细胞淋巴瘤可能不是同质性的疾病，而是包括两组肿瘤：真正的胸腺大B细胞淋巴瘤和起源于纵隔淋巴结的大B细胞淋巴瘤[350,353,379,392]。可能仅前者具有特征性，主要发生于年轻女性，通常缺乏Ig表达。后者就像普通的淋巴结大B细胞淋巴瘤，常常发生于老年男性，Ig通常阳性。在一些病例研究中缺乏女性优势，可能是由于后一组病例所占比例较大。因为研究表明MAL基因表达是纵隔大B细胞淋巴瘤特有的特征，所以需要进一步研究它在界定和诊断这种类型淋巴瘤中的作用[388]。

鉴别诊断

- 大细胞淋巴瘤常被误诊为胸腺瘤或胸腺癌。进一步的研究证实，许多"看上去古怪的"胸腺肿瘤为大细胞淋巴瘤。形成很好的胸腺小体很少出现于胸腺瘤，在恶性肿瘤中出现胸腺小体支持淋巴瘤的诊断。浸润纤维间隔、浸润血管壁以及有显著的多叶核也支持淋巴瘤的诊断。通过白细胞标记物免疫染色容易做出淋巴瘤的明确诊断。细胞角蛋白免疫染色有时能够明确显示突出的陷入或增生的胸腺上皮成分，但常呈片块状分布，不同于胸腺瘤的广泛网状分布。

- 纵隔大B细胞淋巴瘤的巢状结构和透明细胞可能与生殖细胞瘤非常相似。缺乏糖原和核膜显著不规则有助于淋巴瘤的诊断。
- 当硬化明显时，由于皱缩的人为假象使淋巴瘤细胞似乎变小，可导致小细胞淋巴瘤的错误诊断。
- 纵隔大B细胞淋巴瘤与结节硬化性Hodgkin淋巴瘤的合胞体型变异的鉴别有时非常困难。见上面"Hodgkin淋巴瘤"一节。

纵隔灰区淋巴瘤
Mediastinal gray zone lymphoma

灰区淋巴瘤是指不能确定是具有经典Hodgkin淋巴瘤特征还是具有大B细胞淋巴瘤特征的不能分类的肿瘤[342,393-395]。这并不奇怪，因为经典Hodgkin淋巴瘤是B细胞肿瘤，与B细胞非Hodgkin淋巴瘤并不能截然分开。经典Hodgkin淋巴瘤与大B细胞淋巴瘤有如下相似之处：

- 常常缺乏Ⅰ型HLA和Ig基因的功能表达。
- 经典Hodgkin淋巴瘤CD30呈阳性，而纵隔大B细胞淋巴瘤CD30通常也呈阳性。
- 纵隔大B细胞淋巴瘤的一些肿瘤细胞可能类似于经典的Reed-Sternberg细胞和陷窝细胞。
- 基因表达谱广泛重叠。

与纵隔Hodgkin淋巴瘤和纵隔大B细胞淋巴瘤不同，纵隔灰区淋巴瘤男性比女性常见[342,395]。所有患者都表现为大的纵隔肿物。有些病例显示提示结节硬化性Hodgkin淋巴瘤的形态学特征，但是具有大量单核变异细胞，背景炎症细胞减少，CD20染色均匀一致呈强阳性，而且有时CD45有表达。另外一些病例形态学类似于纵隔大B细胞淋巴瘤，但是混有Hodgkin/陷窝细胞，CD20不表达或弱表达，CD15呈阳性。进一步的免疫组化检查发现，其免疫组化表型更类似于纵隔大B细胞淋巴瘤，多数病例表达PAX-5、Oct-2和Bob.1[342]。MAL也常有表达（78%）[342]。

T淋巴母细胞淋巴瘤的前体病变
Precursor T-lymphoblastic lymphoma

临床特征和病理学

T淋巴母细胞淋巴瘤一般发生于青少年和年轻人，表现为由于大的纵隔肿物和（或）胸膜渗出而引起的呼吸窘迫急性发作。锁骨上淋巴结也可肿大。肿瘤生长迅速，本病是一种需要立即治疗的肿瘤科急症[396]。除了活组织检查以外，可以尝试颈部肿物细针吸取或抽取胸腔积液以提供迅速的诊断信息。病理学和免疫细胞化学详见1172页。少数患者在开始治疗的60天内胸部X线检查正常，其预后明显好于伴有持续性纵隔肿块的患者[397]。少数情况下，B细胞或自然杀伤谱系的淋巴母细胞淋巴瘤也可发生于前纵隔[398,399]。

鉴别诊断

- 淋巴母细胞淋巴瘤：可被误诊为富于淋巴细胞的胸腺瘤，尤其是在小的活检标本。即使应用免疫组化检查也可能误诊，因为两者均富有不成熟T细胞（TdT⁺）和细胞角蛋白阳性的胸腺上皮细胞（肿瘤性或陷入的）。对正确诊断淋巴母细胞淋巴瘤有帮助的组织学线索有：
  - 淋巴细胞弥漫浸润纤维间隔和脂肪组织（图21C.67）
  - 缺少明显的小叶结构
  - 染色质细腻及核扭曲（图21C.68）
  - 常见核分裂象。
- 表现为纵隔肿块的粒细胞肉瘤（granulocytic

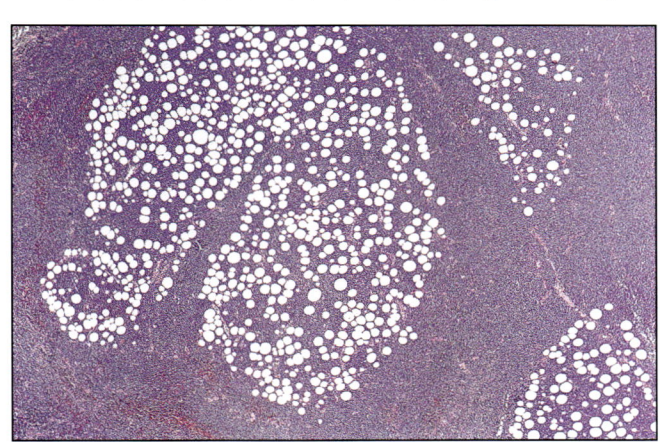

图21C.67 前纵隔T淋巴母细胞性淋巴瘤。一般呈弥漫性浸润，广泛浸润脂肪组织。除了白血病外，这种浸润方式很少见于其他类型的胸腺肿瘤。

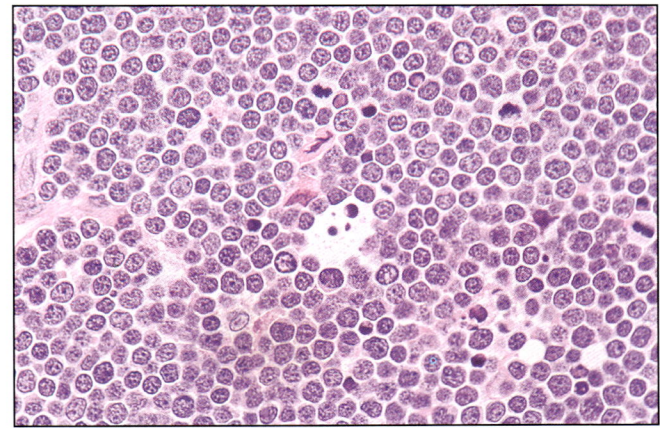

图21C.68 前纵隔T淋巴母细胞性淋巴瘤。淋巴瘤细胞一般中等大小，核膜薄，染色质细腻。

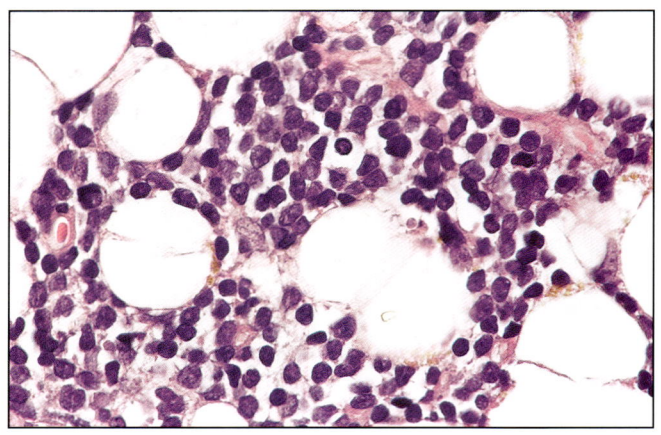

图21C.69 前纵隔T淋巴母细胞性淋巴瘤。纵隔镜活检时人为挤压造成肿瘤细胞小而深染，可能误诊为小淋巴细胞淋巴瘤。仔细观察相对完好区域可以发现，细胞实际上比小淋巴细胞略大。通过TdT免疫染色可能容易确定诊断。

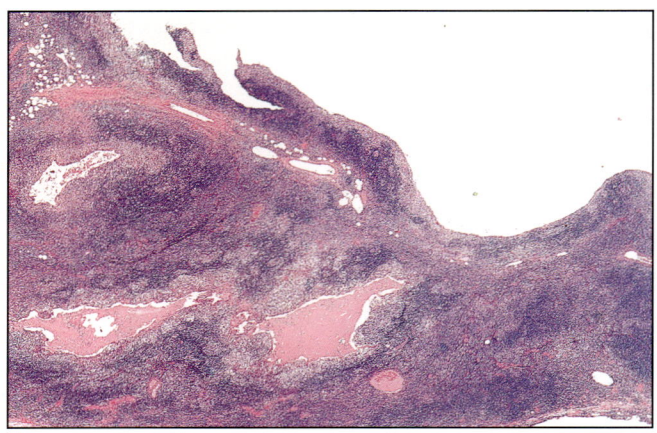

A

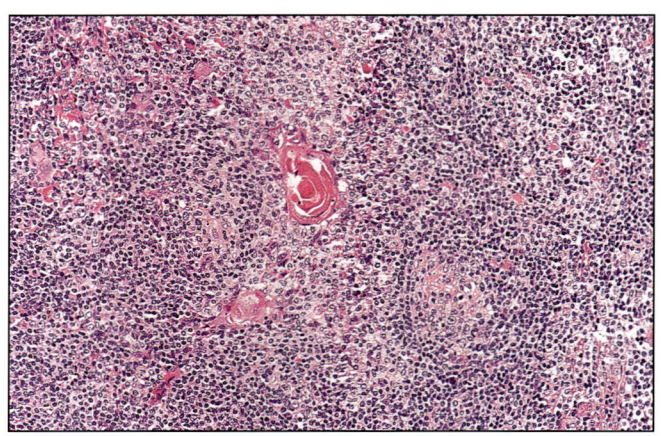

B

图21C.70 胸腺的结外边缘区B细胞淋巴瘤。（A）内衬胸腺上皮的多发性囊腔实际上是这种类型胸腺肿瘤的一个固定特征。由于出现异质性的细胞群，这种类型淋巴瘤一般呈现多样化的表现。囊腔周围的细胞较大，染色较淡，形成囊腔周围淡染环。（B）可见反应性淋巴滤泡（右下方）。淋巴瘤细胞浸润并扩展到视野中心的胸腺小体。淋巴瘤细胞包括类似于小淋巴细胞的细胞、单核细胞样B细胞和某些浆细胞。

sarcoma）：可被误诊为淋巴母细胞淋巴瘤。前者核通常较大，核仁较清楚，具有丰富的胞浆。另外，可以出现散在的嗜酸性髓细胞，为正确诊断进一步提供了线索。

- 小细胞淋巴瘤：在小的活检标本中，因组织固定欠佳或组织切片较厚，淋巴母细胞可以出现小而深染的细胞核，可能被误认为低级别小细胞淋巴瘤（图21C.69）。患者年轻是正确诊断最重要的线索。

黏膜相关淋巴组织型结外边缘区B细胞淋巴瘤
Extranodal marginal zone B-cell lymphoma of MALT type

临床特征

黏膜相关淋巴组织型结外边缘区B细胞淋巴瘤可以是原发性胸腺肿瘤。多数患者为成人（41～50岁和51～60岁年龄组），女性多见。本病在亚洲人群中比较流行。与自身免疫性疾病密切相关（＞50%），尤其是Sjögren综合征和类风湿性关节炎[4,378,404-409]。多数患者无症状，纵隔肿块是在影像学检查时的偶然发现。局部淋巴结可能受累。常见异型蛋白血症（常为IgA）。本病呈惰性经过，预后较好。

病理学

大体上，胸腺常常显示多发性囊肿，后者被褐色鱼肉样肿瘤分开。组织学特征与结外边缘区B细胞淋巴瘤相同。背景中出现反应性淋巴滤泡（图21C.70）。中心细胞样细胞或类似于单核细胞样B细胞的细胞常常形成宽带状或片块状，伴有明显的浸润并蔓延至胸腺上皮和胸腺小体（图21C.70）。常常出现成簇的浆细胞（肿瘤性）。多发性散在的囊肿内衬难以归类的细胞或非角化性复层鳞状上皮，类似于多房性胸腺囊肿。肿瘤细胞表达B细胞系标记物，并且常常合成IgA[409]。

免疫细胞化学特征

- 全B细胞标记物阳性。
- CD5、CD10、CD23和cyclin D1呈阴性。75%以上的病例表达IgA。

遗传学特征

Ig基因克隆性重排，大约半数病例伴有体细胞超突变。没有进行性突变[410]。Ig基因分析显示，V（H）基因倾向于形成V（H）3-30和V（H）3-23片断，自身免疫性B细胞经常表达这两个片断。观察到的V（H）基因利用和突变提示，在胸腺MALT型淋巴瘤的发生和进展中，特异性抗原可能起了病理学相关作用[409,410]。*API2-MALT1* 基因融合是结外边缘区B细胞淋巴瘤独特的分子学特征，在胸腺来源的MALT型淋巴瘤没有观察到这种基因融合[409]。

鉴别诊断

- 胸腺反应性淋巴细胞增生：支持淋巴瘤诊断的主要特征是：淋巴细胞浸润的破坏性本质和在胸腺小体内形成明显的淋巴上皮病变。免疫组化染色证明有大片的B细胞或轻链限制性，可以证实淋巴瘤的诊断。
- 透明血管型Castleman病：前纵隔是Castleman病的好发部位。特征性的透明血管滤泡不同于结外边缘区B细胞淋巴瘤的反应性滤泡。滤泡间区域由小淋巴细胞组成，有许多具有高内皮的小静脉穿过。免疫染色显示B细胞主要局限于滤泡，而滤泡间区主要是T细胞，这与结外边缘区B细胞淋巴瘤滤泡间区出现成片的B细胞形成对比。
- 显示胸腺受累的其他类型小B细胞淋巴瘤。

组织细胞和树突状细胞肿瘤
Histiocytic and dendritic cell tumors

发生在儿童的Langerhans细胞组织细胞增生症（Langerhans cell histiocytosis）可以单独累及胸腺，或作为多器官疾病的一部分。如果受累的部位数目不多，则预后较好[411]。有时可能是重症肌无力患者切除胸腺时的偶然发现[412-415]。组织学上，具有核沟的Langerhans细胞浸润胸腺，伴有胸腺上皮破坏[416]。通过S-100蛋白、CD1a和langerin免疫染色容易确定诊断。

累及胸腺的组织细胞肉瘤（histiocytic sarcoma）和恶性组织细胞增生症（malignant histiocytosis）非常罕见，几乎总是作为纵隔生殖细胞肿瘤的并发症出现[302-304,417]。在少数情况下，前纵隔也可以发生原发性滤泡树突状细胞肿瘤（follicular dendritic cell tumor），可以发生在透明血管型Castleman病的患者中（见第21章第一部分）[418-422]。交错树突状细胞肿瘤（interdigitating dendritic cell tumor）和显示杂合树突状细胞表型的肿瘤也有少数报道[423]。

胸腺和前纵隔间叶性肿瘤
Mesenchymal tumors of the thymus and anterior mediastinum

各种间叶性肿瘤均可发生于前纵隔，虽然常常难以确定肿瘤是起源于胸腺还是起源于纵隔软组织。有些肉瘤可能起源于纵隔生殖细胞肿瘤内[310]。

脂肪瘤 Lipoma

脂肪瘤是纵隔最常见的良性间叶性肿瘤。肿瘤通常较大。与胸腺脂肪瘤（thymolipoma）不同，其不存在散在的胸腺实质成分[424]。

脂肪肉瘤 Liposarcoma

临床特征

脂肪肉瘤可以发生在前纵隔，有时可累及其他部位（如腹膜后和股部）[424-427]。含有胸腺组织的病例可以认为是胸腺脂肪瘤的相应恶性病变（所谓的胸腺脂肪肉瘤，thymoliposarcoma）[428]。

前纵隔脂肪肉瘤患者的平均发病年龄为43岁，男性发病略占优势。肿瘤最常在胸部X线检查时偶然发现，但是有些患者可出现呼吸困难或胸痛。32%的病例发生复发，平均时间间隔为3年。黏液样脂肪肉瘤的预后比高分化脂肪肉瘤差[428]。

病理学

高分化脂肪肉瘤占病例的60%，黏液样脂肪肉瘤占28%，其余12%具有混合性特征。少数病例有大量淋巴浆细胞浸润，类似于淋巴瘤或反应性纤维炎性病变。

胸腺脂肪瘤 Thymolipoma

临床特征

胸腺脂肪瘤又名胸腺脂肪瘤性错构瘤（thymolipomatous hamartoma），是由胸腺和成熟脂肪组织构成的罕见良性肿瘤。至于是肿瘤、错构瘤还是仅仅是增生性胸腺中的脂肪增生，目前还存在争议[4,144]。

患者年龄从2岁到64岁不等（最常见于10～30岁之间），平均年龄为33岁[429-431]。无性别差异。50%以上的患者表现为与肿块性病变相关的症状，或出现少见的瘤外综合征，如重症肌无力、红细胞发育不良、低丙种球蛋白血症、Graves病以及再生障碍性贫血[2,430,432]。肿瘤为良性，手术切除可以治愈。

病理学

胸腺脂肪瘤通常较大，重量超过500克，大小从4.5 cm到36 cm不等[430]。肿瘤界限清楚，切面质软黄色，伴有散在的白色条纹或实性区域。

组织学上，肿瘤由大的成熟脂肪细胞小叶组成，伴有散在的含有胸腺小体的胸腺组织的结构正常，胸腺小

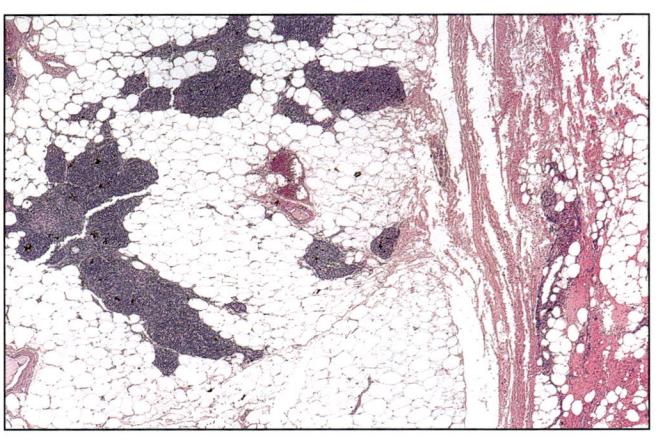

图21C.71 胸腺脂肪瘤。肿瘤界限清楚,由丰富的成熟脂肪组织和散在于其中的灶状胸腺组织构成。

体通常可见囊性变和钙化（图21C.71）[430]。两种成分所占比例差异很大,但是肿瘤中胸腺组织的量通常超过正常情况下对应于患者年龄所应有的胸腺组织的量。少数情况下,可以见到肌样细胞[433]。此外,胸腺脂肪瘤内可以发生胸腺瘤[434]。

胸腺纤维脂肪瘤（thymofibrolipoma）是罕见的变型,间质成分由大量纤维结缔组织和散在的脂肪组织构成。

孤立性纤维瘤 Solitary fibrous tumor

孤立性纤维性肿瘤偶尔可以作为原发性肿瘤发生在前纵隔,与发生于胸膜和软组织的孤立性纤维瘤相同[436-438]。有时可能发生低血糖症。肿瘤是由伴有少量胞浆的梭形细胞构成的,伴有致密的胶原,通常有细胞丰富和细胞稀少区域交替出现。血管外皮细胞瘤性血管结构并不少见。尽管肿瘤看似温和,但是超过一半的病例可出现细胞非典型性、核分裂活性、凝固性坏死乃至明显的肉瘤性区域。肿瘤CD34呈阳性,细胞角蛋白呈阴性。纵隔孤立性纤维瘤的肿瘤侵袭性比发生于其他部位的强,大约50%的病例发生局部复发,25%死亡[10]。

主要应与梭形细胞胸腺瘤鉴别,后者的胶原形成分隔而不是与肿瘤细胞密切混合,而且肿瘤细胞细胞角蛋白染色呈阳性。

滑膜肉瘤 Synovial sarcoma

前纵隔或后纵隔的原发性滑膜肉瘤的发病年龄广泛[439,440]。肿瘤可以局限或浸润周围的解剖学结构。局部复发和远处转移常见[440]。双相性病例的特征是由排列成巢、裂隙状、乳头状和腺样结构的上皮性成分与排列成束的梭形细胞错综混合而成。单相性病例由单一形态的梭形细胞群组成。一些病例出现囊性变、坏死、出血、玻璃样变性和钙化。通过免疫组化研究可以确定诊断,通过证实特征性的SYT-SSX基因融合可以进一步支持诊断。

脉管和相关肿瘤 Vascular and related tumors

淋巴管瘤是儿童前纵隔常见的肿瘤[441-443]。前纵隔血管瘤通常为海绵状血管瘤,但也可以是富于细胞的毛细血管瘤,并可合并Kasabach-Merritt综合征[443-446]。所谓的血管外皮细胞瘤、上皮样血管内皮细胞瘤（可能含有破骨巨细胞）和血管肉瘤也有报道[443,444,447-450]。血管肉瘤常为恶性畸胎瘤的肉瘤性成分而不是单独发生的肿瘤（图21C.59B）[11,310,451,452]。

横纹肌肉瘤 Rhabdomyosarcoma

累及胸腺或前纵隔的横纹肌肉瘤最常以畸胎瘤合并症的形式出现,也就是畸胎瘤伴有另外的恶性成分（图21C.59A）[11,12],或作为胸腺癌肉瘤的一种部分。

少数情况下,胸腺可以发生原发性横纹肌肉瘤[443,453]。通常发生于年轻成人,表现为与纵隔肿块相关的症状。本病具有高度侵袭性的临床经过,通常在6个月内出现复发和转移并引起死亡[453]。组织学上,可以是腺泡状、胚胎性或多形性横纹肌肉瘤[453]。少数病例主要由透明细胞构成[454]。

发生于胸腺的异位肿瘤 Ectopic tumors occurring in the thymus

由于在发育过程中迁移异常,纵隔内可见甲状腺组织[4]。少数情况下,甲状腺肿瘤可以起源于异位甲状腺组织,表现为发生在颈部的一系列的甲状腺肿瘤[445-459]。

因为下极的甲状旁腺与胸腺共同起源于第三咽囊,异位甲状旁腺可以发生于前上纵隔。因此,甲状旁腺腺瘤可发生于纵隔,而且多达22%的患者出现甲状旁腺功能亢进症（图21C.72）（见第18章第二部分）[261,457,459-464]。少数情况下,甲状旁腺癌也可以发生于纵隔[261,464,465]。甲状旁腺肿瘤可能显示以嗜酸细胞或主细胞为主,也可以为混合细胞型[464]。通过甲状旁腺激素免疫染色检查阳性可容易确定甲状旁腺肿瘤的诊断。

胸腺和前纵隔的罕见的肿瘤和瘤样病变 Rare tumors and tumor-like lesions of the thymus and anterior mediastinum

已报道的发生在胸腺或前纵隔的一些罕见肿瘤和瘤样病变包括：浆细胞瘤[466,467]、粒细胞肉瘤（经常伴有硬化）[400,401,468-471]、炎性假瘤[472]、硬化性纵隔炎（特发

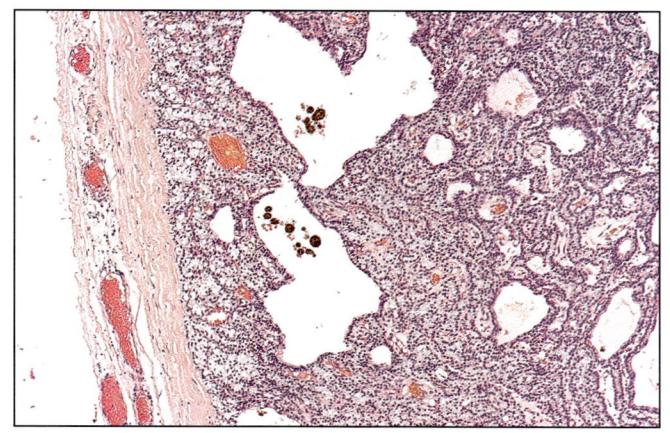

图21C.72 胸腺内异位甲状旁腺腺瘤。辨认甲状旁腺性质的线索是透明细胞和呈栅栏状排列的核。甲状旁腺激素免疫染色可以确定诊断。

性纤维炎症性病变)[473]、副神经节瘤[261,474-476]、室管膜瘤[473]、良性和恶性神经鞘肿瘤(与前纵隔比,后纵隔常见的多)[443,478,479]、恶性Triton瘤[480]、神经母细胞瘤(在成人伴有不适当的抗利尿激素综合征)[481]、神经节母细胞瘤[482]、纤维瘤病[442]、弹力纤维脂肪瘤[483]、巨细胞血管纤维瘤[484]、血管瘤样纤维组织细胞瘤[485]、平滑肌瘤[442]、平滑肌肉瘤(可能起源于支气管囊肿)[486-488]、脂肪平滑肌肉瘤[489]、横纹肌瘤[490]、腺泡状软组织肉瘤[491]、良性间叶瘤[424]、脂肪母细胞瘤病[492]、软骨脂肪瘤[493]、所谓的恶性纤维组织细胞瘤[443,494]、恶性横纹肌样肿瘤[144]、骨肉瘤[495-497]、软骨肉瘤[498]、间皮瘤[424]、肺型硬化性血管瘤[499]和涎腺型混合瘤[500],以及起源于淋巴上皮性囊肿或前肠重复囊肿的腺癌(严格说来不是原发性胸腺上皮肿瘤)[501-503]。

胸腺或前纵隔转移性肿瘤
Metastatic tumors in thymus or anterior mediastinum

除了由邻近器官的肿瘤直接浸润以外,胸腺和前纵隔的淋巴结可发生转移性肿瘤[504]。各种类型的肿瘤均可扩散至这个部位,如甲状腺癌、黑色素瘤、前列腺癌和支气管源性癌[505-507]。

纵隔肿瘤:诊断方法和误区
Mediastinal tumors: diagnostic approach and pitfalls

纵隔肿瘤的组织学分型

纵隔肿瘤切除标本的组织学分型一般并不困难,但由于组织较小,有挤压和压迫的人为假象(细胞表现为小而深染),纵隔镜或穿刺活检的诊断可能出现困难。

在鉴别胸腺瘤和恶性淋巴瘤时,以下特征强烈支持胸腺瘤的诊断:

- 明显的小叶状结构,至少有些小叶伴有成角的轮廓(图21C.7和21C.11)。
- 宽而无细胞的纤维性间隔(图21C.7)。
- 无法解释的散在的大而淡染的细胞,细胞界限不清(图21C.12B和21C.14)。
- 血管周围间隙(图21C.12C和21C.15A)。
- 出现CD20阳性的星状淋巴细胞(星样B细胞)[151]。

另一方面,淋巴瘤的特征是在纤维性间质内呈比较弥漫的生长,并且常常出现核的多分叶状结构。参见"Hodgkin淋巴瘤"一节的特征,有助于鉴别纵隔大B细胞淋巴瘤和结节硬化性Hodgkin淋巴瘤。

胸腺类癌可以与其他类型肿瘤鉴别,如胸腺癌具有明显的纤细的纤维血管间隔(图21C.48),小梁状或巢状排列,常见粉刺样坏死和钙化以及颗粒状胞浆。生殖细胞肿瘤常应该考虑为纵隔的恶性肿瘤。

是胸腺瘤还是胸腺癌?

一个富于上皮的胸腺肿瘤可能引起是胸腺瘤(主要为B3型)还是胸腺癌(鳞状细胞癌)的鉴别诊断问题。下列特征(代表缺少器官型本质)支持胸腺癌的诊断:

- 虽然以轮廓明显光滑为主的肿瘤性上皮岛表面上可能类似于胸腺瘤的特征性小叶结构,但其不同之处在于上皮岛要小,而且至少显示有一些上皮岛轮廓不规则(图21C.37A)。
- 肿瘤细胞岛之间是富于细胞的纤维组织增生性间质,常常伴有淋巴细胞和浆细胞浸润,而不是硬化性间质(图21C.37B)。
- 缺乏真正的血管周围间隙。即使出现,也是血管周围狭窄的间隙,其中含有浆细胞而不是淋巴细胞。
- 广泛的细胞非典型性。

上皮细胞的CD5或CD117免疫反应呈阳性以及缺少TdT阳性的淋巴细胞,支持胸腺癌而不是胸腺瘤的诊断(图21C.45)。

胸腺瘤分类的组织学线索

A型胸腺瘤是一种腺体肿瘤,含有局灶性的腺体结构,而B型胸腺瘤从不形成腺体结构。这样在一个梭形

表21C.8 胸腺瘤分类的形态学线索	
胸腺瘤的形态学特征	可能的组织学类型
以淋巴细胞为主	B1型胸腺瘤、B2型胸腺瘤、AB型胸腺瘤
以上皮细胞为主	A型胸腺瘤、B3型胸腺瘤、类固醇治疗后的B1或B2型胸腺瘤
以梭形细胞为主	A型胸腺瘤、AB型胸腺瘤、有时B3型胸腺瘤
出现腺体	A型胸腺瘤、AB型胸腺瘤
玫瑰花结结构	A型胸腺瘤（包括微结节性胸腺瘤）、AB型胸腺瘤
"A型"胸腺瘤伴有中等量淋巴细胞浸润	AB型胸腺瘤、微结节性胸腺瘤
形态学类似于B细胞慢性淋巴细胞白血病	B1型胸腺瘤

细胞肿瘤中如果发现存在腺体，则可以肯定地做出 A 型胸腺瘤的诊断（图 21C.17）。同样，即使肿瘤细胞为立方形，如果肿瘤细胞混于腺体结构中，也可以诊断为 A 型胸腺瘤（表 21C.8）。

A 型胸腺瘤缺少淋巴细胞。在一个疑似 A 型胸腺瘤的胸腺肿瘤中如果出现富于淋巴细胞的病灶，则主要应该考虑为微结节性胸腺瘤和 AB 型胸腺瘤。在微结节性胸腺瘤中，淋巴细胞间质内部存在细胞角蛋白阳性的上皮细胞（图 21C.29）；而在 AB 型胸腺瘤中，则有细胞角蛋白阳性的网状上皮细胞出现在淋巴细胞中。

在 B 型胸腺瘤谱系中，从 B1 型到 B3 型胸腺瘤，淋巴细胞比例明显减少。B2 型胸腺瘤的上皮细胞不同于 B1 型胸腺瘤，B2 型胸腺瘤上皮细胞核较大并有较明显的核仁。另一方面，B3 型胸腺瘤的上皮细胞形态多样，可为挖空细胞样细胞，或与 B2 型胸腺瘤的细胞相似。有些病例可能显示 B1/B2 或 B2/B3 型胸腺瘤的交界性特征。一般来说，B1 型胸腺瘤的上皮细胞散在分布，而 B2 型胸腺瘤的上皮细胞可能成簇。然而，一旦出现明显的实性上皮细胞巢则必须诊断为 B3 型胸腺瘤。

前纵隔梭形细胞肿瘤的诊断思考

前纵隔梭形细胞肿瘤的鉴别诊断要考虑到各种类型的肿瘤：A 型胸腺瘤、B3 型胸腺瘤的梭形细胞变异、肉瘤样或梭形细胞胸腺癌、梭形细胞类癌、肉瘤样卵黄囊瘤、伴有梭形细胞的纵隔大 B 细胞淋巴瘤、畸胎瘤、发生于畸胎瘤的肉瘤以及各种良性和恶性间叶性肿瘤。

出现由硬化性间隔分隔的小叶结构支持胸腺瘤的诊断。只有所有的梭形细胞表现都温和时，才可以诊断 A 型胸腺瘤。出现散在的内衬矮柱状或扁平细胞的腺体结构时，可以进一步肯定 A 型胸腺瘤的诊断（图

21C.17A），而不是间叶性肿瘤和 B3 型胸腺瘤。如果与富于细胞的孤立性纤维肿瘤鉴别有困难，细胞角蛋白（胸腺瘤阳性）和 CD34（孤立性纤维性肿瘤阳性）免疫染色有助于诊断。如果梭形细胞具有非典型性或出现核分裂象，必须慎重鉴别是梭形细胞 B3 型胸腺瘤还是肉瘤样/梭形细胞胸腺癌（图 21C.27），如果出现器官型结构，可以把 B3 型胸腺瘤与胸腺癌鉴别开来。

通过在肿瘤其他区域辨认比较典型的生长方式，可以很容易地诊断梭形细胞类癌和肉瘤样卵黄囊瘤。神经内分泌标记物和甲胎蛋白免疫染色分别有助于证实两者的诊断。在做出原发性纵隔肉瘤的诊断之前，建议广泛取材以排除发生于生殖细胞肿瘤的体细胞恶性肿瘤和癌肉瘤。

胸腺内囊肿的诊断思考：恶性肿瘤的可能征象

一些良性囊性病变可以发生于胸腺或前纵隔，如单纯性胸腺囊肿、多房性胸腺囊肿、淋巴上皮样囊肿、支气管源性囊肿、体腔囊肿和胃肠囊肿[4,508,509]。胸腺囊肿（thymic cyst）是单房性囊肿，内衬扁平、立方、柱状、纤毛或非角化性复层鳞状上皮，具有伴淋巴细胞浸润的纤维性囊壁[4]。通过在囊壁内找到胸腺组织可以确定诊断。多房性胸腺囊肿（multilocular thymic cyst）的特征是多发性内衬上皮的囊肿，在成人可能是获得性反应性病变，也可发生于免疫缺陷病毒感染的儿童（图 21C.73）[219,510]。囊壁内有不同程度的慢性炎细胞浸润，常有胆固醇裂隙沉积，并伴有异物巨细胞反应[219,511]。偶尔，可出现明显的假上皮瘤性上皮增生，类似于肿瘤性病变[512]。少数情况下，胸腺瘤、胸腺癌以及类癌可以起源于胸腺囊肿或多房性胸腺囊肿的内衬上皮[20,193,218-220,513]。

胸腺发生的各种肿瘤均可伴有囊肿形成，如 Hodgkin 淋巴瘤、非 Hodgkin 淋巴瘤和生殖细胞肿瘤，

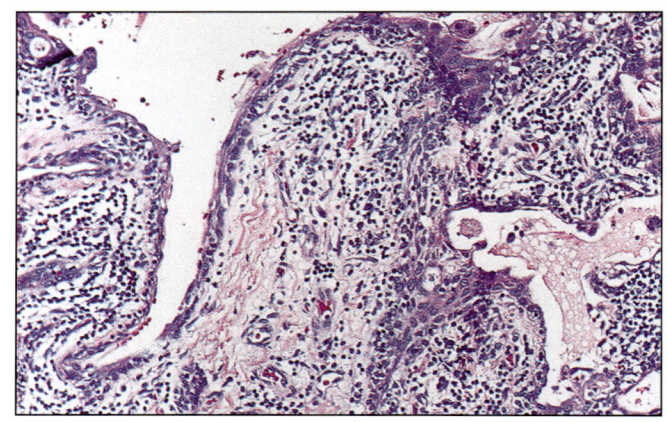

图21C.73 多房性胸腺囊肿。囊肿内衬具有鳞状上皮性质的扁平胸腺上皮。囊壁一般富于淋巴细胞。

囊肿可能非常明显，以至于在组织学检查时可能将肿瘤性成分漏掉。这些内衬上皮的囊肿通常是多发性的，可能是髓质导管上皮衍化而来的结构（包括胸腺小体）在占位性病变的诱导下发生囊性变而形成的（图21C.62和21C.70）[219]。胸腺瘤或胸腺癌也可发生囊性变。因此，每当遇见胸腺囊性病变时，均应充分取材查找肿瘤，尤其是实性区域和增厚的间隔。

显著的反应性胸腺上皮增生与胸腺瘤
Florid reactive thymic epithelial proliferation versus thymoma

各种类型的肿瘤（如淋巴瘤和生殖细胞肿瘤）内或其周围残留的胸腺上皮有时可能显示明显的反应性增生，可能被误诊为胸腺瘤（图21C.56和21C.63）。通过注意多灶性本质、上皮增生程度有限、缺少胸腺瘤特征性的拼图样小叶结构，而且在其他区域出现特殊类型肿瘤的诊断性特征，可以做出正确诊断。

胸腺显著肉芽肿的诊断思考

肉芽肿性反应可以累及胸腺，如结节病和感染（如结核和组织胞浆菌病）。然而，有些胸腺肿瘤可以伴有显著的上皮样肉芽肿性反应，以至于掩盖了肿瘤（图21C.57）。最著名的例子是Hodgkin淋巴瘤（过去被误认为是"肉芽肿性胸腺瘤"）和精原细胞瘤[514]。因此，每当在胸腺内遇到肉芽肿时，必须仔细检查组织以查找这些肿瘤。如果有疑问，免疫染色最有助于诊断：Hodgkin淋巴瘤CD30呈阳性，精原细胞瘤CD117或Oct-3/4呈阳性。

参考文献

1. Rosai J, Levine G D 1976 Tumors of the thymus. Atlas of tumor pathology, 2nd series, Fascicle 13. Armed Forces Institute of Pathology, Washington DC
2. Blossom G B, Steiger Z, Stephenson L W 1997 Neoplasms of the mediastinum. In: DeVita V T J, Hellman S, Rosenberg S A (eds) Cancer, principles and practice of oncology, 5th edn. Lippincott-Raven, Philadelphia, 951–970
3. Suster S, Rosai J 1990 Histology of the normal thymus. Am J Surg Pathol 14: 284–303
4. Shimosato Y, Mukai K 1997 Tumors of the mediastinum. Atlas of tumor pathology, 3rd Series, Fascicle 21. Armed Forces Institute of Pathology, Washington DC
5. Marino M, Muller-Hermelink H K 1985 Thymoma and thymic carcinoma. Relation of thymoma epithelial cells to the cortical and medullary differentiation of thymus. Virchows Arch A Pathol Anat Histopathol 407: 119–149
6. Chan J K, Tsang W Y, Seneviratne S, et al. 1995 The MIC2 antibody 013. Practical application for the study of thymic epithelial tumors. Am J Surg Pathol 19: 1115–1123
7. Isaacson P G, Norton A J, Addis B J 1987 The human thymus contains a novel population of B lymphocytes. Lancet ii: 1488–1491
8. Hofmann W J, Momburg F, Moller P 1988 Thymic medullary cells expressing B lymphocyte antigens. Hum Pathol 19: 1280–1287
9. Calaminici M, Piper K, Lee A M, et al. 2004 CD23 expression in mediastinal large B-cell lymphomas. Histopathology 45: 619–624
10. Rosai J, Sobin L H 1999 Histological typing of tumors of the thymus. WHO international histological classification of tumors. Springer Verlag, Berlin.
11. Moran C A, Suster S 1997 Primary germ cell tumors of the mediastinum: I. Analysis of 322 cases with special emphasis on teratomatous lesions and a proposal for histopathologic classification and clinical staging. Cancer 80: 681–690
12. Moran C A, Suster S 1998 Germ cell tumors of the mediastinum. Adv Anat Pathol 5: 1–15
13. Muller-Hermelink H K, Engel P, Kuo T T, et al. 2004 Tumours of the thymus: Introduction. In: Travis W D, Brambilla E, Muller-Hermelink H K, et al (eds) Pathology and genetics. Tumours of the lung, pleura, thymus and heart. WHO classification of tumours. IARC Press, Lyon, 148–151
14. Walker A N, Mills S E, Fechner R E 1990 Thymomas and thymic carcinomas. Semin Diagn Pathol 7: 250–265
15. Maggi G, Casadio C, Cavallo A, et al. 1991 Thymoma: results of 241 operated cases. Ann Thorac Surg 51: 152–156
16. Kuo T T, Lo S K 1993 Thymoma: a study of the pathologic classification of 71 cases with evaluation of the Muller-Hermelink system. Hum Pathol 24: 766–771
17. Fechner R E 1969 Recurrence of noninvasive thymomas, report of four cases and review of the literature. Cancer 23: 1423–1427
18. Monden Y, Nakahara K, Iioka S, et al. 1985 Recurrence of thymoma: clinicopathological features, therapy, and prognosis. Ann Thorac Surg 39: 165–169
19. Kornstein M J, Curran W J, Turrisi A T, et al. 1988 Cortical versus medullary thymomas: a useful morphologic distinction? Hum Pathol 19: 1335–1339
20. Ritter J H, Wick M R 1999 Primary carcinomas of the thymus gland. Semin Diagn Pathol 16: 18–31
21. Suster S 2005 Thymic carcinoma: update of current diagnostic criteria and histologic types. Semin Diagn Pathol 22: 198–212
22. Suster S, Moran C A 2006 Thymoma classification: current status and future trends. Am J Clin Pathol 125: 542–554
23. Mackay B, Osborne B M, McKenna R J Jr 1985 Atypical thymoma. Ultrastruct Pathol 9: 241–246
24. Suster S, Moran C A 1999 Thymoma, atypical thymoma, and thymic carcinoma. A novel conceptual approach to the classification of thymic epithelial neoplasms. Am J Clin Pathol 111: 826–833
25. Levine G D, Rosai J 1978 Thymic hyperplasia and neoplasia: a review of current concepts. Hum Pathol 9: 495–515
26. Lewis J E, Wick M R, Scheithauer BW, et al. 1987 Thymoma. A clinicopathologic review. Cancer 60: 2727–2743
27. Gray G F, Gutowski W T 1979 Thymoma, a clinicopathologic study of 54 cases. Am J Surg Pathol 3: 235–249
28. Blumberg D, Port J L, Weksler B 1995 Thymoma: a multivariate analysis of factors predicting survival. Ann Thorac Surg 60: 908–914
29. Sperling B, Marschall J, Kennedy R, et al. 2003 Thymoma: a review of the clinical and pathological findings in 65 cases. Can J Surg 46: 37–42
30. Thomas C R, Wright C D, Loehrer PJ 1999 Thymoma: state of the art. J Clin Oncol 17: 2280–2289
31. Masaoka A, Hashimoto T, Shibata K, et al. 1989 Thymomas associated with pure red cell aplasia. Histologic and follow-up studies. Cancer 64: 1872–1878
32. Lyonnais J 1988 Thymoma and pancytopenia. Am J Hematol 28: 195–196
33. Ackland S P, Bur M E, Adler S S 1988 White blood cell aplasia associated with thymoma. Am J Clin Pathol 89: 260–263
34. Marx A, Schultz A, Wilisch A, et al. 1998 Paraneoplastic autoimmunity in thymus tumors. Dev Immunol 6: 129–140
35. Regnard J F, Magdeleinat P, Dromer C, et al. 1996 Prognostic factors and long-term results after thymoma resection: a series of 307 patients. J Thorac Cardiovasc Surg 112: 376–384
36. Detterbeck F C 2006 Clinical value of the WHO classification system of thymoma. Ann Thorac Surg 81: 2328–2334
37. Barton A D 1997 T-cell lymphocytosis associated with lymphocyte-rich thymoma. Cancer 80: 1409–1417
38. de Jong D, Richel D J, Schenkeveld C, et al. 1997 Oligoclonal peripheral T-cell lymphocytosis as a result of aberrant T-cell development in a cortical thymoma. Diagn Mol Pathol 6: 244–248
39. Doll D C, Landreneau R J, List A F 1991 Malignant thymoma associated with peripheral T-cell lymphocytosis. Med Pediatr Oncol 19: 496–498
40. Medeiros L J, Bhagat S K, Naylor P, et al. 1993 Malignant thymoma associated with T-cell lymphocytosis. A case report with immunophenotypic and gene rearrangement analysis. Arch Pathol Lab Med 117: 279–283
41. Shachor Y, Radnay J, Bernheim J, et al. 1988 Malignant thymoma with peripheral blood lymphocytosis. Cancer 61: 1222–1227
42. Tamaoki J, Chiyotani A, Nagai A, et al. 1997 Invasive thymoma with CD4+CD8+ double-positive T cell lymphocytosis. Respiration 64: 176–178
43. Yokoi K, Miyazawa N, Kano Y, et al. 1997 Tumor lysis syndrome in invasive thymoma with peripheral blood T-cell lymphocytosis. Am J Clin Oncol 20: 86–89
44. Otton S H, Standen G R, Ormerod I E 2000 T cell lymphocytosis associated with polymyositis, myasthenia gravis and thymoma. Clin Lab Haematol 22: 307–308
45. McGuire L J, Huang D P, Teoh R, et al. 1988 Epstein–Barr virus genome in thymoma and thymic lymphoid hyperplasia. Am J Pathol 131: 385–390
46. Chan J K C, Yip T T C, Tsang W Y W, et al. 1994 Lack of evidence of pathogenetic role of Epstein–Barr virus in lymphoid hyperplasia and

47. Inghirami G, Chilosi M, Knowles D M 1990 Western thymomas lack Epstein–Barr virus by Southern blotting analysis and by polymerase chain reaction. Am J Pathol 136: 1429–1436
48. Wu T C, Kuo T T 1993 Study of Epstein–Barr virus early RNA 1 (EBER1) expression by in situ hybridization in thymic epithelial tumors of Chinese patients in Taiwan. Hum Pathol 24: 235–238
49. Borisch B, Kirchner T, Marx A, et al. 1990 Absence of the Epstein–Barr virus genome in the normal thymus, thymic epithelial tumors, thymic lymphoid hyperplasia in a European population. Virchows Arch B Cell Pathol 59: 359–365
50. Chen P C, Pan C C, Yang A H, et al. 2002 Detection of Epstein–Barr virus genome within thymic epithelial tumours in Taiwanese patients by nested PCR, PCR in situ hybridization, and RNA in situ hybridization. J Pathol 197: 684–688
51. Pescarmona E, Giardini R, Brisigotti M, et al. 1992 Thymoma in childhood: a clinicopathological study of five cases. Histopathology 21: 65–68
52. Ramon y Cajal S, Suster S 1991 Primary thymic epithelial neoplasms in children. Am J Surg Pathol 15: 466–474
53. Pescarmona E, Rendina E A, Venuta F, et al. 1990 Analysis of prognostic factors and clinicopathological staging of thymoma. Ann Thorac Surg 50: 534–538
54. Dawson A, Ibrahim N B, Gibbs A R 1994 Observer variation in the histopathological classification of thymoma: correlation with prognosis. J Clin Pathol 47: 519–523
55. Bedini A V, Andreani S M, Tavecchio L, et al. 2005 Proposal of a novel system for the staging of thymic epithelial tumors. Ann Thorac Surg 80: 1994–2000
56. Fang W, Chen W, Chen G, et al. 2005 Surgical management of thymic epithelial tumors: a retrospective review of 204 cases. Ann Thorac Surg 80: 2002–2007
57. Kim D J, Yang W I, Choi S S, et al. 2005 Prognostic and clinical relevance of the World Health Organization schema for the classification of thymic epithelial tumors: a clinicopathologic study of 108 patients and literature review. Chest 127: 755–761
58. Masaoka A, Yamakawa Y, Fujii Y 1999 Well-differentiated thymic carcinoma: is it thymic carcinoma or not? J Thorac Cardiovasc Surg 117: 628–630
59. Koga K, Matsuno Y, Noguchi M, et al. 1994 A review of 79 thymomas: modification of staging system and reappraisal of conventional division into invasive and non-invasive thymoma. Pathol Int 44: 359–367
60. Tsuchiya R, Koga K, Matsuno Y, et al. 1994 Thymic carcinoma: proposal for pathological TNM and staging. Pathol Int 44: 505–512
61. Ruffie P, Gory-Delabaere G, Fervers B, et al. 1999 Standards, options and recommendations (SOR) for clinical care of malignant thymoma. Groupe de Travail SOR. Bull Cancer 86: 365–384
62. Graeber G M, Tamim W 2000 Current status of the diagnosis and treatment of thymoma. Semin Thorac Cardiovasc Surg 12: 268–277
63. Gawrychowski J, Rokicki M, Gabriel A, et al. 2000 Thymoma – the usefulness of some prognostic factors for diagnosis and surgical treatment. Eur J Surg Oncol 26: 203–208
64. Verley J M, Hollmann K H 1985 Thymoma. A comparative study of clinical stages, histologic features, and survival in 200 cases. Cancer 55: 1074–1086
65. Salyer W R, Eggleston J C 1976 Thymomas: a clinical and pathological study of 65 cases. Cancer 39: 229–249
66. Curran W J Jr, Kornstein M J, Brooks J J, et al. 1988 Invasive thymoma: the role of mediastinal irradiation following complete or incomplete surgical resection. J Clin Oncol 6: 1722–1727
67. Ruffini E, Mancuso M, Oliaro A, et al. 1997 Recurrence of thymoma: analysis of clinicopathologic features, treatment, and outcome. J Thorac Cardiovasc Surg 113: 55–63
68. Haniuda M, Miyazawa M, Yoshida K, et al. 1996 Is postoperative radiotherapy for thymoma effective? Ann Surg 224: 219–224
69. Bergh N P, Gatzinsky P, Larsson S, et al. 1978 Tumors of the thymus and thymic region: I. Clinicopathological studies on thymomas. Ann Thorac Surg 25: 91–98
70. Rachmaninoff N, Fentress V 1964 Thymoma with metastasis to the brain. Am J Clin Pathol 41: 618–625
71. Gravanis M B 1968 Metastasizing thymoma, report of a case and review of the literature. Am J Clin Pathol 49: 690–696
72. Guillan R A, Zelman S, Smalley R L 1971 Malignant thymoma associated with myasthenia gravis, and evidence of extrathoracic metastasis. Cancer 27: 823–830
73. Nakahara K, Ohno K, Hashimoto J 1988 Thymoma: results with complete resection and adjuvant postoperative irradiation in 141 consecutive patients. J Thorac Cardiovasc Surg 95: 1041–1047
74. Goldel N, Boning L, Fredrik A 1989 Chemotherapy of invasive thymoma, a retrospective study of 22 cases. Cancer 63: 1493–1500
75. Nakagawa K, Asamura H, Matsuno Y, et al. 2003 Thymoma: a clinicopathologic study based on the new World Health Organization classification. J Thorac Cardiovasc Surg 126: 1134–1140
76. Gripp S, Hilgers K, Wurm R, et al. 1998 Thymoma: prognostic factors and treatment outcomes. Cancer 83: 1495–503
77. Mornex F, Resbeut M, Richaud P, et al. 1995 Radiotherapy and chemotherapy for invasive thymomas: a multicentric retrospective review of 90 cases. The FNCLCC trialists. Int J Radiat Oncol Biol Phys 32: 651–659
77a. Strobel P, Bauer A, Puppe B, et al. 2004 Tumor recurrence and survival in patients treated for thymomas and thymic squamous cell carcinomas: a retrospective analysis. J Clin Oncol 22: 1501–1509
78. Arakawa A, Yasunaga T, Saitoh Y 1990 Radiation therapy of invasive thymoma. Int J Radiol Oncol 18: 529–534
79. Fornasiero A, Daniele O, Ghiotto C 1990 Chemotherapy of invasive thymoma. J Clin Oncol 8: 1419–1423
80. Venuta F, Rendina E A, Pescarmona E O, et al. 1997 Multimodality treatment of thymoma: a prospective study. Ann Thorac Surg 64: 1585–1591, 1591–1592
81. Giaccone G 2005 Treatment of malignant thymoma. Curr Opin Oncol 17: 140–146
82. Iwasaki Y, Ohsugi S, Takemura Y, et al. 2002 Multidisciplinary therapy including high-dose chemotherapy followed by peripheral blood stem cell transplantation for invasive thymoma. Chest 122: 2249–2252
83. Langenfeld J, Graeber G M 1999 Current management of thymoma. Surg Oncol Clin North Am 8: 327–339
84. Bernatz P E, Khonsari S, Harrison E G, Jr., Taylor W F: Thymoma: factors influencing prognosis. Surg Clin North Am 53: 885–892, 1973
85. Lattes R 1962 Thymoma and other tumors of the thymus, an analysis of 107 cases. Cancer 15: 1224–1260
86. Bernatz P E, Harrison E G, Clagett O T 1961 Thymoma: a clinicopathologic study. J Thorac Cardiovasc Surg 41: 424–444
87. Pescarmona E, Rendina E A, Venuta F, et al. 1990 The prognostic implication of thymoma histologic subtyping. A study of 80 consecutive cases. Am J Clin Pathol 93: 190–195
88. Batata M A, Martini N, Huvos A G 1974 Thymoma: clinicopathologic features, therapy and prognosis. Cancer 34: 389–396
89. Kornstein M J, Hoxie J A, Levinson A I 1985 Immunohistology of human thymomas. Arch Pathol Lab Med 109: 460–463
90. Monden Y, Uyama T, Taniki T 1988 The characteristics of thymoma with myasthenia gravis: a 28 year experience. J Surg Oncol 38: 151–154
91. Muller-Hermelink H K, Marino M, Palestro G 1986 Pathology of thymic epithelial tumors. Curr Top Pathol 75: 207–268
92. Muller-Hermelink H K, Marx A, Kirchner T 1994 Advances in the diagnosis and classification of thymic epithelial tumors. In: Anthony P P, MacSween R N M (eds) Recent advances in histopathology, Vol. 16. Churchill Livingstone, Edinburgh, 49–72
93. Kirchner T, Muller-Hermelink H K 1989 New approaches to the diagnosis of thymic epithelial tumors. In: Fenoglio-Preiser C M, Wolff M, Rilke F (eds) Progress in surgical pathology. Field & Wood, New York, 167–189
94. Kirchner T, Schalke B, Marx A, et al. 1989 Evaluation of prognostic features in thymic epithelial tumors. Thymus 14: 195–203
95. Yoneda S, Marx A, Heimann S, et al. 1999 Low-grade metaplastic carcinoma of the thymus. Histopathology 35: 19–30
96. Muller-Hermelink H K, Marx A, Kirchner T 1996 Thymus and mediastinum. In: Damjanov I, Linder J (eds) Anderson's pathology. CV Mosby, St Louis, 1218–1243
97. Kirchner T, Schalke B, Buchwald J, et al. 1992 Well-differentiated thymic carcinoma. An organotypical low-grade carcinoma with relationship to cortical thymoma. Am J Surg Pathol 16: 1153–1169
98. Quintanilla-Martinez L, Wilkins E W Jr, Ferry J A, et al. 1993 Thymoma – morphologic subclassification correlates with invasiveness and immunohistologic features: a study of 122 cases. Hum Pathol 24: 958–969
99. Quintanilla-Martinez L, Wilkins E W Jr, Choi N, et al. 1994 Thymoma. Histologic subclassification is an independent prognostic factor. Cancer 74: 606–617
100. Ricci C, Rendina E A, Pescarmona E O, et al. 1989 Correlations between histological type, clinical behaviour, and prognosis in thymoma. Thorax 44: 455–460
101. Ho F C, Fu K H, Lam S Y, et al. 1994 Evaluation of a histogenetic classification for thymic epithelial tumours. Histopathology 25: 21–29
102. Tan P H, Sng I T 1995 Thymoma – a study of 60 cases in Singapore. Histopathology 26: 509–518
103. Engel P, Marx A, Muller-Hermelink H K 1999 Thymic tumours in Denmark. A retrospective study of 213 cases from 1970 to 1993. Pathol Res Pract 195: 565–570
104. Schneider P M, Fellbaum C, Fink U, et al. 1997 Prognostic significance of histomorphologic subclassification for epithelial thymic tumors. Ann Surg Oncol 4: 46–56
105. Pan C C, Wu H P, Yang C F, et al. 1994 The clinicopathological correlation of epithelial subtyping in thymoma: a study of 112 consecutive cases. Hum Pathol 25: 893–899
106. Pan C C, Chen W Y, Chiang H, et al. 1995 A multivariate analysis of prognostic factors in thymoma. Chung Hua I Hsueh Tsa Chih (Taipei) 56: 120–124
107. Blumberg D, Burt M E, Bains M S, et al. 1998 Thymic carcinoma: current staging does not predict prognosis. J Thorac Cardiovasc Surg 115: 303–308, 308–309
108. Suster S, Moran C A 1997 Primary thymic epithelial neoplasms: current concepts and controversies. Anat Pathol 2: 1–19
109. Suster S, Moran C A 1999 Primary thymic epithelial neoplasms: spectrum of differentiation and histological features. Semin Diagn Pathol 16: 2–17
110. Suster S 2006 My approach to the diagnosis of thymoma. J Clin Pathol (in press)
111. Suster S, Moran C A 2005 Problem areas and inconsistencies in the WHO classification of thymoma. Semin Diagn Pathol 22: 188–197

112. Marx A, Strobel P, Zettl A, et al. 2004 Thymomas. In: Travis W D, Brambilla E, Muller-Hermelink H K, et al (eds) Pathology and genetics. Tumours of the lung, pleura, thymus and heart. WHO classification of tumours. IARC Press, Lyon, 152–153
113. Puglisi F, Finato N, Mariuzzi L, et al. 1995 Microscopic thymoma and myasthenia gravis. J Clin Pathol 48: 682–683
114. Kuo T T, Lee M C 1991 Amyloid production in a thymoma. Surg Pathol 4: 69–71
115. Williams D J, MacSween R N M 1989 Peliosis thymoma: association with tuberculosis. [Letter] J Clin Pathol 42: 331
116. Pescarmona E, Rendina E A, Venuta F, et al. 1995 Recurrent thymoma: evidence for histological progression. Histopathology 27: 445–449
117. Fukuda T, Ohnishi Y, Emura I, Tachikawa S 1992 Microcytic variant of thymoma: histological and immunohistochemical findings in two cases. Virchows Arch A Pathol Anat Histopathol 420: 185–189
118. Pescarmona E, Pisacane A, Rendina E A, et al. 1991 'Organoid' thymoma: well-differentiated variant with distinctive clinicopathological features. Histopathology 18: 161–164
119. Suster S, Moran C A 1999 Micronodular thymoma with lymphoid B-cell hyperplasia: clinicopathologic and immunohistochemical study of eighteen cases of a distinctive morphologic variant of thymic epithelial neoplasm. Am J Surg Pathol 23: 955–962
120. Strobel P, Marino M, Feuchtenberger M, et al. 2005 Micronodular thymoma: an epithelial tumour with abnormal chemokine expression setting the stage for lymphoma development. J Pathol 207: 72–82
121. Tateyama H, Saito Y, Fujii Y, et al. 2001 The spectrum of micronodular thymic epithelial tumours with lymphoid B-cell hyperplasia. Histopathology 38: 519–527
122. Marx A, Strobel P, Marino M, et al. 2004 Micronodular thymoma with lymphoid stroma. In: Travis W D, Brambilla E, Muller-Hermelink H K, et al. (eds) Pathology and genetics. Tumours of the lung, pleura, thymus and heart. WHO classification of tumours. IARC Press, Lyon, 167–168
123. Suster S, Moran C A, Chan J K 1997 Thymoma with pseudosarcomatous stroma: report of an unusual histologic variant of thymic epithelial neoplasm that may simulate carcinosarcoma. Am J Surg Pathol 21: 1316–1323
124. Chan J K, Zettl A, Inoue M, et al. 2004 Metaplastic thymoma. In: Travis W D, Brambilla E, Muller-Hermelink H K, et al. (eds) Pathology and genetics. Tumours of the lung, pleura, thymus and heart. WHO classification of tumours. IARC Press, Lyon, 169–170
125. Moran C A, Suster S 1998 Thymoma with prominent cystic and hemorrhagic changes and infarction. [Abstract] Mod Pathol 11: 178A
126. Kuo T T 1994 Sclerosing thymoma – a possible phenomenon of regression. Histopathology 25: 289–291
127. Moran C A, Suster S 2004 'Ancient' (sclerosing) thymomas: a clinicopathologic study of 10 cases. Am J Clin Pathol 121: 867–871
128. Suster S, Rosai J 1992 Cystic thymomas. A clinicopathologic study of ten cases. Cancer 69: 92–97
129. Kobayashi Y, Fujii Y, Yano M, et al. 2006 Preoperative steroid pulse therapy for invasive thymoma: clinical experience and mechanism of action. Cancer 106: 1901–1907
130. Moran C A, Suster S, Koss M N 1994 Plasma cell-rich thymoma. Am J Clin Pathol 102: 199–201
131. Sato T, Tamaoki N 1989 Myoid cells in the human thymus and thymoma revealed by three different immunohistochemical markers for striated muscle. Acta Pathol Jpn 39: 509–519
132. Moran C A, Koss M N Rhabdomyomatous thymoma. Am J Surg Pathol 17: 633–636, 1993
133. Pescarmona E, Rosati S, Pisacane A, et al. 1992 Microscopic thymoma: histological evidence of multifocal cortical and medullary origin. Histopathology 20: 263–266
134. Puglisi F, Di Loreto C, Finato N, et al. 1997 Microscopic thymoma and myasthenia gravis: a clinicopathological and immunohistochemical study of two cases. In: Marx A, Muller-Hermelink H K (eds) Epithelial tumors of the thymus, pathology, biology and treatment. Plenum Press, New York, 75–79
135. Marx A, Chen G, Strobel P, et al. Rare thymomas. In: Travis W D, Brambilla E, Muller-Hermelink H K, et al. (eds) Pathology and genetics. Tumours of the lung, pleura, thymus and heart. WHO classification of tumours. IARC Press, Lyon, 171
136. Rosai J 2004 Rosai and Ackerman's surgical pathology, 9th edn. CV Mosby, Edinburgh
137. Cheuk W, Tsang W Y, Chan J K 2005 Microthymoma: definition of the entity and distinction from nodular hyperplasia of the thymic epithelium (so-called microscopic thymoma). Am J Surg Pathol 29: 415–419
138. Ring N P, Addis B J 1986 Thymoma: an integrated clinicopathological and immunohistochemical study. J Pathol 149: 327–337
139. Kodama T, Watanabe S, Sato Y 1986 An immunohistochemical study of thymic epithelial tumors: epithelial component. Am J Surg Pathol 10: 26–33
140. Lee D, Wright D H 1988 Immunohistochemical study of 22 cases of thymoma. J Clin Pathol 41: 1297–1304
141. Kuo T 2000 Cytokeratin profiles of the thymus and thymomas: histogenetic correlations and proposal for a histological classification of thymomas. Histopathology 36: 403–414
142. Chilosi M, Castelli P, Martignoni G, et al. 1992 Neoplastic epithelial cells in a subset of human thymomas express the B cell-associated CD20 antigen. Am J Surg Pathol 16: 988–997
143. Katzin W E, Fishleder A J, Linden M D 1988 Immunoglobulin and T-cell receptor genes in thymomas: genotypic evidence supporting the nonneoplastic nature of the lymphocytic component. Hum Pathol 19: 232–328
144. Rosai J 1987 The pathology of thymic neoplasia. Monogr Pathol 29: 161–183
145. Ito M, Taki T, Mihaye M 1988 Lymphocyte subsets in human thymoma studied with monoclonal antibodies. Cancer 61: 284–287
146. Chan W C, Zaatari G S, Tabei S, et al. 1984 Thymoma: an immunohistochemical study. Am J Clin Pathol 82: 160–166
147. Eimoto T, Teshima K, Shirakusa T 1986 Heterogeneity of epithelial cells and reactive components in thymomas: an ultrastructural and immunohistochemical study. Ultrastruct Pathol 10: 157–173
148. Mokhtar N, Hsu S M, Lad R P, et al. 1984 Thymoma: lymphoid and epithelial components mirror the phenotype of normal thymus. Hum Pathol 15: 378–384
149. Sato Y, Watanabe S, Mukai K 1986 An immunohistochemical study of thymic epithelial tumors: lymphoid component. Am J Surg Pathol 10: 862–879
150. Kornstein M J, Kay S 1990 B cells in thymomas. Mod Pathol 3: 61–63
151. Taubenberger J K, Jaffe E S, Medeiros L J 1991 Thymoma with abundant L26-positive 'asteroid' cells. A case report with an analysis of normal thymus and thymoma specimens. Arch Pathol Lab Med 115: 1254–1257
152. Martin J M, Randhawa G, Temple W J 1986 Cervical thymoma. Arch Pathol Lab Med 110: 354–357
153. Fukayama M, Maeda Y, Funata N 1988 Pulmonary and pleural thymoma, diagnostic application of lymphocyte markers to the thymoma of unusual site. Am J Clin Pathol 89: 617–621
154. Salter D M, Krajewski A S 1986 Metastatic thymoma: a case report and immunohistological analysis. J Clin Pathol 39: 275–27s8
155. Levine G D, Rosai J, Bearman R M 1975 The fine structure of thymoma, with emphasis on its differential diagnosis. Am J Pathol 81: 49–86
156. Zettl A, Strobel P, Wagner K, et al. 2000 Recurrent genetic aberrations in thymoma and thymic carcinoma. Am J Pathol 157: 257–266
157. Zhou R, Zettl A, Strobel P, et al. 2001 Thymic epithelial tumors can develop along two different pathogenetic pathways. Am J Pathol 159: 1853–1860
158. Inoue M, Starostik P, Zettl A, et al. 2003 Correlating genetic aberrations with World Health Organization-defined histology and stage across the spectrum of thymomas. Cancer Res 63: 3708–3715
159. Inoue M, Marx A, Zettl A, et al. 2002 Chromosome 6 suffers frequent and multiple aberrations in thymoma. Am J Pathol 161: 1507–1513
160. Zisis C, Rontogianni D, Tzavara C, et al. 2005 Prognostic factors in thymic epithelial tumors undergoing complete resection. Ann Thorac Surg 80: 1056–1062
161. Chen G, Marx A, Wen-Hu C, et al. 2002 New WHO histologic classification predicts prognosis of thymic epithelial tumors: a clinicopathologic study of 200 thymoma cases from China. Cancer 95: 420–429
162. Kondo K, Yoshizawa K, Tsuyuguchi M, et al. 2004 WHO histologic classification is a prognostic indicator in thymoma. Ann Thorac Surg 77: 1183–1188
163. Hsu C P, Chen C Y, Chen C L, et al. 1994 Thymic carcinoma. Ten years' experience in twenty patients. J Thorac Cardiovasc Surg 107: 615–620
164. Truong L D, Mody D R, Cagle P T 1990 Thymic carcinoma, a clinicopathologic study of 13 cases. Am J Surg Pathol 14: 151–166
165. Suster S, Rosai J 1991 Thymic carcinoma. A clinicopathologic study of 60 cases. Cancer 67: 1025–1032
166. Chung D A 2000 Thymic carcinoma – analysis of nineteen clinicopathological studies. Thorac Cardiovasc Surg 48: 114–119
167. Suster S, Moran C A 1998 Thymic carcinoma: spectrum of differentiation and histologic types. Pathology 30: 111–122
168. Kuo T T, Chang J P, Lin F J, et al. 1990 Thymic carcinomas: histopathological varieties and immunohistochemical study. Am J Surg Pathol 14: 24–34
169. Negron-Soto J M, Cascade P N 1995 Squamous cell carcinoma of the thymus with paraneoplastic hypercalcemia. Clin Imag 19: 122–124
170. Yoshiike F, Koizumi T, Yoneyama A, et al. 2004 Thymic squamous cell carcinoma producing parathyroid hormone-related protein and CYFRA 21–1. Intern Med 43: 493–495
171. Chalabreysse L, Etienne-Mastroianni B, Adeleine P, et al. 2004 Thymic carcinoma: a clinicopathological and immunohistological study of 19 cases. Histopathology 44: 367–374
172. Carlson R W, Dorfman R F, Sikic B 1990 Successful treatment of metastatic thymic carcinoma with cisplatin, vinblastine, bleomycin, and etoposide chemotherapy. Cancer 66: 2092–2094
173. Lin J T, Wei-Shu W, Yen C C, et al. 2005 Stage IV thymic carcinoma: a study of 20 patients. Am J Med Sci 330: 172–175
174. Kurup A, Loehrer P J Sr 2004 Thymoma and thymic carcinoma: therapeutic approaches. Clin Lung Cancer 6: 28–32
175. Wick M R, Scheithauer B W, Weiland L H, et al. 1982 Primary thymic carcinomas. Am J Surg Pathol 6: 613–630
176. Shimosato Y, Kameya T, Nagai K, et al. 1977 Squamous cell carcinoma of the thymus. An analysis of eight cases. Am J Surg Pathol 1: 109–121
177. Snover D C, Levine G D, Rosai J 1982 Thymic carcinoma. Five distinctive histological variants. Am J Surg Pathol 6: 451–470
178. Chen K T 1984 Squamous carcinoma of the thymus. J Surg Oncol 25: 61–63
179. Morinaga S, Sato Y, Shimosato Y, et al. 1987 Multiple thymic squamous cell carcinomas associated with mixed type thymoma. Am J Surg Pathol 11: 982–988

180. Shimosato Y 1997 Thymic carcinoma. In: Marx A, Muller-Hermelink H K (eds) Epithelial tumors of the thymus, pathology, biology, treatment. Plenum Press, New York, 9–15
181. Katoh Y, Shimamura K, Kakudo K 1990 An autopsy case of a cystic variant of thymic carcinoma mimicking a thymic cyst. Virchows Arch [A] 417: 85–87
182. Leyvraz S, Henle W, Chahinian A P Association of Epstein–Barr virus with thymic carcinoma. N Engl J Med 312: 1296–1299, 1985
183. Dimery I W, Lee J S, Blick M, et al. 1988 Association of the Epstein–Barr virus with lymphoepithelioma of the thymus. Cancer 61: 2475–2480
184. Stephan J L, Galambrun C, Boucheron S, et al. 2000 Epstein–Barr virus-positive undifferentiated thymic carcinoma in a 12-year-old white girl. J Pediatr Hematol Oncol 22: 162–166
185. Mann R B, Wu T C, MacMahon E M E 1992 In-situ localization of Epstein–Barr virus in thymic carcinoma. Mod Pathol 5: 363–366
186. Fujii T, Kawai T, Saito K 1993 EBER-1 expression in thymic carcinoma. Acta Pathol Jpn 43: 107–110
187. Eimoto T, Kitaoka M, Ogawa H, et al. 2002 Thymic sarcomatoid carcinoma with skeletal muscle differentiation: report of two cases, one with cytogenetic analysis. Histopathology 40: 46–57
188. Okudela K, Nakamura N, Sano J, et al. 2001 Thymic carcinosarcoma consisting of squamous cell carcinomatous and embryonal rhabdomyosarcomatous components. Report of a case and review of the literature. Pathol Res Pract 197: 205–210
189. Chan A C L, Chan J K C, Eimoto T, et al. 2004 Sarcomatoid carcinoma. In: Travis W D, Brambilla E, Muller-Hermelink H K, et al. (eds) Pathology and genetics. Tumours of the lung, pleura, thymus and heart. WHO classification of tumours. IARC Press, Lyon, 179–181
190. Nishimura M, Kodama T, Nishiyama H, et al. 1997 A case of sarcomatoid carcinoma of the thymus. Pathol Int 47: 260–263
191. Suarez Vilela D, Salas Valien J S, Gonzalez Moran M A, et al. 1992 Thymic carcinosarcoma associated with a spindle cell thymoma: an immunohistochemical study. Histopathology 21: 263–268
192. Suster S, Moran C A 1999 Spindle cell thymic carcinoma: clinicopathologic and immunohistochemical study of a distinctive variant of primary thymic epithelial neoplasm. Am J Surg Pathol 23: 691–700
193. Moran C A, Suster S 1995 Mucoepidermoid carcinomas of the thymus. A clinicopathologic study of six cases. Am J Surg Pathol 19: 826–834
194. Nonaka D, Klimstra D, Rosai J 2004 Thymic mucoepidermoid carcinomas: a clinicopathologic study of 10 cases and review of the literature. Am J Surg Pathol 28: 1526–1531
195. Yasuda M, Yasukawa T, Ozaki D, et al. 2006 Mucoepidermoid carcinoma of the thymus. Jpn J Thorac Cardiovasc Surg 54: 23–26
196. Hofmann W, Moller P, Manke H G, et al. 1985 Thymoma. A clinicopathologic study of 98 cases with special reference to three unusual cases. Pathol Res Pract 179: 337–353
197. Kawashima O, Kamiyoshihara M, Sakata S, et al. 1999 Basaloid carcinoma of the thymus. Ann Thorac Surg 68: 1863–1865
198. Wolfe J T 3rd, Wick M R, Banks P M, et al. 1983 Clear cell carcinoma of the thymus. Mayo Clin Proc 58: 365–370
199. Stephens M, Khalil J, Gibbs A R 1987 Primary clear cell carcinoma of the thymus gland. Histopathology 11: 763–765
200. Wick M R, Ritter J H, Humphrey P A, et al. 1997 Clear cell neoplasms of the endocrine system and beyond. Semin Diagn Pathol 14: 183–202
201. Hasserjian R P, Klimstra D S, Rosai J 1995 Carcinoma of the thymus with clear-cell features. Report of eight cases and review of the literature. Am J Surg Pathol 19: 835–41
202. Matsuno Y, Morozumi N, Hirohashi S, et al. 1998 Papillary carcinoma of the thymus: report of four cases of a new microscopic type of thymic carcinoma. Am J Surg Pathol 22: 873–880
203. Choi W W, Lui Y H, Lau W H, et al. 2003 Adenocarcinoma of the thymus: report of two cases, including a previously undescribed mucinous subtype. Am J Surg Pathol 27: 124–130
204. Babu M K, Nirmala V 1994 Thymic carcinoma with glandular differentiation arising in a congenital thymic cyst. J Surg Oncol 57: 277–279
205. Kapur P, Rakheja D, Bastasch M, et al. 2006 Primary mucinous adenocarcinoma of the thymus: a case report and review of the literature. Arch Pathol Lab Med 130: 201–204
206. Takahashi F, Tsuta K, Matsuno Y, et al. 2005 Adenocarcinoma of the thymus: mucinous subtype. Hum Pathol 36: 219–223
207. Nonaka D, Rodriguez J, Rollo J L, et al. 2005 Undifferentiated large cell carcinoma of the thymus associated with Castleman disease-like reaction: a distinctive type of thymic neoplasm characterized by an indolent behavior. Am J Surg Pathol 29: 490–495
208. de Queiroga E M, Chikota H, Bacchi C E, et al. 2004 Rhabdomyomatous carcinoma of the thymus. Am J Surg Pathol 28: 1245–1250
209. Falconieri G, Moran C A, Pizzolitto S, et al. 2005 Intrathoracic rhabdoid carcinoma: a clinicopathological, immunohistochemical, and ultrastructural study of 6 cases. Ann Diagn Pathol 9: 279–283
210. Toprani T H, Tamboli P, Amin M B, et al. 2003 Thymic carcinoma with rhabdoid features. Ann Diagn Pathol 7: 106–111
211. Franke A, Strobel P, Fackeldey V, et al. 2004 Hepatoid thymic carcinoma: report of a case. Am J Surg Pathol 28: 250–256
211a. French C A, Kutok J L, Faquin W C et al. 2004 Midline carcinoma of children and young adults with NUT rearrangement. J Clin Oncol 22: 4135–4139
212. Lee A C, Kwong Y I, Fu K H, et al. 1993 Disseminated mediastinal carcinoma with chromosomal translocation (15; 19). A distinctive clinicopathologic syndrome. Cancer 72: 2273–2276
213. Kees U R, Mulcahy M T, Willoughby M L 1991 Intrathoracic carcinoma in an 11-year-old girl showing a translocation t(15; 19). Am J Pediatr Hematol Oncol 13: 459–464
214. Kubonishi I, Takehara N, Iwata J, et al. 1991 Novel t(15; 19)(q15; p13) chromosome abnormality in a thymic carcinoma. Cancer Res 51: 3327–3328
215. Marx A, French C A, Fletcher J A 2004 Carcinoma with t(15; 19) translocation. In: Travis W D, Brambilla E, Muller-Hermelink H K, et al. (eds) Pathology and genetics. Tumours of the lung, pleura, thymus and heart. WHO classification of tumours. IARC Press, Lyon, 185–186
216. Suster S, Moran C A 1996 Primary thymic epithelial neoplasms showing combined features of thymoma and thymic carcinoma. A clinicopathologic study of 22 cases. Am J Surg Pathol 20: 1469–1480
217. Kuo T T, Chan J K 1998 Thymic carcinoma arising in thymoma is associated with alterations in immunohistochemical profile. Am J Surg Pathol 22: 1474–1481
218. Leong A S Y, Brown J H 1984 Malignant transformation of a thymic cyst. Am J Surg Pathol 8: 471–475
219. Suster S, Rosai J 1991 Multilocular thymic cyst: an acquired reactive process. Study of 18 cases. Am J Surg Pathol 15: 388–398
220. Yamashita S, Yamazaki H, Kato T, et al. 1996 Thymic carcinoma which developed in a thymic cyst. Intern Med 35: 215–218
221. Hattori H 2003 High-grade thymic carcinoma other than basaloid or mucoepidermoid type could be associated with multilocular thymic cyst: report of two cases. Histopathology 43: 501–502
222. Dorfman D M, Shahsafaei A, Chan J K 1997 Thymic carcinomas, but not thymomas and carcinomas of other sites, show CD5 immunoreactivity. Am J Surg Pathol 21: 936–940
223. Kornstein M J, Rosai J 1998 CD5 labeling of thymic carcinomas and other nonlymphoid neoplasms. Am J Clin Pathol 109: 722–726
224. Berezowski K, Grimes M M, Gal A, et al. 1996 CD5 immunoreactivity of epithelial cells in thymic carcinoma and CASTLE using paraffin-embedded tissue. Am J Clin Pathol 106: 483–486
225. Hishima T, Fukayama M, Fujisawa M, et al. 1994 CD5 expression in thymic carcinoma. Am J Pathol 145: 268–275
226. Tateyama H, Eimoto T, Tada T, et al. 1999 Immunoreactivity of a new CD5 antibody with normal epithelium and malignant tumors including thymic carcinoma. Am J Clin Pathol 111: 235–240
227. Hishima T, Fukayama M, Hayashi Y, et al. 1998 Neuroendocrine differentiation in thymic epithelial tumors with special reference to thymic carcinoma and atypical thymoma. Hum Pathol 29: 330–338
228. Nakagawa K, Matsuno Y, Kunitoh H, et al. 2005 Immunohistochemical KIT (CD117) expression in thymic epithelial tumors. Chest 128: 140–144
229. Pan C C, Chen P C, Chiang H 2004 KIT (CD117) is frequently overexpressed in thymic carcinomas but is absent in thymomas. J Pathol 202: 375–381
230. Lauriola L, Erlandson R A, Rosai J 1998 Neuroendocrine differentiation is a common feature of thymic carcinoma. Am J Surg Pathol 22: 1059–1066
231. Kuo T T 2000 Frequent presence of neuroendocrine small cells in thymic carcinoma: a light microscopic and immunohistochemical study. Histopathology 37: 19–26
232. Hino N, Kondo K, Miyoshi T, et al. 1997 High frequency of p53 protein expression in thymic carcinoma but not in thymoma. Br J Cancer 76: 1361–1366
233. Chen F F, Yan J J, Jin Y T, et al. 1996 Detection of bcl-2 and p53 in thymoma: expression of bcl-2 as a reliable marker of tumor aggressiveness. Hum Pathol 27: 1089–1092
234. Pich A, Chiarle R, Chiusa L, et al. 1996 p53 expression and proliferative activity predict survival in non-invasive thymomas. Int J Cancer 69: 180–183
235. Stefanaki K, Rontogianni D, Kouvidou C H, et al. 1997 Expression of p53, mdm2, p21/waf1 and bcl-2 proteins in thymomas. Histopathology 30: 549–555
236. Tateyama H, Eimoto T, Tada T, et al. 1995 p53 protein expression and p53 gene mutation in thymic epithelial tumors. An immunohistochemical and DNA sequencing study. Am J Clin Pathol 104: 375–381
237. Weirich G, Schneider P, Fellbaum C, et al. 1997 p53 alterations in thymic epithelial tumours. Virchows Arch 431: 17–23
238. Asamura H, Nakajima T, Mukai K 1988 Degree of malignancy of thymic epithelial tumors in terms of nuclear DNA content and nuclear area, an analysis of 39 cases. Am J Pathol 133: 615–622
239. Kuo T T, Lo S K 1993 DNA flow cytometric study of thymic epithelial tumors with evaluation of its usefulness in the pathologic classification. Hum Pathol 24: 746–749
240. Tseng Y L, Wang S T, Wu M H, et al. 2003 Thymic carcinoma: involvement of great vessels indicates poor prognosis. Ann Thorac Surg 76: 1041–1045
241. Chan J K, Rosai J 1991 Tumors of the neck showing thymic or related branchial pouch differentiation: a unifying concept. Hum Pathol 22: 349–367
242. Shih D F, Wang J S, Tseng H H et al. 1997 Primary pleural thymoma. Arch Pathol Lab Med 121: 79–82
243. Kung I T, Loke S L, So S Y, et al. 1985 Intrapulmonary thymoma: report of two cases. Thorax 40: 471–474
244. Yamashita H, Murakami N, Noguchi S, et al. 1983 Cervical thymoma and incidence of cervical thymus. Acta Pathol Jpn 33: 189–194

245. Mende S, Moschopulos M, Marx A, et al. 2004 Ectopic micronodular thymoma with lymphoid stroma. Virchows Arch 444: 397–399
246. Miller D V, Tazelaar H D, Handy J R, et al. 2005 Thymoma arising within cardiac myxoma. Am J Surg Pathol 29: 1208–1213
247. Fetsch J F, Laskin W B, Michal M, et al. 2004 Ectopic hamartomatous thymoma: a clinicopathologic and immunohistochemical analysis of 21 cases with data supporting reclassification as a branchial anlage mixed tumor. Am J Surg Pathol 28: 1360–1370
248. Travis W D, Colby T V, Corrin B, et al. 1999 Histological typing of lung and pleural tumors. WHO international histological classification of tumors. Springer Verlag, Berlin
249. Beasley M B, Thunnissen F B, Hasleton P S, et al. 2004 Carcinoid tumour. In: Travis W D, Brambilla E, Muller-Hermelink H K, et al. (eds) Pathology and genetics. Tumours of the lung, pleura, thymus and heart. WHO classification of tumours. IARC Press, Lyon, 59–62
250. Klemm K M, Moran C A 1999 Primary neuroendocrine carcinomas of the thymus. Semin Diagn Pathol 16: 32–41
251. Moran C A, Suster S 2000 Neuroendocrine carcinomas (carcinoid tumors) of the thymus: a clinicopathologic analysis of 80 cases. Am J Clin Pathol 114: 100–110
252. Moran C A 2005 Primary neuroendocrine carcinomas of the mediastinum: review of current criteria for histopathologic diagnosis and classification. Semin Diagn Pathol 22: 223–229
253. Marx A, Shimosato Y, Kuo T T, et al. 2004 Thymic neuroendocrine tumours. In: Travis W D, Brambilla E, Muller-Hermelink H K, et al. (eds) Pathology and genetics. Tumours of the lung, pleura, thymus and heart. WHO classification of tumours. IARC Press, Lyon, 188–195
254. Rosai J, Levine G, Weber W R, et al. 1976 Carcinoid tumors and oat cell carcinomas of the thymus. Pathol Annu 11: 201–226
255. Rosai J, Higa E 1972 Mediastinal endocrine neoplasm, of probable thymic origin, related to carcinoid tumor. Clinicopathologic study of 8 cases. Cancer 29: 1061–1074
256. Wick M R, Carney J A, Bernatz P E, et al. 1982 Primary mediastinal carcinoid tumors. Am J Surg Pathol 6: 195–205
257. Wick M R, Scott R E, Li C Y, et al. 1980 Carcinoid tumor of the thymus: a clinicopathologic report of seven cases with a review of the literature. Mayo Clin Proc 55: 246–254
258. Moran C A, Suster S 2000 Neuroendocrine carcinomas (carcinoid tumor) of the thymus. A clinicopathologic analysis of 80 cases. Am J Clin Pathol 114: 100–110
259. Salyer W R, Salyer D C, Eggleston J C 1976 Carcinoid tumors of the thymus. Cancer 37: 958–973
260. Wick M R, Rosai J 1988 Neuroendocrine neoplasms of the thymus. Pathol Res Pract 183: 188–199
261. Wick M R, Rosai J 1991 Neuroendocrine neoplasms of the mediastinum. Semin Diagn Pathol 8: 35–51
262. Teh B T, Zedenius J, Kytola S, et al. 1998 Thymic carcinoids in multiple endocrine neoplasia type 1. Ann Surg 228: 99–105
263. Teh B T 1998 Thymic carcinoids in multiple endocrine neoplasia type 1. J Intern Med 243: 501–504
264. Teh B T, McArdle J, Chan S P, et al. 1997 Clinicopathologic studies of thymic carcinoids in multiple endocrine neoplasia type 1. Medicine (Baltimore) 76: 21–29
265. Zeiger M A, Swartz S E, MacGillivray D C, et al. 1992 Thymic carcinoid in association with MEN syndromes. Am Surg 58: 430–434
266. Ferolla P, Falchetti A, Filosso P, et al. 2005 Thymic neuroendocrine carcinoma (carcinoid) in multiple endocrine neoplasia type 1 syndrome: the Italian series. J Clin Endocrinol Metab 90: 2603–2609
267. Rosai J, Higa E, Davie JM 1972 Mediastinal endocrine neoplasm in patients with multiple endocrine adenomatosis. A previously unrecognized association. Cancer 29: 1075–1083
268. Wang D Y, Chang D B, Kuo S H, et al. 1994 Carcinoid tumours of the thymus. Thorax 49: 357–360
269. Vietri F, Illuminati G, Guglielmi R, et al. 1994 Carcinoid tumour of the thymus gland. Eur J Surg 160: 645–647
270. Mizuno T, Masaoka A, Hashimoto T, et al. 1990 Coexisting thymic carcinoid tumor and thymoma. Ann Thorac Surg 50: 650–652
271. Levine G D, Rosai J 1976 A spindle cell variant of thymic carcinoid tumor. A clinical, histologic, and fine structural study with emphasis on its distinction from spindle cell thymoma. Arch Pathol Lab Med 100: 293–300
272. Moran C A, Suster S 1999 Spindle-cell neuroendocrine carcinomas of the thymus (spindle-cell thymic carcinoid): a clinicopathologic and immunohistochemical study of seven cases. Mod Pathol 12: 587–591
273. Ho F C, Ho J C 1977 Pigmented carcinoid tumour of the thymus. Histopathology 1: 363–369
274. Lagrange W, Dahm H H, Karstens J, et al. 1987 Melanocytic neuroendocrine carcinoma of the thymus. Cancer 59: 484–488
275. Klemm K M, Moran C A, Suster S 1999 Pigmented thymic carcinoids: a clinicopathological and immunohistochemical study of two cases. Mod Pathol 12: 946–948
276. Yamaji I, Iimura O, Mito T, et al. 1984 An ectopic, ACTH producing, oncocytic carcinoid tumor of the thymus: report of a case. Jpn J Med 23: 62–66
277. Moran C A, Suster S 2000 Primary neuroendocrine carcinoma (thymic carcinoid) of the thymus with prominent oncocytic features: a clinicopathologic study of 22 cases. Mod Pathol 13: 489–494
278. Moran C A, Suster S 1999 Oncocytic neuroendocrine carcinoma of the thymus: clinicopathological and immunohistochemical study of 22 cases [Abstract]. Mod Pathol 12: 185A
279. Suster S, Moran C A 1995 Thymic carcinoid with prominent mucinous stroma. Report of a distinctive morphologic variant of thymic neuroendocrine neoplasm. Am J Surg Pathol 19: 1277–1285
280. Moran C A, Suster S 1999 Angiomatoid neuroendocrine carcinoma of the thymus: report of a distinctive morphological variant of neuroendocrine tumor of the thymus resembling a vascular neoplasm. Hum Pathol 30: 635–639
281. Kuo T T 1994 Carcinoid tumor of the thymus with divergent sarcomatoid differentiation: report of a case with histogenetic consideration. Hum Pathol 25: 319–323
282. Paties C, Zangrandi A, Vassallo G, et al. 1991 Multidirectional carcinoma of the thymus with neuroendocrine and sarcomatoid components and carcinoid syndrome. Pathol Res Pract 187: 170–177
283. Herbst W M, Kummer W, Hofmann W, et al. 1987 Carcinoid tumors of the thymus. An immunohistochemical study. Cancer 60: 2465–2470
284. Wick M R, Scheithauer B W 1982 Oat-cell carcinoma of the thymus. Cancer 49: 1652–1657
285. Chan J K, Suster S, Wenig B M, et al. 1997 Cytokeratin 20 immunoreactivity distinguishes Merkel cell (primary cutaneous neuroendocrine) carcinomas and salivary gland small cell carcinomas from small cell carcinomas of various sites. Am J Surg Pathol 21: 226–234
286. Chetty R, Batitang S, Govender D 1997 Large cell neuroendocrine carcinoma of the thymus. Histopathology 31: 274–276
287. Davis R D Jr, Oldham H N Jr, Sabiston DC Jr 1987 Primary cysts and neoplasms of the mediastinum: recent changes in clinical presentation, methods of diagnosis, management, and results. Ann Thorac Surg 44: 229–237
288. Meares E M, Briggs E M 1972 Occult seminoma of the testis masquerading as primary extragonadal germinal neoplasms. Cancer 30: 300–306
289. Nichols C R 1992 Mediastinal germ cell tumors. Semin Thorac Cardiovasc Surg 4: 45–50
290. Lee Y M, Jackson S M 1985 Primary seminoma of the mediastinum. Cancer Control Agency of British Columbia experience. Cancer 55: 450–452
291. Martini N, Golbey R B, Hajdu S I, et al. 1974 Primary mediastinal germ cell tumors. Cancer 33: 763–769
292. Truong L D, Harris L, Mattioli C, et al. 1986 Endodermal sinus tumor of the mediastinum. A report of seven cases and review of the literature. Cancer 58: 730–739
293. Dehner L P 1990 Germ cell tumors of the mediastinum. Semin Diagn Pathol 7: 266–284
294. Weidner N 1999 Germ-cell tumors of the mediastinum. Semin Diagn Pathol 16: 42–50
295. Schlumberger H G 1946 Teratoma of the anterior mediastinum in the group of military age, a study of 16 cases and a review of theories of genesis. Arch Pathol 41: 398–444
296. Gonzalez-Crussi F 1982 Extragonadal teratomas. Atlas of tumor pathology, 2nd series, Fascicle 18. Armed Forces Institute of Pathology, Washington DC
297. Nichols C R, Heerema N A, Palmer C, et al. 1987 Klinefelter's syndrome associated with mediastinal germ cell neoplasms. J Clin Oncol 5: 1290–1294
298. Lachman M F, Kim K, Koo B C 1986 Mediastinal teratoma associated with Klinefelter's syndrome. Arch Pathol Lab Med 110: 1067–1077
299. Bergh N P, Gatzinsky P, Larsson S, et al. 1978 Tumors of the thymus and thymic region: III. Clinicopathological studies on teratomas and tumors of germ cell type. Ann Thorac Surg 25: 107–111
300. Wychulis A R, Payne W S, Clagett O T 1971 Surgical treatment of mediastinal tumors, a 40-year experience. J Thorac Cardiovasc Surg 62: 379–392
301. Dominguez Malagon H, Perez Montiel D 2005 Mediastinal germ cell tumors. Semin Diagn Pathol 22: 230–240
302. Nichols C R, Roth B J, Heerema N, et al. 1990 Hematologic neoplasia associated with primary mediastinal germ-cell tumors. N Engl J Med 322: 1425–1429
303. DeMent S H, Eggleston J C, Spivak J L 1985 Association between mediastinal germ cell tumors and hematologic malignancies. Report of two cases and review of the literature. Am J Surg Pathol 9: 23–30
304. deMent S H 1990 Association between mediastinal germ cell tumors and hematologic malignancies: an update. Hum Pathol 21: 699–703
305. Chariot P, Monnet I, LeLong F, et al. 1991 Systemic mast cell disease associated with primary mediastinal germ cell tumor. Am J Med 90: 381–385
306. Chariot P, Monnet I, Gaulard P, et al. 1993 Systemic mastocytosis following mediastinal germ cell tumor: an association confirmed. Hum Pathol 24: 111–112
307. Orazi A, Neiman R S, Ulbright T M, et al. 1993 Hematopoietic precursor cells within the yolk sac tumor component are the source of secondary hematopoietic malignancies in patients with mediastinal germ cell tumors. Cancer 71: 3873–3881
308. Zon R, Orazi A, Neiman R S, et al. 1994 Benign hematologic neoplasm associated with mediastinal mature teratoma in a patient with Klinefelter's syndrome: a case report. Med Pediatr Oncol 23: 376–379
309. Downie P A, Vogelzang N J, Moldwin R L, et al. 1994 Establishment of a leukemia cell line with i(12p) from a patient with a mediastinal germ cell tumor and acute lymphoblastic leukemia. Cancer Res 54: 4999–5004

310. Manivel C, Wick M R, Abenoza P, et al. 1986 The occurrence of sarcomatous components in primary mediastinal germ cell tumors. Am J Surg Pathol 10: 711–717
311. Wick M R, Perlman E J, Strobel P, et al. 2004 Germ cell tumours with somatic-type malignancy. In: Travis W D, Brambilla E, Muller-Hermelink H K, et al. (eds) Pathology and genetics. Tumours of the lung, pleura, thymus and heart. WHO classification of tumours. IARC Press, Lyon, 188–195
312. Moran C A, Suster S, Przygodzki R M, et al. 1997 Primary germ cell tumors of the mediastinum: II. Mediastinal seminomas – a clinicopathologic and immunohistochemical study of 120 cases. Cancer 80: 691–698
313. Schantz A, Sewall W, Castleman B 1972 Mediastinal germinoma, a study of 21 cases with an excellent prognosis. Cancer 30: 1189–1194
314. Hainsworth J D, Greco F A 1992 Extragonadal germ cell tumors and unrecognized germ cell tumors. Semin Oncol 19: 119–127
315. Moran C A, Suster S, Koss M N 1997 Primary germ cell tumors of the mediastinum: III. Yolk sac tumor, embryonal carcinoma, choriocarcinoma, and combined nonteratomatous germ cell tumors of the mediastinum – a clinicopathologic and immunohistochemical study of 64 cases. Cancer 80: 699–707
316. Moran C A, Suster S 1997 Primary mediastinal choriocarcinomas: a clinicopathologic and immunohistochemical study of eight cases. Am J Surg Pathol 21: 1007–1012
317. Sham J S, Fu K H, Chiu C S, et al. 1989 Experience with the management of primary endodermal sinus tumor of the mediastinum. Cancer 64: 756–761
318. Nichols C R, Saxman S, Williams S D, et al. 1990 Primary mediastinal nonseminomatous germ cell tumors. A modern single institution experience. Cancer 65: 1641–1646
319. Bokemeyer C, Nichols C R, Droz J P, et al. 2002 Extragonadal germ cell tumors of the mediastinum and retroperitoneum: results from an international analysis. J Clin Oncol 20: 1864–1873
320. Schneider D T, Calaminus G, Reinhard H, et al. 2000 Primary mediastinal germ cell tumors in children and adolescents: results of the German cooperative protocols MAKEI 83/86, 89, and 96. J Clin Oncol 18: 832–839
321. Billmire D, Vinocur C, Rescorla F, et al. 2001 Malignant mediastinal germ cell tumors: an intergroup study. J Pediatr Surg 36: 18–24
322. Burns B F, McGaughey W T 1986 Unusual thymic seminomas. Arch Pathol Lab Med 110: 539–541
323. Moran C A, Suster S 1995 Mediastinal seminomas with prominent cystic changes. A clinicopathologic study of 10 cases. Am J Surg Pathol 19: 1047–1053
324. Suda K, Mizuguchi K, Hebisawa A 1984 Pancreatic tissue in teratoma. Arch Pathol Lab Med 108: 835–837
325. Bordi C, De Vita O, Pollice L 1985 Full pancreatic endocrine differentiation in a mediastinal teratoma. Hum Pathol 16: 961–964
326. Southgate J, Slade P R 1982 Teratodermoid cyst of the mediastinum with pancreatic enzyme secretion. Thorax 37: 476–477
327. Lancaster K J, Liang C Y, Myers J C, et al. 1997 Goblet cell carcinoid arising in a mature teratoma of the mediastinum. Am J Surg Pathol 21: 109–113
328. Song S Y, Ko Y H, Ahn G 2005 Mediastinal germ cell tumor associated with histiocytic sarcoma of spleen: case report of an unusual association. Int J Surg Pathol 13: 299–303
329. Went P T, Dirnhofer S, Stallmach T, et al. 2005 Placental site trophoblastic tumor of the mediastinum. Hum Pathol 36: 581–584
330. Moran C A, Suster S 1997 Hepatoid yolk sac tumors of the mediastinum: a clinicopathologic and immunohistochemical study of four cases. Am J Surg Pathol 21: 1210–1214
331. Moran C A, Suster S 1997 Mediastinal yolk sac tumors associated with prominent multilocular cystic changes of thymic epithelium: a clinicopathologic and immunohistochemical study of five cases. Mod Pathol 10: 800–803
332. Moran C A, Suster S 1997 Yolk sac tumors of the mediastinum with prominent spindle cell features: a clinicopathologic study of three cases. Am J Surg Pathol 21: 1173–1177
333. Greco F A, Oldham R K, Fer M F 1982 The extragonadal germ cell cancer syndrome. Semin Oncol 9: 448–455
334. Suster S, Moran C A, Dominguez-Malagon H, et al. 1998 Germ cell tumors of the mediastinum and testis: a comparative immunohistochemical study of 120 cases. Hum Pathol 29: 737–742
335. Arber D A, Tamayo R, Weiss L M 1998 Paraffin section detection of the c-kit gene product (CD117) in human tissues: value in the diagnosis of mast cell disorders. Hum Pathol 29: 498–504
336. Cheng L 2004 Establishing a germ cell origin for metastatic tumors using OCT4 immunohistochemistry. Cancer 101: 2006–2010
337. Yousem S A, Weiss L M, Warnke R A 1985 Primary mediastinal non-Hodgkin's lymphomas: a morphologic and immunologic study of 19 cases. Am J Clin Pathol 83: 676–680
338. Strickler J G, Kurtin P J 1991 Mediastinal lymphoma. Semin Diagn Pathol 8: 2–13
339. Waldron J A Jr, Dohring E J, Farber L R 1985 Primary large cell lymphomas of the mediastinum: an analysis of 20 cases. Semin Diagn Pathol 2: 281–295
340. Kim H C, Nosher J, Haas A 1985 Cystic degeneration of thymic Hodgkin's disease following radiation therapy. Cancer 55: 354–356
341. Casey T T, Cousar J B, Mangum M 1990 Monomorphic lymphomas arising in patients with Hodgkin's disease, correlation of morphologic, immunophenotypic, and molecular genetic findings in 12 cases. Am J Pathol 136: 81–94
342. Traverse-Glehen A, Pittaluga S, Gaulard P, et al. 2005 Mediastinal gray zone lymphoma: the missing link between classic Hodgkin's lymphoma and mediastinal large B-cell lymphoma. Am J Surg Pathol 29: 1411–1421
343. Addis B J, Isaacson P G 1986 Large cell lymphoma of the mediastinum: a B-cell tumour of probable thymic origin. Histopathology 10: 379–390
344. Moller P, Lammler B, Eberlein-Gonska M, et al. 1986 Primary mediastinal clear cell lymphoma of B-cell type. Virchows Arch A Pathol Anat Histopathol 409: 79–92
345. Davis R E, Dorfman R F, Warnke R A 1990 Primary large-cell lymphoma of the thymus: a diffuse B-cell neoplasm presenting as primary mediastinal lymphoma. Hum Pathol 21: 1262–1268
346. Hofmann W J, Momburg F, Moller P, et al. 1988 Intra- and extrathymic B cells in physiologic and pathologic conditions. Immunohistochemical study on normal thymus and lymphofollicular hyperplasia of the thymus. Virchows Arch A Pathol Anat Histopathol 412: 431–442
347. Menestrina F, Chilosi M, Bonetti F, et al. 1986 Mediastinal large-cell lymphoma of B type, with sclerosis: histopathological and immunohistochemical study of eight cases. Histopathology 10: 589–600
348. Menestrina F, Harris N L, Moller P 2004 Primary mediastinal large B-cell lymphoma. In: Travis W D, Brambilla E, Muller-Hermelink H K, et al. (eds) Pathology and genetics. Tumours of the lung, pleura, thymus and heart. WHO classification of tumours. IARC Press, Lyon, 222–224
349. The non-Hodgkin's Lymphoma Classification Project 1997 A clinical evaluation of the International Lymphoma Study Group classification of non-Hodgkin's lymphoma. Blood 89: 3909–3918
350. Suster S 1999 Primary large-cell lymphomas of the mediastinum. Semin Diagn Pathol 16: 51–64
351. Perrone T, Frizzera G, Rosai J 1986 Mediastinal diffuse large-cell lymphoma with sclerosis. A clinicopathologic study of 60 cases. Am J Surg Pathol 10: 176–191
352. Todeschini G, Ambrosetti A, Meneghini V, et al. 1990 Mediastinal large-B-cell lymphoma with sclerosis: a clinical study of 21 patients. J Clin Oncol 8: 804–808
353. Lamarre L, Jacobson J O, Aisenberg A C, et al. 1989 Primary large cell lymphoma of the mediastinum. A histologic and immunophenotypic study of 29 cases. Am J Surg Pathol 13: 730–739
354. Jacobson J O, Aisenberg A C, Lamarre L, et al. 1988 Mediastinal large cell lymphoma. An uncommon subset of adult lymphoma curable with combined modality therapy. Cancer 62: 1893–1898
355. Aisenberg A C 1999 Primary large cell lymphoma of the mediastinum. Semin Oncol 26: 251–258
356. Falini B, Venturi S, Martelli M, et al. 1995 Mediastinal large B-cell lymphoma: clinical and immunohistological findings in 18 patients treated with different third-generation regimens. Br J Haematol 89: 780–789
357. Rohatiner A Z, Whelan J S, Ganjoo R K, et al. 1994 Mediastinal large-cell lymphoma with sclerosis (MLCLS). Br J Cancer 69: 601–604
358. Lazzarino M, Orlandi E, Paulli M, et al. 1997 Treatment outcome and prognostic factors for primary mediastinal (thymic) B-cell lymphoma: a multicenter study of 106 patients. J Clin Oncol 15: 1646–1653
359. Chim C S, Liang R, Chan A C, et al. 1996 Primary B cell lymphoma of the mediastinum. Hematol Oncol 14: 173–179
360. Cazals-Hatem D, Lepage E, Brice P, et al. 1996 Primary mediastinal large B-cell lymphoma. A clinicopathologic study of 141 cases compared with 916 nonmediastinal large B-cell lymphomas, a GELA ('Groupe d'Etude des Lymphomes de l'Adulte') study. Am J Surg Pathol 20: 877–888
361. Lavabre-Bertrand T, Donadio D, Fegueux N, et al. 1992 A study of 15 cases of primary mediastinal lymphoma of B-cell type. Cancer 69: 2561–2566
362. Lazzarino M, Orlandi E, Paulli M, et al. 1993 Primary mediastinal B-cell lymphoma with sclerosis: an aggressive tumor with distinctive clinical and pathologic features. J Clin Oncol 11: 2306–2313
363. Abou-Elella A A, Weisenburger D D, Vose J M, et al. 1999 Primary mediastinal large B-cell lymphoma: a clinicopathologic study of 43 patients from the Nebraska Lymphoma Study Group. J Clin Oncol 17: 784–790
364. Bishop P C, Wilson W H, Pearson D, et al. 1999 CNS Involvement in primary mediastinal large B-cell lymphoma. J Clin Oncol 17: 2479
365. Todeschini G, Secchi S, Morra E, et al. 2004 Primary mediastinal large B-cell lymphoma (PMLBCL): long-term results from a retrospective multicentre Italian experience in 138 patients treated with CHOP or MACOP-B/VACOP-B. Br J Cancer 90: 372–376
366. Zinzani P L, Martelli M, Bertini M, et al. 2002 Induction chemotherapy strategies for primary mediastinal large B-cell lymphoma with sclerosis: a retrospective multinational study on 426 previously untreated patients. Haematologica 87: 1258–1264
367. Zinzani P L, Maretlli M, Magagnoli M, et al. 1999 Treatment and clinical management of primary mediastinal large B-cell lymphoma with sclerosis: MACOP-B regimen and mediastinal radiotherapy monitored by 67-gallium scan in 50 patients. Blood 94: 3289–3293
368. Kirn D, Mauch P, Shaffer K, et al. 1993 Large-cell and immunoblastic lymphoma of the mediastinum: prognostic features and treatment outcome in 57 patients. J Clin Oncol 11: 1336–1343
369. Paulli M, Strater J, Gianelli U, et al. 1999 Mediastinal B-cell lymphoma: a study of its histomorphologic spectrum based on 109 cases. Hum Pathol 30: 178–187

370. Moller P, Lammler B, Herrmann B, et al. 1986 The primary mediastinal clear cell lymphoma of B-cell type has variable defects in MHC antigen expression. Immunology 59: 411–417
371. Moller P, Moldenhauer G, Momburg F, et al. 1987 Mediastinal lymphoma of clear cell type is a tumor corresponding to terminal steps of B cell differentiation. Blood 69: 1087–1095
372. Moller P, Matthaei-Maurer D U, Hofmann W J, et al. 1989 Immunophenotypic similarities of mediastinal clear–cell lymphoma and sinusoidal (monocytoid) B cells. Int J Cancer 43: 10–16
373. Higgins J P, Warnke R A 1999 CD30 expression is common in mediastinal large B-cell lymphoma. Am J Clin Pathol 112: 241–247
374. Suster S, Moran C A 1996 Pleomorphic large cell lymphomas of the mediastinum. Am J Surg Pathol 20: 224–232
375. Suster S 1992 Large cell lymphoma of the mediastinum with marked tropism for germinal centers. Cancer 69: 2910–2916
376. Kanavaros P, Gaulard P, Charlotte F, et al. 1995 Discordant expression of immunoglobulin and its associated molecule mb-1/CD79a is frequently found in mediastinal large B cell lymphomas. Am J Pathol 146: 735–741
377. Pileri S A, Gaidano G, Zinzani P L, et al. 2003 Primary mediastinal B-cell lymphoma: high frequency of BCL-6 mutations and consistent expression of the transcription factors OCT-2, BOB.1, and PU.1 in the absence of immunoglobulins. Am J Pathol 162: 243–253
378. Nakagawa A, Nakamura S, Koshikawa T 1993 Clinicopathologic study of primary mediastinal non-lymphoblastic non-Hodgkin's lymphomas among the Japanese. Acta Pathol Jpn 43: 44–54
379. al-Sharabati M, Chittal S, Duga-Neulat I, et al. 1991 Primary anterior mediastinal B-cell lymphoma. A clinicopathologic and immunohistochemical study of 16 cases. Cancer 67: 2579–2587
380. Copie-Bergman C, Plonquet A, Alonso M A, et al. 2002 MAL expression in lymphoid cells: further evidence for MAL as a distinct molecular marker of primary mediastinal large B-cell lymphomas. Mod Pathol 15: 1172–1180
381. Roberts R A, Wright G, Rosenwald A R, et al. 2006 Loss of major histocompatibility class II gene and protein expression in primary mediastinal large B-cell lymphoma is highly coordinated and related to poor patient survival. Blood 108: 311–318
382. Fraternali-Orcioni G, Falini B, Quaini F, et al. 1999 Beta-HCG aberrant expression in primary mediastinal large B-cell lymphoma. Am J Surg Pathol 23: 717–721
383. Bentz M, Barth T F, Bruderlein S, et al. 2001 Gain of chromosome arm 9p is characteristic of primary mediastinal B-cell lymphoma (MBL): comprehensive molecular cytogenetic analysis and presentation of a novel MBL cell line. Genes Chromos Cancer 30: 393–401
384. Pileri S A, Zinzani P L, Gaidano G, et al. 2003 Pathobiology of primary mediastinal B-cell lymphoma. Leuk Lymphoma 44 Suppl 3: S21–26
385. Tsang P, Cesarman E, Chadburn A, et al. 1996 Molecular characterization of primary mediastinal B cell lymphoma. Am J Pathol 148: 2017–2025
386. Scarpa A, Borgato L, Chilosi M, et al. 1991 Evidence of c-myc gene abnormalities in mediastinal large B-cell lymphoma of young adult age. Blood 78: 780–788
387. Scarpa A, Moore P S, Rigaud G, et al. 1999 Molecular features of primary mediastinal B-cell lymphoma: involvement of p16INK4A, p53 and c-myc. Br J Haematol 107: 106–113
388. Copie-Bergman C, Gaulard P, Maouche-Chretien L, et al. 1999 The MAL gene is expressed in primary mediastinal large B-cell lymphoma. Blood 94: 3567–3575
389. Rosenwald A, Wright G, Leroy K, et al. 2003 Molecular diagnosis of primary mediastinal B cell lymphoma identifies a clinically favorable subgroup of diffuse large B cell lymphoma related to Hodgkin's lymphoma. J Exp Med 198: 851–862
390. Savage K J, Monti S, Kutok J L, et al. 2003 The molecular signature of mediastinal large B-cell lymphoma differs from that of other diffuse large B-cell lymphomas and shares features with classical Hodgkin's lymphoma. Blood 102: 3871–3879
391. Calvo K R, Traverse-Glehen A, Pittaluga S, et al. 2004 Molecular profiling provides evidence of primary mediastinal large B-cell lymphoma as a distinct entity related to classic Hodgkin's lymphoma: implications for mediastinal gray zone lymphomas as an intermediate form of B-cell lymphoma. Adv Anat Pathol 11: 227–238
392. Chadburn A, Frizzera G 1999 Mediastinal large B-cell lymphoma vs classic Hodgkin's lymphoma. Am J Clin Pathol 112: 155–158
393. Muller-Hermelink H K, Rudiger T, Rosenwald A, et al. 2004 Grey zone between Hodgkin's lymphoma and non-Hodgkin's lymphomas (NHL). In: Travis W D, Brambilla E, Muller-Hermelink H K, et al. (eds) Pathology and genetics. Tumours of the lung, pleura, thymus and heart. WHO classification of tumours. IARC Press, Lyon, 233
394. Rudiger T, Jaffe E S, Delsol G, et al. 1998 Workshop report on Hodgkin's disease and related diseases ('grey zone' lymphoma). Ann Oncol 9 Suppl 5: S31–38
395. Garcia J F, Mollejo M, Fraga M, et al. 2005 Large B-cell lymphoma with Hodgkin's features. Histopathology 47: 101–110
396. Nathwani B N, Kim H, Rappaport H 1976 Malignant lymphoma, lymphoblastic. Cancer 38: 964–983, 1976
397. Shepherd S F, A'Hern R P, Pinkerton C R 1995 Childhood T-cell lymphoblastic lymphoma – does early resolution of mediastinal mass predict for final outcome? The United Kingdom Children's Cancer Study Group (UKCCSG). Br J Cancer 72: 752–756
398. Sander C A, Jaffe E S, Gebhardt F C, et al. 1992 Mediastinal lymphoblastic lymphoma with an immature B-cell immunophenotype. Am J Surg Pathol 16: 300–305
399. Koita H, Suzumiya J, Ohshima K, et al. 1997 Lymphoblastic lymphoma expressing natural killer cell phenotype with involvement of the mediastinum and nasal cavity. Am J Surg Pathol 21: 242–248
400. Banerjee D, Silva E 1981 Mediastinal mass with acute leukemia. Myeloblastoma masquerading as lymphoblastic lymphoma. Arch Pathol Lab Med 105: 126–129
401. Kubonishi I, Ohtsuki Y, Machida K I 1984 Granulocytic sarcoma presenting as a mediastinal tumor. Report of a case and cytological and cytochemical studies of tumor cells in vivo and in vitro. Am J Clin Pathol 82: 730–734
402. Au W Y, Ma S K, Chan A C, et al. 1998 Near tetraploidy in three cases of acute myeloid leukemia associated with mediastinal granulocytic sarcoma. Cancer Genet Cytogenet 102: 50–53
403. Wong W S, Loong F, Ooi G C, et al. 2004 Primary granulocytic sarcoma of the mediastinum. Leuk Lymphoma 45: 1931–1933
404. Isaacson P G, Chan J K, Tang C, et al. 1990 Low-grade B-cell lymphoma of mucosa-associated lymphoid tissue arising in the thymus. A thymic lymphoma mimicking myoepithelial sialadenitis. Am J Surg Pathol 14: 342–351
405. Di Loreto C, Mariuzzi L, De Grassi A, et al. 1996 B cell lymphoma of the thymus and salivary gland. J Clin Pathol 49: 595–597
406. Yokose T, Kodama T, Matsuno Y, et al. 1998 Low-grade B cell lymphoma of mucosa-associated lymphoid tissue in the thymus of a patient with rheumatoid arthritis. Pathol Int 48: 74–81
407. Takagi N, Nakamura S, Yamamoto K, et al. 1992 Malignant lymphoma of mucosa-associated lymphoid tissue arising in the thymus of a patient with Sjogren's syndrome. A morphologic, phenotypic, and genotypic study. Cancer 69: 1347–1355
408. Yamasaki S, Matsushita H, Tanimura S, et al. 1998 B-cell lymphoma of mucosa-associated lymphoid tissue of the thymus: a report of two cases with a background of Sjögren's syndrome and monoclonal gammopathy. Hum Pathol 29: 1021–1024
409. Inagaki H, Chan J K, Ng J W, et al. 2002 Primary thymic extranodal marginal-zone B-cell lymphoma of mucosa-associated lymphoid tissue type exhibits distinctive clinicopathological and molecular features. Am J Pathol 160: 1435–1443
410. Yoshida M, Okabe M, Eimoto T, et al. 2006 Immunoglobulin VH genes in thymic MALT lymphoma are biased toward a restricted repertoire and are frequently unmutated. J Pathol 208: 415–422
411. Siegal G P, Dehner L P, Rosai J 1985 Histiocytosis X (Langerhans' cell granulomatosis) A clinicopathologic study of four childhood cases. Am J Surg Pathol 9: 117–124
412. Pescarmona E, Rendina E A, Ricci C, et al. 1989 Histiocytosis X and lymphoid follicular hyperplasia of the thymus in myasthenia gravis. Histopathology 14: 465–470
413. Bramwell N H, Burns B F 1986 Histiocytosis X of the thymus in association with myasthenia gravis. Am J Clin Pathol 86: 224–227
414. Novak I, Castro C Y, Listinsky C M 2003 Multiple Langerhans cell nodules in an incidental thymectomy. Arch Pathol Lab Med 127: 218–220
415. Lee B H, George S, Kutok J L 2003 Langerhans cell histiocytosis involving the thymus. A case report and review of the literature. Arch Pathol Lab Med 127: e294–297
416. Bove K E, Hurtubise P, Wong K Y 1985 Thymus in untreated systemic histiocytosis X. Pediatr Pathol 4: 99–115
417. Takahashi S, Asamoto M, Nakazawa T, et al. 1994 Robb–Smith type malignant histiocytosis associated with a mediastinal germ cell tumor. Jpn J Clin Oncol 24: 327–330
418. Perez-Ordoñez B, Erlandson R A, Rosai J 1996 Follicular dendritic cell tumor: report of 13 additional cases of a distinctive entity. Am J Surg Pathol 20: 944–955
419. Chan J K, Fletcher C D, Nayler S J, et al. 1997 Follicular dendritic cell sarcoma. Clinicopathologic analysis of 17 cases suggesting a malignant potential higher than currently recognized. Cancer 79: 294–313
420. Fassina A, Marino F, Poletti A, et al. 2001 Follicular dendritic cell tumor of the mediastinum. Ann Diagn Pathol 5: 361–367
421. Guettier C, Validire P, Emilie D, et al. 2006 Follicular dendritic cell tumor of the mediastinum: expression of fractalkine and SDF-1alpha as mast cell chemoattractants. Virchows Arch 448: 218–222
422. Krober S M, Marx A, Aebert H, et al. 2004 Sarcoma of follicular dendritic cells in the dorsal mediastinum. Hum Pathol 35: 259–263
423. Dillon K M, Hill C M, Cameron C H, et al. 2002 Mediastinal mixed dendritic cell sarcoma with hybrid features. J Clin Pathol 55: 791–794
424. Patcher M R, Lattes R 1963 Mesenchymal tumors of the mediastinum: tumors of fibrous tissue, adipose tissue, smooth muscle and striated muscle. Cancer 16: 74–94
425. Havlicek F, Rosai J 1984 A sarcoma of thymic stroma with features of liposarcoma. Am J Clin Pathol 82: 217–224
426. Standerfer R J, Armistead S H, Paneth M 1981 Liposarcoma of the mediastinum: report of two cases and review of the literature. Thorax 36: 693–694
427. Jones H, Yaman M, Penn C R, et al. 1993 Primary stromal sarcoma of the thymus with areas of liposarcoma. Histopathology 23: 81–82
428. Klimstra D S, Moran C A, Perino G, et al. 1995 Liposarcoma of the anterior mediastinum and thymus. A clinicopathologic study of 28 cases. Am J Surg Pathol 19: 782–791

429. Rosado de Christenson M L, Pugatch R D, Moran C A, et al. 1994 Thymolipoma: analysis of 27 cases. Radiology 193: 121–126
430. Moran C A, Rosado de Christenson M, Suster S 1995 Thymolipoma: clinicopathologic review of 33 cases. Mod Pathol 8: 741–744
431. Ringe B, Dragojevic D, Frank G, et al. 1979 Thymolipoma – a rare, benign tumor of the thymus gland two case reports and review of the literature. Thorac Cardiovasc Surg 27: 369–374
432. Takamori S, Hayashi A, Tayama K, et al. 1997 Thymolipoma associated with myasthenia gravis. Scand Cardiovasc J 31: 241–242
433. Iseki M, Tsuda N, Kishikawa M, et al. 1990 Thymolipoma with striated myoid cells. Histological, immunohistochemical, and ultrastructural study. Am J Surg Pathol 14: 395–398
434. Argani P, de Chiocca I C, Rosai J 1998 Thymoma arising with a thymolipoma. Histopathology 32: 573–574
435. Moran C A, Zeren H, Koss M N 1994 Thymofibrolipoma. A histologic variant of thymolipoma. Arch Pathol Lab Med 118: 281–282
436. Chan J K 1997 Solitary fibrous tumour – everywhere, and a diagnosis in vogue. Histopathology 31: 568–576
437. Witkin G B, Rosai J 1989 Solitary fibrous tumor of the mediastinum. A report of 14 cases. Am J Surg Pathol 13: 547–557
438. Weidner N 1991 Solitary fibrous tumor of the mediastinum. Ultrastruct Pathol 15: 489–492
439. Witkin G B, Miettinen M, Rosai J 1989 A biphasic tumor of the mediastinum with features of synovial sarcoma. A report of four cases. Am J Surg Pathol 13: 490–499
440. Suster S, Moran C A 2005 Primary synovial sarcomas of the mediastinum: a clinicopathologic, immunohistochemical, and ultrastructural study of 15 cases. Am J Surg Pathol 29: 569–578
441. Brown L R, Reiman H M, Rosenow E C et al. 1986 Intrathoracic lymphangioma. Mayo Clin Proc 61: 882–892
442. Patcher M R, Lattes R 1963 Mesenchymal tumors of the mediastinum: tumors of lymph vascular origin. Cancer 16: 108–117
443. Swanson P E 1991 Soft tissue neoplasms of the mediastinum. Semin Diagn Pathol 8: 14–34
444. Patcher M R, Lattes R 1963 Mesenchymal tumors of the mediastinum: tumors of blood vascular origin. Cancer 16: 95–107
445. Moran C A, Suster S 1995 Mediastinal hemangiomas: a study of 18 cases with emphasis on the spectrum of morphological features. Hum Pathol 26: 416–421
446. Hiraiwa H, Hamazaki M, Tsuruta S, et al. 1998 Infantile hemangioendothelioma of the thymus with massive pleural effusion and Kasabach–Merritt syndrome: histopathological, flow cytometrical analysis of the tumor. Acta Paediatr Jpn 40: 604–607
447. Lamovec J, Sobel H J, Zidar A, et al. 1990 Epithelioid hemangioendothelioma of the anterior mediastinum with osteoclast-like giant cells. Light microscopic, immunohistochemical, and electron microscopic study. Am J Clin Pathol 93: 813–817
448. Suster S, Moran C A, Koss M N 1994 Epithelioid hemangioendothelioma of the anterior mediastinum. Clinicopathologic, immunohistochemical, and ultrastructural analysis of 12 cases. Am J Surg Pathol 18: 871–881
449. Gibbs A R, Johnson N F, Giddings J C, et al. 1984 Primary angiosarcoma of the mediastinum: light and electron microscopic demonstration of Factor VIII-related antigen in neoplastic cells. Hum Pathol 15: 687–691
450. Kardamakis D, Bouboulis N, Ravazoula P, et al. 1996 Primary hemangiosarcoma of the mediastinum. Lung Cancer 16: 81–86
451. Saito A, Watanabe K, Kusakabe T, et al. 1998 Mediastinal mature teratoma with coexistence of angiosarcoma, granulocytic sarcoma and a hematopoietic region in the tumor: a rare case of association between hematological malignancy and mediastinal germ cell tumor. Pathol Int 48: 749–753
452. Ulbright T M, Clark S A, Einhorn L H 1985 Angiosarcoma associated with germ cell tumors. Hum Pathol 16: 961–964
453. Suster S, Moran C A, Koss M N 1994 Rhabdomyosarcomas of the anterior mediastinum: report of four cases unassociated with germ cell, teratomatous, or thymic carcinomatous components. Hum Pathol 25: 349–356
454. Begin L R, Schurch W, Lacoste J, et al. 1994 Glycogen-rich clear cell rhabdomyosarcoma of the mediastinum. Potential diagnostic pitfall. Am J Surg Pathol 18: 302–308
455. Lindskog B I, Malm A 1965 Diagnostic and surgical considerations on mediastinal (intrathoracic) goiter. Dis Chest 47: 201–207
456. Wick M R 1990 Mediastinal cysts and intrathoracic thyroid tumors. Semin Diagn Pathol 7: 285–294
457. Strollo D C, Rosado de Christenson M L, Jett J R 1997 Primary mediastinal tumors. Part 1: tumors of the anterior mediastinum. Chest 112: 511–522
458. Dominguez-Malagon H, Guerrero-Medrano J, Suster S 1995 Ectopic poorly differentiated (insular) carcinoma of the thyroid. Report of a case presenting as an anterior mediastinal mass. Am J Clin Pathol 104: 408–412
459. Chan J K 2004 Ectopic thyroid and parathyroid tumours. In: Travis W D, Brambilla E, Muller-Hermelink H K, et al. (eds) Pathology and genetics. Tumours of the lung, pleura, thymus and heart. WHO classification of tumours. IARC Press, Lyon, 246
460. Clark O H 1988 Mediastinal parathyroid tumors. Arch Surg 123: 1096–1100
461. Nathaniels E K, Nathaniels A M, Wang C A 1970 Mediastinal parathyroid tumors: a clinical and pathological study of 84 cases. Ann Surg 171: 165–170
462. Kelly M D, Sheridan B F, Farnsworth A E, et al. 1994 Parathyroid carcinoma in a mediastinal sixth parathyroid gland. Aust NZ J Surg 64: 446–449
463. Conn J M, Goncalves M A, Mansour K A, et al. 1991 The mediastinal parathyroid. Am Surg 57: 62–66
464. Moran C A, Suster S 2005 Primary parathyroid tumors of the mediastinum: a clinicopathologic and immunohistochemical study of 17 cases. Am J Clin Pathol 127: 749–754
465. Murphy M N, Glennon P G, Diocee M S, et al. 1986 Nonsecretory parathyroid carcinoma of the mediastinum. Light microscopic, immunocytochemical, and ultrastructural features of a case, and review of the literature. Cancer 58: 2468–2476
466. Arbona G I, Lloyd T V, Lucas J 1980 Mediastinal extramedullary plasmacytoma. South Med J 73: 670–671
467. Moran C A, Suster S, Fishback N F, et al. 1995 Extramedullary plasmacytomas presenting as mediastinal masses: clinicopathologic study of two cases preceding the onset of multiple myeloma. Mod Pathol 8: 257–259
468. Garaventa A, Dallorso S, Savioli C, et al. 1989 Granulocytic sarcoma presenting as an isolated mediastinal mass. A difficult diagnostic problem. Acta Paediatr Scand 78: 473–475
469. McCluggage W G, Boyd H K, Jones F G, et al. 1998 Mediastinal granulocytic sarcoma: a report of two cases. Arch Pathol Lab Med 122: 545–547
470. Hishima T, Fukayama M, Hayashi Y, et al. 1999 Granulocytic sarcoma of the thymus in a nonleukaemic patient. Virchows Arch 435: 447–451
471. Nounou R, Al-Zahrani H H, Ajarim D S, et al. 2002 Extramedullary myeloid cell tumours localised to the mediastinum: a rare clinicopathological entity with unique karyotypic features. J Clin Pathol 55: 221–225
472. Harpaz N, Gribetz A R, Krellenstein D J, et al. 1986 Inflammatory pseudotumor of the thymus. Ann Thorac Surg 42: 331–333
473. Flieder D B, Suster S, Moran C A 1999 Idiopathic fibroinflammatory (fibrosing/sclerosing) lesions of the mediastinum: a study of 30 cases with emphasis on morphologic heterogeneity. Mod Pathol 12: 257–264
474. Pachter M R 1963 Mediastinal nonchromaffin paraganglioma, a clinicopathologic study based on eight cases. J Thorac Cardiovasc Surg 45: 152–160
475. Moran C A, Suster S, Fishback N, et al. 1993 Mediastinal paragangliomas. A clinicopathologic and immunohistochemical study of 16 cases. Cancer 72: 2358–2364
476. Yoshino N, Hisayoshi T, Maruyama Y, et al. 2004 Paraganglioma of the posterior mediastinum diagnosed by immunohistochemical staining. Jpn J Thorac Cardiovasc Surg 52: 217–220
477. Doglioni C, Bontempini L, Iuzzolino P, et al. 1988 Ependymoma of the mediastinum. Arch Pathol Lab Med 112: 194–196
478. Davidson K G, Walbaum P R, McCormack R J M 1978 Intrathoracic neural tumors. Thorax 33: 359–367
479. Marchevsky A M 1999 Mediastinal tumors of peripheral nervous system origin. Semin Diagn Pathol 16: 65–78
480. Otani Y, Morishita Y, Yoshida I, et al. 1996 A malignant Triton tumor in the anterior mediastinum requiring emergency surgery: report of a case. Surg Today 26: 834–836
481. Argani P, Erlandson R A, Rosai J 1997 Thymic neuroblastoma in adults: report of three cases with special emphasis on its association with the syndrome of inappropriate secretion of antidiuretic hormone. Am J Clin Pathol 108: 537–543
482. Asada Y, Marutsuka K, Mitsukawa T, et al. 1996 Ganglioneuroblastoma of the thymus: an adult case with the syndrome of inappropriate secretion of antidiuretic hormone. Hum Pathol 27: 506–509
483. De Nictolis M, Goteri G, Campanati G, et al. 1995 Elastofibrolipoma of the mediastinum. A previously undescribed benign tumor containing abnormal elastic fibers. Am J Surg Pathol 19: 364–367
484. Fukunaga M, Ushigome S 1998 Giant cell angiofibroma of the mediastinum [Letter]. Histopathology 32: 187–189
485. Asakura S, Tezuka N, Inoue S, et al. 2001 Angiomatoid fibrous histiocytoma in mediastinum. Ann Thorac Surg 72: 283–285
486. Sunderrajan E V, Luger A M, Rosenholtz M J, et al. 1984 Leiomyosarcoma in the mediastinum presenting as superior vena cava syndrome. Cancer 53: 2553–2556
487. Bernheim J, Griffel B, Versano S 1980 Mediastinal leiomyosarcoma in the wall of a bronchial cyst [Letter]. Arch Pathol Lab Med 104: 221
488. Eroglu A, Kurkcuoglu C, Karaoglanoglu N, et al. 2002 Primary leiomyosarcoma of the anterior mediastinum. Eur J Cardiothorac Surg 21: 943–945
489. Gomez-Roman J J, Val-Bernal J F 1997 Lipoleiomyosarcoma of the mediastinum. Pathology 29: 428–430
490. Miller R, Kurtz S M, Powers J M 1978 Mediastinal rhabdomyoma. Cancer 42: 1983–1988
491. Flieder D B, Moran C A, Suster S 1997 Primary alveolar soft-part sarcoma of the mediastinum: a clinicopathological and immunohistochemical study of two cases. Histopathology 31: 469–473
492. Dudgeon D L, Haller J A J 1984 Pediatric lipoblastomatosis, two unusual cases. Surgery 95: 371–373
493. Lim Y C 1980 Mediastinal chondrolipoma. Am J Surg Pathol 4: 407–409
494. Chen W, Chan C W, Mok C 1982 Malignant fibrous histiocytoma of the mediastinum. Cancer 50: 797–800
495. Ikeda T, Ishihara T, Yoshimatsu H, et al. 1974 Primary osteogenic sarcoma of the mediastinum. Thorax 29: 582–588
496. Valderrama E, Kahn L B, Wind E 1983 Extraskeletal osteosarcoma arising in an ectopic hamartomatous thymus. Report of a case and review of the literature. Cancer 51: 1132–1137

497. Greenwood S M, Meschter S C 1989 Extraskeletal osteogenic sarcoma of the mediastinum. Arch Pathol Lab Med 113: 430–433
498. Phillips G W, Choong M 1991 Chondrosarcoma presenting as an anterior mediastinal mass. Clin Radiol 43: 63–64
499. Sakamoto K, Okita M, Kumagiri H, et al. 2003 Sclerosing hemangioma isolated to the mediastinum. Ann Thorac Surg 75: 1021–1023
500. Feigin G A, Robinson B, Marchevsky A 1986 Mixed tumor of the mediastinum. Arch Pathol Lab Med 110: 80–81
501. Ishimaru Y, Shibata Y, Ohkawara S, et al. 1989 Lymphoepithelial cystic lesion related to adenocarcinoma in the mediastinum. Am J Clin Pathol 92: 808–813
502. Chuang M T, Barba F A, Kaneko M 1981 Adenocarcinoma arising in an intrathoracic duplication cyst of foregut origin: a case report with review of the literature. Cancer 47: 1887–1890
503. Olsen J B, Clemmensen O, Andersen K 1991 Adenocarcinoma arising in a foregut cyst of the mediastinum. Ann Thorac Surg 51: 497–499
504. McLoud T C, Meyer J E 1982 Mediastinal metastasis. Radiol Clin North Am 20: 453–468
505. McLoud T C, Kalisher L, Stark P 1978 Intrathoracic lymph node metastases from extrathoracic neoplasms. Am J Roentgenol 131: 403–407
506. Middleton G 1966 Involvement of the thymus by metastatic neoplasms. Br J Cancer 20: 41–46
507. Lindell M M, Doubleday L C, von Eschenbach A C 1982 Mediastinal metastasis from prostatic carcinoma. J Urol 128: 331–334
508. Rosai J 1996 Ackerman's Surgical Pathology, 8th edn. CV Mosby, St Louis
509. Wick M R 2005 Cystic lesions of the mediastinum. Semin Diagn Pathol 22: 241–253

造血系统肿瘤
Tumors of the hematopoietic system

22

Jeffery L. Kutok 著

陈定宝 译　回允中 校

骨髓增生异常综合征	1363
急性骨髓性白血病	1370
前体B细胞淋巴母细胞性白血病/	
淋巴母细胞性淋巴瘤	1386
前体T细胞淋巴母细胞性白血病/	
淋巴母细胞性淋巴瘤	1389
慢性骨髓增生性病变	1390
慢性骨髓性白血病	1391
慢性嗜酸性粒细胞性白血病/	
嗜酸性粒细胞增多综合征	1394
真性红细胞增多症	1396
特发性血小板增多症	1398

慢性特发性骨髓纤维化	1399
浆细胞性骨髓瘤	1401
成人T细胞性白血病/淋巴瘤	1404
毛细胞性白血病	1406
B细胞慢性淋巴细胞性白血病/	
小淋巴细胞性淋巴瘤	1408
前B细胞淋巴细胞性白血病	1409
前T细胞淋巴细胞性白血病	1410
T细胞大颗粒淋巴细胞性白血病	1412
肥大细胞疾病	1413

　　识别重现性染色体异常相关基因对血液病理学领域的影响比诊断病理学其他任何领域的影响都要深远。对造血系统疾病尤其如此，后者被不确切地定义为淋巴造血系统疾病，最常累及骨髓和外周血。与其他遗传性或后天性改变一样，这些遗传学异常可导致细胞程序改变，与特征性的形态学以及或许是更重要的与特殊的临床行为和预后有关。这些分子学发现对肿瘤分类影响极大，导致过去十年以来造血系统恶性肿瘤的分类发生了几次重大的转变。过去基于常见的形态学、细胞化学和免疫表型特征进行分类的疾病，现在常常通过单一的遗传学缺陷特征与其他疾病鉴别开来。例如，在目前的WHO分类方案中，识别特殊的细胞遗传学异常能最准确地界定慢性骨髓性白血病（CML）、急性前骨髓性白血病（APL）、伴有嗜酸性粒细胞增多的急性骨髓单核细胞性白血病（AMML）以及一些骨髓增生异常相关性综合征。除了预测临床行为和预后外，临床医生还依靠发现这些细胞遗传学异常来指导应用独特而有效的针对异常蛋白的靶向治疗，例如应用甲磺酸伊马替尼（Gleevec）治疗慢性骨髓性白血病，以及应用全反式视黄酸（ATRA）治疗急性前骨髓性白血病。这些遗传学缺陷也为识别新的和持续存在的疾病提供了良好的标记物。分子诊断技术，包括Southern印迹、聚合酶链式反应（PCR）、荧光原位杂交（FISH）和常规核型分析，在造血系统肿瘤的分类中已经得到广泛应用。虽然这种造血系统恶性肿瘤分类的不断变化对于普通外科病理医生适应而言确实形成了挑战，但其目的不是造成混乱而是更好地界定这些疾病，即基于新的可识别的特征以提供有用的治疗和预后信息。本章将讨论最常见的造血系统肿瘤类型的现代观点，包括骨髓增生异常综合征（MDS）、急性白血病、慢性骨髓增生性疾病（CMPD）以及成熟淋巴细胞性白血病（mature lymphoid leukemias）。

骨髓增生异常综合征
Myelodysplastic syndromes

定义和分类

　　骨髓增生异常综合征（MDS）是异源性克隆的骨髓干细胞疾病的总称，均具有分化异常，导致无效造血、骨髓衰竭和正常外周血细胞减少。增生异常（dysplasia）这一术语是指骨髓细胞的形态学改变，是由干细胞缺陷引起的。受累的骨髓细胞可能包括红细胞系、巨核细胞系和粒细胞系，可单独受累也可联合受累。重要的是，除了外周血细胞计数减少以外，这些疾病常常伴有骨髓原始细胞成分增多。原始细胞增多与进展为急性白血病的危险性有关。最近，WHO修改了应用已久的法国-美国-英国（French-American-British, FAB）的MDS分类方法（表22.1和22.2）。修改后的WHO分类方案试图提出几个已经发现的问题，包括：（1）越来越多的资料表明，骨髓原始细胞计数＞20%的患者的生存率类似急性骨髓性白血病患者[1]；（2）在难治性贫血（RA）、伴有环形铁粒原始红细胞的难治性贫血（RARS）以及伴有原始细胞过多的难治性贫血（RAEB）的患者中，预后具有异质性；（3）慢性骨髓单核细胞性白血病（CMML）和伴有孤立性缺失（5q）的MDS具有独特的临床和形态学特征[2-4]。有鉴于此，新的WHO分类方案是：（1）将诊断急性骨髓性白血病（AML）的原始细胞的百分率从30%降至20%，删去了FAB分类中的伴有原始细胞过多转化的难治性贫血（RAEB-T）；（2）根据出现多系（两种或三种髓细胞系）或是单系（主要是红系）增生异常，将难治性贫血和伴有环形铁粒原始红细胞的难治性贫血分为两个主要的类型；（3）将伴有原始细胞过多的难治性贫血（RAEB）再分为两种类型：RAEB-1

表22.1 骨髓增生异常综合征的FAB（French-American-British）分类：血液和骨髓所见

疾病	外周血原始细胞计数	骨髓原始细胞计数
难治性贫血（RA）	＜1%	＜5%
伴有环形铁粒原始红细胞的难治性贫血（RARS）	＜1%	＜5%；环形铁粒原始红细胞＞15%
伴有原始细胞过多的难治性贫血（RAEB）	＜5%；没有奥尔小体（Auer rods）	5%～20%；没有奥尔小体
伴有原始细胞过多转化的难治性贫血（RAEB-T）	原始细胞＞5%，或伴有奥尔小体	20%～30%，或5%～20%但伴有奥尔小体
慢性骨髓单核细胞性白血病	单核细胞＞1×10⁹/L；原始细胞计数不定	上述任意一种

表22.2 WHO骨髓增生异常综合征分类：血液和骨髓所见

疾病	外周血所见		骨髓所见		
	血细胞减少	原始细胞计数	增生异常	原始细胞计数	环形铁粒原始红细胞
难治性贫血（RA）	贫血	没有或极少	仅仅红系增生异常	＜5%	＜15%
伴有多系发育异常的难治性血细胞减少（RCMD）[a]	两系或全血细胞减少	没有或极少；没有奥尔小体	两种或多种骨髓细胞系（＞10%的细胞）	＜5%；没有奥尔小体	＜15%
伴有环形铁粒原始红细胞的难治性贫血（RARS）	贫血	没有	仅仅红系增生异常	＜5%	＞15%
伴有多系发育异常和环形铁粒原始红细胞的难治性血细胞减少（RCMD-RS）[a]	两系或全血细胞减少	没有或极少；没有奥尔小体	两种或多种骨髓细胞系（＞10%的细胞）	＜5%；没有奥尔小体	＞15%
伴有原始细胞过多的难治性贫血-1（RAEB-1）[a]	单系、两系或全血细胞减少	＜5%；没有奥尔小体	单系或多系	5%～9%；没有奥尔小体	＜15%
伴有原始细胞过多的难治性贫血-2（RAEB-2）[a]	单系、两系或全血细胞减少	＜5%；或者如果骨髓原始细胞＜10%，则为5%～19%；可能出现奥尔小体	单系或多系	10%～19%；可能出现奥尔小体	＜15%
骨髓增生异常综合征，不能分类（MDS-U）	单系、两系或全血细胞减少	没有或极少；没有奥尔小体	单系	5%；没有奥尔小体	＜15%
伴有孤立性缺失（5q）的MDS	巨红细胞性贫血；血小板计数正常或增多	＜5%；没有奥尔小体	异常，分叶少的巨核细胞	＜5%；没有奥尔小体	＜15%

Adapted from Brunning et al.[5]
[a] 单核细胞计数必须少于1×10⁹/L，否则必须考虑慢性骨髓单核细胞性白血病。

（骨髓原始细胞占5%～9%）和RAEB-2（骨髓原始细胞占10%～19%）；（4）将慢性骨髓单核细胞性白血病从MDS种类中删去，放入新近提出的骨髓疾病范畴内，后者具有与MDS和骨髓增生性疾病重叠的特征；以及（5）将伴有（5q）缺失综合征的MDS患者看做是单独的染色体异常，作为一个独立的群体（表22.2）[5,6]。虽然有关MDS的诊断标准尚有争议[6-8]，但是很多应用最新发布的指南的研究[5]认为，WHO的分类方案在预测预后方面优于FAB分类。的确，如同有关MDS新的知识在不断增长一样，新的WHO分类方案也会不断得到改善。另外，WHO分类方案界定危险群体的能力不会妨碍其他好的预后评分系统的应用，例如国际预后评分系统（IPSS）[9a,10]，其主要依赖临床特征。

总的临床和实验室特征

MDS或表现为原发性疾病或作为化疗或放疗之后发生的一种继发性疾病。其主要发生于老年患者，中位年龄为72岁；但是年龄范围广泛（16～96岁）[9]。MDS可发生于儿童，尤其是有遗传性DNA修复缺陷疾病背景者，例如Fanconi贫血。MDS的发病率随着年龄的增长而稳定上升；总体发病率大约为每年为4～12例/100 000人，但在70岁以上的患者，其总体发病率比此比例高3～4倍[11,12]。MDS的发病率近年似乎有所增加，这种发现可能反映了人口的老龄化，更多的内科医生已意识到这种疾病，并在老年患者中应用了诊断程序[12]。应用强烈化疗达到痊愈或长期缓解的癌症患者似乎是继发性MDS发病率升高的原因。这是遗传毒性治疗的一种悲剧性后果，因为继发性MDS的生存时间明显短于原发性MDS。在多种类型的MDS中，男性的发病率略高，孤立性缺失（5q）综合征是个例外。

MDS的临床特征与骨髓衰竭有关，包括继发于贫血的疲劳、继发于中性白细胞减少的感染以及继发于血小板减少的出血。根据定义，MDS的贫血反映了红细胞生成的固有缺陷，对补血药治疗无反应或不显疗效。贫血常常是巨幼细胞性贫血。血小板增多可见于孤立性缺失（5q）患者，但从不见于其他患者。死亡可发生于骨髓衰竭相关性并发症、转化为急性白血病，或偶尔发生于输血治疗造成的铁过量并发症。髓外受累少见，应该考虑另外一种最初诊断，或在已证实患有骨髓增生异常的患者，应该考虑髓外的白血病转化。

MDS的一般形态学特征

一旦临床上疑为MDS，应仔细评估外周血和骨髓形态学异常特征以利诊断。在缺乏克隆性细胞遗传学异常的情况下（见下文），诊断主要依靠形态学所见。对于确切评估MDS，在新鲜分离的标本上制备完好的Wright-Giemsa染色的外周血或骨髓抽吸涂片是重要的。这种所见的主观特性可能造成诊断困难，即使出现这种表现，"增生异常"的形态学也可能与MDS无关，而与营养缺乏、接触毒物和感染因素有关。因此，MDS的诊断和分类需要仔细将形态学所见与其他临床及实验室资料联系起来。

红细胞生成障碍性异常
Dyserythropoietic abnormalities

成熟性无核外周血红细胞常见的形态学异常包括：大红细胞症、红细胞大小不一和异形红细胞症、点状嗜碱细胞增多症以及细胞双形性。在骨髓内，红细胞前体核的形态学异常最为常见，包括巨幼红细胞样成熟（核与胞浆成熟之间不同步）、多核及核碎片以及搭桥或出芽（图22.1）。胞浆空泡形成、环形铁粒原始红细胞（有核红细胞至少具有5个普鲁士蓝染色的核周铁颗粒，围绕核的1/3以上[13]）（图22.2）及胞浆PAS阳性颗粒也常可见到。

粒细胞生成障碍性异常
Dysgranulopoietic abnormalities

在粒细胞中，形态学异常最常见于中性粒细胞系，包括外周血中性粒细胞呈颗粒减少[继发性颗粒和髓过氧化物酶（MPO）染色丢失]、分叶过少（hyposegmentation），包括假性Pelger-Huet形成（双核中性粒细胞伴有染色质凝聚）（图22.3），甚或出现分叶过多（hypersegmentation）。在骨髓内，颗粒细胞前体——正常情况下沿骨小梁骨内膜表面排列——可形成簇，与骨小梁不相延续。这些骨髓前体细胞显示核与胞浆的成熟之间缺乏同步，分叶过少（图22.4），原发性或继发性颗粒减少，以及巨大的原始颗粒。

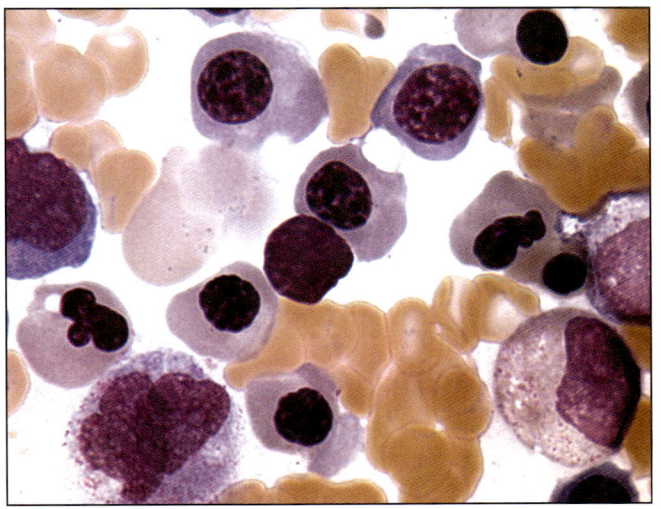

图22.1 骨髓抽吸涂片显示难治性贫血患者的明显的红细胞生成障碍。注意晚幼红细胞核明显不规则。（Wright-Giemsa染色）

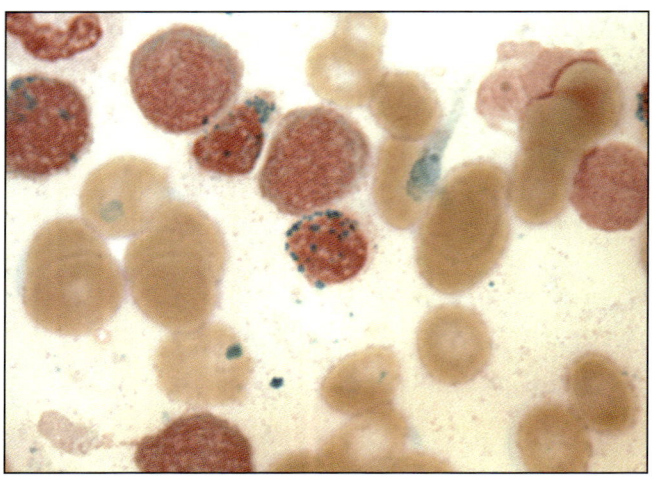

图22.2 骨髓增生异常（难治性贫血）的骨髓抽吸涂片显示2个环形铁粒原始红细胞。（铁染色）

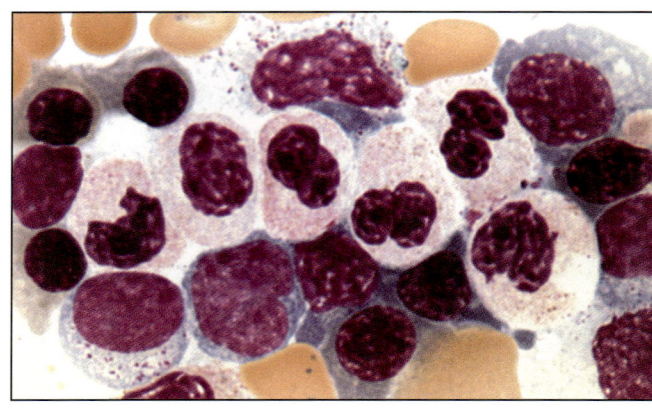

图22.4 骨髓抽吸涂片显示难治性贫血患者的明显的粒细胞生成障碍，伴有多系发育异常。注意中性粒细胞分叶过少。（Wright-Giemsa染色）

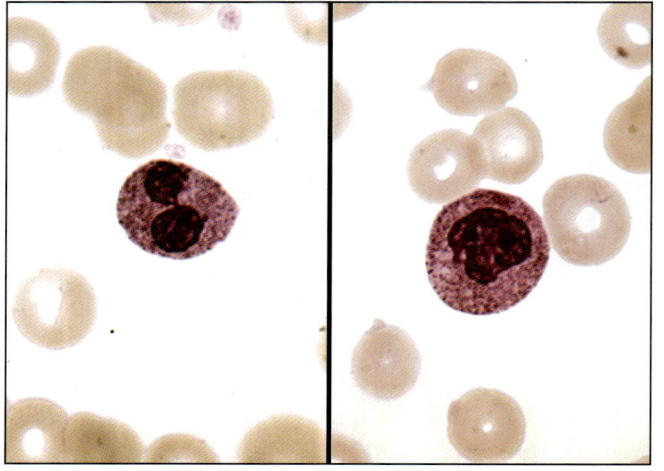

图22.3 MDS。外周血象显示成熟中性粒细胞发育异常。假性-Pelger-Huet形成（左）和未分叶的中性粒细胞（右）。（Wright-Giemsa染色）

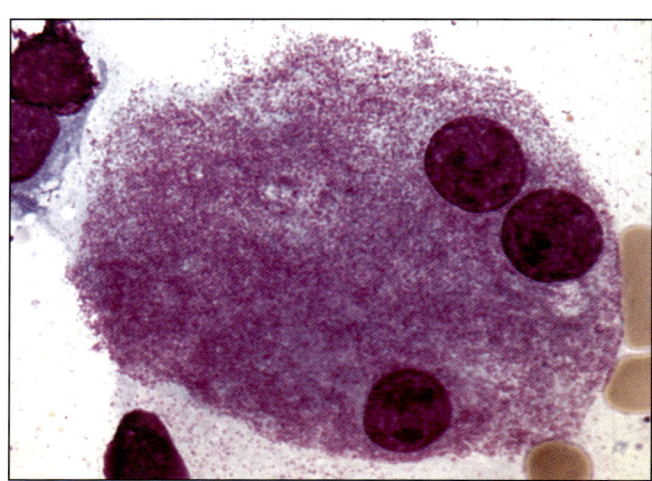

图22.5 伴有多系发育异常的难治性血细胞减少症的骨髓抽吸涂片，显示发育异常的巨核细胞伴有所谓的"典当球"样外观。（Wright-Giemsa染色）

巨核细胞生成障碍性异常
Dysmegakaryopoietic abnormalities

在MDS中，巨核细胞常常显示最明显的发育异常性改变，包括小的分叶减少的"微小巨核细胞"形成，核的分叶减少，或反之呈多倍体化，以及间隙宽广、不连续的核分叶[所谓的"典当球"（pawn ball）核，反映其类似于古时候当铺老板的3个球的典当商符号[14]（图22.5和22.6）。

难治性贫血（RA）（又称"单纯性"红细胞生成障碍性难治性贫血或伴有单系发育异常的难治性贫血）
Refractory anemia (RA) (a.k.a. "pure" dyserythropoietic refractory anemia or refractory anemia with unilineage dysplasia)

这是骨髓增生异常的一种少见亚型，大约占所有

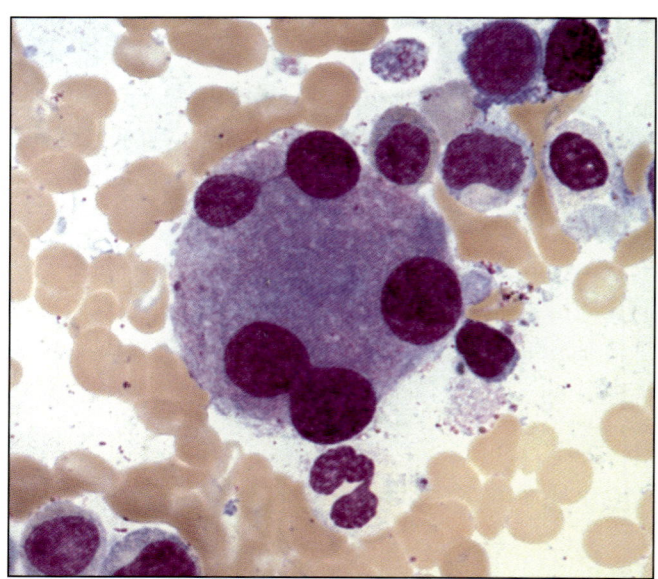

图22.6 一例伴有过多原始细胞的难治性贫血患者的骨髓抽吸涂片，显示发育异常的巨核细胞。（Wright-Giemsa染色）

MDS 病例的 9%[9]。患者表现为孤立性贫血，外周血没有其他异常。外周红细胞血色素通常正常，或者是正常红细胞，或者是巨红细胞。骨髓常常是正常细胞或细胞增多，少数病例显示增生低下的表现。在抽吸涂片中，红细胞增生异常可从轻微到明显的异常，巨幼红细胞样分化常见（图 22.1、22.7 和 22.8）。在多数活检标本中可能容易见到红细胞前体的核的不规则性。在难治性贫血中，见不到粒细胞或巨核细胞成分的形态学异常，母细胞在骨髓细胞成分中所占不足 5%。普鲁士蓝染色常常显示铁的含量正常或增多，只是偶尔（< 15%）可见环形铁粒原始红细胞（图 22.2）。大约 25% 的病例可见异常的核型，其中多数病例属于低危险预后类别（见下）[9]。

白血病转化的危险性低（约为 8%），中位生存期为 69 个月[9]。

伴有环形铁粒原始红细胞的难治性贫血（RARS）[又称单纯性（红细胞生成障碍性）铁粒原始红细胞贫血（PSA）]
Refractory anemia with ringed sideroblasts (RARS) [a.k.a. pure (dyserythropoietic) sideroblastic anemia (PSA)]

WHO 将这种获得性原发性铁粒原始红细胞性贫血定义为单纯性红细胞生成障碍性疾病，类似于难治性贫血；然而不同的是其可出现 > 15% 的环形铁粒原始红细胞。RARS 大约占 MDS 的 11%[9]。多数为老年患者（中位年龄为 73 岁），没有性别差异，表现为中度贫血[15]。外周血所见各异。有时外周血涂片显示为具有正常血色素细胞和低血色素细胞两种特性细胞群；或者可见正常血色素性、巨红细胞性或正常红细胞性贫血[16]。骨髓细胞成分可由正常细胞到明显细胞增多，并且最常见的是红细胞系增生伴巨幼红细胞样改变[15]（图 22.9）。根据定义，可见许多环形铁粒原始红细胞（在一些大型研究中显示有核红细胞成分的中位数为 40%）[15]（图 22.10）。略少于 10% 的病例可见 PAS 阳性的有核红细胞[15]。骨髓成髓细胞数目少于 5%，见不到粒细胞或巨核细胞增生异常。克隆性染色体异常在这种类型的 MDS 中最不常见（< 10% 的病例），与进展为白血病的比例极低有关（2%）[9]。其总体生存率与难治性贫血的相同[9]。

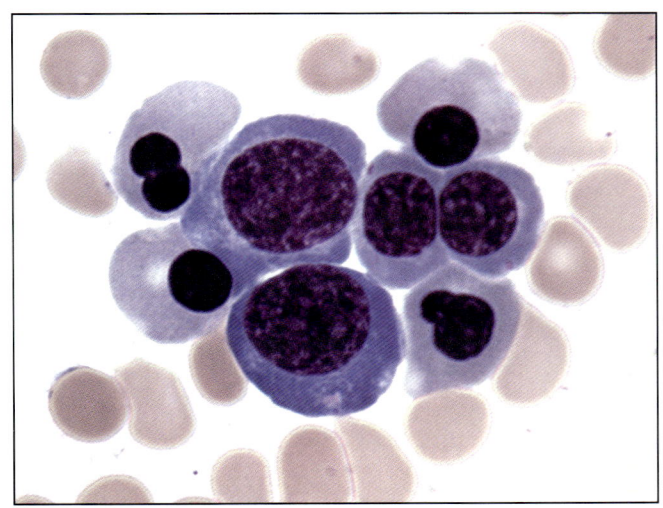

图22.7　难治性贫血（RA）的骨髓抽吸涂片，显示巨幼红细胞样红细胞分化和核的不规则性。非红系缺乏增生异常，本例的诊断符合难治性贫血、又称"单纯性"红细胞生成障碍性难治性贫血，或伴有单系增生异常的难治性贫血。（Wright-Giemsa染色）

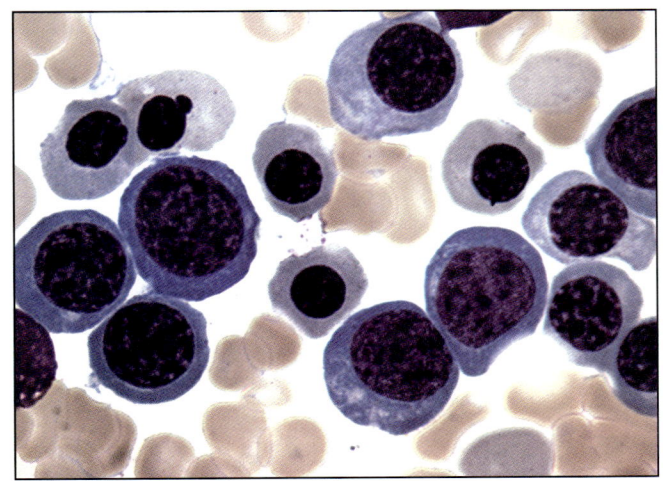

图22.8　难治性贫血（RA）的骨髓抽吸涂片，显示红细胞系增生，核仅有轻微的不规则性。（Wright-Giemsa染色）

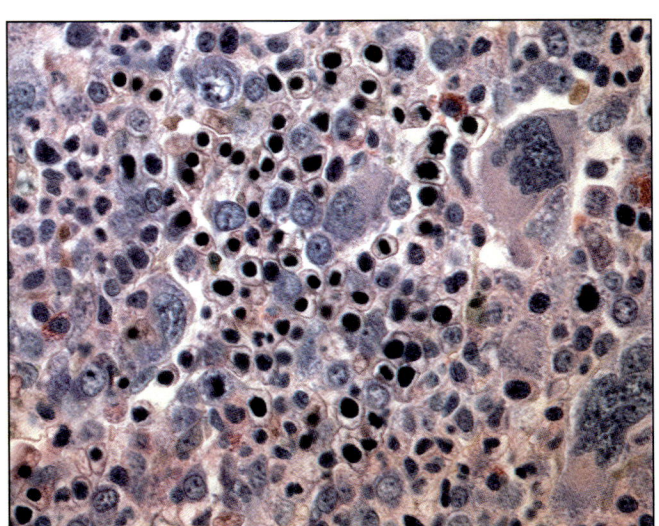

图22.9　伴有环形铁粒原始红细胞的难治性贫血（RARS）患者的骨髓芯针活检标本的组织学切片，显示伴有核异常的红细胞系增生，明显见于晚幼红细胞。铁染色和环形铁粒原始红细胞（见图22.10）的识别有助于这种类型的骨髓增生异常与难治性贫血的鉴别。（Giemsa染色）

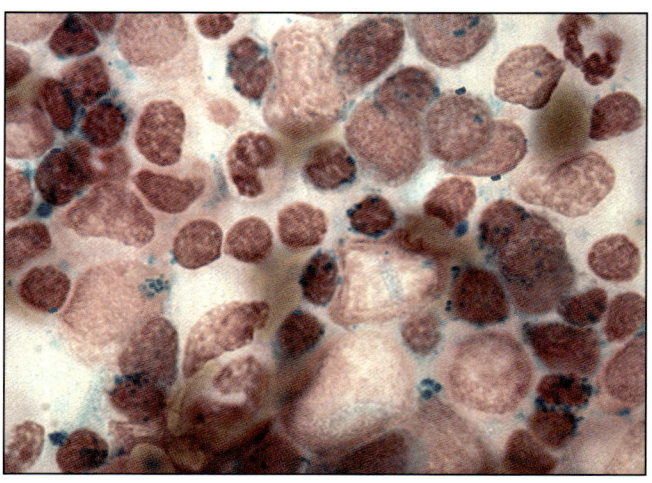

图22.10 难治性贫血伴有环形铁粒原始红细胞（RARS）的骨髓抽吸涂片显示大量环形铁粒原始红细胞，占有核红细胞样成分的15%以上。（铁染色）

伴有多系增生异常的难治性贫血（RCMD）和伴有多系增生异常和环形铁粒原始红细胞的难治性贫血（RCMD-RS）
Refractory cytopenia with multilineage dysplasia (RCMD) and refractory cytopenia with multilineage dysplasia and ringed sideroblasts (RCMD-RS)

这两种类型的MDS具有类似的临床特征，在WHO分类中被归类在一起[1]。它们分别大约占MDS的25%(RCMD)和15%（RCMD-RS）[9]。在这两种病变中，外周血必须显示两系或全血细胞减少，骨髓必须显示两种或多种髓细胞系>10%的细胞具有增生异常的特征[17]（图22.4、22.5和22.11）。唯一的鉴别特征是环形铁粒原始红细胞的百分比，RCMD<15%，而RCMD-RS>15%。在外周血中见不到原始细胞（<1%），骨髓的原始细胞也不增加（<5%）。

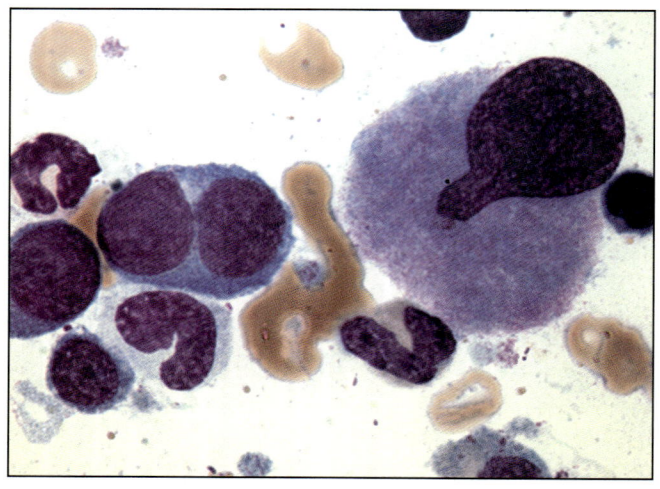

图22.11 难治性血细胞减少症伴有多系增生异常的骨髓抽吸涂片显示巨核细胞增生异常，分叶减少，双核，嗜碱性有核红细胞，以及巨大嗜中性粒细胞带形成。（Wright-Giemsa染色）

见不到奥尔小体（Auer rods）。Germing等[9]通过WHO的大型研究进一步细化了RCMD或RCMD-RS中异型增生的定义。如果一个细胞系中10%或以上的细胞其胞浆颗粒减少和（或）核分叶减少或增多，则考虑存在粒细胞生成障碍（dysgranulopoiesis）。如果在至少25个巨核细胞中有10个或以上表现为微小巨核细胞，或具有多个分开的细胞核，或为单个无分叶的细胞核，则诊断为巨核细胞生成障碍（dysmegakaryopoiesis）。重要的是，难治性贫血和RCMD之间的血液学特征、细胞遗传学异常、进展为急性骨髓性白血病（AML）的比例以及总体生存率明显不同[4,9,18,19]。异常核型见于37%的RCMD病例，进展为急性白血病的发生率大约为11%。总体中位生存率为33个月[9]。

已经得到公认，基于FAB分类系统所定义的RARS在临床上是一种异质性疾病[15,20,21]。多年来越来越多的证据表明，与仅有红细胞增生异常和环形铁粒原始红细胞增加的患者相比，多系细胞减少和多系增生异常（与RCMD所见相同）以及环形铁粒原始红细胞增加（有核红细胞>15%）的患者进展为急性白血病的比例较高，且生存率降低[15]。为了区分这些临床上不同的疾病，符合RCMD-RS标准的病例被归入WHO分类方案中RCMD的范畴[17]。大的研究已经证实，RARS和RCMD-RS的预后不同，而RCMD和RCMD-RS的预后类似[9,15,18]。RCMD-RS克隆性细胞遗传学异常的发生率类似于RCMD（RCMD-RS为50%，RCMD为37%，而RARS仅为9%）。另外，RCMD-RS转化为急性骨髓性白血病的比例几乎比RARS的高10倍，这是总体生存率明显不同的原因(RCMD-RS的中位生存期为32个月，而RARS的则为69个月）[9]。相反，RCMD和RCMD-RS的中位生存期几乎相同[9]。

伴有原始细胞过多的难治性贫血（RAEB）
Refractory anemia with excess blasts (RAEB)

这种类型的MDS的主要特征是：在骨髓中可见形态学增生异常和5%～19%的原始细胞[22]。原始细胞成分的增加与进行性骨髓衰竭和进展为急性骨髓性白血病的比例增高有关[9]。另外，在骨髓原始细胞占5%～9%的患者和占10%～19%的患者之间，已经证实其进展为急性白血病与总体生存期明显不同[7,9,10]。因此，WHO分类将RAEB分为两种亚类，RAEB-1（骨髓原始细胞占5%～9%）（图22.12）和RAEB-2（骨髓原始细胞占10%～19%）（图22.13）[22]。外周血具有明显的原始细胞（5%～19%）但骨髓原始细胞少于10%的患者暂时归入RAEB-2的范畴。这些RAEN-2患者的生存期可能类似于急性骨髓性白血病，然而，对这样的病例应

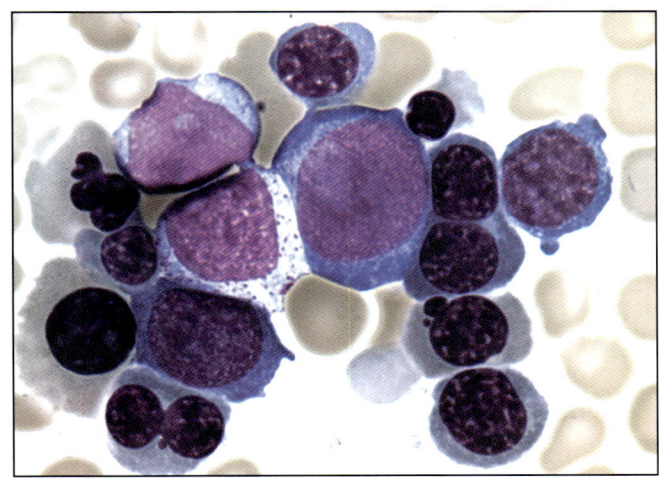

图22.12 伴有原始细胞过多-1（RAEB-1）的难治性贫血的骨髓抽吸涂片，显示红细胞系增生异常和一个骨髓原始细胞（左上）。（Wright-Giemsa染色）

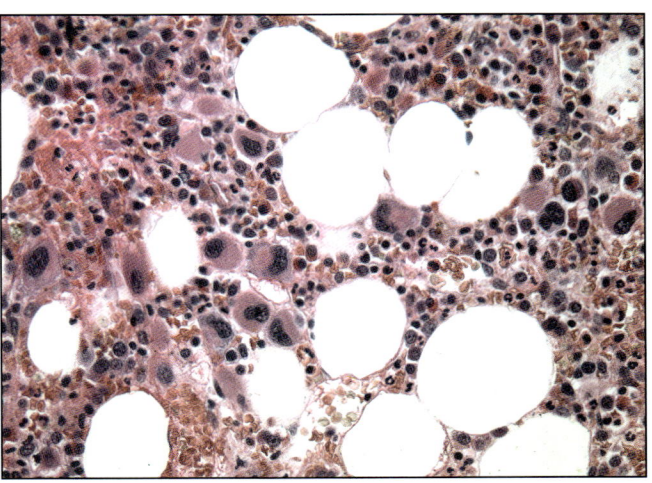

图22.14 伴有孤立性（5q）缺失的骨髓增生异常综合征的骨髓芯针活检的组织学切片。注意可见多量分叶减少的巨核细胞。（HE染色）

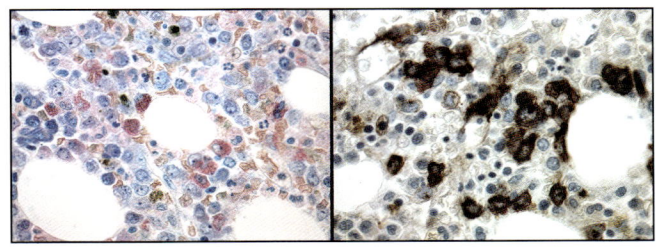

图22.13 伴有原始细胞过多-2（RAEB-2）的难治性贫血的骨髓芯针活检组织学切片，显示间质内原始细胞成分增多，染色质分散，核仁小而明显（左图，Giemsa染色），CD34免疫染色则易于计数（右图）。

该仔细考虑治疗的选择[1]。奥尔小体（Auer rods）的意义也是争议的根源。根据 FAB 的标准，不管原始细胞计数多少，只要出现奥尔小体就将患者归入 RAEB-T 的范畴[1a]。RAEB-T 已从 WHO 分类中删除，其中大多数患者重新分类为急性骨髓性白血病。在 WHO 的分类中，将具有奥尔小体且骨髓原始细胞少于 20% 的患者归入 RAEB-2 的范畴，有研究认为其临床结果类似于前两组患者[1]。RAEB 的临床症状常常比其他类型的 MDS 严重，具有与骨髓衰竭有关的特征。增生异常的特征往往明显，而且常常累及所有三个髓系。大约 35% 的 RAEB-1 的病例和 42% 的 RAEB-2 的病例显示核型异常，21% 的 RAEB-1 和 35% 的 RAEB-2 进展为急性骨髓性白血病[9]。虽然总体生存率差，但 RAEB-1 与 RAEB-2 之间的生存期却有显著性差异（分别为 18 个月和 10 个月）[9]。

伴有孤立性（5q）缺失（5q综合征）的骨髓增生异常综合征
Myelodysplastic syndrome associated with an isolated del (5q) (5q-syndrome)

5q 综合征是一种相对少见的病变，仅仅占所有 MDS 的 2%[9]。这种临床病理学独特的疾病与单基因异常有关，是一种 5 号染色体长臂远侧区大小不等的中间缺失，涉及 q13-q33 带。5q 综合征主要但并不是全部发生于中年女性（中位年龄为 68 岁；男女比例为 3:7），与先前接受化疗和放疗无关[23]。巨红细胞性贫血是最常见的特征，见于 80% 的患者[23]。贫血常常伴有血小板计数增高和中度白细胞减少，中性粒细胞减少明显，血小板减少或许罕见。骨髓细胞成分通常增多，其特征是巨核细胞数目明显增多，巨核细胞小，分叶减少（图 22.14）。可见红系和粒系不同程度的增生异常。外周血和骨髓的原始细胞数均少于 5%。伴有孤立性（5q）缺失的患者预后非常好（随访 20 年以上，中位生存率为 116 个月），少数病例进展为急性骨髓性白血病（8%）[9]。表现为其他染色体异常或原始细胞 > 5% 的患者不应该归入这个范畴，因为这些所见伴有更加明显的侵袭性临床经过[9,23,24]。

MDS 的细胞遗传学所见

在大约 40% 的 MDS 患者中，应用标准核型分析可

表22.3 骨髓增生异常综合征的常见核型异常

染色体异常	发生率（%）
5 号染色体全部或部分丢失	13
7 号染色体全部或部分丢失	5
8 号染色体 3 体	5
X 或 Y 染色体丢失	2
(20q) 缺失	2
(17p) 缺失	< 1

Adapted from Heaney ML, Golde DW.1999 Myelodysplasia. N Engl J Med 340:1649-1660.

检测到克隆性染色体异常[9,10]，应用高分辨率方法检测的数目甚至更高（79%）[25]。FISH 在检测 MDS 克隆性细胞遗传学异常中并未显示具有更大的应用价值[26,27]。原发性 MDS 最常见的异常在表 22.3 中列出。其他较少的重复性染色体畸变包括：平衡的染色体易位，失衡性结构异常（缺失和重复），以及染色体数目异常。克隆性遗传学缺陷在治疗相关性 MDS 病例中也是典型的，几乎发生于 100% 的病例，常常累及 5 号和 7 号染色体[28,29]。在适当的临床情况下，辨认克隆性细胞遗传学畸变可以证实 MDS 的诊断并为内科医生提供重要的预后信息。广为接受的关于 MDS 的 IPSS（International scoring system for evaluating prognosis in myelodysplastic syndrome）[10]已形成一种新的细胞遗传学分级系统，并可很好地描述其亚组的预后。在这个系统中，一个正常核型、孤立性（5q）缺失、（20q）缺失或 -Y 缺失被认为是低度危险性异常，具有良好的预后。除了累及 7 号染色体以外，具有任何一种或两种其他染色体异常均被认为是中度危险性异常。高度危险性是指具有复杂的(三种以上)重排或任何累及 7 号染色体的异常。复杂性细胞遗传学异常还与进展为急性白血病的危险性较高以及生存期缩短有关[30]。

鉴别诊断

如前所述，在由 B12 和叶酸缺乏（图 22.15）、接触包括化疗在内的毒物以及某些感染性因子引起的巨幼红细胞性贫血中，形态学增生异常是常见的特征。必须排除这些形态学增生异常的常见原因才能作出诊断。MDS 还需要与急性骨髓性白血病鉴别，原始细胞大于 20% 的病例应该考虑急性骨髓性白血病。对于抽吸涂片不充分的病例，在芯针活检中对原始细胞成分进行 CD34 免疫染色有利于确定原始细胞；然而，可见缺乏 CD34 表达的骨髓原始细胞（图 22.13）。在有核红细胞成分占细胞构成 50% 以上的增生异常的骨髓中，非红细胞系的原始细胞计数＞20%，最好诊断为急性骨髓性白血病（红系/粒系亚型）而不是 MDS。具有重要的临床意义是：鉴别伴有骨髓细胞成分减少（发生于大约 15% 的病例）的 MDS[31]与获得性再生障碍性贫血或再生不良性急性骨髓性白血病。仔细检查增生异常细胞核的形态学特征（在再生障碍性贫血中一般缺乏）和准确的原始细胞计数可能有助于这种鉴别。

最后，现在已将慢性骨髓单核细胞性白血病（chronic myelomonocytic leukemia，CMML）从单纯性 MDS 类别中排除，而将其看成是一种与 MDS 和骨髓增生性疾病具有重叠特征的疾病。WHO 将 CMML 界定为克隆性干细胞异常，特征是外周血（单核细胞＞1×10^9/L）和骨髓有明显的单核细胞增生，伴有累及一种或多种髓系的增生异常[31a]（图 22.16）。原始细胞在骨髓细胞成分中不超过 20%。在诊断 CMML 之前，必须除外其他类型的骨髓增生性疾病，尤其是慢性骨髓性白血病。如果缺乏骨髓增生异常或骨髓增生轻微，而符合其他的要求，仍然可以作出 CMML 的诊断，条件是：（1）骨髓细胞出现获得性克隆性细胞遗传学异常；（2）单核细胞增生至少持续 3 个月；以及（3）单核细胞增生的其他原因已被排除[31a]。

急性骨髓性白血病
Acute myeloid leukemia

定义和分类

急性骨髓性白血病（AML）的特征是骨髓、血和其

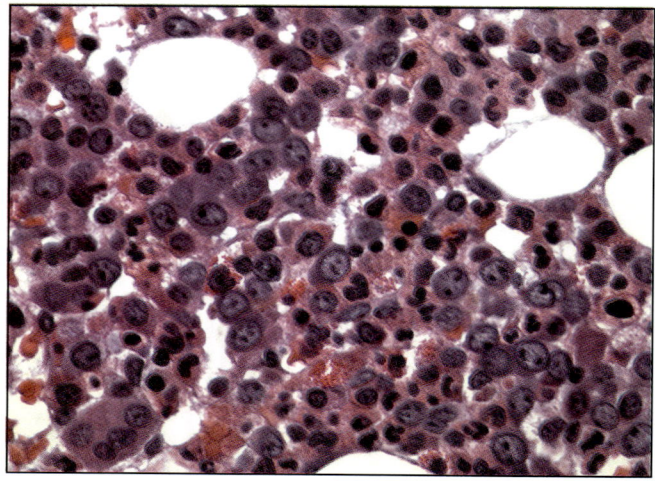

图 22.15 一例患有严重叶酸缺乏和巨幼红细胞性贫血的患者的骨髓芯针活检的组织学切片，类似于骨髓增生异常综合征。（HE 染色）

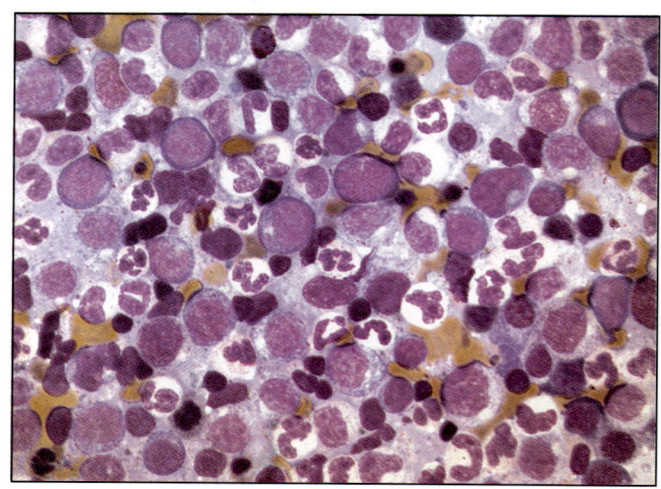

图 22.16 慢性骨髓单核细胞性白血病患者的骨髓抽吸涂片，显示常见中性粒细胞、早期和晚期单核细胞成分，而骨髓原始细胞少见。（Wright-Giemsa 染色）

表22.4 急性骨髓性白血病的FAB分类

FAB亚型	形态学	细胞化学	免疫表型
M0	无颗粒，没有奥尔小体的原始表现的原始细胞＞30%；与淋巴母细胞常常难以区分	MPO、SBB或NSE阳性的原始细胞＜3%	CD117⁺、CD13⁺、CD33⁺、CD11b⁺、HLA-DR⁺、CD34⁺、CD7⁻/⁺、CD2⁻/⁺、CD19⁻/⁺
M1	原始细胞＞30%；骨髓有核细胞＜10%，为前髓细胞或较成熟的中性粒细胞；可见奥尔小体	MPO、SBB阳性的原始细胞＞3%	CD117⁺、CD13⁺、CD33⁺、HLA-DR⁺
M2	原始细胞＞30%，骨髓有核细胞＞10%，为前髓细胞或较成熟的中性粒细胞；可见奥尔小体	MPO、SBB阳性的原始细胞＞3%	CD117⁺、CD13⁺、CD33⁺[在t(8;21)病例CD19⁻/⁺、TDT⁻/⁺]
M3	原始细胞或伴有许多嗜苯胺蓝大颗粒的异常前髓细胞＞30%；可见伴有多个奥尔小体的束状细胞（faggot cell）；双叶或哑铃形核，尤其是在微小颗粒亚型（M3v）	原始细胞和前髓细胞MPO和SBB呈强阳性	CD13⁺、CD33⁺、HLA-DR⁻、CD34⁻/⁺、CD2⁻/⁺、CD117⁺
M4	骨髓原始细胞、原始单核细胞、前单核细胞＞30%；骨髓中单核细胞＞20%但＜80%；骨髓中中性粒细胞和粒细胞前体＞20%	单核细胞NSE呈阳性；骨髓原始细胞MPO、SBB呈阳性	不同比例的原始细胞和单核细胞：CD13⁺、CD33⁺、CD11b⁺、CD14⁺、CD117⁻/⁺、CD34⁻/⁺
M4Eo	骨髓原始细胞、原始单核细胞、前单核细胞＞30%；骨髓中单核细胞＞20%但＜80%；骨髓中性粒细胞和前体细胞＞20%；骨髓出现嗜酸性粒细胞，包括伴有大的嗜碱性颗粒的异常嗜酸性粒细胞	单核细胞NSE呈阳性；骨髓原始细胞MPO、SBB呈阳性；嗜酸性粒细胞CAE和PAS呈阳性	不同比例的原始细胞和单核细胞：CD13⁺、CD33⁺、CD11b⁺、CD14⁺、CD117⁻/⁺、CD34⁻/⁺、CD2±
M5	单核细胞＞80%[或以原始单核细胞为主，＞80%（M5a），或以前单核细胞为主，伴有原始单核细胞＜80%（M5b）]	单核细胞NSE呈阳性，MPO、SBB呈阴性	CD13⁺、CD33⁺、CD11b⁺、CD14⁺、CD4⁺、CD34⁻
M6	红系前体细胞和（或）原始红细胞＞50%；＞30%的非红系前体细胞是骨髓原始细胞；奥尔小体可出现在骨髓原始细胞内	骨髓原始细胞MPO、SBB呈阳性；红系原始细胞PAS呈阳性	髓系前体细胞：CD13⁺、CD33⁺、HLA-DR⁺、CD34±、红系前体细胞：血型糖蛋白（glycophorin）⁺和血红蛋白（hemoglobin）⁺
M7	原始细胞＞30%，形态学、免疫表型或电子显微镜研究证实巨核细胞衍化＞50%	MPO、SBB呈阴性；巨核细胞PAS常常阳性	HLA-DR⁺、CD33⁺、CD34⁺、CD61⁺、CD41⁺、vWf⁺、CD42⁺

⁺：阳性；⁻：阴性；±：常常阳性；⁻/⁺：常常阴性。
MPO：髓过氧化物酶；SBB：苏丹黑B；NSE：非特异性酯酶；CAE：氯乙酸酯酶；PAS：过碘酸-Schiff反应；vWf：von Willebrand因子。

他器官中骨髓原始细胞或前体细胞克隆性增加（占骨髓细胞成分的20%以上）。这些骨髓成分包括中性粒细胞、嗜酸性粒细胞和嗜碱性粒细胞系的细胞，以及单核细胞、红系和巨核细胞系的细胞。在有残留的正常造血情况下，不成熟的骨髓成分增加，常常导致造血不足（即粒细胞减少症、贫血和血小板减少症）。急性这一术语表示在无任何治疗的情况下，疾病呈迅速进展的临床经过。多年来，FAB分类已提供了可重复的白血病类型的亚分类[1a]（表22.4），但其对于预后的实用价值有限。虽然FAB的某些形态学亚型，如急性前骨髓性白血病（acute promyelocytic leukemia，APL）(FAB M3)和伴有嗜酸性粒细胞增多（FAB M4Eo）的急性骨髓单核细胞性白血病（AMML）具有独特的临床病理学特征，但是这些特征与累及特异性关键基因的经常发生的遗传学异常的关系似乎更为密切。基于这些异常的存在来进行的AML分类加大了其在预测临床行为和逐渐增加的治疗指导方面的重要性。已经发现，AML具有四种独特而明显的遗传学异常[即t(8;21)(q22;q22)、inv(16)(p13q22)或t(16;16)(p13;q22)、t(15;17)(q22;q22)以及11q23异常]，或者需要特殊的治疗或者与临床预后密切相关。伴有这些异常的AML分别被归入不同的组别，作为通向AML分子分类系统的第一步（表22.5）。除了上述遗传学亚型，基于其临床相关性，WHO建立了新的AML亚型，认可先前存在的MDS或先前化疗对预后的重要性。相对来说，

急性骨髓性白血病

表22.5	WHO的急性骨髓性白血病分类

伴有多发性遗传学异常的急性骨髓性白血病
- t(8;21)(q22;q22); (*AML1/ETO*)
- inv(16)(p13q22) 或 t(16;16)(p13;q22); (*CBFβ/MYH11*)
- t(15;17)(q22;q12) (*PML/RARα*)
- 11q23 异常 (*MLL*)

伴有多系增生异常的急性骨髓性白血病
- 继 MDS 或 MDS/MPD 之后
- 先前没有 MDS

急性骨髓性白血病，治疗相关的
- 烷基化因素
- 拓扑异构酶 II 型抑制物
- 其他因素

急性骨髓性白血病，非其他类别的
- 急性骨髓性白血病，分化较少
- 急性骨髓性白血病，没有成熟性成分
- 急性骨髓性白血病，伴有成熟性成分
- 急性骨髓单核细胞性白血病
- 急性原始单核细胞性和单核细胞性白血病
- 急性红白血病
- 急性原始巨核细胞性白血病
- 急性嗜碱细胞性白血病
- 急性全骨髓增生伴有骨髓纤维化
- 粒细胞肉瘤

表22.6	急性骨髓性白血病的FAB亚型及其相应的WHO类型
FAB亚型	**WHO类型**
M0	急性骨髓原始细胞性白血病，分化较少
M1	急性骨髓原始细胞性白血病不伴有成熟性成分
M2	急性骨髓原始细胞性白血病伴有成熟性成分
M3	急性前骨髓性白血病伴有 t(15;17)(q22;q12)
M4	急性骨髓单核细胞性白血病
M4-Eo	急性骨髓性白血病，伴有 inv(16)(p13q22) 或 t(16;16)(p13;q22)
M5	急性原始单核细胞性或单核细胞性白血病
M6	急性红白血病
M7	急性原始巨核细胞性白血病
–	急性嗜碱细胞性白血病
–	急性全骨髓增生伴有骨髓纤维化
–	髓细胞肉瘤

WHO 的其余 AML 类别（非特异性）与对应的 FAB 类别相比没有什么改变（表 22.6）；然而，其发现了作为附加的、具有临床意义的白血病遗传学标记物（如 FLT3 长度突变和 MLL 部分串联重复），随着经常发生的遗传学异常，新的分子亚型有可能加到 AML 的列表中。

AML 的一般临床和实验室特征

虽然 AML 与先前接受放疗、细胞毒性化疗和诸如苯等某些环境毒物之间具有明显的联系，但是绝大多数 AML 病例是特发性的。AML 可发生于任何年龄，但主要发生于年龄较大的成人（中位年龄为 60 岁）。对于男性和女性来说，在 25~65 岁之间其发生率上升 10 倍以上（1.0~10.6/100 000 人口），而在 70~74 岁之间达到每年 15.7/100 000 人口[32]。60 岁以上，男性发病率增高；年龄较小时则没有性别差异。

AML 的临床病理学特征与骨髓中原始细胞增生及其浸润到诸如肝和脾等正常组织有关。在骨髓中最常见的后果是正常造血成分被替代，导致血细胞减少。由于贫血、中性粒细胞减少和血小板减少，分别可能发生乏力、苍白和劳累时呼吸困难、感染和发热以及出血[33]。几乎总是可以出现贫血和血小板减少。播散性血管内凝血的实验室证据常常与急性前骨髓性白血病（APL）或原始单核胞性白血病有关。多数患者白细胞计数增高（>10×10^9/L）；白细胞计数 > 100×10^9/L 发生于 15%~20% 的患者（最常见于单核细胞性白血病）[34-36]。白细胞计数 > 150×10^9/L 可以导致白细胞停滞，即白血病细胞在不同器官的微血管内聚集（尤其是脑和肺），导致危及生命的组织梗死和出血[35,37-39]。白细胞减少可见于年龄较大的患者，也可见于颗粒增多的 APL 或伴有多系增生异常、阵发性夜间血红蛋白尿或 Fanconi 贫血的 AML[40,41]。外周血常常可以见到原始细胞，但在多达 10% 的患者中缺乏原始细胞（所谓的非白血病性表现，aleukemic presentation）[36]。

其他组织（淋巴结、皮肤、牙龈和脑脊膜）发生浸润少见，最常见的是白血病伴有单核细胞分化。少数情况下，AML 可以作为孤立性的肿块发生，这种病例通常被命名为"粒细胞肉瘤"（granulocytic sarcoma），或者因为出现髓过氧化酶（MPO）而呈绿色，称为"绿色瘤"（chloroma）（也见第 21 章）。这种肿瘤可在有任何其他 AML 证据之前数月甚或几年就被发现，也可能是复发的第一个证据。易于侵犯的部位是骨（尤其是颅骨和面骨）、乳腺、睾丸、卵巢和脑。

AML 的一般形态学特征

大多数病例骨髓细胞成分增加，主要由原始细胞和（或）不成熟性粒细胞或单核细胞组成。成熟中的粒细胞成分和巨核细胞有相应程度的减少（有少数明显例外的情况）。红系前体细胞的数目差异较大；红系成分增多常常见于急性红白血病或起源于 MDS 的 AML。按照 WHO 的指南，原始细胞应占有核细胞的 20% 以上，典型的病例这一数字大于 50%。为了诊断的目的，急性前骨髓性白血病（APML）的非典型性前髓细胞、急性原始单核细胞性/单核细胞性白血病的原始单核细胞和前

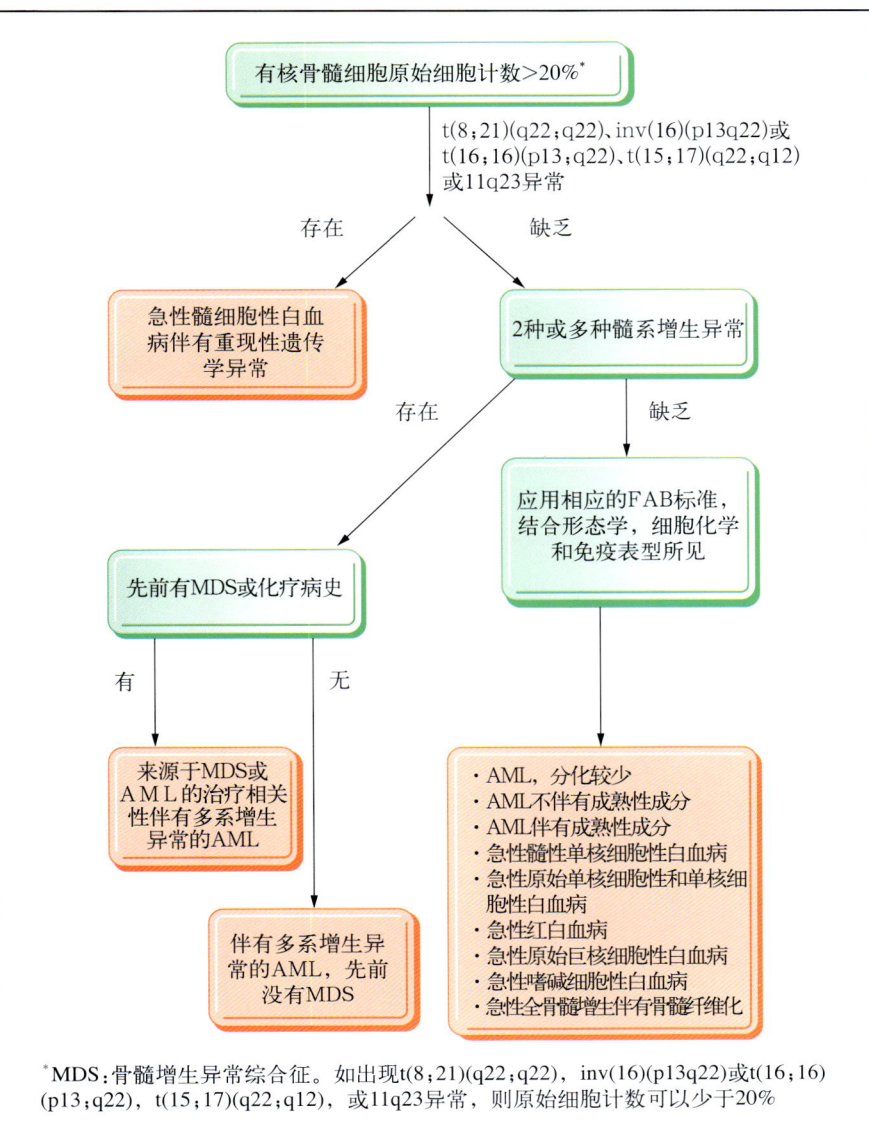

图22.17 应用WHO标准诊断急性骨髓性白血病（AML）的流程图。

*MDS：骨髓增生异常综合征。如出现t(8;21)(q22;q22)，inv(16)(p13q22)或t(16;16)(p13;q22)，t(15;17)(q22;q12)，或11q23异常，则原始细胞计数可以少于20%

单核细胞以及急性原始巨核细胞性白血病的原始巨核细胞都可以作为原始细胞计数。除了罕见的"单纯性"急性原始红细胞白血病外，原始红细胞不包括在原始细胞的计数之中。其他例外情况发生于伴有 t(8;21)(q22;q22)、inv(16)(p13q22) 或 t(16;16)(p13;q22)、t(15;17)(q22;q12)或11q23异常的病例；在这种情况下，做出 AML 的诊断的原始细胞数目不需要＞20%。在所有其他亚型中，一旦确立原始细胞计数＞20%，细胞化学、免疫表型和临床病史都要用于最后的亚分类（图22.17）。

骨髓原始细胞是相对大的细胞（14～18μm），伴有单个圆形至卵圆形的细胞核，染色质纤细，分布均匀，有一个至多个清楚的核仁（图22.18）。核被中等量的嗜碱性胞浆围绕，其中常常含有几个嗜苯胺蓝性颗粒。有些病例，可见许多胞浆颗粒，或胞浆颗粒融合形成杆状结构（奥尔小体）（图22.18）。奥尔小体只出现在骨髓衍生的原始细胞。对于较少分化的 AML，原始细胞常常较小且核仁不明显，有少量缺乏颗粒的胞浆，使细胞

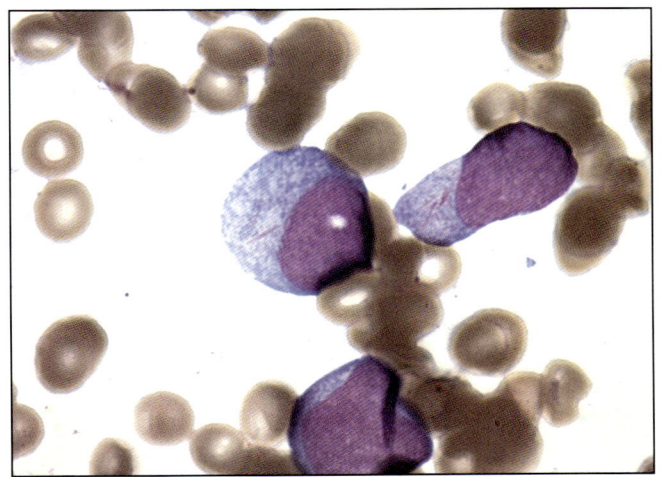

图22.18 AML。骨髓抽吸涂片显示骨髓原始细胞伴有易于识别的奥尔小体。（Wright-Giemsa染色）

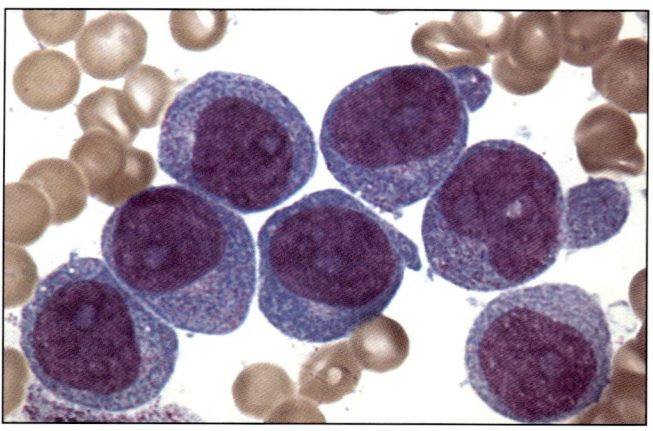

图22.19 AML。骨髓抽吸涂片显示原始单核细胞，核呈圆形，核仁明显，胞浆细颗粒状。（Wright-Giemsa染色）

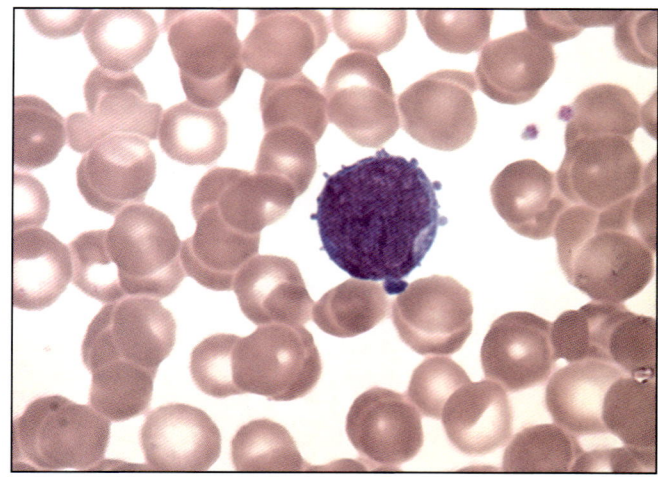

图22.21 AML。骨髓抽吸涂片显示一个孤立的原始巨核细胞，核浆比例高，胞浆内有小的空泡。（Wright-Giemsa染色）

在形态上难以与淋巴母细胞鉴别。

原始单核细胞是大细胞（15～20μm），核呈圆形，常有明显单个的核仁，胞浆丰富，嗜碱性，伴有纤细至粗大的分布均匀的嗜苯胺蓝颗粒，偶有空泡（图22.19）。胞浆可呈"空泡状"或有伪足形成。前单核细胞核呈分叶状，伴有纤细的皱褶或折痕，核仁不明显，胞浆丰富，蓝灰色，颗粒稀少，常常有空泡形成。

原始红细胞是中等至大的细胞，核呈圆形，染色质纤细分散，核仁一个至多个，胞浆深度嗜碱性，偶见空泡（图22.20），含有PAS阳性物质。

原始巨核细胞是中等至大的细胞，核呈圆形至不规则形，偶见双叶核，染色质纤细，分散，核仁明显，1～3个（图22.21）。细胞具有丰富淡染嗜碱性胞浆，通常缺乏颗粒，常常可见突起或伪足。

AML的细胞化学所见

造血系统的细胞化学染色是利用细胞的特异性酶

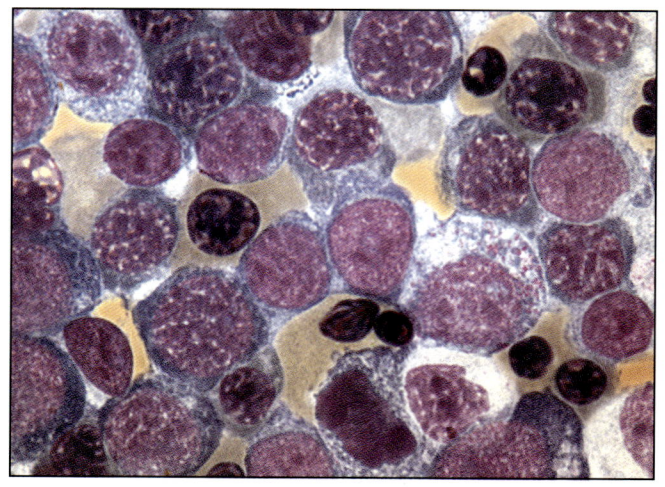

图22.20 AML。骨髓抽吸涂片显示包括原始红细胞在内的红系前体细胞，核呈圆形，染色质纤细，胞浆强嗜碱性。（Wright-Giemsa染色）

和细胞的化学特性。未经固定的标本，如风干的抽吸涂片或印片，一般用这种试验。一般来说，髓过氧化物酶（myeloperoxidase，MPO）、苏丹黑B（Sudan black B，SBB）和特异性脂酶（specific esterase，SE）染色有助于识别骨髓的粒细胞成分；而非特异性酯酶（non-specific esterase，NSE）着染单核系的细胞（表22.7）。PAS呈阳性可证实红白血病中原始红细胞的存在，可以鉴别伴有较少分化成分的AML中的原始细胞（PAS呈阴性）和前体B细胞性淋巴母细胞（PAS呈块状阳性）。

AML的免疫表型所见

免疫表型分析结合形态学和细胞遗传学试验非常有用（表22.8）。对于免疫表型来说，宁愿选择流式细胞分析这项技术，因为其具有特异性[42]、多参数变量以及可以应用多种抗体试剂。虽然AML亚型存在很大程度的免疫表型异质性，但是仍存在着某些特征性的形态[如t(15;17)急性前骨髓性白血病中HLA-DR呈阴性，t(8;21)AML中CD19/CD56呈阳性]。另外，两系或两种表型的白血病的确切诊断需要进行免疫表型研究。

AML的分子遗传学所见

如同已经强调的一样，为了弄清可疑的AML的特性，需要进行细胞遗传学和其他分子遗传学研究。理想的是，所有病例均应进行常规核型分析，而FISH或反转录酶聚合酶链式反应（RT-PCR）可以用于证实MLL存在t(8;21)、inv(16)或t(16;16)、t(15;17)或异常。另外，出现MDS的特征性的遗传学改变可能有助于继发性AML的诊断。伴有t(8;21)、t(15;17)或inv(16)的AML具有相对良好的预后（也见下文）[43]。在没有这些有利改变的患者，出现复杂性的核型、5号染色体单体、(5q)缺失、7号染色体单体或3q异常，与相对较差的预后有

表22.7	正常和肿瘤性造血细胞的细胞化学染色	
染色	正常细胞阳性	肿瘤细胞阳性
髓过氧化物酶（MPO）（原始颗粒）	早期骨髓原始细胞（弱阳性） 骨髓原始细胞→中性粒细胞 嗜酸性粒细胞单核细胞（几无颗粒）	骨髓原始细胞 前髓细胞（强阳性）
苏丹黑 B（SBB）（原始颗粒和细胞内脂质）	早期骨髓原始细胞（弱阳性） 骨髓原始细胞→中性粒细胞 嗜酸性粒细胞单核细胞（几无颗粒）	骨髓原始细胞 前髓细胞（强阳性）
特异性酯酶（SE）（原始颗粒） 萘基 AS-D 氯乙酸酯酶（CAE/Leder）	早期骨髓原始细胞（弱阳性） 骨髓原始细胞→前髓细胞肥大细胞单核细胞（几无颗粒）	骨髓原始细胞（弱阳性） 前髓细胞（强阳性） 原始单核细胞（±，颗粒纤细散在） 伴有 inv(16) 或 t(16;16) 的 AML 中的嗜酸性粒细胞
非特异性酯酶（NSE） α-萘基乙酸酯酶（ANA）	单核细胞和巨噬细胞（可被氟化钠抑制） 颗粒细胞（阴性至弱阳性） 巨核细胞	原始单核细胞（可被氟化钠抑制） APL 中的前髓细胞（25%） 淋巴母细胞（多灶性点状或 Golgi 形态） 原始巨核细胞和原始红细胞（多灶性点状） T-PLL 中的幼稚淋巴细胞
α-萘基丁酸酯酶（ANB）	单核细胞和巨噬细胞 颗粒细胞（阴性至弱阳性） 巨核细胞（弱阳性）	原始单核细胞 淋巴母细胞（多灶性点状）
过碘酸-Schiff 反应（PAS）	中性粒细胞（弥漫性颗粒形态） 单核细胞（几无颗粒）	淋巴母细胞（核周，粗大，块状颗粒形态） 红白血病（原始细胞和红系前体细胞呈块状阳性）

AML：急性骨髓性白血病；APL：急性前骨髓性白血病；T-PLL：T 细胞性幼稚淋巴细胞性白血病。

关[44]。伴有 +8、+21、+22、(9q) 缺失、(7q) 缺失或其他多种结构或数目缺陷的患者，不包括在有利或低危险人群中，具有中等程度的预后[44]。

伴有多发性遗传学异常的急性骨髓性白血病 t(8;21)(q22;q22)、(AML1/ETO) 或 (RUNX1/MTG8)

定义：这种平衡性染色体易位大约占所有 AML 病例的 10%，几乎占伴有成熟成分的 AML（FAB M2 亚型）病例的 40%[45,46]。易位连接于 21 号染色体上的 *AML1* 或 *RUNX1* 基因的 5' 部分和 8 号染色体上的 *ETO* (eight-twenty-one) 或 *MTG8* 基因的 3' 末端部分。形成的 AML1-ETO 融合蛋白抑制 AML1 靶基因的转录激活，AML1 靶基因在正常情况下负责粒细胞的分化[47-52]。t(8;21) 可以通过标准的核型分析检测（图 22.22），而且可以通过 FISH 加以证实（图 22.23）。伴有这种异常的 AML 常见于较年轻的患者，在应用多周期高剂量阿糖胞苷（cytarabine）化疗后一般具有良好的治疗反应，完全消退比例高，而且可以长期生存[53,54]。

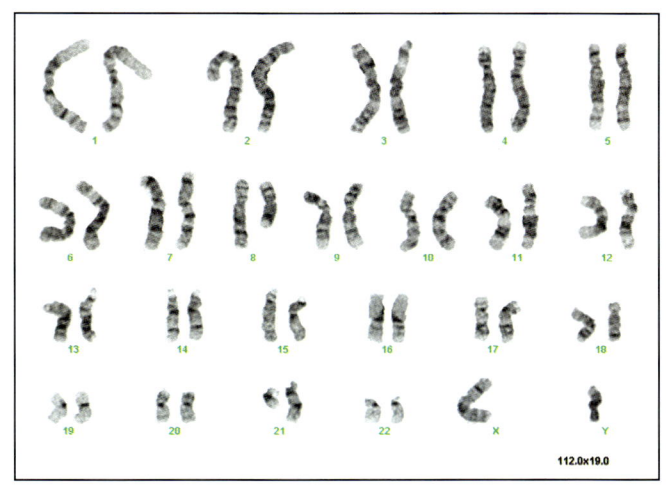

图22.22 核型分析显示8;21平衡性染色体易位。（Courtesy of Paola Dal Cin PhD and Cynthia Mclaughlin BS, Brigham & Women's Hospital, Boston, MA.）

表22.8 选择性流式细胞术和免疫组化标记物

抗原或CD	造血细胞反应	流式细胞术检测	免疫组化检测 未固定	免疫组化检测 固定
造血系统前体细胞				
CD45（dim）	原始白细胞	+	+	+
CD117	原始白细胞（原始单核细胞±），肥大细胞	+	+	+
CD34	原始白细胞	+	+	+
TdT	B 和 T 淋巴母细胞，某些骨髓原始细胞	+	+	+
HLA-DR	B 淋巴母细胞，骨髓原始细胞（非前髓细胞）	+	+	–
骨髓单核细胞				
CD33	CFU-GEMM 至前髓细胞，单核细胞	+	–	–
CD13	CFU-GM 至粒细胞，单核细胞	+	–	–
CD14	单核细胞	+	–	–
CD68	单核细胞，巨噬细胞	–	+	+
CD15	粒细胞	+	+	+
髓过氧化物酶（MPO）	中性粒细胞，嗜酸性粒细胞	–	+	+
溶菌酶（Lysozyme）	骨髓单核细胞	–	+	+
巨核细胞				
CD41（GPIIb/IIIa）	血小板和巨噬细胞	+	+	+
CD42（GPIb）	血小板和巨噬细胞	+	+	–
CD61（GPIIIa）	血小板和巨噬细胞	+	+	+
von Willebrand 因子	血小板和巨噬细胞	–	+	+
红系				
血型糖蛋白 A	红细胞及前体细胞	+	+	+
血红蛋白	红细胞及前体细胞	–	+	+
B 淋巴细胞				
CD20	B 淋巴细胞	+	+	+
CD19	B 淋巴细胞	+	+	–
CD10	B 淋巴细胞亚类，粒细胞	+	+	+
CD23	B 淋巴细胞	+	+	+
表面免疫球蛋白（sIg）	成熟 B 淋巴细胞	+	+	–
胞浆免疫球蛋白（cIg）	浆细胞	+	+	+
CD138	浆细胞	+	+	+
T 淋巴细胞				
CD2	T 淋巴细胞，肿瘤性肥大细胞	+	+	+
CD3	T 淋巴细胞	+	+	+
CD5	T 淋巴细胞	+	+	+
CD4	辅助型 T 淋巴细胞	+	+	+
CD8	细胞毒性 T 淋巴细胞	+	+	+
CD1a	胸腺细胞，Langerhans 细胞	–	+	+

CD：分化群；TdT：末端脱氧核苷转移酶；CFU-GEMM：集落组成单位-粒细胞-红细胞-巨噬细胞-巨核细胞；CFU-GM：集落组成单位-粒细胞-单核细胞；GP：糖蛋白。

Modified from Fleming MD, Kutok J L, Skarin AT 2002 Examination of the bone marrow. In: Handin R I, Lux S E, Stossel T P（eds）Blood: principles and practice of hematology. Lippincott, Williams and Wilkins Philadelphia, p59-79.

病理学所见：伴有 t(8;21) 的病例的最常见的骨髓形态学表现是：急性骨髓原始细胞性白血病伴有超出原始细胞阶段的成熟性成分（图 22.24）。偶尔可能缺乏成熟成分，或在少数情况下呈单核细胞分化。原始细胞一般具有明显的嗜苯胺蓝颗粒，而且容易发现奥尔小体。成熟性粒细胞常常可见明显的胞浆或核的异常，包括颗粒增多、异常的团块状颗粒（类似于 Chediak-Higashi 异常）或假性 Pelger-Huet 核的异常。重要的是要认识到，这些改变可见于伴有 t(8;21) 的 AML，而且这些改变并不代表先前存在 MDS。少数情况下，分化程度可能达到原始细胞仅占细胞成分的 20% 以下。在这种情况下，仍可做出 AML t(8;21) 的诊断。

细胞化学和免疫表型所见：在不伴有单核细胞分化的病例，原始细胞一般显示 MPO 和 SBB 不同强度的染色。然而，在有些伴有异常颗粒形成的病例缺乏这种染色。大多数病例表达 CD34、CD13、CD33 和 HLA-DR。有趣的是，在这种疾病中（81% 的儿童病例），B 细胞标

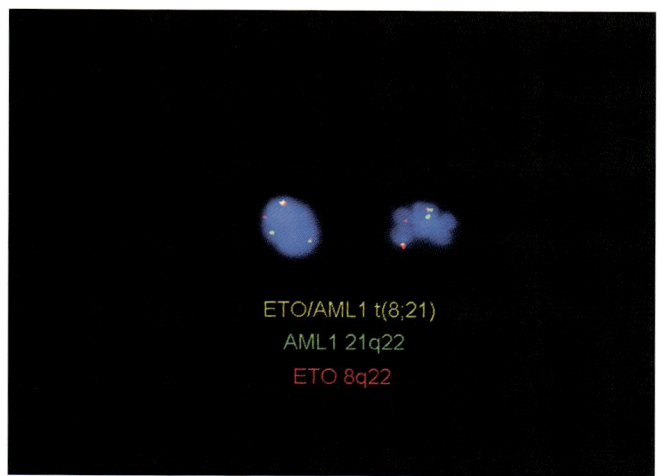

图22.23 应用检测染色体21q22（绿色）的AML1和染色体8q22（红色）的ETO的探针进行分裂间期核的荧光原位杂交（FISH），显示融合信号（黄色），代表8;21染色体平衡性易位。（Courtesy of Paola Dal Cin PhD and Cynthia Mclaughlin BS, Brigham & Women's Hospital, Boston, MA.）

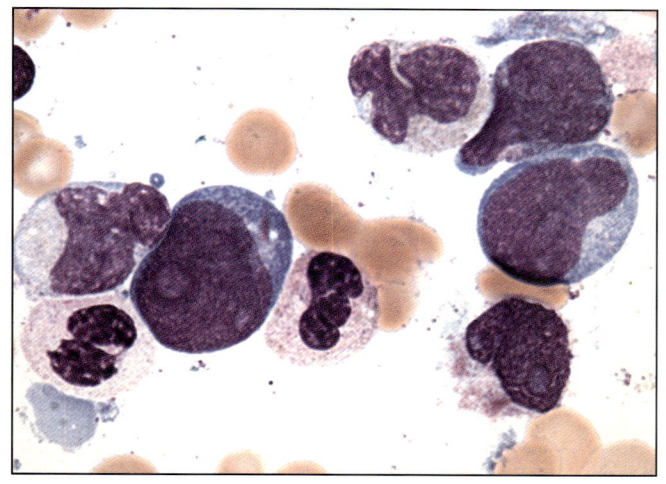

图22.24 伴有t(8;21)的急性骨髓性白血病病例的骨髓抽吸涂片。显示几个骨髓原始细胞，其中一个具有胞浆奥尔小体（左中），混有成熟性粒细胞成分。（Wright-Giemsa染色）

记物CD19常常在原始细胞成分中共同表达，而CD19/CD56共同表达对于这种染色体异常相当特异[55]。在50%以上的病例中少数原始细胞末端脱氧核苷转移酶（TdT）可能呈阳性[56]。

Inv(16)(p13q22)或t(16;16)(p13,q22)：(CBFβ/MYH11)

定义：这种异常可以导致急性骨髓单核细胞性白血病（AMML），伴有明显的骨髓嗜酸性粒细胞增多。遗传学缺陷涉及位于染色体16q22的 CBFβ 基因和位于染色体16p13的平滑肌肌浆球蛋白重链基因。染色体倒位或易位可导致这些基因断裂或再结合，形成框内融合基因产物（CBFβ/MYH11）。CBFβ是AML1的正常异源二聚体的配体 [这种蛋白质参与t(8;21)]，而

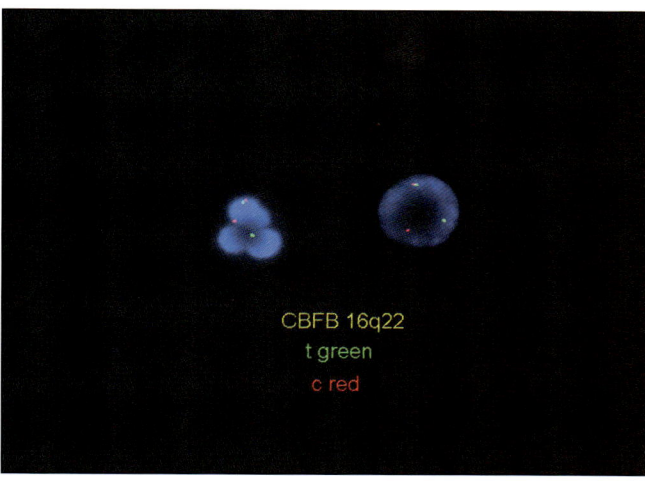

图22.25 应用由染色体16q22的CBFβ的着丝粒（红色）和端粒（绿色）区的探针进行分裂间期核的荧光原位杂交，显示红色和绿色信号分裂开，代表伴有嗜酸性粒细胞增多的急性骨髓单核细胞性白血病，或存在inv16或t(16;16)。（Courtesy of Paola Dal Cin PhD and Cynthia Mclaughlin BS, Brigham & Women's Hospital, Boston, MA.）

MYH11融合可导致AML1介导的骨髓细胞分化的抑制[48,52]。如同t(8;21)一样，inv(16)(p13q22)比较常见于较年轻的患者，大约占所有AML病例的10%~12%。在常规核型分析中检测inv(16)(p13q22)常常是困难的；RT-PCR或FISH方法有利于检测CBFβ/MYH11融合（图22.25）。出现这种遗传学异常与应用多周期高剂量阿糖胞苷治疗具有良好的临床反应和长期生存有关[53,57]；然而，伴有 inv(16)(p13q22) 的患者可能比经类似治疗的t(8;21)患者具有较高的复发危险性[54]。

病理学所见：骨髓显示骨髓原始细胞、原始单核细胞和前单核细胞混合存在，占骨髓细胞成分的20%以上（图22.26和22.27）。在大多数病例，嗜酸性粒细胞增多，在所有的病例均出现异常嗜酸性粒细胞。具有特征性的异常包括：在早期前体嗜酸性粒细胞中可见大的嗜酸性颗粒，更为明显的是，在前体嗜酸性粒细胞内可见大的嗜碱性颗粒 [所谓的"嗜酸-嗜碱性"(eo-basos)]（图22.27）。奥尔小体常常可见。虽然大多数具有这些特征的病例相当于 FAB M4Eo 类别，但是伴有 inv(16)(p13q22) 的病例偶尔缺乏嗜酸性粒细胞增多，只有通过细胞遗传学或分子生物学检查才能辨认。

细胞化学和免疫表型所见：在多数病例，嗜酸性粒细胞显示不典型的PAS细胞化学反应且萘酚AS-D氯乙酸酯酶呈阳性（表22.7）[58]。另外，MPO阳性见于3%以上的骨髓原始细胞，而单核细胞成分NSE呈弱阳性反应。通过免疫表型分析还可见到单核细胞分化的证据，包括

急性骨髓性白血病

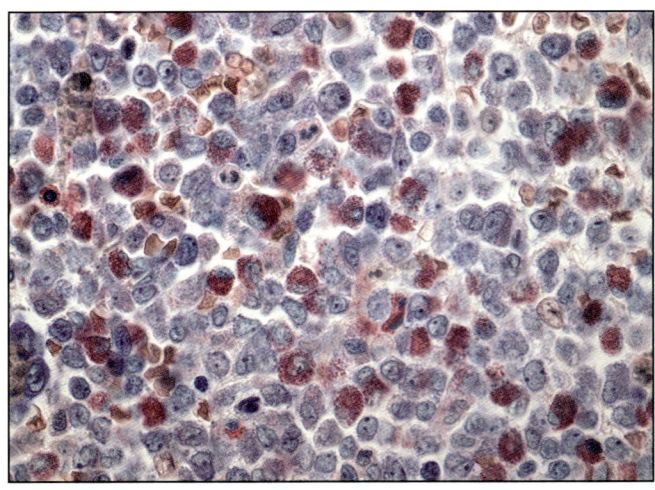

图22.26 伴有嗜酸性粒细胞增多和inv(16)的急性骨髓单核细胞白血病的骨髓芯针活检的组织学切片。显示多量原始细胞，核呈圆形，核仁明显，胞浆量少，常常混有嗜酸性粒细胞成分。（Giemsa染色）

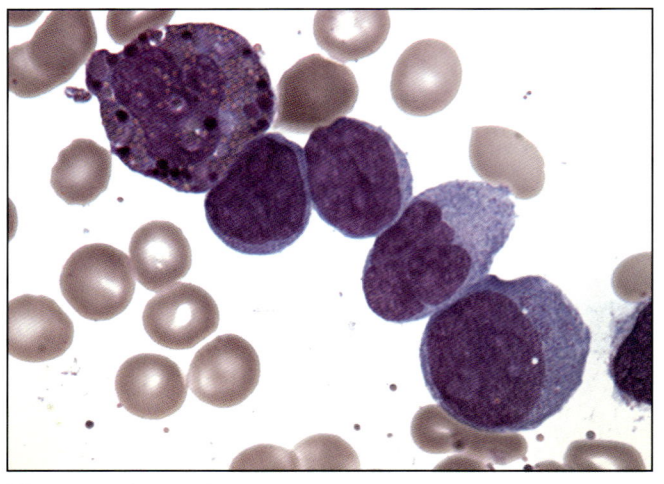

图22.27 伴有嗜酸性粒细胞增多和inv(16)的急性骨髓单核细胞白血病的骨髓抽吸涂片。显示骨髓原始细胞和原始单核细胞（右下），伴有明显大的嗜碱性颗粒的异常嗜酸性粒细胞成分（左上，所谓的嗜酸-嗜碱性）。（Wright-Giemsa染色）

CD14、CD11b、CD4、CD36，而单核细胞样成分有溶菌酶的表达。典型的骨髓抗原、CD13和CD33也可见于原始细胞内。虽然不特异，但T细胞标记物CD2在骨髓原始细胞中常有共同表达，应该及时寻找inv(16)(p13q22)[59]。

t(15;17)(q22;q12)；（PML/RAR和变型）

定义：t(15;17)(q22;q12)和其他较少见的累及17q12位点的RARα重排与APL有关，其特征是非典型性前髓细胞在骨髓内聚集。APL最常见于成年患者，占所有AML类型的5%~10%[36,60-62]。在所有APL病例中有98%可见t(15;17)(q22;q12)异常，融合17号染色体上的RARα基因和15号染色体上的PML基因，产生PML-RARα融合蛋白[62-66]。PML-RARα融合蛋白抑

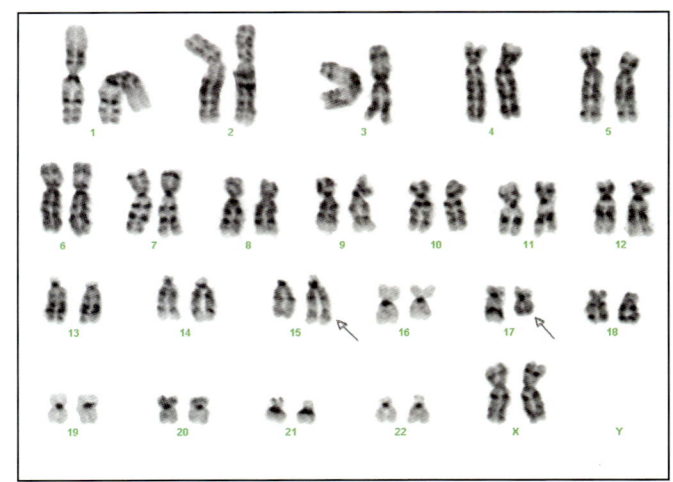

图22.28 核型分析显示15;17染色体平衡易位。（Courtesy of Paola Dal Cin PhD and Cynthia Mclaughlin BS, Brigham & Women's Hospital, Boston，MA.）

制RARα的功能，这是正常髓细胞发生的关键，导致阻止前髓细胞阶段的分化[62]。这种异常可被药理学剂量的ATRA或三氧化二砷克服，后者可诱导肿瘤性前髓细胞分化并凋亡[67-70]。ATRA疗法连同蒽环类药，使长期生存的可能性提高[70]。在少数病例，可见交替性染色体平衡易位，导致新的RARα融合基因[62,64]。可变性的配体蛋白包括前髓细胞白血病锌指（PLZF）、核磷蛋白（NPM）、核分裂器（NUMA）和STAT5b[71-74]。重要的是，具有上述一些可变性融合蛋白（PLZF-RARα和STAT5b-RARα）的肿瘤对于ATRA分化疗法没有反应[63]。有趣的是，除了t(15;17)以外，30%以上的APL病例也具有内部串联重复（ITD）或酪氨酸激酶受体FLT3的Asp835突变[75]，其不仅在疾病的发病机制中起作用，而且是第二个有利的治疗靶点[76-78]。标准核型分析已常规应用于APL的诊断（图22.28），FISH和RT-PCR亦然（图22.29）。RT-PCR检测PML-RARα融合转录在监测残留的少数病变中特别有用。值得注意的是，APL常常伴有播散性血管内凝血样出血性素质，这可能与纤维蛋白溶解增高状态有关，后者同时发生血液凝固系统激活受限[79,80]。

病理学所见：APL有两种形态学亚型，即较常见的颗粒增多或"典型的"变型和较少见的"微小颗粒"变型[81,82]。各种RARα重排与颗粒增多或微小颗粒亚型之间无相关性。颗粒增多变型常常伴有白细胞减少，而微小颗粒变型较常伴有白细胞增多。骨髓芯针活检一般显示细胞成分明显增多，终末骨髓分化受限，伴有多量非典型性前髓细胞（图22.30）。在抽吸涂片中，颗粒增多的APL的非典型性前髓细胞显示核的大小和形状变化很大，常常伴有双叶或锯齿状。胞浆充满许多大的鲜粉色/红色至紫红色的颗粒，

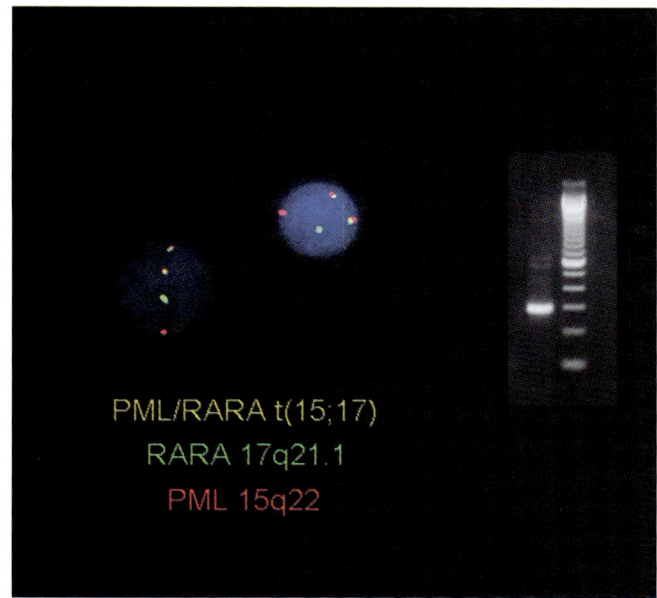

图22.29 左：应用针对17号染色体上RARα（绿色）和染色体15q22上PML（红色）的探针进行分裂间期核的荧光原位杂交，显示融合信号（黄色），代表15;17染色体平衡性易位。右：琼脂糖凝胶证实一例伴有t(15;17)的前骨髓性白血病存在PML-RARα融合转录（左侧泳道；右侧泳道为1kb梯度），与应用反转录酶聚合链式反应（RT-PCR）技术检查到的一样。（Courtesy of Paola Dal Cin PhD and Cynthia Mclaughlin BS, Brigham & Women's Hospital, Boston, MA.）

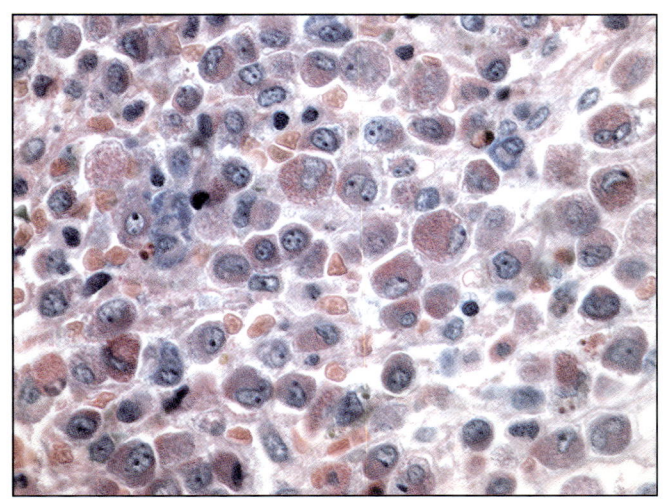

图22.30 一例颗粒增多性伴有t(15;17)的急性前骨髓性白血病的骨髓芯针活检组织学切片，显示成片的非典型性前髓细胞，伴有明显的嗜酸性胞浆颗粒。（Giemsa染色）

这些颗粒可能掩盖细胞核（图22.31）。可见多量奥尔小体，偶尔其大量聚集，类似于成捆的木棒（所谓的"柴捆"细胞，"faggot" cells）（图22.32）。在微小颗粒变型的APL中，嗜苯胺蓝颗粒是亚显微性的（大小 < 200nm），光学显微镜下不易识别[61, 81]。这些病例的颗粒呈灰尘状或不明显，而比较容易见到显示明显双叶状或哑铃形的细胞核（图22.33）。仔细检查时，在微小颗粒性APL中可见少量较典型的颗粒增多的成分以及奥尔小体。

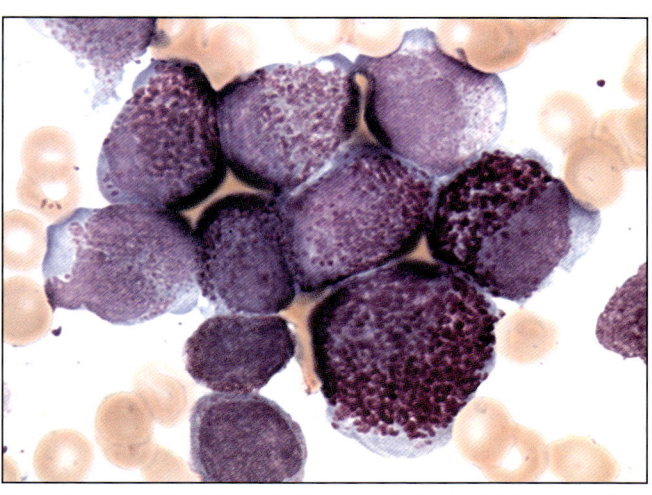

图22.31 一例颗粒增多性伴有t(15;17)的急性前骨髓性白血病的骨髓抽吸涂片，显示大的非典型性前髓细胞，细胞核偏心，胞浆充满多量覆盖细胞核的深染的颗粒。（Wright-Giemsa染色）

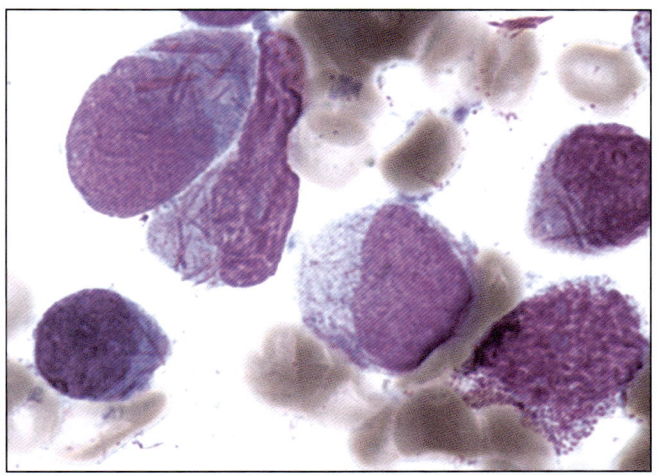

图22.32 一例颗粒增多性伴有t(15;17)的急性前骨髓性白血病的骨髓抽吸涂片，显示前髓细胞伴有多量奥尔小体，类似于成捆的木棒（所谓的"柴捆细胞"）。（Wright-Giemsa染色）

细胞化学和免疫表型所见：在颗粒增多和微小颗粒性病变中，MPO 均呈强阳性（图 22.34）。这种表现应该促使 *PML-RARα* 融合的检查，尤其是在微小颗粒性病例。流式细胞检查发现 CD33 呈均一阳性，CD31 表达不一。其特征是缺乏 HLA-DR，CD34 通常呈阴性。CD15 很少有表达，从未见到 CD34/CD15 双重阳性细胞[83,84]。首选 T 细胞标记物 CD2 常常表达[85,86]。如果出现 CD34、HLA-DR 和 CD2 的表达，常常需要注意有无微小颗粒性 APL[85-87]。

鉴别诊断：由于微小颗粒性变型具有颗粒不明显的性质，所以这种疾病容易被漏掉。重要的线索包括：MPO 强阳性染色，缺乏 HLA-DR 表达，或偶尔可见颗粒增多或含有奥尔小体的成分。一般来说，这种病例的形态学特征提示单核细胞性白血病，通过组织化学或

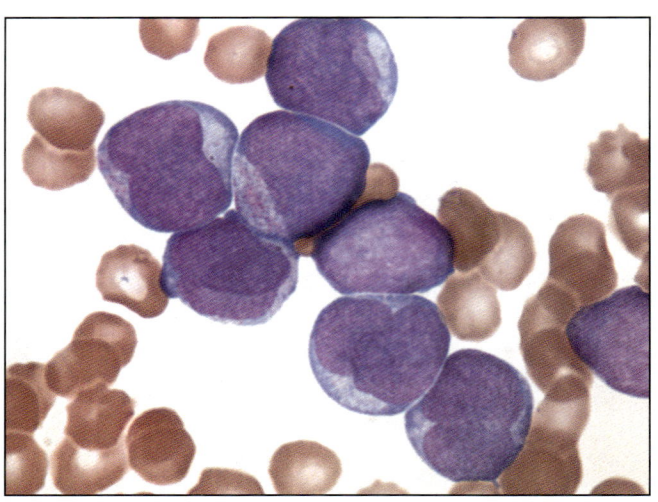

图22.33 一例微小颗粒性伴有t(15;17)的急性前骨髓性白血病的骨髓抽吸涂片，显示非典型性前髓细胞，伴有折叠或双叶的细胞核，胞浆颗粒不清楚到不能发现。（Wright-Giemsa染色）

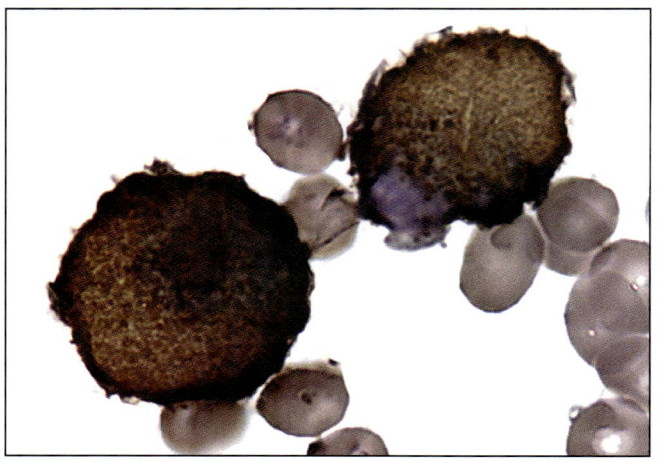

图22.34 一例伴有t(15;17)的急性前骨髓性白血病的骨髓髓过氧化物酶组织化学染色，显示颗粒含有的过氧化物酶强阳性染色。

免疫表型检查可以排除。在大多数病例，通过细胞遗传学、FISH 和 RT-PCR 可以检测 *PML-RARα* 融合，证实 APL 的诊断。偶尔，药物诱导的粒细胞缺乏或大颗粒淋巴细胞性白血病可能类似于 APL，由于在前髓细胞阶段成熟停止。这些病例可以通过缺乏非典型性前髓细胞及缺乏奥尔小体加以鉴别。

11q23（MLL）异常

定义：11q23异常见于6% ~ 8%的原发性AML病例[46]。受累的基因是人类同源性果蝇基因（*Drosophila trithorax* gene），也叫混合谱系白血病（mixed-lineage leukemia, *MLL*）。最常见的异常表现为平衡性染色体易位。在*MLL*易位中观察到40种以上不同的配体基因[88]。

在新形成的 AML，11q23 异常最常见于婴儿 AML；然而，绝大多数 *MLL* 重排与先前化疗有关（见下文）。常常通过普通的细胞遗传学检测 *MLL* 重排（图 22.35）。当质量好的细胞分裂中期获得时，FISH 并不会增加检测产出，但当染色体制备不是最佳或出现复杂的重排时，FISH 是有用的（图 22.36）[89]。与 t(8;21) 或 inv(16) 相关性 AML 相比，新形成的伴有 11q23 异常的 AML 病例具有中等预后[44]。

病理学、细胞化学和免疫表型所见：虽然没有界定出现伴有 11q23 异常的 AML 的特殊形态学，但这些缺陷常常伴有原始单核细胞或骨髓单核细胞的形态学、免疫表型和细胞化学所见。偶尔，11q23 异常可见于伴有或不伴有成熟性成分的 AML。与单核细胞分化密切相关，这与易于发生黏膜或皮肤等髓外受累有关。在与先前化疗无关的病例，增生异常的特征是少见的。

伴有多系增生异常的急性骨髓性白血病
Acute myeloid leukemia with multilineage dysplasia

定义

这种类型的 AML 最常见于老年人，定义为血液或骨髓中出现 > 20% 的原始细胞，伴有 > 50% 的两种或多种髓系细胞的增生异常[90,91]。在伴有新形成的 AML 或具有已知 MDS 病史的患者可以作出这种诊断。在任何情况下出现多系增生异常均会对完全缓解和无病生存的机会带来不利影响[44,91,92]。

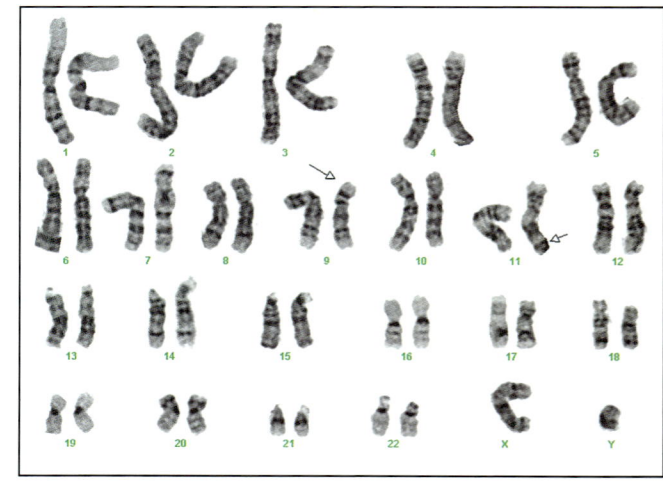

图22.35 核型分析证实9;11平衡性染色体易位，提示急性骨髓性白血病具有混合谱系白血病（MLL）重排。（Courtesy of Paola Dal Cin PhD and Cynthia Mclaughlin BS, Brigham & Women's Hospital, Boston, MA.）

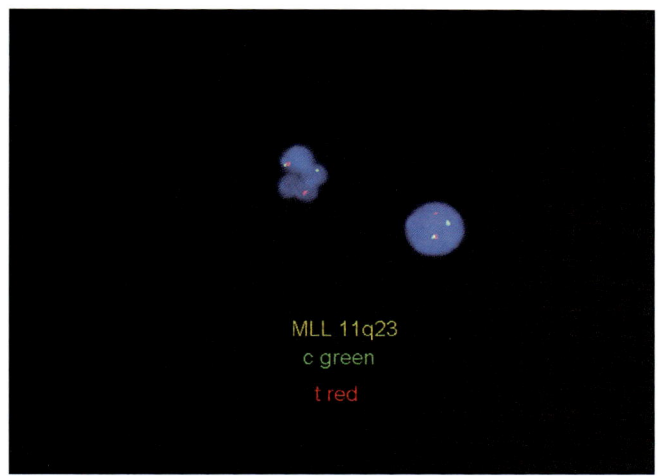

图22.36 分裂间期核荧光原位杂交，应用的探针为位于染色体11q23的混合谱系白血病（MLL）基因的着丝粒（红色）和端粒（绿色）区，显示红色和绿色信号分开，提示白血病涉及MLL基因的重排。(Courtesy of Paola Dal Cin PhD and Cynthia Mclaughlin BS, Brigham & Women's Hospital, Boston, MA.)

急性骨髓性白血病 / 骨髓增生异常综合征，治疗相关性
Acute myeloid leukemia/myelodysplastic syndromes, therapy-related

这些类型的 AML 和 MDS 直接来源于先前接触细胞毒剂和（或）放射治疗。由于其预后差并对治疗有不利影响，所以认识这些疾病非常重要。不利的药剂包括烷基化药物、γ 射线和 DNA 拓扑异构酶 II 抑制剂（例如鬼臼毒素、依托泊苷和替你泊苷）。分类可根据适当对应的 WHO 分类，附加上"治疗相关性"这一术语来表示这种病因学联系。

烷基化药物和放射相关性 AML 通常发生于治疗后 5 年以上，危险性与患者的年龄和治疗的累加剂量有关[93,94]。另外，最常见的是先前有增生异常期，伴有细胞减少和骨髓衰竭（常常表现为 RCMD 或 RAEB1 或 RAEB2）。骨髓原始细胞或骨髓单核细胞性 AML 最常见。有些病例表现为急性全骨髓增生伴有骨髓纤维化（见下文）。虽然对烷基化或放射治疗没有遗传学特异性，但是核型分析常常显示 5 号或 7 号染色体部分或完全缺失[95,96]。许多应用高剂量烷基化药物治疗的患者也出现 11q23 和 21q22 异常[97]。

应用 DNA 拓扑异构酶 II 抑制剂治疗后的 AML 显示到疾病发作有一个短的间隔（1～3 年），而且缺乏先前 MDS 的病史。还能见到伴有 t(4;11) 的急性淋巴母细胞性白血病（ALL）。DNA 拓扑异构酶 II 抑制剂相关性 AML 比其他类型的治疗相关性 AML 少见，通常显示单核细胞性或骨髓单核细胞性分化，常常伴有 11q23 异常[93,94,98]。许多 11q23 的易位配体已被识别；t(6;11)(q27;q23)、t(9;11)(p21-22;q32)、t(10;11)(p12;q23) 和 t(11;19)(q23;p13.1-p13.3) 异常最常见[95,99-104]。在这种情况下其他异常也已被描述，包括 t(8;21)、inv(16) 和 t(15;17)[98,105]。治疗相关性 MDS/AML 的总体生存率差，尤其是伴有 11q23 异常的患者[97]。

病理学和免疫表型所见

患者一般表现为严重的全血细胞减少。骨髓细胞成分常常减少。原始细胞计数常常在 20%～50% 之间。见于典型 MDS 的增生异常在成熟成分中也可注意到，最常影响巨核细胞；CD34 染色有助于辨认原始细胞，原始细胞同时表达髓系抗原 CD13 和（或）CD33。常常可见 CD7 或 CD56 的异常表达。

细胞遗传学所见

常常可见与 MDS 中所见相同的染色体异常，包括 5 和 7 号染色体单体；(5q)、(7q)、(9q)、(20q) 缺失；8、21 和 22 号染色体三体；以及 3q 异常[44]。有趣的是，3q 畸变常常伴有血小板增多症。

鉴别诊断

伴有 t(8;21) 的 AML 病例常常显示增生异常的形态学改变。这些病例先前没有 MDS 病史，不应该归类为伴有多系增生异常的 AML。红白血病或伴有明显红系增生的 MDS 也常常包括在鉴别诊断中。如果红系前体细胞数目 > 50%，原始细胞占非红系细胞的 20% 以上，并且不出现多系增生异常，则应诊断为红白血病。当原始细胞增多，但占非红系成分的 20% 以下，而且出现增生异常时，诊断 RAEB 是恰当的。

急性骨髓性白血病，非特异性
Acute myeloid leukemia, not otherwise categorized

不符合前述分类的病例被放入这种 WHO 亚型中（表 22.9 和图 22.37 至 22.51），大部分相当于从前的 FAB 分类（表 22.6）。WHO 分类的主要变化是要求骨髓中原始细胞组成 > 20%，而不是 FAB 分类要求的 30%。几种新的病变也包括在"非特异性"组中，包括急性嗜碱细胞性白血病和伴有骨髓纤维化的急性全骨髓增生症（表 22.9）。后一种疾病的特征是所有髓系成分扩大，骨髓纤

表22.9　WHO急性骨髓性白血病（AML），非特异性（NOS）

WHO亚型	形态学	细胞化学	免疫表型
AML，极少分化	>20%无颗粒，中等大小，原始表现，没有奥尔小体；常常难以与淋巴母细胞鉴别	MPO、SBB、SE或NSE阳性的原始细胞<3%	CD117$^±$、CD13$^±$、CD33$^±$、TdT$^±$、HLA-DR$^+$、CD34$^+$、CD7$^{-/+}$、CD2$^{-/+}$、CD19$^{-/+}$
AML，没有成熟成分	骨髓原始细胞>20%；<10%的骨髓有核细胞是前髓细胞或较成熟的粒细胞成分；可见奥尔小体	MPO、SBB阳性的原始细胞>3%	CD117$^+$、CD13$^+$、CD33$^+$、HLA-DR$^+$、CD34$^+$
AML，伴有成熟成分	>20%骨髓原始细胞 ± 嗜苯胺蓝颗粒；>10%的骨髓有核细胞是前髓细胞或较成熟的粒细胞成分；可见典型的奥尔小体	MPO、SBB阳性的原始细胞>3%	CD13$^+$、CD33$^+$、CD15$^+$、CD34$^±$、CD117$^±$、HLA-DR$^±$
急性骨髓单核细胞性白血病	骨髓原始细胞、原始单核细胞、前单核细胞>20%；单核细胞和前体单核细胞>20%；中性粒细胞和粒细胞前体细胞>20%	单核细胞NSE呈阳性；骨髓原始细胞MPO、SBB呈阳性	不同比例的骨髓原始细胞或原始单核细胞和单核细胞以及粒细胞：CD13$^+$、CD33$^+$、CD11b$^+$、CD14$^+$、CD4$^+$、CD117$^±$、CD34$^±$
AML，伴有单核细胞分化	单核细胞>80%（或原始单核细胞为主，>80%；或前单核细胞为主，原始细胞<80%）	单核细胞NSE呈阳性，MPO、SBB呈阴性	CD13$^±$、CD33$^+$、CD117$^±$、CD34$^-$、CD36$^+$、CD11b$^+$、CD14$^±$、CD4$^+$
急性红白血病（红系/髓系）	红系前体细胞和（或）原始红细胞>50%；>20%的非红系前体细胞是骨髓原始细胞；骨髓原始细胞中可见奥尔小体	骨髓原始细胞MPO、SBB呈阳性；原始红细胞PAS呈阳性	髓系前体细胞：CD13$^+$、CD33$^+$、HLA-DR$^+$、CD34$^±$ 红系前体细胞：血型糖蛋白$^+$、血红蛋白$^+$
急性红白血病（单纯红系）	红系前体细胞和（或）原始红细胞>80%没有明显的骨髓原始细胞成分	原始红细胞ANA和PAS呈阳性	红系前体细胞：血型糖蛋白$^±$（较分化的成分表达较强）、血红蛋白$^+$、CD34$^-$、HLA-DR$^-$
急性原始巨核细胞性白血病	原始细胞>20%，通过形态学、免疫表型或电镜检查显示：>50%为巨核细胞来源	MPO、SBB呈阴性；巨核细胞PAS±	HLA-DR$^+$、CD33$^+$、CD34$^+$、CD61$^+$、CD41$^+$、vWf$^+$、CD42$^+$
急性嗜碱性粒细胞性白血病	>20%的细胞中等大小，核呈卵圆形或至双叶，核仁1个或3个，胞浆嗜碱性，伴有多个粗大的嗜碱性颗粒	异染性甲苯胺蓝染色、酸性磷酸酶呈阳性	CD13$^+$、CD33$^+$、CD34$^+$、HLA-DR$^+$、CD9$^+$、TdT$^±$
急性全骨髓增生伴有骨髓纤维化	全骨髓增生伴有成簇的原始细胞，包括增生异常的巨核细胞，背景为明显的网状纤维化	前体粒细胞MPO呈阳性；原始巨核细胞PAS±	原始细胞CD117$^+$、CD13$^+$、CD33$^+$、MPO$^+$；前体巨核细胞CD41$^+$、CD61和vWf$^+$

$^+$：阳性；$^-$：阴性；$^±$：常常阳性；$^{-/+}$：常常阴性。
MPO：髓过氧化物酶；SBB：苏丹黑B；NSE：非特异性酯酶；CD：分化群；TdT：末端脱氧核苷转移酶；PAS：过碘酸Schiff反应；ANA：α萘基乙酸酯酶；vWf：vov Willebrand因子。

维化明显，以及原始细胞增多。尚未确定这是一种独特的疾病还是一组异源性的疾病，包括原发性或继发性纤维增生性MDS，罕见的伴有纤维化的原发性AML，甚或不常见的毒性骨髓病[106,107]。

虽然不存在特异性细胞遗传学异常，但是有些所见常常与特别的表型或形态学有关（表22.10）。这些所见包括在伴有成熟的AML或伴有嗜碱性粒细胞增多的AMML中，有12p异常或t(6;9)(p23;q34)；以及在婴儿急性原始巨核细胞性白血病中见到的t(1;22)，后者常常伴有骨髓浸润的形态，类似于转移性肿瘤[109]。急性原始巨核细胞性白血病还与Down综合征有关，因此肿瘤细胞存在21三体。这些病例没有t(1;22)易位，但常常显示多种其他染色体异常，包括8号染色体三体以及GATA基因突变。

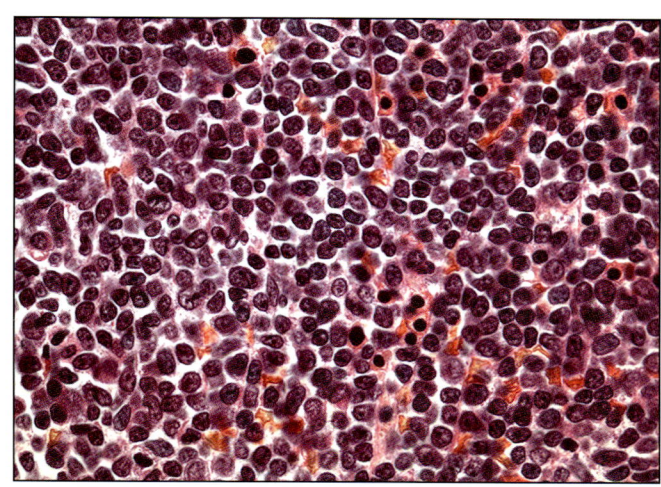

图22.37 一例极少分化的AML病例的骨髓芯针活检组织学切片,显示小的原始细胞成分,伴有不同程度的清楚的核仁,胞浆稀少。这种组织学表现几乎与急性淋巴母细胞性白血病相同(见图22.52),确切诊断为急性骨髓性白血病,需要进行免疫表型检查。(HE染色)

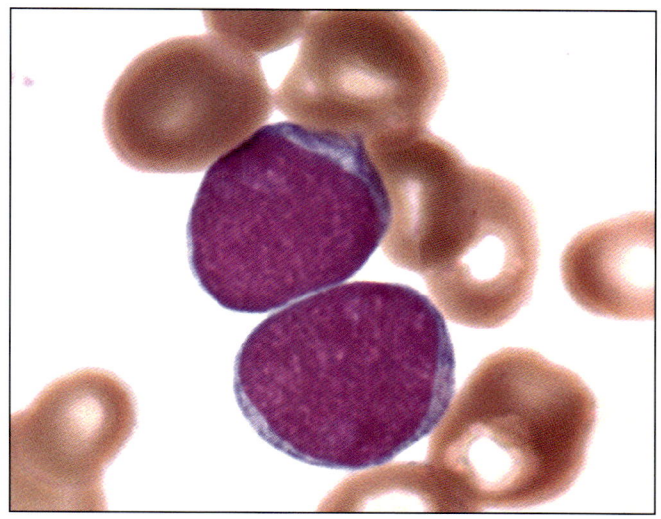

图22.38 极少分化的AML的骨髓抽吸涂片,显示骨髓原始细胞(由免疫表型确定),核呈圆形,含有均一的染色质,没有明显的核仁,仅有一圈少量的无颗粒的嗜碱性胞浆。(Wright-Giemsa染色)

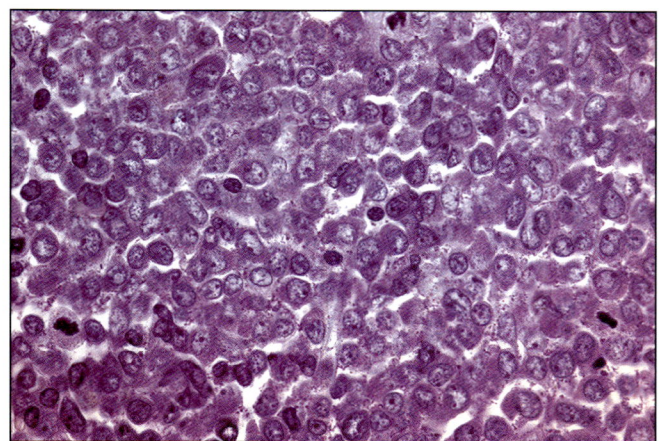

图22.39 一例没有成熟成分的AML病例的骨髓芯针活检组织学切片,显示片状骨髓原始细胞,伴有中等量的颗粒状胞浆。见不到原始细胞阶段之后的分化。(Giemsa染色)

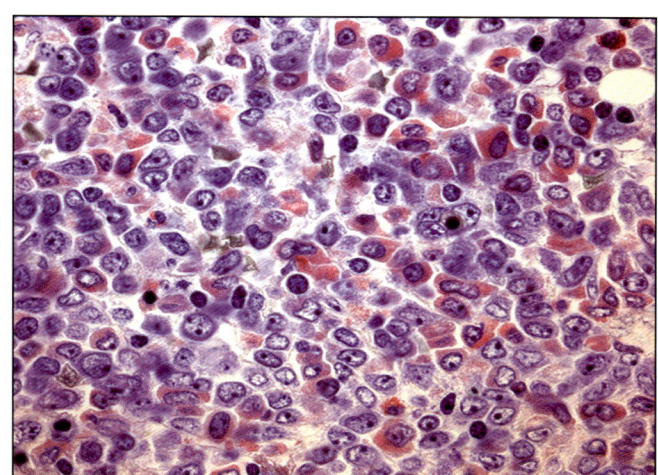

图22.40 一例伴有成熟成分的AML病例的骨髓芯针活检组织学切片,显示具有散在染色质,有小而明显核仁的骨髓原始细胞,以及中等数量的伴有较丰富嗜酸性颗粒状胞浆的前髓细胞和髓细胞混合存在。(Giemsa染色)

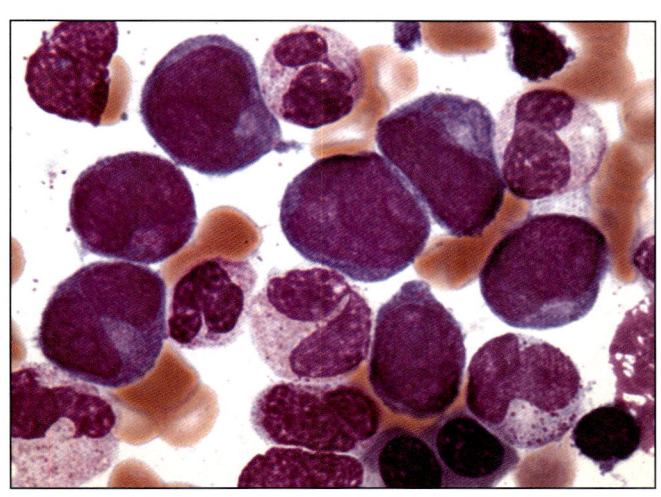

图22.41 例伴有成熟成分的AML的骨髓抽吸涂片,显示骨髓原始细胞和混合的较成熟的粒细胞成分。(Wright-Giemsa染色)

急性骨髓性白血病

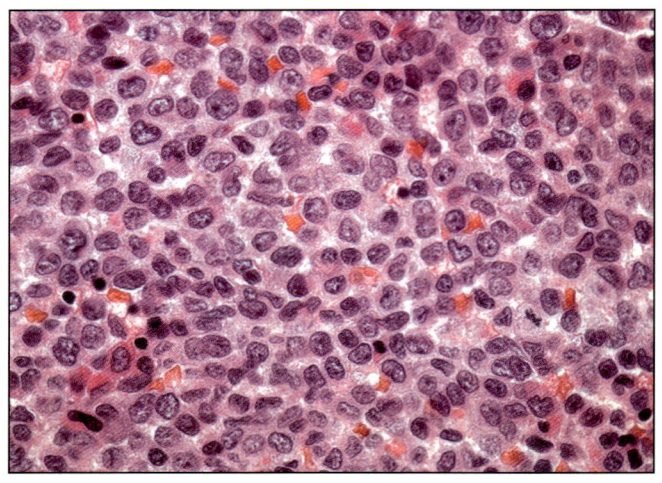

图22.42　一例急性骨髓单核细胞性白血病病例的骨髓芯针活检的组织学切片，显示伴有圆核和明显核仁的骨髓原始细胞成分，混合有较不规则的和有折叠核的单核细胞成分。（HE染色）

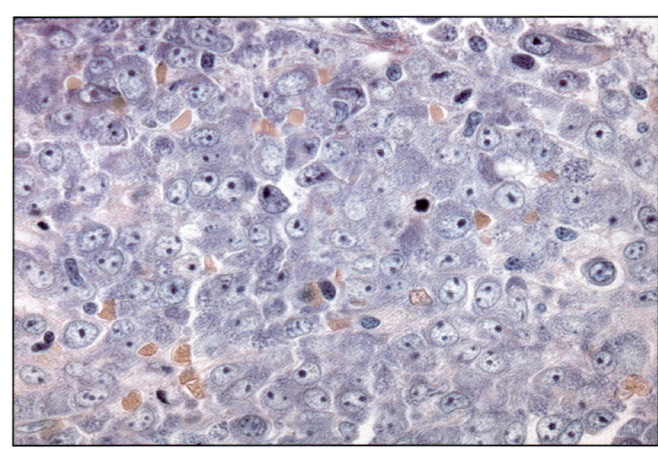

图22.44　一例急性原始单核细胞性白血病病例的骨髓芯针活检组织学切片，显示片状原始单核细胞，伴有圆形核，散在染色质，1～2个明显核仁和中等量的双嗜性胞浆。（Giemsa染色）

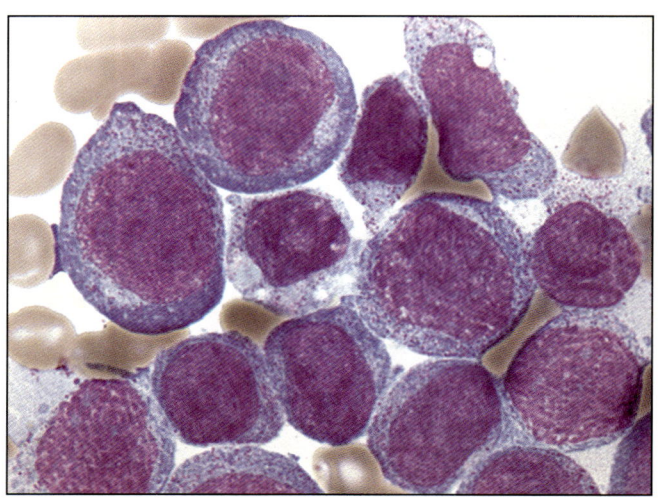

图22.43　急性骨髓单核细胞性白血病的骨髓抽吸涂片，显示伴有圆形核、明显核仁和嗜碱性胞浆的大的单核细胞成分（左上），以及伴有圆形核、不明显核仁和少量胞浆的较小的骨髓原始细胞成分（中下）。（Wright-Giemsa染色）

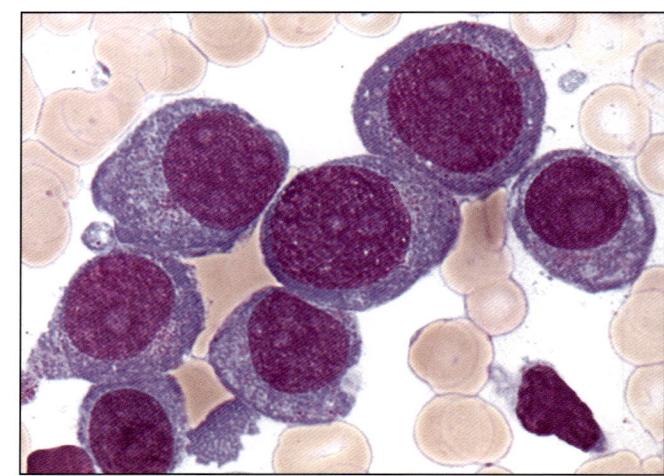

图22.45　急性原始单核细胞性白血病的骨髓抽吸涂片，显示大的原始单核细胞成分，核呈圆形，核仁明显，胞浆嗜碱性。注意可见少量嗜酸性胞浆颗粒，后者是原始单核细胞的特征。（Wright-Giemsa染色）

图22.46　（右）一例急性单核细胞性白血病病例的骨髓芯针活检组织学切片，显示片状前单核细胞，核不规则，折叠，核仁不明显，胞浆中等量，粉红色。（HE染色）

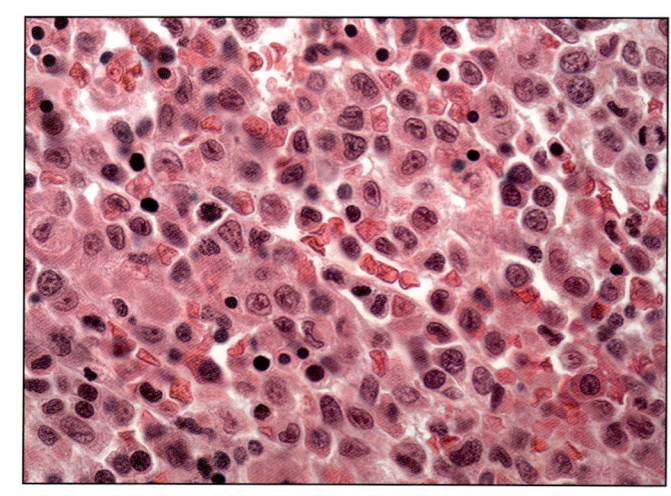

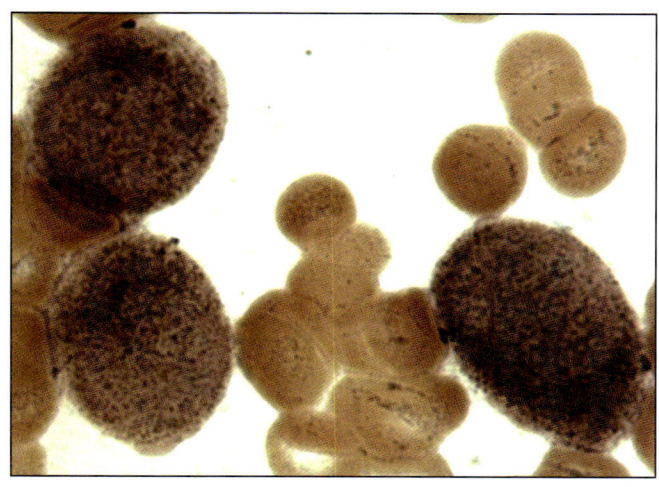

图22.47 一例急性单核细胞性白血病病例的骨髓抽吸涂片，非特异性酯酶组织化学染色显示胞浆成分呈强阳性。

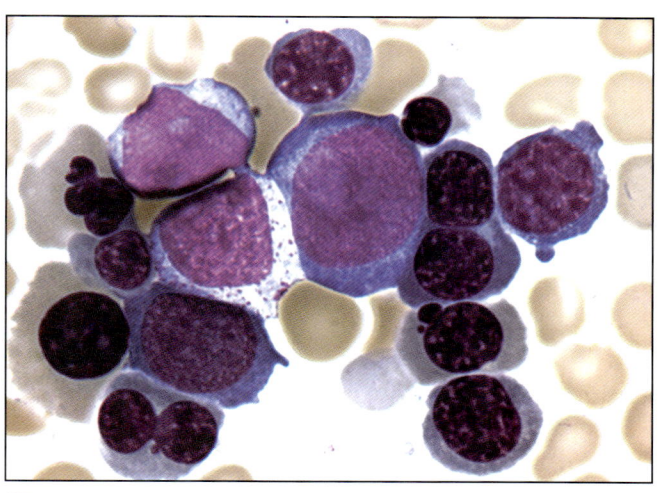

图22.49 红白血病的骨髓抽吸涂片，显示骨髓原始细胞成分和大量增生异常的红系成分。本例尽管有显著数目的红系成分，骨髓原始细胞的百分率＞20%的非红系成分是诊断为红白血病（红系-粒系型）的根据。（Wright-Giemsa染色）

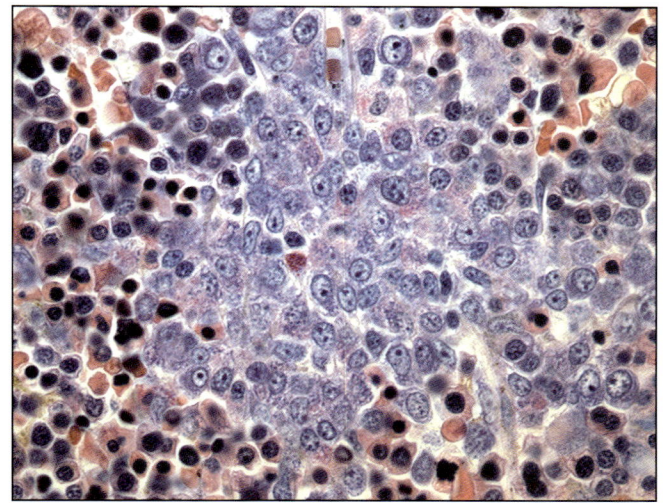

图22.48 一例红白血病（红系-粒系型）病例的骨髓芯针活检组织学切片，中央显示一大片骨髓原始细胞成分，周围是增生异常的红系成分。（Giemsa染色）

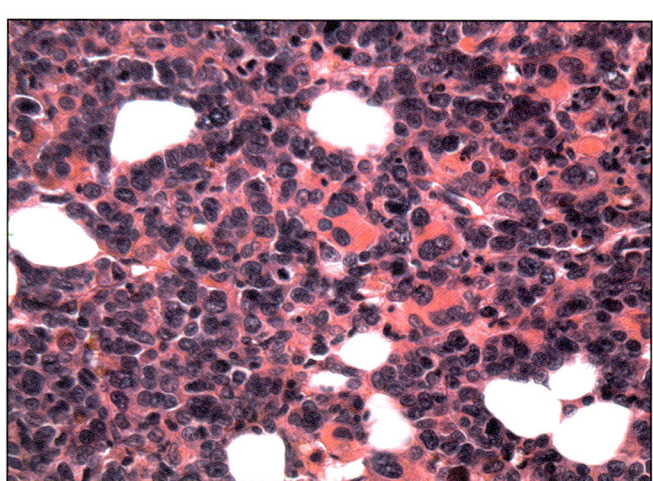

图22.50 一例急性原始巨核细胞性白血病病例的骨髓芯针活检组织学切片，显示成片的大的原始巨核细胞，混合有大的非典型性巨核细胞。（HE染色）

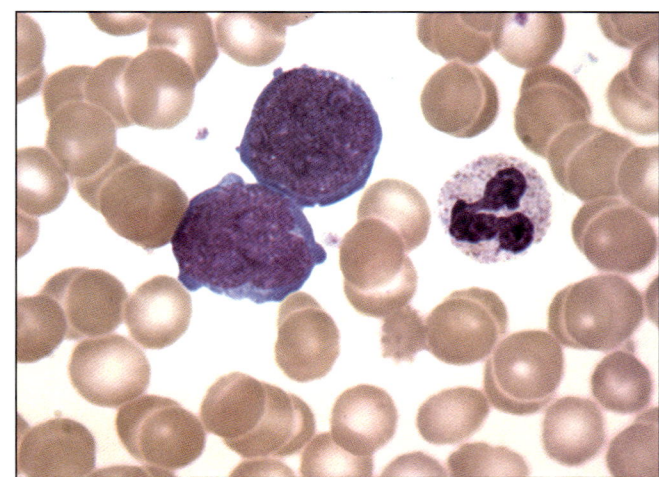

图22.51 （右）急性原始巨核细胞性白血病的骨髓抽吸涂片，显示2个原始巨核细胞和少量嗜碱性胞浆，伴有明显的膜空泡。（Wright-Giemsa染色）

表22.10	WHO非特异性急性骨髓性白血病（AML）伴随的细胞遗传学异常
WHO分类	细胞遗传学异常
急性骨髓原始细胞性白血病，极少分化	+4、+8、+13、-7
急性骨髓原始细胞性白血病，没有成熟成分	inv(3)(q21;q26)
急性骨髓原始细胞性白血病，伴有成熟成分	12p异常，t(6;9)(p23;q34)-嗜碱性粒细胞增多
急性骨髓单核细胞性白血病	12p异常，t(6;9)(p23;q34)-嗜碱性粒细胞增多
急性原始单核细胞或单核细胞性白血病	t(8;16)(p11;p13)、t(8;16)(q34;p13)
急性红白血病	核型复杂和（或）5号和7号染色体异常
急性原始巨核细胞性白血病	t(1;22)(p13;q13)、inv(3)(q21;q26)
急性全骨髓增生伴有骨髓纤维化	5号和7号染色体异常

前体B细胞淋巴母细胞性白血病/淋巴母细胞性淋巴瘤
Precursor B-cell lymphoblastic leukemia/lymphoblastic lymphoma

定义

前体B细胞淋巴母细胞性白血病/淋巴母细胞性淋巴瘤（B-ALL/LBL）是一种属于B细胞谱系的不成熟淋巴细胞（B淋巴母细胞）的克隆性肿瘤。大多数病例主要累及血和骨髓（90%的病例），最好称为B-细胞急性淋巴母细胞性白血病（B-cell acute lymphoblastic leukemia，B-ALL）。其余的病例表现为髓外肿块，伴有或不伴有骨髓受累（如果伴有骨髓受累，占骨髓细胞成分<25%），称为B细胞淋巴母细胞性淋巴瘤（B-cell lymphoblastic lymphoma，B-LBL）[110]。两种表现是否具有不同的生物学基础尚不清楚，而且因为B-ALL和B-LBL在形态学和免疫表型方面不易区分，所以应用任何一种名称在某种程度上都是武断的。在WHO分类中，这种分类没有将对应于早期B细胞不同成熟阶段的前体淋巴细胞肿瘤分开（即早期前体B-ALL、常见的B-ALL和前体B-ALL）。然而，伴有表面免疫球蛋白轻链表达的较成熟的B细胞肿瘤和Burkitt或Burkitt样形态（以前的ALL FAB L3亚型）不再归入此类。

一般临床和实验室特征

大多数ALL病例具有前体B细胞的表型（80%~85%），其余为T细胞来源（见下文）。在美国，每年大约有3000个病例被诊断为ALL[111]。所有类型的ALL经年龄校正后的发生率为1.5例/100 000人口[32]。这个发生率随年龄而有很大变化，儿童年龄组发生率最高（从出生到19岁为2.7例/100 000人口），第二个高峰是年龄较大者（65岁以后为1.4例/100 000人口）[112]。总的来说，ALL是一种主要发生在儿童的疾病，所有病例中有3/4发生于6岁以下的患者[113]。男性病例稍多，高加索人和西班牙人的发病率较高。

同AML病例一样，大多数症状与正常骨髓成分被原始细胞进行性替代的结果有关。这包括由中性粒细胞减少引起的非特异性感染、贫血引起的乏力和嗜睡，以及继发于血小板减少的黏膜皮肤出血。白细胞计数常常在正常范围，但可以降低或升高。循环中的原始细胞成分和成熟性淋巴细胞占外周血细胞成分的绝大部分。常常可见骨和关节疼痛、全身淋巴结肿大和（或）肝脾大。诊断时，2%的病例可见明显的睾丸受累[114]。在B-ALL中，常见中枢神经系统（CNS）受累[115]，需要进行积极的CNS预防性治疗并经常监测脑脊液细胞学。复发常常发生于髓外组织（CNS、睾丸、卵巢或肾），先于骨髓复发。如前所述，先前应用依托泊苷疗法治疗的患者容易罹患伴有MLL异常的B-ALL。

根据定义，B-LBL累及髓外部位；最常见的是皮肤、骨和软组织，较少见的是淋巴结（也见第21章）。这种状况并不常见，大约仅占所有LBL病例的10%~15%[116]。与T-LBL不同（见下文），B-LBL很少表现为纵隔肿物[110]。如果B-LBL中出现骨髓受累，则占其细胞成分不足25%（根据定义），比较典型者为<5%[110]。

外周血、抽吸和活检所见

外周血和抽吸涂片对于准确辨认淋巴母细胞成分是重要的。当白血病细胞充满骨髓时，可能难以抽吸，偶尔导致涂片不充分。对于这些病例需要进行芯针活检检查。B淋巴母细胞有些不同的表现，从同质性的小细胞群到较为异质性的较大的细胞群，小细胞核呈圆形至轻度不规则形，染色质致密，核仁不明显，而较大的细胞核不规则，有核裂或有切迹，染色质分布不均一，有一个或多个明显的核仁（图22.52）。胞浆稀少至中等量，可略呈嗜碱性，当细胞增大时可呈深度嗜碱性。有时可见小的空泡，并可见少数粗大的颗粒。偶尔，原始细胞的特征是出现不对称的被称为尾足的

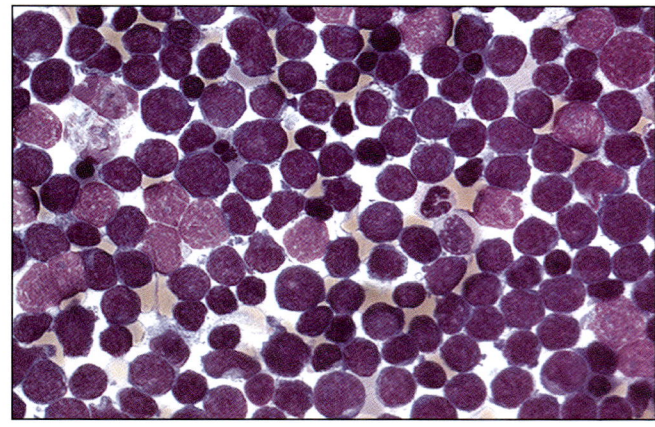

图22.52 前体B细胞性急性淋巴母细胞性白血病的骨髓抽吸涂片，显示肿瘤以小淋巴母细胞为主，染色质均匀，胞浆稀少，无颗粒，嗜碱性。（Wright-Giemsa染色）

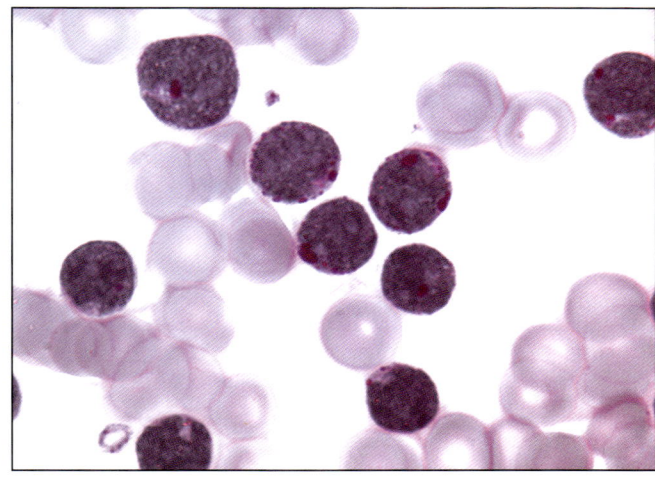

图22.54 一例前体B细胞急性淋巴母细胞性白血病骨髓抽吸涂片的过碘酸-Schiff（PAS）组织化学染色，显示明显的块状胞浆染色。

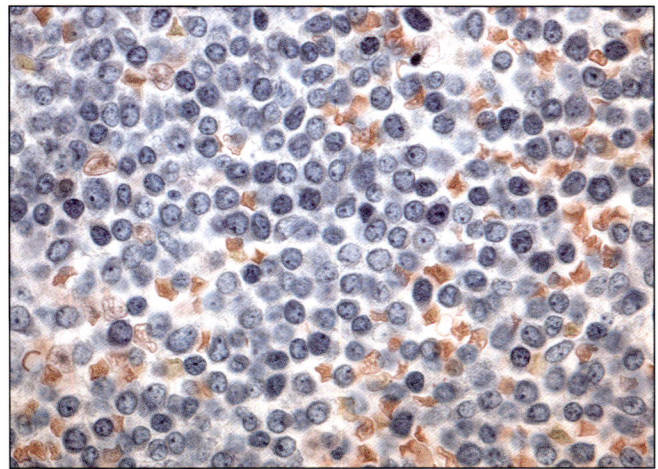

图22.53 前体B细胞性急性淋巴母细胞性白血病的骨髓芯针活检组织学切片，显示小的原始淋巴细胞弥漫性累及骨髓，染色质细而散在，核仁不清楚，胞浆稀少。（Giemsa染色）

胞浆突起，形成所谓的"手镜"细胞（"hand mirror" cells）[117]。

芯针活检或组织切片一般富于细胞，显示多量排列紧密的淋巴母细胞，核呈圆形至不规则形，偶尔呈脑回状，染色质稀少或散在，核仁小，几乎见不到胞浆（图22.53）。在骨髓芯针活检标本，如果有明显残留的造血细胞，则其形态学是正常的。在B-ALL，常见坏死区，膨胀性瘤块可引起溶骨性病变。核分裂象通常多见，有时在B-LBL累及的组织中，可见含有可染小体的巨噬细胞（形成"星空"表现，"starry-sky" appearance）。

细胞化学和免疫表型所见

前B淋巴母细胞的形态学表现可能类似于见于极少分化的AML的骨髓原始细胞。另外，在组织学切片中，小B淋巴母细胞与前T淋巴母细胞相同，可能难以与成熟的小淋巴细胞鉴别。有鉴于此，诊断和分类需要进行细胞化学和免疫表型特征的检查。淋巴母细胞胞浆糖原PAS染色呈阳性，位于核周，呈粗大块状结构（图22.54和表22.7）。淋巴母细胞MPO呈阴性，SBB仅有微弱染色。可见多灶性、点状或Golgi形态的NSE反应，但通常远比原始单核细胞微弱。

流式细胞分析是检查白血病原始细胞免疫分型最有用的方法。TdT和HLA-DR几乎总是见于B-ALL/LBL，而表面免疫球蛋白轻链表达阴性具有特征性。B-ALL/LBL内可见几种独特形式的抗原表达，与肿瘤细胞的分化程度有关（早期前体细胞常见，或为前体B-ALL）（表22.11）。另外，一些常见的细胞遗传学所见，包括涉及MLL基因的t(4;11)，而t(1;19)和t(12;21)与特征性的免疫表型有关（表22.11）。值得注意的是，MLL异常常伴有骨髓抗原的出现，比如CD15、CD13或CD33，而B系结构提示早期前体B细胞表型。t(1;19)异常显示典型的前体B细胞免疫表型，见于25%的具有这种免疫表型的病例。t(12;21)特征性地显示CD10和HLA-DR的高水平表达。流式细胞分析也可用于监测微小的残留病变，用于鉴别正常的骨髓前B细胞（原始血细胞）和白血病细胞（见下文）。石蜡切片TdT免疫染色可能有助于证实器官和软组织内存在白血病浸润。

分子遗传学所见

特异性遗传学异常见于60%～75%的病例的原始细胞[118]。核型分析及其他分子遗传学技术有时有助于诊断，并可提供预后信息（图22.55）。儿童B-ALL的最常见的染色体异常如表22.12所示。标准的核型分析

表22.11 B细胞淋巴母细胞性白血病/淋巴母细胞性淋巴瘤（B-ALL/LBL）不同分化阶段的免疫表型所见和基因型

抗原	早期前体细胞	普通细胞	前体细胞	t(4;11)	t(1;19)	t(12;21)
TdT	+	+	+	+	+	+
HLA-DR	+	+	+	+	+	+
CD10	−	+	+	−	+	+
CD19	+	+	+	+	+	+
CD20	−	−	−	−	−/+	−
cCD22	+	+	+	±	+	+
cCD79a	+	+	+	+	+	+
cμ-Ig	−	−	+	−	+	+
sIg	−	−	−	−	−	−
CD34	+	+	−	+	−	−
CD15	−	−	−	+	−	−
CD24	+	+	+	−	+	+

+：阳性；−：阴性；±：常常阳性；−/+，常常阴性。
TdT：末端脱氧核苷转移酶；cCD22：胞浆CD22；cCD79a：胞浆CD79a；cμ-Ig：胞浆μ免疫球蛋白重链；sIg：表面免疫球蛋白。

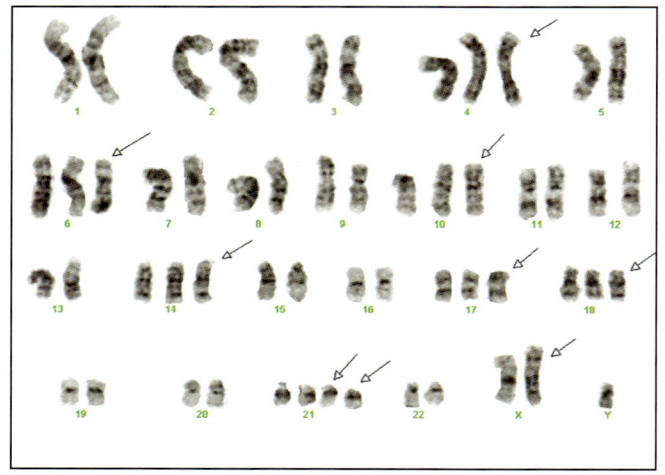

图22.55 一例前体B细胞急性淋巴母细胞性白血病的核型分析，显示超二倍体（n=55）。(Courtesy of Paola Dal Cin PhD and Cynthia McLaughlin BS, Brigham & Women's Hospital, Boston, MA.)

足以发现大多数这些异常，t(12;21)是个例外。这种融合涉及 *TEL* 和 *AML1* 基因，在普通的核型分析中不能发现，必须应用RT-PCR、Southern印迹或FISH检测[119]。另外，*FLT3* 的活化性环状突变见于20%的伴有 *MLL* 异常的B-ALL，以及25%的伴有超二倍体的B-ALL，这些可以作为引人注意的治疗靶点[120-122]。

在成人B-ALL，t(9;22)(q34;q11)见于25%的病例，另外10%可见 *MLL* 重排，而小儿B-ALL的典型异常[超二倍体，t(1;19)或t(12;21)]仅仅见于少部分病例[123-125]。除了细胞遗传学所见以外，年龄、白细胞计数、性别和最初对治疗的反应对于儿童危险性分级具有重要作用。

与儿童相比，成人B-ALL/LBL一般情况下是一种预后差的疾病，应用现代治疗的治愈率在儿童可达80%，而在成人仅为40%[118,126]。这似乎部分地反映了相对而言常常出现风险大的细胞遗传学异常而不常出现风险小的细胞遗传学异常。然而，迄今为止，成人ALL的生物学尚未得以广泛研究[127]。

鉴别诊断

除了显然要与AML和T-ALL鉴别以外，B-ALL偶尔可能与儿童的伴有骨髓受累的许多小圆形蓝染细胞肿瘤混淆，尤其是当临床上没有明显的肿物时。检查骨髓抽吸涂片标本中的肿瘤细胞团，其特征是非造血性肿瘤，而用抽吸和芯针活检标本的免疫表型通常足以作出正确的诊断。病毒感染时，外周血中可见非典型性淋巴细胞，通过其成熟的染色质结构、核与胞浆比例低以及核仁明显，可与白血病的原始细胞鉴别。最后，在婴儿和小儿，淋巴细胞可占骨髓细胞成分的

表22.12	儿童B细胞淋巴母细胞性白血病/淋巴母细胞性淋巴瘤（B-ALL/LBL）的遗传学改变和预后意义		
非随机性染色体异常	受累基因	发生率（%）	预后意义
超二倍体	>50但<65的染色体	25	良好
t(12;21)(p13;q22)	TEL、AML1	22	良好
MLL重排[例如t(4;11)、t(11;19)、t(9;11)]	AF-4、ENL、AF-9、MLL	8	不良
t(1;19)(q23;p13)	PBX1、E2A	5	没有意义
t(9;22)(q34;q11)	ABL、BCR	3	不良
低二倍体	<45的染色体	1	不良

Adapted from Pui and Evans.[118]

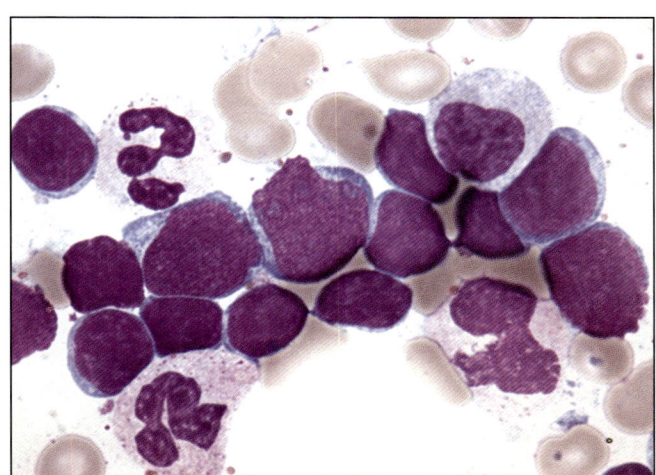

图22.56 骨髓抽吸涂片显示非肿瘤性、功能性B细胞前体（原始血细胞）增多。注意形态学表现类似于肿瘤性B淋巴母细胞（图22.52）。细胞大小和染色质形态的不同及其特征性的免疫表型谱系是辨认这些原始血细胞的线索。（Wright-Giemsa染色）

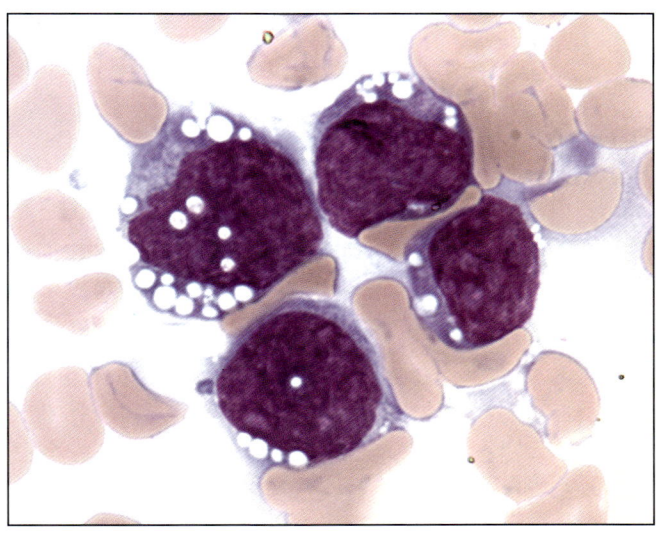

图22.57 Burkitt淋巴瘤/白血病的骨髓抽吸涂片。与前体B细胞急性淋巴母细胞性白血病相比，这些细胞较大，核染色较深，并可见明显的胞浆空泡。（Wright-Giemsa染色）

50%。在小儿，这些淋巴细胞的亚群具有一系列不成熟淋巴细胞的形态学表现，小到常常较大的圆形细胞核，染色质细，形态不成熟，胞浆缺乏到有少量嗜碱性胞浆（图22.56）。这些功能性B淋巴细胞前体（"原始血细胞"，hematogone）可能难以与恶性淋巴母细胞鉴别。在化疗后尤为如此，即使在成年患者，此时原始血细胞数量极度增多[128]。许多表现，尤其是出现显示全程B细胞分化的异源性前B细胞群（包括成熟B细胞），异源性黏附分子表达，以及非成簇的骨髓结构性分布，可能有助于辨认正常的原始血细胞[129,130]。另外，反应性不成熟性淋巴细胞增生不出现细胞遗传学异常和异常的免疫表型标记物。

在淋巴组织，B-LBL必须与T-LBL、髓细胞肉瘤、Burkitt淋巴瘤/白血病（图22.57）和套细胞淋巴瘤的原始细胞样变型鉴别。

前体T细胞淋巴母细胞性白血病/淋巴母细胞性淋巴瘤
Precursor T-cell lymphoblastic leukemia/lymphoblastic lymphoma

定义

前体T细胞淋巴母细胞性白血病/淋巴母细胞性淋巴瘤（T-ALL/LBL）是B-ALL/LBL的T系对应病变，是一种不成熟的T细胞祖细胞（T淋巴母细胞）的克隆性肿瘤。T-ALL和T-LBL所应用的术语和定义与B-ALL或B-LBL的相同。

一般临床和实验室特征

T-ALL占儿童急性淋巴母细胞性白血病病例的15%，占成人病例的25%[127,131]。根据定义，血和骨髓是主要的受累部位。与 B-ALL 相比，T-ALL 患者的平均中位年龄较大，以男性为主[132]。伴有血白细胞计数增高，大多数病例出现前纵隔肿物，并常常累及中枢神经系统[131,132]。

T 细胞淋巴母细胞性肿瘤的最常见症状与 T-LBL 的一样，大约占所有 LBL 类型的 85%[116]。T-LBL 也最常累及青少年男性，典型表现为前纵隔（胸腺）肿物（大约为 50% 的病例），骨髓受累 < 25%（根据定义）。外周淋巴结、肝、脾、皮肤、性腺和中枢神经系统是可能受累的其他部位。

少数情况下，T-LBL 伴有明显的血液学疾病，特征是由 T-LBL、外周血和（或）骨髓嗜酸性粒细胞增多以及骨髓增生和（或）白血病构成的三联征。这种综合征与 (8;13)(p11;q11) 染色体易位有关，在淋巴细胞和骨髓细胞中均可见到（见图 22.67）[133-135]。

外周血、抽吸和活检所见

如前所述，T-ALL 和 T-LBL 都伴有白细胞增多（常常高于 50×10^9/L)，循环血中可见原始细胞。骨髓抽吸和活检可见细胞增多，但与 B-ALL 相比，较常显示残留的正常造血成分。T-ALL、T-LBL 和 B-ALL/LBL 之间的形态学区别微小，而且是不可靠的（见上文）。与 B 淋巴母细胞相比，T 淋巴母细胞核的沟回和核深染更加明显[136]（图 22.58）。骨髓活检或组织切片的核分裂比例常常很高。

细胞化学和免疫表型所见

90% 以上的 T-ALL 病例的白血病细胞胞浆显示核周灶状酸性磷酸酶强阳性染色[136]。PAS、MPO、SE 或 NSE 染色呈阴性。T 淋巴母细胞常常表达与不同 T 细胞分化阶段相当的标记物。TdT 染色细胞核总是呈阳性，最有助于证实浸润成分的不成熟本质。T 细胞/胸腺细胞标记物 CD1a、CD2、CD3（胞浆）、CD4、CD5、CD7、CD8 和 CD99 可有不同程度地表达。常常可见 CD4/CD8 双阳性的淋巴母细胞，偶尔可见 CD10 表达。有趣的是，与 T-ALL 相比，T-LBL 更容易表达较成熟的胸腺细胞的免疫表型[116]。尽管 T 系 ALL/LBL 具有分化成类似于正常胸腺细胞的能力，但这种分化还不具有治疗意义[118]。骨髓分化的标记物可见于高达 1/3 的成人和 1/4 的儿童 ALL 病例[137,138]。这种特征没有临床意义，但可能有助于免疫监测残留的微小病变[118]。具有双相表型的白血病细胞的白血病患者表达淋巴细胞相关分子和髓细胞性限制性分子，治疗可能需要针对两种谱系[118,137]。

分子遗传学所见

已经发现三种主要类型的遗传学异常与 T-ALL/LBL 有关，其发生率几乎相同。这些异常包括：(1) 多种基因的易位，伴有 7q35 位点的 β T 细胞受体、14q11.2 位点的 α T 细胞受体和 δ T 细胞受体，或 7p14-15 位点的 γ T 细胞受体；(2) 9p 缺失，导致 *CDKN2A* 肿瘤抑制因子丢失；或 (3) 核型分析不易检测到的 *TAL1* 基因 5' 调节区的缺失。

最近有研究表明，在所有人类 T-ALL 中，有 50% 具有激活的 *NOTCH1* 突变[139]。这些突变提供了 NOTCH1 的功能获得，一种对早期 T 细胞发生起关键作用的蛋白，对 T-ALL 的 NOTCH1 失调具有重要作用。与在 B-ALL/LBL 观察到的与多种细胞遗传学异常相关的危险分级相比，迄今为止，T-ALL/LBL 尚没有与遗传学改变相应的临床影响的报道。

慢性骨髓增生性病变
Chronic myeloproliferative disorders

定义和分类

慢性骨髓增生性病变（CMPD）包括五种主要的临床病理学病变：(1) CML；(2) 慢性嗜酸性粒细胞白血病/特发性嗜酸性粒细胞增多综合征（CEL/HES）；(3) 真性红细胞增多症（polycythemia vera, PV）；(4) 特发性血小板增多症（ET）；以及 (5) 慢性特发性骨髓纤维化（CIMF）。如病名提示的那样，这些增生性干细胞病变的特征是：骨髓中成熟骨髓成分产物增多，表现为特

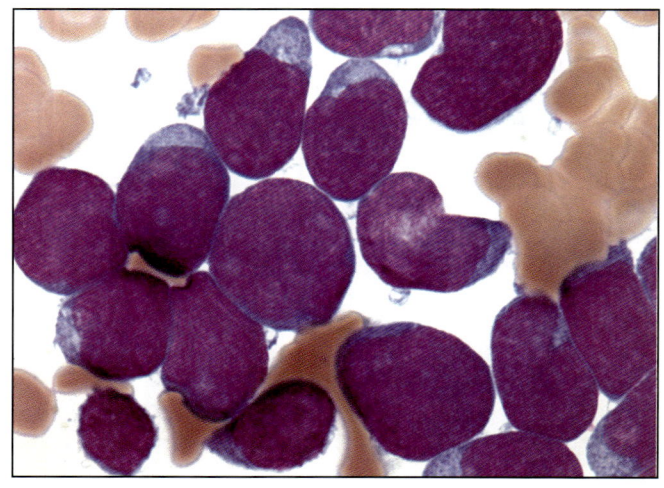

图 22.58 前体 T 细胞急性淋巴母细胞性白血病的骨髓抽吸涂片，显示多量淋巴母细胞，核不规则，染色质散在，偶见清楚的核仁，伴有少量无颗粒的嗜碱性胞浆。（Wright-Giemsa 染色）

征性的外周血和实验室检查表现。组织学特征常常有重叠，而且在许多病例中，进行骨髓检查仅仅是为了支持最初总体的临床病理学表现，而不是为了严格诊断的目的。这些病变的分子基础尚不清楚，一个出现的常见的问题是：这些疾病是酪氨酸激酶驱动的非细胞因子依赖性疾病。在这些非细胞因子依赖性骨髓增生性疾病中，促使细胞增生和抗凋亡途径的遗传学异常（CML 中的 *BCR-ABL* 融合，CEL/HES 中的 *FIP1L1-PDGFR*α 融合，以及 PV、ET 和 CIMF 中的 *JAK2V617F* 突变）可以通过细胞遗传学和分子诊断技术检测而有助于正确诊断。分子诊断对于这些疾病尤为重要，因为特异性治疗针对的是 ABL 和血小板源性生长因子受体 α（PDGFRα）酪氨酸激酶的存在。一旦诊断确立，骨髓检查最常进行，以评估治疗效果、检测原始细胞转化和骨髓纤维化的存在，或获得材料以监测残留的微小病变。

表22.13 Ph染色体阴性或"非典型性"慢性骨髓性白血病的遗传学异常

细胞遗传学异常	酪氨酸激酶融合蛋白
t (8;22) (p11;q11)	BCR-FGFR1
t (4;22) (q12; q11)	BCR-PDGFRα
t (9;12) (q34;p13)	TEL-ABL
t (9;12) (p24;p13)	TEL-JAK2
t (9;22) (p24;q11)	BCR-JAK2

BCR：断裂点簇部位；FGFR1：纤维母细胞生长因子受体 1；PDGFRα：血小板衍生生长因子受体 α；TEL：易位 E26 转化特异性白血病蛋白；JAK2：Janus 激酶 2。
Adapted from Goldman and Melo.[168]

慢性骨髓性白血病
Chronic myelogenous leukemia

定义

慢性骨髓性白血病（CML）是白血病中第一个被识别的独特疾病。CML 是现代分子肿瘤学的疾病原型。这种克隆性干细胞疾病被定义为出现 Ph 染色体（Philadelphia chromosome），一种累及 9 号和 22 号染色体的交互性易位，可导致 *BCR-ABL* 融合基因。现在认为这种融合基因的基本激酶活性是引起慢性期临床疾病的主要原因。其重要性的证据部分来自应用 BCR-ABL 激酶抑制剂明显有效的经验。虽然已经清楚肿瘤性克隆是粒细胞、单核细胞、红系细胞、巨核细胞以及淋巴细胞谱系的祖细胞，但是这种疾病最初的特征是成熟中的粒细胞和血小板增生。如果不治疗，这种慢性疾病最终将进展为较为侵袭性的阶段（通常在 3～5 年），称为急性期和原始细胞期（转化为急性髓细胞性或淋巴细胞性白血病）。少部分病例在临床和形态学上不易与存在的 CML 区别（在一项大型研究中占 3.5%[140]），CML 缺乏 *BCR-ABL* 融合基因。目前，这些病例被称为"非典型性"CML。非典型性一词用于强调缺乏 Ph 染色体，而不是指与 CML 有重叠的血液学或组织学特征。这些疾病以 *BCR-ABL* 相似的方式，也涉及细胞遗传学异常，导致酪氨酸激酶蛋白表达失调（表 22.13）。同 ABL 酪氨酸激酶一样，其许多失调的激酶通过激酶抑制剂具有抑制反应，例如 Gleevec，因此应该注意识别这种缺陷，而不是仅仅将其归入"非典型性 CML"类中。Ph 染色体阳性的 CML 与非典型性 CML 是相似的。

临床特征

在美国，在所有人种的成人中，CML 的发病率大约为每年 1.5～2 例 /100 000 人口[32]。此发病率随着年龄的增长逐渐增加，71～80 岁时达到 6～7 例 /100 000 人口。诊断时的中位年龄一般在 41～50 岁[140-142]，但是 CML 可以发生于任何年龄。大多数病例（85%）是在疾病的慢性期诊断的[141]。男性比女性稍多[140]。目前，这种疾病偶尔可在没有症状的患者的外周血检查时发现，大约占 20%～40% 的病例[34,140,141]。在其余病例，最常见的症状是疲劳或嗜睡，随后出现出血、体重下降、脾区不适或腹胀、盗汗和骨痛[140,141]。50%～75% 的患者可触及脾，但是肝大不常见[140,141]。紫癜出现在 15% 的病例[140]。急性期和原始细胞危象一般伴有骨髓衰竭的相关症状。另外，原始细胞危象（blast crisis）可出现于髓外部位，包括淋巴结、脾、皮肤及其他部位。

外周血所见

慢性骨髓性白血病-慢性期
CML-chronic phase（CML-CP）

白细胞总数显示一定范围的数值增高，50%～70% 的患者白细胞计数 > 100 个细胞 ×10^9/L[140,141]。外周血涂片检查，以分叶核中性粒细胞和中性粒细胞前体（带状核和骨髓细胞）为主，仅见少数原始细胞成分[143]。嗜碱性粒细胞增多常常见于 CML，也可见到嗜酸性粒细胞增多。大多数病例可见血小板增多[140]，一般可以出现贫血，45%～60% 患者的血红蛋白水平 < 12.0g/dl[141]。

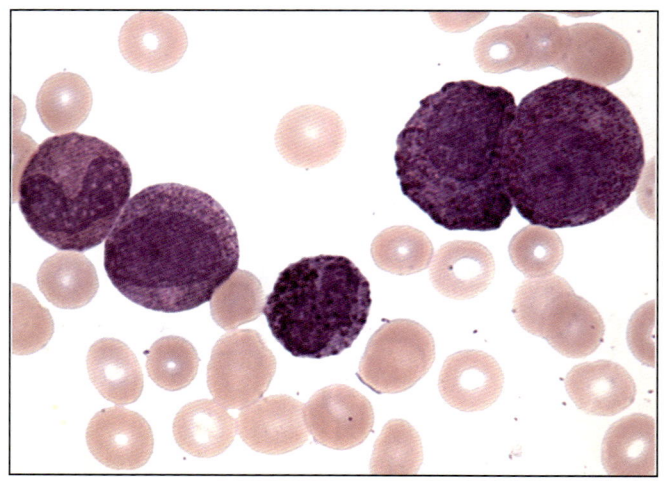

图22.59 慢性骨髓性白细胞-急性期外周血涂片，显示不成熟颗粒增多的骨髓细胞前体和明显的嗜碱性粒细胞增多。（Wright-Giemsa染色）

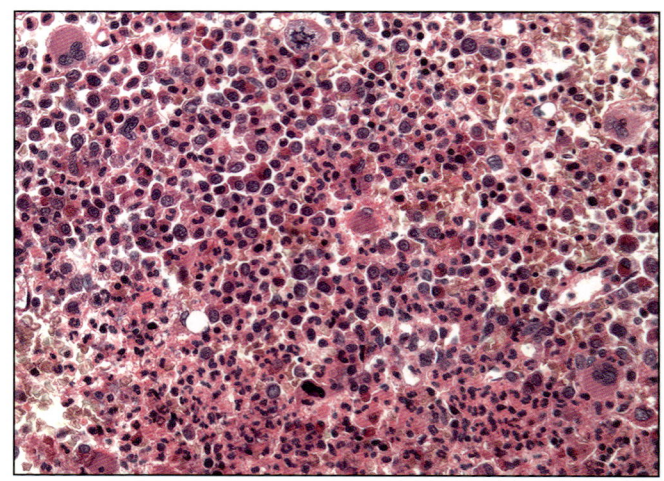

图22.60 一例慢性骨髓性白血病慢性期骨髓芯针活检的组织学切片，显示细胞成分增多，粒细胞成分增多型，包括成熟的中性粒细胞和嗜酸性粒细胞以及多量小的分叶减少的巨核细胞。（HE染色）

慢性骨髓性白血病-急性期
CML-accelerated phase（CML-AP）

出现以下一种或多种外周血特征提示进展至急性期：嗜碱性粒细胞增多，>20%，原始细胞占白细胞的10%～19%，和（或）持续性血小板减少（<100个细胞×10^9/L）或血小板增多（>1000个细胞×10^9/L）（图22.59）[144]。

骨髓和抽吸涂片所见

慢性骨髓性白血病-慢性期（CML-CP）

未经治疗的稳定期 CML 骨髓活检的组织学检查显示：细胞成分明显增多（细胞成分>95%），伴有受压而不明显的窦隙（图22.60）。细胞成分以成熟粒细胞（中性粒细胞、嗜酸性粒细胞和嗜碱性粒细胞）和巨核细胞为主，但粒细胞前体（髓细胞、后髓细胞和前髓细胞）也有相应的增加（图22.61和22.62）。这些早期成分常常在骨小梁附近聚集成3～5个细胞厚度的同心层，有点类似于正常粒细胞的分化。原始细胞成分没有增多，出现片块状原始细胞，或骨小梁旁不成熟细胞层明显增厚，这些均应怀疑疾病进展（即急性期或原始细胞期）。嗜碱性粒细胞在芯针活检标本中不易见到，因为颗粒在处理过程中丢失，最好用抽吸涂片标本评估。红系细胞数量减少，髓系与红系的比例一般大于10:1。髓系与红系均为有序分化，没有明显的增生异常。巨核细胞数量可以正常，但最常见的是数量增多，常常可见小的分叶减少并伴有胞浆减少的细胞（图22.63）。常见密集排列的成簇的巨核细胞，这种表现不常见于伴有反应性继发性巨核细胞增生患者的骨髓。海蓝组织细胞（sea-blue

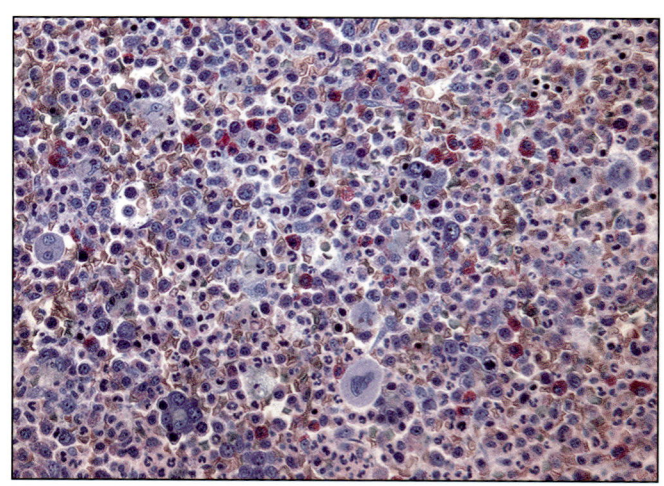

图22.61 慢性骨髓性白血病慢性期骨髓芯针活检Giemsa染色，显示许多粒细胞成分，胞浆粉色至红色，呈颗粒状，混有泡沫样伴有淡染或"海"蓝色胞浆的组织细胞。（Giemsa染色）

histiocyte，又叫假 Gaucher 细胞，pseudo-Gaucher cell）可见于大多数病例，继发于由细胞循环增多而引起的过多膜脂质的吞噬作用。疾病的早期可见网状纤维不同程度的增多。

脾显示由粒细胞前体增多而导致的红髓髓索膨胀，其中嗜中性骨髓细胞通常占大多数。白髓相应减少，脾窦内可见髓外造血。还可见到脾索的网状纤维纤维化，新生的造血灶加之血流受损常常可引起梗死。

甲磺酸伊马替尼（Imatinib mesylate，Gleevec）治疗可导致的骨髓改变，包括细胞成分减少、髓系与红系的比例（常常伴有红系相对增生）下降以及网状纤维纤维化减少[145,146]。在 Gleevec 治疗的骨髓中还常常出现淋巴细胞浸润数目增多。

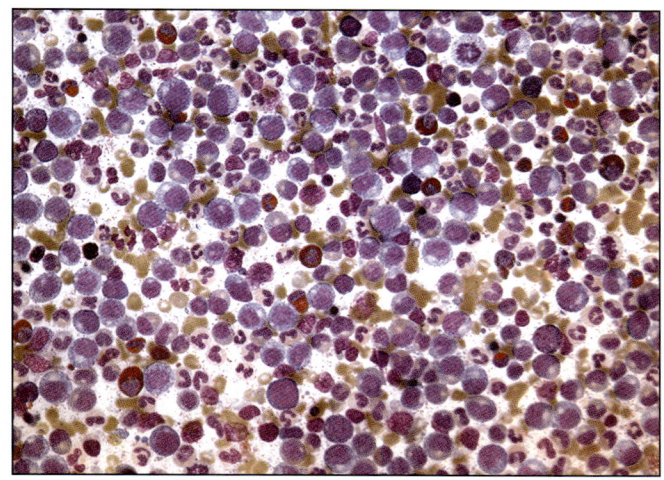

图22.62 慢性骨髓性白血病慢性期的骨髓抽吸涂片，显示细胞成分增多和粒细胞生成左移，包括多量骨髓细胞和后髓细胞，伴有明显的胞浆核窝和嗜碱性胞浆。还可见到混合的成熟中性粒细胞和嗜酸性粒细胞。（Wright-Giemsa染色）

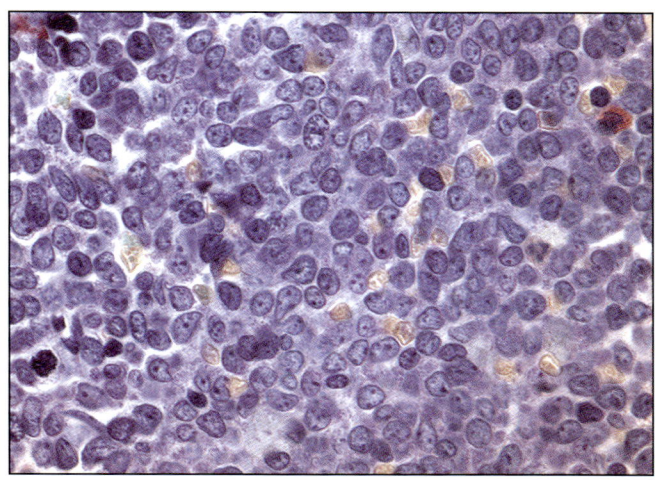

图22.64 慢性骨髓性白血病原始细胞危象骨髓芯针活检的组织学切片，显示成片小的原始细胞和偶尔混合的粒细胞。本例免疫表型分析显示为混合性淋巴性和骨髓细胞表型。（Giemsa染色）

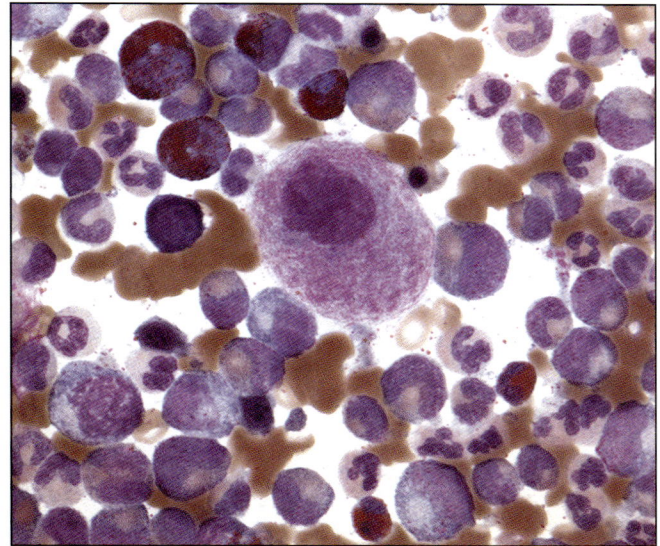

图22.63 慢性骨髓性白血病慢性期的骨髓抽吸涂片，显示主要为成熟中的粒细胞成分和小的分叶少的巨核细胞。（Wright-Giemsa染色）

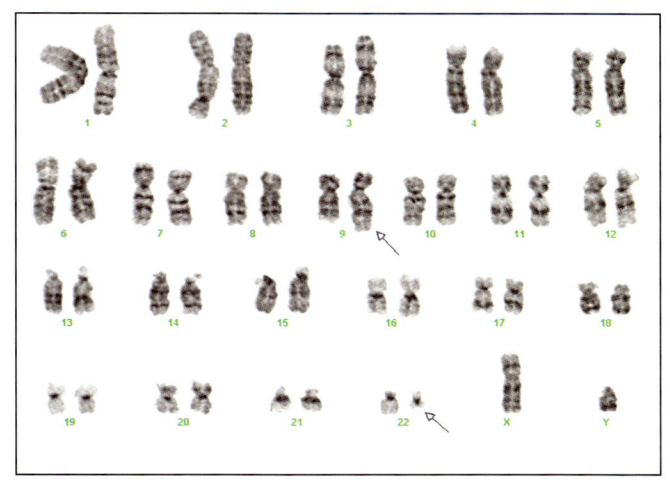

图22.65 核型分析显示9；22染色体平衡性易位，这是慢性骨髓性白血病的特征。衍生的22号染色体被称为Ph染色体。（Courtesy of Paola Dal Cin PhD and Cynthia Mclaughlin BS, Brigham & Women's Hospital, Boston, MA.）

慢性骨髓性白血病-急性期（CML-AP）

除了上述外周血特征以外，疾病进展至急性期还包括原始细胞成分或前髓细胞的数目增多（尤其是骨小梁旁或窦隙旁区），对治疗没有反应的脾增大，或获得额外的克隆性遗传学异常[144]。大片巨核细胞，伴有网状纤维或胶原纤维纤维化或粒细胞增生异常，也与进展至急性期有关，虽然这些还没有被接受为独立的诊断标准[144]。

慢性骨髓性白血病-原始细胞期（CML-blast phase）

在原始细胞期（骨髓原始细胞成分＞20%），原始细胞可能是髓细胞性（大约80%）、淋巴细胞性（大约20%）或偶尔为二者混合性（双系）。进展为髓细胞性或淋巴细胞性白血病的能力强烈支持存在Ph阳性转化的多潜能干细胞。原始细胞转化常常在骨髓甚或在髓外部位呈片状结构（图22.64）。当怀疑急性期或灶状原始细胞转化时，CD34免疫组织化学染色可能有助于评估骨髓的原始细胞成分。

分子遗传学所见

如前所述，CML与染色体平衡性易位（9；22）(q34;q11)有关，涉及22号染色体上的 *BCR* 基因和9号染色体上的 *ABL* 酪氨酸激酶基因。异常的22号染色体含有功能性融合基因，将其长臂相当的一部分丢失给9号染色体，被称为 Ph 染色体（图22.65）。CML 中的 *BCR-ABL* 杂合基因的常见产物是 210kDa 蛋白，显示具有启动和维持白血病表型的激酶活性和功能失调。少数情况下，从伴有明显外周血中性粒细胞增多患者的一种变型 t(9;22) 中可检测到 230kDa 的 BCR-ABL 融合蛋白。核型分析和确证性 FISH 是证实 CML 诊断所必需的初始检查（图22.66）。另外，RT-PCR 检查有助于识别伴有隐匿性或复杂性易位的病例。*BCR-ABL* 转录水平的定量 RT-PCR 有助于随后评估治疗效果并监测可能存在的复发。进展至急性期或原始细胞危象与特征性的遗传学异常有关，包括 Ph 染色体、8、19 号染色体三体或 i (17q) 的复制[147]。

鉴别诊断

反应性骨髓增生（reactive myeloid hyperplasia）或白血病样反应（leukemoid reaction）必须与 CML 相鉴别。可以通过识别引起这种病变的相关状况以及证实 CML 缺乏 t(9;22) 或与非典型性 CML 相关的其他易位来进行这种鉴别（表22.13）。

其他形式的慢性骨髓增生也必须除外，根据缺乏其他临床、病理学和分子遗传学特征。

与 8p11 骨髓增生综合征有关的骨髓增生与 CML 具有某些相似之处[130-135,148]。其特征是保留分化能力的骨髓细胞生成过多，但缺乏嗜碱性粒细胞增多并倾向于在诊断的 1-2 年内进展为 AML（图22.67）。这种病例大约 70% 表现为或发生淋巴母细胞性淋巴瘤，主要是原始 T 细胞表型。髓细胞和淋巴瘤细胞都具有 8p11 易位，证实本病来自造血干细胞。

慢性嗜酸性粒细胞性白血病/嗜酸性粒细胞过多综合征
Chronic eosinophilic leukemia/ hypereosinophilic syndrome

定义

这种少见的异源性病变的特征是骨髓中嗜酸性粒细胞生成过多，导致明显的持续性外周血嗜酸性粒细胞增多。在许多病例，疾病的慢性过程和嗜酸性粒细胞浸润器官可导致组织长期接触嗜酸性粒细胞的颗粒成分，而最终造成多系统组织损伤。WHO 定义的慢性嗜酸性粒细胞性白血病（CEL）/嗜酸性粒细胞过多综合征（HES）的诊断标准要求（1）血液持续性嗜酸性粒细胞增多 > 1.5×10^9/L，达 6 个月以上；（2）骨髓嗜酸性粒细胞增多；以及（3）血液或骨髓中骨髓原始细胞 < 20%。另外，必须除外继

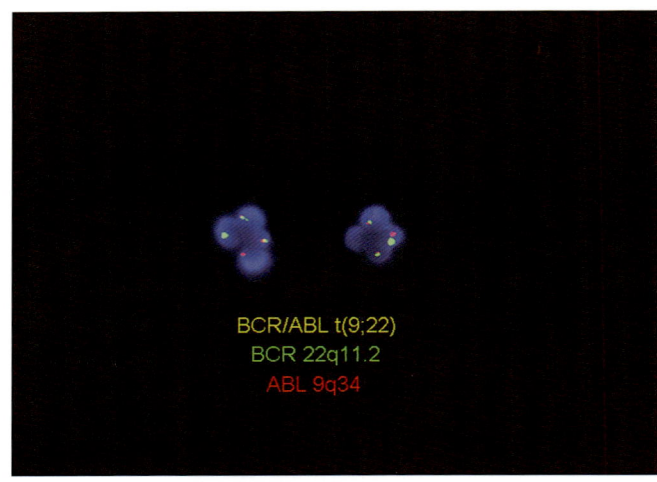

图22.66 应用针对22q11染色体*BCR*（绿色）和9q34染色体*ABL*（红色）的探针进行分裂间期核的荧光原位杂交，显示代表慢性骨髓性白血病的9;22染色体平衡性易位的融合信号（黄色）。（Courtesy of Paola Dal Cin PhD and Cynthia Mclaughlin BS, Brigham & Women's Hospital, Boston, MA.）

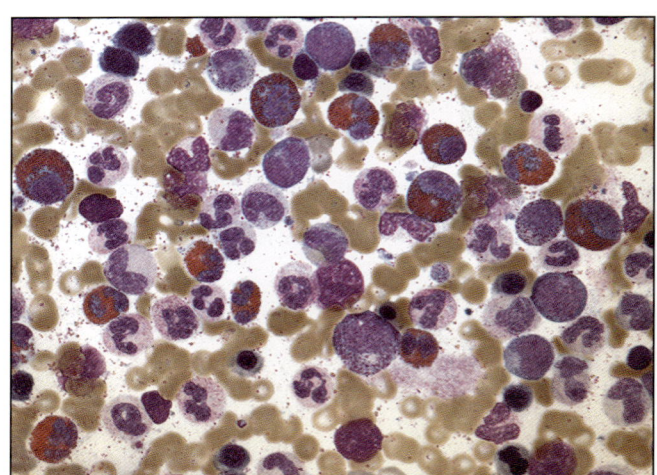

图22.67 骨髓抽吸涂片显示与具有t(8;13)的干细胞异常有关的骨髓增生障碍。这种特征与慢性骨髓性白血病的慢性期几乎不能区别。（Wright-Giemsa染色）

发性嗜酸性粒细胞增多的已知原因，例如反应性病因和伴有嗜酸性粒细胞增多的肿瘤性疾病，包括其他克隆性骨髓病变（如 CML）、Hodgkin 淋巴瘤以及克隆性或异常的 T 细胞群（表22.14）。根据 WHO 标准，CEL 和 HES 之间的鉴别是根据是否存在克隆性遗传学或核型异常，或外周血（> 2%）或骨髓（> 5% 但 < 19%）原始细胞是否增多。如果符合两条之中的任何一条，则建议诊断 CEL 而不是诊断 HES。确定嗜酸性粒细胞增多症病例的克隆性存在困难，可能低估 CEL 病例。

另外，新近在少数伴有嗜酸性粒细胞过多的病例中证实：存在一种常见的克隆性分子遗传学缺陷，说明本病的分子学分类可能具有比较重要的作用。这种发现来自于甲磺酸伊马替尼（Imatinib mesylate，Gleevec）

表22.14	与慢性嗜酸性粒细胞性白血病/特发性嗜酸性粒细胞过多综合征不同的嗜酸性粒细胞增多的原因

伴有非克隆性嗜酸性粒细胞的反应性嗜酸性粒细胞增多
　过敏性病变
　高敏状态
　寄生虫或非寄生虫感染
　结缔组织疾病
　肺综合征

伴有非克隆性嗜酸性粒细胞的肿瘤性病变
　T细胞淋巴瘤（血管免疫母细胞性淋巴结病、外周T细胞性淋巴瘤、蕈样霉菌病）
　Hodgkin淋巴瘤
　急性淋巴母细胞性白血病/淋巴瘤

伴有克隆性嗜酸性粒细胞的肿瘤性骨髓造血性疾病
　系统性肥大细胞增多症，伴有嗜酸性粒细胞增多和 FIP1L1-PDGFRα 融合
　慢性骨髓性白血病
　急性骨髓单核细胞性白血病伴有 inv(16) 或 t(16;16)(p13;q22)
　急性淋巴母细胞性白血病伴有 t(5;14)(q31;q32)
　CMML 样疾病伴有 t(5;12)(q33;p13)
　8p11 骨髓增生综合征（干细胞性白血病/淋巴瘤）
　真性红细胞增多症
　特发性血小板增多症
　慢性特发性骨髓纤维化

PDGFRα：血小板衍生生长因子受体α；
CMML：慢性骨髓单核细胞性白血病

治疗有效的 CEL 或 HES 患者。这些患者具有 4q12 染色体长臂的一个区域缺失，可导致两种侧位基因的融合，即酪氨酸激酶、PDGFRα 和 FIP1L1[149]。融合基因（FIP1L1-PDGFRα）导致 PDGFRα 蛋白的组成性激活和嗜酸性粒细胞生长因子独立性增生。这种融合与 BCR-ABL 融合基因非常类似，因此可以解释其对 Gleevec 治疗的敏感性。然而，似乎还存在其他分子异常，因为大约 40% 对 Gleevec 有反应的患者缺乏 FIP1L1-PDGFRα 融合[149]。

临床和实验室所见

CEL/HES 男性比女性常见，中位年龄范围在 20 岁到 50 岁之间[150]。大约 10% 的患者没有症状，其嗜酸性粒细胞增多是一种偶然的发现。最常见的体征和症状（以发生率递减的顺序）是：虚弱和乏力、咳嗽、呼吸困难、肌痛、血管水肿、发热或皮疹以及鼻炎[150]。器官受累常常发生，导致组织直接损伤和许多继发性并发症。明显的心血管并发症发生于半数以上的患者，不是 CEL/HES 所特有的，因为它们可以见于许多伴有嗜酸性粒细胞增多的疾病[150]。常见的并发症包括心肌内膜炎、心脏附壁血栓、心内膜心肌纤维化、限制性心肌病和瓣膜功能不全[150-154]。其他常见的浸润部位包括：皮肤、中枢神经系统、肺、脾和胃肠道[150,151,155-159]。实验室检查可能显示白细胞碱性磷酸酶水平异常，或者升高或者降低[160]，以及血清维生素 B_{12} 和维生素 B_{12} 连接蛋白异常，可以正常或升高[160-163]。CEL 和 HES 之间没有界限清楚的临床和实验室区别；然而，一项研究显示，明显升高的维生素 B_{12} 血清水平和脾大与患者分类为 CEL 而不是 HES 有关[163]。

外周血所见

白细胞总数常常中等程度增多（即 $20\sim30\times10^9/L$），伴有嗜酸性粒细胞增多，最常见的范围是 30%～70%[160]；然而，白细胞计数明显增高（＞$50\times10^9/L$）也已有报道[163,164]。外周血中可见伴有不同程度形态学改变的成熟性和不成熟性嗜酸性粒细胞。另外，可见包括早期中性粒细胞前体细胞的中性粒细胞增多、嗜碱性粒细胞轻度增多和伴有有核红细胞的轻度贫血[157,165]。

骨髓和抽吸所见

骨髓最常见的是细胞成分增多，主要是由于所有分化阶段的嗜酸性粒细胞增生所致（图 22.68 和 22.69）。成熟性嗜酸性粒细胞的形态学改变包括：体积增大，胞浆空泡形成或透明，以及核的分叶改变[166]。通常出现 Charcot-Leyden 结晶，常常位于巨噬细胞内。红细胞生成和巨核细胞生成通常是正常的，但有时可见巨核细胞数目减少。WHO 诊断 CEL 的标准是出现骨髓原始细胞增多（5%～19%）；然而重要的是，嗜酸性粒细胞增生是活检的显著特征。有趣的发现是，大多数病例中常见散在聚集的肥大细胞，提示其与肥大细胞疾病具有某些

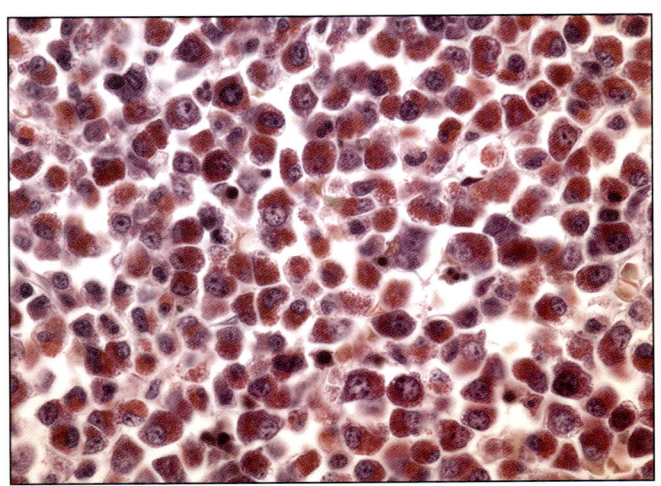

图22.68　一例慢性嗜酸性粒细胞性白血病伴有（4q）缺失导致 FIP1L1-PDGFRα 基因融合病例的骨髓芯针活检的组织学切片。注意成片的成熟性和不成熟性嗜酸性粒细胞成分，含有明显的嗜酸性颗粒，缺乏中性粒细胞成分。（Giemsa染色）

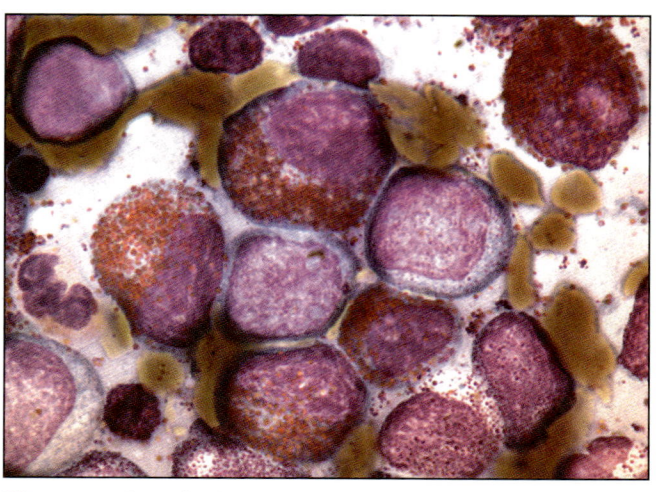

图22.69 伴有（4q）缺失导致FIP1L1-PDGFRα融合基因的慢性嗜酸性粒细胞性白血病的骨髓抽吸涂片。几个嗜酸性骨髓细胞伴有大的橘红色胞浆颗粒，可见典型的骨髓原始细胞（中央）。（Wright-Giemsa染色）

表22.15	WHO诊断真性红细胞增多症的标准
A1：	红细胞量增加在平均正常预期值25%以上，或男性血红蛋白 > 18.5g/dl，女性血红蛋白 > 16.5g/dl
A2：	除外继发性红细胞增多的原因
A3：	脾大
A4：	克隆性细胞遗传学异常，除外Ph染色体或BCR/ABL融合基因
A5：	体外内源性红系集落形成
B1：	血小板增多 > 400×10^9/L
B2：	白细胞 > 12×10^9/L
B3：	骨髓活检显示全骨髓增生，伴有明显的红系和巨核细胞增生
B4：	血清红细胞生成素水平低

以下情况可诊断为真性红细胞增多症：（1）A1+A2以及出现任何其他类别的A；或（2）A1+A2以及出现任何两种类别的B。

共同特征[167]。增生异常的特征可以见于其他细胞系的细胞，在某些病例还可见到骨髓纤维化。

分子遗传学所见

如上所述，在增生性嗜酸性粒细胞中出现克隆性遗传学改变是CEL的标志。不能证实克隆性和原始细胞成分没有增加的病例被称为HES。导致部分CEL病例FIP1L1-PDGFRα融合的（4q12）缺失太少，以致通过标准核型分析不能识别，必须应用FISH检测。

鉴别诊断

CEL/HES的诊断必须排除所有其他反应性或肿瘤性继发性嗜酸性粒细胞增多的原因（表22.14）。如上所述，有些类型的骨髓肿瘤形式显然是累及所有髓系的干细胞病变，包括嗜酸性粒细胞系。在可作出选择性诊断的病例，建议将这些独特的疾病与CEL分别归类[168,169]。最后，有一部分患者具有系统性肥大细胞增多症（SM）的临床和病理学特征，也表现为嗜酸性粒细胞增多且具有FIP1L1-PDGFRα融合（见1415页）[167,170]。这些病例诊断为肥大细胞增多症或CEL可能有点武断，主要取决于突出的临床特征。最重要的是要识别FIP1L1-PDGFRα融合基因，因为这些患者对甲磺酸伊马替尼（Gleevec）治疗有效[167]。

真性红细胞增多症　Polycythemia vera

定义

真性红细胞增多症（PV）是起源于多潜能造血祖细胞的一种干细胞病变，可导致红细胞、血小板和粒细胞生成增多。红细胞量的增加是这种疾病的临床标志，它是一种独立于红细胞生成调节正常通路的膨胀，与其他可辨认的继发性红细胞增多的原因无关。这些细胞的增多，尤其是见于红系细胞的增多，是细胞对生长因子（如红细胞生成素和血小板生成素）依赖性减少、细胞因子高敏感性和对凋亡信号的抑制共同起作用的结果[171]，可能是新近识别的Janus激酶2（Janus kinase 2, JAK2）基因的JH2假性激酶域突变的结果[171a-e]。迄今为止，还没有发现这种疾病有单一特异性的遗传学缺陷或标记物。诊断PV依靠临床和实验室所见，主要是要排除红细胞增多的继发性原因（表22.15）。

临床和实验室所见

据报道，PV的发病率为每年0.8～2.3例/100 000人口，在某些种族人群中报道的发病率甚至更低[172-174]。PV主要是发生于老年人的疾病，诊断时的中位年龄大约为60岁，仅有少数患者在40岁之前作出诊断[175,176]。男性患者略多[174-176]，犹太血统的患者稍多[177]。发病和死亡的最大原因是血液黏滞性过高的结局，原因是这些患者常常具有红细胞量增加和血栓形成（静脉或动脉）的趋势[175,176,178-180]。其并发症包括：高血压、雷诺现象（Raynaud phenomenon）、跛行、末梢坏疽、Budd-Chiari综合征、心肌梗死和卒中。少数情况下也可发生出血并发症[175,178]。另外，多数患者主诉头痛、头晕、瘙痒或与脾大有关的腹部症状，大多数患者出现脾大。

外周血、骨髓和抽吸涂片所见

在所谓的真性红细胞增多症的红细胞增多期或早

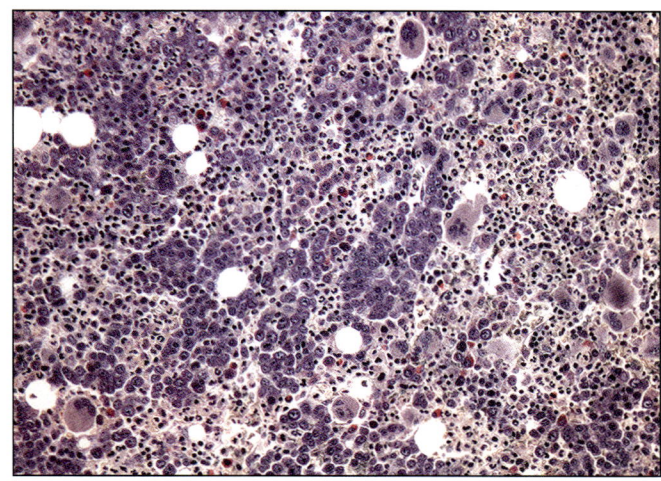

图22.70 一例早期真性红细胞增多症的骨髓芯针活检的组织学切片，显示细胞成分增多和全骨髓增生，伴有片块状嗜碱性红系前体细胞，散在粒细胞前体和巨核细胞。（Giemsa染色）

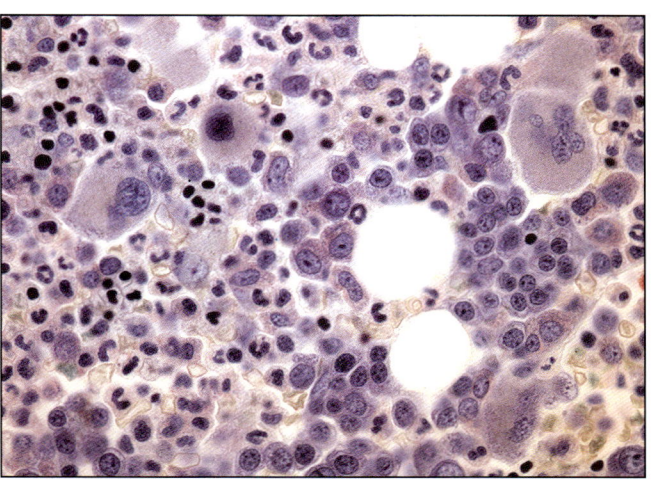

图22.71 一例富于细胞期真性红细胞增多症的骨髓芯针活检的组织学切片，显示所有三系增生，包括伴有圆形核和嗜碱性胞浆的不成熟性红系成分增多，以及核分叶少的小巨核细胞和核分叶多的较大的巨核细胞。（Giemsa染色）

期，外周血的最初评估显示：红细胞量增多，红细胞计数、血红蛋白和血细胞比容相应增加。大多数患者白细胞计数也轻度升高，平均计数为 $10\times10^9/L$[176]。所有粒细胞成分，包括嗜碱性粒细胞和嗜酸性粒细胞，均可显示中度增多。大多数患者的血小板倾向于轻度增多。骨髓组织学检查显示：由于全系（粒系、红系和巨核细胞系）增多，引起细胞成分增多（图22.70），巨核细胞松散聚集，呈多形性，包括伴有多分叶核的巨大巨核细胞和微小巨核细胞（图22.71），网状纤维轻度增多，铁的含量减少[181-183]。在疾病的早期，原始细胞成分并不增多。

PV 常常显示类似于 CIMF 所见的晚期造血系统并发症，包括贫血、骨髓纤维化、髓外造血（骨髓化生）以及急性白血病；然而，在缺乏先前细胞毒性治疗的情况下，这些并发症的真正发病率及其临床意义尚无定论[171,184]。当出现这些并发症时，外周血显示白红原始细胞图像，伴有泪滴状红细胞、粒细胞前体和有核红细胞。相关的骨髓表现包括：细胞成分多样，细胞常常稀少，骨髓伴有明显的网状纤维甚或胶原纤维化，红系和粒系生成减少，常常显示异型增生细胞核特征的巨核细胞持续性存在，以及偶尔可见骨质硬化的骨（图22.72）。可见骨髓生成障碍和早期骨髓成分数量增多；然而，原始细胞增多应该怀疑进展为急性白血病。骨髓增生异常或 AML 是最严重的晚期并发症[184-186]。

脾所见

脾常常增大，在广泛骨髓纤维化的患者脾大最为明显。在疾病的早期，脾显示明显的红髓充血，白髓难以觉察。髓外造血仅仅在疾病晚期（骨髓化生）明显，伴有骨髓纤维化[187]。

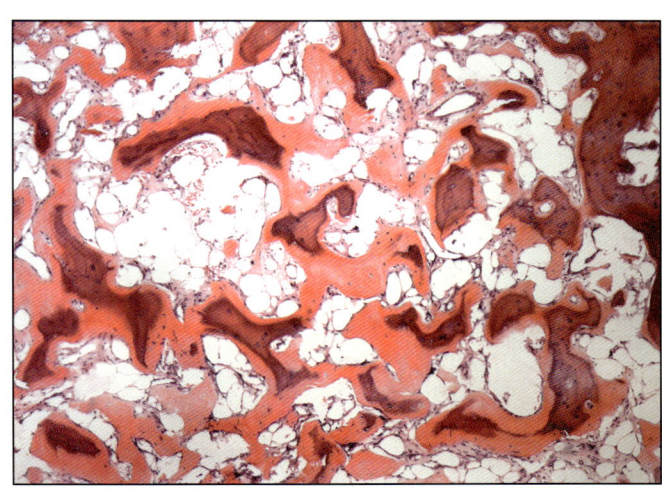

图22.72 一例处于疾病晚期的真性红细胞增多症的骨髓芯针活检的组织学切片，显示明显的骨质硬化和骨髓间隙细胞成分减少，伴有纤细的网状纤维。（HE染色）

分子遗传学所见

最近，在80%以上的PV患者以及大约40%的ET和CIMF患者中发现非受体酪氨酸激酶——JAK2（V617F 置换）——克隆性体细胞突变[171a-e]。在一种鼠模型中，最终产物的活化可诱导红细胞增生并增加对细胞因子的高度敏感性[171c]。虽然尚未建立实验方案，但是显然，检测 JAK2 V617F 突变不久将对 CMPD 的诊断产生重要的影响。由于缺乏特异性所见以及在诊断时获得的资料相对少（仅仅占13%～18%的患者），核型诊断的价值往往有限[188-190]。1p、8号和9号染色体三体以及13q和20q染色体缺失常常可能遇到，似乎与先前的治疗无关[188-190]。与未经治疗或单独应用 phelobotomy 治疗的患者

特发性血小板增多症
Essential thrombocythemia

相比，其他染色体异常经常见于进行化疗的患者（59%与18%）[188]。另外，最初出现的细胞遗传学异常似乎不能预测骨髓纤维化、骨髓化生或白血病的发生[188,190]。

定义

特发性血小板增多症（ET）是一种克隆性慢性骨髓增生性干细胞疾病，其本身主要表现在巨核细胞系的细胞。本病的特征是外周血血小板持续性增多（> 600×10^9/L）和相应的骨髓巨核细胞增生。同PV一样，其临床经过由于血栓出血性素质而变得十分复杂。考虑到血小板增多有许多继发性原因以及在其他慢性骨髓增生性疾病也可有血小板增多，准确地诊断这种疾病常常非常困难。然而，*JAK2* V617F突变可发生于近50%的ET病例，其识别非常有助于排除血小板增多的一些其他原因[171b]。过去，如真性红细胞增多症研究小组（PVSG）命名的那样，ET的诊断主要是排除性诊断[191,192]。但在新近的WHO分类中，现在将骨髓活检表现包括在内作为主要的诊断标准（表22.16）。似乎PVSG的标准可能导致许多早期或纤维化前期的CIMF误诊为ET[193]。有鉴于此，从前文献报道的ET的临床和实验室特征必须谨慎解释。同其他许多慢性骨髓增生性疾病一样，ET的详细发病机制仍不清楚；但是，调节正常血小板生成的JAK2信号通路紊乱可能是主要的致病因素[194]。其他可能的发病机制来自对少数家族性ET病例的研究。近期发现，某些家族存在血小板生成素基因5'端未翻译区[195]和血小板生成素受体基因（c-MPL）[196]突变，可导致血小板生成素生成过多或受体功能亢进。然而，有必要进行进一步的检查，因为迄今为止，在获得性病变中并未证实有同样的突变[197]。

临床和实验室所见

ET的发病率估计大约在每年2.5例/100 000人[198]，但在普通人群中，真正的发病率尚未进行系统的研究。诊断时中位年龄的范围在60和70岁之间，但ET可发生于儿童[191,198,199]。大约一半的患者没有症状，表现为偶然发现血小板计数升高[200-202]。中位血小板计数一般接近 1000×10^9/L，范围在 $600 \sim 1700 \times 10^9$/L 之间[198]。有症状的患者常常出现与周围小血管血栓形成有关的症状[203]。这些症状包括头痛、头晕、视觉障碍、一过性缺血发作以及指（趾）末梢缺血。危及生命的并发症包括脑梗死或肝静脉血栓形成。当发生出血时，最常见的是黏膜部位，例如胃肠道，可导致明显的铁缺乏性贫血。严重出血少见，通常发生于血小板计数最高或服用抗血小板药物的患者。轻度至中度脾大仅仅见于少部分患者[202]。肝大更为少见，其发生总是伴有脾大。

外周血、骨髓和抽吸所见

外周血涂片显示血小板数目增多，包括大的和颗粒减少的成分。可见中性粒细胞增多或嗜碱性粒细胞增多，但典型地为轻度增多。骨髓细胞成分常常轻度增多，但也有细胞成分正常甚或减少的病例[183]。巨核细胞的数目和大小明显增加，且常常排列成簇状（图22.73）。巨核细胞的分叶增多，但染色质和胞浆正常，成熟性没有改变[183,204]。缺乏胶原纤维化，网状纤维纤维化或者缺乏，或者至多是出现轻微网状纤维纤维化。红系和粒细胞前体细胞的数目和形态通常正常。转化为骨髓增生异常或急性白血病的少见，似乎常常与先前的化疗有关[198,200,205]。如出现脾大，是由于大量的血小板充满了红髓的脾索，常常呈灰白色。

分子遗传学所见

如上所述，大约40%～50%的ET病例显示*JAK2* V617F突变[171b,171e]。此外，X失活研究显示，大多数病例具有克隆性造血[206,207]。其他细胞遗传学异常在诊断时并不常见，大约发生于5%的患者[208,209]。几种反复

表22.16	WHO的特发性血小板增多症的诊断标准

确定标准

1. 血小板计数持续性大于 600×10^9/L
2. 骨髓活检标本显示主要为巨核细胞系增生，伴有增大的成熟巨核细胞数目增多

否定标准

1. 没有真性红细胞增多症的证据：红细胞量正常，或男性血红蛋白 < 18.5g/dl，女性血红蛋白 < 16.5g/dl；骨髓可见铁染色，血清铁蛋白正常，或平均血球容积正常；如果不符合前两种情况，铁治疗不能使红细胞量或血红蛋白水平增加到真性红细胞增多症的程度
2. 没有慢性骨髓性白血病（CML）的证据：没有Ph染色体且没有*BCR/ABL*融合基因
3. 没有慢性特发性骨髓纤维化的证据：缺乏胶原纤维化，网状纤维纤维化轻微或缺乏
4. 没有骨髓增生异常综合征的证据：没有del(5q)、t(3;3)(q21;q26)、inv(3)(q21q26)
5. 没有因潜在的炎症、感染、肿瘤或先前脾切除引起的反应性血小板增多的证据

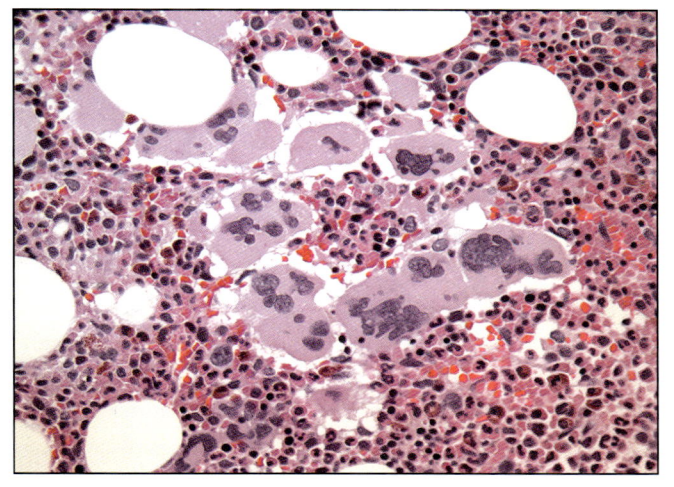

图22.73 特发性血小板增多症的骨髓芯针活检组织学切片，显示大而成簇的巨核细胞，细胞大小增大和核的分叶增加。（HE染色）

表22.17	与骨髓纤维化有关的病变

血液学疾病

骨髓疾病
 慢性特发性骨髓纤维化
 急性骨髓性白血病
 急性骨髓纤维化/急性原始巨核细胞性白血病
 慢性骨髓性白血病
 骨髓增生异常或骨髓增生异常/骨髓增生综合征
 真性红细胞增多症
 慢性骨髓单核细胞性白血病
 慢性嗜酸性粒细胞性白血病
 系统性肥大细胞性疾病

淋巴组织疾病
 毛细胞性白血病
 Hodgkin淋巴瘤
 非Hodgkin淋巴瘤
 多发性骨髓瘤
 急性淋巴母细胞性白血病

非血液学疾病

转移性肿瘤
结缔组织疾病
人类免疫缺陷病毒感染
肾病性骨营养不良
结核
甲状旁腺功能亢进
维生素D缺乏（佝偻病）
Gray血小板综合征

出现的细胞遗传学异常已被描述，似乎最有可能与先前化疗有关[205,210,211]。

鉴别诊断

为了作出ET诊断，必须除外反应性血小板增多症的潜在原因。后者包括由于感染、炎症、铁缺乏性贫血、肿瘤或先前脾切除而引起的血小板计数增多。与反应性血小板增多症相比，巨核细胞明显成簇是CMPD较常伴有的特征，但对于任何亚型的CMPD都不是特异性的。

为了排除其他类型的CMPD，应该仔细检查骨髓巨核细胞的形态学特征，巨核细胞一般增大，但具有正常的成熟。这不同于出现在CML中的小的分叶减少的巨核细胞；在CIMF中，则是大而奇异或成熟异常的巨核细胞；在PV中是成熟正常但大小不同的巨核细胞[183,204]。缺乏明显的网状纤维纤维化有助于鉴别ET和慢性特发性骨髓纤维化（CIMF）[212]。重要的是，虽然10%以上的ET患者可见少量的网状纤维纤维化，但是并不能预测将来会发生骨髓纤维化或骨髓化生[213]。

几种具有特异性染色体异常的MDS均伴有明显的血小板增多，包括del(5q)、t(3;3)(q21;q26.2)或inv(3)(q21;q26.2)，需要与ET进行鉴别。对于出现在这些MDS类型中的粒细胞增生异常或小巨核细胞进行核型分析和评估有助于作出鉴别诊断。另外，一种类型的获得性环形铁粒原始红细胞性贫血可能表现为血小板增多症[214]。后者在临床上不同于ET，其行为似乎类似于混合性骨髓增生/MDS。本病骨髓环形铁粒原始红细胞铁染色丰富，而ET缺乏铁染色，由此可鉴别这两种病变。

慢性特发性骨髓纤维化
Chronic idiopathic myelofibrosis

定义

慢性特发性骨髓纤维化（CIMF）也称为"原因不明的骨髓化生"或"骨髓纤维化伴有骨髓化生"，是一种克隆性干细胞疾病，其特征为巨核细胞异常增生，不成熟性粒细胞相对增多，红细胞生成无效，骨髓内反应性网状纤维或胶原沉积（骨髓纤维化），以及脾或其他器官的髓外造血（骨髓化生）。其他CMPD或MDS可见这些特征的不同程度的明显的重叠（尤其是骨髓纤维化），因此，诊断CIMF的依据是排除其他可能具有这些表现的克隆性和非克隆性病变（表22.17）。重要的是，相当一部分患者处于所谓的疾病纤维化前期，几乎没有其晚期的血液、骨髓或髓外表现，难以作出准确的诊断[193,215,216]。这种病变的克隆性干细胞的本质已经确立[217,218]，而且大约40%的病例涉及JAK2 V617F突变[171e]。然而，确切的发病机制尚不清楚。骨髓微环境的特征性改变不仅包括纤维化，还包括血管形成、骨质硬化的增加以及增生的间质细胞增多，这可能是由克隆性增生的细胞成分产生的细胞因子介导的反应性病变[219]。

临床和实验室特征

CIMF 是一种少见病变，所报告的发病率为每年 0.3 和 1.5 例/100 000 人[198,220,221]。它主要是一种老年人的疾病，诊断时的中位年龄为 65 岁，只有大约 10% 的患者小于 46 岁[222-225]。许多患者最初没有症状，当常规检查发现脾增大或血计数异常时才引起注意。主诉常常与脾大有关（如早期饱满感、外周水肿、腹胀）或出现"B"症状，如乏力、体重减轻、盗汗和低热[219]。出现症状时，90% 以上的病例因髓外造血而呈现脾大[226]，而且脾随着疾病的进展进行性增大。肝大也是常见的最初表现（65%）。髓外造血也可发生于脾或肝以外的部位，尤其是在疾病晚期或姑息性脾切除之后。常常受累的组织包括淋巴结、浆膜面、泌尿生殖系统、肺、肾上腺、皮肤以及脊柱旁和硬膜下或硬膜外间隙[219,227-230]。

外周血、骨髓和抽吸所见

纤维化前期　Prefibrotic phase

本病的富于细胞期呈现有限的骨髓纤维化，常常被误诊为其他的 CMPD，例如 ET[193]。可能有轻度贫血以及不同程度的白细胞增多和血小板增多。缺乏或仅有轻微的本病明确的特征性的表现，如成白红细胞增多症（leukoerythroblastosis）、脾大和骨髓纤维化。仔细检查骨髓活检标本常常显示某些特征性表现：混合性粒细胞和巨核细胞增生，红系再生不良，间质水肿，以及浆细胞和淋巴细胞增加（图 22.74）。巨核细胞常常成簇，显示明显的正常成熟异常，如不典型性甚至是奇异形的核分叶，染色质粗块状或致密，以及核的大小变化很大（图 22.75）[183,215,231]。巨核细胞还常常可见于扩张的窦隙内。还常常可见到没有胞浆的"裸露的"巨核细胞核。如果在这个阶段见到网状纤维，则主要局限于血管周围区域[232]。

纤维化期　Fibrotic phase

本期的特征是骨髓内网状纤维和胶原广泛沉积，相应地出现骨髓痨（myelophthisic）或成白红细胞增多症的外周血象。外周血涂片显示有核红细胞、前体粒细胞和泪滴状红细胞（泪细胞，dacrocyte）（图 22.76）。应用银浸染或三色染色最易评估纤维化的程度（图 22.77）。另外，骨髓显示细胞成分减少（常常呈片状分布），巨核细胞增生异常，骨质硬化伴骨梁骨胶原增加，以及扩张的窦隙伴有腔内造血。原始细胞计数一般少于 10%，粒细胞或红系增生异常并不明显。外周血或骨髓可见 10%～19% 的原始细胞，代表疾病处于急性期并

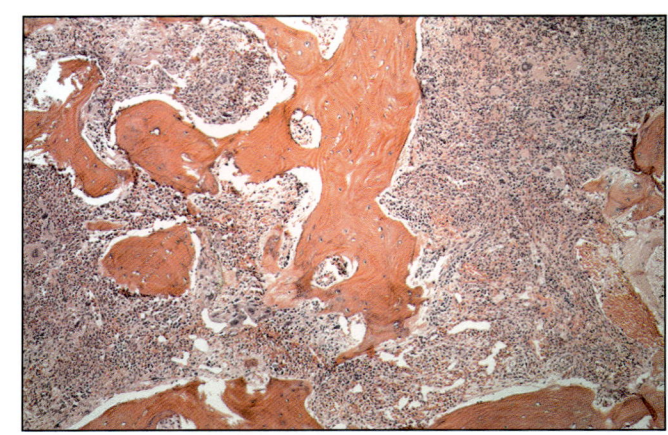

图22.74　一例慢性特发性骨髓纤维化的早期骨髓芯针活检的组织学切片，显示骨中等增厚，骨髓腔细胞成分增多，以及轻度的网状纤维纤维化。在这个时期，其难以与其他类型的慢性骨髓增生性病变鉴别，尤其是真性红细胞增多症和特发性血小板增多症。（HE染色）

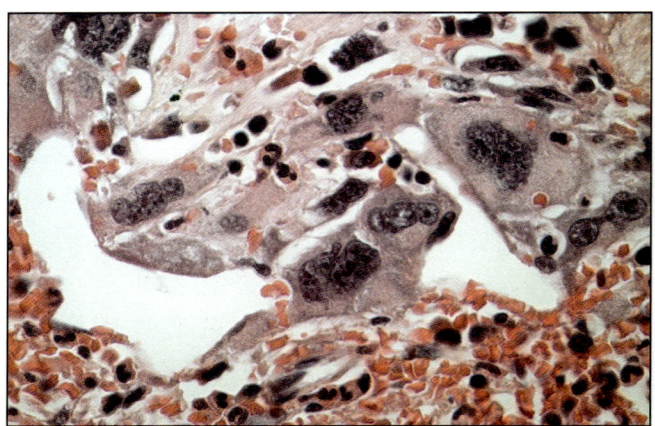

图22.75　一例慢性特发性骨髓纤维化的骨髓芯针活检的组织学切片，显示扩张的窦隙内有成簇的巨核细胞。巨核细胞核显示非典型性特征，包括分叶不同和深染。（HE染色）

向急性白血病进展。有明显的髓外造血，导致明显的脾大和肝大。在脾内，红系前体细胞一般成簇排列在红髓窦隙内。异常巨核细胞出现在红髓窦隙及脾索内，有时呈大的簇状结构。红髓脾索内可见粒细胞前体，但常规染色难以辨认。

分子遗传学特征

JAK2 V617F 突变可见于大约 40% 的病例[171e]，缺乏 Ph 染色体。与 ET 和 PV 不同，35%～60% 的病例在诊断 CIMF 时显示核型异常[219,222,233,234]。CIMF 可见三种细胞遗传学异常：del(13q)、del(20q) 以及部分 1q 三体[219,222,233,234]。也与骨髓增生异常有关且可能是治疗相关的其他表现包括：8、9 和 21 号染色体三体，以及 del(5)、del(7) 和 del(8)[219,222,234]。伴有异常核型的患者生

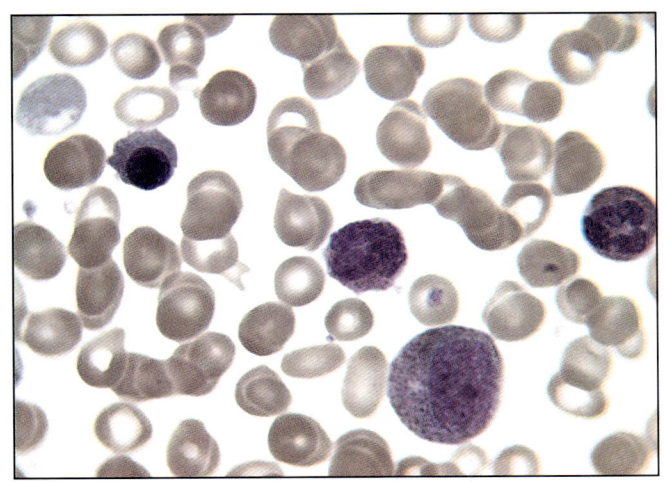

图22.76 一例晚期慢性特发性骨髓纤维化患者的外周血涂片，显示成白红细胞增多症。注意这张图的左上方可见有核红细胞，右下方可见晚期骨髓细胞。（Wright-Giemsa染色）。（Courtesy of Adam Kuten MD, Brigham & Women's Hospital, Boston, MA.）

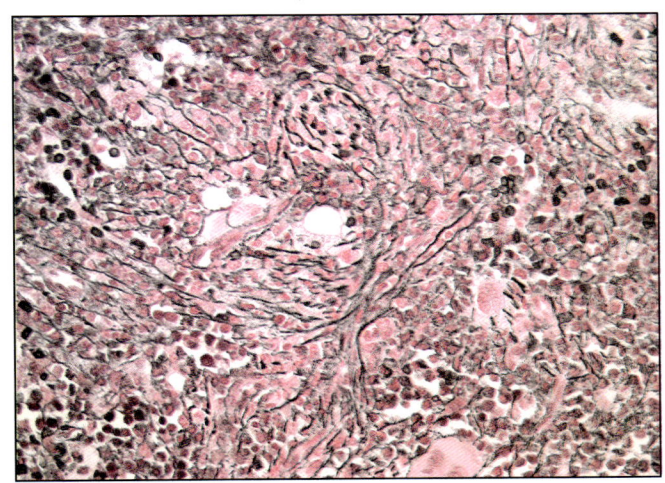

图22.77 一例慢性特发性骨髓纤维化病例的骨髓芯针活检组织学切片，网状纤维染色显示间质网状纤维明显增加（呈棕-黑色）。（核固红复染）。

存期短[222,235]，尤其是伴有与骨髓增生异常有关的细胞遗传学所见者[234]。

鉴别诊断

如上所述，必须除外骨髓纤维化、髓外造血和成白红细胞增多症（leukoerythroblastosis）的其他原因（表22.17）。虽然纤维化前期CIMF非常类似于ET，但CIMF的预后极差[193]。支持CIMF的特征包括：巨核细胞伴有核成熟异常、窦隙内造血、成白红细胞增多症和脾大。急性骨髓纤维化（WHO分类又称急性全骨髓增生伴有骨髓纤维化）是一种罕见类型的AML，它也具有CIMF的某些特征；最有帮助的鉴别点是缺乏明显的脾大，以及出现骨髓增生异常和不成熟的骨髓细胞数目增多。这是一种迅速进展的急性白血病，伴有突出的不成熟细胞，骨髓细胞增生异常，伴有散在染色质的没有分叶或分叶减少的巨核细胞，缺乏或仅有轻度脾大。骨髓增生异常伴有骨髓纤维化还可能类似于CIMF，但一般可见增生异常和原始细胞计数增多。

浆细胞性骨髓瘤 Plasma cell myeloma

定义

浆细胞性骨髓瘤（PCM）是终末分化的B淋巴细胞（浆细胞或"骨髓瘤"细胞）的克隆性肿瘤性增生，主要以多灶性方式累及骨骼系统（因此过去称为"多发性骨髓瘤"）。浆细胞病（plasma cell dyscrasias）还包括其他几种独特的临床疾病：不明意义的单克隆性γ-球蛋白病（monoclonal gammopathy of uncertain significance, MGUS）（图22.78）、慢燃性骨髓瘤（smoldering myeloma）、惰性骨髓瘤、非分泌性骨髓瘤以及一种被称为浆细胞性白血病的侵袭性骨髓瘤（表22.18）。MGUS随机进展为PCM的比率是每年0.6%～3%，取决于单克隆免疫球蛋白的水平。MGUS与骨髓瘤具有许多共同的遗传学异常，支持它是一种前体病变的想法。诊断PCM或其变型需要将病理学与临床、实验室和放射学所见联系起来（表22.18和22.19）。

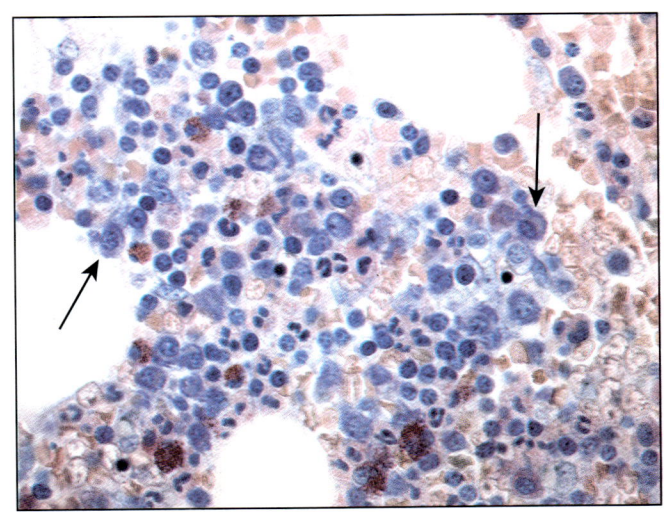

图22.78 一例不明意义的单克隆性γ-球蛋白病患者的骨髓芯针活检的组织学切片，显示少量成熟表现的间质内浆细胞（箭头所示）。κ和λ免疫球蛋白轻链和免疫球蛋白重链免疫组化染色显示，这些浆细胞的免疫球蛋白Gκ为单克隆性，与患者的克隆性血清副蛋白有关。（Giemsa染色）。

表22.18	WHO对不明意义的单克隆性γ-球蛋白病（MGUS）和浆细胞性骨髓瘤的其他临床类型的诊断标准

MGUS
1. 单克隆免疫球蛋白的峰值低于骨髓瘤水平
2. 骨髓浆细胞增多症的细胞成分＜10%
3. 没有溶骨性病变或骨髓瘤相关性症状

慢燃性骨髓瘤
1. 骨髓浆细胞增多症的细胞成分占10%～30%
2. 单克隆性免疫球蛋白的峰值与骨髓瘤水平相同
3. 没有溶骨性病变或骨髓瘤相关性症状（贫血、肾功能不全、高钙血症）

惰性骨髓瘤
诊断标准与浆细胞性骨髓瘤相同，除了：
1. M成分：免疫球蛋白G＜7g/dl，免疫球蛋白A＜5g/dl
2. 溶骨性病变少见（≤3），没有压迫性骨折
3. 血红蛋白、血清钙和肌酸酐正常
4. 没有感染

非分泌性骨髓瘤
诊断标准与浆细胞性骨髓瘤相同，除了：
1. 血清或尿中检测不到单克隆性免疫球蛋白

浆细胞性白血病
1. 外周循环血中浆细胞＞2×10⁹/L或外周血白细胞为20%

表22.19	WHO的浆细胞性骨髓瘤诊断标准

主要标准
1. 组织活检为浆细胞瘤
2. 骨髓浆细胞增生症的细胞成分＞30%
3. 单克隆免疫球蛋白的峰值：
   1) 血清电泳IgG＞3.5g/dl或IgA＞2g/dl，或
   2) 24小时尿电泳κ或λ链分泌物＞1.0g

次要标准
1. 骨髓浆细胞增生症的细胞成分占10%～30%
2. 单克隆免疫球蛋白的峰值低于主要标准所要求的峰值
3. 溶骨性病变
4. 正常IgM＜50mg/dl，IgA＜100mg/dl或IgG＜600mg/dl

诊断需要一项主要标准和一项次要标准，或必须包括（1）和（2）在内的三项次要标准。

临床特征

PCM是第二种最常见的造血系统恶性肿瘤（占造血系统肿瘤的10%）和最常见的浆细胞病。其主要发生于老年人，诊断时的中位年龄为66岁。仅仅2%的病例发生于40岁以下的个体[236]。发病率约为每年5.5例/100 000人，男性发病率略高，黑人比白人的发病率增加2倍[32]。2001年，美国共有14 000个病例报告，占所有癌症相关死亡的2%[237]。

PCM的临床后果与以下因素有关：多发性骨病变的占位性和破坏性本质，存在高水平的克隆性血清免疫球蛋白，以及伴有正常体液免疫的改变。膨胀性肿瘤吸收骨髓骨并侵蚀骨皮质，形成溶骨性病变。这种病变伴有严重的骨痛（最常出现的症状），常常由运动诱发。其他并发症包括病理性骨折和高钙血症；脊椎塌陷常见。最常见的受累部位包括脊椎、肋骨、颅骨、骨盆、股骨、锁骨和肩胛骨。大约70%的多发性骨髓瘤患者有髓外病变。最常侵犯的器官是肝、脾和淋巴结，但是，器官肿大少见[236]。骨或软组织的孤立性病变（浆细胞瘤，plasmacytoma）可见于5%的浆细胞肿瘤，是诊断PCM的主要标准（表22.19）。

常见乏力，与贫血有关，见于3/4的患者。白细胞减少症和血小板减少症不常见。贫血的基础是多因素的，骨髓红系成分被替代或由于肾衰竭造成的红细胞生成素生成减少是重要的原因。肾衰竭是导致集合管和远端肾小管中单克隆性轻链沉淀（称为Bence Jones蛋白）的最常见原因（骨髓瘤肾，myeloma kidney）。有些患者发生肾AL型淀粉样变。肌酸酐水平和红细胞沉积率常常增加。

大多数患者的正常血清免疫球蛋白水平减少，原因是对细菌感染过于敏感。单克隆性血清免疫球蛋白见于80%的患者，几乎相同数量的患者尿中可见单克隆轻链[236]。在1/4的患者，单克隆免疫球蛋白轻链仅仅可在尿中检测到（Bence Jones蛋白尿）。总的来说，接近99%的PCM病例血清和尿中可见单克隆蛋白；其余为数不多的肿瘤被称为非分泌性骨髓瘤（non-secretory myeloma）。大多数PCM产生IgG或IgA。分泌IgM、IgD或IgE的肿瘤也可发生，但极其少见。

PCM的预后一般较差。治疗后可以明显缓解，但中位生存率仅仅大约为3年。目前正在评估新的药物对这种疾病的长期疗效，例如蛋白酶体抑制剂，bortezomib（Velcade）。

外周血、骨髓和抽吸所见

PCM外周血比较独特的一种特征是形成钱串状红细胞。表现为红细胞呈线状排列，类似于堆起来的钱币，是由高水平的浆细胞免疫球蛋白导致的。在少数病例，或作为终末病变，循环血中可见肿瘤性浆细胞（浆细胞性白血病，plasma cell leukemia）。

大体上，多发性骨髓瘤的骨病变表现为胶状灰色至红色的结节。绝大多数患者骨髓浆细胞＞10%（中位数为50%）[236]。骨髓活检可见不同形态的浆细胞浸润，包括骨梁和血管周围小簇状排列，间质内大量聚集，或片块状弥漫性取代骨髓（图22.79）。破骨性活性通常增

强。抽吸涂片中浆细胞的形态学变化多样，从以成熟表现的浆细胞为主，到较不成熟或浆母细胞成分（图22.80和22.81）。偶尔以间变性浆细胞样成分为主。成熟浆细胞具有圆形或卵圆形偏位的细胞核，染色质呈团块状形似"钟表表面"，胞浆丰富，嗜碱性，核旁高尔基体明显淡染（"核窝"）（图22.80）。浆母细胞较大，具有大而偶尔位于中心的细胞核，核仁明显，胞浆嗜碱性（图22.81）。常常可见多核细胞和胞浆免疫球蛋白包涵体。包涵体的形态表现呈多样性。最具有特征性的包涵体包括：单个大的嗜酸性折光性胞浆（Russell小体）包涵体或假性核（Dutcher小体）包涵体；多个淡蓝色葡萄状小滴（所谓的桑葚状细胞，显示其形态类似于早期胚胎）；以及杆样晶状或原纤维性胞浆包涵体。表达Ig的肿瘤伴有高糖含量，有时具有红色/绯红色的胞浆，这种表现被称为"火焰细胞"（flame cell）。核仁的出现对于肿瘤性浆细胞是最特异的，因为多核或胞浆包涵体可以见于反应性浆细胞增多症。

其他组织

骨外病变常常由骨病变的直接蔓延而发生，通常来自肋骨或椎体。在脾，浸润充满红髓髓窦并压迫白髓。肝受累常见，但仅在少数情况下才引起症状；浸润累及肝窦状隙，尤其是门脉系统。淋巴结受累也常见，伴有片状浆细胞弥漫性浸润；网状纤维特征性地围绕单个浆细胞。

免疫表型所见

浆细胞表达表面CD38、CD79a和CD138（syndecan-1），流式细胞检查有助于辨认。与正常浆细胞不同，肿瘤性浆细胞常常表达CD56/58。通过免疫组化检查，CD138可有助于估计活检标本中的浆细胞数目。另外，石蜡切片中的胞浆免疫球蛋白重链或轻链易于识别，对于评估浆细胞浸润的单一型免疫球蛋白表达极其有用（图22.82）。在骨髓瘤，主要表达轻链的细胞与轻微表达轻链细胞的比例（即肿瘤性浆细胞与非肿瘤性浆细胞的比例）几乎总是大于16:1[238]。

分子遗传学所见

免疫球蛋白基因（Ig）重排的分子诊断研究（Southern印迹、PCR）一般显示单一单克隆性重排的Ig带；然而，少数病例可见多条重排带。通过常规分析，核型异常的发生率为30%～50%[239-243]，但是这种增生低下的肿瘤难以进行核型分析，染色体畸变的真正发生率可能较高。

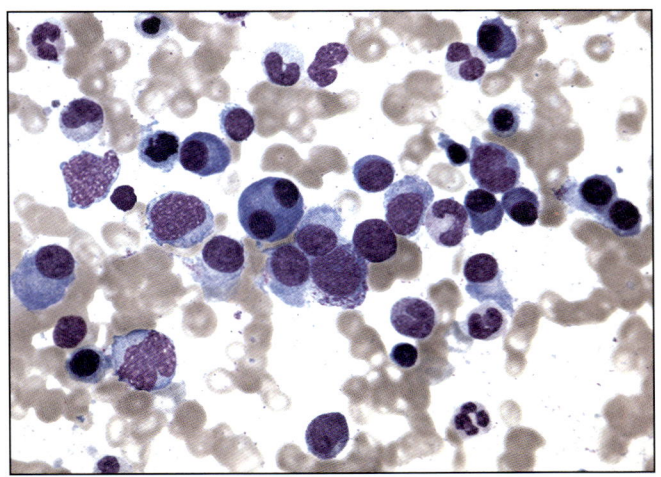

图22.80　一例浆细胞性骨髓瘤轻度受累患者的骨髓抽吸涂片，显示增生异常的浆细胞增多，核偏位，染色质致密，胞浆嗜碱性，核旁高尔基区明显，含有双核浆细胞（中央）和不成熟表现的有核成分（左中）。（Wright-Giemsa染色）。

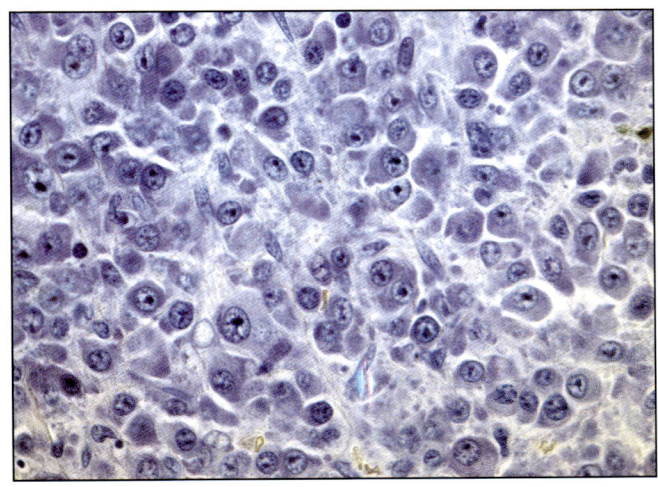

图22.79　一例浆细胞性骨髓瘤患者的骨髓芯针活检组织学切片，显示大的肿瘤性浆细胞成片排列，含有多核细胞和明显的核仁。（Giemsa染色）

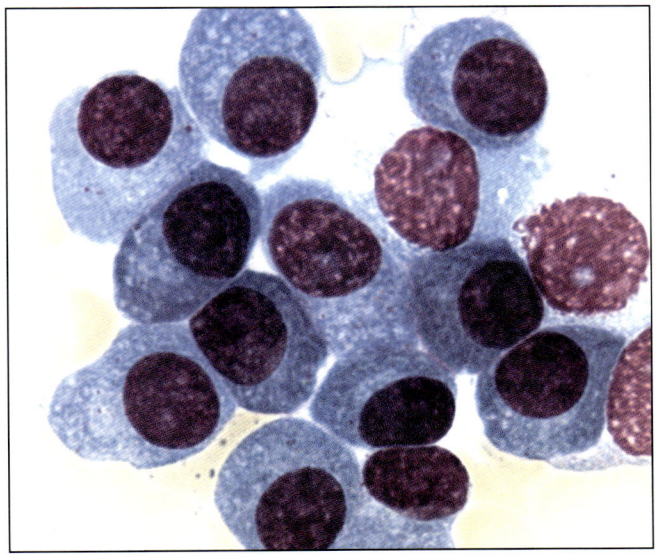

图22.81　一例浆细胞性骨髓瘤广泛受累的患者的骨髓抽吸涂片，显示肿瘤性浆细胞，包括不成熟表现的成分，伴有接近中央的细胞核，明显的核仁和少量胞浆。（Wright-Giemsa染色）。

特征性的数目异常是染色体 13、13q14、8、14 和 X 的丢失，以及染色体 3、5、7、9、11、15、19 和 21 的获得[244,245]。累及免疫球蛋白重链（IgH）位点的易位发生率高（占 50%～70% 的病例）。其中 40% 的病例，易位的配偶体是以下五个位点之一：11q13（bcl-1/cyclin D1 位点）、6p21（cyclin D3）、4p16（纤维母细胞生长因子受体 3 和多发性骨髓瘤 SET 结构域）、16q23（c-maf）和 20q11（mafB）[244-246]。有趣的是，累及这些位点的 IgH 易位较常发生于亚二倍体（例如染色体 13 丢失），而不是超二倍体异常[247,248]。累及 IgH 位点的其余易位涉及多种其他染色体的配偶体。

鉴别诊断

在临床和病理学特征方面，浆细胞性骨髓瘤（PCM）与不明意义的单克隆性 γ-球蛋白病（MGUS）、慢燃性骨髓瘤、惰性骨髓瘤、非分泌性骨髓瘤和浆细胞性白血病的鉴别点列于表 22.18。另外，几种其他重要的疾病必须与克隆性浆细胞病鉴别。

骨髓反应性浆细胞增生症的细胞成分很少超过 20%；然而有些慢性炎症性病变却可见到大量浆细胞。虽然反应性浆细胞（尤其是多核细胞）中可见一些细胞学非典型性，但这些细胞很少具有浆母细胞的特征。免疫表型或血清学检查证实：单克隆性 γ-球蛋白病对于诊断是至关重要的。

有些弥漫性大细胞性淋巴瘤的浆细胞样免疫母细胞可能极其类似于组织切片中的浆母细胞。在困难的病例，免疫组化检查可能会有所帮助；与浆母细胞不同，免疫母细胞的单克隆抗体染色一般表达白细胞共同抗原（CD45）和 B 细胞抗原，例如 CD20 和 CD19，而且可能表达 IgM 和 IgG。另外，弥漫性大 B 细胞性淋巴瘤几乎从不伴有明显的 M 波峰。

偶尔，PCM 在形态学上极其类似于淋巴浆细胞性淋巴瘤，后者由数量不等的小淋巴细胞、浆细胞样淋巴细胞和成熟浆细胞组成（图 22.83）（见第 21 章）。淋巴浆细胞性淋巴瘤的临床特征类似于其他淋巴瘤，包括淋巴结肿大、肝大和脾大。没有浆细胞骨髓瘤样溶骨性病变和病理学特征。IgM 副蛋白是淋巴浆细胞性淋巴瘤最典型的特征（即 Waldenström 巨球蛋白血症），而在 PCM 却很少见。

出现孤立性浆细胞瘤，或在骨或在髓外部位（见第 21 章），都必须与系统性 PCM 患者出现的一个明显的肿物鉴别。为了作出这种在临床上具有重要意义的鉴别诊断，有必要进行骨髓活检和抽吸涂片检查。

成人T细胞性白血病/淋巴瘤
Adult T-cell leukemia/lymphoma

定义

成人 T 细胞性白血病/淋巴瘤（ATLL）是 CD4 阳性的 T 淋巴细胞的克隆性肿瘤，伴有人类 T 细胞白血病反转录病毒 1 型（HTLV-1）感染[249]。ATLL 包括在世界卫生组织的外周 T 细胞和自然杀伤（NK）细胞性肿瘤分类中。ATLL 最常见于世界上 HTLV-1 感染流行的区域，包括日本西南部、西非和中非以及加勒比。它还散在地发生于中美和南美、中东和美国东南部。HTLV-1 与人类免疫缺陷病毒（HIV-1）或获得性免疫缺陷综合征（AIDS）病毒有关，同 HIV-1 一样，HTLV-1 具有 CD4 阳性 T 细胞的趋向性。虽然确切的分子机制尚未完全清楚，但仅出现在 HTLV-1 反转录病毒的 TAX 基因产

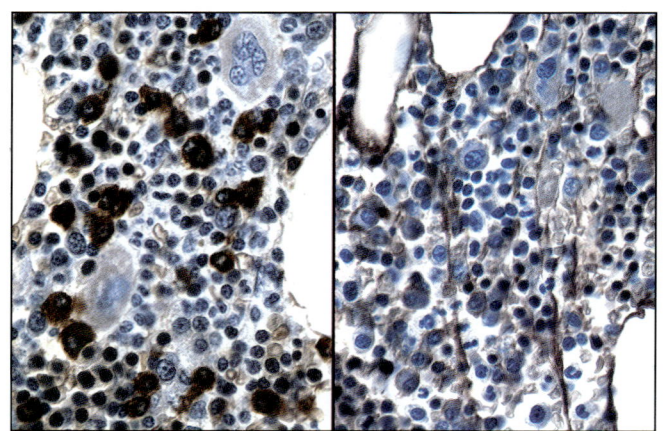

图22.82　一例浆细胞性骨髓瘤患者的骨髓芯针活检的组织学切片，免疫球蛋白 κ（左）和 λ（右）轻链免疫染色显示，浆细胞主要为胞浆 κ 染色，符合存在克隆性浆细胞病。（苏木素复染）。

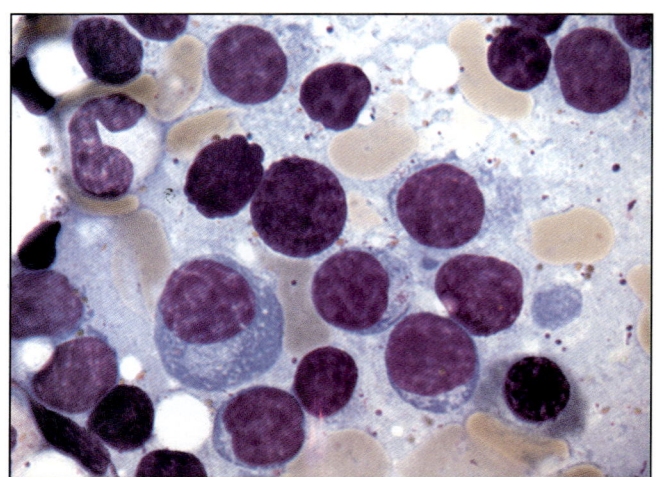

图22.83　一例淋巴浆细胞性淋巴瘤（Waldenström 巨球蛋白血症）患者的骨髓抽吸涂片，显示小淋巴细胞，具有偏位核和少量嗜碱性胞浆的淋巴浆细胞样细胞，并显示较大而典型的浆细胞混合存在。（Wright-Giemsa染色）。

物似乎可以通过扩展非恶性细胞群来启动致病事件，即多克隆 HTLV-1 感染 CD4 阳性的 T 细胞。最后，通过另外的突变和基因组不稳定性，在这种前体细胞群中形成单克隆肿瘤性 T 细胞群。在 ATLL 肿瘤细胞内出现克隆性 HTLV-1 原病毒支持这种模式的发病机制[252]。

临床特征

全世界有 1.5～2 千万人通过接触血液、血液制品或母乳感染 HTLV-1，但 ATLL 仅仅发生于少数感染个体（累积发生率为 2.5%）[250-252]。尽管在流行地区感染发生于很小的年龄，ATLL 还是在很长的潜伏期之后才发生，疾病发病的中位年龄为 55 岁。

ATLL 伴有特征性的系统性临床症状，包括循环血中出现肿瘤细胞（白血病）、高钙血症、淋巴结肿大、肝脾大、皮肤病变和溶骨性病变[253]。结外或髓外的其他受累部位包括胃肠道、肺和中枢神经系统。血清检查 HTLV-1 对于确定诊断是关键的。四种变型的 ATLL 已被描述，鉴别根据循环血中肿瘤性 T 细胞的数量、血清钙水平和其他临床特征进行。ATLL 类型包括最常见的急性型、淋巴瘤型、慢性型和慢燃型。这些变型的临床表现见表 22.20。急性型和淋巴瘤型似乎比慢性型或慢燃型更具有侵袭性。

外周血、骨髓和抽吸所见

除了慢燃型以外，其他类型的成人 T 细胞性白血病/淋巴瘤均有明显的白细胞增多，由中等大到大的多形性肿瘤性 T 淋巴细胞组成，常常可见显著的多分叶核或脑回状核。核的表现被描述为"花状"或"三叶草叶状"（图 22.84）。大多数细胞核染色质致密，偶尔深染，并有不同程度的明显的核仁；少数细胞具有较原始细胞核的表现，染色质散在，核仁明显。胞浆一般稀少至中等量，嗜碱性。慢燃型和慢性型患者的肿瘤细胞的非典型性常不明显。贫血和血小板减少的出现与骨髓浸润的程度有关。

骨髓受累程度各异；斑片状受累最常见，但偶尔可见弥漫性取代骨髓。骨髓标本中一种突出的表现是：出现明显的破骨性和成骨性活性，导致显著的骨吸收，这是高钙血症的原因。

其他病理学所见

皮肤受累见于大约 60% 的患者[249, 254]，可能非常类似于蕈样霉菌病（mycosis fungoides，MF），包括诸如灶状亲表皮性和 Pautrier 微脓肿等特征。

淋巴结受累呈典型的白血病结构，肿瘤细胞集中在淋巴窦内和淋巴窦周围的组织中。少数情况下，淋巴结内可见 EB 病毒阳性的 Reed-Sternberg 样细胞，同在其

表 22.20　成人 T 细胞性白血病/淋巴瘤（ATLL）变型的临床特征

急性型 ATLL
- 白血病期（白细胞计数增高）
- 皮疹，丘疹性或结节性，偶尔为表皮剥脱性
- 淋巴结肿大
- 肝脾大
- 高钙血症，有或无溶骨性病变
- 发热、不适
- 乳酸脱氢酶增高
- T 细胞免疫缺陷
- 侵袭性临床经过（生存期一般少于 1 年）

淋巴瘤型 ATLL
- 淋巴结肿大明显
- 没有外周血受累
- 其他症状类似于急性型 ATLL
- 生存期类似于急性型 ATLL

慢性型 ATLL
- 白细胞计数增高，肿瘤细胞 > 10%
- 没有高钙血症
- 轻度淋巴结肿大和肝脾大
- 皮肤病变的形式为表皮剥脱性皮疹
- 乳酸脱氢酶轻度增高
- 生存期 > 2 年

慢燃型 ATLL
- 白细胞计数正常，肿瘤细胞 < 5%
- 常见皮肤和肺病变
- 钙和乳酸脱氢酶正常
- 没有淋巴结肿大和肝脾大
- 生存期 > 2 年

他 T 细胞免疫性疾病一样，如伴有异常蛋白血症的血管免疫母细胞性淋巴结病（AILD）。

免疫表型所见

在绝大多数病例，肿瘤细胞表达 T 细胞相关性标记物 CD2、CD3、CD5、CD4 和 CD25。CD7 常常缺乏。与细胞的 CD4 阳性 T 辅助细胞表型一致，细胞毒性 T 细胞颗粒标记物 TIA-1 和粒酶 B（granzyme B）呈阴性。

分子遗传学所见

在大多数病例，应用 Southern 印迹或 PCR 检查可显示肿瘤细胞为克隆性 T 细胞受体基因重排。如上所述，可存在克隆性 HTLV-1 原病毒。在 ATLL 中没有发现特异性染色体异常。

鉴别诊断

分叶增多的 ATLL 细胞非常类似于 MF/Sézary 综合

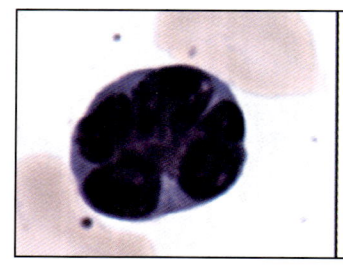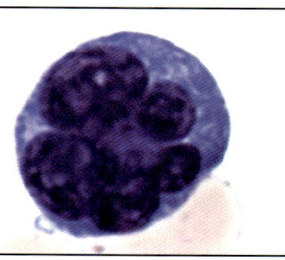

图22.84 成人T细胞性白血病/淋巴瘤的外周血涂片，显示两个不同肿瘤细胞的明显的非典型性形态学改变。注意核呈高度分叶状，形成类似于花瓣状的结构。（Wright-Giemsa染色）

征的脑回状细胞，单独依靠形态学可能难以鉴别，尤其是在皮肤。肿瘤性浸润的免疫表型也不是很有帮助；只有缺乏CD25染色（一种ATLL中总出现的标记物，但是也常常见于MF）支持MF而不是ATLL。临床和实验室特征，包括患者的出生地、HTLV-1血清学和钙水平，在鉴别这些疾病时最有用。

毛细胞性白血病　Hairy cell leukemia

定义

毛细胞性白血病（HCL）是一种惰性、克隆性、成熟性B细胞淋巴组织增生性疾病，表现在骨髓、脾和外周血液。这种肿瘤的一种正常B细胞的类似物难以辨认，有些证据提示，这种细胞来源于生发中心后的B细胞[255-258]。准确诊断是重要的，因为HCL对特异性化疗高度敏感（如对2-氯脱氧腺苷，干扰素-α或2-脱氧柯福霉素），但对标准的非Hodgkin淋巴瘤的治疗不敏感[259]。

临床和实验室所见

HCL少见，大约占成人淋巴细胞性白血病的1%～2%，在美国每年有600～800例[260-261]。好发于中年男性，诊断时的中位年龄为50岁，男女比例大约为4:1[262-264]。

大多数病例中，HCL伴有全血细胞减少[262-266]。因此，患者通常表现为与贫血有关的虚弱和乏力，与中性粒细胞减少有关的感染发作，或与血小板减少有关的出血综合征[263,264,267]。有趣的是，单核细胞减少几乎总是HCL的特征[262,266]。

由中度或明显的脾大引起的腹胀是常见的症状[262-264]。肝大仅仅见于20%的患者，淋巴结肿大少见[263,264,268]。在其他病例，HCL是在血液检查时偶尔发现的[262,264]。

外周血、骨髓和抽吸所见

患者很少表现为症状明显的白血病，循环血中常常仅有少数肿瘤细胞，仔细检查才能识别。抽吸涂片可能有助于评估细胞形态学，但是毛细胞浸润总是伴有网状纤维增生，常常造成"干抽"（dry taps）。毛细胞具有卵圆形至锯齿状或肾形细胞核和小而不明显的核仁（图22.85）。染色质分布较均匀，异染色质比正常淋巴细胞的少，具有"海绵喷画"的性质。毛细胞最引人注意的特征在其胞浆：胞浆丰富，透明至浅蓝色，边缘呈不规则的波浪状，形成"凹凸不平的"、"毛发状"或"树突状"突起。这些胞浆突起可能难以见到，因为这些突起纤细，最好应用相差显微镜辨认。在抽吸涂片中常常可见淡蓝色的胞浆碎片。少数情况下，胞浆中可见平行的嗜碱性带，相当于电子显微镜检查见到的核糖体-层状复合体[269]。

骨髓芯针活检制片中，HCL的表现实际上具有诊断性。大多数病例的骨髓细胞成分增多，但是细胞成分可能正常或减少[268]。受累的形态各异，或为斑片状和浸润间质，或为弥漫性；见不到结节性聚集，如果结节性聚集出现，则高度提示其他诊断。细胞核呈卵圆形至肾形，核仁不明显，其特征是胞浆宽阔，具有明显的边缘，呈现所谓的"煎蛋"样外观（图22.86）。伴有弥漫性骨髓浸润的病例易于诊断；然而，在细胞成分正常和减少的病例，脂肪细胞和残留的造血成分与浸润的细胞混合存在，造成检测数量少的毛细胞显得困难（图22.87）。如上所述，网状纤维网常常伴有毛细胞浸润，应用网状纤维染色易于辨认。

脾所见

脾实质被HCL累及（也见第21章）总是呈同质性暗红色；结节从不明显[265]。组织学上，肿瘤浸润蔓延至脾的红髓髓索。称为"血湖"的充满血液的假性窦隙（即内衬肿瘤细胞而不是内皮细胞的含有红细胞的腔隙）极具特征性。与大多数小B细胞肿瘤不同，这种肿瘤不累及白髓，而是压迫白髓，有时白髓完全消失[265]。

细胞化学和免疫表型所见

耐酒石酸酸性磷酸酶细胞化学染色（TRAP染色）呈弥漫阳性[270]，但在很大程度上已被免疫表型所取代。流式细胞术免疫表型分析显示B细胞表型（CD20+、CD19+、CD22+和CD79a+），而且共同表达CD103、CD25（IL-2受体α）、FMC-7和CD11c。

在石蜡包埋组织切片中，HCL细胞对DAB.44这种标记物高度敏感，发现本病所有非变型的病例均有免疫

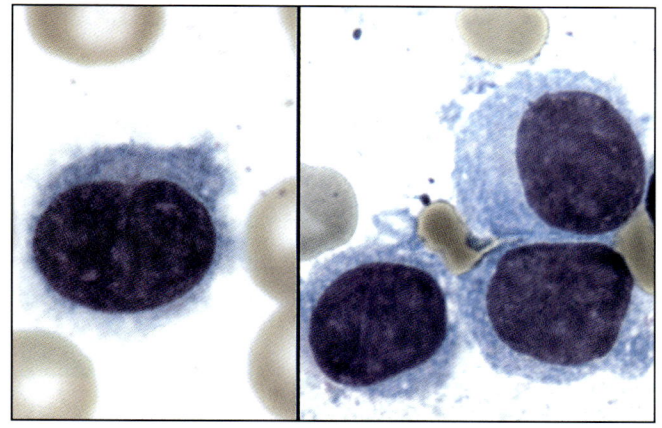

图22.85 毛细胞性白血病外周血涂片，显示几个细胞具有圆形至有切迹的细胞核，胞浆丰富，胞浆边缘不规则或凹凸不平（"毛发状"）。（Wright-Giemsa染色）

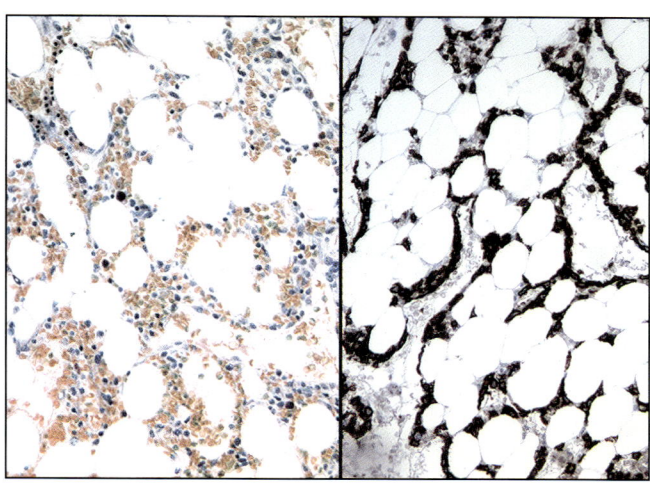

图22.87 一例细胞成分减少的毛细胞性白血病病例的骨髓芯针活检的组织学切片，显示淋巴细胞浸润不明显（左图，Giemsa染色）。同一病例的CD20免疫组化染色（右图，苏木素复染），显示大多数细胞成分由肿瘤细胞组成。

反应[271]。然而，DAB.44表达对于毛细胞并不特异，可见于许多其他造血系统恶性肿瘤。在临床怀疑HCL骨髓增生低下的患者，应该常规进行CD20或DAB.44染色，因为在常规染色切片中，白血病浸润的范围乃至是否存在很可能被误诊（图22.87）。

分子遗传学所见

迄今为止，尚未发现HCL具有特异性的细胞遗传学异常。可见克隆性免疫球蛋白重链和轻链基因重排。

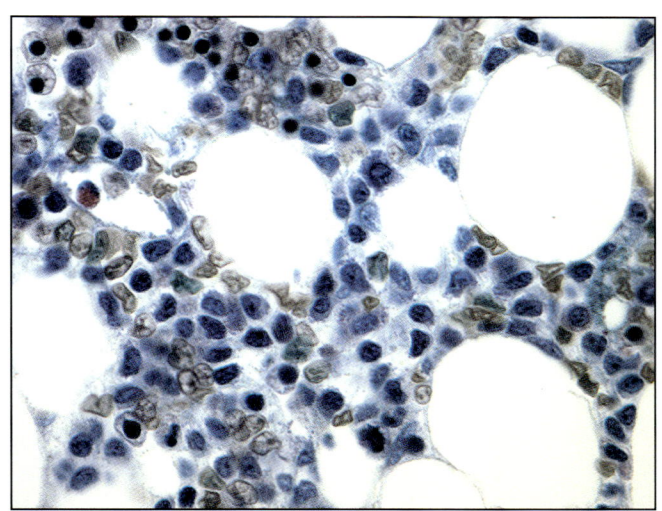

图22.86 毛细胞性白血病的骨髓芯针活检的组织学切片，显示淋巴细胞浸润间质。细胞核呈卵圆形至不规则形，中等量的细胞胞浆收缩与周围细胞分开，导致特征性的宽间隙排列。（Giemsa染色）

鉴别诊断

毛细胞白血病变型
Hairy cell leukemia variant

一种罕见的HCL变型已有描述，它具有某些独特的形态学、临床和免疫表型特征。同HCL一样，这种HCL受累患者出现贫血、血小板减少和脾大，但是不同的是，其白细胞计数增高，证实有许多毛细胞，见不到单核细胞减少[272,273]。其肿瘤细胞比典型的毛细胞稍大，核呈圆形至卵圆形，有时为双叶形，染色质粗，核仁明显，胞浆嗜碱性，这种特征类似于前B淋巴细胞。然而，其胞浆突起类似于典型毛细胞突起。与典型的HCL不同，其骨髓内的网状纤维仅有中等量增多，抽吸涂片常常易于获得[273]。细胞通常（但不总是）TRAP呈阴性，CD25或CD103常常没有表达。重要的是，这些细胞抗IFN-α[273]。

伴有绒毛状淋巴细胞的脾淋巴瘤（splenic lymphoma with villous lymphocytes, SLVL）是一种小B细胞性淋巴细胞增生异常，可能是脾边缘区淋巴瘤的一种变型（见第21章）。其循环血中淋巴细胞的胞浆比毛细胞的少，并有短的绒毛状胞浆突起，这些突起可能有极性。其骨髓受累表现为结节性聚集，而且与HCL明显不同，其脾的病变可累及白髓。最后，SLVL的肿瘤细胞一般没有CD25或CD103表达，TRAP常常呈阴性。

伴有脾大的其他小淋巴细胞增生的形态学和免疫表型特征均不同于HCL（见第21章）。

B细胞慢性淋巴细胞性白血病/小淋巴细胞性淋巴瘤
B-cell chronic lymphocytic leukemia/small lymphocytic lymphoma

定义

B细胞慢性淋巴细胞性白血病/小淋巴细胞性淋巴瘤（B-CLL/SLL）是一种成熟的、表达CD5、幼稚的或生发中心后记忆性B淋巴细胞的惰性克隆性肿瘤性疾病。CLL/SLL在形态学、免疫表型和基因型上是同源性的，但具有宽广的临床谱系；范围从以外周淋巴结、脾和肝受累为主，几乎不伴有骨髓和血液累及（称为SLL），到主要表现为骨髓和外周血的伴有轻微的淋巴结和脾累及的疾病（称为CLL）。淋巴结和脾病变的特征在第21章讨论。骨髓和外周血的特征将在这里详细讨论。

临床和实验室特征

B-CLL占慢性淋巴细胞性白血病的绝大多数，世界范围内的发病率为 < 1～5.5例/100 000人[274]。其好发于中老年人（中位年龄为65～70岁），男女比例为2:1[275]。大多数患者在诊断时没有症状；其他患者伴有乏力、体重减轻、慢性感染或与器官肿大有关的症状。诊断时常常可见某种程度的血和骨髓受累；孤立性髓外疾病非常少见。尽管有些武断，淋巴细胞计数大于 $10 \times 10^9/L$ 仍被用作鉴别CLL和SLL的特征。晚期由于骨髓浸润可发生贫血和血小板减少。肿瘤常常不同程度地累及淋巴结、脾和肝。

低γ-球蛋白血症常见，这促成了对感染的高度敏感。免疫失调还表现在容易发生自身免疫介导性溶血性贫血或血小板减少。有些患者具有血清副蛋白（或为IgM，或为IgG），但与多发性骨髓瘤和Waldenström巨球蛋白血症不同，其浓度很低。疾病经过漫长，但由于骨髓替代和继发性免疫缺陷，最终可导致健康逐渐恶化[274]。治疗仅仅针对症状明显或有疾病进展组织学证据的患者。有时可以转化为弥漫性大细胞性淋巴瘤(所谓的Richter转化)或前B淋巴细胞性白血病(B-PLL)(见下文)，通常预示更具侵袭性的临床经过。

外周血、骨髓和抽吸检查

在B-CLL患者，外周血和抽吸涂片常常含有小圆形淋巴细胞，核呈圆形，染色质呈块状，胞浆稀少淡染，没有颗粒（图22.88）。偶尔还常常可见较大的淋巴细胞，伴有较明显的核仁和较丰富的胞浆（所谓的前淋巴细胞），但在外周血，淋巴细胞所占比例不足15%（见下文有关B-PLL的标准）。常常可见许多伴有碎裂或胞浆中有模糊细胞核的细胞（所谓的破碎细胞，smudge cell），是在制片过程中受到损伤的易碎的肿瘤细胞。破碎细胞可用于诊断，因为很少见于其他慢性淋巴细胞增生性疾病。仔细观察抽吸涂片可以辨认单形性淋巴细胞聚集，反映在骨髓中存在结节状肿瘤浸润。

在骨髓活检中可见结节状、混合性或弥漫性间质受累（图22.89和22.90）[276,277]。一般来说，出现B-CLL弥漫性替代骨髓与晚期和较迅速进展过程有关[276,277]。随着弥漫性骨髓受累，中心增生常常较为明显（图22.89）。前淋巴细胞弥漫性或片状浸润是前淋巴细胞转化的标志，这些细胞核呈圆形至轻度不规则形，核仁明显，胞浆中等量（图22.91）。在大B细胞转化时，骨髓受累通常发生于病程的晚期，并且常常在尸检时发现[278]。大细胞常常类似于免疫母细胞或显示明显的多形性，核不规则，偶尔呈双核或多核，弥漫性替代骨髓。

免疫表型所见

流式细胞术对于明确B-CLL中淋巴细胞浸润的免疫表型最为有用，但是随着抗原修复的改善，石蜡包埋组织切片免疫组化检查被证实可用性也在增加[279]。肿瘤细胞表达B细胞相关抗原CD19、CD20（弱）和CD79a，并共同表达CD5、CD23和CD43。不表达CD10和cyclin D1。其特征是可见单一类型的低水平表面免疫球蛋白（常常为IgM和IgD）。

分子遗传学所见

最常见的异常包括13q12-14、11q或17p缺失和12q三体[280]（图22.92）。少数B-CLL/SLL具有免疫球

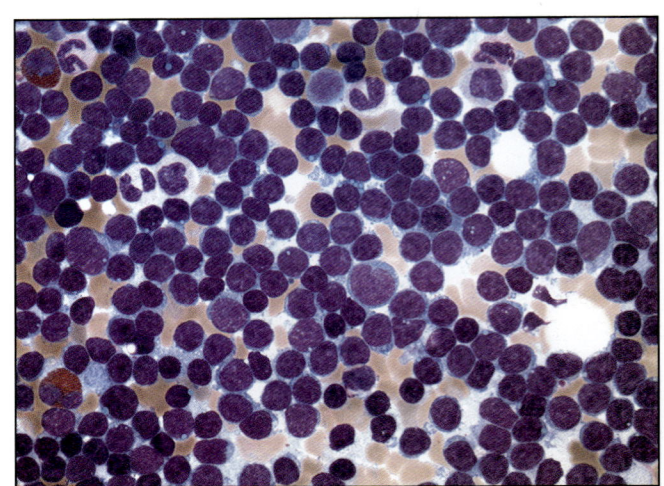

图22.88 一例B细胞性慢性淋巴细胞性白血病/小淋巴细胞性淋巴瘤病例的骨髓抽吸涂片，显示片状的小的具有成熟表现的肿瘤性淋巴细胞，与小B淋巴细胞几乎不能区分。（Wright-Giemsa染色）

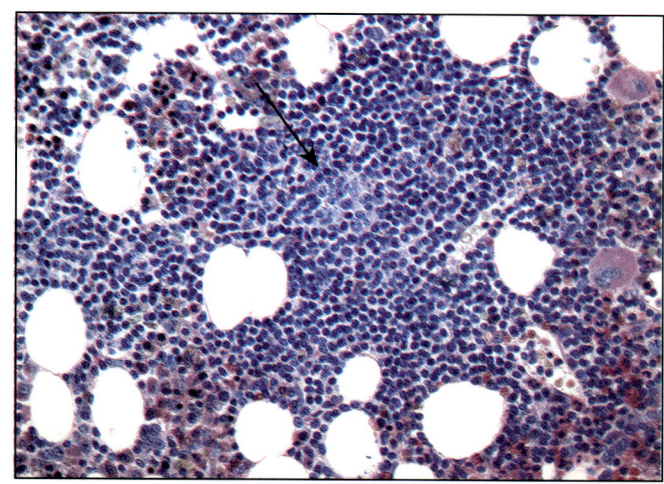

图22.89 一例B细胞性慢性淋巴细胞性白血病/小淋巴细胞性淋巴瘤的骨髓芯针活检的组织学切片，显示大片聚集的小肿瘤细胞取代正常脂肪细胞。箭头指示增生的中心含有核分裂象和核仁较大的前淋巴细胞。（Giemsa染色）

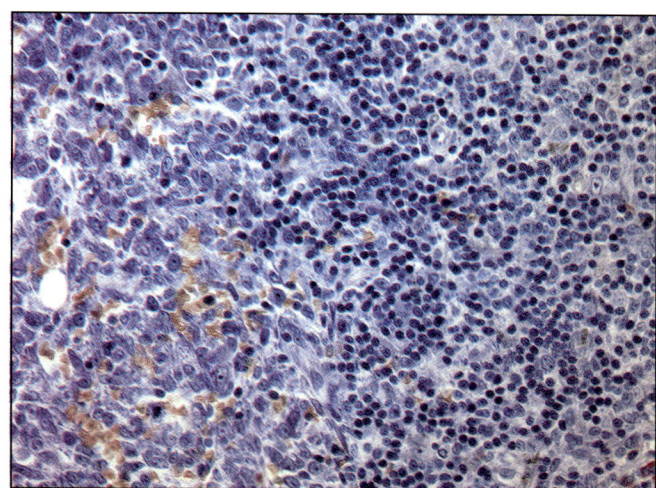

图22.91 一例B细胞性慢性淋巴细胞性白血病/小淋巴细胞性淋巴瘤的骨髓芯针活检的组织学切片，显示组织学转化。视野的右侧是典型的B细胞慢性淋巴细胞性白血病的小淋巴细胞浸润，而切片的左侧被具有较大的不规则核和明显核仁的细胞取代。（Giemsa染色）

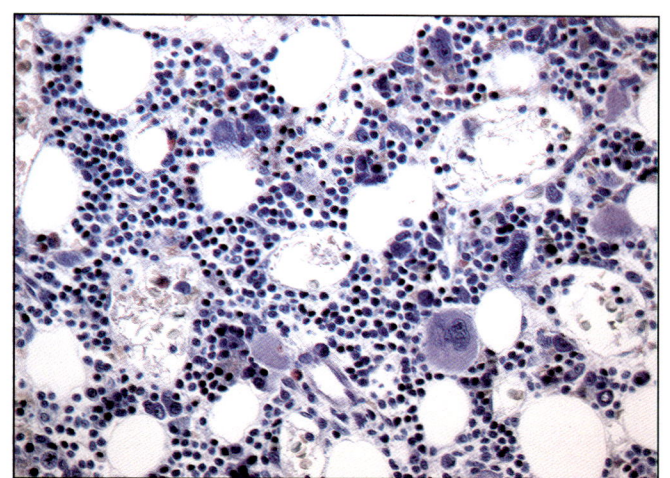

图22.90 一例B细胞性慢性淋巴细胞性白血病/小淋巴细胞性淋巴瘤的骨髓芯针活检的组织学切片，显示骨髓间质受累。（Giemsa染色）

蛋白重链可变区（IgVH）基因体细胞超突变，符合生发中心后记忆性B细胞来源[281]。其余病例没有显示IgVH基因体细胞超突变，与幼稚B细胞来源相一致。有趣的是，这些未突变的肿瘤预后似乎较差[282,283]。近期报告，ZAP-70蛋白的表达与未突变的IgVH状态、疾病的迅速进展和生存率差有关[284,285]。p53缺失或突变者预后似乎也差[283]。

鉴别诊断

鉴别诊断包括反应性淋巴细胞增多症以及其他B系和T系慢性淋巴细胞增生性疾病。已证实克隆性B细胞群对于鉴别早期CLL和反应性淋巴细胞增多症有用。

外周血液形态学上最常与CLL混淆的病变是SLVL、淋巴浆细胞性淋巴瘤和前T淋巴细胞性白血病（T-PLL）的小细胞变型。鉴别特征包括外周血形态学和骨髓受累结构的微小区别，但明确诊断（在缺乏淋巴结活检提示特异病征性增生中心的情况下）需要进行免疫表型分析。

当CLL有前淋巴细胞转化时，鉴别诊断包括新形成的B-PLL或T-PLL。转化的CLL的前淋巴细胞在数量上比PLL中的少，通常不超过白血病细胞的55%，而且比B-PLL更具多形性。通过形态学和免疫表型检查不能区分CLL的大细胞转化（Richter综合征）与新形成的大细胞淋巴瘤；这种诊断需要确定的CLL病史，或在诊断时发现伴随的CLL。大细胞成分的基因重排以及先前或并存的典型CLL可能为这种病变的克隆相关性提供明确证据。

前B细胞淋巴细胞性白血病
B-cell prolymphocytic leukemia

定义

前B细胞淋巴细胞性白血病（B-PLL）是一种成熟性淋巴细胞的肿瘤性病变，特征是骨髓、外周血和脾明显受累，但肝大或淋巴结肿大轻微。外周血肿瘤性前B淋巴细胞占全部淋巴细胞的比例超过55%[286]。前淋巴细胞数量在11%~55%之间的患者被称为B-CLL/PLL。这种异质性病变的临床和免疫表型特征介于CLL和PLL之间，至少可能包括两种类型的B-CLL：一种

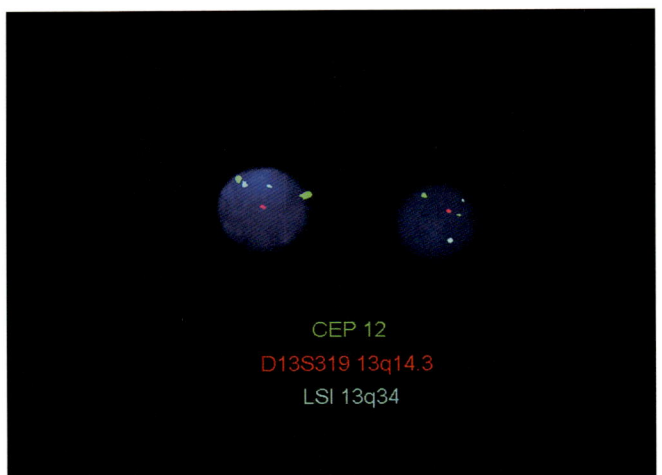

图22.92 B细胞性慢性淋巴细胞性白血病/小淋巴细胞性淋巴瘤间期核的FISH检测,应用的探针针对染色体12(绿色)和染色体13:13q14.3(红色)和13q34(蓝色)的两个位点。注意两个肿瘤细胞均缺乏两个红色信号,代表13q14.3缺失。相反,可见针对染色体12和较远部位的染色体13q34的13q的探针的两个信号。(Courtesy of Paola Dal Cin PhD and Cynthia Mclaughlin BS, Brigham & Women's Hospital, Boston, MA.)

伴有前淋巴细胞比例增多,但在其他方面是典型的病变,另外一种为"前淋巴细胞"转化。前淋巴细胞计数在这个范围(11%~55%)的患者可以排除新形成的B-PLL的诊断。B-PLL是一种侵袭性的疾病,在所有分期中其生存期都短[287,288]。

临床和实验室特征

B-PLL是一种少见的白血病,通常发生于老年人。平均的发病年龄为64~70岁,以男性为主[286,289]。白细胞计数通常明显增高,常常超过100×10^9/L[287,289,290]。常常可见贫血和血小板减少。

外周血、骨髓活检和抽吸所见

涂片中占优势的细胞比CLL细胞大,具有中等量的高度嗜碱性的胞浆[291](图22.93)。核呈圆形至卵圆形,染色质中等程度凝聚,介于成熟淋巴细胞和原始细胞之间。有单个明显的核仁。在骨髓内,通常有弥漫性或混合性结节状和间质性前淋巴细胞浸润。另外,还可见到较大的细胞,具有空泡状核和非常突出的大核仁,称为副免疫母细胞。

在脾,肿瘤细胞弥漫性浸润红髓髓索并使白髓膨胀。所有病例的脾的红髓髓索均有弥漫性浸润的白血病细胞。另外,有核仁的前淋巴细胞和副免疫母细胞集中在边缘区,而较小的细胞位于白髓中央,形成反转的假滤泡或增生中心样结构。在病程的早期,淋巴结受累通常为局灶性而且轻微,但最终可能发生弥漫性取代淋巴结。

免疫表型所见

B-PLL的免疫表型在几个方面均不同于B-CLL。在B-PLL中较常有表面免疫球蛋白CD20和FMC-7的高水平表达。另外,CD23呈阴性,CD5仅有不同程度的表达。

分子遗传学所见

据描述,B-PLL与涉及bcl-1的t(11;14)(q13;q32)和免疫球蛋白重链基因有关;然而,现在似乎最好将这些病例看做是少见类型的套细胞性淋巴瘤[292]。有趣的是,在任何B细胞的恶性肿瘤中,p53突变的发生率在B-PLL(53%)最高,而且可能是这种疾病疗效不好的原因[293]。另外,13q14和11q23缺失常常见于B-PLL[294]。

鉴别诊断

主要应与B-CLL/PLL和CLL的前淋巴细胞转化进行鉴别诊断。有些转化的CLL病例保留了特征性的CLL免疫表型,这一点是有用的。但是,其他一些病例获得了类似于B-PLL的非典型性表面膜标记物,可能只有通过病史或持续存在的形态学及免疫表型典型的CLL细胞来鉴别。

前T细胞淋巴细胞性白血病
T-cell prolymphocytic leukemia

定义

前T细胞淋巴细胞性白血病(T-PLL)是一种成熟

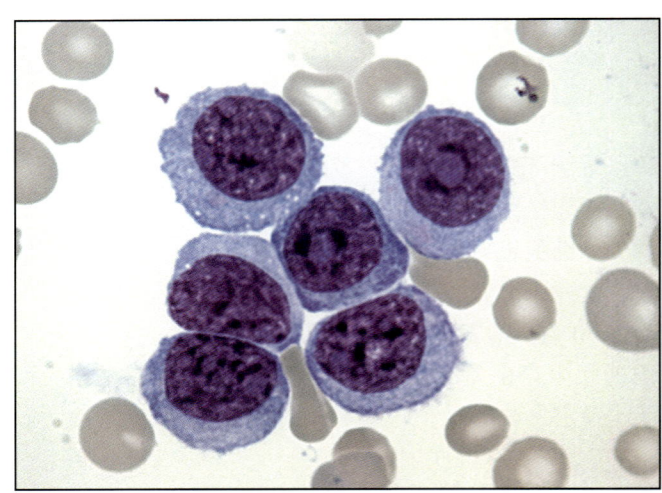

图22.93 一例前B淋巴细胞性白血病患者的外周血涂片。细胞比B细胞性慢性淋巴细胞性白血病/小淋巴细胞性淋巴瘤的细胞大,而且具有明显的核仁和中等量的嗜碱性胞浆。(Wright-Giemsa染色)

性胸腺后 T 细胞的肿瘤性增生，与 B-PLL 具有许多共同的的临床特征。在新近的 WHO 分类中，T-PLL 还包括前面提到的 T 细胞慢性淋巴细胞性白血病（T-CLL），尽管有某些形态学差异（即细胞较小），但其在临床和遗传学上均类似于 T-PLL。因此，在 WHO 分类中没有 T-CLL 单独的分类。

临床和实验室特征

T-PLL 大约占所有成熟 T 细胞白血病的 1/3，但当与成熟 B 细胞淋巴细胞性白血病比较时，则较为少见。这种疾病主要发生于老年患者（中位年龄为 69 岁），特征是脾大、淋巴结肿大、皮肤浸润、浆液性渗出和白细胞计数增高（通常大于 $100 \times 10^9/L$）[295]。外周血白细胞 90% 以上是非典型性前 T 淋巴细胞（见下文），半数患者可见贫血和血小板减少[295]。皮肤可出现全身性或局灶性斑丘疹性皮疹，但没有红皮病。虽然大多数 T-PLL 散发发生，但是伴有共济失调性毛细血管扩张症（ataxia telangiectasia，AT）的患者的 T-PLL 发病率增高，这与共济失调性毛细血管扩张症突变的（ATM）基因出现突变有关[295-299]。一般情况下，T-PLL 是一种侵袭性疾病；中位生存期少于 1 年。

外周血和骨髓所见

在制备完好的外周血涂片中，肿瘤细胞是小至中等大小的细胞，显示某些前淋巴细胞的特征，但在病例内和不同病例之间形态学差异可能很大。最常见的细胞具有圆形至卵圆形的细胞核，染色质中等密集，有单个明显的核仁，少量强嗜碱性无颗粒的胞浆，常常伴有胞浆空泡和突起（图 22.94）。在少数病例，细胞不规则，呈脑回状或有折叠现象。许多病例显示明显的多形性，这是由于形态规则和不规则的细胞核混合存在造成的[300]。最后，还可发生被有些作者称为"小细胞型 T-PLL"的病例[295]（占 15% 的病例）。后者的细胞相对小，核浆比例高，核仁不明显，有一小圈嗜碱性的胞浆。

骨髓的肿瘤细胞可呈间质性、结节性或弥漫性浸润结构，与 B-PLL 不能区分。一般见不到仅仅是局灶性或结节性的结构。在浸润的区域，网状纤维通常增多。

其他组织累及

脾受累常见，呈现弥漫性红髓浸润和白髓消失。常常可见淋巴结浸润，或弥漫性破坏淋巴结结构，或部分累及淋巴结副皮质区。与 B-PLL 不同，见不到增生中心，类似于其他淋巴结 T 细胞病变，常常有明显的内衬内皮细胞的小静脉。

与 ATLL 或 MF 不同，皮肤受累表现为明显的皮肤浸润，常常累及皮肤附件，有时蔓延至皮下脂肪，但不损害表皮。

免疫表型所见

在绝大多数病例，肿瘤细胞表达 CD2、CD3（程度不同）、CD5 和 CD7。T 细胞亚型标记物分析显示，大多数肿瘤细胞单独表达 CD4；然而，大约 20% 的病例表达 CD4 和 CD8。TdT 呈阴性，可能有助于排除 T-ALL/T-LBL。仅有少数病例（10%）单独表达 CD8[295]。NK 或 T-LGL 标记物表达罕见[295]。细胞化学上，应用 α-萘基醋酸盐作为底物，这些细胞可能显示 NSE 呈灶状或点状阳性（表 22.7）[300]。

分子遗传学所见

在诊断时通常存在多种共存的细胞遗传学改变。最一致的异常涉及染色体 14q11-q32 区（占 70% ~ 90% 的病例）。在大多数病例，这种异常表现为 inv(14)(q11q32)，其余的病例显示 t(14;14)(q11;q32)[295,301]。这些异常可通过将其置于 TCR-α/β 调控成分控制之下，激活 TCL1 位点的四种癌基因（TCL1、TCL1b、TNG1 和 TNG2）[302-304]。有趣的是，其中有些类似的异常在有 AT 患者的扩展的恶性前期 T 细胞克隆中已有描述[305]。AT 和 T-PLL 之间进一步的联系来自于对散发性 T-PLL 病例的研究，显示在大多数 T-PLL 患者中，ATM 基因失活（在染色体 11q22.3-23.1 的部位）是由大的缺失或点突变造成的[297-299]。最后，接近 80% 的 T-PLL 还显示同时伴有 8 号染色体的异常，主要是由 i(8)(q10) 导致的 8q 三体[295,301]。

鉴别诊断

B-PLL 和 B-CLL 是 T-PLL 鉴别诊断中最常见的疾

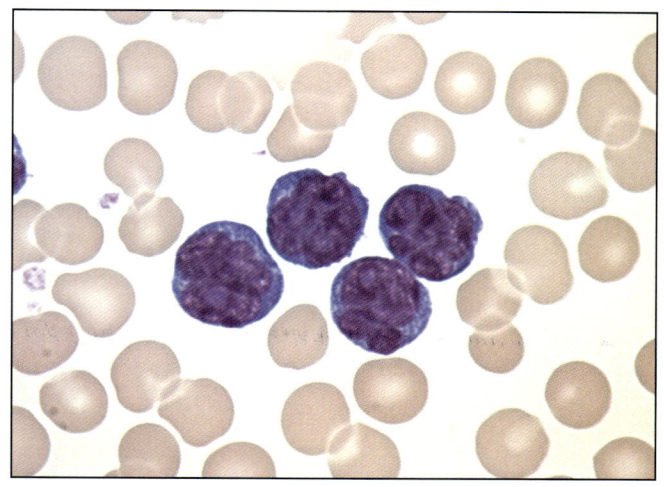

图22.94 前 T 细胞淋巴细胞性白血病的外周血涂片，显示 4 个前淋巴细胞，比 B 系前淋巴细胞性白血病的细胞小，核形状不规则，核仁不太明显，胞浆量少。（Wright-Giemsa 染色）

病，最好通过免疫表型检查排除。ATLL 和 MF 也包括在鉴别诊断中，尤其是当 T-PLL 累及皮肤时。这些疾病的形态学可能具有共同特征，特别是当 T-PLL 细胞呈高度脑回状时。CD7 表达的出现有助于 T-PLL 与 ATLL 和 MF 的鉴别，因为后两种疾病 CD7 表达常常丢失。CD25 表达和 HTLV-1 血清学检查也有利于鉴别 ATLL 和 T-PLL。最后，14q11-q32 的异常是 T-PLL 的特征，有助于与其他 T 细胞性淋巴组织增生进行鉴别诊断。

T细胞大颗粒淋巴细胞性白血病
T-cell large granular lymphocyte leukemia

定义

T 细胞大颗粒淋巴细胞性（T-LGL）白血病是一种异质性的疾病，特征是外周血中细胞毒性 T 细胞性大颗粒淋巴细胞持续增高。许多疾病的患者其外周血中的大颗粒淋巴细胞（large granular lymphocytes, LGL）都可能短暂性增多，包括病毒感染甚或其他血液性疾病。持续性的不能解释的 LGL 增多（$> 2 \times 10^9/L$）超过 6 个月，可将 T-LGL 白血病与短暂的反应性 LGL 增多区分开来。另外，当应用分子遗传学技术仔细检查时，T-LGL 白血病一般显示克隆性 T 细胞受体重排。细胞表达表面 CD3 和一种 T 细胞受体（通常是 TCRαβ），可将其与 NK 细胞增生鉴别开来，在 WHO 分类中 NK 细胞增生是单独分类（见下文）。

临床特征

T-LGL 白血病最常发生于中年人；中位年龄是 60 岁（范围是 4～88 岁）[306]。没有性别差异。淋巴细胞的增生范围一般为 $2 \times 10^9/L \sim 20 \times 10^9/L$；90% 的患者 LGL 计数大于 $1 \times 10^9/L$（正常 LGL 计数 $= 0.5 \times 10^9/L$）[306]。2/3 的患者在诊断时有症状。最初的许多临床特征与中性粒细胞减少有关，这种病变常常伴有中性粒细胞减少[307,308]。有些研究显示，中性粒细胞减少可发生于高达 47% 的患者，并可导致反复发生的细菌感染[306,309]。贫血也很常见，有时可见轻度的血小板减少。

全身性症状也常见，例如发热、盗汗和体重减轻。中度脾大是最常见的体检所见；肝大和淋巴结肿大有时也可出现，但通常并不明显。自身免疫性疾病的发生常常伴有 T-LGL 白血病。相当比例的 T-LGL 白血病患者患有类风湿性关节炎（25%），当同时伴有中性粒细胞减少和脾大时，这种疾病非常类似于 Felty 综合征[306,308]。其他自身免疫现象也有描述，如出现类风湿因子、抗核抗体和抗血小板抗体、多克隆性高 γ-球蛋白血症和循环性免疫复合体[306]。T-LGL 白血病还可能是真性红细胞再生障碍最常见的原因[310,312]。

外周血、骨髓活检和抽吸检查

形态学所见最好在外周血和抽吸涂片中评估。肿瘤细胞是大的淋巴细胞，核呈圆形至肾形，染色质致密，缺乏核仁，胞浆中等量，弱嗜碱性至透明，含有数量不等的纤细至粗大的嗜苯胺蓝颗粒。

骨髓细胞常常丰富，含有少量局灶性的间质性淋巴细胞浸润。偶尔可见明显的弥漫性浸润。细胞大，染色质致密，胞浆丰富；在组织学切片中颗粒不明显。伴随的中性粒细胞减少可能反映在骨髓中粒细胞前体减少，有时是因为骨髓细胞阶段成熟停止[310]。中性粒细胞减少的程度一般与 T-PLL 白血病累及骨髓的范围无关，符合免疫性病因学。红系成分常常相对增多。

其他组织所见

当淋巴结受累时，浸润主要累及副皮质区和髓索。脾受累发生于接近所有病例的一半，其特征是红髓浸润，伴有白髓反应性滤泡增生。肝的浸润可见于肝门区和窦状隙区域。

免疫表型所见

大多数病例显示表面 CD3 阳性，并表达 TCRαβ、CD8、CD16 和 CD57。T-LGL 白血病细胞还表达称为 B220 的同种型 CD45[313]。细胞毒性 T 细胞标记物通常也有表达，如穿孔素（perforin）、粒酶 B（granzyme B）、TIA-1、FAS（CD95）和 FAS 配体（CD178）。少数病例表达 CD4，伴有或不伴有 CD8 的共同表达。伴有 TCRγδ 表达的罕见病例也已有描述[314]。

分子遗传学所见

应用 Southern 印迹或 PCR 发现克隆性 TCRβ 或 γ 基因重排的证据对于鉴别反应性多克隆 LGL 增生与 T-LGL 白血病至关重要。偶尔可见克隆性细胞遗传学异常，但这些异常并不反复出现，并且尚未发现与 T-LGL 白血病有关的特征性遗传学异常。

鉴别诊断

T-LGL 白血病细胞与正常大颗粒淋巴细胞在形态学上通常没有区别。因此，重要的是与大颗粒淋巴细胞反应性增多进行鉴别诊断。大颗粒淋巴细胞反应性增多常与病毒感染（肝炎、EB 病毒、巨细胞病毒）、某些皮肤疾病、骨髓或实体器官移植、非 Hodgkin 淋巴瘤以及噬

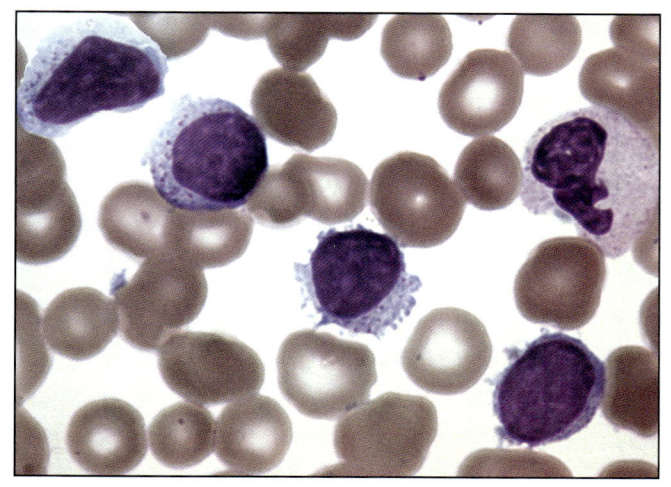

图22.95 大颗粒性淋巴细胞性白血病的外周血涂片，显示4个大的淋巴细胞，胞浆丰富透明，含有明显的嗜苯胺蓝颗粒。（Wright-Giemsa染色）

血细胞综合征有关[306]。在这些情况下，淋巴细胞增多是一过性的，而且随着原来疾病的消除而消退。因此，在没有提示白血病的血细胞减少或病理学特征的患者，为了排除T-LGL白血病，可能需要观察一段时间。如果淋巴细胞持续性增多，克隆性分析将有助于评估其是否为肿瘤性疾病。

LGL浸润在芯针活检组织学切片上难以察觉，需要与其他淋巴组织增生性病变鉴别，如CLL。免疫表型标记物可以用于辨认浸润的细胞毒性T细胞本质。在这些情形下，结合外周血检查所见是非常重要的。

惰性NK细胞淋巴组织增生性疾病 Indolent NK-cell lymphoproliferative disorder

这种淋巴组织增生性疾病在形态学上不易与T-LGL白血病区分，但可显示NK免疫表型，最常见的特征是：缺乏表面CD3而存在CD56和CD16[315]。与侵袭性NK细胞白血病不同（见下文），它具有惰性、非进展性经过，类似于T-LGL白血病[316]。这些患者不出现脾大、肝大或淋巴结肿大，且没有明显的自身免疫性表现。T细胞受体分析不显示T细胞受体重排；然而，分子学研究的确显示X染色体失活的单克隆性结构[317]。

侵袭性NK细胞白血病 Aggressive NK-cell leukemia

这种疾病的淋巴瘤对应病变在第21章详细讨论。不同于上面描述的惰性NK细胞LGL白血病，这种疾病存在一种免疫表型类似、但临床上不相称的侵袭性疾病，称为侵袭性NK细胞白血病。这种疾病与鼻型NK/T细胞淋巴瘤具有许多共同特征，侵袭性NK细胞性白血病很可能是同一种疾病的一种白血病形式[318]。

患者为青少年和年轻人。在亚洲人中比在高加索人中有较大的流行趋势。大多数患者显示侵袭性系统性疾病的体征，伴有发热、肝脾大、淋巴结肿大、凝血病和多器官衰竭。皮肤受累少见。对传统治疗几乎没有反应，这些患者一般呈现迅速致死的经过。

白血病的外周血象常见，但循环血中肿瘤细胞的数目相差很大，形态学也是如此，从表现类似于典型的T-LGL到大的非典型细胞，伴有粗染色质，明显的核仁和粗大的嗜苯胺蓝颗粒。骨髓受累也有很大差异，从弥漫性破坏至局灶性片块状受累（图22.96）。

肥大细胞疾病 Mast cell disease

肥大细胞是骨髓成分，几乎存在于所有富有血管的组织中，参与机体的防御和IgE介导的免疫反应[319]。肥大细胞疾病（肥大细胞增多症）被定义为肥大细胞在一个或多个组织部位异常聚集，导致多种临床表现。肥大细胞疾病的特征在第21章讨论。这一部分集中讨论本病的骨髓所见，在新近的WHO分类中是确立系统性肥大细胞增多症（SM）诊断的关键（表22.21）。在有些病例，骨髓和外周受累非常明显，以致有理由命名为肥大细胞性白血病（MCL）（表22.22）。另外，SM可能常常伴有其他克隆性血液学疾病。

系统性肥大细胞增多症 Systemic mastocytosis

虽然有限的皮肤受累是肥大细胞病最常见的表现，但是10%的肥大细胞病变是系统性疾病，最常累及骨髓、脾、淋巴结、肝和胃肠道。大约半数系统性疾病还可见到皮肤受累。由于骨髓受累非常常见（有些研究中为75%~90%），当怀疑肥大细胞增多症时，应该进行骨髓检查[320]。几种类型的骨髓受累已有描述。最常见的是片状或灶状血管周围和骨梁周围浸润[321]（图22.97）。浸润部位常常伴有明显的网状纤维纤维化，可能被淋巴细胞围绕，常常可见嗜酸性粒细胞。偶尔可见骨小梁旁区片状浸润，伴有纤维化和骨质硬化。间插的部位常常含有正常脂肪和骨髓造血成分；然而，在有些病例，有细胞成分增多和粒细胞生成增多，伴有分化异常[321]。偶尔可见弥漫性受累，最常伴有肥大细胞性白血病（见下文）。

活检标本中肥大细胞的细胞学特征有些差异。在HE染色切片，肥大细胞常常显示圆形至卵圆形细胞核，染色质成熟，胞浆丰富，含有小的嗜酸性颗粒。还可见

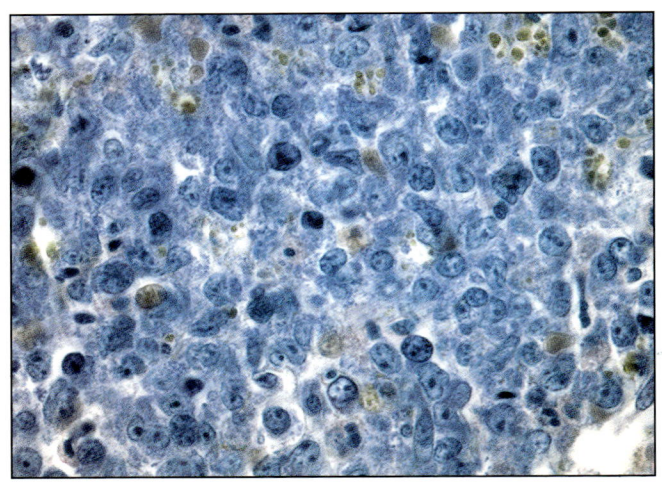

图22.96 一例侵袭性T自然杀伤细胞性白血病的骨髓芯针活检组织学切片。骨髓有弥漫性中到大的淋巴细胞巢浸润，核呈多形性，核仁清楚程度不同，胞浆中等量。在组织切片中没有见到胞浆颗粒。（Giemsa染色）

表22.21	WHO的系统性肥大细胞增多症的诊断标准

主要标准[a]

肥大细胞呈多灶性密集浸润或聚集，经免疫组化或特殊染色证实，出现在骨髓和（或）其他非皮肤器官（肥大细胞聚集应含有 15 个以上肥大细胞）

次要标准[a]

1. 组织切片中 25% 以上的肥大细胞是梭形细胞或非典型性细胞，包括骨髓；或骨髓抽吸涂片中 25% 以上的肥大细胞是不成熟的或具有非典型性
2. 在 816 号密码子可见 c-KIT 点突变
3. 肥大细胞共同表达 CD117 以及 CD2 和（或）CD25
4. 血清总类胰蛋白酶 > 20ng/ml（缺乏可能与这种测量混淆的骨髓疾病）

[a] 有一项主要标准和一项次要标准，或有三项次要标准即可以诊断为系统性肥大细胞增多症。

表22.22	肥大细胞性白血病（MCL）的WHO诊断标准

符合系统性肥大细胞增多症的标准，加上：
- 肥大细胞弥漫性浸润骨髓间质
- 骨髓抽吸涂片显示肥大细胞 > 20%
- 外周白细胞中肥大细胞计数 > 10%（如果 < 10%，则诊断为肥大细胞性白血病的非白血病性变型）

到梭形细胞形态改变，核的两端变细，胞浆淡染，颗粒不明显（图 22.97）。这些细胞可能类似于纤维母细胞，尤其是在纤维性的骨小梁旁区浸润时，确定这些细胞为肥大细胞是困难的（图 22.97）。增强识别异染性颗粒的特殊染色（Giemsa 和甲苯胺蓝）对于证实肥大细胞的存在非常重要。萘酚 AS-D 氯乙酸酯酶（CAE）细胞化学在含有成熟颗粒的肥大细胞也呈阳性反应。另外，免疫组化标记物具有很大价值，如肥大细胞类胰蛋白酶或 CD117（存在于正常的或肿瘤性肥大细胞）以及 CD2 和 CD25（仅仅存在于肿瘤性肥大细胞）（表 22.8）。由于骨髓纤维化，常常难以获得足够的抽吸涂片，因此价值有限。肥大细胞常常在骨针之间呈簇状排列，在这些区域内肥大细胞明显增多可能是芯针活检标本总体增多的一个线索。

分子学研究已显示，绝大多数 SM 病例在 *KIT* 基因的 816 号密码子具有 Asp → Val 置换，导致这种生长因子受体的组成性激活[322]。

肥大细胞性白血病　Mast cell leukemia

肥大细胞性白血病（MCL）是一种侵袭性的系统性肥大细胞疾病，其特征是非典型性、常常是不成熟肥大细胞广泛累及骨髓和外周血（表 22.22）。骨髓抽吸常常显示大颗粒性肥大细胞数目明显增多（> 20%）（图 22.98）。有些非典型性核的特征在 MCL 比 SM 常见，包括多核和出现明显的核仁或缺乏胞浆颗粒。

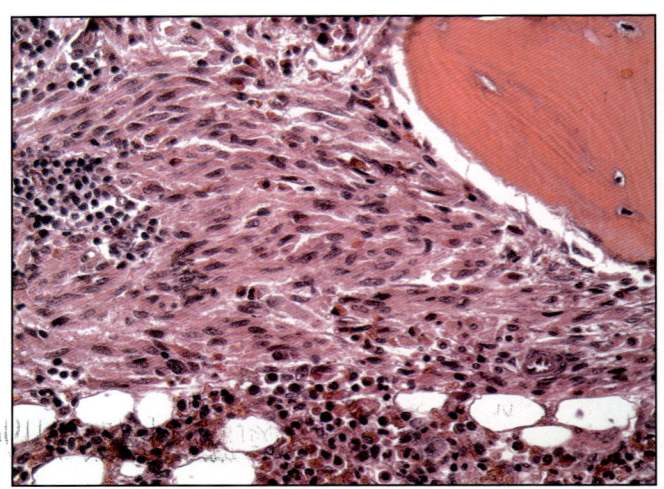

图22.97 系统性肥大细胞增多症的骨髓芯针活检组织学切片。骨小梁旁区可见多量异常肥大细胞，显示细长或梭形形态学改变。在HE染色切片上不易识别肥大细胞颗粒，明确评估需要进行Giemsa特殊染色或免疫组化检查。

伴有克隆性血液学非肥大细胞系疾病的系统性肥大细胞增多症
Systemic mastocytosis with associated clonal hematologic non-mast cell lineage disease（SM-AHNMD）

应该注意的是，SM 的诊断特征可见于符合许多其他血液学疾病的 WHO 诊断标准的患者。其中包括其他 CMPD、MDS、AML 和非 Hodgkin 淋巴瘤。虽然散在的非典型性表现的肥大细胞常常可能与许多血液学病变有关，但如果见到免疫表型异常的肥大细胞聚集，则可作出 SM-AHNMD 的诊断。

伴有嗜酸性粒细胞增多的系统性肥大细胞增多症
Systemic mastocytosis with eosinophilia

如前所述，少数存在典型 SM 症状的患者伴有外周血和骨髓嗜酸性粒细胞增多。虽然其中有些病例具有与其他类型的 SM 同样的 *KIT* 突变，少数病例具有 del4q 异常，导致与 CEL/HES 所见相同的 *FIP1L1/PDGFRα* 融合基因[167]。骨髓显示界限不清的肥大细胞松散集聚，伴有密集的嗜酸性粒细胞增多，不同于仅仅见于 SM 的

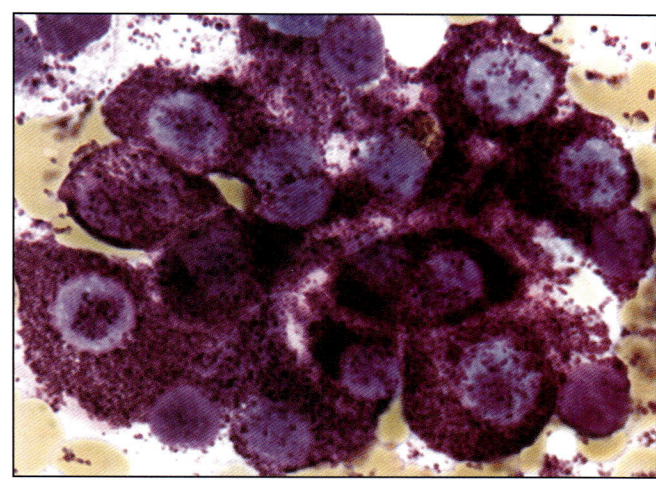

图22.98 一例肥大细胞性白血病患者的骨髓抽吸涂片，显示许多大的肥大细胞，核呈圆形，位于中央，可见明显的粉色胞浆颗粒。（Wright-Giemsa染色）

大的、界限清楚的血管周围聚集。重要的是，与伴有 *KIT* 点突变的 SM 不同，伴有 *FIP1L1/PDGFRα* 突变的患者对甲磺酸伊马替尼（Gleevec）治疗有反应。有鉴于此，对伴有明显嗜酸性粒细胞增多的 SM 患者应该进行 FISH 或 RT-PCR 检查以分析 4q 间质缺失[167]。

参考文献

1. Strupp C, Gattermann N, Giagounidis A et al. 2003 Refractory anemia with excess of blasts in transformation: analysis of reclassification according to the WHO proposals. Leuk Res 27: 397–404
1a. Bennett JM, Catovsky D, Daniel MT et al. 1976. Proposals for the classification of the acute leukemias. French-American-British (FAB) Co-operative Group. Br J Haematol 33: 451–458
2. Michaux J L, Martiat P 1993 Chronic myelomonocytic leukaemia (CMML) – a myelodysplastic or myeloproliferative syndrome? Leuk Lymphoma 9: 35–41
3. Germing U, Gattermann N, Minning H et al. 1998 Problems in the classification of CMML – dysplastic versus proliferative type. Leuk Res 22: 871–878
4. Cermak J, Michalova K, Brezinova J et al. 2003 A prognostic impact of separation of refractory cytopenia with multilineage dysplasia and 5q-syndrome from refractory anemia in primary myelodysplastic syndrome. Leuk Res 27: 221–229
5. Brunning R, Bennett J, Flandrin G et al. 2001 Myelodysplastic syndromes: Introduction. In: Jaffe E S, Harris N L, Stein H et al. (ed) World Health Organization classification of tumours. Pathology and genetics of tumours of haematopoietic and lymphoid tissues. IARC Press, Lyon, p 63–67
6. Bennett J M, Brunning R D, Vardiman J W 2002 Myelodysplastic syndromes: from French–American–British to World Health Organization: a commentary. Blood 99: 3074–3075
7. Nosslinger T, Reisner R, Koller E et al. 2001 Myelodysplastic syndromes, from French–American–British to World Health Organization: comparison of classifications on 431 unselected patients from a single institution. Blood 98: 2935–2941
8. Greenberg P, Anderson J, de Witte T et al. 2000 Problematic WHO reclassification of myelodysplastic syndromes. Members of the International MDS Study Group. J Clin Oncol 18: 3447–3452
9. Germing U, Gattermann N, Strupp C et al. 2000 Validation of the WHO proposals for a new classification of primary myelodysplastic syndromes: a retrospective analysis of 1600 patients. Leuk Res 24: 983–992
9a. Muller-Berndorff H, Haas PS, Kunzmann R et al. 2006. Comparison of five prognostic scoring systems, the French-American-British (FAB) and World Health Organization (WHO) classifications in patients with myelodysplastic syndromes: results of a single center analysis. Ann Hematol – in press.
10. Greenberg P, Cox C, LeBeau M M et al. 1997 International scoring system for evaluating prognosis in myelodysplastic syndromes. Blood 89: 2079–2088
11. Williamson P J, Kruger A R, Reynolds P J et al. 1994 Establishing the incidence of myelodysplastic syndrome. Br J Haematol 87: 743–745
12. Aul C, Gattermann N, Schneider W 1992 Age-related incidence and other epidemiological aspects of myelodysplastic syndromes. Br J Haematol 82: 358–367
13. Juneja S K, Imbert M, Sigaux F et al. 1983 Prevalence and distribution of ringed sideroblasts in primary myelodysplastic syndromes. J Clin Pathol 36: 566–569
14. Steensma D P 2003 "Pawn ball megakaryocytes": from the marvellous Medici and dear old saint Nick to the unsanctified marrow of myelodysplasia. Hematology 8: 11–18

15. Germing U, Gattermann N, Aivado M et al. 2000 Two types of acquired idiopathic sideroblastic anaemia (AISA): a time-tested distinction. Br J Haematol 108: 724–728
16. Brunning R D, Bennett J M, Flandrin G et al. 2001 Refractory anaemia with ringed sideroblasts. In: Jaffe E S, Harris N L, Stein H et al. (ed) World Health Organization classification of tumours. Pathology and genetics of tumours of haematopoietic and lymphoid tissues. IARC Press, Lyon, 2001
17. Brunning R D, Bennett J M, Flandrin G et al. 2001 Refractory cytopenia with multilineage dysplasia. In: Jaffe E S, Harris N L, Stein H et al. (ed) World Health Organization classification of tumours. Pathology and genetics of tumours of haematopoietic and lymphoid tissues. IARC Press, Lyon, p 70
18. Rosati S, Mick R, Xu F et al. 1996 Refractory cytopenia with multilineage dysplasia: further characterization of an 'unclassifiable' myelodysplastic syndrome. Leukemia 10: 20–26
19. Matsuda A, Jinnai I, Yagasaki F et al. 1998 Refractory anemia with severe dysplasia: clinical significance of morphological features in refractory anemia. Leukemia 12: 482–485
20. Gattermann N, Aul C, Schneider W 1990 Two types of acquired idiopathic sideroblastic anaemia (AISA). Br J Haematol 74: 45–52
21. Gattermann N, Aul C, Schneider W et al. 1990 Risk of leukemic transformation in two types of acquired idiopathic sideroblastic anemia. Haematol Blood Transfus 33: 374–381
22. Brunning R D, Bennett J M, Flandrin G et al. 2001 Refractory anaemia with excess blasts. In: Jaffe E S, Harris N L, Stein H et al. (ed) World Health Organization classification of tumours. Pathology and genetics of tumours of haematopoietic and lymphoid tissues. IARC Press, Lyon, p 71
23. Mathew P, Tefferi A, Dewald G W et al. 1993 The 5q- syndrome: a single-institution study of 43 consecutive patients. Blood 81: 1040–1045
24. Boultwood J, Lewis S, Wainscoat J S 1994 The 5q- syndrome. Blood 84: 3253–3260
25. Yunis J J, Rydell R E, Oken M M et al. 1986 Refined chromosome analysis as an independent prognostic indicator in de novo myelodysplastic syndromes. Blood 67: 1721–1730
26. Romeo M, Chauffaille M de L, Silva M R et al. 2002 Comparison of cytogenetics with FISH in 40 myelodysplastic syndrome patients. Leuk Res 26: 993–996
27. Ketterling R P, Wyatt W A, VanWier S A et al. 2002 Primary myelodysplastic syndrome with normal cytogenetics: utility of 'FISH panel testing' and M-FISH. Leuk Res 26: 235–240
28. Michels S D, McKenna R W, Arthur D C et al. 1985 Therapy-related acute myeloid leukaemia and myelodysplastic syndrome: a clinical and morphologic study of 65 cases. Blood 65: 1364–1372
29. Le Beau M M, Albain K S, Larson R A et al. 1986 Clinical and cytogenetic correlations in 63 patients with therapy-related myelodysplastic syndromes and acute nonlymphocytic leukemia: further evidence for characteristic abnormalities of chromosomes no. 5 and 7. J Clin Oncol 4: 325–345
30. Jacobs R H, Cornbleet M A, Vardiman J W et al. 1986 Prognostic implications of morphology and karyotype in primary myelodysplastic syndromes. Blood 67: 1765–1772
31. Rios A, Canizo M C, Sanz M A et al. 1990 Bone marrow biopsy in myelodysplastic syndromes: morphological characteristics and contribution to the study of prognostic factors. Br J Haematol 75: 26–33
31a. Vardiman JW, Pierre R, Bain B et al. 2001. Chronic myelomonocytic leukemia. In: Jaffe ES, Harris NL, Stein H, Vardiman JW (eds). World Health Organization Classification of Tumors. Pathology and genetics of tumors of hematopoietic and lymphoid tissues. Lyon, IARC Press, pp. 49–52
32. Surveillance E, and End Results (SEER) Program SEER*Stat Databases 2003 Incidence – SEER 11 regs + AK public-use, Nov 2003 sub for expanded races (1992–2001) and incidence – SEER 11 regs public-use, Nov 2003 sub for Hispanics (1992–2001). In: National Cancer Institute, DCCPS, Surveillance Research Program, Cancer Statistics Branch; released April 2004, based on the November 2003 submission. Available online at: www.seer.cancer.gov
33. Burns C P, Armitage J O, Frey A L et al. 1981 Analysis of the presenting features of adult acute leukemia: the French–American–British classification. Cancer 47: 2460–2469
34. Rowe J M 1983 Clinical and laboratory features of the myeloid and lymphocytic leukemias. Am J Med Technol 49: 103–109
35. Creutzig U, Ritter J, Budde M et al. 1987 Early deaths due to hemorrhage and leukostasis in childhood acute myelogenous leukemia. Associations with hyperleukocytosis and acute monocytic leukemia. Cancer 60: 3071–3079
36. Stanley M, Mckenna R W, Ellinger G et al. 1985 Classification of 358 cases of acute myeloid leukemia by FAB criteria: analysis of clinical and morphologic features. In: Bloomfield C D (ed) Chronic and acute leukemias in adults. Martinus Nihoff, Boston, p 147–174
37. Dutcher J P, Schiffer C A, Wiernik P H et al. 1987 Hyperleukocytosis in adult acute nonlymphocytic leukemia: impact on remission rate and duration, and survival. J Clin Oncol 5: 1364–1372
38. McKee L C Jr, Collins R D 1974 Intravascular leukocyte thrombi and aggregates as a cause of morbidity and mortality in leukemia. Medicine (Baltimore) 53: 463–478
39. Ventura G J, Hester J P, Smith T L et al. 1988 Acute myeloblastic leukemia with hyperleukocytosis: risk factors for early mortality in induction. Am J Hematol 27: 34–37
40. Howe R B, Bloomfield C D, McKenna R W 1982 Hypocellular acute leukemia. Am J Med 72: 391–395
41. Needleman S W, Burns C P, Dick F R et al. 1981 Hypoplastic acute leukemia. Cancer 48: 1410–1414
42. Arber D A, Jenkins K A 1996 Paraffin section immunophenotyping of acute leukemias in bone marrow specimens. Am J Clin Pathol 106: 462–468
43. Arber D A, Stein A S, Carter N H et al. 2003 Prognostic impact of acute myeloid leukemia classification. Importance of detection of recurring cytogenetic abnormalities and multilineage dysplasia on survival. Am J Clin Pathol 119: 672–680
44. Grimwade D, Walker H, Oliver F et al. 1998 The importance of diagnostic cytogenetics on outcome in AML: analysis of 1612 patients entered into the MRC AML 10 trial. The Medical Research Council Adult and Children's Leukaemia Working Parties. Blood 92: 2322–2333
45. Peterson L F, Zhang D E 2004 The 8;21 translocation in leukemogenesis. Oncogene 23: 4255–4262
46. Lowenberg B, Downing J R, Burnett A 1999 Acute myeloid leukemia. N Engl J Med 341: 1051–1062
47. Hiebert S W, Lutterbach B, Amann J 2001 Role of co-repressors in transcriptional repression mediated by the t(8;21), t(16;21), t(12;21), and inv(16) fusion proteins. Curr Opin Hematol 8: 197–200
48. Hiebert S W, Lutterbach B, Durst K et al. 2001 Mechanisms of transcriptional repression by the t(8;21), t(16;21), t(12;21), and inv(16) fusion proteins. Cancer Chemother Pharmacol 48 (suppl 1): S31–S34
49. Amann J M, Nip J, Strom D K et al. 2001 ETO, a target of t(8;21) in acute leukemia, makes distinct contacts with multiple histone deacetylases and binds mSin3A through its oligomerization domain. Mol Cell Biol 21: 6470–6483
50. Meyers S, Lenny N, Hiebert S W 1995 The t(8;21) fusion protein interferes with AML-1B-dependent transcriptional activation. Mol Cell Biol 15: 1974–1982
51. Westendorf J J, Yamamoto C M, Lenny N et al. 1998 The t(8;21) fusion product, AML-1-ETO, associates with C/EBP-alpha, inhibits C/EBP-alpha-dependent transcription, and blocks granulocytic differentiation. Mol Cell Biol 18: 322–333
52. Marcucci G, Caligiuri M A, Bloomfield C D 2000 Molecular and clinical advances in core binding factor primary acute myeloid leukemia: a paradigm for translational research in malignant hematology. Cancer Invest 18: 768–780
53. Bloomfield C D, Lawrence D, Byrd J C et al. 1998 Frequency of prolonged remission duration after high-dose cytarabine intensification in acute myeloid leukemia varies by cytogenetic subtype. Cancer Res 58: 4173–4179
54. Bloomfield C D, Ruppert A S, Mrozek K et al. 2004 Core binding factor acute myeloid leukemia. Cancer and Leukemia Group B (CALGB) study 8461. Ann Hematol 83 (suppl 1): S84–S85
55. Hurwitz C A, Raimondi S C, Head D et al. 1992 Distinctive immunophenotypic features of t(8;21)(q22;q22) acute myeloblastic leukemia in children. Blood 80: 3182–3188
56. Schachner J, Kantarjian H, Dalton W et al. 1988 Cytogenetic association and prognostic significance of bone marrow blast cell terminal transferase in patients with acute myeloblastic leukemia. Leukemia 2: 667–671
57. Mrozek K, Heinonen K, de la Chapelle A et al. 1997 Clinical significance of cytogenetics in acute myeloid leukemia. Semin Oncol 24: 17–31
58. Bitter M A, Le Beau M M, Larson R A et al. 1984 A morphologic and cytochemical study of acute myelomonocytic leukemia with abnormal marrow eosinophils associated with inv(16)(p13q22). Am J Clin Pathol 81: 733–741
59. Jennings C D, Foon K A 1997 Recent advances in flow cytometry: application to the diagnosis of hematologic malignancy. Blood 90: 2863–2892
60. French registry of acute leukemia and myelodysplastic syndromes 1987 Age distribution and hemogram analysis of the 4496 cases recorded during 1982–1983 and classified according to FAB criteria. Groupe Français de Morphologie Hématologique. Cancer 60: 1385–1394
61. Castoldi G L, Liso V, Specchia G et al. 1994 Acute promyelocytic leukemia: morphological aspects. Leukemia 8 (suppl 2): S27–S32
62. Melnick A, Licht J D 1999 Deconstructing a disease: RARalpha, its fusion partners, and their roles in the pathogenesis of acute promyelocytic leukemia. Blood 93: 3167–3215
63. Zelent A, Guidez F, Melnick A et al. 2001 Translocations of the RARalpha gene in acute promyelocytic leukemia. Oncogene 20: 7186–7203
64. Sirulnik A, Melnick A, Zelent A et al. 2003 Molecular pathogenesis of acute promyelocytic leukaemia and APL variants. Best Pract Res Clin Haematol 16: 387–408
65. de The H, Chomienne C, Lanotte M et al. 1990 The t(15;17) translocation of acute promyelocytic leukaemia fuses the retinoic acid receptor alpha gene to a novel transcribed locus. Nature 347: 558–561
66. Chang K S, Stass S A, Chu D T et al. 1992 Characterization of a fusion cDNA (RARA/myl) transcribed from the t(15;17) translocation breakpoint in acute promyelocytic leukemia. Mol Cell Biol 12: 800–810
67. Tallman M S 1996 Differentiating therapy in acute myeloid leukemia. Leukemia 10: 1262–1268
68. Tallman M S 1994 All-trans-retinoic acid in acute promyelocytic leukemia and its potential in other hematologic malignancies. Semin Hematol 31 (suppl 5): 38–48
69. Avvisati G, Tallman M S 2003 All-trans retinoic acid in acute promyelocytic leukaemia. Best Pract Res Clin Haematol 16: 419–432
70. Tallman M S 2004 Acute promyelocytic leukemia as a paradigm for targeted therapy. Semin Hematol 41 (suppl 4): 27–32

71. Redner R L, Rush E A, Faas S et al. 1996 The t(5;17) variant of acute promyelocytic leukemia expresses a nucleophosmin-retinoic acid receptor fusion. Blood 87: 882–886
72. Chen S J, Zelent A, Tong J H et al. 1993 Rearrangements of the retinoic acid receptor alpha and promyelocytic leukemia zinc finger genes resulting from t(11;17)(q23;q21) in a patient with acute promyelocytic leukaemia. J Clin Invest 91: 2260–2267
73. Wells R A, Catzavelos C, Kamel-Reid S 1997 Fusion of retinoic acid receptor alpha to NuMA, the nuclear mitotic apparatus protein, by a variant translocation in acute promyelocytic leukaemia. Nat Genet 17: 109–113
74. Arnould C, Philippe C, Bourdon V et al. 1999 The signal transducer and activator of transcription STAT5b gene is a new partner of retinoic acid receptor alpha in acute promyelocytic-like leukaemia. Hum Mol Genet 8: 1741–1749
75. Shih L Y, Kuo M C, Liang D C et al. 2003 Internal tandem duplication and Asp835 mutations of the FMS-like tyrosine kinase 3 (FLT3) gene in acute promyelocytic leukemia. Cancer 98: 1206–1216
76. Gilliland D G, Griffin J D 2002 Role of FLT3 in leukemia. Curr Opin Hematol 9: 274–281
77. Gilliland D G, Griffin J D 2002 The roles of FLT3 in hematopoiesis and leukemia. Blood 100: 1532–1542
78. Kelly L M, Kutok J L, Williams I R et al. 2002 PML/RARalpha and FLT3-ITD induce an APL-like disease in a mouse model. Proc Natl Acad Sci USA 99: 8283–8288
79. Avvisati G, ten Cate J W, Sturk A et al. 1988 Acquired alpha-2-antiplasmin deficiency in acute promyelocytic leukaemia. Br J Haematol 70: 43–48
80. Avvisati G, Lo Coco F, Mandelli F 2001 Acute promyelocytic leukemia: clinical and morphologic features and prognostic factors. Semin Hematol 38: 4–12
81. Golomb H M, Rowley J D, Vardiman J W et al. 1980 "Microgranular" acute promyelocytic leukemia: a distinct clinical, ultrastructural, and cytogenetic entity. Blood 55: 253–259
82. Savage R A, Hoffman G C, Lucas F V Jr 1981 Morphology and cytochemistry of "microgranular" acute promyelocytic leukemia (FAB M3). Am J Clin Pathol 75: 548–552
83. Orfao A, Chillon M C, Bortoluci A M et al. 1999 The flow cytometric pattern of CD34, CD15 and CD13 expression in acute myeloblastic leukemia is highly characteristic of the presence of PML-RARalpha gene rearrangements. Haematologica 84: 405–412
84. Rizzatti E G, Portieres F L, Martins S L et al. 2004 Microgranular and t(11;17)/PLZF-RARalpha variants of acute promyelocytic leukemia also present the flow cytometric pattern of CD13, CD34, and CD15 expression characteristic of PML-RARalpha gene rearrangement. Am J Hematol 76: 44–51
85. Biondi A, Luciano A, Bassan R et al. 1995 CD2 expression in acute promyelocytic leukemia is associated with microgranular morphology (FAB M3v) but not with any PML gene breakpoint. Leukemia 9: 1461–1466
86. Lin P, Hao S, Medeiros L J et al. 2004 Expression of CD2 in acute promyelocytic leukemia correlates with short form of PML-RARalpha transcripts and poorer prognosis. Am J Clin Pathol 121: 402–407
87. Piedras J, Lopez-Karpovitch X, Cardenas R 1998 Light scatter and immunophenotypic characteristics of blast cells in typical acute promyelocytic leukemia and its variant. Cytometry 32: 286–290
88. Mitelman F, Johansson B, Mertens F 2001 Mitelman database of chromosome aberrations in cancer, 7/2001 update. Available online at: http://cgap.nci.nih.gov/Chromosomes/Mitelman
89. Cox M C, Panetta P, Venditti A et al. 2003 Comparison between conventional banding analysis and FISH screening with an AML-specific set of probes in 260 patients. Hematol J 4: 263–270
90. Brunning R D, Matutes E, Harris N L et al. 2001 Acute myeloid leukemia with multilineage dysplasia. In: Jaffe E S, Harris N L, Stein H et al. (ed) World Health Organization classification of tumours. Pathology and genetics of tumours of haematopoietic and lymphoid tissues. IARC Press, Lyon, p 88–89
91. Gahn B, Haase D, Unterhalt M et al. 1996 De novo AML with dysplastic hematopoiesis: cytogenetic and prognostic significance. Leukemia 10: 946–951
92. Head D R 1996 Revised classification of acute myeloid leukemia. Leukemia 10: 1826–1831
93. Ellis M, Ravid M, Lishner M 1993 A comparative analysis of alkylating agent and epipodophyllotoxin-related leukemias. Leuk Lymphoma 11: 9–13
94. Rund D, Ben-Yehuda D 2004 Therapy-related leukemia and myelodysplasia: evolving concepts of pathogenesis and treatment. Hematology 9: 179–187
95. Pedersen-Bjergaard J, Philip P, Larsen S O et al. 1993 Therapy-related myelodysplasia and acute myeloid leukemia. Cytogenetic characteristics of 115 consecutive cases and risk in seven cohorts of patients treated intensively for malignant diseases in the Copenhagen series. Leukemia 7: 1975–1986
96. Pedersen-Bjergaard J, Andersen M K, Christiansen D H 2000 Therapy-related acute myeloid leukemia and myelodysplasia after high-dose chemotherapy and autologous stem cell transplantation. Blood 95: 3273–3279
97. Bloomfield C D, Archer K J, Mrozek K et al. 2002 11q23 balanced chromosome aberrations in treatment-related myelodysplastic syndromes and acute leukemia: report from an international workshop. Genes Chromos Cancer 33: 362–378
98. Andersen M K, Johansson B, Larsen S O et al. 1998 Chromosomal abnormalities in secondary MDS and AML. Relationship to drugs and radiation with specific emphasis on the balanced rearrangements. Haematologica 83: 483–488
99. Aguiar R C, Chase A, Coulthard S et al. 1997 Abnormalities of chromosome band 8p11 in leukemia: two clinical syndromes can be distinguished on the basis of MOZ involvement. Blood 90: 3130–3135
100. Harrison C J, Cuneo A, Clark R et al. 1998 Ten novel 11q23 chromosomal partner sites. European 11q23 Workshop participants. Leukemia 12: 811–822
101. Swansbury G J, Slater R, Bain B J et al. 1998 Hematological malignancies with t(9;11)(p21-22;q23) – a laboratory and clinical study of 125 cases. European 11q23 Workshop participants. Leukemia 12: 792–800
102. Lillington D M, Young B D, Berger R et al. 1998 The t(10;11)(p12;q23) translocation in acute leukaemia: a cytogenetic and clinical study of 20 patients. European 11q23 Workshop participants. Leukemia 12: 801–804
103. Martineau M, Berger R, Lillington D M et al. 1998 The t(6;11)(q27;q23) translocation in acute leukaemia: a laboratory and clinical study of 30 cases. EU Concerted Action 11q23 Workshop participants. Leukemia 12: 788–791
104. Secker-Walker L M, Moorman A V, Bain B J et al. 1998 Secondary acute leukemia and myelodysplastic syndrome with 11q23 abnormalities. EU Concerted Action 11q23 Workshop. Leukemia 12: 840–844
105. Quesnel B, Kantarjian H, Bjergaard J P et al. 1993 Therapy-related acute myeloid leukemia with t(8;21), inv(16): a report on 25 cases and review of the literature. J Clin Oncol 11: 2370–2379
106. Thiele J, Kvasnicka H M, Schmitt-Graeff A 2004 Acute panmyelosis with myelofibrosis. Leuk Lymphoma 45: 681–687
107. Thiele J, Kvasnicka H M, Zerhusen G et al. 2004 Acute panmyelosis with myelofibrosis: a clinicopathological study on 46 patients including histochemistry of bone marrow biopsies and follow-up. Ann Hematol 83: 513–521
108. Alsabeh R, Brynes R K, Slovak M L et al. 1997 Acute myeloid leukemia with t(6;9) (p23;q34): association with myelodysplasia, basophilia, and initial CD34 negative immunophenotype. Am J Clin Pathol 107: 430–437
109. Carroll A, Civin C, Schneider N et al. 1991 The t(1;22) (p13;q13) is nonrandom and restricted to infants with acute megakaryoblastic leukemia: a Pediatric Oncology Group study. Blood 78: 748–752
110. Lin P, Jones D, Dorfman D M et al. 2000 Precursor B-cell lymphoblastic lymphoma: a predominantly extranodal tumor with low propensity for leukemic involvement. Am J Surg Pathol 24: 1480–1490
111. Cortes J E, Kantarjian H M 1995 Acute lymphoblastic leukemia. A comprehensive review with emphasis on biology and therapy. Cancer 76: 2393–2417
112. Xie Y, Davies S M, Xiang Y et al. 2003 Trends in leukemia incidence and survival in the United States (1973–1998). Cancer 97: 2229–2235
113. Sandler D P, Ross J A 1997 Epidemiology of acute leukemia in children and adults. Semin Oncol 24: 3–16
114. Gajjar A, Ribeiro R C, Mahmoud H H et al. 1996 Overt testicular disease at diagnosis is associated with high risk features and a poor prognosis in patients with childhood acute lymphoblastic leukemia. Cancer 78: 2437–2442
115. Homans A C, Barker B E, Forman E N et al. 1990 Immunophenotypic characteristics of cerebrospinal fluid cells in children with acute lymphoblastic leukemia at diagnosis. Blood 76: 1807–1811
116. Weiss L M, Bindl J M, Picozzi V J et al. 1986 Lymphoblastic lymphoma: an immunophenotype study of 26 cases with comparison to T cell lymphoblastic leukemia. Blood 67: 474–478
117. Schumacher H R, Champion J E, Thomas W J et al. 1979 Acute lymphoblastic leukemia – hand mirror variant. An analysis of a large group of patients. Am J Hematol 7: 11–7
118. Pui C H, Evans W E 1998 Acute lymphoblastic leukemia. N Engl J Med 339: 605–615
119. Romana S P, Poirel H, Leconiat M et al. 1995 High frequency of t(12;21) in childhood B-lineage acute lymphoblastic leukemia. Blood 86: 4263–4269
120. Armstrong S A, Staunton J E, Silverman L B et al. 2002 MLL translocations specify a distinct gene expression profile that distinguishes a unique leukemia. Nat Genet 30: 41–47
121. Armstrong S A, Kung A L, Mabon M E et al. 2003 Inhibition of FLT3 in MLL. Validation of a therapeutic target identified by gene expression based classification. Cancer Cell 3: 173–183
122. Armstrong S A, Mabon M E, Silverman L B et al. 2004 FLT3 mutations in childhood acute lymphoblastic leukemia. Blood 103: 3544–3546
123. Groupe Français de Cytogenétique Hématologique. 1996 Cytogenetic abnormalities in adult acute lymphoblastic leukemia: correlations with hematologic findings outcome. A Collaborative Study of the Group Français de Cytogénétique Hématologique. Blood 87: 3135–3142
124. Wetzler M, Dodge R K, Mrozek K et al. 1999 Prospective karyotype analysis in adult acute lymphoblastic leukemia: the cancer and leukemia group B experience. Blood 93: 3983–3993
125. Pui C H, Relling M V, Downing J R 2004 Acute lymphoblastic leukemia. N Engl J Med 350: 1535–1548
126. Pui C H, Cheng C, Leung W et al. 2003 Extended follow-up of long-term survivors of childhood acute lymphoblastic leukemia. N Engl J Med 349: 640–649
127. Copelan E A, McGuire E A 1995 The biology and treatment of acute lymphoblastic leukemia in adults. Blood 85: 1151–1168

128. Davis R E, Longacre T A, Cornbleet P J 1994 Hematogones in the bone marrow of adults. Immunophenotypic features, clinical settings, and differential diagnosis. Am J Clin Pathol 102: 202–211
129. Rimsza L M, Larson R S, Winter S S et al. 2000 Benign hematogone-rich lymphoid proliferations can be distinguished from B-lineage acute lymphoblastic leukemia by integration of morphology, immunophenotype, adhesion molecule expression, and architectural features. Am J Clin Pathol 114: 66–75
130. Longacre T A, Foucar K, Crago S et al. 1989 Hematogones: a multiparameter analysis of bone marrow precursor cells. Blood 73: 543–552
131. Pui C H, Behm F G, Singh B et al. 1990 Heterogeneity of presenting features and their relation to treatment outcome in 120 children with T-cell acute lymphoblastic leukemia. Blood 75: 174–179
132. Sen L, Borella L 1975 Clinical importance of lymphoblasts with T markers in childhood acute leukemia. N Engl J Med 292: 828–832
133. Xiao S, Nalabolu S R, Aster J C et al. 1998 FGFR1 is fused with a novel zinc-finger gene, ZNF198, in the t(8;13) leukaemia/lymphoma syndrome. Nat Genet 18: 84–87
134. Somers G R, Slater H, Rockman S et al. 1997 Coexistent T-cell lymphoblastic lymphoma and an atypical myeloproliferative disorder associated with t(8;13)(p21;q14). Pediatr Pathol Lab Med 17: 141–158
135. Inhorn R C, Aster J C, Roach S A et al. 1995 A syndrome of lymphoblastic lymphoma, eosinophilia, and myeloid hyperplasia/malignancy associated with t(8;13)(p11;q11): description of a distinctive clinicopathologic entity. Blood 85: 1881–1887
136. McKenna R W, Parkin J, Brunning R D 1979 Morphologic and ultrastructural characteristics of T-cell acute lymphoblastic leukemia. Cancer 44: 1290–1297
137. Pui C H, Raimondi S C, Head D R et al. 1991 Characterization of childhood acute leukemia with multiple myeloid and lymphoid markers at diagnosis and at relapse. Blood 78: 1327–1337
138. Pui C H, Behm F G, Crist W M 1993 Clinical and biologic relevance of immunologic marker studies in childhood acute lymphoblastic leukemia. Blood 82: 343–362
139. Weng A P, Ferrando A A, Lee W et al. 2004 Activating mutations of NOTCH1 in human T cell acute lymphoblastic leukemia. Science 306: 269–271
140. Savage D G, Szydlo R M, Goldman J M 1997 Clinical features at diagnosis in 430 patients with chronic myeloid leukaemia seen at a referral centre over a 16-year period. Br J Haematol 96: 111–116
141. Faderl S, Talpaz M, Estrov Z et al. 1999 Chronic myelogenous leukemia: biology and therapy. Ann Intern Med 131: 207–219
142. Bergsagel D E 1967 The chronic leukemias: a review of disease manifestations and the aims of therapy. Can Med Assoc J 96: 1615–1620
143. Spiers A S, Bain B J, Turner J E 1977 The peripheral blood in chronic granulocytic leukaemia. Study of 50 untreated Philadelphia-positive cases. Scand J Haematol 18: 25–38
144. Vardiman J W, Pierre R, Thiele J et al. 2001 Chronic myelogenous leukaemia. In: Jaffe E S, Harris N L, Stein H et al. (ed) World Health Organization classification of tumours. Pathology and genetics of tumours of haematopoietic and lymphoid tissues. IARC Press, Lyon, p 20–26
145. Frater J L, Tallman M S, Variakojis D et al. 2003 Chronic myeloid leukemia following therapy with imatinib mesylate (Gleevec). Bone marrow histopathology and correlation with genetic status. Am J Clin Pathol 119: 833–841
146. Hasserjian R P, Boecklin F, Parker S et al. 2002 STI571 (imatinib mesylate) reduces bone marrow cellularity and normalizes morphologic features irrespective of cytogenetic response. Am J Clin Pathol 117: 360–367
147. Sessarego M, Panarello C, Coviello D A et al. 1987 Karyotype evolution in CML: high frequency of translocations other than the Ph. Cancer Genet Cytogenet 25: 73–80
148. Chen J, Deangelo D J, Kutok J L et al. 2004 PKC412 inhibits the zinc finger 198-fibroblast growth factor receptor 1 fusion tyrosine kinase and is active in treatment of stem cell myeloproliferative disorder. Proc Natl Acad Sci USA 101: 14479–14484
149. Cools J, DeAngelo D J, Gotlib J et al. 2003 A tyrosine kinase created by fusion of the PDGFRA and FIP1L1 genes as a therapeutic target of imatinib in idiopathic hypereosinophilic syndrome. N Engl J Med 348: 1201–1214
150. Weller P F, Bubley G J 1994 The idiopathic hypereosinophilic syndrome. Blood 83: 2759–2779
151. Fauci A S, Harley J B, Roberts W C et al. 1982 NIH conference. The idiopathic hypereosinophilic syndrome. Clinical, pathophysiologic, and therapeutic considerations. Ann Intern Med 97: 78–92
152. Tanino M, Kitamura K, Ohta G et al. 1983 Hypereosinophilic syndrome with extensive myocardial involvement and mitral valve thrombus instead of mural thrombi. Acta Pathol Jpn 33: 1233–1242
153. Ommen S R, Seward J B, Tajik A J 2000 Clinical and echocardiographic features of hypereosinophilic syndromes. Am J Cardiol 86: 110–113
154. Radford D J, Garlick R B, Pohlner P G 2002 Multiple valvar replacements for hypereosinophilic syndrome. Cardiol Young 12: 67–70
155. Gotlib J, Cools J, Malone J M et al. 2003 The FIP1L1-PDGFRα fusion tyrosine kinase in hypereosinophilic syndrome and chronic eosinophilic leukemia: implications for diagnosis, classification, and management. Blood 103: 2879–2891
156. Brito-Babapulle F 1997 Clonal eosinophilic disorders and the hypereosinophilic syndrome. Blood Rev 11: 129–145
157. Spry C J, Davies J, Tai P C et al. 1983 Clinical features of fifteen patients with the hypereosinophilic syndrome. Q J Med 52: 1–22
158. Spry C J 1982 The hypereosinophilic syndrome: clinical features, laboratory findings and treatment. Allergy 37: 539–551
159. Schooley R T, Flaum M A, Gralnick H R et al. 1981 A clinicopathologic correlation of the idiopathic hypereosinophilic syndrome. II. Clinical manifestations. Blood 58: 1021–1026
160. Chusid M J, Dale D C, West B C et al. 1975 The hypereosinophilic syndrome: analysis of fourteen cases with review of the literature. Medicine (Baltimore) 54: 1–27
161. Ghosh K, Shome D K, Marwaha N et al. 1985 Normal plasma levels of B12 binding proteins in hypereosinophilic syndrome and secondary hypereosinophilia. Blood 65: 510–511
162. Zittoun J, Farcet J P, Marquet J et al. 1984 Cobalamin (vitamin B12) and B12 binding proteins in hypereosinophilic syndromes and secondary eosinophilia. Blood 63: 779–783
163. Vandenberghe P, Wlodarska I, Michaux L et al. 2004 Clinical and molecular features of FIP1L1-PDGFRA (+) chronic eosinophilic leukemias. Leukemia 18: 734–742
164. Parrillo J E, Fauci A S, Wolff S M 1978 Therapy of the hypereosinophilic syndrome. Ann Intern Med 89: 167–172
165. Flaum M A, Schooley R T, Fauci A S et al. 1981 A clinicopathologic correlation of the idiopathic hypereosinophilic syndrome. I. Hematologic manifestations. Blood 58: 1012–1020
166. Brunning R D, McKenna R W 1994 Tumors of the bone marrow. Hypereosinophilic syndrome. In: Atlas of Tumor Pathology, third series. Armed Forces Instititute of Pathology, Washington, D C, p 246–250
167. Pardanani A, Brockman S R, Paternoster S F et al. 2004 FIP1L1-PDGFRA fusion: prevalence and clinicopathologic correlates in 89 consecutive patients with moderate to severe eosinophilia. Blood 104: 3038–3045
168. Goldman J M, Melo J V 2003 Chronic myeloid leukemia – advances in biology and new approaches to treatment. N Engl J Med 349: 1451–1464
169. Bain B 2004 The idiopathic hypereosinophilic syndrome and eosinophilic leukemias. Haematologica 89: 133–137
170. Pardanani A, Ketterling R P, Brockman S R et al. 2003 CHIC2 deletion, a surrogate for FIP1L1-PDGFRA fusion, occurs in systemic mastocytosis associated with eosinophilia and predicts response to imatinib mesylate therapy. Blood 102: 3093–3096
171. Spivak J L 2002 Polycythemia vera: myths, mechanisms, and management. Blood 100: 4272–4290
171a. Baxter EJ, Scott LM, Campbell PJ et al. 2005. Acquired mutation of the tyrosine kinase JAK2 in human myeloproliferative disorders. Lancet 365: 1054–1061
171b. Levine RL, Wadleigh M, Cools J et al. 2005. Activating mutation in the tyrosine kinase JAK2 in polycythemia vera, essential thrombocythemia and myeloid metaplasia with myelofibrosis. Cancer Cell 7: 387–397
171c. James C, Ugo V, Le Couedic JP et al. 2005. A unique clonal JAK2 mutation leading to constitutive signalling causes polycythemia vera. Nature 434: 1144–1148
171d. Kralovics R, Passamonti F, Buser AS et al. 2005. A gain-of-function mutation of JAK2 in myeloproliferative disorders. N Engl J Med 352: 1779–1790
171e. Jones AV, Kreil S, Zoi K et al. 2005. Widespread occurrence of the JAK2 V617F mutation in chromic myeloproliferative disorders. Blood 106: 2162–2168
172. Tefferi A 2003 Polycythemia vera: a comprehensive review and clinical recommendations. Mayo Clin Proc 78: 174–194
173. Modan B 1965 An epidemiological study of polycythemia vera. Blood 1965;26: 657–667
174. Najean Y, Rain J D, Billotey C 1998 Epidemiological data in polycythaemia vera: a study of 842 cases. Hematol Cell Ther 40: 159–165
175. Gruppo Italiano Studio Policitemia 1995 Polycythemia vera: the natural history of 1213 patients followed for 20 years. Ann Intern Med 123: 656–664
176. Landolfi R, Marchioli R, Kutti J et al. 2004 Efficacy and safety of low-dose aspirin in polycythemia vera. N Engl J Med 350: 114–124
177. Najean Y, Rain J D 1997 The very long-term evolution of polycythemia vera: an analysis of 318 patients initially treated by phlebotomy or 32P between 1969 and 1981. Semin Hematol 34: 6–16
178. Orlandi E, Castelli G, Brusamolino E et al. 1989 Hemorrhagic and thrombotic complications in polycythemia vera. A clinical study. Haematologica 74: 45–49
179. Michiels J J, van Genderen P J, Lindemans J et al. 1996 Erythromelalgic, thrombotic and hemorrhagic manifestations in 50 cases of thrombocythemia. Leuk Lymphoma 22 (suppl 1): 47–56
180. Murphy S 1999 Diagnostic criteria and prognosis in polycythemia vera and essential thrombocythemia. Semin Hematol 36 (suppl 2): 9–13
181. Thiele J, Zankovich R, Schneider G et al. 1988 Primary (essential) thrombocythemia versus polycythemia vera rubra. A histomorphometric analysis of bone marrow features in trephine biopsies. Anal Quant Cytol Histol 10: 375–382
182. Thiele J, Kvasnicka H M, Zankovich R et al. 2001 The value of bone marrow histology in differentiating between early stage polycythemia vera and secondary (reactive) polycythemias. Haematologica 86: 368–374
183. Thiele J, Kvasnicka H M, Fischer R 1999 Histochemistry and morphometry on bone marrow biopsies in chronic myeloproliferative disorders – aids to diagnosis and classification. Ann Hematol 78: 495–506

184. Perkins J, Israels M C G, Wilkinson J F 1964 Polycythemia vera: clinical studies on a series of 127 patients managed without radiation therapy. Q J Med 33: 499–518
185. Modan B, Lilienfeld A M 1965 Polycythemia vera and leukemia – the role of radiation treatment. A study of 1222 patients. Medicine (Baltimore) 44: 305–344
186. Landaw S A 1986 Acute leukemia in polycythemia vera. Semin Hematol 23: 156–165
187. Wolf B C, Banks P M, Mann R B et al. 1988 Splenic hematopoiesis in polycythemia vera. A morphologic and immunohistologic study. Am J Clin Pathol 89: 69–75
188. Diez-Martin J L, Graham D L, Petitt R M et al. 1991 Chromosome studies in 104 patients with polycythemia vera. Mayo Clin Proc 66: 287–299
189. Rege-Cambrin G, Mecucci C, Tricot G et al. 1987 A chromosomal profile of polycythemia vera. Cancer Genet Cytogenet 25: 233–245
190. Swolin B, Weinfeld A, Westin J 1988 A prospective long-term cytogenetic study in polycythemia vera in relation to treatment and clinical course. Blood 72: 386–395
191. Murphy S, Iland H, Rosenthal D et al. 1986 Essential thrombocythemia: an interim report from the Polycythemia Vera Study Group. Semin Hematol 23: 177–182
192. Murphy S, Peterson P, Iland H et al. 1997 Experience of the Polycythemia Vera Study Group with essential thrombocythemia: a final report on diagnostic criteria, survival, and leukemic transition by treatment. Semin Hematol 34: 29–39
193. Thiele J, Kvasnicka H M 2003 Chronic myeloproliferative disorders with thrombocythemia: a comparative study of two classification systems (PVSG, WHO) on 839 patients. Ann Hematol 82: 148–152
194. Tefferi A 2001 Chronic myeloid disorders: classification and treatment overview. Semin Hematol 38 (suppl 2): 1–4
195. Kondo T, Okabe M, Sanada M et al. 1998 Familial essential thrombocytemia associated with one-base deletion in the 5′-untranslated region of the thrombopoietin gene. Blood 92: 1091–1096
196. Ding J, Komatsu H, Wakita A et al. 2004 Familial essential thrombocytemia associated with a dominant-positive activating mutation of the c-MPL gene, which encodes for the receptor for thrombopoietin. Blood 103: 4198–4200
197. Allen A J, Gale R E, Harrison C N et al. 2001 Lack of pathogenic mutations in the 5′-untranslated region of the thrombopoietin gene in patients with non-familial essential thrombocythaemia. Eur J Haematol 67: 232–237
198. Mesa R A, Silverstein M N, Jacobsen S J et al. 1999 Population-based incidence and survival figures in essential thrombocythemia and agnogenic myeloid metaplasia: an Olmsted County Study, 1976–1995. Am J Hematol 61: 10–15
199. Dror Y, Zipursky A, Blanchette V S 1999 Essential thrombocythemia in children. J Pediatr Hematol Oncol 21: 356–363
200. Fenaux P, Simon M, Caulier M T et al. 1990 Clinical course of essential thrombocythemia in 147 cases. Cancer 66: 549–556
201. Bellucci S, Janvier M, Tobelem G et al. 1986 Essential thrombocythemias. Clinical evolutionary and biological data. Cancer 58: 2440–2447
202. Jantunen E, Juvonen E, Ikkala E et al. 1998 Essential thrombocythemia at diagnosis: causes of diagnostic evaluation and presence of positive diagnostic findings. Ann Hematol 77: 101–106
203. Colombi M, Radaelli F, Zocchi L et al. 1991 Thrombotic and hemorrhagic complications in essential thrombocythemia. A retrospective study of 103 patients. Cancer 67: 2926–2930
204. Michiels J J 2004 Bone marrow histopathology and biological markers as specific clues to the differential diagnosis of essential thrombocythemia, polycythemia vera and prefibrotic or fibrotic agnogenic myeloid metaplasia. Hematol J 5: 93–102
205. Sterkers Y, Preudhomme C, Lai J L et al. 1998 Acute myeloid leukemia and myelodysplastic syndromes following essential thrombocythemia treated with hydroxyurea: high proportion of cases with 17p deletion. Blood 91: 616–622
206. el Kassar N, Hetet G, Li Y et al. 1995 Clonal analysis of haemopoietic cells in essential thrombocythaemia. Br J Haematol 90: 131–137
207. el-Kassar N, Hetet G, Briere J et al. 1998 Clonality analysis of hematopoiesis and thrombopoietin levels in patients with essential thrombocythemia. Leuk Lymphoma 30: 181–188
208. Mitelman F 1981 The Third International Workshop on Chromosomes in Leukemia. Lund, Sweden, July 21–25, 1980. Introduction. Cancer Genet Cytogenet 4: 96–98
209. Sessarego M, Defferrari R, Dejana A M et al. 1989 Cytogenetic analysis in essential thrombocythemia at diagnosis and at transformation. A 12-year study. Cancer Genet Cytogenet 43: 57–65
210. Elis A, Amiel A, Manor Y et al. 1996 The detection of trisomies 8 and 9 in patients with essential thrombocytosis by fluorescence in situ hybridization. Cancer Genet Cytogenet 92: 14–17
211. Swolin B, Safai-Kutti S, Anghem E et al. 2001 No increased frequency of trisomies 8 and 9 by fluorescence in situ hybridization in untreated patients with essential thrombocythemia. Cancer Genet Cytogenet 126: 56–59
212. Thiele J, Kvasnicka H M 2003 Diagnostic differentiation of essential thrombocythaemia from thrombocythaemias associated with chronic idiopathic myelofibrosis by discriminate analysis of bone marrow features – a clinicopathological study on 272 patients. Histol Histopathol 18: 93–102
213. Tefferi A 1999 Risk-based management in essential thrombocytemia. In: Schechter G P, Hoffman R, Schrier S L (ed) Hematology 1999: American Society of Hematology education program book. American Society of Hematology, Washington, D C, p 172–177
214. Gupta R, Abdalla S H, Bain B J 1999 Thrombocytosis with sideroblastic erythropoiesis: a mixed myeloproliferative myelodysplastic syndrome. Leuk Lymphoma 34: 615–619
215. Thiele J, Kvasnicka H M, Boeltken B et al. 1999 Initial (prefibrotic) stages of idiopathic (primary) myelofibrosis (IMF) – a clinicopathological study. Leukemia 13: 1741–1748
216. Buhr T, Georgii A, Choritz H 1993 Myelofibrosis in chronic myeloproliferative disorders. Incidence among subtypes according to the Hannover classification. Pathol Res Pract 189: 121–132
217. Jacobson R J, Salo A, Fialkow P J 1978 Agnogenic myeloid metaplasia: a clonal proliferation of hematopoietic stem cells with secondary myelofibrosis. Blood 51: 189–194
218. Buschle M, Janssen J W, Drexler H et al. 1988 Evidence for pluripotent stem cell origin of idiopathic myelofibrosis: clonal analysis of a case characterized by a N-ras gene mutation. Leukemia 2: 658–660
219. Tefferi A 2000 Myelofibrosis with myeloid metaplasia. N Engl J Med 342: 1255–1265
220. McNally R J, Rowland D, Roman E 1997 Age and sex distributions of hematological malignancies in the UK. Hematol Oncol 15: 173–189
221. Ridell B, Carneskog J, Wedel H et al. 2000 Incidence of chronic myeloproliferative disorders in the city of Goteborg, Sweden 1983–1992. Eur J Haematol 65: 267–271
222. Dupriez B, Morel P, Demory J L et al. 1996 Prognostic factors in agnogenic myeloid metaplasia: a report on 195 cases with a new scoring system. Blood 88: 1013–1018
223. Cervantes F, Pereira A, Esteve J et al. 1997 Identification of 'short-lived' and 'long-lived' patients at presentation of idiopathic myelofibrosis. Br J Haematol 97: 635–640
224. Cervantes F, Barosi G, Hernandez-Boluda J C et al. 2001 Myelofibrosis with myeloid metaplasia in adult individuals 30 years old or younger: presenting features, evolution and survival. Eur J Haematol 66: 324–327
225. Cervantes F, Barosi G, Demory J L et al. 1998 Myelofibrosis with myeloid metaplasia in young individuals: disease characteristics, prognostic factors and identification of risk groups. Br J Haematol 102: 684–690
226. Thiele J, Steinberg T, Zankovich R et al. 1989 Primary myelofibrosis-osteomyelosclerosis (agnogenic myeloid metaplasia): correlation of clinical findings with bone marrow histopathology and prognosis. Anticancer Res 9: 429–435
227. Tzankov A, Krugmann J, Steurer M et al. 2002 Idiopathic myelofibrosis with nodal, serosal and parenchymatous infiltration. Case report and review of the literature. Acta Haematol 107: 173–176
228. Stahl S M, Ellinger G, Baringer J R 1979 Progressive myelopathy due to extramedullary hematopoiesis: case report and review of the literature. Ann Neurol 5: 485–489
229. Oesterling J E, Keating J P, Leroy A J et al. 1992 Idiopathic myelofibrosis with myeloid metaplasia involving the renal pelves, ureters and bladder. J Urol 147: 1360–1362
230. Brown J A, Gomez-Leon G 1984 Subdural hemorrhage secondary to extramedullary hematopoiesis in postpolycythemic myeloid metaplasia. Neurosurgery 14: 588–591
231. Thiele J, Kvasnicka H M, Zankovich R et al. 2001 Clinical and morphological criteria for the diagnosis of prefibrotic idiopathic (primary) myelofibrosis. Ann Hematol 80: 160–165
232. Thiele J, Kvasnicka H M, Zankovich R et al. 2002 Early-stage idiopathic (primary) myelofibrosis – current issues of diagnostic features. Leuk Lymphoma 43: 1035–1041
233. Reilly J T, Snowden J A, Spearing R L et al. 1997 Cytogenetic abnormalities and their prognostic significance in idiopathic myelofibrosis: a study of 106 cases. Br J Haematol 98: 96–102
234. Tefferi A, Mesa R A, Schroeder G et al. 2001 Cytogenetic findings and their clinical relevance in myelofibrosis with myeloid metaplasia. Br J Haematol 113: 763–771
235. Demory J L, Dupriez B, Fenaux P et al. 1988 Cytogenetic studies and their prognostic significance in agnogenic myeloid metaplasia: a report on 47 cases. Blood 72: 855–859
236. Kyle R A, Gertz M A, Witzig T E et al. 2003 Review of 1027 patients with newly diagnosed multiple myeloma. Mayo Clin Proc 78: 21–33
237. Greenlee R T, Hill-Harmon M B, Murray T et al. 2001 Cancer statistics, 2001. CA Cancer J Clin 51: 15–36
238. Peterson L C, Brown B A, Crosson J T et al. 1986 Application of the immunoperoxidase technique to bone marrow trephine biopsies in the classification of patients with monoclonal gammopathies. Am J Clin Pathol 85: 688–693
239. Dewald G W, Kyle R A, Hicks G A et al. 1985 The clinical significance of cytogenetic studies in 100 patients with multiple myeloma, plasma cell leukemia, or amyloidosis. Blood 66: 380–390
240. Gould J, Alexanian R, Goodacre A et al. 1988 Plasma cell karyotype in multiple myeloma. Blood 71: 453–456
241. Lai J L, Zandecki M, Mary J Y et al. 1995 Improved cytogenetics in multiple myeloma: a study of 151 patients including 117 patients at diagnosis. Blood 85: 2490–2497
242. Sawyer J R, Waldron J A, Jagannath S et al. 1995 Cytogenetic findings in 200 patients with multiple myeloma. Cancer Genet Cytogenet 82: 41–49
243. Ferti A, Panani A, Arapakis G et al. 1984 Cytogenetic study in multiple myeloma. Cancer Genet Cytogenet 12: 247–253

244. Hideshima T, Bergsagel P L, Kuehl W M et al. 2004 Advances in biology of multiple myeloma: clinical applications. Blood 104: 607–618
245. Hallek M, Bergsagel P L, Anderson K C 1998 Multiple myeloma: increasing evidence for a multistep transformation process. Blood 91: 3–21
246. Bergsagel P L, Kuehl W M 2001 Chromosome translocations in multiple myeloma. Oncogene 20: 5611–5622
247. Smadja N V, Leroux D, Soulier J et al. 2003 Further cytogenetic characterization of multiple myeloma confirms that 14q32 translocations are a very rare event in hyperdiploid cases. Genes Chromosomes Cancer 38: 234–239
248. Fonseca R, Debes-Marun C S, Picken E B et al. 2003 The recurrent IgH translocations are highly associated with nonhyperdiploid variant multiple myeloma. Blood 102: 2562–2567
249. Blayney D W, Jaffe E S, Fisher R I et al. 1983 The human T-cell leukemia/lymphoma virus, lymphoma, lytic bone lesions, and hypercalcemia. Ann Intern Med 98: 144–151
250. Yamaguchi K, Watanabe T 2002 Human T lymphotropic virus type-I and adult T-cell leukemia in Japan. Int J Hematol 76 (suppl 2): 240–245
251. Yamaguchi K 1994 Human T-lymphotropic virus type I in Japan. Lancet 343: 213–216
252. Mahieux R, Gessain A 2003 HTLV-1 and associated adult T-cell leukemia/lymphoma. Rev Clin Exp Hematol 7: 336–361
253. Bunn P A Jr, Schechter G P, Jaffe E et al. 1983 Clinical course of retrovirus-associated adult T-cell lymphoma in the United States. N Engl J Med 309: 257–264
254. Jaffe E S, Blattner W A, Blayney D W et al. 1984 The pathologic spectrum of adult T-cell leukemia/lymphoma in the United States. Human T-cell leukemia/lymphoma virus-associated lymphoid malignancies. Am J Surg Pathol 8: 263–275
255. Forconi F, Sahota S S, Raspadori D et al. 2004 Hairy cell leukemia: at the cross road of somatic mutation and isotype switch. Blood 104: 3312–3317
256. Basso K, Liso A, Tiacci E et al. 2004 Gene expression profiling of hairy cell leukemia reveals a phenotype related to memory B cells with altered expression of chemokine and adhesion receptors. J Exp Med 199: 59–68
257. Maloum K, Magnac C, Azgui Z et al. 1998 VH gene expression in hairy cell leukaemia. Br J Haematol 101: 171–178
258. Wagner S D, Martinelli V, Luzzatto L 1994 Similar patterns of V kappa gene usage but different degrees of somatic mutation in hairy cell leukemia, prolymphocytic leukemia, Waldenström's macroglobulinemia, and myeloma. Blood 83: 3647–3653
259. Tallman M S, Peterson L C, Hakimian D et al. 1999 Treatment of hairy-cell leukemia: current views. Semin Hematol 36: 155–163
260. Schiller G, Said J, Pal S 2003 Hairy cell leukemia and sarcoidosis: a case report and review of the literature. Leukemia 17: 2057–2059
261. Staines A, Cartwright R A 1993 Hairy cell leukaemia: descriptive epidemiology and a case-control study. Br J Haematol 85: 714–717
262. Bouroncle B A 1979 Leukemic reticuloendotheliosis (hairy cell leukemia). Blood 53: 412–436
263. Golomb H M, Catovsky D, Golde D W 1978 Hairy cell leukemia: a clinical review based on 71 cases. Ann Intern Med 89: 677–683
264. Flandrin G, Sigaux F, Sebahoun G et al. 1984 Hairy cell leukemia: clinical presentation and follow-up of 211 patients. Semin Oncol 11 (suppl 2): 458–471
265. Burke J S, Byrne G E Jr, Rappaport H 1974 Hairy cell leukemia (leukemic reticuloendotheliosis). I. A clinical pathologic study of 21 patients. Cancer 33: 1399–1410
266. Frassoldati A, Lamparelli T, Federico M et al. 1994 Hairy cell leukemia: a clinical review based on 725 cases of the Italian Cooperative Group (ICGHCL). Italian Cooperative Group for Hairy Cell Leukemia. Leuk Lymphoma 13: 307–316
267. Golomb H M, Hadad L J 1984 Infectious complications in 127 patients with hairy cell leukemia. Am J Hematol 16: 393–401
268. Burke J S, Rappaport H 1984 The diagnosis and differential diagnosis of hairy cell leukemia in bone marrow and spleen. Semin Oncol 11: 334–346
269. Brunning R D, McKenna R W 1994 Tumors of the bone marrow. Hairy cell leukemia. In: Atlas of Tumor Pathology, third series. Armed Forces Institutte of Pathology, Washington, D C, p 276–287
270. Paoletti M, Bitter M A, Vardiman J W 1988 Hairy-cell leukemia. Morphologic, cytochemical, and immunologic features. Clin Lab Med 8: 179–95
271. Hasserjian R P, Pinkus G P 1994 DBA.44. An effective marker for detection of hairy cell leukemia in bone marrow biopsies. Appl Immunohisto 2: 197–204
272. Cawley J C, Burns G F, Hayhoe F G 1980 A chronic lymphoproliferative disorder with distinctive features: a distinct variant of hairy-cell leukemia. Leuk Res 4: 547–559
273. Sainati L, Matutes E, Mulligan S et al. 1990 A variant form of hairy cell leukemia resistant to alpha-interferon: clinical and phenotypic characteristics of 17 patients. Blood 76: 157–162
274. Redaelli A, Laskin B L, Stephens J M et al. 2004 The clinical and epidemiological burden of chronic lymphocytic leukaemia. Eur J Cancer Care (Engl) 13: 279–287
275. Muller-Hermelink H K, Catovsky D, Montserrat E et al. 2001 Chronic lymphocytic leukaemia/small lymphocytic lymphoma. In: Jaffe E S, Harris N L, Stein H et al. (eds) World Health Organization classification of tumours. Pathology and genetics of tumours of haematopoietic and lymphoid tissues. IARC, Lyon, p. 127–130
276. Pangalis G A, Roussou P A, Kittas C et al. 1984 Patterns of bone marrow involvement in chronic lymphocytic leukemia and small lymphocytic (well differentiated) non-Hodgkin's lymphoma. Its clinical significance in relation to their differential diagnosis and prognosis. Cancer 54: 702–708
277. Lipshutz M D, Mir R, Rai K R et al. 1980 Bone marrow biopsy and clinical staging in chronic lymphocytic leukemia. Cancer 46: 1422–1427
278. Harousseau J L, Flandrin G, Tricot G et al. 1981 Malignant lymphoma supervening in chronic lymphocytic leukemia and related disorders. Richter's syndrome: a study of 25 cases. Cancer 48: 1302–1308
279. Chen C C, Raikow R B, Sonmez-Alpan E et al. 2000 Classification of small B-cell lymphoid neoplasms using a paraffin section immunohistochemical panel. Appl Immunohistochem Mol Morphol 8: 1–11
280. Juliusson G, Oscier DG, Fitchett M et al. 1990 Prognostic subgroups in B-cell chronic lymphocytic leukemia defined by specific chromosomal abnormalities. N Engl J Med 323: 720–724
281. Fais F, Ghiotto F, Hashimoto S et al. 1998 Chronic lymphocytic leukemia B cells express restricted sets of mutated and unmutated antigen receptors. J Clin Invest 102: 1515–1525
282. Hamblin T J, Davis Z, Gardiner A et al. 1999 Unmutated Ig V(H) genes are associated with a more aggressive form of chronic lymphocytic leukemia. Blood 94: 1848–1854
283. Oscier DG, Gardiner AC, Mould SJ et al. 1997 Multivariate analysis of prognostic factors in CLL: clinical stage, IGVH gene mutational status and loss or mutation of the p53 gene are independent prognostic factors. Blood 100: 1177–1184
284. Rassenti LZ, Huynh L, Toy TL et al. 2004 ZAP-70 compared with immunoglobulin heavy-chain gene mutation status as a predictor of disease progression in chronic lymphocytic leukemia. N Engl J Med 351: 893–901
285. Crespo M, Bosch F, Villamor N et al. 2003 ZAP-70 expression as a surrogate for immunoglobulin-variable-region mutations in chronic lymphocytic leukemia. N Engl J Med 348: 1764–1775
286. Melo J V, Catovsky D, Galton D A 1986 The relationship between chronic lymphocytic leukaemia and prolymphocytic leukaemia. I. Clinical and laboratory features of 300 patients and characterization of an intermediate group. Br J Haematol 63: 377–387
287. Stone R M 1990 Prolymphocytic leukemia. Hematol Oncol Clin North Am 4: 457–471
288. Melo J V, Catovsky D, Gregory W M et al. 1987 The relationship between chronic lymphocytic leukaemia and prolymphocytic leukaemia. IV. Analysis of survival and prognostic features. Br J Haematol 65: 23–29
289. Galton D A, Goldman J M, Wiltshaw E et al. 1974 Prolymphocytic leukaemia. Br J Haematol 27: 7–23
290. Bearman R M, Pangalis G A, Rappaport H 1978 Prolymphocytic leukemia: clinical, histopathological, and cytochemical observations. Cancer 42: 2360–2372
291. Melo J V, Wardle J, Chetty M et al. 1986 The relationship between chronic lymphocytic leukaemia and prolymphocytic leukaemia. III. Evaluation of cell size by morphology and volume measurements. Br J Haematol 64: 469–478
292. Ruchlemer R, Parry-Jones N, Brito-Babapulle V et al. 2004 B-prolymphocytic leukaemia with t(11;14) revisited: a splenomegalic form of mantle cell lymphoma evolving with leukaemia. Br J Haematol 125: 330–336
293. Lens D, De Schouwer P J, Hamoudi R A et al. 1997 p53 abnormalities in B-cell prolymphocytic leukemia. Blood 89: 2015–2023
294. Lens D, Matutes E, Catovsky D et al. 2000 Frequent deletions at 11q23 and 13q14 in B cell prolymphocytic leukemia (B-PLL). Leukemia 14: 427–432
295. Matutes E, Brito-Babapulle V, Swansbury J et al. 1991 Clinical and laboratory features of 78 cases of T-prolymphocytic leukemia. Blood 78: 3269–3274
296. Matutes E 1998 T-cell Prolymphocytic leukemia. Cancer Control 5: 19–24
297. Stoppa-Lyonnet D, Soulier J, Lauge A et al. 1998 Inactivation of the ATM gene in T-cell prolymphocytic leukemias. Blood 91: 3920–3926
298. Stilgenbauer S, Schaffner C, Litterst A et al. 1997 Biallelic mutations in the ATM gene in T-prolymphocytic leukemia. Nat Med 3: 1155–1159
299. Vorechovsky I, Luo L, Dyer M J et al. 1997 Clustering of missense mutations in the ataxia-telangiectasia gene in a sporadic T-cell leukaemia. Nat Genet 17: 96–99
300. Matutes E, Garcia Talavera J, O'Brien M et al. 1986 The morphological spectrum of T-prolymphocytic leukaemia. Br J Haematol 64: 111–124
301. Maljaei S H, Brito-Babapulle V, Hiorns L R et al. 1998 Abnormalities of chromosomes 8, 11, 14, and X in T-prolymphocytic leukemia studied by fluorescence in situ hybridization. Cancer Genet Cytogenet 103: 110–116
302. Pekarsky Y, Hallas C, Croce C M 2001 Molecular basis of mature T-cell leukemia. JAMA 286: 2308–2314
303. Pekarsky Y, Hallas C, Isobe M et al. 1999 Abnormalities at 14q32.1 in T cell malignancies involve two oncogenes. Proc Natl Acad Sci USA 96: 2949–2951
304. Virgilio L, Narducci M G, Isobe M et al. 1994 Identification of the TCL1 gene involved in T-cell malignancies. Proc Natl Acad Sci USA 91: 12530–12534
305. Narducci M G, Virgilio L, Isobe M et al. 1995 TCL1 oncogene activation in preleukemic T cells from a case of ataxia-telangiectasia. Blood 86: 2358–2364
306. Lamy T, Loughran T P Jr 2003 Clinical features of large granular lymphocyte leukemia. Semin Hematol 40: 185–195

307. Loughran T P Jr, Kadin M E, Starkebaum G et al. 1985 Leukemia of large granular lymphocytes: association with clonal chromosomal abnormalities and autoimmune neutropenia, thrombocytopenia, and hemolytic anemia. Ann Intern Med 102: 169–175
308. Loughran T P Jr, Starkebaum G 1987 Large granular lymphocyte leukemia. Report of 38 cases and review of the literature. Medicine (Baltimore) 66: 397–405
309. Pandolfi F, Loughran T P Jr, Starkebaum G et al. 1990 Clinical course and prognosis of the lymphoproliferative disease of granular lymphocytes. A multicenter study. Cancer 65: 341–348
310. Dhodapkar M V, Lust J A, Phyliky R L 1994 T-cell large granular lymphocytic leukemia and pure red cell aplasia in a patient with type I autoimmune polyendocrinopathy: response to immunosuppressive therapy. Mayo Clin Proc 69: 1085–1088
311. Kouides P A, Rowe J M 1995 Large granular lymphocyte leukemia presenting with both amegakaryocytic thrombocytopenic purpura and pure red cell aplasia: clinical course and response to immunosuppressive therapy. Am J Hematol 49: 232–236
312. Kwong Y L, Wong K F 1998 Association of pure red cell aplasia with T large granular lymphocyte leukaemia. J Clin Pathol 51: 672–675
313. Bleesing J J, Janik J E, Fleisher T A 2003 Common expression of an unusual CD45 isoform on T cells from patients with large granular lymphocyte leukaemia and autoimmune lymphoproliferative syndrome. Br J Haematol 120: 93–96
314. Morikawa K, Oseko F, Hara J et al. 1990 Functional analysis of clonally expanded CD8, TCR gamma delta T cells in a patient with chronic T-gamma lymphoproliferative disease. Leuk Res 14: 581–592
315. Morice W G, Kurtin P J, Leibson P J et al. 2003 Demonstration of aberrant T-cell and natural killer-cell antigen expression in all cases of granular lymphocytic leukaemia. Br J Haematol 120: 1026–1036
316. Rabbani G R, Phyliky R L, Tefferi A 1999 A long-term study of patients with chronic natural killer cell lymphocytosis. Br J Haematol 106: 960–966
317. Tefferi A, Greipp P R, Leibson P J et al. 1992 Demonstration of clonality, by X-linked DNA analysis, in chronic natural killer cell lymphocytosis and successful therapy with oral cyclophosphamide. Leukemia 6: 477–480
318. Chan J K 1998 Natural killer cell neoplasms. Anat Pathol 3: 77–145
319. Galli S J 1993 New concepts about the mast cell. N Engl J Med 328: 257–265
320. Lawrence J B, Friedman B S, Travis W D et al. 1991 Hematologic manifestations of systemic mast cell disease: a prospective study of laboratory and morphologic features and their relation to prognosis. Am J Med 91: 612–624
321. Horny H P, Parwaresch M R, Lennert K 1985 Bone marrow findings in systemic mastocytosis. Hum Pathol 16: 808–814
322. Longley B J, Metcalfe D D, Tharp M et al. 1999 Activating and dominant inactivating c-KIT catalytic domain mutations in distinct clinical forms of human mastocytosis. Proc Natl Acad Sci USA 96: 1609–1614

皮肤肿瘤
Tumors of the skin

23

Daniel J. Santa Cruz 著

钱利华 译　回允中 校

引言	1423
表皮肿瘤	1423
附件肿瘤	1442
皮肤囊肿	1465
Merkel 细胞（神经内分泌）癌	1465
黑色素细胞肿瘤	1466
间叶性肿瘤	1484
淋巴组织肿瘤	1495
转移	1505

引言

与病理学其他领域一样，皮肤肿瘤的命名经常在改变。有些新提出的术语并没有对先前较普及的术语加以改进。有些名称尽管显然不够准确，但是由于根深蒂固，替代性术语接受起来非常缓慢；如蕈样霉菌病和化脓性肉芽肿分别被皮肤 T 细胞性淋巴瘤和分叶状毛细血管瘤替代。为了避免混淆，本章采用目前最为常用的术语，避免使用不再应用的旧的名称。

本章讨论皮肤肿瘤和瘤样病变得以诊断的基本特征。为了便于组织，本章讨论的病变按照从表皮到皮下的顺序排序。最为常见于软组织肿瘤在第 24 章讨论。

表皮肿瘤　Tumors of the epidermis

表皮肿瘤，皮肤表面的病变，可为良性，亦可为恶性，除了角化细胞以外，也可含有黑色素细胞、Langerhans 细胞或 Merkel 细胞。

良性表皮肿瘤和瘤样病变
Benign epidermal tumors and tumor-like conditions

表皮能够发生一系列角化细胞病变，其病因学常常并不清楚。本组少数病变的特征是细胞学的多形性而不是生物学进展。临床和组织学表现有相当程度的重叠。因此，为了客观地确定其先后关系，必须考虑临床病理之间的联系。表 23.1 比较全面地列举了这些增生性疾病，其中一些在本章将进一步描述（如鳞状细胞乳头状瘤和表皮痣）。

脂溢性角化症　Seborrheic keratosis

脂溢性角化症的定义为主要由单形性基底细胞样角化细胞构成的良性表皮增生，以一种或多种生长方式为特征。

临床上，病变常常为多发性，最常发生于中年成人，没有性别差异。一般发生于躯干和头颈部，少数发生于生殖器。几乎从不发生于手掌或足底。病变质软至较硬，取决于角化物质的数量，并且外生性病变具有油滑的、"贴上去"的外观。颜色呈肉色、黄色到黑色。称为"黑色素棘皮瘤"（melanoacanthoma）病变的临床表现和部位类似于脂溢性角化症，但是有些也可发生于口腔[1]或生殖器皮肤[2]；这些病变被认为是脂溢性角化症的相对常见亚型[3]。所有脂溢性角化症的病变均可通过单纯切除、刮除或冷冻方法治愈。临床诊断一般比较容易；然而，如果色素较深或出现炎症和退化的区域，有些病变可能会与恶性黑色素瘤混淆。

组织学上，肿瘤在邻近表皮的水平上通常呈对称性分布。一般呈隆起状，表现为外生性膨胀（图 23.1）。一系列的结构形态包括棘皮增厚、过度角化、网状和疣状类型。这些一般性的结构形态具有多种生长方式，在任何单个病变中可呈均一或混合性表现。这些生长方式包括单一形态、多形性、克隆性、成束以及棘层松解等表现[4]。一般可出现角质及假性角质囊肿，后者是正常角化的微小囊腔，可位于增厚的病变内（角质囊肿，horn cysts）或聚集在表面（假性角质囊肿，pseudohorn cysts）（图 23.2）。任何特定的病变，尤其是如果病变较薄时，可以没有这些表现。三维重建显示，这些囊腔可为孤立性囊肿或为隧道样结构。这些微小囊腔被认为是来源于病变附近或其下方的毛囊皮脂腺单位[5]。

表皮肿瘤

| 表23.1 | 表皮良性棘皮症性病变 |

原发性——特发性

临床系列

孤立性
棘层松解
　疣状角化不良瘤
淡染（透明）细胞棘皮瘤（棘皮症）
表皮痣和综合征
内翻性毛囊角化症（内翻性脂溢性角化症）
乳头状瘤[带蒂的脂溢性角化症和（或）软垂疣]
脂溢性角化症

多发性（包括综合征）
疣状肢端角化症
黑色丘疹性皮病
淡染（透明）细胞棘皮瘤（棘皮症）
表皮痣和综合征
乳头和乳晕过度角化症
屈部网状色素沉着异常（Dowling-Degos病）
脂溢性角化症
出疹性（Leser-Trélat征）
多发性和（或）家族性
灰泥样角化症

组织学系列

脂溢性角化症一类
结构形态（可以混合）
　棘皮症性
　过度角化性
　内翻性
　网状（腺样）
　疣状
细胞生长形态（可以混合）
　棘层松解
　克隆性
　束状（"激惹性"），伴有或不伴有消退
　黑色素沉着性（黑色素棘皮瘤）
　单形性
　多形性
细胞学特征（可以混合）
　角化细胞
　小的基底细胞样细胞 ⇆ 大的角化细胞 ⇆ 凋亡
　嗜双色至透明性（不常见）胞浆
　梭形至星形角化细胞
　任何类型的色素性角化细胞
　伴有（黑色素棘皮瘤）或不伴有树突状黑色素细胞
透明细胞类
　淡染细胞棘皮瘤（透明细胞棘皮瘤）
　克隆性，伴有导管成分（汗孔瘤类）（见附件肿瘤）
　外毛根鞘瘤（见附件肿瘤）

其他类
棘层松解性棘皮瘤
克隆性病变，伴有导管成分（末端汗管瘤或汗孔瘤类）
　（见附件肿瘤）
表皮松解性棘皮瘤
内翻性毛囊角化症（内翻性脂溢性角化症）
大细胞棘皮瘤（通常单独分类，日光性或光化性角化症）
苔藓样角化症（通常单独分类，日光性或光化性角化症）
疣状黄色瘤（归入黄色瘤）

继发性——病毒引起的

组织学系列

疣状增生
寻常疣——HPV
跖疣——HPV
尖锐湿疣——HPV
传染性软疣（伴有毛囊受累）——痘病毒

表皮增生，伴有或不伴有轻度疣状改变
扁平疣——HPV
扁平湿疣——HPV
羊痘疮——副痘病毒
疣状表皮发育不良——HPV（伴有细胞学多形性）
Bowen样丘疹病——HPV（伴有细胞学多形性）

继发性——反应性棘皮症性病变，伴有或不伴有基础病变

组织学系列

表皮增生，伴有角化细胞成熟
　痒疹形态——单纯性苔藓结构
　结节性痒疹
　裂隙性棘皮瘤
　慢性结节性耳轮软骨皮炎
　皮肤纤维瘤（中线皮肤部位）

假癌性结构
　假癌性增生（伴有附件受累）
　颗粒细胞瘤
　血管角质瘤
　Spitz痣
　黑色素瘤（某些）
　神经肿瘤（某些）
　痒疹形态病变（有时）

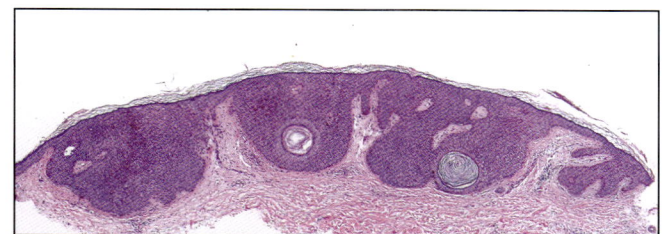

图23.1 脂溢性角化症,网状型。外生性角化性病变。

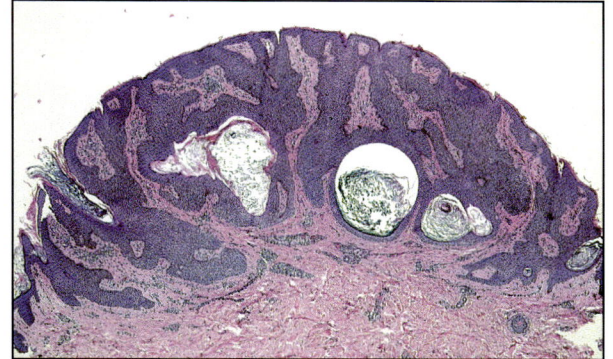

图23.2 脂溢性角化症,均匀一致的角化细胞,伴有角质囊肿和假性角质囊肿。

脂溢性角化症有时也可伴有肿瘤,包括基底细胞癌[6]、Bowen病、外毛根鞘瘤[7,8]、角化棘皮瘤以及恶性黑色素瘤。在一项有100例脂溢性角化症切除的病例的研究中,伴有非黑色素瘤性恶性肿瘤的发生率为4.6%[9]。由此可认为,对临床表现非同寻常的脂溢性角化症进行组织学检查是非常重要的。脂溢性角化症样表皮增生常常伴有黑色素细胞痣。

本文作者将激惹性角化症和炎性脂溢性角化症进行了区分。炎性脂溢性角化症(inflamed seborrheic keratoses)含有大量的苔藓样炎症细胞浸润,可以出现上述各种生长结构,但是此外尚有一般由单核细胞、噬黑色素细胞或两者组成的炎症浸润(图23.3)。在有些特殊的病例,整个脂溢性角化症出现退化现象,表现为原有

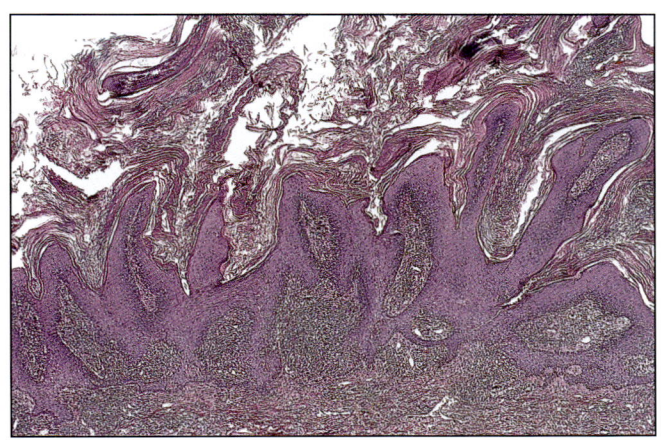

图23.3 激惹性脂溢性角化症。外生性疣状病变,病变基底部可见明显的宿主反应。

病变残留以及有病变变化的临床病史。

"激惹性"脂溢性角化症("irritated" seborrheic keratoses)是由创伤引起的[10],常常由于患者抠挖造成。它们与人乳头状瘤病毒(HPV)感染无关[11]。激惹性脂溢性角化症可以含有角质及假性角质囊肿,呈一系列角化表现,从完全正常的角化到混合性直至角化不全。棘层松解在这些病变中相对常见[4,12]。可以见到鳞状"漩涡",可有许多核分裂象。这些病变有时很难与高分化鳞状细胞癌区分。

黑色素棘皮瘤(melanoacanthoma):其组织学表现不同于脂溢性角化症谱系中的其他病变;其特征为无色素的角化细胞与树突状黑色素细胞散在分布[13]。上皮厚度不一,但一般厚于相邻的皮肤。单个病变中的角化细胞常常类似于激惹性或克隆性脂溢性角化症的细胞(图23.4A)。一般缺乏微小角质囊腔,但是可以出现在任何特定的病变中。

细胞学上,任何一种类型的脂溢性角化症的肿瘤细胞均为一致的基底细胞样细胞,彼此由易于见到的细胞间桥相互连接,表面为正常角化的角质,除非有继发创伤。在有些病变中可见单个角化细胞成熟,其特征为胞浆显著嗜酸、角化、凋亡或所有这些特征同时出现。在一些病变中,这些成熟的角化细胞密集而有序地排列,形成巢状结构或"漩涡",如常见于激惹性脂溢性角化症的病变。有些脂溢性角化症含有梭形或星形角化细胞,常常在病变内呈束状排列("丛状")。这种特征常见于激惹性脂溢性角化症以及黑色素棘皮瘤。在克隆性脂溢性角化中,球状的角化细胞团形态表现一致,被细胞形态轻度多形性的角化细胞小梁分隔。棘层松解性脂溢性角化症的角化细胞含有松散的桥粒。黑色素性脂溢性角化症含有多量基底细胞样色素性角化细胞,与黑色素棘皮瘤不同,后者的树突状黑色素细胞中含有黑色素(图23.4B)。在其他病变中,多形性脂溢性角化症[14]可见许多角化细胞具有核分裂象,其意义并不完全明了;然而,我们推测这可能为激惹性病变的特征,或可能发生在有进展性生物学潜能的病变。

主要的鉴别诊断包括寻常疣[12]、内翻性毛囊角化症(被认为是脂溢性角化症的变型,见下文)、表皮松解性棘皮瘤、浅染细胞棘皮瘤(pale cell acanthoma)、大细胞棘皮瘤、疣状黄色瘤、一些外毛根鞘瘤以及末端汗管瘤(汗孔瘤)的一些病变。

内翻性毛囊角化症(inverted follicular keratosis)[15] 定义为一种良性的、一般为对称性的成熟鳞状细胞内陷性(内翻性)增生,可以是外生性的,也可以内生性的。其组织学特征为出现密集排列的同心圆形层状鳞状细胞漩

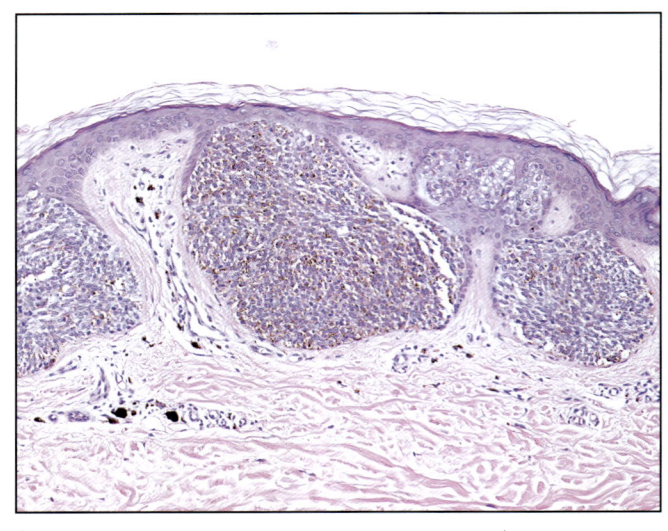
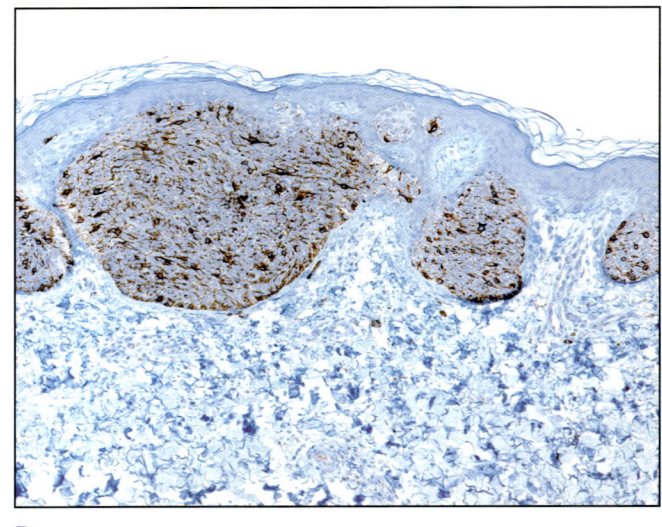

图23.4 （A）脂溢性角化症，黑色素棘皮瘤变型。角化细胞重度色素沉着，整个黑色素细胞数量增加。（B）病变主要由角化细胞构成，而且含有许多树突状黑色素细胞。Melan A染色。

涡，伴有向心性成熟，即所谓的"鳞状漩涡"（squamous eddies）。虽然在概念上一直存在显著的争议[16,17]，但是我们将其视为脂溢性角化症的一个变型。

临床上，内翻性毛囊角化症通常为孤立性病变，直径不足1 cm，一般累及中年白种人，没有性别差异[16,18,19]。这种病变几乎总是发生于有毛发的皮肤。最常发生于面部[20]，包括眼睑[21]和唇部[22]，但是也可见于肢体或躯干[23]。病变各异，可从光滑、丘疹至疣状，从皮肤颜色至色素沉着，以及从正常角化至角化过度。生物学上，病变为良性，但如果切除不完全，少数病例可以复发[24]。鉴别诊断包括寻常疣、脂溢性角化症以及其他各种丘疹或角化性病变[25]。

组织学上，内翻性毛囊角化症有两个基本特征：内翻性结构形态（图23.5）和鳞状漩涡（图23.6）。这里的内翻是指向深部真皮内生长，不管整个病变是外生性的还是内生性的。常常出现角化过度，可以是正常角化、角化不全或两者混合。从表面或窄或宽地向下延伸，垂直于鳞状细胞索，最深处边缘钝圆。多数病例的病变下方或病变内没有毛囊[26]。然而，在极少数情况下，毛囊穿过病变，出现于病变表面；在其他一些情况下，毛囊终止于病变内[25]。鳞状漩涡是靶样结构，可见于病变的任何区域，但在病变的深部最为明显。如果出现角化，常常为局灶性的且轻微，远远不如脂溢性角化症的典型的充满角质的微囊或角质囊肿或鳞状细胞癌的角化不全性微囊（"角珠"）常见。偶尔，皮脂腺细胞与鳞状漩涡紧密附着[20]，类似于皮脂腺导管[27]。鳞状漩涡之间病变

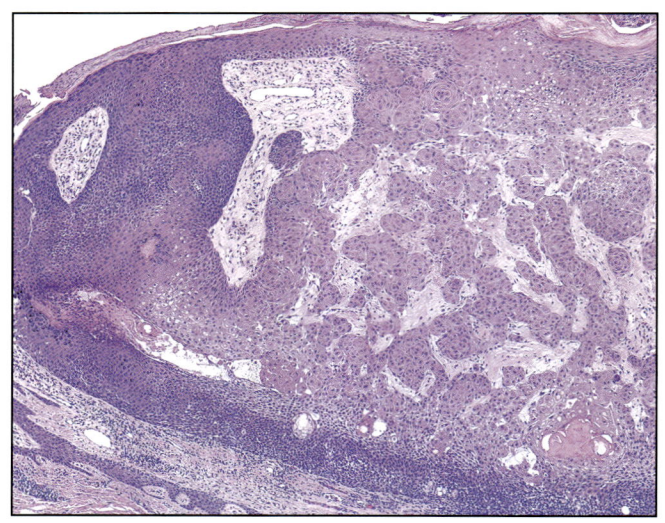
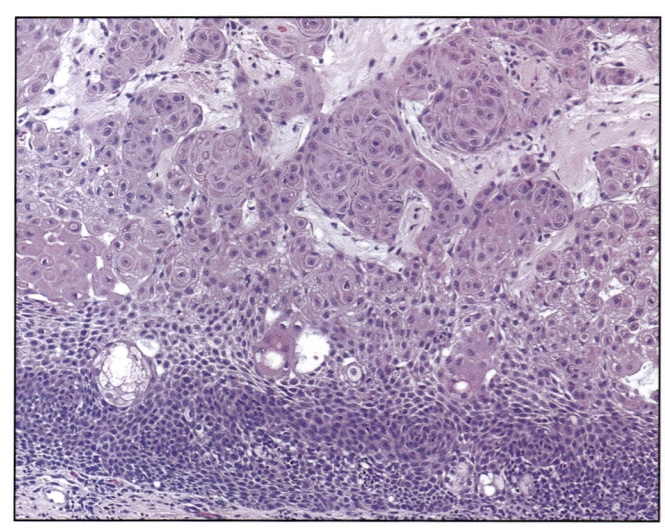

图23.5 内翻性毛囊角化症（内翻性脂溢性角化症）。伴有鳞状漩涡的内生性角化细胞病变。

图23.6 内翻性毛囊角化症（内翻性脂溢性角化症）。病变向下生长，含有大量小的鳞状漩涡。

细胞的特征为圆形和基底细胞样至梭形细胞，常见核分裂象[26]。黑色素可见于某些病变的角化细胞当中。有些病例的角化细胞 PAS 反应呈阳性。迄今，应用抗 HPV 共同抗原的抗体检测发现，仅有个别病例呈阳性[28]，多数为阴性[29]。间质一般为纤维性，缺乏黏液，使人联想到基底细胞癌的间质。间质内可见单核细胞浸润，有时可见嗜酸性粒细胞。鉴别诊断包括脂溢性角化症、外毛根鞘瘤、鳞状细胞癌、角化棘皮瘤和寻常疣[16]，偶尔还要与漏斗部肿瘤鉴别[30]。

棘层松解性棘皮瘤[31-34]
Acantholytic acanthoma

棘层松解性棘皮瘤定义为角化细胞增生，其中角化细胞的连接、桥粒的完整性减弱，导致棘层松解。临床上，这种病变可发生于任何性别的成年人，表现为大小为 1 cm 左右的角化性丘疹。除了某些例外的情况，病变一般位于躯干部。临床诊断各异，从基底细胞癌、日光性角化症乃至脂溢性角化症。患者缺乏 Grover 病（短暂性棘层松解性角化不良）、Darier 病或 Hailey-Hailey 病（家族性良性天疱疮）病史。

组织学上，病变特征为一系列的上皮增生以及某一（任何）水平或表皮内的棘层松解（图 23.7）。病变可能出现角质层下、角质层内、基底层上部裂隙或各种部位裂隙混合出现，并可类似于其他棘层松解性或大疱性病变。然而，棘层松解性棘皮瘤缺少单一形态的细胞学表现以及脂溢性角化症中充满角质的微囊。

棘层松解性棘皮瘤的一种特殊亚型为"疣状角化不良瘤"（warty dyskeratoma）[32,35-37]，临床表现为疣状、丘疹或囊性病变。显微镜下，病变呈火山口形或囊状结构（图 23.8）。出现乳头状过度角化性生长，并伴有棘层松解和绒毛形成（图 23.9）。棘层松解通常位于基底层上部，但也可扩展至表皮生发层。表皮内可见大量单个细胞角化不良以及有核或无核（"圆形小体"和"谷粒"）细胞，

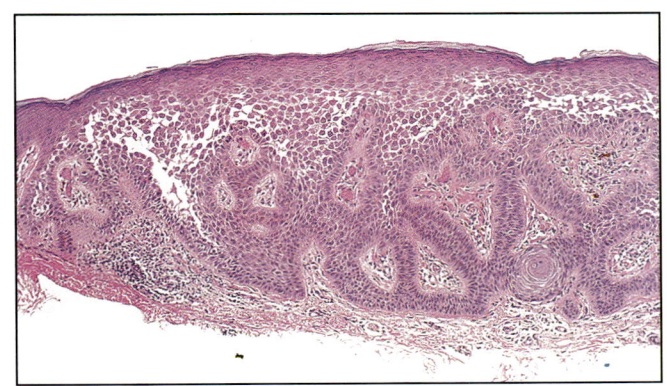

图 23.7 棘层松解性棘皮瘤。这个病变类似于脂溢性角化症，但棘层松解遍及整个表皮。

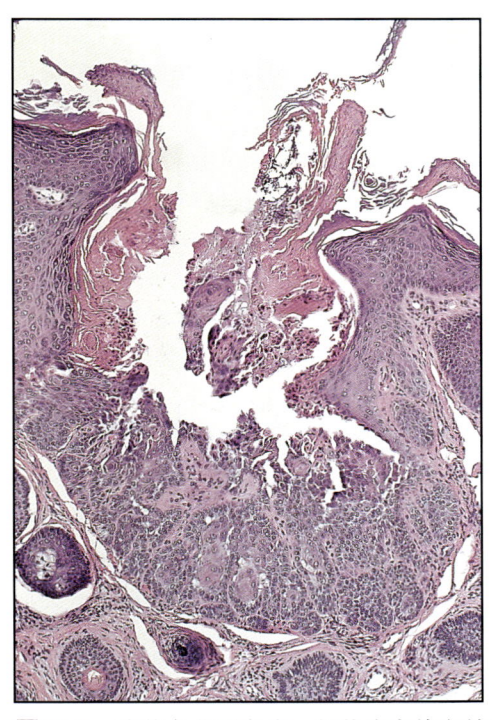

图 23.8 疣状角化不良瘤。杯状病变伴有棘层松解和绒毛，类似于 Darier 病。

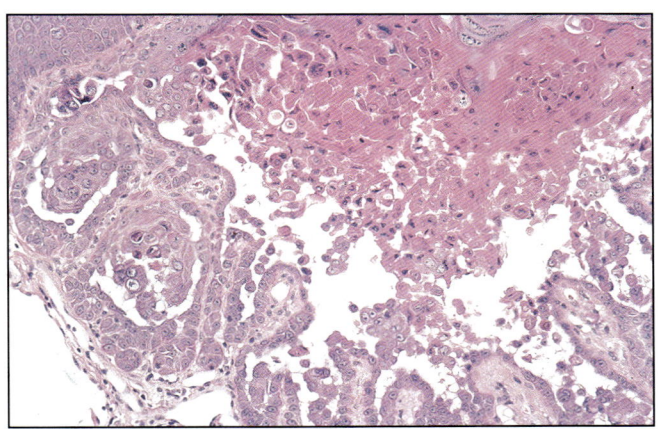

图 23.9 疣状角化不良瘤。注意内衬表皮的真皮乳头状突起（"绒毛"）。

其结构类似于 Darier 病。虽然多数病变具有疣状结构，但其他一些病变表现为囊性滤泡结构。这些组织学改变与较复杂性的临床病变可能难以区分，如 Darier 病、短暂性棘层松解性角化不良症以及线性表皮痣。在黑色素瘤和基底细胞癌再次切除的较大的手术标本中发现棘层松解性角化不良症极为常见。在缺乏播散性皮病或其他临床上明显病变的情况下，没有临床相关性。

淡染细胞棘皮瘤（透明细胞棘皮瘤）
Pale cell acanthoma（clear cell acanthoma）

淡染细胞棘皮瘤[38]的定义为散在的特发性银屑病样病变，由大而淡染的非角化性含有糖原的单形性角化细胞组成，伴有中性粒细胞。病变与相邻的表皮以及包含

的任何附件成分界限清楚。

临床上，这种没有症状的病变常常在数月至数年后发现。几乎均发生于成人，两种性别受累均等，最多见于下肢，但也可见于躯干和面部[39]。一般为单发，但也可为多发性和（或）出疹性的[40-46]。单个病变呈丘疹[47,48]至息肉状，皮色至红色到棕色，取决于血管形成的数量。病变大小一般为1～2 cm或较大[50,51]。仔细检查可以发现细小的毛细血管，加压时皮肤变白；然而临床极少有出血，不同于肢端汗腺瘤（acrospiroma）。病变表面一般光滑至圆凸状，湿润且有光泽，但有些病例表面可为细腻的"薄片状"鳞屑[48]。局部切除或损毁[50,52]一般可以治愈，但极少数病例可以复发[53]。临床上需与分叶状毛细血管瘤（化脓性肉芽肿）、溃疡性外生性基底细胞癌、外生性纤维组织细胞瘤以及光滑的脂溢性角化症鉴别。其他病变，诸如息肉样恶性黑色素瘤，在少数情况下也要与本病鉴别。

组织学上，病变一般呈对称性，与周围皮肤相比有不同程度的隆起，但其基底部常常位于邻近正常表皮网脊的下方（图23.10）[47]。病变的网脊从宽基底到银屑病样乃至网状；通常呈向心性[54]，但不同病例之间差异很大，包括一种罕见的囊性结构[55]。病变表面为正常角化并有局灶性角化不全，而颗粒层减少或消失。具有特征性的改变是：病变细胞与相邻正常表皮之间界限分明。另外，病变内包含的任何附件结构均被明显的分界线分开，一般为几个细胞厚度。细胞学上，病变内的上皮细胞为单形性，含有大量淡染的嗜酸性胞浆（图23.11）；常常出现轻度的细胞间水肿。大多数病例几乎没有核分裂象；极个别的病例伴有核分裂象，可能是与淡染细胞棘皮瘤有形态学重叠的透明细胞鳞状细胞癌[56]。应用和不用淀粉酶消化的PAS染色显示：病变细胞内有大量的

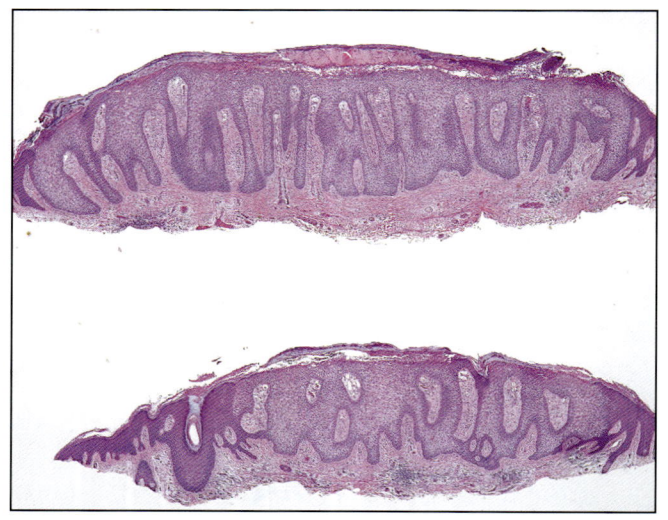

图23.10 淡染（透明）细胞棘皮瘤。淡染角化细胞的外生性病变，含有丰富的糖原。

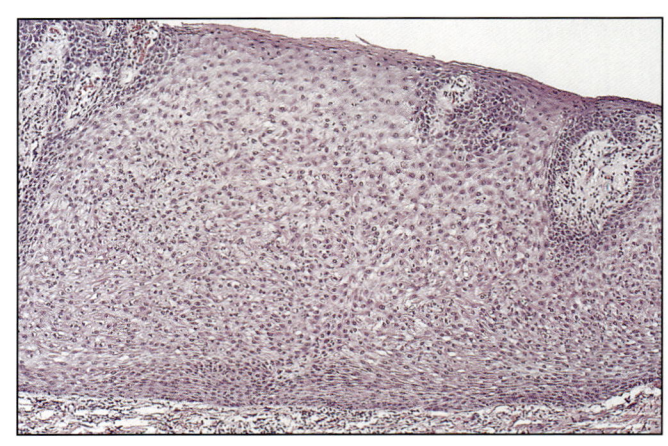

图23.11 淡染（透明）细胞棘皮瘤。高倍镜下显示透明（淡染）的角化细胞。

胞浆内糖原[57]。与汗腺不同，淡染细胞棘皮瘤磷酸化酶染色呈阴性[57]。病变内的黑色素细胞数量不等，并且是唯一含有黑色素颗粒的细胞类型[58-60]。在罕见的情况下，角化细胞内可以见到黑色素沉积（melanization）[61]。然而，在这种情况下，病变内的黑色素沉积也可认为是混杂的黑色素棘皮瘤（hybrid of melanoacanthoma）。细胞角蛋白和内皮蛋白（involucrin）的免疫过氧化物酶染色[53,62]以及多种凝集素（lectins）的形态[63]支持表面上皮分化，而病变CEA染色呈阴性[53]。超微结构检查其主要特征为：大量胞浆内糖原以及溶酶体样颗粒[64]。见于多数病变的令人难以理解的特征是：病变表皮内有中性粒细胞积聚。中性粒细胞可以完整或为碎片，可为单个或成簇分布。中性粒细胞常常位于表皮的各个层面，不同于银屑病的海绵状脓疱[65]。

真皮乳头常有水肿；真皮乳头的毛细血管一般较为显著，有时呈扭曲状。通常存在淋巴细胞、浆细胞或两者的单核细胞浸润。极少数情况下还可以出现嗜酸性粒细胞[54]。病变下方的汗腺导管增生可有可无。有一例伴有小汗腺纤维腺瘤（eccrine syringofibroadenoma）的报告[66]。

组织学上的鉴别诊断包括表皮内的肢端汗腺瘤、外毛根鞘瘤、毛囊漏斗部肿瘤、脂溢性角化症和银屑病。有时淡染细胞棘皮瘤的组织学改变并不伴有显著的肿瘤，而可能为一种反应性表现。

表皮松解性棘皮瘤[67,68]
Epidermolytic acanthoma

表皮松解性棘皮瘤[69]的定义为散在的特发性角化细胞病变，伴有表皮松解性过度角化症的组织学改变。

伴有表皮松解性角化过度症组织学特征的病变对应于一系列的临床改变。这些表现可能不同，从孤立性斑片（局灶性表皮松解性角化过度症）到瘤样病变、囊肿、

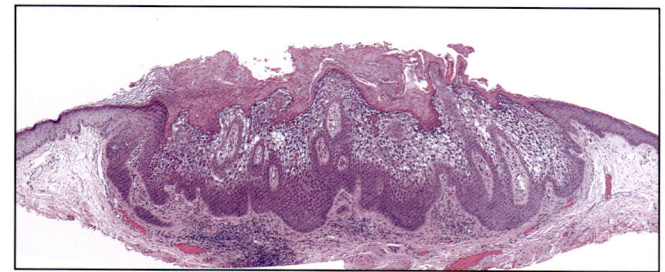

图23.12　表皮松解性棘皮瘤。这个疣状病变可见明显的表皮松解性过度角化。

掌跖过度角化症、表皮痣、脂溢性角化症以及先天性鱼鳞病样红皮病。病变发生于两种性别的儿童或成人，表现为面部、肢体或肛门生殖区的孤立性[67,69-71]、多发性[72,73]或播散性[74]散在分布的病变。临床鉴别诊断包括疣、传染性软疣、毛囊炎或软"纤维瘤"。

组织学上，病变以一系列的角化细胞成熟改变为特征，出现细胞核境界不清的透明细胞，棘层和颗粒层有明显的角质透明颗粒，表面不规则，密集的正常角化呈镶嵌样结构（图23.12）[70]。另外，这些组织学改变可以见于许多其他的病变，如脂溢性角化症或鳞状细胞癌。在这些病变中没有检测出HPV[75]，但有人提示其发病机制可能为角蛋白K1和K10基因突变[67]。超微结构检查，基本改变为棘层出现异常的张力丝束，颗粒层下方可见异常增大的角质透明颗粒以及明显的细胞间水肿[73]。主要的组织学鉴别诊断包括表皮松解性日光角化症以及掌跖疣（蚁冢状疣，myrmecia）。

病毒诱导的病变　Virally-induced lesions

可能易于发现病毒的多数表皮病变是与人乳头状瘤病毒和痘病毒有关的病变。这些病变的组织学标志为疣状增生：表皮和真皮呈锥状增生，呈现一系列的乳头状乃至指状的表现。

HPV相关性病变　HPV-associated lesions

HPV普遍存在，差不多有80种类型，HPV感染是由一种或多种这种DNA病毒引起的[76-79]。然而，HPV感染可能并非总是伴有临床病变[80]，相反，各种类似于含有HPV的特殊的临床病变可能并不含有病毒。组织学上，目前我们认为是HPV感染的单个病变仅仅是根据部位和临床病理学特征。发生于皮肤的病变常常列在术语疣（verruca）的项下。见于肛门生殖部位黏膜的病变通常放在术语湿疣（condyloma）项下[81]。皮肤HPV感染不常见的形态学亚型是伴有细胞学多形性的鳞状上皮病变，如Bowen样丘疹病和疣状表皮发育不良（epidermodysplasia verruciformis）。

寻常疣（verruca vulgaris）（普通疣，common wart）定义为由各种类型的HPV引起的皮肤角化细胞疣状增生，尤其是由HPV 1、2、4、7和26-29引起的[77]。临床上这种病变可以累及所有年龄患者的各种皮肤区域，但最常累及儿童和青少年手指的甲周区域和膝部。这种病变是对称性的并呈乳头状。如果除去病变表面的角质，一般可出现点状出血。鉴别诊断包括疣状脂溢性角化症以及许多其他表面偶尔出现疣状增生的病变。

组织学上，基本特征为外生性对称性疣状增生，表面为角化不全的柱状角质层（图23.13）。上皮突起一般为宽大圆形到指状（图23.14），伴有广泛扩张的真皮乳头毛细血管。细胞学上，特征性的表现为挖空细胞形成、浅表颗粒层增厚和细胞核的均一性，常常伴有多核细胞。然而，这些改变并非总是见于每个病例，尤其是在衰老

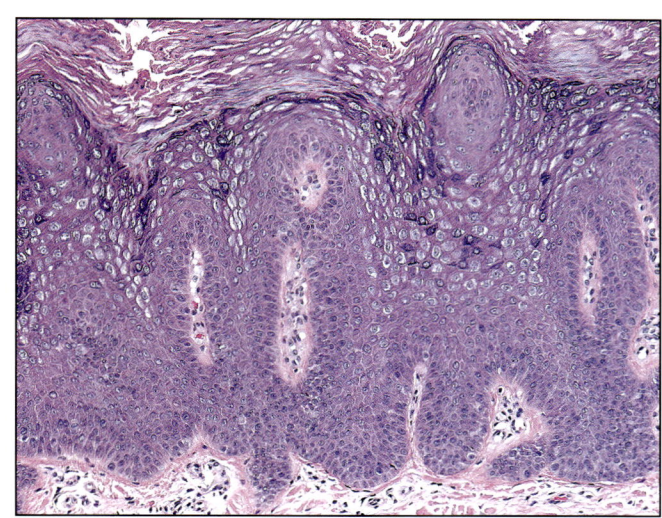

图23.13　寻常疣。外生-内生性乳头状瘤样生长方式。

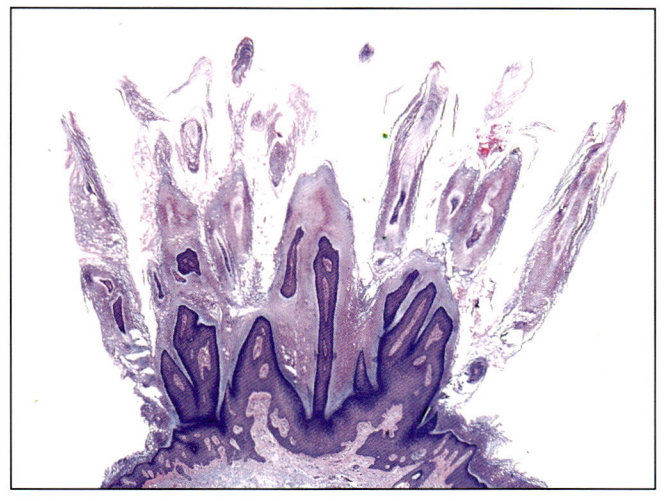

图23.14　寻常疣。显著的外生性丝状乳头。

的疣。一般来说，通常寻找不到病毒颗粒，可能需要一些特殊技术，如免疫过氧化物酶染色、原位杂交、电子显微镜检查、聚合酶链反应或所有这些技术，但是在这种情况下很少有必要应用这些技术。

疣的亚型（variants of verruca）。不常活检的疣的其他亚型包括扁平疣（veruca plana）和掌疣或跖疣（蚁冢状疣或掌跖疣，myrmecia or palmoplantar wart）。临床上，前者通常为多发性的，几乎全部位于面部、颈部或肢体，而且正如命名所意指的，病变扁平到略呈丘疹状。后者通常见于青少年的掌部或跖部，一般为内生性的且有疼痛。组织学上，扁平疣通常对称并轻度增生，但疣状改变和角化不全较轻。挖空细胞或轻度细胞学多形性可能是一些病例的唯一线索。蚁冢状疣不同于其他类型的疣，一般为对称性和内生性的（图 23.15）。常常出现表皮增生，伴有袋样疣状改变，位于较宽的角化细胞基底之上。细胞学上，浅表角化细胞含有较大的胞浆内角质透明颗粒。表面的角质层通常不规则，角化不全，并且具有镶嵌结构，不同于正常掌跖角质层的均一性紧密排列的正常角化。HPV 及疣状改变也可见于毛囊囊肿[82-86]。

湿疣（condyloma）定义为由一种或多种类型的 HPV 引起的发生于肛门生殖器部位黏膜的角化细胞病变[77]。其疣状型是一系列称为尖锐湿疣（condyloma acuminatum）的病变，而丘疹或扁平型称为扁平湿疣（condyloma planum）。

临床上，所有类型的湿疣均可发生于任何年龄的人[87,88]，但最常见于有多个性伴侣的性活跃的成人。临床病变各异，从不足 5 mm 的小丘疹到少见的大块瘤样病变，可能环绕整个肛门生殖器部位。鉴别诊断包括原位癌、Bowen 样丘疹病以及脂溢性角化症。治疗必须个性化，但局部化疗、手术、干燥或联合疗法已经取得了不同程度成功。遗憾的是，多数病变疗效不好。

组织学上，尖锐湿疣为增生性疣状病变，其中匍行性的表皮集中并经过宽的前沿与真皮毗连[81]。扁平湿疣为没有疣状改变的棘层增厚性病变。两种类型的湿疣的浅表部分一般均有挖空细胞形成（图 23.16）、颗粒层增生，细胞核从均匀一致到脑回状，可为多核细胞。在许多病例中，下层细胞出现深染的细胞核，常常出现核分裂象。其中有些病例在组织学上可能类似于原位鳞状细胞癌，不要与鬼白树脂治疗效应混淆[89]。有些湿疣伴有鳞状细胞癌[90-93]，明确提示为连续性病变，尤其是在 Bowen 样丘疹病[94-96]。

表皮发育不良性疣（epidermodysplasia verruciformis）[97,98]是一种罕见的病变，定义为播散性扁平或丘疹性疣及斑点，发生于 1 岁以内并持续终生。通常有家族史。另外，这种病变可能发生恶性肿瘤，如原位鳞状细胞癌和鳞状细胞癌。许多类型 HPV，尤其是 HPV 5[77]，常常与表皮发育不良性疣有关，甚至可以出现在发生恶性肿瘤的情况下[99]。推测其他未知的免疫学因素也参与本病的发生。如有报告称与器官移植以及人免疫缺陷病毒（HIV）感染有关[100]。

组织学上，扁平疣性表皮发育不良性疣类似于普通的扁平疣，但有些可出现脂溢性角化症样改变[101]。可有轻度疣状增生，靠近表皮尖端伴有空泡状胞浆空晕。常常伴有细胞增大[102]。可见细胞核固缩以及网篮状的正常

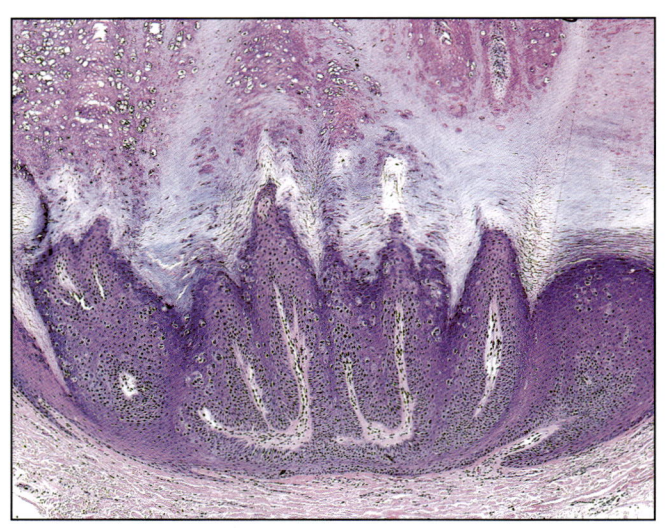

图 23.15　跖疣。内生性乳头状瘤样病变，伴有颗粒层增厚。

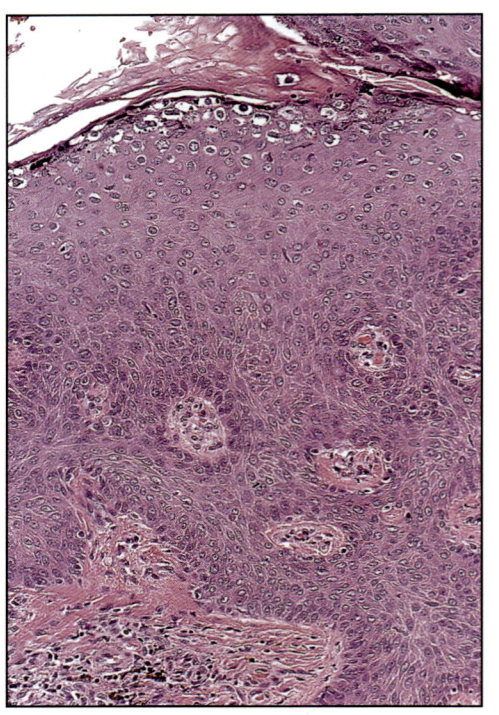

图 23.16　尖锐湿疣。注意浅表的挖空细胞。还有各种形态的成熟角化细胞。

角化和角化不全[103]。超微结构检查可以见到细胞核内病毒颗粒。

痘病毒相关性病变
Pox virus-associated lesions

传染性软疣（molluscum contagiosum）[104]。痘病毒类中的一种 DNA 病毒是传染性软疣的致病因子[105,106]。其定义为在临床上出现丘疹样、圆顶形瘤样病变，组织学特征为出现"软疣小体"或 Henderson-Patterson 小体，为病毒颗粒的球形聚集。

临床上，病变发生于年轻人或免疫抑制患者，如 HIV 感染群体[107]，可以表现为播散性病变，治疗困难。病变直径通常 3～6 mm（较大的病变罕见），为脐凹形丘疹，基底呈红斑样。挤压病变可出现白色物质，为混有角质的积聚的软疣小体。治疗通过局部破坏，但有的病变在临床上可能类似于基底细胞癌，这样的病变可能需要活检[108]。

组织学上，病变的特征为一系列杯状至囊性病变，含有许多诊断性软疣小体，每个细胞一个（图 23.17）。从深部毛囊上皮到表浅部分，软疣小体从嗜酸性变为嗜碱性。伴随这种情况出现的是单个细胞核受压以及颗粒层增厚。最终，软疣小体与角质碎片一起被挤到表面。这种组织学表现是独特的，没有其他需要考虑的鉴别诊断。极少数情况下，传染性软疣病变可能伴有不同寻常的炎症细胞浸润，其中有些在组织学上可能非常显著，但在生物学上为良性病变[109-111]。

假癌性（假上皮瘤样）增生[112]
Pseudocarcinomatous（pseudoepitheliomatous）hyperplasia

这种良性病变最好被定义为表皮增生，伴有附件上皮明显的鳞状化（毛囊、导管或两者），导致类似于浸润性鳞状细胞癌的瘤样病变[113]。当导管受累远远超过毛囊受累时，常常称为鳞状汗腺化生（squamous syringometaplasia）或汗腺鳞状化生（syringosquamous metaplasia）[114-121]。

假癌性增生本身并不是一种临床疾病，而是由多种伴有皮肤损伤的临床状况引起的结果，其中包括手术后创伤[122]、结节性痒疹、结节性耳轮软骨皮炎以及裂隙性棘皮瘤等多种疾病。另外，假癌性增生也可见于对下部病变的反应，如颗粒细胞瘤[113]、Spitz 痣[123]、孤立性限局性神经瘤[124]以及包括着色真菌病、孢子丝菌病和芽生菌病在内的深部真菌感染，以及卤素皮病（halogenoderma）。

组织学上，假癌性增生一般呈对称性，具有一系列生长方式，从近乎一致的增生性漏斗结构，到出现漏斗以及岛状终末导管鳞状化两种结构，乃至仅有岛状导管鳞化（图 23.18）。其边界一般局限，但有浸润。如果有微囊出现，其内可充满正常角化、角化不全或两种类型的角质；然而，正常角化的角质较为常见。这种病变并不累及皮下组织，除非出现深的窦道。假癌性增生有轻度或没有细胞学的多形性表现；然而，有些病例可见凋亡的角化细胞。

相反，鳞状细胞癌常常出现细胞学多形性，包括表面以及病变的浸润部分，并且通常有许多角化不全性微囊[125]。另外，鳞状细胞癌除非很小，一般呈非对称性。虽然绝大多数伴有神经周围浸润的鳞状上皮病变为鳞状细胞癌，但是偶尔这种变化可以见于与肿瘤无关的活检部位[126]。因此，在假癌性增生的诊断中似乎有理由认为应该优先考虑病变的结构特征。

表 23.2 比较了这两种病变的异同。

角化棘皮瘤[127,128] Keratoacanthoma

角化棘皮瘤是指一系列良性的、杯形角化细胞肿瘤，肿物生长迅速，并可自行消退。本病包括在鳞状细胞癌

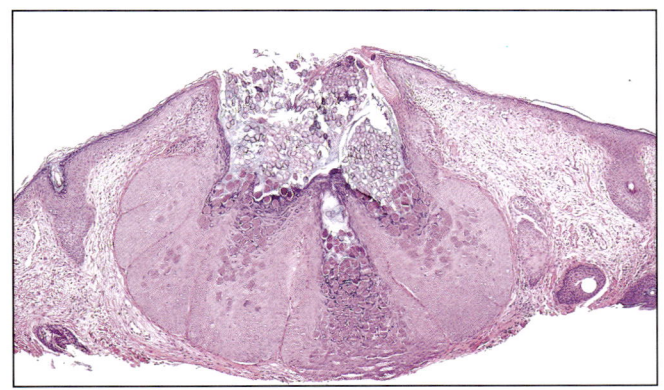

图 23.17 传染性软疣。内生性上皮伴有多量球形软疣（Henderson-Patterson）小体，出现在毛囊的浅表部位。

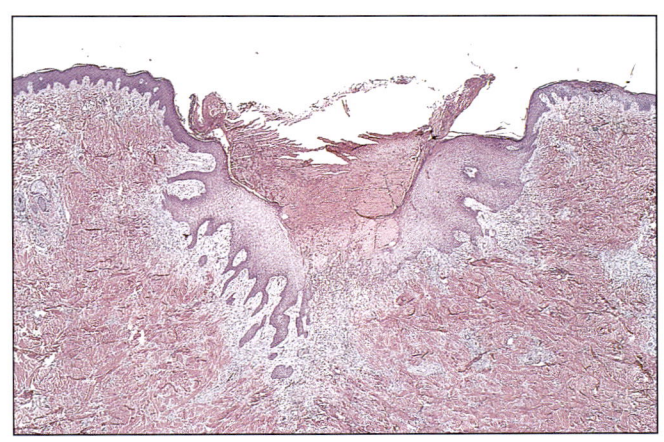

图 23.18 假癌性增生。垂直分布，球状增厚的鳞状上皮位于真皮浅层，伴有肉芽组织。

表23.2　假癌性增生与鳞状细胞癌

标准	假癌性增生	鳞状细胞癌
生长速度	不定，多为创伤后或手术后	生长缓慢（数月或数年）
对称性	通常对称	不对称，轻度隆起或溃疡
中央角质栓	一般没有，有时有侵蚀	罕见
移行区	病变与邻近表皮截然分开	正常表皮逐步移行为多形性鳞状细胞乃至肿瘤
边缘	浸润性	不定，清楚或为浸润性，或两者兼有
微囊	如果出现，则为正常角化，角化不全罕见	如果出现，通常为角化不全
附件受累	病变的特征或为毛囊或为导管，或两者兼有	可有可无
细胞学多形性	罕见	常见
胞浆	丰富，常为"玻璃"或透明样	丰富或稀少
凋亡角化细胞	不常见	常见
炎症浸润	不定，但通常轻微	不定
神经周围浸润	罕见	不常见
皮下受累	从无	较大的肿瘤并不少见
纤维化	如果出现，位于病变附近或病变内	如果出现，位于肿瘤巢周围
消退	缓慢	不经治疗干预不会消退
转移	从不	罕见，但如有深部浸润，就可以发生

的鉴别诊断之中，两者的比较见表23.3。其形态学表现类似于鳞状细胞癌，而且实际上可能为顿挫性癌（abortive carcinoma）[129]。关于角化棘皮瘤的性质，存在不同的观点。有些作者完全抛弃这一诊断[130]，而其他一些作者（包括我们）认为应用这个诊断需要慎重，而且必须用于适当的临床状况和组织学改变。

临床上，角化棘皮瘤为对称性病变，常常发生于中年以上或免疫抑制患者暴露于日光的皮肤，没有性别差异[132]。病变一般为外生性，中心含有角栓。不常见的亚型包括：发生于非阳光暴露部位皮肤的病变、巨大的病变（边缘性角化棘皮瘤，keratoacanthoma marginatum centrifugum）、多发性和综合征性[133]以及甲下棘皮瘤[134-136]。角化棘皮瘤可以通过切除来治疗，也可以在确定组织学诊断后进行密切的临床随访。

组织学上，角化棘皮瘤为对称性病变，深部出现球状鳞状细胞小叶，含有丰富的嗜酸性半透明胞浆，一般称为"玻璃样"胞浆。病变周边可见正常表皮"唇"，向中心的角化性火山口延伸（图23.19）。整个角化性小叶常常有丰富的角质。凋亡的角化细胞通常出现在角化性小叶中（图23.20）。角质也可见于微小的囊腔中；此时常常为角化不全，并且常常伴有微小脓肿（图23.21）以及弹力纤维和胶原纤维[137]。病变周边常可见淋巴细胞和嗜酸性粒细胞浸润；浆细胞罕见。神经周围受累可以见到，对鉴别角化棘皮瘤和鳞状细胞癌没有特别的帮助[138, 139]。血管侵犯偶可发生，但并不一定伴有预后不良[140]。少数病例中，组织学检查病变为典型的角化棘皮瘤，但可能

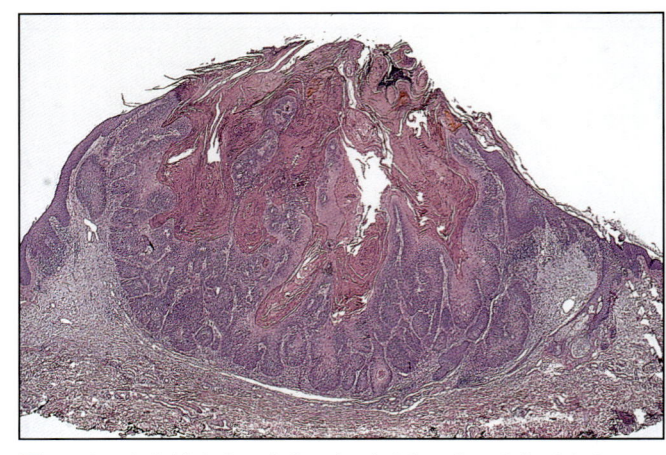

图23.19　角化棘皮瘤。病变呈杯形对称，中心为角质火山口。

表23.3	角化棘皮瘤与鳞状细胞癌	
标准	角化棘皮瘤	鳞状细胞癌
生长速度	生长迅速（数周至数月）	生长缓慢（数月至数年）
对称性	对称性隆起，伴有突出的"唇"	非对称性，轻度隆起或溃疡
角质栓	中心，常见	罕见
移行区	肿瘤和表皮之间突然转化	正常表皮逐步移行至多形性鳞状细胞乃至肿瘤
细胞学多形性	不定，有些病变多形性非常显著	比较常见
胞浆	丰富，常为"玻璃样"或透明样	丰富或较少
肿瘤深部不全角化的微囊内中性粒细胞脓肿	常见	罕见
弹力纤维	常见于周围肿瘤巢	周围肿瘤巢中不常见
吞噬弹力纤维	常见	罕见
炎症浸润	常为苔藓样	不定
嗜酸性粒细胞	常见	罕见
浆细胞	罕见	常见
神经周围浸润	罕见	罕见
皮下受累	在大的肿瘤并不少见	在大的肿瘤并不少见
纤维化	当出现时，位于病变深部	当出现时，围绕肿瘤巢
消退	自行	不进行治疗，不会消退
转移	从不，如果出现，就不是角化棘皮瘤	罕见，如有深部浸润，就可以发生

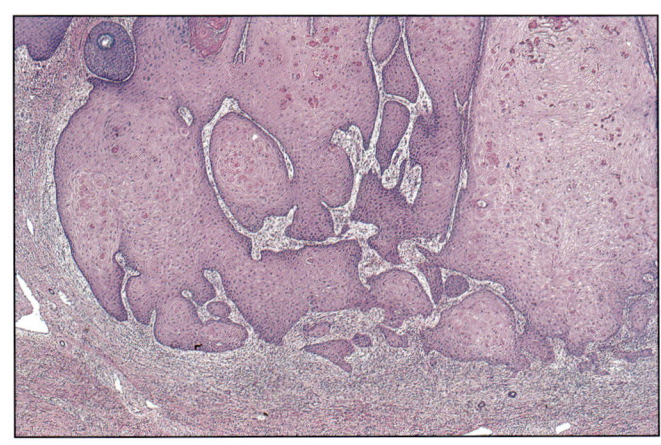

图23.20　角化棘皮瘤。这些"玻璃样"鳞状小叶通常含有凋亡的角化细胞。

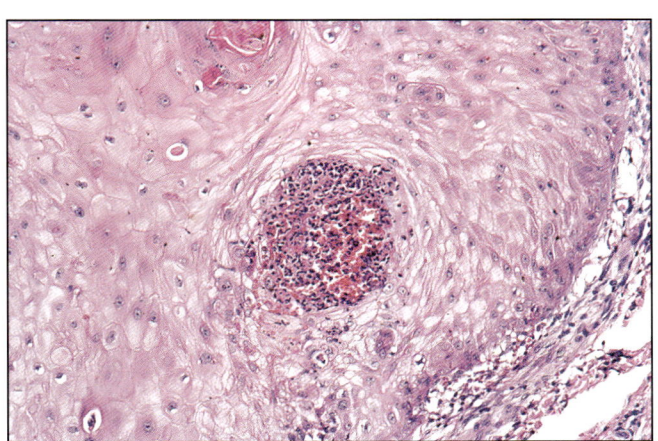

图23.21　角化棘皮瘤。微小脓肿常见于病变的进展性边缘。

会出现侵袭性的临床经过，提示最初病变的诊断并不正确，或通过常规显微镜和临床病理关系并不是总能将其与一些鳞状细胞癌鉴别开来[130]。

细胞学上，角化细胞从良性一致性表现到多形性并伴有多量核分裂象不等，但这些特征均无助于明确诊断。结构特征对于明确诊断比细胞学特征更有帮助。

曾尝试应用现代技术（不是临床病理的相互关系）找到一种鉴别角化性棘皮瘤和鳞状细胞癌的方法，这些尝试尚未取得重大进展[141]。如曾有尝试性研究认为，*p*53的表达可以区分两种病变[129,142,143]。然而，即使是对照性病变也表达p53，如假癌性增生。突变型或野生型p53蛋白表达好像代表细胞未成熟性和增生的能力，并非肿瘤或恶性的标志[143]。bcl-2的表达——一种被认为参与保护细胞从而避免出现凋亡的原癌基因——与鳞状细胞癌相比，在角化性棘皮瘤中减少，提示角化性棘皮瘤发生不明原因的程序化退化[144]，但很难仅仅基于这一参数来作出诊断。增生性抗原Ki-67在两种类型的病变中均有表达，不能用来进行鉴别[129,142]。其他方法，如免疫组织化学方法显示桥粒糖蛋白（desmosomal glycoproteins）[145]，可以用于辅助诊断，但不能确定诊断。

我们仍然认为角化性棘皮瘤是一个有用的诊断，如果应用于适当的临床病变，可以服务于患者并指导患者的临床治疗。角化性棘皮瘤和鳞状细胞癌是可以明确区分的，尤其是当为病理医生提供了足够的活检组织时。

日光性角化症和日光性原位癌[146-148]
The actinic keratoses and actinic carcinomas in situ

日光性角化症是一类角化细胞病变，伴有不同的细胞形态学表现，局限于表皮，是皮肤长期暴露于紫外线而发生的继发性改变。这些病变包括与日光照射有关的病变，但并不局限于日光照射。其亚型相对有限（表23.4），在此仅深入讨论老年性雀斑、大细胞性棘皮瘤以及日光性角化症。苔藓样角化症与日光性角化症一并讨论。播散性表浅性日光性汗孔角化症不在本章的讨论范围，在其他部分讨论[149-151]。在本章的讨论中，普通的日光性角化症被认为是原位癌的一种形式[146]，但是否所有类型的日光性角化症都应该包括在原位癌中尚有待于确定。

日光性雀斑（老年性雀斑）[152,153]
Solar lentigo (lentigo senilis)

这是日光暴露部位皮肤的一种境界不规则的色素性斑点或薄的斑片，其组织学特征为上皮脚间断性的变长以及色素增加，伴有一些（数量不等）皮肤日光性弹力组织变性。在HE染色切片上，黑色素细胞增生并不明显[154]。

临床上，病变一般为多发性的，发生于中老年人面部和臂部尚好的皮肤。斑点呈散在或融合性表现，一般为1.0 cm或更小，有一定程度的色素沉着，常常呈黑色。病变为良性的，不需特殊治疗。临床上，鉴别诊断包括单纯性雀斑、恶性雀斑、较薄的脂溢性或日光性角化症。

组织学上，病变境界清楚，整个病变均匀一致。可见上皮脚间断性变长和色素增加，呈"棒状"结构（图23.22）。一般没有角化不全。多数色素细胞为角化细胞；然而，黑色素细胞确有轻度增加，需要特殊技术来进行定量[155]，不同于雀斑或单纯性雀斑。细胞学上，色素增加的角化细胞一般大小一致，没有核分裂象。

唯一具有意义的组织学鉴别诊断包括黏膜黑色素性斑点[156,157]、雀斑以及单纯性雀斑，尽管日光性雀斑的改变可以伴有其他病变，如苔藓样角化症以及网状脂溢性角化症[158]。

表23.4　日光性角化症

不常伴随癌
　日光性雀斑（老年性雀斑）
　苔藓样（日光性）角化症
　大细胞性棘皮瘤
　播散性浅表性日光性汗孔角化症

常常伴随癌（原位癌）
　日光性角化症系列（结构和细胞学可以混合）
　　增厚
　　　萎缩（再生不良）
　　　正常营养（易机化的）
　　　肥大（增生）
　　生长结构
　　　没有上皮脚
　　　出芽，线性至宽基底
　　　疣状
　　　腺样
　　　Paget样
　　细胞学
　　　轻度或基底部多形性
　　　多形性，伴有成熟
　　　Bowen样，伴有或不伴有广泛角化
　　　伴有或不伴有色素沉着
　　　透明细胞

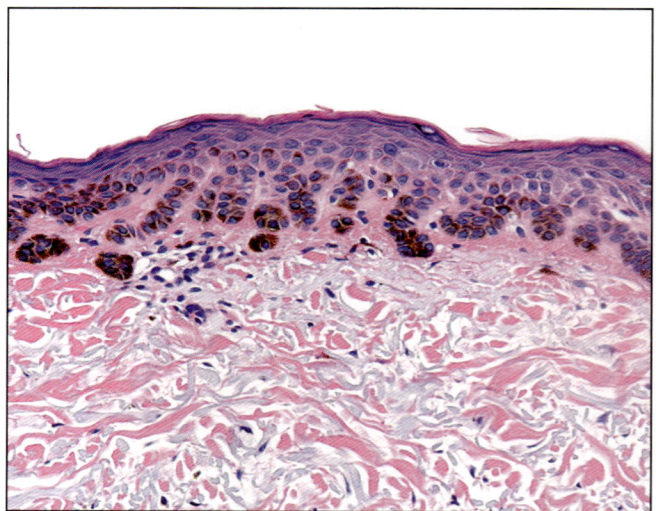

图23.22　日光性雀斑。日光累及的皮肤上可见棒状表皮色素增加。

大细胞性棘皮瘤 [159-169]
Large cell acanthoma

大细胞性棘皮瘤定义为发生于暴露于阳光的皮肤部位的斑状病变，其组织学特征为大而境界清楚的、相对一致的多倍体性角化细胞[161,162]，表现为颗粒层增厚，角化正常，分化成熟，其中通常有残留的毛囊皮脂腺上部（acrotrichium）和汗腺上部（acrosyringium）细胞或两者，这些细胞可以穿过病变。其中一些病变类似于脂溢性角化症，而另一些具有原位癌的特征[166]。

临床上[164]，大细胞性棘皮瘤多发生于女性。从黄色至棕色，或（极少数）为无色的[159]对称性斑片，伴有轻度的角质鳞屑。直径一般为 0.5～1.0 cm，多位于面部，但也可发生于肢体或躯干。少数情况下可以多发[166,170]。生物学上其呈惰性，诊断之前可以存在数十年[168]，可通过手术或冷冻疗法治疗。临床鉴别诊断包括日光性雀斑、脂溢性角化症、日光性角化症以及基底细胞癌。

组织学上[164]，周围正常表皮与病变分界清楚（图23.23）。低倍镜下，病变从正常到轻度增厚乃至疣状[159,166]；病变对称，常常出现基底细胞色素增加。上皮脚有改变，从没有上皮脚到出现均匀一致的上皮脚，常常伴有"方波"或"棒状"结构，见于大约半数的病例。角化细胞穿过轻度乃至可能显著增厚的颗粒层，出现成熟性表现。当颗粒层呈轻度增厚以及出现层状正常角化时，表面显示网篮状正常角化；当颗粒层显著增厚时，则类似于某些脂溢性角化症。在极少数病例，角质出现镶嵌样结构，类似于跖疣。病变上半部的角化细胞中常可见到糖原。基底部黑色素细胞的数量没有增加，不同于单纯性雀斑。

细胞学上，病变中的基底细胞大小大约是正常基底细胞的两倍；细胞核通常位于顶端，靠近基底膜的胞浆丰富。黑色素颗粒可以形成一个"帽"，盖在基底细胞核的上方。病变内的任何附件通常内衬正常大小的细胞，常常可用于比较，但也有例外[166]。核分裂象或细胞凋亡不常见，但在有些病例可出现于基底层上部，由此提出了是否有原位癌的问题[166]。真皮常常出现一定程度的日光性弹性组织变性、毛细血管扩张、慢性炎症或所有这些特征的混合出现。鉴别诊断包括日光性雀斑以及日光性角化症，这些形态可能共同存在于某种特殊的病变中。

日光性角化症 [146-148,171]
Actinic (solar) keratosis

日光性角化症定义为一种多形性角化细胞病变，出现于表皮中的一层或多层，可以表现为真皮乳头内不规则的出芽样扩展，并不向网状真皮内延伸。类似的唇部病变称为日光性唇炎（actinic cheilitis）[172]。

这些病变的发生率尚不确定，患者多数为肤色白皙的中年或老年人，在阳光暴露部位可见多发性病变，可为红斑性、局限性鳞屑片块或皮肤角质[173]。肥大性病变常见于手上[174]。不常见的临床表现常见于面部，如播散性色素沉着，可能与恶性雀斑或脂溢性角化症混淆[175]。有些例外情况，如复发性病变随后发生鳞状细胞癌的病例报告。日光性角化症在生物学上属于惰性或进展缓慢的病变，通过冷冻[176]或化疗可有效地治疗。不能否认，日光性角化症不经治疗完全能够发展成鳞状细胞癌，从这个意义上讲，它是原位鳞状细胞癌的一种类型[146]。

这种病变的组织学变异非常多样[177,178]，多种组织学结构常常共存于一个病变中。病变范围可从萎缩性（图23.24）到肥大性（增生性）（图23.25）[174]。可出现单层多形性角化细胞乃至全层（Bowen样）多形性改变（图23.26）。其生长方式可能不同，从均一性到

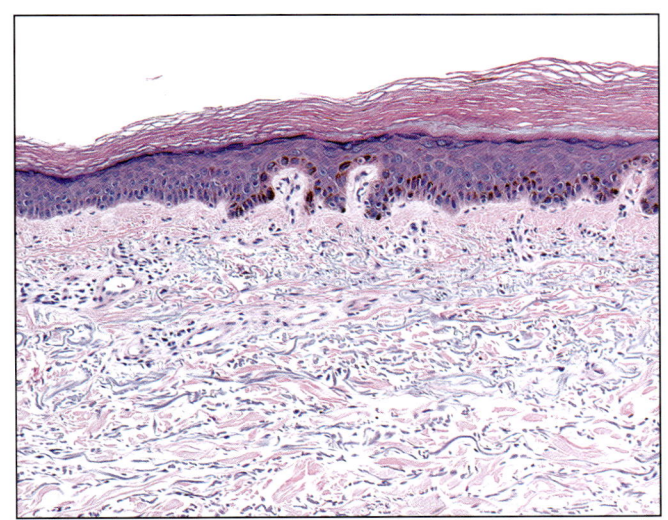

图23.23 大细胞性角化棘皮瘤。右半部分皮肤增厚，含有大小大约为正常两倍的角化细胞。表面为正常角化。

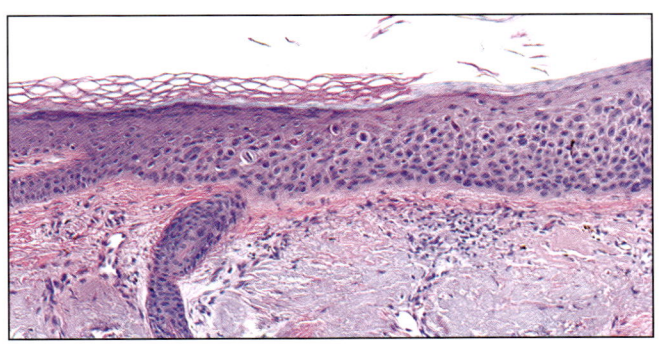

图23.24 日光性角化症。在日光性弹力组织变性的背景中，鳞状细胞呈非典型性，表面角化不全。

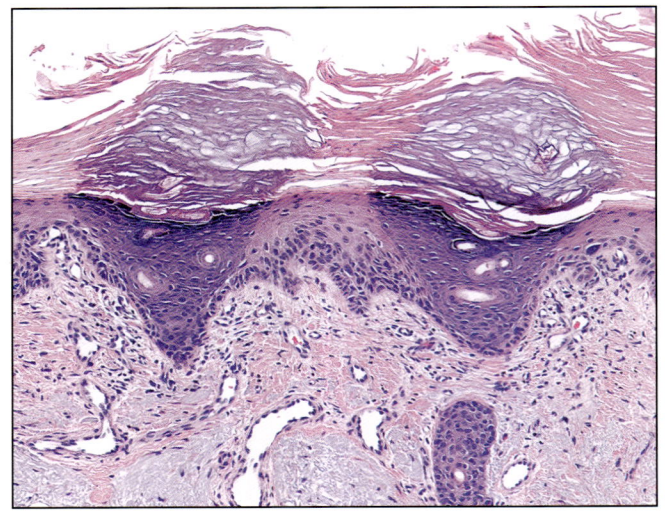

图23.25 日光性角化症,肥大性。显著的角化不全性过度角化。注意汗腺导管上方正常角化。

非均一性和表皮松解性[179]、Paget样、腺样(棘层松解性或"Darier样";假腺样)[180]。典型病例的特征为角化细胞成熟杂乱,颗粒层缺失,以及出芽样扩展至真皮乳头。

在HE切片中,日光性角化症的典型组织学特征为保留皮肤附件。普通的基底细胞结构被增大或多形性的鳞状细胞所替代,这种改变仅在毛囊或导管的开口被阻断。表面角质角化不全反映了角化细胞成熟异常;然而,附件角化细胞及角质得以保留,除了有些周围出现增大或多形性角化细胞外套的病例以外[177]。上述改变导致附件出现纤细且垂直的柱状正常角化和表面宽大的角化不全性角质交替出现。交替改变的频繁程度取决于附件的密度以及病变产生角质的数量,角化

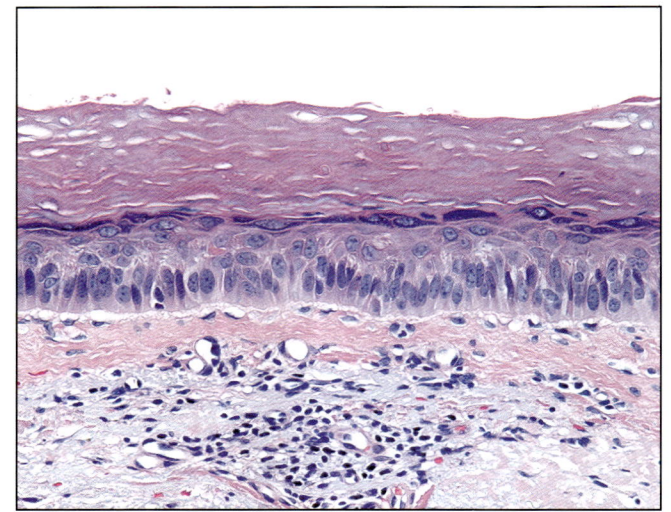

图23.26 日光性角化症,Bowen样型。在日光累及的皮肤中,全层鳞状上皮出现非典型性。这个病变也为肥大性。

不全层也可狭窄且呈柱状。

细胞学上,角化细胞的变化范围从单形性至多形性,嗜酸性至透明细胞,以及有色素型至无色素型。许多角化细胞具有丰富的嗜酸性胞浆;一些可为多核细胞,而另一些可呈凋亡改变。病变有色素时,角化细胞和噬黑色素细胞内可见黑色素[175]。

日光性角化症的真皮浸润从近乎没有到较为广泛。一般为单核细胞,但偶尔可见嗜酸性粒细胞和中性粒细胞,尤其是当病变继发擦伤或穿破时。有些作者应用"苔藓样日光性角化症"一词来表示与扁平苔藓极为类似但具有角质层的角化不全以及一定程度的角化细胞增大或多形性的孤立性病变。有些作者对这一概念提出质疑,并将这些病变简单地称为良性苔藓样角化症或"苔藓样角化症",并将它们归入良性角化细胞增生中[181]。我们发现后一种命名比较实用,并且比较符合临床。

组织学鉴别诊断主要为浅表性鳞状细胞癌。我们认为,日光性角化症与鳞状细胞癌的主要区别在于:后者的纤维性网状真皮内出现异常角化细胞以及独立的角化症灶。然而,其他作者在确定早期浸润方面有不同的标准[182]。

Bowen病和其他Bowen样病变[183]
Bowen's disease and other bowenoid lesions

我们应用Bowen病一词来表示一种类型的鳞状细胞原位癌,后者表现为一系列的类似于鳞状细胞癌的病变,常常累及表皮全层,但没有侵犯真皮。这种病变在有些病例中可伴有浸润性癌成分。

尽管这些病变发生浸润癌的几率相对较低,但发生在黏膜部位的病变则相反,如在阴茎龟头部或外阴[184]。因此,我们认为原位鳞状细胞癌这一概念只要运用得当还是有用的。

依据我们的定义,有几种特殊的临床状况需要鉴别。最具特征性的病变是Bowen病,它常常可与鳞状细胞原位癌交替使用。Bowen病临床表现为大片红斑,常常发生于躯干。当类似病变发生于外阴、阴茎龟头或口腔时,则采用增殖性红斑(erythroplasia)一词。有些化学药物,如砷剂,也与这种病变的发生有关。当具有类似组织学改变的病变发生于暴露于日光的部位时,常常应用Bowen样日光性角化症(bowenoid actinic keratosis)一词。发生于年轻人肛门生殖器部位部位的散在性色素性丘疹,称为Bowen样丘疹病(bowenoid papulosis)[186-196]。后者常常伴有多株HPV中的一种[77,95,197],进展为癌的并不多见[95,198,199]。

组织学上，鳞状细胞原位癌的范围较广[200]。低倍镜下的形态可为扁平至疣状，并从萎缩性到增生性。所有病变均有全层鳞状细胞成熟异常（图23.27）。有些病变有巢状（克隆性）结构（图23.28）；有些病变出现透明细胞改变（图23.29），并且有些结构可能类似于Paget病或恶性黑色素瘤的典型表皮内结构（图23.30）。许多病例毛囊皮脂腺上部和毛囊漏斗受累。

鳞状细胞原位癌常常出现显著的角化细胞多形性。一般可见多量核分裂象或凋亡细胞。然而，少数病例出现从深部至浅部的有序成熟。发生于黑皮肤个体的病变色素分布不规则，有时为树突状黑色素细胞。角质层常常出现特征性的融合性角化不全，但Bowen样日光性角化症的表面常常为伴有"跳跃区域"的角质，类似于典型的日光性角化症。

鳞状细胞原位癌下方的间质炎症浸润不同，从正常到致密的单核细胞浸润，有些病例可呈苔藓样浸润。个别情况下，可以出现噬黑素细胞性皮炎（melanophagic dermatitis）及病变消退。有时可见丰富的血管网，类似于毛细血管瘤。有些病例可出现淀粉样物，尤其是伴有单核细胞浸润的病例。极少数病例类似于附件肿瘤[201]。

Bowen样丘疹病（bowenoid papulosis）在组织学上类似于鳞状细胞原位癌，但有轻微的差异[191]。典型病变与正常皮肤分界清楚，如果活检包括整个病变，典型病变的组织学表现呈外生性生长或隆起于正常皮肤表面（图23.31）。出现表皮增生，伴有颗粒层增生和表面角化不全，以出现含有包涵体样小体的细

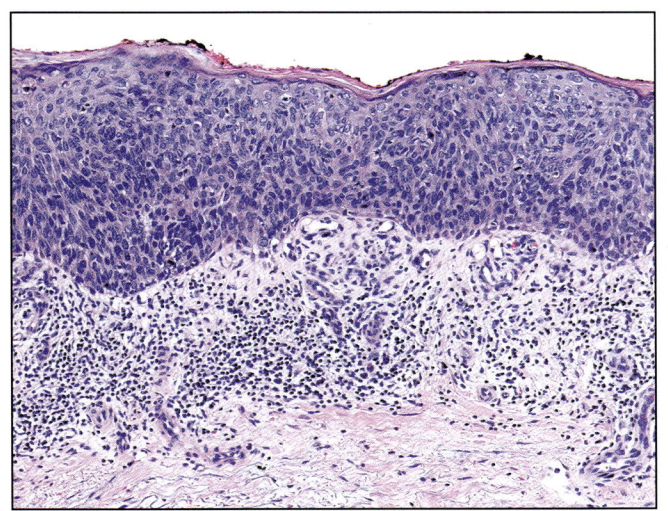

图23.27 鳞状细胞原位癌（Bowen病）。表皮全层非典型性，通常位于非阳光照射部位。

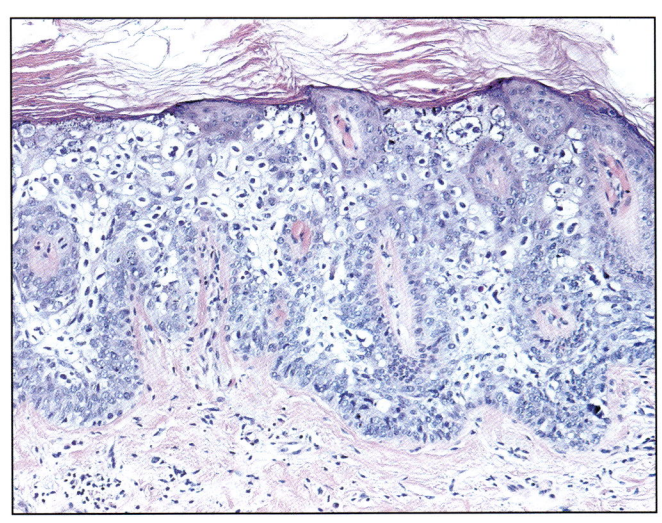

图23.29 鳞状细胞原位癌（Bowen病），透明细胞型。浅表性透明细胞见于典型的Bowen病。

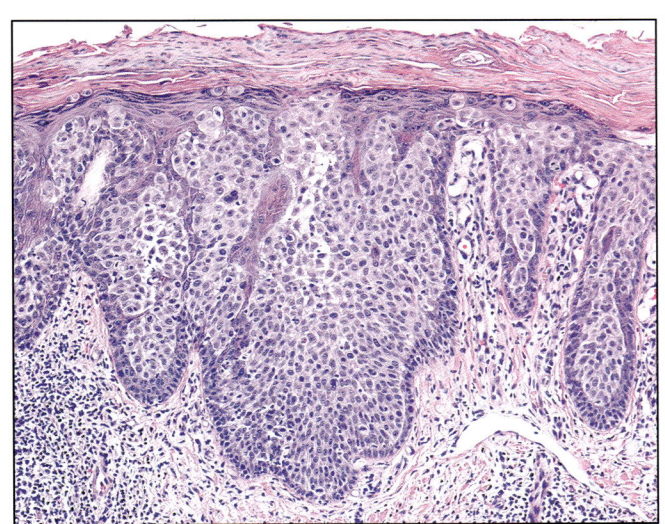

图23.28 Bowen病，克隆性。未成熟的角化细胞"克隆"可与导管病变混淆。

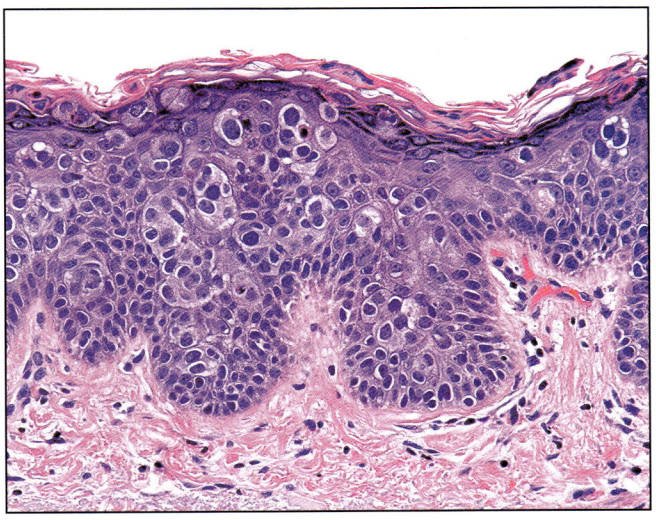

图23.30 鳞状细胞原位癌（Bowen病），Paget样型。孤立的细胞遍布表皮，类似于Paget病和浅表播散性黑色素瘤。也可见少数非典型性细胞克隆。

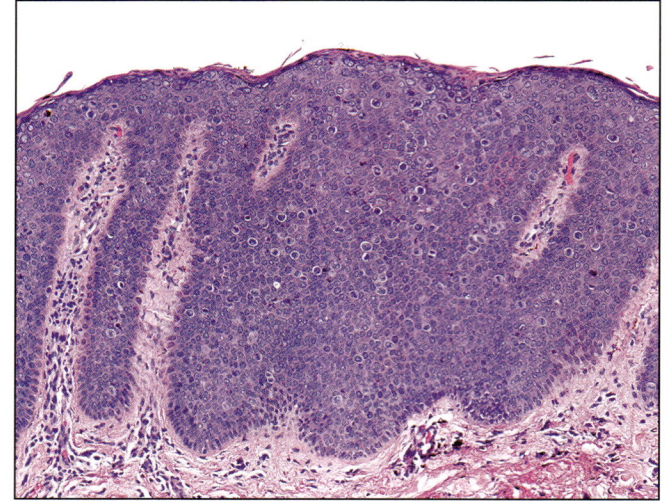

图23.31　Bowen样丘疹病。单个或成团的丘疹全层呈非典型性，保留成熟性结构。

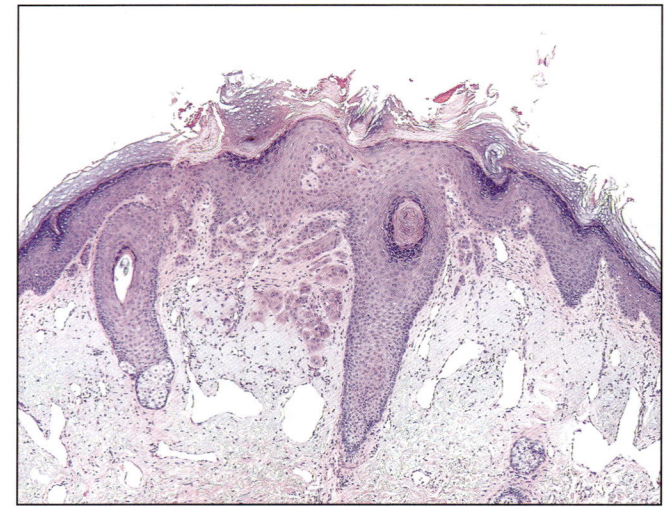

图23.32　鳞状细胞癌，普通型。病变中可见分枝状鳞状细胞小叶从表面溃疡处向外扩展。

胞为特征。也可出现角化细胞密集、非均一性表现以及轻度成熟改变，与Bowen病的一般概念即上皮的基底和顶端部分表现类似不同。一般说来，Bowen样丘疹病不累及毛囊皮脂腺上部和毛囊漏斗，但汗腺上部以及皮肤小汗腺或顶泌汗腺导管可能受累。这一点不同于Bowen病，后者表现通常相反。常可见到巨大的多核以及凋亡的角化细胞。角化细胞核分裂可以见于整个表皮。人乳头状瘤病毒共同抗原免疫过氧化酶染色一般为阳性，但差异较大[202]。真皮内常出现明显的毛细血管扩张。这种病变常常伴有单核细胞浸润。

鳞状细胞癌[203]　Squamous cell carcinoma

鳞状细胞癌指由异常鳞状细胞构成的超出原位生长阶段的一系列的肿瘤。诊断时病变可位于真皮内或超出真皮范围，包括转移到其他部位的肿瘤。

临床上，鳞状细胞癌常常表现为中年人日光暴露部位的皮肤病变。病变表现不同，从皮肤颜色或色素沉着性斑片到带有鳞屑的结节或溃疡性肿瘤。有些病例与日光照射没有明显关系。其亚型包括疣状癌（见下文）和化学物质相关性鳞状细胞癌，如与接触砷有关的肿瘤。生物学上，鳞状细胞癌一般呈惰性表现，除非病变深达汗腺螺管水平以及病变持续时间较长[204]；厚度小于2 mm的病变统计学上没有转移的危险[205,206]，而厚度大于4 mm或有深度浸润的病变则有明显转移的危险性[207]。疣状癌一般位于黏膜，如口腔黏膜、宫颈或阴茎龟头（巨大湿疣）；皮肤病变常常位于足部跖面。可出现局部破坏[208]，但仅有个别病例播散至原发部位以外。一般情况下，日光暴露部位病变

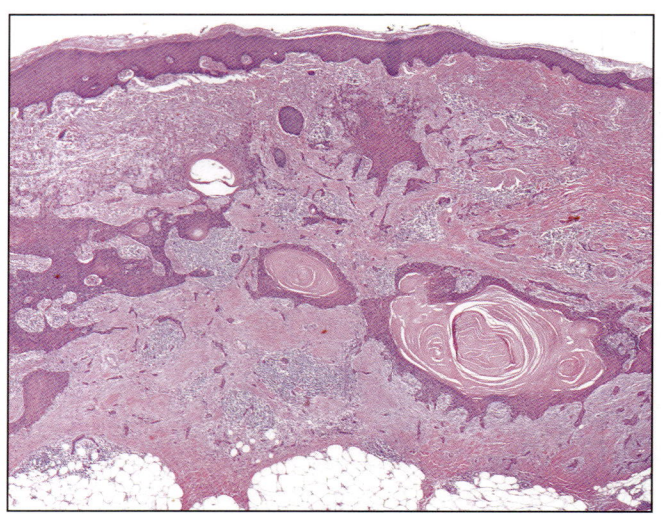

图23.33　鳞状细胞癌，普通型。病变中可见明显的角化不全性角质囊肿（"角珠"）。

的鉴别诊断仅仅限于角化棘皮瘤和基底细胞癌，但有些病变可与脂溢性角化症混淆，对于色素性病变，需要与恶性黑色素瘤鉴别。疣状癌需要与跖疣（verruca plantaris）鉴别。

组织学上，最常见的结构为伴有明显角化的浸润性鳞状细胞小叶。常常有中度至重度的细胞学多形性，其特征不仅是核/浆比例较高，而且还有凋亡细胞以及具有典型性及非典型性核分裂象的细胞。早期浸润性病变可以表现为单个细胞浸润真皮乳头（图23.32）。高分化鳞状细胞癌出现相对成熟的角化（图23.33，23.34）。有些高分化的病例可能很难与角化棘皮瘤鉴别（见表23.3）。在假腺体的亚型中[209]，分叶状结构完整，

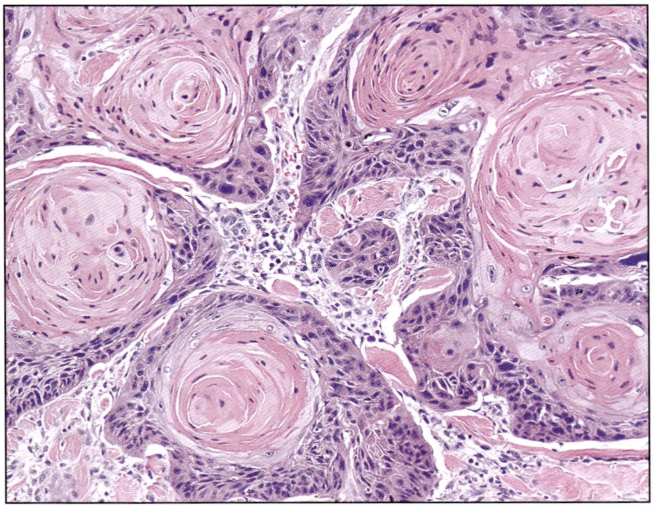

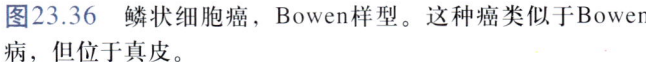

图23.34 伴有"角珠"的鳞状细胞癌。这是浸润性鳞状细胞癌。

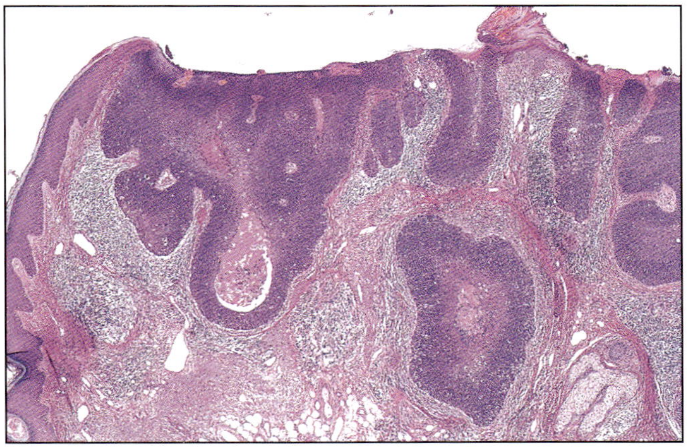

图23.36 鳞状细胞癌，Bowen样型。这种癌类似于Bowen病，但位于真皮。

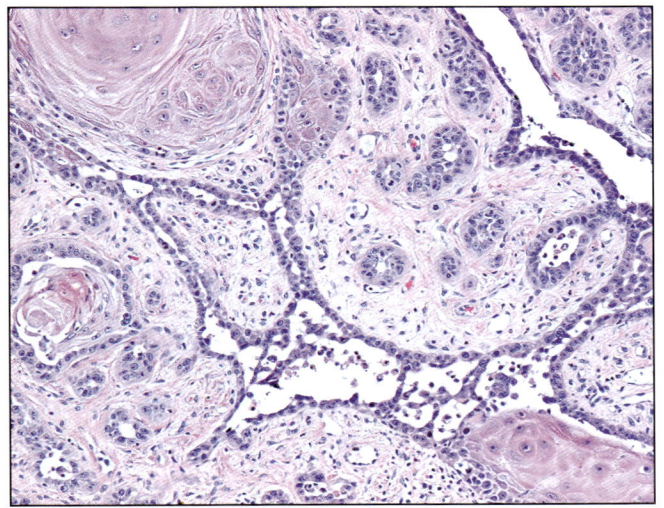

图23.35 鳞状细胞癌，假腺体型。复杂的腺样结构可能与腺癌以及血管肉瘤混淆。

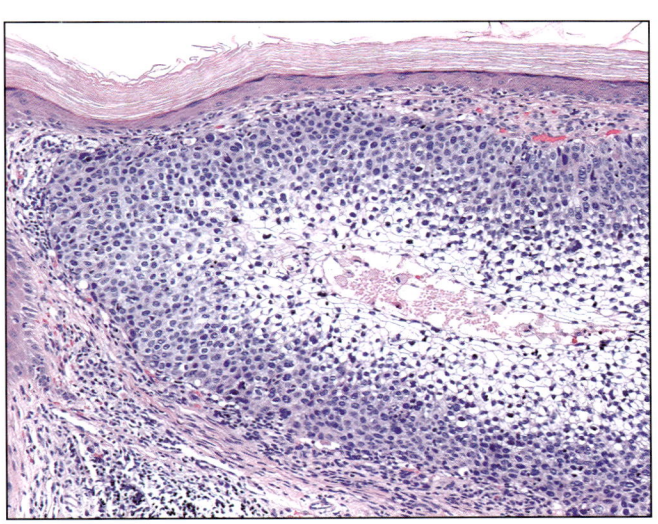

图23.37 鳞状细胞癌，透明细胞型。非角化型鳞状细胞癌小叶，中央呈透明细胞表现。

但鳞状细胞失去黏附或出现棘层松解（图23.35）。这就导致类似于腺体肿瘤，如腺癌、附件导管癌甚或血管肉瘤[210,211]。侵袭性较强的病例其生长方式表现为浸润性鳞状细胞条索或单个鳞状细胞浸润，而非鳞状细胞小叶。这样的病例出现神经周围或血管浸润非常常见，并且预后不良。有些病例出现非常显著的间质纤维组织增生（使人联想起硬化性基底细胞癌），这种结构也与较为侵袭性的生物学行为有关。鳞状细胞癌不常见的细胞类型包括Bowen样（图23.36）、透明细胞（图23.37）、印戒细胞[212,213]、基底细胞样细胞以及梭形细胞（图23.38），分别可与腺体肿瘤、基底细胞癌以及其他梭形细胞肿瘤混淆。

免疫组织化学染色，鳞状细胞癌一般AE1/AE3细胞角蛋白和上皮膜抗原（EMA）为阳性，但CAM5.2和BER-EP4一般为阴性。通常情况下，这些病变S-100蛋白和间叶性标记物为阴性。

鳞状细胞癌的其他生长方式包括类似于原位癌的肿瘤，但是或出现深层真皮侵犯或呈外生性乳头状结构[214]，而不是浸润性生长。化生性（癌肉瘤样）亚型含有不常见的同源性（梭形细胞）和异源性（特殊的肉瘤性）成分，但可能与预后不良无关[215]。

疣状癌（verrucous carcinoma）[216-219]为细胞学呈良性表现的鳞状细胞癌。结构上类似于寻常疣，不同点在于：其具有局灶性破坏性生长方式，可以包括骨的侵犯（图23.39）[208]。鳞状细胞小叶排列紧密，沿着病变进展的前部常常含有微小脓肿，因此得名隧道癌（carcinoma cuniculatum）。在绝大多数病例中，免疫组织化学检查尚未检测出病毒相关性抗原，但在极少数

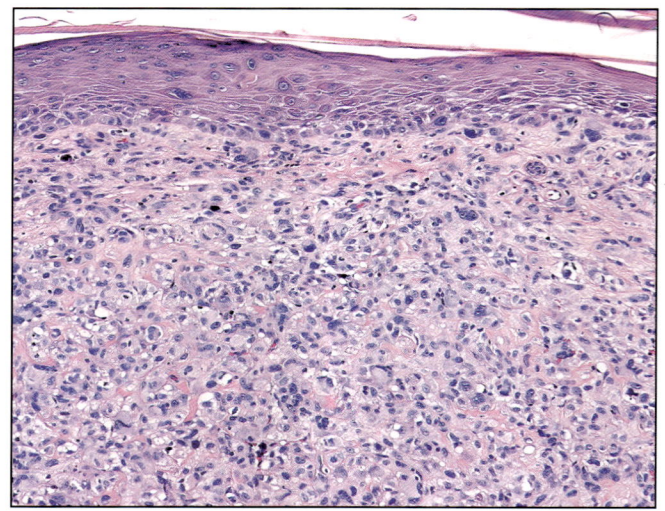

图23.38 鳞状细胞癌,梭形细胞型。病变表现为成片的高度多形性的细胞,没有明显的角化。病变与非典型性纤维黄色瘤极为类似,但肿瘤细胞角蛋白呈阳性。

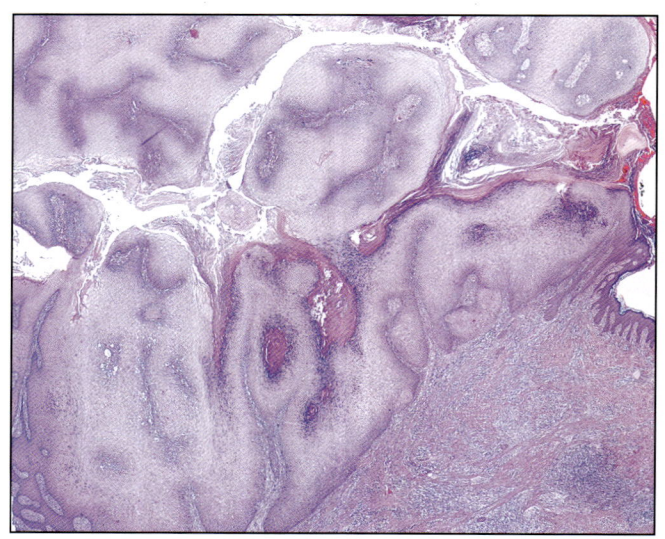

图23.39 鳞状细胞癌,疣状型。注意低倍镜下类似于寻常疣。

病例已经发现 HPV[93,220,221]。浅表性活检评估疣状癌病例特别困难。因此,对于任何组织学呈良性以及临床上存在数月乃至数年的深在性疣状鳞状细胞病变,都应怀疑到疣状癌的诊断。与临床的相互关系,包括放射学检查,对于作出诊断都十分重要。

基底细胞癌[220,222] Basal cell carcinoma

基底细胞癌是指一系列呈惰性生物学行为的皮肤上皮性肿瘤,由具有不同形态结构的深染的基底细胞样细胞构成,分布于可能为反应性的或诱导产生的特征性纤维黏液样间质中。基底细胞癌是皮肤最常见的恶性肿瘤。

临床上,基底细胞癌多发生于暴露日光的部位,尤其是在白种成人的面部。然而,它们可以发生于任何种族的任何皮肤部位。发生在年轻人的属极个别现象,除了皮脂腺痣或痣样基底细胞癌综合征以外[223,224]。通过单纯切除绝大多数可以治愈,但少数深层浸润的病变由于广泛性硬化掩盖了其浸润性生长方式或由于神经周围浸润等因素而难以切除。鉴别诊断一般包括日光性角化症、脂溢性角化症、Bowen病、鳞状细胞癌以及(在少数情况下)恶性黑色素瘤。

组织学上,基底细胞癌有多种生长方式[225-228]。岛屿状结构最具特征性,占临床结节性表现的大多数。镜下可见大小不一的散在性或融合性、囊性或实性基底细胞样细胞岛(图23.40),周围常常有栅栏状排列的外层细胞,可能与间质分隔开,形成所谓的"人工收缩假象"(图23.41)。邻近的间质为纤维组织增生性、黏液样或两者并存。肿瘤内或间质内或两者均可出现黏液(图23.42)。任何一个肿瘤中均可见其他结构,

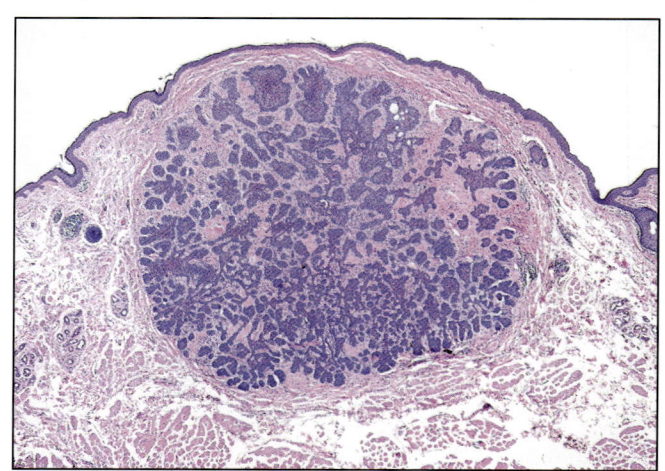

图23.40 基底细胞癌,普通型。可见由岛屿状基底细胞样细胞构成的结节。

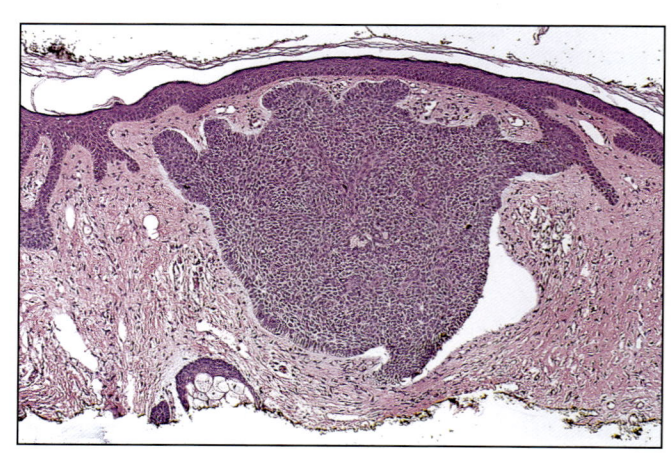

图23.41 基底细胞癌,注意人工收缩假象。

如小岛状、网状缎带样或小梁状、巢状腺泡状，或这些结构混合出现。偶尔可以见到继发性淀粉样变[229-231]或坏死区；肿瘤小叶或其邻近的间质中常常可见黑色素。另外，可以见到来自下方的导管结构进入肿瘤组织，并含有浓缩的嗜酸性物质。有时可以出现充满角化不全性物质的漏斗或"毛膜"（tricholemmal）角质的微小囊腔。极少数情况下可见钙化灶[232]。

细胞学上，绝大多数肿瘤含有小而一致的细胞，其中多数为凋亡细胞。个别细胞可见核分裂象。少数病例出现瘤巨细胞、透明细胞[233,234]、腺体细胞[235,236]、印戒细胞[237-239]或肌上皮样细胞[240,241]聚集区。

基底细胞癌的其他生长方式包括浅表多中心性以及硬化性亚型。

浅表性基底细胞癌临床上一般表现为斑块，常常需要与Bowen病鉴别。组织学上，基底细胞样细胞岛为不连续的半岛状，自表皮呈出牙状扩展，仅仅延伸到真皮浅层（图23.43）。常可见到炎症性宿主反应，可为浅表活检病变的诊断提供线索。浅表性基底细胞癌可出现分叶状浸润性成分。因此它会使人认为，浅表性变型为原位性病变。

硬化性结构在临床上为扁平瘢痕样斑片。组织学上，胶原性间质占据50%以上肿瘤成分。基底细胞样细胞一般排列成细线条索状。间质一般致密，呈反应性（图23.44）。对于这种肿瘤，在诊断切缘阴性的时候要格外小心，因为肿瘤细胞和皮肤附件均可受挤压，彼此之间具有相似性。这些病变的鉴别诊断非常重要，包括纤维组织增生性毛发上皮瘤、微囊性癌以及转移性乳腺癌[242]。

有些基底细胞癌可出现局灶性的特征性肿瘤分化结构，在生物学行为以及组织学表现方面不同于基底细胞癌。如伴有导管[243]、皮脂腺（图23.45）、毛囊[244,245]

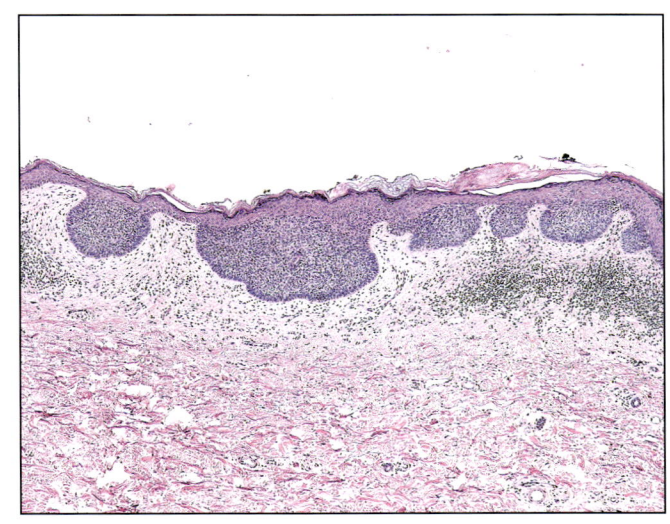

图23.43 基底细胞癌，浅表性。出芽状基底细胞样细胞巢通过较宽的前缘与表皮相连。

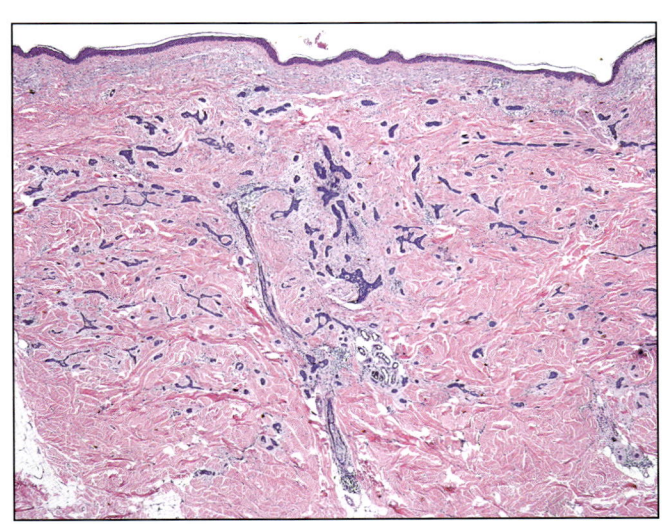

图23.44 基底细胞癌，硬化性。纤维组织增生性间质中可见纤细的基底细胞样条带。

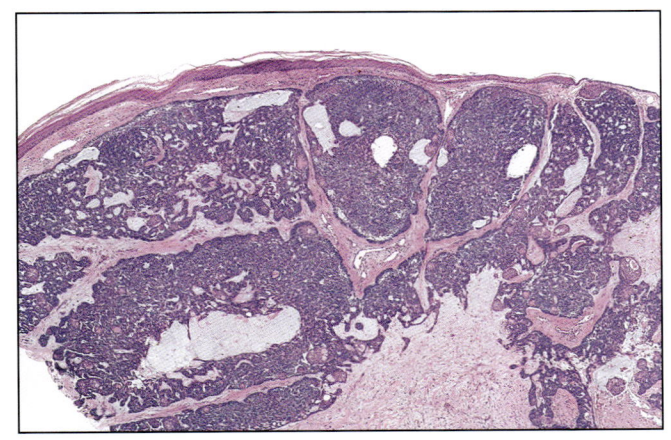

图23.42 基底细胞癌，黏液性。病变的间质部分可见黏液性区域。

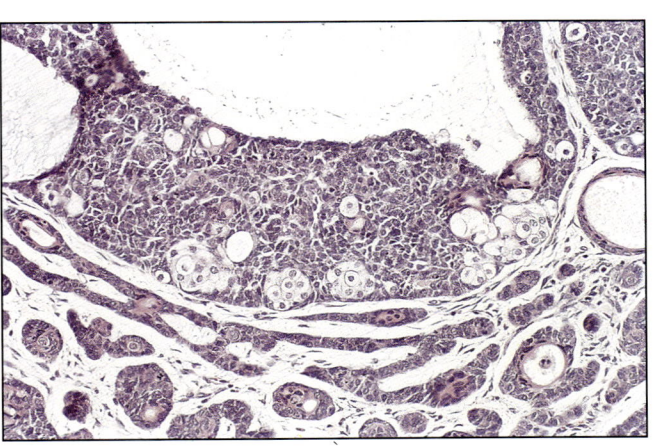

图23.45 基底细胞癌，伴有皮脂腺性区域。这种不常见的亚型可被纳入低级别皮脂腺肿瘤中。

或伴有增厚基底膜的角化性分化区的基底细胞癌[246]，或所有这些形式。有些病例甚至可出现神经内分泌特征[247,248]。除了角化性肿瘤以外，我将所有这些生长方式上属于普通基底细胞癌范畴的肿瘤纳入基底细胞癌。例外的情况是：各种肿瘤形态共存的病例预后可能较差，如所谓的小汗腺上皮瘤，尽管没有什么特别的特征，但或许应当将其并入附件癌中。角化性基底细胞样肿瘤多被归入基底细胞癌中，除非出现广泛角化和少见的浸润性生长方式，这样的病例应用基底细胞样癌这一术语比较合适；其他作者将其称为基底细胞鳞状细胞癌[249,250]。

由于多数基底细胞癌为惰性的，90%的病例可通过局部切除而得到长期治愈，尤其是采用特殊的技术，如Mohs手术[251,252]，即使肿瘤巨大[253]。在冰冻切片的诊断误区中，毛囊中心基底细胞样细胞区或外套瘤（mantleomas）[254]或毛囊小瘤可类似于硬化性基底细胞癌，必须将它们区别开[255]。

多数基底细胞癌病例可通过HE切片诊断。极少数病例可能需要免疫组织化学染色来与鳞状细胞癌鉴别。可以应用抗Ber-EP4抗体[256]，因为它可标记基底细胞癌中的基底细胞，而鳞状细胞癌不被标记。然而Ber-EP4是非特异性的，必须用于缩小诊断范围[257]。有些资料提示，CD34可能有助于鉴别毛囊肿瘤和基底细胞癌的间质，多数毛囊肿瘤间质CD34呈阳性，而基底细胞癌间质为阴性[258]。然而，应用这些抗体时需要谨慎[257]。

有极少数转移性病变被纳入了基底细胞癌[249,259,260]。这些病例大约2/3来自面部。直径在3cm以上的病变大约1.9%出现转移，硬化性基底细胞癌的总的转移率不足1%。对伴有T3和T4肿瘤的患者最好随访10年或更长，因为有远期转移的可能性[260]。然而，实际上多数基底细胞癌并不发生转移，至少多数病例在没有转移的时候就已诊断和治疗。

附件肿瘤　Adnexal tumors

附件肿瘤定义为伴有与一种或多种类型的正常皮肤可见的附件上皮（以及相应间质）相似的分化的良性或恶性病变。病变可为单发性或多发性。有些可以是某一综合征的成分，既可以是自发性的，也可以有家族性背景。

这些病变一般按照皮肤中确认的四种附件结构即毛囊、皮脂腺、顶泌汗腺和小汗腺进行讨论。然而，必须了解的是，任何一种病变都可能出现一种或多种分化系列。一般依照主要成分来进行肿瘤分类。

毛囊肿瘤　Tumors of the hair follicle

皮质毛囊肿瘤可以看做是一类类似于一种或多种毛囊成分的病变[261-263]，由毛胚芽、基质、皮质、毛球下的内外根鞘以及从毛球至表面的毛鞘组成。另外，有些肿瘤有比较明显的毛囊周围纤维鞘。

毛痣　Hair nevi

这里的痣或错构瘤是指：毛发出现在皮肤内，但其形态学异常，或与相邻正常皮肤的关系出现异常改变[264-267]。毛痣涵盖了一大类病变，从小的瘤样病变[268]到大的斑片的不同形态学类型的毛[269-270]。

毛囊瘤　Trichofolliculoma

这些肿瘤是由小的毛囊组成的，小毛囊围绕一个或多个常常开口于皮肤表面的囊样扩张的间隙呈放射状排列。一般表现为皮肤颜色的面部小结节，中央可以出现小的表皮开口。病变可能出现白须；少数情况下，整个表面可以长出较大的毛发。毛囊瘤可以发生于任何年龄，但通常在11～20岁时做出诊断[271-275]。因为许多病变为结节性，而且没有开口，所以临床上应与各种肿瘤和瘤样病变进行鉴别诊断。

组织学上，多数毛囊瘤是由内衬鳞状上皮的囊肿构成的，中心扩张，偶尔与表皮相连（图23.46）。中心囊腔含有正常角化的层状角质，内衬上皮颗粒层明显。囊腔内常见毛发。尽管多数病变仅有一个囊腔，但有些病变呈多房性。这些囊肿呈分枝状，形成"车轮"样可见多数毫毛，伴有或不伴有明显的皮脂腺成分[276]。这些结构的小的毛胚可能出芽，其内的Merkel细胞容易识别[277]。偶

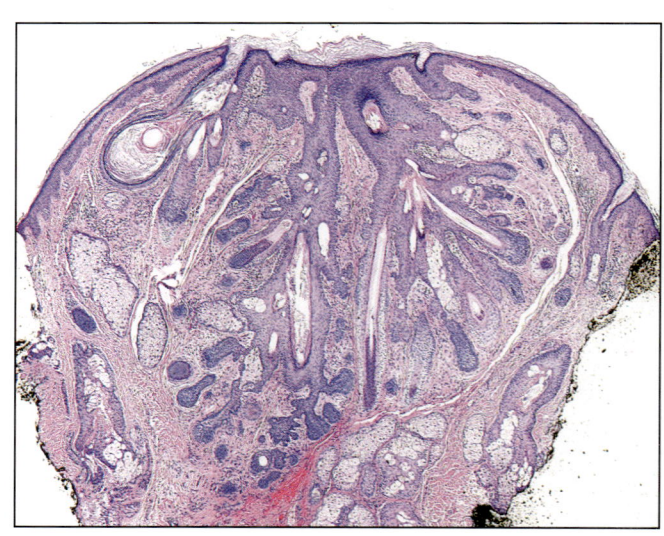

图23.46　毛囊瘤。可见囊肿，其周围有放射状排列的毫毛。

尔出现明显的皮脂腺小叶，产生皮样囊肿样结构，称为皮脂腺毛囊瘤（sebaceous trichofolliculoma）[278,279]。称为毛囊皮脂腺囊性错构瘤（folliculosebaceous cystic hamartoma）的病变也包含在这个范畴中[280,281]。这类病变的另一端则基本见不到毛发。病变部位可出现单纯性鳞状细胞条索或出芽。

毛发上皮瘤组（毛母细胞瘤）
Trichoepithelioma group (trichoblastomas)

毛发上皮瘤是指含有上皮结构的一系列良性毛囊上皮-间质肿瘤，类似于毛囊和（或）毛胚芽的一部分或多个部分。本病涵盖的范围极为广泛，因为它包括了所有细胞系的分化，于向毛胚芽、毛发或毛囊特殊定向分化的其他毛发和（或）毛囊肿瘤不同。我们喜欢将这些病变分类为经典性（毛胚芽、毛鞘和毛发）、毛母细胞性（主要为毛胚芽）、毛-"腺瘤"（主要为漏斗或峡部毛鞘）以及纤维组织增生性（一种特殊的伴有硬化性间质的毛胚芽、毛发和毛鞘病变）。

经典性毛发上皮瘤（classic trichoepithelioma）[282-284]：这种类型的肿瘤可为家族性多发性病变（腺样囊性上皮瘤，epithelioma adenoids cysticum），也可表现为孤立性病变。多发性病变多见于青春期或成年人，常常分布于面部中央。孤立性肿瘤可见于任何部位的有毛发被覆的皮肤，但以头颈部最为多见。极少数毛发上皮瘤可伴有其他附件肿瘤和综合征[285-301]。

组织学上，经典性毛发上皮瘤为对称性病变（图23.47），含有混合性上皮成分，包括伴有间叶性乳头状小体（毛囊乳头）的毛胚芽（图23.1）[302]到小的角质囊肿，乃至花边样网状基底细胞样结构，以及成熟的毛发（极少）。含有这些结构的间质一般为纤维化性间质，不同区域之间结构均一，并且近邻肿瘤，不同于基底细胞癌的

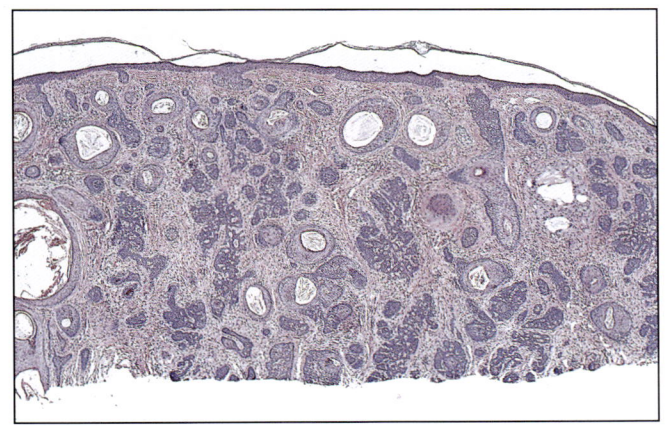

图23.47 经典性毛发上皮瘤。注意病变对称性、囊肿以及多种基底细胞样上皮成分。

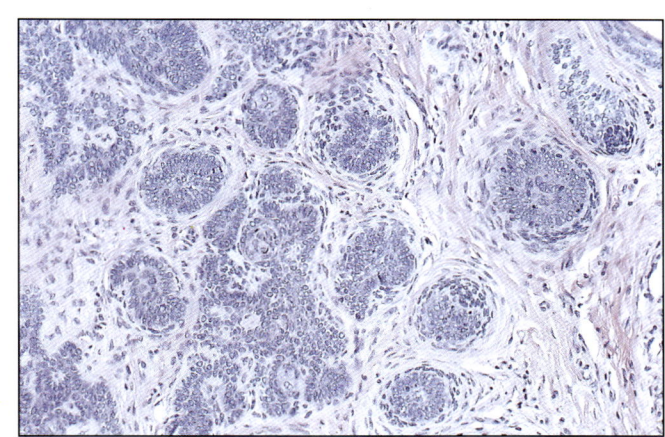

图23.48 经典性毛发上皮瘤。纤维性间质中可见数个伴有乳头状间叶小体的毛胚芽。

人工收缩假象。在有些病变中，角质囊肿破裂可能继而发生诸如角质肉芽肿等反应性病变。极少数情况下，这些病变可伴有基底细胞癌[303]。

毛母细胞肿瘤（trichoblastic tumors）[304]：这是一类上皮成分以毛胚芽（毛母细胞）为主并常常伴有较少至多量间质成分的肿瘤。这类肿瘤命名的变化取决于间质的多少、毛胚芽的数量以及出现在病变中的任何其他上皮成分。这类病变也可依照大小以及基底细胞样成分的结构特征来分类。

临床上，病变为孤立性的，有时位于真皮深层或皮下组织，肢体、躯干或盆腔部位较常见[305]，但有些可位于头颈部。多数病变的最大径不足1 cm，但少数可较大，直径可达数个厘米[306,307]。病变一般容易剥除，而且局部切除可以治愈。临床一般没有特别的鉴别诊断。

组织学上，这些病变的境界几乎总是非常清楚。肿瘤中极少含有角质囊肿，与经典的毛发上皮瘤不同。最原始的病变为毛母细胞瘤（trichoblastoma）[296,304]，仅含有基底细胞样的毛胚芽，没有间质和间叶性诱导[308]。具有中度成熟程度的病变，如具有间质分化以及伴有间叶性诱导的毛胚芽，被称为毛母细胞纤维瘤（trichoblastic fibroma）（图23.49）[309-313]。这些病变的范围从仅有毛胚芽和间质[314]到仅有间质、毛胚芽、基底细胞样细胞条索以及花边样的上皮成分[311]。最成熟的肿瘤称为毛源性毛母细胞瘤（trichogenic trichoblastoma）[315,316]，后者类似于毛母细胞瘤，但是此外它还含有完整的毛囊[304]。皮肤不常见的也含有毛胚芽的黏液性病变有时称为毛源性黏液瘤（trichogenic myxoma，又叫浅表性血管黏液瘤，见第24章）[317]。对于各种这类病变来说，主要的鉴别诊断为经典性毛发上皮瘤和基底细胞癌。

纤维上皮瘤（fibroepithelioma，又叫Pinkus瘤）[318]：临床上表现为丘疹或斑片，一般位于躯干背部。组织学上，

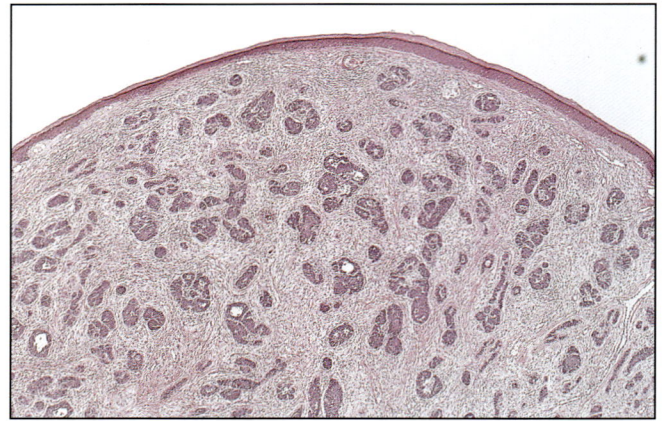

图23.49 毛母细胞纤维瘤。多量毛母细胞或毛胚芽分布于纤维性间质中。我们将这种病变视为毛发上皮瘤系列中的未成熟性亚型。

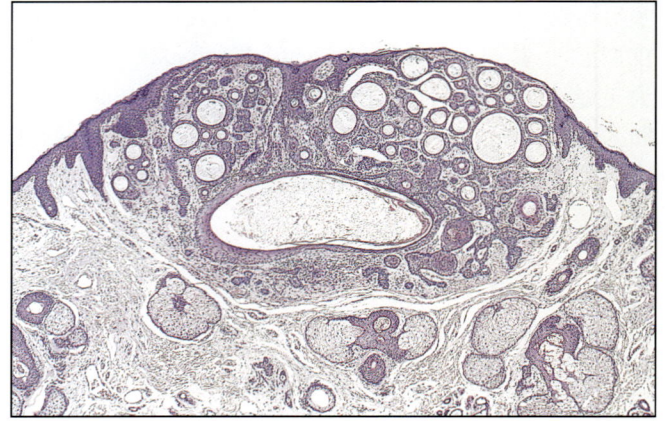

图23.51 毛发腺瘤。多量角质囊肿和基底细胞样细胞条索位于纤维性基质中。我们将其视为毛发上皮瘤系列中的成熟或终末亚型。

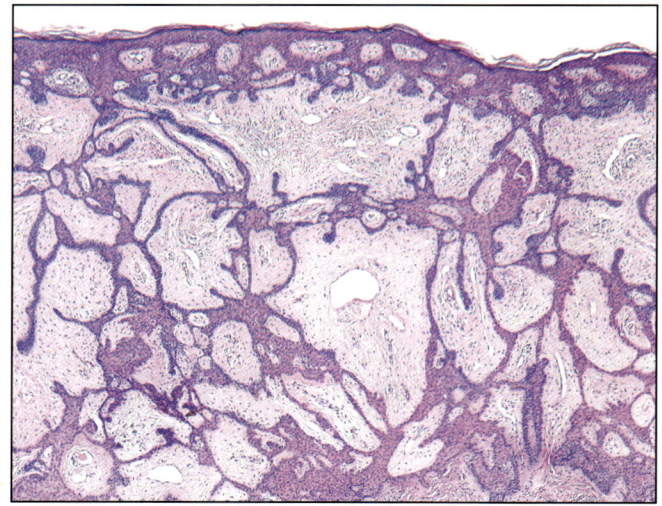

图23.50 纤维上皮瘤（Pinkus瘤）。网状基底细胞样细胞条索与表面相连，偶尔含有毛胚芽。

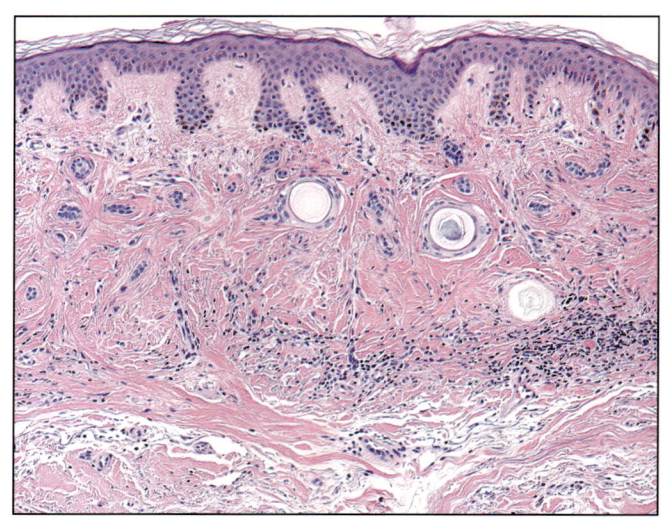

图23.52 纤维组织增生性毛发上皮瘤。纤细的基底细胞样细胞条索和小的角质囊肿位于纤维组织增生性间质中。

可见均匀分布的网状结构，伴有明显的纤维性间质（图23.50）。这些病变生物学行为上呈惰性，不同于典型的基底细胞癌，最好纳入毛囊附件肿瘤系列。

毛发-"腺瘤" [tricho-"adenoma"(Nikolowski)] [319,320]：定义为毛发上皮瘤伴有局限于纤维性间质内的明显的囊腔；它并非为腺瘤。这些病变类似于毛囊的漏斗部分，而不是生发部分。临床上，毛发腺瘤一般为结节状至疣状。

组织学上，毛发腺瘤（trichoadenoma）为对称性病变，伴有混合性的角质囊肿，可以通过基底细胞样细胞条索彼此相连，也可以不相连（图23.51）。如果角质囊肿破裂，偶尔可见角质肉芽肿。个别病例表面呈疣状增生 [321]。

纤维组织增生性毛发上皮瘤（desmoplastic trichoepithelioma）[242,322]：是一类对称性、境界清楚的肿瘤，由位于纤维组织增生性真皮内的受压的毛囊上皮构成。不论范围多大，皮下组织均不受累。

临床上，这些病变一般为孤立性病变，但在个别情况下可为多发性病变。两种类型的家族性病例均有报道 [323,324]。肿瘤一般见于女性的面颊。多数直径不足1cm，并且出现中央小凹 [325]。局部切除可以治愈。主要的临床鉴别诊断是硬化性基底细胞癌和微囊性附件癌。

组织学上，这些病变为对称性病变，伴有境界清楚的纤维化区域，将肿瘤与正常皮肤分隔开（图23.52）。除了受压的上皮条索外，浅表部位可见小的角质囊肿，如果囊肿破裂，可以出现角质肉芽肿。在深处偶尔可见小的毛胚芽。虽然小汗腺及导管可以出现在肿瘤之中，但这些仅为继发性受累。有证据提示，这些病变含有Merkel细胞，而硬化性基底细胞癌中没有这些成分 [326]。基质分解素-3（stromelysin-3）为基质金属蛋白酶，在纤维组织增生性毛发上皮瘤的间质中呈阴性，但在一些硬化性基底细胞癌中呈阳性 [327]；因此，这个标记物可以用于诊断。

鉴别诊断包括硬化性基底细胞癌、微囊性附件癌和转移癌，尤其是来自乳腺的转移癌，所有这些病变均可出现非对称性和非均一性的真皮硬化性结构，并且诊断时有皮下组织受累。然而，评估表浅刮除活检标本时应当谨慎，因为这种活检标本可能含有不能区分是惰性抑或较为侵袭性的肿瘤区域。

皮肤淋巴腺瘤　Cutaneous lymphadenoma

皮肤淋巴腺瘤是伴有多量淋巴细胞和其他单核细胞浸润的基底细胞样细胞良性肿瘤。有些肿瘤具有类似于毛囊皮脂腺结构的区域[328,329]。少数肿瘤还有某种程度的导管分化[330,331]。

这种病变最常见于年轻成人的面部。有些病例可能有超过20年的缓慢生长的病史，支持其具有良性的生物学行为和自限性的本质。临床上，皮肤浸润表现为境界不清的肉色区域。

组织学上，真皮内出现多发性上皮性小叶，与表皮常常没有明显的连接（图23.53）。病变出现分化成熟的、相对无细胞的纤维性间质，几乎没有炎症细胞。上皮性小叶外周可见明显的立方性或扁平角化细胞层，并有少数角化漩涡灶形成。这些上皮性小叶中央的细胞较大，细胞核大，核仁明显，并且有多量嗜双色性胞浆，混有多量小淋巴细胞（图23.54）。尽管淋巴细胞似乎选择性地位于上皮内，但有些淋巴细胞可以进入间质。通过S-100蛋白染色可以证实上皮小叶内有许多树突状细胞。曾有争议，有人认为这种类型的病变是"成釉性"毛母质瘤（"adamantinoid" trichoblastoma）[332]。我认为这些病变可能表现为毛囊分化，对于这些病变我也避免应用"成釉性"一词。我认为这些病变在结构上非常接近纤维组织增生性毛发上皮瘤（desmoplastic trichoepithelioma）[333]，但在一些病变中出现一些导管和（或）皮脂腺结构，正如我们在自己的病例中所见到的，这一事实导致最初"皮肤淋巴腺瘤"一词的出现。鉴别诊断包括基底细胞癌，毫无疑问，在出现皮肤淋巴腺瘤这种概念之前，通常都被诊断为基底细胞癌[228]。

毛囊漏斗肿瘤[334-341]
Tumor of the follicular infundibulum

不管这类病变在历史上被赋予什么名称，它们都是由成片的合体细胞样粉染细胞条索构成的，类似于毛囊峡部。这些细胞条索平行于皮肤表面排列，并间断性地与之相连。临床上，这种病变为小的丘疹或斑片，可为单发或多发[342-344]，多发性病变可伴有综合征或其他肿瘤[335,345]。病变常常局限于头颈部，但也可见于躯干。临床鉴别诊断包括基底细胞癌、花斑性糠疹或播散性浅

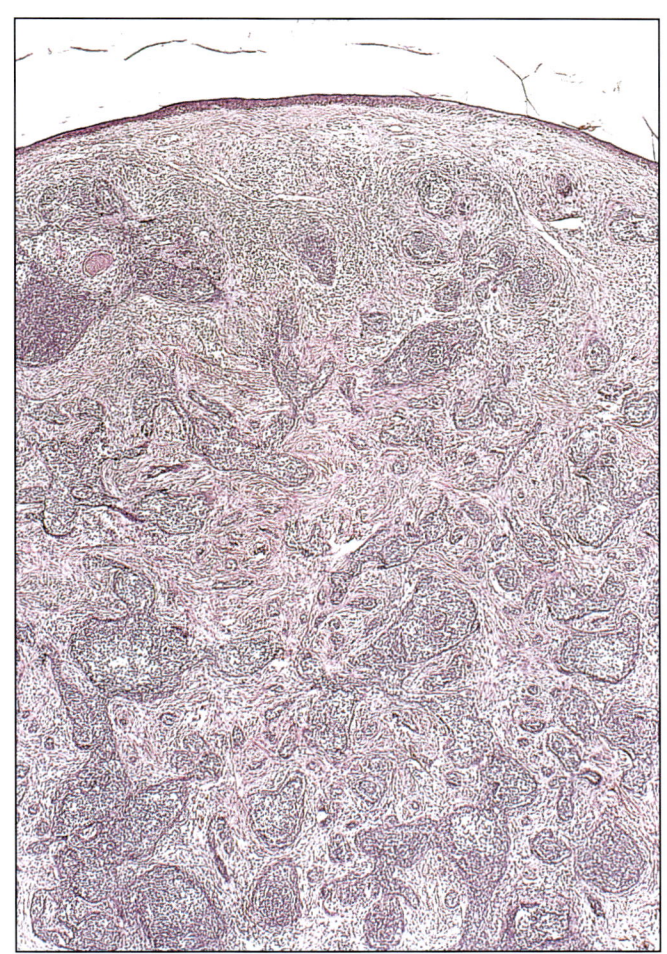

图23.53　淋巴腺瘤。这种病变由周围有基底细胞样细胞的小岛构成。小岛内含有多量淋巴细胞和组织细胞。

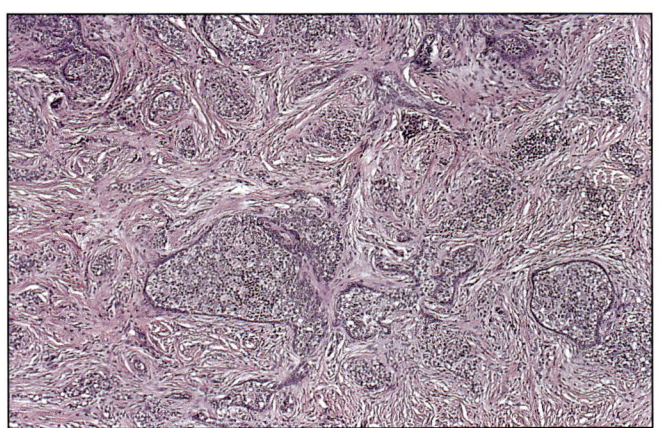

图23.54　淋巴腺瘤。图中可见上皮内有单核细胞浸润。注意硬化性间质。

表日光性汗孔角化病。

组织学上，肿瘤呈对称性、片状生长方式，细胞含有均匀一致细胞核和粉染的胞浆，类似于峡部上皮细胞，尽管历史上其名称为漏斗瘤（infundibuloma）（图23.55）。病变周围有增厚的PAS阳性的基底膜围绕，其下真皮内可见致密的弹力纤维网[335]。病变中可见小的角化正常的微腔或导管。整个病变多层次的重新构建显

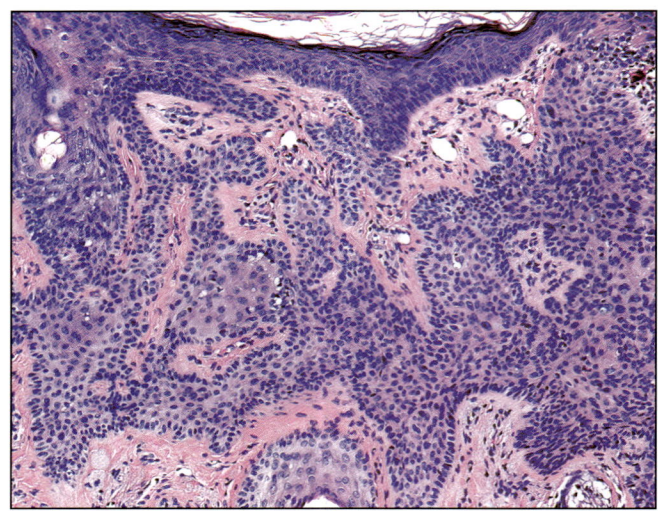

图23.55 毛囊漏斗肿瘤。鳞状细胞呈片状生长，与表面上皮平行。

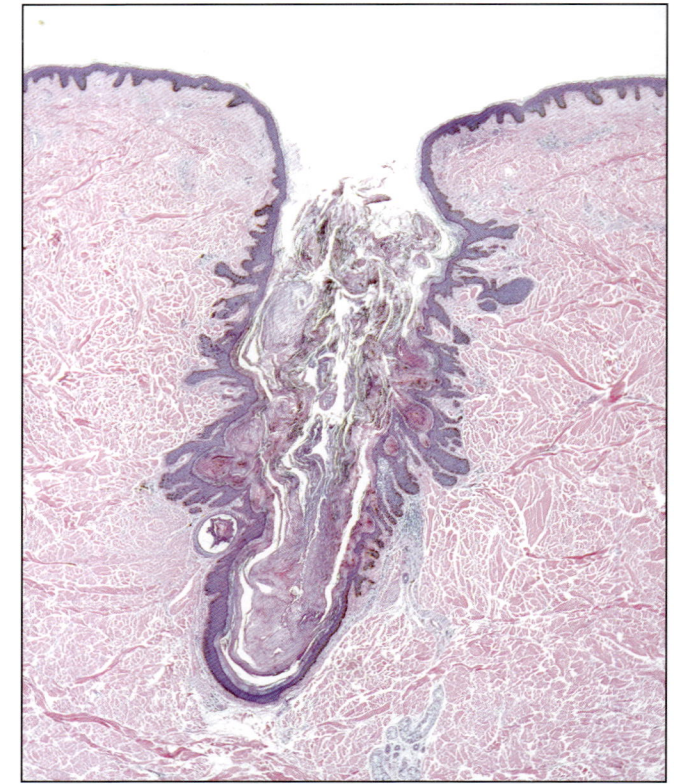

图23.56 毛囊孔扩张（Winer）。内陷并增宽的开口充满正常角化的角质。

示有多数孔隙与表皮相连。鉴别诊断包括斑状脂溢性角化病、日光性角化病以及浅表性基底细胞癌。

毛囊孔扩张[346,347]
Dilated pore（Winer）

这种病变是指大小不一的孤立性毛囊孔扩张性病变，通常发生于成人的上唇，但在少数情况下也可以见于其他部位。组织学上为单一的漏斗形结构，深达真皮内，但开口于表面（图 23.56）。病变内衬漏斗上皮，其内充满致密层状角质。囊内衬可见一大片棘皮症结构，但并不突出。一种不常见的含有毛发皮脂样角质栓的亚型被称为毛发皮质粉刺（hair cortex comedo），也有可能被纳入皮质肿瘤中[348]。临床鉴别诊断包括粉刺和基底细胞癌；组织学上要与粉刺鉴别。

毛鞘棘皮瘤[349-353]
Pilar sheath acanthoma

这是一种孤立性病变，通常位于成人的面部，尤其是唇部。病变可透过膨胀的开口与表面相连，并且可含有成片的类似于漏斗和峡部的上皮，由中心孔向外呈放射状排列（图23.57）。切面可以出现小囊肿，取决于切面水平。有些病例可有导管结构，但多数为实性的。极少数情况下可以见到毛囊的其他部分甚至皮脂腺成分。临床上的鉴别诊断包括粉刺、毛囊孔扩张以及毛囊囊肿。组织学上要与毛囊孔扩张、毛囊瘤（trichofolliculoma）以及肢端汗腺瘤（acrospiroma）鉴别。

外毛根鞘瘤[354] Tricholemmoma

外毛根鞘瘤以单发性或多发性丘疹为特征，组织学上由含糖原的透明上皮细胞组成，上皮细胞周围有明显

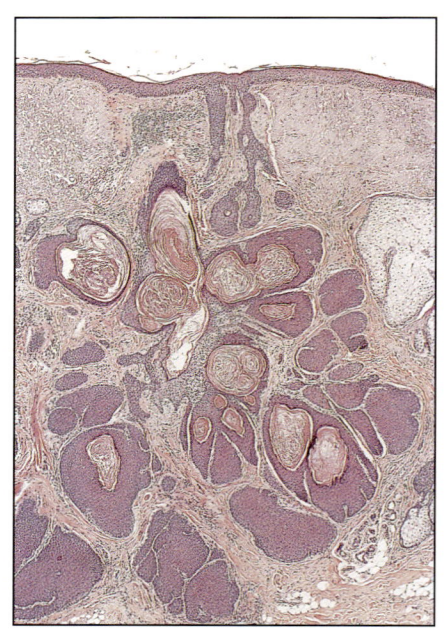

图23.57 毛鞘棘皮瘤。多数形态单一的鳞状上皮芽伴有角质囊肿，由中央向外呈放射状排列，可与表面相连。

的透明层，类似于毛囊过渡部分的外壳，即主要是毛球部分。

临床上，病变一般发生于老年人，但患者年龄范围可从11～20岁到81～90岁不等。单个病变一般为圆

顶形的肤色丘疹，直径不足 5 mm。多数位于面部，特别是在鼻部，但眼睑、唇以及口腔也可受累[355-357]。临床上外毛根鞘瘤的鉴别诊断包括疣、反转性脂溢性（"毛囊"）角化病以及基底细胞癌。

多发性外毛根鞘瘤的特征是伴有 Cowden 综合征（多发性错构瘤综合征）[358]，定义为一系列多发性皮肤错构瘤（外毛根鞘瘤、疣状角化细胞病变以及纤维瘤）[359-364]、内脏错构瘤[365]和（或）内脏癌（尤其是乳腺癌）[358]。它是一种外显率高的常染色体显性遗传性病[366]。Cowden 综合征面部病变的临床鉴别诊断包括病毒性疣、Darier 病、结节性硬化、毛发上皮瘤、神经纤维瘤病、痣样基底细胞癌综合征、汗腺腺瘤以及圆柱瘤[360]。肢端病变的鉴别诊断包括疣状表皮发育不良、扁平疣、疣状肢端角化病、灰泥样角化病以及点状皮肤角化病[360]。治疗上应当个性化[367]，因为病变数量较多，不可能手术切除或局部破坏所有的病变。

组织学上，外毛根鞘瘤为对称性病变，一般呈球形，边缘清楚，被明显的 PAS 阳性的透明膜包绕（图23.58）。外毛根鞘瘤通常具有结构上的变异，从毛囊样垂直分布的病变到分叶状球形没有导管的肢端汗管瘤样病变甚至疣状病变。在许多病例可见与表面有广泛的连接。细胞易形成外周栅栏状排列，尤其是在位置较深的部分。不一致的表现为鳞状细胞漩涡或角化正常的微囊，类似于内翻性脂溢性角化病。纤维组织增生性外毛根鞘瘤[368]可出现大量间质，围绕上皮周边，常分布于肿瘤结节的中央（图 23.59）。这种亚型含有梭形细胞成分，肿瘤细胞与间质相互混杂，类似于癌。也可以见到大片嗜酸性无定形、alcian 蓝和 PAS 淀粉酶阳性的物质；这可能为基底膜物质。有些病例中可以检测出内皮蛋白（involucrin）[369]。外毛根鞘瘤的细胞和毛球的外鞘部分一般 CD34 呈阳性[370]。间质含有波形蛋白，细胞外基质含有肌腱蛋白（tenascin）和 I 型胶原 I[371]。极少数病例伴有基底细胞癌[372]和皮脂腺痣[373]。

在有些外毛根鞘瘤中可以见到单个毛囊与之相连；在毛囊中部出现明显透明细胞上皮增生。有不等量的纤维性间质，类似于毛鞘；有些病例可见单核炎症细胞浸润。

一些肿瘤主要位于表皮下，而另一些可呈疣状[374,375]。有人提出，外毛根鞘瘤，尤其是呈疣状结构的病变，为老年疣（aged warts）[376,377]。有人支持这种见解，有人反对[378-381]。在外毛根鞘瘤中确认病毒颗粒或抗原的尝试除极个别者[382]均未成功[203,260]。

细胞学上，上皮细胞含有丰富的透明胞浆，其中含有糖原，很容易通过淀粉酶敏感性 PAS 染色来证实[354]。有些病变含有嗜酸性"中间型"细胞，缺乏典型病变的透明细胞表现。有人将这些病变叫做"毛囊

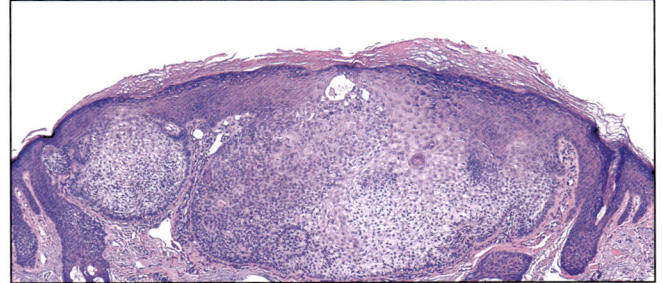

图23.58　外毛根鞘瘤。芽样透明细胞肿瘤位于增厚的玻璃样基底膜上。

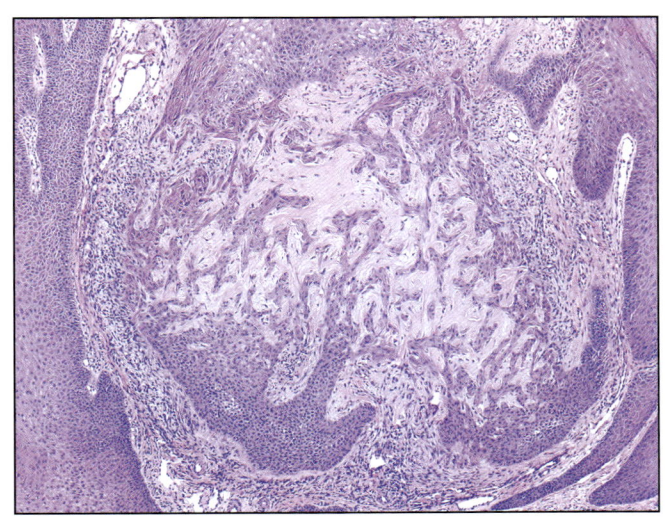

图23.59　外毛根鞘瘤，纤维组织增生性。复杂的淡染细胞条索和玻璃样间质。

口瘤"（"acrotrichomas"）或"毛囊汗孔瘤"（"follicular poromas"）[384]。

最为困难的鉴别诊断是与透明细胞肢端汗腺瘤（汗孔瘤）的鉴别，后者含有导管腔并缺乏外毛根鞘瘤的外周栅栏状结构以及玻璃样基底膜成分。以中间型细胞为主的肿瘤与基底细胞癌或内翻性脂溢性角化病的鉴别可能有困难[246]。纤维组织增生性外毛根鞘瘤还有与其他恶性肿瘤即与梭形细胞鳞状细胞癌和纤维组织增生性基底细胞癌混淆的危险。

漏斗囊肿（表皮样囊肿）
Infundibular cyst（epidermoid cyst）

这是最常见的毛囊囊肿（大约占 80%）。临床上，病变可位于任何有毛发的皮肤部分，但一般见于头、颈或躯干部[385]。大小从 2 mm 到 5 cm，可以通过单纯切除治疗或仅仅是观察。临床上鉴别诊断较多。与结肠息肉、硬纤维瘤以及骨瘤同时发生的多发性漏斗囊肿被称为 Gardner 综合征[386]。

组织学上，囊肿一般与表面并不相连，但偶尔可见小的连接。囊肿内衬成熟至颗粒层的复层鳞状上皮，并

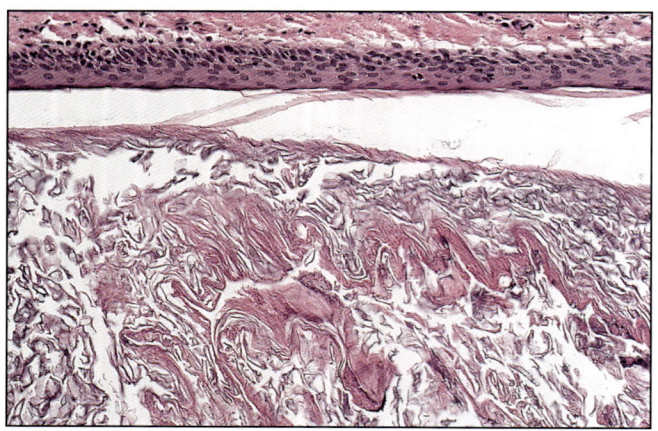

图23.60　角质囊肿，漏斗型。纤细的角质与表面类似。

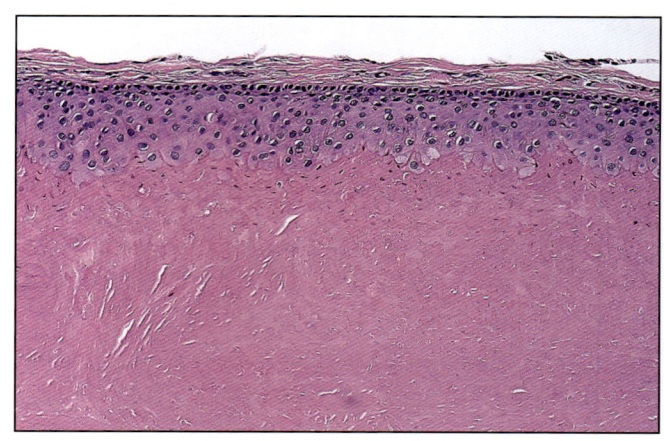

图23.61　角质囊肿，外毛根鞘型。致密的角质类似于毛发，没有颗粒细胞层。

形成网篮状以及角化正常的层状鳞片，类似于表皮（图23.60）。偶尔，囊肿色素增加，一般见于黑皮肤的患者。在极少数情况下，可出现诸如原位癌、传染性软疣、棘层松解性角化不良以及HPV诱导的疣状改变。如果囊肿壁有破裂，可出现异物肉芽肿性角质反应。

色素性毛囊囊肿[387-391]
Pigmented follicular cyst

这是一种极为少见的内衬复层鳞状上皮的囊肿，含有层状角质以及多量毛干。临床上病变位于头、颈、躯干部，极个别位于肢体。直径一般小于2 cm，常常由于Tyndall效应而呈黑色。临床鉴别诊断包括蓝痣、汗腺囊瘤以及囊性基底细胞瘤。

组织学上，病变在表面有一个窄的开口。病变内衬成熟至颗粒层的复层鳞状上皮，而且囊腔内含有层状角质以及多量毛发。典型的病变并不伴有其他的附件。组织学上需要与发疹性毫毛囊肿鉴别。

外毛根鞘（毛发：峡部-毛发生长中期）囊肿
Tricholemmal (pilar: isthmus-catagen) cyst

这是第二个最常见的毛囊囊肿（大约占10%～15%的病例），历史上曾称为皮脂腺囊肿，尽管过去对各种组织学类型的囊肿不恰当地采用过多种名称。临床上，外毛根鞘囊肿几乎均发生于头皮，但躯干或肢体其他部位也可受累[385]。女性比男性更常见。单纯切除可以治愈。需要与多种皮肤肿瘤进行鉴别诊断。

组织学上，上皮内衬显示角化细胞成熟不及颗粒层。内衬细胞较大，靠近顶部含有多量胞浆，类似于毛囊生长中期的峡部角化。角化突然出现且致密，不同于漏斗囊肿的层状角化（图23.61）。有些病例出现内衬上皮增生，类似于增生性外毛根鞘囊肿（毛发肿瘤）（图23.62），这是主要的鉴别诊断。

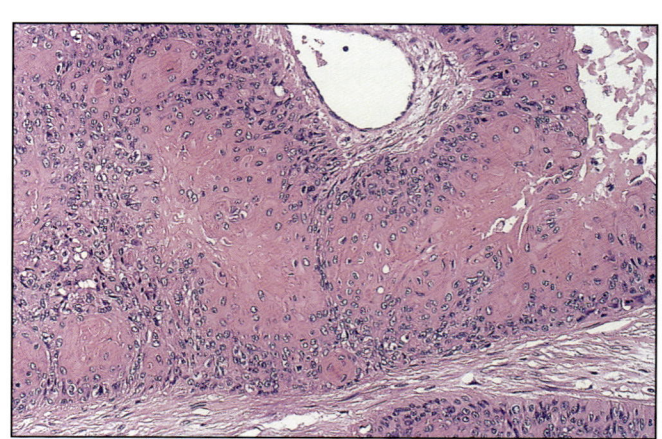

图23.62　增生性外毛根鞘囊肿，与外毛根鞘囊肿类似，但上皮结构较为复杂，并且位于真皮中层和深部。

混合性毛囊囊肿
Hybrid (mixed) follicular cyst

这是一种含有两种或两种以上内衬上皮类型的囊肿，如漏斗和外毛根鞘上皮[392]，但可包含非常宽泛的范围并已有文献记载[393-397]。这种变化可能有助于认识下面的一些综合征，如Gardner综合征中的多发性囊肿，其中有些囊肿的内衬上皮类似于漏斗和毛母质上皮，这些是它的一种属性[398]。如果仔细检查所有的囊肿，常常可以发现微妙的混合性改变，但在单个病变中发现独特的不同类型的上皮并不多见。

发疹性毫毛囊肿[399-406]
Eruptive vellus hair cyst

这是一种罕见的现象，由多发性小囊肿组成，常常迅速生长，显示漏斗、皮脂腺导管以及局灶性峡部-毛发生长中期的成熟表现，并且含有毫毛。有些作者认为这些病变只不过是皮脂腺囊瘤的亚型[399]。

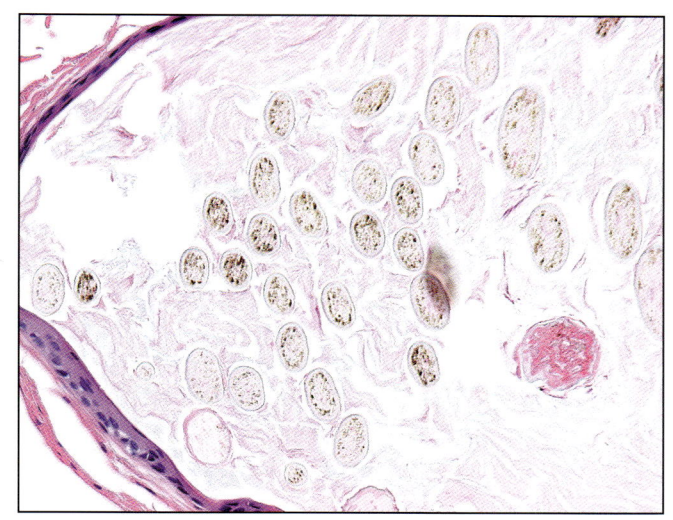

图23.63 发疹性毫毛囊肿。上皮较薄，含有小的毛干以及不等量的角质。

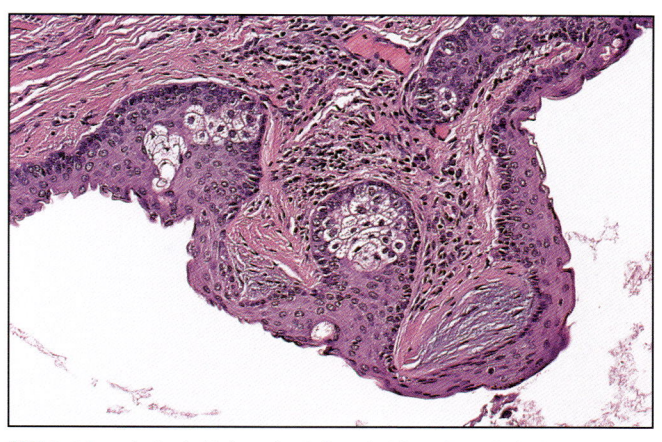

图23.64 皮脂腺囊瘤。囊肿表面起皱，囊壁内含有皮脂腺。与发疹性毫毛囊肿的特征有重叠。

临床上，囊肿一般在30岁以前变得明显，白种人主要在20岁以前，东方人在11～30岁。有些受累患者具有血缘关系，提示有些病例与遗传有关[407-409]。这些病变为颜色不同的丘疹，大小为直径1～4 mm，有些病变可见中央脐凹。未见到Köbner现象伴随本病发生的报道。没有性别差异。病变出现的部位依照递减的顺序为胸壁、上肢、面部[410]和小腿。累及胸部的病例中半数没有其他部位受累。临床鉴别诊断包括粉刺、多发性皮脂腺囊瘤、毛囊炎、毛发角化病、毛囊多毳角栓病、穿孔性病变以及粟粒疹。多数病变顽固，难以治疗，但有少数采用二氧化碳激光[411]和维甲酸[412]治疗成功的病例报告。

组织学上，漏斗成熟达颗粒层，但是偶尔囊肿内衬起皱，类似于皮脂腺导管，或其部分内衬类似于峡部-毛发生长中期囊肿。囊内可见多数小毛干（图23.63）。偶尔有终期毛囊，极少数情况下可以见到皮脂腺和（或）平滑肌。组织学鉴别诊断包括皮脂腺囊瘤[413,414]、漏斗囊肿以及色素性毛囊囊肿。

皮脂腺囊瘤（皮脂腺导管囊肿）[399,406,413,415-423]
Steatocystoma（sebaceous duct cyst）

这是一种小囊肿，其内衬上皮类似于皮脂腺导管有皱褶的上皮。皮脂腺常常伴有这种囊肿。

临床上，这些囊肿常常发生于11～20岁至31～40岁，最多见于青春期或青春期前后。一般表现为肤色到蓝色乃至黑色的丘疹，大小从几个毫米到几个厘米。如果切开囊肿，常可见白色液体流出。囊肿一般为多发性的（多发性皮脂腺囊瘤），但也可为孤立性的（单发性皮脂腺囊瘤）。病变多位于胸部，但也可见于面部、背部、肢体以及其他少数部位。如果囊肿呈多发性，通常为常染色体显性遗传类型。有时皮脂腺囊瘤伴有外胚层发育不良。对于多发性病变，鉴别诊断包括发疹性毫毛囊肿、Gardner综合征以及聚合性痤疮。孤立性病变的鉴别诊断包括多种囊肿和肿瘤。除了异维甲酸[424]和冷冻手术[425]外，其他疗法一般均不成功。

组织学上，皮脂腺囊瘤为空腔，匍行的囊壁衬以薄层鳞状上皮，表面上皮起皱（图23.64）。几乎没有颗粒层[418,419]。可见发育不全的上皮从囊肿延续至表皮表面。皮脂腺常常与之相邻或与囊肿壁直接延续[417]。囊肿内偶尔可见毫毛[426]；极少数情况下，囊壁内可见毫毛芽[419]。鉴别诊断包括发疹性毫毛囊肿、皮样囊肿、囊性皮脂腺增生以及色素性毛囊囊肿。

毛母质瘤（钙化性上皮瘤；毛母质瘤）[427-432]
Pilomatricoma（calcifying epithelioma；trichomatricoma）

这是一种良性皮肤和（或）皮下肿瘤，组织学上类似于基线以上毛球水平的毛母质部分。临床上，多数病变为分布于头、颈或上肢的孤立性结节。结节可能质韧或质硬，且较平，直径一般从5 mm到2 cm。极少数情况下可为多发性[433]，有穿孔和（或）迅速进展。常常发生于20岁以内，但也可见于任何年龄[434]。临床鉴别诊断较多，除非病变较平。极个别病例伴有强直性肌营养不良[435,436]。单纯切除可以治愈。

组织学上，病变的特征是基底细胞样小叶，周围可见混有角质的嗜酸性衰老细胞；后者称为"影"细胞（"shadow" cells）（图23.65）。基底细胞样细胞一般呈均一性，形态一致，大小类似于基底细胞癌的基底细胞样细胞。任何组织学视野内均可见许多处于核分裂的细胞。影细胞无细胞核，但基本上保留了基底细胞样细胞的形

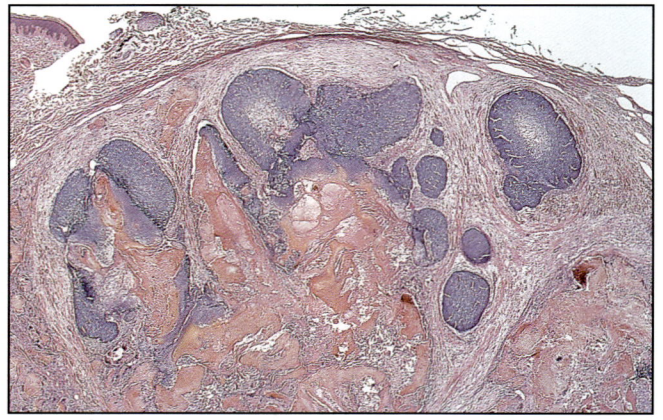

图23.65 毛母质瘤。肿瘤由基底细胞样细胞构成，伴有粉染的影细胞。

态（图23.66）。作为一种继发性现象，通常还可出现巨细胞浸润和营养不良性钙化，据推测是宿主对影细胞和角质的反应。含有相当数量基底细胞样细胞的病变可为囊性；没有基底细胞样细胞的病变一般为由影细胞、钙化以及巨细胞反应组成的实性肿瘤。与普通的毛母质瘤相比，称为母质瘤（matricoma）[437]的病变倾向于较大并保留较多的基底细胞样细胞。另一种亚型称为增生性毛母质瘤，由大的分叶状基底细胞样细胞增生构成，伴有或大或小的影细胞灶[438]。在 Gardner 综合征的囊肿中[439,440]以及在极少数器官样（皮脂腺）痣[441]中已经观察到毛母质瘤样改变。组织化学[442]和超微结构上[443]，毛母质瘤类似于毛基质。组织学鉴别诊断包括基底细胞癌、神经内分泌癌以及母质癌（matrical carcinoma）。毛母质瘤一般容易诊断，除非整个病变由基底细胞样细胞构成，最初无需考虑鉴别诊断。

复合性毛囊肿瘤 Complex follicular tumors

这些病变为混合性肿瘤，目前很难将其纳入任何其他诊断类别。这些肿瘤常常以病变中占主导的上皮类型来命名。含有不同毛囊装置部分的肿瘤称为全毛囊瘤（panfolliculoma）[444]。

毛发和毛囊癌
Carcinomas of the hair and hair follicle

与毛发和（或）毛囊成分相类似的癌极为少见，多为单个病例报告。这些病变大致可以按照类似于峡部、毛囊移行部位的外毛根鞘或基质结构的癌来进行分类，因此称为外毛根鞘癌或母质癌。

外毛根鞘癌（trocholemmal carcinoma）[445-447]：这些肿瘤从形态学上很难界定，主要是由于难以与普通的透明细胞性鳞状细胞癌区分[448]。如果将透明细胞性恶性顶端汗腺腺瘤（顶端汗腺癌、汗孔癌）考虑在鉴别诊断中，则情况更为复杂。外毛根鞘癌为多分叶性肿瘤，伴有多量透明细胞分化（图23.67）。病变具有良性对应肿瘤的囊性-分叶状生长方式，但伴有明显的细胞学多形性、结构紊乱以及浸润性生长（图23.68）。在同一张切片中伴有良性成分（即显示增生性特征的所谓的增生性毛瘤，proliferating pilar tumor）的并不少见。也有的毛囊癌在结构上类似于或明显起源于增生性外毛根鞘囊肿[449-454]。甚至有人认为所有的增生性外毛根鞘囊肿都是癌[455]。

母质癌（matrical carcinomas）[456-460]：这些病变类似于毛母质瘤的形态学特征，伴有细胞学多形性、浸润性生长、体积较大以及转移潜能。

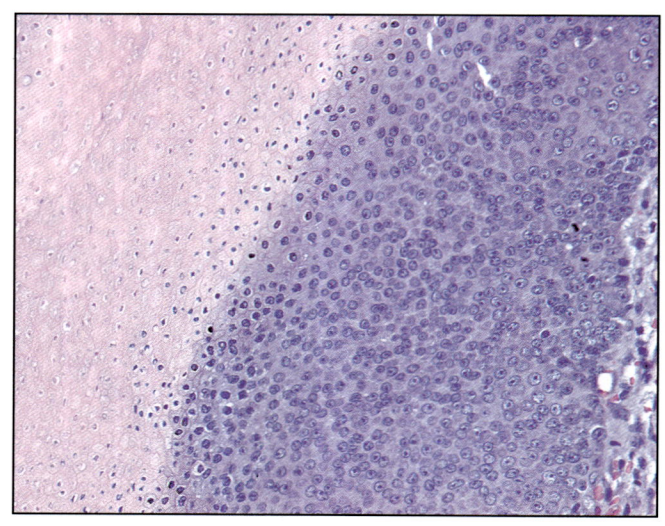

图23.66 毛母质瘤。基底细胞样细胞向影细胞移行。

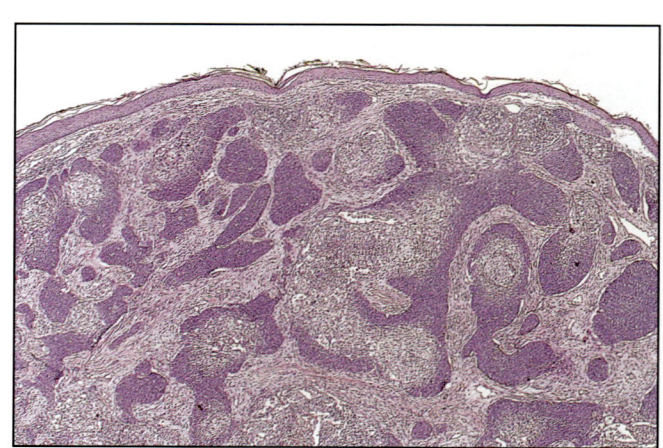

图23.67 外毛根鞘癌。肿瘤由含有透明细胞的小叶构成。

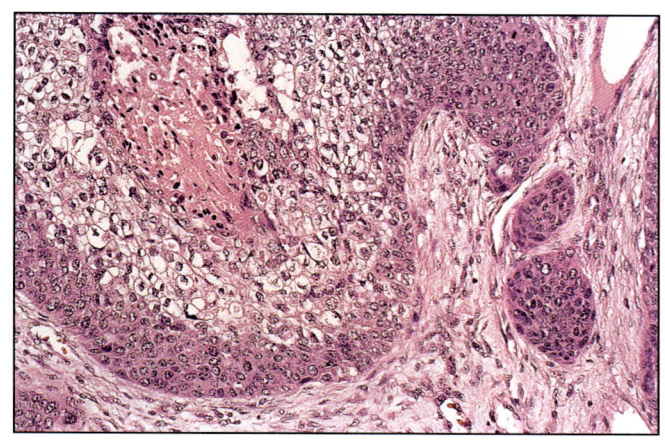

图23.68 外毛根鞘癌。这个小叶有些类似于毛球部位的外毛囊鞘。

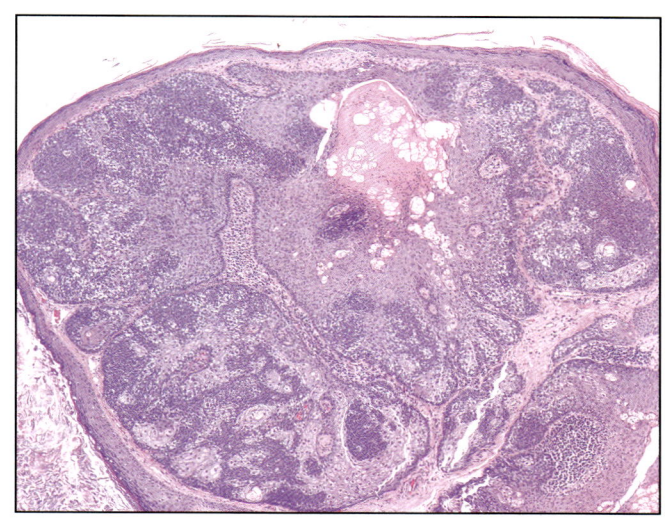

图23.69 皮脂腺腺瘤。皮脂腺细胞小叶含有生发细胞。这个病变含有皮脂腺细胞小叶，伴有轻度终末性分化。

皮脂腺肿瘤　Sebaceous neoplasms

与非常常见的皮脂腺增生不同，皮脂腺肿瘤相对少见。组织学上，这些肿瘤包括皮脂腺腺瘤、皮脂腺瘤、皮脂腺母质瘤、皮脂腺上皮瘤以及皮脂腺癌。其他病变，诸如分泌皮脂的腺瘤（sebocrine adenomas）[461]、皮肤淋巴腺瘤[329]以及伴有皮脂腺分化的浅表性上皮瘤[462]，可出现在皮脂腺细胞区域，可以包括在这个家族内。我们进一步发现，多种基底细胞样细胞肿瘤均可出现在皮脂腺细胞灶，包括基底细胞癌、圆柱瘤以及汗腺腺瘤。从实用角度讲，可将多数皮脂腺肿瘤分为两个大类：皮脂腺腺瘤和皮脂腺癌。

皮脂腺腺瘤[463,464]　Sebaceous adenoma

这是一组含有皮脂腺细胞和明显生发层的分叶状肿瘤。病变一般散在分布，具有自限性。在一些情况下，伴有这种肿瘤的患者可出现内脏恶性肿瘤，主要是结肠的（Muir-Torre综合征）[465-469]。

临床上，多数皮脂腺腺瘤为黄色病变，表现为成人头部的孤立性肿瘤。多数病变直径不足1 cm，单纯切除可以治愈。

组织学上表现多样，从主要由成熟皮脂腺以及一至两层生发上皮构成的小肿瘤到主要由多数基底细胞样生发上皮和极少数成熟皮脂腺细胞构成的肿瘤（图23.69，23.70）。后一种类型的皮脂腺腺瘤可能出现皮脂腺导管和小囊。这种分类中的所有肿瘤均缺少癌所特有的间质浸润这一特征。鉴别诊断包括基底细胞癌和皮脂腺癌。

皮脂腺癌[470-472]　Sebaceous carcinoma

这是一类少见的、类似于皮脂腺腺瘤的皮肤肿瘤，但通常伴有某种程度的间质浸润，生物学上呈进行性临

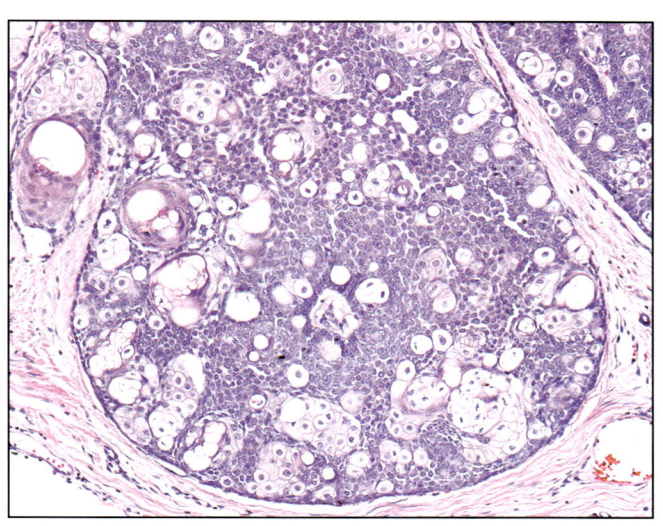

图23.70 皮脂腺腺瘤。皮脂腺细胞小叶伴有生发细胞。这个病变含有皮脂腺细胞，伴有明显的生发结构。

床经过。历史上将这些肿瘤分为眼部（眼睑）[473,474]和眼外（非眼睑）两类[475]，前一种最常见（见第29章）。这些肿瘤具有复发和转移的潜能，但现有资料尚不足以提供更多的结论。

组织学上，这种病变类似于良性皮脂腺肿瘤，除了可出现浸润性区域以及常常含有多形性透明和实性细胞团外（图23.71和23.72）。Paget样播散有时为眼部肿瘤的特征，不要误诊为是小汗腺和顶泌汗腺导管癌、黑色素瘤或Merkel细胞癌[476]。在有些病例中，免疫染色对诊断可能有帮助，因为这些癌中的皮脂腺细胞EMA和人乳脂球蛋白呈阳性，但S-100蛋白、CEA或乳腺相关抗原GCDFP-15为阴性[477]。其中一些抗原基底细胞样

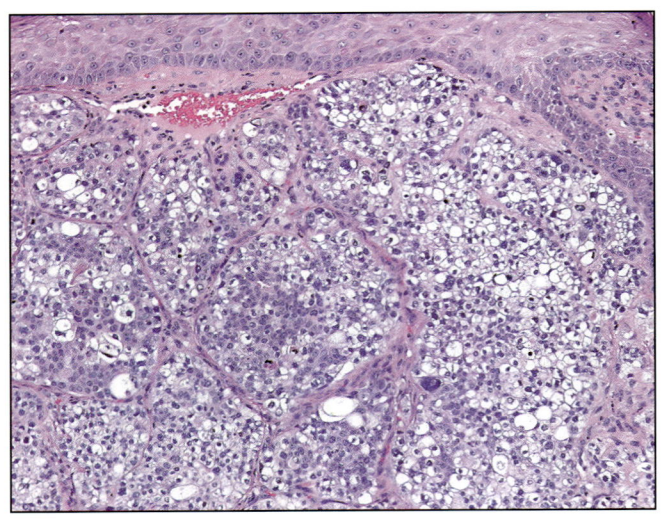

图23.71 皮脂腺癌。低倍镜下，皮脂腺小叶丧失其规则结构。

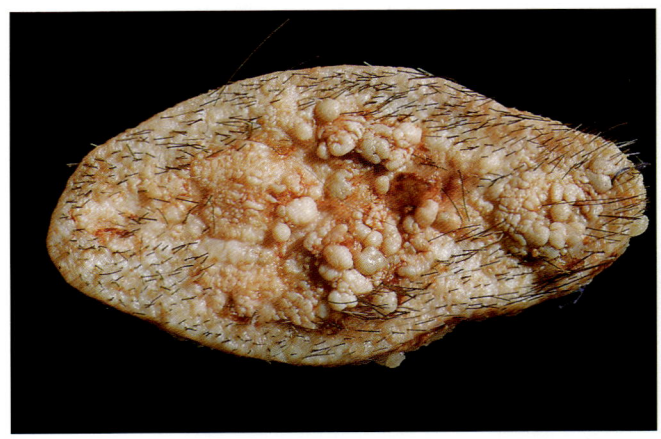

图23.73 器官样痣。大体表现为没有毛发的圆形隆起性疣状病变。

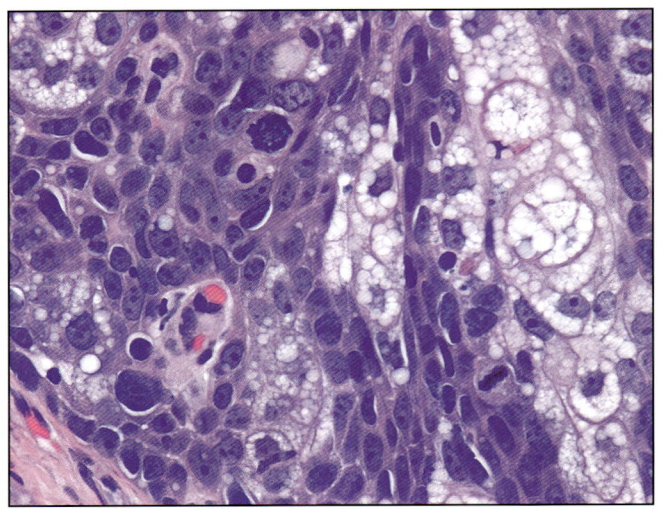

图23.72 皮脂腺癌。肿瘤细胞明显多形性，但仍可见皮脂腺分化。

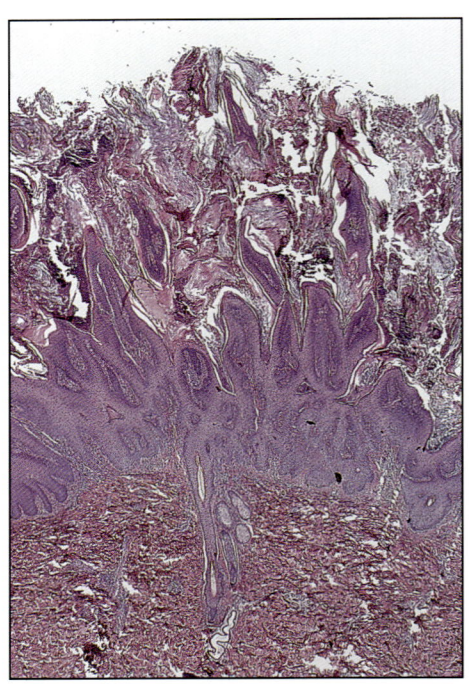

图23.74 器官样痣。疣状亚型一般见于年轻人。注意病变下方缺少附件结构。

成分着色不好，因此应用时应当多加小心。近来有学说提示，许多曾经被称为皮脂腺腺瘤的病变，现在依据病变出现不对称性、囊性变、融合性坏死以及细胞学多形性应当称为皮脂腺癌[470,472]。

一些附件肿瘤具有类似于毛囊、皮脂腺以及导管（器官样痣）的特征。有流行病学证据表明，另一些肿瘤与毛囊具有相关性，如圆柱瘤和汗腺腺瘤，但组织学表现却不一样。

器官样痣（Jadassohn皮脂腺痣）[478-482]
Organoid nevus（nevus sebaceous of Jadassohn）

这一术语涵盖了一系列的错构瘤，伴有主要是成熟的、所有附件分化谱系的成分。基底细胞样细胞增生相对常见，多数为毛母细胞性[483]，极少数可以发生恶性变。

临床上，器官样痣一般见于头颈部，尤其是头皮，多数呈黄色至肉色，无毛发，为先天性斑片、斑块和线样病变，或为散在的疣状肿瘤（图23.73）。一般有三个生长阶段：早期（儿童）、中期（青春期）以及晚期（青春期后）。治疗为手术切除，除非是美容方面的疑难病例。

组织学上，早期肿瘤由表皮增生伴小灶皮脂腺、毛发雏形以及少量导管或腺体成分构成（图23.74）。中期肿瘤保留表皮增生；另外，常见基底细胞样细胞增生，同顶泌汗腺小叶一样（图23.75）。在其晚期，器官样痣可能伴有其他肿瘤。最常见表现可能为基底细胞样错构瘤或毛母细胞瘤（见1443页）[483,484]，经常与基底细胞癌混淆。另外，几乎每一种其他类型的附件肿瘤在皮脂

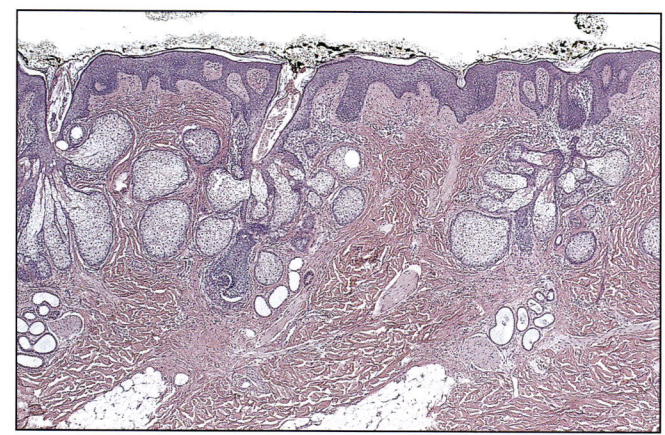

图23.75 器官样痣。注意毛囊变小，还要注意皮脂腺中的孔洞，后者是许多器官样痣的特征性改变。

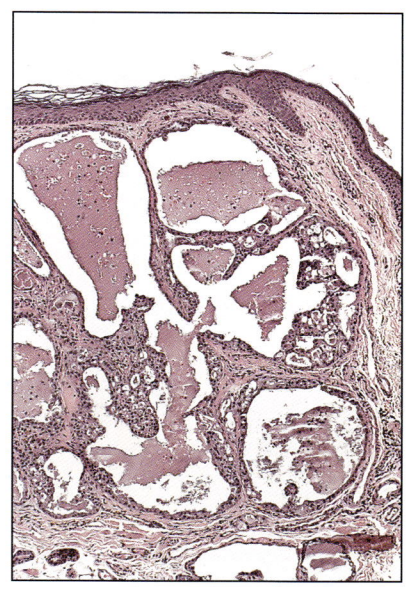

图23.76 顶泌汗腺汗腺囊瘤。浸润性小管伴有顶泌汗腺型内衬和细胞学非典型性。

腺痣中均有描述。其中较常见的是外毛根鞘瘤[373]、汗腺腺瘤[485]、毛发上皮瘤以及汗腺囊瘤。实际上可以想象，任何类型的附件肿瘤均可见于这些畸形当中。

汗腺肿瘤　Sweat gland neoplasms

组织学上，汗腺肿瘤分为顶泌汗腺肿瘤和小汗腺肿瘤。区别顶泌汗腺和小汗腺并非都那么容易。每一种类型的汗腺的导管都是相同的。顶泌汗腺尖端"去头式"分泌与汗腺导管乳头状反应性改变很难区分。事实上，与其他某些错构瘤不同的是，小汗腺分泌分化难以准确表示。另外，对于发生在青春期之后的作为正常腺体结构的大小汗腺（apoeccrine glands）的描述可能也是悬而未决的问题。有些肿瘤出现明显的顶泌汗腺分泌分化，而其他肿瘤具有明显的导管成分，还有一些肿瘤没有定型分化。

顶泌汗腺肿瘤　Apocrine neoplasms

顶泌汗腺痣（apocrine nevus）[486-488]：这是一类极其少见的错构瘤，含有成熟的顶泌汗腺小叶，呈瘤样生长方式。一般见于成人，多数病变发生于腋窝、胸部或头皮。

顶泌汗腺囊瘤/囊腺瘤（apocrine hidrocystoma/cystadenoma）[489,490]：这是一类从内衬单层顶泌汗腺的充满液体的囊肿到含有内衬顶泌汗腺乳头状结构的多房性囊肿的病变。

临床上，病变一般见于老年人的面部和头部，男女均可发生。其他部位也可受累，如躯干和肛门生殖区。病变多数为孤立性的，呈肤色或带蓝黑色[491]，直径一般不足2 cm。有时可为多发性病变。临床鉴别诊断包括基底细胞癌以及一些黑色素细胞病变，如蓝痣。手术治疗可以治愈。

大体上，病变为单房性或多房性囊状结构，含有清亮或棕色液体。组织学上，囊肿内衬一层高柱状细胞，伴有多量嗜酸性颗粒状胞浆和圆形位于基底部的细胞核（图23.76）。常常出现"断头式"分泌。如果出现乳头状结构，则被覆顶泌汗腺上皮。极少数情况下，内衬上皮可形成筛状[489]或微囊性[492]结构。如果生长过度，上皮增生可类似于乳头状汗腺腺瘤或乳头状汗管囊腺瘤[493]。然而，在其他区域可以内衬单层立方上皮。顶泌汗腺细胞常常含有PAS阳性的抗淀粉酶颗粒，可能是脂褐素。在某些病例中，上皮细胞下可见肌上皮细胞[490]。免疫组织化学染色，GCDFP-15为阳性，不同于所谓的小汗腺汗囊瘤（见下文）[494]。超微结构上，内衬细胞类似于正常顶泌汗腺[495]。鉴别诊断包括所谓的小汗腺汗囊瘤、大小汗腺[496]、皮肤纤毛囊肿[497]以及阴茎中线囊肿。

"小汗腺"汗腺囊瘤（"eccrine" hidrocystoma）[498-500]：是指小的、有时为多发性的（Robinson型）内衬单层上皮的导管囊肿。常常发生于成人头颈部区域。

临床上，白种人一般为成年女性受累。囊肿较小，直径一般从1～3 mm，透明至蓝色。多发性病变一般见于面部；而单发性病变还可见于颈部、胸部及躯干。多发性囊肿的鉴别诊断包括晶状粟疹、多发性皮脂腺囊瘤以及发疹性毫毛囊肿。单发性病变的鉴别诊断包括顶泌汗腺囊腺瘤、囊性基底细胞癌以及皮肤纤毛囊肿。单

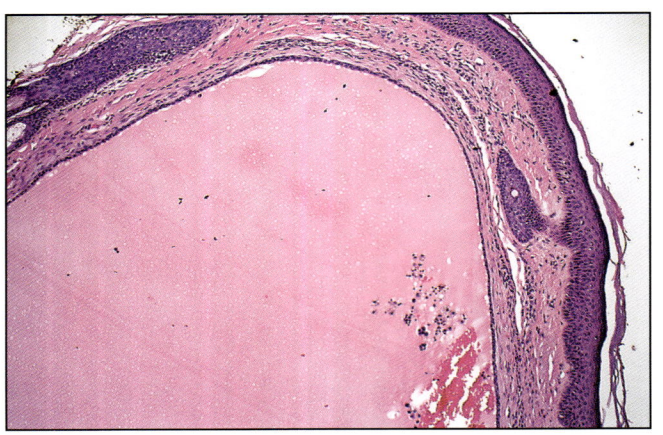

图23.77 小汗腺汗腺囊瘤。内衬单排细胞的单房性囊肿。

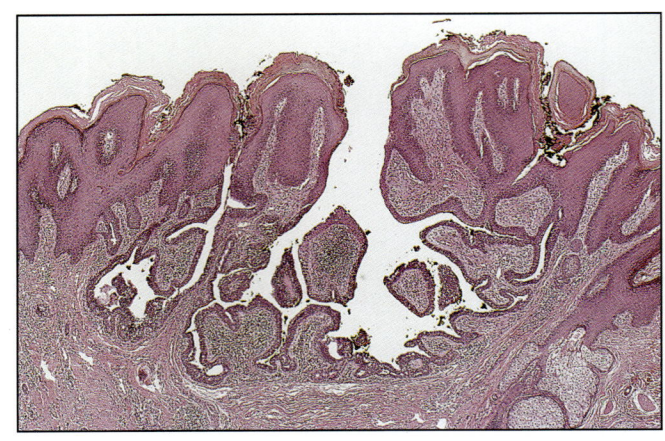

图23.78 乳头状汗管腺瘤。疣状肿瘤伴有顶泌汗腺型内衬，常常开口于表面。常常见于器官样痣当中。

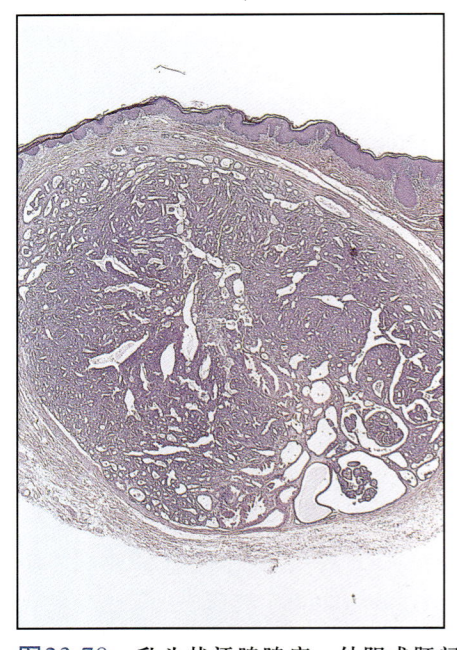

图23.79 乳头状汗腺腺瘤。外阴或肛门周围境界清楚的病变，由管状乳头状腺体组成，类似于乳腺导管。

发性囊肿可手术切除。多发性病变药物治疗可能有效[501]。

组织学上，囊肿为单房，内衬单层立方细胞，没有肌上皮层[500,502]（图23.77）。小汗腺小叶一般排列紧密[502,503,504]，偶尔可见导管进入囊肿[499,504,505]。可以想象，有些病变为顶泌汗腺囊瘤变性[494,506,507]。没有断头式分泌或胞浆内PAS阳性颗粒[500]，不同于顶泌汗腺囊腺瘤。有些病例S-100蛋白和CEA呈阳性[508]，但GCDFP-15为阴性[509]。超微结构上，内衬细胞类似于小汗腺或顶泌汗腺导管上皮细胞[502,510,511]。鉴别诊断包括顶泌汗腺或大小汗腺囊肿或囊腺瘤。

小管性顶泌汗腺腺瘤（tubular apocrine adenoma）[512-516]：这是一系列的小结节状肿瘤，由伴有顶泌汗腺特征的小管组成。病变见于成人，有些可能发生在皮脂腺痣的患者。组织学上，病变境界清楚，由扩张的小管构成，常常内衬一层或多层细胞，顶部为顶泌汗腺细胞。小管成分常常被纤维性间质分隔。当这些病变混杂有缺少顶泌汗腺上皮的区域时，有人称之为"管状乳头状汗腺腺瘤"（tubulo-papillary hidradenomas）[517]。

乳头状汗管腺瘤（乳头状汗管囊腺瘤）[papillary syringadenoma (syringocystadenoma papilliferum)][518-520]：这是一组通常见于成人头皮的良性肿瘤，表面呈颗粒状，可有血性渗出液。多数病变直径不足2cm。有些伴有皮脂腺痣。组织学上，病变呈内陷性，常常暴露于表面，尽管有些可为囊性及闭合性。一般来说，内陷（或囊肿）含有多量圆形乳头状真皮轴心，周围有两层上皮细胞，可以出现也可以不出现断头式分泌（图23.78）。乳头轴心可含有多量浆细胞，尤其是在开口于表面的病例。

乳头状汗腺腺瘤[papillary hidradenoma (hidradenoma papilliferum)][521-523]：这是一组良性外阴或肛周肿瘤，主要发生于成年女性，一般为结节状，极少数可开口于表面。累及其他解剖学部位者极为少见[524]。多数病变为1cm或更小。组织学上，多数肿瘤境界清楚（图23.79），且为实性；另一些肿瘤可为囊性。生长方式为由小管以及被覆两层细胞的乳头状丛混合而成，两层细胞为顶部的立方细胞和深部的肌上皮细胞（图23.80）。部分肿瘤内常可见特殊的顶泌汗腺改变，尽管存在较大差异。嗜酸细胞改变并不少见[525]。一个重要的鉴别诊断是腺癌，通过辨认乳头状汗腺腺瘤的低倍镜下生长方式、顶泌汗腺改变以及两层上皮细胞，几乎都能将腺癌排除在外。

乳头腺瘤（乳头导管乳头状瘤病）[nipple adenoma (florid papillomatosis of the nipple ducts)][526-534]：这是一种罕见的乳头良性病变，几乎均发生于女性。病变直径

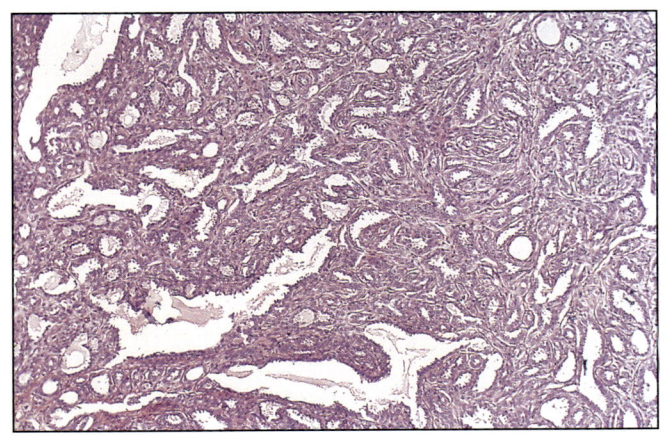

图23.80 乳头状汗腺腺瘤。复杂的小管和乳头。

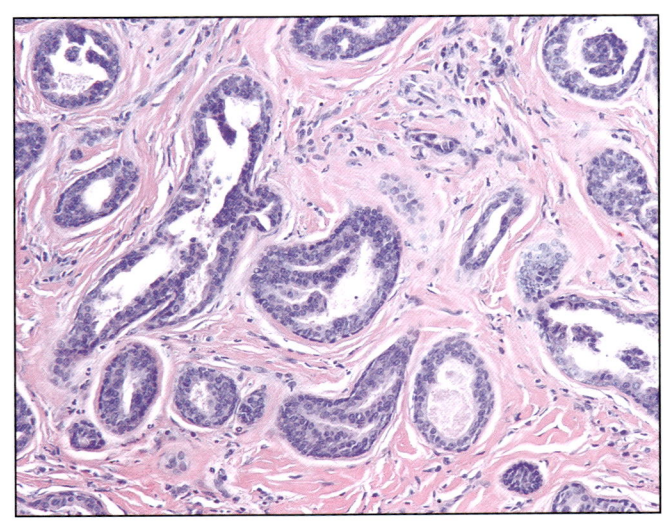

图23.82 乳头腺瘤。乳头腺瘤的上皮增生，不要与癌混淆。

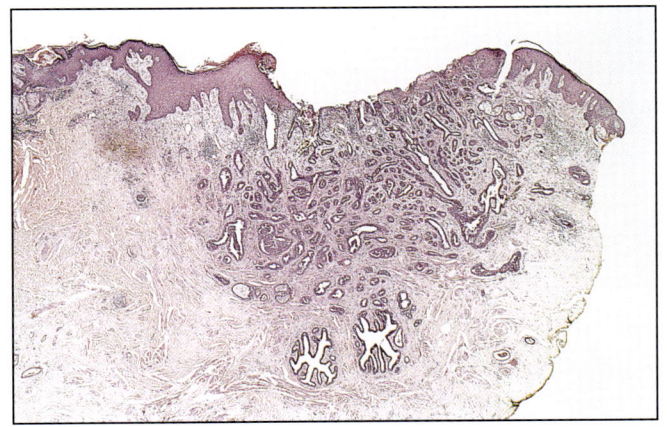

图23.81 乳头腺瘤。乳头真皮内境界清楚的病变，由类似于乳腺组织的导管构成。

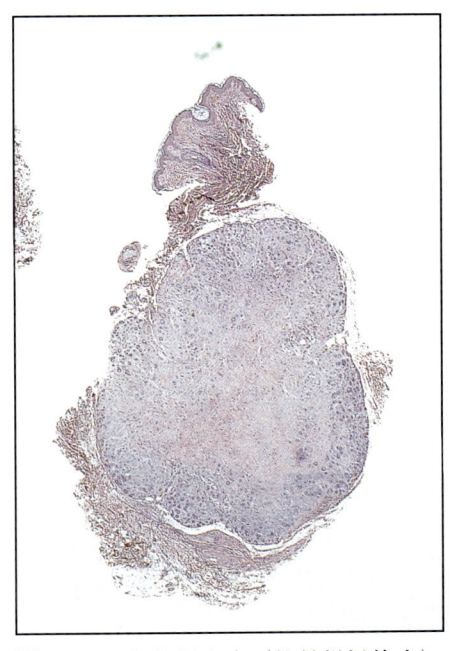

图23.83 良性混合瘤（软骨样汗管瘤）。境界清楚的含有小管的玻璃样病变。

一般小于1cm，几乎均为单侧发生，多数有结痂，或有表面湿润，呈浆液性或血性，必须与乳头Paget病鉴别。组织学上，多数乳头腺瘤为境界清楚的结节，由多数导管样结构构成，内层衬以导管型上皮，外层为肌上皮层（图23.81）。可见导管、腺样或小管状结构，伴有或不伴有上皮增生（图23.82）。可以见到数量不等的硬化、顶泌汗腺化生或鳞状上皮化生。有些病例伴有导管内乳头状瘤。在少数情况下，这种病变可能伴有癌[534]。有些病例中可见汗管瘤样结构[535,536]；组织学上类似于微囊性附件癌。

混合瘤（软骨样汗管瘤）[527-542]
Mixed tumor（chondroid syringoma）

这是一类伴有复杂小管状上皮成分以及黏液样或软骨样间质的良性导管肿瘤。这种肿瘤组织学上与发生于涎腺（见第7章）或软组织（见第24章）的类似肿瘤相同，但皮肤病变切除之后仅有少数复发。主要或完全由梭形或卵圆形肌上皮细胞构成的病变称为皮肤肌上皮瘤（cutaneous myoepithelioma）[542a]。

临床上，这些肿瘤几乎均为孤立性结节，见于成人的头颈部。少数发生于远端肢体。受累患者中女性稍多于男性，没有特殊的临床表现。

组织学上，病变境界清楚，位于真皮或皮下组织，与表皮并不相连（图23.83）。病变含有微管（图23.84）或分支管状的混合性上皮结构（图23.85）。上皮为导管性，伴有或不伴有顶泌汗腺分泌区域[543]。在极少数情况下，有些肿瘤中可见影细胞、毛囊其他成分以及皮脂腺细胞[543,544]。其他一些病变可能由极其透明的细胞构成[545,546]。极少见的表现包括出现许多胶原小体[547]。间质为纤维母细胞性、黏液样、黏液软骨样，或在极少数情况下为骨样组织[548,549]，并且具有类似于肋软骨的特征[541]。

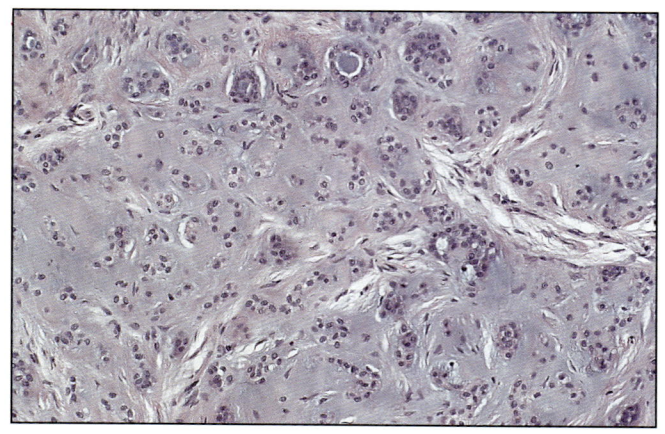

图23.84 良性混合瘤（软骨样汗管瘤）。导管型细胞和肌上皮细胞位于黏液样间质中。

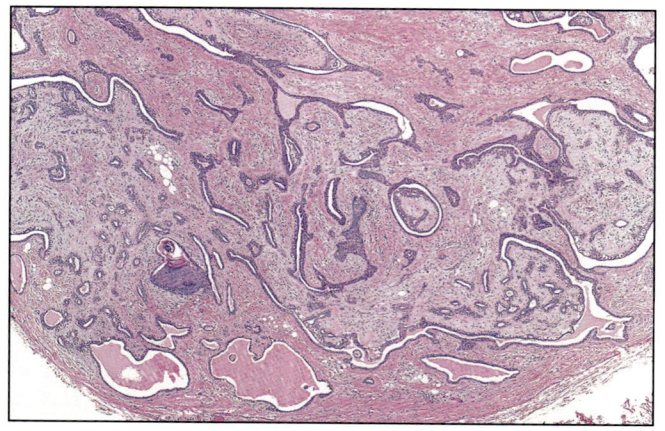

图23.85 良性混合瘤。这种病变具有分支管状结构。

免疫组化检查，一致的表现为肌上皮细胞 S-100 以及多种角蛋白标记物呈阳性[550,551]，包括 CAM5.2。顶泌汗腺型上皮 GCDFP-15 和 EMA 也常常为阳性。

小汗腺肿瘤 Eccrine neoplasms

多数历史上定义为"小汗腺"的肿瘤实际上为导管肿瘤。在一个附件肿瘤中见到小汗腺腺泡分化非常少见；即多数病变内含有导管成分，但是缺乏看起来像小汗腺分泌部分的结构。这个范畴的肿瘤包含历史上分类为"小汗腺"的肿瘤，记住先前的陈述。

小汗腺痣（eccrine nevi）：为极为少见的良性病变，与毛发痣相似。病变定义为位于真皮内的小汗腺导管或腺泡结构，表现为数量过多或相互之间以及与其他皮肤结构之间的关系出现异常。有三种主要类型：小汗腺血管瘤性错构瘤、汗孔角化性"小汗腺"口和真皮导管痣以及"小汗腺"汗管纤维腺瘤。

小汗腺血管瘤性错构瘤（eccrine angiomatous hamartoma）[552-559]：这是一组散在的孤立性或多发性、常常有痛感且多汗的[556,560]病变，常常发生于年轻人的手、足或躯干。组织学上，可见小汗腺分泌小叶数量增加，其周围（以及其内）毛细血管大小的血管数量增加，其中有些血管可能扩张。免疫组织化学上，有 S-100 蛋白、CEA、CD34、CD44、人神经生长因子受体以及 Ulex europaeus 抗原呈阳性的报道[561,562]。为了减轻疼痛，有些病例可能需要局部切除，包括手指（脚趾）截除术[563]。

汗孔角化性"小汗腺"口及皮肤导管痣（porokeratotic "eccrine" ostial and dermal duct nevus）[564-572]：是指从局限性到线形的针尖大小的角化性丘疹，除了少数病例外[573]均为先天性病变。一般发生于掌部、足底、手指或脚趾，但其他部位也可受累[574-577]。组织学上，丘疹相当于角样板（cornoid lamellae），位于许多增生性导管口的附近，可能与小汗腺有关，因为可见小汗腺腺体的分泌部分与某些导管融合。有报告称导管的腔面 CEA 呈阳性[578]。极少数情况下，毛囊开口也可受累[579]。小汗腺螺管不受累。

汗管纤维腺瘤（顶端汗管痣）[syringofibroadenoma (acrosyringeal nevus)][117,580-587]：其临床特征为一系列的孤立性或多发性丘疹、斑块或肿瘤，可呈线形或簇状分布。有些病变湿润，触之有海绵感。多数病变发生于老年人；有些可能伴有出汗性外胚层发育不良（hidrotic ectodermal dysplasia）[588,589]，而且有人提出，在一些情况下本病是 Schöpf 综合征（眼睑汗囊瘤、少毛、牙发育不全以及指甲异常）的一个标志[590]。对于孤立性病变，治疗为局部切除，但对于多发性病变的患者，必须采用个性化治疗。

组织学上，可见伴有导管分化的纤细且相互吻合的上皮索条，从表皮向外扩展（图 23.86）。常常出现复杂的网状结构（图 23.87）。明显的表皮分化也常出现。有些病变中有较为明显的黏液样间质。具有这种形态的少数病变与癌有关，由此提出这些病变会不会是癌的

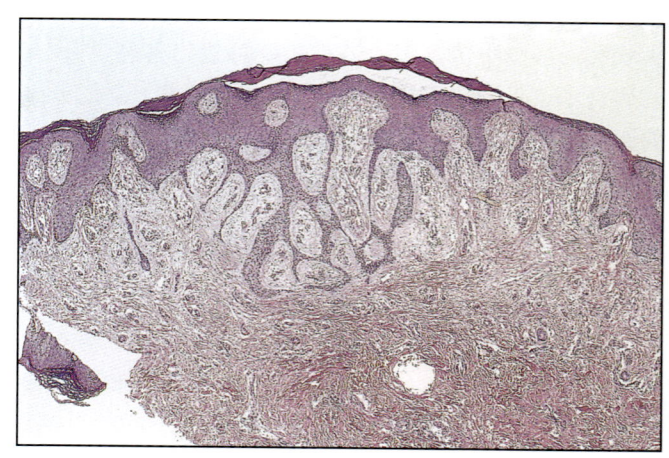

图23.86 小汗腺汗管纤维腺瘤。汗腺的顶端汗管部分呈网状延长。

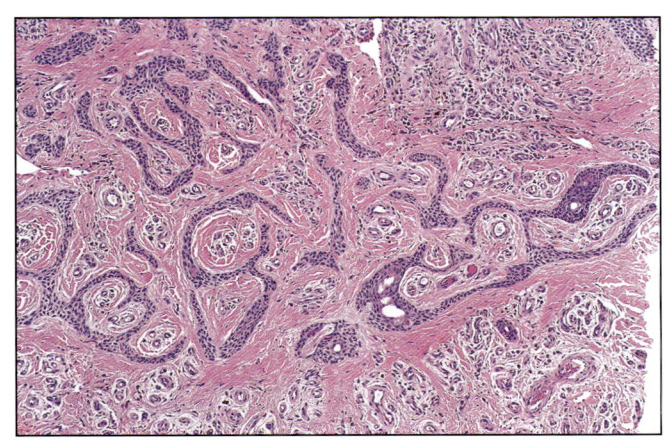

图23.87 汗管纤维腺瘤。可见网状结构。注意导管。

说法[591,592]。其他学说提示，至少在某些情况下这些病变只不过是溃疡周围少见的增生表现或其他类型的肿瘤[593,594]。

汗管瘤[595]　Syringoma

这是一组以复杂的扭曲导管为特征的良性肿瘤。临床上，肿瘤一般发生于成人的头颈部，但任何部位均可受累。本病好发于眼睑，一般呈皮肤颜色。比较独特的表现是发疹性汗管瘤，通常发生于青春期，并且没有特别的好发部位。有些汗管瘤患者伴有21号染色体三体[596]。

组织学上，汗管瘤为交错排列的巢状、条索状及小囊状结构，位于真皮上半部分（图23.88）。病变很少与表皮相连，而是包埋于致密的胶原性间质当中。当病变与表皮相连时，其管腔常常与小的角化性囊状结构相通。汗管瘤的导管由一层或两层立方细胞构成，极少数病变出现透明细胞改变。有些肿瘤仅有少数上皮结构，而其他一些具有增生性囊性结构，囊腔内伴有层状角化。囊肿破裂后常常发生对角质的异物反应。

免疫组织化学上，EMA阳性见于导管外周细胞，CK10表达见于中间细胞，CK6、CK19和CEA表达见于腔面细胞[597]。雌激素、孕激素[598]以及雄激素[599]受体为阴性。普通型与透明细胞型汗管瘤的免疫表型好像没有差异[600]。鉴别诊断主要局限于微囊性附件癌（见1462页），有可能成为诊断误区，尤其是在浅表刮除活检时。

乳头状小汗腺腺瘤[601-607]　Papillary eccrine adenoma

这些良性导管肿瘤由内衬乳头状两层立方形细胞的小管组成，而且被纤维性间隔分开。临床上，少数报告显示这些病变好发于上肢，但是没有特殊表现。

组织学上，病变为境界清楚、没有包膜的真皮肿物，紧邻表皮下方。病变由大小不一的扩张扭曲的导管构成。导管有明显的乳头，内衬导管腔的细胞为排列成双层的均一的立方细胞（图23.89）。多数导管细胞的细胞核规则，呈圆形或卵圆形，伴有小的核仁。除了极少数的病例以外，核分裂象罕见或缺乏[608]。导管腔内偶尔含有颗粒状或无定形的嗜酸性物质。纤维胶原性间质围绕导管周围。

主要的鉴别诊断为管状顶泌汗腺腺瘤。有人认为这两种病变同属于一个范畴，称为"管状乳头状汗腺瘤"（tubulopapillary hidradenoma）[517]。

顶端汗管瘤（汗孔瘤）[609]　Acrospiroma（poroma）

这是一组良性、形态相对一致的导管肿瘤，可与皮肤表面连接也可不连接。

临床上，顶端汗管瘤或汗孔瘤"家族"从孤立性斑块（汗腺棘皮瘤类）到外生性丘疹（"小汗腺"汗孔瘤类）乃至真皮结节（真皮顶端汗管瘤类）。这些肿瘤一般发生于成人。"小汗腺"汗孔瘤类的病变常常发生于足底，并有渗出或出血，而这一类中的另外一些病变可发生于任何部位，并且常常较干燥或有皮肤被覆。

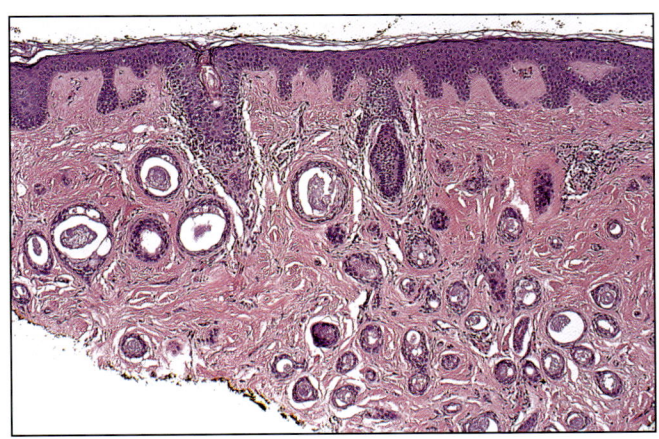

图23.88 汗管瘤。小而复杂的小管聚集，由于正切的原因，上皮向下延伸（"逗号尾巴"）。

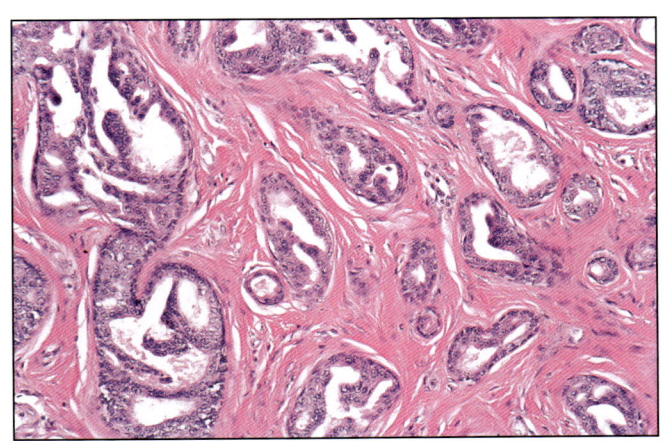

图23.89 乳头状（小汗腺）腺瘤。导管具有两层细胞，且腔内有小的乳头状突起。

组织学上，这些病变依照肿瘤与表皮的相关部位可进一步分类。肿瘤主要限于表皮内成巢分布的称为表皮顶端汗管瘤（epidermal acrospiroma）或汗腺棘皮瘤（hidroacanthoma）（图23.90）[610]。累及表皮和真皮的病变称为近表皮顶端汗管瘤（juxtaepidermal acrospiroma）或诊断为汗孔瘤（poroma）或小汗腺汗孔瘤（eccrine poroma）（图23.91和23.92）[611,612]。完全局限于真皮或仅与表皮有轻微连接的病变称为真皮顶端汗管瘤（dermal acrospiroma），但又曾被称为汗腺腺瘤（hidradenoma）（图23.93和23.94）；伴有显著导管的病变称为真皮导管肿瘤（dermal duct tumors）（图23.95和23.96）[613]。

顶端汗管瘤的特征是：结构和细胞类型明显多样，经常在一个肿瘤之内。在一个肿瘤当中可见多少不等的明显的大体或镜下囊肿和管腔。多数囊腔内衬立方或柱状上皮，有时显示不同程度的黏液性（杯状细胞）分化。局灶性鳞状上皮化生也可出现。这些腔隙内可见无定形、

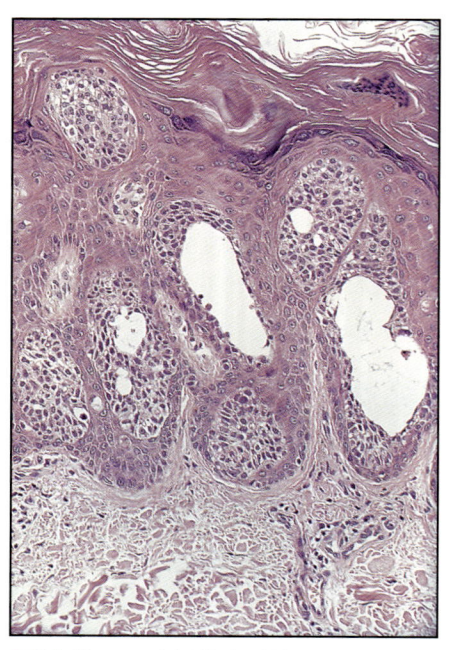

图23.90 顶端汗管瘤（单纯性汗腺棘皮瘤亚型）。表皮内汗孔瘤细胞克隆性结构，伴有导管。

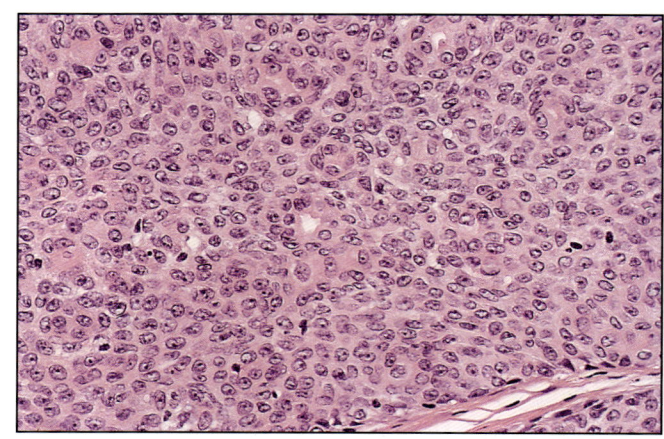

图23.92 顶端汗管瘤（小汗腺汗孔瘤亚型）。"汗孔样"细胞形态一致，不相重叠。可见少数小导管。

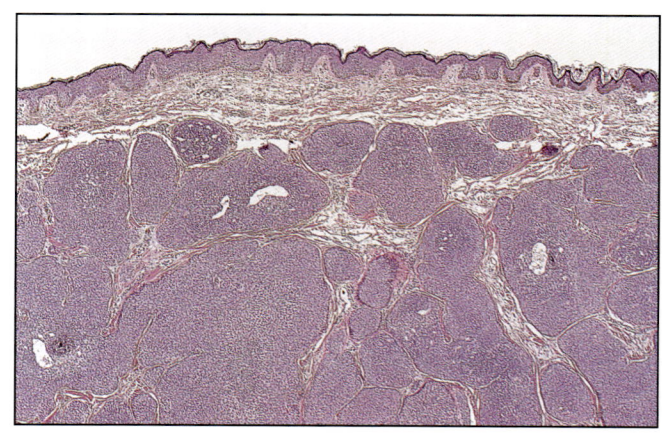

图23.93 顶端汗管瘤（汗腺瘤亚型）。低倍镜下，大大小小的导管细胞小叶形成实性岛。

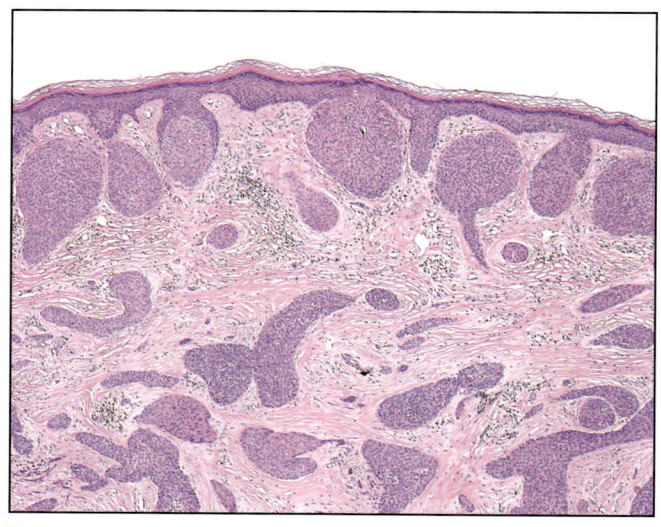

图23.91 顶端汗管瘤（小汗腺汗孔瘤亚型）。病变与表面相连，但向深处真皮扩展。

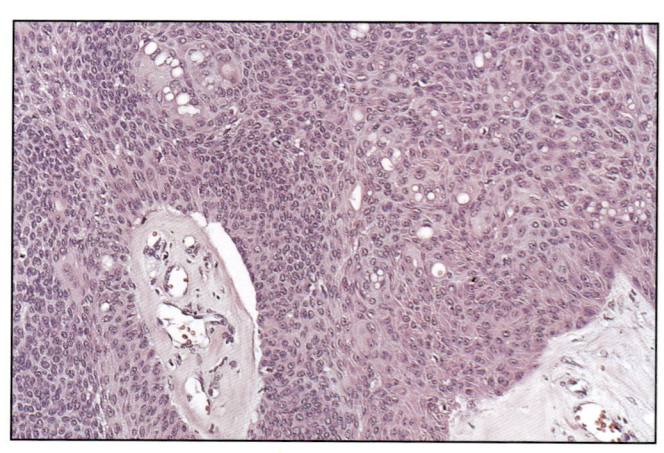

图23.94 顶端汗管瘤（汗腺瘤亚型）。肿瘤细胞类似于小汗腺汗孔瘤的细胞。可见多数导管。

蛋白样嗜酸性成分。伴有与表皮连接的肿瘤常常具有实性成片的小的立方细胞，细胞核一致，有少量的嗜碱性胞浆。偶尔可含有中等至多量的黑色素[614]。相似的细胞类型在多数实性肿瘤中占主导地位。

顶端汗管瘤的任何亚型一般均含有较大的多角形细胞，伴有多量嗜酸性胞浆以及鳞状细胞特征。肿瘤细胞倾向于聚集在一起，呈同心性排列。聚集细胞的中央常常形成管腔，并且伴有表皮分化。与之交替出现的是一些位于中央的细胞，可见胞浆空泡，代表胞浆内腔隙形成，再现了导管的胚胎发生。

有些肿瘤出现成片的多角形细胞，伴有多量透明胞浆（PAS 呈阳性且淀粉酶敏感），核位于中央，细胞膜明显。这种类型的细胞可以构成肿瘤的一部分，或占据肿瘤的大部。当这种类型的细胞比较显著时，这种病变常常被称为汗腺腺瘤（hidradenoma）或汗孔样汗腺腺瘤（poroid hidradenoma）。

这些病变的免疫组化特征差异很大。一般说来，广谱细胞角蛋白和 CEA（尤其是导管部分）呈阳性。可以出现极少数的 S-100 蛋白阳性的细胞灶（一般为树突细胞性）。GCDFP-15 一般为阴性[621-623]。

间质由纤细的胶原纤维组成，较具特征性的是嗜酸性玻璃样胶原成分。极为少见的是肿瘤小叶周边有炎症浸润。有些肿瘤中央含有小的坏死区，可见核固缩以及嗜酸性颗粒状胞浆。

核分裂象并不少见，在一些肿瘤中可以较多。尽管细胞核一般极其规则且为空泡状，伴有细颗粒状染色质，但有些肿瘤含有少数大细胞，细胞核具有多形性。可以理解，这种表现会引起一些关注；然而，它几乎总是局限于少数细胞，似乎没有什么预后意义[624]。少数病例出现小而纤细的索条和巢状结构。其他一些病例可见圆形的小而规则的基底细胞样细胞巢，伴有汗孔瘤样表皮内成分。许多细胞巢中心有囊肿，管腔样腔隙内含有嗜酸性颗粒样物质。

圆柱瘤[625-628]　Cylindroma

这是一种良性基底细胞样细胞肿瘤，具有镶嵌样结构，自然病史为惰性，但有时会造成损害。虽然对其组织发生尚有争议，但在临床上这个家族中的病变被认为具有毛囊皮脂腺分布。

临床上，圆柱瘤可为单发性或多发性，多见于成人。单发性病变最为常见；为头皮、头颈部或躯干出现的红斑性或皮肤颜色的病变。病变表面毛细血管扩张，但其他可呈肉色。有些病变有疼痛。多发性病变一般被称为头巾样瘤（turban tumor），因为它可覆盖整个头皮。在极少数情况下，它可能伴有毛发上皮瘤（Brooke-Spiegler 综合征）以及汗管瘤[287,629]。如果为家族性的，则为常染色体显性遗传类型。切除后局部复发极为少见。令人信服的组织学恶性的圆柱瘤极其少见。

组织学上，肿瘤为境界清楚的、没有包膜的真皮内结节，由基底细胞样细胞构成的细胞岛及索条构成，周围绕以增厚的玻璃样变的 PAS 阳性基膜。细胞排列成连锁的"拼图样"结构（图 23.97）。肿瘤细胞岛可有腔隙或假腔隙形成。一般描述有两种类型的细胞：第一种是小而深染的细胞，常常位于肿瘤结节的外周；第二种是较大而淡染的细胞，构成细胞索的中央部分。

汗腺腺瘤[626,630-632]　Spiradenoma

这个术语代表一系列的良性真皮肿瘤，由两种基底细胞样细胞群构成。有些病例可能与圆柱瘤共存[629]。

临床上，这种肿瘤发生于成人，通常见于躯干，但极少数可发生于头皮。手掌和足底一般不会发生。有些病变有疼痛。

组织学上，汗腺腺瘤由一个或多个常常呈卵圆形至球形的清楚的小叶组成，位于真皮深层或皮下组织。低

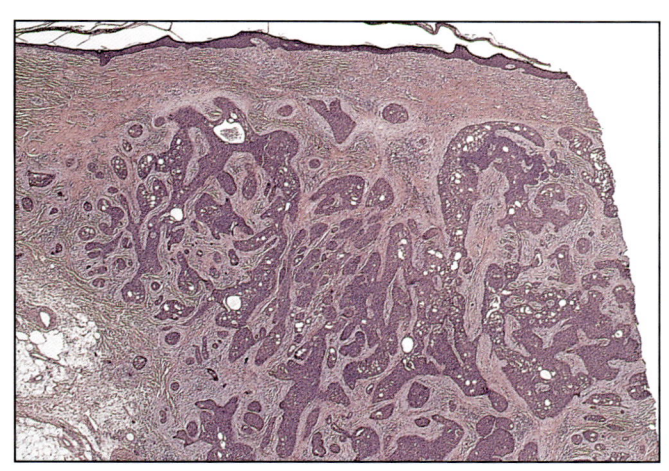

图 23.95　顶端汗管瘤（真皮导管瘤亚型）。这种病变具有一些浸润性，含有许多导管，即使在低倍镜下也可见到。

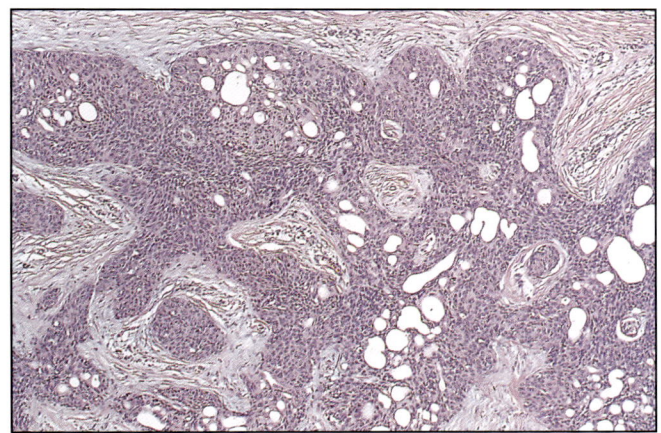

图 23.96　顶端汗管瘤（真皮导管瘤亚型）。可见许多导管，使得这种病变容易确认为顶端汗管瘤。

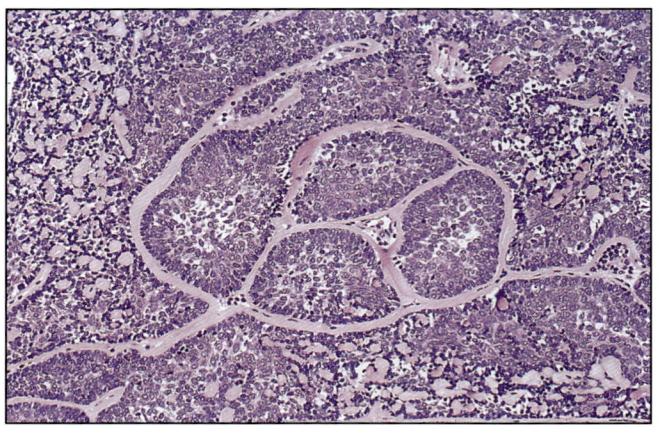

图23.97 圆柱瘤。注意肿瘤岛的"拼图样"结构及其周围的玻璃样物质。

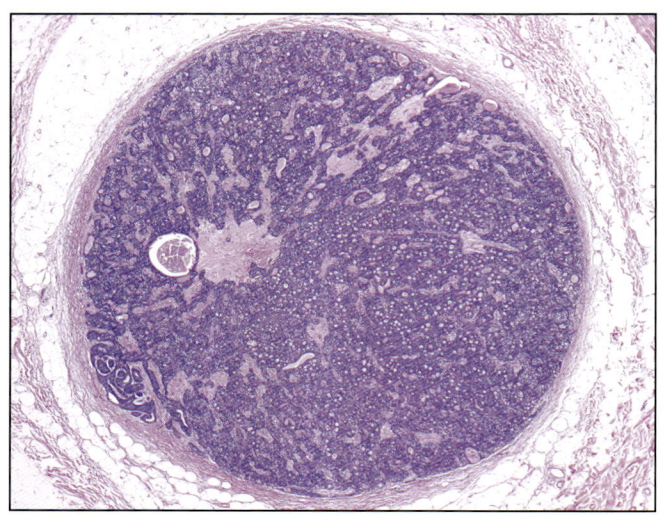

图23.98 汗腺腺瘤。境界清楚的基底细胞样肿瘤,内部可见纤维血管成分。

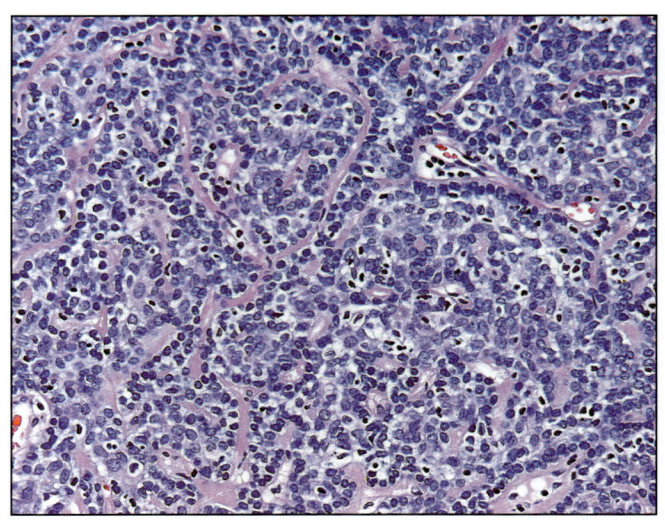

图23.99 汗腺腺瘤。两种类型的基底细胞样细胞群。

在萎缩的腺体小叶周围出现明显的嗜酸性基底膜样物质沉积。这种物质 PAS 为阳性,类似于见于圆柱瘤中的玻璃样物质。

小汗腺和(或)顶泌汗腺腺癌[635]
Adenocarcinomas of eccrine and/or apocrine glands

小汗腺和(或)顶泌汗腺腺癌包含一大类生长结构多样以及生物学潜能不同的肿瘤。这里列出的病变结合了传统的病变分类,即顶泌汗腺、小汗腺及混合性导管类型。

顶泌汗腺腺癌(除外了乳腺外的 Paget 病或耵聍腺癌)[apocrine adenocarcinoma[636-638] (excluding cases of extramammary Paget's disease or ceruminous carcinoma)]:这是一种文献记录及研究极少的附件腺癌,一般发生于成人腋窝或腹股沟区,两种性别均可受累。多数为孤立性肿瘤,呈结节性表现。这种肿瘤患者多数有漫长的临床经过;局部肿瘤切除及淋巴结清除可以治愈,即使是在已有转移的患者。

组织学上,病变由含有顶泌汗腺("断头式")分泌上皮的小管组成。生长结构可呈乳头状、实性或混合性表现(图 23.100)。有时可出现从良性到多形性的过渡性区域。极少数病例可含有成片的印戒细胞[639]。核分裂指数变化可能很大,在有些情况下对于确立诊断并无帮助。浸润性生长方式是有助于诊断的特征,特别是在细胞学表现均一的病例。

组织化学和免疫组织化学方面,病变中形成腔隙的细胞一般含有 PAS 阳性抗淀粉酶物质。肿瘤细胞 GCDFP-15 一般呈阳性。上皮共同抗原(细胞角蛋白、CEA 和 EMA)一般也有表达。S-100 蛋白仅有极少数呈阳性。

倍镜下,病变呈均一嗜碱性,围以完整的纤维性包膜(图23.98)。极少数常常是较大的肿瘤,可部分或几乎整个呈囊性,含有嗜酸性蛋白性成分或红细胞,类似于血管肿瘤[633,634]。有些肿瘤出现广泛纤维化,使常见的均一性结构出现扭曲。

肿瘤结节由紧密排列的细胞构成,形成弥漫性、"腺泡状"或假玫瑰花结结构。一般出现两种类型的细胞:大细胞和小细胞(图23.99)。大细胞含有相当大的空泡状细胞核以及颗粒状染色质,而且常常有明显的核仁;胞浆不多。小细胞含有浓缩的细胞核;这些细胞常常位于大细胞的周边。两种类型的细胞均可出现"腺泡状"结构。有些肿瘤含有数量不等的排列成小管的细胞,一般位于病变的周边;小管细胞一般较大,含有嗜酸性胞浆。偶尔,肿瘤实质内可见导管成分。

有些肿瘤出现明显的变性改变、纤维化以及囊肿形成。有些较大的肿瘤可部分或全部坏死,仅有一薄层肿瘤细胞。在血管类型的肿瘤中可见血栓形成。有些肿瘤

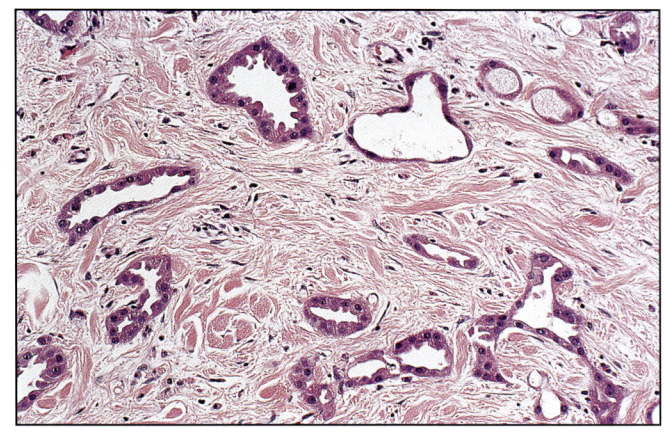

图23.100 顶泌汗腺腺癌。多形性细胞形成管状及筛状结构，含有嗜酸性胞浆。

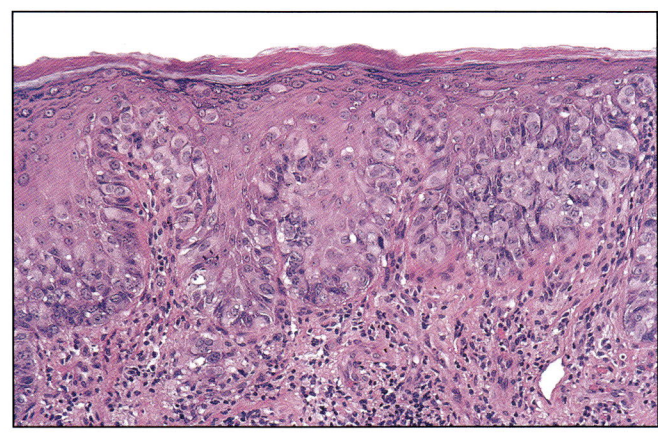

图23.102 乳腺外Paget病。基底层可见明显的上皮样细胞，并散在分布于整个表皮。

超微结构方面，当与正常顶泌汗腺进行比较时，原发性和继发性顶泌汗腺癌显示分化丧失，尤其是继发性病变[636]。

乳腺外 Paget 病(extramammary Paget's disease)[640,641]：这是一种原位腺癌类型，常常伴有某种程度的顶泌汗腺分化，组织学上类似于乳腺 Paget 病（见第 16 章）。乳腺外 Paget 病这一术语只能严格用于开始发生于表皮（图 23.101）或附件且可以（极少数）扩展至真皮的原位腺癌[642]。如果这些表皮特征伴有内脏的癌，如直肠[643]、前列腺[644]、膀胱[645]或转移性癌，那么应当将其视为原发性肿瘤向表皮的 Paget 样播散[642]。如果 Paget 样播散伴有明显的附件腺癌，而且仅仅是少数细胞呈原位腺癌表现，则应当称为来自附件腺癌的 Paget 样播散[646]。

临床上，乳腺外 Paget 病一般见于成人肛门生殖区、腋窝、眼睑或外耳部分，表现为从红斑区到渗出性的结痂性斑块乃至肿瘤。常为多灶性，治疗海绵层细胞间水肿性皮炎的常规方法对其无效。

除了表皮内细胞显示顶泌汗腺腺癌改变等基本组织学特征以外（图 23.102），附件上皮也可出现 Paget 样细胞。少数区域可出现小管结构，这不同于乳腺 Paget 病，后者上皮内小管罕见。对于某些病例，还有可能通过免疫过氧化酶染色来区别继发性 Paget 样播散[647]。我们知道，乳腺外 Paget 病的免疫表型包括 CK 7 呈阳性、CK 20 呈阴性以及 GCDFP-15 呈阳性[643,648,649]。相反，伴有 Paget 样播散的直肠腺癌的免疫表型为 CK 7 和 CK 20 呈阳性，而 GCDFP-15 为阴性[643,649]。CAM5.2（图23.103）、AE1/AE3、CEA 以及 EMA 也为阳性。

令人遗憾的是，最初诊断时并非总能知道是否存在真皮部分或深在的原发癌，除非采用特殊的方法，有时难以查出。调查发现，12%（但一般也是较高比例）的病例具有这种相关性，即在检查原位成分的同时存在内脏病变的证据[645,650]。值得注意但并非异乎寻常的

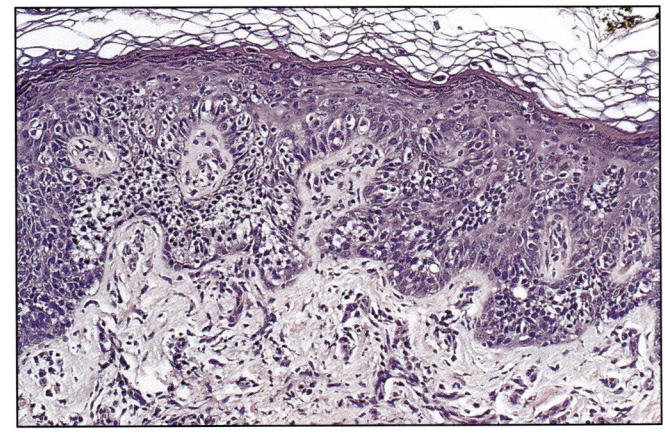

图23.101 乳腺外Paget病。表皮内可见成簇及单个分布的腺癌细胞。

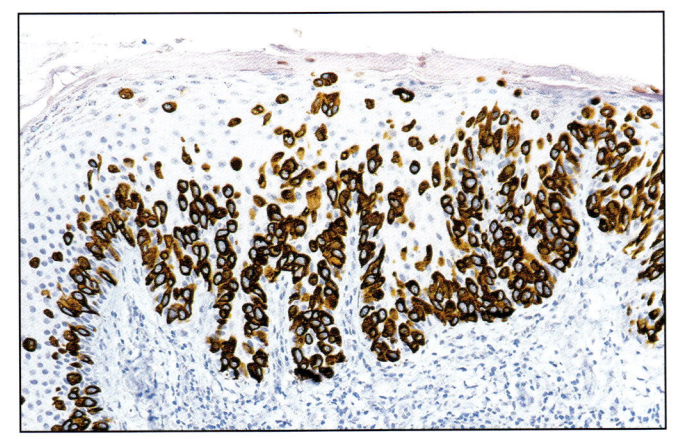

图23.103 乳腺外Paget病，角蛋白CAM5.2染色。这是一个可靠的标记物，但并不完全特异。

表23.5 乳腺外Paget病与其他显示Paget样播散的病变

病变	PAS不伴有淀粉酶	PAS伴有淀粉酶	黏液卡红	Alcian蓝	CEA	CK(AE1/3)	Cam5.2(CK8/18)	CK7	CK20	S100	HMB-45	GCDFP-15	PSA	EMA	突触素	溶菌酶	CD15
Paget病	+/-	+/-	+/-	+/-	+/-	+	+	+	-	-	-	+	-	+	n/a	n/a	n/a
乳腺外Paget病	+	+	+	+	+	+	+	+	+/-(50%)	-	-	+	-	+	n/a	-	-
直肠癌Paget样播散	+	+	+	+	+	+	+	+	+	-	-	-	-	+	n/a	n/a	-
黑色素瘤Paget样播散	+/-	+/-	-	-	-	-	-	-	-	+	+	-	-	-	n/a	n/a	-
神经内分泌癌Paget样播散	n/a	n/a	n/a	n/a	-	+/-	+核旁"圆点"	n/a	+	-	-	-	-	+	+	n/a	n/a
前列腺癌Paget样播散	+/-	+/-	+/-	+/-	-	-	+	-	n/a	n/a	-	-	+	-	+	n/a	n/a
Paget样Bowen病	+/-	+/-	+/-	+/-	-	+/-	+/-	-	n/a	-	-	-	-	n/a	-	n/a	n/a

PAS：过碘酸Schiff；GCDFP-15：大囊肿病液体蛋白；CK：细胞角蛋白；PSA：前列腺特异性抗原；EMA：上皮膜抗原；n/a：没有得到。

是，当内脏癌出现Paget样播散时，这些癌的位置通常靠近原位成分[650]。对于等待进一步检查的病例，直到检查完成并最终明确病变范围，Paget现象（Paget phenomenon）一词被当作过渡性术语。

鉴别诊断包括恶性黑色素瘤[651]、Bowen病、处于表皮阶段的神经内分泌癌[652]以及内脏癌的Paget样播散。表23.5将乳腺外的Paget病与其他出现Paget样播散的病变进行了对比。

微囊性附件癌[258,653-657]
Microcystic adnexal carcinoma

这是一种浸润性肿瘤，由位于纤维性间质中的小囊腔、导管以及基底细胞样细胞条索构成（图23.104）。临床上，病变最常发生于成人的面部。一般为皮肤颜色的硬结性斑块，但也可以是肿胀。病变一般仅为局部侵袭性，局部切除可以治愈，前提是完全切除肿瘤。

组织学上，浅表部位通常可见微小角质囊肿。实性基底细胞样细胞条索与囊肿交替出现；其中有些可能含有导管和微小钙化，尽管有些病变可含有明显的腔隙、实性索条、透明细胞改变以及分枝状小管。在真皮中层，基底细胞样细胞条索和导管比较明显，而微小角质囊肿减少。除了导管以外，有些病例还含有皮脂腺细胞以及毛囊分化的证据[655,656]。在较深的部位，间质纤维组织增生一般更为明显，上皮成分可减少至三两个细胞的小巢（图23.105）。常常有神经和骨骼肌浸润。细胞学上，多数病变含有大小相对一致的细胞；极少有细胞出现核分裂象。伴有明显腺体成分的病变也可见到，被称为硬化性汗腺导管癌（sclerosing sweat duct carcinoma）或恶性汗管瘤（malignant syringoma）[653]。

免疫组织化学检查，这些病变的腺腔表达CEA，并且表达各种细胞角蛋白，但是间质缺乏CD34染色，在有些病例中这一点可能有助于与纤维组织增生性毛发上

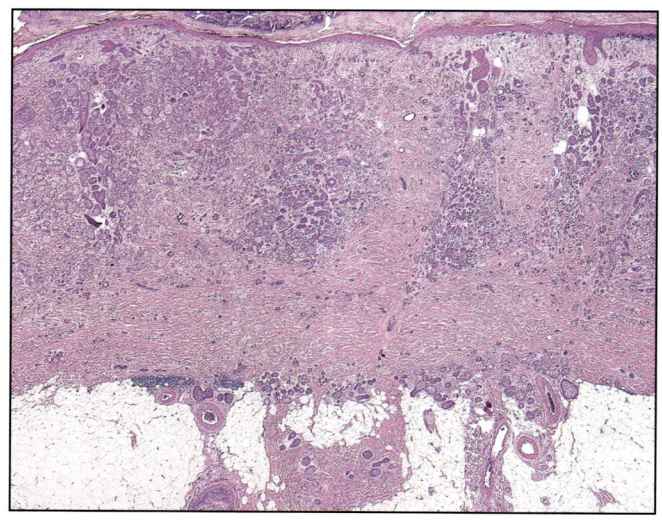

图23.104 微囊性附件癌。浸润性基底细胞样肿瘤呈长条索状、囊状及导管结构。

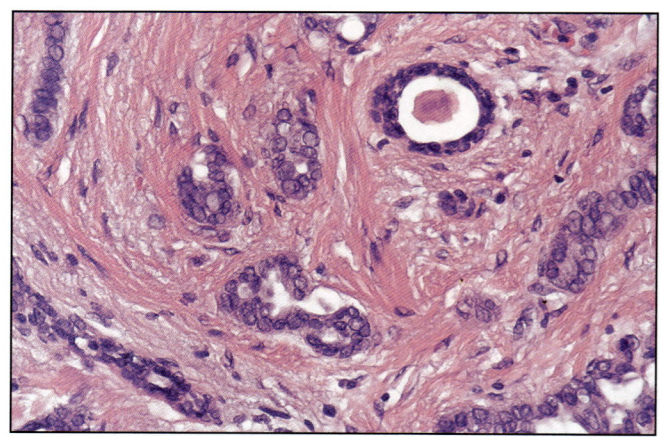

图23.105 微囊性附件癌。小管内衬单层细胞。真皮内可见一些单个细胞浸润。

皮瘤（可能含有CD34阳性的间质细胞）鉴别[258,655]。

鉴别诊断包括纤维组织增生性毛发上皮瘤、硬化性基底细胞癌、转移性乳腺癌、汗管瘤以及乳头状小汗腺腺瘤。

黏液癌[658-661]　Mucinous carcinoma

这是一种低级别的癌，以大的黏液湖中含有分泌黏液的上皮细胞团为特征。其形态学表现与乳腺黏液癌极为相似（见第16章）。

临床上，病变一般为3cm或较小，肉质样，呈灰色或蓝色。多数发生于头部，尤其是眼睑周围。这种肿瘤常常累及老年人；黑人似乎容易发生。复发常见，但转移性播散极为少见。

组织学上，多数肿瘤呈分叶状，呈膨胀性生长结构（图23.106）。实际上并不出现间质反应。极少数病例除了特征性的黏液湖以外，还可出现实性区域。这些肿瘤细胞在细胞学上呈温和的均匀一致的表现，没有核分裂象（图23.107）。与乳腺相应病变相似，许多病例显示病变周边有异型增生或原位癌的特征[661]。

黏液湖为PAS阳性，并且抗淀粉酶，与涎黏蛋白一致。免疫组织化学上，病变多种细胞角蛋白染色均呈阳性，尤其低分子量角蛋白。CEA和GCDFP-15在有些病例中有表达，少数病例S-100蛋白呈阳性[662]。雌激素和孕激素受体见于少数病例，进一步体现了与乳腺肿瘤极为类似[663]。少数病例出现神经内分泌分化[664,665]。肌肉肌动蛋白在这些病变中极少有表达[666]。一例DNA分析显示主要为二倍体DNA成分，伴有少数多倍体细胞[667]。

鉴别诊断为转移性黏液癌和一些黏液性基底细胞癌（罕见），其PAS染色为阴性。

恶性顶端汗管瘤（顶端汗管癌、汗孔癌、所谓的恶性小汗腺汗孔瘤；透明细胞汗腺癌）[635,668-671]　Malignant acrospiroma (acrospirocarcinoma, porocarcinoma, so-called malignant eccrine poroma; clear cell hidradenocarcinoma)

恶性顶端汗管瘤包括一组罕见的表皮、近表皮以及真皮导管的癌，其特征是非角化性，但细胞学呈多形性的细胞巢和细胞岛（图23.108）。常见透明细胞变病灶以及明显的导管成分。不要过分强调这些病变罕见，尽管在一项历时超过8年的75万例的大宗实验室检查中，仅仅发现5例这样的病变[672]。

临床上，汗孔瘤样（近表皮）病变表现为硬结性或疣状斑块，极个别病例覆盖大片表面。顶端汗管瘤样（真皮）病变可以表现为息肉、斑块或结节。多数病变发生于老年人，主要位于下肢[671]。

组织学上，原位或近表皮的病变从表皮内多形性实性细胞巢（图23.109）或伴有腔隙的透明细胞（汗腺腺癌）到伴有中央坏死区以及神经周围和淋巴管浸润的表皮和（或）真皮病变。增殖率高以及淋巴血管浸润与较侵袭性的经过有关[671]。极少数病例出现嗜表皮性播散[673,674]。真皮顶端汗管瘤样病变表现类似，但完全属于真皮肿瘤，可出现岛状、硬化性或粉刺型组织学表现。

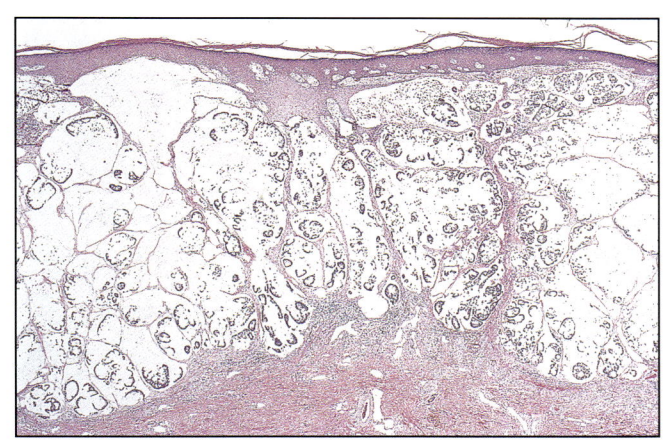

图23.106　黏液腺癌。大的黏液湖含有单个和成簇的肿瘤细胞。

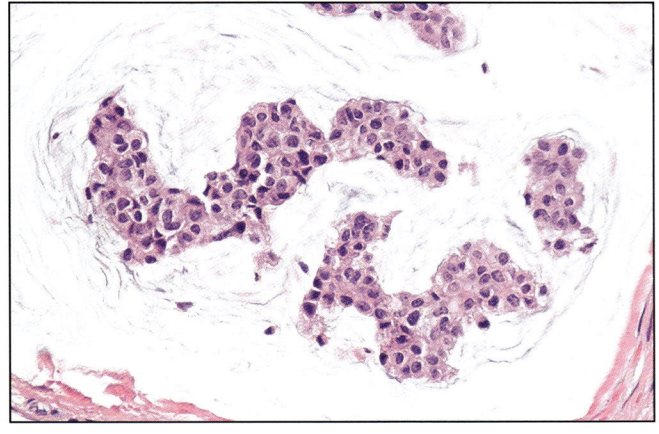

图23.107　黏液腺癌。肿瘤细胞呈温和的均一性表现，通常缺少核分裂象。

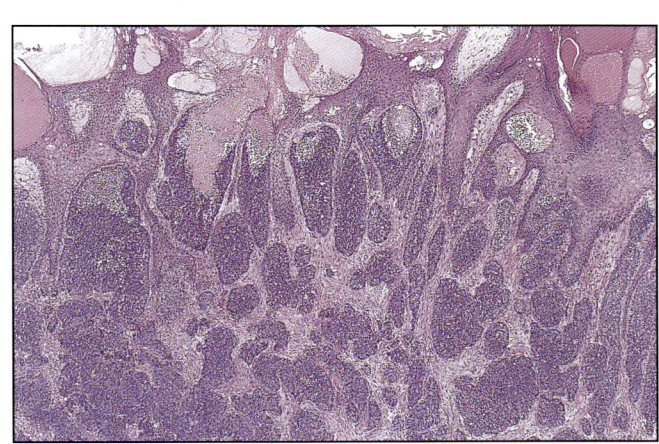

图23.108　恶性顶端汗管瘤（顶端汗管癌）。成巢的多形性基底细胞样细胞和导管，可与（如同本例）或不与表面相连。

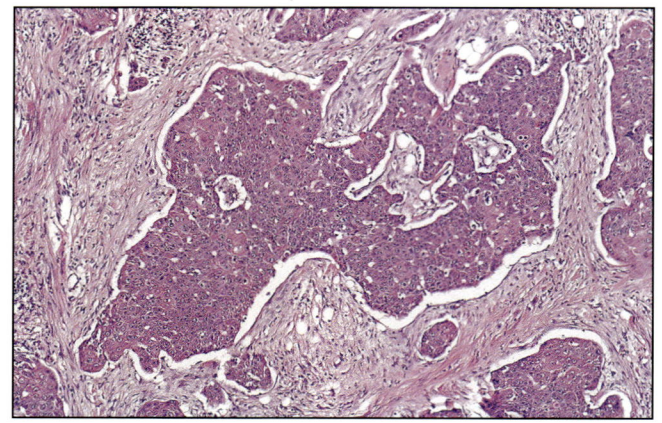

图23.109 恶性顶端汗管瘤（顶端汗管癌）。肿瘤细胞相对一致，但细胞岛呈浸润性。

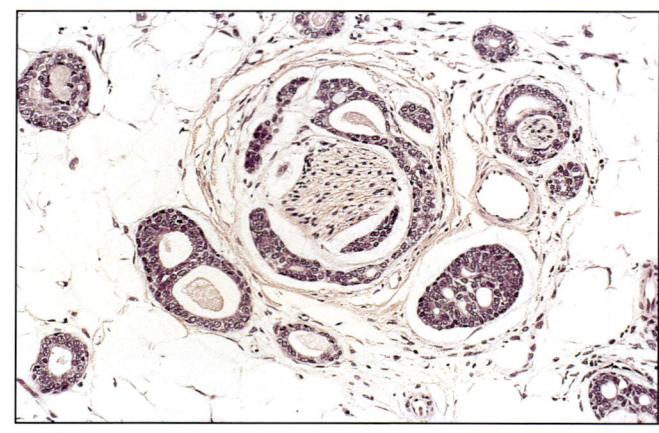

图23.111 腺样囊性癌。这些病变中常常有明显的神经周围以及神经内浸润。

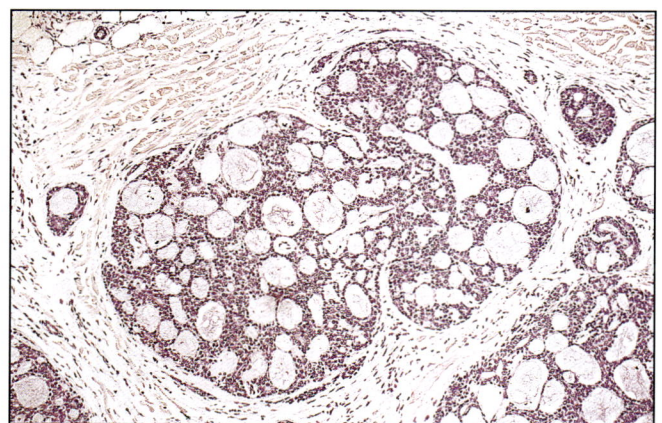

图23.110 腺样囊性癌。肿瘤细胞岛含有筛状区域。

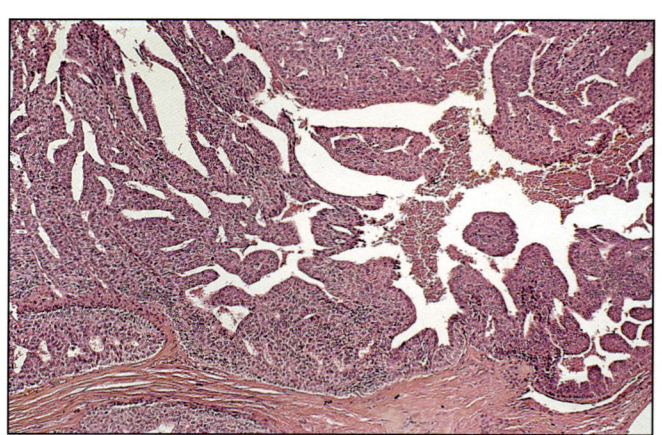

图23.112 指（趾）乳头状腺癌。病变由乳头状丛构成。

免疫组织化学上，病变呈一系列的细胞角蛋白阳性染色，尤其是低分子量角蛋白。病变的导管腔 CEA 呈阳性。在一些病变中可以检测出雌激素和孕激素受体[675,676]。DNA 分析显示病变为多倍体[677]。

腺样囊性癌[678-684] Adenoid cystic carcinoma

腺样囊性癌为浸润性病变，一般发生于头皮。组织学表现类似于涎腺（见第 7 章）和其他部位的相应病变（图 23.110）。筛状、腺管样及基底细胞样细胞结构也可见到。与在其他部位一样，皮肤腺样囊性癌也有明显的神经周围浸润（图 23.111）。

指（趾）乳头状腺癌[685,686] Digital papillary adenocarcinoma

这些肿瘤最常发生于老年人的指趾以及手掌和足底附近的组织。病变容易出现深层局部浸润和复发。大约 15% 的患者出现转移性疾病，尤其是当肿瘤有骨侵犯时。组织学上，病变呈乳头状结构（图 23.112 和 23.113），伴有灶状实性腺样及梭形细胞区域。实性区域的特征

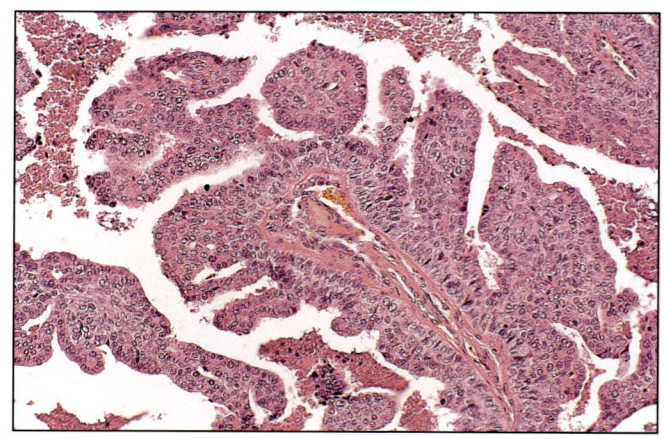

图23.113 指（趾）乳头状腺癌，乳头状丛含有纤维血管轴心。

是出现筛状结构（图 23.114），而且可有鳞状上皮化生。免疫组织化学染色，肿瘤细胞角蛋白、CEA 和 S-100 蛋白呈阳性。虽然其中有些病变过去被认为是腺瘤，但目前认为所有这些病变均为腺癌，即使有些病变仅有轻度

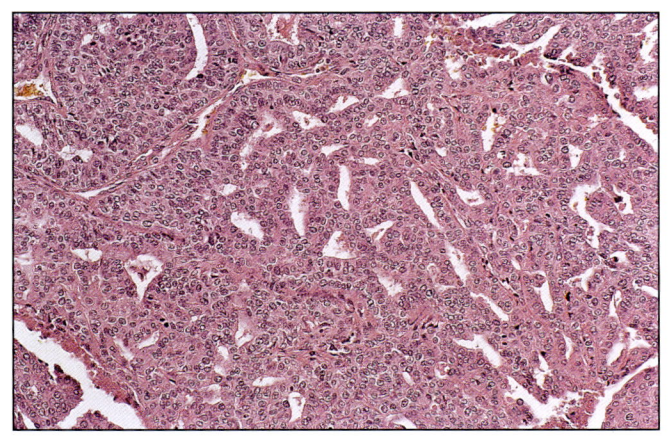

图23.114 指（趾）乳头状腺癌。筛状区域常常比较明显。可见细胞学多形性。

细胞学多形性[687]。

其他附件癌　Miscellaneous adnexal caecinomas

这些涵盖一系列极为少见的皮肤恶性肿瘤，包括印戒细胞癌[688-690]、恶性混合瘤[550,691-693]、圆柱癌[694-696]、汗管腺癌[697-700]、乳头状汗管腺癌[701,702]、黏液表皮样癌[703-706]、小汗腺上皮瘤[707-709]、淋巴上皮瘤样癌[710-718]、小细胞汗腺癌[719]以及非特异性导管腺癌[637]。

皮肤囊肿　Cutaneous cysts

皮肤囊肿定义为发生于真皮及少数发生于皮下的囊性结构。皮肤囊肿可以也可以不与表面或其他附件结构连接，具有一种或多种类型的内衬上皮，含有一种或多种附件结构，或为单发性，或为多发性，并可伴有临床综合征。

我们一般将直径大于2 mm的囊肿与粟粒疹分开[720]。创伤种植性囊肿的内衬几乎总是类似于表皮，除此以外的皮肤囊肿被认为是特发性囊性畸形，即错构瘤，一般按照出现在囊肿壁上的主要上皮类型来命名，尽管其他成分也可出现在单个病例中。

一般来说，皮肤附件囊肿可以大致分为毛囊、皮脂腺导管（皮脂腺囊瘤）或小汗腺/顶泌汗腺导管或混合性囊肿，取决于囊肿上皮内衬与其正常对应结构的相似性。另外，本章其他部分所描述的特殊类型的病变也可以以囊性为主，如汗孔扩张（Winer）、毛囊瘤、纤维毛囊瘤、毛母质瘤以及顶端汗管瘤（汗孔瘤）。

皮样囊肿　Dermoid cyst

这是一种不常见的先天性囊肿，其内衬在组织学上类似于皮肤，通常位于头颈部的皮下，沿胚胎闭合线分布[722]。组织学上，囊肿内衬漏斗上皮以及一种或多种附件结构。然而，任何特别的囊肿均可含有所有类型的上皮（即小汗腺、顶泌汗腺、毛囊和皮脂腺）。平滑肌成分也可出现。皮样囊肿不同于畸胎瘤，后者含有由三个胚层衍化而来的组织。

不常见的皮肤囊肿　Uncommon cutaneous cysts

各种不常见的或罕见的皮肤囊肿已有报道，包括鳃裂囊肿[723]、支气管源性囊肿（支气管源性迷芽瘤）[724]、纤毛囊肿[497]、囊性畸胎瘤[725,726]、子宫内膜异位症[727]和输卵管内膜异位[728]、指（趾）黏液性囊肿[729]、毛囊皮脂腺囊性错构瘤[280]、阴茎中缝囊肿[730,731]、化生性滑膜囊肿[732,733]、黏液囊肿[734,735]、脐肠系膜导管囊肿（脐部息肉）[736-738]、呼吸道囊肿[739]、胸腺囊肿[740]以及甲状舌管囊肿[741]。

Merkel细胞（神经内分泌）癌　Merkel cell (neuroendocrine) carcinoma

皮肤的神经内分泌癌以一系列的小蓝细胞肿瘤为特征，多见于真皮内。

神经内分泌癌最常发生于老年人，且好发于身体上部。尽管躯干和下肢也可受累。组织学上，类似的病变有发生于涎腺、软组织甚至淋巴结的罕见病例报告。临床鉴别诊断是非特异的。肿瘤的预后各异；有关肿瘤的大小和深度与临床预后相互关系的资料纯属经验之谈，因为这种肿瘤极为少见。临床分期似乎是最重要的预后因素[742]。近些年来所积累的、主要为尚未发表的资料提示，这些肿瘤总体上为侵袭性肿瘤，容易反复复发，多数病例最终出现转移[743]。

组织学上，可见一系列的小梁状、岛状或弥漫性生长结构，其中任何一种或所有这些表现可共存于同一个肿瘤当中。病变常常累及整个真皮，表皮一般因薄层Grenz带而免于受累（图23.115）。不常见表现包括亲表皮性[653,744,745]，伴有角化细胞多形性类似于Bowen病[746,747]，以及导管成分。细胞学上，肿瘤细胞一般呈单一形态。胞浆通常稀少，且为嗜双色至嗜酸性。细胞核相对一致，呈灰色，并可出现细胞核变形，类似于内脏小细胞癌（图23.116）；然而，与多数内脏小细胞癌病例不同的是，皮肤神经内分泌癌容易辨认，缺少因挤压造成的人工假象。染色质呈细颗粒状及"粉尘"状；可见小核仁。组织化学上，银染色一般为阴性，与肿瘤细胞缺乏神经分泌颗粒相符合。免疫组织

黑色素细胞肿瘤 Melanocytic tumors

黑色素细胞病变包含一大类肿瘤，从小的斑状雀斑性增生到先天性或后天性黑色素细胞痣乃至黑色素细胞瘤[759]。表 23.6 将这些病变进行了对比。

良性黑色素细胞病变 Benign melanocytic lesions

黑色素细胞痣定义为生物学稳定的临床斑点、斑块、丘疹或息肉，实际上 100% 的浅肤色的个体均可发生，而且组织学上几乎均为对称性的表皮、真皮或两者内的黑色素细胞数量增加。诊断名称依据黑色素细胞在皮肤中所处的部位。另外，黑色素细胞的细胞学类型（即其细胞核和细胞浆的特征）在黑色素细胞痣的命名中起着重要的作用。

临床上，黑色素细胞痣可为先天性或后天性。前者可从直径不足 1 cm 的小病变到累及大部皮肤表面区域的所谓的躯干下部痣（bathing trunk nevi）[760,761]。其中有些痣可出现不常见的临床表现，如眼睑先天性分裂痣[762]或不规则性色素性病变，如"斑痣"（nevus spilus）[763,764]。后天性黑色素细胞痣可发生于任何年龄，临床上一般表现为明显的小的斑点。其中有些病变最终变为斑块、丘疹或息肉。虽然这一序列并非见于每一个黑色素细胞痣，但是这一原则适用于多数病例。不同病变之间色素沉着差异很大；可从皮肤颜色到褐色、棕色至黑色。有些后天性黑色素细胞痣可类似于[765]或伴有[766]脂溢性角化症，而另一些病变可呈分叶状[767]或带蒂[768]。这些病变绝大多数不需要进行活检。鉴别诊断一般为脂溢性角化症或恶性黑色素瘤。

组织学上，多数良性黑色素细胞病变为对称性（将一侧病变与另一侧比较时，出现镜影表现），包括临床检查及低倍镜下扫描的组织学表现。另外，几乎所有直径小于 3.0 mm 的黑色素细胞病变均为良性[769]。然而，最后证明某一病变是否为良性总是需要临床随访。

黑色素细胞痣一般的诊断分类包括单纯性雀斑、交界性黑色素细胞痣、复合性黑色素细胞痣以及真皮黑色素细胞痣，下面分别对每一种进行讨论[770]。

单纯性雀斑 Lentigo simplex

临床上这是一种色素沉着性（棕色至黑色）斑点，其组织学特征为雀斑样黑色素细胞增生以及角化细胞色素沉着过多，伴有或不伴有上皮脚延长（图 23.117）[156]。临床鉴别诊断为所有类型的色素沉着过多性斑点。组织学鉴别诊断为老年雀斑和交界性黑色素细胞痣。前者光学显微镜检查可见角化细胞色素沉着过多以及黑色素细胞轻度增生。后者可能含有类似于单纯性雀斑的区域，

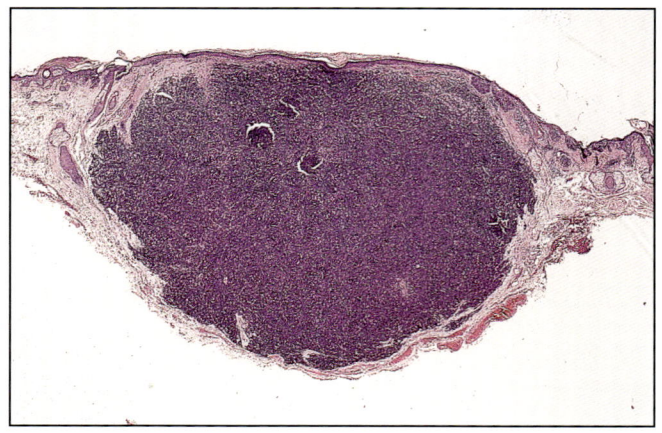

图 23.115　神经内分泌癌。低倍镜下为基底细胞样小细胞肿瘤。

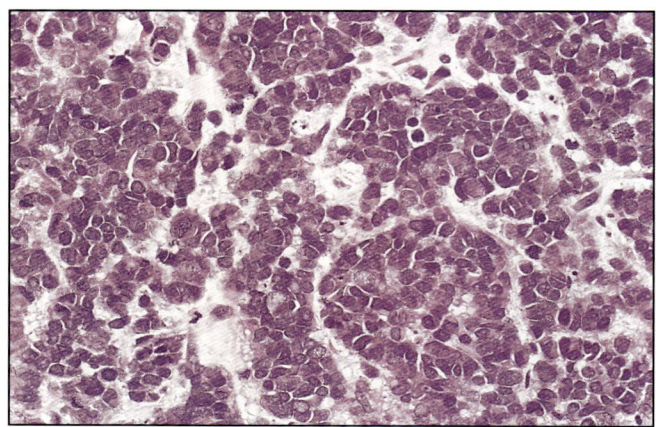

图 23.116　神经内分泌癌。多数肿瘤呈巢状及索条状生长结构。

化学染色上[684,748,749]，常常出现一致性的表现；包括核旁"点状"聚集的细丝，低分子量角蛋白表现为阳性，如 AE1/AE3、CAM 5.2 或 CK 20[750]。点状神经细丝蛋白阳性也常见。CK20 呈阳性有助于与其他类型的小细胞癌的鉴别[751]。在多数病例中，EMA（上皮膜抗原）、NSE（神经元特异性烯醇化酶）、神经细丝、嗜铬素以及 BER-EP4 也呈阳性[752]。S-100 蛋白、CEA 和淋巴细胞标记物总是呈阴性。超微结构检查，肿瘤细胞之间通过粘着斑点彼此相连。可见特征性的核旁细丝呈现环状聚集[753-757]。在固定较好的标本中还可以见到 80～120 nm 大小的神经分泌颗粒。

组织学鉴别诊断通常有限，包括小细胞性恶性黑色素瘤、皮肤淋巴瘤[758]、神经内分泌性基底细胞癌（极少见）[247]、转移性小细胞癌以及 Ewing 肉瘤。在这些肿瘤当中，与转移性小细胞癌的鉴别常常最为困难，建议仔细查问临床病史，并提议行胸部放射学检查，尽管 CK 20 和 CK 7 免疫染色一般可以鉴别[751]。

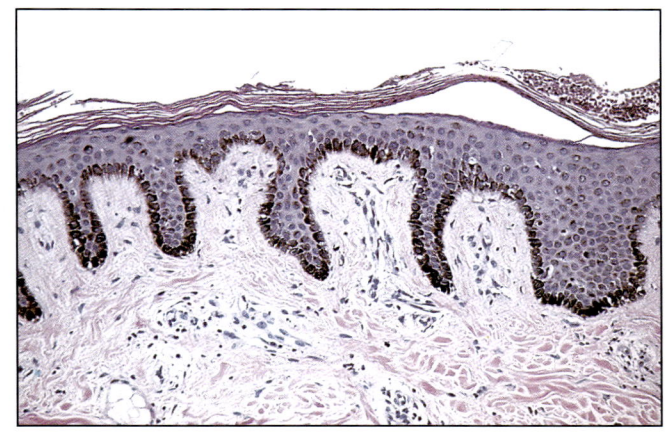

图23.117 单纯性雀斑。真皮与表皮交界处出现线样色素沉着过多和黑色素细胞增生。

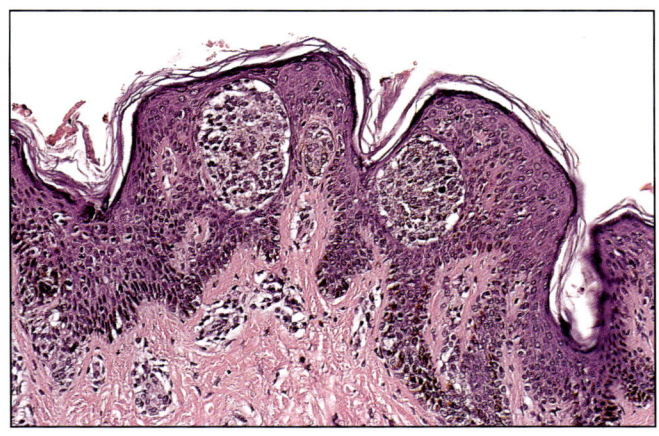

图23.119 黑色素细胞痣，交界型。表皮内黑色素细胞性痣细胞团。没有真皮成分。

但除此以外还可出现表皮黑色素细胞性痣细胞团。

黏膜黑色素斑 [156,157,771-774]
Mucosal melanotic macule

这是一类口腔或生殖器黏膜的色素沉着斑，组织学特征为表皮基底层细胞色素沉着增加（图23.118），一般呈扁平状。黑色素细胞的数量通常没有明显增加，但黑色素细胞常常为树突样，并且在 HE 染色切片中明显可见。单个病变可以表现为局灶性黑色素细胞增生。当然，生殖器的病变与日光照射没有直接关系。

普通黑色素细胞痣 Common melanocytic nevi

交界性黑色素细胞痣（junctional melanocytic nevi）：病变特征为一类小的斑点状病变，组织学上为分布均匀的黑色素细胞性痣细胞团和（或）雀斑性黑色素细胞增生，混合有程度不一的角化细胞色素沉着过多（图23.119）。此时的"痣细胞团"（theque）是指在 HE 染色的切片上，表皮内有 3 个或 3 个以上的呈巢状聚集的黑色素细胞团。在交界性黑色素细胞痣中，痣细胞团大小一般类似，但在周边可逐步变小。在有些病变中，HE 染色切片上的痣细胞团可以"相连"。连续切片可以证实这些痣细胞团为偏心性。交界性黑色素细胞痣的一个明确的特征是病变局限。"局限"是指病变最外周的部分出现交界性痣细胞团，不同于交界性雀斑性黑色素细胞痣或恶性黑色素瘤，后者的病变周边通常以单个（不成团的）细胞定界。痣细胞团之间可见单个或成对的黑色素细胞。有些黑色素细胞在真皮与表皮交界处连续（雀斑性分布），但也可见到跳跃性分布。真皮乳头间质的改变轻微，可有也可没有浅表血管周围单核细胞浸润。如果出现间质改变，一般表现为同心圆性纤维化，即真皮乳头纤维化在单个上皮脚处密集排列。主要的组织学鉴别诊断为单纯性雀斑和交界性雀斑性黑色素细胞痣，单纯性雀斑缺少痣细胞团，而交界性雀斑性黑色素细胞痣为非局限性病变。

复合性黑色素细胞痣（compound melanocytic nevus）：病变的临床特征为一大类隆起的、常常为色素沉着性的丘疹及息肉，具有交界性黑色素细胞性痣细胞团以及真皮内黑色素细胞团（图23.120）。这些病变的真皮成分表现多样，但是从观察许多这样的病变中可以得出几条有用的原则。

组织学上，几乎所有的真皮成分均为对称性，低倍镜下具有均匀一致的生长方式。这类病变的生长方式可有明显不同，但在同一个特殊的病变中，生长方式一般较为一致。可能引起诊断混淆的许多组织学人工假象也可见于这些病变。收缩人工假象是：真皮细胞巢明显位于"淋巴管"腔内；而分离人工假象是：细胞巢内的黑色素细胞条索是分离的，类似于血管腔隙[775,776]。其他不常见的特征也有描述[777]。

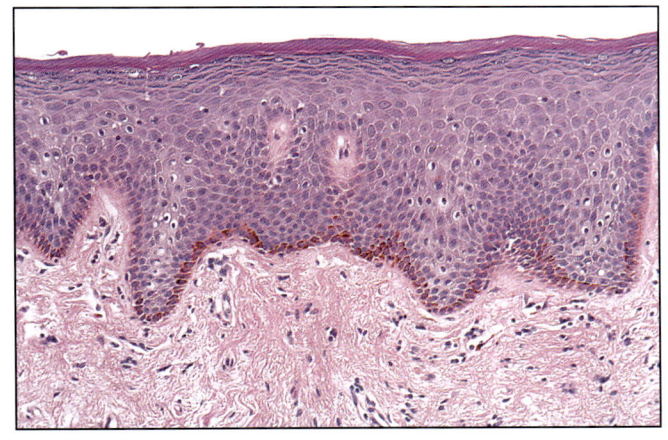

图23.118 黏膜黑色素斑。上皮基底层可见明显的色素沉着过多。

黑色素细胞肿瘤

表23.6 黑色素细胞病变

类型	发生率	大小	对称性	表皮内境界	黑色素细胞部位	黑色素细胞巢团	黑色素性巢细胞团的周围性	巢细胞团以外的黑色素细胞	黑色素细胞形状及DE jxn性质	真皮内黑色素细胞	成熟	内部一致性	色素沉着	黑色素细胞核分裂象	S-100	MelanA	细胞角蛋白
单纯性雀斑	常见	小 <5mm	是	清楚	表皮在DE jxn	无	n/a	全部	上皮样，一致，周期性分布	无	n/a	是	一致，如有	无	+	+/−	−
黑色素细胞痣，交界性	不常见	小 <5mm	是	清楚	表皮在DE jxn	有	一致	无	上皮样，巢细胞团内一致	无	n/a	是	一致，如有	无	+	+/−	−
雀斑样黑色素细胞痣，交界性	不常见	一般 <5mm 有时较大	是	不清	表皮在DE jxn	有	一致，桥状，下部纤维化，常见	许多在DE jxn	上皮样，一致，周期性分布	无	n/a	是	一致，如有	无	+	+/−	−
Spitz痣，交界性	不常见	一般 <5mm	是	清楚	表皮在DE jxn	有	一致，有时痣细胞团替代表皮	许多在DE jxn，但数量一般少于痣细胞团	上皮样（或）梭形，常有多量粉色胞浆伴有假性包涵体	无	n/a	是	一致，如有	常见	+	+/−	−
色素性梭形细胞痣，交界性	不常见	一般 <5mm	是	清楚	表皮在DE jxn	有	一致	极少在DE jxn	梭形，常有多量粉色胞浆有假性包涵体	无	n/a	是	一致，常为存噬黑色素性皮炎	极为常见	+	+/−	−
肢端黑色素细胞痣，交界性	不常见	一般 <5mm	是	清楚	表皮在DE jxn	有	一致	许多在DE jxn	上皮样，梭形，细胞小于Spitz	无	n/a	是	一致，如有	无	+	+/−	−
黑色素细胞痣，复合性	常见	一般 <5mm	是	清楚	表皮和真皮	有	一致	极少在DE jxn	上皮样，梭形，巢细胞团内一致	通常表皮以及巢状	通常	通常	一致，如有	无	+	+/−	−
雀斑样黑色素细胞痣，（复合性）	常见	一般 <5mm 有时较大	是	不清	表皮和真皮	有	一致，桥状，下部纤维化，常见	许多在DE jxn	上皮样，一致，周期性分布	表皮样形，有时梭形，一般呈巢状，有时弥漫	通常	通常	一致，如有	无	+	+/−	−
先天性黑色素细胞痣	不常见	一般 >5mm	是	清楚	表皮和真皮	有	一致	极少在DE jxn	上皮样，胞浆中等粉红色胞浆伴有假性包涵体	一般呈巢状，有时弥漫，通常累积附属器性	通常	通常	一致，如有	极少	+	+/−	−
黑色素细胞痣，伴有空泡现象	不常见	一般 <5mm	是	不清	表皮和真皮	有	一致	许多在DE jxn	通常黑色素细胞难以识别	一般呈巢状，难以与淋巴细胞鉴别	通常	通常	一致，如有	无	+	+/−	−
Spitz痣复合性	不常见	一般 <5mm 有时较大	是	清楚	表皮和真皮	有	一致，有时痣细胞团一般少于痣细胞团	许多在DE jxn 但数量一般少于痣细胞团	上皮样（或）梭形，常有多量粉红色胞浆伴有假包涵体	上皮样，有时梭形，一般多量胞浆，巢状和单个孤立细胞，后各较深	通常	通常	一般没有	常见	+	+/−	−
色素性梭形细胞痣，复合性	极少见	一般 <5mm 有时较大	是	清楚	表皮和真皮	有	一致	极少在DE jxn	梭形，常有多量粉红色胞浆有假性包涵体	梭形，巢状，有时弥漫真皮乳头	通常	通常	一致，常为存噬黑色素性皮炎	常为	+	+/−	−
黑色素细胞痣，（生殖部位性）	不常见	一般 <5mm 有时较大	是	不清	表皮和真皮	有	一致	许多在DE jxn	上皮样，一致，周期性分布，常常呈小"巢"	上皮样，有时梭形，一般呈巢状，有时弥漫	通常	通常	一致，如有	无	+	+/−	−
肢端黑色素痣，复合性	常见	一般 <5mm 有时较大	是	不清	表皮和真皮	有	一致	许多在DE jxn	上皮样（或）梭形，细胞小于Spitz	上皮样，梭形，一般呈巢状，有时弥漫	通常	通常	一致，如有	无	+	+/−	−

表23.6 黑色素细胞病变（续）

类型	发生率	大小	对称性	表皮内境界	黑色素细胞部位	黑色素巢细胞团	黑色素性巢细胞团的周期性	巢细胞团以外的黑色素细胞	黑色素细胞形状及DE jxn性质	真皮内黑色素细胞	成熟	内部一致性	色素沉着	黑色素细胞核分裂象	S-100	MelanA	细胞角蛋白
黑色素细胞痣，真皮内	常见	一般<5mm 有时较大	是	n/a	真皮	无	n/a	全部	n/a	上皮样，一般呈巢状	通常	通常	一致，如有	无	+	+/-	-
肢端黑色素细胞痣，真皮内	极少	一般<5mm 有时较大	是	n/a	真皮	无	n/a	全部	n/a	上皮样，一般呈巢状，有时弥漫性	通常	通常	一致，如有	无	+	+/-	-
Spitz痣，真皮内	极少	一般<5mm	是	n/a	真皮	无	n/a	全部	n/a	上皮样和（或）梭形，常有多胞胞浆，巢状和孤立单个细胞，后者部位深	通常	通常	一半没有	常见	+	+	-
Spitz痣，纤维化/组织增生性	极少	一般<5mm	是	n/a	真皮	无	n/a	全部	n/a	梭形细胞伴有多量胞浆，与纤维性间质混杂	有时	通常	一半没有	常见	+	+/-	-
蓝痣，普通型	常见	一般<5mm 有时较大	是	n/a	真皮	无	n/a	全部	n/a	树突状，弥漫性伴有纤维化	否	通常	一致，如有	无	+	+	-
蓝痣，上皮样型	不常见	一般<5mm 有时较大	是	n/a	真皮	无	n/a	全部	n/a	上皮样，巢状，有时见"细胞球"结构	否	通常	一致，如有，常见多量噬黑素细胞	极少，如有黑色素瘤	+	+	-
深部浸润性黑色素细胞痣	常见	一般<5mm 有时较大	是	n/a	真皮	无	n/a	全部	n/a	上皮样，巢状或弥漫，深部浸入真皮	有时	通常	一致，如有	极少	+	+	-
原位黑色素瘤	常见	不一，从小到很大	否	不清	表皮	常见	不规则	许多在DE jxn	上皮样或呈梭形	n/a	n/a	少见	不规则，如有	不少	+	+	-
黑色素瘤，Paget样	常见	不一，从小到很大	否	不清	表皮和真皮	常见	不规则	许多在DE jxn，整个真皮伴有Paget样结构	一般上皮样	一般上皮样	少见	少见	不规则，如有	常见	+	+	-
黑色素瘤，雀斑	常见	不一，从小到很大	否	不清	表皮和真皮	有时	不规则	许多在DE jxn	一般呈梭形	上皮样或梭形	少见	少见	不规则，如有	不少	+	+	-
结节状黑色素瘤	不常见	不一，从小到很大	否	不清	表皮和真皮	有时	不规则	有时见于表皮	上皮样或梭形	上皮样或梭形	少见	少见	不规则，如有	较常见	+	+	-
黑色素瘤，雀斑样	极少	不一，从小到很大	常见	有时清晰	表皮和真皮	有时	有时规则	有时见于表皮	上皮样或梭形	上皮样或梭形	有时	有时	有时一致	不常见	+	+	-
黑色素瘤，胶样	极少	不一，从小到很大	否	不清	表皮和真皮	有时	不规则	许多在DE jxn	一般呈梭形	一般呈梭形	少见	少见	不规则，如有	常见	+	+	-
黑色素瘤，纤维组织增生性	极少	不一，从小到很大	否	不清	表皮和真皮	有时	不规则	有时见于表皮	一般呈梭形	一般呈梭形	少见	少见	不规则，如有	不常见	+	+/-	-
黑色素瘤，嗜神经性	极少	不一，从小到很大	否	不清	表皮和真皮	有时	不规则	有时见于表皮	一般呈梭形	一般呈梭形	少见	少见	不规则，如有	不常见	+	+/-	-
黑色素瘤，蓝痣样	极少	不一，从小到很大	否	n/a	真皮	无	n/a	n/a	n/a	一般上皮样	少见	少见	不规则，如有	常见	+	+/-	-

DE jxn: 真皮表皮交界; n/a: 没有得到。

皮肤肿瘤

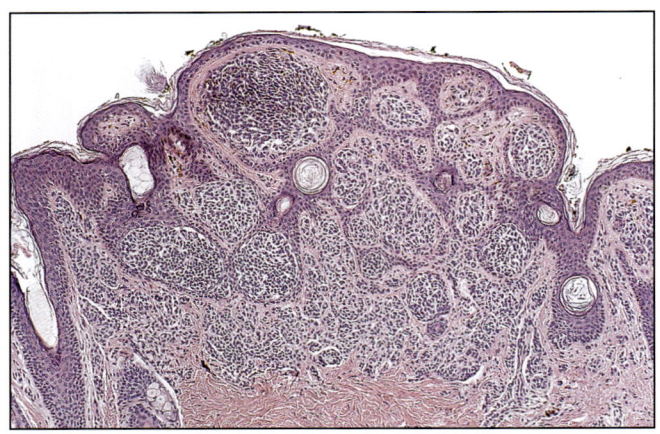

图23.120 黑色素细胞痣，复合性。可见表皮和真皮成分。

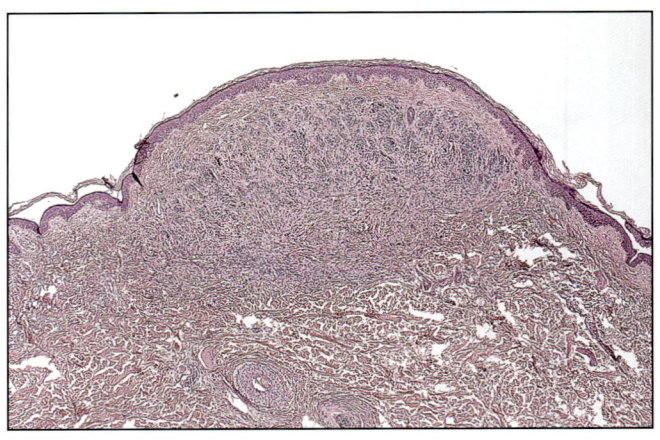

图23.121 黑色素细胞痣，真皮内型。完全位于真皮内的黑色素细胞对称性增生。

"成熟"（衰老）[778] 一般见于复合痣和真皮黑色素细胞痣；它是指在真皮不同水平中黑色素细胞的大小和形状不同。在真皮乳头或浅层，一般为圆形或上皮样的色素沉着性黑色素细胞（A 型）。在真皮中部，黑色素细胞呈淋巴细胞样（B 型）。最深部的细胞为无黑色素性的神经样或梭形细胞，类似于神经鞘细胞或触觉小体（Meissner corpuscles）（C 型）[779]。以退化为主的病变可与神经纤维瘤极为类似。其他公认的退行性改变包括出现多核细胞、脂肪变[780] 以及化生性骨化。

不同病变之间胞浆内色素沉着不同；然而，在一个单个痣内，浅表部分的黑色素通常较重，而较深部分黑色素逐步减少。除了先天性黑色素细胞痣、梭形和（或）上皮样细胞痣（Spitz）以及色素沉着性梭形细胞痣（Reed）外，附件周围或真皮外膜一般并不受累。

免疫组织化学上，黑色素细胞痣 S-100 蛋白染色实际上胞浆和细胞核总是呈阳性。另外，胞浆常有微管蛋白（tubulin）表达[781]。黑色素瘤相关性抗体也可标记病变的一些部分，一般为真皮与表皮交界处的黑色素细胞[782]。神经鞘细胞相关性抗体标记所谓的 C 型黑色素细胞[783]；然而，其他学者注意到，这些细胞缺乏与神经成分的相似之处。超微结构检查发现，细胞含有黑色素小体。

除了多数复合性黑色素细胞痣中出现的特征性 A-C 型黑色素细胞外，某些特殊类型的病变以具有明显不同类型的黑色素细胞为特征，这些细胞多数为大的上皮样和（或）梭形细胞，分别见于 Spitz 痣和 Reed 痣。这些将在下面详细讨论。

真皮黑色素细胞痣（dermal melanocytic nevus）：这是一类缺乏表皮交界处痣细胞团的良性黑色素细胞痣，可能具有多种生长方式，包括伴有某种成熟性的典型的浅表性上皮样黑色素细胞结构（图 23.121）、伴有假血管腔隙的结构（图 23.122）、伴有广泛神经样细胞的结构（图 23.123）以及伴有脂肪组织的结构（图 23.124）。

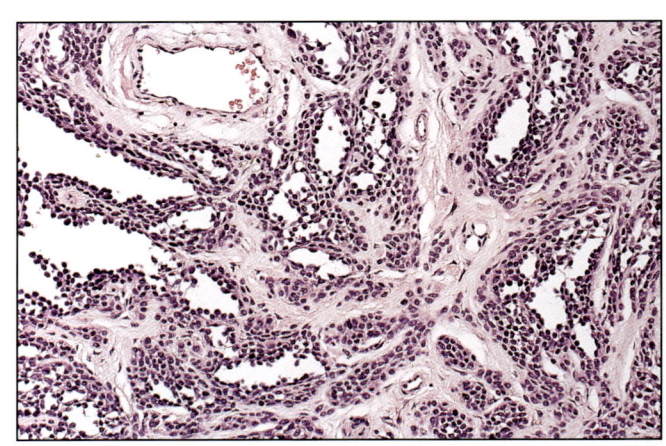

图23.122 黑色素细胞痣，真皮内型。在某些病变中，假血管腔隙可较为明显。

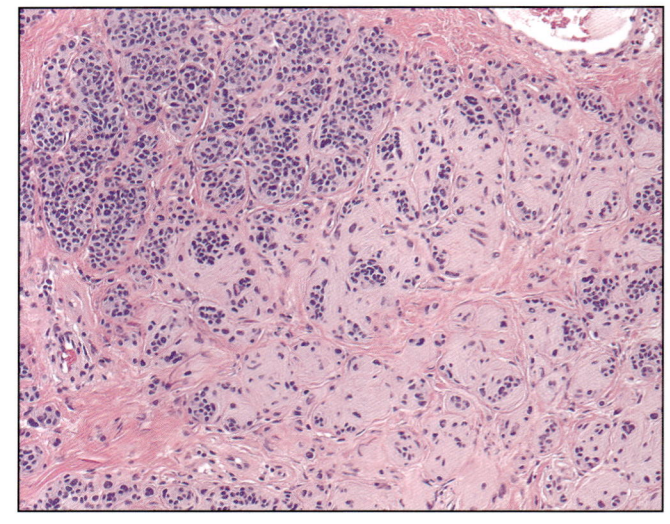

图23.123 黑色素细胞痣，真皮内型。出现浅表性的上皮样细胞以及深层的神经样细胞（成熟）。

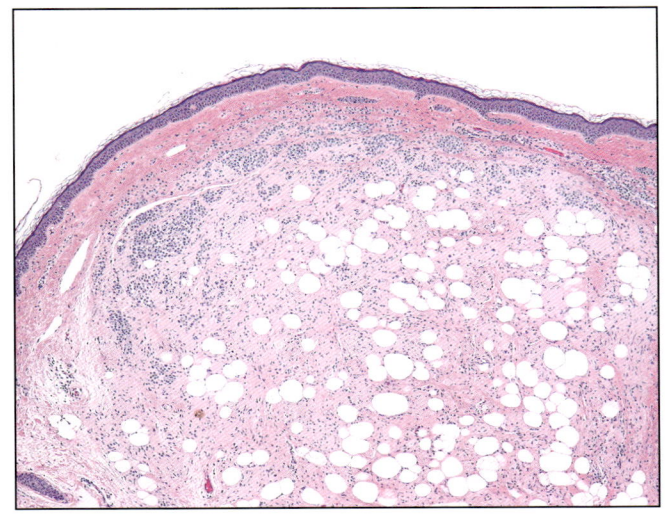

图23.124 黑色素细胞痣，真皮内型。病变内可见脂肪组织。有时这种病变称为"脂肪神经痣"。

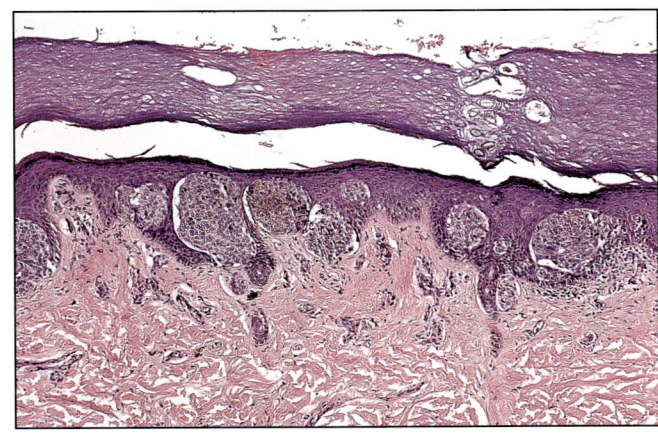

图23.125 肢端黑色素细胞痣，病变小而对称，伴有表面角质层角化过度。

虽然典型的病例类似于复合性黑色素细胞痣的真皮成分（如上所述），但是其他类型差异较大，即所谓的真皮黑色素瘤类：蓝痣、Ota痣[784-786]和Ito痣[786]以及胎斑（Mongolian spot）[787,788]。

黑色素细胞痣的特殊亚型
Specific variants of melanocytic nevi

有些黑色素细胞痣在与恶性黑色素瘤的鉴别诊断中意义重大，尤其是上皮样和（或）梭形细胞痣（Spitz）、色素性梭形细胞痣（Reed）、蓝痣（Tièche）以及雀斑性黑色素细胞痣，这些将在这部分之后详细讨论。

肢端黑色素细胞痣（acral melanocytic nevus）[789,790]在黑人中最常见，可为交界性、复合性或真皮性痣。这种痣的交界性成分的主要成分为雀斑性单个细胞结构（图23.125）。另外，这些病变的恶变率常常被错误地认为比通常的恶变率高，由于黑色素细胞易于进入表皮上部，可能引起诊断上的高度关注。

类似的评述适用于外阴或生殖器黑色素细胞痣（vulvar or genital melanocytic nevi）[791,792]，后者最常见于年轻人，尽管这样命名，这些病变不仅见于外阴，也可见于会阴，而且在极少数情况下可见于阴阜及腋窝。它们还可发生于男性生殖器，但不常见[793]。诊断常常困难，因为这些病变显示常常见于黑色素瘤的组织学特征，值得注意的是，上皮脚集中（图23.126），其中含有黑色素细胞小"巢"（图23.127），后者也可见于附件上皮。

气球细胞痣（balloon cell nevus）[794-796]的多数黑色素细胞出现惊人的透明细胞表现，加之病变一般为无色素性，使得诊断更具有挑战性。

先天性黑色素细胞痣（congenital melanocytic nevi）[761,797-799]为常见亚型，出生时或出生后不久出现。

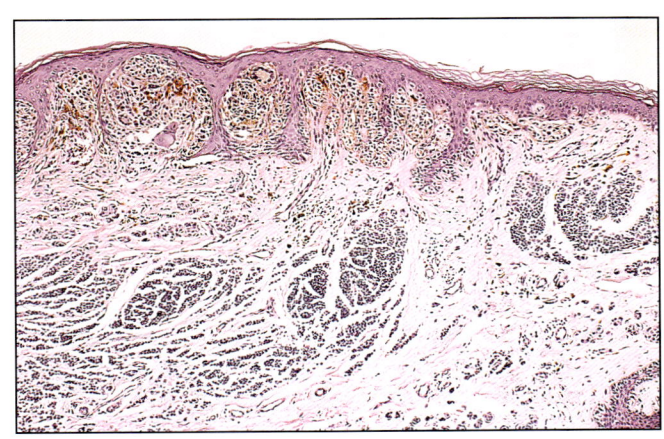

图23.126 外阴黑色素细胞痣（生殖器型）。这些病变常常出现雀斑样结构，伴有多核黑色素细胞。注意真皮内成熟表现。

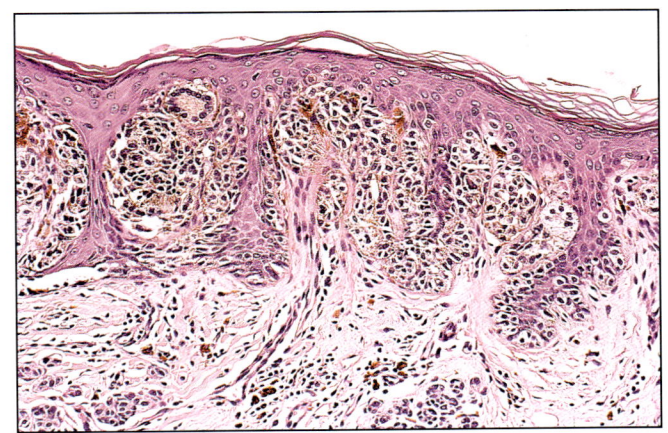

图23.127 外阴黑色素细胞痣（生殖器型）。在真皮与表皮交界处，注意花环状黑色素细胞及黑色素细胞"巢"，与常常见于普通痣的大的痣细胞团不同。

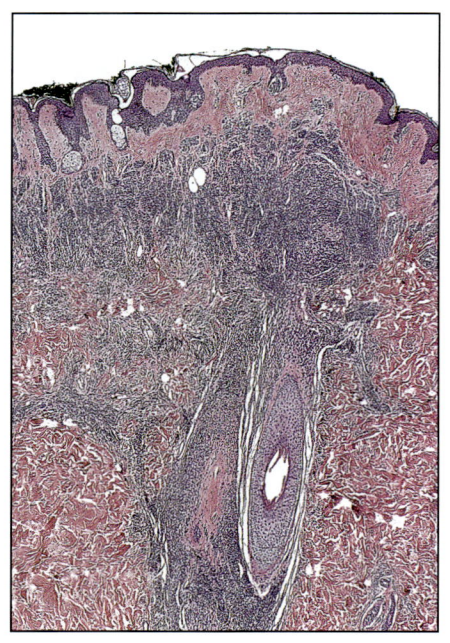

图23.128 先天性黑色素细胞痣。注意这个病变明显累及附件。

先天性黑色素细胞痣的特征是还容易累及真皮深层。易于浸润或累及毛囊、皮脂腺、汗腺导管、毛囊肌肉以及血管的内皮下部分(图23.128)。当出现任何这些特征时，常常遍及整个病变。

深部穿透性痣（deep penetrating nevus）[800-802]是一种发生于年轻人的黑色素细胞性肿瘤，由索条状和巢状上皮样黑色素细胞组成，并向深部扩展进入网状真皮（图23.129）。病变色素沉着过多，从概念上可被认为是上皮样细胞与蓝痣之间的交杂。一种类似的病变为丛状梭形细胞痣（plexiform spindle cell nevus）[803,804]。它具有梭形细胞痣和深层穿透性痣的共同特征。

晕痣（halo nevi）[805]为黑色素细胞病变，临床上表现为病变周围无黑色素环。组织学上，这些病变出现大量淋巴细胞浸润，可能掩盖黑色素细胞成分（图23.130）。在病变的晚期阶段，可能难以找到由于病变进展而消失的黑色素细胞。黑色素细胞可呈多形性表现，有时可以出现上皮样细胞（Spitz样）改变[806]。有些黑色素细胞痣具有晕痣的组织学特征，但在临床上可能没有无黑色素区改变；空晕现象用来描述这种病变的组织学改变。相反，偶尔临床上诊断的晕痣可能没有特征性的炎症性组织学改变；对于具有这种组织学改变的病变，并没有提出特殊的命名，但它强调了采用晕痣这一名称事实上是来源于临床观察，当组织学所见与临床表现不符合时，应当在病理报告中予以澄清。

混合痣（combined nevus）这一命名表示痣具有混合性的细胞结构。在常见的亚型中，肥胖的色素沉着性梭形细胞在普通的痣细胞巢中成束状分布。在其他亚型中可出现一种或几种黑色素细胞成分，具有蓝痣或Spitz痣的细胞学特征。在 Pulitzer 及其同事[807]研究的95例病例中，49%为普通型。大体上，多数病变为色素沉着的深的丘疹或结节。3/4的病例临床诊断为痣、蓝痣或黑色素瘤。15%的病例伴有"黑色素细胞异型增生性"组织学特征，这些病变多数为普通类型。对于常见亚型来说，其细胞学特征、伴有明显的浸润性生长方式以及程度不等的非典型交界性成分的特征，常常会导致病理医生误诊并错误地预示其生物学潜能。黑色素细胞痣细胞表型的多样性以及遗传学的不稳定性在混合痣中均有表现。

这些痣亚型还需要更好地了解，因为其很可能被误诊为黑色素瘤[808]。混合痣切面上一般呈非对称性——黑色素瘤的标志之一。这一点加上一些细胞学改变，如

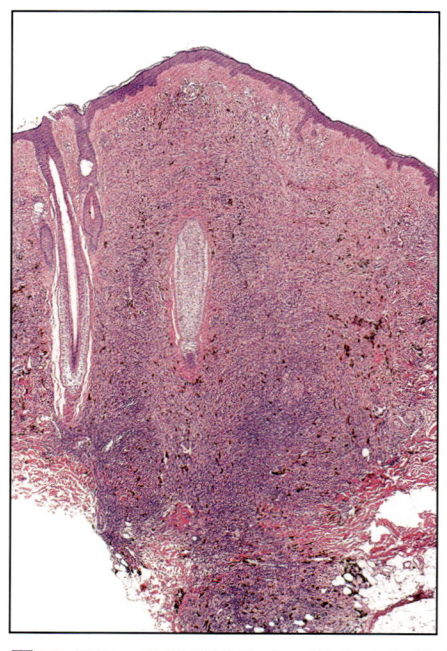

图23.129 深部穿透性痣。这个病变具有明显的垂直性生长方式。

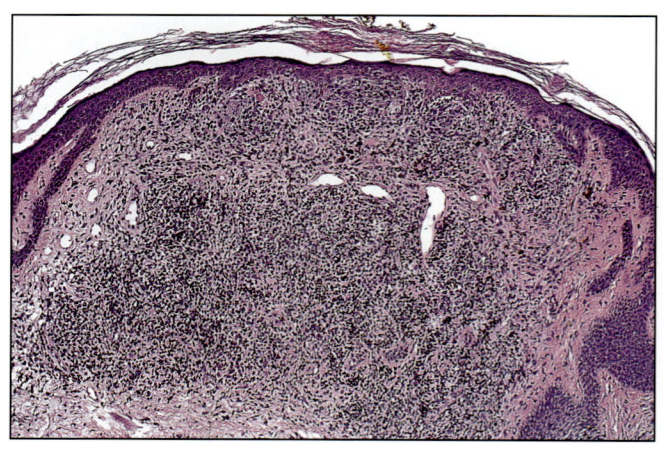

图23.130 晕痣。显著的宿主反应使得原本的黑色素细胞增生模糊不清。

反转性黑色素生成方式以及炎症反应，可造成组织学图像混淆（图 23.131）。

复发性/持续性痣（recurrent/persistent nevus）：色素痣如果切除不完全，常常出现复发，偶尔会引起患者和临床医生的关注。这种病变最初是于 1975 年由 Komberg 和 Ackerman 描述的[809]。Park 等研究了 175 例病例并制定了诊断标准[810]。复发性痣一般为残留在皮肤附件汗腺和毛囊结构内的痣细胞巢的再度生长。在其再度生长结构中，黑色素细胞将再生的表皮作为支架，沿表皮底层生长。其生长方式可为巢状，但最常见的是雀斑样结构。细胞排列紊乱，一般色素沉着较重，给人以黑色素瘤的印象。病变排列成三个区域：表皮内成分、真皮瘢痕以及深层的残留性痣（图 23.132）。用于诊断的组织学标准为：相对缺乏细胞学非典型性。最为重要的标准可能为：复发性色素沉着以及黑色素细胞增生仅限于瘢痕部位，并不超出原有痣的边界。如有可能，病理医生应尽量审查最初的活检，因为当初未被破坏的黑色素细胞病变应当明显为良性。值得引起注意的是应该记住，部分性刮除的黑色素瘤也可复发。并非所有复发性黑色素细胞病变均为良性[811,812]。

梭形细胞和（或）上皮样细胞痣（Spitz痣）[813-823]
Spindle and/or epithelioid cell nevus (Spitz nevus)

这是一种良性的、散在分布的、对称性的境界清楚的黑色素细胞病变，组织学上由梭形细胞、较大的上皮样细胞或两者构成。这种病变可以是交界性、复合性或真皮性。

这些黑色素细胞痣相对常见。临床上，这种病变一般发生于头颈部，但任何皮肤表面均可出现[818,824]。极少数情况下可出现眼部[825]或黏膜[826]受累。尽管多见于 20 岁以内的患者[820]，但也常常发生于成人[818,827]。所有种族均可受累[828]。肿瘤一般散在分布，境界清楚，呈圆顶形，尽管有些病变可呈斑点状。多数病变直径不足 1cm[823]。一般情况下病变呈皮肤颜色至红色或棕色。多为单发性，但也可出现多发性病变[829]，病变可为成簇[830-838]、线样[839]或播散性分布[840-842]。孤立性病变在临床上的鉴别诊断通常有限；可能需要考虑其他类型的黑色素细胞痣、皮肤纤维瘤、分叶状毛细血管瘤、幼年性黄色肉芽肿、肥大细胞瘤或恶性黑色素瘤[820]。对于多发性病变，应当考虑多种鉴别诊断，包括附件肿瘤、播散性黄色肉芽肿、新生儿肌纤维瘤病或其他"组织细胞性"病变。治疗为单纯性切除并带有窄的边缘。如果诊断正确，即使肿瘤未被完整切除，病变也不会转移[843]。然而，未完整切除的病变可持续存在，如果再度活检，可能很难与恶性黑色素瘤鉴别[844]。

组织学上，Spitz 痣几乎总是呈对称性，而且境界清楚（图 23.133）。同其他黑色素细胞痣一样，尽管病变可呈交界性、复合性或真皮性，但从概念上讲它是复合性病变，因为最常见且最易识别。覆盖这种病变的表皮极少正常；一般出现某种程度的棘层增厚。常常出现上皮脚变细，并与痣细胞团和真皮痣细胞巢紧密并行排列（图 23.134）。在有些病例中，上皮脚形成网状结构；而在其他病例中，表皮增生类似于见于颗粒细胞瘤或溃疡部位的假癌性增生[123,846,847]。

复合性 Spitz 痣的表皮部分一般呈规则性分布，垂直变长的痣细胞团由梭形和（或）上皮样黑色素细胞构成（图 23.135）。在许多痣细胞团中，邻近表皮处或痣细胞团的表浅部位可见新月形腔隙，其内有"覆盖的"黑色素细胞。痣细胞团也可见于附件上皮内。孤立性黑色素细胞或痣细胞团可见于表皮较高的部位，甚至可以

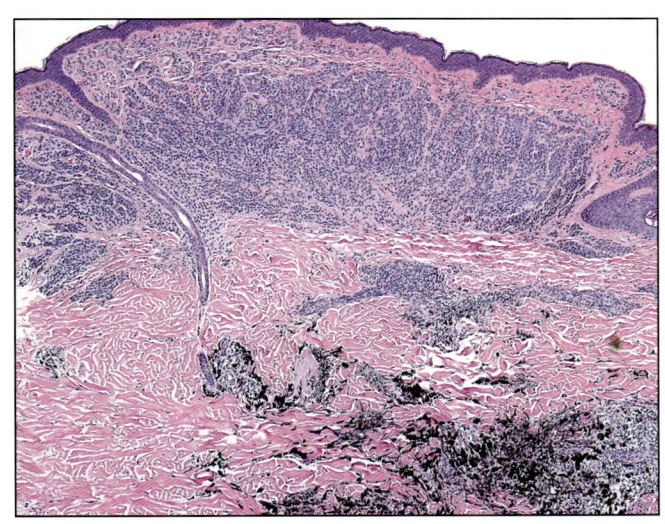

图 23.131　混合痣。浅层为规则的真皮痣，而较深部分为蓝痣成分。

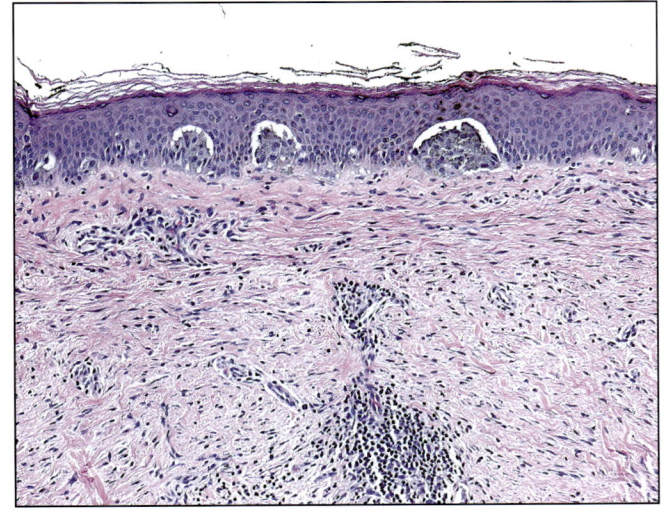

图 23.132　复发性/持续性痣。分层的黑色素细胞病变，伴有较深部分的残留性真皮痣。中心可见瘢痕，并有复发性不规则的表皮内成分。

黑色素细胞肿瘤

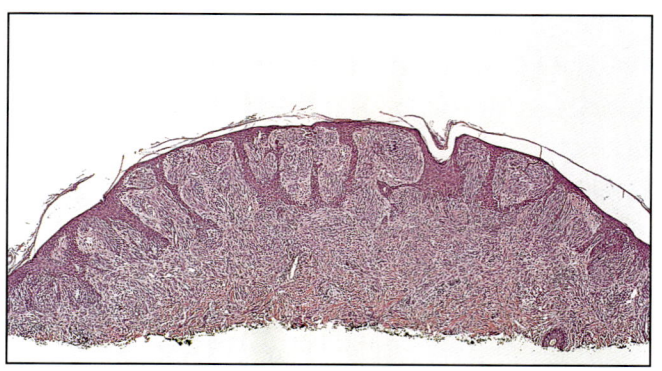

图23.133　Spitz痣。注意这种病变的对称性。具有某种成熟的表现。表皮增生可见并常见于这些病变中。

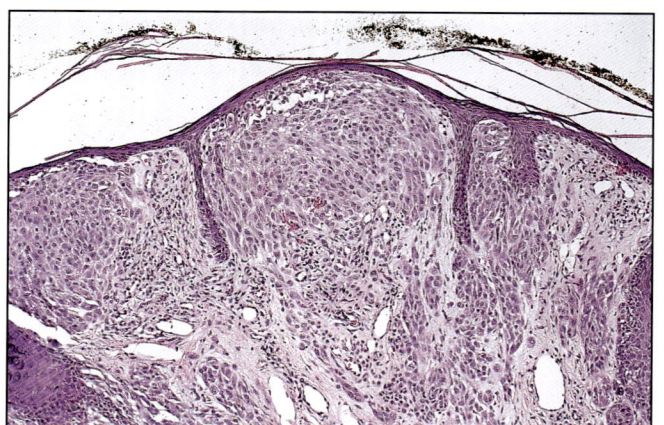

图23.134　Spitz痣。病变由大而粉红的上皮样细胞和梭形细胞构成。

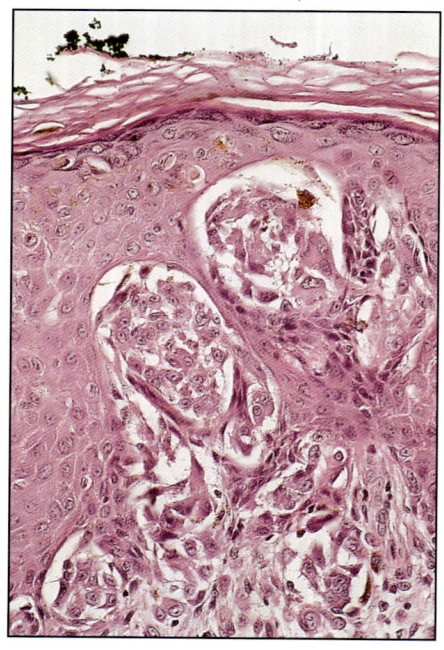

图23.135　Spitz痣。表皮内的痣细胞团常常在其浅表部位出现新月形裂隙。

出现于角质层内；事实上，整个痣细胞团可使表皮结构消失[848,849]。然而，无规则分布的表皮内结构（Paget样播散）通常也可见于浅表播散性恶性黑色素瘤，而在大多数Spitz痣病例中没有这种结构。一种极少见的Paget样Spitz痣的亚型已有报道；不过，做出这样一种诊断必须非常小心[850,851]。嗜酸性小体或所谓的Kamino小体可见于许多痣细胞团内或其周围[852-854]。这些PAS阳性、抗淀粉酶的玻璃样结构由层粘连蛋白（laminin）、Ⅳ型和Ⅶ型胶原[855]以及纤维粘连蛋白（fibronectin）[856,857]构成，在其他物质中，没有证据表明这些为变性的基底细胞或黑色素细胞[857]。虽然在单个病例中出现这些表现并不能完全除外恶性黑色素瘤，但是出现大量Kamino小体则非常不利于黑色素瘤的诊断。

真皮部分可以出现成巢的和单个孤立的黑色素细胞，但极少见到带状及"小管"结构[858]。当从浅层至深层扫描病变时，可见细胞巢一般主要位于浅层，而在较深部位，逐渐变为单个黑色素细胞。病变与病变之间可出现不同程度的色素沉着，但在同一病变内一般呈均匀分布。与真皮成分有关的间质反应轻微是其特征。当发生间质纤维化时，一般普遍呈均一表现，不同于多数恶性黑色素瘤的真皮成分。毛细血管扩张性血管腔隙常见。单核细胞浸润常常散在分布于病变内及病变周围，而且这种表现可以很明显，以至于可以类似于晕的改变[806]，但某一病变内及其周围出现明显的噬黑色素细胞性皮炎并不多见，除了色素沉着性梭形细胞亚型。极少数情况下，黑色素细胞团可明显位于血管[846]及淋巴管腔内[859]。亲神经和（或）亲立毛肌（pilomyotropism）也可见到。所有这些表现如果脱离病变背景，均不能视为恶性指征。

细胞学上[823]，痣细胞团和痣细胞巢内的黑色素细胞相似。不论是梭形还是上皮样黑色素细胞，在低倍镜下不同视野之间形态通常单一，虽然在高倍镜下存在明显的差异，尤其是上皮样黑色素细胞之间。上皮样黑色素细胞具有一系列的形态学表现，从伴有多量嗜酸性胞浆（伴有或不伴有黑色素）到伴有"肌母细胞样"逗号样尾巴的上皮样黑色素细胞（图23.136）。有些可为多核细胞[824]，并且可能类似于Touton巨细胞。上皮样细胞的细胞核呈空泡状，伴有小而明显的核仁；单个细胞内可有也可没有假包涵体[860]，即细胞核的胞浆内陷[861]，这些特征没有一个具有明确的诊断意义。梭形细胞常常均匀一致，在痣细胞团和痣细胞巢内排列紧密。在表皮痣细胞团内，梭形细胞常常沿相邻表面或附件上皮分布。在真皮细胞巢中，一般呈束状排列（"丛集"或"鱼群"）。两种类型的细胞均可以出现核分裂象；但核分裂象一般稀少，通常为正常核分裂象，如果出现核分裂象，则多见于病变的浅表区域。

免疫组织化学上，Spitz痣S-100蛋白染色一般胞浆

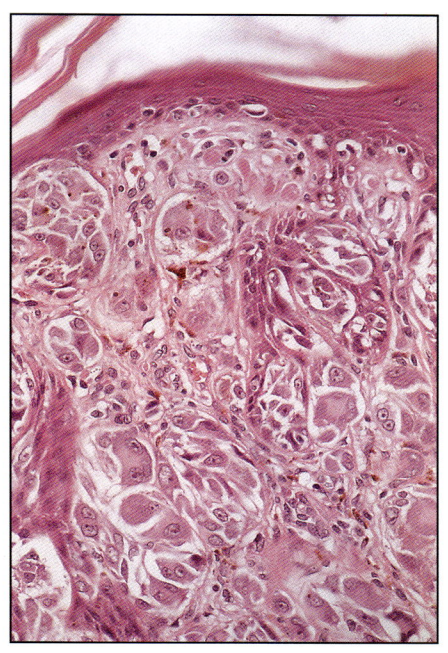

图23.136 Spitz痣。黑色素细胞常常呈奇异大小和形状，包括这种肌母细胞样类型。

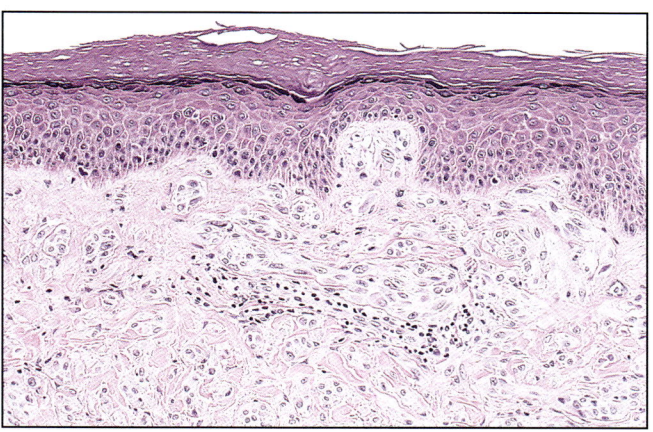

图23.137 Spitz痣，真皮型。没有表皮成分，但细胞学与普通型Spitz痣类似。真皮病变常伴有间质纤维组织增生。

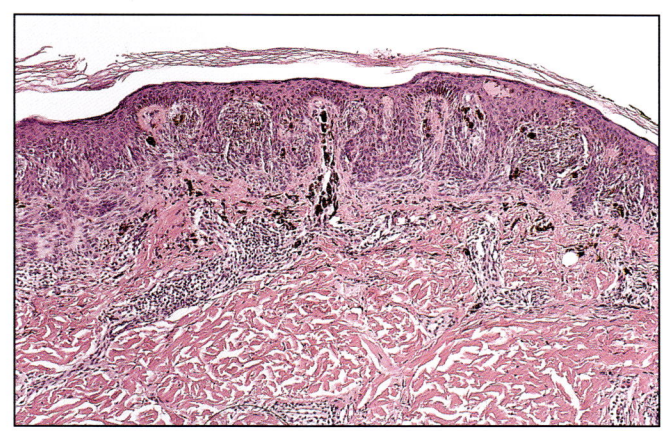

图23.138 色素性梭形细胞痣（Reed）。这是一种由梭形细胞构成的浅表性复合性黑色素细胞痣。注意真皮内色素沉着。

和细胞核呈阳性。Melan A在Spitz痣为阳性[862-864]。动力学研究显示，Spitz痣具有低MIB-1和bcl-2评分，不同于作为对照的黑色素瘤[865]。DNA分析显示Spitz痣为二倍体，与常常为多倍体的黑色素瘤不同[866]。

还可见到另外两种组织学类型的Spitz痣。这些应该分别被看做是Spitz痣概念序列中的两端：交界性Spitz痣和真皮Spitz痣。

交界性Spitz痣（junctionl Spitz nevi）组织学上类似于复合痣所见的表皮部分。然而，如果黑色素细胞完全为梭形细胞并具有"推挤性"边缘，则不能与色素性梭形细胞痣（Reed）区分；事实上，由于这个原因，后者被认为是特殊类型的Spitz痣[867]。

真皮Spitz痣（dermal Spitz nevi）缺少表皮成分，组织学上可类似于复合性Spitz痣的真皮部分（图23.137）或呈纤维组织增生性表现[868]。鉴别诊断包括皮肤纤维瘤、网状组织细胞瘤以及纤维组织增生性恶性黑色素瘤。

色素性梭形细胞痣 [867,869-877]
Pigmented spindle cell nevus（Reed）

色素性梭形细胞痣定义为由梭形黑色素细胞组成的良性、对称性、交界性或复合性黑色素细胞痣，其下方几乎总是伴有明显的噬黑色素细胞聚集。色素性梭形细胞痣被认为是一种特殊类型的梭形和（或）大的上皮样细胞痣（Spitz）。

临床上，色素性梭形细胞痣边界清楚，对称性或轮廓不规则，呈暗棕色到黑色。直径通常不足1cm，多见于21～30岁的年轻妇女的肢体[874,876]，尤其是大腿[870]。

鉴别诊断包括非特异性黑色素细胞痣、Spitz痣、雀斑性黑色素细胞痣、恶性黑色素瘤以及纤维组织细胞瘤[877]。单纯切除可以治愈。

组织学上，病变为交界性或复合性的[874]；不仅周边的表皮痣细胞团界限清楚，而且深层真皮的边界也清楚（图23.138）[872]。真皮与表皮交界处极少出现单个的黑色素细胞[877]。可有表皮增生，但通常不如Spitz痣明显。尽管痣细胞团可使表皮消失，并且在一些病例的表皮内可见单个黑色素细胞，但没有Paget样播散（图23.139）。Kamino小体通常可见于多数病例[874,878]。组织结构的嗜酸性属性常常被黑色素沉积所掩盖。有真皮成分时，黑色素细胞巢排列密集，呈束状生长方式，并且占据少部分真皮，深度一般不超过真皮乳头[874]。在有些病例中，痣细胞团可见于毛囊或小汗腺或顶泌汗腺的导管上皮[874]。细胞巢之间胶原稀疏，有少数单个细胞浸润胶原。这种形态不同于多数Spitz痣，后者在胶原纤维之间常常可见单个黑色素细胞。与典型的Spitz痣病例不同的是，色素性梭形细胞痣的特征是：基底部可见宽大的色素较重的噬黑色素

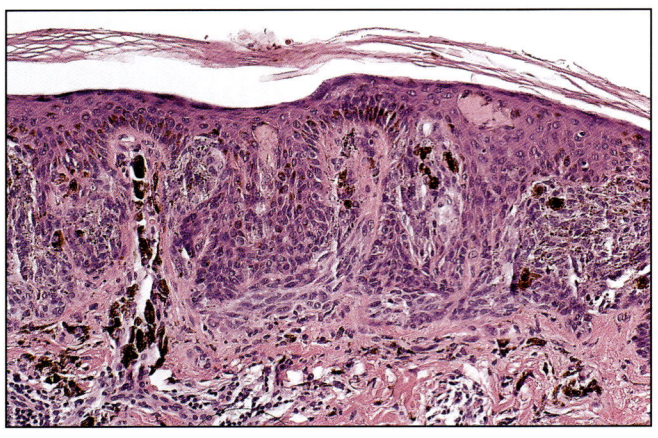

图23.139 色素性梭形细胞痣（Reed）。注意右侧梭形细胞如何排列。可见噬黑色素细胞性皮炎。

一般发生于臀部和头颈部[881]，而且可能伴有Carney综合征[887-889]。不过，任何部位均可能受累。单纯切除可以治愈。鉴别诊断包括结节性恶性黑色素瘤、Spitz痣、色素性毛囊囊肿、顶泌汗腺汗囊瘤/囊腺瘤、动脉瘤性纤维组织细胞瘤以及囊性基底细胞癌。

组织学上，树突性（普通型）蓝痣为真皮内不明显到明显的弥漫性细胞团（图23.140）。仅有个别病例出现交界性成分[890]。典型者有Grenz带。黑色素细胞为双极树突状（图23.141），色素较细，伴有不同数量的含有大量黑色素的吞噬细胞。可见小的黑色素细胞巢，病变内及其周围的胶原成分一般类似于邻近非病变部位的胶原。偶尔出现黑色素减退[891,892]，以至于与皮肤纤细胞和淋巴细胞带。不过，没有浆细胞成分[874]。作者曾经见过位于整个真皮的类似病变。这些病变在结构和细胞学特征上与较普通的色素性梭形细胞痣极为类似，并且通常含有少量黑色素。

细胞学上，这些病变完全由黑色素细胞构成，伴有梭形或偏心性的细胞核，类似于Spitz痣的梭形细胞区域[874]。然而，在多数色素性梭形细胞痣，核分裂象少见。免疫组织化学特征类似于Spitz痣（见上文）。

主要的鉴别诊断为恶性黑色素瘤。不同之处在于：色素性梭形细胞痣为境界清楚的对称性病变。然而有些病例的鉴别诊断可能较为困难。

蓝痣[879-882] Blue nevus

这是一种局限性的先天性或后天性黑色素细胞痣，临床表现为一系列的蓝色病变，组织学上有几种生长方式。病变从弥漫性对称性的真皮内色素性树突状黑色素细胞团（普通型），到混合性树突状黑色素细胞和均匀一致的上皮样黑色素细胞伴硬化性间质（混合型），乃至上皮样黑色素细胞伴硬化性间质（富于细胞或上皮样型）。从概念上讲，Ota痣、Ito痣及胎斑处于蓝痣组织学系列的普通蓝痣的"末端"；然而在临床上，它们是独特的病变，通常可以与局限性蓝痣区分开来。人的蓝痣可与马的黑色素性疾病相比[883]。

蓝痣的临床表现不同，从对称性斑片到丘疹、斑块[884]或圆顶形肿瘤，直径很少大于2 cm。富于细胞型蓝痣常常大于普通型蓝痣[881,885]。颜色一般为蓝色至黑色（由于Tyndall效应），取决于黑色素在真皮内所处的位置。任何性别及年龄均可受累，包括新生儿[886]。然而，11～20岁至31～40岁的年轻人最容易受累[881]。普通型蓝痣最常发生于上肢和头颈部，而富于细胞型蓝痣

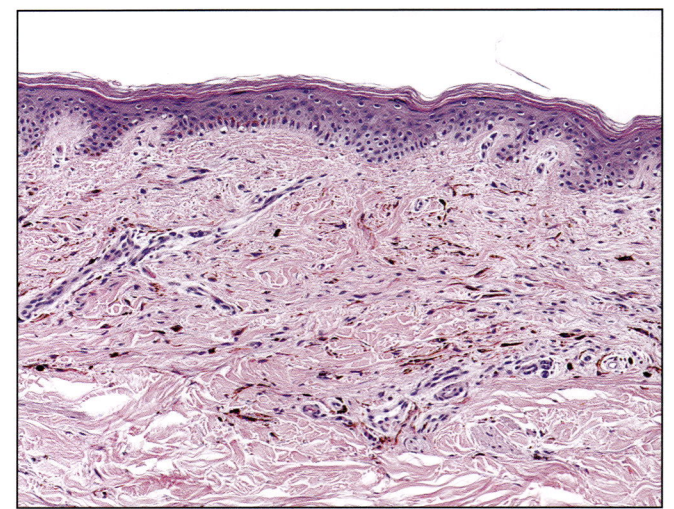

图23.140 蓝痣（普通型）。真皮内病变为硬化性和色素沉着性。

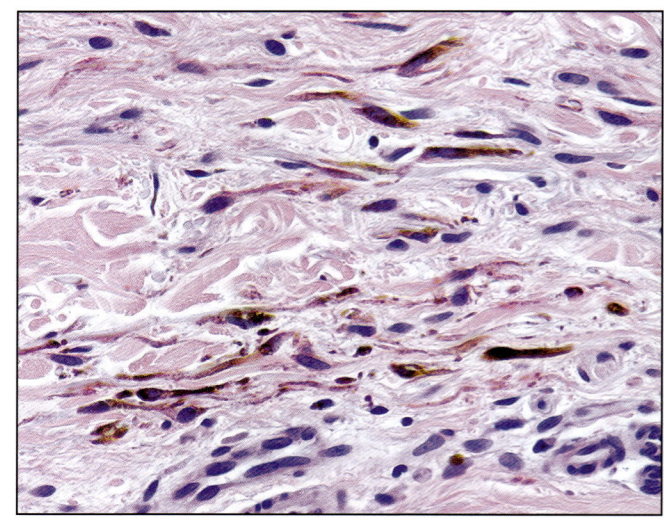

图23.141 蓝痣（普通型）。色素位于树突状黑色素细胞和巨噬细胞内。

维瘤难以鉴别。一般的鉴别诊断包括 Ito 痣、Ota 痣和胎斑。

低倍镜下，富于细胞性蓝痣为明显的对称性和纤维性病变（图 23.142）。较深的部分一般境界清楚，可以扩展至皮下组织。如果非常靠近诸如骨等固定组织，有些病变则可以出现局部破坏[893]。病变生长方式不同，从弥漫性至巢状[881]。巢状结构类似于类癌中描述的"细胞球"（zellballen）（图 23.143）。其他作者应用束状[894,895]和"腺泡状"[896]等词语来描述黑色素细胞巢。这些病变甚至被称为"环层小体神经纤维瘤"（pacinian neurofibromas）[897]。偶尔可能有细胞巢分离，出现黏液样[897]或动脉瘤样间隙，其中可能充满血液。除非了解这一特性，当见到这样的区域时，有可能误诊为恶性黑色素瘤伴血管浸润[879,898]。富于细胞性蓝痣大多为无黑色素性[899]，有时可引起与透明细胞肉瘤混淆。超微结构上，富于细胞性蓝痣的一些细胞可类似于神经鞘细胞，尽管也可以见到黑色素生成[900]。

细胞学上，高度富于细胞性蓝痣与普通性蓝痣不同，前者的细胞含有圆形或椭圆形而不是梭形的细胞核。黑色素细胞一般具有丰富的嗜酸性胞浆，HE 切片上可呈合体细胞样表现。胞浆内可见色素性微小黑色素小体和巨大黑色素小体以及无黑色素的巨大黑色素小体[901]。应用特殊染色仍然可以见到树突状突起，类似于普通蓝痣，而不同于非特异性黑色素细胞痣。

免疫组织化学上，蓝痣 S-100 蛋白和 melan A 染色呈阳性，与黑色素瘤不能区分[864,902,903]。然而重要的是，富于细胞性蓝痣 S-100 呈阴性非常常见，但 HMB-45 为阳性[904]。一项研究报告，组织学上呈多形性的富于细胞性蓝痣有 DNA 异常，这些蓝痣极少有核分裂象，应用 MIB-1 和 PCNA 染色显示其增生指数升高，但 bcl-2 较低[905]；所有患者在随访过程中均没有疾病出现。这只是强调对于这些病变，临床和病理相互联系是非常重要的。

高度富于细胞性蓝痣的鉴别诊断包括恶性黑色素瘤、纤维组织细胞瘤、色素性隆凸性皮肤纤维肉瘤以及神经鞘瘤。

蓝痣的其他组织学亚型包含一大类伴有两种组织学结构的病变，即混合性蓝痣。有些蓝痣混合有类似于非特异性细胞学类型的黑色素细胞痣区域，或伴有有时见于 Spitz 痣的大的上皮样细胞和"肌母细胞样"细胞[879,888,896,906]。有些蓝痣可含有树突状交界性成分[890]。

在有些皮肤蓝痣病例中，局部淋巴结内可见到类似于皮肤病变的细胞[896,907]。对于这些生物学上惰性的病例，尚不清楚哪一种病变最先发生。对于任何病例，都必须考虑同时发生的可能性。显然，对这些患者最好进行细致的随访。

各种类型的蓝痣恶变，即发生于蓝痣内的恶性黑色素瘤，已有少数报道。事实上，具有临床随访的客观报告较少。我们接触到的极少数病例具有以下特征：患者临床上有长期稳定的蓝痣的病史，近来临床上病变发生改变，病理学检查出现良性和恶性两种特征，而且随访足够时间出现显著的患病率或因转移性病变而死亡。组织学上，病变的相关部位出现坏死、细胞学多形性以及处于核分裂的细胞[908,909,909a]。随访时间不够但出现一致性和多形性两种组织学特征的病变很可能是发生了恶变的病变[908,910,911]。文献中这样报告的几种其他病变可能是一些例子，但不太像[912-915]。这些病变被认为是原发性恶性黑色素瘤伴类似于富于细胞性蓝痣的细胞学特征[909a]。

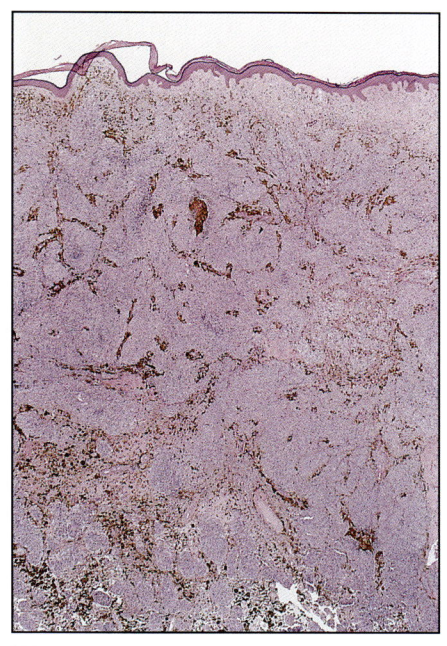

图 23.142　蓝痣，富于细胞型。分叶状的卵圆形黑色素细胞境界不清，伴有噬黑色素细胞性皮炎。

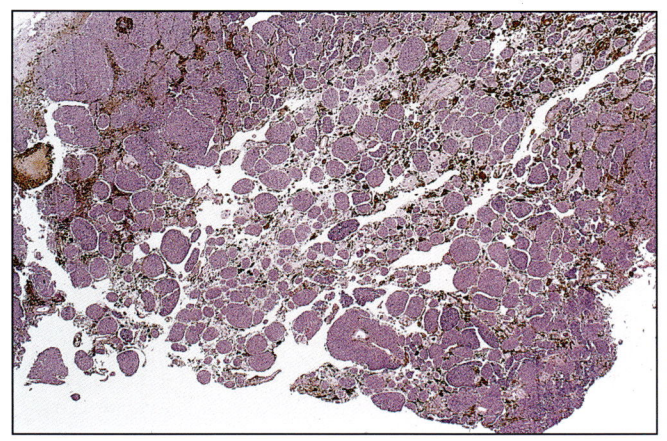

图 23.143　蓝痣，富于细胞型。在较大的肿瘤中，成巢的肿瘤细胞有时呈孤立性分布。

黑色素细胞肿瘤

雀斑性黑色素细胞痣（B-K 痣和综合征[916]；异型增生性痣和综合征[917,918]；家族性非典型性多发性痣 - 黑色素瘤综合征[919]；非典型性痣综合征[920]，伴有结构紊乱的痣）
Lentiginous melanocytic nevus (B-K mole and syndrome; dysplastic nevus and syndrome; familial atypical multiple mole-melanoma syndrome; atypical mole syndrome, nevus with architectural disorder)

这是一种组织学上定义为一类对称性、水平排列的交界性或复合性黑色素细胞痣，伴有炎症和纤维性间质改变。虽然伴有不规则的或异质性临床特征的病变可能是雀斑性黑色素细胞痣，但是完全相同的临床病变也可以是其他形态学类型的痣和黑色素瘤。尽管有各种名称来描述这些病变[921]，但本文作者根据组织学标准并没有将"异型增生性"痣（"dysplastic"nevus）纳入这个类别。异型增生性痣这一名称如果具有任何含义的话，也只是一个临床用词，并非组织学术语[922]。另外，结构紊乱的黑色素细胞痣一词也不适于用来描述这些病变，因为实际上这些病变排列有序[923]，不能将这个术语作为这些病变的一个类别；而且，这一术语并没有明确描述什么是雀斑性黑色素细胞痣，什么不是雀斑性黑色素细胞痣。

从历史上看，在 Clark 等[916] 称之为 B-K 痣综合征[916]，及 Lynch 等[919] 称之为家族性非典型性多发性痣 - 黑色素瘤综合征（FAMMM）[919] 的病变中，在伴有恶性黑色素瘤并有多个家族成员患有恶性黑色素瘤的个体，或在有多量痣而没有恶性黑色素瘤（自发性成熟）的个体，或在恶性黑色素瘤伴有多量黑色素细胞痣（家族性或自发性）的个体，多发性黑色素细胞痣已有描述。因为这些黑色素细胞痣其中许多在组织学上为雀斑性痣，而且在某些方面类似于浅表播散性恶性黑色素瘤，所以它们被称为"异型增生性"痣[918]。

下面讨论的有关"异型增生性"痣和"异型增生性痣综合征"的争论主要是在组织学水平上，因为组织学上应用的"非典型性"（atypia）或"异型增生"（dysplasia）的标准并不一致，而且具有随意性[768,924-926]。虽然保留了这种命名法，但是许多作者对"异型增生"在组织学上究竟意味着什么存在相当大的差异[927-936]。

用于这类病变的描述性命名已有选择，因为的确没有必要暗示任何发生黑色素瘤的可能性。组织学上，我们宁愿选择雀斑性黑色素细胞痣用于诊断一系列对称性黑色素细胞病变；这些病变为交界性或复合性；在真皮与表皮交界处的雀斑性结构中可见圆形、轻度不规则性或梭形的交界性黑色素细胞痣细胞团以及单个黑色素细胞；而且如果存在的话，可以从两侧延伸到真皮黑色素细胞成分以外（肩膀现象，shoulder phenomenon）（图

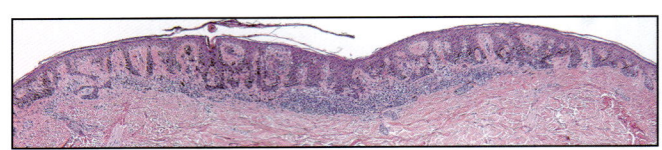

图23.144　雀斑性黑色素细胞痣。宽大的对称性黑色素病变，周围区域较薄。

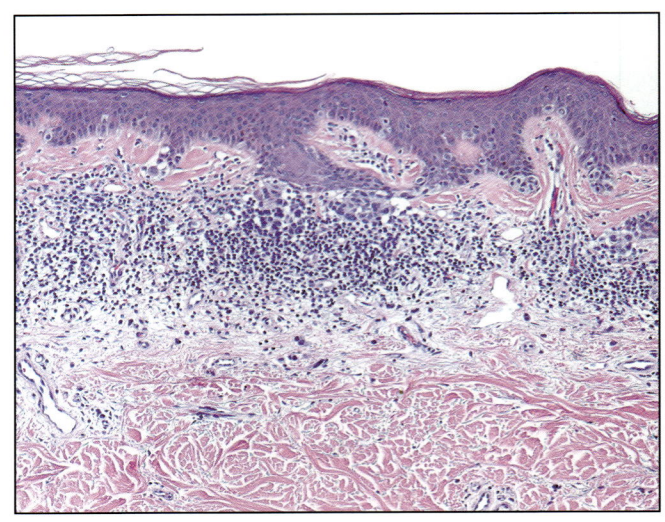

图23.145　雀斑性黑色素细胞痣。交界性成分伴有真皮乳头内炎症浸润。

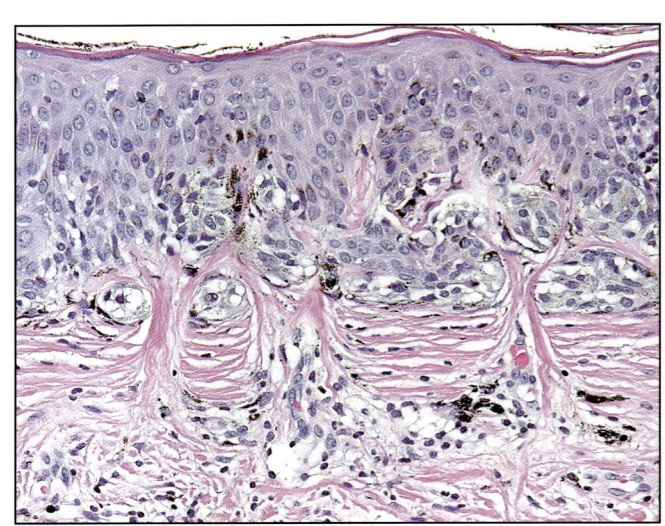

图23.146　雀斑性黑色素细胞痣。黑色素细胞呈雀斑性增生，真皮乳头伴有层状纤维化。

23.144）[937]。这些病变缺乏单个或成团黑色素细胞在表皮各层内杂乱分布的表皮结构，这一特征为许多恶性黑色素瘤的特征性表皮改变。在许多情况下，雀斑性黑色素细胞痣的黑色素细胞具有丰富的双染性至嗜酸性的胞浆；有些细胞可能含有分布均匀的细腻的胞浆内黑色素（"粉尘状"）。细胞核可为均一性或非均一性，上皮样和（或）梭形。通常小于角化细胞的细胞核，但有些细胞核可以较大（图 23.145 和 23.146）。黑色素细胞没有核分裂象。如果存在真皮成分，则可从真皮乳头扩展至网状真皮；"成熟"通常可见，尽管有些可以出现"成熟

阻滞"。有些病变可有少量到多量的血管周围淋巴细胞浸润，伴有或不伴有噬黑色素细胞，但是后者一般稀少；的确，如果出现广泛性的黑色病（噬黑色素细胞性皮炎），则应当重新考虑支持恶性黑色素瘤的诊断。真皮乳头纤维化可以不同，从轻度到广泛，但在不同病变之间一般比较一致，不同于皮肤恶性黑色素瘤。纤维化可为同心性（围绕上皮脚）或层状（在表皮下）；两种结构均可出现。鉴别诊断包括浅表播散性黑色素瘤和一些先天性黑色素细胞痣。

如果伴有上述组织学结构的病变出现临床表现，可见一系列的改变，从极少数到许许多多的病变，任何一个病变的最大径可为几个毫米乃至一个厘米。另外，伴有各种数量的这种病变的患者均可发生恶性黑色素瘤，尽管伴有各种组织学类型的多数病变的个体或具有家族性黑色素瘤病史的个体出现黑色素瘤的危险性可能较高[938]。较大病变的特征是边界不规则、色素沉着不均匀以及病变周围色素逐步消退，临床上可以类似于恶性黑色素瘤[939]。较小的病变一般较为平淡，临床可发生于正常的患者[940]，即在正常情况下不需活检。

在一项有关组织学呈雀斑性黑色素细胞痣改变的黑色素细胞痣的研究中，不论临床上观察的痣的大小，对53%的临床上正常（对照组）的患者进行了活检[941]。另外，通过比较黑色素瘤和雀斑性黑色素细胞痣患者以及正常对照患者，发现每组患者之间的组织学差异没有统计学意义[942]。这些资料高度提示，对于单个患者来说，雀斑性黑色素细胞痣与发生恶性黑色素瘤的关系可能不大。事实上，任何一个雀斑性黑色素细胞痣仅仅代表了它的一个生长时期[943]，在少数多次活检后的复发性雀斑性黑色素细胞痣[944]以及肾移植后的发疹性雀斑性黑色素细胞痣[945]或HIV感染[946]病例已有描述。尽管目前还不清楚，但我们推测研究者将会显示任何类型的所有痣都可能与其他临床或环境因素有关（如日光照射），在单个患者，应用统计学评估其发生恶性黑色素瘤的潜在可能性或许是最有效的参数[947,948]。

临床病理间的相互联系对于这些痣极其重要，但对患者个体仍然是一个次要的问题。临床医生只有怀疑是黑色素瘤时才进行活检，除非患者由于个人原因要求手术切除。鉴于同样的原因和目的，在诊断中也要注意神经纤维瘤与神经纤维瘤病或结肠管状腺瘤与家族性多发性息肉病的相互关系。临床病理之间的相互联系是用来除外某一病变为恶性，并非用来确立综合征的诊断。

黑色素瘤 Melanoma

原位恶性黑色素瘤[949-952] Malignant melanoma in situ

原位恶性黑色素瘤表示一组上皮样、梭形或两种类

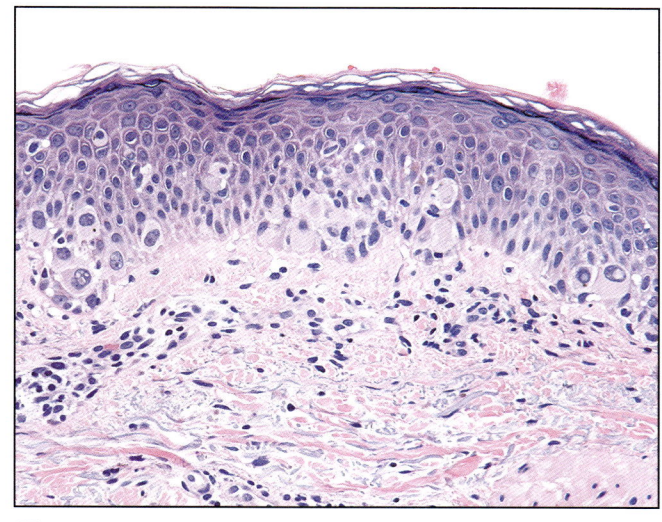

图23.147 原位黑色素瘤，雀斑型。在真皮与表皮交界处可见融合性黑色素细胞增生。

型混合的黑色素细胞随机分布于表皮各层（Paget样播散）的皮肤病变，在阳光损害皮肤的真皮与表皮交界处呈雀斑性结构（恶性雀斑）或呈混合性结构。虽然有些作者对这种定义持有异议，但是本文作者发现，这种定义对于从形态学上诊断缺少真皮成分的黑色素瘤是一个实用的方法。

临床上，原位恶性黑色素瘤类似于扁平或轻度隆起的恶性黑色素瘤病变，这些病变需要活检鉴别[953]。除了缺乏真皮成分以外，组织学上病变与恶性黑色素瘤完全相同（图23.147）。还应当记住的是，来自其他部位的黑色素瘤的嗜表皮性转移可与原位黑色素瘤极其类似[954]。主要的鉴别诊断包括乳腺外Paget病、Paget样Bowen病以及色素性日光性角化症，不采用melan A免疫染色很难与后者鉴别，原位黑色素瘤melan A呈阳性。

诊断原位黑色素瘤是有用的，只要：

1. 其可以理解，形态学所见并不一定意味着生物学上具有致死性的结果。
2. 确认这样的病变将导致其被完整切除。

一种特殊情况是，在先前没有经过活检的病变中发现原位恶性黑色素瘤和真皮消退现象。恒定不变的问题是：真皮曾经有过肿瘤吗？统计学上，伴有消退的原位黑色素瘤的患者黑色素瘤复发的危险性好像较大。与原位病变不伴有消退表现的病例相比，这些病变应当被纳入更需要关注的一类。

浸润性黑色素瘤 Invasive melanoma

浸润性恶性黑色素瘤定义为一系列累及表皮和真皮或单独累及真皮的可能致死的黑色素细胞病变。所有原发性皮肤黑色素瘤的进展至少通过两个生长阶段中的一

种。组织学上，这些生长阶段被称为放射状和垂直性生长。前一种术语相当于临床上的大小不等的斑点；后一种术语相当于结节。组织学上，放射状或斑点状生长阶段呈水平状或与表皮平行；然而，垂直性（所有方向）或结节性生长阶段则向各个方向扩展，包括垂直于表皮的方向。垂直性生长阶段的重要性在于：它与真皮浸润不是同义词，常常伴有显著的细胞结构改变和非典型性[955]。

在多数病例中，从时间上讲，斑点状（放射状）生长阶段发生在结节性（垂直性）生长阶段之前。众所周知这是正确的，因为如果追述患者的临床病变过程，其病史一般为一个增大的色素沉着性斑点开始出现颜色改变、出血或两者均有。在一些未经治疗的患者，多数已经观察到在斑点内已形成结节。

组织学上，原始型斑点状生长阶段为原位恶性黑色素瘤加细胞学上类似于表皮成分的真皮乳头黑色素细胞成分（图23.148）[956]。这些表现可以伴有或不伴有其他改变，如非对称性间质纤维组织增生以及或多或少的广泛性炎症反应，伴有或不伴有消退。通常免疫组织化学表现为S-100蛋白和melan A阳性，尤其是上皮样黑色素瘤。细胞角蛋白一般为阴性，但并非一成不变。有些病变的发生似乎与先前存在的黑色素细胞痣密切相关，提示恶性转变，但多数病例可能为新形成的肿瘤。

尽管黑色素瘤的诊断依赖于识别异常的黑色素细胞，但伴随斑点状生长阶段的间质及炎症改变也具有重要的诊断意义。炎症浸润出现于真皮浅层，呈带状及融合性表现，特征性地交错分布于非典型性黑色素细胞之间，宿主可能是在试图限制肿瘤的生长。在推测的早期生长阶段，炎症浸润稀疏，呈苔藓样表现。随后表皮内（或真皮）的黑色素瘤可能被破坏，留下萎缩的表皮。浅表真皮由于或多或少的胶原沉积而呈纤维化表现。这些改变构成了消退性（regression）区域，加上病变的非对称性形态学表现，为诊断提供了有价值的线索（图23.149）。人们可能推断消退性表现对患者具有保护作用，但并非如此。部分甚或全部具有消退性表现的患者随后均可能出现转移性病变或死亡。然而，消退并非黑色素瘤所特有。良性黑色素细胞病变也可含有淋巴细胞浸润伴消退性表现。这些病变包括晕痣、Spitz痣以及后天性痣。有些黑色素瘤可出现明显的黏液样间质，不论其生长阶段[957]。

斑点状生长阶段的恶性黑色素瘤的特征性诊断标准如下：

1. 宽大的、非对称性黑色素细胞病变
2. 周围没有界限
3. 非典型性黑色素细胞
4. 单个黑色素细胞多于成巢黑色素细胞
5. 单个黑色素细胞分布于表皮各层（Paget样或"大粒散弹"结构）
6. 附件有类似的"大粒散弹"浸润
7. 融合性真皮炎症浸润
8. 融合性真皮纤维化
9. 消退区域。

必须注意的是，这些标准中的任何一个偶尔也可见于良性病变，但出现多数这些指标非常支持黑色素瘤的诊断。结节性生长阶段的恶性黑色素瘤定义为病变出现下面一种组织学参数：

1. 斑点状生长阶段的黑色素瘤内出现膨胀性结节（有时较小）。
2. 一个孤立性的膨胀性恶性黑色素瘤结节伴有少量或不伴有周围表皮内成分（经典的结节性黑色素瘤）（图23.150）。
3. 一个外生性恶性黑色素瘤息肉。

一般情况下，识别一个恶性黑色素瘤结节比较容易，

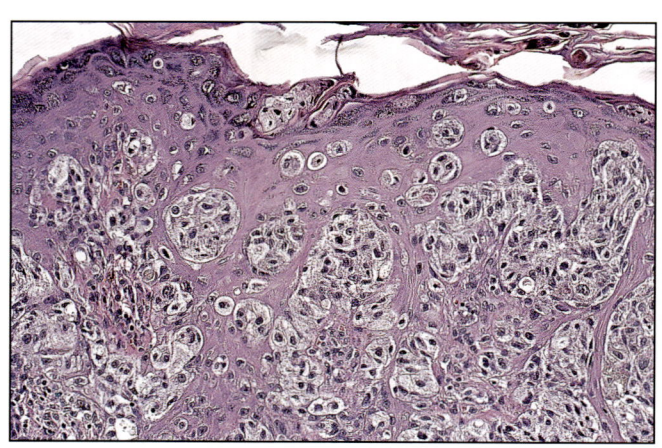

图23.148 恶性黑色素瘤，Paget样播散。表皮各层含有随机分布的非典型性黑色素细胞。

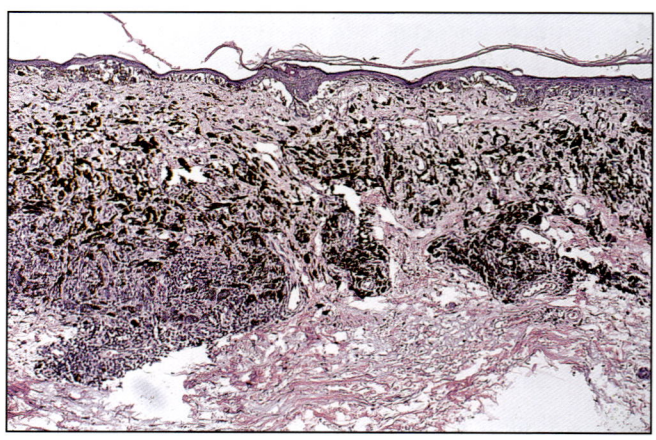

图23.149 恶性黑色素瘤伴有"消退"。注意充满黑色素的巨噬细胞带以及雀斑性黑色素瘤下方的慢性炎症和纤维化。

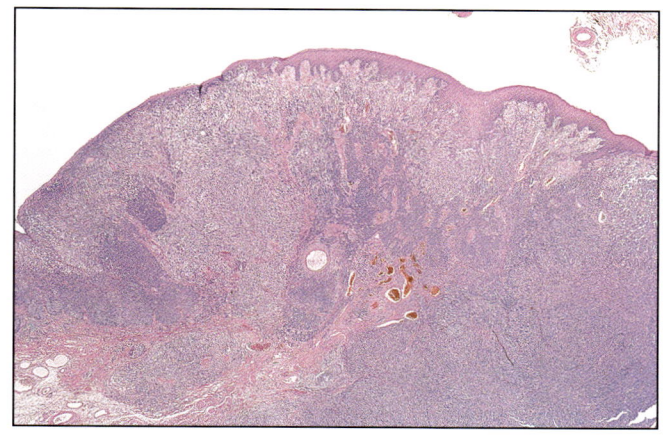

图23.150 恶性黑色素瘤，结节性。没有Paget样播散。肿瘤表现为外生性真皮结节。

尤其是如果是孤立性且细胞呈多形性的病变，如果放射状（斑点状或水平性）生长阶段的黑色素瘤背景中出现膨胀性结节，或如果呈息肉样表现时。诊断中的难点在于：当病变为孤立性、III级或较深以及细胞学表现均一时。如果这种肿瘤也为对称性的，而且缺乏显著的间质反应，则可与某些黑色素细胞痣混淆。因此，这一类别的病变被称为"痣样黑色素瘤"（图23.151和23.152）[958-960]，但在应用这一术语之前常常被称为"微小偏离性黑色素瘤"[961-964]。这些病变被认为是一系列的结节状、组织学上类似于黑色素细胞痣的恶性黑色素瘤。然而，我们认为这些病变与厚度相同的经典组织学形态的恶性黑色素瘤具有相同的致死潜能。被称为"痣样黑色素瘤"（nevoid melanoma）或"微小偏离性黑色素瘤"（minimal deviation melanoma）的肿瘤还没有得到广泛而系统性的研究；多数研究是经验性的，没有足够的随访。这一类别的肿瘤的预后是否的确好于其他同等厚度的黑色素瘤，尚需进一步调查予以证实。

对于确诊为斑点状生长阶段的恶性黑色素瘤，有些病变中存在一个或少数几个稍大的真皮黑色素瘤细胞巢；这些可被视作"小的"膨胀性结节。我将这些病变当作结节性生长阶段的成分。作为一个实际问题，对于这些区域，我在病理学诊断报告中不给予任何特殊的命名，而其他作者会给予任何特殊的命名[953]。结节性生长阶段的黑色素瘤常常显示与分布于类似水平上的相邻肿瘤细胞巢的不同的细胞学特征。因而，在一些病变中可见上皮样和小细胞聚集或色素性和无黑色素性细胞巢并排分布。这种现象被称为病变内转变，被认为是克隆性或表型差异的证据，为恶性肿瘤的典型表现。

原发性恶性黑色素瘤的镜下分期（microstaging）是关注的重点，因为它们是最初评估这些患者的金标准[965]。组织学上，Clark及其同事提出的分级系统[966]如下：

I 级：原位；所有肿瘤细胞均位于基底膜之上的表皮内。
II 级：真皮乳头受累，包括附件周围受累，但并未充满真皮乳头。个别细胞条索或小巢可扩展至网状真皮。
III 级：肿瘤占据真皮乳头和网状真皮之间的交界面。孤立性的细胞条索可侵入网状真皮。
IV 级：明确浸润网状真皮。
V 级：皮下组织受累。

尽管这种方法有益于传达肿瘤在皮肤内的解剖学定位，并能定量评估肿瘤的预后，但是基于公制计量的Breslow深度系统是为更加可靠的方法[967]。大体上，Breslow法需要从垂直于皮肤表面的一点测量肿瘤的最厚部分。测量包括从表皮颗粒层的顶端到真皮肿瘤的底部，以毫米表示（近似至百分之一毫米）。累及任何

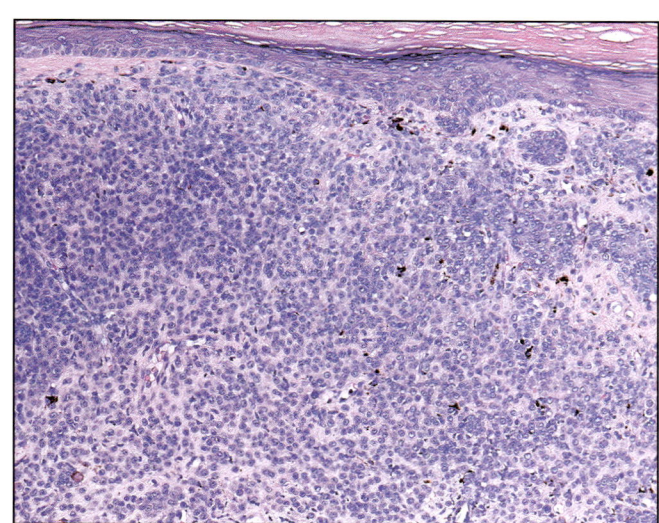

图23.151 痣样黑色素瘤。病变具有广泛的真皮黑色素细胞性成分，伴有一定程度的垂直性成熟。

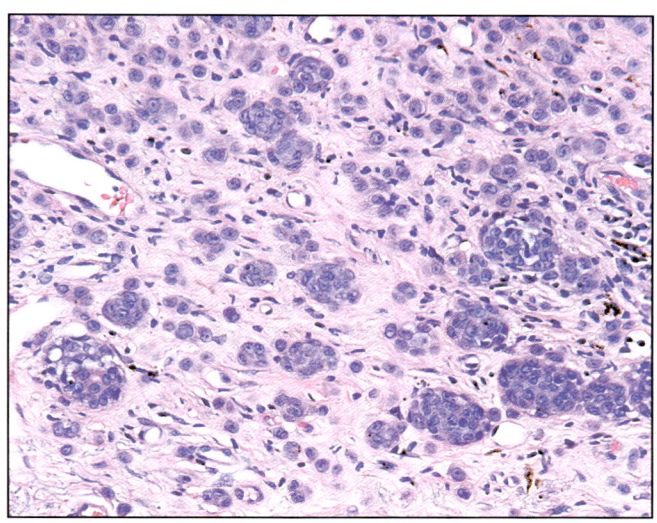

图23.152 痣样黑色素瘤。病变由非常类似于真皮痣的黑色素细胞构成。具有轻度多形性。

附件周围真皮的肿瘤应该避免测量在内，因为它会错误地增加肿瘤的厚度。对于特殊的病例，如病变伴有溃疡，位于溃疡基底部的存活的肿瘤可作为表皮测量的起始点。对于伴有消退区域的肿瘤，照常应该进行这种测量，但要附加有消退存在的陈述。对于出现显微镜下卫星灶的病例，我建议将其视为微小转移，并选择一个模拟点进行测量。一般来说，黑色素瘤小于 0.75 mm 厚时预后极好，鲜有例外情况。Clark 及其同事将 Breslow 模式整合到一个数据集中，其中包括肿瘤厚度以及其他组织学参数，如核分裂指数、肿瘤淋巴细胞浸润、消退、瘤体部位以及性别[953]。其他大型研究已经证实了解剖学部位和肿瘤厚度对于预后的重要性，尽管对于性别的相关性存在较大争议[968,969]。在薄的（≤1mm）黑色素瘤中，患者的年龄和性别似乎具有预后相关性[970]。作为一个实际问题，我将 Breslow 和 Clark 分级作为最低的报告标准；如果出现卫星性转移、消退或血管或神经周围浸润等表现，也应当报告。其他作者建议，黑色素瘤诊断报告应当只根据具有治疗和预后重要性的相关参数加以简化，如黑色素瘤伴有亲神经性、黑色素瘤伴有卫星转移以及黑色素瘤伴有广泛消退[971]。而作为黑色素瘤的另一个极端，解剖和外科病理学主任协会建议：在常规报告中要提供广泛的信息[972]。

恶性黑色素瘤有不同的分类方法，主要是强调一种或另一种特征[973]。这里不涉及发生于眼（见第 29 章）、内脏器官或原发灶不明的转移性黑色素瘤（后者占病例的 5%～10%）。最为流行的一种分类是依据斑点状生长阶段的特征。这种分类是将皮肤黑色素瘤称为浅表播散性黑色素瘤、雀斑性黑色素瘤（恶性雀斑黑色素瘤）、肢端雀斑性黑色素瘤以及肛门生殖部位黑色素瘤。如果出现结节而没有可以证实的斑点状阶段，则称为结节性黑色素瘤。这种分类受到挑战，因为可重复性差[974]，主要是因为细胞学有重叠。这种分类方法对于某些病例是准确的，鉴于这些肿瘤之间存在临床病理学差异，它仍不失为一种有用的分类方法。

浅表播散性黑色素瘤（superficial spreading melanoma）：这些病变的特征为非典型性黑色素细胞增生伴有成巢生长倾向，细胞学上呈上皮样表现，并且表皮内有明显的呈 Paget 样分布的单个细胞群（"大粒散弹"播散）。黑色素沉积多少不等，呈"粉末状"表现。炎症浸润一般沿真皮浅层呈带状分布。纤维化程度不一但呈融合性。浅表播散性黑色素瘤也可出现结节状成分，常常保留上皮样和成巢的细胞学特征。鉴别诊断包括乳腺外和乳腺 Paget 病、伴有表皮内 Paget 样结构的鳞状细胞癌以及极少数伴有亲表皮性的神经内分泌癌。这些黑色素瘤 S-100 蛋白和 melan A 几乎总是呈阳性，而其他病变一般为阴性。

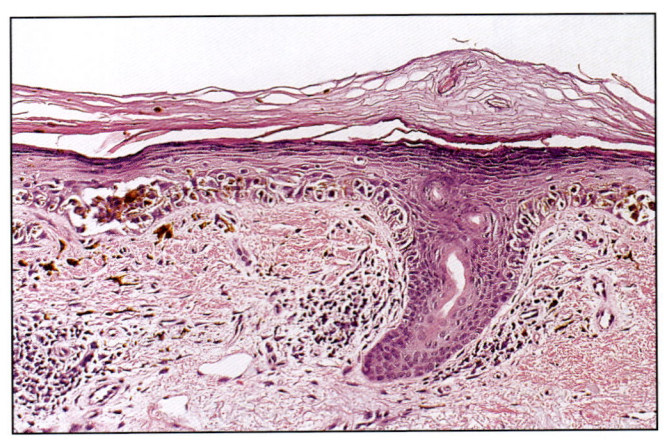

图23.153 雀斑性黑色素瘤。这种特殊的病变出现特征性的附件受累。其他部位出现真皮浸润。

雀斑性黑色素瘤（lentiginous melanoma）：这些黑色素瘤常常发生于面部阳光暴晒的部位，但也可见于躯干上部（图 23.153）。组织学上，病变特征为黑色素细胞增生，常常伴有梭形细胞学表现，沿表皮基底层分布。黑色素细胞倾向于沿毛囊上部生长，直到皮脂腺导管水平为止。细胞学上，黑色素细胞较小，伴有少量胞浆和不明显的细胞核。树突状突起和细胞周围由于固定而引起的收缩人工假象为其特征性表现。黑色素细胞和周围的角化细胞通常均有明显的色素沉着。少数情况下，黑色素细胞可呈较明显的上皮样表现，并且可能有巢状生长方式。真皮浅层常常出现明显的日光性损伤，但也可为正常表现。可以出现程度不一的炎症或纤维化，并且常常穿透真皮浅层。雀斑性黑色素瘤的真皮部分常常出现梭形细胞形态。S-100 蛋白和 melan A 在鉴别这些病变和伴有类似特征的鳞状细胞癌时非常有用。

肢端雀斑性黑色素瘤（acral lentiginous melanoma）：这些病变的特征是位于足底表面[975-977]，但这个名称也适用于甲下的病变[978,979]。组织学上，这些肿瘤的生长方式具有上皮样和雀斑性黑色素瘤的混合性特征（图 23.154）。细长的树突状黑色素细胞为特征性表现，而且常见梭形细胞结构。与传统的 Paget 样（浅表播散性）黑色素瘤相比，其间质及炎症反应不甚明显。形成不好的病变可能难以与肢端黑色素细胞痣鉴别。极少数肢端雀斑性黑色素瘤病例的原发性病变中或淋巴结转移中可能有肿瘤性骨的结构[980]。有兴趣的是，少数肢端黑色素瘤显示活化的 KIT 突变[980a]。

结节性黑色素瘤（nodular melanoma）：根据定义，这些黑色素瘤几乎没有明显的斑点状生长阶段[981]。最为常见的细胞学特征为上皮样表现，类似于 Paget 样（浅表播散性）黑色素瘤。结节性黑色素瘤是较厚的病变，预后较差。

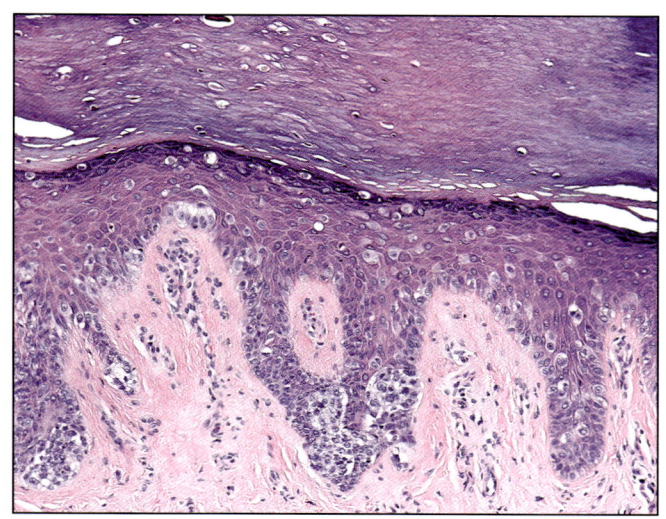

图23.154 肢端雀斑性黑色素瘤。表皮内的痣细胞团和单个黑色素细胞。这个病变中可见轻度真皮浸润。

其中有些病变开始可能为伴有 Paget 样或雀斑性成分的黑色素瘤，出现过度结节状生长。或许没有真正的"结节性"黑色素瘤，只不过是有些黑色素瘤含有结节而已。换句话说，一个黑色素瘤结节可能为许多类型的黑色素瘤的共同的最后结果，而并非一个特殊的"类型"。

肛门生殖部位黑色素瘤（anogenital melanoma）：这些病变也具有混合性上皮样和雀斑性特征，尤其是外阴黑色素瘤。外阴黑色素瘤常常出现多核黑色素细胞，这种表现极少见于其他部位的原发性黑色素瘤。区别这些解剖部位的良性和恶性黑色素细胞病变在诊断上是比较棘手的问题[791-793]。

不常见的黑色素瘤 Unusual melanomas

虽然黑色素瘤通常根据斑点状生长阶段来分类，但是有些黑色素瘤的结节状（多方向）生长阶段可以出现显著的表型差异。以下的形态学亚型存在鉴别诊断问题和明显的诊断误区。

纤维组织增生性黑色素瘤（desmoplastic melanoma）[982-988]：这种黑色素瘤亚型一般形成大的肿块，常常为无黑色素性肿瘤（图 23.155）。尽管有些病变为新发生的纤维组织增生，但多数为持续性病变。纤维组织增生性黑色素瘤常常伴有雀斑性黑色素瘤。肿瘤细胞主要为梭形细胞，均匀一致，周围有丰富的胶原性基质。可见核分裂象，即使是细胞稀少的肿瘤。其生长方式可为杂乱、束状或席纹状排列，非常类似于多种软组织肿瘤。黑色素沉积一般较少，有时在常规 HE 切片中难以发现。常常出现成片的淋巴细胞浸润。几乎所有的病变 S-100 蛋白染色均为阳性，melan A 在表皮内及真皮浅层部分

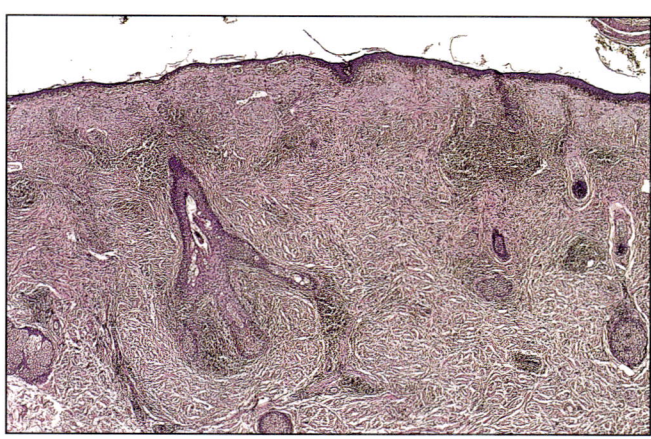

图23.155 纤维组织增生性黑色素瘤。低倍镜下，肿瘤由良性梭形细胞构成，其上为雀斑性结构。

呈局灶阳性，而多数病变的深部区域常常呈阴性。纤维组织增生性黑色素瘤一词只能用于细胞学特征均一的病变。鉴别诊断包括神经纤维瘤、纤维组织细胞瘤、瘢痕组织以及纤维组织增生性痣。高级别的细胞学上呈多形性的病变应当称为多形性梭形细胞黑色素瘤（pleomorphic spindle cell melanomas），因为这些病变可能具有较差的预后（图 23.156-23.158）。后者的鉴别诊断包括梭形细胞癌、非典型性纤维黄色瘤以及恶性外周神经鞘肿瘤。

亲神经性黑色素瘤（neurotropic melanoma）[989-995]：这种亚型与纤维组织增生性黑色素瘤关系密切；常常出现混合性结构。这两种病变倾向于发生在类似的临床状况下，尤其是发生在头颈部。组织学上，肿瘤细胞排列呈束状生长方式，类似于外周神经鞘肿瘤（图 23.159）。细胞学多形性极少出现，但可见核分裂象。肿瘤细胞常常侵入或围绕神经束，因而称为亲神经性黑色素瘤。神经受累可能轻微；有时少数增大的或异型的细胞核是正确诊断的唯一线索。鉴别诊断包括多种良性神经和黑色素细胞病变，包括纤维组织增生性黑色素细胞痣、神经纤维瘤以及恶性外周神经鞘肿瘤。

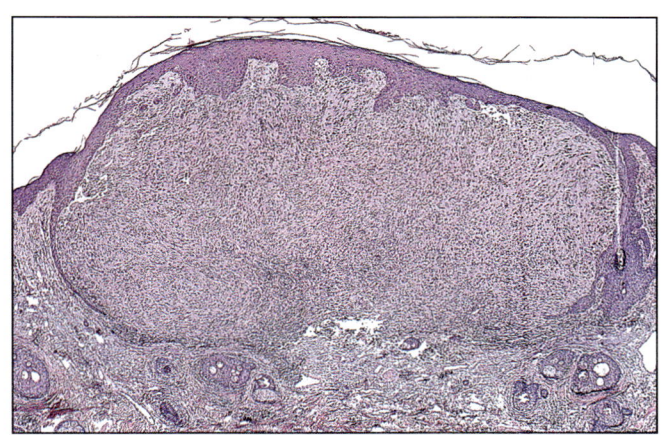

图23.156 梭形细胞黑色素瘤。低倍镜下显示为非对称性肿瘤。

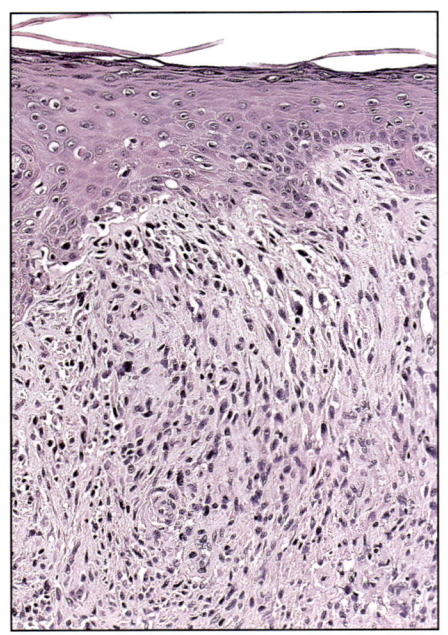

图23.157　梭形细胞黑色素瘤。这个病变没有交界性或表皮成分。

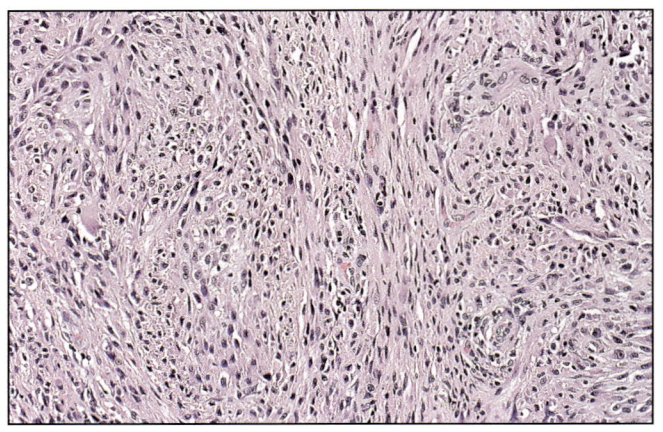

图23.158　梭形细胞黑色素瘤。细胞学上，病变类似于梭形细胞鳞状细胞癌或非典型性纤维黄色瘤。

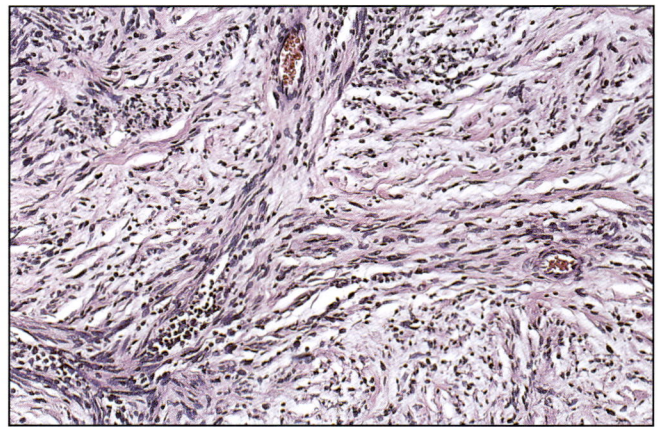

图23.159　亲神经性黑色素瘤。黑色素瘤与神经混合存在（中央）。

气球样细胞黑色素瘤（balloon cell melanoma）[996-999]：这种类型的黑色素瘤的特征为黑色素细胞大，伴有丰富的透明胞浆（图23.160）。这些病变通常没有细胞学多形性，核分裂数可以忽略不计，因而可误诊为气球样黑色素细胞痣。当病变也为无黑色素时，鉴别诊断包括黄色瘤、透明细胞附件肿瘤以及转移性疾病，最值得注意的是来自肾细胞癌的转移。

印戒细胞黑色素瘤（signet-cell melanoma）[1000-1002]：这是一种细胞学亚型，肿瘤细胞具有多量嗜酸性乃至透明的胞浆，伴有偏位的细胞核。这种类型的黑色素瘤极易与其他伴有印戒细胞表现的肿瘤混淆，主要为产生黏液的腺癌。

蓝痣样黑色素瘤（恶性蓝"痣"）[blue nevus-like melanoma（malignant blue nevi）][896,908,1003]：这些黑色素细胞肿瘤常常发生于头皮，广泛生长于网状真皮内，缺少表皮成分。仔细检查标本有时在附近可能发现蓝痣区域，提示为恶性变，至少有些病变是这样。鉴别诊断包括富于细胞性蓝痣和转移性黑色素瘤。

横纹肌样恶性黑色素瘤（rhabdoid malignant melanoma）[1004-1006]：这是一种相对少见的恶性黑色素瘤（尽管所占比例在转移性病变中较高，可能多达10%），以横纹肌样表现为其主要特征，出现圆形上皮样细胞形态学改变，伴有大的空泡状细胞核以及玻璃样嗜酸性胞浆包涵体。这种形态进一步证实了肾外肿瘤的非特异性横纹肌样形态学表现（见第24章），可能引起诊断困难，因为横纹肌样成分S-100蛋白和melan A免疫染色可能呈阴性，因此需要仔细寻找非横纹肌样区域或交界性/表皮内成分。

间叶性肿瘤 Mesenchymal tumors

真皮肿瘤为一大类病变，主要由类似于真皮结缔组织、

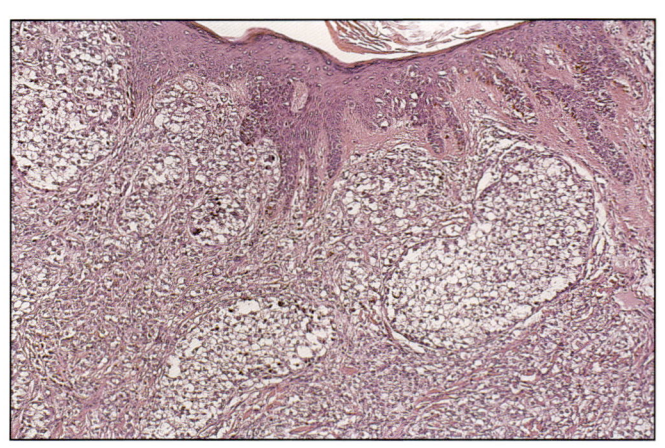

图23.160　黑色素瘤的气球细胞改变。这种透明细胞形态可为局灶性或遍布整个病变。

血管、神经、平滑肌或骨骼肌的细胞构成。有些肿瘤由通常认为不属于真皮的细胞组成，如具有骨髓或淋巴表型的细胞，也可出现明显的真皮成分，这些均包括在这一部分中。

皮肤间质肿瘤　Tumors of dermal stroma

纤维组织细胞瘤（皮肤纤维瘤）[1007-1012]　Fibrous histiocytoma (dermatofibroma)

这种病变定义为一类良性、境界清楚的皮肤肿瘤，由单核和（或）多核细胞构成，伴有吞噬细胞和（或）肌纤维母细胞特征，具有多种生长方式。

纤维组织细胞瘤的病因学不清[1010]，没有令人信服的物理学证据将其与昆虫叮咬[1013]或其他创伤联系起来，尽管许多作者推论存在这样一种相互关系。细胞遗传学资料显示，至少有些病变为克隆性[1014]，支持为肿瘤性病变。临床上，纤维组织细胞瘤一般发生于成人，但儿童也可受累[1015]。通常情况下，病变为无痛性的，多见于肢体和躯干。多数直径在 5 mm 至 2 cm 之间，特征为皮肤颜色到棕色乃至紫色的光滑斑块、结节或息肉，表面被覆完整的、常常是增厚的皮肤。有些病变出现中央小凹。任何类型的纤维组织细胞瘤均可通过将其捏在指间并发现肿瘤固定于皮内而受到高度疑似。多数病例通过切除可以治愈。只有比较富于细胞、动脉瘤样或深部浸润的病例持续存在或有较高的复发率[1016,1017]。有个别转移至局部淋巴结和肺的病例报告，但是根据形态学表现可能难以预测[1018-1020]。鉴别诊断为囊肿和附件肿瘤。黑色的息肉样病变有时可被误认为是恶性黑色素瘤。

组织学上，纤维组织细胞瘤通常为一类对称性、主要位于真皮的局限性病变，边缘可以清楚也可以呈浸润性（图 23.161 和 23.162）。组织学结构为弥漫性、网状、血管瘤样乃至瘢痕瘤样。然而，典型的特征是见于多数病例的席纹状、车轮状或花饰样结构。细胞学上，病变由不同程度的卵圆至梭形、单核至多核细胞构成，伴有两染性胞浆。有些病例可见泡沫样巨噬细胞和巨细胞，包括 Touton 细胞。可以出现较多的含铁血黄素[1021]、红细胞或脂质[1022,1023]（图 23.163）。如果用偏振光显微镜观察纤维组织细胞瘤，那么在病变中可以见到双折光性胶原，不同于隆凸性皮肤纤维肉瘤[1024]。免疫染色 XIIIa 因子常常可以标记纤维组织细胞瘤的树突状细胞，尽管区别病变细胞与先前存在的非肿瘤性真皮细胞常常比较困难[1009,1025,1026]。另外，伴有泡沫样胞浆的上皮样细胞（多半是非肿瘤性组织细胞）一般 HAM56、CD68 以及波形蛋白呈阳性。有些病例结蛋白[1027]或 HHF-35 可能呈阳性。超微结构上，病变可出现纤维母细胞和含有脂质组织细胞的细胞学特征[1028]。皮肤纤维瘤 CD34 通常（并

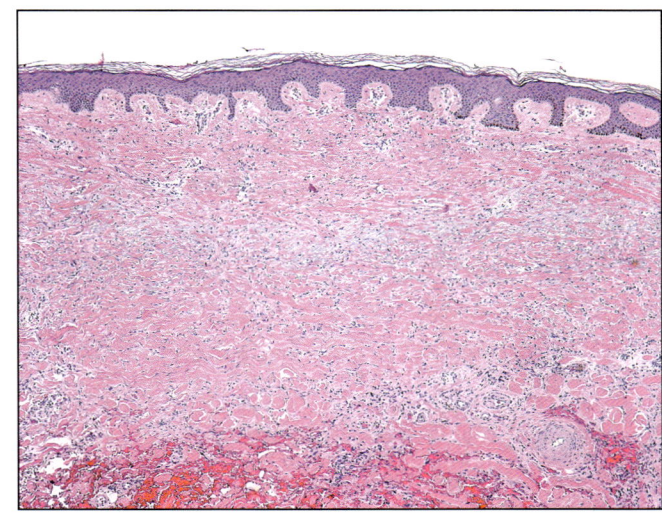

图23.161　皮肤纤维瘤（纤维组织细胞瘤）。病变为外生性丘疹，伴有表皮增生。

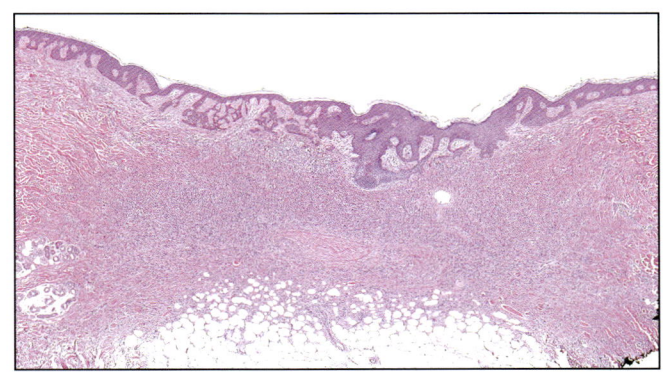

图23.162　皮肤纤维瘤（纤维组织细胞瘤）。病变临床上呈萎缩表现，但仍保留有表皮增生。

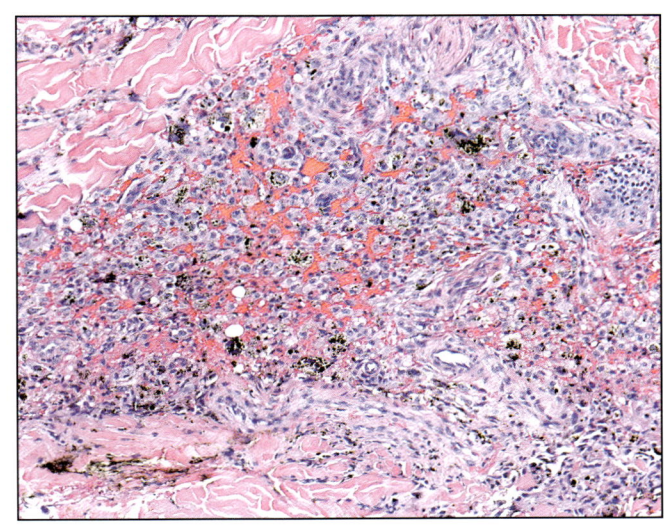

图23.163　皮肤纤维瘤（纤维组织细胞瘤），含铁血黄素型。这些病变可含有血细胞、含铁血黄素和泡沫细胞。

不总是）呈阴性，不同于隆凸性皮肤纤维肉瘤[1026,1029]。

具有许多不同的特征，单一病例中可以出现也可以不出现，但是如果出现，则为典型的诊断线索。这些特征包括：病变上方的对称性表皮增生、席纹状生长方式以及病变周边梭形细胞周围有（或"陷入"）玻璃样胶原纤维（所谓的胶原瘢痕形成）。

单个纤维组织细胞瘤病变可以以混合性的结构和细胞学形态为特征，或可以以一种类型为主。当出现后一种情况时，则采用特殊的命名，如下文所述。

动脉瘤性（血管瘤样）纤维组织细胞瘤 [aneurysmal (angiomatoid) fibrous histiocytoma][1030-1033]：这种病变主要发生于年轻人，可出现迅速生长。这些病变一般比普通纤维组织细胞瘤大，伴有囊性质地、色素沉着或血管样表现。组织学上，可见多量充满血液的海绵状腔隙，没有内皮衬覆，分布于富于细胞的含铁血黄素性纤维组织细胞瘤的背景中（见下文）。常常可见显著的含铁血黄素沉着、多数噬铁细胞和巨细胞以及中等数量的处于核分裂的细胞。通常有某种程度的细胞多形性，病变周围的玻璃样胶原束被肿瘤细胞包围。多数病例病变上方可有一定程度的表皮增生[1030]，这使病变具有血管和梭形细胞形态（图23.164）。可以理解的是，动脉瘤性纤维组织细胞瘤有时可能类似于Kaposi肉瘤的结节期。鉴别诊断还包括动脉瘤样恶性纤维组织细胞瘤（见第24章）、梭形细胞血管瘤（见第3章）以及梭形细胞黑色素瘤。

非典型性纤维组织细胞瘤[1034,1035]**、伴有畸形细胞的皮肤纤维瘤**[1036,1037]**、多形性纤维瘤**[1038] **以及"假肉瘤性"纤维组织细胞瘤**[1039] （atypical fibrous histiocytoma, dermatofibroma with monster cells, pleomorphic fibroma, and "pseudosarcomatous" fibrous histiocytoma）：这些术语用来描述一种临床上非特异性亚型，即在典型的纤维组织细胞瘤组织学背景中出现多形性细胞。这种细胞学多形性的特征为奇异深染的巨细胞以及伴有大的空泡状细胞核的组织细胞样细胞（图23.165）。有些病例可能含有非典型性核分裂象。这些病变常常被误诊为肉瘤，但绝大多数病例呈良性经过[1035]。

上皮样纤维组织细胞瘤（epithelioid fibrous histiocytoma）[1040-1043]：这也是一种需要注意的伴有特殊上皮样细胞形态学表现的亚型（图23.166和23.167）。病变常常呈息肉样结构。肿瘤细胞含有丰富的嗜酸性胞浆，因而类似于上皮样细胞痣（Spitz），并且有些是双核细胞。这些病变一般为外生性，没有交界性成分，不形成痣细胞团。可以含有大的血管腔隙而可能类似于血管病变[1041]。S-100蛋白和melan A呈阴性，而XIIIa因子和波形蛋白可为阳性[1042,1043]。肿瘤细胞CD31、CD34和VIII因子呈阴性，但可突出血管成分[1041]。

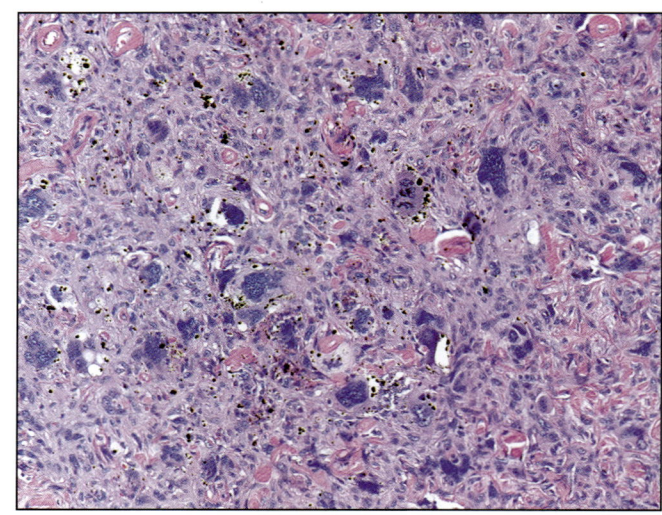

图23.165 非典型性纤维组织细胞瘤。奇异形巨细胞和极为肥胖的组织细胞样细胞。

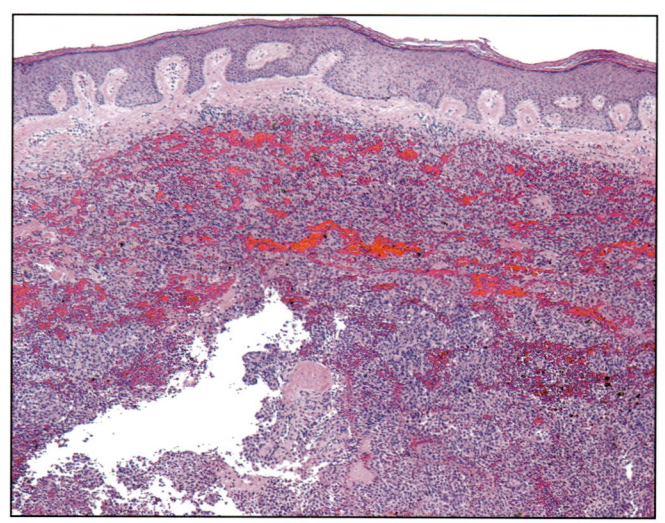

图23.164 动脉瘤性纤维组织细胞瘤。这个病变中可见几个充满血液的腔隙。有些病变中可见丰富的含铁血黄素沉着。

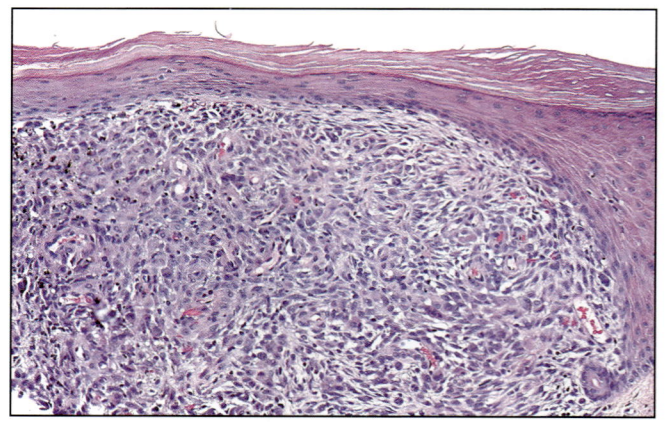

图23.166 上皮样良性纤维组织细胞瘤。低倍镜下，病变类似于黑色素细胞痣。

富于细胞性纤维组织细胞瘤 [（hyper）cellular fibrous histiocytoma][1016,1018,1019,1044]：这种类型的纤维组织细胞瘤大约占病例的 5%，由于其形态相对单一且呈束状排列（图 23.168），容易被误认为是恶性病变。扩展至浅层皮下组织以及小的中央坏死区相对常见。这种亚型多达 20% 的病例有持续性病变或出现复发。

纤维组织细胞瘤的其他亚型包括透明细胞[1045,1046]和颗粒细胞[1047-1049]皮肤纤维瘤、深部穿透性皮肤纤维瘤[1050]、胆固醇性纤维组织细胞瘤[1022]、脂质性纤维组织细胞瘤[1023]、纤维组织细胞瘤伴有（碰撞？）基底细胞癌[1051]或伴有血管平滑肌瘤[1052]、孤立性[1053]或播散性皮肤树突细胞瘤[1054]、含铁血黄素性纤维组织细胞瘤[1055]、多核细胞血管纤维组织细胞瘤[1056-1058]、栅栏状纤维组织细胞瘤[1059]以及硬化性血管瘤[1060]，这些亚型可以作为这些病变的再分类，并要与具有侵袭性生物学行为的肿瘤鉴别。然而，许多形态学亚型有可能是见于任何纤维组织细胞瘤的不同阶段，其证据是常常见到混合性病变。

由此看来，所谓的硬化性血管瘤、含铁血黄素性纤维组织细胞瘤以及动脉瘤性纤维组织细胞瘤是一个连续的谱系。

鉴别诊断包括瘢痕、瘢痕瘤、硬化性纤维瘤[1061-1063]、一些血管瘤、巨细胞纤维母细胞瘤、皮肤结节性"筋膜炎"[1064]、储脂性皮肤树突细胞错构瘤[1065]、皮肤肌纤维瘤[1066]、非典型性纤维黄色瘤以及隆凸性皮肤纤维肉瘤[1067]。区分后者在生物学上最具重要性，因为它可以复发和（或）伴有纤维肉瘤性区域。然而，皮肤纤维肉瘤在细胞学上形态比较单一，浸润脂肪组织呈现独特的蜂窝状结构，而且 CD34 呈阳性[1068]。纤维组织细胞瘤与隆凸性皮肤纤维肉瘤的对比见表 23.7。

巨细胞纤维母细胞瘤 [1069-1071]
Giant cell fibroblastoma

巨细胞纤维母细胞瘤为生物学上低级别的皮肤和（或）皮下肿瘤，由梭形细胞、多核细胞以及内衬多核细胞的所谓的血管扩张样腔隙构成。

临床上，这些病变主要累及 10 岁以内的男孩[1070]，但也可发生于成人。常见部位为躯干，少数可见于下肢[1072]，但其他部位也有报告[1073]。病变直径大约为 1～8 cm，有个别例外[1074]，表面皮肤通常正常。切除一般可以治愈，但如果没有完整切除，多达 1/3 的病变持续存在并再度生长。临床没有特别的鉴别诊断。

组织学上，病变境界不清，表现为在致密到疏松的胶原性基质中有丰富的细胞至黏液性改变（图 23.169）。结构形态呈弥漫性、束状和（或）混合性结构。一般情况下可见较宽的窦样"血管扩张样"腔隙；然而，这些为假性血管，缺少真正的内皮细胞内衬（图 23.170）。细胞学上，多数呈弥漫性排列的细胞为梭形或星状细胞。也可见到多核巨细胞，其中多数呈花环结构[1072]。伴有多核的细胞常常内衬血管扩张样腔隙。核分裂指数低

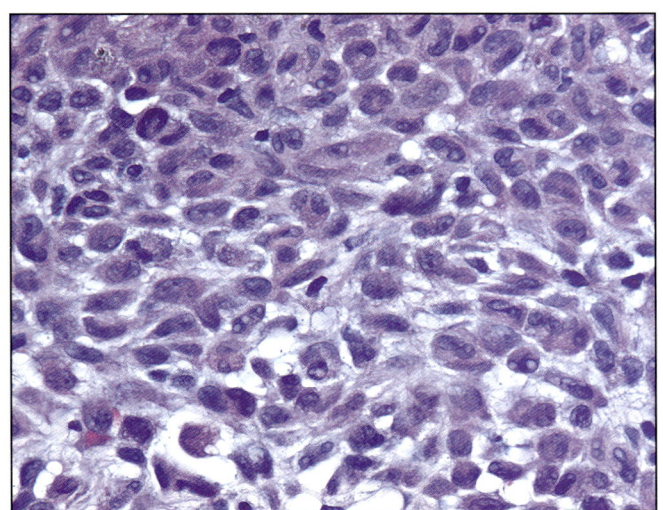

图 23.167 上皮样良性纤维组织细胞瘤。由良性的、常常是双核的上皮样细胞组成。

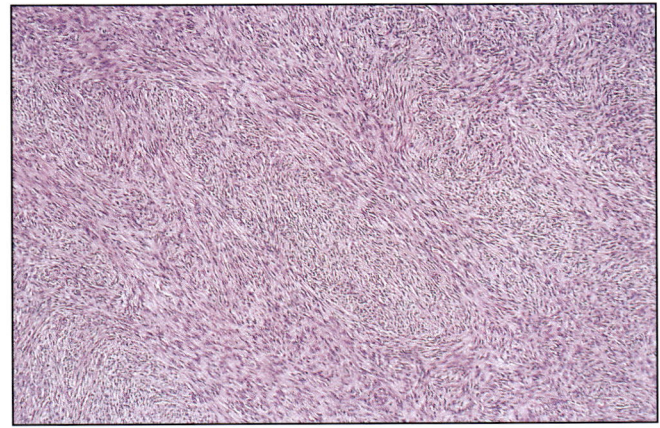

图 23.168 富于细胞性良性纤维组织细胞瘤。病变细胞丰富，主要呈束状结构。

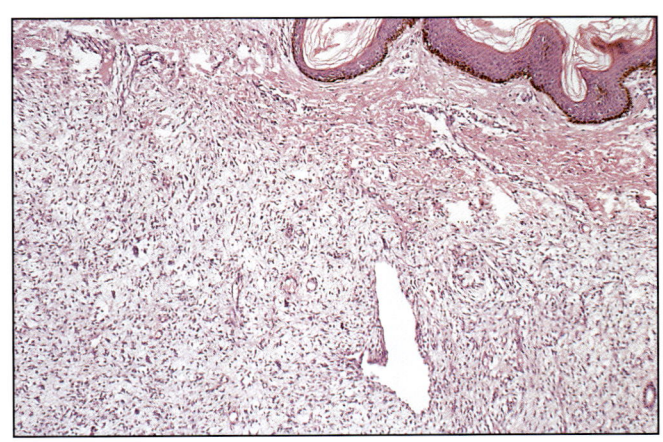

图 23.169 巨细胞纤维母细胞瘤。富于细胞区。

表23.7	纤维组织细胞瘤与隆凸性皮肤纤维肉瘤	
特征	纤维组织细胞瘤（皮肤纤维瘤）	隆凸性皮肤纤维肉瘤
年龄	从21～30岁开始	一般21～50岁
性别	均可	均可
部位	肢体常见，有时躯干	上部躯干，背部常见，其他部位罕见，不发生于手掌或足底
大小范围	多数<1 cm，极少数较大	常常>1 cm，有时很大
单个病变	通常，多发性罕见	通常
临床结节	通常为单个结节	常为多发性结节
多发性病变	有时	罕见
表皮改变	通常增生，有时没有改变	萎缩或没有改变
对称性	是	不是
在真皮的部位	通常充满真皮	常常充满真皮
在皮下的部位	浅表，如果有皮下成分	实际上所有病例为浸润表现
病变边界	浸润性，但是规则	浸润性，但不规则
周边胶原"陷入"	有，常伴有"瘢痕瘤"结构	无
细胞构成	通常较少，但可为瘢痕样到极其富于细胞	通常富于细胞
生长方式	席纹状或弥漫性	通常为弥漫性和席纹状，个别呈纤维肉瘤的人字形结构
附件陷入病变内	不常见	常见
病变上部附件变形	偶尔可见	从无
偏振光显微镜见病变内胶原双折光	有	无
细胞学多样性	常见，从纤维细胞到组织细胞乃至混合性	不常见，通常为规则的小的梭形细胞
病变细胞核分裂象	不常见	常见
少见形态或伴随改变	含铁血黄素性，动脉瘤性，胆固醇性，席纹状，有时伴有多形性巨细胞（见正文）	色素性（Bednar瘤），有时伴有巨细胞纤维母细胞瘤和（或）纤维肉瘤
波形蛋白	+	+
CD34	−或+/−	+或+/−
XIIIa因子	+	−
S-100	−	−
HMB-45	−	−
HAM56	+	−或+/−
HHF-35	+到+/−	−到+/−
SMA	+/−	−
结蛋白	+/−	−
细胞角蛋白	−	−
p53蛋白	−	+
持续存在/复发	不常见	常见
转移潜能	无/非常罕见（见正文）	典型病变较小，如果出现纤维肉瘤结构15%

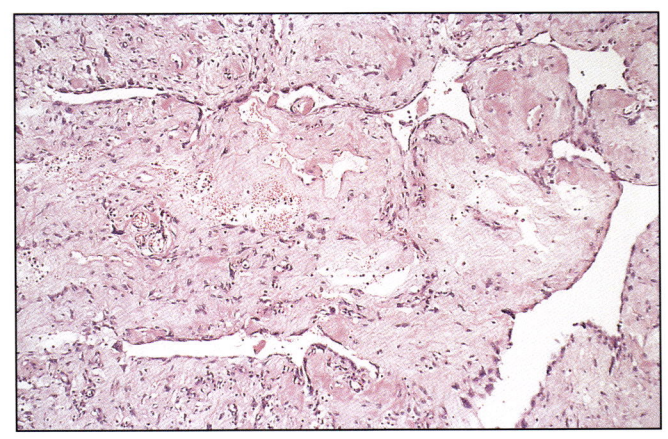

图23.170 巨细胞纤维母细胞瘤。血管扩张样腔隙内衬单核和多核细胞。

（<1个/10HFP）。包括内衬血管扩张样腔隙的细胞在内，免疫染色显示波形蛋白[1072,1075,1076]和CD34[1075,1077]呈阳性，但内皮、神经以及肌肉标记物通常为阴性[1069,1073]。极少数病例HHF-35和HAM-56呈阳性[1069,1072]。超微结构检查，肿瘤细胞类似于纤维母细胞，称为褶皱细胞（veil cells）[1078]。细胞遗传学分析发现，这些肿瘤出现明显的与皮肤纤维肉瘤完全相同的可复制的核型异常（涉及17和22号染色体）[1079]。

鉴别诊断包括浅表或深部幼年性黄色肉芽肿、纤维组织细胞瘤以及神经肿瘤，所有这些均可通过临床病理和（或）免疫组织化学方法来鉴别。从概念上讲，巨细胞纤维母细胞瘤与隆凸性皮肤纤维肉瘤密切相关[1071,1079,1080]，因为两者有许多类似的临床病理学特征；主要的鉴别点在于：典型的巨细胞纤维母细胞瘤病例的年龄较轻并出现明显的血管扩张样区域。然而，伴有混合性特征（图23.171）的巨细胞纤维母细胞瘤病例也有报道[1080]，而且巨细胞纤维母细胞瘤病例可以复发成为皮肤纤维肉瘤[1081]，反过来也是一样[1082]。伴有色素性皮肤纤维肉瘤的也有报道[1083]。

隆凸性皮肤纤维肉瘤[1084,1085]
Dermatofibrosarcoma protuberans

隆凸性皮肤纤维肉瘤是一种形态相对单一的单核梭形细胞病变，累及真皮和皮下组织。肿瘤可局部复发，但极少有转移。除了某些例外情况以外，这些病变的细胞对多数神经和巨噬细胞标记物呈阴性，超微结构上与纤维母细胞类似。

临床上，隆凸性皮肤纤维肉瘤通常发生于成人，主要在20～50岁之间，两种性别及所有种族均可受累。病变常常始于儿童期[1086]；实际上，在儿童期确诊的病例少见[1087,1088]。诊断之前病变持续的时间常常超过5年，有些病例为10年[1089]。多数病变发生于躯干、腹股沟或下肢，但许多病例发生在头颈部[1090]。手掌及足底部不受累。病变表现各异，从斑块到小的孤立性肿物，到成簇的结节，直径从几个厘米[1091]乃至巨大的带蒂的肿瘤，直径超过20 cm[1092]。外生性生长一般代表持续时间较长。有些病变可为色素减少或色素增加[1093]；极少数可出现溃疡[840]。需要切除病变且切缘要干净以防止复发，尽管有些广泛切除后仍有复发。对于一些经过挑选的病例，据说Mohs手术有助于保证切缘的干净[1094,1095]，但由于病变常常出现复杂分支样皮下组织浸润，一般并不提倡应用这种技术。极少数病例可转移至局部淋巴结或内脏[1092,1096-1104]，但发生转移的病例似乎远远低于0.5%。

组织学上，出现一系列结构和细胞学表现，最具特征性的改变是病变境界不清，形态一致的梭形细胞团排列成单种形态的席纹状结构[1086]，并且向皮下组织扩展（图23.172），常常呈花边和（或）线状浸润或围绕脂肪组织小叶（图23.173）。病变上方的表皮一般正常或萎缩，并且通过Grenz带与肿瘤分隔。皮肤附件常常陷于肿瘤

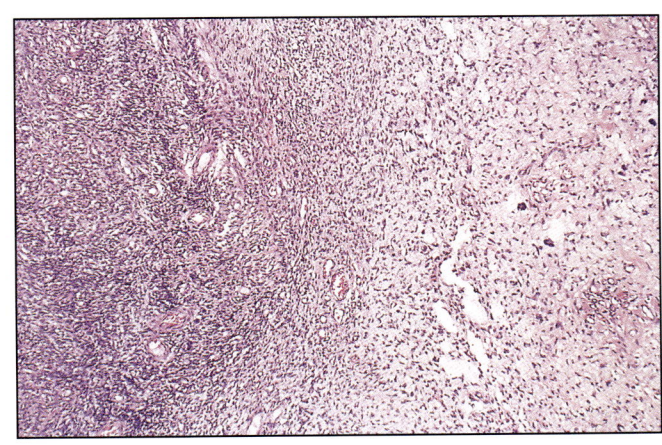

图23.17 混合性皮肤纤维肉瘤（左）和巨细胞纤维母细胞瘤（右）。

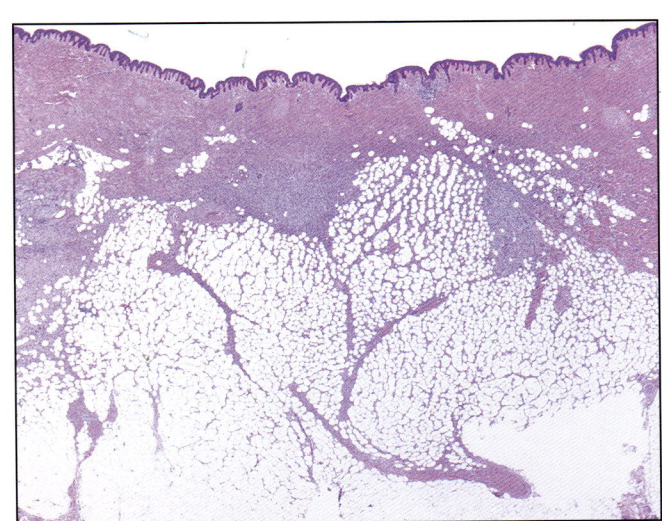

图23.172 隆突性皮肤纤维肉瘤。注意真皮和皮下组织广泛受累，呈蜂窝样结构。

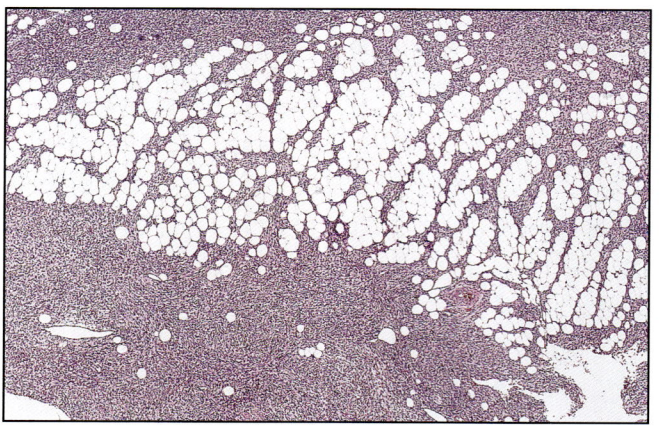

图23.173 隆凸性皮肤纤维肉瘤。注意脂肪组织明显浸润为这些病变常见的特征。

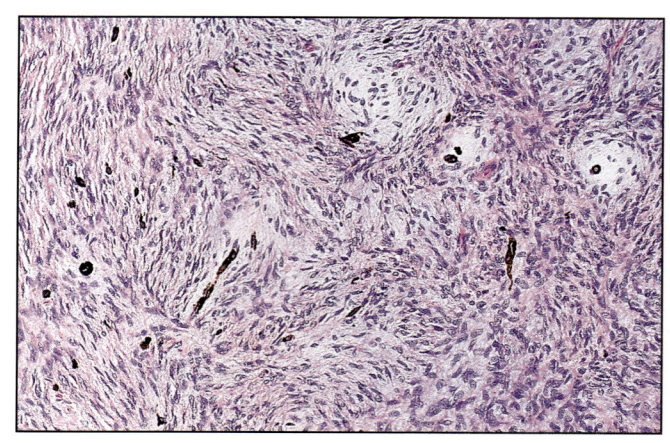

图23.175 色素性皮肤纤维肉瘤（Bednár瘤）。注意树突性黑色素细胞。

内，不同于纤维组织细胞瘤。隆凸性皮肤纤维肉瘤还缺乏偏振化的胶原[1024]，这也有别于纤维组织细胞瘤。其他形态也可以见于单个病变当中，如弥漫性、束状、黏液样[1086,1092,1105]、巨细胞纤维母细胞瘤样[1083,1097,1102,1103]、萎缩性[1088,1106-1110]、硬化性[1111]或皮下病变[1112]，并且这些形态可以混合出现。可以有富于细胞成分的人字形结构，伴有核分裂数目增加，类似于纤维肉瘤（图23.174）[1113-1116]以及肌样结节[1117]和类似于恶性纤维组织细胞瘤的区域[1118]，而别处伴有皮肤纤维肉瘤的典型改变。这种纤维肉瘤改变较常发生在初发的而不是持续性（复发性）的病变。与单纯性低级别肿瘤相比，这些病变在临床上更具侵袭性病程；发生转移的危险性大约为10%～15%[1114,118a]。

细胞学上，肿瘤细胞为梭形，伴有两染性至嗜酸性胞浆，细胞核细长。可出现轻度细胞多形性或细胞核深染。极少数情况下可见泡沫细胞、Touton细胞[1119]和（或）颗粒细胞[1120]。核分裂指数一般较低，每10个高倍视野极少超过5个核分裂象。在一些病变中偶尔可见含有多量黑色素的树突性梭形细胞，即所谓的Bednár瘤（图23.175）[1121]，后者在隆凸性皮肤纤维肉瘤中所占的比例不到5%[1122]。这种病例较常见于黑人，但临床上并没有其他特殊表现。间质玻璃样变范围和程度不一。

除了波形蛋白和CD34以外，多数隆凸性皮肤纤维肉瘤病例免疫组织化学染色均为阴性[1026,1029,1123-1125]，而波形蛋白和CD34在几乎所有的病例中均为阳性。在多数情况下，CD34阳性对于与富于细胞性良性纤维组织细胞瘤鉴别具有价值。与皮肤纤维瘤不同，p53蛋白表达已经见于隆凸性皮肤纤维肉瘤[1126]，新近发现的一种新的标记物——Apo D也是如此[1127]。个别隆凸性皮肤纤维肉瘤病例表达HAM56或HHF-35。实际上，S-100蛋白、溶菌酶、α1-抗胰蛋白酶和α1-抗糜蛋白酶以及金属硫蛋白（metallothionein）在每一个病例均为阴性[1128]，但有个别例外。

超微结构上，隆凸性皮肤纤维肉瘤出现一系列改变。主要改变是细胞类似于纤维母细胞[1129-1134]，但有些作者发现，肿瘤细胞周围有不连续的基底膜成分，提示与神经束膜细胞类似[1135,1136]。

通过细胞遗传学分析已经发现，隆凸性皮肤纤维肉瘤病例有由17和22号染色体易位部分构成的环状染色体，而且一致的基因融合产物具有克隆性[1079,1137-1139]。环状染色体好像是多种低级别软组织恶性肿瘤所共有的特征。

隆凸性皮肤纤维肉瘤必须与纤维组织细胞瘤鉴别（见表23.7），后者一般较小，对称，特征为异原性单核细胞群，常常含有脂质和（或）含铁血黄素。有些皮肤纤维瘤可以出现深部浸润，但一般不会有明显的脂肪组织浸润[1050]。非典型性纤维黄色瘤和所谓的恶性纤维组织细胞瘤（MFH）容易与隆凸性皮肤纤维肉瘤鉴别，因为它们具有明显的细胞学多形性。典型的纤维肉瘤一般是深在的肿瘤，仅有极少数扩展至真皮；核分裂指数通常远远大于皮肤纤维肉瘤。真皮[1064]或皮下筋膜炎可通过

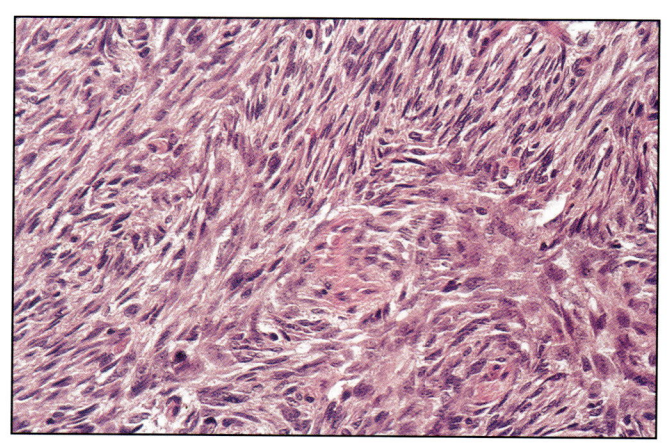

图23.174 隆凸性皮肤纤维肉瘤。少数病变出现纤维肉瘤样结构。

其均一的"组织培养"的生长方式来鉴别。黏液样脂肪肉瘤和黏液纤维肉瘤与黏液性隆凸性皮肤纤维肉瘤的不同点：在于前者可见脂母细胞，而后者出现多形性细胞。

非典型性纤维黄色瘤 [1140-1143]
Atypical fibroxanthoma

非典型性纤维黄色瘤（AFX）（从前也叫奇异性皮肤纤维肉瘤[1144]、假肉瘤性皮肤纤维瘤[1145]以及假肉瘤性网状组织细胞瘤[1146]）是指一组发生于成人的一般呈惰性经过的皮肤肿瘤，其组织学特征为由梭形、上皮样以及巨大多形性细胞群构成的肿瘤，核分裂象多见，有些细胞的胞浆内出现明显的脂质成分。有些作者将非典型性纤维黄色瘤视为所谓的恶性纤维组织细胞瘤（MFH）的浅表性亚型，尽管实事上还没有明确证据表明非典型性纤维黄色瘤会发生转移，而且恶性纤维组织细胞瘤也不是一种独特的病变。

临床上，非典型性纤维黄色瘤常常表现为迅速增大或外生性息肉，一般为孤立性的，发生于老年人头颈部日光损害部位的皮肤。溃疡并不常见。极少数情况下也可累及其他部位[1147,1148]。多数患者有长期日光照射的病史；少数病例先前有创伤[1149]。也有人说年龄较轻患者的病变常常位于非日光照射部位[1140]，但我们怀疑其中有些可能是伴有多形性细胞的纤维组织细胞瘤，如在不常见的纤维组织细胞瘤亚型中描述的（见1486页）。非典型性纤维黄色瘤的大小从直径1 cm到大于6 cm，但多数病变为1～2 cm。如果病变完整，其被覆皮肤光滑，并可能呈黄色表现。临床鉴别诊断包括鳞状细胞癌、恶性黑色素瘤以及分叶状血管瘤（化脓性肉芽肿）[1140]。实际上局部切除对于所有病例来说均可治愈。浅表性病变极少复发[1150]，有少数转移的病例报告[1140,1151-1154]，但那些病例的诊断标准一点也不可信，许多病例缺乏免疫组织化学染色。

组织学上，非典型性纤维黄色瘤可呈对称性或非对称性。境界一般清楚，但也可以向两侧浸润。息肉样病变可出现环状鳞状上皮或皮肤附件[1142]。许多病变可见Grenz区（图23.176），但有些病变与表皮邻接。有些病变扩展至浅表皮下组织，但程度非常有限。比较深的层面可能围以单核炎症细胞浸润[1142]。这些肿瘤的结构生长方式可为杂乱的、席纹状或束状。间质富于网织纤维。个别病例可出现软骨样物质[1155]，也可出现骨或骨样组织。如果发现附件位于肿瘤内，则一般不受累及[1142]。整个病变中可以出现从不甚明显至扩张的毛细血管；有些病例可含有出血区域[1156]，但缺乏明确的坏死。没有血管和神经周围浸润；如果出现上述表现，应当怀疑为较为侵袭性的病变。据认为，与侵袭性行为和转移相关

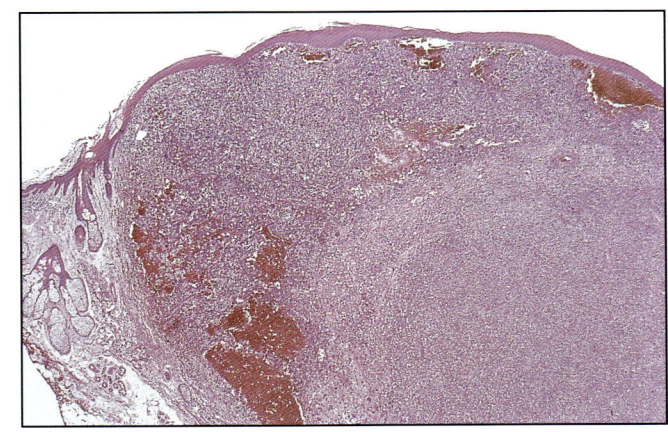

图23.176　非典型性纤维黄色瘤。典型的息肉样、境界清楚的病变。

的因子为血管浸润、复发、深部组织浸润、肿瘤坏死，可能还有宿主抵抗力有缺陷或降低[1156]。现今多数作者并不接受非典型性纤维黄色瘤的定义内包括皮下播散、血管浸润或坏死。

细胞学上，肿瘤细胞具有连续性的改变，从以梭形细胞为主到以圆形细胞为主，伴有或不伴有多形性，并且混有多少不等的巨细胞。细胞胞浆一般丰富，从嗜酸性到两染性。许多细胞可能充满微泡状脂质，通过油红O染色容易发现[1140]。细胞核的大小及形状差异很大（图23.177），从没有核仁到可见几个明显的核仁，而且细胞核可类似于Reed-Sternberg细胞[1142]。典型性或非典型性（多极）核分裂象均可见到[1140]；核分裂指数在每个高倍视野一个的范围内。病变内的多核巨细胞可出现单形性和（或）多形性的细胞核[1142,1155]。偶尔可见Touton巨细胞[1148]。许多病例几乎完全为单形性的梭形细胞并呈束状分布（图23.178）[1157]；这种病例常常被

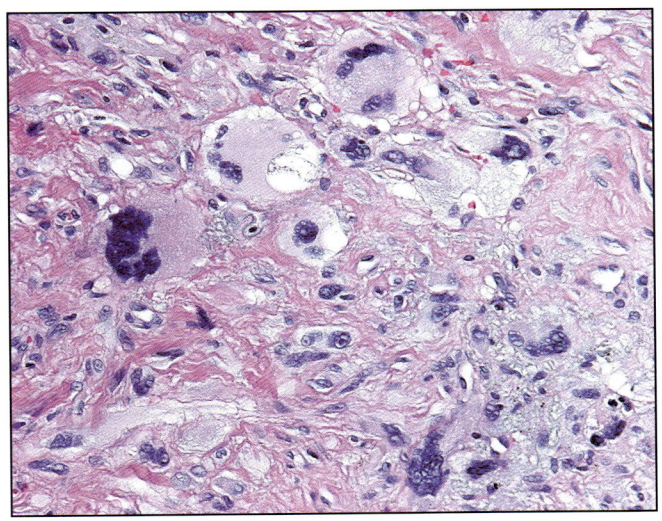

图23.177　非典型性纤维黄色瘤。肿瘤由多形性的多角形和梭形细胞组成，伴有奇异性核分裂象，类似于软组织的所谓的恶性纤维组织细胞瘤。

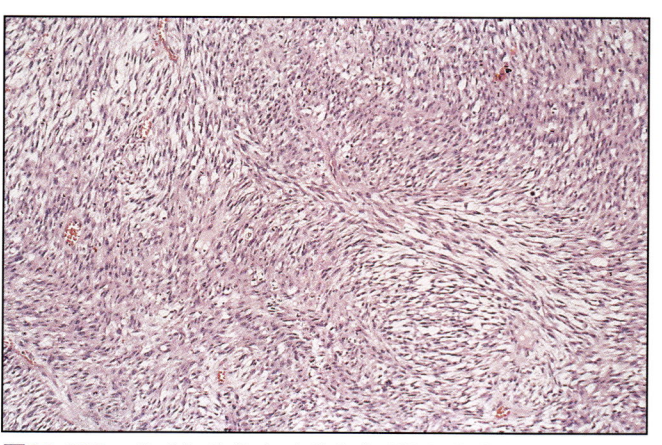

图23.178　梭形细胞非多形型非典型性纤维黄色瘤。这个病变类似于梭形细胞黑色素瘤或平滑肌肉瘤。

误认为是恶性。极个别病例含有破骨细胞样巨细胞[1102,1155,1158-1160]。透明细胞亚型[1161]、颗粒细胞[1162]以及"色素性"亚型[1163]已有报道。

免疫组织化学染色上，非典型性纤维黄色瘤的细胞波形蛋白、HAM56、α1-抗胰蛋白酶、α1-抗糜蛋白酶以及组织蛋白酶B几乎总是呈阳性，尽管这些抗原大部分为非特异性的[1164,1165]。在一些非典型性纤维黄色瘤中，已经证实有对单核细胞较特异的标记物[1166,1167]，但这些资料尚存疑问。大约半数的病变肌动蛋白呈阳性[1167]。重要的是，S-100蛋白、melan A、结蛋白以及细胞角蛋白为阴性[1165-1171]。在这些病变中常可见到S-100阳性的非肿瘤性树突状细胞。

超微结构上，细胞具有丰富的胞浆，内含线状伪足[1172]、大量含有吞噬物质的溶酶体、脂质空泡以及数量不等的胞浆内细丝[1173]。没有基底膜，也没有胞饮空泡以及诊断性包涵体。极个别病例有胞浆内含有Langerhans样颗粒的细胞[1174]，可能为混入肿瘤当中的非肿瘤性Langerhans细胞。

流式细胞DNA分析显示，非典型性纤维黄色瘤多数为二倍体DNA，不同于所谓的恶性纤维组织细胞瘤，后者通常为非整倍体[1175]。然而在所有的非典型性纤维黄色瘤中，DNA图像分析均发现有非整倍体细胞[1176]，提示组织学发现的多形性细胞与非典型性纤维黄色瘤的非整倍体区域密切相关。

主要的鉴别诊断包括梭形细胞鳞状细胞癌、恶性黑色素瘤、平滑肌肉瘤以及所谓的恶性纤维组织细胞瘤（不能分类的多形性肉瘤），所有这些病变在常规组织学检查时均可相似。除了表皮或交界性成分以外，鳞状细胞癌可通过其细胞角蛋白阳性、黑色素瘤可通过具有S-100蛋白及少数病例melan A阳性以及平滑肌肉瘤可通过结蛋白阳性或超微结构特征来鉴别。多形性肉瘤，常常是指恶性纤维组织细胞瘤，只有通过充分了解临床关系才

有可能得到鉴别；预后差的深部软组织病变偶尔可以扩展至真皮。一般来说，真皮和浅层皮下组织的肉瘤相对比较惰性，包括细胞学呈多形性的病变，尽管文献中报告的病例选择的是非同寻常的表现。隆凸性皮肤纤维肉瘤可以除外，因为其特征为单形性的细胞学表现。恶性巨细胞肿瘤可以除外，因为它有呈良性细胞学改变的破骨细胞样巨细胞并混合有多形性单核细胞，尽管有些人将位于浅表部位的这些病变纳入非典型性纤维黄色瘤的范畴[1155,1177]。网状组织细胞瘤可通过其一致性的上皮样细胞伴有丰富的"毛玻璃样"胞浆来鉴别。

类似于非典型性纤维黄色瘤的改变也可见于接受照射的皮肤[1178,1179]。分子遗传学证据提示，紫外线照射是形成非典型性纤维黄色瘤的触发点[1180,1181]。

其他纤维瘤性病变
Miscellaneous fibromatous lesions

皮肤的其他各种纤维性病变已有描述，多数在第24章有较详细的描述。其中有些常见，有些少见或罕见。这些病变包括瘢痕疙瘩[1182]、肥厚性瘢痕[1182]、皮肤"筋膜炎"[1064,1183,1184]、结缔组织痣[1184-1187]、硬化性纤维瘤[1061-1063,1188-1194]、腱鞘纤维瘤[1195,1196]、腱鞘巨细胞瘤[1197]、成人肌纤维瘤病和肌纤维瘤[1198-1206]、皮肤肌纤维瘤[1066,1207-1210]、退化性或隔离性脑脊膜膨出或错构瘤（迷芽瘤）[1211-1217]（见第27章）以及纤维上皮性息肉（软垂疣、软纤维瘤、外阴阴道息肉、息肉样肌纤维母细胞瘤）[1218-1221]。许多人认为，如果没有多核间质细胞出现，则所谓的"多形性纤维瘤"[1038]非常类似于纤维上皮性息肉或与之密切相关。鼻（面）部的纤维性丘疹（fibrous papule）表现为皮色丘疹，其组织学上在层状纤维化背景中含有特征性的"星形"细胞，伴有薄壁扩张的血管

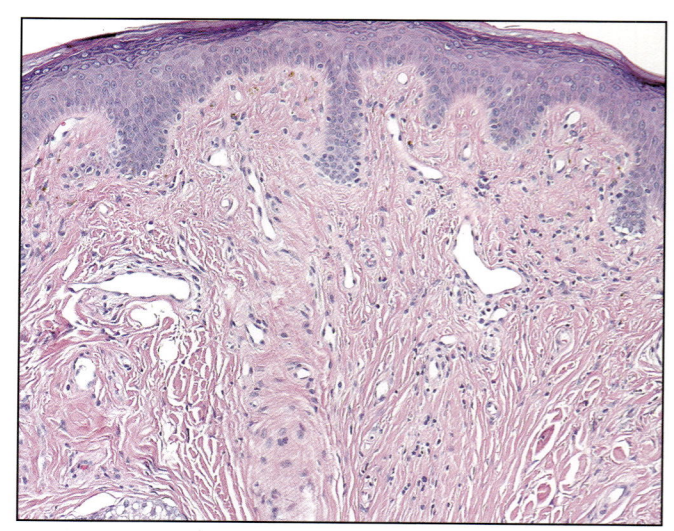

图23.179　纤维性丘疹。有纤维化，伴有明显的血管和星形单核细胞。

（图23.179）[1025,1222-1229]。纤维性丘疹的组织学亚型包括上皮样、透明细胞、颗粒细胞以及炎症亚型[1230,1231]。其他病变包括获得性（指趾）纤维角化瘤[1225,1232-1235]、儿童[1236-1241]或成人指趾纤维瘤（包括躯体纤维瘤病）[1242]、婴儿纤维性错构瘤[1243-1248]、白色纤维性丘疹病[1249,1250]、幼年性玻璃样纤维瘤病[1251]以及皮肤炎性假瘤[1252,253]。

"组织细胞性"病变 "Histiocytic" lesions

黄色肉芽肿（幼年型或成人型）[1254-1256] Xanthogranuloma (juvenile or adult)

黄色肉芽肿（过去称为痣黄色内皮瘤，naevoxanthoendothelioma）[1257]是指一组良性、自限性皮肤和（或）皮下病变，组织学特征为单核脂质细胞弥漫性生长，但境界清楚。病变中常常含有Touton巨细胞以及淋巴细胞、嗜酸性粒细胞、浆细胞和不同程度的纤维化。

临床上，黄色肉芽肿一般为皮肤病变，男女均等受累，并且不伴有血清脂质异常。20%的病例出生时就出现病变，但通常发生于6~24个月之间。成年人受累大约见于15%的病例[1258-1261]。病变大小一般不足1cm（尽管有些可以很大）[1262]，多数位于头颈部，但也可见于其他部位的皮肤，包括眼眶周围组织[1263,1264]、软组织以及骨骼肌[1256,1265-1269]。单发性与多发性病变的比例大约为2:1；后者可以成簇分布。内脏器官受累有极个别报告[1256,1270,1271]。病变通常为自限性的，可以自发性消退，但有个别例外。

黄色肉芽肿的组织学标志为弥漫性的、均匀一致的成团的单核吞噬细胞，混合有Touton巨细胞、嗜酸性粒细胞以及浆细胞，每种成分所占比例可有不同。病变被覆的表皮一般正常或萎缩，但少数可以形成溃疡。细胞团一般与表皮邻接，但有些病例可出现Grenz区。黄色肉芽肿常常含有皮肤固有结构，如皮肤附件，这不同于纤维组织细胞瘤，后者一般没有这些结构。

细胞学表现较为宽泛，从伴有多量Touton细胞（图23.180）和（或）纤维化的富含脂质的单核细胞，到没有Touton巨细胞、仅含同质性胞浆内含有微泡状脂质的单核细胞[1272-1275]。偶尔可见扇贝形细胞[1276]和"畸形细胞"[1277]。早期病变的细胞浆可能以嗜酸性表现为主。可以见到核分裂象，有时数量惊人[1272-1275]。

组织学上，黄色肉芽肿的单核细胞内可见胞浆内脂质。病变内网织纤维丰富，围绕小簇细胞分布。少数情况下可含铁血黄素。免疫组织化学染色显示，黄色肉芽肿表达波形蛋白、HHF-35、HAM56、CD68、组织蛋白酶B以及XIIIa因子[1266,1274,1278-1280]。S-100蛋白标记病变周边的树突状细胞，但据说单核细胞没有表达[1279]，

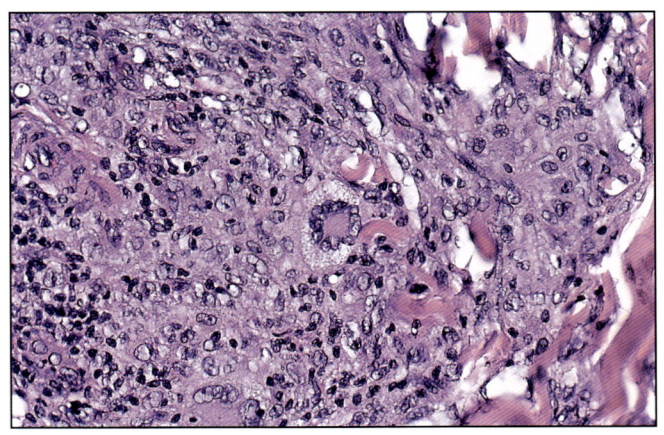

图23.180　黄色肉芽肿。这个病变的特征为细胞脂质较少。可见Touton细胞以及散在嗜酸性粒细胞。

尽管新近资料提示并非如此[1280]。其他阴性标记物包括MAC387（L1抗原）、Leu-M1（CD15）、结蛋白、平滑肌特异性肌动蛋白以及CD34[1279]。超微结构上，黄色肉芽肿的单核细胞类似于所谓的纤维组织细胞、巨噬细胞或肌纤维母细胞[1281-1284]。

黄色肉芽肿的鉴别诊断包括Langerhans细胞组织细胞增生症——其S-100蛋白和CD1a呈阳性以及其他非Langerhans细胞组织细胞增生症[1285]、纤维组织细胞瘤、网状组织细胞瘤和黄色瘤，所有这些均可通过临床和（或）形态学表现来鉴别。

网状组织细胞瘤 Reticulohistiocytoma

网状组织细胞瘤为少见的皮肤病变，主要累及年轻人或中年人，以女性为主，可以是孤立性的[1286,1286a]或多发性的[1287-1289]。多中心性病变可能伴有破坏性关节炎，主要累及手指。有些患者还有黄斑瘤（xanthelasma），大约30%的患者伴有恶性肿瘤[1287]或系统性血管炎。皮肤病变表现为生长缓慢的结节，一般小于1cm，主要位于头颈部或躯干上部，但是孤立性网状组织细胞瘤并没有特异的发生部位，而多中心性网状组织细胞瘤的病变多位于肢端。病变可以消退和再生长，目前一般认为，网状组织细胞瘤（或多中心性网状组织细胞瘤病）是免疫介导的反应性疾病而不是肿瘤。

组织学上，皮肤和滑膜病变类似于幼年性黄色肉芽肿的浅表性病变，只是多核细胞比较明显，这些细胞可见特殊的嗜酸性毛玻璃样胞浆，而且细胞核主要位于周边（图23.181）。这些细胞还混合有单核上皮样细胞、组织细胞以及混合性的炎症细胞（图23.182）。与黄色肉芽肿不同的是，巨细胞胞浆内含有PAS阳性的抗淀粉酶物质。免疫组织化学染色显示明确的单核细胞/巨噬细胞分化[1286a,1290]。另外，有些证据表明，应用XIIIa因

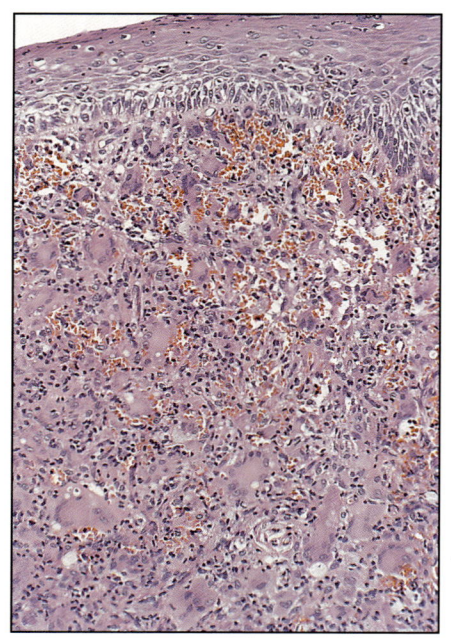

图23.181 网状组织细胞瘤。典型的真皮病变，为大的多核细胞，伴有明显的嗜酸性毛玻璃样胞浆。

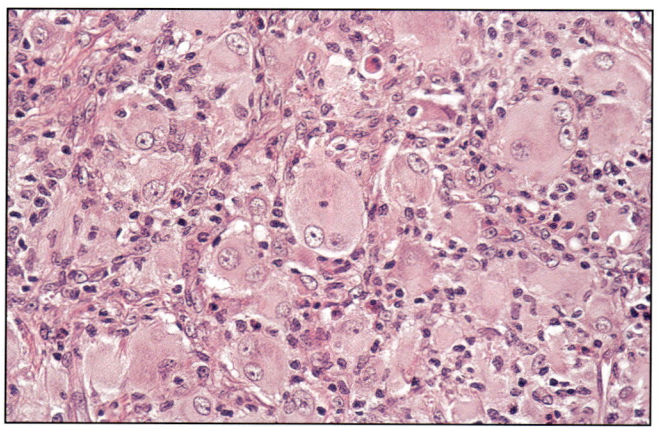

图23.182 网状组织细胞瘤。多核巨细胞极为明显，高倍镜下可见玻璃样胞浆。

子和HHF-35染色可将网状组织细胞瘤与多中心性网状组织细胞病鉴别开来。在网状组织细胞瘤，这两种标记物均为阳性，而在多中心性网状组织细胞病的病变，这两种标记物均为阴性[1291]。

神经肿瘤　Neural tumors

皮肤神经肿瘤在皮肤病理诊断中极为常见。这些病变临床上多数为难以归类的结节，只有通过组织学检查才能鉴别。一般来说，皮肤神经肿瘤的组织学特征与其他部位的类似（见第27章）。诊断的主要类型为：神经瘤，或为创伤性或为局限型；神经纤维瘤，或为孤立性或为神经纤维瘤病的多发性病变；神经鞘瘤；颗粒细胞瘤；以及皮肤神经鞘黏液瘤。除此以外，还有非常罕见的外周神经鞘恶性肿瘤，少数情况下可以发生在皮肤。所有这些病变均在第27章详细讨论，此处简要叙述局

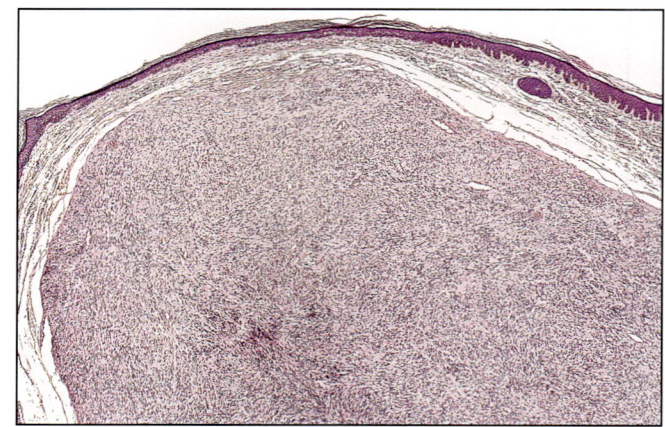

图23.183 栅栏状有包膜的神经瘤。真皮内的局限性病变。注意病变内的束状结构。有些病变出现神经鞘瘤样结构。

限性神经瘤和皮肤神经鞘黏液瘤。

栅栏状有包膜的神经瘤（孤立性局限性神经瘤）[1292-1299]
Palisaded encapsulated neuroma (solitary circumscribed neuroma)

这是一种较小的肉色的肿瘤，一般发生于成年男性和女性的面部，其他部位极为少见[1300]。病变一般是孤立性的，不伴有von Recklinghausen病（也见第27章）。局部切除可以治愈。

组织学上，病变界限非常清楚，由大小和形状不一的束状结构组成（图23.183）。主要细胞类型为梭形细胞，胞浆细长，细胞核椭圆形，两端变细，但也有上皮样亚型[1301]。这种增生的神经鞘细胞S-100呈阳性，并且混有多量小的轴突，可通过经典的组织化学染色以及神经细丝（neurofilament）或外周蛋白（peripherin）[1298]免疫染色来识别，外周蛋白是一种神经元的免疫组织化学标记物[1302]。神经鞘细胞和轴突的数量不一[1298]。过去将这种病变误认为是介于神经鞘瘤和神经纤维瘤之间的病变，但目前公认它是一种特殊病变。尽管原来这样命名，但是这些病变常常没有栅栏状结构，而且只有部分包膜。

皮肤神经鞘黏液瘤
Neurothekeoma (dermal nerve sheath myxoma)

这是一类小的良性肿瘤，一般发生于年轻人的头颈部以及身体的上半部。这种黏液样病变主要向神经鞘分化（也见第27章），而富于细胞的皮肤神经鞘黏液瘤的肿瘤性本质还不甚清楚。

临床上，多数神经鞘黏液瘤的大小为1 cm或更小，一般持续存在数月至数年。女性更为多见。临床鉴别诊断是非特异性的，不伴有任何神经嵴病（neurocristopathy）。局部复发极为少见。

组织学上，典型的形态为上皮样至梭形细胞，排列成小叶或"细胞球"（cell balls）分布于黏液样基质当中。小叶中的细胞呈上皮样至梭形，相当一致。多数小叶中可见丰富的 alcian 蓝阳性的黏液样基质。然而，根据报告病变可从伴有大量黏液而细胞成分较少[1303]至伴有少量黏液而高度富于细胞——即所谓的"富于细胞性"神经鞘黏液瘤[1304-1306]。富于细胞性神经鞘黏液瘤曾经被认为是毛肌瘤（pilar myomas）的亚型[1307]，但是随着混合类型的发现[1304]，即在同一病变中出现黏液样和富于细胞的结构，富于细胞性神经鞘黏液瘤被认为可能是神经鞘黏液瘤谱系中的一部分[1308]。不过，几乎没有证据表明富于细胞性神经鞘黏液瘤有神经鞘分化。有人提出可以将富于细胞性（上皮样）神经鞘黏液瘤放在上皮样皮肤纤维瘤范畴内，因为其生长方式和细胞学特征彼此类似[1309]，但缺乏其他支持性依据。

细胞学上，富于细胞区域的肿瘤细胞一般含有两染性胞浆以及相对一致的细胞核，细胞之间大小稍有不同。有些病例含有多核细胞。细胞排列成巢状及束状，位于玻璃样胶原带之间。这些肿瘤易见核分裂象，不应当作为恶性指征。极少数富于细胞性病变可出现显著的细胞学多形性，伴有多量核分裂象、深部扩展以及血管浸润，但迄今为止，短期随访尚未见有复发[1310]。

免疫组织化学染色显示，典型的黏液性病变 S-100 蛋白[1311]、IV 型胶原和波形蛋白通常呈阳性，而 EMA 不同程度呈阳性，一般位于小叶的周边。平滑肌特异性肌动蛋白、NSE 以及 Leu-7 呈阴性[1304]。富于细胞性病变 NKI/C3 和波形蛋白通常呈阳性，而 NSE 和平滑肌肌动蛋白不同程度呈阳性[1308,1310]。S-100 蛋白、melan A、细胞角蛋白、结蛋白、CD34、CD68、蛋白基因产物 9.5[1304,1305,1308,1310,1311] 和 EMA 呈阴性[1312]。

病变细胞的超微结构特征依据来自富于细胞性病变的资料主要分为四种类型。I 型细胞为多角形，伴有卵圆形细胞核、胞浆微丝以及个别微丝相关性致密小体。这些细胞的大多数，即大约 90% 为富于细胞性神经鞘黏液瘤，显示局灶性细胞浆膜致密，个别区域出现基底膜样物质。II 型细胞分化比较明显，为卵圆形或梭形细胞，胞浆内含有多量细丝。这些细胞被连续的基底膜包绕。这些细胞符合神经鞘细胞的特征，出现在典型的和混合性神经鞘黏液瘤中，或许也可出现在极少数富于细胞性神经鞘黏液瘤中。III 型细胞具有神经束膜细胞的特征，在典型的黏液性神经鞘黏液瘤中相对少见。IV 细胞类似于纤维母细胞，在所有亚型的神经鞘黏液瘤中均可见到。这些细胞类型支持如下假说，即典型的神经鞘黏液瘤具有神经（主要为神经鞘细胞）分化，而富于细胞性神经鞘黏液瘤主要由不完全分化的细胞构成，多数具有提示肌纤维母细胞分化的特征[1315]。

因此，HE 染色和超微结构表现的广泛多样性可能反映了这些病变的异质性。富于细胞性神经鞘黏液瘤的最为重要的鉴别诊断是 Spitz 痣和黏液样，或富于细胞性恶性黑色素瘤。后一种病变在多数情况下可通过病变结构均一性、境界清楚、缺少纤维化以及免疫染色来鉴别。然而，黏液性神经鞘黏液瘤一般 S-100 呈阳性，易于与大多数其他皮肤黏液样梭形细胞病变区分。

肌肉肿瘤　Tumors of muscle

平滑肌肿瘤以及极个别的骨骼肌肿瘤可见于皮肤。这些肿瘤中绝大多数为错构瘤、毛平滑肌瘤（毛囊平滑肌瘤）、生殖部位平滑肌瘤或血管平滑肌瘤。皮肤原发性平滑肌肉瘤少见，不过其形态学上的奇异性表现与侵袭性经过似乎并不相关。这些病变在第 24 章中详细讨论。

血管肿瘤　Vascular tumors

皮肤血管肿块、畸形或肿瘤，包含一系列的临床和组织学改变。一般来说，这些病变由内衬内皮的毛细血管大小的腔隙、海绵样大小的腔隙组成或两者混合存在。腔隙内充满血液、淋巴液或两者。血管肿瘤也可以是以实性为主的肿瘤，伴有一系列从良性到中间性乃至恶性的生物学行为。组织学上多数皮肤病变类似于软组织或内脏中所见的表现，包括 Kaposi 肉瘤，可见第 3 章中的描述。

淋巴组织肿瘤　Lymphoid tumors

皮肤淋巴组织肿瘤在临床上及组织学上一般难以归类，尤其是在表皮、真皮或两者中仅有少量淋巴细胞的阶段。

从历史上看，皮肤淋巴瘤的诊断范畴来源于最早出现皮肤体征的患者、蕈样霉菌病或皮肤 T 细胞性淋巴瘤的患者。直到最近几年，除了蕈样霉菌病之外，皮肤淋巴瘤才应用来自淋巴结淋巴瘤的诊断标准。

估计皮肤淋巴瘤的年发生率为每年 0.5/10 万～1/10 万人[1316]。皮肤 T 细胞性淋巴瘤（蕈样霉菌病）大约占原发性皮肤淋巴瘤的 60%，其中 20% 为 B 细胞性淋巴瘤。大约 10% 的病例为罕见的或不常见的其他淋巴组织增生性疾病[1317]。

近年来有人尝试将皮肤淋巴瘤分类标准化。表 23.8 对比了重新整合的 WHO-EORTC[1318]、WHO[1319,1320]、欧洲癌症研究和治疗组织（EORTC）[1317]以及修正的欧洲-美国（REAL）的皮肤淋巴瘤分类。这一节除了讨论蕈样霉菌病，还将讨论罕见的和不常见的皮肤淋巴瘤亚型的特征。读者也可参考第 21 章有关皮肤以外淋巴瘤和

表23.8　WHO-EORTC[1318]、WHO[1319,1320]、EORTC[1317]以及REAL皮肤淋巴瘤分类

T或B细胞	WHO-EORTC（2005）	WHO（2001）	EORTC（1997）	REAL（1994）
T细胞和NK	蕈样霉菌病（MF） 　亲毛囊MF 　Paget样网状细胞增多MF 　芽肿性皮肤松弛症MF	蕈样霉菌病（MF） 　MF相关性毛囊黏液病亚型 　Paget样网状细胞增多MF亚型 　肉芽肿性皮肤松弛症MF亚型	蕈样霉菌病（MF） 　MF相关性毛囊黏液病 　Paget样网状细胞增多 　肉芽肿性皮肤松弛症 　（暂时）	蕈样霉菌病（MF）
	Sézary综合征	Sézary综合征	Sézary综合征	Sézary综合征
	成人T细胞白血病淋巴瘤	未列	未列	未列
	原发性皮肤CD30+ 淋巴组织增生性疾病 　淋巴瘤样丘疹病 原发性皮肤间变 大细胞淋巴瘤	淋巴瘤样丘疹病 （恶性潜能未定的T细胞增生） 外周T细胞淋巴瘤	淋巴瘤样丘疹病 CD30+大T细胞淋巴瘤 　间变性 　多形性 　免疫母细胞性 CD30+大T细胞淋巴瘤 　多形性大细胞 　免疫母细胞性	未列 间变性大细胞淋巴瘤 外周T细胞淋巴瘤 非特殊性 外周T细胞淋巴瘤 非特殊性 未列
	皮下脂膜炎性 T细胞淋巴瘤	皮下脂膜炎样 T细胞淋巴瘤	皮下脂膜炎样 T细胞淋巴瘤（暂时）	皮下脂膜炎性 T细胞淋巴瘤
	结外NK/T细胞 淋巴瘤，鼻型	外周T细胞淋巴瘤	未列	
	原发性皮肤外周 T细胞淋巴瘤，非特殊性 　原发性皮肤侵袭性亲 　表皮CD8阳性T细 　胞淋巴瘤（暂时） 　皮肤γ/δT细胞淋巴瘤 　（暂时） 　原发性皮肤CD4+ 　小/中等大小多形性 　T细胞淋巴瘤（暂时）		多形性小/中等大小 细胞（暂时）	外周T细胞淋巴瘤， 非特殊性

白血病的讨论。

淋巴组织增生（假淋巴瘤、皮肤淋巴细胞瘤）
Lymphoid hyperplasia（pseudolymphoma, lymphocytoma cutis）

淋巴组织增生表示一系列的异原性淋巴细胞浸润，在组织学的某些方面上可能类似于恶性淋巴瘤，但并不出现淋巴瘤的临床表现及生物学行为，尽管有些病变可能顽固，可能是低级别淋巴瘤。

病变由多种原因导致的反应性T和B淋巴细胞增生组成。炎症浸润呈带样、结节状或弥漫性，主要由淋巴细胞构成，但也可出现其他炎症细胞。皮肤淋巴组织增生根据浸润的主要细胞类型分为T细胞和B细胞型。皮肤T细胞增生包括特发性淋巴瘤样药物反应、淋巴瘤样接触性皮炎、持续性结节状节肢动物叮咬反应、结节状疥疮、光化性类网状细胞增多症以及不常见的对传染性软疣的反应。有些人还将淋巴瘤样丘疹病纳入这一组，但EORTC将这种疾病归为低级别淋巴瘤。皮肤B细胞增生包括特发性病变、螺旋体性皮肤淋巴细胞瘤、文身所致的皮肤淋巴细胞瘤、带状疱疹后瘢痕皮肤淋巴细胞瘤以及一些持续性结节状节肢动物叮咬反应[1321]。

组织学上，病变结构可为结节状或弥漫性，一般局

表23.8 WHO-EORTC[1318]、WHO[1319,1320]、EORTC[1317]以及REAL皮肤淋巴瘤分类（续）

T或B细胞	WHO-EORTC（2005）	WHO（2001）	EORTC（1997）	REAL（1994）
B细胞	原发性皮肤滤泡中心淋巴瘤	滤泡性淋巴瘤	滤泡中心细胞淋巴瘤（主要位于头部和躯干）	滤泡中心淋巴瘤 I. 小细胞为主 II. 大小细胞混合 III. 大细胞为主 弥漫大B细胞淋巴瘤
	原发性皮肤边缘区B细胞淋巴瘤	结外边缘区B细胞淋巴瘤（MALT型）	免疫细胞瘤/边缘区B细胞淋巴瘤	结外边缘区B细胞淋巴瘤（MALT型）
	未列	浆细胞瘤	浆细胞瘤（暂时）	浆细胞瘤
	原发性皮肤弥漫大B细胞淋巴瘤，下肢型	弥漫大B细胞淋巴瘤	下肢大B细胞淋巴瘤	弥漫大B细胞淋巴瘤
	原发性皮肤弥漫大B细胞淋巴瘤，其他			
	血管内大B细胞淋巴瘤	血管内大B细胞淋巴瘤	血管内大B细胞淋巴瘤	未列
前驱病变	CD4+/CD56+皮肤造血系统肿瘤（母细胞性NK细胞淋巴瘤）	未列	未列	未列

限于真皮上部，即所谓"头重脚轻的"（top heavy）表现。许多病例中可出现次级生发中心，而且免疫表型为多形性，包括丰富的多克隆B细胞和T辅助细胞以及少数CD30+细胞。在许多病例中，出现嗜酸性粒细胞和含有可染小体的组织细胞。具有κ和λ轻链的浆细胞常常出现。然而，也可发生克隆性过度生长，提示有些病例有可能进展为淋巴瘤[1322]。

鉴别诊断包括皮肤淋巴瘤或淋巴瘤扩展至皮肤。一些其他病变也可出现明显的混合性细胞浸润，如伴有嗜酸细胞增多的血管淋巴组织增生（上皮样血管瘤）。极少数情况下，上皮性肿瘤可以伴有淋巴细胞浸润。这些病变包括淋巴（腺）瘤（见1445页）以及淋巴上皮瘤样癌。

有关其他疾病变讨论[1323]，如光化性类网状细胞增多症、药物诱发的假淋巴瘤、接触性淋巴组织病变、叮咬反应、特发性假淋巴瘤以及炎性假瘤[1253]等，在其他皮肤病理学文献中详细讨论。下面讨论的病变，如淋巴瘤样丘疹病等，曾经被纳入这个范畴，但现在被认为是低级别的皮肤淋巴瘤。

淋巴瘤 Lymphoma

这一部分对EORTC提出的皮肤淋巴瘤做一简要概括。表23.9对这些病变的主要特征进行了比较，读者可以从这个表以及文献中[1317]了解这些类型的淋巴瘤的许多详细内容。

皮肤T细胞性淋巴瘤[1324]
Cutaneous T-cell lymphomas

蕈样霉菌病以及Sézary综合征大约占所有皮肤原发性T细胞性淋巴瘤的一半[1325]。这里描述的许多不常见类型的T细胞性淋巴瘤与EORTC分类概括的一样。读者可以参阅本书第21章或可以累及皮肤的不常见的T细胞性淋巴组织增生性病变的文献，如淋巴瘤样肉芽肿病，它可以发生于皮肤，表现为血管中心性淋巴瘤，但它是一种系统性病变，还常常累及肺和中枢神经系统[1326,1327]。

蕈样霉菌病[1328] Mycosis fungoides

这是一组常常被称为蕈样霉菌病的皮肤肿瘤，尽管在本质上是淋巴组织肿瘤而不是真菌感染。病变表现为亲表皮和（或）由肿瘤性淋巴细胞构成的Pautrier微脓肿。

临床上，患者一般为成人，常常伴有长期顽固性脱屑和（或）红斑病史，或最终发生肿瘤。临床预后差异很大，病史一般较长；EORTC的一组278例患者中5年生存率为87%[1317]。暴发性病程极为少见，除非在典型蕈样霉菌病的基础上发生大细胞性T细胞性淋巴瘤[1329]。

组织学上，常常出现轻度表皮海绵层细胞间水肿。如果临床表现典型，可以确诊为蕈样霉菌病的明确的特征包括：表皮内出现特征性的小团扭曲的淋巴细胞聚集，称为Pautrier微脓肿（图23.184）。其他确诊的病例在基底膜上方可以出现较为明显的淋巴细胞，其细胞核扭曲，排列成线样（图23.185）。其他病例在表皮的各层均可

淋巴组织肿瘤

表 23.9 皮肤淋巴瘤的主要特征的比较

T或B细胞	EORTC分类	临床特征	组织病理学	免疫表型	遗传学特征	5年生存率	评论
T细胞	蕈样霉菌病	斑片疹，数年后最终发展为肿瘤，一般见于成人（"Alibert-Bazin"型）。有些患者晚期可发生肿瘤、淋巴结和内部器官	伴有曲形（脑状）细胞核的小至中等大小淋巴细胞亲表皮性和（或）Pautrier微脓肿可以见到。单个细胞或晚期肿瘤期呈弥漫性侵润	CD3+, CD4+, CD45RO+, CD8-, CD30-。极少数CD3+, CD4-, CD8+。肿瘤期常出现T细胞抗原缺失	多数病例有T细胞受体基因重排，包括斑片期病变，所见并不一致。	87%（基于278例患者）	病变晚期可出现CD30阳性或弥漫大细胞淋巴瘤，并提示侵袭性病程
T细胞	蕈样霉菌病相关性毛囊黏蛋白沉积症	头颈部毛囊疹丘疹及肿瘤，有些伴有脱发。瘢样以外部位不出现病变	蕈样霉菌样表现，但没有显著的毛囊浸润，代之以表皮囊泡及毛囊黏蛋白沉积	与蕈样霉菌病相同	多数病例有T细胞受体基因重排，有助于与黏蛋白脱发相鉴别	70%（基于30例患者）	早期可不被识别，因为缺乏亲表皮性，并被错误视归为多形性CTCL
T细胞	Paget样网织细胞增多症	生长缓慢的角化过度性斑块，一般位于肢体远端。皮肤以外部位不出现病变	表皮增生，含有大的淋巴细胞呈Paget样结构以及表皮呈巢状生长	CD3+, CD4+, CD8- 或 CD3+, CD4-, CD8+，有些病例表达CD30	某些病例具有克隆性T细胞基因重排	极好，惰性病变	Worringer-Kolopp病是Paget样网织细胞增多症的同义词，所谓Ketron-Goodman型应视其为多形性蕈样霉菌病
T细胞	肉芽肿性皮肤松弛症（暂时）	腋窝或腹股沟局部皮肤下垂。男性发病率大于女性。1/3的病例伴发Hodgkin病或蕈样霉菌病	弥漫肉芽肿性浸润，伴有多形性T细胞以及多核巨细胞，有弹力纤维溶解	肿瘤细胞CD3+, CD4+, CD8-	具有TCR基因重排	多数病例为惰性	
T细胞	淋巴瘤样丘疹病	弥漫丘疹、丘疹坏死或结节中等不同发展阶段的皮肤病变不消长，单个病变一般在6个星期内出现消退。10%~20%的患者可出现另一种类型的淋巴瘤，通常为蕈样霉菌病、CD30+大T细胞淋巴瘤或Hodgkin病	依据活检病变的时期不同而差异较大。A型：楔形病变，非亲表皮，伴有大的CD30+多形性细胞，核似Reed-Sternberg样，嗜酸细胞以及小淋巴细胞也可见到。B型：蕈样霉菌样表现，伴亲表皮。可与A型共存。C型：CD30+大细胞淋巴瘤样，极少伴有发疹性细胞	A型和C型：CD30+, CD2+/-, CD3+, CD4+/-, CD5+/-, CD8-, CD15-, EMA+。B型：CD3+, CD4+, CD8-, CD30-，小的脑状细胞类似于蕈样霉菌病	克隆性重排见于60%的病例，包括那些伴发淋巴瘤的病例	100%（基于70例患者）	文献报道表示，淋巴瘤样丘疹病中有10%~20%的患者伴发淋巴瘤
T细胞	CD30+大T细胞淋巴瘤	一般为成人。男女比为3:2。多数表现为溃疡性结节。自发性消退见于25%的病例，25%出现局部淋巴结受累	弥漫、非亲表皮浸润。多数病例中，肿瘤细胞明显多形性。常有明显核仁以及大量母细胞表现，极少数情况下，细胞呈免疫母细胞形态表现。有些出现LyP样表现。有些可见多反应性淋巴细胞。嗜酸细胞以及中性粒细胞	75%以上的细胞CD30+。而全T细胞抗原通常CD4+（CD2, CD3, CD5）缺失，不足5%为CD8+。多数EMA和CD15为阴性	克隆性T细胞基因重排见于多数病例。对于（2:5）易位见于儿童淋巴瘤，它常见CD30+间变性大细胞淋巴瘤，也可发生于这些病变	90%（基于57例患者）	蕈样霉菌患者发生CD30+大T细胞淋巴瘤通常预后较差
T细胞	多形性，小中等大小细胞（暂时）	单发或多发性结节或肿瘤，没有蕈样霉菌病的斑片病点	小至中等大小多形性T细胞弥漫性浸润，可以浸润皮下组织。可CD30+大T细胞的鉴别表现。以及CD30-大T细胞以上的大肿瘤细胞	CD4+, 而全T标记物（CD2, CD3, CD5）缺失。有些病例CD8+	常出现克隆性T细胞基因重排	62%（基于18例患者）	与蕈样霉菌病的鉴别困难。出现多量CD8+T细胞，并伴有CD20+B细胞和组织细胞提示不限性T细胞淋巴瘤。小中等大小多形性T细胞可见到。CD8+的病例更具侵袭性
T细胞	皮下脂膜炎样T细胞淋巴瘤（暂时）	皮下结节或斑片，一般位于下肢部。患者可出现全身性体征，噬血细胞综合征常伴有迅速致死性病程。皮损播散不常见	皮下浸润类似于脂膜炎，形性T细胞以及巨噬细胞，核碎裂，以及噬红细胞表现	CD3+, CD4+, CD8+或CD3+, CD4-, CD8+。多数病例CD56-，极少数病例表达γ/δ	大约50%的病例出现克隆性T细胞基因重排	较差，即使进行了冲击治疗	α/β且CD8+的病例程较长，不伴有皮外播散或噬血综合征

表 23.9 皮肤淋巴瘤的主要特征的比较（续）

T或B细胞	EORTC分类	临床特征	组织病理学	免疫表型	遗传学特征	5年生存率	评论
T细胞	CD30⁻大T细胞淋巴瘤	单发、局限或广泛的斑块、结节或肿瘤	中等大小至大的多形性T细胞弥漫浸润，伴有曲状细胞核和免疫母细胞，占肿瘤细胞的30%以上。可以出现亲表皮性和血管中心结构表现	异常CD4⁺T细胞表型，全T标记物（CD2, CD3, CD5）缺失。CD30⁻散在阳性细胞	克隆性T细胞基因重排见于多数病例	15%（基于36例患者）	可类似于蕈样霉菌病伴有大T细胞淋巴瘤转化，但先前没有蕈样霉菌病病史。如果大T细胞占80%以上，则多数预后较差。CD30⁻大T细胞血管中心型淋巴瘤也包括在此
T细胞	Sézary综合征	瘙痒性红皮病伴有脑状细胞。淋巴结肿大、脱发、指甲营养不良以及掌跖过度角化病常见。但淋巴结、骨髓可含有肿瘤细胞，但浸润一般没有肿瘤细胞成分	Sézary细胞可见于皮肤或淋巴结，但不很明显	CD3⁺, CD4⁺, CD45RO⁺, CD8⁻或CD30⁻	TCR基因重排见于多数病例。克隆性T细胞可见于外周血	11%（基于12个病例）	EORTC认为确诊这种综合征依据出现CD4⁺细胞扩增以及外周血CD4/CD8比例大于10%
B细胞	滤泡中心细胞淋巴瘤（主要位于头颈部）	非结痂性丘疹、斑块及肿瘤。一般位于头、颈及躯干。病变不治疗，病变可生长数年，但极少扩展至皮肤之外	结节状或弥漫性浸润，一般不累及表皮。肿瘤细胞为中心细胞（细胞较小、小裂细胞）和中心母细胞（细胞较大、核不明显）。可有残留的生发中心。较晚期病变为升和，中心细胞数量增加，中心晚期反应性T细胞，较晚期病变中心和反应性T细胞，极少有反应性T细胞	表达B细胞抗原（CD19⁺, CD20⁺, CD22⁺, CD79a⁺）。可出现单一型sIg表达，但在肿瘤性病变为阴性的病变为CD5⁻和CD10⁻	克隆性见于多数病例。不伴有t(14;18)易位。bcl-2蛋白一般为阴性	97%（基于84例患者）	最常见的皮肤B细胞淋巴瘤类型，位于头颈部的病变在生物学反应形态学方面不同于发生在腿部的病变，并且被单独分类
B细胞	免疫细胞瘤/边区B细胞淋巴瘤	单发或多发性皮肤皮下肿瘤，一般位于皮肤	结节状或弥漫性浸润，由特征性的小淋巴样细胞和浆细胞和免疫母细胞构成。有时可以见到中心浆细胞样细胞浸润单核样淋巴浆细胞样细胞常位于小静脉周边。可以见到小的CD20⁺B细胞核以反应性滤泡。PAS阳性胞核内包涵体常见	细胞呈单一型cIg, CD79⁺, CD5⁻浆细胞CD20⁻	可出现克隆性Ig基因重排。没有已知的特殊易位	100%（基于12个病例）	皮肤免疫细胞瘤被称为低度恶性皮肤相关淋巴组织B细胞淋巴瘤或皮肤粘膜相关淋巴瘤
B细胞	腿部大B细胞淋巴瘤	一般发生于老年患者，大约80%的患者在70岁以上。男女比例为1.3～1.4。病变为红色至蓝色的结节，位于一侧腿部，极少为两侧腿部	大B细胞非亲表皮性真皮浸润，伴有数量不等的中心母细胞。大中心细胞以及免疫母细胞。可见极少数的小裂细胞和炎症细胞	表达单一型sIg和（或）cIg, CD19⁺, CD20⁺, CD22⁺以及CD79a⁺。bcl-2蛋白高表达	可出现克隆性Ig基因重排。Bcl-2蛋白表达不伴有t(14;18)	58%（基于18个病例）	
B细胞	血管内大B细胞淋巴瘤	紫色质硬的斑片或斑块，位于下腿部下方或躯干	真皮内扩张血管，皮下含有大的淋巴样细胞，可以导致小静脉、毛细血管以及小动脉血管阻塞，20%的病例血也可出现血管外浸润	CD19⁺, CD20⁻, CD22⁺, CD79a⁺, 单一型sIg⁺, 极少数伴有T细胞表型病例有报告	可出现克隆性Ig基因重排	50%（基于4例患者）	可以累及中枢神经系统和皮肤，通常预后较差
B细胞	浆细胞瘤（暂时）	单发或多发性紫红色至紫色皮肤或皮下结节，没有特别的发生部位	结节状或弥漫性真皮浸润，几乎完全由成熟浆细胞构成，包括多核细胞，缺乏克隆性淋巴细胞，与免疫细胞瘤相同	单一型cIg⁺和CD38⁺，但CD20和LCA阴性		此型病变没有死亡报告	极为少见，只占髓外浆细胞瘤的4%

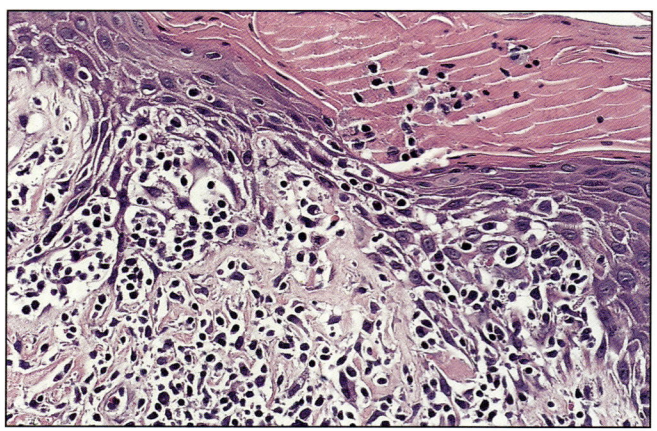

图23.184 恶性淋巴瘤，T细胞型（蕈样霉菌病）。表皮内Pautrier微脓肿。

出现散在的单个非典型性淋巴细胞。有些病例可出现混合性结构，包括伴有大细胞性淋巴瘤特征的细胞[1330]。发现任何明显的上述结构可为确定诊断增添极为重要的砝码；然而，如果缺乏明显的组织学表现或足够的临床证据，诊断蕈样霉菌病应该谨慎。许多蕈样霉菌病病例也可出现特征性的带状真皮乳头纤维化，真皮乳头血管可呈"丝环状"硬化。这些病例常常伴有细胞核扭曲的淋巴细胞以及浆细胞，偶尔可见嗜酸性粒细胞。

免疫表型方面，蕈样霉菌病 CD3、CD4、CD45RO（UCHL1）通常呈阳性，CD8 和 CD30 呈阴性。T 细胞抗原在肿瘤阶段可以丢失[1331]。这些病变常常可见 T 细胞受体基因重排，即使是在早期阶段[1332]。

如果浸润不太明显，尤其是缺乏表皮浸润时，则不能明确预测一个病例在临床上是否会有进展。这些患者中有些很可能既可出现蕈样霉菌病，也可经过一段时间后发生最终的病变。如果活检主要为炎症表现，我们并不主张应用过于积极的诊断方法，因为目前对于了解本病的自然病史并没有实际意义。可能会导致不必要和过早的治疗。

依据临床和组织学背景进行分类的皮肤 T 细胞性淋巴瘤的少见亚型包括：疣状、脓疱性、大疱性、亲汗腺性、黑色棘皮症样、色素减少性、色素增加性以及色素性紫癜样皮肤 T 细胞性淋巴瘤。主要根据组织学进行分类的亚型包括：棘细胞层水肿性、黏液性、单纯皮肤性以及慢性单纯性苔藓样类型。这些亚型中没有一种具有预后意义。

蕈样霉菌病相关性毛囊黏蛋白沉积症（mycosis fungoides-associated follicular mucinosis）[1333]：这种类型的蕈样霉菌病的特征是：普通类型的细胞可见于亲表皮性蕈样霉菌病中但局限于毛囊，并且伴有毛囊黏蛋白沉积症。

临床上，多数病变表现为发生于头颈部的斑片或斑块。可以伴有脱发。EORTC 患者的 5 年存活率大约为 70%[1317]。

组织学上，出现亲毛囊性浸润，毛囊壁伴有轻度改变（图23.186）。浸润的细胞形态通常单一，含有脑回状的 CD4+ 的淋巴细胞（图23.187），其表型类似于普通的蕈样霉菌病病例。I 型细胞间黏附分子（ICAM）在其毛囊中心浸润前部毛囊球的角化细胞可表达，但在表皮或缺乏淋巴瘤的对照组——毛囊黏蛋白沉积症患者的毛囊没有表达。另外，亲毛囊表现见于一些缺乏毛囊黏蛋白沉积症的蕈样霉菌病患者。其遗传学表现类似于普通的蕈样霉菌病[1334]。

Sézary 综合征（Sézary's syndrome）[1335-1337]：是 T 细胞性淋巴瘤/白血病，定义为弥漫性红皮病，伴有淋巴结病，在皮肤、淋巴结以及外周血中可见扭曲的 T 细胞（Sézary 细胞）。

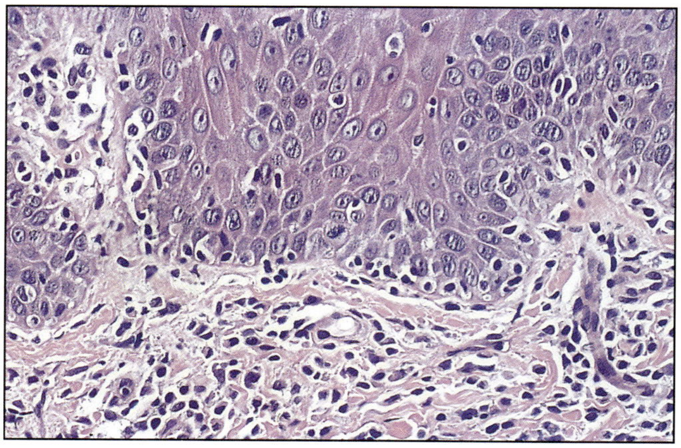

图23.185 恶性淋巴瘤，T细胞型（蕈样霉菌病）。淋巴细胞亲表皮表现。

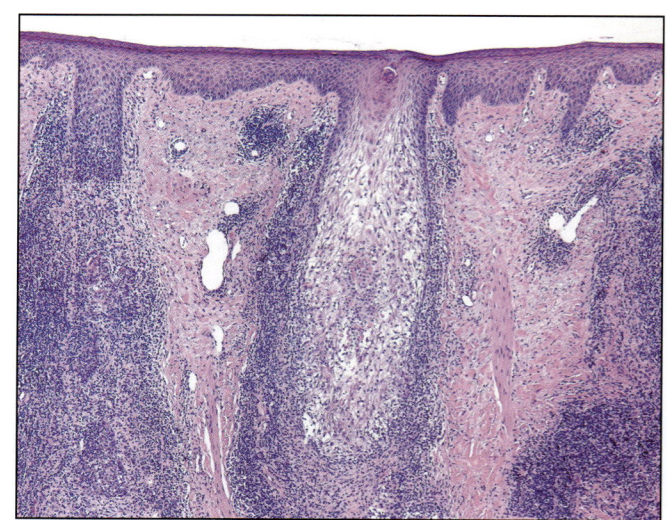

图23.186 蕈样霉菌病相关性毛囊黏蛋白沉积症。毛囊中心性浸润表现为毛囊黏液性膨胀。

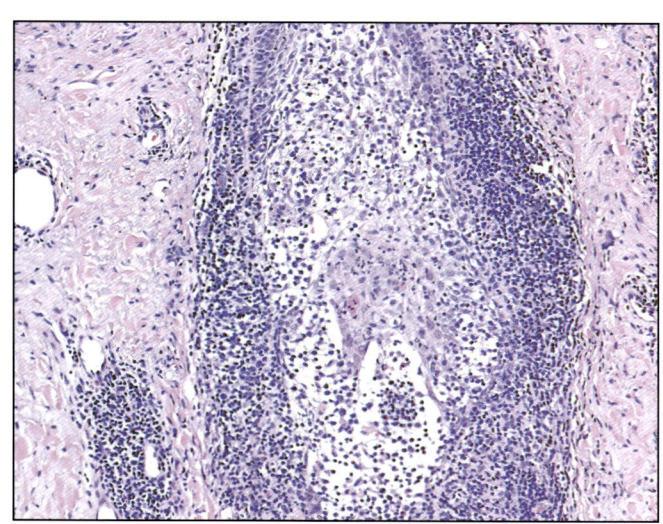

图23.187 蕈样霉菌病相关性毛囊黏蛋白沉积症。可见多形性淋巴细胞浸润。注意毛囊上皮广泛受累。

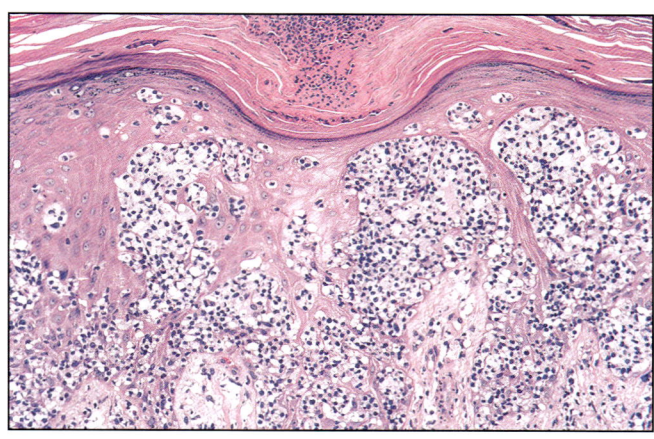

图23.188 Paget样网状细胞增多症。这种亲表皮性淋巴细胞浸润有Paget样播散,真皮有轻度浸润。

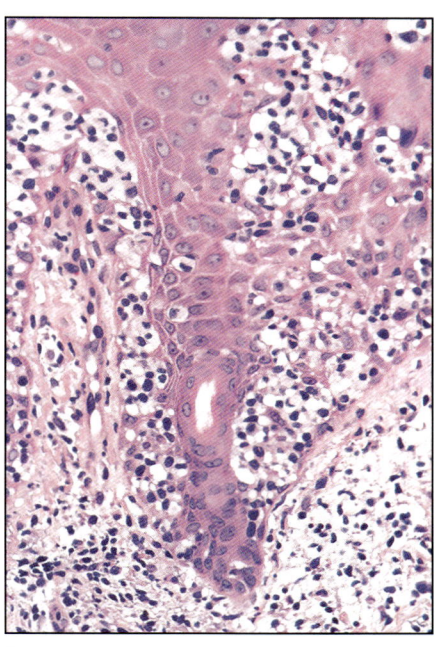

图23.189 Paget样网状细胞增多症。附件也可被多形性淋巴细胞浸润穿透。

临床上,患者一般表现为弥漫性红皮病、掌跖角化过度、脱发以及瘙痒。存活率一般较差。EORTC 患者的 5 年生存率为 11%[1317]。

组织学上,其表现可类似于蕈样霉菌病,但肿瘤细胞常常缺乏亲表皮表现,而且形态常常比典型的蕈样霉菌病单一[1338,1339]。在一项研究中[1340],来自 41 例伴有循环血中 Sézary 细胞以及 T 细胞 β 受体(TCR)基因重排检测出克隆性 T 细胞的 79 个皮肤活检标本显示:26/79(33%)标本有慢性皮炎,证实非特异性的组织学表现较为常见。41 例患者中有 11 例红皮病性皮肤缺乏 CTCL 表现。这些患者的生存率与其余 30 个患者没有明显差异,后者的活检显示诊断性的 CTCL,诸如伴有非典型性淋巴细胞的皮肤淋巴细胞带(18/79,23%)或蕈样霉菌病样浸润(30/79,38%)。

其免疫表型类似于蕈样霉菌病:CD3+、CD4+、CD45RO+、CD8- 和 CD30-。基因重排可见于多数病例。

Paget 样网状细胞增多症(Woringer-Kolopp 病)[pagetoid reticulosis (Woringer-Kolopp disease)][1341]:蕈样霉菌病的这种亚型一般表现为肢体疣状斑块,临床上并不会有进展。如果为多发性病变或出现皮肤的广泛播散(即所谓的 Ketron-Goodman 型),则不应将其视为 Paget 样网状细胞增多症,而应视为普通的蕈样霉菌病。Paget 样网状细胞增多症预后极好,没有与疾病相关的死亡报告。

组织学上,可见表皮增生、过度角化以及明显的扭曲单核细胞呈 Paget 样浸润(图 23.188),伴有或不伴有表皮内成簇的肿瘤细胞巢。附件结构也可受累(图 23.189)。

免疫表型方面,这些细胞 CD3+、CD4+、CD8- 或 CD3+、CD4-、CD8+,伴有或不伴有 CD30 阳性[134,1343]。克隆性 TCR 基因重排也已经确定[1344]。

在鉴别诊断中,除了普通的蕈样霉菌病以外,有些病例可能还需要除外恶性黑色素瘤。

CD30+ 皮肤大细胞性 T 细胞性淋巴瘤[1345,1346]
CD30+ cutaneous large T-cell lymphoma

这是一类少见的皮肤大细胞性多形性淋巴瘤,最初被称为非典型性消退性组织细胞增生症,Kiel 和 REAL 分类将其划归为间变性大细胞性淋巴瘤(见第 21 章)。目前认为,这些病变中的大多数肿瘤细胞表达 CD30,并且预后极好,在 EORTC 的患者中,5 年生存率达到 90%。

临床上,任何年龄或性别均可受累,男女比例为 3:2。先前没有其他类型淋巴瘤或淋巴瘤样丘疹病病史。25% 的患者可以发生肿瘤消退。但这对预后并不产生明显影响[1345]。

组织学上，这些病变由非亲表皮性、弥漫分布的多形性单核细胞和巨细胞组成，伴有单个嗜酸性核仁或多个核仁。少数情况下，肿瘤细胞具有免疫母细胞的形态学特征。常常伴有小的反应性淋巴细胞、巨噬细胞以及嗜酸性粒细胞浸润。被覆病变的表皮可有显著的增生。

免疫组织化学方面，75%以上的肿瘤细胞CD30（Ber-H2、Ki-1）呈阳性。可以出现全T细胞标记物（即CD2、CD3、CD5）的缺失。CD8在有些病例中可为阳性。这些病变多数为EMA和CD15阴性。多数病例出现TCR基因重排[1347]。多数原发性皮肤病变为ALK-1阴性，后者阳性则提示有并存的系统性淋巴瘤。

由于这些病变的细胞可呈多形性表现，诊断时必须保持高度警惕。对于某一具体病例，可能还要考虑到多形性癌、黑色素瘤和肉瘤，包括上皮样血管肉瘤。

淋巴瘤样丘疹病 [1346,1348,1349]
Lymphomatoid papulosis

淋巴瘤样丘疹病为一类自限性的、多发性丘疹性至结节状的淋巴细胞病变，通常发生于年轻人，但极少数也可发生于儿童和老年人。多数病变可自行消退，但在大约10%~20%的病例，患者随后可发生其他类型的淋巴瘤，如蕈样霉菌病、CD30⁺大细胞性T细胞性淋巴瘤或Hodgkin淋巴瘤。

临床上，病变为丘疹或丘疹坏死性表现。不同病变一般处于不同的发展阶段，而且病变可以持续不同的时间，一般呈良性经过[1317]。单个病变持续时间极少超过6周[1348,1350]。

组织学上，单个病变的特征为多形性的大单核细胞和小单核细胞呈楔形浅表及深层浸润，可混有中性粒细胞、巨噬细胞以及数量不等的嗜酸性粒细胞（图23.190）。这些细胞浸润一般造成表皮消失，常常导致坏死或溃疡形成。这些病变常常被分为三种不同的形态学类型，A、B或C型[1347,1351-1353]。这些"类型"可以混合，并且可以发生于同一患者或同一病变当中。"A"型由伴有组织细胞样特征的、类似于Reed-Sternberg细胞的多形性细胞构成（图23.191），呈楔形浸润，这些细胞CD30⁺，并散在有嗜酸性粒细胞、中性粒细胞以及小淋巴细胞。其他标记物可以呈阳性也可以呈阴性，诸如CD2、CD3、CD4和CD5。CD8和CD15为阴性。"B"型具有小淋巴细胞性蕈样霉菌病样结构，并且其免疫表型表达类似于典型的蕈样霉菌病。"C"型由单一形态的大T细胞组成，伴有类似于"A"型的表型，但是没有混合性炎症表现。T细胞受体基因重排发生于大约60%的病例，单个病变可以是单克隆性的也可以是多克隆性的。而且，单克隆性增生并不一定代表这个患者将会发生淋巴瘤。组织学上鉴别诊断包括苔藓豆疹样糠疹、蕈样霉菌病以及CD30⁺大细胞性T细胞性淋巴瘤。对于这些患者，诊断必须结合临床相关性表现。

CD30⁻大细胞性T细胞性淋巴瘤
CD30⁻ large T-cell lymphoma

这一组淋巴瘤是由大的CD30⁻多形性T细胞组成，先前或目前没有蕈样霉菌病。

临床上，患者常常表现为孤立性肿瘤或肿瘤性斑块，可以迅速进展为普遍性的皮肤病变。存活率较差。EORTC研究的36例患者中，估计5年生存率为15%[1317]。组织学上，病变由占30%以上的多形性单核细胞弥漫性浸润皮肤组成。可有也可没有扭曲的细胞核以及亲表皮现象。其中有些病变可为血管中心性的，是引起血管内淋巴瘤的原因。

免疫表型方面，肿瘤性大细胞为CD30⁻，并且CD2⁻、CD3⁻、CD4⁺。少数散在细胞CD30可呈阳性，但

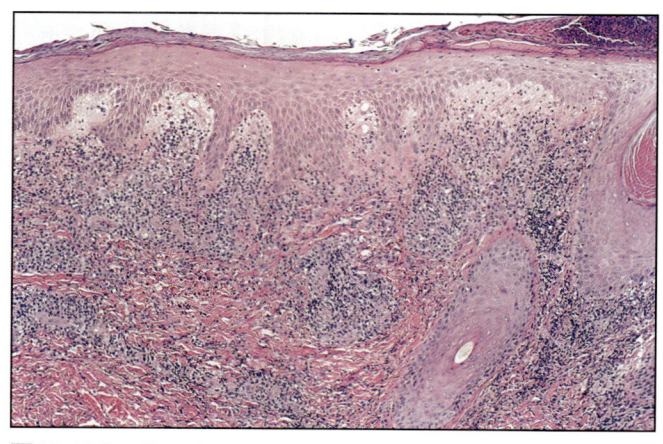

图23.190　淋巴瘤样丘疹病。楔形单核细胞浸润，含有多形性淋巴细胞。

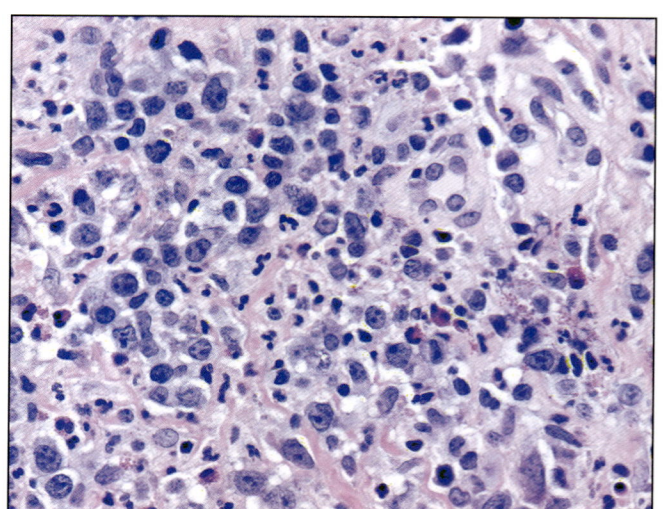

图23.191　淋巴瘤样丘疹病。这个病变中的大的多形性细胞为CD30呈阳性（A型）。

并不能说明肿瘤为 CD30 阳性。克隆性 TCR 基因重排可见于多数病例。多形性细胞或免疫母细胞成分超过 80% 的病例预后最差。

必须与多形性癌、黑色素瘤以及肉瘤进行鉴别诊断。

多形性小/中等大小细胞性淋巴瘤 [1354]
Pleomorphic small/medium-sized cell lymphoma

这在 EORTC 分类中是一个暂时性类别。它由小至中等大小的多形性 T 细胞构成。其临床表现与典型的蕈样霉菌病稍有不同。临床上，患者表现为丘疹或结节，但缺乏斑块。小样本量患者研究显示，5 年生存率大约为 60%。

组织学上，淋巴细胞在皮肤或皮下呈弥漫性生长。有些病例可出现亲表皮表现。与大细胞性 CD30 阴性淋巴瘤的不同在于其浸润性的大的多形性肿瘤细胞所占比例少于 30%。有些病例可能具有血管中心性结构；伴有多数 CD8$^+$ 细胞的血管中心性病例预后可能较差。

免疫表型方面，肿瘤细胞 CD4$^+$，但 CD2、CD3 和 CD5 表达减少或常常丧失。在少数病例中，CD8 可为阳性。CD30 呈阴性。全 B 细胞抗原 CD19、CD20 和 CD22 也为阴性。通常可见 TCR 基因克隆性重排。

鉴别诊包括普通的蕈样霉菌病，当肿瘤中混有多量 CD8$^+$ 和 CD20$^+$ 的细胞时，还应与皮肤淋巴组织增生鉴别。

肉芽肿性皮肤松弛症 [1355-1357]
Granulomatous slack skin

在 EORTC 指南中，这只是一个暂时性名称[1317]。病变为腋窝和腹股沟区皮肤缓慢形成松弛区域，主要发生于男性，预后较好。

临床上，大约 1/3 的受累患者存在 Hodgkin 淋巴瘤，但有些患者可有典型的蕈样霉菌病。

组织学上，可见弥漫性单核细胞浸润，偶尔可见多核巨细胞以及伴有扭曲细胞核的 T 淋巴细胞。皮肤弹力纤维溶解是临床特征性表现的原因（图 23.192）。

其免疫表型类似于典型的蕈样霉菌病，克隆性 TCR 重排已被证实。

由于这些患者具有明显的临床表现，因此临床相关表现对于作出正确诊断极为重要。

皮下脂膜炎样 T 细胞性淋巴瘤 [1358,1359]
Subcutaneous panniculitis-like T-cell lymphoma

在 EORTC 的分类方案中，这是一个临时性分类[1317]，由位于皮下组织的 T 细胞性淋巴瘤构成，可能伴有噬血细胞综合征。

临床上，患者表现为皮下结节及斑块，一般位于腿

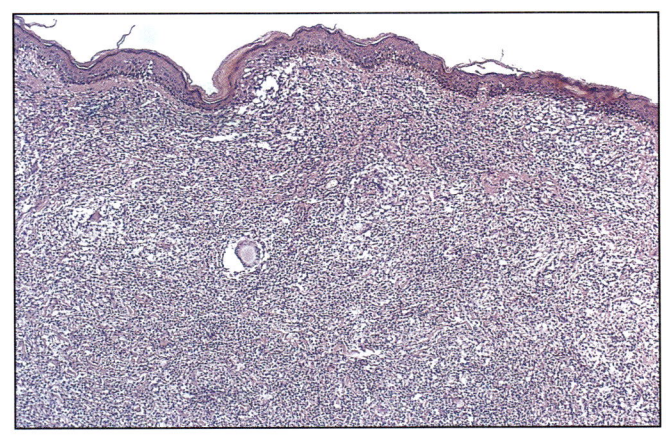

图 23.192　T 细胞型恶性淋巴瘤，肉芽肿亚型。伴有巨细胞的罕见的弥漫性结构，临床上为皮肤松弛症。

部或躯干。这种病变可能伴有诸如发热和体重减轻等征象。出现噬血细胞综合征常常预示着有迅速进展的临床经过。预后较差。伴有 CD8$^-$ 的 α/β 表型具有长期的临床经过，而不出现皮肤外播散或噬血细胞综合征。γ/δ 表型见于某些病例。这些淋巴瘤倾向于具有比较侵袭性的临床经过。在新的 WHO/EORTC 分类中，只有 γ/δ 被认为是皮下脂膜炎样 T 细胞性淋巴瘤，而 α/β T 细胞表型被纳入皮肤 α/β T 细胞性淋巴瘤的范畴[1318]。

组织学上，多形性肿瘤细胞弥漫性浸润皮下组织，并且伴有巨噬细胞以及噬红细胞表现。极少出现皮下组织以外的播散。

免疫表型为 CD3$^+$、CD4$^+$、CD8$^-$ 或 CD3$^+$、CD4$^-$、CD8$^+$。CD56 在多数病例中为阴性。TCR 基因克隆性重排可见于大约 50% 的病例。

皮肤 B 细胞性淋巴瘤　Cutaneous B-cell lymphoma

大约 20%～25% 的皮肤原发性淋巴瘤为 B 细胞性淋巴瘤。其中少数病变，尤其是边缘带型淋巴瘤，好像与博氏疏螺旋体（Borrelia Burgdorferi）感染有关，至少在英国是这样[1353a]。然而，累及皮肤的多数 B 细胞性淋巴瘤常常伴有内脏或淋巴结病变。皮肤 B 细胞性淋巴瘤的典型临床表现为斑块或结节，可为单发，也可成簇，发生于成人。组织学上，B 细胞性淋巴瘤为结节状或弥漫性（图 23.193），一般为单一形态，皮肤较深部位常常伴有多量淋巴细胞成分（"底部重"），并且常常出现皮下浸润。细胞学表现与淋巴结相应病变完全一致（见第 21 章）。令人遗憾的是，单独 HE 切片不能区分这些淋巴瘤与许多类似的良性病变，包括某些叮咬反应、反应性增生（所谓的假淋巴瘤）、某些感染性因素、某些 T 细胞性淋巴瘤、白血病浸润以及某些少见的浆细胞浸润。除非 HE 切片证据非常明确，对于多数病例来说，获得淋巴结活检或皮肤活检应用特殊染色对于确定病变类型非常有

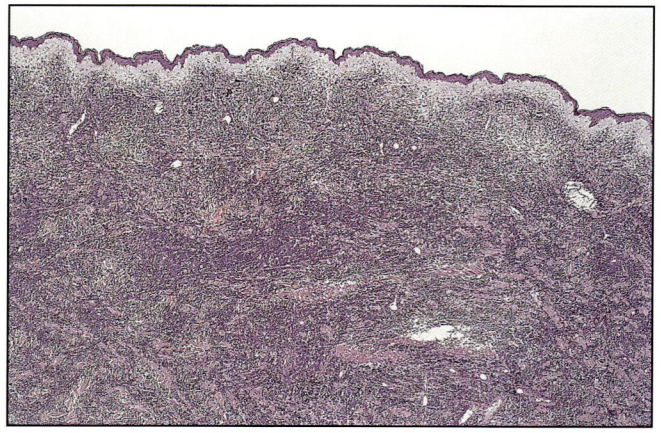

图23.193 恶性淋巴瘤,B细胞型。真皮弥漫性浸润,伴有Grenz带。

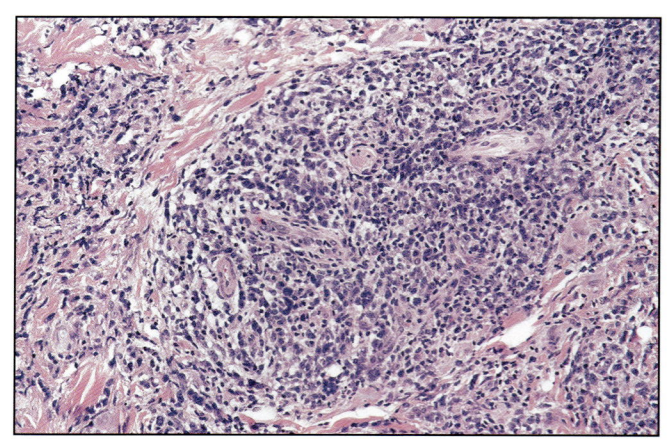

图23.195 原发性皮肤滤泡中心细胞性淋巴瘤。这个结节类似于一个生发中心。

用,如免疫球蛋白标记物、轻链以及B或T细胞系标记物[1331]。对于有些病例,基因重排分析可能有所帮助。

EORTC将皮肤原发性B细胞性淋巴瘤分为五组,他们认为其中两组为暂时性的[1317]。其他人发现REAL分类同样有用[1360]。EORTC分类亚型的特征如下:

原发性皮肤滤泡中心细胞性淋巴瘤 (primary cutaneous follicle center cell lymphoma)[1361-1364]:这是一种由滤泡中心细胞、中心细胞以及中心母细胞组成的淋巴瘤。它是原发性皮肤B细胞性淋巴瘤中的最常见类型,其临床和生物学表现均不同于发生于腿部的大细胞病变(见下文)。

临床上,患者表现为结节、丘疹、斑块和肿瘤,一般位于头颈或躯干上部。生存率一般较好,5年生存率接近100%,并且皮肤外病变并不常见。

组织学上,皮肤浸润呈结节状或弥漫性,表皮通常不受侵犯(图23.194)。结节性病变类似于淋巴结的生发中心(图23.195)。早期病变主要为中心细胞,含有或小或大的有裂细胞核,伴有少数较大的含有明显核仁的中心母细胞(图23.196)。在浸润的细胞中可以混有反应性T细胞,并且可以见到残留的反应性生发中心。晚期病变以肿瘤性表现为特征,可见大量的中心母细胞和少数反应性T细胞。迅速生长的病变可能有单一形态的中心细胞以及多分叶细胞和免疫母细胞浸润。

免疫表型方面,这些是表达CD19、CD20、CD22和CD79a的B细胞。在一些病变,这种病变可以显示也可以缺乏表面免疫球蛋白(sIg)。缺乏CD5和CD10表达。多数病例可能显示克隆性Ig基因重排。与原发性淋巴结病变不同的是:这些病例没有(14;18)易位[1365],而且通常缺乏bcl-2蛋白。

原发性皮肤免疫细胞瘤(边缘区B细胞性淋巴瘤) (primary cutaneous immunocytoma (marginal zone B-cell lymphoma)[1366-1368]:在石蜡切片中,这是一种小淋巴浆细胞样细胞、小淋巴细胞以及含有单形性胞浆免疫球蛋白(cIg)的浆细胞的淋巴瘤。它们被认为是MALT型(或皮肤相关淋巴组织型)淋巴瘤[1369]或REAL分类中的结外边缘区淋巴瘤。

临床上,患者表现为肢体的孤立性或多发性皮肤或

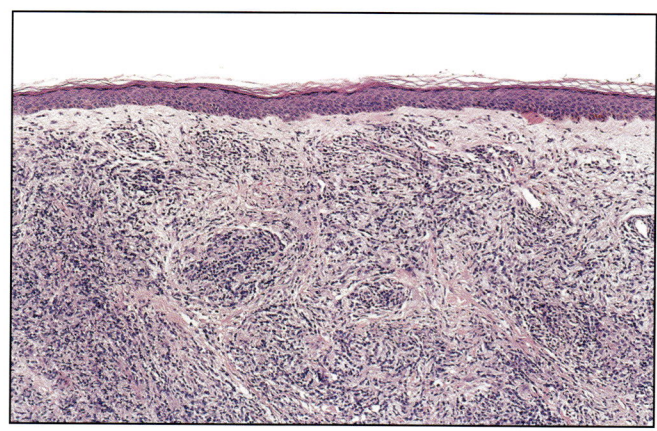

图23.194 原发性皮肤滤泡中心细胞性淋巴瘤。注意结节状生长方式。表皮不受累。

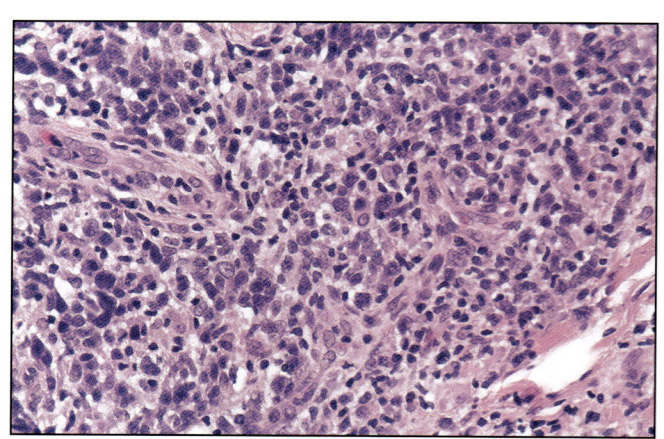

图23.196 原发性皮肤滤泡中心细胞性淋巴瘤。中心细胞性和中心母细胞性淋巴细胞。

皮下组织肿瘤。预后较好，估计 5 年生存率为 100%。

组织学上，小淋巴浆细胞样细胞、小淋巴细胞以及浆细胞呈结节状或弥漫性浸润，可以伴有中心细胞和中心母细胞。淋巴浆细胞样细胞和浆细胞一般位于浸润灶的周边，并且具有单形性表现。其中一些细胞可见 PAS 阳性的核内包涵体。

免疫表型方面，细胞含有单形性的胞浆免疫球蛋白、CD79a、CD5 呈阴性。Bcl-2 呈阳性，bcl-6 和 CD10 呈阴性[1370]。浆细胞 CD20 呈阴性。克隆性 Ig 基因重排可以见于这些病变。

腿部大 B 细胞性淋巴瘤（large B-cell lymphoma of the leg）[1371]：这些淋巴瘤位于腿部，主要含有中心母细胞和免疫母细胞。发生于腿部的皮肤弥漫性大 B 细胞性淋巴瘤比发生于其他部位的更具侵袭性[1372]。

临床上，患者一般为 71 ~ 80 岁或年纪更大的女性。病变表现为腿部的红色至蓝色的结节。尽管其组织学表现类似于滤泡中心细胞性淋巴瘤，但其预后较差，原因不明。

组织学上，病变由弥漫性浸润的非亲表皮性中心母细胞、大的中心细胞以及免疫母细胞组成，其表现类似于软组织或骨的原发性大细胞性淋巴瘤。

免疫表型为 CD19、CD20、CD22 和 CD79a 阳性。可以出现单形性的血清 Ig 和胞浆 Ig。这些病变 bcl-2 蛋白呈阳性，不同于头部和躯干的滤泡中心细胞性淋巴瘤。

血管内大 B 细胞性淋巴瘤（intravascular large B-cell lymphoma）[1373-1375]：这是 EORTC 确定的一个临时性名称，曾经被认为是一种血管内皮的病变（所谓的恶性血管内皮瘤病），但是现在知道它是血管内 B 细胞性淋巴瘤，5 年生存率相对较差，尤其是有皮肤以外部位受累的患者。患者表现为腿部和躯干的紫色斑片和斑块，常常被认为是皮下病变。

组织学上，真皮和皮下血管扩张，其内充满有些多形性的肿瘤细胞。有些病例也可出现血管外浸润。

免疫表型方面，肿瘤细胞 CD19、CD20、CD22 和 CD79a 呈阳性，伴有单形性的表面 Ig。也可有克隆性的 Ig 基因重排。

浆细胞瘤（plasmacytoma）[1376]：这是 EORTC 确定的一个临时性名称，病变发生于皮肤，表现为浆细胞呈克隆性膨胀性生长，缺乏多发性骨髓瘤。这种肿瘤极为少见，仅占髓外浆细胞瘤的 4%[1377]。临床上，病变表现为孤立性或多发性的红色至紫色的皮肤或皮下肿瘤。预后极好。

组织学上，出现成熟浆细胞以及多核浆细胞弥漫性浸润。没有克隆性淋巴细胞出现。

免疫表型为单一类型的胞浆 Ig，CD38 呈阳性。CD20 和 LCA 呈阴性。

转移　Metastasis

皮肤恶性肿瘤转移至其他部位
Malignancies of the skin metastatic to other sites

常见的皮肤恶性肿瘤，尤其是癌，只要在病变较小或较薄时将其完全切除，发生转移的机会并不很高。基底细胞癌几乎从不转移，除非病变存在多年且较大或出现深部浸润[249,260]。另一方面，鳞状细胞癌容易出现转移，尤其是当原发性病变部位较深或出现血管浸润时。当发生转移时，在广泛播散之前病变常常沿局部淋巴管引流部位转移[249,260]。如果出现播散，可以累及骨和内脏器官，如肺等[249]。

附件癌容易出现局部深层浸润，但极少发生转移性病变。容易出现转移的病变是恶性顶端汗管瘤（顶端汗腺癌）、乳头状指（趾）部腺癌[685,687]、皮脂腺癌以及 Merkel 细胞癌[752,754]。

有关黑色素瘤向局部以外播散文献中已有大量报道。切除黑色素瘤的前哨淋巴结可以相对预测多数黑色素瘤发生局部淋巴结播散，尽管尚未证实这种方法是否会影响长期生存率[1378-1380]。虽然黑色素瘤常常首先播散至局部淋巴结这一点是明确的，但是有些病例难以预料，可以发生出人意料的广泛播散。另外，有时这些病变在发现原发性肿瘤并予以治疗之后多年发生转移。

间叶性恶性肿瘤常常只出现局部侵袭。诸如皮肤纤维肉瘤或皮肤平滑肌肉瘤等极少出现继发性病变。然而，皮肤血管肉瘤常常发生转移。

恶性肿瘤转移至皮肤[1381,1382]
Malignancies metastatic to the skin

有关各种类型的恶性肿瘤转移至皮肤已有上千例报告，但多数为回顾性研究，极少有进行系统性分析确定的独特的转移类型。

估计所有癌症患者发生皮肤转移的不足 10%，但难以对不同作者的研究进行比较[1383-1385]。在 Brownstein 和 Helwig 的研究中[1383,1386,1387]，对美军病理学会（AFIP）的 724 例患者的活检进行了组织学检查。在男性，最为常见的原发性恶性肿瘤为肺癌（24%）、大肠癌（19%）、黑色素瘤（13%）以及口腔鳞状细胞癌（12%）。在女性，最为常见的原发性恶性肿瘤为乳腺癌（69%）、大肠癌（9%）、黑色素瘤（5%）以及卵巢癌（4%），尽管这项研究是在女性肺癌发生率显著增高之前进行的。躯干前部为转移性肿瘤的常见部位，而下肢皮肤受累并不常见。男性大约75%的转移性病变位于头颈前部区域，而女性75%的病变见于前胸和腹部。如果原发性肿瘤为肺癌或肾癌，转移性病变常常相对先于原发性肿瘤而被发现，但乳腺癌或口腔鳞状细胞癌极少发生这种情况。

组织学上[1382-1383]，转移性病变可以类似于原发性肿瘤，或可能有明显的多形性，以至为了提示原发肿瘤的起源需要进行免疫组织化学或超微结构分析，尤其是在不知道原发性肿瘤的情况下。一些肿瘤的生长结构比其他肿瘤更具特征性；这些肿瘤包括绒毛膜癌、肝细胞癌、精原细胞瘤、Leydig 细胞瘤以及肾细胞癌[1382]。另外，免疫组织化学对于鉴别黑色素瘤（S-100 蛋白和melan A 呈阳性）和癌（细胞角蛋白一般为阳性）可能特别有用，尤其是当应用一组试剂时。有些病变具有特征性的抗原，如前列腺腺癌（PSA）和甲状腺癌（甲状腺球蛋白、TTF-1 和降钙素），有助于鉴别诊断。超微结构分析可能有助于辨认恶性肿瘤，但目前应用不如前些年多，原因是对于免疫组织化学的依赖程度增加（见第 31 章）。如癌中可见桥粒，腺癌可见胞浆之间或胞浆内腔隙，黑色素瘤可见黑色素小体，以及类癌和神经内分泌癌中可见致密核心颗粒，这些类型的细胞器和结构可能有助于确立诊断。

尽管应用辅助技术有助于辨认特殊的病变，但是临床相关性以及密切随访也是极为重要的辅助手段，尤其是当转移性病变表现为一种体征时，因为有些原发性病变（尤其在肺）可能难以发现[1382,1383]。一旦发现了皮肤转移性病变，其预后一般极差。

参考文献

1. Goode R K, Crawford B E, Callihan M D et al. 1983 Oral melanoacanthoma. Review of the literature and report of ten cases. Oral Surg Oral Med Oral Pathol 56: 622–628
2. Vion B, Mérot Y 1989 Melanoacanthoma of the penis shaft. Dermatologica 179: 87–89
3. Simón P, Requena L, Sánchez Yus E 1991 How rare is melanoacanthoma? Arch Dermatol 127: 583–584
4. Chen M, Shinmori H, Takemiya M et al. 1990 Acantholytic variant of seborrheic keratosis. J Cutan Pathol 17: 27–31
5. Sanderson K V 1968 The structure of seborrhoeic keratoses. Br J Dermatol 80: 588–593
6. Mikhail G R, Mehregan A H 1982 Basal cell carcinoma in seborrheic keratosis. J Am Acad Dermatol 6: 500–506
7. Burgess J T, Smith W B, Keeling J H 1994 Seborrheic keratosis with trichilemmomas masquerading as melanoma. Cutis 54: 351–353.
8. Diaz Cascajo C, Reichel M, Sánchez J L 1996 Malignant neoplasms associated with seborrheic keratoses. An analysis of 54 cases. Am J Dermatopathol 18(3): 278–282
9. Maize J C, Snider R L 1995 Nonmelanoma skin cancers in association with seborrheic keratoses. Clinicopathologic correlations. Dermatol Surg 21(11):960–962
10. Mevorah B, Mishima Y 1965 Cellular response of seborrheic keratosis following croton oil irritation and surgical trauma. With special reference to melanoacanthoma. Dermatologica 131: 452–464
11. Zhu W Y, Leonardi C, Kinsey W et al. 1991 Irritated seborrheic keratoses and benign verrucous acanthomas do not contain papillomavirus DNA. J Cutan Pathol 18: 449–452
12. Tagami H, Yamada M 1978 Seborrheic keratosis: an acantholytic variant. J Cutan Pathol 5: 145–149
13. Mishima Y, Pinkus H 1960 Benign mixed tumor of melanocytes and malpighian cells. Melanoacanthoma: its relationship to Bloch's benign non-nevoid melanoepithelioma. Arch Dermatol 81: 539–550
14. Rahbari H 1979 Bowenoid transformation of seborrhoeic verrucae (keratoses). Br J Dermatol 101: 459–463
15. Helwig E B 1955 Inverted follicular keratosis. In: Proceedings, twentieth seminar of the American Society of Clinical Pathologists, International Congress of Clinical Pathology, 1954. American Society of Clinical Pathologists, Washington, DC
16. Spielvogel R L, Austin C, Ackerman A B 1983 Inverted follicular keratosis is not a specific keratosis but a verruca vulgaris (or seborrheic keratosis) with squamous eddies. Am J Dermatopathol 5: 427–442
17. Lund H Z 1983 The nosologic position of inverted follicular keratosis is still unsettled. Am J Dermatopathol 5: 443–445
18. Moehlenbeck F W 1983 Inverted follicular keratosis. A morbis sui generis? Am J Dermatopathol 5: 471–472
19. Möhlenbeck F W 1975 Inverted follicular keratosis. Hautarzt 26: 21–24
20. Azzopardi J G, Laurini R 1975 Inverted follicular keratosis. J Clin Pathol 28: 465–471
21. Boniuk M, Zimmerman L E 1963 Eyelid tumors with reference to lesions confused with squamous cell carcinoma. II. Inverted follicular keratosis. Arch Ophthalmol 69: 698–707
22. Adrian J C 1984 Inverted follicular keratosis of the lip. Oral Surg Oral Med Oral Pathol 57(6): 625–630
23. Mehregan A H 1964 Inverted follicular keratosis. Arch Dermatol 89: 229–235
24. Schweitzer J G, Yanoff M 1987 Inverted follicular keratosis. A report of two recurrent cases. Ophthalmology 94: 1465–1468
25. Mehregan A H 1983 Inverted follicular keratosis is a distinct follicular tumor. Am J Dermatopathol 5: 467–470
26. Sim-Davis D, Marks R, Wilson-Jones E 1976 The inverted follicular keratosis. A surprising variant of seborrheic wart. Acta Dermato-Venereol 56: 337–344
27. Draluck J C, Ackerman A B 1990 Squamous eddies are spirals of sebaceous ducts [abstract]. Am J Dermatopathol 12: 309
28. Hori K 1991 Inverted follicular keratosis and papillomavirus infection. Am J Dermatopathol 13: 145–151
29. Mehregan A H, Nadji M 1984 Inverted follicular keratosis and verruca vulgaris. An investigation for the papillomavirus common antigen. J Cutan Pathol 11: 99–102
30. Findlay G H 1989 Multiple infundibular tumours of the head and neck. Br J Dermatol 120: 33–638
31. Barnette D J Jr, Cobb M 1995 A solitary, erythematous, hyperkeratotic papule. Acantholytic acanthoma. Arch Dermatol 131(2): 211–212, 214–215
32. Brownstein M H 1985 The benign acanthomas. J Cutan Pathol 12(3–4): 172–188
33. Brownstein M H 1988 Acantholytic acanthoma. J Am Acad Dermatol 19(5 Pt 1): 783–786
34. Megahed M, Scharffetter-Kochanek K 1993 Acantholytic acanthoma. Am J Dermatopathol 15(3): 283–285
35. Griffiths T W, Hashimoto K, Sharata H H et al. 1997 Multiple warty dyskeratomas of the scalp. Clin Exp Dermatol 22:89–191
36. Panja R K 1977 Warty dyskeratoma. J Cutan Pathol 4(4): 194–200
37. Rubenstein M H, Harrist T J 1981 Pathology quiz case 1: warty dyskeratoma. Arch Dermatol 117(11): 746–748
38. Degos R, Delort J, Civatte J et al. 1962 Tumeur épidermique d'aspect particulier: Acanthome a cellules claires. Ann Dermatol Syphiligr (Paris) 89: 361–371
39. Degos R, Civatte J 1970 Clear-cell acanthoma. Experience of 8 years. Br J Dermatol 83: 248–254
40. Burg G, Wursch T, Fah J et al. 1994 Eruptive hamartomatous clear-cell acanthomas. Dermatology 189(4): 437–439
41. Desmons F, Breullard F, Thomas P et al. 1977 Multiple clear-cell acanthoma (Degos): histochemical and ultrastructural study of two cases. Int J Dermatol 16: 203–213
42. Goette DK, Diakon NC 1983 Multiple clear cell acanthomas. Arch Dermatol 119(4): 359–361
43. Innocenzi D, Barduagni F, Cerio R et al. 1994 Disseminated eruptive clear cell acanthoma – a case report with review of the literature. Clin Exp Dermatol 19(3): 249–253
44. Naeyaert J M, de Bersaques J, Geerts M L et al. 1987 Multiple clear cell acanthomas. A clinical, histological, and ultrastructural report. Arch Dermatol 123(12): 1670–1673
45. Trau H, Fisher B K, Schewach-Millet M 1980 Multiple clear cell acanthomas. Arch Dermatol 116: 433–434
46. Williams R E A, Lever R, Seywright M 1989 Multiple clear cell acanthomas – treatment by cryotherapy. Clin Exp Dermatol 14: 300–301

47. Zak F G, Martinez M, Statsinger A L 1966 Pale cell acanthoma. Arch Dermatol 93(6): 674–678
48. Fine R M, Chernosky M E 1969 Clinical recognition of clear-cell acanthoma (Degos'). Arch Dermatol 100: 559–562
49. Petzelbauer P, Konrad K 1990 Polypous clear cell acanthoma. Am J Dermatopathol 12: 393–395
50. Grossin M, Mazer J-M, Auffret N et al. 1983 Formes rares de l'acanthome a cellules claires. Ann Dermatol Syphiligr (Paris) 110: 721–722
51. Roytman M, Frumkin A, Everett M A 1987 Giant clear cell acanthoma. J Am Acad Dermatol 17: 513–514
52. Betti R, Bruscagin C, Inselvini E et al. 1995 Successful cryotherapic treatment and overview of multiple clear cell acanthomas. Dermatol Surg 21(4): 342–344
53. Hashimoto T, Inamoto N, Nakamura K 1988 Two cases of clear cell acanthoma: an immunohistochemical study. J Cutan Pathol 15: 27–30
54. Brownstein M H, Fernando S, Shapiro L 1973 Clear cell acanthoma: clinicopathologic analysis of 37 new cases. Am J Clin Pathol 59: 306–311
55. Hamaguchi T, Penneys N 1995 Cystic clear cell acanthoma. J Cutan Pathol 22(2): 188–190
56. Grunwald M H, Rothem A, Halevy S 1991 Atypical clear cell acanthoma. Int J Dermatol 30(12): 848–850
57. Wells C G, Wilson-Jones E 1967 Degos' acanthoma (acanthome à cellules claires). Br J Dermatol 79: 249–258
58. Fanti P A, Passarini B, Varotti C 1990 Melanocytes in clear cell acanthoma. Am J Dermatopathol 12: 373–376
59. Langer K, Wuketich S, Konrad K 1994 Pigmented clear cell acanthoma. Am J Dermatopathol 16(2): 134–139
60. Pierard G E 1991 Melanocytes in clear cell acanthoma (letter; comment). Am J Dermatopathol 13(4): 430
61. Pierard G E 1986 Mélanoacanthome a cellules claires. Ann Dermatol Venereol 113: 253–255
62. Ohnishi T, Watanabe S 1995 Immunohistochemical characterization of keratin expression in clear cell acanthoma. Br J Dermatol 133(2): 186–193
63. Akiyama M, Hayakawa K, Watanabe Y et al. 1990 Lectin binding sites in clear cell acanthoma. J Cutan Pathol 17: 197–201
64. Hu F, Sisson J K 1969 The ultrastructure of the pale cell acanthoma. J Invest Dermatol 52: 185–188
65. Wilson Jones E, Wells G C 1966 Degos' acanthoma (acanthome a cellules claires). A clinical and histological report of nine cases. Arch Dermatol 94: 286–294
66. Cramer H-J 1971 Klarzellenakanthom (Degos) mit syringomatösen und naevus-sebaceus-artigen anteilen. Dermatologica 143: 265–270
67. Cohen P R, Ulmer R, Theriault A et al. 1997 Epidermolytic acanthomas: clinical characteristics and immunohistochemical features. Am J Dermatopathol 19(3): 232–241
68. Reichel M 1999 Hypergranulotic dyscornification. A distinctive histologic pattern of maturation of epidermal epithelium present in solitary keratoses. Am J Dermatopathol 21(1): 21–24
69. Shapiro L, Baraf C S 1970 Isolated epidermolytic acanthoma. A solitary tumor showing granular degeneration. Arch Dermatol 101: 220–223
70. Ackerman A B 1970 Histopathologic concept of epidermolytic hyperkeratosis. Arch Dermatol 102: 253–259
71. Niizuma K 1979 Isolated epidermolytic acanthoma. A histological study. Dermatologica 159: 30–36
72. DeConinck A, Willemsen M, DeDobbeleer G et al. 1986 Vulvar localisation of epidermolytic acanthoma. A light- and electron-microscopic study. Dermatologica 172: 276–278
73. Hirone T, Fukushiro R 1973 Disseminated epidermolytic acanthoma. Nonsystematized multiple verrucoid lesions showing granular degeneration. Acta Dermato-Venereol 53: 393–402
74. Knipper J E, Hud J A, Cockerell C J 1993 Disseminated epidermolytic acanthoma. Am J Dermatopathol 15(1): 70–72
75. Leonardi C, Zhu W, Kinsey W et al. 1991 Epidermolytic acanthoma does not contain human papillomavirus DNA. J Cutan Pathol 18: 103–105
76. Beutner K R 1989 Human papillomavirus infection. J Am Acad Dermatol 20: 114–123
77. Cobb M W 1990 Human papillomavirus infection. J Am Acad Dermatol 22: 547–566
78. zur Hausen H 1996 Papillomavirus infections – a major cause of human cancers. Biochim Biophys Acta 1288(2) F55–F78
79. Stanley M 2003 Genital human papillomavirus infections – current and prospective therapies. J Natl Cancer Inst Monogr (31): 117–124
80. Nuovo G J, Hochman H A, Eliezri Y D et al. 1990 Detection of human papillomavirus DNA in penile lesions histologically negative for condyloma. Am J Surg Pathol 14(9): 829–836
81. Li J, Ackerman A B 1994 "Seborrheic keratoses" that contain human papillomavirus are condylomata acuminata. Am J Dermatopathol 16(4): 398–405; discussion 406–408
82. Aloi F, Tomasini C, Pippione M 1992 HPV-related follicular cysts. Am J Dermatopathol 14(1): 37–41
83. Egawa K, Honda Y, Inaba Y et al. 1995 Detection of human papillomaviruses and eccrine ducts in palmoplantar epidermoid cysts. Br J Dermatol 132(4): 533–542
84. Egawa K, Kitasato H, Honda Y et al. 1998 Human papillomavirus 57 identified in a plantar epidermoid cyst. Br J Dermatol 138(3): 510–514
85. Kato N, Ueno H 1992 Two cases of plantar epidermal cyst associated with human papillomavirus. Clin Exp Dermatol 17(4): 252–256
86. Soyer H P, Schadendorf D, Cerroni L et al. 1993 Verrucous cysts: histopathologic characterization and molecular detection of human papillomavirus-specific DNA. J Cutan Pathol 20(5): 411–417
87. Cohen B A, Honig P, Androphy E 1990 Anogenital warts in children. Clinical and virologic evaluation for sexual abuse. Arch Dermatol 126: 1575–1580
88. Obalek S, Jablonska S, Favre M et al. 1990 Condylomata acuminata in children: frequent association with human papillomaviruses responsible for cutaneous warts. J Am Acad Dermatol 23(2 Pt 1): 205–213
89. Wade T R, Ackerman A B 1984 The effects of resin of podophyllin on condyloma acuminatum. Am J Dermatopathol 6: 109–122
90. Beckman A M, Daling J R, Sherman K J et al. 1989 Human papillomavirus infection and anal cancer. Int J Cancer 43: 1042–1049
91. Duggan M A, Boras V F, Inoue M et al. 1989 Human papillomavirus DNA determination of anal condylomata, dysplasias, and squamous carcinomas with in situ hybridization. Am J Clin Pathol 92: 16–21
92. Gal A A, Saul S H, Stoler M H 1989 In situ hybridization analysis of human papillomavirus in anal squamous cell carcinoma. Mod Pathol 2: 439–443
93. Valente P T, Hurt M A, Jelen I 1991 Human papillomavirus-associated vulvar verrucous carcinoma in a 20-year-old with an intact hymen. A case report. J Reprod Med 36: 213–216
94. Lupulescu A, Mehregan A H, Rahbari H et al. 1977 Venereal warts vs Bowen disease. J Am Med Assoc 237: 2520–2522
95. Park K-C, Kim K-H, Youn S-W. 1998 Heterogeneity of human papillomavirus DNA in a patient with Bowenoid papulosis that progressed to squamous cell carcinoma. Br J Dermatol 139: 1087–1091
96. Steffen C 1982 Concurrence of condylomata acuminata and bowenoid papulosis. Confirmation of the hypothesis that they are related conditions. Am J Dermatopathol 4: 5–8
97. Majewski S, Jablonska S 1995 Epidermodysplasia verruciformis as a model of human papillomavirus-induced genetic cancer of the skin. Arch Dermatol 131(11): 1312–1318.
98. Majewski S, Jablonska S 1997 Human papillomavirus-associated tumors of the skin and mucosa. J Am Acad Dermatol 36(5 Pt 1): 659–685
99. Ostrow R S, Bender M, Niimura M et al. 1982 Human papillomavirus DNA in cutaneous primary and metastasized squamous cell carcinomas from patients with epidermodysplasia verruciformis. Proc Natl Acad Sci USA 79: 1634–1638
100. Berger T G, Sawchuk W S, Leonardi C et al. 1991 Epidermodysplasia verruciformis-associated papillomavirus infection complicating human immunodeficiency virus disease. Br J Dermatol 124: 79–83
101. Tomasini C, Aloi F, Pippione M 1993 Seborrheic keratosis-like lesions in epidermodysplasia verruciformis. J Cutan Pathol 20(3): 237–241
102. Feuerman E J, Sandbank M, David M 1979 Two siblings with epidermodysplasia verruciformis with large clear cells in the epidermis: electron microscope and immunological findings. Acta Dermato-Venereol 59: 513–520
103. Jablonska S, Orth G, Jarzabek-Chorzelska M et al. 1979 Epidermodysplasia verruciformis versus disseminated verrucae planae: is epidermodysplasia verruciformis a generalized infection with wart virus? J Invest Dermatol 72: 114–119
104. Epstein W L 1992 Molluscum contagiosum. Semin Dermatol 11(3): 184–189
105. Mehregan A H 1961 Molluscum contagiosum. A clinicopathological study. Arch Dermatol 84: 123–127
106. Reed R J, Parkinson R P 1977 The histogenesis of molluscum contagiosum. Am J Surg Pathol 1: 161–166
107. Lombardo P C 1985 Molluscum contagiosum and the acquired immunodificiency syndrome. Arch Dermatol 121: 834–835
108. Fivenson D P, Weltman R E, Gibson S H 1988 Giant molluscum contagiosum presenting as basal cell carcinoma in an acquired immunodeficiency syndrome patient. J Am Acad Dermatol 19: 912–914
109. Ackerman A B, Tanski E V 1977 Pseudoleukemia cutis: report of a case in association with molluscum contagiosum. Cancer 40: 813–817
110. de Diego J, Berridi D, Saracibar N et al. 1998 Cutaneous pseudolymphoma in association with molluscum contagiosum. Am J Dermatopathol 20(5): 518–521
111. Guitart J, Hurt M A 1999 Pleomorphic T-cell infiltrate associated with molluscum contagiosum. Am J Dermatopathol 21(2): 178–180
112. Freeman R G 1974 On the pathogenesis of pseudoepitheliomatous hyperplasia. J Cutan Pathol 1: 231–237
113. Grunwald M H, Lee J Y-Y, Ackerman A B 1988 Pseudocarcinomatous hyperplasia. Am J Dermatopathol 10: 95–103
114. Bhawan J, Malhotra R 1990 Syringosquamous metaplasia. A distinctive eruption in patients receiving chemotherapy. Am J Dermatopathol 12(1): 1–6
115. Cribier B, Lipsker D, Grosshans E 1993 Squamous syringometaplasia: an original manifestation of pathomimesis. Ann Dermatol Venereol 120(12): 900–903
116. Helton J L, Metcalf J S 1995 Squamous syringometaplasia in association with annular elastolytic granuloma. Am J Dermatopathol 17(4): 407–409
117. Hurt M A, Igra-Serfaty H, Stevens C S 1990 Eccrine syringofibroadenoma (Mascaró). An acrosyringeal hamartoma. Arch Dermatol 126(7): 945–949
118. Rios-Buceta L, Penas P F, Dauden-Tello E et al. 1995 Recall phenomenon with the unusual presence of eccrine squamous syringometaplasia. Br J Dermatol 133(4): 630–632

119. Rongioletti F, Rebora A 1992 Eccrine squamous syringometaplasia in chemotherapy-induced acral erythema (letter to the editor). J Am Acad Dermatol 26(2 Pt 1): 284
120. Serrano T, Saez A, Moreno A 1993 Eccrine squamous syringometaplasia. A prospective clinicopathologic study. J Cutan Pathol 20(1): 61–65
121. Valks R, Fraga J, Porras-Luque J et al. 1997 Chemotherapy-induced eccrine squamous syringometaplasia. A distinctive eruption in patients receiving hematopoietic progenitor cells. Arch Dermatol 133(7): 873–878
122. Weber P J, Johnson B L, Dzubow L M 1989 Pseudoepitheliomatous hyperplasia following Mohs micrographic surgery. J Dermatol Surg Oncol 15: 557–560
123. Scott G, Chen K T K, Rosai J 1989 Pseudoepitheliomatous hyperplasia in Spitz nevi. A possible source of confusion with squamous cell carcinoma. Arch Pathol Lab Med 113: 61–63
124. Alexander J, Theaker J M 1991 An unusual solitary circumscribed neuroma (palisaded encapsulated neuroma) of the skin – with observations on the nature of pseudo-epitheliomatous hyperplasia. Histopathology 18: 175–177
125. DiLeonardo M 1996 Pseudocarcinomatous hyperplasia vs. squamous-cell carcinoma. Dermatopathol Pract Concept 2(1): 45
126. Stern J B, Haupt H M 1990 Reexcision perineural invasion. Not a sign of malignancy. Am J Surg Pathol 14: 183–185
127. Kern W H, McCray M K 1980 The histopathologic differentiation of keratoacanthoma and squamous cell carcinoma. J Cutan Pathol 7: 318–325
128. Rook A, Whimster I 1979 Keratoacanthoma – a thirty year retrospect. Br J Dermatol 100: 41–47
129. Cain C T, Niemann T H, Argenyi Z B 1995 Keratoacanthoma versus squamous cell carcinoma. An immunohistochemical reappraisal of p53 protein and proliferating cell nuclear antigen expression in keratoacanthoma-like tumors. Am J Dermatopathol 17(4): 324–331
130. Hodak E, Jones R E, Ackerman A B 1993 Solitary keratoacanthoma is a squamous-cell carcinoma: three examples with metastases. Am J Dermatopathol 15(4): 332–342
131. Dufresne R G, Marrero G M, Robinson-Bostom L 1997 Seasonal presentation of keratoacanthomas in Rhode Island. Br J Dermatol 136(2): 227–229
132. Reed R J 1972 Actinic keratoacanthoma. Arch Dermatol 106: 858–864
133. Schnitzler L, Schubert B, Verret J-L et al. 1977 Épithéliomatose familiale de Ferguson-Smith. Ann Dermatol Venereol 104: 206–216
134. Allen C A, Stephens M, Steel W M 1994 Subungual keratoacanthoma. Histopathology 25(2): 181–183
135. Oliwiecki S, Peachey R D, Bradfield J W et al. 1994 Subungual keratoacanthoma – a report of four cases and review of the literature. Clin Exp Dermatol 19(3): 230–235
136. Stoll D M, Ackerman A B 1980 Subungual keratoacanthoma. Am J Dermatopathol 2(3): 265–271
137. King D F, Barr R J 1980 Intraepithelial elastic fibers and intracytoplasmic glycogen: diagnostic aids in differentiating keratoacanthoma from squamous cell carcinoma. J Cutan Pathol 7: 140–148
138. Cooper P H, Wolfe J T III 1988 Perioral keratoacanthomas with extensive perineural invasion and intravenous growth. Arch Dermatol 124(9): 1397–1401
139. Lapins N A, Helwig E B 1980 Perineural invasion by keratoacanthoma. Arch Dermatol 116: 791–793
140. Calonje E, Wilson Jones E 1992 Intravascular spread of keratoacanthoma. An alarming but benign phenomenon. Am J Dermatopathol 14(5): 414–417
141. LeBoit P E 1995 Is keratoacanthoma a variant of squamous cell carcinoma. New insights into an old controversy… soon? Am J Dermatopathol 17(4): 319–320
142. Kerschmann R L, McCalmont T H, LeBoit P E 1994 p53 oncoprotein expression and proliferation index in keratoacanthoma and squamous cell carcinoma. Arch Dermatol 130(2): 181–186
143. Lee Y S, Teh M 1994 p53 expression in pseudoepitheliomatous hyperplasia, keratoacanthoma, and squamous cell carcinoma of skin. Cancer 73(9): 2317–2323
144. Sleater J P, Beers B B, Stephens C A et al. 1994 Keratoacanthoma: a deficient squamous cell carcinoma? Study of bcl-2 expression. J Cutan Pathol 21(6): 514–519
145. Krunic A L, Garrod D R, Smith N P et al. 1996 Differential expression of desmosomal glycoproteins in keratoacanthoma and squamous cell carcinoma of the skin: an immunohistochemical aid to diagnosis. Acta Dermato-Venereol 76(5): 394–398
146. Ackerman A B, Parsons L 1997 Respect at last for solar keratosis (editorial). Dermatopathol Pract Concept 3(2): 101–103
147. Schwartz R A 1996 Premalignant keratinocytic neoplasms. J Am Acad Dermatol 35(2 Pt 1): 223–242
148. Schwartz R A 1997 The actinic keratosis. A perspective and update. Dermatol Surg 23(11): 1009–1019; quiz 1020–1021
149. Chernosky M E, Freeman R G 1967 Disseminated superficial actinic porokeratosis (DSAP). Arch Dermatol 96: 611–624
150. Shumack S, Commens C, Kossard S 1991 Disseminated superficial actinic porokeratosis. A histological review of 61 cases with particular reference to lymphocytic inflammation. Am J Dermatopathol 13: 26–31
151. Shumack S P, Commens C A 1989 Disseminated superficial actinic porokeratosis: a clinical study. J Am Acad Dermatol 20: 1015–1022
152. Cawley E P, Curtis A C, Staib G 1950 Lentigo senilis. Arch Dermatol Syphilol (Chicago) 62: 635–641
153. Miescher G, Häberlin L, Guggenheim L 1936 Über fleckförmige alterspigmenteirungen: ihre beziehungen zur melanotischen präcancerose und zur senilen warze. Arch Dermatol Syph 174: 105–125
154. Hodgson C 1963 Senile lentigo. Arch Dermatol 87: 197–207
155. Montagna W, Hu F, Carlisle K 1980 A reinvestigation of solar lentigines. Arch Dermatol 116: 1151–1154
156. DiLeonardo M 1998 Simple lentigo vs. labial lentigo vs. reticulated melanotic macule. Dermatopathol Pract Concept 4(2): 142–143
157. Sánchez J 1998 A unifying concept of melanotic macule. Dermatopathol Pract Concept 4(2): 120–123
158. Mehregan A H 1975 Lentigo senilis and its evolutions. J Invest Dermatol 65: 429–433
159. Ambrojo P, Aguilar A, Requena L et al. 1990 Achromic verrucous large cell acanthoma. J Cutan Pathol 17: 182–184
160. Argenyi Z B, Huston B M, Argenyi E E et al. 1994 Large-cell acanthoma of the skin. A study by image analysis cytometry and immunohistochemistry. Am J Dermatopathol 16(2): 140–144
161. Fand S B, Pinkus H K B 1970 Polyploidy in benign epidermal neoplasia [abstract]. J Cell Biol 47: 59a–60a
162. Pinkus H 1970 Epidermal mosaic in benign and precancerous neoplasia (with special reference to large-cell acanthoma). Acta Dermatol (Kyoto) 65: 75–81
163. Rabinowitz A D, Inghirami G 1992 Large-cell acanthoma. A distinctive keratosis. Am J Dermatopathol 14(2): 136–138
164. Rahbari H, Pinkus H 1978 Large cell acanthoma. One of the actinic keratoses. Arch Dermatol 114: 49–52
165. Roewert H J, Ackerman A B 1992 Large-cell acanthoma is a solar lentigo. Am J Dermatopathol 14(2): 122–132
166. Sánchez Yus E, de Diego V, Urrutia S 1988 Large cell acanthoma. A cytologic variant of Bowen's disease? Am J Dermatopathol 10: 197–208
167. Sánchez Yus E, del Rio E, Requena L 1992 Large-cell acanthoma is a distinctive condition. Am J Dermatopathol 14(2): 140–147
168. Sherertz E F, Hess S P, White W L 1991 Perplexing pigmented papules simulating malignant melanoma [large cell acanthoma]. Cutis 47: 97–100
169. Weinstock M A 1992 Large-cell acanthoma. Am J Dermatopathol 14(2): 133–134
170. Rabinowitz A D 1983 Multiple large cell acanthomas. J Am Acad Dermatol 8: 840–845
171. Freundenthal W 1926 Verruca senilis und keratoma senilis. Arch Dermatol Syph 152: 505–528
172. Nicolau S G, Balus L 1964 Chronic actinic cheilitis and cancer of the lower lip. Br J Dermatol 76: 278–289
173. Marks R 1990 Solar keratoses. Br J Dermatol Suppl 35: 49–54
174. Billano R A, Little W A 1982 Hypertrophic actinic keratosis. J Am Acad Dermatol 7: 484–489
175. James M P, Wells G C, Whimster I W 1978 Spreading pigmented actinic keratoses. Br J Dermatol 98: 373–379
176. Lubritz R R, Smolewski S A 1982 Cryosurgery cure rate of actinic keratosis. J Am Acad Dermatol 7: 631–632
177. Pinkus H 1958 Keratosis senilis. A biologic concept of its pathogenesis and diagnosis based on the study of normal epidermis and 1730 seborrheic and senile keratoses. Am J Clin Pathol 29: 193–207
178. Wade T R, Ackerman A B 1978 The many faces of solar keratoses. J Dermatol Surg Oncol 4: 730–734
179. Ackerman A B, Reed R J 1973 Epidermolytic variant of solar keratosis. Arch Dermatol 107: 104–106
180. Carapeto F J, García-Pérez A 1974 Acantholytic keratosis. Dermatologica 148: 233–239
181. Frigy A F, Cooper P H 1985 Benign lichenoid keratosis. Am J Clin Pathol 83: 439–443
182. Jones R E Jr 1984 Questions to the editorial board and other authorities. What is the boundary that separates a thick solar keratosis and a thin squamous-cell carcinoma? Am J Dermatopathol 6: 301–306
183. Bowen J T 1983 Centennial paper. May 1912 (J Cutan Dis Syph 1912 30: 241–255). Precancerous dermatoses: a study of two cases of chronic atypical epithelial proliferation. By John T. Bowen, MD, Boston. Arch Dermatol 119(3): 243–260
184. Degos R, Civatte J, Belaich S et al. 1976 Maladie de Bowen cutanée ou muqueuse. A propos de 243 cas. Ann Dermatol Syphiligr (Paris) 103(1): 5–14
185. Ackerman A B 1979 Carcinoma in situ. Hum Pathol 10: 127–128
186. DiLeonardo M 1997 Solar keratosis vs. Bowen's disease vs. Bowenoid papulosis. Dermatopathol Pract Concept 3(2): 130–131
187. Feldman S B, Sexton F M, Glenn J D et al. 1989 Immunosupression in men with bowenoid papulosis. Arch Dermatol 125: 651–654
188. Kwittken J 1982 Genital keratinocytic dysplasia. Mt Sinai J Med 49: 289–296
189. Lloyd K M 1970 Multicentric pigmented Bowen's disease of the groin. Arch Dermatol 101: 48–51
190. Obalek S, Jablonska S, Beaudenon S et al. 1986 Bowenoid papulosis of the male and female genitalia: risk of cervical neoplasia. J Am Acad Dermatol 14: 433–444
191. Patterson J W, Kao G F, Graham J H et al. 1986 Bowenoid papulosis. A clinicopathologic study with ultrastructural observations. Cancer 57: 823–836
192. Schwartz R A, Janniger C K 1991 Bowenoid papulosis. J Am Acad Dermatol 24: 261–264

193. Sweidan N A A, Salman S M, Zaynoun S T et al. 1990 Linear bowenoid papulosis of the genitalia. Int J Dermatol 29: 430–431
194. Wade T R, Kopf A W, Ackerman A B 1978 Bowenoid papulosis of the penis. Cancer 42: 1890–1903
195. Wade T R, Kopf A W, Ackerman A B 1979 Bowenoid papulosis of the genitalia. Arch Dermatol 115: 306–308
196. Weitzner J M, Fields K W, Robinson M J 1989 Pediatric bowenoid papulosis: risks and management. Pediatr Dermatol 6: 303–305
197. Rüdlinger R, Grob R, Yu Y X et al. 1989 Human papillomavirus-35-positive bowenoid papulosis of the anogenital area and concurrent human papillomavirus-35-positive verruca with bowenoid dysplasia of the periungual area. Arch Dermatol 125: 655–659
198. Bonnekoh B, Mahrle G, Steigleder G K 1986 Übergang in kutanes plattenepithelkarzinom bei zwei patienten mit bowenoider papulose (HPV-16). Z Hautkr 62: 773–785
199. Rüdlinger R, Buchmann P 1989 HPV 16-positive bowenoid papulosis and squamous-cell carcinoma of the anus in an HIV-positive man. Dis Colon Rectum 32: 1042–1045
200. Strayer D S, Santa Cruz D J 1980 Carcinoma in situ of the skin: a review of histopathology. J Cutan Pathol 7: 244–259
201. Fulling K H, Strayer D S, Santa Cruz D J 1981 Adnexal metaplasia in carcinoma in situ of the skin. J Cutan Pathol 8: 79–88
202. Penneys N S, Mogollon R J, Nadji M et al. 1984 Papillomavirus common antigens. Papillomavirus antigen in verruca, benign papillomatous lesions, trichilemmoma, and bowenoid papulosis: an immunoperoxidase study. Arch Dermatol 120: 859–861
203. Kane C L, Keehn C A, Smithberger E et al. 2004 Histopathology of cutaneous squamous cell carcinoma and its variants. Semin Cutan Med Surg 23(1): 54–61
204. Perez G L, Randle H W 1995 Natural history of squamous cell carcinoma of the skin: case report. Cutis 55(1): 34–36
205. Breuninger H, Black B, Rassner G 1990 Microstaging of squamous cell carcinomas. Am J Clin Pathol 94: 624–627
206. Ghiselli R W 1990 On the microstaging of skin cancer. Am J Clin Pathol 94: 661–662
207. Clayman G L, Lee J J, Holsinger F C et al. 2005 Mortality risk from squamous cell skin cancer. J Clin Oncol 23: 759–765
208. Yip K M H, Lin-Yip J, Kumta S et al. 1997 Subcutaneous ("inverted") verrucous carcinoma with bone invasion. Am J Dermatopathol 19(1): 83–86
209. Nappi O, Pettinato G, Wick M R 1989 Adenoid (acantholytic) squamous cell carcinoma of the skin. J Cutan Pathol 16: 114–121
210. Cockayne S E, Shah H, Slater D N et al. 1998 Spindle and pseudoglandular squamous cell carcinoma arising in lichen sclerosus of the vulva. Br J Dermatol 138(4): 695–697
211. Nappi O, Wick M R, Pettinato G et al. 1992 Pseudovascular adenoid squamous cell carcinoma of the skin. A neoplasm that may be mistaken for angiosarcoma. Am J Surg Pathol 16: 429–438
212. Cramer S F, Heggeness L M 1989 Signet-ring squamous cell carcinoma. Am J Clin Pathol 91: 488–491
213. McKinley E, Valles R, Bang R et al. 1998 Signet-ring squamous cell carcinoma: a case report. J Cutan Pathol 25(3): 176–181
214. Landman G, Taylor R M, Friedmen K J 1990 Cutaneous papillary squamous cell carcinoma. J Cutan Pathol 17: 105–110
215. Patel N K, McKee P H, Smith N P et al. 1997 Primary metaplastic carcinoma (carcinosarcoma) of the skin. A clinicopathologic study of four cases and review of the literature. Am J Dermatopathol 19(4): 363–372
216. Brownstein M H, Shapiro L 1976 Verrucous carcinoma of skin. Cancer 38: 1710–1716
217. Kao G F, Graham J H, Helwig E B 1982 Carcinoma cuniculatum (verrucous carcinoma of the skin). A clinicopathologic study of 46 cases with ultrastructural observations. Cancer 49: 2395–2403
218. McKee P H, Wilkinson J D, Black M M et al. 1981 Carcinoma (epithelioma) cuniculatum: a clinico-pathological study of nineteen cases and review of the literature. Histopathology 5: 425–436
219. Prioleau P G, Santa Cruz D J, Meyer J S et al. 1980 Verrucous carcinoma. A light and electron microscopic, autoradiographic, and immunofluorescence study. Cancer 45: 2849–2857
220. Cuesta K H, Palazzo J P, Mittal K R 1998 Detection of human papillomavirus in verrucous carcinoma from HIV-seropositive patients. J Cutan Pathol 25: 165–170
221. Noel J C, Peny M O, Goldschmidt D et al. 1993 Human papillomavirus type 1 DNA in verrucous carcinoma of the leg. J Am Acad Dermatol 29(6): 1036–1038
222. Miller S J 1991 Biology of basal cell carcinoma (part I). J Am Acad Dermatol 24: 1–13
223. Howell J B, Anderson D E 1982 "The basal-cell nevus" by Howell and Caro, January 1959. Commentary: The nevoid basal cell carcinoma syndrome. Arch Dermatol 118(10): 813–826
224. Howell J B, Caro M R 1959 The basal-cell nevus. A.M.A. Arch Dermatol 79(1): 67–80
225. Horlock N M, Wilson G D, Daley F M et al. 1997 Cellular proliferation characteristics of basal cell carcinoma: relationship to clinical subtype and histopathology. Eur J Surg Oncol 23(3): 247–252
226. Lowe L, Rapini R P 1991 Newer variants and simulants of basal cell carcinoma. J Dermatol Surg Oncol 17: 641–648
227. Sexton M, Jones D B, Maloney M E 1990 Histologic pattern analysis of basal cell carcinoma. Study of a series of 1039 consecutive neoplasms. J Am Acad Dermatol 23: 1118–1126
228. Wade T R, Ackerman A B 1978 The many faces of basal-cell carcinoma. J Dermatol Surg Oncol 4: 23–28
229. Looi L M 1983 Localized amyloidosis in basal cell carcinoma. A pathologic study. Cancer 52: 1833–1836
230. Satti M B, Azzopardi J G 1990 Amyloid deposits in basal cell carcinoma of the skin. A pathologic study of 199 cases. J Am Acad Dermatol 22: 1082–1087
231. Weedon D, Shand E 1979 Amyloid in basal cell carcinoma. Br J Dermatol 101: 141–146
232. Walsh J, Perniciaro C, Randle H 1999 Calcifying basal cell carcinomas Dermatol Surg 25: 49–51
233. Oliver G F, Winkelmann R K 1988 Clear-cell basal cell carcinoma: histopathological, histochemical, and electron microscopic findings. J Cutan Pathol 15: 404–408
234. Starink T M, Blomjous C E, Stoof T J et al. 1990 Clear cell basal cell carcinoma. Histopathology 17: 401–405
235. Barr R J, Graham J H 1979 Granular cell basal cell carcinoma. A distinct histopathologic entity. Arch Dermatol 115(9): 1064–1967
236. Mrak R E, Baker G F 1987 Granular cell basal cell carcinoma. J Cutan Pathol 14(1): 37–42
237. Cohen R E, Zaim M T 1988 Signet-ring clear-cell basal cell carcinoma. J Cutan Pathol 15(3): 183–187
238. Seo I S, Warner T F C S, Priest J B 1979 Basal cell carcinoma-signet ring type. Ultrastructural study. J Cutan Pathol 6: 101–107
239. White G M, Barr R J, Liao S Y 1991 Signet ring cell basal cell carcinoma. Am J Dermatopathol 13(3): 288–292
240. Sahin A A, Ro J Y, Grignon D J et al. 1989 Basal cell carcinoma with hyaline inclusions. Arch Pathol Lab Med 113: 1015–1018
241. Suster S, Cajal R 1991 Myoepithelial differentiation in basal cell carcinoma. Am J Dermatopathol 13: 350–357
242. Brownstein M H, Shapiro L 1977 Desmoplastic trichoepithelioma. Cancer 40: 2979–2986
243. Nogita T, Ohta A, Hidano A et al. 1995 Basal cell carcinoma with eccrine differentiation. J Dermatol (Tokyo) 22(2): 111–115
244. Hunt S J, Abell E 1991 Malignant hair matrix tumor ("malignant trichoepithelioma") arising in the setting of multiple hereditary trichoepithelioma. Am J Dermatopathol 13(3): 275–281
245. Walsh N, Ackerman A B 1990 Infundibulocystic basal cell carcinoma: a newly described variant. Mod Pathol 3: 599–608
246. El-Shabrawi L, LeBoit P E 1997 Basal cell carcinoma with thickened basement membrane: a variant that resembles some benign adnexal neoplasms. Am J Dermatopathol 19(6): 568–574
247. George E, Swanson P E, Wick M R 1989 Neuroendocrine differentiation in basal cell carcinoma. An immunohistochemical study. Am J Dermatopathol 11(2): 131–135
248. Visser R, Bosman F T 1985 Neuroendocrine differentiation in basal cell carcinomas: a retrospective immunohistochemical and ultrastructural study. J Cutan Pathol 12: 117–124
249. Farmer E R, Helwig E B 1980 Metastatic basal cell carcinoma: a clinicopathologic study of seventeen cases. Cancer 46(4): 748–757
250. Lopes de Faria J, Nunes P H 1988 Basosquamous cell carcinoma of the skin with metastases. Histopathology 12(1): 85–94
251. Rowe D E, Carroll R J, Day C L Jr 1989 Long-term recurrence rates in previously untreated (primary) basal cell carcinoma: implications for patient follow-up. J Dermatol Surg Oncol 15: 315–328
252. Rowe D E, Carroll R J, Day C L Jr 1989 Mohs surgery is the treatment of choice for recurrent (previously treated) basal cell carcinoma. J Dermatol Surg Oncol 15: 424–431
253. Canterbury T D, Wheeler W E, Madan E 1990 Giant basal cell carcinoma of the back. West Virginia Med J 86: 291–292
254. Steffen C 1993 Mantleoma. A benign neoplasm with mantle differentiation. Am J Dermatopathol 15(4): 306–310
255. Leshin B, White W L 1990 Folliculocentric basaloid proliferation. The bulge (der Wulst) revisited. Arch Dermatol 126: 900–906, 1598
256. Jimenez F J, Burchette J L Jr, Grichnik J M et al. 1995 Ber-EP4 immunoreactivity in normal skin and cutaneous neoplasms. Mod Pathol 8(8): 854–858
257. Swanson P E, Fitzpatrick M M, Ritter J H et al. 1998 Immunohistologic differential diagnosis of basal cell carcinoma, squamous cell carcinoma, and trichoepithelioma in small cutaneous biopsy specimens. J Cutan Pathol 25(3): 153–159
258. Kirchmann T T, Prieto V G, Smoller B R 1995 Use of CD34 in assessing the relationship between stroma and tumor in desmoplastic keratinocytic neoplasms. J Cutan Pathol 22(5): 422–426
259. Lo J S, Snow S N, Reizner G T et al. 1991 Metastatic basal cell carcinoma: report of twelve cases with a review of the literature. J Am Acad Dermatol 24(5 Pt 1): 715–719
260. Snow S N, Sahl W, Lo J S et al. 1994 Metastatic basal cell carcinoma. Report of five cases. Cancer 73(2): 328–335
261. McCalmont T H 1996 A call for logic in the classification of adnexal neoplasms (editorial). Am J Dermatopathol 18(2): 103–109
262. McCalmont T H 1998 Analysis of the anatomic distribution of adnexal neoplasms suggests a preponderance of lesions of folliculosebaceous lineage (abstract). J Cutan Pathol 25(9): 504

263. Rosen L B 1990 A review and proposed new classification of benign acquired neoplasms with hair follicle differentiation. Am J Dermatopathol 12(5): 496–516
264. Ban M, Kamiya H, Yamada T et al. 1997 Hair follicle nevi and accessory tragi: variable quantity of adipose tissue in connective tissue framework. Pediatr Dermatol 14(6): 433–436
265. Davis D A, Cohen P R 1996 Hair follicle nevus: case report and review of the literature. Pediatr Dermatol 13(2): 135–138
266. Labandeira J, Peteiro C, Toribio J 1996 Hair follicle nevus. Case report and review. Am J Dermatopathol 18(1): 90–93
267. Sousa M A J, Fonseca J C M, Ackerman A B 1998 Hair follicle nevus. Dermatopathol Pract Concept 4(3): 231–232
268. Pippione M, Aloi F, Depaoli M A 1984 Hair-follicle nevus. Am J Dermatopathol 6(3): 245–247
269. Haneke E 1979 The dermal component in melanosis naeviformis Becker. J Cutan Pathol 6: 53–58
270. Reda A M, Rogers R S III, Peters M S 1990 Woolly hair nevus. J Am Acad Dermatol 22(2 Pt 2): 377–380
271. Duperrat B, Mascaro J M, Lambergeon S 1964 Naevus annexiel en "Soie Floche": Trichofolliculome de Miescher. Bull Soc Franc Dermatol Syphiligr 71: 318–320
272. Gray H R, Helwig E B 1962 Trichofolliculoma. Arch Dermatol 86: 619–625
273. Hyman A B, Clayman S J 1957 Hair follicle nevus. Report of a case and a review of the literature concerning this lesion and some related conditions. Arch Dermatol 75: 678–684
274. Ishii N, Kawaguchi H, Takahashi K et al. 1992 A case of congenital trichofolliculoma. J Dermatol (Tokyo) 19(3): 195–196
275. Kligman A M, Pinkus H 1960 The histogenesis of nevoid tumors of the skin. The folliculoma – a hair follicle tumor. Arch Dermatol 81(6): 922–930
276. Kato N, Ueno H 1991 A pedunculated follicular hamartoma: a case showing a central trichofolliculoma-like tumor with multiple trichogenic tumors. J Dermatol (Tokyo) 18(8): 465–471
277. Hartschuh W, Schulz T 1999 Immunohistochemical investigation of the different developmental stages of trichofolliculoma with special reference to the Merkel cell. Am J Dermatopathol 21(1): 8–15
278. Nomura M, Hata S 1990 Sebaceous trichofolliculoma on scrotum and penis. Dermatologica 181(1): 68–70
279. Plewig G 1980 Sebaceous trichofolliculoma. J Cutan Pathol 7: 394–403
280. Kimura T, Miyazawa H, Aoyagi T et al. 1991 Folliculosebaceous cystic hamartoma. A distinctive malformation of the skin. Am J Dermatopathol 13(3): 213–220
281. Yamamoto O, Suenaga Y, Bhawan J 1994 Giant folliculosebaceous cystic hamartoma. J Cutan Pathol 21(2): 170–172
282. Brooke H G 1892 Epithelioma adenoides cysticum. Br J Dermatol 4: 269–286
283. Fordyce J A 1892 Multiple benign cystic epithelioma of the skin. J Cutan Genito-Urinary Dis 10: 459–473
284. Gray H R, Helwig E B 1963 Epithelioma adenoides cysticum and solitary trichoepithelioma. Arch Dermatol 87: 142–154
285. Binkley G W, Johnson H H Jr 1951 Epithelioma adenoides cysticum: basal cell nevi, agenesis of the corpus callosum and dental cysts. Arch Dermatol 63: 73–82
286. Brownstein M H, Starink T M 1987 Desmoplastic trichoepithelioma and intradermal nevus: a combined malformation. J Am Acad Dermatol 17(3): 489–492
287. Burrows N P, Russell Jones R, Smith N P 1992 The clinicopathological features of familial cylindromas and trichoepitheliomas (Brooke-Spiegler syndrome): a report of two families. Clin Exp Dermatol 17(5): 332–336
288. Cramers M 1981 Trichoepithelioma multiplex and dystrophia unguis congenita: a new syndrome? Acta Dermato-Venereol 61(4): 364–365
289. Gerretsen A L, Beemer F A, Deenstra W et al. 1995 Familial cutaneous cylindromas: investigations in five generations of a family. J Am Acad Dermatol 33(2 Pt 1): 199–206
290. Gottschalk H R, Graham J H, Aston E E IV 1974 Dermal eccrine cylindroma, epithelioma adenoides cysticum of Brooke, and eccrine spiradenoma. Arch Dermatol 110: 473–474
291. Gross P P 1953 Epithelioma adenoides cysticum with follicular cysts of maxilla and mandible. J Oral Surg 11: 160–165
292. Headington J T, Batsakis J G, Beals T F et al. 1977 Membranous basal cell adenoma of parotid gland, dermal cylindromas, and trichoepitheliomas. Comparative histochemistry and ultrastructure. Cancer 39: 2460–2469
293. Ingels E M 1935 Epithelioma adenoides cysticum with features of syringoma. Arch Dermatol Syphilol (Chicago) 32: 75–85
294. Lloyd K M, Lloyd J R, Fatteh S 1990 Palmar pits and multiple trichoepitheliomas: an association. J Am Acad Dermatol 22(6 Pt 1): 1109–1110
295. Michaëlsson G, Olsson E, Westermark P 1981 The Rombo syndrome: A familial disorder with vermiculate atrophoderma, milia, hypotrichosis, trichoepitheliomas, basal cell carcinomas and peripheral vasodilation with cyanosis. Acta Dermato-Venereol 61: 497–503
296. Puig L, Nadal C, Fernandez-Figueras M T et al. 1998 Brooke-Spiegler syndrome variant: segregation of tumor types with mixed differentiation in two generations. Am J Dermatopathol 20(1): 56–60
297. Rasmussen J E 1975 A syndrome of trichoepitheliomas, milia, and cylindromas. Arch Dermatol 111: 610–614

298. Schirren C G, Wörle B, Kind P et al. 1995 A nevoid plaque with histological changes of trichoepithelioma and cylindroma in Brooke-Spiegler syndrome. J Cutan Pathol 22(6): 563–569
299. Starink T M, Lane E B, Meijer C J 1986 Generalized trichoepitheliomas with alopecia and myasthenia gravis: clinicopathologic and immunohistochemical study and comparison with classic and desmoplastic trichoepithelioma. J Am Acad Dermatol 15(5 Pt 2): 1104–1112
300. Welch J P, Wells R S, Kerr C B 1968 Ancell-Spiegler cylindromas (turban tumors) and Brooke-Fordyce trichoepitheliomas: evidence for a single genetic entity. J Med Genet 5(1): 29–35
301. Weyers W, Nilles M, Eckert F et al. 1993 Spiradenomas in Brooke-Spiegler syndrome. Am J Dermatopathol 15(2): 156–161
302. Brooke J D, Fitzpatrick J E, Golitz L E 1989 Papillary mesenchymal bodies: a histologic finding useful in differentiating trichoepitheliomas from basal cell carcinomas. J Am Acad Dermatol 21(3 Pt 1): 523–528
303. Wallace M L, Smoller B R 1997 Trichoepithelioma with an adjacent basal cell carcinoma, transformation or collision? J Am Acad Dermatol 37(2 Pt 2): 343–345
304. Headington J T 1970 Differentiating neoplasms of hair germ. J Clin Pathol 23: 464–471
305. Tatnall F M, Wilson Jones E 1986 Giant solitary trichoepitheliomas located in the perianal area: a report of three cases. Br J Dermatol 115(1): 91–99
306. Czernobilsky B 1972 Giant solitary trichoepithelioma. Arch Dermatol 105(4): 587–588
307. Filho G B, Toppa N H, Miranda D et al. 1984 Giant solitary trichoepithelioma. Arch Dermatol 120(6): 797–798
308. Headington J T 1976 Tumors of the hair follicle. A review. Am J Pathol 85(2): 480–514
309. Altman D A, Mikhail G R, Johnson T M et al. 1995 Trichoblastic fibroma. A series of 10 cases with report of a new plaque variant. Arch Dermatol 131(2): 198–201
310. Gilks C B, Clement P B, Wood W S 1989 Trichoblastic fibroma. A clinicopathologic study of three cases. Am J Dermatopathol 11(5): 397–402
311. Grouls V, Hey A 1988 Trichoblastic fibroma (fibromatoid trichoepithelioma). Pathol Res Pract 183(4): 462–468
312. Requena L, Renedo G, Sarasa J et al. 1990 Trichoblastic fibroma. J Cutan Pathol 17(6): 381–384
313. Watanabe S, Torii H, Matsuyama T et al. 1996 Trichoblastic fibroma. A case report and an immunohistochemical study of cytokeratin expression. Am J Dermatopathol 18(3): 308–313
314. Long S A, Hurt M A, Santa Cruz D J 1988 Immature trichoepithelioma: report of six cases. J Cutan Pathol 15(6): 353–358
315. Requena L, Requena I, Romero E et al. 1990 Trichogenic trichoblastoma. An unusual neoplasm of hair germ. Am J Dermatopathol 12(2): 175–181
316. Torii H, Ohnishi T, Matsuyama T et al. 1997 Trichogenic trichoblastoma arising on the supraclavicular fossa with an immunohistochemical study of cytokeratin expression. Clin Exp Dermatol 22(4): 183–188
317. Allen P W, Dymock R B, MacCormac L B 1988 Superficial angiomyxomas with and without epithelial components. Report of 30 tumors in 28 patients. Am J Surg Pathol 12(7): 519–530
318. Pinkus H 1953 Premalignant fibroepithelial tumors of skin. A.M.A. Arch Dermatol Syphilol 67: 598–615
319. Nikolowski W 1958 "Tricho-adenom" (organoides follikel-hamartom). Arch Klin Exp Derm 207: 34–45
320. Rahbari H, Mehregan A, Pinkus H 1977 Trichoadenoma of Nikolowski. J Cutan Pathol 4: 90–98
321. Jaqueti G, Requena L, Sánchez Yus E 1989 Verrucous trichoadenoma. J Cutan Pathol 16(3): 145–148
322. MacDonald D M, Wilson Jones E, Marks R 1977 Sclerosing epithelial hamartoma. Clin Exp Dermatol 2: 153–160
323. Dervan P A, O'Hegarty M, O'Loughlin S et al. 1985 Solitary familial desmoplastic trichoepithelioma. A study by conventional and electron microscopy. Am J Dermatopathol 7(3): 277–282
324. Shapiro P E, Kopf A W 1991 Familial multiple desmoplastic trichoepitheliomas. Arch Dermatol 127(1): 83–87
325. Blanc D, Zahouani H, Rochefort A et al. 1990 Desmoplastic trichoepithelioma nosology. Reappraisal about a case developed on a varicella scar. Dermatologica 180(1): 44–47
326. Hartschuh W, Schulz T 1995 Merkel cells are integral constituents of desmoplastic trichoepithelioma: an immunohistochemical and electron microscopic study. J Cutan Pathol 22(5): 413–421
327. Thewes M, Worret W-I, Engst R et al. 1998 Stromelysin-3: a potent marker for histopathologic differentiation between desmoplastic trichoepithelioma and morphealike basal cell carcinoma. Am J Dermatopathol 20(2): 140–142
328. Civatte J, Moulonguet-Michau I, Marinho E et al. 1990 Tumeur épithélio-lympho-histocytaire. A propos de 3 cas. Ann Dermatol Venereol 117: 441–444
329. Santa Cruz D J, Barr R J, Headington J T 1991 Cutaneous lymphadenoma. Am J Surg Pathol 15(2): 101–110
330. Requena L, Sánchez Yus E 1992 Cutaneous lymphadenoma with ductal differentiation. J Cutan Pathol 19(5): 429–433
331. Tsang W Y, Chan J K C 1991 So-called cutaneous lymphadenoma: a lymphotropic solid syringoma? Histopathology 19(4): 382–385
332. Soyer H P, Kutzner H, Jacobson M et al. 1996 Cutaneous lymphadenoma is adamantinoid trichoblastoma. Dermatopathol Pract Concept 2(1): 32–38
333. Schroh R G 1997 Cutaneous lymphadenoma with desmoplastic trichoepitheliomatoid features (abstract). J Cutan Pathol 24(2): 123

334. Casas J G, Palacios A M, Schroh R G et al. 1981 Tumor del infundibulo folicular. Rev Argent Dermatol 62: 223–224
335. Cribier B, Grosshans E 1995 Tumor of the follicular infundibulum: a clinicopathologic study. J Am Acad Dermatol 33(6): 979–984
336. Horn T D, Vennos E M, Bernstein B D et al. 1995 Multiple tumors of follicular infundibulum with sweat duct differentiation. J Cutan Pathol 22(3): 281–287
337. Kolenik S A III, Bologna J L, Castiglione F M Jr et al. 1996 Multiple tumors of the follicular infundibulum. Int J Dermatol 35(4): 282–284
338. Mehregan A H 1971 Tumor of follicular infundibulum. Dermatologica 142: 177–183
339. Mehregan A H 1984 Infundibular tumors of the skin. J Cutan Pathol 11(5): 387–395
340. Mehregan A H, Butler J D 1961 A tumor of follicular infundibulum. Arch Dermatol 83: 924–927
341. Trunnell T N, Watsman M 1979 Tumor of the follicular infundibulum. Cutis 24: 317–318
342. Kossard S, Finley A G, Poyzer K et al. 1989 Eruptive infundibulomas. A distinctive presentation of the tumor of follicular infundibulum. J Am Acad Dermatol 21(2 Pt 2): 361–366
343. Kossard S, Kocsard E, Poyzer K G 1983 Infundibulomatosis. Arch Dermatol 119(3): 267–268
344. Mehregan A H, Baker S 1985 Basaloid follicular hamartoma: three cases with localized and systematized unilateral lesions. J Cutan Pathol 12(1): 55–65
345. Schnitzler L, Civatte J, Robin F et al. 1987 Tumeurs multiples de l'infundibulum pilaire avec dégénérescence baso-cellulaire. A propos d'un cas. Ann Dermatol Venereol 114: 551
346. Winer L H 1954 The dilated pore. A trichoepithelioma. J Invest Dermatol 23: 181–188
347. Klovekorn G, Klovekorn W, Plewig G et al. 1983 [Giant pore and hair-shaft acanthoma. Clinical and histologic diagnosis]. Hautarzt 34(5): 209–216
348. Toshitani A, Imayama S, Urabe A et al. 1996 Hair cortex comedo. Am J Dermatopathol 18(3): 322–325
349. Ackerman A B, de Viragh P A, Chongchitnant N et al. 1993 Pilar sheath acanthoma (chapter 22). In: Neoplasms with Follicular Differentiation. Lea & Febiger, Philadelphia, p 509–529
350. Bhawan J 1979 Pilar sheath acanthoma. A new benign follicular tumor. J Cutan Pathol 6: 438–440
351. DiLeonardo M 1996 Dilated pore vs. pilar sheath acanthoma vs. trichofolliculoma. Dermatopathol Pract Concept 2(2): 108
352. Hurt M A 1996 Pilar sheath acanthoma (lobular infundibuloisthmicoma) (abstract). Am J Dermatopathol 18(4): 435
353. Mehregan A H, Brownstein M H 1978 Pilar sheath acanthoma. Arch Dermatol 114: 1495–1497
354. Headington J T, French A J 1962 Primary neoplasms of the hair follicle. Histogenesis and classification. Arch Dermatol 86: 430–441
355. Brownstein M H, Shapiro L 1973 Trichilemmoma. Analysis of 40 new cases. Arch Dermatol 107(6): 866–869
356. Ingrish F M, Reed R J 1968 Tricholemoma. Dermatol Int 7: 182–184
357. Möhlenbeck F W 1974 Trichilemmom. Eine studie von 100 fällen. Z Hautkr 49: 791–795
358. Lloyd K M, Dennis M 1963 Cowden's disease: A possible new symptom complex with multiple system involvement. Ann Intern Med 58: 136–142
359. Brownstein M H, Mehregan A H, Bikowski J B 1977 Trichilemmomas in Cowden's disease. J Am Med Assoc 238: 26
360. Brownstein M H, Mehregan A H, Bikowski J B et al. 1979 The dermatopathology of Cowden's disease. Br J Dermatol 100: 667–673
361. Johnson B L, Kramer E M, Lavker R M 1987 The keratotic tumors of Cowden's disease: an electronmicroscopic study. J Cutan Pathol 14(5): 291–298
362. Starink T M, Hausman R 1984 The cutaneous pathology of extrafacial lesions in Cowden's disease. J Cutan Pathol 11(5): 338–344
363. Starink T M, Hausman R 1984 The cutaneous pathology of facial lesions in Cowden's disease. J Cutan Pathol 11(5): 331–337
364. Starink T M, Meijer C J, Brownstein M H 1985 The cutaneous pathology of Cowden's disease: new findings. J Cutan Pathol 12(2): 83–93
365. Carlson G J, Nivatvongs S, Snover D C 1984 Colorectal polyps in Cowden's disease (multiple hamartoma syndrome). Am J Surg Pathol 8(10): 763–770
366. Starink T M, van der Veen J P W, Arwert F et al. 1986 The Cowden syndrome: a clinical and genetic study in 21 patients. Clin Genet 29(3): 222–233
367. Wheeland R G, McGillis S T 1989 Cowden's disease – treatment of cutaneous lesions using carbon dioxide laser vaporization: a comparison of conventional and superpulsed techniques. J Dermatol Surg Oncol 15(10): 1055–1059
368. Hunt S J, Kilzer B, Santa Cruz D J 1990 Desmoplastic trichilemmoma: histologic variant resembling invasive carcinoma. J Cutan Pathol 17(1): 45–52
369. Hashimoto T, Inamoto N, Nakamura K et al. 1987 Involucrin expression in skin appendage tumours. Br J Dermatol 117(3): 325–332
370. Poblet E, Jimenez-Acosta F, Rocamora A 1994 QBEND/10 (anti-CD34 antibody) in external root sheath cells and follicular tumors. J Cutan Pathol 21(3): 224–228
371. Massi D, Franchi A 1997 Desmoplastic trichilemmoma: a case report with immunohistochemical characterization of the extracellular matrix components. Acta Dermato-Venereol 77(5): 347–349
372. Crowson A N, Magro C M 1996 Basal cell carcinoma arising in association with desmoplastic trichilemmoma. Am J Dermatopathol 18(1): 43–48
373. Rosón E, Gómez Centeno P et al. 1998 Desmoplastic trichilemmoma arising within a nevus sebaceus. Am J Dermatopathol 20(5): 495–497
374. Brownstein M H, Shapiro E E 1979 Trichilemmomal horn: cutaneous horn overlying trichilemmoma. Clin Exp Dermatol 4: 59–63
375. Kimura S 1983 Trichilemmal keratosis (horn): a light and electron microscopic study. J Cutan Pathol 10(1): 59–67
376. Ackerman A B 1977 Trichilemmoma (letter). Arch Dermatol 114: 286
377. Ackerman A B, Wade T R 1980 Tricholemoma. Am J Dermatopathol 2(3): 207–224
378. Brownstein M H 1980 Trichilemmoma. Benign follicular tumor or viral wart? Am J Dermatopathol 2(3): 229–231
379. Headington J T 1980 Trichilemmoma. To be or not to be? Am J Dermatopathol 2(3): 225–226
380. Reed R J 1980 Trichilemmoma. A cutaneous hamartoma. Am J Dermatopathol 2(3): 227–228
381. Richfield D F 1980 Tricholemoma. True and false types. Am J Dermatopathol 2(3): 233–234
382. Schaller J, Rohwedder A, Keminer O et al. 1997 Detection of HPV-DNA in trichilemmomas by polymerase chain reaction (abstract). Dermatopathol Pract Concept 3(1): 5
383. Duperrat B, Mascaró J M 1963 Une tumeur bénigne developpée aux dépens de l'acrotrichium du partie intraépidermique du follicule pilaire: Porome folliculaire (acanthome folliculaire intraépidermique; acrotrichoma). Dermatologica 126: 291–310
384. Oswald F H 1971 On benign intraepidermal follicular acanthomas. Dermatologica 142: 29–44
385. McGavran M H, Binnington B 1966 Keratinous cysts of the skin. Arch Dermatol 94: 499–508
386. Leppard B, Bussey H J R 1975 Epidermoid cysts, polyposis coli and Gardner's syndrome. Br J Surg 62: 387–393
387. Mehregan A H, Medenica M 1982 Pigmented follicular cysts. J Cutan Pathol 9(6): 423–427
388. Pavlidakey G P, Mehregan AH, Hashimoto K 1986 Pigmented follicular cysts. Int J Dermatol 25: 174–177
389. Requena Caballero L, Sánchez Yus E 1989 Pigmented follicular cyst. J Am Acad Dermatol 21(5 Pt 2): 1073–1075
390. Salopek T G, Lee S K, Jimbow K 1996 Multiple pigmented follicular cysts: a subtype of multiple pilosebaceous cysts. Br J Dermatol 134(4): 758–762
391. Sandoval R, Urbina F 1994 Pigmented follicular cyst. Br J Dermatol 131(1): 130–131
392. Brownstein M H 1983 Hybrid cyst: a combined epidermoid and trichilemmal cyst. J Am Acad Dermatol 9: 872–875
393. Ahn S K, Chung J, Lee W S et al. 1996 Hybrid cysts showing alternate combination of eruptive vellus hair cyst, steatocystoma multiplex, and epidermoid cyst, and an association among the three conditions. Am J Dermatopathol 18(6): 645–649
394. Requena L, Sánchez Yus E 1991 Follicular hybrid cysts. An expanded spectrum. Am J Dermatopathol 13(3): 228–233
395. Satoh T, Mitoh Y, Katsumata M et al. 1989 Follicular cyst derived from hair matrix and outer root sheath. J Cutan Pathol 16(2): 106–108
396. Stevens CS 1985 Follicular cysts: how should we name them? (letter). J Am Acad Dermatol 12: 367–368
397. Young E, Orentreich N, Ackerman AB 1976 The "vanilla fudge" cyst. Cutis 18: 513–515
398. Cooper P H, Fechner R E 1983 Pilomatricoma-like changes in the epidermal cysts of Gardner's syndrome. J Am Acad Dermatol 8(5): 639–644
399. Ackerman A B 1995 Eruptive vellus hair cyst? In: Ackerman's resolving quandaries in dermatology, pathology, and dermatopathology. Promethean Medical Press, Ltd, Philadelphia, p 111–113
400. Benoldi D, Allegra F 1989 Congenital eruptive vellus hair cysts. Int J Dermatol 28(5): 340–341
401. Esterly N B, Fretzin D F, Pinkus H 1977 Eruptive vellus hair cysts. Arch Dermatol 113: 500–503
402. Kiene P, Hauschild A, Christophers E 1996 Eruptive vellus hair cysts and steatocystoma multiplex. Variants of one entity? Br J Dermatol 134(2): 365–367
403. Lee S, Kim J-G 1979 Eruptive vellus hair cyst. Arch Dermatol 115: 744–746
404. Lee S, Kim J-G, Kang JS 1984 Eruptive vellus hair cysts. Arch Dermatol 120(9): 1191–1195
405. Sánchez Yus E, Simón RS, Herrera M et al. 1997 The many faces of steatocystoma-vellus hair cyst hamartoma (abstract). J Cutan Pathol 24(2): 121
406. Tomková H, Fujimoto W, Arata J 1997 Expression of keratins (K10 and K17) in steatocystoma multiplex, eruptive vellus hair cysts, and epidermoid and trichilemmal cysts. Am J Dermatopathol 19(3): 250–253
407. Mayron R, Grimwood R E 1988 Familial occurrence of eruptive vellus hair cysts. Pediatr Dermatol 5: 94–96
408. Piepkorn M W, Clark L, Lombardi D L 1981 A kindred with congenital vellus hair cysts. J Am Acad Dermatol 5: 661–665
409. Stiefler R E, Bergfeld W F 1980 Eruptive vellus hair cysts – an inherited disorder. J Am Acad Dermatol 3: 425–429
410. Kumakiri M, Takashima I, Iju M et al. 1982 Eruptive vellus hair cysts – a facial variant. J Am Acad Dermatol 7: 461–467

411. Huerter C J, Wheeland R G 1987 Multiple eruptive vellus hair cysts treated with carbon dioxide laser vaporization. J Dermatol Surg Oncol 13: 260–263
412. Fisher D A, Bergfeld W F 1981 Retinoic acid in the treatment of eruptive vellus hair cysts. J Am Acad Dermatol 5: 221–222
413. Sánchez-Yus E, Aguilar-Martínez A, Cristóbal-Gil M C et al. 1988 Eruptive vellus hair cyst and steatocystoma multiplex: two related conditions? J Cutan Pathol 15: 40–42
414. Sexton M, Murdock D K 1989 Eruptive vellus hair cysts. A follicular cyst of the sebaceous duct (sometimes). Am J Dermatopathol 11(4): 364–368
415. Abdel Aziz A M, El-Khashab M M 1972 Steatocystoma multiplex: histologic studies and histogenesis. J Egypt Med Assoc 55: 292–311
416. Bosellini P L 1898 Beitrag zur Lehre von den multipeln folliculären hautzysten. Arch Dermatol Syph 45: 81
417. Brownstein M H 1982 Steatocystoma simplex. A solitary steatocystoma. Arch Dermatol 118(6): 409–411
418. Kimura S 1981 An ultrastructural study of steatocystoma multiplex and the normal pilosebaceous apparatus. J Dermatol (Tokyo) 8(6): 459–465
419. Plewig G, Wolff H H, Braun-Falco O 1982 Steatocystoma multiplex: anatomic reevaluation, electron microscopy, and autoradiography. Arch Dermatol Res 272(3–4): 363–380
420. Pringle J J 1899 A case of peculiar multiple sebaceous cysts (steatocystoma multiplex). Br J Dermatol 11: 381–388
421. Requena L, Martin L, Renedo G et al. 1993 A facial variant of steatocystoma multiplex. Cutis 51(6): 449–452
422. Rohde B, Jänner M, Post B et al. 1974 Steatocystoma multiplex. Hautarzt 25: 29–34
423. Setoyama M, Mizoguchi S, Usuki K et al. 1997 Steatocystoma multiplex. A case with unusual clinical and histological manifestation. Am J Dermatopathol 19(1): 89–92
424. Moritz D L, Silverman R A 1988 Steatocystoma multiplex treated with isotretinoin: a delayed response. Cutis 42(5): 437–439
425. Notowicz A 1980 Treatment of lesions of steatocystoma multiplex and other epidermal cysts by cryosurgery. J Dermatol Surg Oncol 6: 98–99
426. Contreras M A, Costello M J 1957 Steatocystoma multiplex with embryonal hair formation. Case presentation and consideration of pathogenesis. Arch Dermatol 76: 720–725
427. Ch'in K-Y 1933 Calcified epithelioma of the skin. Am J Pathol 9: 497–524
428. Forbis R Jr, Helwig E B 1961 Pilomatrixoma (calcifying epithelioma). Arch Dermatol 83(4): 606–618
429. Kaddu S, Soyer H P, Hödl S et al. 1996 Morphological stages of pilomatricoma. Am J Dermatopathol 18(4): 333–338
430. Marrogi A J, Wick M R, Dehner L P 1992 Pilomatrical neoplasms in children and young adults. Am J Dermatopathol 14(2): 87–94
431. Martins A G 1956 Tumor mumificado de Malherbe. Arq Pathol (Lisboa) 28: 123–204
432. Moehlenbeck F W 1973 Pilomatrixoma (calcifying epithelioma). A statistical study. Arch Dermatol 108: 532–534
433. Wilson Jones E, Schellander F G 1972 Multifocal pilomatrixoma. Part of a follicular malformation. Trans St John's Hosp Dermatol Soc 58: 182–185
434. Kaddu S, Soyer H P, Cerroni L et al. 1994 Clinical and histopathological spectrum of pilomatricomas in adults. Int J Dermatol 33(10): 705–708
435. Chiaramonti A, Gilgor R S 1978 Pilomatricomas associated with myotonic dystrophy. Arch Dermatol 114: 1363–1365
436. Ribera M, Calderon P, Barranco C et al. 1989 Pilomatrixomas múltiples asociados a distrofia miotónica y a carcinoma medular de tiroides. Med Cutan Iber Lat Am 17: 395–398
437. Ackerman A B, de Viragh P A, Chongchitnant N et al. 1993 Pilomatricoma and matricoma (chapter 21). In: Neoplasms with Follicular Differentiation. Lea & Febiger, Philadelphia p 477–506
438. Kaddu S, Soyer H P, Wolf I H et al. 1997 Proliferating pilomatricoma: a histopathologic simulator of matrical carcinoma. J Cutan Pathol 24(4): 228–234
439. Cooper P H, Fechner R E 1983 Pilomatricoma-like changes in the epidermal cysts of Gardner's syndrome. J Am Acad Dermatol 8(5): 639–644
440. Leppard B J, Bussey H J R 1976 Gardner's syndrome with epidermoid cysts showing features of pilomatrixomas. Clin Exp Dermatol 1: 75–82
441. Aloi FG, Boalino G, Pippione M 1984 Sindrome del nevo epidermico di Solomon. Nevo verruco-sebaceo con siringocistoadenoma papillfero e pilomatricoma. G Ital Dermatol Venereol 119(6): 401–405
442. Hashimoto K, Nelson R G, Lever W F 1966 Calcifying epithelioma of Malherbe. Histochemical and electron microscopic studies. J Invest Dermatol 46: 391–408
443. McGavran M H 1965 Ultrastructure of pilomatrixoma (calcifying epithelioma). Cancer 18: 1445–1456
444. Schirren C G, Rutten A, Plewig C 1996 Panfolliculoma. Clinical and immunohistochemical findings in 4 cases. Hautarzt 47: 610–615
445. Boscaino A, Terracciano L M, Donofrio V et al. 1992 Tricholemmal carcinoma: a study of seven cases. J Cutan Pathol 19(2): 94–99
446. Swanson P E, Marrogi A J, Williams D J et al. 1992 Tricholemmal carcinoma: clinicopathologic study of 10 cases. J Cutan Pathol 19(2): 100–109
447. Wong T-Y, Suster S 1994 Tricholemmal carcinoma. A clinicopathologic study of 13 cases. Am J Dermatopathol 16(5): 463–473
448. Headington J T 1992 Tricholemmal carcinoma [editorial]. J Cutan Pathol 19(2): 83–84
449. Batman P A, Evans H J R 1986 Metastasising pilar tumour of scalp. J Clin Pathol 39: 757
450. Mori O, Hachisuka H, Sasai Y 1990 Proliferating trichilemmal cyst with spindle cell carcinoma. Am J Dermatopathol 12(5): 479–484
451. Noto G, Pravatà G, Aricò M 1997 Malignant proliferating trichilemmal tumor (letter to the editor). Am J Dermatopathol 19(2): 202–204
452. Saida T, Oohara K, Hori Y et al. 1983 Development of a malignant proliferating trichilemmal cyst in a patient with multiple trichilemmal cysts. Dermatologica 166: 203–208
453. Takenaka H, Kishimoto S, Shibagaki R et al. 1998 Recurrent malignant proliferating trichilemmal tumour: local management with ethanol injection. Br J Dermatol 139(4): 726–729
454. Weiss J, Heine M, Grimmel M et al. 1995 Malignant proliferating trichilemmal cyst. J Am Acad Dermatol 32(5 Pt 2): 870–873
455. Mones J M, Ackerman A B 1998 Proliferating trichilemmal cyst is squamous-cell carcinoma. Dermatopathol Pract Concept 4(4): 295–310
456. Green D E, Sanusi I D, Fowler M R 1987 Pilomatrix carcinoma. J Am Acad Dermatol 17: 264–270
457. McCulloch T A, Singh S, Cotton D W K 1996 Pilomatrix carcinoma and multiple pilomatrixomas. Br J Dermatol 134(2): 368–371
458. Rahbari H, Mehregan A H 1993 Pilary complex carcinoma: an adnexal carcinoma of the skin with differentiation towards the components of the pilary complex. J Dermatol (Tokyo) 20(10): 630–637
459. Sau P, Lupton G P, Graham J H 1993 Pilomatrix carcinoma. Cancer 71(8): 2491–2498
460. Tateyama H, Eimoto T, Tada T et al. 1992 Malignant pilomatricoma. An immunohistochemical study with antihair keratin antibody. Cancer 69(1): 127–132
461. Zaim M T 1988 Sebocrine adenoma. An adnexal adenoma with sebaceous and apocrine poroma-like differentiation. Am J Dermatopathol 10(4): 311–318
462. Friedman K J, Boudreau S, Farmer E R 1987 Superficial epithelioma with sebaceous differentiation. J Cutan Pathol 14(4): 193–197
463. Rulon D B, Helwig E B 1974 Cutaneous sebaceous neoplasms. Cancer 33: 82–102
464. Troy J L, Ackerman A B 1984 Sebaceoma. A distinctive benign neoplasm of adnexal epithelium differentiating toward sebaceous cells. Am J Dermatopathol 6(1): 7–13
465. Cohen P R, Kohn S R, Davis D A et al. 1995 Muir-Torre syndrome. Dermatol Clin 13(1): 79–89
466. Cohen P R, Kohn S R, Kurzrock R 1991 Association of sebaceous gland tumors and internal malignancy: the Muir-Torre syndrome. Am J Med 90(5): 606–613
467. Muir E G, Yates Bell A J, Barlow K A 1967 Multiple primary carcinomata of the colon, duodenum and larynx associated with keratoacanthomata of the face. Br J Surg 54: 191–195
468. Schwartz R A, Torre D P 1995 The Muir-Torre syndrome: A 25 year retrospect. J Am Acad Dermatol 33(1): 90–104
469. Torre D 1968 Multiple sebaceous tumors (Society Transactions). Arch Dermatol 98(5): 549–551
470. DiLeonardo M, Ackerman A B 1998 Sebaceous carcinoma revisited. Dermatopathol Pract Concept 4(3): 214–215
471. Nelson B R, Hamlet K R, Gillard M et al. 1995 Sebaceous carcinoma. J Am Acad Dermatol 33(1): 1–15
472. Nussen S, Ackerman A B 1998 Sebaceous "adenoma" is sebaceous carcinoma. Dermatopathol Pract Concept 4(1): 5–14
473. Doxanas M T, Green W R 1984 Sebaceous gland carcinoma. Review of 40 cases. Arch Ophthalmol 102(2): 245–249
474. Wolfe J T III, Yeatts R P, Wick M R et al. 1984 Sebaceous carcinoma of the eyelid. Errors in clinical and pathologic diagnosis. Am J Surg Pathol 8(8): 597–606
475. Wick M R, Goellner J R, Wolfe J T III et al. 1985 Adnexal carcinomas of the skin. II. Extraocular sebaceous carcinomas. Cancer 56(5): 1163–1172
476. Russell W G, Page D L, Hough A J et al. 1980 Sebaceous carcinoma of meibomian gland origin. The diagnostic importance of pagetoid spread of neoplastic cells. Am J Clin Pathol 73(4): 504–511
477. Ansai S, Hashimoto H, Aoki T et al. 1993 A histochemical and immunohistochemical study of extra-ocular sebaceous carcinoma. Histopathology 22(2): 127–133
478. Domingo J, Helwig E B 1979 Malignant neoplasms associated with nevus sebaceus of Jadassohn. J Am Acad Dermatol 1: 545–556
479. García Hernández M J, Muñoz Pérez M A, Rios J J et al. 1996 Nevus sebaceus: clinical-pathological study (abstract). J Cutan Pathol 23(1): 74
480. Mehregan A H, Pinkus H 1965 Life history of organoid nevi. Arch Dermatol 91: 574–588
481. Morioka S 1985 The natural history of nevus sebaceus. J Cutan Pathol 12(3–4): 200–213
482. Wilson Jones E, Heyl T 1970 Nevus sebaceus. A report of 140 cases with special regard to the development of secondary malignant tumors. Br J Dermatol 82: 99–117
483. Ackerman A B 1995 Basal-cell carcinoma in nevus sebaceus? In: Ackerman's Resolving Quandaries in Dermatology, Pathology, and Dermatopathology. Promethean Medical Press, Ltd, Philadelphia, p 31–32
484. Kaddu S, Schappi H, Kerl H et al. 1999 Trichoblastoma and sebaceoma in nevus sebaceus. Am J Dermatopathol 21: 552–556

485. Yoon D H, Jang I G, Kim T Y et al. 1997 Syringocystadenoma papilliferum, basal cell carcinoma and trichilemmoma arising from nevus sebaceus of Jadassohn. Acta Dermato-Venereol 77(3): 242–243
486. Ando K, Hashikawa Y, Nakashima M et al. 1991 Pure apocrine nevus. A study of light-microscopic and immunohistochemical features of a rare tumor. Am J Dermatopathol 13(1): 71–76
487. Herrmann J J, Eramo L R 1995 Congenital apocrine hamartoma: an unusual clinical variant of organoid nevus with apocrine differentiation. Pediatr Dermatol 12(3): 248–251
488. Kim J H, Hur H, Lee C W et al. 1988 Apocrine nevus (letter). J Am Acad Dermatol 18(3): 579–581
489. Mehregan A H 1964 Apocrine cystadenoma. A clinicopathologic study with special reference to the pigmented variety. Arch Dermatol 90: 274–279
490. Smith J D, Chernosky M E 1974 Apocrine hidrocystoma (cystadenoma). Arch Dermatol 109: 700–702
491. Veraldi S, Gianotti R, Pabisch S et al. 1991 Pigmented apocrine hidrocystoma – a report of two cases and review of the literature. Clin Exp Dermatol 16(1): 18–21
492. Hunter G A, Donald G F 1970 Apocrine cystadenoma. Aust J Dermatol 11: 82–86
493. Schewach-Millet M, Trau H 1984 Congenital papillated apocrine cystadenoma: a mixed form of hidrocystoma, hidradenoma papilliferum, and syringocystadenoma papilliferum. J Am Acad Dermatol 11(2 Pt 2): 374–376
494. de Viragh P A, Szeimies R M, Eckert F 1997 Apocrine cystadenoma, apocrine hidrocystoma, and eccrine hidrocystoma: three distinct tumors defined by expression of keratins and human milk fat globulin 1. J Cutan Pathol 24(4): 249–255
495. Hassan M O, Khan M A, Kruse T V 1979 Apocrine cystadenoma. An ultrastructural study. Arch Dermatol 115: 194–200
496. Sato K, Leidal R, Sato F 1987 Morphology and development of an apoeccrine sweat gland in human axillae. Am J Physiol 252: R166–R180
497. Farmer E R, Helwig E B 1978 Cutaneous ciliated cysts. Arch Dermatol 114: 70–73
498. Dostrovsky A, Sagher F 1942 Experimentally induced disappearance and re-appearance of lesions of hidrocystoma. J Invest Dermatol 5: 167–172
499. Robinson A R 1893 Hidrocystoma. J Cutan Genito-Urinary Dis 11: 293–303
500. Smith J D, Chernosky M E 1973 Hidrocystomas. Arch Dermatol 108: 676–679
501. Clever H W, Sahl W J 1991 Multiple eccrine hidrocystomas: a nonsurgical treatment (letter). Arch Dermatol 127(3): 422–424
502. Sperling L C, Sakas E L 1982 Eccrine hidrocystomas. J Am Acad Dermatol 7(6): 763–770
503. Cordero A A, Montes L F 1976 Eccrine hidrocystoma. J Cutan Pathol 3: 292–294
504. Wolf M, Brownstein M H 1973 Eccrine hidrocystoma (society transactions). Arch Dermatol 108: 850
505. Adam J 1895 Hidrocystoma. Br J Dermatol 7: 169–174
506. Simón R S, Sánches Yus E 1998 Does eccrine hidrocystoma exist? (letter to the editor). J Cutan Pathol 25: 182–183
507. Tellechea O, Reis J P 1998 Immunohistochemical analysis of 18 cases of hidrocystoma (abstract). Am J Dermatopathol 20(6): 596
508. Tokura Y, Takigawa M, Inoue K et al. 1986 S-100 protein-positive cells in hidrocystomas. J Cutan Pathol 13(2): 102–110
509. Mazoujian G, Margolis R 1988 Immunohistochemistry of gross cystic disease fluid protein (GCDFP-15) in 65 benign sweat gland tumors of the skin. Am J Dermatopathol 10(1): 28–35
510. Ebner H, Erlach E 1975 Ekkrine hidrozyste. Dermatol Monatsschr 161: 739–744
511. Hassan M O, Khan M A 1979 Ultrastructure of eccrine cystadenoma. A case report. Arch Dermatol 115: 1217–1221
512. Ansai S, Watanabe S, Aso K 1989 A case of tubular apocrine adenoma with syringocystadenoma papilliferum. J Cutan Pathol 16(4): 230–236
513. Civatte J, Belaich S, Lauret P 1979 Adénome tubulaire apocrine (quatre cas). Ann Dermatol Venereol 106: 665–669
514. Landry M, Winkelmann R K 1972 An unusual tubular apocrine adenoma. Histochemical and ultrastructural study. Arch Dermatol 105: 869–879
515. Tellechea O, Reis J P 1998 Immunohistochemical analysis of 12 cases of tubular apocrine adenoma (TAA) and papillary eccrine adenoma (PEA) (abstract). Am J Dermatopathol 20(6): 597
516. Umbert P, Winkelmann R K 1976 Tubular apocrine adenoma. J Cutan Pathol 3: 75–87
517. Fox S B, Cotton D W K 1992 Tubular apocrine adenoma and papillary eccrine adenoma. Entities or unity? Am J Dermatopathol 14(2): 149–154
518. Helwig E B, Hackney V C 1955 Syringadenoma papilliferum. Arch Dermatol 71: 361–372
519. Niizuma K 1976 Syringocystadenoma papilliferum. Light and electron microscopic studies. Acta Dermato-Venereol 56: 327–336
520. Tellechea O, Reis J P 1998 Immunohistochemical analysis of 15 cases of syringocystadenoma papilliferum (abstract). Am J Dermatopathol 20(6): 597
521. Anderson N P 1950 Hidradenoma of the vulva. Arch Dermatol Syphilol (Chicago) 62: 873–892
522. Meeker J H, Neubecker R D, Helwig E B 1962 Hidradenoma papilliferum. Am J Clin Pathol 37: 182–195
523. Woodworth H J, Dockerty M B, Wilson R B et al. 1971 Papillary hidradenoma of the vulva: A clinicopathologic study of 69 cases. Am J Obstet Gynecol 110: 501–508
524. Santa Cruz D J, Prioleau P G, Smith M E 1981 Hidradenoma papilliferum of the eyelid. Arch Dermatol 117(1): 55–56
525. Kazakov D V, Mikyskova I, Kutzner H et al. 2005 Hidradenoma papilliform with oxyphilic metaplasia. A clinicopathologic study of 18 cases, including detection of human papillomavirus. Am J Surg Pathol 27: 102–110
526. Brownstein M H, Phelps R G, Magnin P H 1985 Papillary adenoma of the nipple: analysis of fifteen new cases. J Am Acad Dermatol 12(4): 707–715
527. Diaz N M, Palmer J O, Wick M R 1992 Erosive adenomatosis of the nipple: histology, immunohistology, and differential diagnosis. Mod Pathol 5(2): 179–184
528. Jones D B 1955 Florid papillomatosis of the nipple ducts. Cancer 8: 315–319
529. Miller L, Tyler W, Maroon M et al. 1997 Erosive adenomatosis of the nipple: a benign imitator of malignant breast disease. Cutis 59(2): 91–92
530. Montemarano A D, Sau P, James W D 1995 Superficial papillary adenomatosis of the nipple: A case report and review of the literature. J Am Acad Dermatol 33(5 Pt 2): 871–875
531. Montemarano A D, Sau P, James W D 1997 Superficial papillary adenomatosis of the nipple (correspondence). J Am Acad Dermatol 36(1): 133
532. Moulin G 1997 Superficial papillary adenomatosis of the nipple (correspondence). J Am Acad Dermatol 36(1): 133
533. Myers J L, Mazur M T, Urist M M et al. 1990 Florid papillomatosis of the nipple: Immunohistochemical and flow cytometric analysis of two cases. Mod Pathol 3(3): 288–293
534. Rosen P P, Caicco J A 1986 Florid papillomatosis of the nipple. A study of 51 patients, including nine with mammary carcinoma. Am J Surg Pathol 10: 87–101
535. Jones M W, Norris H J, Snyder R C 1989 Infiltrating syringomatous adenoma of the nipple. A clinical and pathological study of 11 cases. Am J Surg Pathol 13(3): 197–201
536. Rosen P P 1983 Syringomatous adenoma of the nipple. Am J Surg Pathol 7: 739–745
537. Abenoza P, Ackerman A B, DiLeonardo M 1990 Mixed tumors (chapter 11). In: Neoplasms with Eccrine Differentiation. Lea & Febiger, Philadelphia, p 285–309
538. Hara K 1995 Mixed tumours of the skin: a histopathological, enzyme-histochemical and immunohistochemical study. Histopathology 26(2): 145–152
539. Hassab-El-Naby H M, Tam S, White W L et al. 1989 Mixed tumors of the skin. A histological and immunohistochemical study. Am J Dermatopathol 11(5): 413–428
540. Headington J T 1961 Mixed tumors of the skin: eccrine and apocrine types. Arch Dermatol 84: 989–996
541. Hirsch P, Helwig E B 1961 Chondroid syringoma. Mixed tumor of the skin of salivary gland type. Arch Dermatol 84(5): 835–847
542. Stout A P, Gorman J G 1959 Mixed tumors of the skin of the salivary gland type. Cancer 12: 537–543
542a. Hornick JL, Fletcher CDM 2004 Cutaneous myoepithelioma: a clinicopathologic and immunohistochemical study of 14 cases. Hum Pathol 35: 14–24
543. Gianotti R, Coggi A, Alessi E 1998 Cutaneous apocrine mixed tumor: derived from the apocrine duct of the folliculo-sebaceous-apocrine unit? Am J Dermatopathol 20(3): 323–325
544. Requena L, Sánchez Yus E, Santa Cruz D J 1992 Apocrine type of cutaneous mixed tumor with follicular and sebaceous differentiation. Am J Dermatopathol 14(3): 186–194
545. Argényi Z B, Goeken J A, Balogh K 1989 Hyaline cells in chondroid syringomas. A light-microscopic, immunohistochemical, and ultrastructural study. Am J Dermatopathol 11(5): 403–412
546. Ferreiro J A, Nascimento A G 1995 Hyaline-cell rich chondroid syringoma. A tumor mimicking malignancy. Am J Surg Pathol 19(8): 912–917
547. Argenyi Z B, Balogh K 1991 Collagenous spherulosis in chondroid syringomas. Am J Dermatopathol 13(2): 115–121
548. Akasaka T, Onodera H, Matsuta M 1997 Cutaneous mixed tumor containing ossification, hair matrix, and sebaceous ductal differentiation. J Dermatol (Tokyo) 24(2): 125–131
549. Shimizu S, Han-Yaku H, Fukushima S et al. 1996 Immunohistochemical study of mixed tumor of the skin with marked ossification. Dermatology 193(3): 255–257
550. Bates A W, Baithun S I 1998 Atypical mixed tumor of the skin: histologic, immunohistochemical, and ultrastructural features in three cases and a review of the criteria for malignancy. Am J Dermatopathol 20(1): 35–40
551. Ohnishi T, Watanabe S 1997 Histogenesis of mixed tumor of the skin, apocrine type: immunohistochemical study of keratin expression. Am J Dermatopathol 19(5): 456–461
552. Challa V R, Jona J 1977 Eccrine angiomatous hamartoma: a rare skin lesion with diverse histological features. Dermatologica 155: 206–209
553. Donati P, Amantea A, Balus L 1989 Eccrine angiomatous hamartoma: a lipomatous variant. J Cutan Pathol 16(4): 227–229
554. Hyman A B, Harris H, Brownstein M H 1968 Eccrine angiomatous hamartoma. NY State J Med 68(21): 2803–2806

555. Kikuchi I, Kuroki Y, Inoue S 1982 Painful eccrine angiomatous nevus on the sole. J Dermatol (Tokyo) 9(4): 329–332
556. Kwon O-C, Oh S-T, Kim S-W et al. 1998 Eccrine angiomatous hamartoma. Int J Dermatol 37(10): 787–789
557. Velasco J A, Almeida V 1988 Eccrine-pilar angiomatous nevus. Dermatologica 177(5): 317–322
558. Vilanova X, Piñol Aguadé J, Castells A 1963 Hamartome angiomateux sudoripare sécrétant. Dermatologica 127: 9–16
559. Wolf R, Krakowski A, Dorfman B et al. 1989 Eccrine angiomatous hamartoma. A painful step. Arch Dermatol 125(11): 1489–1490
560. Mayou S C, Black M M, Jones R R 1988 Sudoriferous hamartoma. Clin Exp Dermatol 13(2): 107–108
561. Smith V C, Montesinos E, Revert A et al. 1996 Eccrine angiomatous hamartoma: report of three patients. Pediatr Dermatol 13(2): 139–142
562. Sulica R L, Kao G F, Sulica V I et al. 1994 Eccrine angiomatous hamartoma (nevus): immunohistochemical findings and review of the literature. J Cutan Pathol 21(1): 71–75
563. Gabrielsen T-Ø, Elgjo K, Sommerschild H 1991 Eccrine angiomatous hamartoma of the finger leading to amputation. Clin Exp Dermatol 16(1): 44–45
564. Abell E, Read S I 1980 Porokeratotic eccrine ostial and dermal duct naevus. Br J Dermatol 103: 435–441
565. Aloi F G, Pippione M 1986 Porokeratotic eccrine ostial and dermal duct nevus. Arch Dermatol 122(8): 892–895
566. Balato N, Cusano F, Lembo G et al. 1986 Naevus sudoral eccrine porokératosique pseudo-coméedonien palmaire et plantaire. Ann Dermatol Venereol 113: 921
567. Civatte J, Jeanmougin M, Denisart M et al. 1986 Naevus sudoral eccrine palmaire pseudo-comédonien. Ann Dermatol Venereol 113: 923–924
568. Driban N E, Cavicchia J C 1987 Porokeratotic eccrine ostial and dermal duct nevus. J Cutan Pathol 14(2): 118–121
569. Fernández-Redondo V, Toribio J 1988 Porokeratotic eccrine ostial and dermal duct nevus. J Cutan Pathol 15(6): 393–395
570. Marsden R A, Fleming K, Dawber R P R 1979 Comedo naevus of the palm – a sweat duct naevus? Br J Dermatol 101: 717–722
571. Moreno A, Pujol R M, Salvatella N et al. 1988 Porokeratotic eccrine ostial and dermal duct nevus. J Cutan Pathol 15(1): 43–48
572. Warren K J, Baselga E, Fleming M G et al. 1998 Keratotic papules on the palm of a 12-year-old boy (porokeratotic eccrine ostial and dermal duct nevus). Pediatr Dermatol 15(2): 140–142
573. Stoof T J, Starink T M, Nieboer C 1989 Porokeratotic eccrine ostial and dermal duct nevus. Report of a case of adult onset. J Am Acad Dermatol 20(5 Pt 2): 924–927
574. Beer K, Medenica M 1996 Solitary truncal porokeratotic eccrine ostial and dermal duct nevus in a sixty-year-old man. Int J Dermatol 35(2): 124–125
575. Cobb M W, Vidmar D A, Dilaimy M S 1990 Porokeratotic eccrine ostial and dermal duct nevus: a case of systematized involvement. Cutis 46(6): 495–497
576. Leung C S, Tang W Y M, Lam W Y et al. 1998 Porokeratotic eccrine ostial and dermal duct naevus with dermatomal trunk involvement: literature review and report on the efficacy of laser treatment. Br J Dermatol 138: 684–688
577. Murata Y, Nogita T, Kawashima M et al. 1991 Unilateral, systematized, porokeratotic eccrine ostial and dermal duct nevi. J Am Acad Dermatol 24(2 Pt 1): 300–301
578. Soloeta R, Yanguas I, Lozano M et al. 1996 Immunohistochemical study of porokeratotic eccrine nevus. Int J Dermatol 35(12): 881–883
579. Coskey R J, Mehregan A H, Hashimoto K 1982 Porokeratotic eccrine duct and hair follicle nevus. J Am Acad Dermatol 6(5): 940–943
580. Abenoza P, Ackerman A B, DiLeonardo M 1990 Fibroadenomas (chapter 10). In: Neoplasms with Eccrine Differentiation. Lea & Febiger, Philadelphia, p 275–284
581. Eckert F, Betke M, Schmoeckel C et al. 1992 Myoepithelial differentiation in benign sweat gland tumors. Demonstrated by a monoclonal antibody to alpha-smooth muscle actin. J Cutan Pathol 19(4): 294–301
582. Fretzin D F, Sloan J B, Beer K et al. 1995 Eccrine syringofibroadenoma. A clear-cell variant. Am J Dermatopathol 17(6): 591–593
583. Ishida-Yamamoto A, Iizuka H 1996 Eccrine syringofibroadenoma (Mascaro). An ultrastructural and immunohistochemical study. Am J Dermatopathol 18(2): 207–211
584. Mascaró J-M 1963 Considérations sur les tumeurs fibroépithéliales: le syringofibradénome eccrine. Ann Dermatol Syph (Paris) 90: 143–153
585. Mehregan A H, Marufi M, Medenica M 1985 Eccrine syringofibroadenoma (Mascaro). Report of two cases. J Am Acad Dermatol 13(3): 433–436
586. Ohnishi T, Suzuki T, Watanabe S 1995 Eccrine syringofibroadenoma. Report of a case and immunohistochemical study of keratin expression. Br J Dermatol 134: 449–454
587. Weedon D, Lewis J 1977 Acrosyringeal nevus. J Cutan Pathol 4: 166–168
588. Nordin H, Månsson T, Svensson Å 1988 Familial occurrence of eccrine tumours in a family with ectodermal dysplasia. Acta Dermato-Venereol 68(6): 523–530
589. Simpson E L, Styles A R, Cockerell C J 1998 Eccrine syringofibroadenomatosis associated with hidrotic ectodermal dysplasia. Br J Dermatol 138(5): 879–884
590. Starink T M 1997 Eccrine syringofibroadenoma: multiple lesions representing a new cutaneous marker of the Schöpf syndrome, and solitary nonhereditary tumors. J Am Acad Dermatol 36(4): 569–576
591. González-Serva A, Pró-Rísquez M A, Oliver M et al. 1997 Syringofibrocarcinoma versus squamous cell carcinoma involving syringofibroadenoma: is there a malignant counterpart of Mascaró's syringofibroadenoma? Am J Dermatopathol 19(1): 58–65
592. Lele S M, Gloster E S, Heilman E R et al. 1997 Eccrine syringofibroadenoma surrounding a squamous cell carcinoma: A case report. J Cutan Pathol 24(3): 193–196
593. Requena L, Sánchez Yus E, Simón P et al. 1996 Induction of cutaneous hyperplasias by altered stroma. Am J Dermatopathol 18(3): 248–268
594. Winter J A, Shea C R 1996 Eccrine syringofibroadenoma associated with unusual clinicopathologic features (abstract). J Cutan Pathol 23(1): 98
595. Patrizi A, Neri I, Marzaduri S et al. 1998 Syringoma: a review of twenty-nine cases. Acta Dermato-Venereol 78(6): 460–462
596. Butterworth T, Strean L P, Beerman H et al. 1964 Syringoma and mongolism. Arch Dermatol 90: 483–487
597. Demirkesen C, Hoede N, Moll R 1995 Epithelial markers and differentiation in adnexal neoplasms of the skin: an immunohistochemical study including individual cytokeratins. J Cutan Pathol 22(6): 518–535
598. Flanagan S, Elgart G, Badiavas E et al. 1996 Expression of estrogen and progesterone receptors in syringomas (abstract). J Cutan Pathol 23(1): 73
599. Shikata N, Kurokawa I, Andachi H et al. 1995 Expression of androgen receptors in skin appendage tumors: an immunohistochemical study. J Cutan Pathol 22(2): 149–153
600. Ohnishi T, Watanabe S 1997 Immunohistochemical analysis of keratin expression in clear cell syringoma. A comparative study with conventional syringoma. J Cutan Pathol 24(6): 370–376
601. Abenoza P, Ackerman A B, DiLeonardo M 1990 Papillary tubular adenomas (chapter 13). In: Neoplasms with Eccrine Differentiation. Lea & Febiger, Philadelphia, p 353–370
602. Ambo M, Kumakiri M, Kobayashi H et al. 1997 Papillary eccrine adenoma with a pomegranate-like appearance. J Dermatol (Tokyo) 24(12): 773–776
603. Elpern D J, Farmer E R 1978 Papillary eccrine adenoma (letter). Arch Dermatol 114: 1241
604. Jerasutus S, Suvanprakorn P, Wongchinchai M 1989 Papillary eccrine adenoma: an electron microscopic study. J Am Acad Dermatol 20(6): 1111–1114
605. Rulon D B, Helwig E B 1977 Papillary eccrine adenoma. Arch Dermatol 113: 596–598
606. Sexton M, Maize J C 1988 Papillary eccrine adenoma. A light microscopic and immunohistochemical study. J Am Acad Dermatol 18(5 Pt 1): 1114–1120
607. Tellechea O, Reis J P, Marques C et al. 1995 Tubular apocrine adenoma with eccrine and apocrine immunophenotypes or papillary tubular adenoma? Am J Dermatopathol 17(5): 499–505
608. Panet-Raymond G, Johnson W C 1973 Adenocarcinoma of the eccrine sweat glands. Arch Dermatol 107: 94–96
609. Johnson B L, Helwig E B 1969 Eccrine acrospiroma. A clinicopathologic study. Cancer 23: 641–657
610. Smith J L S, Coburn J G 1956 Hidroacanthoma simplex. An assessment of a selected group of intraepidermal basal cell epitheliomata and of their malignant homologues. Br J Dermatol 68: 400–418
611. Hyman A B, Brownstein M H 1969 Eccrine poroma. An analysis of forty-five new cases. Dermatologica 138: 29–38
612. Pinkus H, Rogin J R, Goldman P 1956 Eccrine poroma. Tumors exhibiting features of the epidermal sweat duct unit. Arch Dermatol 74: 511–521
613. Winkelmann R K, McLeod W A 1966 The dermal duct tumor. Arch Dermatol 94(1): 50–55
614. Wilson Jones E 1971 Pigmented nodular hidradenoma. Arch Dermatol 104: 117–123
615. Ban M, Yoneda K, Kitajima Y 1997 Differentiation of eccrine poroma cells to cytokeratin 1- and 10-expressing cells, the intermediate layer cells of eccrine sweat duct, in the tumor cell nests. J Cutan Pathol 24(5): 246–248
616. Biernat W, Kordek R, Wozniak L 1996 Phenotypic heterogeneity of nodular hidradenoma. Immunohistochemical analysis with emphasis on cytokeratin expression. Am J Dermatopathol 18(6): 592–596
617. Gianotti R, Alessi E 1997 Clear cell hidradenoma associated with the folliculo-sebaceous-apocrine unit. Am J Dermatopathol 19(4): 351–357
618. Metze D, Grunert F, Neumaier M et al. 1996 Neoplasms with sweat gland differentiation express various glycoproteins of the carcinoembryonic antigen (CEA) family. J Cutan Pathol 23(1): 1–11
619. Ohnishi T, Watanabe S 1997 Histogenesis of clear cell hidradenoma: immunohistochemial study of keratin expression. J Cutan Pathol 24(1): 30–36
620. Wollina U, Castelli E, Rulke D 1995 Immunohistochemistry of eccrine poroma and porocarcinoma – more than acrosyringeal tumors? Recent Results Cancer Res 139: 303–316
621. Komatsu T 1989 An immunohistochemical study of cutaneous tumors using an antibody to the breast cyst fluid protein (GCDFP-15). Nippon Hifuka Gakkai Zasshi 99(9): 991–997
622. Mazoujian G 1990 Immunohistochemistry of GCDFP-24 and zinc alpha2 glycoprotein in benign sweat gland tumors. Am J Dermatopathol 12(5): 452–457
623. Mazoujian G, Margolis R 1988 Immunohistochemistry of gross cystic disease fluid protein (GCDFP-15) in 65 benign sweat gland tumors of the skin. Am J Dermatopathol 10(1): 28–35
624. Cooper P H 1987 Mitotic figures in sweat gland adenomas. J Cutan Pathol 14(1): 10–14

625. Crain R C, Helwig E B 1961 Dermal cylindroma (dermal eccrine cylindroma). Am J Clin Pathol 35: 504–515
626. Meybehm M, Fischer H-P 1997 Spiradenoma and dermal cylindroma: comparative immunohistochemical analysis and histogenetic considerations. Am J Dermatopathol 19(2): 154–161
627. Munger B L, Graham J H, Helwig E B 1962 Ultrastructure and histochemical characteristics of dermal eccrine cylindroma (turban tumor). J Invest Dermatol 39: 577–595
628. Urbach F, Graham J H, Goldstein J et al. 1963 Dermal eccrine cylindroma. A histochemical, electron microscopic, and therapeutic (x-ray) study. Arch Dermatol 88: 880–894
629. DiLeonardo M 1998 Spiradenoma, cylindroma, and overlap of them. Dermatopathol Pract Concept 4(4): 322–323
630. Hashimoto K, Gross B G, Lever W F 1966 Eccrine spiradenoma. Histochemical and electron microscopic studies. J Invest Dermatol 46: 347–365
631. Kersting D W, Helwig E B 1956 Eccrine spiradenoma. Arch Dermatol 72: 199–227
632. Mambo N C 1983 Eccrine spiradenoma: clinical and pathologic study of 49 tumors. J Cutan Pathol 10(5): 312–320
633. Cotton D W, Slater D N, Rooney N et al. 1986 Giant vascular eccrine spiradenomas: a report of two cases with histology, immunohistology and electron microscopy. Histopathology 10(10): 1093–1099
634. Senol M, Ozcan A, Sasmaz S et al. 1998 Giant vascular eccrine spiradenoma. Int J Dermatol 37(3): 221–223
635. Santa Cruz D J 1987 Sweat gland carcinomas: a comprehensive review. Semin Diagn Pathol 4(1): 38–74
636. Paties C, Taccagni G L, Papotti M et al. 1993 Apocrine carcinoma of the skin. A clinicopathologic, immunocytochemical, and ultrastructural study. Cancer 71(2): 375–381
637. Warkel R L, Helwig E B 1978 Apocrine gland adenoma and adenocarcinoma of the axilla. Arch Dermatol 114(2): 198–203
638. Yamamoto O, Haratake J, Hisaoka M et al. 1993 A unique case of apocrine carcinoma on the male pubic skin: histopathologic and ultrastructural observations. J Cutan Pathol 20(4): 378–383
639. Kuno Y, Numata T, Kanzaki T 1999 Adenocarcinoma with signet ring cells of the axilla showing apocrine features: a case report. Am J Dermatopathol 21(1): 37–41
640. Helwig E B, Graham J H 1963 Anogenital (extramammary) Paget's disease: a clinicopathologic study. Cancer 16: 387–403
641. Jones R E Jr, Austin C, Ackerman A B 1979 Extramammary Paget's disease: a critical reexamination. Am J Dermatopathol 1(2): 101–132
642. Ackerman A B 1995 Mammary and extramammary Paget's disease? In: Ackerman's Resolving Quandaries in Dermatology, Pathology, and Dermatopathology. Promethean Medical Press, Ltd, Philadelphia, p 181–183
643. Goldblum J R, Hart W R 1998 Perianal Paget's disease: a histologic and immunohistochemical study of 11 cases with and without associated rectal adenocarcinoma. Am J Surg Pathol 22(2): 170–179
644. Allan S J R, McLaren K, Aldridge R D 1998 Paget's disease of the scrotum: a case exhibiting positive prostate-specific antigen staining and associated prostatic adenocarcinoma. Br J Dermatol 138: 689–691
645. Battles O E, Page D L, Johnson J E 1997 Cytokeratins, CEA, and mucin histochemistry in the diagnosis and characterization of extramammary disease. Am J Clin Pathol 108(1): 6–12
646. Hurt M A, Hardarson S, Stadecker M J et al. 1992 Fibroepithelioma-like changes associated with anogenital epidermotropic mucinous carcinoma. Fibroepitheliomatous Paget phenomenon. J Cutan Pathol 19(2): 134–141
647. Kohler S, Smoller B R 1996 Gross cystic disease fluid protein-15 reactivity in extramammary Paget's disease with and without associated internal malignancy. Am J Dermatopathol 18(2): 118–123
648. Goldblum J R, Hart W R 1997 Vulvar Paget's disease: a clinicopathologic and immunohistochemical study of 19 cases. Am J Surg Pathol 21(10): 1178–1187
649. Nowak M A, Guerriere-Kovach P, Pathan A et al. 1998 Perianal Paget's disease. Distinguishing primary and secondary lesions using immunohistochemical studies including gross cystic disease fluid protein-15 and cytokeratin 20 expression. Arch Pathol Lab Med 122(12): 1077–1081
650. Chanda J J 1985 Extramammary Paget's disease: prognosis and relationship to internal malignancy. J Am Acad Dermatol 13(6): 1009–1014
651. Glasgow B J, Wen D R, Al-Jitawi S et al. 1987 Antibody to S-100 protein aids the separation of pagetoid melanoma from mammary and extramammary Paget's disease. J Cutan Pathol 14(4): 223–226
652. Gillham S L, Morrison R G, Hurt M A 1991 Epidermotropic neuroendocrine carcinoma. Immunohistochemical differentiation from simulators, including malignant melanoma. J Cutan Pathol 18(2): 120–127
653. Cooper P H, Mills S E, Leonard D D et al. 1985 Sclerosing sweat duct (syringomatous) carcinoma. Am J Surg Pathol 9(6): 422–433
654. Goldstein D J, Barr R J, Santa Cruz D J 1982 Microcystic adnexal carcinoma: a distinct clinicopathologic entity. Cancer 50(3): 566–572
655. LeBoit P E, Sexton M 1993 Microcystic adnexal carcinoma of the skin. A reappraisal of the differentiation and differential diagnosis of an underrecognized neoplasm. J Am Acad Dermatol 29(4): 609–618
656. Pujol R M, LeBoit P E, Su W P D 1997 Microcystic adnexal carcinoma with extensive sebaceous differentiation. Am J Dermatopathol 19(4): 358–362
657. Wick M R, Cooper P H, Swanson P E et al. 1990 Microcystic adnexal carcinoma. An immunohistochemical comparison with other cutaneous appendage tumors. Arch Dermatol 126(2): 189–194
658. Mendoza S, Helwig E B 1971 Mucinous (adenocystic) carcinoma of the skin. Arch Dermatol 103(1): 68–78
659. Snow S N, Reizner G T 1992 Mucinous eccrine carcinoma of the eyelid. Cancer 70(8): 2099–2104
660. Wright J D, Font R L 1979 Mucinous sweat gland adenocarcinoma of eyelid. A clinicopathological study of 21 cases with histochemical and electron microscopic observations. Cancer 44: 1757–1768
661. Kazakov D V, Suster S, LeBoit P E et al. 2005 Mucinous carcinoma of the skin, primary and secondary. A clinicopathologic study of 63 cases with emphasis on the morphologic spectrum of primary cutaneous forms: homologies with mucinous lesions in the breast. Am J Surg Pathol 29: 764–782
662. Carson H J, Gattuso P, Raslan W F et al. 1995 Mucinous carcinoma of the eyelid. An immunohistochemical study. Am J Dermatopathol 17(5): 494–498
663. Hanby A M, McKee P, Jeffrey M et al. 1998 Primary mucinous carcinomas of the skin express TFF1, TFF3, estrogen receptor, and progesterone receptors. Am J Surg Pathol 22(9): 1125–1131
664. Banerjee S S, Eyden B P 1996 Neuroendocrine differentiation in eccrine carcinoma (correspondence). Histopathology 29(4): 389–390
665. Rahilly M A, Beattie G J, Lessells A M 1995 Mucinous eccrine carcinoma of the vulva with neuroendocrine differentiation. Histopathology 27(1): 82–86
666. Wach F, Hein R, Kuhn A et al. 1994 Immunohistochemical demonstration of myoepithelial cells in sweat gland carcinomas. Br J Dermatol 130(4): 432–437
667. Katoh N, Hirano S, Hosokawa Y et al. 1994 Mucinous carcinoma of the skin: report of a case with DNA cytofluorometric study. J Dermatol (Tokyo) 21(2): 117–121
668. Mehregan A H, Hashimoto K, Rahbari H 1983 Eccrine adenocarcinoma. A clinicopathologic study of 35 cases. Arch Dermatol 119(2): 104–114
669. Poiares Baptista A, Tellechea O, Reis J P et al. 1993 Porocarcinome eccrine. Revue de 24 cas. Ann Dermatol Venereol 120(1): 107–115
670. Shaw M, McKee P H, Lowe D et al. 1982 Malignant eccrine poroma: a study of twenty-seven cases. Br J Dermatol 107(6): 675–680
671. Robson A, Greene J, Ansari N et al. 2001 Eccrine porocarcinoma (malignant eccrine poroma). A clinicopathologic study of 69 cases. Am J Surg Pathol 25: 710–720
672. Abenoza P, Ackerman A B, DiLeonardo M 1990 Porocarcinomas (chapter 15). In: Neoplasms with eccrine differentiation. Lea & Febiger, Philadelphia, p 415–431
673. Landa N G, Winkelmann R K 1991 Epidermotropic eccrine porocarcinoma. J Am Acad Dermatol 24(1): 27–31
674. Pinkus H, Mehregan A H 1963 Epidermotropic eccrine carcinoma. A case combining features of eccrine poroma and Paget's dermatosis. Arch Dermatol 88: 597–606
675. Swanson P E, Mazoujian G, Mills S E et al. 1991 Immunoreactivity for estrogen receptor protein in sweat gland tumors. Am J Surg Pathol 15(9): 835–841
676. Wallace M L, Smoller B R 1995 Estrogen and progesterone receptors and anti-gross cystic disease fluid protein 15 (BRST-2) fail to distinguish metastatic breast carcinoma from eccrine neoplasms. Mod Pathol 8(9): 897–901
677. Hagler J, Trattner A, Nativ O et al. 1996 Benign and malignant eccrine poroma – a flow cytometric comparison. Isr J Med Sci 32(12): 1151–1153
678. Cooper P H, Adelson G L, Holthaus W H 1984 Primary cutaneous adenoid cystic carcinoma. Arch Dermatol 120(6): 774–777
679. Eckert F, Pfau A, Landthaler M 1994 Das adenoid-zystische schweißdrüsenkarzinom. Eine klinisch-pathologische und immunhistochemische studie. Hautarzt 45(5): 318–323
680. Fukai K, Ishii M, Kobayashi H et al. 1990 Primary cutaneous adenoid cystic carcinoma: ultrastructural study and immunolocalization of types I, III, IV, V collagens and laminin. J Cutan Pathol 17(6): 374–380
681. Kato N, Yasukawa K, Onozuka T 1998 Primary cutaneous adenoid cystic carcinoma with lymph node metastasis. Am J Dermatopathol 20(6): 571–577
682. Matsumura T, Kumakiri M, Ohkawara A et al. 1993 Adenoid cystic carcinoma of the skin – an immunohistochemical and ultrastructural study. J Dermatol (Tokyo) 20(3): 164–170
683. van der Kwast TH, Vuzevski VD, Ramaekers F et al. 1988 Primary cutaneous adenoid cystic carcinoma: case report, immunohistochemistry, and review of the literature. Br J Dermatol 118(4): 567–577
684. Wick M R, Swanson P E 1986 Primary adenoid cystic carcinoma of the skin. A clinical, histological, and immunocytochemical comparison with adenoid cystic carcinoma of salivary glands and adenoid basal cell carcinoma. Am J Dermatopathol 8(1): 2–13
685. Kao G F, Helwig E B, Graham J H 1987 Aggressive digital papillary adenoma and adenocarcinoma. A clinicopathological study of 57 patients, with histochemical, immunopathological, and ultrastructural observations. J Cutan Pathol 14(3): 129–146
686. Smith K J, Skelton H G, Holland T T 1992 Recent advances and controversies concerning adnexal neoplasms. Dermatol Clin 10(1): 117–160
687. Duke W, Lupton G 2000 Aggressive digital papillary adenocarcinoma (aggressive digital papillary adenoma and adenocarcinoma revisited). Am J Sur Pathol 24: 775–784

688. Grizzard W S, Torczynski E, Edwards W C 1976 Adenocarcinoma of the eccrine sweat glands. Arch Ophthalmol 94: 2112–2123
689. Jakobiec F A, Austin P, Iwamoto T et al. 1983 Primary infiltrating signet ring carcinoma of the eyelids. Ophthalmology 90(3): 291–299
690. Rosen Y, Kim B, Yermakov V A 1975 Eccrine sweat gland tumor of clear cell origin involving the eyelids. Cancer 36: 1034–1041
691. Ishimura E, Iwamoto H, Kobashi Y et al. 1983 Malignant chondroid syringoma. Report of a case with widespread metastasis and review of the pertinent literature. Cancer 52(10): 1966–1973
692. Metzler G, Schaumburg-Lever G, Hornstein O et al. 1996 Malignant chondroid syringoma. Immunohistopathology. Am J Dermatopathol 18(1): 83–89
693. Trown K, Heenan P J 1994 Malignant mixed tumor of the skin (malignant chondroid syringoma). Pathology 26: 237–243
694. Gerretsen A L, van der Putte S C, Deenstra W et al. 1993 Cutaneous cylindroma with malignant transformation. Cancer 72(5): 1618–1623
695. Navarro V, Monteagudo C, Calduch L et al. 1998 Well-differentiated malignant solitary dermal cylindroma. An immunohistochemical study (abstract). Am J Dermatopathol 20(6): 598
696. Rockerbie N, Solomon A R, Woo T Y et al. 1989 Malignant dermal cylindroma in a patient with multiple dermal cylindromas, trichoepitheliomas, and bilateral dermal analogue tumors of the parotid gland. Am J Dermatopathol 11(4): 353–359
697. Argenyi Z B, Nguyen A V, Balogh K et al. 1992 Malignant eccrine spiradenoma. A clinicopathologic study. Am J Dermatopathol 14(5): 381–390
698. Cooper P H, Frierson H F Jr, Morrison A G 1985 Malignant transformation of eccrine spiradenoma. Arch Dermatol 121(11): 1445–1448
699. Herzberg A J, Elenitsas R, Strohmeyer C R 1995 An unusual case of early malignant transformation in a spiradenoma. Dermatol Surg 21(8): 731–734
700. Granter S R, Seeger K, Calonje E et al. 2000 Malignant eccrine spiradenoma (spiradenocarcinoma): a clinicopathologic study of 12 cases. Am J Dermatopathol 22(2): 97–103
701. Bondi R, Urso C 1996 Syringocystadenocarcinoma papilliferum. Histopathology 28(5): 475–477
702. Seco Navedo M A, Fresno Forcelledo M, Orduna Domingo A et al. 1982 Syringocystadenome papillifere a evolution maligne. Presentation d'un cas. Ann Dermatol Venereol 109(8): 685–689
703. Friedman R J 1989 Low-grade primary cutaneous adenosquamous (mucoepidermoid) carcinoma. Report of a case and review of the literature. Am J Dermatopathol 11(1): 43–50
704. Landman G, Farmer E R 1991 Primary cutaneous mucoepidermoid carcinoma: report of a case. J Cutan Pathol 18(1): 56–59
705. Wenig B L, Sciubba J J, Goodman R S et al. 1983 Primary cutaneous mucoepidermoid carcinoma of the anterior neck. Laryngoscope 93(4): 464–467
706. Yen A, Sanchez R L, Fearneyhough P et al. 1997 Mucoepidermoid carcinoma with cutaneous presentation. J Am Acad Dermatol 37(2 Pt 2): 340–342
707. Freeman R G, Winkelmann R K 1969 Basal cell tumor with eccrine differentiation (eccrine epithelioma). Arch Dermatol 100(2): 234–242
708. McKee P H, Fletcher C D M, Rasbridge S A 1990 The enigmatic eccrine epithelioma (eccrine syringomatous carcinoma). Am J Dermatopathol 12(6): 552–561
709. Sánchez N P, Winkelmann R K 1982 Basal cell tumor with eccrine differentiation (eccrine epithelioma). J Am Acad Dermatol 6(4 Pt 1): 514–518
710. Axelsen S M, Stamp I M 1995 Lymphoepithelioma-like carcinoma of the vulvar region. Histopathology 27: 281–282
711. Ko T, Muramatsu T, Shirai T 1997 Lymphoepithelioma-like carcinoma of the skin. J Dermatol (Tokyo) 24(2): 104–109
712. Maruyama M, Miyauchi S, Ohtsuka H et al. 1995 Lymphoepithelioma-like carcinoma originating on the eyelid. J Dermatol (Tokyo) 22(3): 218–222
713. Ortiz-Frutos F J, Zarco C, Gil R et al. 1993 Lymphoepithelioma-like carcinoma of the skin. Clin Exp Dermatol 18(1): 83–86
714. Requena L, Sanchez Yus E, Jimenez E et al. 1994 Lymphoepithelioma-like carcinoma of the skin: a light-microscopic and immunohistochemical study. J Cutan Pathol 21(6): 541–548
715. Shek T W H, Leung E Y F, Luk I S C et al. 1996 Lymphoepithelioma-like carcinoma of the skin. Am J Dermatopathol 18(6): 637–644
716. Swanson S A, Cooper P H, Mills S E et al. 1988 Lymphoepithelioma-like carcinoma of the skin. Mod Pathol 1(5): 359–365
717. Takayasu S, Yoshiyama M, Kurata S et al. 1996 Lymphoepithelioma-like carcinoma of the skin. J Dermatol (Tokyo) 23(7): 472–475
718. Wick M R, Swanson P E, LeBoit P E et al. 1991 Lymphoepithelioma-like carcinoma of the skin with adnexal differentiation. J Cutan Pathol 18(2): 93–102
719. Busam K J, Gellis S, Shimamura A et al. 1998 Small cell sweat gland carcinoma in childhood. Am J Surg Pathol 22(2): 215–220
720. Epstein W, Kligman A M 1956 The pathogenesis of milia and benign tumors of the skin. J Invest Dermatol 26: 1–10
721. King E S J 1933 Post-traumatic epidermoid cysts of hands and fingers. Br J Surg 21: 29–43
722. Brownstein M H, Helwig E B 1973 Subcutaneous dermoid cysts. Arch Dermatol 107: 237–239
723. Bhaskar S N, Bernier J L 1959 Histogenesis of branchial cysts. A report of 468 cases. Am J Physiol 35: 407–423
724. Fraga S, Helwig E B, Rosen S H 1971 Bronchogenic cysts in the skin and subcutaneous tissue. Am J Clin Pathol 56(2): 230–238
725. Camacho F 1982 Benign cutaneous cystic teratoma. J Cutan Pathol 9(5): 345–351
726. Moreno A, Muns R 1985 A cystic teratoma in skin. Am J Dermatopathol 7(4): 383–386
727. Tidman M J, MacDonald D M 1988 Cutaneous endometriosis. A histopathologic study. J Am Acad Dermatol 18(2 Pt 1): 373–377
728. Doré N, Landry M, Cadotte M et al. 1980 Cutaneous endosalpingiosis. Arch Dermatol 116: 909–912
729. Johnson W C, Graham J H, Helwig E B 1965 Cutaneous myxoid cyst. J Am Med Assoc 191: 15–20
730. Asarch R G, Golitz L E, Sausker W F et al. 1979 Median raphe cysts of the penis. Arch Dermatol 115: 1084–1086
731. Cole L A, Helwig E B 1976 Mucoid cysts of the penile skin. J Urol 115: 397–400
732. Gonzalez J G, Ghiselli R W, Santa Cruz D J 1987 Synovial metaplasia of the skin. Am J Surg Pathol 11: 343–350
733. Stern D R, Sexton F M 1988 Metaplastic synovial cyst after partial excision of nevus sebaceus. Am J Dermatopathol 10(6): 531–535
734. Cohen L 1965 Mucoceles of the oral cavity. Oral Surg Oral Med Oral Pathol 19: 365–372
735. Jensen J L 1990 Superficial mucoceles of the oral mucosa. Am J Dermatopathol 12(1): 88–92
736. Moore T C 1956 Omphalomesenteric duct anomalies. Surg Gynecol Obstetr 103: 569–580
737. Nix T E, Young C J 1964 Congenital umbilical anomalies. Arch Dermatol 90: 160–165
738. Steck W D, Helwig E B 1964 Cutaneous remnants of the omphalomesenteric duct. Arch Dermatol 90: 463–470
739. Eggert J E, Harris G J, Caya J G 1988 Respiratory epithelial cyst of the orbit. Ophthal Plast Reconstr Surg 4: 101–104
740. Sanusi I D, Carrington P R, Adams D N 1982 Cervical thymic cyst. Arch Dermatol 118(2): 122–124
741. Allard R H B 1982 The thyroglossal cyst. Head Neck Surg 5: 134–146
742. Allen P J, Bowne W B, Jaques D P et al. 2005 Merkel cell carcinoma: prognosis and treatment of patients from a single institution. J Clin Oncol 23: 2300–2309
743. Goessling W, McKee P H, Mayer R J 2002 Merkel cell carcinoma. J Clin Oncol 20: 588–598
744. Hashimoto K, Lee M W, D'Annunzio D R et al. 1998 Pagetoid Merkel cell carcinoma: epidermal origin of the tumor. J Cutan Pathol 25(10): 572–579
745. LeBoit P E, Crutcher W A, Shapiro P E 1992 Pagetoid intraepidermal spread in Merkel cell (primary neuroendocrine) carcinoma of the skin. Am J Surg Pathol 16(6): 584–592
746. Ohnishi Y, Murakami S, Ohtsuka H et al. 1997 Merkel cell carcinoma and multiple Bowen's disease: incidental association of possible relationship to inorganic arsenic exposure? J Dermatol (Tokyo) 24(5): 310–316
747. Tang C-K, Toker C, Nedwich A et al. 1982 Unusual cutaneous carcinoma with features of small cell (oat cell-like) and squamous cell carcinomas. A variant of malignant Merkel cell neoplasm. Am J Dermatopathol 4(6): 537–548
748. Layfield L, Ulich T, Liao S et al. 1986 Neuroendocrine carcinoma of the skin: an immunohistochemical study of tumor markers and neuroendocrine products. J Cutan Pathol 13(4): 268–273
749. Sibley R K, Dahl D 1985 Primary neuroendocrine (Merkel cell?) carcinoma of the skin. II. An immunocytochemical study of 21 cases. Am J Surg Pathol 9: 109–116
750. Scott M P, Helm K F 1999 Cytokeratin 20: a marker for diagnosing Merkel cell carcinoma. Am J Dermatopathol 21(1): 16–20
751. Chan J K, Suster S, Wenig B M et al. 1997 Cytokeratin 20 immunoreactivity distinguishes Merkel cell (primary cutaneous neuroendocrine) carcinomas and salivary gland small cell carcinomas from small cell carcinomas of various sites. Am J Surg Pathol 21(2): 226–234
752. Skelton H G, Smith K J, Hitchcock C L et al. 1997 Merkel cell carcinoma: analysis of clinical, histologic, and immunohistologic features of 132 cases with relation to survival. J Am Acad Dermatol 37(5 Pt 1): 734–739
753. Haneke E 1985 Electron microscopy of Merkel cell carcinoma from formalin-fixed tissue. J Am Acad Dermatol 12: 487–492
754. Sibley R K, Dehner L P, Rosai J 1985 Primary neuroendocrine (Merkel cell?) carcinoma of the skin. I. A clinicopathologic and ultrastructural study of 43 cases. Am J Surg Pathol 9(2): 95–108
755. Sidhu G S, Mullins J D, Feiner H et al. 1980 Merkel cell neoplasms. Histology, electron microscopy, biology, and histogenesis. Am J Dermatopathol 2(2): 101–119
756. Tang C-K, Toker C 1978 Trabecular carcinoma of the skin. An ultrastructural study. Cancer 42: 2311–2321
757. Wick M R, Goellner J R, Scheithauer B W et al. 1983 Primary neuroendocrine carcinomas of the skin (Merkel cell tumors). A clinical, histologic, and ultrastructural study of thirteen cases. Am J Clin Pathol 79: 6–13
758. Wick M R, Kaye V N, Sibley R K et al. 1986 Primary neuroendocrine carcinoma and small-cell malignant lymphoma of the skin. A discriminant immunohistochemical comparison. J Cutan Pathol 13(5): 347–358
759. Magana-Garcia M, Ackerman A B 1990 What are nevus cells? Am J Dermatopathol 12: 93–102

760. Egan C L, Oliveria S A, Elenitsas R et al. 1998 Cutaneous melanoma risk and phenotypic changes in large congenital nevi: a follow-up study of 46 patients. J Am Acad Dermatol 39(6): 923–932
761. Mark G J, Mihm M C, Liteplo M G et al. 1973 Congenital melanocytic nevi of the small and garment type: clinical, histologic, and ultrastructural studies. Hum Pathol 4: 395–418
762. McDonnell P J, Mayou B J 1988 Congenital divided naevus of the eyelids. Br J Ophthalmol 72: 98–201
763. Cohen H J, Minkin W, Frank S B 1970 Nevus spilus. Arch Dermatol 102(4): 433–437
764. Rhodes A R 1996 Nevus spilus: a potential precursor of cutaneous melanoma worthy of aggressive surgical excision? Pediatr Dermatol 13(3): 250–252
765. Gurbuz O, Hurwitz R M 1990 Keratotic melanocytic nevus. Int J Dermatol 29: 713–715
766. Requena L, Sánchez M, Requena C 1989 Simultaneous occurrence of junctional nevus and seborrheic keratosis. Cutis 44: 465–466
767. Cho K H, Lee A Y, Suh D H et al. 1991 Lobulated intradermal nevus. Report of three cases. J Am Acad Dermatol 24: 74–77
768. Ackerman A B, Magana-Garcia M, DiLeonardo M 1990 Naming acquired melanocytic nevi. Unna's, Miescher's, Spitz's, Clark's. Am J Dermatopathol 12: 193–209
769. Ackerman A B 1982 Signs that stamp pigmented melanocytic nevi as benign. Am J Dermatopathol 4: 461–466
770. Brodell R T, Sims D M, Zaim M T 1988 Natural history of melanocytic nevi. Am Fam Phys 38: 93–101
771. Barnhill R L, Albert L S, Shama S K et al. 1990 Genital lentiginosis: a clinical and histopathologic study. J Am Acad Dermatol 22: 453–460
772. Gupta G, Williams R E A, Mackie R M 1997 The labial melanotic macule: a review of 79 cases. Br J Dermatol 136: 772–775
773. Maize J C 1988 Mucosal melanosis. Dermatol Clin 6: 283–293
774. Spann C R, Owen L G, Hodge S J 1987 The labial melanotic macule. Arch Dermatol 123: 1029–1031
775. Sagebiel R W 1972 Histologic artifacts of benign pigmented nevi. Arch Dermatol 105: 691–693
776. Söderström K-O 1987 Angiomatous type of intradermal nevi. Am J Dermatopathol 9: 549–551
777. Weedon D 1982 Unusual features of nevocellular nevi. J Cutan Pathol 9: 284–292
778. Goovaerts G, Buyssens N 1988 Nevus cell maturation or atrophy? Am J Dermatopathol 10: 20–27
779. Suzuki T, Ajioka Y, Kogure S 1988 Monoclonal S-100 immunocytochemistry of pigmented naevi with tactile-like corpuscles. J Pathol 155: 121–126
780. Eng W, Cohen P R 1998 Nevus with fat: clinical characteristics of 100 nevi containing mature adipose cells. J Am Acad Dermatol 39(5 Pt 1): 704–711
781. Smolle J, Soyer H-P, Kerl H 1990 Tubulin expression in melanocytic skin tumors. An immunohistochemical study. Am J Dermatopathol 12: 17–24
782. Paul E, Cochran A J, Wen D-R 1988 Immunohistochemical demonstration of S-100 protein and melanoma-associated antigens in melanocytic nevi. J Cutan Pathol 15: 161–165
783. Aso M, Hashimoto K, Eto H et al. 1988 Expression of schwann cell characteristics in pigmented nevus. Immunohistochemical study using monoclonal antibody to schwann cell associated antigen. Cancer 62: 938–943
784. Cole H N Jr, Hubler W R, Lund H Z 1950 Persistent, aberrant Mongolian spots. Arch Dermatol Syphilol (Chicago) 61: 244–260
785. Kopf A W, Weidman A I 1962 Nevus of Ota. Arch Dermatol 85: 195–208
786. Mishima Y, Mevorah B 1961 Nevus Ota and nevus Ito in American Negroes. J Invest Dermatol 36: 133–154
787. Dorsey C S, Montgomery H 1954 Blue nevus and its distinction from Mongolian spot and nevus of Ota. J Invest Dermatol 22: 225–236
788. Kikuchi I 1989 The biological significance of the Mongolian spot. Int J Dermatol 28: 513–514
789. Han K-H 1998 Acral lentiginous nevus. J Dermatol (Tokyo) 25: 23–27
790. Kerl H, Trau H, Ackerman A B 1984 Differentiation of melanocytic nevi from malignant melanomas in palms, soles, and nail beds solely by signs in the cornified layer of the epidermis. Am J Dermatopathol 6(Supplement 1): 159–160
791. Christensen W N, Friedman K J, Woodruff J D et al. 1987 Histologic characteristics of vulvar nevocellular nevi. J Cutan Pathol 14: 87–91
792. Friedman R J, Ackerman A B 1981 Difficulties in the histologic diagnosis of melanocytic nevi on the vulvae of premenopausal women (chapter 8). In: Ackerman AB (ed) Pathology of malignant melanoma. Masson, New York, p 119–127
793. Clark W H Jr, Hood A F, Tucker M A et al. 1998 Atypical melanocytic nevi of the genital type with a discussion of reciprocal parenchymal-stromal interactions in the biology of neoplasia. Hum Pathol 29(1 Suppl 1): S1–S24
794. Goette D K, Doty R D 1978 Balloon cell nevus. Summary of the clinical and histologic characteristics. Arch Dermatol 114(1): 109–111
795. Schrader W A, Helwig E B 1967 Balloon cell nevi. Cancer 20: 1502–1514
796. Wilson Jones E, Sanderson K V 1963 Cellular naevi with peculiar foam cells. Br J Dermatol 75: 47–54
797. Clemmensen O J, Kroon S 1988 The histology of "congenital features" in early acquired melanocytic nevi. J Am Acad Dermatol 19: 742–746
798. DiLeonardo M 1997 Congenital melanocytic nevi. Dermatopathol Pract Concept 3(3): 250–251
799. Everett M A 1989 Histopathology of congenital pigmented nevi. Am J Dermatopathol 11:1–12
800. Mehregan D A, Mehregan A H 1993 Deep penetrating nevus. Arch Dermatol 129(3): 328–331
801. Seab J A, Graham J H, Helwig E B 1989 Deep penetrating nevus. Am J Surg Pathol 13: 39–44
802. Robson A, Morley-Quante M, Hempel H et al. 2003 Deep penetrating nevus: clinicopathological study of 31 cases with further delineation of histological features allowing distinction from other pigmented benign melanocytic lesions and melanoma. Histopathology 43: 529–537
803. Barnhill R L, Mihm M C Jr, Magro C M 1991 Plexiform melanocytic spindle cell naevus: a distinctive variant of plexiform melanocytic naevus. Histopathology 18: 243–247
804. Cooper P H 1992 Deep penetrating (plexiform spindle cell) nevus. A frequent participant in combined nevus. J Cutan Pathol 19(3): 172–180
805. Wayte D M, Helwig E B 1968 Halo nevi. Cancer 22: 69–90
806. Harvell J D, Meehan S A, LeBoit P E 1997 Spitz's nevi with halo reaction: a histopathologic study of 17 cases. J Cutan Pathol 24(10): 611–619
807. Pulitzer D R, Martin P C, Cohen A P et al. 1991 Histologic classification of the combined nevus. Analysis of the variable expression of melanocytic nevi. Am J Surg Pathol 15(12): 1111–1122
808. Rogers G S, Advani H, Ackerman A B 1985 A combined variant of Spitz's nevi. How to differentiate them from malignant melanomas. Am J Dermatopathol 7 Suppl: 61–78
809. Kornberg R, Ackerman A B 1975 Pseudomelanoma. Recurrent melanocytic nevus following partial surgical removal. Arch Dermatol 111: 1588–1590
810. Park H K, Leonard D D, Arrington J H III et al. 1987 Recurrent melanocytic nevi: clinical and histologic review of 175 cases. J Am Acad Dermatol 17: 285–292
811. Arrese Estrada J, Pierard-Franchimont C, Pierard G E 1990 Histogenesis of recurrent nevus. Am J Dermatopathol 12(4): 370–372
812. Sexton M, Sexton C W 1991 Recurrent pigmented melanocytic nevus. A benign lesion, not to be mistaken for malignant melanoma. Arch Pathol Lab Med 115(2): 122–126
813. Casso E M, Grin-Jorgensen C M, Grant-Kels J M 1992 Spitz nevi (see comments). J Am Acad Dermatol 27(6 Pt 1): 901–913
814. Coskey R J, Mehregan A 1973 Spindle cell nevi in adults and children. Arch Dermatol 108: 535–536
815. Cramer S F 1998 The melanocyte differentiation pathway in Spitz nevi. Am J Dermatopathol 20(6): 555–570
816. Gartmann H, Ganser M 1985 Der Spitz-naevus. Spindelzellen-und/oder epitheloidzellennaevus – eine klinische analyse von 652 tumoren. Z Hautkr 60: 22–28
817. Gartmann H, Ganser M 1985 Der Spitz-naevus. Spindelzellen-und/oder epitheloidzellennaevus – eine histologische analyse von 652 tumoren. Z Hautkr 60: 29–42
818. Kernen J A, Ackerman L V 1960 Spindle cell nevi and epithelioid cell nevi (so-called juvenile melanomas) in children and adults. A clinicopathological study of 27 cases. Cancer 13: 612–625
819. Ko C B, Walton S, Wyatt E H et al. 1993 Spitz nevus. Int J Dermatol 32(5): 354–357
820. Paniago-Pereira C, Maize J C, Ackerman A B 1978 Nevus of large spindle and/or epithelioid cells (Spitz nevus). Arch Dermatol 114: 1811–1823
821. Spitz S 1948 Melanomas of childhood. Am J Pathol 24: 591–609
822. Weedon D 1984 The Spitz nevus. Clin Oncol 3: 493–507
823. Weedon D, Little J H 1977 Spindle and epithelioid cell nevi in children and adults. A review of 211 cases of the Spitz nevus. Cancer 40: 217–225
824. McWhorter H E, Woolner L B 1954 Pigmented nevi, juvenile melanomas, and malignant melanomas in children. Cancer 7: 564–585
825. Kantelip B, Boccard R, Nores J M et al. 1989 A case of conjunctival Spitz nevus: review of literature and comparison with cutaneous locations. Ann Ophthalmol 21: 176–179
826. Nikai H, Miyauchi M, Ogawa I et al. 1990 Spitz nevus of the palate. Report of a case. Oral Surg Oral Med Oral Pathol 69: 603–608
827. Echevarria R, Ackerman L V 1967 Spindle and epithelioid cell nevi in the adult. Clinicopathologic report of 26 cases. Cancer 20: 175–189
828. Carr E M, Heilman E, Prose N S 1990 Spitz nevi in black children. J Am Acad Dermatol 23: 842–845
829. Prose N S, Heilman E, Felman Y M et al. 1983 Multiple benign juvenile melanoma. J Am Acad Dermatol 9: 236–242
830. Brownstein W E 1972 Multiple agminated juvenile melanoma. Arch Dermatol 106: 89–91
831. Goldberg N S, Shapiro L R, Weiss S S et al. 1989 Agminated Spitz nevus in a boy with blepharophimosis syndrome. Cutis 44: 385–387
832. Gould D J, Bleehen S S 1980 Multiple agminate juvenile melanoma. Clin Exp Dermatol 5: 63–65
833. Hamm H, Happle R, Bröcker E-B 1987 Multiple agminate Spitz naevi: review of the literature and report of a case with distinctive immunohistological features. Br J Dermatol 117: 511–522
834. Krakowski A, Tur E, Brenner S 1981 Multiple agminated juvenile melanoma: a case with a sunburn history, and a review. Dermatologica 163: 270–275
835. Kriner J, Mehregan A H 1978 Multiple agminate juvenile melanoma. J Cutan Pathol 5: 90–91

836. Lancer H A, Muhlbauer J E, Sober A J 1983 Multiple agminated spindle cell nevi: unique clinical presentation and review. J Am Acad Dermatol 8: 707–711
837. Paties C T, Borroni G, Rosso R et al. 1987 Relapsing eruptive multiple Spitz nevi or metastatic Spitzoid malignant melanoma? Am J Dermatopathol 9: 520–527
838. Renfro L, Grant-Kels J M, Brown S 1989 Multiple agminate Spitz nevi. Pediatr Dermatol 6: 114–117
839. Guillot B, Barneon G 1988 Naevomatose juvénile de Spitz. Forme profuse linéaire. Ann Dermatol Venereol 115: 345–347
840. Burkhardt B R, Soule E H, Winkelmann R K 1966 Dermatofibrosarcoma protuberans. Study of fifty-six cases. Am J Surg 111: 638–644
841. Capetanakis J 1975 Juvenile melanoma disseminatum. Br J Dermatol 92: 207–211
842. Dawe R S, Wainwright N J, Evans A T et al. 1998 Multiple widespread eruptive Spitz naevi. Br J Dermatol 138(5): 872–874
843. Kaye V N, Dehner L P 1990 Spindle and epithelioid cell nevus (Spitz nevus). Natural history following biopsy. Arch Dermatol 126: 1581–1583
844. Omura E F, Kheir S M 1984 Recurrent Spitz's nevus. Am J Dermatopathol 6(Suppl 1): 207–212
845. Binder S W, Asnong C, Paul E et al. 1993 The histology and differential diagnosis of Spitz nevus. Semin Diagn Pathol 10(1): 36–46
846. Allen A C 1963 Juvenile melanomas. Ann NY Acad Sci 100: 29–48
847. Burket J M 1979 Multiple benign juvenile melanoma. Arch Dermatol 115: 229
848. Merot Y 1988 Transepidermal elimination of nevus cells in spindle and epithelioid cell (Spitz) nevi. Arch Dermatol 124: 1441–1442
849. Mérot Y, Frenk E 1989 Spitz nevus (large spindle cell and/or epithelioid cell nevus). Age-related involvement of the suprabasal epidermis. Virchow's Arch A Pathol Anat Histopathol 415: 97–101
850. Busam K J, Barnhill R L 1995 Pagetoid Spitz nevus. Intraepidermal Spitz tumor with prominent pagetoid spread. Am J Surg Pathol 19(9): 1061–1067
851. Haupt H M, Stern J B 1995 Pagetoid melanocytosis. Histologic features in benign and malignant lesions. Am J Surg Pathol 19(7): 792–797
852. Arbuckle S, Weedon D 1982 Eosinophilic globules in the Spitz nevus. J Am Acad Dermatol 7: 324–327
853. Kamino H, Misheloff E, Ackerman A B et al. 1979 Eosinophilic globules in Spitz's nevi. New findings and a diagnostic sign. Am J Dermatopathol 1: 319–324
854. Moreno A, Salvatella N, de Moragas J M 1984 Glóbulos eosinofílicos en el "nevus" de Spitz. Med Cutan Ibero-Lat-Am 12: 91–93
855. Schmoeckel C, Stolz W, Burgeson R et al. 1990 Identification of basement membrane components in eosinophilic globules in a case of Spitz's nevus. Am J Dermatopathol 12(3): 272–274
856. Kamino H, Jagirdar J 1984 Fibronectin in eosinophilic globules of Spitz's nevi. Am J Dermatopathol 6(Suppl 1): 313–316
857. Wesselmann U, Becker L R, Bröcker E B et al. 1998 Eosinophilic globules in Spitz nevi: no evidence for apoptosis. Am J Dermatopathol 20(6): 551–554
858. Burg G, Kempf W, Höchli M et al. 1998 "Tubular" epithelioid cell nevus: a new variant of Spitz's nevus. J Cutan Pathol 25(9): 475–478
859. Howat A J, Variend S 1985 Lymphatic invasion in Spitz nevi. Am J Surg Pathol 9: 125–128
860. Rose D S 1995 Nuclear pseudoinclusions in melanocytic naevi and melanomas. J Clin Pathol 48(7): 676–677
861. Sakamoto F, Ito M, Sato Y 1990 Ultrastructural study of nuclear inclusions in spindle and epithelioid cell nevus cells. J Cutan Pathol 17: 82–86
862. Bergman R, Dromi R, Trau H et al. 1995 The pattern of HMB-45 antibody staining in compound Spitz nevi. Am J Dermatopathol 17(6): 542–546
863. Palazzo J P, Duray P H 1988 Congenital agminated Spitz nevi: immunoreactivity with a melanoma-associated monoclonal antibody. J Cutan Pathol 15: 166–170
864. Skelton H Gd, Smith K J, Barrett T L et al. 1991 HMB-45 staining in benign and malignant melanocytic lesions. A reflection of cellular activation. Am J Dermatopathol 13(6): 543–550
865. Kanter-Lewensohn L, Hedblad M-A, Wejde J et al. 1997 Immunohistochemical markers for distinguishing Spitz nevi from malignant melanomas. Mod Pathol 10: 917–920
866. Winokur T S, Palazzo J P, Johnson W C et al. 1990 Evaluation of DNA ploidy in dysplastic and Spitz nevi by flow cytometry. J Cutan Pathol 17(6): 342–347
867. Küchler A, Ackerman A B 1995 Pigmented spindle cell tumor is Spitz's nevus. Dermatopathol Pract Concept 1(2): 121–129
868. Barr R J, Morales R V, Graham J H 1980 Desmoplastic nevus. A distinct histologic variant of mixed spindle cell and epithelioid cell nevus. Cancer 46: 557–564
869. Barnhill R L, Barnhill M A, Berwick M et al. 1991 The histologic spectrum of pigmented spindle cell nevus: a review of 120 cases with emphasis on atypical variants. Hum Pathol 22: 52–58
870. Barnhill R L, Mihm M C Jr 1989 Pigmented spindle cell naevus and its variants: distinction from melanoma. Br J Dermatol 121: 717–726
871. Gartmann H 1981 Der pigmentierte spindelzellentumor (PSCT). Z Hautkr 56: 862–876
872. Reed R J, Ichinose H, Clark W H Jr et al. 1975 Common and uncommon melanocytic nevi and borderline melanomas. Semin Oncol 2: 119–147
873. Requena L, Sánchez Yus E 1990 Pigmented spindle cell naevus. Br J Dermatol 123: 757–763
874. Sagebiel R W, Chinn E K, Egbert B M 1984 Pigmented spindle cell nevus. Clinical and histologic review of 90 cases. Am J Surg Pathol 8: 645–653
875. Sau P, Graham J H, Helwig E B 1984 Pigmented spindle cell nevus (abstract). Arch Dermatol 120: 1615
876. Sau P, Graham J H, Helwig E B 1993 Pigmented spindle cell nevus: a clinicopathologic analysis of ninety-five cases. J Am Acad Dermatol 28(4): 565–571
877. Smith N P 1987 The pigmented spindle cell tumor of Reed: an underdiagnosed lesion. Semin Diagn Pathol 4: 75–87
878. Wistuba I, Gonzalez S 1990 Eosinophilic globules in pigmented spindle cell nevus. Am J Dermatopathol 12: 268–271
879. Gonzalez-Cámpora R, Galera-Davidson H et al. 1994 Blue nevus: classical types and new related entities. A differential diagnostic review. Pathol Res Pract 190(6): 627–635
880. Montgomery H, Kahler J E 1939 The blue nevus (Jadassohn-Tieche): its distinction from ordinary moles and malignant melanomas. Am J Cancer 36: 527–539
881. Rodriguez H A, Ackerman L V 1968 Cellular blue nevus. Clinicopathologic study of forty-five cases. Cancer 21: 393–405
882. Tièche M 1906 Über benigne melanome ("chromatophorome") der haut – "blaue naevi". Virchow's Archiv Pathol Anat 186: 212–229
883. Levene A 1980 On the natural history and comparative pathology of the blue naevus. Ann Roy Coll Surg Eng 62: 327–334
884. Heymann W R, Yablonsky T M 1991 Congenital appearance of plaque-type blue nevi. Arch Dermatol 127: 587
885. Schleicher S M, Milstein H J, Cola C D 1991 Stump the experts (cellular blue nevus). J Dermatol Surg Oncol 17: 408, 476
886. Radentz W H 1990 Congenital common blue nevus. Arch Dermatol 126: 124–125
887. Carney J A 1995 Carney complex: the complex of myxomas, spotty pigmentation, endocrine overactivity, and schwannomas. Semin Dermatol 14(2): 90–98
888. Carney J A, Stratakis C A 1998 Epithelioid blue nevus and psammomatous melanotic schwannoma: the unusual pigmented skin tumors of the Carney complex. Semin Diagnost Pathol 15(3): 216–224
889. Carney J A, Ferreiro J A 1996 The epithelioid blue nevus. A multicentric familial tumor with important associations, including cardiac myxoma and psammomatous melanotic schwannoma. Am J Surg Pathol 20(3): 259–272
890. Kamino H, Tam S T 1990 Compound blue nevus: a variant of blue nevus with an additional junctional dendritic component. Arch Dermatol 126: 1330–1333
891. Bolognia J L, Glusac E J 1998 Hypopigmented common blue nevi (letter to the editor). Arch Dermatol 134(6): 754–756
892. Carr S, See J, Wilkinson B et al. 1997 Hypopigmented common blue nevus. J Cutan Pathol 24(8): 494–498
893. Silverberg G D, Kadin M E, Dorfman R F et al. 1971 Invasion of the brain by a cellular blue nevus of the scalp. A case report with light and electron microscopic studies. Cancer 27: 349–355
894. Gartmann H 1965 Neuronaevus bleu Masson – cellular blue nevus Allen. Arch Klin Exp Dermatol 221: 109–121
895. Masson P 1950 Neuro-nevi "bleu". Arch de Vecchi Anat Pat 14: 1–28
896. Temple-Camp C R E, Saxe N, King H 1988 Benign and malignant cellular blue nevus. A clinicopathological study of 30 cases. Am J Dermatopathol 10: 289–296
897. Prichard R W, Custer R P 1952 Pacinian neurofibroma. Cancer 5: 297–301
898. Allen A C 1949 A reorientation on the histogenesis and clinical significance of cutaneous nevi and melanomas. Cancer 2: 28–56
899. Zembowicz A, Granter S R, McKee P H et al. 2002 Amelanotic cellular blue nevus: a hypopigmented variant of the cellular blue nevus: clinicopathologic analysis of 20 cases. Am J Surg Pathol 26: 1493–1500
900. Mishima Y 1970 Cellular blue nevus. Melanogenic activity and malignant transformation. Arch Dermatol 101: 104–110
901. Tschen J A, Cartwright J, Font R L 1989 Nonmelanized macromelanosomes in a cellular blue nevus. Light and electron microscopic observations. Arch Dermatol 125: 809–812
902. Sun J, Morton T H Jr, Gown A M 1990 Antibody HMB-45 identifies the cells of blue nevi. An immunohistochemical study on paraffin sections. Am J Surg Pathol 14: 748–751
903. Wood W S, Tron V A 1991 Analysis of HMB-45 immunoreactivity in common and cellular blue nevi. J Cutan Pathol 18(4): 261–263
904. Dei Tos A P, Khurana J S, Kurtin P J et al. 1999 Absence of S100 protein immunoreactivity in cellular blue nevus: a potential diagnostic pitfall. Appl Immunohistochem Molec Morphol 7: 255–259
905. Tran T A, Carlson J A, Basaca P C et al. 1998 Cellular blue nevus with atypia (atypical cellular blue nevus): a clinicopathologic study of nine cases. J Cutan Pathol 25(5): 252–258
906. Avidor I, Kessler E 1977 "Atypical" blue nevus – a benign variant of cellular blue nevus. Presentation of three cases. Dermatologica 154: 39–44
907. Lambert W C, Brodkin R H 1984 Nodal and subcutaneous cellular blue nevi. A pseudometastasing pseudomelanoma. Arch Dermatol 120: 367–370
908. Connelly J, Smith J L Jr 1991 Malignant blue nevus. Cancer 67(10): 2653–2657
909. Merkow L P, Burt R C, Hayeslip D W et al. 1969 A cellular and malignant blue nevus: a light and electron microscopic study. Cancer 24(5): 888–896

909a. Granter S R, McKee P H, Calonje E et al. 2001 Melanoma associated with blue nevus and melanoma mimicking cellular blue nevus: a clinicopathologic study of 10 cases on the spectrum of so-called 'malignant blue nevus'. Am J Surg Pathol 25: 316–323
910. Gonzalez-Campora R, Diaz-Cano S, Vazquez-Ramirez F et al. 1996 Cellular blue nevus with massive regional lymph node metastases. Dermatol Surg 22(1): 83–87
911. Modly C, Wood C, Horn T 1989 Metastatic malignant melanoma arising from a common blue nevus in a patient with subacute cutaneous lupus erythematosus. Dermatologica 178: 171–175
912. Fisher E R 1956 Malignant blue nevus. A.M.A. Arch Dermatol 74: 227–231
913. Hernandez F J 1973 Malignant blue nevus. A light and electron microscopic study. Arch Dermatol 107: 741–744
914. Kwittken J, Negri L 1966 Malignant blue nevus. Case report of a Negro woman. Arch Dermatol 94: 64–69
915. Reiss R F, Gray G F Jr 1975 Malignant blue nevus. Occurrence with aggressive behavior. NY State J Med 75(10): 1749–1751
916. Clark W H J, Reimer R R, Greene M et al. 1978 Origin of familial malignant melanomas from heritable melanocytic lesions. The B-K mole syndrome. Arch Dermatol 114: 732–738
917. Elder D E 1985 The dysplastic nevus. Pathology17: 291–297
918. Elder D E, Greene M H, Bondi E E et al. 1981 Acquired melanocytic nevi and melanoma. The dysplastic nevus syndrome. (Chapter 11). In: Ackerman AB (ed) Pathology of malignant melanoma. Masson, New York, p 185–215
919. Lynch H T, Frichot B C III, Lynch J F 1978 Familial atypical multiple mole-melanoma syndrome. J Med Genet (Engl) 15(5): 352–356
920. Kopf A W, Friedman R J, Rigel D S 1990 Atypical mole syndrome. J Am Acad Dermatol 22: 117–118
921. Frazier R, Massi D, Ackerman A B 1996 "Dysplastic nevus": terminology between 1976 and 1996. Dermatopathol Pract Concept 2(2): 87–89
922. Shapiro P E 1992 Making sense of the dysplastic nevus controversy. A unifying perspective. Am J Dermatopathol 14(4): 350–356
923. Weinstock M A, Barnhill R L, Rhodes A R et al. 1997 Reliability of the histopathologic diagnosis of melanocytic dysplasia. The Dysplastic Nevus Panel. Arch Dermatol 133(8): 953–958
924. Ackerman A B 1988 What nævus is dysplastic, a syndrome and the commonest precursor of malignant melanoma? A riddle and an answer. Histopathology 13: 241–256
925. Clark W H Jr, Ackerman A B 1989 An exchange of views regarding the dysplastic nevus controversy. Semin Dermatol 8: 229–250
926. Seywright M M, Doherty V R, MacKie R M 1986 Proposed alternative terminology and subclassification of so called "dysplastic naevi". J Clin Pathol 39: 189–194
927. Barnhill R L, Roush G C, Duray P H 1990 Correlation of histologic architectural and cytoplasmic features with nuclear atypia in atypical (dysplastic) nevomelanocytic nevi. Hum Pathol 21: 51–58
928. Black W C, Hunt W C 1990 Histologic correlations with the clinical diagnosis of dysplastic nevus. Am J Surg Pathol 14: 44–52
929. Clemente C, Cochran A J, Elder D E et al. 1991 Histopathologic diagnosis of dysplastic nevi: concordance among pathologists convened by the World Health Organization melanoma programme. Hum Pathol 22: 313–319
930. Cook M G, Fallowfield M E 1990 Dysplastic naevi – an alternative view. Histopathology 16: 29–35
931. Jones R E Jr 1989 Questions to the editorial board and other authorities (dysplastic nevus). Am J Dermatopathol 11: 276–284
932. Mehregan A H 1988 Dysplastic nevi: a histopathological investigation. J Cutan Pathol 15: 276–281
933. Rhodes A R, Mihm M C Jr, Weinstock M A 1989 Dysplastic melanocytic nevi: a reproducible histologic definition emphasizing cellular morphology. Mod Pathol 2: 306–319
934. Roth M E, Grant-Kels J M, Ackerman A B et al. 1991 The histopathology of dysplastic nevi. Continued controversy. Am J Dermatopathol 13: 38–51
935. Sagebiel R W 1989 The dysplastic melanocytic nevus. J Am Acad Dermatol 20: 496–501
936. Urso C, Bondi R 1994 The histological spectrum of acquired nevi. An analysis of the intraepidermal melanocytic proliferation in common and dysplastic nevi. Pathol Res Pract 190(6): 609–614
937. Rivers J K, Cockerell C J, McBride A et al. 1990 Quantification of histologic features of dysplastic nevi. Am J Dermatopathol 12: 42–50
938. Albert L S, Rhodes A R, Sober A J 1990 Dysplastic melanocytic nevi and cutaneous melanoma: markers of increased melanoma risk for affected persons and blood relatives. J Am Acad Dermatol 22: 69–75
939. Greene M H, Clark W H Jr, Tucker M A et al. 1986 Acquired precursors of cutaneous malignant melanoma. The familial dysplastic nevus syndrome. New Engl J Med 312: 91–97
940. Klein L J, Barr R J 1990 Histologic atypia in clinically benign nevi. A prospective study. J Am Acad Dermatol 22: 275–282
941. Piepkorn M, Meyer L J, Goldgar D et al. 1989 The dysplastic melanocytic nevus: a prevalent lesion that correlates poorly with clinical phenotype. J Am Acad Dermatol 20: 407–415
942. Ahmed I, Piepkorn M W, Rabkin M S et al. 1990 Histopathologic characteristics of dysplastic nevi. J Am Acad Dermatol 22: 727–733
943. Piepkorn M 1990 A hypothesis incorporating the histologic characteristics of dysplastic nevi into the normal biological development of melanocytic nevi. Arch Dermatol 126: 514–518
944. Barnes L M, Nordlund J J 1987 The natural history of dysplastic nevi. A case history illustrating their evolution. Arch Dermatol 123: 1059–1061
945. Barker J N W N, MacDonald D M 1988 Eruptive dysplastic naevi following renal transplantation. Clin Exp Dermatol 13: 123–125
946. Duvic M, Lowe L, Rapini R P et al. 1989 Eruptive dysplastic nevi associated with human immunodeficiency virus infection. Arch Dermatol 125: 397–401
947. Grob J J, Gouvernet J, Aymar D et al. 1990 Count of benign melanocytic nevi as a major indicator of risk for nonfamilial nodular and superficial spreading melanoma. Cancer 66: 387–395
948. Weiß J, Garbe C, Bertz J et al. 1990 Risikofaktoren für die entwicklung maligner melanome in der Bundesrepublik Deutschland. Hautarzt 41: 309–313
949. Ackerman A B 1998 Melanoma in situ and matters that transcend it. Hum Pathol 29(1): 4–5
950. Ackerman A B, Borghi S 1991 "Pagetoid melanocytic proliferation" is the lastest evasion from a diagnosis of "melanoma in situ". Am J Dermatopathol 13: 583–604
951. Dubow B E, Ackerman A B 1990 Ideas in pathology. Malignant melanoma in situ: the evolution of a concept. Mod Pathol 3(6): 734–744
952. Weyers W, Bonczkowitz M, Weyers I et al. 1996 Melanoma in situ versus melanocytic hyperplasia in sun-damaged skin. Assessment of the significance of histopathologic criteria for differential diagnosis. Am J Dermatopathol 18(6): 560–566
953. Clark W H Jr, Elder D E, Guerry D IV et al. 1989 Model predicting survival in stage I melanoma based on tumor progression. J Natl Cancer Inst 81: 1893–1904
954. Abernethy J L, Soyer H P, Kerl H et al. 1994 Epidermotropic metastatic malignant melanoma simulating melanoma in situ. A report of 10 examples from two patients. Am J Surg Pathol 18(11): 1140–1149
955. Wick M R 1998 Prognostic factors for cutaneous melanoma (editorial). Am J Clin Pathol 110(6): 713–718
956. Barnhill R L, Mihm M C Jr 1993 The histopathology of cutaneous malignant melanoma. Semin Diagnost Pathol 10(1): 47–75
957. Hitchcock M G, McCalmont T H, White W L 1999 Cutaneous melanoma with myxoid features: twelve cases with differential diagnosis. Am J Surg Pathol 23(12): 1506–1513
958. McNutt N S 1998 "Triggered trap": nevoid malignant melanoma. Semin Diagn Pathol 15(3): 203–209
959. Wong T Y, Suster S, Duncan L M et al. 1995 Nevoid melanoma: a clinicopathological study of seven cases of malignant melanoma mimicking spindle and epithelioid cell nevus and verrucous dermal nevus. Hum Pathol 26(2): 171–179
960. Zembowicz A, McCusker M, Chiarelli C et al. 2001 Morphological analysis of nevoid melanoma: a study of 20 cases with a review of the literature. Am J Dermatopathol 23: 167–175
961. Muhlbauer J E, Margolis R J, Mihm M C Jr et al. 1983 Minimal deviation melanoma: a histologic variant of cutaneous malignant melanoma in its vertical growth phase. J Invest Dermatol 80 Suppl: 63s–65s
962. Phillips M E, Margolis R J, Merot Y et al. 1986 The spectrum of minimal deviation melanoma: a clinicopathologic study of 21 cases. Hum Pathol 17(8): 796–806
963. Reed R J 1988 Minimal deviation melanoma. Monogr Pathol (30): 110–152
964. Reed R J, Webb S V, Clark W H Jr 1990 Minimal deviation melanoma (halo nevus variant). Am J Surg Pathol 14(1): 53–68
965. Hurt M A, Santa Cruz D J 1994 Malignant melanoma microstaging. History, premises, methods, and recommendations – a call for standardization. Pathol Ann 29(Pt 2): 51–74
966. Clark W H Jr, From L, Bernardino E A et al. 1969 The histogenesis and biologic behavior of primary human malignant melanomas of the skin. Cancer Res 29: 705–726
967. Breslow A 1980 Progress in cutaneous melanoma. Tumor thickness as a guide to treatment. Pathol Ann 15(Pt 1): 1–22
968. Garbe C, Buttner P, Bertz J et al. 1995 Primary cutaneous melanoma. Identification of prognostic groups and estimation of individual prognosis for 5093 patients. Cancer 75(10): 2484–2491
969. Sahin S, Rao B, Kopf A W et al. 1997 Predicting ten-year survival of patients with primary cutaneous melanoma: corroboration of a prognostic model. Cancer 80(8): 1426–1431
970. Leiter U, Buettner P G, Eigentler T K et al. 2004 Prognostic factors of thin cutaneous melanoma: an analysis of the central malignant melanoma registry of the German Dermatological Society. J Clin Oncol 22: 3660–3667
971. Dewan M, Ackerman A B 1998 Simplifying classification of primary cutaneous melanoma. Dermatopathol Pract Concept 4(4): 351–354
972. Cochran A J, Bailly C, Cook M et al. 1998 Recommendations for the reporting of tissues removed as part of the surgical treatment of cutaneous melanoma. Am J Clin Pathol 110(6): 719–722
973. Perniciaro C 1997 Dermatopathologic variants of malignant melanoma. Mayo Clinic Proc 72(3): 273–279
974. Ackerman A B 1980 Malignant melanoma: a unifying concept. Hum Pathol 11(6): 591–595
975. Arrington J H III, Reed R J, Ichinose H et al. 1977 Plantar lentiginous melanoma: a distinctive variant of human cutaneous malignant melanoma. Am J Surg Pathol 1(2): 131–143
976. Dwyer P K, Mackie R M, Watt D C et al. 1993 Plantar malignant melanoma in a white Caucasian population. Br J Dermatol 128(2): 115–120

977. Lin C S, Wang W J, Wong C K 1990 Acral melanoma. A clinicopathologic study of 28 patients. Int J Dermatol 29(2): 107–112
978. Patterson R H, Helwig E B 1980 Subungual malignant melanoma: a clinical-pathologic study. Cancer 46(9): 2074–2087
979. Rigby H S, Briggs J C 1992 Subungual melanoma: a clinico-pathological study of 24 cases. Br J Plastic Surg 45(4): 275–278
980. Lucas D R, Tazelaar H D, Unni K K et al. 1993 Osteogenic melanoma. A rare variant of malignant melanoma. Am J Surg Pathol 17(4): 400–409
980a. Curtin J A, Busam J, Pinkel D, Bastian B C 2006 Somatic activation of KIT in distinct subtypes of melanoma. J Clin Oncol 24: 4340–4346
981. Heenan P J, Holman C D 1982 Nodular malignant melanoma: a distinct entity or a common end stage? (letter to the editor). Am J Dermatopathol 4(5): 477–478
982. Ackerman A B, Davis-Daneshfar A 1996 Desmoplastic melanoma. Dermatopathol Pract Concept 2(3): 150–155
983. Anstey A, Cerio R, Ramnarain N et al. 1994 Desmoplastic malignant melanoma. An immunocytochemical study of 25 cases. Am J Dermatopathol 16(1): 14–22
984. Anstey A, McKee P, Wilson Jones E 1993 Desmoplastic malignant melanoma: a clinicopathological study of 25 cases. Br J Dermatol 129(4): 359–371
985. Bruijn J A, Salasche S, Sober A J et al. 1992 Desmoplastic melanoma: clinicopathologic aspects of six cases. Dermatology 185(1): 3–8
986. Conley J, Lattes R, Orr W 1971 Desmoplastic malignant melanoma (a rare variant of spindle cell melanoma). Cancer 28(4): 914–936
987. Kaneishi N K, Cockerell C J 1998 Histologic differentiation of desmoplastic melanoma from cicatrices. Am J Dermatopathol 20(2): 128–134
988. Longacre T A, Egbert B M, Rouse R V 1996 Desmoplastic and spindle-cell malignant melanoma. An immunohistochemical study. Am J Surg Pathol 20(12): 1489–1500
989. Baer S C, Schultz D, Synnestvedt M et al. 1995 Desmoplasia and neurotropism. Prognostic variables in patients with stage I melanoma. Cancer 76(11): 2242–2247
990. Carlson J A, Dickersin G R, Sober A J et al. 1995 Desmoplastic neurotropic melanoma. A clinicopathologic analysis of 28 cases. Cancer 75(2): 478–494
991. Crotty K A, Quinn M, Thompson J et al. 1998 Desmoplastic and desmoplastic neurotropic melanoma: the Sydney melanoma unit experience with 280 patients (abstract). J Cutan Pathol 25(9): 492
992. Kanik A B, Yaar M, Bhawan J 1996 p75 nerve growth factor receptor staining helps identify desmoplastic and neurotropic melanoma. J Cutan Pathol 23(3): 205–210
993. Quinn M J, Crotty K A, Thompson J F et al. 1998 Desmoplastic and desmoplastic neurotropic melanoma: experience with 280 patients. Cancer 83(6): 1128–1135
994. Reed R J, Leonard D D 1979 Neurotropic melanoma. A variant of desmoplastic melanoma. Am J Surg Pathol 3(4): 301–311
995. Smithers B M, McLeod G R, Little J H 1990 Desmoplastic, neural transforming and neurotropic melanoma: a review of 45 cases. Aust NZ J Surg 60(12): 967–972
996. Aloi F G, Coverlizza S, Pippione M 1988 Balloon cell melanoma: a report of two cases. J Cutan Pathol 15(4): 230–233
997. Kao G F, Helwig E B, Graham J H 1992 Balloon cell malignant melanoma of the skin. A clinicopathologic study of 34 cases with histochemical, immunohistochemical, and ultrastructural observations. Cancer 69(12): 2942–2952
998. Nowak M A, Fatteh S M, Campbell T E 1998 Glycogen-rich malignant melanomas and glycogen-rich balloon cell malignant melanomas. Frequency and pattern of PAS positivity in primary and metastatic melanomas. Arch Pathol Lab Med 122: 353–360
999. Peters M S, Su W P D 1985 Balloon cell malignant melanoma. J Am Acad Dermatol 13(2 Pt 2): 351–354
1000. al-Talib R K, Theaker J M 1991 Signet-ring cell melanoma: light microscopic, immunohistochemical and ultrastructural features. Histopathology 18(6): 572–575
1001. LiVolsi V A, Brooks J J, Soslow R et al. 1992 Signet cell melanocytic lesions. Mod Pathol 5(5): 515–520
1002. Sheibani K, Battifora H 1988 Signet-ring cell melanoma. A rare morphologic variant of malignant melanoma. Am J Surg Pathol 12(1): 28–34
1003. Boni R, Panizzon R, Huch Boni RA et al. 1996 Malignant blue naevus with distant subcutaneous metastasis. Clin Exp Dermatol 21(6): 427–430
1004. Borek B T, McKee P H, Freeman J A et al. 1998 Primary malignant melanoma with rhabdoid features: a histologic and immunocytochemical study of three cases. Am J Dermatopathol 20(2): 123–127
1005. Bittesini L, Dei Tos A P, Fletcher C D 1992 Metastatic malignant melanoma showing a rhabdoid phenotype: further evidence of a non-specific histological pattern. Histopathology 20(2): 167–170
1006. Chang E S, Wick M R, Swanson P E et al. 1994 Metastatic malignant melanoma with "rhabdoid" features. Am J Clin Pathol 102(4): 426–431
1007. Black W C, McGavran M H, Graham P 1969 Nodular subepidermal fibrosis. A clinical pathologic study emphasizing the frequency of clinical misdiagnoses. Arch Surg 98: 296–300
1008. Gonzalez S, Duarte I 1982 Benign fibrous histiocytoma of the skin. A morphologic study of 290 cases. Pathol Res Pract 174: 379–391
1009. Li D F, Iwasaki H, Kikuchi M et al. 1994 Dermatofibroma: superficial fibrous proliferation with reactive histiocytes. A multiple immunostaining analysis [see comments]. Cancer 74(1): 66–73
1010. Nestle F O, Nickoloff B J, Burg G 1995 Dermatofibroma: an abortive immunoreactive process mediated by dermal dendritic cells? Dermatology 190(4): 265–268
1011. Niemi K M 1970 The benign fibrohistiocytic tumours of the skin. Acta Dermato-Venereol 50(Suppl 63): 7–42
1012. Vilanova J R, Flint A 1974 The morphological variations of fibrous histiocytomas. J Cutan Pathol 1: 155–164
1013. Evans J, Clarke T, Mattacks C A et al. 1989 Dermatofibromas and arthropod bites: is there any evidence to link the two? Lancet 2: 36–37
1014. Vanni R, Fletcher C D, Sciot R et al. 2000 Cytogenetic evidence of clonality in cutaneous benign fibrous histiocytomas: a report of the CHAMP study group. Histopathology 37(3): 212–217
1015. Marrogi A J, Dehner L P, Coffin C M et al. 1992 Benign cutaneous histiocytic tumors in childhood and adolescence, excluding Langerhans' cell proliferations. A clinicopathologic and immunohistochemical analysis. Am J Dermatopathol 14(1): 8–18
1016. Calonje E, Mentzel T, Fletcher C D M 1994 Cellular benign fibrous histiocytoma. Clinicopathologic analysis of 74 cases of a distinctive variant of cutaneous fibrous histiocytoma with frequent recurrence. Am J Surg Pathol 18(7): 668–676
1017. Franquemont D W, Cooper P H, Shmookler B M et al. 1990 Benign fibrous histiocytoma of the skin with potential for local recurrence: a tumor to be distinguished from dermatofibroma. Mod Pathol 3: 158–163
1018. Colby T V 1997 Metastasizing dermatofibroma (letter to the editor). Am J Surg Pathol 21(8): 976
1019. Colome-Grimmer M I, Evans H L 1996 Metastasizing cellular dermatofibroma. A report of two cases. Am J Surg Pathol 20(11): 1361–1367
1020. Guillou L, Gebhard S, Salmeron M et al. 2000 Metastasizing fibrous histiocytoma of the skin: a clinicopathologic and immunohistochemical analysis of three cases. Mod Pathol 13: 654–660
1021. Requena L, Aguilar A, Lopez Redondo M J et al. 1990 Multinodular hemosiderotic dermatofibroma. Dermatologica 181(4): 320–323
1022. Hunt S J, Santa Cruz D J, Miller C W 1990 Cholesterotic fibrous histiocytoma. Its association with hyperlipoproteinemia. Arch Dermatol 126: 506–508
1023. Iwata J, Fletcher C D 2000 Lipidized fibrous histiocytoma: clinicopathologic analysis of 22 cases. Am J Dermatopathol 22(2): 126–134
1024. Barr R J, Young E M, King D F 1986 Non-polarizable collagen in dermatofibrosarcoma protuberans: a useful diagnostic aid. J Cutan Pathol 13: 339–346
1025. Cerio R, Rao B K, Spaull J et al. 1989 An immunohistochemical study of fibrous papule of the nose: 25 cases. J Cutan Pathol 16(4): 194–198
1026. Hsi E D, Nickoloff B J 1996 Dermatofibroma and dermatofibrosarcoma protuberans: an immunohistochemical study reveals distinctive antigenic profiles. J Dermatol Sci 11(1): 1–9
1027. Soini Y 1990 Cell differentiation in benign cutaneous fibrous histiocytomas. An immunohistochemical study with antibodies to histiomonocytic cells and intermediate filament proteins. Am J Dermatopathol 12: 134–140
1028. Candiani P, Rainoldi R, Sideri M et al. 1981 Ultrastructural aspects of the dermatofibroma. Tumori 67: 249–252
1029. Goldblum J R, Tuthill R J 1997 CD34 and factor-XIIIa immunoreactivity in dermatofibrosarcoma protuberans and dermatofibroma. Am J Dermatopathol 19(2): 147–153
1030. Calonje E, Fletcher C D M 1995 Aneurysmal benign fibrous histiocytoma: clinicopathologic analysis of 40 cases of a tumour frequently misdiagnosed as a vascular neoplasm. Histopathology 26(4): 323–331
1031. Hairston M A, Reed R J 1966 Aneurysmal sclerosing hemangioma of skin. Arch Dermatol 93: 439–442
1032. Santa Cruz D J, Kyriakos M 1981 Aneurysmal ("angiomatoid") fibrous histiocytoma of the skin. Cancer 47: 2053–2061
1033. Yang P, Hirose T, Hasegawa T et al. 1995 Aneurysmal fibrous histiocytoma of the skin. A histological, immunohistochemical, and ultrastructural study. Am J Dermatopathol 17(2): 179–184
1034. Leyva W H, Santa Cruz D J 1986 Atypical cutaneous fibrous histiocytoma. Am J Dermatopathol 8: 467–471
1035. Kaddu S, McMenamin M E, Fletcher C D M 2002 Atypical fibrous histiocytoma of the skin: clinicopathologic analysis of 59 cases with evidence of infrequent metastasis. Am J Surg Pathol 26: 35–46
1036. Setoyama M, Fukumaru S, Kanzaki T 1997 Case of dermatofibroma with monster cells: a review and an immunohistochemical study. Am J Dermatopathol 19(3): 312–315
1037. Tamada S, Ackerman A B 1987 Dermatofibroma with monster cells. Am J Dermatopathol 9: 380–387
1038. Kamino H, Lee J Y-Y, Berke A 1989 Pleomorphic fibroma of the skin: A benign neoplasm with cytologic atypia. A clinicopathologic study of eight cases. Am J Surg Pathol 13(2): 107–113
1039. Beham A, Fletcher C D M 1990 Atypical "pseudosarcomatous" variant of cutaneous benign fibrous histiocytoma: report of eight cases. Histopathology 17: 167–169
1040. Glusac E J, Barr R J, Everett M A et al. 1994 Epithelioid cell histiocytoma. A report of 10 cases including a new cellular variant. Am J Surg Pathol 18(6): 583–590
1041. Glusac E J, McNiff J M 1999 Epithelioid cell histiocytoma: a simulant of vascular and melanocytic neoplasms. Am J Dermatopathol 21(1): 1–7

1042. Singh Gomez C, Calonje E, Fletcher C D M 1994 Epithelioid benign fibrous histiocytoma of skin: clinico-pathological analysis of 20 cases of a poorly known variant. Histopathology 24(2): 123–129
1043. Wilson Jones E, Cerio R, Smith N P 1989 Epithelioid cell histiocytoma: a new entity. Br J Dermatol 120: 185–195
1044. Vanni R, Marras S, Faa G et al. 1997 Cellular fibrous histiocytoma of the skin: evidence of a clonal process with different karyotype from dermatofibrosarcoma. Genes Chromos Cancer 18(4): 314–317
1045. Wambacher-Gasser B, Zelger B, Zelger B G et al. 1997 Clear cell dermatofibroma. Histopathology 30(1): 64–69
1046. Zelger B W, Steiner H, Kutzner H 1996 Clear cell dermatofibroma. Case report of an unusual fibrohistiocytic lesion. Am J Surg Pathol 20(4): 483–491
1047. Soyer H P, Metze D, Kerl H 1997 Granular cell dermatofibroma. Am J Dermatopathol 19(2): 168–173
1048. Val-Bernal J F, Mira C 1996 Dermatofibroma with granular cells. J Cutan Pathol 23(6): 562–565
1049. Zelger B G, Steiner H, Kutzner H et al. 1997 Granular cell dermatofibroma. Histopathology 31(3): 258–262
1050. Zelger B, Sidoroff A, Stanzl U et al. 1994 Deep penetrating dermatofibroma versus dermatofibrosarcoma protuberans. A clinicopathologic comparison. Am J Surg Pathol 18(7): 677–686
1051. Goette D K, Helwig E B 1975 Basal cell carcinomas and basal cell carcinoma-like changes overlying dermatofibromas. Arch Dermatol 111: 589–592
1052. Requena L, Ortiz S, Sánchez M et al. 1990 Angioleiomyoma within a histiocytoma. J Cutan Pathol 17: 278–280
1053. Gray M H, Smoller B R, McNutt N S et al. 1990 Giant dermal dendrocytoma of the face: a distinct clinicopathologic entity. Arch Dermatol 126: 689–690
1054. Nickoloff B J, Wood G S, Chu M et al. 1990 Disseminated dermal dendrocytomas. A new cutaneous fibrohistiocytic proliferative disorder? Am J Surg Pathol 14: 867–871
1055. Bernstein J C 1939 Hemosiderin histiocytoma of the skin. Arch Dermatol Syphilol (Chicago) 40: 390–396
1056. Smith N P, Wilson Jones E 1985 Multinucleate cell angiohistiocytoma – a new entity. Br J Dermatol 113(Suppl 29): 15
1057. Smolle J, Auboeck L, Gogg-Retzer I et al. 1989 Multinucleate cell angiohistiocytoma: a clinicopathological, immunohistochemical and ultrastructural study. Br J Dermatol 121: 113–121
1058. Wilson Jones E, Cerio R, Smith N P 1990 Multinucleate cell angiohistiocytoma: an acquired vascular anomaly to be distinguished from Kaposi's sarcoma. Br J Dermatol 122: 651–663
1059. Schwob V S, Santa Cruz D J 1986 Palisading cutaneous fibrous histiocytoma. J Cutan Pathol 13: 403–407
1060. Gross R E, Wolback S B 1943 Sclerosing hemangiomas. Their relationship to dermatofibroma, histiocytoma, xanthoma and to certain pigmented lesions of the skin. Am J Pathol 19: 533–551
1061. Lo W L, Wong C K 1990 Solitary sclerotic fibroma. J Cutan Pathol 17: 269–273
1062. Metcalf J S, Maize J C, LeBoit P E 1991 Circumscribed storiform collagenoma (sclerosing fibroma). Am J Dermatopathol 13: 122–129
1063. Rapini R P, Golitz L E 1989 Sclerotic fibromas of the skin. J Am Acad Dermatol 20: 266–271
1064. Goodlad J R, Fletcher C D M 1990 Intradermal variant of nodular "fasciitis". Histopathology 17: 569–571
1065. Bork K, Gabbert H, Knop J 1990 Fat-storing hamartoma of dermal dendrocytes. Clinical, histologic, and ultrastructural study. Arch Dermatol 126: 794–796
1066. Kamino H, Reddy V B, Gero M et al. 1992 Dermatomyofibroma. A benign cutaneous, plaque-like proliferation of fibroblasts and myofibroblasts in young adults. J Cutan Pathol 19: 85–93
1067. Kamino H, Jacobson M 1990 Dermatofibroma extending into the subcutaneous tissue. Differential diagnosis from dermatofibrosarcoma protuberans. Am J Surg Pathol 14: 1156–1164
1068. Abenoza P, Lillemoe T 1993 CD34 and factor XIIIa in the differential diagnosis of dermatofibroma and dermatofibrosarcoma protuberans. Am J Dermatopathol 15(5): 429–434
1069. Fletcher C D M 1988 Giant cell fibroblastoma of soft tissue: a clinicopathological and immunohistochemical study. Histopathology 13: 499–508
1070. Shmookler B M, Enzinger F M 1982 Giant cell fibroblastoma: a peculiar childhood tumor. Lab Invest 46: 76A
1071. Shmookler B M, Enzinger F M, Weiss S W 1989 Giant cell fibroblastoma. A juvenile form of dermatofibrosarcoma protuberans. Cancer 64: 2154–2161
1072. Hirose T, Sasaki M, Shintaku M et al. 1990 Giant cell fibroblastoma. A case report. Acta Pathol Jpn 40: 540–544
1073. Barr R J, Young E M, Liao S-Y 1986 Giant cell fibroblastoma: an immunohistochemical study. J Cutan Pathol 13: 301–307
1074. Rosen L B, Amazon K, Weitzner J et al. 1989 Giant cell fibroblastoma. A report of a case and review of the literature. Am J Dermatopathol 11: 242–247
1075. Weiss S W, Nickoloff B J 1993 CD-34 is expressed by a distinctive cell population in peripheral nerve, nerve sheath tumors, and related lesions. Am J Surg Pathol 17(10): 1039–1045
1076. Pinto A, Hwang W-S, Wong A L et al. 1992 Giant cell fibroblastoma in childhood: immunohistochemical and ultrastructural study. Mod Pathol 5: 639–642
1077. Diaz-Cascajo C, Borrego L, Bastida-Inarrea J et al. 1996 Giant cell fibroblastoma. New histological observations. Am J Dermatopathol 18(4): 403–408
1078. Abdul-Karim F W, Evans H L, Silva E G 1985 Giant cell fibroblastoma: a report of three cases. Am J Clin Pathol 83: 165–170
1079. Rubin B P, Fletcher J A, Fletcher C D M 1997 The histologic, genetic, and biological relationships between dermatofibrosarcoma protuberans and giant cell fibroblastoma: an unexpected story. Adv Anat Pathol 4(5): 336–341
1080. Beham A, Fletcher C D M 1990 Dermatofibrosarcoma protuberans with areas resembling giant cell fibroblastoma: report of two cases. Histopathology 17: 165–167
1081. Alguacil-Garcia A 1991 Giant cell fibroblastoma recurring as dermatofibrosarcoma protuberans. Am J Surg Pathol 15(8): 798–801
1082. Coyne J, Kaftan S M, Craig R D 1992 Dermatofibrosarcoma protuberans recurring as a giant cell fibroblastoma. Histopathology 21(2): 184–187
1083. Zamecnik M, Michal M 1994 Giant-cell fibroblastoma with pigmented dermatofibrosarcoma protuberans component. Am J Surg Pathol 18(7): 736–740
1084. Darier J 1924 Dermatofibromes progressifs et récidivants ou fibrosarcomes de la peau. Ann Dermatol Syph (Paris) 5: 545–562
1085. Hoffmann E 1925 Über das knollentreibende fibrosarkom der haut (dermatofibrosarkoma protuberans). Dermatol Zeitschr 43: 1–28
1086. Taylor H B, Helwig E B 1962 Dermatofibrosarcoma protuberans. A study of 115 cases. Cancer 15: 717–725
1087. Bouyssou-Gauthier M-L, Labrousse F, Longis B et al. 1997 Dermatofibrosarcoma protuberans in childhood. Pediatr Dermatol 14(6): 463–465
1088. Martin L, Combemale P, Dupin M et al. 1998 The atrophic variant of dermatofibrosarcoma protuberans in childhood: a report of six cases. Br J Dermatol 139(4): 719–725
1089. McMaster P E 1934 Sarcomatoid fibroma of the skin (progressive and recurring dermatofibroma). Ann Surg 99: 338–347
1090. Barnes L, Coleman JA, Johnson JT 1984 Dermatofibrosarcoma protuberans of the head and neck. Arch Otolaryngol 110: 398–404
1091. Gentele H 1951 Malignant, fibroblastic tumors of the skin (chapter 6). In: Malignant, fibroblastic tumors of the skin. Clinical and pathological-anatomical studies of 129 cases of malignant fibroblastic tumors from the cutaneous and subcutaneous layers observed at Radiumhemmet during the period 1927–1947. Acta Dermato-Venereol 31(Suppl 27): 91–132
1092. McPeak C J, Cruz T, Nicastri A D 1967 Dermatofibrosarcoma protuberans: An analysis of 86 cases – five with metastasis. Ann Surg 166: 803–816
1093. Bednár B 1957 Storiform neurofibromas of the skin, pigmented and nonpigmented. Cancer 10: 368–376
1094. Goldberg D J, Maso M 1990 Dermatofibrosarcoma protuberans in a 9-year-old child: treatment by Mohs micrographic surgery. Pediatr Dermatol 7: 57–59
1095. Robinson J K 1985 Dermatofibrosarcoma protuberans resected by Mohs' surgery (chemosurgery). A 5-year prospective study. J Am Acad Dermatol 12: 1093–1098
1096. Adams J T, Saltzstein S L 1963 Metastasizing dermatofibrosarcoma protuberans: report of two cases. Am Surg 29: 879–886
1097. Binkley G W 1939 Dermatofibrosarcoma protuberans. Report of six cases. Arch Dermatol Syphilol (Chicago) 40: 578–594
1098. Bonnabeau R C Jr, Stoughton W B, Armanious A W et al. 1974 Dermatofibrosarcoma protuberans. Report of a case with pulmonary metastasis and multiple intrathoracic recurrences. Oncology 29(1): 1–12
1099. Brenner W, Schaefler K, Chhabra H et al. 1975 Dermatofibrosarcoma protuberans metastatic to a regional lymph node. Cancer 36: 1897–1902
1100. Hausner R J, Vargas-Cortes F, Alexander R W 1978 Dermatofibrosarcoma protuberans with lymph node involvement. A case report of simultaneous occurrence with an atypical fibroxanthoma of the skin. Arch Dermatol 114: 88–91
1101. Kahn L B, Saxe N, Gordon W 1978 Dermatofibrosarcoma protuberans with lymph node and pulmonary metastases. Arch Dermatol 114: 599–601
1102. Penner D W 1951 Metastasizing dermatofibrosarcoma protuberans. Cancer 4: 1083–1086
1103. Przybora L A, Wojnerowicz C 1959 Malignancy of dermatofibrosarcoma protuberans and report of 2 cases with lymph gland metastases. Oncologia 12: 236–254
1104. Volpe R, Carbone A 1983 Dermatofibrosarcoma protuberans metastatic to lymph nodes and showing a dominant histiocytic component. Am J Dermatopathol 5: 327–334
1105. Frierson H F, Cooper P H 1983 Myxoid variant of dermatofibrosarcoma protuberans. Am J Surg Pathol 7: 445–450
1106. Ashack R J, Tejada E, Parker C et al. 1992 A localized atrophic plaque on the back. Dermatofibrosarcoma protuberans (DFSP) (Atrophic variant). Arch Dermatol 128: 549, 552
1107. Davis D A, Sánchez R L 1998 Atrophic and plaquelike dermatofibrosarcoma protuberans. Am J Dermatopathol 20(5): 498–501
1108. Lambert W C, Abramovits W, Gonzalez-serva A et al. 1985 Dermatofibrosarcoma non-protuberans: description and report of five cases of morpheaform variant of derrmatofibrosarcoma. J Surg Oncol 28: 7–11
1109. Page E A, Assaad D M 1987 Atrophic dermatofibroma and dermatofibrosarcoma protuberans. J Am Acad Dermatol 17: 947–950

1110. Zelger B W, Ofner D, Zelger B G 1995 Atrophic variants of dermatofibroma and dermatofibrosarcoma protuberans. Histopathology 26(6): 519–527
1111. Diaz-Cascajo C, Weyers W, Borghi S 1998 Sclerosing dermatofibrosarcoma protuberans. J Cutan Pathol 25(8): 440–444
1112. Diaz-Cascajo C, Weyers W, Rey-Lopez A et al. 1998 Deep dermatofibrosarcoma protuberans: a subcutaneous variant. Histopathology 32(6): 552–555
1113. Ding J, Hashimoto H, Enjoji M 1989 Dermatofibrosarcoma protuberans with fibrosarcomatous areas. A clinicopathologic study of nine cases and a comparison with allied tumors. Cancer 64: 721–729
1114. Mentzel T, Beham A, Katenkamp D et al. 1998 Fibrosarcomatous ("high-grade") dermatofibrosarcoma protuberans. Clinicopathologic and immunohistochemical study of a series of 41 cases with emphasis on prognostic significance. Am J Surg Pathol 22(5): 576–587
1115. Wrotnowski U, Cooper P H, Shmookler B M 1988 Fibrosarcomatous change in dermatofibrosarcoma protuberans. Am J Surg Pathol 12: 287–293
1116. Connelly J H, Evans H L 1992 Dermatofibrosarcoma protuberans: a clinicopathological review with emphasis on fibrosarcomatous areas. Am J Dermatopathol 16: 921–925
1117. Calonje E, Fletcher C D M 1996 Myoid differentiation in dermatofibrosarcoma protuberans and its fibrosarcomatous variant: clinicopathologic analysis of 5 cases. J Cutan Pathol 23(1): 30–36
1118. O'Dowd J, Laidler P 1988 Progression of dermatofibrosarcoma protuberans to malignant fibrous histiocytoma: report of a case with implications for tumor histogenesis. Hum Pathol 19: 368–370
1118a. Abbott J J, Oliveira A M, Nascimento A G 2006 The prognostic significance of fibrosarcomatous transformation in dermatofibrosarcoma protuberans. Am J Surg Pathol 30: 436–443.
1119. Fletcher C D M, Evans B J, Macartney J C et al. 1985 Dermatofibrosarcoma protuberans: a clinicopathological and immunohistochemical study with a review of the literature. Histopathology 9: 921–938
1120. Banerjee S S, Harris M, Eyden B P et al. 1990 Granular cell variant of dermatofibrosarcoma protuberans. Histopathology 17: 375–378
1121. Dupree W B, Langloss J M, Weiss S W 1985 Pigmented dermatofibrosarcoma protuberans (Bednar tumor). Am J Surg Pathol 9: 630–639
1122. Fletcher C D M, Theaker J M, Flanagan A et al. 1988 Pigmented dermatofibrosarcoma protuberans (Bednar tumour): melanocytic colonization or neuroectodermal differentiation? A clinicopathological and immunohistochemical study. Histopathology 13: 631–643
1123. Aiba S, Tabata N, Ishi H et al. 1992 Dermatofibrosarcoma protuberans is a unique fibrohistiocytic tumor expressing CD34. Br J Dermatol 127(2): 79–84
1124. Brathwaite C, Suster S 1994 Dermatofibrosarcoma protuberans. A critical reappraisal of the role of immunohistochemical stains for diagnosis. Appl Immunohistochem 2(1): 36–41
1125. Cohen P R, Rapin R P, Farhood A I 1994 Dermatofibroma and dermatofibrosarcoma protuberans: differential expression of CD34 and factor XIIIa. Am J Dermatopathol 16(6): 573–574
1126. Diaz-Cascajo C, Bastida-Inarrea J, Borrego L et al. 1995 Comparison of p53 expression in dermatofibrosarcoma protuberans and dermatofibroma: lack of correlation with proliferation rate. J Cutan Pathol 22(4): 304–309
1127. West R B, Harvell J, Linn S C et al. 2004 Apo D in soft tissue tumors: a novel marker of dermatofibrosarcoma protuberans. Am J Surg Pathol 28: 1063–1069
1128. Nakamura T, Ogata H, Katsuyama T 1987 Pigmented dermatofibrosarcoma protuberans. Report of two cases as a variant of dermatofibrosarcoma protuberans with partial neural differentiation. Am J Dermatopathol 9: 18–25
1129. Auböck L 1975 Zur ultrastruktur fibröser und histiocytärer hauttumoren (dermatofibrom, dermatofibrosarcoma protuberans, fibroxanthom und histiocytom). Virchow's Arch A Pathol Anat Histopathol 368: 253–274
1130. Dominguez-Malagon H R, Ordonez N G, Mackay B 1995 Dermatofibrosarcoma protuberans: ultrastructural and immunocytochemical observations. Ultrastruct Pathol 19(4): 281–289
1131. Escalona-Zapata J, Alvarez Fernandez E, Llorca Escuin F 1981 The fibroblastic nature of dermatofibrosarcoma protuberans. A tissue culture and ultrastructural study. Virchow's Arch A Pathol Anat Histopathol 391: 165–175
1132. Ozzello L, Hamels J 1976 The histiocytic nature of dermatofibrosarcoma protuberans. Tissue culture and electron microscopic study. Am J Clin Pathol 65: 136–148
1133. Schmoeckel C, Albini A, Krieg T et al. 1985 The fibroblastic nature of dermatofibrosarcoma protuberans: morphological investigations in vivo and in vitro. Arch Dermatol Res 278: 138–147
1134. Tremblay M, Bonenfant J-L, Cliche J 1970 Le dermatofibrosarcome protubérant étude clinico-pathologique de trente cas avec l'ultrastructure de deux cas. Union Med Can 99: 871–876
1135. Alguacil-Garcia A, Unni K K, Goellner J R 1978 Histogenesis of dermatofibrosarcoma protuberans. An ultrastructural study. Am J Clin Pathol 69: 427–434
1136. Hashimoto K, Brownstein M H, Jakobiec F A 1974 Dermatofibrosarcoma protuberans. A tumor with perineural and endoneural cell features. Arch Dermatol 110: 874–885
1137. Bridge J A, Neff J R, Sandberg A A 1990 Cytogenetic analysis of dermatofibrosarcoma protuberans. Cancer Genet Cytogenet 49: 199–202
1138. Naeem R, Lux M L, Huang S F et al. 1995 Ring chromosomes in dermatofibrosarcoma protuberans are composed of interspersed sequences from chromosomes 17 and 22. Am J Pathol 147(6): 1553–1558
1139. Stephenson C F, Berger C S, Leong S P et al. 1992 Ring chromosome in a dermatofibrosarcoma protuberans. Cancer Genet Cytogenet 58: 52–54
1140. Fretzin D F, Helwig E B 1973 Atypical fibroxanthoma of the skin. A clinicopathologic study of 140 cases. Cancer 31(6): 1541–1552
1141. Helwig E B 1963 Tumor seminar (case 6) (atypical fibroxanthoma). Texas St J Med 59: 652–689
1142. Kempson R L, McGavran M H 1964 Atypical fibroxanthomas of the skin. Cancer 17(11): 1463–1471
1143. Reed R J 1967 Atypical fibroxanthomas and spindle-cell carcinomas of the skin. Bull Tulane Univ Med Fac 26: 75–89
1144. Bourne R G 1963 Paradoxical fibrosarcoma of skin (pseudosarcoma): a review of 13 cases. Med J Aust 1: 504–510
1145. Levan N E, Kwong M Q 1963 Pseudosarcomatous dermatofibroma. Arch Dermatol 88: 908–912
1146. Gordon H W 1964 Pseudosarcomatous reticulohistiocytoma. A report of four cases. Arch Dermatol 90: 319–325
1147. Noede N, Korting G W 1968 Pseudosarkomatöses xanthofibrom. Arch Klin Exp Dermatol 232: 119–126
1148. Vargas-Cortes F, Winkelmann R K, Soule E H 1973 Atypical fibroxanthomas of the skin. Further observations with 19 additional cases. Mayo Clinic Proc 48: 211–218
1149. Tapernoux B, Jeanneret J P, Delacrétaz J 1971 Fibroxanthome atypique. Dermatologica 142: 93–98
1150. Kroe J, Pitcock J A 1969 Atypical fibroxanthoma of the skin. Report of ten cases. Am J Clin Pathol 51(4): 487–492
1151. Dahl I 1976 Atypical fibroxanthoma of the skin. A clinico-pathological study of 57 cases. Acta Pathol Microbiol Scand A 84: 183–197
1152. Glavin F L, Cornwell M L 1985 Atypical fibroxanthoma of the skin metastatic to a lung. Report of a case, features by conventional and electron microscopy, and a review of relevant literature. Am J Dermatopathol 7(1): 57–63
1153. Helwig E B, May D 1986 Atypical fibroxanthoma of the skin with metastasis. Cancer 57(2): 368–376
1154. Kemp J D, Stenn K S, Arons M et al. 1978 Metastasizing atypical fibroxanthoma. Coexistence with chronic lymphocytic leukemia. Arch Dermatol 114(10): 1533–1535
1155. Wilson P R, Strutton G M, Stewart M R 1989 Atypical fibroxanthoma: two unusual variants. J Cutan Pathol 16(2): 93–98
1156. Hudson A W, Winkelmann R K 1972 Atypical fibroxanthoma of the skin: a reappraisal of 19 cases in which the original diagnosis was spindle-cell squamous carcinoma. Cancer 29(2): 413–422
1157. Calonje E, Wadden C, Wilson Jones E et al. 1993 Spindle-cell non-pleomorphic atypical fibroxanthoma: analysis of a series and delineation of a distinctive variant. Histopathology 22(3): 247–254
1158. Tomaszewski M M, Lupton G P 1997 Atypical fibroxanthoma. An unusual variant with osteoclast-like giant cells. Am J Surg Pathol 21(2): 213–218
1159. Val-Bernal J F, Corral J, Fernandez F et al. 1994 Atypical fibroxanthoma with osteoclast-like giant cells. Acta Dermato-Venereol 74(6): 467–470
1160. Val-Bernal J F, Fernandez F A 1997 Atypical fibroxanthoma with osteoclastlike giant cells (letter). Am J Surg Pathol 21(11): 1393
1161. Requena L, Sangueza O P, Sanchez Yus E et al. 1997 Clear-cell atypical fibroxanthoma: an uncommon histopathologic variant of atypical fibroxanthoma. J Cutan Pathol 24(3): 176–182
1162. Rudisaile S N, Hurt M A, Santa Cruz D J 2005 Granular cell atypical fibroxanthoma. J Cutan Pathol 32(4): 314–317
1163. Diaz-Cascajo C, Borghi S, Bonczkowitz M 1998 Pigmented atypical fibroxanthoma. Histopathology 33(6): 537–541
1164. Leong A S-Y, Milios J 1987 Atypical fibroxanthoma of the skin: a clinicopathological and immunohistochemical study and a discussion of histogenesis. Histopathology 11(5): 463–475
1165. Silvis N G, Swanson P E, Manivel J C et al. 1988 Spindle-cell and pleomorphic neoplasms of the skin. A clinicopathologic and immunohistochemical study of 30 cases, with emphasis on "atypical fibroxanthomas". Am J Dermatopathol 10(1): 9–19
1166. Eckert F, Burg G, Braun-Falco O et al. 1989 Immunostaining in atypical fibroxanthoma of the skin. Pathol Res Pract 184(1): 27–34
1167. Longacre T A, Smoller B R, Rouse R V 1993 Atypical fibroxanthoma. Multiple immunohistologic profiles. Am J Surg Pathol 17(12): 1199–1209
1168. Eusebi V, Ceccarelli C, Piscioli F et al. 1984 Spindle cell tumours of the skin of debatable origin. An immunocytochemical study. J Pathol 144(3): 189–199
1169. Ma C K, Zarbo R J, Gown A M 1992 Immunohistochemical characterization of atypical fibroxanthoma and dermatofibrosarcoma protuberans. Am J Clin Pathol 97(4): 478–483
1170. Ricci A R Jr, Cartun R W, Zakowski M F 1988 Atypical fibroxanthoma. A study of 14 cases emphasizing the presence of Langerhans' histiocytes with implications for differential diagnosis by antibody panels. Am J Surg Pathol 12(8): 591–598
1171. Winkelmann R K, Peters M S 1985 Atypical fibroxanthoma. A study with antibody to S-100 protein. Arch Dermatol 121(6): 753–755
1172. Barr R J, Wuerker R B, Graham J H 1977 Ultrastructure of atypical fibroxanthoma. Cancer 40(2): 736–743
1173. Woyke S, Domagala W, Olszewski W et al. 1974 Pseudosarcoma of the skin. An electron microscopic study and comparison with the fine

structure of the spindle-cell variant of squamous carcinoma. Cancer 33(4): 970–980
1174. Carson J W, Schwartz A, McCandless C M et al. 1984 Atypical fibroxanthoma of the skin. Report of a case with Langerhans-like granules. Arch Dermatol 120(2): 234–239
1175. Worrell J T, Ansari M Q, Ansari S J et al. 1993 Atypical fibroxanthoma: DNA ploidy analysis of 14 cases with possible histogenetic implications. J Cutan Pathol 20(3): 211–215
1176. Michie B A, Reid R P, Fallowfield M E 1994 Aneuploidy in atypical fibroxanthoma: DNA content quantification of 10 cases by image analysis. J Cutan Pathol 21(5): 404–407
1177. Gould E, Albores-Saavedra J, Rothe M et al. 1989 Malignant giant cell tumor of soft parts presenting as a skin tumor. Am J Dermatopathol 11: 197–201
1178. Kemmett D, Gawkrodger D J, McLaren K M et al. 1988 Two atypical fibroxanthomas arising separately in X-irradiated skin. Clin Exp Dermatol 13(6): 382–384
1179. Rachmaninoff N, McDonald J R, Cook J C 1961 Sarcoma-like tumors of the skin following irradiation. Am J Clin Pathol 36(5): 427–437
1180. Dei Tos A P, Maestro R, Doglioni C et al. 1994 Ultraviolet-induced p53 mutations in atypical fibroxanthoma. Am J Pathol 145(1): 11–17
1181. Sakamoto A, Oda Y, Itakura E et al. 2001 Immunoexpression of ultraviolet photoproducts and p53 mutation analysis in atypical fibroxanthoma and superficial malignant fibrous histiocytoma. Mod Pathol 14: 581–588
1182. Rockwell W B, Cohen I K, Ehrlich H P 1989 Keloids and hypertrophic scars: a comprehensive review. Plastic Reconstruct Surg 84: 827–837
1183. Price S K, Kahn L B, Saxe N 1993 Dermal and intravascular fasciitis. Unusual variants of nodular fasciitis. Am J Dermatopathol 15(6): 539–543
1184. Uitto J, Santa Cruz D J, Eisen A Z 1980 Connective tissue nevi of the skin. Clinical, genetic, and histopathologic classification of hamartomas of the collagen, elastin, and proteoglycan type. J Am Acad Dermatol 3: 441–461
1185. Fork H E, Sanchez R L, Wagner R F Jr, et al. 1991 A new type of connective tissue nevus: isolated exophytic elastoma. J Cutan Pathol 18(6): 457–463
1186. Pierard G E, Lapiere C M 1985 Nevi of connective tissue. A reappraisal of their classification. Am J Dermatopathol 7(4): 325–333
1187. Trau H, Dayan D, Hirschberg A et al. 1991 Connective tissue nevi collagens. Study with picrosirius red and polarizing microscopy. Am J Dermatopathol 13(4): 374–377
1188. Chapman M S, Perry A E, Baughman R D 1998 Cowden's syndrome, Lhermitte–Duclos disease, and sclerotic fibroma. Am J Dermatopathol 20(4): 413–416
1189. García-Doval I, Casas L, Toribio J 1998 Pleomorphic fibroma of the skin, a form of sclerotic fibroma: an immunohistochemical study. Clin Exp Dermatol 23(1): 22–24
1190. McCalmont T H 1994 Sclerotic fibroma: a fossil no longer. J Cutan Pathol 21(1): 82–85
1191. Nahass G 1998 Sclerotic fibroma-like changes in dermatofibrosarcoma protuberans (abstract). J Cutan Pathol 25(9): 507
1192. Pujol R M, de Castro F, Schroeter A L et al. 1996 Solitary sclerotic fibroma of the skin: a sclerotic dermatofibroma? Am J Dermatopathol 18(6): 620–624
1193. Shitabata P K, Crouch E C, Fitzgibbon J F et al. 1995 Cutaneous sclerotic fibroma. Immunohistochemical evidence of a fibroblastic neoplasm with ongoing type I collagen synthesis. Am J Dermatopathol 17(4): 339–343
1194. Zelger B G, Zelger B, Steiner H et al. 1997 Sclerotic lipoma: lipomas simulating sclerotic fibroma. Histopathology 31(2): 174–181
1195. Chung E B, Enzinger F M 1979 Fibroma of tendon sheath. Cancer 44: 1945–1954
1196. Cooper P H 1984 Fibroma of tendon sheath. J Am Acad Dermatol 11: 625–628
1197. Sapra S, Prokopetz R, Murray A H 1989 Giant cell tumor of tendon sheath. Int J Dermatol 28: 587–590
1198. Beham A, Badve S, Suster S et al. 1993 Solitary myofibroma in adults: clinicopathological analysis of a series. Histopathology 22(4): 335–341
1199. Chung E B, Enzinger F M 1981 Infantile myofibromatosis. Cancer 48: 1807–1818
1200. Daimaru Y, Hashimoto H, Enjoji M 1989 Myofibromatosis in adults (adult counterpart of infantile myofibromatosis). Am J Surg Pathol 13: 859–865
1201. Granter S R, Badizadegan K, Fletcher C D M 1998 Myofibromatosis in adults, glomangiopericytoma, and myopericytoma. A spectrum of tumors showing perivascular myoid differentiation. Am J Surg Pathol 22(5): 513–525
1202. Guitart J, Ritter J H, Wick M R 1996 Solitary cutaneous myofibromas in adults: report of six cases and discussion of differential diagnosis. J Cutan Pathol 23(5): 437–444
1203. Jennings T A, Duray P H, Collins F S et al. 1984 Infantile myofibromatosis. Evidence for an autosomal-dominant disorder. Am J Surg Pathol 8: 529–538
1204. Kutzner H, Requena L, Hügel H et al. 1996 Adult myofibroma: an acquired neoplasm of vascular (myopericytic) character. Dermatopathol Pract Concept 2(3): 190–195
1205. Requena L, Kutzner H, Hugel H et al. 1996 Cutaneous adult myofibroma: a vascular neoplasm. J Cutan Pathol 23(5): 445–457
1206. Smith K J, Skelton H G, Barrett T L et al. 1989 Cutaneous myofibroma. Mod Pathol 2(6): 603–609
1207. Colome M I, Sanchez R L 1994 Dermatomyofibroma: report of two cases. J Cutan Pathol 21(4): 371–376
1208. Hugel H 1993 Plaque-like dermal fibromatosis/dermatomyofibroma. J Cutan Pathol 20(1): 9
1209. Mentzel T, Calonje E, Fletcher C D M 1993 Dermatomyofibroma: additional observations on a distinctive cutaneous myofibroblastic tumour with emphasis on differential diagnosis. Br J Dermatol 129(1): 69–73
1210. Tani M, Komura A, Ichihashi M 1997 Dermatomyofibroma (plaqueförmige dermale fibromatose). J Dermatol (Tokyo) 24(12): 793–797
1211. Bale P M, Hughes L, de Silva M 1990 Sequestrated meningoceles of scalp: extracranial meningeal heterotopia. Hum Pathol 21: 1156–1163
1212. Berry A D III, Patterson J W 1991 Meningoceles, meningomyeloceles, and encephaloceles: a neuro-dermatopathologic study of 132 cases. J Cutan Pathol 18(3): 164–177
1213. Commens C, Rogers M, Kan A 1989 Heterotropic brain tissue presenting as bald cysts with a collar of hypertrophic hair. The "hair collar" sign. Arch Dermatol 125: 1253–1256
1214. Lopez D A, Silvers D N, Helwig E B 1974 Cutaneous meningiomas. A clinicopathologic study. Cancer 34: 728–744
1215. Sibley D A, Cooper P H 1989 Rudimentary meningocele: a variant of "primary cutaneous meningioma". J Cutan Pathol 16: 72–80
1216. Suster S, Rosai J 1990 Hamartoma of the scalp with ectopic meningothelial elements. A distinctive benign soft tissue lesion that may simulate angiosarcoma. Am J Surg Pathol 14: 1–11
1217. Theaker J M, Fletcher C D M, Tudway A J 1990 Cutaneous heterotopic meningeal nodules. Histopathology 16: 475–479
1218. Hartmann C-A, Sperling M, Stein H 1990 So-called fibroepithelial polyps of the vagina exhibiting an unusual but uniform antigen profile characterized by expression of desmin and steroid hormone receptors but no muscle-specific actin or macrophage markers. Am J Clin Pathol 93: 604–608
1219. Mucitelli D R, Charles E Z, Kraus F T 1990 Vulvovaginal polyps. Histologic appearance, ultrastructure, immunocytochemical characteristics, and clinicopathologic correlations. Int J Gynecol Pathol 9: 20–40
1220. Östör A G, Fortune D W, Riley C B 1988 Fibroepithelial polyps with atypical stromal cells (pseudosarcoma botryoides) of vulva and vagina. A report of 13 cases. Int J Gynecol Pathol 7: 351–360
1221. Nucci M R, Young R H, Fletcher C D 2000 Cellular pseudosarcomatous fibroepithelial stromal polyps of the lower female genital tract: an underrecognized lesion often misdiagnosed as sarcoma. Am J Surg Pathol 24(2): 231–240
1222. Ackerman A B, de Viragh P A, Chongchitnant N et al. 1993 Fibrous papule (chapter 12). In: Neoplasms with Follicular Differentiation. Lea & Febiger, Philadelphia, p 207–229
1223. Graham J H, Sanders J B, Johnson W C et al. 1965 Fibrous papule of the nose: a clinicopathologic study. J Invest Dermatol 45: 194–203
1224. Guitart J, Bergfeld W F, Tuthill R J 1991 Fibrous papule of the nose with granular cells: two cases. J Cutan Pathol 18(4): 284–287
1225. Nemeth A J, Penneys N S, Bernstein H B 1988 Fibrous papule: a tumor of fibrohistiocytic cells that contain factor XIIIa. J Am Acad Dermatol 19: 1102–1106
1226. Rosen L B, Suster S 1988 Fibrous papules. A light microscopic and immunohistochemical study. Am J Dermatopathol 10(2): 109–115
1227. Santa Cruz D J, Prioleau P G 1979 Fibrous papule of the face. An electron-microscopic study of two cases. Am J Dermatopathol 1(4): 349–352
1228. Saylan T, Marks R, Wilson Jones E 1971 Fibrous papule of the nose. Br J Dermatol 85(2): 111–118
1229. Soyer H P, Kutzner H, Metze D et al. 1997 Fibrous papule with clear fibrocytes. Dermatopathol Pract Concept 3(2): 110–113
1230. Bansal C, Stewart D, Li A et al. 2005 Histologic variants of fibrous papule. J Cutan Pathol 32(6): 424–428
1231. Lee A N, Stein S L, Cohen L M 2005 Clear cell fibrous papule with NKI/C3 expression: clinical and histologic features in six cases. Am J Dermatopathol 27: 296–300
1232. Bart R S, Andrade R, Kopf A W et al. 1968 Acquired digital fibrokeratomas. Arch Dermatol 97: 120–129
1233. Hare P J, Smith P A J 1969 Acquired (digital) fibrokeratoma. Br J Dermatol 81: 667–670
1234. Kint A, Baran R, De Keyser H 1985 Acquired (digital) fibrokeratoma. J Am Acad Dermatol 12: 816–821
1235. Verallo V V M 1968 Acquired digital fibrokeratomas. Br J Dermatol 80: 730–736
1236. Choi K C, Hashimoto K, Setoyama M et al. 1990 Infantile digital fibromatosis. Immunohistochemical and immunoelectron microscopic studies. J Cutan Pathol 17: 225–232
1237. Ishii N, Matsui K, Ichiyama S et al. 1989 A case of infantile digital fibromatosis showing spontaneous regression. Br J Dermatol 121: 129–133
1238. Mukai M, Torikata C, Iri H et al. 1992 Immunohistochemical identification of aggregated actin filaments in formalin-fixed, paraffin-embedded sections. I. A study of infantile digital fibromatosis by a new pretreatment. Am J Surg Pathol 16(2): 110–115
1239. Reye R D K 1965 Recurring digital fibrous tumors of childhood. Arch Pathol 80: 228–231
1240. Santa Cruz D J, Reiner C B 1978 Recurrent digital fibroma of childhood. J Cutan Pathol 5: 339–346
1241. Zhu W Y, Xia M Y, Huang Y F et al. 1991 Infantile digital fibromatosis: ultrastructural human papillomavirus and herpes simplex virus DNA observation. Pediatr Dermatol 8(2): 137–139

1242. Viale G, Doglioni C, Iuzzolino P et al. 1988 Infantile digital fibromatosis-like tumour (inclusion body fibromatosis) of adulthood: report of two cases with ultrastructural and immunocytochemical findings. Histopathology 12: 415–424
1243. Aberer E, Maintiz M, Entacher U et al. 1988 Fibrous hamartoma of infancy – infantile subcutaneous myofibroblastoma. Dermatologica 176: 46–51
1244. Enzinger F M 1965 Fibrous hamartoma of infancy. Cancer 18: 241–248
1245. Fletcher C D M, Powell G, van Noorden S et al. 1988 Fibrous hamartoma of infancy: a histochemical and immunohistochemical study. Histopathology 12: 65–74
1246. Greco M A, Schinella R A, Vuletin J C 1984 Fibrous hamartoma of infancy. An ultrastructural study. Hum Pathol 15: 717–723
1247. Paller A S, Sherman J O 1989 Fibrous hamartoma of infancy. Eight additional cases and a review of the literature. Arch Dermatol 125: 88–91
1248. Reye R D K 1956 A consideration of certain subdermal "fibrous tumors" of infancy. J Pathol Bacteriol 72: 149–154
1249. Cerio R, Gold S, Wilson Jones E 1991 White fibrous papulosis of the neck. Clin Exp Dermatol 16: 224–225
1250. Shimizu H, Kimura S, Harada T et al. 1989 White fibrous papulosis of the neck: A new clinicopathologic entity? J Am Acad Dermatol 20: 1073–1077
1251. Kan A E, Rogers M 1989 Juvenile hyaline fibromatosis: an expanded clinicopathologic spectrum. Pediatr Dermatol 6: 68–75
1252. El-Shabrawi L, Kerl K, Cerroni L et al. 1998 Inflammatory pseudotumor of the skin (abstract). J Cutan Pathol 25(9): 494
1253. Hurt M A, Santa Cruz D J 1990 Cutaneous inflammatory pseudotumor. Lesions resembling "inflammatory pseudotumors" or "plasma cell granulomas" of extracutaneous sites. Am J Surg Pathol 14: 764–773
1254. Helwig E B, Hackney V C 1954 Juvenile xanthogranuloma (nevoxantho-endothelioma) (abstract). Am J Pathol 30: 625–626
1255. Hernandez-Martin A, Baselga E, Drolet B A et al. 1997 Juvenile xanthogranuloma. J Am Acad Dermatol 36(3 Pt 1): 355–367
1256. Dehner L P 2003 Juvenile xanthogranulomas in the first two decades of life: a clinicopathologic study of 174 cases with cutaneous and extracutaneous manifestations. Am J Surg Pathol 27: 579–593
1257. McDonagh J E R 1912 A contribution to our knowledge of the nævo-xantho-endotheliomata. Br J Dermatol 24: 85–99
1258. Cohen B A, Hood A 1989 Xanthogranuloma: report on clinical and histologic findings in 64 patients. Pediatr Dermatol 6: 262–266
1259. Rodriguez J, Ackerman A B 1976 Xanthogranuloma in adults. Arch Dermatol 112: 43–44
1260. Sonoda T, Hashimoto H, Enjoji M 1985 Juvenile xanthogranuloma. Clinicopathologic analysis and immunohistochemical study of 57 patients. Cancer 56: 2280–2286
1261. Tahan S R, Pastel-Levy C, Bhan A K et al. 1989 Juvenile xanthogranuloma. Clinical and pathologic characterization. Arch Pathol Lab Med 113: 1057–1061
1262. Resnick S D, Woosley J, Azizkhan R G 1990 Giant juvenile xanthogranuloma: exophytic and endophytic variants. Pediatr Dermatol 7: 185–188
1263. Chang M W, Frieden I J, Good W 1996 The risk of intraocular juvenile xanthogranuloma: survey of current practices and assessment of risk. J Am Acad Dermatol 34(3): 445–449
1264. Zimmerman L E 1965 Ocular lesions of juvenile xanthogranuloma. Am J Ophthalmol 60: 1011–1035
1265. de Graaf J H, Timens W, Tamminga R Y et al. 1992 Deep juvenile xanthogranuloma: a lesion related to dermal indeterminate cells. Hum Pathol 23(8): 905–910
1266. Janney C G, Hurt M A, Santa Cruz D J 1991 Deep juvenile xanthogranuloma. Subcutaneous and intramuscular forms. Am J Surg Pathol 15: 150–159
1267. Nascimento A G 1997 A clinicopathologic and immunohistochemical comparative study of cutaneous and intramuscular forms of juvenile xanthogranuloma. Am J Surg Pathol 21(6): 645–652
1268. Sanchez Yus E, Requena L, Villegas C et al. 1995 Subcutaneous juvenile xanthogranuloma. J Cutan Pathol 22(5): 460–465
1269. White W, Garen P 1991 Juvenile xanthogranuloma of the paravertebral soft tissue in infancy: a report of two cases. Pediatr Pathol 11: 105–113
1270. Botella-Estrada R, Sanmartín O, Grau M et al. 1993 Juvenile xanthogranuloma with central nervous system involvement. Pediatr Dermatol 10(1): 64–68
1271. Freyer D R, Kennedy R, Bostrom B C et al. 1996 Juvenile xanthogranuloma: forms of systemic disease and their clinical implications. J Pediatr 129(2): 227–237
1272. Claudy A L, Misery L, Serre D et al. 1993 Multiple juvenile xanthogranulomas without foam cells and giant cells. Pediatr Dermatol 10(1): 61–63
1273. Newman C C, Raimer S S, Sánchez R L 1997 Nonlipidized juvenile xanthogranuloma: a histologic and immunohistochemical study. Pediatr Dermatol 14(2): 98–102
1274. Shapiro P E, Silvers D N, Treiber R K 1991 Juvenile xanthogranuloma with inconspicuous or absent foam cells and giant cells. J Am Acad Dermatol 24: 1005–1009
1275. Tanz W S, Kim Y A, Schwartz R A et al. 1995 Juvenile xanthogranuloma with inconspicuous foam cells and giant cells. Int J Dermatol 34(9): 653–655
1276. Zelger B G, Orchard G, Rudolph P et al. 1998 Scalloped cell xanthogranuloma. Histopathology 32(4): 368–374
1277. Ackerman A B 1995 Xanthogranuloma with "monster" cells. Dermatopathol Pract Concept 1(4): 267, 280
1278. Sangueza O P, Salmon J K, White C R Jr et al. 1995 Juvenile xanthogranuloma: a clinical, histopathologic and immunohistochemical study. J Cutan Pathol 22(4): 327–335
1279. Zelger B, Cerio R, Orchard G et al. 1994 Juvenile and adult xanthogranuloma. A histological and immunohistochemical comparison. Am J Surg Pathol 18(2): 126–135
1280. Kraus M D, Haley J C, Ruiz R et al. 2001 Juvenile xanthogranuloma: an immunophenotypic study with a reappraisal of histogenesis. Am J Dermatopathol 23: 104–111
1281. Bhawan J, Majno G 1989 The myofibroblast. Possible derivation from macrophages in xanthogranuloma. Am J Dermatopathol 11: 255–258
1282. Gonzalez-Crussi F, Campbell R J 1970 Juvenile xanthogranuloma ultrastructural study. Arch Pathol Lab Med 89: 65–72
1283. Seifert H W 1981 Membrane activity in juvenile xanthogranuloma. J Cutan Pathol 8: 25–33
1284. Seo I S, Min K W, Mirkin L D 1986 Juvenile xanthogranuloma. Ultrastructural and immunocytochemical studies. Arch Pathol Lab Med 110: 911–915
1285. Winkelmann R K, Oliver G F 1989 Subcutaneous xanthogranulomatosis: an inflammatory non-X histiocytic syndrome (subcutaneous xanthomatosis). J Am Acad Dermatol 21: 924–929
1286. Purvis W E, Helwig E B 1954 Reticulohistiocytic granuloma ("reticulohistiocytoma") of the skin. Am J Clin Pathol 24: 1005–1015
1286a. Miettinen M, Fetsch J F 2006 Reticulohistiocytoma (solitary epithelioid histiocytoma): a clinicopathologic and immunohistochemical study of 44 cases. Am J Sug Pathol 30: 521–528
1287. Barrow M V, Holubar K 1969 Multicentric reticulohistiocytosis. A review of 33 patients. Medicine (Baltimore) 48(4): 287–305
1288. Oliver G F, Umbert I, Winkelmann R K et al. 1990 Reticulohistiocytoma cutis – review of 15 cases and an association with systemic vasculitis in two cases. Clin Exp Dermatol 15(1): 1–6
1289. Suwabe H, Tsutsumi Y 1996 Reticulohistiocytoma involving the skin, subcutaneous tissue and a regional lymph node. Pathol Int 46(7): 531–537
1290. Salisbury J R, Hall P A, Williams H C et al. 1990 Multicentric reticulohistiocytosis. Detailed immunophenotyping confirms macrophage origin. Am J Surg Pathol 14(7): 687–693
1291. Zelger B, Cerio R, Soyer H P et al. 1994 Reticulohistiocytoma and multicentric reticulohistiocytosis. Histopathologic and immunophenotypic distinct entities. Am J Dermatopathol 16(6): 577–584
1292. Albrecht S, Kahn H J, From L 1989 Palisaded encapsulated neuroma: an immunohistochemical study. Mod Pathol 2(4): 403–406
1293. Argenyi Z B 1990 Immunohistochemical characterization of palisaded, encapsulated neuroma. J Cutan Pathol 17(6): 329–335
1294. Argenyi Z B, Cooper P H, Santa Cruz D 1993 Plexiform and other unusual variants of palisaded encapsulated neuroma. J Cutan Pathol 20(1): 34–39
1295. Dakin M C, Leppard B, Theaker J M 1992 The palisaded, encapsulated neuroma (solitary circumscribed neuroma). Histopathology 20(5): 405–410
1296. Dover J S, From L, Lewis A 1989 Palisaded encapsulated neuromas. A clinicopathologic study. Arch Dermatol 125(3): 386–389
1297. Fletcher C D M 1989 Solitary circumscribed neuroma of the skin (so-called palisaded, encapsulated neuroma). A clinicopathologic and immunohistochemical study. Am J Surg Pathol 13(7): 574–580
1298. Kossard S, Kumar A, Wilkinson B 1999 Neural spectrum: palisaded encapsulated neuroma and verocay body poor dermal schwannoma. J Cutan Pathol 26(1): 31–36
1299. Reed R J, Fine R M, Meltzer H D 1972 Palisaded, encapsulated neuromas of the skin. Arch Dermatol 106(6): 865–870
1300. Megahed M 1994 Palisaded encapsulated neuroma (solitary circumscribed neuroma). A clinicopathologic and immunohistochemical study. Am J Dermatopathol 16(2): 120–125
1301. Tsang W Y, Chan J K 1992 Epithelioid variant of solitary circumscribed neuroma of the skin. Histopathology 20(5): 439–441
1302. Prieto V G, McNutt N S, Lugo J et al. 1997 Differential expression of the intermediate filament peripherin in cutaneous neural lesions and neurotized melanocytic nevi. Am J Surg Pathol 21(12): 1450–1454
1303. Gallager RL, Helwig EB 1980 Neurothekeoma: a benign cutaneous tumor of neural origin. Am J Clin Pathol 74(6): 759–764
1304. Argenyi Z B, LeBoit P E, Santa Cruz D et al. 1993 Nerve sheath myxoma (neurothekeoma) of the skin: light microscopic and immunohistochemical reappraisal of the cellular variant. J Cutan Pathol 20(4): 294–303
1305. Barnhill R L, Mihm M C Jr 1990 Cellular neurothekeoma. A distinctive variant of neurothekeoma mimicking nevomelanocytic tumors. Am J Surg Pathol 14(2): 113–120
1306. Rosati L A, Fratamico F C, Eusebi V 1986 Cellular neurothekeoma. Appl Pathol 4(3): 186–191
1307. Calonje E, Wilson Jones E, Smith N P et al. 1992 Cellular "neurothekeoma": an epithelioid variant of pilar leiomyoma? morphological and immunohistochemical analysis of a series. Histopathology 20(5): 397–404
1308. Mentzel T, Calonje E, Fletcher C D M 1996 Cellular "neurothekeoma": correction of a mistaken hypothesis. Dermatopathol Pract Concept 2(4): 237–240
1309. Zelger B G, Steiner H, Kutzner H et al. 1998 Cellular "neurothekeoma": an epithelioid variant of dermatofibroma? Histopathology 32(5): 414–422

1310. Busam K J, Mentzel T, Colpaert C et al. 1998 Atypical or worrisome features in cellular neurothekeoma. A study of 10 cases. Am J Surg Pathol 22(9): 1067–1072
1311. Barnhill R L, Dickersin G R, Nickeleit V et al. 1991 Studies on the cellular origin of neurothekeoma: clinical, light microscopic, immunohistochemical, and ultrastructural observations. J Am Acad Dermatol 25(1 Pt 1): 80–88
1312. Ariza A, Bilbao J M, Rosai J 1988 Immunohistochemical detection of epithelial membrane antigen in normal perineurial cells and perineurioma. Am J Surg Pathol 12(9): 678–683
1313. Angervall L, Kindbloom L G, Haglid K 1984 Dermal nerve sheath myxoma: A light and electron microscopic, histochemical and immunohistochemical study. Cancer 53(8): 1752–1759
1314. Aronson P J, Fretzin D F, Potter B S 1985 Neurothekeoma of Gallager and Helwig (dermal nerve sheath myxoma variant): Report of a case with electron microscopic and immunohistochemical studies. J Cutan Pathol 12(6): 506–519
1315. Argenyi Z B, Kutzner H, Seaba M M 1995 Ultrastructural spectrum of cutaneous nerve sheath myxoma/cellular neurothekeoma. J Cutan Pathol 22(2): 137–145
1316. Weinstock M A, Horn J W 1988 Mycosis fungoides in the United States: increasing incidence and descriptive epidemiology. J Am Med Assoc 260: 42–46
1317. Willemze R, Kerl H, Sterry W et al. 1997 EORTC classification for primary cutaneous lymphomas: a proposal from the Cutaneous Lymphoma Study Group of the European Organization for Research and Treatment of Cancer. Blood 90(1): 354–371
1318. Willemze R, Jaffe E S, Burg G et al. 2005 WHO-EORTC classification for cutaneous lymphomas. Blood 105(10): 3768–3785
1319. Russell Jones R 2003 World Health Organization classification of hematopoietic and lymphoid tissues: implications for dermatology. J Am Acad Dermatol 48(1): 93–102
1320. Sander C A, Flaig M J, Jaffe E S 2001 Cutaneous manifestations of lymphoma: a clinical guide based on the WHO classification. World Health Organization. Clin Lymphoma 2(2): 86–100
1321. Ploysangam T, Breneman D L, Mutasim D F 1998 Cutaneous pseudolymphomas. J Am Acad Dermatol 38(6 Pt 1): 877–895
1322. Nihal M, Mikkola D, Horvath N et al. 2003 Cutaneous lymphoid hyperplasia: a lymphoproliferative continuum with lymphomatous potential. Hum Pathol 34: 617–622
1323. Rijlaarsdam U, Willemze R 1991 Cutaneous pseudo-T-cell lymphomas. Semin Diagn Pathol 8: 102–108
1324. Willemze R 2003 Cutaneous T-cell lymphoma: epidemiology, etiology, and classification. Leuk Lymphoma 44(3): S49–54
1325. Kempf W, Dummer R, Burg G 1999 Approach to lymphoproliferative infiltrates of the skin. The difficult lesions. Am J Clin Pathol 111(Suppl 1): s84–s93
1326. Brodell R T, Miller C W, Eisen A Z 1986 Cutaneous lesions of lymphomatoid granulomatosis. Arch Dermatol 122(3): 303–306
1327. Liebow A A, Carrington C R, Friedman P J 1972 Lymphomatoid granulomatosis. Hum Pathol 3(4): 457–558
1328. LeBoit P E 1991 Variants of mycosis fungoides and related cutaneous T-cell lymphomas. Semin Diagn Pathol 8: 73–81
1329. Vergier B, de Muret A, Beylot-Barry M et al. 2000 Transformation of mycosis fungoides: clinicopathological and prognostic features of 45 cases. French Study Group of Cutaneous Lymphomas. Blood 95(7): 2212–2218
1330. Cerroni L, Rieger E, Hödl S et al. 1992 Clinicopathologic and immunologic features associated with transformation of mycosis fungoides to large-cell lymphoma. Am J Surg Pathol 16: 543–552
1331. Ralfkiaer E 1991 Immunohistological markers for the diagnosis of cutaneous lymphomas. Semin Diagn Pathol 8: 62–72
1332. Wood G S, Tung R M, Haeffner A C et al. 1994 Detection of clonal T-cell receptor gamma gene rearrangements in early mycosis fungoides/Sezary syndrome by polymerase chain reaction and denaturing gradient gel electrophoresis (PCR/DGGE). J Invest Dermatol 103(1): 34–41
1333. Vergier B, Beylot-Barry M, Beylot C et al. 1996 Pilotropic cutaneous T-cell lymphoma without mucinosis. A variant of mycosis fungoides? French Study Group of Cutaneous Lymphomas. Arch Dermatol 132(6): 683–687
1334. Zelickson B D, Peters M S, Muller S A et al. 1991 T-cell receptor gene rearrangement analysis: cutaneous T cell lymphoma, peripheral T cell lymphoma, and premalignant and benign cutaneous lymphoproliferative disorders. J Am Acad Dermatol 25(5 Pt 1): 787–796
1335. Foulc P, N'Guyen J M, Dreno B 2003 Prognostic factors in Sezary syndrome: a study of 28 patients. Br J Dermatol 149(6): 1152–1158
1336. Sézary A, Bouvrain Y 1938 Erythrodermie avec presence de cellules monstrueuses dans le derme et dans le sang circulant. Bull Soc Fr Dermatol Syphiligr 45: 254
1337. Wieselthier J S, Koh H K 1990 Sezary syndrome: diagnosis, prognosis, and critical review of treatment options. J Am Acad Dermatol 22(3): 381–401
1338. Kohler S, Kim Y H, Smoller B R 1997 Histologic criteria for the diagnosis of erythrodermic mycosis fungoides and Sezary syndrome: a critical reappraisal. J Cutan Pathol 24(5): 292–297
1339. Diwan A H, Prieto V G, Herling M et al. 2005 Primary Sezary syndrome commonly shows low grade cytologic atypia and an absence of epidermotropism. Am J Clin Pathol 123: 510–515
1340. Trotter M J, Whittaker S J, Orchard G E et al. 1997 Cutaneous histopathology of Sezary syndrome: a study of 41 cases with a proven circulating T-cell clone. J Cutan Pathol 24(5):86–291
1341. Smoller B R, Bishop K, Glusac E et al. 1995 Reassessment of histologic parameters in the diagnosis of mycosis fungoides. Am J Surg Pathol 19(12): 1423–1430
1342. Burns M K, Chan L S, Cooper K D 1995 Woringer-Kolopp disease (localized pagetoid reticulosis) or unilesional mycosis fungoides? An analysis of eight cases with benign disease. Arch Dermatol 131(3): 325–329
1343. Mielke V, Wolff H H, Winzer M et al. 1989 Localized and disseminated pagetoid reticulosis. Diagnostic immunophenotypical findings. Arch Dermatol 125(3): 402–406
1344. Wood G S, Weiss L M, Hu C H et al. 1988 T-cell antigen deficiencies and clonal rearrangements of T-cell receptor genes in pagetoid reticulosis (Woringer–Kolopp disease). New Engl J Med 318(3): 164–167
1345. Beljaards R C, Kaudewitz P, Berti E et al. 1993 Primary cutaneous CD30-positive large cell lymphoma: definition of a new type of cutaneous lymphoma with a favorable prognosis. A European Multicenter Study of 47 patients. Cancer 71(6): 2097–2104
1346. Kaudewitz P, Burg G 1991 Lymphomatoid papulosis and Ki-1 (CD-30) positive cutaneous large cell lymphomas. Semin Diagn Pathol 8: 117–124
1347. Banerjee S S, Heald J, Harris M 1991 Twelve cases of Ki-1 positive anaplastic large cell lymphoma of skin. J Clin Pathol 44(2): 119–125
1348. Macaulay W L 1968 Lymphomatoid papulosis. A continuing self-healing eruption, clinically benign – histologically malignant. Arch Dermatol 97(1): 23–30
1349. Le Boit P E 1996 Lymphomatoid papulosis and cutaneous CD30+ lymphoma. Am J Dermatopathol 18(3): 221–235
1350. Willemze R 1985 Lymphomatoid papulosis. Dermatol Clin 3(4): 735–747
1351. Karp D L, Horn T D 1994 Lymphomatoid papulosis. J Am Acad Dermatol 30(3): 379–395; quiz 396–398
1352. Willemze R, Beljaards R C 1993 Spectrum of primary cutaneous CD30 (Ki-1)-positive lymphoproliferative disorders. A proposal for classification and guidelines for management and treatment. J Am Acad Dermatol 28(6): 973–980
1353. Willemze R, Meyer C J, Van Vloten W A et al. 1982 The clinical and histological spectrum of lymphomatoid papulosis. Br J Dermatol 107(2): 131–144
1354. Friedmann D, Wechsler J, Delfau M-H et al. 1995 Primary cutaneous pleomorphic small T-cell lymphoma. A review of 11 cases. The French Study Group on Cutaneous Lymphomas. Arch Dermatol 131(9): 1009–1015
1355. Argenyi Z B, Goeken J A, Piette W W et al. 1992 Granulomatous mycosis fungoides. Clinicopathologic study of two cases. Am J Dermatopathol 14: 200–210
1356. LeBoit P E 1994 Granulomatous slack skin. Dermatol Clin 12(2): 375–389
1357. LeBoit P E, Zackheim H S, White C R Jr 1988 Granulomatous variants of cutaneous T-cell lymphoma. The histopathology of granulomatous mycosis fungoides and granulomatous slack skin. Am J Surg Pathol 12(2): 83–95
1358. Gonzalez C L, Medeiros L J, Braziel R M et al. 1991 T-cell lymphoma involving subcutaneous tissue. A clinicopathologic entity commonly associated with hemophagocytic syndrome. Am J Surg Pathol 15(1): 17–27
1359. Wang C-YE, Su W P D, Kurtin P J 1996 Subcutaneous panniculitic T-cell lymphoma. Int J Dermatol 35(1): 1–8
1359a. Goodlad J R, Davidson M M, Hollowood K et al. 2000 Primary cutaneous B-cell lymphoma and Borrelia burgdorferi infection in patients from the Highlands of Scotland. Am J Surg Pathol 24: 1279–1285
1360. Yang B, Tubbs R R, Finn W et al. 2000 Clinicopathologic reassessment of primary cutaneous B-cell lymphomas with immunophenotypic and molecular genetic characterization. Am J Surg Pathol 24(5): 694–702
1361. Berti E, Alessi E, Caputo R 1991 Reticulohistiocytoma of the dorsum (Crosti's disease) and other B-cell lymphomas. Semin Diagn Pathol 8: 82–90
1362. Garcia C F, Weiss L M, Warnke R A et al. 1986 Cutaneous follicular lymphoma. Am J Surg Pathol 10(7): 454–463
1363. Santucci M, Pimpinelli N, Arganini L 1991 Primary cutaneous B-cell lymphoma: a unique type of low-grade lymphoma. Clinicopathologic and immunologic study of 83 cases. Cancer 67(9): 2311–2326
1364. Willemze R, Meijer C J, Sentis H J et al. 1987 Primary cutaneous large cell lymphomas of follicular center cell origin. A clinical follow-up study of nineteen patients. J Am Acad Dermatol 16(3 Pt 1): 518–526
1365. Goodlad J R, Krajewski A S, Batstone P J et al. 2002 Primary cutaneous follicular lymphoma. A clinicopathologic and molecular study of 16 cases in support of a distinct entity. Am J Surg Pathol 26: 733–741
1366. Baldassano M F, Bailey E M, Ferry J A et al. 1999 Cutaneous lymphoid hyperplasia and cutaneous marginal zone lymphoma. Comparison of morphologic and immunophenotypic features. Am J Surg Pathol 23(1): 88–96
1367. Cerroni L, Signoretti S, Hofler G et al. 1997 Primary cutaneous marginal zone B-cell lymphoma: a recently described entity of low-grade malignant cutaneous B-cell lymphoma. Am J Surg Pathol 21(11): 1307–1315
1368. Rijlaarsdam J U, van der Putte S C, Berti E et al. 1993 Cutaneous immunocytomas: a clinicopathological study of 26 cases. Histopathology 23(2): 117–125
1369. Mayou S C, Cotter F E, Norton A J et al. 1991 A cutaneous B-cell lymphoma of novel immunophenotype. Br J Dermatol 125(4): 373–376
1370. de Leval L, Harris N L, Longtine J A et al. 2001 Cutaneous B cell lymphomas of follicular and marginal zone types: use of Bcl-6, CD10,

Bcl-2 and CD21 in differential diagnosis and classification. Am J Surg Pathol 25: 732–741

1371. Vermeer M H, Geelen F A, van Haselen C W et al. 1996 Primary cutaneous large B-cell lymphomas of the legs. A distinct type of cutaneous B-cell lymphoma with an intermediate prognosis. Dutch Cutaneous Lymphoma Working Group. Arch Dermatol 132(11): 1304–1308
1372. Goodlad J R, Krajewski A S, Batstone P J et al. 2003 Primary cutaneous diffuse large B-cell lymphoma. Prognostic significance of clinicopathological subtypes. Am J Surg Pathol 27: 1538–1545
1373. Bhawan J 1987 Angioendotheliomatosis proliferans systemisata: an angiotropic neoplasm of lymphoid origin. Semin Diagn Pathol 4: 18–27
1374. Perniciaro C, Winkelmann R K, Daoud M S et al. 1995 Malignant angioendotheliomatosis is an angiotropic intravascular lymphoma. Immunohistochemical, ultrastructural, and molecular genetics studies. Am J Dermatopathol 17(3): 242–248
1375. Wick M R, Mills S E 1991 Intravascular lymphomatosis: clinicopathologic features and differential diagnosis. Semin Diagn Pathol 8: 91–101
1376. Torne R, Su W P, Winkelmann R K et al. 1990 Clinicopathologic study of cutaneous plasmacytoma. Int J Dermatol 29(8): 562–566
1377. Wiltshaw E 1976 The natural history of extramedullary plasmacytoma and its relation to solitary myeloma of bone and myelomatosis. Medicine (Baltimore) 55(3): 217–238
1378. Brady M S, Coit D G 1997 Sentinel lymph node evaluation in melanoma. Arch Dermatol 133(8): 1014–1020
1379. Glass F L, Cottam J A, Reintgen D S et al. 1998 Lymphatic mapping and sentinel node biopsy in the management of high-risk melanoma. J Am Acad Dermatol 39(4 Pt 1): 603–610
1380. Szymanski M B, Ackerman A B 1998 Sentinel lymph node biopsy? Dermatopathol Pract Concept 4(3): 253–257
1381. Schwartz R A 1995 Cutaneous metastatic disease. J Am Acad Dermatol 33(2 Pt 1): 161–182
1382. Schwartz R A 1995 Histopathologic aspects of cutaneous metastatic disease. J Am Acad Dermatol 33(4): 649–657
1383. Brownstein M H, Helwig E B 1973 Spread of tumors to the skin. Arch Dermatol 107(1): 80–86
1384. Gates O 1937 Cutaneous metastases of malignant disease. Am J Cancer 30(4): 718–730
1385. Reingold I M 1966 Cutaneous metastases from internal carcinoma. Cancer 19(2): 162–168
1386. Brownstein M H, Helwig E B 1972 Patterns of cutaneous metastasis. Arch Dermatol 105(6): 862–868
1387. Brownstein M H, Helwig E B 1972 Metastatic tumors of the skin. Cancer 29(5): 1298–1307

软组织肿瘤
Soft tissue tumors

24

Christopher D. M. Fletcher 著

王功伟 译　钱利华 校

引言	1527
脂肪细胞肿瘤	1528
纤维性肿瘤	1539
反应性病变	1539
错构瘤性病变	1543
良性肿瘤	1545
纤维瘤病	1550
纤维母细胞肉瘤	1554

纤维组织细胞肿瘤（所谓的）	1557
平滑肌肿瘤	1562
骨骼肌肿瘤	1566
软骨–骨肿瘤	1570
其他良性病变	1570
中间性生物学潜能的其他病变	1573
其他恶性病变	1576

引言

软组织发生的肿瘤尽管在临床上并不具有特异性，但却是一类复杂多样的病变，可出现多种分化。软组织病变的形态学表现常常掩盖其真正的生物学潜能，在一定程度上需要通过淋巴结的病理学改变来判断：假恶性甚至假良性病变大量存在。仅由于这个原因，在缺乏明确组织学诊断的情况下，对软组织肿瘤可能的临床过程进行预测（或"猜测"）通常是危险的。重要的是要认识到，这些病变即使在组织学上和临床上已理解，即使不是大多数，这些肿瘤的组织学发生概念也并不可靠，而且大多没有意义。有可能例外的是皮下脂肪瘤或良性平滑肌肿瘤，有关这些病变起源于它们相应成熟（分化）组织的证据极少。多数脂肪肉瘤发生在没有脂肪组织的部位，横纹肌肉瘤大多发生于缺乏自主性肌肉的部位，这些事实充分解释了这一观点，这与存在骨外骨肉瘤的意义相同。然而，除了方便以外，同样没有意义的是使用原始间叶干细胞这个概念作为这些肿瘤的祖先，因为很少或没有证据能够证明在出生之前胚胎阶段的躯体间叶组织内存在这样的细胞。然而，有些（或许多）病变有可能起源于骨髓来源的干细胞。要记住的是，所有二倍体细胞携带有遗传信息，呈不同程度表达或抑制，表现出几乎所有的细胞系分化，控制不同间叶细胞系分化的基因极有可能是密切相关的，并且能够在间叶组织发育中的某个点"开启"，除此之外，诸如"上皮性基因"已经不可逆性"关闭"，因此似乎有理由推测：几乎所有的间叶性肿瘤都可以起源于任何间叶细胞。剩下的主要任务或问题是确定在特殊细胞系分化过程中，究竟是什么影响肿瘤形成的因素在起决定性作用（和如何起作用）。现在，诸如骨骼肌 *MyoD* 家族等特殊分化基因的特征及在特殊类型的软组织肿瘤中与肿瘤形成过程有关的基因表达方式正在进行证实[1,2]，在不久的将来其中的一些问题有可能可以回答；然而，在软组织肿瘤形成中，基因表达资料更多是用来证实新型标记物[3]，并没有给基础肿瘤生物学带来希望。

我们所了解的软组织肿瘤分子遗传学的快速发展的一个重要起点（并且在这些相对少见的肿瘤中是一个对有关研究兴趣的主要影响因素）是：许多肿瘤类型显示重复性的细胞遗传学异常。在良性软组织肿瘤中（良性神经鞘瘤也同样，见第 27 章），似乎有共同的基因通路，不管分化细胞系如何，其中许多涉及高死亡率基因[4,5]，主要是 12 号染色体的 *HMGA2* 和 6 号染色体的 *HMGA1*。相反，许多类型的软组织肉瘤（类似于白血病）则以特殊的细胞遗传学突变为特征，最常见的是相应的染色体易位，它们具有相关的肿瘤特异性，因此具有诊断意义[6,7]。表 24.1 中列出了软组织肉瘤的特异性染色体异常。遗憾的是，许多较常见的肉瘤（老年人的高级别梭形细胞和多形性肉瘤）具有较为复杂的核型，缺乏特异的组织类型特征[8,9]。

表24.1　软组织肉瘤细胞遗传学突变

肿瘤类型	细胞遗传学改变	基因重排
Ewing肉瘤/原始外周神经外胚层肿瘤	t(11;22)(q24;q12) t(21;22)(q22;q12) t(7;22)(p22;q12) t(17;22)(q12;q12) t(2;22)(q33;q12)	FLI-1-EWSR1 ERG-EWSR1 ETV1-EWSR1 EIAF-EWSR1 FEV-EWSR1
腺泡状横纹肌肉瘤	t(2;13)(q35;q14) t(1;13)(p36;q14)	PAX3-FOXO1A PAX7-FOXO1A
黏液样/圆形细胞脂肪肉瘤	t(12;16)(q13;q11) t(12;22)(q13;q11-12)	DDIT3-FUS DDIT3-EWSR1
纤维组织增生性小圆细胞肿瘤	t(11;22)(p13;q12)	WT1-EWSR1
滑膜肉瘤	t(x;18)(p11.2;q11.2)	SSX1-SYT SSX2-SYT
透明细胞肉瘤	t(12;22)(q13;q12)	ATF-1-EWSR1
骨骼肌外黏液样软骨肉瘤	t(9;22)(q22;q12) t(9;17)(q22;q11)	NR4A3-EWSR1 NR4A3-RBP56
隆突性皮肤纤维肉瘤/巨细胞纤维母细胞瘤	t(17;22)(q22;q13)	PDGFB-COL1A1
婴儿纤维肉瘤	t(12;15)(p13;q25)	ETV6-NTRK3
腺泡状软组织肉瘤	t(x;17)(p11;q25)	ASPL-TFE3
低级别纤维黏液样肉瘤	t(7;16)(q33;p11)	FUS-CREB3L2
血管瘤样"MFH"		ATF-1重排
非典型脂肪瘤样肿瘤/高分化脂肪肉瘤	12q环和巨型标记物	HMGA(2)、CDK4和MDM2扩增

通常，光镜形态学加相关辅助技术仍然是软组织肿瘤分类和诊断的基础。值得注意的是，在临床上这些基础牢固的技术仍有助于确定以前常规方法不能明确的肿瘤。

软组织肉瘤的分级是许多重要肿瘤分期系统（如AJCC）的一个特征之一，并且越来越成为制订肿瘤治疗方案的关键性信息之一。目前还没有一个理想的组织学分级系统，并且令人失望的是，对于处理大量病例的中心来说，凭借经验的"目测"等陈旧方式似乎与应用各种较为客观的方案同样有效。两个最著名的分类体系是 NCI[10] 和法国肉瘤分类[11,12]，其中法国体系（以分化、核分裂象以及坏死为依据）更受欢迎[13]，因为这个体系更具可重复性，并且把极少数患者纳入某种程度上有些无助的"中间级别"一类。软组织肉瘤的分级仍然存在极为主观和不能令人满意的地方[14]，遗憾的是，还没有一个更为"科学"的指标（诸如通过免疫组化检测增殖指数、DNA 流式细胞学或癌基因状况）能够提供可重复的、对传统形态学评价有所改良的办法。值得注意的是，看起来综合评判肿瘤大小、血管浸润和肿瘤坏死（组织学确定）对于预测肿瘤的预后与肿瘤分级同样有效[14a]。

除了这些一般性考虑以外，需要提示读者的是，血管性肿瘤和外周神经外胚层肿瘤在单独的章节中讨论。同样，发生在内脏部位或主要发生于皮肤的间叶性病变在相应的章节讨论。

脂肪细胞肿瘤　Adipocytic tumors

脂肪细胞肿瘤是软组织肿瘤中最大类中的一组，主要是由于良性皮下脂肪瘤的发病率高。此外，脂肪肉瘤（包括非典型脂肪瘤样肿瘤）是原发性恶性软组织肿瘤中最常见的一种类型。除了脂肪母细胞瘤和个别脂肪瘤以外，绝大多数脂肪性肿瘤发生在成人。通常，免疫组化及电镜等辅助诊断技术的作用有限，或只是偶尔有用，因为多数病例的诊断仅仅依靠光镜形态学。以前将脂肪

表24.2	脂肪细胞肿瘤中常见的染色质异常
肿瘤类型	最常见的细胞遗传学异常
孤立性脂肪瘤	易位，涉及12q13-15 13q重排 重排，涉及6p21-33
梭形细胞/多形性脂肪瘤	16单体或16q部分性缺失伴13q不平衡突变
脂肪母细胞瘤/脂肪母细胞瘤病	重排，涉及8q11-13
冬眠瘤	重排，涉及11q13、10q22
软骨样脂肪瘤	重排，涉及11q13
血管脂肪瘤	正常核型
非典型脂肪瘤样肿瘤（高分化脂肪肉瘤）	环形染色体以及12q13-15的长臂染色体标记物
去分化脂肪肉瘤	环形染色体以及来自12q13-15的长臂染色体标记物；许多病变中有其他复杂异常
黏液样/圆形细胞脂肪肉瘤	t(12;16)(q13;p11) t(12;22)(q13;q11-12)
多形性脂肪肉瘤	复杂重排，通常伴有染色体数量显著增加

母细胞作为脂肪肉瘤的主要诊断标准，现在的做法已经发生改变，不仅是由于绝大多数非典型脂肪性肿瘤（高分化脂肪肉瘤）和黏液样脂肪肉瘤缺乏脂肪母细胞，而且由于现在脂肪母细胞在多形性脂肪瘤、软骨样脂肪瘤、脂肪母细胞瘤以及少数梭形细胞脂肪瘤中也被认为是一种常规所见。值得提醒的是，由于有些肿瘤可以侵犯和吞噬脂肪，脂肪的特殊染色（如油红O和苏丹黑）极少具有诊断价值，现在几乎已不再用于诊断，尤其是它们也容易出现技术假象。在脂肪细胞肿瘤的分类和诊断中，与这些老技术相比，目前细胞遗传学分析的作用越来越重要，尤其是当肿瘤位置较深时，因为其中许多肿瘤具有相对组织特异性的核型异常[15]（表24.2）。

良性脂肪瘤　Benign lipoma

临床特征

良性脂肪瘤极其常见，最常见于皮下组织[16-19]。多数见于30岁以上的成人，不同性别的发生率一致，分布部位广泛。躯干和近端肢体是最常见部位，手足部位的脂肪瘤极少见。多数为单发，生长缓慢，质软，无痛，

然而，2%～3%的患者有多发性病变。儿童脂肪瘤不常见，但并非像有时说的特别少见。尽管可以发生深在的良性脂肪瘤（见下文），但对于腹部或后腹膜，似乎成熟的脂肪肿瘤应当有所怀疑，因为多数被证明是高分化脂肪肉瘤。皮下脂肪瘤单纯切除后出现局部复发的病例不超过1%～2%。

病理学特征

多数脂肪瘤界限清楚，有薄层被膜并呈分叶状。大小不一，但很少超过10cm。对于大于此数值的病例，应当仔细取材，因为实际上这些病例大多为非典型脂肪瘤样肿瘤（见下文）。在多数病例中，肿瘤切面为成熟脂肪组织，个别混有纤维或黏液样区域或脂肪坏死区域。组织学上，多数肿瘤仅由成熟的单泡脂肪细胞构成，细胞大小稍有变化，细胞边缘可见不甚明显、被挤压的小细胞核。常可见短带状、相对无细胞的胶原纤维组织，或泡沫细胞聚集伴有散在巨细胞成分，提示镜下脂肪坏死。后者可引起脂肪细胞大小不等。出现广泛纤维性成分时可命名为"纤维脂肪瘤"，其纤维组织背景中细胞成分较少，以胶原为主。同样，偶尔可以见到小灶黏液样变性，如果黏液变性较为广泛且出现融合，则有时采用"黏液脂肪瘤"一词。这样的病变中血管常常较多，至少局部容易见到良性梭形细胞成分和粗大胶原束，建议最好将这些病变看做黏液型梭形细胞脂肪瘤。5%的病例有骨或软骨化生，通常位于致密纤维组织区域内；传统上，这样病变并不称为"良性间叶瘤"，该术语是用于少见的、含有明显软骨-骨和血管成分的病变[20]，尽管"软骨脂肪血管瘤"这个术语可能更为恰当。以作者的经验，这些病变最常见于四肢（尤其是远端）和肩带周围，是完全良性病变。皮下脂肪瘤（在多数病例中）表现为重复性核型异常，最常累及染色体12q13-15部分[22,23]，尽管还没有证据表明这些表现与临床病理特征有关联。

脂肪瘤的变型　Variants of lipoma

"皮肤脂肪瘤"（dermal lipoma）[24,25]　一词有时用于描述那些多为单发、有蒂的皮肤病变，主要发生在年轻成人，很可能是以脂肪组织为主的纤维上皮性息肉的一型（"皮肤乳头状瘤"）。过去，有些作者认为，脂肪组织息肉样病变为皮内黑色素细胞痣的偶然性改变。只有当这些病变为多发且聚集于下肢周围时，才应当使用"浅表性脂肪瘤样痣"一词。后者容易累及较年轻的患者，其在发生上被看做是错构瘤性。

滑膜脂肪瘤（synovial lipoma）[26]　也被看做是树枝状脂肪瘤，其特征是滑膜下聚集的成熟脂肪组织呈绒

毛状突入关节腔。绒毛被覆增生性、伴有不同程度炎症的滑膜。这些病变主要发生在成人，最常累及膝部，常常与半月板或关节变性改变有关；如此看来，其本质几乎可以肯定是反应性改变。极少数见于儿童或青少年的边界清楚的滑膜脂肪瘤已有报道。

肌内脂肪瘤（intramuscular lipoma）[27-29] 不同于较为浅表的脂肪瘤，多数界限不清，呈浸润性，如果切除不完全，20%的病例可有局部复发。一般发生于中年人，没有性别差异，表现为生长缓慢的深在性肿物；股部和躯干是最常见的受累部位。组织学上，多数病例由成熟脂肪细胞构成，呈不规则分枝状，分布于不同程度萎缩的肌纤维之间（图24.1）。血管成分极少，通常如毛细血管大小，不同于肌内血管瘤（见第3章）。病变内肌纤维的数量或范围在大体上通常并不明显。处理所有深在性肿瘤时，必须仔细排除非典型性脂肪瘤（见下文），按照目前的诊断标准，后者可能比肌内脂肪瘤更常见。继发或化生性改变的范围与皮下脂肪瘤（见上文）相同。大约10%的肌内脂肪瘤界限清楚，呈非浸润性，这些病变不会复发[29]。与肌内脂肪瘤密切相关的是肌间脂肪瘤（intermuscular lipoma），后者只有依靠精确的放射学和术中病变部位进行诊断。此型脂肪瘤最常见于前腹壁，局部复发率较低。深在性脂肪瘤的其他少见发生部位包括腱鞘（通常在手足周围）、精索、纵隔或骨旁部位。

脂肪瘤病（lipomatosis）[30-35] 是一种少见病变，特征是脂肪组织呈弥漫性过度生长，主要累及成年男性，其表现呈四种主要类型中的一种：

1. 多发对称性脂肪瘤病[31,34]：是最常见形式，主要累及颈部和肩部（Madelung 病或 Launois-Bensaude 腺脂肪瘤病），通常与周围性神经病、酗酒和高脂血症有关。类似的临床特征也可见于接受 HIV-1 蛋白酶抑制因子治疗的患者。
2. 非对称性脂肪瘤病[32]：分布随意；缺乏明显的临床相关性。
3. 盆腔脂肪瘤病[30,35]：发生在直肠和膀胱周围，具有特征性的放射学特点，可以导致尿路梗阻和尿毒症。
4. 纵隔腹部脂肪瘤病[33] 也与酗酒、高脂血症和成熟期发病的糖尿病有关。

组织学上，所有类型的脂肪组织均界限不清，完全成熟，可以出现局部纤维化。神经脂肪瘤病，以前被称为神经的纤维脂肪瘤性错构瘤，在第27章中描述。

脂肪母细胞瘤　Lipoblastoma

临床特征

脂肪母细胞瘤[36-38]主要为新生儿肿瘤，主要累及3岁以内的男孩，尽管也遇到过极少数7岁或8岁病例。多数病例表现为肢体浅表性的、界限清楚的、生长缓慢的肿物；平均直径大约为5cm。深部病变往往更大，有时可呈弥漫性浸润，在后者，它们被称为脂肪母细胞瘤病。切除后局部复发并不常见，一般仅见于浸润性类型。

组织学特征

界限清楚的和弥漫性的两种类型都具有分叶状结构，由不同程度的成熟的和不成熟的脂肪细胞构成，并被纤维间隔所分隔。较不成熟的小叶由原始间叶细胞、脂肪母细胞和小毛细血管构成，所有成分均位于黏液样间质当中，除了缺乏细胞核非典型性以外，非常类似于黏液样脂肪肉瘤（图24.2）。较成熟的小叶类似于脂肪瘤，除了脂肪细胞的细胞核更加明显以及脂肪细胞大小有些变化以外。即使在不成熟的区域，核分裂象也不常见。个别小叶可出现类似于棕色脂肪（冬眠瘤样）的表现，小的髓外造血灶极其常见[37]。复发性病变经常显示向单纯性脂肪瘤成熟的表现。脂肪母细胞瘤通常出现一致性的8q11-13染色体异常，导致 *PLAG1* 基因重排[39]。组织学上脂肪母细胞瘤与黏液样脂肪肉瘤的鉴别具有重要意义，后者在10岁以下儿童极其少见；识别脂肪母细胞瘤的主要线索是：出现明显的小叶结构、较大范围的分化/成熟以及缺乏细胞核非典型性。在极少数病例中，根据患者年龄在形态学上进行区分几乎是不可能的（或至少是武断的），但这种鉴别并没有临床意义，因为年龄在10～20岁患者的黏液样脂肪肉瘤似乎都是极低级别的。

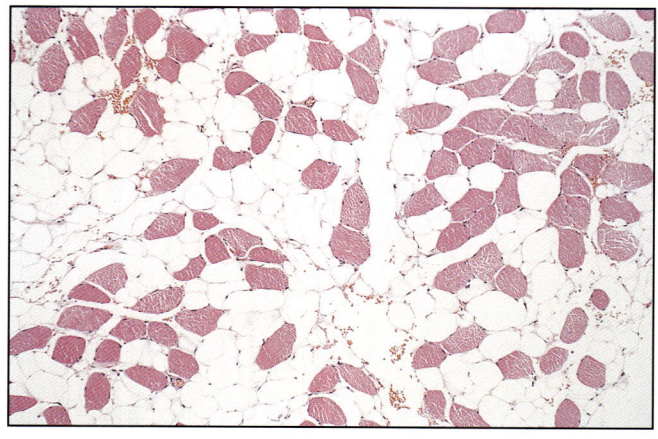

图24.1　肌内脂肪瘤。典型病例显示肌纤维之间有成熟脂肪细胞浸润。

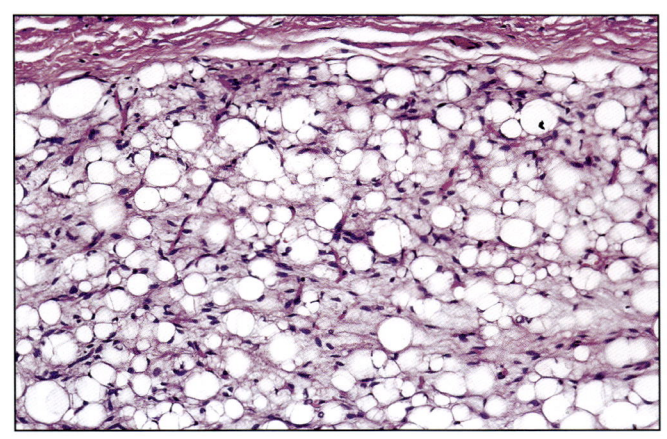

图24.2 脂肪母细胞瘤。注意缺乏细胞核非典型性、黏液样间质和鸡爪样血管。

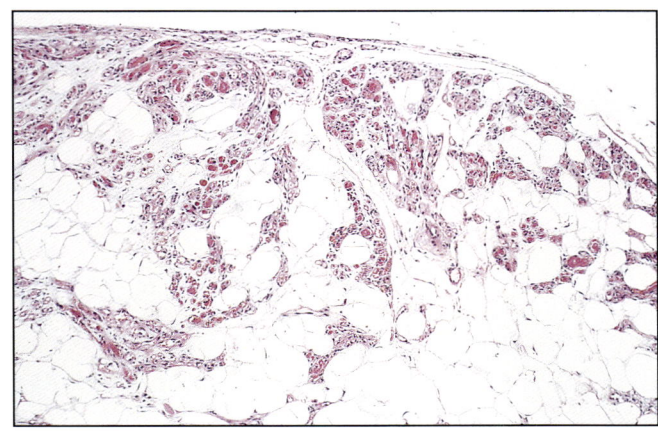

图24.3 血管脂肪瘤。注意血管主要位于周边,含有纤维素性微血栓。

血管脂肪瘤 Angiolipoma

临床特征

血管脂肪瘤[40,41]是极为常见的良性病变,几乎均位于皮下,50%以上的病例为多发性的。有非常明显的男性倾向,最多见于青年时期。解剖分布广泛,但上肢(尤其是前臂)和躯干最常受累。大约一半的患者主诉疼痛和压痛,如果病变太多而不能直接切除,在临床治疗上会比较麻烦。可能是由于病变常常没有症状,切除时大多不足2cm。没有局部复发倾向,但在其他部位可有新病变继续出现。

组织学特征

血管脂肪瘤不同于普通脂肪瘤的地方在于其另外还有薄壁小毛细血管样血管成分,大多分布在肿瘤周边(图24.3)。较为经典的是,这些毛细血管(至少是局部的)含有小的纤维素性血栓,常常是对诊断有帮助的一个特征:实际上,缺乏这个特征可强烈质疑该诊断。病变中血管成分的多少差异较大,可以达到90%或更多,对于这样的病例,有时使用"细胞性血管脂肪瘤"[42]一词。这些细胞较为丰富的病变可以出现明显梭形内皮细胞表现,加上毛细血管周围明显的管周细胞表面上可以类似于Kaposi肉瘤或原发性毛细血管性血管瘤。识别病变内的脂肪细胞和微血栓有助于鉴别诊断。时间较长的血管脂肪瘤常常出现退行性特征,其形式有血管周围纤维化、玻璃样变性以及间质黏液样变性。有趣的是(与多数其他脂肪性肿瘤比较),血管脂肪瘤都具有正常的核型。深在性的肌内病变过去被称为"浸润性血管脂肪瘤"[43],目前已划归为肌内血管瘤伴明显的脂肪细胞成分(见第3章);由于肌内血管瘤的局部复发率较高,因此这种区分很重要。

肌脂肪瘤 Myolipoma

肌脂肪瘤是一种少见肿瘤,其特征是成熟脂肪组织和平滑肌以不同比例混合[44];最常见的是以肌肉成分为主(图24.4)。这些肿瘤通常较大,盆腔和腹部最常见,女性稍多见。迄今为止,随访资料有限,但其临床过程呈良性。重要的鉴别诊断是血管肌脂肪瘤(见下文)以及伴有异源性平滑肌成分的高分化脂肪肉瘤。

软骨样脂肪瘤 Chondroid lipoma

软骨样脂肪瘤与肌脂肪瘤同样不常见,容易被误诊为肉瘤,因为其主要的细胞成分与脂肪母细胞和软骨母细胞极为类似[45,46](图24.5)。最常累及成年女性,解剖学分布广泛,尽管多数病例位于皮下。有包膜的病变不易局部复发。关键的形态学特征是:在黏液透明变性的假软骨样基质中混有成熟脂肪细胞,细胞核呈良性表现的脂肪母细胞,以及冬眠瘤

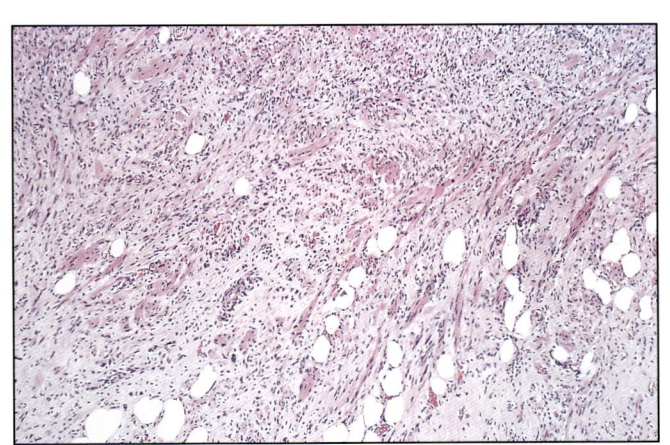

图24.4 肌脂肪瘤。典型的平滑肌细胞和脂肪细胞混合。

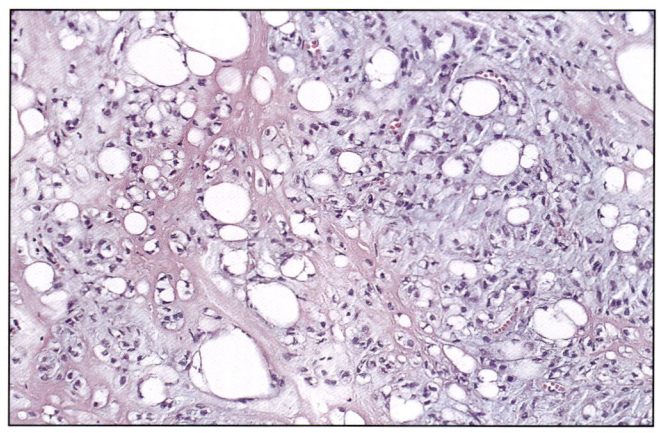

图24.5 软骨样脂肪瘤。软骨母细胞与脂肪母细胞难以鉴别。

样细胞。超微结构检查出现特征性的结节样胞浆突起[46]，细胞遗传学分析显示11q13异常，不同于冬眠瘤[47]。

肾外血管肌脂肪瘤
Extrarenal angiomyolipoma

血管肌脂肪瘤在第12章中有详细描述。极少数也可以发生在腹膜后或盆腔软组织[48,49]，此时常常有奇异性表现的平滑肌和脂肪细胞成分更容易被误诊为恶性。特征性的厚壁血管以及特殊的平滑肌细胞免疫组化HMB45或melan-A（被认为是黑色素瘤抗原）染色阳性应有助于正确诊断[49]。与更为常见的肾同种肿瘤相同，肾外的病变可能与结节性硬化有关。此外，我们已经遇到过新近明确的（所谓的）软组织"恶性上皮样血管肌脂肪瘤"[50]病例。此类病变在PEComa中讨论（见1575页）。

肾上腺外髓脂肪瘤
Extra-adrenal myelolipoma

髓脂肪瘤在第19章中有更详细的描述。在肾上腺外及肝外已有不足40例报道[51,53]，几乎均见于成年女性，骶前或后腹膜最为常见。极少数病例呈多中心性[52]。其与任何血液疾病均无关，与所谓髓外造血性"肿瘤"的区别在于：存在明显的脂肪成分，以及髓脂肪瘤中缺乏红系增生。

梭形细胞和多形性脂肪瘤
Spindle cell and pleomorphic lipoma

梭形细胞和多形性脂肪瘤在同一标题下描述，是因为相当一部分的病例出现重叠性的临床形态学特征，因此目前将它们看做是同一种病变的变型。

临床特征

梭形细胞和多形性脂肪瘤[54,57]最常发生在中老年人，以男性为主。临床上这些病变大多与普通脂肪瘤不能鉴别，但是80%以上的病例发生在背部上方，遍及一侧肩部或颈后。10%发生在头颈部比较靠前的区域，包括面部，个例报告有口腔[58]或更少见的眼眶[59]。少数完全位于皮内的病变其解剖学分布更为广泛，令人诧异的是以女性为主[60]。肿瘤通常单发，无痛性，生长缓慢，直径很少超过5cm。个别患者出现多发性病变，可能为家族性的[61]。局部切除后极少复发，还没有证据表明，梭形细胞或多形性脂肪瘤具有去分化能力（与非典型性脂肪性肿瘤相比，见下文）。主要原因是这些病变基本上为皮下（或个别真皮）来源，由于深部组织发生的少数组织学上类似的病变容易出现复发，最好划归为非典型性脂肪肿瘤，通常也有核型的支持。发生于少见解剖部位的病例也应该被视为质疑诊断。

病理学特征

梭形细胞和多形性脂肪瘤界限清楚，被膜较薄，可呈分叶状。与普通脂肪瘤相比，其切面较灰白、质硬，偶尔出现明显的双相（脂肪/纤维）性表现。组织学上，梭形脂肪瘤的特征是成熟性脂肪细胞和短梭形未分化细胞混合，细胞核呈均一性，胞浆淡染，边界不清（图24.6）。这些细胞没有（或仅有极少数）核分裂象，排列成短束状；细胞核可呈栅栏状，与良性Schwann细胞瘤极为相似。这些细胞位于数量不等的纤维黏液样间质中，后者以轻度嗜酸的玻璃样胶原纤维和多量肥大细胞为特征。脂肪细胞和梭形细胞成分的相对比例差异极大（图24.7）。这些病变中的血管成分也多少不等[57]，有时出现分枝状薄壁血管，类似于所谓的"血管周细胞瘤"。间质黏液变常见，可以较明显和呈弥漫性（图24.8），以至有可能被认为是"黏液样脂肪瘤"；个别病变可以出现纤细的鸡爪样血管，类似于黏液样脂肪肉瘤。"树突状纤维黏液脂肪瘤"[62]名下所描述的病变似乎代表了黏液样梭形细胞脂肪瘤。伴有广泛黏液变性的极少数病例可出现明显的假血管样变性，特征是肿瘤组织呈绒毛状突入貌似的空腔[63]（图24.9）。

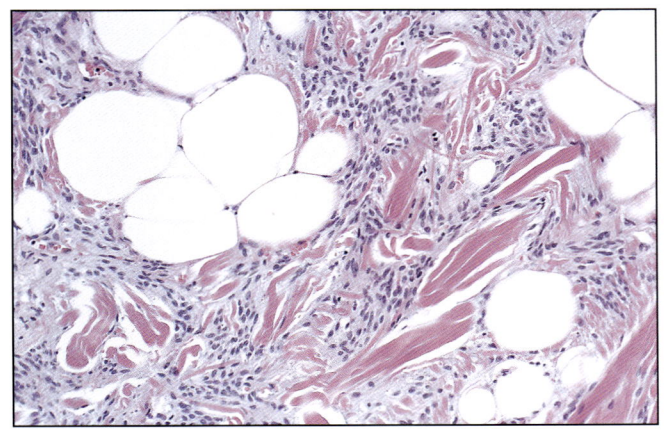

图24.6 梭形细胞脂肪瘤。注意典型的脂肪细胞、良性未分化梭形细胞和玻璃样胶原束混合。

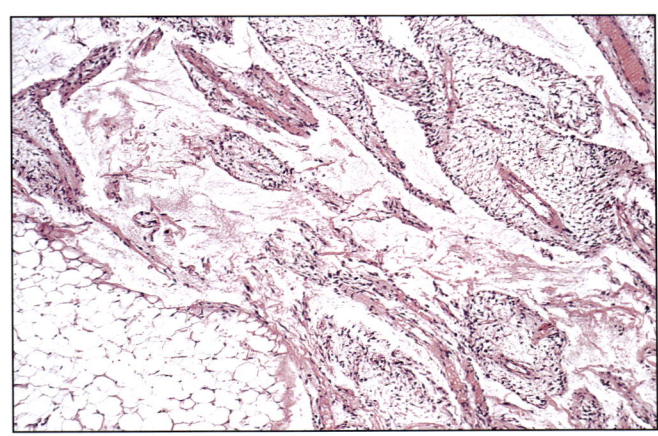

图24.9 梭形细胞脂肪瘤。显著的黏液样变性可以导致绒毛状的淋巴血管瘤样表现。

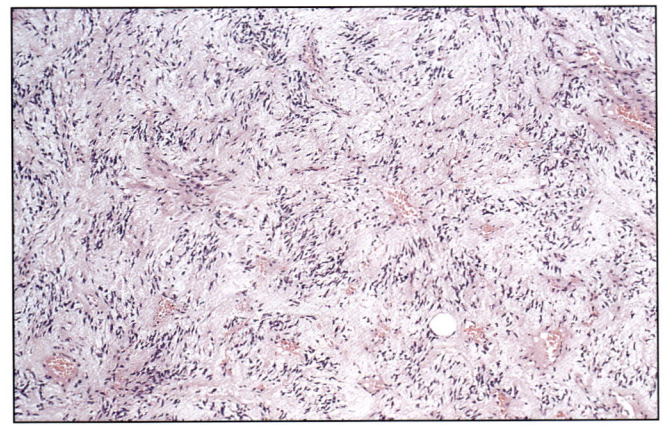

图24.7 梭形细胞脂肪瘤。病变以梭形细胞为主，类似于Schwann细胞瘤。

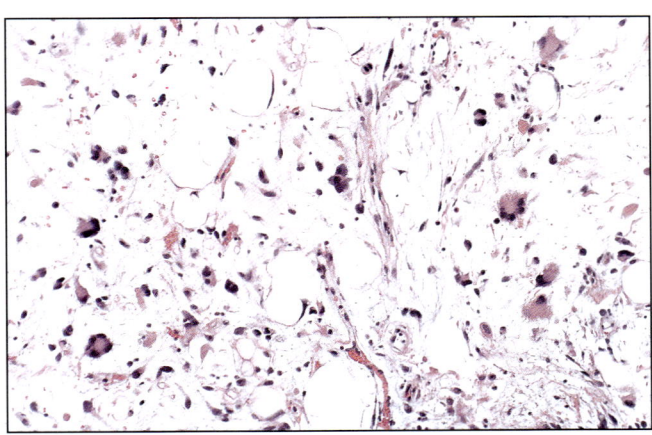

图24.10 多形性脂肪瘤。典型的花样巨细胞以及浓染的间质细胞。

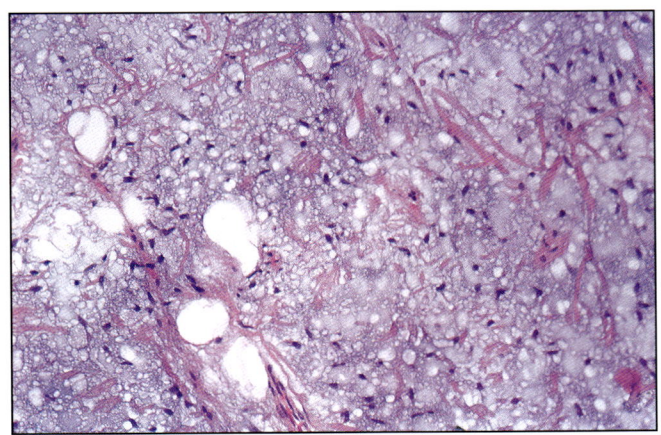

图24.8 黏液样梭形细胞脂肪瘤。间质显著黏液变性极为常见，有时会与黏液样脂肪肉瘤混淆。

经典型多形性脂肪瘤由成熟脂肪细胞混以数量不等的奇异型深染的且常为多核的间质细胞构成（图24.10）。多核细胞常常表现为细胞核分布于外周，呈环状（花状）围绕嗜酸性胞浆排列。在这些病变中出现少数多泡性脂肪母细胞并不少见，有时也可以见到核分裂象（可以是异常表现）。间质有数量不等的胶原。比这种"经典型"多形性脂肪瘤更为常见的是：病变出现混杂性表现；此种病变除了存在数量不等的奇异性或多核间质细胞以外，常常与梭形细胞脂肪瘤非常相似。

梭形细胞为主型（图24.7）与Schwann细胞瘤的鉴别在于识别内部的脂肪细胞，并且梭形细胞S-100呈阴性。与高分化脂肪肉瘤鉴别（通常是多形性脂肪瘤）主要依靠解剖部位和位置浅表等细致的临床病理相关性。另外，与高分化脂肪肉瘤相比，梭形细胞或多形性脂肪瘤中脂肪细胞的大小一般差异很小，并且脂肪细胞的核异型性较轻。梭形细胞脂肪瘤出现一致性的13q和16q染色体异常[15,64]，与非典型脂肪瘤样肿瘤中出现的环形染色体明显不同（见表24.2）。

冬眠瘤　Hibernoma

临床特征

冬眠瘤是一种并不常见的肿瘤，可显现棕色脂肪分化[65-67]。几乎全部发生在成人，没有性别差异，发病高峰年龄为20～50岁。儿童病例非常少见。最常见的部位是股部、肩部、肩胛间区或颈后，但整体上解剖分布非常广泛。病变一般生长极为缓慢，无痛性；术前病变常常存在5年以上。尽管多数病例位于皮下，但有10%的病例位于肌内（尤其是股部），病变大小通常为5～10cm。不易出现局部复发，尚没有明确的恶性冬眠瘤报道。

病理学特征

冬眠瘤界限清楚，有被膜，切面常常呈棕黑色。组织学上，病变由多少不等的以下成分混合而成：（1）大圆形细小空泡细胞，胞浆嗜酸性，呈颗粒状；（2）同样的大细胞，稍呈嗜酸性，但有较大的（脂肪母细胞样）脂肪空泡；以及（3）成熟性单一空泡的脂肪细胞，在多数病例中大约占所有细胞的40%～50%（图24.11）。有些病例以成熟脂肪细胞或多泡性脂肪母细胞样细胞为主。所有这些细胞都具有良性、常常位于周边的小核仁。肿瘤分叶一般比较明显。偶尔可见髓外造血。个别病例可以有明显的黏液样间质，极少数病例出现类似于梭形细胞脂肪瘤的梭形细胞成分[65]。细胞遗传学方面，这些病变出现11q13和（不见的）10q22基因重排[15]。11q13异常最多见的是导致MEN-1基因位点缺失[68]。不存在实际上的鉴别诊断，因为脂肪细胞成分与所有类型的颗粒细胞肿瘤都很容易鉴别。然而，应该记住的是，黏液样脂肪肉瘤含有冬眠瘤样细胞极其常见。

脂肪肉瘤　Liposarcoma

按照作者的观点，脂肪肉瘤是唯一最常见的软组织肉瘤，至少占所有成人肉瘤的20%。有三种主要类型：高分化（去分化型是一个亚型）、黏液样（圆形细胞型是一个亚型）和多形性。传统上，主要的诊断特征是出现脂肪母细胞，但是确定高分化（非典型脂肪瘤样）病变（见下文）还有其他可选择的标准。脂肪特殊染色和免疫组化一般没有根本性作用，除了个别时候S-00蛋白染色可以突出多泡的脂肪母细胞以及圆形细胞性脂肪肉瘤中的肿瘤细胞常常为S-100阳性。此外，MDM2和CDK4染色在诊断非典型脂肪瘤样肿瘤以及去分化脂肪肉瘤方面具有一定作用（见下文）。单泡性（印戒）脂肪母细胞尽管十分常见，但容易与横切的小血管或有空泡的内皮细胞混淆，因此，多泡性脂肪母

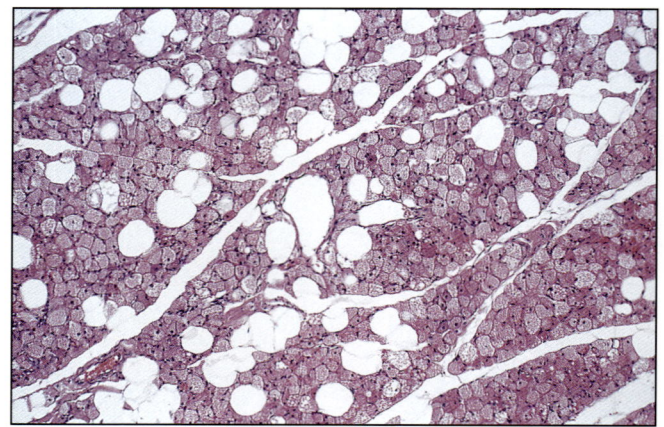

图24.11　冬眠瘤。注意分叶状结构以及颗粒状嗜酸性细胞和脂肪细胞混合。

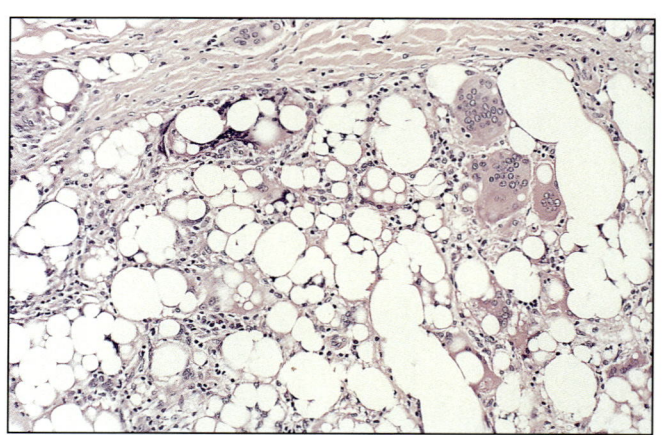

图24.12　硅胶肉芽肿。出现异物巨细胞是有用的诊断线索。

细胞是诊断所需的主要成分。这些细胞有两个或多个边缘清晰的、通常较大的胞浆空泡，其中含有锯齿或扇贝状非典型浓染细胞核。多核极为常见。模糊或界限不清的小"泡"，尤其是当伴有良性或位于中央的小细胞核时，通常不能算数！与这些多泡（不同于印戒）细胞真正类似的病变是硅胶肉芽肿，最常见于乳腺植入或其他组织扩张器周围（图24.12）。与脂肪肉瘤的鉴别一般比较容易，因为高分化病变不会出现这么多的"脂肪母细胞"。

临床特征

脂肪肉瘤为成人肿瘤，男性稍多见。总体上，发病高峰年龄是41～70岁。儿童脂肪肉瘤极其罕见，通常局限于10～15岁年龄组[69]；最常见的是黏液型，预后极好。在成人，临床特征随着组织学类型不同而稍有不同[70-73]，但总体上绝大多数病例病变部位深在，其生长速度与组织学分级平行。与其他类型相比，黏液样肿瘤主要累及稍年轻的成人（21～50岁）。病史

较长的大肿物近期迅速生长通常提示去分化或黏液样病变进展为高级别（圆形细胞）类型。在作者的资料中，35%的脂肪肉瘤发生在下肢（尤其是股部），22%位于躯干或肢体带周围，15%位于上肢，15%位于后腹膜，8%位于头颈部或纵隔，5%位于精索。当将肿瘤部位与组织学类型相连时，黏液样、圆形细胞和多形性脂肪肉瘤以四肢为主；高分化病变通常平均分布于四肢和腹膜后；去分化病变最常见于腹膜后。脂肪肉瘤的多中心倾向已有报道，但反映的是惰性软组织转移（黏液亚型的一个特征），多数这样的患者最终发展为播散性病变。总体上，5年生存的可能性不如主要依靠诊断标准那么精确；大概的5年生存率是：高分化病变90%（10年是60%，反映了腹膜后病变的局部复发常常不可控制）；去分化病变为60%~70%（10年40%~50%）（同样，多数死于腹膜后的局部复发）；单纯性黏液样病变为90%；黏液样和"圆形细胞"（富于细胞）病变为40%~50%；单纯"圆形细胞"（高级别黏液样）病变为25%；以及多形性病变大约为50%~60%。

病理学特征

高分化脂肪肉瘤[73-76] 也被称为非典型脂肪瘤样肿瘤（见下文描述），主要有两种形式：脂肪细胞型（脂肪瘤样）和硬化型，前者更常见。两者占脂肪肉瘤的比例大约为40%~50%。在腹膜后，肿瘤常常出现混合类型。硬化型在腹膜后和精索比在其他部位更常见。病变往往较大，界限清楚，粗大结节状；硬化型较灰白、质硬。少数病例的边缘显示不规则性浸润邻近肌肉。

脂肪细胞型（脂肪瘤样）脂肪肉瘤主要由相对成熟的单泡脂肪细胞构成，细胞大小不一，至少有部分细胞含有非典型的、浓染细胞核（图24.13）。这些细胞中混有散在的奇异的、常常是多核的间质细胞以及多少不等的纤维性间隔，其中含有浓染的梭形细胞以及个别奇异型细胞（见上文）（图24.14）。非典型梭形或多核细胞也可见于病变内的大血管壁内。脂肪母细胞瘤的数量不等。这些细胞不再是诊断所必需，但在纤维间隔附近常常容易发现；有些病例中缺乏或难以发现这些细胞（见下文）。病变较大、病史较长时，常见有脂肪坏死区域。个别病例含有骨化生或散在的大的横纹肌母细胞成分，或出现部分平滑肌分化；后一种成分可以是"成熟性"[77]或肉瘤性，尽管分化较好[78]。与硬化型脂肪肉瘤不同的是：后者主要由胶原纤维组织构成，会有些纤细的纤维样表现。纤维组织内有散在的成熟脂肪细胞和通常为多核的奇异的、浓染间质细胞（图24.15）；在多数病例中很难发现脂肪

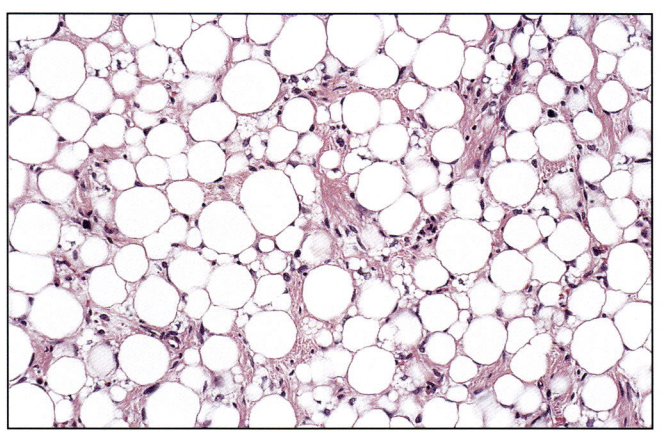

图24.13 高分化脂肪细胞型脂肪肉瘤。注意脂肪细胞大小不等，细胞核浓染，有散在的脂肪母细胞。

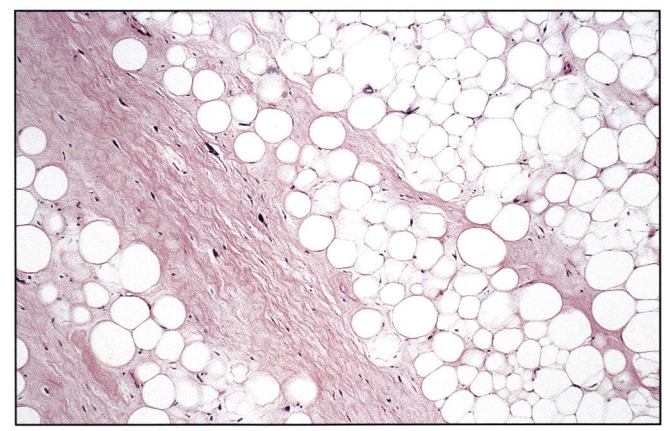

图24.14 高分化脂肪细胞型脂肪肉瘤。纤维性间隔内常常含有奇异性间质细胞。

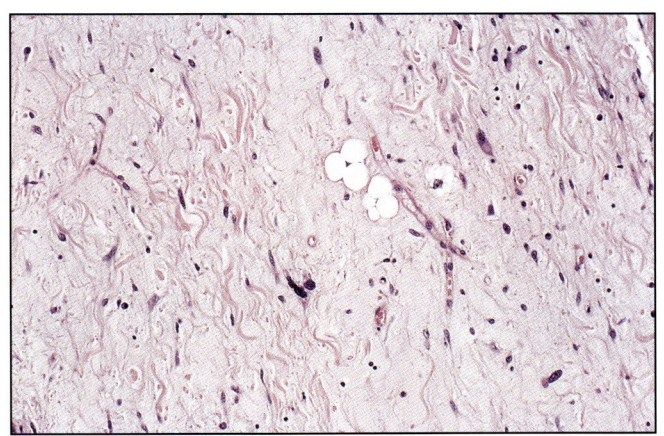

图24.15 高分化硬化型脂肪肉瘤。注意纤维性胶原和少量脂肪母细胞。

母细胞。对于脂肪细胞型和硬化型脂肪肉瘤，取材应该仔细、充分，一般大体上应密集连续切片，以便可以除外有去分化成分（见下文）。

其他两种高分化脂肪肉瘤极少遇到：炎症型[79,80]，几乎都位于腹膜后，其中大量淋巴浆细胞聚集可类似于炎性假瘤（图24.16）；梭形细胞型[81,82]，皮下十分常见，主要发生在肢体和躯干，容易误诊为神经鞘肿瘤（图24.17）。

考虑到组织学上纯粹的高分化脂肪肉瘤不发生转移，以及接受扩大手术切除的病变（通常是除腹膜后以外的病变）容易治愈等事实，Evans 等采用了"非典型脂肪瘤"一词[75]。进一步明确的是，出现脂肪细胞和（或）间质细胞异型而缺乏脂肪母细胞的深在性脂肪肿瘤在行为上与高分化脂肪肉瘤完全相同；换句话说，如果沿肿瘤边缘切除或切除不彻底，常有局部复发，而对于复发（尤其是反复出现），从理论上讲有去分化风险（<5%）存在，因此存在转移潜能。不管病变的位置和深度如何，其生物学潜能是相同的，尽管皮下非典型脂肪肿瘤较小且大多更容易充分切除，例如，

与腹膜后病变相比，去分化更为少见。同样重要的是，要注意非典型脂肪肿瘤不管位置如何，以及是否含有脂肪母细胞，其特征性的核型是源自12号染色体长臂的环状（或长标）染色体[83,84]。这些环状或标记性染色体含有无数的基因复制（即扩增），包括 *MDM2*、*CDK4* 和 *HMGA (2)*。而导致的 MDM2 蛋白过表达近来已被建议作为高分化和去分化病变有用的免疫组化标记物[85]。非典型脂肪瘤样肿瘤这个概念极具可行性，但必须密切临床与病理之间的联系，以免不了解情况的外科医生对如此诊断的意义估计不足。作者仅仅对于腹膜后、精索和纵隔的病变喜欢使用"高分化脂肪肉瘤"一词，因为这些病变可以通过局部作用和局部复发致死，而对于外科容易切除部位（主要是肢体和躯干）的病变,使用"非典型脂肪瘤样肿瘤"一词，并在病理报告中对其生物学行为加以注释，这就避免了"肉瘤"诊断所带来的不必要的显著的社会和心理影响。

关于高分化脂肪肉瘤与出现变性或萎缩改变的脂肪瘤、脂肪坏死区域、硬化性炎性病变的鉴别，重点应该放在识别脂肪细胞的细胞核非典型性和找到奇异、浓染的间质细胞。

去分化脂肪肉瘤（dedifferentiated liposarcoma）[86,87]占脂肪肉瘤的10%，经典的定义是：不论是原发还是复发的肿瘤，高分化脂肪肉瘤显示突然转化为高级别的非脂肪源性肉瘤（图24.18）。个别病例可出现局灶性两种成分混合。大概90%的病例为原发病例，10%见于复发病例。迄今为止，去分化脂肪肉瘤在腹膜后最常见，实际上占该部位梭形细胞和多形性肉瘤的大多数。大体上，两种成分大多容易区别，但存在着危险：如果取材只是针对实性、外观上更可怕的高级别区域，就有可能忽视高分化成分；实际上，高分化区域

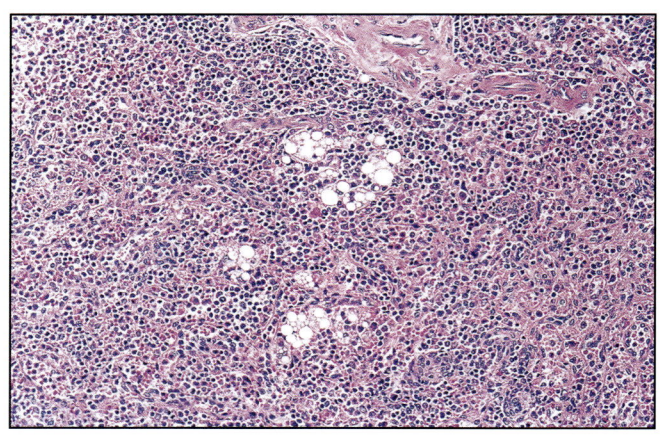

图24.16　高分化炎症型脂肪肉瘤。慢性炎症细胞背景中可见小团脂肪母细胞。

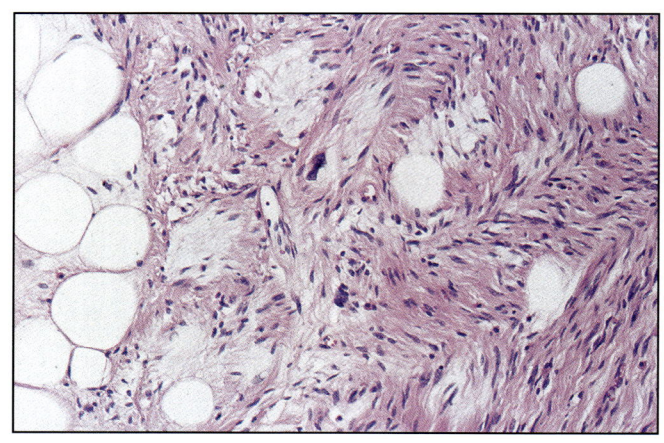

图24.17　出现梭形细胞特征的非典型脂肪瘤性肿瘤。注意脂肪细胞大小不一，有散在的非典型间质细胞。

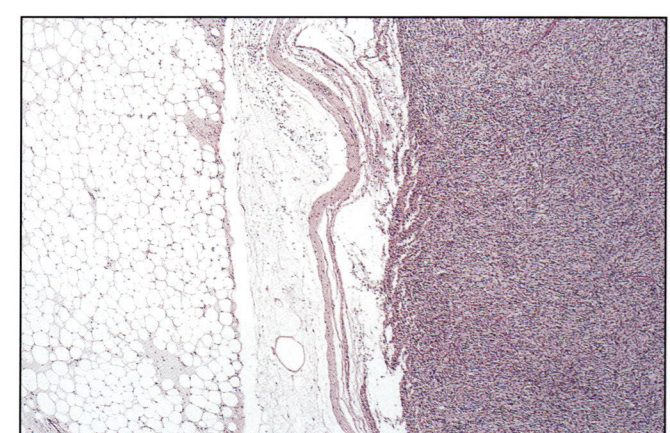

图24.18　去分化脂肪肉瘤。两种成分之间的突然过渡很常见。

可以非常微小或局限，以致外科医生在切除时可能不慎遗留这些成分。去分化成分的组织学类型多样，但大多类似于席纹状/多形性 MFH（所谓的恶性纤维组织细胞瘤，malignant fibrous histiocytoma；图 24.19）、黏液纤维肉瘤（黏液样 MFH）或非特异性肉瘤（NOS）。有些病例出现明显的中性粒细胞浸润[88]，多数肿瘤是以前所谓的炎性 MFH。少部分病例出现多结节失去黏附性的去分化方式，至少有时表明是一种力场改变现象。在多数病例中，非脂肪性的高级别组织学成分没有特殊分化的形态学证据，尽管常有局灶结蛋白阳性，可能反映了肌纤维母细胞分化。与高分化病变相比，去分化脂肪肉瘤显示更为一致的 MDM2 和 CDK4[85] 免疫染色阳性。随着对脂肪肉瘤亚型的认识更为精确，很明显大概 10% 的病例出现异源性分化，最常见的是横纹肌肉瘤（图 24.20）、平滑肌肉瘤或骨肉瘤[86,87,89,90]；这些成分多少不等，似乎对预后没有明显影响。此类肿瘤在过去常常诊断为恶性间质瘤。在一些病例中，一种更为特殊的结构是出现微结节性（脑膜瘤样）梭形细胞漩涡，常常伴有钙化[91,92]。另外一个重要进展是已经认识到，去分化成分在形态学上可以是低级别的，通常由非脂肪性富于细胞的梭形细胞区域构成，呈不甚明显的束状生长结构。此类病例中，细胞学非典型性不很明显，没有坏死。低级别和高级别去分化病变在预后方面没有显著差异，两者的 5 年转移风险仅为 20%～25%。

黏液样脂肪肉瘤（myxoid liposarcoma）和其高级别类型（通常称为圆细胞脂肪肉瘤）大约占脂肪肉瘤的 30%～35%，不论级别如何，其特征是特异性染色体相互易位，可以是 t(12;16)(q13;p11) 或少见的 t(12;22)(q13;q11-12)，两者均可导致 DDIT3 基因重

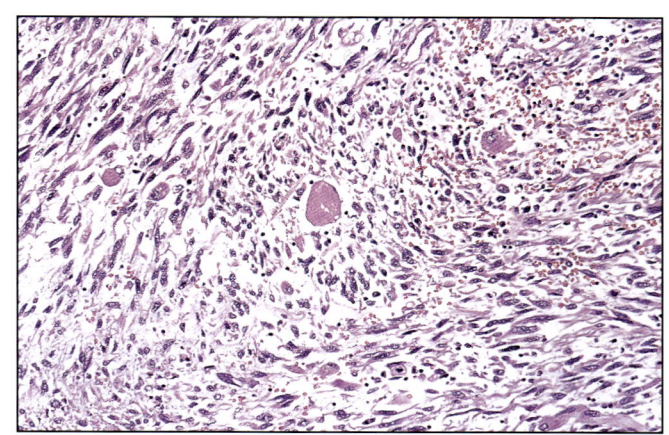

图 24.20　伴有异源性横纹肌肉瘤成分的去分化脂肪肉瘤。注意大多角形的横纹肌母细胞。

排[93-96]，即脂肪细胞分化中的一个翻译因子。在低级别类型中，肿瘤呈凝胶状，呈一些红色，常常含有似乎是较成熟脂肪组织梗死的区域。大约 5% 的病例位于皮下。组织学成分单一时，肿瘤由未分化的难以归类的小梭形细胞和小脂肪母细胞构成（主要为单泡），背景是大量黏液样基质（由透明质酸构成），内有众多细小分枝状薄壁毛细血管，被描述为"牛角"或"鸡爪"形态（图 24.21）。诊断性的多泡脂肪母细胞（通常小于高分化脂肪肉瘤中的细胞）在肿瘤周边的被膜下区域最容易见到。核分裂象极其稀少。常常出现间质黏液池，产生大量腔隙，有假淋巴管瘤样或假腺泡样表现（图 24.22）。此病变的变型包括伴有颗粒状嗜酸性（冬眠瘤样）细胞、出现广泛成熟脂肪细胞分化和极少数以梭形细胞表现为主的病例。个别病例出现局灶软骨化生，极少数病例含有散在的多形性、常为多核的细胞，但是这些似乎没有预

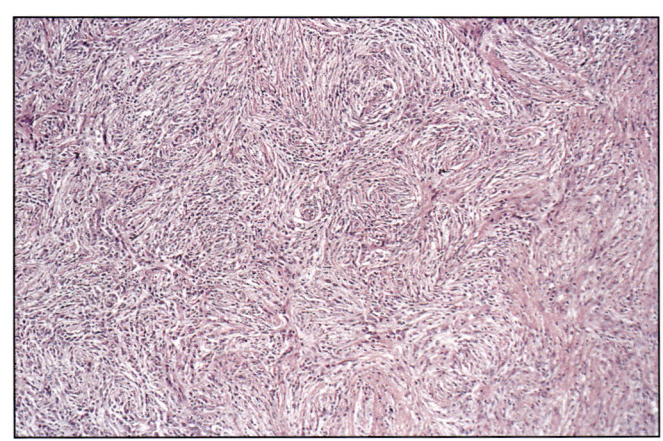

图 24.19　去分化脂肪肉瘤。去分化最常见的结构为席纹状，但并非特别多形性。

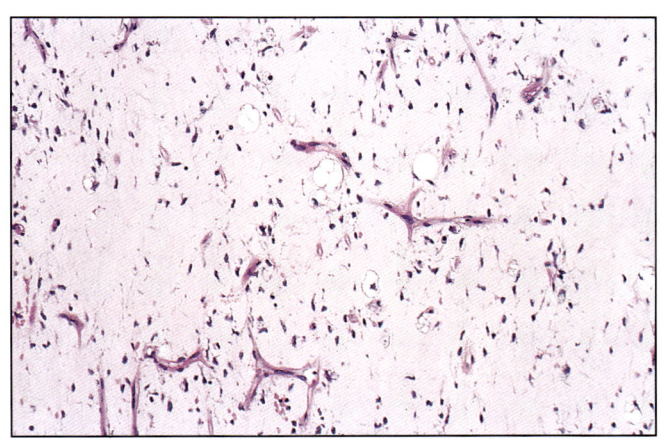

图 24.21　黏液样脂肪肉瘤。特征性的牛角样血管，未分化的小细胞和脂肪母细胞。

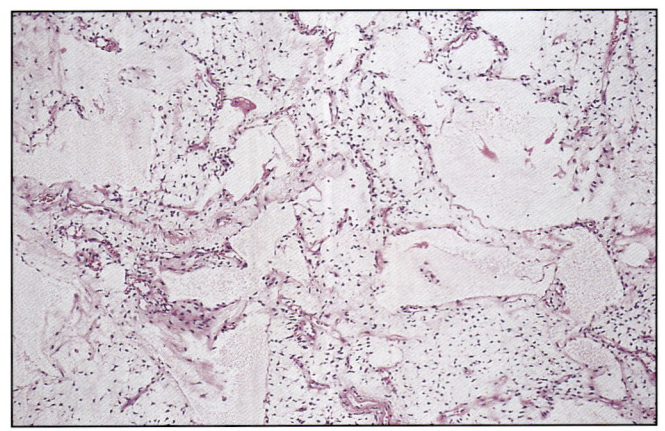

图24.22 黏液样脂肪肉瘤。黏液池常见。

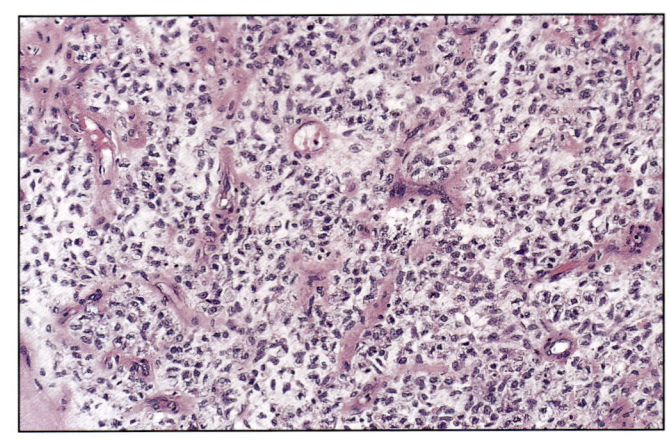

图24.24 圆形细胞脂肪肉瘤。注意仍可见到牛角样血管。

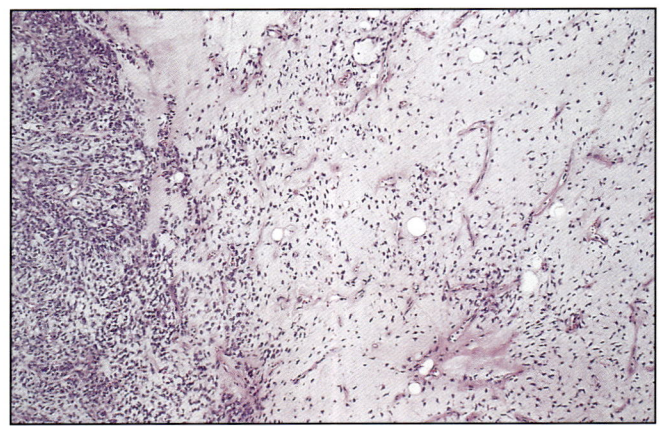

图24.23 黏液样和圆形细胞脂肪肉瘤。注意向更加富于细胞的高级别区域过渡。

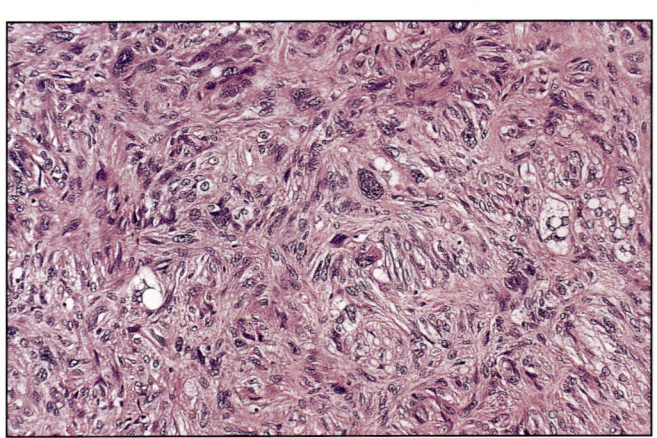

图24.25 多形性脂肪肉瘤。除了有散在的脂肪母细胞外，肿瘤与所谓的MFH不能区分。

后意义。

更为重要的是出现细胞较丰富的区域，常常称为圆细胞分化，意味着其行为更具侵袭性。与黏液性脂肪肉瘤的良性梭形细胞相比，这些细胞有时含有较大、较圆和更为浓染的细胞核，尽管其胞浆依旧不很明显（图24.23），但多数病例高度富于细胞，并且没有真正的圆形细胞形态学表现。仅有少部分病例出现完全性的未分化圆形细胞形态学表现（容易被误认为是其他多种类型的肿瘤）。核分裂象相对更常见。这些细胞所占检测面积的大小变化很大：如果是75%或更多，通常采用"圆细胞脂肪肉瘤"一词（图24.24）。多数病例呈中间性表现，可称为混合性黏液性和圆细胞脂肪肉瘤，或高级别黏液性脂肪肉瘤[72,73,97]。由于高度富于细胞性和圆细胞分化的程度改变呈连续性谱系，从轻度到广泛，有关什么程度具有预后意义仍存在很大的不确定性[98]。当然，任何病变出现10%或更多的高度富于细胞性和圆形细胞区域时应该定为中等级别，被认为具有很大的转移风险；如果这种成分占25%或更多，则应该定为高级别。

富于细胞程度较轻的病例，其预后没有明确的特征，然而，应当保持警惕[98]。

黏液性脂肪肉瘤依据其存在较丰富的血管和脂肪母细胞可与肌内黏液瘤鉴别，与黏液纤维肉瘤的鉴别依据后者出现较为显著的浓染细胞核、多形性以及容易出现较多弯曲的血管。以圆形细胞为主的病变可能很难与几乎所有的间变性圆形细胞恶性肿瘤（包括转移癌）鉴别，但是即使在多数高级别病例，有用的线索仍然存在，即出现牛角样血管和小的黏液池区域。仔细寻找脂肪母细胞应该是很有成效的。有趣的是，尽管多种类型的脂肪性肿瘤中的非脂肪性梭形或多形性细胞 S-100 呈阴性，但黏液性和圆形细胞脂肪肉瘤中的未分化圆形细胞和一些梭形细胞常常出现胞浆（和胞核）S-100 蛋白呈阳性，与脂肪细胞和脂肪母细胞相同[99]。

多形性脂肪肉瘤（pleomorphic liposarcoma）[100,101]大约占脂肪肉瘤的5%。与其他高级别多形性肉瘤（"MFH样"家族）的鉴别只能依据存在多泡性脂肪母细胞（图24.25）。这些细胞可能数量很少或相当局限，所以为了确认其存在，需要仔细取材。其他病例十分类似于黏液纤维肉瘤，或出现明显的片状的大的奇异性脂肪母细胞，少数病例出现明显的上皮样细胞形态学改变[100-102]。除了非常明显的细胞多形性之外，一个常见但并不特异的表现是：出现众多胞浆内嗜酸性小体或小滴，关于其确切本质，尚有争议，尽管最有可能是溶酶体来源。

另外，极少数的脂肪肉瘤为混合型或非特异型病变。混合型病变包括高分化加圆形细胞成分，或黏液性加多形性成分。有些病例过去被分类为"混合型"，现在可能被重新划归为某种去分化的脂肪肉瘤[103]。此类病变的行为和预后很不确定，最好依据肿瘤中的最高级别成分来判断。

纤维性肿瘤　Fibrous tumors

纤维性肿瘤包括一组异源性反应性病变、一般认为的错构瘤性病变以及良性、局灶侵袭性或恶性肿瘤。对于伴有良性临床过程的病变应该纳入哪个确切的生物学类别，常常并不确定。从组织学观点来说，除了极少数以外，这些肿瘤通常由不同比例的纤维母细胞和肌纤维母细胞混合而成；两者比例在疾病的不同阶段会有所变化。这是由两种细胞类型之间的极为密切的生物学关系决定的，实质上代表了一种结构和功能的连续轨迹。纤维母细胞和肌纤维母细胞之间或肌纤维母细胞和平滑肌细胞之间没有明确的定义和公认的分界点，所以如此区分通常是武断的。

反应性病变　Reactive leisions

瘢痕疙瘩　Keloid scar

瘢痕疙瘩[104-106]最常见于青少年和年轻成人，尤其常见于黑人患者。因局部创伤所致，可发生在任何解剖位置，头颈部好发，尤其是耳垂部位。典型病变发痒、隆起和发亮，被覆毛细血管扩张性皮肤，并且超出最初组织损伤的界限。治疗困难，50%的病例在尝试切除后出现局部复发。组织学上，这些常见病变由成熟的、细胞相对稀少的纤维瘢痕组织构成，其内可见宽大带状或结节状嗜酸性透明胶原。后者是诊断的必要条件。瘢痕疙瘩的发病机制尚不明确，但是似乎代表了正常瘢痕组织形成过程中对生长因子过度反应的遗传倾向。

肥厚性瘢痕　Hypertrophic scar

肥厚性瘢痕[105,107]为异常过度瘢痕化的另一种形式。临床上其不同于瘢痕疙瘩的是其比较少见，没有种族倾向，局限于原有的组织损伤部位，局部复发倾向较小。组织学上，与瘢痕疙瘩相比，这些病变由细胞更为丰富的瘢痕组织构成，往往具有结节状结构。与普通瘢痕完全区分一般需要临床病理相互联系。

结节性筋膜炎　Nodular fasciitis

临床特征

典型的结节性筋膜炎[108-111]表现为迅速增大的、常常有疼痛或压痛的皮下结节，最常累及年轻人，以上肢为主，尤其是前臂。尽管持续时间不等，但多数病例病史不足10～12周。几乎所有解剖部位均可受累，少数儿童病例以头颈部为主[112]。病变深度也有所不同：大约10%的病例完全位于肌肉内，少部分发生于骨膜（骨旁筋膜炎）[113]或皮肤（皮内筋膜炎）[114,115]。来源于头部的骨旁病变常出现明显的骨破坏，称为颅骨筋膜炎，儿童最常见[112,116]。另外一种不常见的亚型可累及血管，主要是静脉，呈多结节样，通常位于上肢或头颈部，称为血管内筋膜炎[115,117]。极少数病例可累及关节内。尽管传统上认为其是反应性病变，但不断积累的证据（主要来自细胞遗传学分析）表明，结节性筋膜炎及其相关亚型为克隆增生。

就临床行为而言，这些病变无论结构怎样，均为良性过程，临床上病程具有自限性；如果不进行治疗，病变会自发性萎缩。局部复发（或持续性生长）极为少见，可见于大约2%的病例，几乎都是由于生长活跃期间进行的零碎的、大体切除不彻底造成。对于多数病例，沿病变边缘局灶切除已足够，镜下残留的病变组织经过自行磨耗，一般情况下很少或不会遗留有瘢痕。

病理学特征

多数病变界限清楚，但没有被膜，直径多数小于3cm。切面随生长时间不同而有差异，但可以是黏液样的，中心呈囊性或纤维性。不论部位如何，组织学上具有特征性和可重复性[109-111,118]。与流行的观点不同，多数病例边界清楚，不超过10%的病例出现不规则的浸润性或分枝状生长。典型病例由富于细胞的纤维母细胞增生构成，伴有肥胖的细胞核，偶尔可见核仁，其背景是疏松胶原性间质，出现不同程度的黏液变，一般呈微囊性（图24.26）。正常核分裂象可以很多，但梭形细胞的胞核均无浓染或多形。梭形细胞排

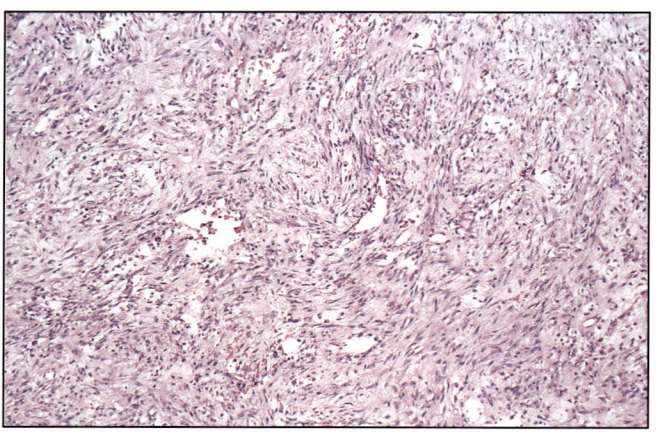

图24.26 结节性筋膜炎。典型的羽毛状表现伴有微囊性变性。

列成相互交织的短束；加上相对淡染的疏松间质组织，使之呈羽毛状表现。偶尔，细胞较丰富的病例出现席纹状结构。间质含有纤细的薄壁毛细血管、外渗红细胞以及散在的炎细胞成分，主要是淋巴细胞和少数中性粒细胞。10%的病例含有多核巨细胞，最常见的类型是破骨细胞（图24.27）。

在有些病例，尤其是在儿童，其间质出现显著的弥漫性黏液变，病变持续时间较长则容易出现进行性间质玻璃样变性，甚至瘢痕疙瘩样改变。少部分病例出现反应性新生骨形成，伴有肥胖的骨母细胞，类似于骨化性肌炎表现（见第25章）；此类病例有时称为骨化性筋膜炎[119]（也见下文纤维-骨性假瘤部分）。

免疫组化方面，与所有肌纤维母细胞性病变所预期的一样，多数细胞呈全肌肉肌动蛋白和SMA阳性，而结蛋白一般为阴性。至于鉴别诊断，在相应的临床背景下，只有少数会有问题。一般来说，极少数的梭形细胞肉瘤生长迅速，如同结节性筋膜炎一样，这些病变几乎都出现显著的细胞核多形性和坏死区域。纤维瘤病可出现类似筋膜炎的区域，尤其是发生于腹腔或乳腺时，但不同的是：显著的浸润性生长、束状结构较长以及更为均一性的胶原性间质含有极少数炎症细胞。纤维瘤病β-连环蛋白免疫染色也常常呈阳性。良性纤维组织细胞瘤在细胞学上形态更为多样，具有更为一致性的席纹或漩涡状生长结构，常常出现局灶性肌动蛋白阳性。

增生性筋膜炎　Proliferative fasciitis

临床特征

与结节性筋膜炎相比，增生性筋膜炎[120,121]通常累及年龄稍大的成人，发病高峰年龄是51～60岁。在儿童极为少见[122]。上肢好发的程度不如结节性筋膜炎明显，有相当部分的病例发生在下肢。除了这些差别以外，临床状况包括极少复发、病史短和病变大小等与经典的结节性筋膜炎极为相同（见上文）。

组织学特征

由于增生性筋膜炎本质上为结节性筋膜炎的一个亚型，因此具有许多共同特征。可以用来区分这一亚型的主要和特异性的差异在于：增生性筋膜炎中存在大的圆形或多角形细胞，伴有双染性或显著嗜碱性胞浆，有一个或两个泡状核，有明显的核仁（图24.28）；这些细胞通常被描述为节细胞样。病变中这些细胞的比例整体上是有差异的，但当其数量较多时，常常与肉瘤混淆，尤其是横纹肌肉瘤。其他与结节性筋膜炎差异较小的是：其间质更为黏液样，可含有纤维素样物质成分。薄壁血

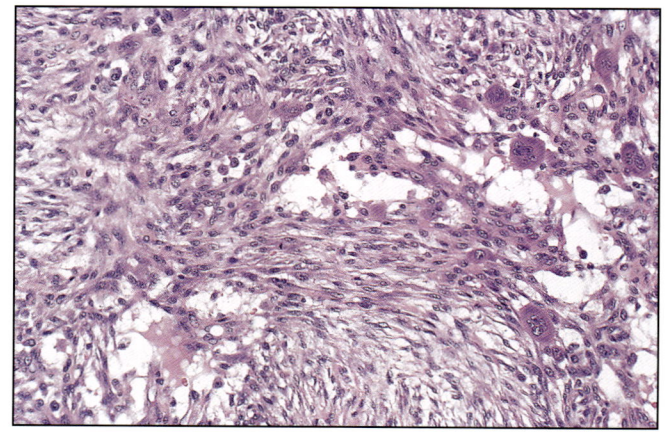

图24.27 结节性筋膜炎。肥胖、具有核分裂活性的肌纤维母细胞为此病变的特征。注意此病例中破骨细胞样的巨细胞。

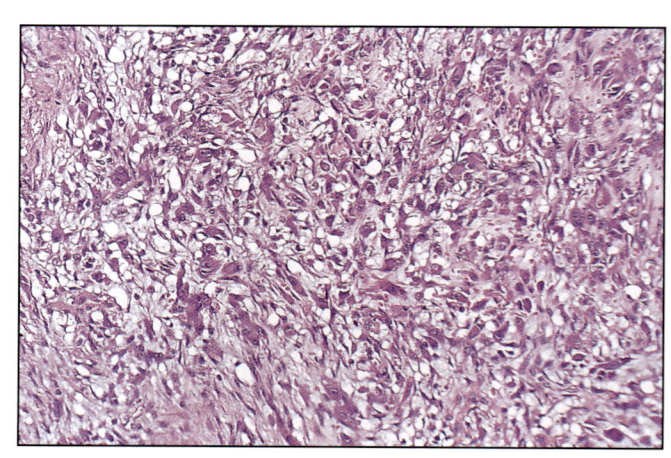

图24.28 增生性筋膜炎。注意肥胖、嗜碱性的神经节样细胞。

管可尤其明显，更加类似于肉芽组织。一般来说，与结节性筋膜炎相比，增生性筋膜炎的病变边缘更为不清。双染性的大细胞被认为是纤维母细胞，有趣的是，尽管有丰富的胞浆，但这些细胞肌动蛋白常常为阴性，不同于与之混杂的梭形肌纤维母细胞。可能唯一实际的鉴别诊断是多形性横纹肌肉瘤。然而，后者极少位于皮下，并且可出现更为显著的细胞非典型性和多形性，常常出现非典型核分裂象。

增生性肌炎　Proliferative myositis

增生性肌炎[123]本质上是增生性筋膜炎的肌内病变。与后者一样，它主要累及老年人，但好发于肩胛带和躯干上部。儿童病例极为少见[122]。临床病史常常少于4周。与其他所有反应性肌纤维母细胞增生一样，其前景极好，复发极为少见。其组织学构成与增生性筋膜炎相同，包括大的节细胞样细胞。这种反应性病变的一个特征性和特殊的结构特征是沿纤维间隔、在单个肌纤维之间扩展，使后者保持完整（图24.29）。这使筋膜炎间质背景中众多被单个分开的嗜酸性肌纤维出现一种所谓"棋盘样"外观。这种生长方式与实际中各种肉瘤都容易鉴别，与更为局限的、不保留肌纤维的骨化性肌炎也容易鉴别（见第25章）。然而，与后者一样，至少10%～20%的增生性肌炎病例含有小灶骨或软骨化生。免疫组化和电镜证实：这些病变本质上为纤维母细胞和肌纤维母细胞混合。

纤维-骨性假瘤　Fibro-osseous pseudotumor

纤维-骨性假瘤[124]有时也被称为富炽性反应性骨膜炎[125]，是类似于筋膜炎的另外一种肌纤维母细胞增生；不同之处仅仅在于：几乎都位于指（趾）部以及容易出现新骨形成。多数受累患者为年轻成人，尤其是女性，表现为迅速增大的痛性肿物，常常位于指（趾）骨旁。放射学方面，常常有病变钙化和显著骨膜反应。与同一部位也可出现纤维性成分的奇特性骨旁骨软骨瘤样增生（Nora病）相比，纤维-骨性假瘤不附着在下方的骨上（见第25章）。组织学方面，其本质上呈筋膜炎表现，另外还有灶状、不规则的类骨质、骨形成，有时有软骨形成（图24.30）。骨或类骨质表面为肥胖的骨母细胞，骨化性肌炎中病变的带状成熟方式（见第25章）在这些病例中见不到，因此被误诊为骨肉瘤的风险增加。始终应该牢记的是，手部无论是骨、还是软组织来源的骨肉瘤极其罕见。

骨化性肌炎　Myositis ossificans

骨化性肌炎在第25章描述，其与这里所描述的筋膜炎家族病变的关系非常密切。值得注意的是，组织学上可与之相比的病变也可发生在肠系膜[126]，常常发生在手术之后。

缺血性筋膜炎　Ischemic fasciitis

缺血性筋膜炎[127]在最初的报告中被称为"非典型褥疮性纤维组织增生"[128]，是一种特殊的反应性纤维母细胞性病变，最常发生在骨性突起的上方，尤其是（但不都是）在不活动的、通常较虚弱的患者。这种病变最常发生于深部皮下组织，尤其是髋部周围或骶骨区。组织学上，此类病例的特征是：宽带状纤维素样坏死，周围是血管炎性肉芽组织，其中可以见到肥胖的、具有核分裂活性的纤维母细胞和肌纤维母细胞，与增生性筋膜炎相似（图24.31）。附近受累的脂肪组织常出现梗死。这些病变的原因被认为是缺血性变性，与褥疮性溃疡相

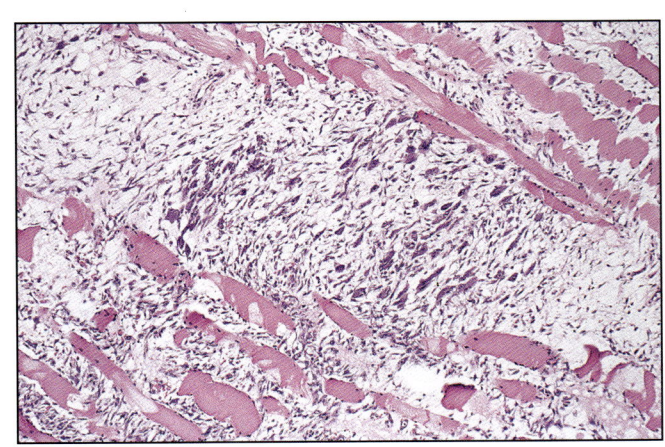

图24.29　增生性肌炎。注意肌纤维相对保留。

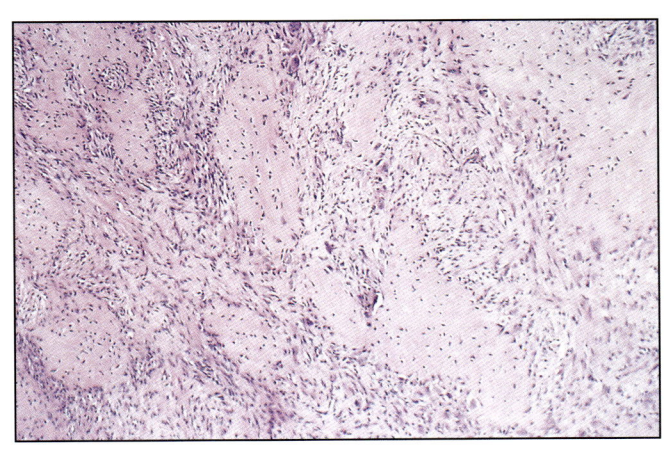

图24.30　纤维-骨性假瘤。此类似筋膜炎的病变伴有不规则类骨质沉积。

反应性病变

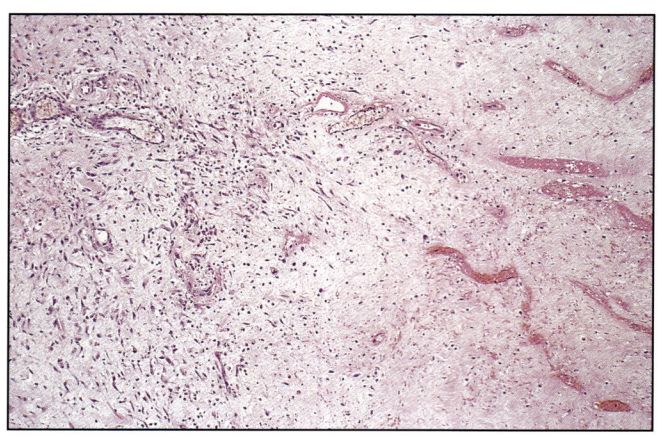

图24.31　缺血性筋膜炎。注意非特征性的纤维素样变性。

似。有些病例切除后可出现局部复发，最有可能是发病诱因持续存在。

内脏反应性肌纤维母细胞增生
Reactive myofibroblastic proliferations at visceral locations

近些年来，发生于内脏的、组织学特征与结节性或增生性筋膜炎极为类似的病变的数量在增加，尤其是在泌尿生殖道[129-132]（图24.32）。以作者的经验，其他比较少见的部位包括喉部和鼻窦。尽管最初认为是损伤后（通常是手术后）出现，但现在认识到，多数此类病例显然是自发性的。这些临床上良性的病变在第12章有更详细的描述。其与炎症性肌纤维母细胞瘤的不同在于其临床情况，以及后者容易出现更为明显的慢性炎症成分，尤其是浆细胞，并且可以出现一定程度的细胞核非典型性。此外，炎症性肌纤维母细胞瘤的局部复发率极高，甚至可以出现恶性病程。

弹力纤维瘤　Elastofibroma

临床特征

弹力纤维瘤[133-135]是相对并不常见的病变，通常发生在老年人的一侧或两侧肩胛下，女性明显多见。常见表现是生长缓慢的、界限不清的肿物，附着于肋骨骨膜，尽管多数病例是由于胸部CT影像学应用的增加而偶然发现的。长期以来，这种病变被认为是肩胛和胸部之间组织由于长期反复外伤所致，尽管所预期的与重体力劳动的关系并未证实可信，但明显的病例群体提示，尤其是在日本的一些地方较明显，至少在一些病例中存在遗传倾向[136]。此外，新近的细胞遗传学和有关分子资料表明，这些病变是克隆性的[137,138]。极少数病例发生在下肢，组织学上类似的病变发生在胃肠道也有报道。病变没有局部复发倾向。

病理学特征

弹力纤维瘤几乎均为界限极其不清，与周围正常组织相互融合，大小可以达到10cm。切面类似于致密纤维脂肪组织。组织学检查显示不规则的致密胶原纤维组织条带，细胞相当稀少，其中有大量嗜酸性弹力纤维（图24.33）。弹力纤维染色可以突出这些物质，排列成粗大串珠样或锯齿状纤维或球形团块（图24.34），非常类似于皮肤弹力纤维假黄色瘤中所见。以前对于这些成分是真正的弹力纤维还是胶原出现弹性组织变性存在很多争议，现已有充分证据表明，这些是真正的弹力蛋白，最有可能来源于骨膜细胞[139]。另外值得注意的是其发病机制，除了双侧以外，无论左利或右利，受累患者内脏可出现类似弹力纤维瘤样改变[140]，再次提示有遗传倾向的可能性。

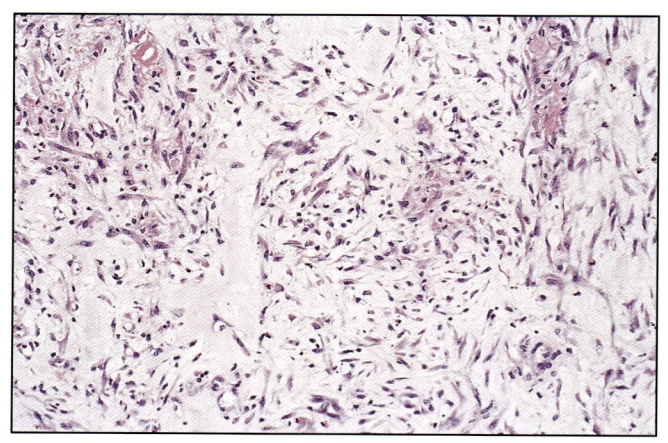

图24.32　内脏反应性肌纤维母细胞增生。这个类似筋膜炎的病变部位靠近胰腺，随后自行消退。

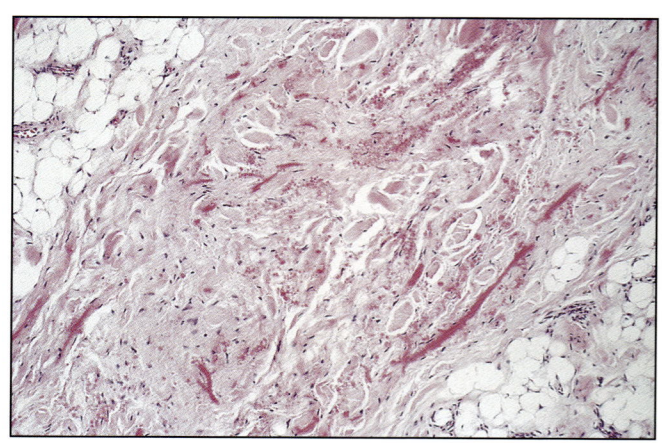

图24.33　弹力纤维瘤。注意嗜酸性的弹力纤维。

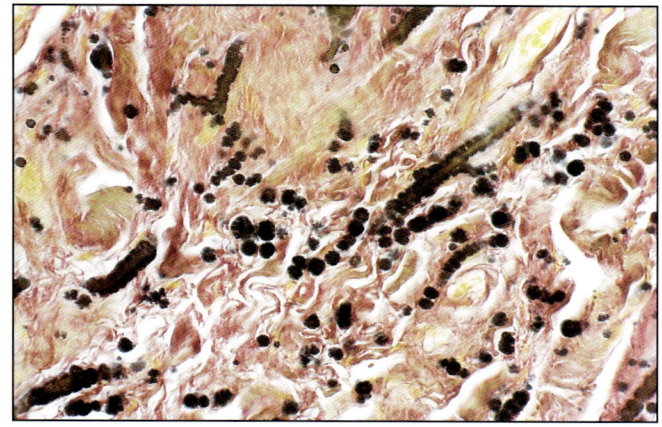

图24.34 弹力纤维瘤。弹力van Gieson染色突出了串珠样和小球状的弹力纤维。

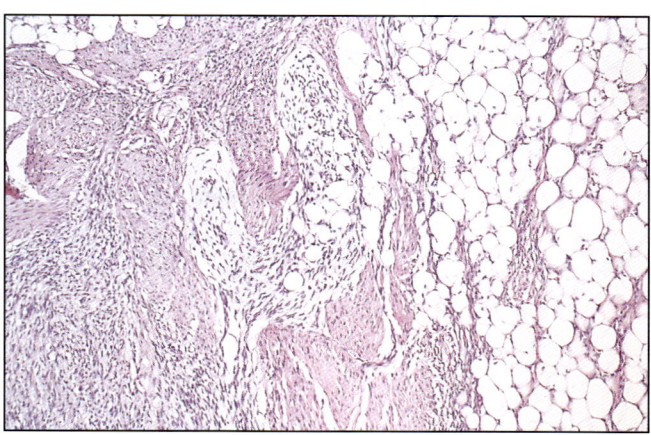

图24.35 婴儿纤维性错构瘤。在这个视野中,所有四种成分都可以见到。

错构瘤性病变　Hamartomatous lesions

错构瘤性病变的分类中包括纤维性病变,似乎具有发育或遗传性基础,几乎完全发生在婴幼儿,基本上是非侵袭性的生长方式。许多传统分类上所谓的"错构瘤"(在所有部位)的病变具有侵袭性,出现克隆性增生(即最有可能是肿瘤性的),所以在不远的将来有可能从本质上对这个概念重新加以评价。

婴儿纤维性错构瘤
Fibrous hamartoma of infancy

临床特征

婴儿纤维性错构瘤[141,142]几乎都发生在2岁以内,有明显的男性倾向。最常见的部位是腋窝、前臂和肩部,但个别病例报道所描述的部位比较广泛。患儿常常出现质硬的、生长缓慢的皮下肿物,大多可以活动,大小一般小于5cm。在个别病例中[142,143],可以出现一个以上的病变。极少数可有局部复发;这些病变一般不复发,然而也没有确切的自行消退倾向[144]。

病理学特征

婴儿纤维性错构瘤为局限性纤维脂肪性肿瘤,但界限不清,质硬,位于真皮深部和皮下。肌肉受累极其少见。组织学方面[141,145,146],四种主要成分的相对比例不同(图24.35):

- 轻度嗜酸性的、肌动蛋白阳性的棒槌状肌纤维母细胞束,细胞核往往逐渐变细并呈波浪状
- 小的圆形和卵圆形未分化梭形或星形细胞巢,背景是含有纤细血管的黏液样间质(图24.36)

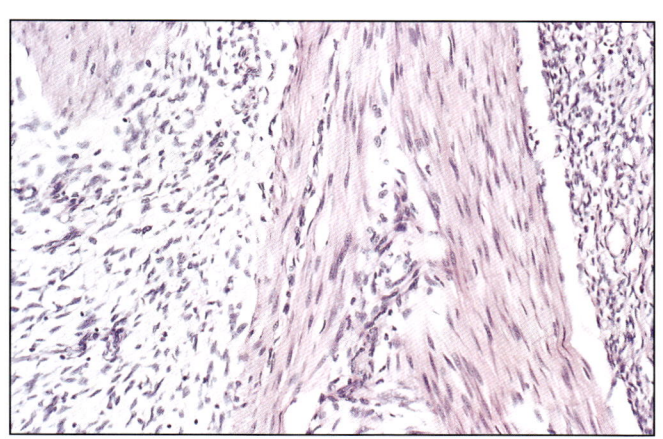

图24.36 婴儿纤维性错构瘤。束状成分是肌纤维母细胞。黏液样的区域表现较为原始。

- 杂乱的胶原纤维组织区域中含有血管和炎性细胞
- 成熟脂肪细胞岛。

一般来说,两种不同的纤维成分占主要部分,有些病例可以出现明显的玻璃样变性。这些病变的器官样生长结构和组织发生尚不能解释。没有实际的鉴别诊断。

婴儿肌纤维瘤病　Infantile myofibroamtosis

正如第3章(见72页)所述,不同类型的纤维瘤(病)可能是血管周围收缩细胞增生("肌周细胞瘤")[147],但由于这是一种相对近期的概念性变化,刚刚开始得到广泛接受,仍在较传统的命名下来描述这些病变。

临床特征

婴儿肌纤维瘤(病)[148-150]以前被称为先天性全身性纤维瘤病,一般发生在2岁之前,先天性病例达30%,显示有中度男性好发倾向。最多10%的患者有

错构瘤性病变

多发性病变，尽管认为这个数字在过去更高。大多数病变发生在皮肤和浅表软组织，尤其是头颈部和躯干，但是骨病变也十分常见[151]（见第 25 章），并且在多的中心病例中可有极个别累及内脏，尤其是胃肠道或肺。作者也遇到过极其少见的孤立性内脏病变。少部分病例是遗传性的，但其机制是常染色体显性遗传还是隐性遗传还不清楚[152,153]。软组织和骨病变的临床过程完全为良性，局部复发罕见。很大一部分病变可自行消退。与之相比，极为少见的多发性内脏病变可能具有致死性预后[148]。老年患者的孤立性病变单独进行讨论（见下文）。

病理学特征

多数病变大小不足 3～4cm。大多边界清楚，但无被膜，切面质硬。组织学可见两种成分，所占比例明显不同。包括嗜酸性梭形细胞漩涡和细胞束，伴有良性、肌样特征性表现，以及由小圆及梭形细胞构成的更为原始的区域，有少量嗜酸性胞浆，细胞核更圆（图 24.37）。这些分化较差的细胞常常围绕分枝状血管外皮细胞瘤样小血管排列（图 24.38）。嗜酸性梭形细胞区域往往主要在周边，常常随着时间的延长出现玻璃样变性，间质呈嗜碱性和假软骨样表现。两种细胞类型的核分裂象极为常见。比较原始的区域常常出现坏死，也可有钙化。血管浸润（更准确地说是内皮下血管周围梭形细胞增生）很常见。在两种类型的细胞中，至少有局灶性肌动蛋白阳性，保持了作为肌纤维母细胞和肌膜细胞的本质，但在梭形细胞中最为显著。在小婴儿病变的活检当中，尤其是在多中心性病变，通常以原始血管外皮细胞瘤样成分为主（图 24.39）。其结果加上其临床特征相同，很显然所谓的"婴儿血管外皮细胞瘤"最可能代表了婴儿肌纤维瘤病谱系的一端[154]，不值得将其作为一个独立性疾病来命名（见第 3 章）。婴儿肌纤维瘤病典型病例中具有的特征性的双相表现使其很少会有鉴别诊断问题。

颈纤维瘤病 Fibromatosis colli

颈部纤维瘤病[155-157]在临床上也称为胸骨乳突瘤或斜颈，是一种不常见的病变，特征为一侧胸锁乳突肌被弥漫性纤维组织取代，右侧最常见。双侧病变十分罕见。该病可发生在任何性别的新生儿，最常发生在臀位和产钳分娩之后，出现颈部不对称和绷紧。许多病例可自行缓解（或在物理治疗帮助下），仅有 15%～20% 的病例继续发展成为真性斜颈（斜颈畸形）。出生之前在子宫中所处位置似乎在最初发病当中起重要作用。组织学显示，骨骼肌成分被细胞相对稀少、常常明显玻璃样变性

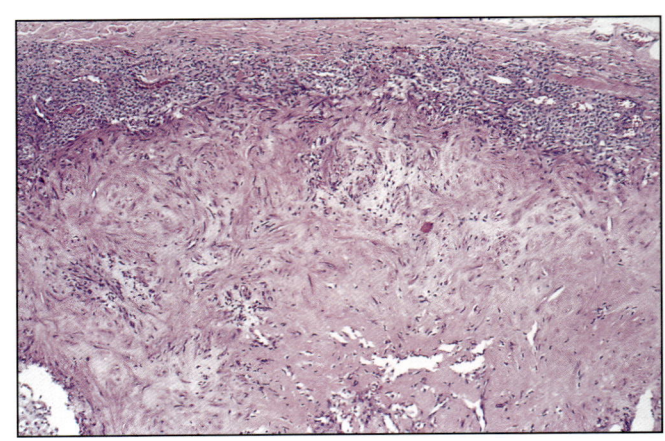

图 24.37　婴幼儿肌纤维瘤病。肌纤维母细胞性梭形细胞的经典性突然过渡为周边较为原始的圆形细胞。

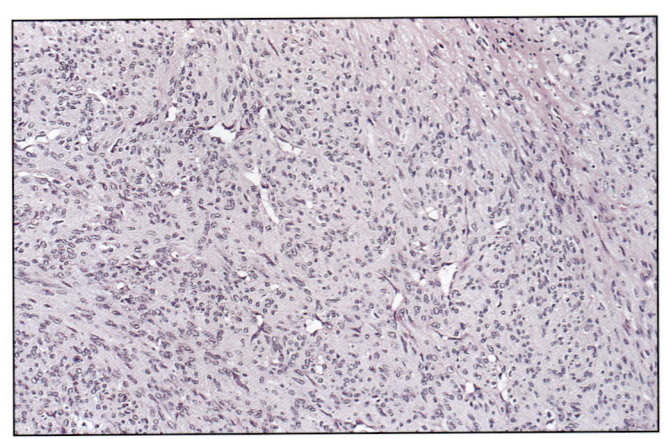

图 24.38　婴儿肌纤维瘤病。此病例中分化较差的区域由圆形细胞构成，伴有嗜酸性胞浆，围绕着分枝状血管组织排列。

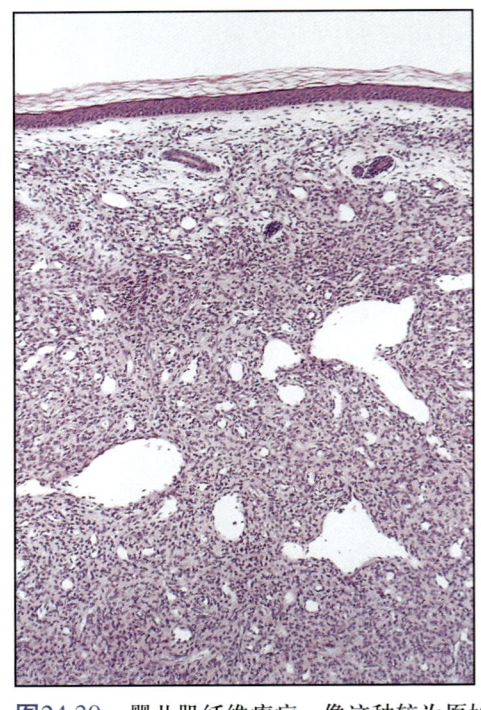

图 24.39　婴儿肌纤维瘤病。像这种较为原始的病变常常被称为"婴儿血管外皮细胞瘤"。

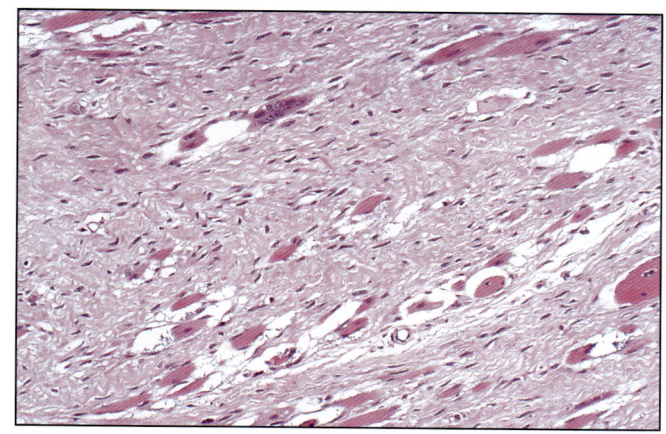

图24.40 颈纤维瘤病。形态学上，这些病变类似于伴有变性肌肉成分的细胞性瘢痕组织。

的纤维组织弥漫性浸润和替代（图24.40）。这些组织在单个肌纤维之间及其周围扩展，后者出现明显变性或反应性改变。组织学上整个病变中出现受损肌纤维有助于与韧带样型纤维瘤病鉴别。

幼年性玻璃样纤维瘤病
Juvenile hyaline fibromatosis

幼年性玻璃样纤维瘤病[158,159]是婴儿和儿童极其少见的病变，为常染色体隐性遗传。其特征是多发性生长缓慢的真皮或皮下肿物，尤其是在头颈部和上部躯干，常常伴有牙龈肥大、重度肢体屈曲挛缩以及骨病。没有智力低下。组织学方面，这些病变由大量嗜酸性均质物质构成，含有良性的、分散不均的纤维母细胞（周围有人工回缩假象）和个别薄壁血管。早期切除的病变细胞相对更丰富。嗜酸性玻璃样物质的确切本质还不清楚。长久以来推断在胶原合成中存在遗传代谢异常；尽管有些资料支持III型胶原合成异常[160]，但编码毛细血管形态发生蛋白2的 *CMG2* 突变最近已经证实是这种疾病的病因[161]，表明基底膜的异常可能决定表型。

良性肿瘤　Benign neoplasms

良性肿瘤类别中多数的纤维性病变为后天性的，主要累及成年人，复发不常见，呈非侵袭性方式。不加限制地使用"纤维瘤"这个诊断是没有意义的，应该避免，不仅仅是由于会纵容诊断的乏味，而且会时不时地（主要是以前）将这个诊断几乎用于本章内的每一种疾病！在此分类中，有些病变更适合在本书的其他章节进行描述：淋巴结肌纤维母细胞瘤在第21章，乳腺肌纤维母细胞瘤在第16章，鼻咽血管纤维瘤在第4章，多形性纤维瘤和巨细胞性纤维母细胞在第23章。

腱鞘纤维瘤　Fibroma of tendon sheath

临床特征

腱鞘纤维瘤[162-164]是一种相对不常见的病变，通常发生在年轻成人或中年人，以男性为主，表现为质硬的结节，大多位于上臂，尤其是手指。通常附着于肌腱。个别病例可见于膝部周围。沿边缘切除或切除不彻底的，高达20%的病变可局部复发，有时不止一次。

病理学特征

腱鞘纤维瘤为界限清楚的、分叶状纤维性结节，大小一般小于2cm。由良性纤维母细胞和肌纤维母细胞构成，胞浆轻度嗜酸性，细胞核逐渐变细，排列成大小不等的短束状，胶原性间质内含有薄壁的、裂隙样血管（图24.41）。细胞构成差异极大，从类似于筋膜炎表现至几乎完全玻璃样变。核分裂活性与细胞丰富程度平行。出现炎症细胞和黏液样间质提示有些病例可能与筋膜炎有关[164]，个别病例出现极少数破骨巨细胞或泡沫细胞也提示与腱鞘巨细胞瘤同属一个谱系[165]，尽管这些病变中出现的细胞遗传学异常[166]不同于巨细胞肿瘤。腱鞘纤维瘤与纤维瘤病的区别在于其局限性和明显的裂隙样血管。纤维组织增生性纤维母细胞瘤（见下文）的特点为星状纤维母细胞以及常常缺少腱鞘起源。这些病变不发生在皮肤，过去如此描述的病变如今最好称为席纹状胶原瘤（见下文）。

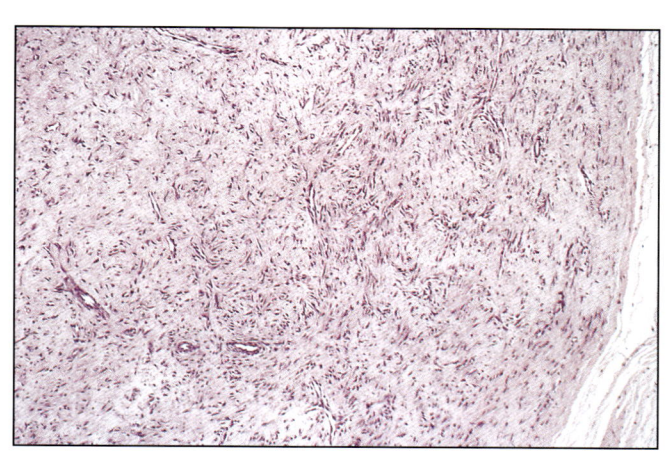

图24.41 腱鞘纤维瘤。裂隙样血管具有特征性。

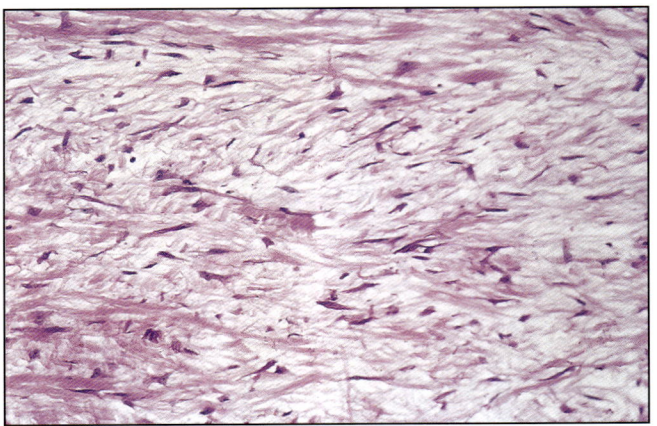

图24.42 纤维组织增生性纤维母细胞瘤。注意星芒状的细胞形态学表现和多少不等的纤维黏液样间质。

纤维组织增生性纤维母细胞瘤（胶原性纤维瘤）
Desmoplastic fibroblastoma (collagenous fibroma)

纤维组织增生性纤维母细胞瘤[167-169]是相对常见的病变，表现为生长缓慢的无痛性皮下肿物，主要见于成人。多数病变小于4cm，解剖部位分布广泛。局部复发非常少见。组织学方面，这些病变界限清楚，但没有被膜，局灶浸润性边缘，陷入周围脂肪细胞或骨骼肌组织。通常位于筋膜组织中央，由星状、双极或梭形纤维母细胞构成，背景为丰富的胶原或局灶黏液样基质，极少含有血管（图24.42）。在病变描述方面，这些病变类似于晚期筋膜炎，但其病史较长且筋膜炎可自行消退可除外筋膜炎可能。通常没有细胞核非典型性，很难找到核分裂象。免疫组织化学方面，病变细胞出现不同程度的肌动蛋白阳性。细胞遗传学方面，这些病变与腱鞘纤维瘤具有相同的t(2;11)易位[170]。

席纹状胶原瘤（硬化性纤维瘤）
Storiform collagenoma (sclerotic fibroma)

席纹状胶原瘤[171,172]是直径小于1cm的孤立性皮下结节，其发生在成人，有广泛的解剖学分布。局部切除后不复发。组织学上为界限清楚的真皮结节，由没有细胞成分的玻璃样胶原条带状交错排列（席纹状）构成（图24.43）。这些胶原束间隔以裂隙，含有极少数不明显的纤维母细胞。其组织学表现与Cowden综合征中所见的多发性纤维瘤基本相同。类似的组织学改变也可见于个别时间较长的（消退性）皮肤纤维组织细胞瘤、孤立性肌纤维瘤、甚至某些炎症病变，提示这一病变可能是一种共同的结构表现，而并非一种特殊的病变[173]。

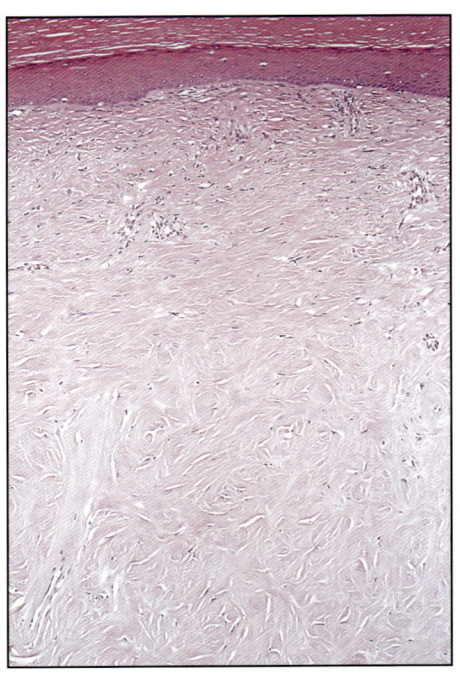

图24.43 席纹状胶原瘤。注意裂隙状、几乎没有细胞的胶原。

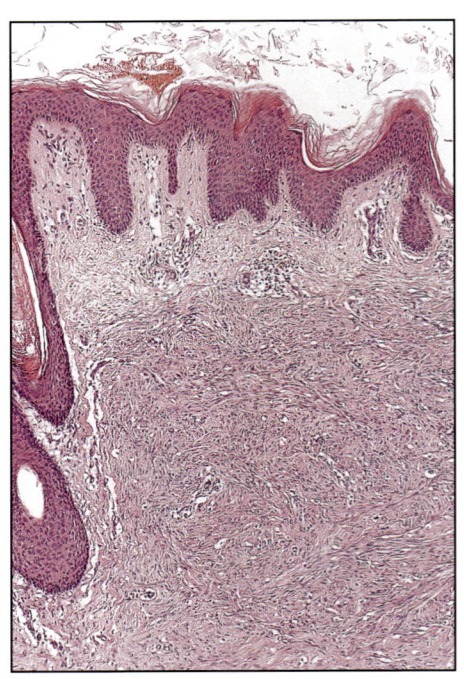

图24.44 皮肤肌纤维瘤。典型的肌纤维母细胞斑块位于网状真皮内。

皮肤肌纤维瘤　Dermatomyofibroma

皮肤肌纤维瘤[174-176]临床上表现为孤立的粉红色至白色的皮肤斑块，直径可达5cm。病变主要累及青少年或年轻人，有非常明显的女性倾向，以躯干上部为主。持续的、非破坏性生长可以延续多年，但切除后复发似乎极其少见。组织学方面，其表现十分独特。病变由带状增生的轻度嗜酸性肌纤维母细胞构成，在网状真皮内呈束状排列（图 24.44）。束状生长结构平行于表皮，被 Grenz 带分隔，皮肤附属器保留完整。病变可以浅表性地扩散至皮下组织。个别病例具有明显的间质血管和出血，因此有可能与 Kaposi 肉瘤混淆[177]。与皮肤纤维肉瘤（见第 23 章）斑片期的区别在于：皮肤肌纤维瘤缺少席纹样生长方式，浸润方式更为局限，以及肌动蛋白呈阳性，CD34 呈阴性。

孤立性肌纤维瘤　Solitary myofibroma

孤立性肌纤维瘤[178-180]本质上是婴儿肌纤维瘤病在成人的相应病变。这种病变没有性别差异，解剖学分布广泛，以头颈部为主（包括口腔[181]），有时可发生于青少年。病变表现为质硬的皮下结节，可有疼痛。成人的内脏和骨病变尚未见报道。真正的复发极为少见，但目前认为成人病变也可以多发[147]，大多见于单个解剖学部位，提示场变（field-change）现象。组织学表现与婴儿肌纤维瘤病相同，除了原始血管外皮细胞瘤样的区域一般较小和不明显以外。与婴儿病变一样，可以出现较明显的内皮下增生（类似于血管浸润），但没有临床意义。

颈项型纤维瘤　Nuchal-type fibroma

颈项型纤维瘤[182,183]是不常见的病变，主要发生在成年男性的颈后，但偶尔也可见于其他部位。在 30%～40% 的患者中明显与糖尿病相关。病变表现为境界不清的皮下或深部真皮肿胀，可局部复发，可能反应了诱发因素的持续存在。组织学上，病变由致密的、细胞成分稀少的胶原组织构成，含有内陷的脂肪细胞和数量增加的小神经。在形态学上与 Gardner 纤维瘤（见下文）有重叠。发病机制尚不明确，但此病变为非破坏性过程。

Gardner 纤维瘤　Gardner fibroma

Gardner 纤维瘤[184,185]是不常见的病变，大多见于儿童和青少年，躯干多发，尤其是脊柱旁区域。在多数患者中，这些病变与家族性腺瘤样息肉病伴发，尽管它们常常在息肉发生之前。多数病变界限不清，大小小于 5cm。重要的是，复发极为常见，表现为韧带样纤维瘤病，或其发生领先于其他一处或多处硬纤维瘤。组织学上，这些病变由大量的细胞稀少的玻璃样胶原条带构成，可见人工裂隙样腔隙（图 24.45）。病变细胞呈良性纤维母细胞表现，病变边缘有周围正常组织内陷。免疫组织化学方面，通常有细胞核 β-连环蛋白阳性，与韧带样纤维瘤病相同（见下文）。形态学上与颈项型纤维瘤存在重叠（见上文），并且同样病变在该标题下已有报道[186]；然而，Gardner 纤维瘤中一般没有小神经成分数量增加，也没有明显的脂肪陷入。

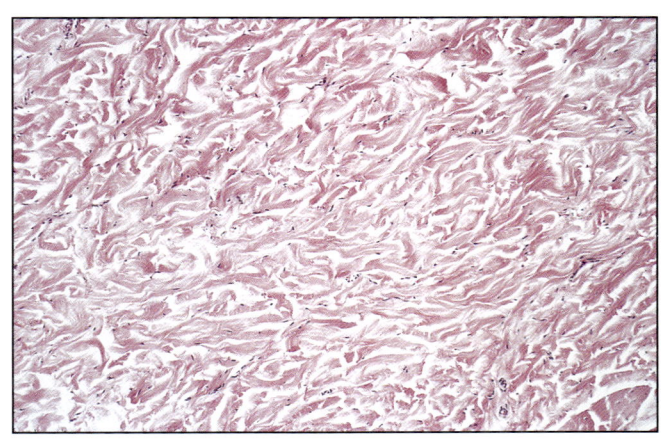

图 24.45　Gardner 纤维瘤。这些极为玻璃样变的病变是家族性腺瘤性息肉病的重要标志。

包涵体纤维瘤病　Inclusion body fibromatosis

临床特征

包涵体纤维瘤病[187,188]更多被称为婴儿指（趾）部纤维瘤病，最常表现为小婴儿指（趾）部小结节，没有性别差异。在高达 1/3 患者中，病变是先天性的，大约同样比例的病变为多发的，累及手或足。令人不可思议的是，拇指和大足趾似乎总能免于受累。没有任何家族倾向的证据。局部切除后常有复发，原因是随后有新病变发生。然而，一旦作出诊断，仅仅是有症状的患者需要治疗，因为多数病例最终可自行消退。有关这一病变的命名，现已认识到，类似病变有时可发生在成人[189,190]或非指（趾）部[191,192]。有趣的是，几乎所有成人病例似乎都位于指（趾）部以外。

病理学特征

病变为灰白、质硬、界限不清的结节，直径小于 1cm，通常附着于皮肤。组织学上为真皮内浸润性肿物，即轻度嗜酸的肌纤维母细胞分布于数量不等的胶原性间质中。病变可向下蔓延至骨膜。诊断的必要条件（并不是都容易见到）是出现胞浆内圆形嗜酸性包涵体，常常靠近细胞核（图 24.46）。这些包涵体比红细胞稍大，在三色染色中呈鲜红色，肌动蛋白呈阳性。也可以通过免疫电镜证实其由肌动蛋白构成[193]。有趣的是，同样的包涵体在其他病变的肌纤维母细胞或平滑肌成分中很少遇到[194]。

血管肌纤维母细胞瘤　Angiomyofibroblastoma

血管肌纤维母细胞瘤[195-197]是不常见的肿瘤，主要发生在育龄女性的外阴阴道部位。然而，极少数类似

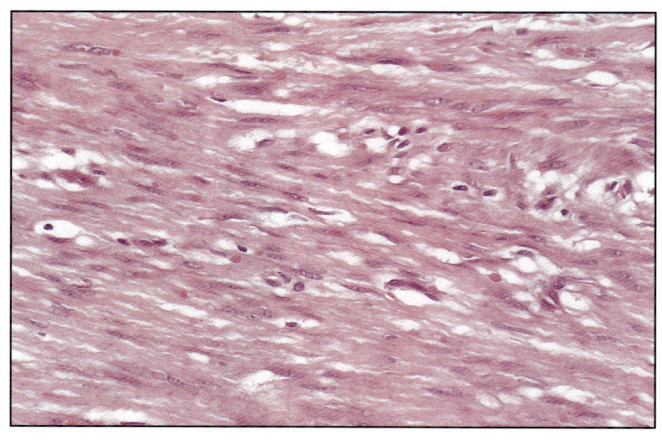

图24.46 包涵体纤维瘤病。典型的指（趾）部肌纤维母细胞病变，伴有多量嗜酸性包涵体。

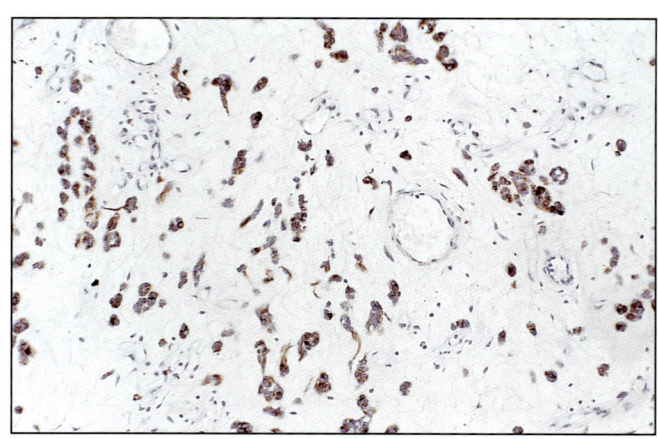

图24.48 血管肌纤维母细胞瘤。结蛋白均为阳性。

的病变也可见于男性。临床上，血管肌纤维母细胞瘤常常被误诊为 Bartholin 囊肿，重要的是，局部切除后很少复发，因此需要与侵袭性血管黏液瘤鉴别（见第13章）。血管肌纤维母细胞瘤病变界限清楚，通常直径小于5cm，由肥胖的圆形、卵圆形或梭形细胞构成，背景为大量水肿样基质，含有多量毛细血管大小的血管。肿瘤细胞常常以血管周围分布为主，具有嗜酸性胞浆，可有双核或多核（图24.27）。偶尔排列成更为实性的细胞巢，极少数病例可有明显的变性浓染细胞核。个别病例含有内在的脂肪细胞成分[195,197]，可以较明显[198]，有些可呈明显上皮样。已经有一例出现肉瘤变的报道[199]。具有特征性的是，在多数病例中，肥胖的纤维母细胞呈结蛋白阳性、肌动蛋白阴性表型（图24.48），但此免疫表型与该部位的侵袭性血管黏液瘤[200]和纤维上皮间质性息肉相同，所以对于鉴别诊断没有帮助。极少数病例出现与侵袭性血管黏液瘤不能区别的区域，提示这两种病变可能有关[200]。

细胞型血管纤维瘤　Cellular angiofibroma

细胞型血管纤维瘤是新近认识的病变，发生在成人外阴、骨盆会阴或睾丸旁区域，没有性别差异[201,202]。在男性，这些病变被简要地称为"血管肌纤维母细胞瘤样肿瘤"[203]。盆腔内及男性的病变往往比外阴的大，最大直径常常超过5cm。发生于女性的病变往往界限清楚，而男性病变通常界限不清。很少局部复发。组织学上，病变由一致性的梭形细胞构成，胞浆境界不清，钝圆或波浪状细胞核呈短束状排列，伴有纤细胶原束、数量众多的常常为厚壁的小血管、散在的脂肪细胞以及多量间质内肥大细胞（图24.49）。持续时间较长的病例可出现间质玻璃样变、水肿，以及有时出现退行变性细胞核非典型性。核分裂象易见，但通常没有细胞学非典型性。然而，作者已遇到极少数病例出现只能诊断为多形性肉瘤的显微镜下病灶，其临床意义尚不清楚。免疫组织化学方面，出现不同程度的 CD34 阳性，可有局灶肌动蛋

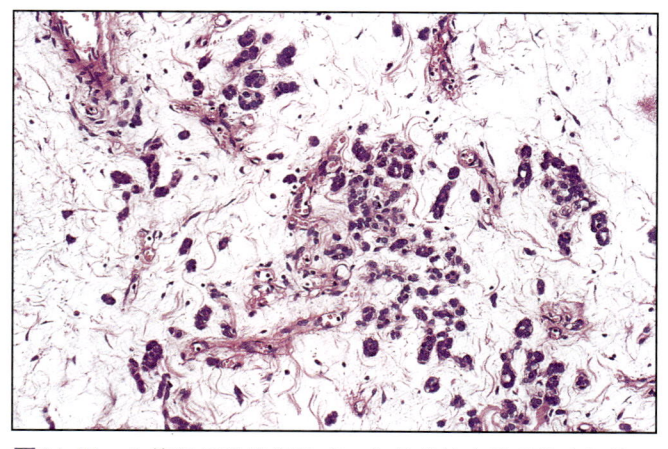

图24.47 血管肌纤维母细胞瘤。与侵袭性血管黏液瘤相比，其细胞更大，更圆。

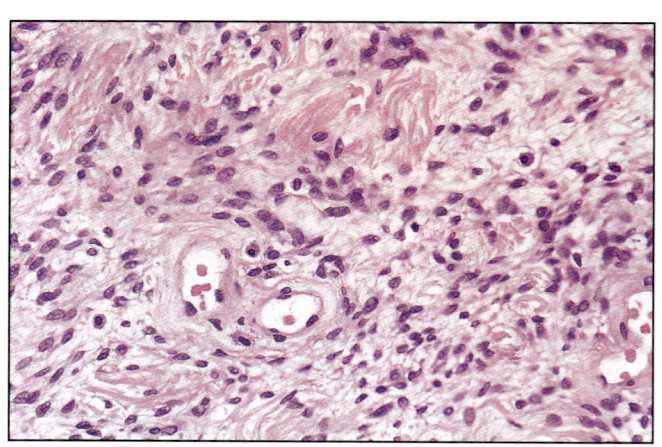

图24.49 细胞型血管纤维瘤。良性短梭形细胞分布于胶原性间质中，其中含有厚壁小血管。

白和结蛋白阳性，与纤维母细胞/肌纤维母细胞病变相同。主要的鉴别诊断包括血管肌纤维母细胞瘤和平滑肌肿瘤。

巨细胞血管纤维瘤　　Giant cell angiofibroma

巨细胞血管纤维瘤最初见于眼眶[204]，但随后的个人（以及其他作者）经验表明，病变几乎可以发生在任何软组织部位，尽管成人头颈部区域最为常见。局部非破坏性复发并不常见。组织学方面，病变界限清楚，无结构样病变由圆形或梭形细胞构成，胞浆淡染、不清，细胞核肥胖，常有褶皱，背景是多少不等的胶原或黏液基质，其中含有多量小血管（管壁常有玻璃样变）。也可见形状不规则的假血管腔，内衬单核或多核肿瘤细胞；多核细胞也常常见于实性细胞区域。肿瘤细胞 CD34 均呈阳性。与巨细胞性纤维母细胞瘤的不同在于其临床状况、缺乏浸润性边缘以及有明显的血管成分。这些病变可能为孤立性纤维性肿瘤（见下文）伴有退变的一个亚型，因而这一命名有可能被废弃。

钙化性腱膜纤维瘤　Calcifying aponeurotic fibroma

依据作者经验，钙化性腱膜纤维瘤是极少见的软组织肿瘤之一，值得注意的是，在过去 30 年中，仅有一组真正的病例发表[206]。病变主要累及儿童和青少年，男性多见，表现为较小的肿物，大多位于手部（尤其是手掌），尽管总体上的解剖学分布广泛[206,208]。局部复发常见，因为病变呈浸润性生长方式，且常常分布于较敏感的解剖部位，使得手术比较保守。然而，随着时间的延长，病变生长似乎停止。组织学上，与韧带样纤维瘤病（见下文）非常相似，但是纤维母细胞成分出现局灶的上皮样细胞形态学表现，细胞核肥胖、泡状，呈平行排列。更为显著的差别在于一定有钙化灶存在，周围是较肥胖的细胞（图 24.50），有些呈软骨母细胞和破骨细胞性巨细胞表现。在持续时间较长的病例中，这些病灶可被比较明显的软骨组织所取代。

钙化性纤维性肿瘤　Calcifying fibrous tumor

钙化性纤维性肿瘤[209-211]以前称为钙化性纤维性假瘤，是一个有些难以理解的病变，主要累及儿童、青少年和年轻成人，尽管发病部位较为广泛，但以腹内和胸膜多见。患者可有多发性病变，极个别病例是家族性的[212]。非破坏性局部复发并不少见。这些病变界限清楚，由细胞相对稀少的玻璃样纤维组织构成，其中可见片状淋巴浆细胞浸润及钙化，常常呈沙粒体

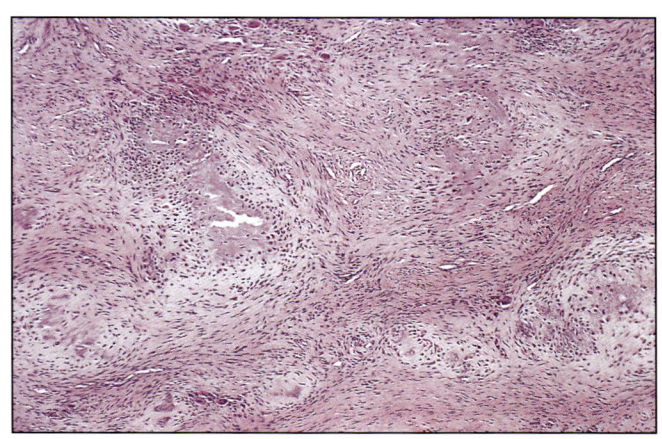

图24.50　钙化性腱膜纤维瘤。注意圆形细胞围绕钙化区呈栅栏状排列。

表现。在病变描述方面，这些病变类似"燃尽"的炎症性肌纤维母细胞性肿瘤，但有关这两个肿瘤之间的关系还有争议[211,213,214]。尽管钙化性纤维性假瘤通常 ALK 呈阴性，但毋庸置疑的是，个别病例在同一解剖部位可同时或不同时地发生两种类型的病变。

孤立性纤维性肿瘤　Solitary fibrous tumor

根据 2002 年 WHO 的分类[215]，多数以前称为血管外皮细胞瘤的病变现在划归为孤立性纤维性肿瘤（也见第 3 章 72 页），主要是因为其本质上明显为纤维母细胞而非外皮细胞[216]。

临床特征

孤立性纤维性肿瘤可以发生在除胸膜[217]以外的许多部位，包括腹膜[217,218]、纵隔[219]、腹膜后、上呼吸道[220]、眼眶[221]、躯体软组织[222-225]、口腔软组织[226]和几乎所有器官[227]（见其他相关章节），实际上现已明确，胸膜外病变比在第 5 章讨论的胸膜病变更为常见。胸膜外病变不论部位如何，几乎都发生在成人，没有性别差异，表现为没有特征的、缓慢增大的肿物，常常位于深部软组织。相关的系统性特征如杵状指或低血糖不常见。多数病例的临床过程为良性；然而，在胸膜，5%～10% 的发生在软组织的病例具有恶性行为[288,289]。在有些病例中，依靠形态学很难预测，因此需要谨慎的是，不要把任何此类病例完全看做良性。

病理学特征

软组织的孤立性纤维性肿瘤常常很大，位置较深，界限清楚，呈分叶状表现。切面一般为灰白色，质硬。组织学表现类似于发生在胸膜的肿瘤，常常称作"无

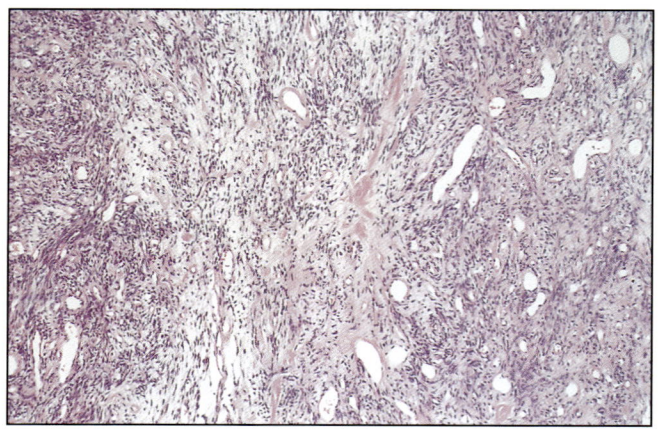

图24.51　孤立性纤维性肿瘤。注意细胞丰富程度的不同和外皮瘤样血管成分。

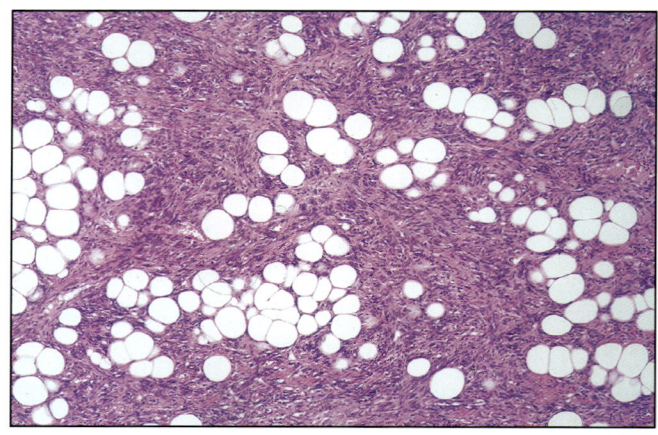

图24.53　脂肪形成性孤立性纤维性肿瘤。这些病变除了有成熟脂肪成分以外，与普通的孤立性纤维性肿瘤无法区别。

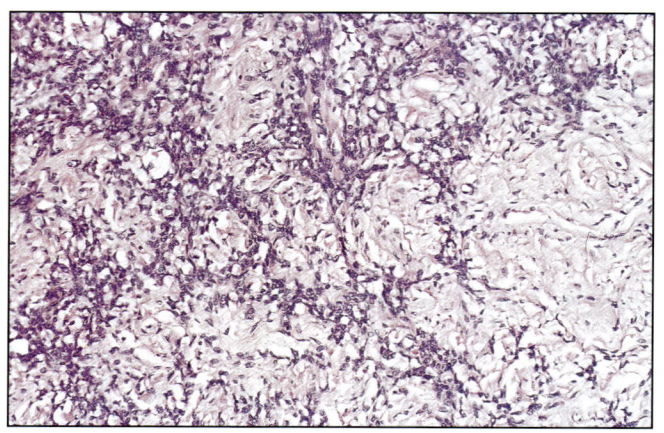

图24.52　孤立性纤维性肿瘤。肿瘤细胞通常穿插于胶原束之间。

结构样"。其显著特征在于：细胞丰富程度变化明显（图24.51），常常出现局灶致密、几乎为瘢痕样的玻璃样变性区域；其中形态学良性的纤维母细胞成分隐藏在胶原束之间（图24.52）；常可见分枝状血管外皮瘤样血管结构，血管周围玻璃样变性常见。局灶黏液样间质也常见，极少数病例出现弥漫黏液样变性[230]。在多数胸膜外病例中，核分裂象往往散在，坏死极为少见。然而，最好将每10个高倍视野多于4个核分裂象的病例视为恶性[228,229]，出现非典型特征，如细胞核多形性或坏死同样令人担忧。在此特殊形态学表现中，肿瘤细胞几乎均为CD34和CD99阳性，但通常S-100、肌动蛋白、结蛋白和角蛋白呈阴性，常常能够为诊断提供有价值的支持。然而，重要的是要知道，这些肿瘤的一个重要亚型可以出现上皮膜抗原（EMA）阳性，极少数病例结蛋白或S-100蛋白可呈阳性。有趣的是，很大一部分病例表现为细胞核β-连环蛋白阳

性[231]。

这些肿瘤中也有另外一部分出现数量不等的脂肪成分（图24.53）。这些病变最初被命名为"脂肪瘤样血管外皮细胞瘤"[232,233]，但是由于后一种名称相对没有意义（见第3章），"脂肪形成性孤立性纤维性肿瘤"应该更为准确[234]。这样的病例主要累及中年人，没有性别差异，在非内脏的软组织中分布广泛。尽管常常较大，但复发并不常见。形态学恶性的病例极其少见。

纤维瘤病　Fibromatoses

依照本章节的概述，纤维瘤病是一组具有局部侵袭性的肿瘤。它们具有浸润、破坏能力，常常有复发，但不转移[235,236]。通常把它们细分为浅表性（掌和跖）和深部（硬纤维瘤）两类。

掌部纤维瘤病（Dupuytren挛缩）
Palmar fibromatosis (Dupuytren's contracture)

临床特征

掌部纤维瘤病[237-239]几乎均局限于成人，发病率随着年龄增长而升高，最终累及4%的个体。的确有极少数儿童病例。男性受累多于女性，有些作者认为其与癫痫和酗酒有些关系的。有些病例明确为家族性的，有些与跖部纤维瘤病或指关节垫有关。与创伤或职业无关。双侧常见。患者最初为在手掌或近端指骨的屈侧面出现小结节，随着时间的延长似乎向纤维带内扩展。此后40%的患者出现进行性屈曲挛缩，累及一个或多个手指，只有通过手掌筋膜切除术才能缓解。极少数情况下，类似病变可发生在手背或手指。沿边

缘切除或切除不完全时，常有局部复发，尤其是在结节性（细胞较丰富）生长阶段。

病理学特征

切除纤维组织的组织学表现取决于病变所处的时期[239-241]。在早期生长"活跃"阶段，临床上对应为结节性表现，病变主要由核分裂活跃、略呈嗜酸性的肌纤维母细胞构成，肥胖的细胞核呈空泡状，呈束状排列，浸润筋膜和皮下组织。随着时间的推移，细胞成分进行性减少，间质胶原成分增多，所以病变最终玻璃样变极为显著。在晚期病变中，细胞胞浆不明显，细胞核变窄，变尖，核分裂不活跃，呈纤维母细胞表现。在此阶段，肌动蛋白一般为阴性。极少数病例可出现骨化生。病变中期，在同一个标本的不同区域，细胞成分变化显著（图24.54）。细胞遗传学方面，这些病变均出现7和8染色三体[242]。与韧带样纤维瘤病相比，这些病变缺乏β-连环蛋白或APC突变[243]。没有实际的鉴别诊断。

跖部纤维瘤病（Ledderhose 病） Plantar fibromatosis (Ledderhose's disease)

跖纤维瘤病[240,244]除了年龄范围较广以外，临床上与手掌同类病变极为相似，发生在5～15岁年龄组十分常见，并不会导致挛缩畸形。双侧不常见，但术后局部复发比掌纤维瘤病更常见。组织学上，跖部纤维瘤病往往呈多结节状，与掌部纤维瘤病相比，细胞较丰富，似乎并不出现同样程度的进行性玻璃样变性。极个别病例可出现明显多核巨细胞[245]。存在与掌部纤维瘤病类似的细胞遗传学异常[246]。

指节垫 Knuckle pad

指节垫[247]据说与掌部纤维瘤病密切相关，由真皮内良性富于细胞的纤维组织构成，被覆上皮过度角化。这些病变不需要治疗。

阴茎纤维瘤病（Peyronie 病） Penile fibromatosis (Peyronie's disease)

尽管传统上将阴茎纤维瘤病与掌跖纤维瘤病联系起来，但这些病变可能并不相关。受累患者年龄主要在40～60岁，表现为阴茎海绵体纤维性斑块，引起勃起时疼痛和弯曲[248,249]。组织学检查，切除组织表现为细胞稀少的胶原性瘢痕组织，含有慢性炎细胞灶（图24.55）。有些病例有先前血管炎的证据，有人认为炎症可能为其发病机制，尽管这些病变也表现出克隆性细胞遗传学异常[250]。瘢痕组织内骨化生十分常见。

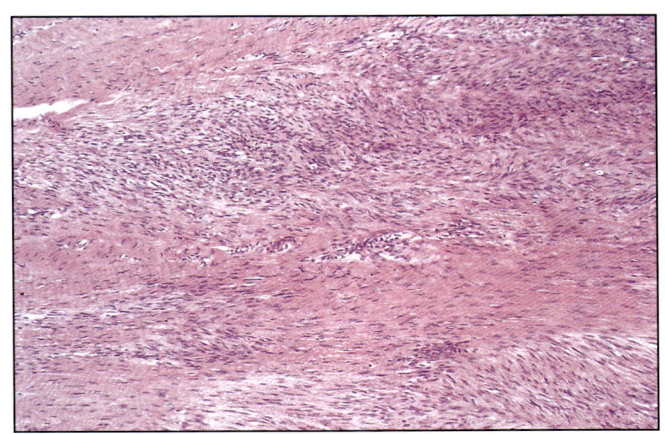

图24.54 掌部纤维瘤病。病变生长中期，细胞成分常常有明显差异。

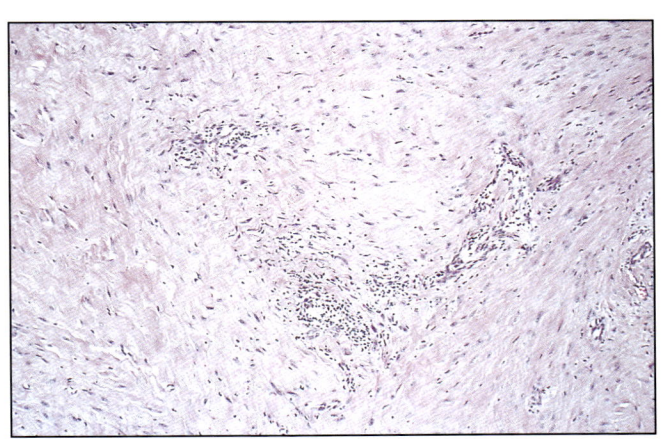

图24.55 Peyronie 病。这些病变比普通纤维瘤病的细胞少，常常含有炎症细胞。

韧带样纤维瘤病 Desmoid fibromatosis

临床特征

韧带样纤维瘤病是一组临床表现多样的深在性纤维性肿瘤。其可分为三个主要生物学类型：散发型、与家族性腺瘤性息肉（FAP）相关的家族型以及多中心型。有些作者喜欢将婴儿和儿童病例单独分类。解剖学方面有三个主要亚型：腹外型（60%的病例）、腹壁型（25%）以及腹内型（15%）。所有这些组别中发病高峰年龄为11～40岁，尽管总体上年龄变化较大。女性比男性多发，比例是2:1。不论在什么部位，所有病例都容易形成较大的浸润性肿物，如果切缘未净，可以反复复发[251-253]。然而，这些病变没有转移潜能，对于所有广泛切除术，必须权衡其影响，要考虑到功能保留问题，尤其是近来有证据表明，对于复发来说，切缘情况并不是可靠的预测因素。非特定比例（但似乎为少数）的病例可通过雌激素拮抗剂（不论性别或激素受体情况如何）、非类固醇抗炎药物或小剂量化疗来成功缓解，但这种反应并不一致。对于成果不甚满意的手术，也可采用放疗加以补充，可以提高局部控制率。近来有少部分患者对伊马替尼（Gleevec）治疗有效果，但其生物学基础尚不明确，可以肯定与 KIT 突变或活化无关[254]。

在临床类型方面，散发型大多为腹外型，最常见部位是肢体带或肢体远端[253,255,256]。与 FAP（Gardner 综合征）有关的病例主要（但并不绝对）发生在腹部，尤其是肠系膜，受累病人以前大多经历过结肠切除[257-259]。有些 FAP 患者可发生多部位的硬纤维瘤[257]。30 岁以下的患者如出现腹内硬纤维瘤，都应当考虑和除外 FAP（或消减型）。少数非 FAP 患者出现多发性腹外硬纤维瘤，大多局限于单一肢体[256,260]。现已明确在 FAP 或家族性非 FAP 基础上容易发生硬纤维瘤的原因，与 5 号染色体长臂上 APC 基因突变有关[261-263]，事实上突变部位与临床表型密切相关[262-265]。对于前腹壁硬纤维瘤来说，这些肿瘤尤其常见于女性，并且在妊娠期间或妊娠后不久十分常见[266]。产后发生的肿瘤常常见于先前的瘢痕中（如剖宫产）。一般来说，现有证据表明，此时高雌激素水平为病变生长的推动因素（并非启动因素）[267]，可能是通过雌激素 β- 受体实现。与腹壁病变一样，其他部位发生的硬纤维瘤中有少部分发生在先前的瘢痕（所谓的"瘢痕性纤维瘤病"）或先前受照射的组织。发生于幼儿的硬纤维瘤在头颈部极为常见[269]，常常不能充分切除，需要进行化疗。

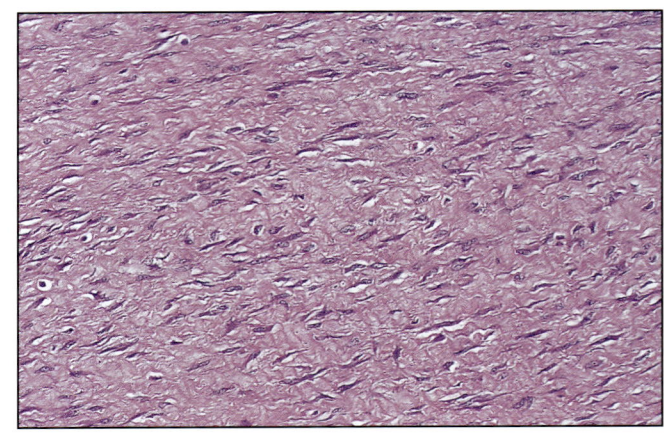

图24.56 韧带样纤维瘤病。注意程度不同的两端细长且肥胖的肌纤维母细胞的细胞核。

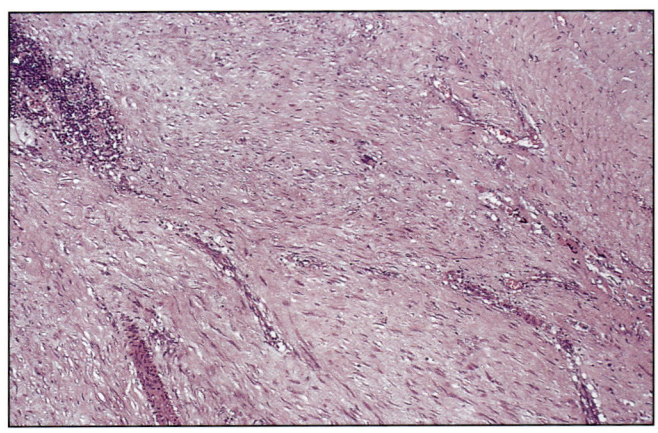

图24.57 韧带样纤维瘤病。浸润性边缘可见典型的淋巴细胞聚集和退变的肌膜样细胞核。

病理学特征

上面提到的所有临床亚型都具有相同的特征。根据部位，病变往往较大，几乎都超过 5cm，切面呈灰白色、旋涡状、纤维性、边缘不规则。组织学上，硬纤维瘤由轻度嗜酸性的纤维母细胞和具有细长或肥胖泡状核的肌纤维母细胞构成（图 24.56）。在单个肿瘤内和肿瘤之间细胞成分和核分裂活性方面差异较大，有些病例可出现局灶性的显著玻璃样变性。总体的生长方式呈宽大的长束状。间质为数量不等的胶原或呈局灶黏液性，含有数量不等的血管，与筋膜炎相比，其血管壁较厚。有些作者提出，血管成分与成人[270]和婴儿[271]病例的复发危险呈正相关，尽管对单个病例尚不具有预测性。筋膜炎中常见的星状细胞学表现、疏松黏液样间质和出血通常并非纤维瘤病的特征，但腹内和乳腺病变除外，其形态学上常常有重叠。然而，纤维瘤病常常出现较长的束状结构。在肿瘤的进展性边缘，常可见淋巴细胞聚集和伴有奇异形肌膜样细胞核的变性骨骼肌细胞（图 24.57）。高达 10% 的病例出现明显的瘢痕疙瘩样玻璃样变，此表现大多见于腹内病变以及黑人患者。较为罕见的是，可以出现骨化生或软骨形成。

肿瘤细胞通常肌动蛋白呈阳性，染色程度与细胞丰富程度呈正相关；依据作者的经验，结蛋白和 S-100 蛋白在少部分确切的肿瘤细胞中通常也呈阳性。重要的是要注意，这些病变 KIT 几乎都是阴性的[272]。超微结构检查容易证实纤维母细胞和肌纤维母细胞的特征。从发病机制角度看，韧带样纤维瘤病有明确的克隆性证据（细胞遗传学[236,273]和 X- 染色体失活[274]分析）；因此，结合其破坏性复发的倾向，有关其是反应性病变的过时观点已经不再成立。现已证实，APC 突变（也存在于散发型病变中）在这些病变中通过 β- 连环蛋白上调来发挥其纤维增生性作用[275]，β- 连环蛋白染色（聚集于细胞核）已被推荐作为有用的诊断性标记物[251,276]，尽管不是所有病例都呈阳性。细胞遗传学方面，这些病变可出现 8 和 20 号三体综合征[277]。

与结节性筋膜炎的鉴别上面已经提到。其他鉴别诊断包括细胞性神经纤维瘤或低级别恶性外周神经鞘瘤，通过比较一致的波浪状细长的细胞核以及更为显著的 S-100 阳性来鉴别，或许要与纤维肉瘤鉴别。许多年以来，韧带样纤维瘤病通常被当作 I 级纤维肉瘤，但由于它们缺乏转移潜能，在今天看来这样并不恰当。胶原成分较多且分化较好、类似于纤维瘤病的真正纤维肉瘤罕见，多数此类病例可能为低级别肌纤维母细胞肉瘤或低级别纤维黏液样肉瘤（见下文）。腹内病变有时可被误诊为胃肠道间质瘤（GIST）。然而，GIST 缺乏长束状结构和硬纤维瘤的胶原性间质，典型病例具有较为嗜酸性的纤维性合胞体胞浆，以及比较一致的卵圆形或梭形细胞核。在很少一部分的婴儿纤维瘤病病例，其细胞成分是如此丰富以至于其与纤维肉瘤几乎难以鉴别。然而，在这个年龄组中，通常没有哪个类型为致死性的，在这些类别之间似乎存在密切的分子遗传学联系，至少在有些病例中是如此，区分这些病变几乎没有什么意义[278]。

脂肪纤维瘤病　Lipofibromatosis

脂肪纤维瘤病[279]是一种少见病变，几乎都发生在小婴儿，发病具有男性倾向。这些病变大多表现为肢体远端的生长缓慢的肿物，有时伴有巨指。肿瘤边界不清，低倍镜下似乎具有丛状结构。肿瘤由细胞学上较一致的纤维母细胞/肌纤维母细胞混合而成，主要排列成束状结构，通常沿原有的纤维隔分布，伴有明显的成熟脂肪组织。成团的微泡状脂肪细胞常常见于纤维和脂肪细胞成分之间。这些肿瘤过去有时被称为"婴儿纤维瘤病"，非破坏性的局部复发率较高。

炎性肌纤维母细胞瘤
Inflammatory myofibroblastic tumor

对于大多数过去称为炎性假瘤、浆细胞肉芽肿、网膜-肠系膜黏液样错构瘤以及炎性纤维肉瘤的病变来说，现在普遍接受的名称为炎性肌纤维母细胞瘤。这种一体化是基于它们在形态学以及临床表现方面有相当程度的重叠，并且结合了临床及其肿瘤本质的遗传学证据[280]。

临床特征

肺外的病变主要发生在儿童和青少年，女性发病略多，明显好发于腹腔[281,282]，尽管总体上的年龄范围和解剖学分布十分广泛，实际上到目前为止，这些病变可见于任何解剖部位。大约 10%～20% 的病例伴有发热、体重减轻、ESR 升高以及有时伴有贫血。肿瘤大小不等，取决于其所在部位，但大多在 5～10cm 范围内。切除后，10%～25% 的患者出现局部复发，可以反复发生。现在也已明确存在低风险性（<5%）转移，尽管这在形态学上很难预测。

病理学特征

该肿瘤基本上是富于细胞性的束状纤维母细胞/肌纤维母细胞增生，伴有显著的慢性炎细胞浸润，尤其是浆细胞（图 24.58）。这一特征是和与之有重叠表现的筋膜炎和纤维瘤病最为明显的不同。少部分病例中细胞成分较少，玻璃样变性更为显著。梭形细胞成分常常是肥胖的、具有不同程度非典型性的细胞核，核分裂数量有差异（图 24.59）。个别病例出现坏死和钙化。极少数原

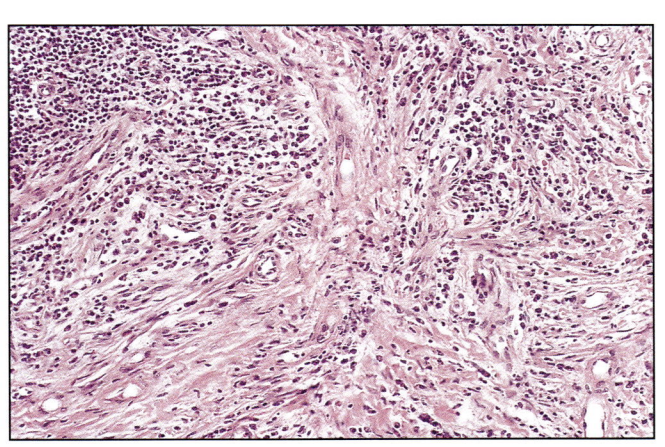

图 24.58　炎性肌纤维母细胞瘤。纵隔病变由细胞丰富的纤维胶原组织构成，含有大量慢性炎性细胞，以浆细胞为主。

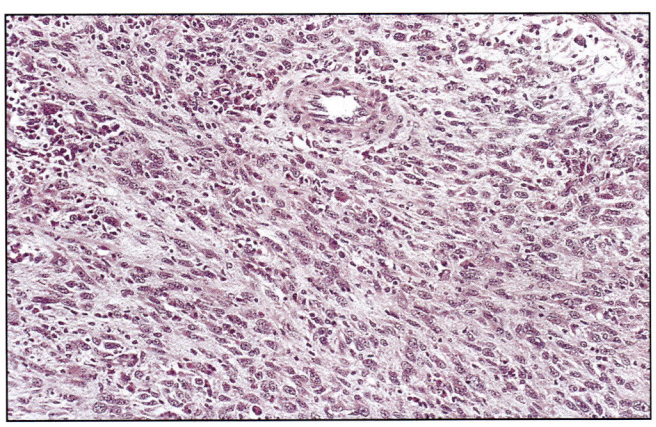

图 24.59　炎性肌纤维母细胞瘤。注意肥胖、具有一定非典型性的纤维母细胞的细胞核以及明显的浆细胞成分。此盲肠旁病变转移到了肝。

纤维母细胞肉瘤

发或复发病例可出现明显恶性细胞形态学表现（通常仅为局灶性的），呈大的组织细胞样细胞或奇异形梭形细胞表现。免疫组织化学上，与其他肌纤维母细胞性病变一样，这些病变通常肌动蛋白呈阳性，结蛋白和角蛋白也呈阳性。细胞遗传学和分子遗传学分析显示 *ALK* 基因重排/易位，具有与间变性大细胞淋巴瘤相似的染色体改变[283,284]。然而，这种遗传学异常只是30%～40%的病例的特征性表现，主要为儿童患者。这些 *ALK* 基因重排常常导致ALK蛋白过度表达（与间变性大细胞淋巴瘤相同），这在有些病例中通过免疫组化方法检测可有助于诊断[285]。从预测行为的角度来看，那些具有明显非典型细胞形态学表现的病例可被认为是恶性的（"炎性纤维肉瘤"），但有极少数细胞学呈良性表现的病变也有转移或复发时出现形态学进展，因此，最好将所有病例看做是低级别肉瘤。有趣的是，有转移的病变似乎 *ALK* 大多为阴性[286]。

低级别肌纤维母细胞肉瘤 Low-grade myofibroblastic sarcoma

低级别肌纤维母细胞肉瘤[287-289]是一个新近认识的病变，过去称为低级别纤维肉瘤，或其他可与韧带样纤维瘤病混淆的病变。病变最常累及年轻人或中年人，没有性别差异。解剖学分布广泛，尽管有20%～25%的病例发生于头颈部（尤其是口腔和舌部）。局部复发常见，长期随访，个别病例出现转移。组织学上，这些病变类似纤维瘤病（图24.60），除了下列表现：（a）细胞的密集较为弥漫；（b）至少出现局灶的轻度细胞核非典型性；以及（c）常常出现骨骼肌内弥漫浸润（类似于增生性肌炎）。免疫组织化学方面，大约65%的病例结蛋白呈弥漫阳性，同样数量的病例（尽管未必是相同的病例）平滑肌肌动蛋白呈阳性。

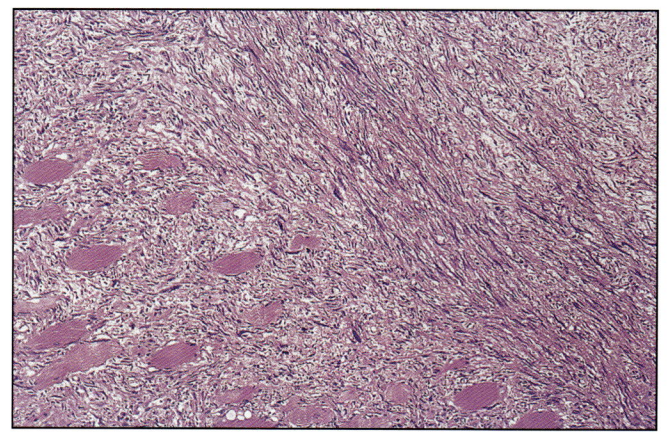

图24.60 低级别肌纤维母细胞肉瘤。注意细胞丰富，轻度细胞核非典型性以及肌肉弥漫性受累。

纤维母细胞肉瘤 Fibroblastic sarcomas

普通型纤维肉瘤 Conventional fibrosarcoma

在20世纪50年代及60年代，纤维肉瘤被广义的定义为有胶原产生的肉瘤，这是一个非常普通的诊断。随着电镜和免疫组织化学的应用，加上严格诊断标准的需求增加，目前纤维肉瘤已非常少见。以前的多数病例目前已划归为恶性外周神经鞘肿瘤或单相型滑膜肉瘤。

临床特征

普通型纤维肉瘤分为两个主要组别，即成人型和婴儿型，两者都极为少见。在作者的资料中，婴儿型病变比成人病变常见。成人型纤维肉瘤[290-292]通常发生于31～60岁，表现为痛性、深在性肿物。男性好发，股部和躯干最常见。根据其组织学分级和手术是否充分，总体5年生存率不超过40%[292]。婴儿型纤维肉瘤[291,293-295]通常发生在2岁以内，常常是先天性的。多数病例发生在四肢，尤其是远端部分，男性多见。与成人型明显不同的是，其5年生存率可能超过80%，辅以新式化疗可能还会更高。转移极其少见，有关这些病例的疾病分类争议较大。

病理学特征

两组病变在大体和形态学上差别不大，尽管成人病变通常略大。多数病变界限清楚，直径不超过10cm，成人病变几乎都为深在性的（筋膜下），很大一部分的婴儿病变位于皮下。所有病例均由形态相对单一的梭形细胞团构成，胞浆淡染，界限不清，细胞核细长，两端尖细，呈典型鱼骨样束状排列（图24.61）。核分裂象多少不等，多形性程度较轻。有些儿童病例的病变由较原始的、稍呈圆形的、较一致的细胞构成；另外，大约30%的病例中可见分枝状血管外皮细胞瘤样血管结构（图24.62）。成人和婴儿病例中，胶原的产生通常有限，这些一般为细胞丰富的肿瘤。过去描述的极为胶原性病例目前最有可能划归为韧带样纤维瘤病或低级别纤维黏液样肉瘤。

纤维肉瘤基本上是一个排除性诊断，从定义上，S-100蛋白、EMA（上皮膜抗原）、角蛋白和结蛋白应当为阴性。有些儿童病例出现局灶肌动蛋白阳性。电镜只能证实纤维母细胞和或许的肌纤维母细胞分化。细胞遗传学也可为婴儿病例的诊断提供支持，因为这些病变具有特异性的 t(12;15)(p13;q25) 易位[297]，导致 *ETV6-NTRK3* 融合，与中胚叶肾瘤一致[298]。

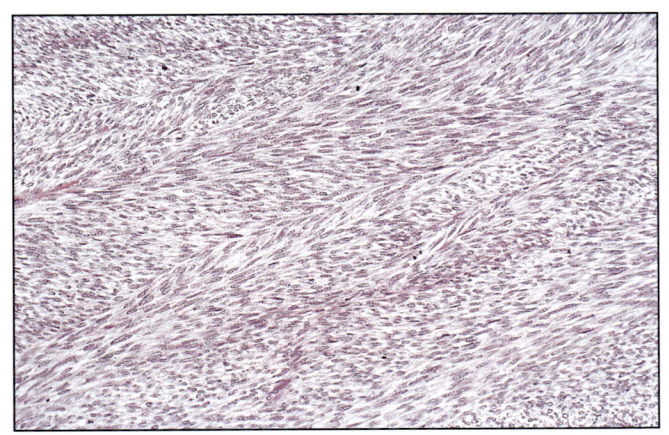

图24.61 成人纤维肉瘤。注意鱼骨样结构。

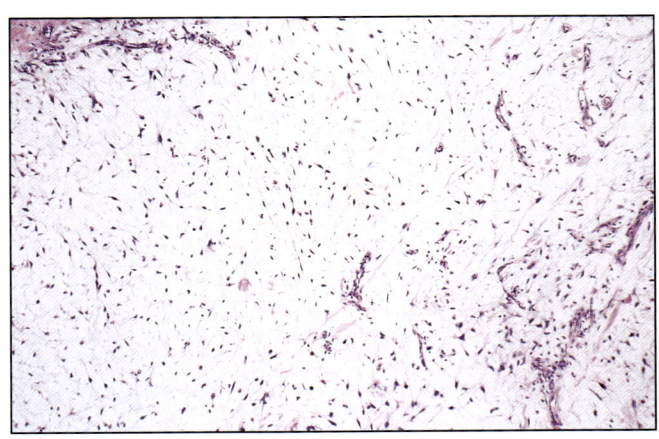

图24.63 低级别黏液样纤维肉瘤。注意细胞成分稀少、纤细的血管成分和细胞核非典型性。

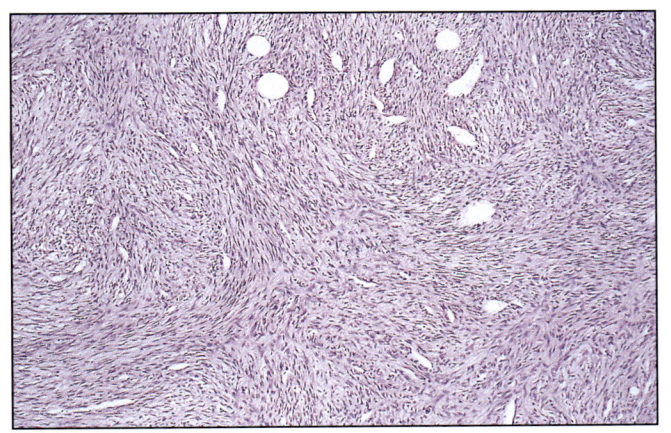

图24.62 婴儿纤维肉瘤。注意束状生长方式和外皮细胞瘤样血管。

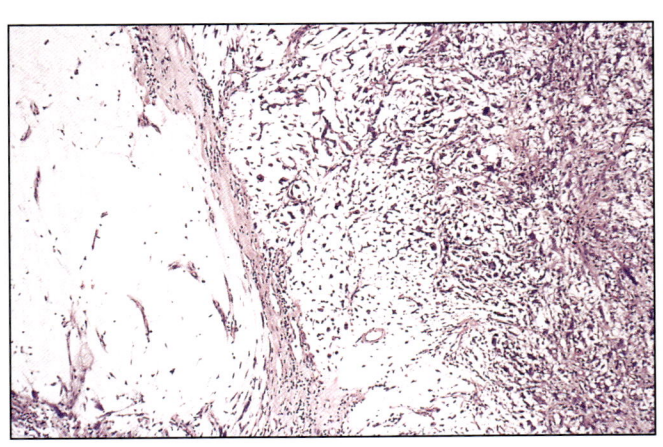

图24.64 高级别黏液样纤维肉瘤。注意从低级别肿瘤（左）到更为多形性的MFH样组织的过渡。

黏液性纤维肉瘤　Myxofibrosarcoma

黏液性纤维肉瘤[299-302]先前称为黏液性MFH，是一种黏液性的特殊病变，组织学级别表现宽泛。是老年人最常见的软组织肉瘤。该谱系中的高级别、低分化端在细胞丰富程度、非典型性以及多形性方面类似于所谓的多形性MFH，这就是为什么用黏液样MFH一词的缘由。然而现在确信，这些病变具有明确的纤维母细胞属性，命名为黏液性纤维肉瘤更为恰当[215]。

临床特征

尽管总体上发病年龄范围较广泛，但黏液性纤维肉瘤主要累及51～80岁的成人。男性稍多见。绝大部分肿瘤发生在四肢；极少发生在腹膜后。如果腹腔内肿瘤出现这种形态学改变，应仔细考虑去分化脂肪肉瘤的诊断。尤其要注意的是，大约2/3的病例发生在皮下，而非深部组织。容易出现多结节和弥漫浸润性生长，其真正的解剖学范围常常被低估，尤其是浅表性肿瘤。生存率与组织学分级有关，但总体5年生存率是60%～70%。级别最低的病变没有转移能力，但可以向高级别转变，因此复发的病变具有转移潜能。高级别病变除了肺和骨播散以外，少数还具有明确的淋巴结转移倾向。

病理学特征

所有级别肿瘤都具有的主要特征是：细胞成分较少的区域内含有薄壁弯曲的血管，其中可见非典型浓染的小梭形细胞和星状细胞，细胞界限不清，有时可见空泡状胞浆（图24.63）。这些小空泡含有酸性黏蛋白而不是脂质（"假性脂母细胞"）。这些病变中的细胞成分和多形性程度与组织学分级平行（图24.64），但通常至少有5%～10%的具有明显黏液样间质的肿瘤符合这一诊

纤维母细胞肉瘤

断。然而，在小活检中可能并非如此。极少数肿瘤（通常是高级别）可出现明显上皮样形态学表现[302a]。基质中主要的酸性黏多糖是透明质酸。梭形和星形细胞具有纤维母细胞的超微结构特征，偶尔可以是肌纤维母细胞[301,303,304]，这反映在有些病例出现肌动蛋白局灶阳性，尤其是伴有更为实性区域的较高级别的病变。波形蛋白一致阳性，CD34一般呈阳性，但其他常用标记物一般为阴性。在高级别病变中，肿瘤区域与非特异性多形性MFH（见下文）无法区分。在超微结构方面，这些奇异性细胞可呈未分化或"组织细胞样"表现。尽管这些肿瘤缺乏任何特殊的核型特征，但随着肿瘤分级的增加（或复发肿瘤出现进展），随之出现的复杂细胞遗传学异常也在增加，可能与遗传学不稳定性有关[305]。

主要的鉴别诊断是黏液性脂肪肉瘤、肌内黏液瘤以及浅表性血管黏液瘤。黏液性脂肪肉瘤不出现这等程度的细胞核非典型性和多形性，其血管成分具有分枝状（鸡爪）结构，并且病变中含有脂肪母细胞。肌内黏液瘤几乎都不含有血管，并且没有细胞核非典型性。还有一组病变，其表现介于肌内黏液瘤和低级别黏液性纤维肉瘤之间，被称为细胞性黏液瘤（见1571页）。不同点在于它们缺乏细胞核非典型性或深染。浅表性血管黏液瘤没有细胞核非典型或多形性，常常具有上皮性成分。黏液型神经鞘或平滑肌肿瘤一般多形性程度较轻，大多具有特殊细胞系分化的免疫组化证据。下面对低级别纤维黏液肉瘤逐个进行描述。

低级别纤维黏液样肉瘤最初是由Evans描述[306,307]，其在临床和形态学方面与名称类似的低级别黏液纤维肉瘤差别很大。病变主要累及21~50岁的成人，发生在分布广泛的软组织筋膜或筋膜下，主要是下肢肢带周围[307-309]。在儿童，皮下部位似乎较为多见[310]。肿瘤大小不等。组织学上，明显良性表现的梭形细胞肿瘤由均一的纤维母细胞构成，大多呈漩涡状排列，伴有不等量的致密胶原（图24.65）或黏液样（图24.66）基质。在黏液性区域中，血管呈薄壁拱桥状排列，但在胶原性区域中较为稀少。核分裂活性少见。复发时细胞成分会更加丰富，常常反复复发。免疫组化染色，大多仅有波形蛋白呈阳性；多数病例中，肌动蛋白、结蛋白、CD34和S-100染色呈阴性，因此有助于除外其他肌纤维母细胞或schwann细胞病变，尽管有些病变可出现局灶CD34或肌动蛋白阳性。然而，重要的是，至少有30%的病例表现为EMA阳性[311]，有可能会导致与神经束膜瘤混淆。最近这些肿瘤显示具有特殊的t(7;16)(q34;p11)易位[311,312]，常常导致FUS-CREB3L2融合性癌基因产生[311]。就最常见的鉴别诊断而言，低级别黏液纤维肉瘤的血管较丰富，黏液更均匀，细胞

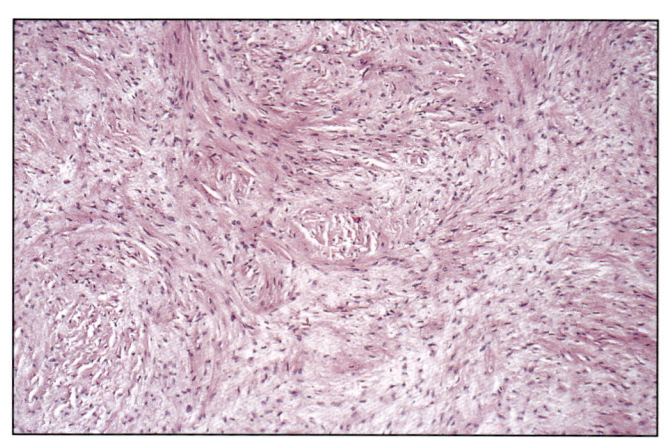

图24.65　低级别纤维黏液样肉瘤。常见有漩涡状胶原表现。

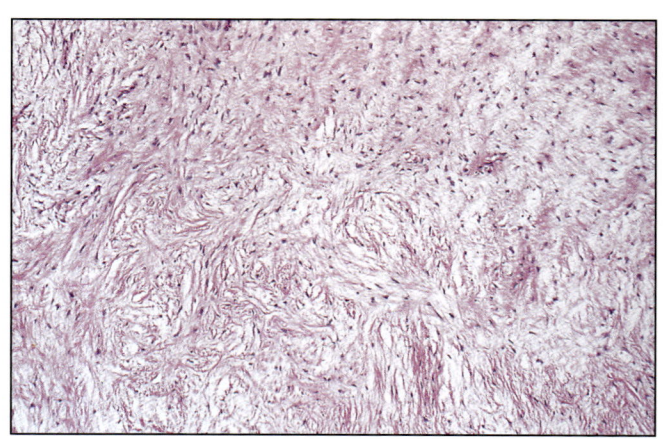

图24.66　低级别纤维黏液样肉瘤。黏液性区域往往范围比较局限。注意良性细胞学表现。

核浓染及多形性更为显著。尽管形态学上普通，这种肿瘤的重要特征在于：多达30%的病例（可能更多）最终出现转移，在10~30年间呈现致死性的临床过程。极具特征的是这些转移为延迟型，并且其他软组织播散也是一个显著特征。

玻璃样梭形细胞肿瘤伴有巨大花环[309,313]，这一诊断术语现已被废弃，仅为低级别纤维黏液样肉瘤的一个形态学类型，不同点只在于出现明显的玻璃样变结节，周围围以呈花环状轴向排列的圆形或卵圆形肿瘤细胞（图24.67）。这些肿瘤与普通低级别纤维黏液样肉瘤具有相同的细胞遗传学异常[311,312]，并且具有完全相同的生物学潜能。

硬化性上皮样纤维肉瘤[314-316]极其少见，并且难以确诊，主要累及年轻人和中年人，没有性别差异，表现为四肢或躯干部位的深在性肿瘤。至少有50%的患者出现局部复发和（或）转移，但系统播散常常延迟5年或更长时间。组织学方面，这些病变由相对较小的、呈巢状、条索和带状的上皮样细胞构成，常常具有透明的细胞浆，其背景为广泛玻璃样变的胶原性

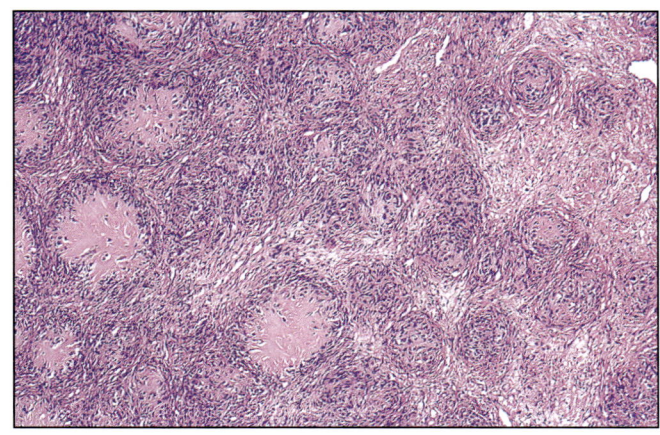

图24.67 低级别纤维黏液样肉瘤伴有巨型花环。形态学表现十分独特。

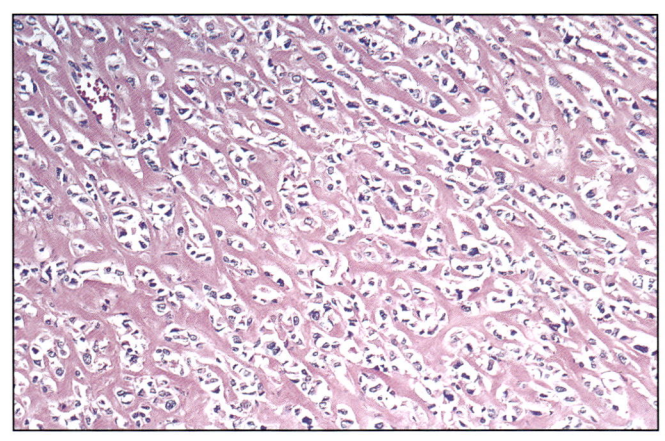

图24.68 硬化性上皮样纤维肉瘤。上皮样细胞索分布于致密胶原性基质中。

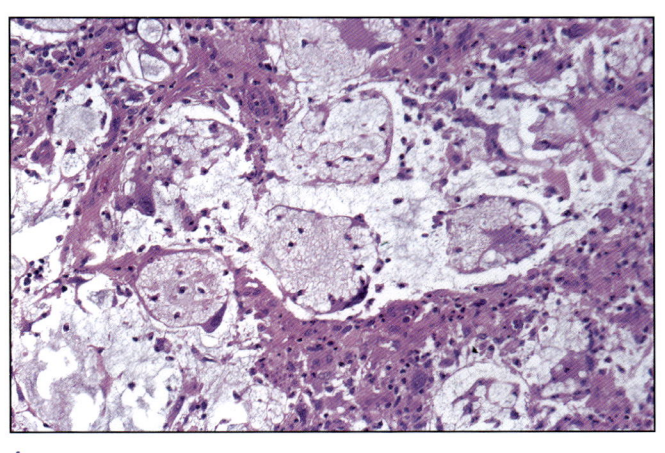

A

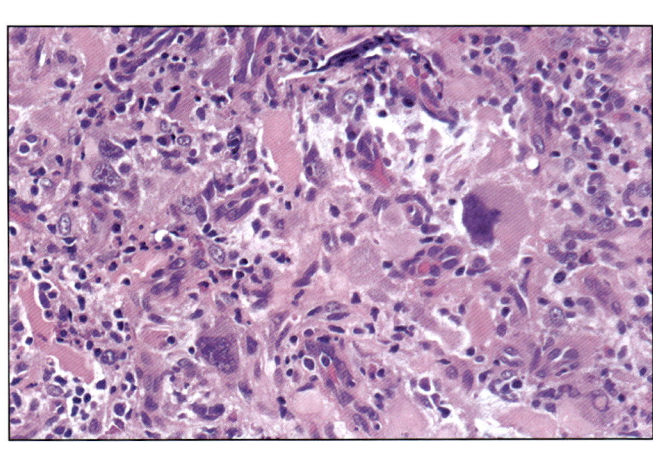

B

图24.69 黏液炎症性纤维母细胞肉瘤。常伴有大的假性脂母细胞成分的黏液性区域（A）与含有细胞核呈干瘪状的Reed-Sternberg样细胞成分的实性区域混合。

间质（图24.68）。通常可以见到类似普通纤维肉瘤束状结构的病灶。多形性不明显，核分裂率一般较低。除波形蛋白以外，有些病例免疫组织化学染色EMA呈阳性，极少数角蛋白和S-100蛋白为阳性；因此需要密切联系临床，除外转移癌。

肢端黏液炎症性纤维母细胞肉瘤[317,318]也被称为炎症性黏液玻璃样肿瘤，主要（但不是全部）发生在成人肢体远端，尤其是手部。其特征是常常反复复发，一般需要进行一定程度的截肢，但是转移似乎（迄今为止）极不常见。组织学上，这些病变的表现与黏液纤维肉瘤十分类似（图24.69a）（见上文），除了出现较多纤维实性区域、比较明显的混合炎性浸润以及Reed-Sternberg样、伴有奇异细胞核和包涵体样核仁的大的上皮样细胞（图24.69b）。后一种细胞大多干瘪。在黏液性区域中常见大的空泡状假性脂母细胞。免疫组化对诊断没有切实的帮助。

纤维组织细胞瘤（所谓的）
Fibrohistiocytic tumors (so-called)

纤维组织细胞分化的概念是基于有些肿瘤是由类似于纤维母细胞和伴有泡圆形细胞核的较肥胖细胞以及类似于组织细胞的细胞所构成的前提之下；这些病变常常具有混合性炎症成分，包括泡沫性巨细胞和破骨细胞性巨细胞；组织培养时，这些病变出现阿米巴样生长和吞噬特性。这些零散的证据现在普遍被认为是误判，一般认为，此分类当中实际上并没有任何一种病变出现真正的组织细胞分化。毫无疑问，"纤维组织细胞"一词属于用词不当，是将一组异源性病变错误地放在一起，其中许多病变可能并不相关。然而，至少在目前这个术语仍被保留，目的是为了诊断的一致性以及更容易表达这些肿瘤的主要概念演化，其中以"恶性纤维组织细胞瘤"（MFH）最具代表性（见下文），2002年WHO分类将其编码化[215]。此类中的皮肤病变包含第23章中描述的隆突性皮肤纤维肉瘤和非典型性纤维黄色瘤。

局限性腱鞘巨细胞瘤
Localized giant cell tumor of tendon sheath

临床特征

局限性巨细胞瘤[319-321]过去常常被称为良性滑膜瘤或局限性结节性腱鞘炎，极为常见，实质上局限于手指（足趾）。手指病变在数量上要多于足趾，比例几乎是10:1，发病高峰年龄是20～40岁，女性占优势，比例为2:1。多数病例表现为无痛性生长缓慢的结节，直径不超过2～3cm，手指（足趾）的任何一面均可受累。局部切除后有10%的病例出现局部复发，但与弥漫型相比，大多累及较大的关节（见第25章），不发生局部侵袭和骨浸润。所谓的"恶性腱鞘巨细胞瘤"[322,323]与大关节弥漫型腱鞘巨细胞瘤密切相关，也在第25章讨论；累及手指（足趾）的类似病变非常罕见。

病理学特征

局限性巨细胞瘤大多为多结节、分叶状肿物，切面黄白色不等。其组成包括不同比例的具有圆形嗜酸性泡状核的单核细胞、破骨性多核巨细胞、泡沫样吞噬细胞、吞噬含铁血黄素细胞以及慢性炎细胞成分（图24.70）。间质为胶原性，具有不同程度的玻璃样变性；通常含有含铁血黄素沉积，有时可见胆固醇裂隙。病变中的细胞多少差异极大；细胞较丰富的病例一般极少有破骨细胞，核分裂比例可以较高，每10个高倍视野常常超过10个。在玻璃样变比较显著的病变中，单核细胞可呈泡状和有些上皮样，破骨细胞稀少。弥漫类型巨细胞瘤一般见不到裂隙样腔隙（见

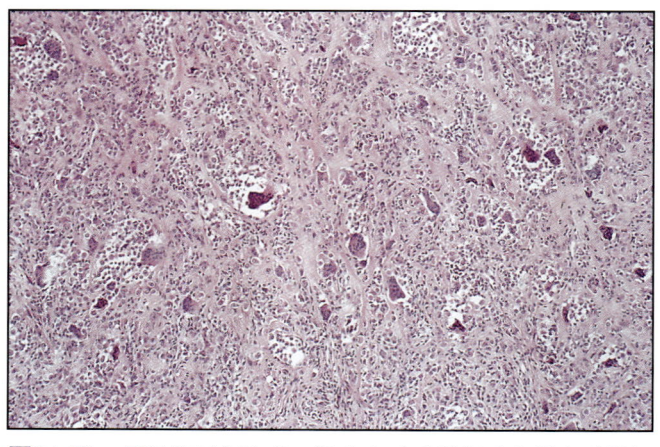

图24.70 局限性巨细胞瘤。注意在玻璃样间质中混有破骨细胞、单核细胞和慢性炎细胞。

第25章）。少部分病例有局灶坏死。

免疫组化方面，多核巨细胞 CD68 均呈阳性，并且表达真正破骨细胞的其他表型特征[324]，至少有一组亚型的单核细胞也为 CD68 阳性表现。单核细胞与正常滑膜细胞非常相似[325,326]，被认为与组织细胞关系密切。另外，一个常见特征是出现结蛋白阳性的树突细胞[327]，本质上可能与淋巴结的所谓的"纤维母细胞性网状细胞"相似。这些病变是否为真正的克隆性肿瘤尚有争议，但对于多数观察者来说似乎很有可能。毋庸置疑的是，这些病变常常表现出克隆性细胞遗传学异常，多数累及1p染色体[328]，而X染色体失活分析表明其为多克隆性[329]。然而，由于这些病变中混有明确的非肿瘤性炎细胞，对于这种X染色体失活研究的正确性还存在疑问，新近 CSF1 基因重排在绝大多数这样的肿瘤中已被证实[330]。尽管有些病例与鞘纤维瘤的特征有重叠[165]，但没有实际的鉴别诊断。

以前被称为色素性绒毛结节性滑膜炎，在第25章中描述。现在一般认为是肿瘤性病变（并且极少数甚至可以转移），具有特殊的细胞遗传学异常，类似于局限性巨细胞瘤[328]。重要的是要记住，此型病变可以完全是关节外的，并且位置远离滑膜结构[323]。

深部良性纤维组织细胞瘤
Deep benign fibrous histocytoma

临床特征

良性纤维组织细胞瘤有一小部分（<2%）全部发生于皮下组织、骨骼肌或腹腔内[331]。尽管总体的发病年龄范围广泛，但此肿瘤主要累及中年人，男性为主。下肢和头颈部是最常见发病部位。多数病变直径为4cm或更大。20%～30%的肿瘤有局部复发，尤其是那些仅边缘性切除或切除不彻底的肿瘤。

病理学特征

与更为常见的皮肤同种病变（见第23章）相比，深在性纤维组织细胞瘤一般界限清楚，有假包膜。偶尔可见中心出血或囊性变表现。不同于皮肤病变的另外一个主要方面在于：细胞多形性一般较轻；多数病例主要由嗜酸性梭形细胞构成，伴有细长或肥胖的泡状核，细胞排列成席纹状结构（图24.71），混有少量淋巴细胞。泡沫细胞和巨细胞不常见。核分裂象常见，但数量一般少于5个/10HPF，有时可见小灶坏死。一个更具假恶性的特征是：偶尔出现血管浸润，与皮肤病变偶尔出现的一样。对于间质，可出现局灶玻璃样变性或黏液变性，血管周围玻璃样变性和血管外皮细胞瘤样血管成分十分

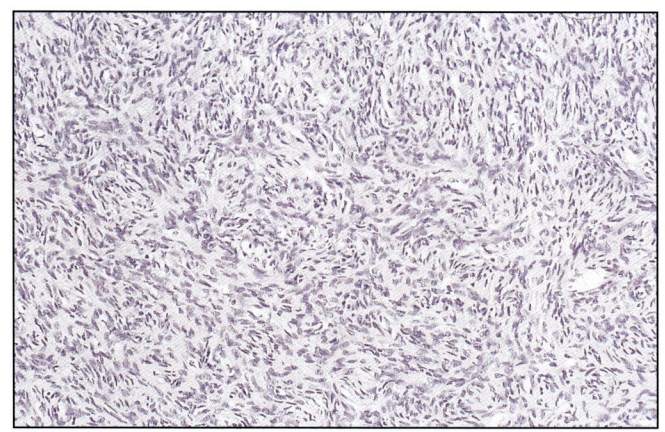

图24.71　深部良性纤维组织细胞瘤。这种界限清楚的皮下病变呈单一性的席纹状表现。

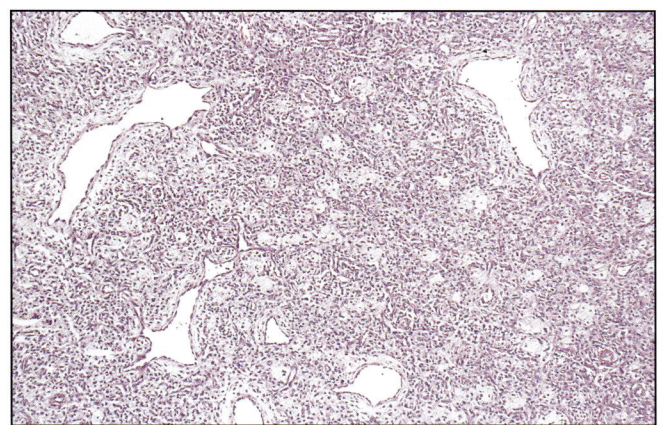

图24.72　深部良性纤维组织细胞瘤。此病例出现分枝状血管外皮细胞瘤样血管成分，还含有多量黄瘤细胞。

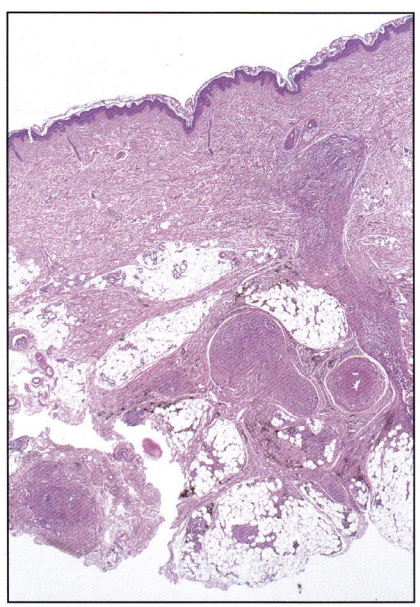

图24.73　丛状纤维组织细胞瘤。这些病变最常见于真皮和皮下交界部位。

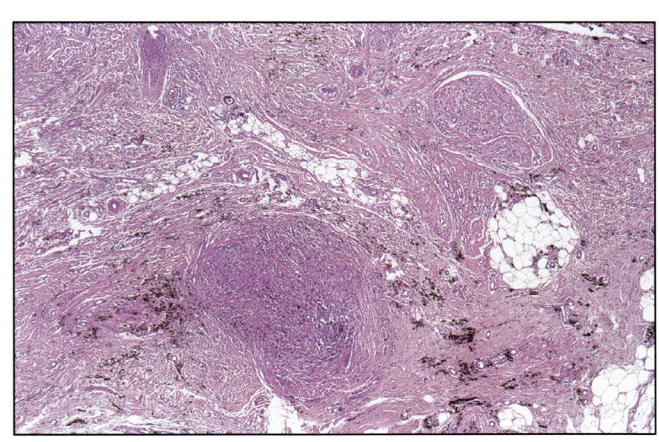

图24.74　丛状纤维组织细胞瘤。注意梭形细胞束和结节状组织细胞样的细胞团混合。

常见（图24.72）。

免疫组化对于诊断并没有积极作用。事实上，新近的经验表明，这些病变往往CD34呈阳性，少数SMA呈阳性。与皮肤纤维肉瘤鉴别最有力的支持是后者位于真皮、特征性的浸润生长方式、胞浆淡染及细胞学形态单一。神经束膜瘤（见第27章）与深部良性纤维组织细胞瘤极为类似，不同点在于免疫组化染色EMA呈阳性。

丛状纤维组织细胞瘤
Plexiform fibrohistocytic tumor

临床特征

丛状纤维组织细胞瘤[332-334]不常见，多数发生于儿童和青少年，有明显的女性倾向。尽管个别病例几乎可以发生于任何部位，但上肢和肢带最常受累。多数病例位于真皮/皮下，深在性病变较少见，多数小于3cm。

边缘性切除或切除不彻底常有局部复发。在最初的最大一组病例中，有2例出现淋巴结转移[325]，但随后的经验表明，可以发生肺转移[327]，尽管还不知道这种现象在其他转诊中心的发生情况。

病理学特征

这些病变通常集中在真皮/皮下交界处，具有明显的丛状/浸润性结构（图24.73）。肿瘤由数量不等的细胞学表现一致的轻度嗜酸性纤维母细胞（类似纤维瘤病）束和结节状组织细胞样细胞团组成，常常混有破骨性巨细胞（图24.74）。对于伴有少量组织细胞样细胞成分的病例，后一种细胞可呈单个散在分布，或在肌纤维母细胞成分中呈小巢状分布。没有非典型性或多形性，但

20%的病例可见血管浸润，由此可以解释其转移倾向。免疫染色，梭形细胞成分 SMA 呈阳性，组织细胞样成分 CD68 呈不同程度阳性，主要见于破骨细胞。

部位表浅、丛状结构以及至少局部有明显的组织细胞样成分表现这些可与纤维瘤病鉴别。有些病例也可能与细胞性神经鞘黏液瘤（neurothekeoma）混淆，但是后者极少呈丛状结构，且缺乏组织细胞样结节，代之以轻度嗜酸性的卵圆形或梭形细胞束和细胞巢，分布于真皮玻璃样胶原束之间。

软组织巨细胞瘤　Giant cell tumor of tissue

软组织巨细胞瘤[335-337]尽管首次描述已经很久远，但多年以来，这种病变被纳入现已废弃的所谓巨细胞 MFH（见下文）一类当中。这些病变大多发生在四肢（少数为躯干）的真皮或皮下，发病年龄范围较广，但成人最常见。肿瘤一般界限清楚，常常小于 5cm。不大常见的深在性病变可以较大。此类肿瘤一般为良性，但可局部复发。极少数病例（出现细胞核多形性和非典型性，核分裂比率一般较高）可出现转移。组织学上，多数肿瘤的特征为多发性小肿瘤结节，组织学上与骨的巨细胞瘤（见第 25 章）无法区分，后者由卵圆形单核细胞和破骨性巨细胞构成（图 24.75）。这些结节分布于细胞丰富的纤维母细胞间质中，有不同程度的出血。有些病例出现明显的反应性成骨，一般位于病变周边。肿瘤细胞通常核分裂象较多。

恶性纤维组织细胞瘤（所谓的）　Malignant fibrous histiocytoma (so-called)

恶性纤维组织细胞瘤（MFH）作为一种流行诊断已超过 25 年，并且被许多人认为是软组织肉瘤中最常见的类型。尽管已有五种亚型，即多形性、黏液样、巨细胞、炎症性及血管瘤样，但现在已逐渐认识到，该组中的"最初成员"，即多形性类型并非为一种独立病变，并且所有亚型之间的关系很小。当然现在已不再认为任何这些病变具有真正的组织细胞分化。在最新的 WHO 分类[215]中，所谓的多形性 MFH 已不再被认为是明确的肿瘤类型，代之以同义的未分化多形性肉瘤，为排除性诊断，不超过成人肉瘤的 5%。所谓黏液样 MFH 现在已被命名为黏液纤维肉瘤，被视为一种纤维母细胞性病变（见 1555 页）。毋庸置疑，所谓血管瘤样 MFH 是一种独立性病变，现在被划分为不能确定细胞系类别的病变（见 1574）。

多形性 MFH/未分化多形性肉瘤　Pleomorphic MFH/undiffentiated pleomorphic sarcoma

尽管以前被认为是唯一最常见的肉瘤，但多形性 MFH 已不再被视为一个病变实体[215,339-341]。现在，它代表着一大类同有大的间变性形态表现的其他肿瘤，其中多数病例具有特殊细胞系分化。或许重新评价多形性 MFH 的最重要线索是要认识到：没有可重复的阳性标准存在，基本上是排除性诊断。传统上被纳入此"废纸篓"的多数肿瘤发生于成人深部软组织，年龄超过 40 岁发病率逐步上升。如果难以确定肿瘤的分化，此时最常见的组织学类型是多形性脂肪肉瘤、平滑肌肉瘤和横纹肌肉瘤[339]，尽管几乎所有肉瘤偶尔都会出现这种形态学表现。重要的是要注意到，有些癌、黑色素瘤和淋巴瘤也可以出现同样的形态学表现；明确这一点具有重要的临床和治疗意义。已日益明确多形性肉瘤亚型具有直接的临床相关性。例如，目前资料已经表明，多形性横纹肌肉瘤尤其具有侵袭性[342,343]，而与其他多形性肉瘤相比，去分化脂肪肉瘤相对呈惰性[86,87]。事实上，一项大型的所谓 MFH 病例的重新回顾已经表明，任何肌源性分化的多形性肉瘤出现转移是非肌源性病变的两倍；这些病变转移也较早[344-346]。只有当病理医生依照常规进行这样的分类才会使预后和治疗的差别显现出来。

从形态学观点看，所有命名为所谓多形性 MFH 的病变一般较大，常伴有坏死区。无论其特殊分化如何（图 24.76），它们几乎都具有显著的细胞学多形性，出现奇异的多核细胞，常见席纹状结构，并有含有数量不等的慢性炎细胞的胶原性间质，且常伴有泡沫状巨噬细胞。只有通过全面取材，结合明智地应用免疫组化和（或）电镜，方可准确分类[339,340,344]。不可避免地，仍有一组至少目前还不能分类的高级别多形性软组织

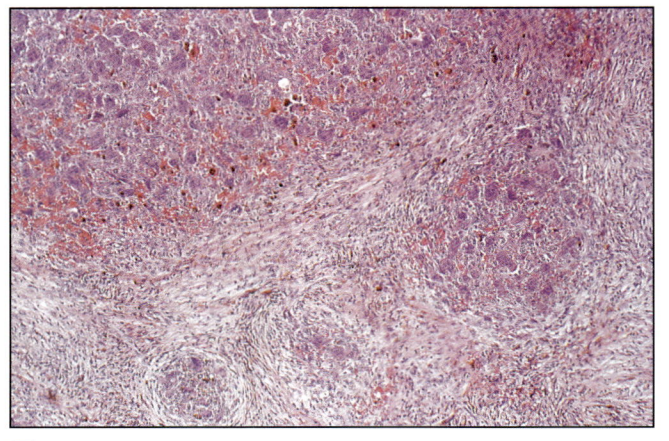

图 24.75　软组织巨细胞瘤。注意典型的多结节性表现。

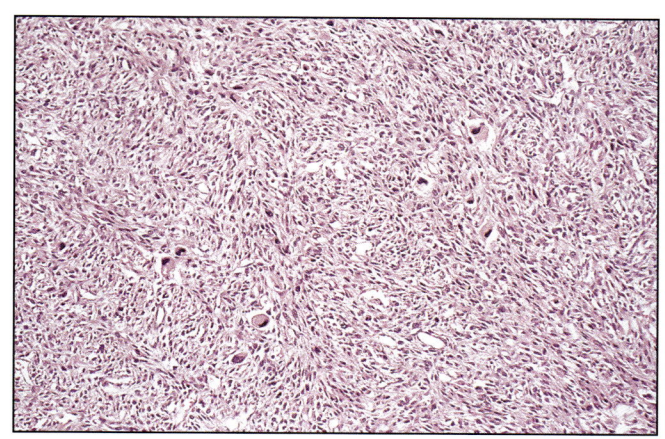

图24.76 高级别多形性肉瘤。席纹状、多形性肿瘤被证实具有Schwann细胞分化。

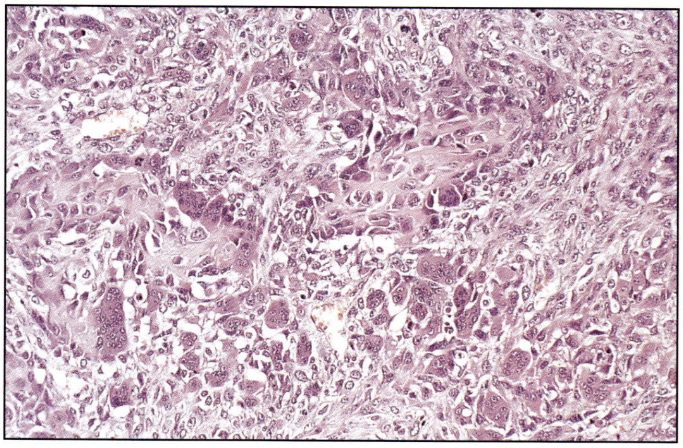

图24.77 富于巨细胞的软组织骨肉瘤。此病变以前常常被称为所谓的巨细胞性"MFH"。

肿瘤。其中有些本质上几乎肯定是纤维母细胞或肌纤维母细胞性，但有一小部分难以确定。对于这些病例，应继续充分研究，但目前只能称其为未分化多形性肉瘤。在未来几年，MFH名称很有可能会完全消失。

巨细胞性MFH/伴有巨细胞的未分化多形性肉瘤
Giant cell MFH/undifferentiated pleomorphic sarcoma with giant cells

巨细胞性MFH是另一组不能准确定义的异源性病变。其中每一种病变常常表现为多结节性生长方式，并出现大量良性破骨细胞样巨细胞成分。这个家族中的大多数病变以累及老年人为主，主要发生在四肢，一般位于浅表软组织内[347,348]。发生在深部（筋膜下）组织的肿瘤多数具有侵袭性行为，而浅表性病变预后一般较好[347]，主要是因为现今后者中多数被重新分类为软组织巨细胞瘤[335,336]（见下文）。

即使在最初的描述中[347]已明确描述，在恶性病变中至少有50%存在骨组织成分，而骨或骨样组织其本质上是肿瘤性的。因此，这些病变从逻辑上应分类为富于巨细胞的软组织骨肉瘤亚型（图24.77）。除了常见的软组织良性巨细胞瘤外，巨细胞性MFH家族中第二大亚型为伴有多量破骨细胞样的巨细胞平滑肌肉瘤[349]（图24.78），其行为与普通平滑肌肉瘤相同。几乎所有其他类型的肉瘤都可以偶尔出现少数破骨细胞，无论其特殊细胞系分化如何，有时破骨细胞的数量多得足以类似于所谓的巨细胞性MFH[350]；另外，不应忘记的是：伴有明显破骨细胞反应的癌，尤其是在甲状腺、胰腺和肺，可以极其类似于所谓的巨细胞

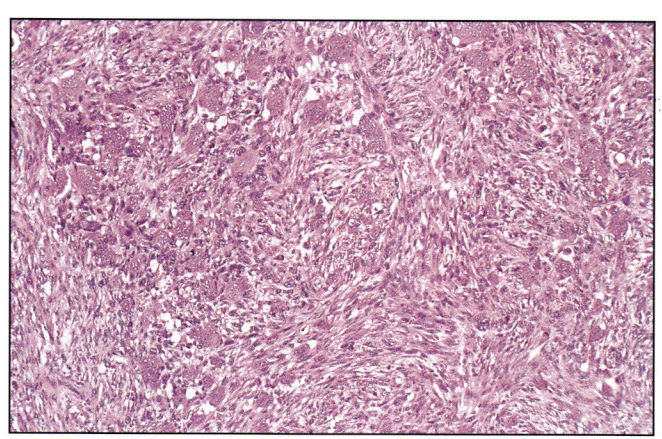

图24.78 类似于所谓的巨细胞性"MFH"的平滑肌肉瘤。注意病变中嗜酸性束状成分，其被证实结蛋白呈阳性。

性MFH，恶性黑色素瘤也可如此（极少见）。

炎性MFH/未分化的多形性肉瘤伴明显炎症
Inflammatory MFH/undifferentiated pleomorphic sarcoma with prominent inflammation

具有所谓炎性MFH表现的病变极为少见。这些病变首次描述于1976年[351]，主要累及成人，以腹膜后或其他内脏软组织为主，可伴有白细胞增多症[352]。形态学上，以大的黄瘤性细胞为主要特征，细胞核呈不同程度的非典型性，混有多量与坏死无关的多形性中性粒细胞（图24.79）。另外还混有多形性或多核细胞，有些可呈Reed-Sternberg样，肿瘤中至少有小部分区域具有梭形细胞席纹样表现，这是其最初被命名为MFH的原因。

经验（与全面取材同样）表明，实际上这些肿瘤多数为去分化脂肪肉瘤[88]，其中高分化成分常常被忽

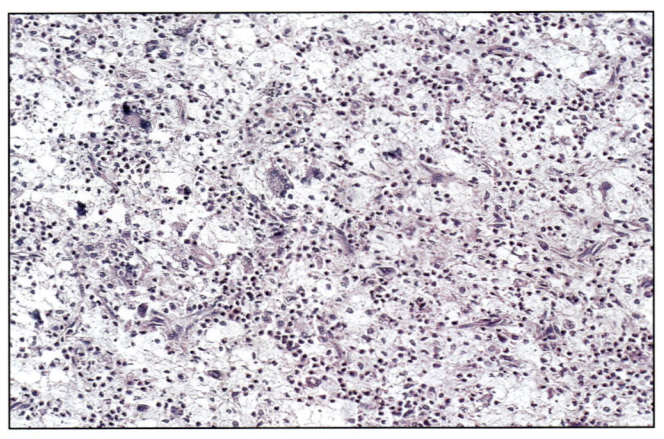

图24.79 去分化脂肪肉瘤。肿瘤的高级别区域表现为泡沫细胞、中性粒细胞和奇异形多核巨细胞混合，这种结构以前被称为炎症性"MFH"。

略。另外，其他可以出现这种结构的肿瘤为低分化癌，尤其是在肺或胃肠道的癌、间变性大细胞性淋巴瘤甚至更为少见的恶性黑色素瘤。鉴别诊断包括黄色瘤样肾盂肾炎、Erdheim-Chester 病以及其他具有明显黄色瘤细胞成分（通常是非肿瘤性的）的肉瘤。"腹膜后黄色肉芽肿"（Oberling）这一概念作为一个病变似乎已经作废。

所谓的血管瘤样 MFH 仍然是一种独立的明确病变，与上面描述的病变没有关系，现在认为属于不明分化系的肿瘤类别（见1574）。

平滑肌肿瘤 Smooth muscle tumors

良性平滑肌肿瘤常见，发生部位广泛。与多数软组织肿瘤相比，多数病例似乎来源于正常组织中的相对应部分。非内脏的软组织平滑肌肉瘤过去认为十分罕见，据估计不超过软组织肉瘤的 5%～7%。发生率的计算主要根据所应用的诊断标准（见下文），但依据作者的资料，平滑肌肉瘤较常见，至少占成人肉瘤的15%。播散性腹膜平滑肌瘤病在第15章描述，静脉内平滑肌瘤病在第13章描述。

先天性平滑肌错构瘤
Congenital smooth muscle hamartoma

先天性平滑肌错构瘤[353-355]是一种罕见的皮肤病变，可见于新生儿，以男婴为主，表现为稍硬的、不同程度色素沉着的斑疹，被覆的毛发一般比正常厚；然而，有些病例临床呈萎缩性表现[355]。多数病例的病变发生在躯干或肢体近端。组织学上，真皮内分化成熟的平滑肌束的数量增多，排列杂乱。毛发的数量实际上并没有增加，但被覆上皮有角化过度和色素沉着。临床上与 Becker 痣有重叠，后者为获得性病变。

毛发平滑肌瘤 Pilar leiomyoma

临床特征

皮肤毛发平滑肌瘤发生于立毛肌，多发比单发更常见，主要见于年轻成人，没有性别差异，表现为小的痛性粉红色丘疹，主要位于四肢和躯干[356-358]。有些病例为家族性的[358-359]，其中一些伴有延胡索酸水合酶种系突变的患者也容易发生子宫平滑肌瘤和乳头状肾细胞癌[360]。乳头孤立性平滑肌瘤不常见，临床病理上与毛发平滑肌瘤无法鉴别。多发性病变的患者常常持续多年发生无数的新病变，控制疼痛可能是个难题；然而，似乎并没有真正的局部复发。

组织学特征

毛发平滑肌瘤是由分化好的平滑肌细胞束构成，胞浆丰富、嗜酸性，细胞核尾端圆钝，雪茄样，有些呈空泡状，不规则地排列于网状真皮内（图 24.80）。被覆表皮常有增生。这些平滑肌束和毛囊的关系密切，形成界限不清、没有包膜的肿物，成分枝状排列于真皮胶原束之间。小部分病例形成界限较清楚的结节。可以出现局灶退行性轻度细胞核异型，核分裂象可达到 1 个 /10HPF，对临床行为似乎没有影响[358]。传统

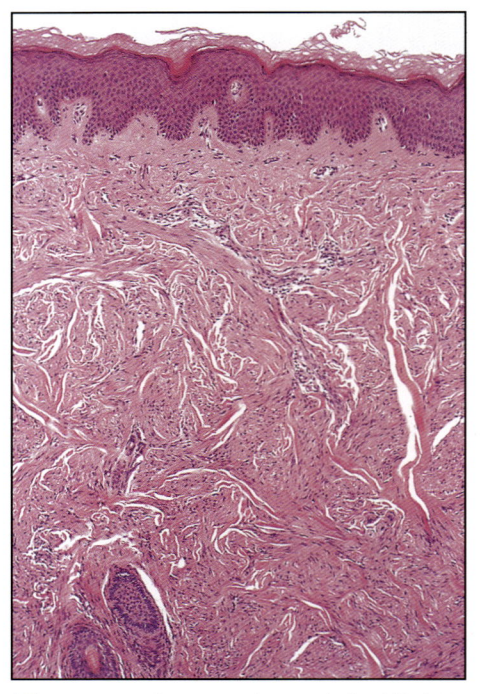

图24.80 毛发平滑肌瘤。一个典型的边界不清的真皮病变。

上任何较多的核分裂象均提示皮肤平滑肌肉瘤的诊断，尽管有关该名称是否正确还有疑问（见下文），因为后者似乎从不转移。在所有病例中，肿瘤细胞肌动蛋白和结蛋白均为阳性。

血管平滑肌瘤
Angioleiomyoma (vascular leiomyoma)

临床特征

血管平滑肌瘤[356,362-363]比毛发平滑肌瘤常见，通常为孤立性的。发病高峰为31～60岁，女性具有中度倾向，尽管整体上解剖学分布广泛，但50%以上位于小腿。极少数病例病变可发生于内脏，以上部呼吸消化道最常见。大概一半病例伴有疼痛或肿胀。切除后局部复发极其少见。

病理学特征

血管平滑肌瘤界限清楚，有被膜，直径常常小于3cm。在浅表皮下组织比在深部真皮更为常见，手术一般易于剔除。肿瘤似乎发生于静脉壁，由成熟平滑肌细胞构成，围绕明显的或不明显的、缝隙状或扩张的厚壁血管，排列成束状和漩涡状结构（图24.81）。通常缺乏核分裂象。退行性变常见，包括血管血栓形成、间质玻璃样或黏液样变性、营养不良性钙化以及固缩性的细胞核异型。大概2%的病例含有成熟脂肪细胞团，这似乎代表了一种退行性化生形态。此种病变与任何其他部位（如肾脏）发生的血管平滑肌脂肪瘤都无关。疼痛在实性、血管较少的病变中似乎最为常见[363,364]，有些作者证实，在这些病例中，病变内存在大量的小神经纤维[364]。鉴别诊断一般不成问题，包括良性Schwann细胞瘤或腱鞘纤维瘤。

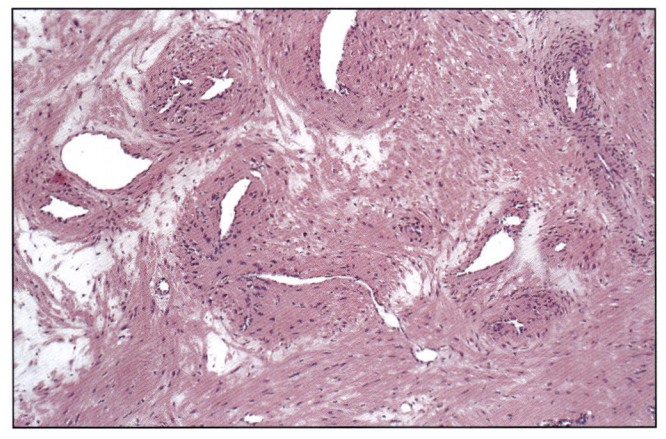

图24.81 血管平滑肌瘤。注意血管壁薄厚不均。此病例还出现了黏液样变性。

深部平滑肌瘤　Deep leiomyoma

临床特征

深部软组织平滑肌瘤[365-367]很少见，只在近些年才有确切的报道。其主要发生在中年人，腹膜后最常见，其次是四肢或躯干。这些病变与平滑肌肉瘤区分的诊断标准依据患者性别和解剖部位[368,369]（见下文）。发生于深部大血管的良性平滑肌瘤几乎不存在。深部平滑肌瘤一般为孤立性的，无痛，生长缓慢，直径通常超过5cm。如果诊断严谨，没有明确的局部复发倾向。

病理学特征

深部平滑肌瘤界限清楚，呈分叶状。尽管由经典性成熟的嗜酸性平滑肌细胞组成，但有些病例，通常是在四肢，其特征表现是容易出现显著的退行性改变，主要为玻璃样变性、黏液变、营养不良性钙化和个别细胞核异型，与某些Schwann细胞瘤相似。极个别病例出现上皮样细胞形态学表现。在所有这些病变中，细胞学非典型性和肿瘤坏死超过轻度的均提示恶性。然而，有关核分裂象的情况比较复杂。除了患者性别以外，对于四肢的病变，核分裂象的数量超过1个/50HPF则具有恶性行为潜能。出现任何核分裂象都应当引起至少是轻度的关注。相反腹膜后的病变多数发生于女性（图24.82a），呈良性表现的病变中核分裂象少于10个/50HPF似乎为良性。此类病变通常雌激素和孕激素受体呈阳性（图24.82b），似乎与子宫平滑肌瘤有很大的相似性[366,367]。迄今为止，有关男性腹膜后病变的资料还不够充分，在此情况下诊断平滑肌瘤应极为慎重。由成熟平滑肌和脂肪构成的深部病变被称为肌脂肪瘤，在1531页描述。

生殖器平滑肌瘤
Genital leiomyoma

"生殖器平滑肌瘤"一词长期以来用于描述乳头、外阴或阴囊发生的平滑肌瘤；作为一组病变，它们常常被纳入毛发平滑肌瘤的亚型。这对于乳头部的病变是完全合理的，但对于外阴和阴囊肿瘤则完全不同[361,370]。阴囊肿瘤累及成人，发生于肌膜，常常较大。这些肿瘤容易出现局灶浸润，常常伴有淋巴细胞聚集。这些肿瘤比外阴病变更为富于细胞，在第13章有详细描述。典型的外阴病变界限清楚，常常具有不同程度的黏液及玻璃样变性。尽管阴囊病变与其他深部软组织平滑肌瘤一样，偶尔出现退行性细胞核异型[371]，但任何核分裂象的出现最好被视为潜在恶性行为的证据。我们以及其他作者[372]曾经遇到过极个别的成人阴囊平

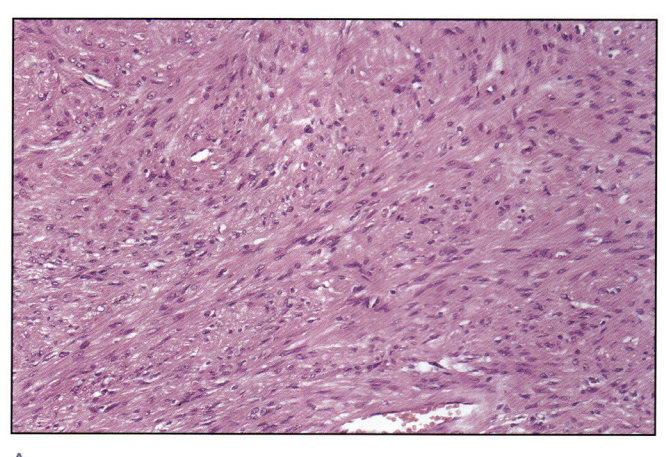 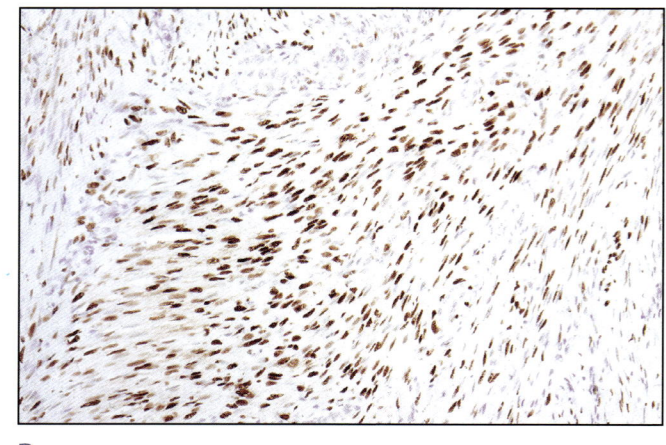

图24.82 深部平滑肌瘤。形态学上富于细胞但为良性的平滑肌肿瘤（A）见于女性腹膜后，表现为弥漫细胞核ER阳性（B）。

滑肌错构瘤性增生；最好通过完全缺乏非典型性和组织学上不形成独立的肿物等来确诊。阴囊平滑肌显著增生也可见于淋巴水肿的患者[373]。

平滑肌肉瘤
Leiomyosarcoma

临床特征

尽管具有许多相同的组织学特征，但从临床观点上看，软组织平滑肌肉瘤被分成四个主要组别。腹内平滑肌肉瘤[374-376]：发生于腹膜后、肠系膜或网膜，占病例的40%~45%，一般见于41~70岁，女性好发。这些肿瘤往往很大，常常不能广泛切除。主要转移到肺和肝，总体5年生存率是20%~30%。四肢皮下或深部软组织平滑肌肉瘤[374,377-380]：占病例的30%~35%；同样主要累及成人年龄组，但男性稍多。股部是最常见部位。大概50%的病例最终出现转移，总体5年生存率是60%~65%。所谓的皮肤平滑肌肉瘤[378,381,382]：大约占病例的15%~20%，主要累及年轻人，男性为主。四肢、尤其是小腿为好发部位，这些病变常常为痛性的。尽管局部复发常见，并且手术不充分可以重复发生，但几乎见不到转移；事实上，普遍认为皮肤平滑肌肉瘤从不转移，无论组织学特征如何。在此特殊情况下使用"肉瘤"一词会引发严重问题，"非典型皮内平滑肌肿瘤"更受欢迎。血管平滑肌肉瘤[374,380,383-385]：大约占病例的5%，通常发生于下腔静脉或下肢的大静脉。主要累及老年人，下腔静脉病变具有极为明显的女性倾向。总体5年生存率大约为20%，尽管发生在较小及较远端静脉的病例预后似乎较好[377,384]。

独立于这四个主要分类的是外生殖器平滑肌肉瘤[361,370]；乳头部病变类似于皮肤病变，外阴或阴囊肿瘤尽管在组织学上类似于皮肤病变，但往往预后相对较好，少有转移。儿童平滑肌肉瘤[386-388]极少见，可发生于内脏或躯体软组织。软组织病例中似乎女性稍多见，且解剖学分布广泛，皮肤和深部组织受累的几率相同。多数真正的儿童软组织病例似乎预后极好，极少有转移，主要因为多数病例形态学上属低级别[388]。有趣的是，一定比例的内脏（颅内同样）平滑肌肿瘤（多数为平滑肌肉瘤）与免疫抑制有关，主要见于HIV感染者[389-391]，其次是器官移植后[391]。这些肿瘤在病因学上与EB病毒有关，最常见于儿童，行为差异极大。

病理学特征

一般来说，深在性的平滑肌肉瘤往往较大，出现的坏死比浅表性肿瘤的更多。除了皮肤病变以外，多数肿瘤界限清楚，有薄的假包膜。组织学表现依分化程度而不同，但是最低标准是：至少局部存在轻度嗜酸性梭形细胞束，细胞核呈空泡状、圆形或雪茄形（图24.83），SMA和（或）结蛋白一致呈强阳性，或超微结构上出现确切的平滑肌分化证据，尤其是纵向长丝，伴有局部致密、明显、几乎连续的外板以及吞饮小泡。总体上，不超过70%~80%的平滑肌肉瘤结蛋白呈阳性（常常只是局灶性的），这不仅反映了分化缺失，也反映了正常平滑肌的表型改变[392-395]。另外，大约60%~65%的平滑肌肉瘤也表现为钙调素结合蛋白（caldesmon）阳性。

重要的是（尤其在鉴别诊断时），所有部位的平滑肌肉瘤中，30%~40%的免疫染色CK和EMA呈阳

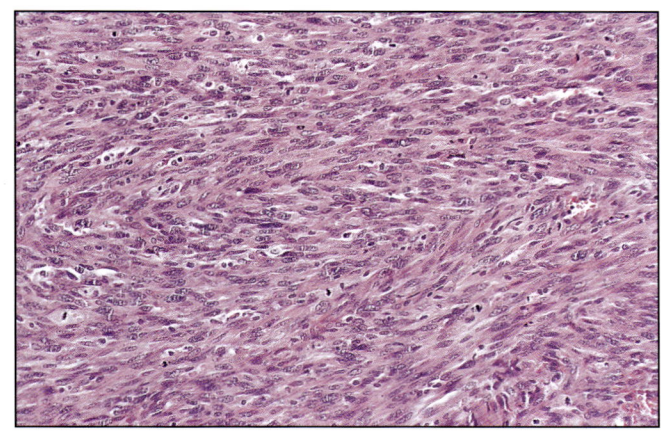

图24.83 平滑肌肉瘤。出现典型细胞学表现的中等级别病变。

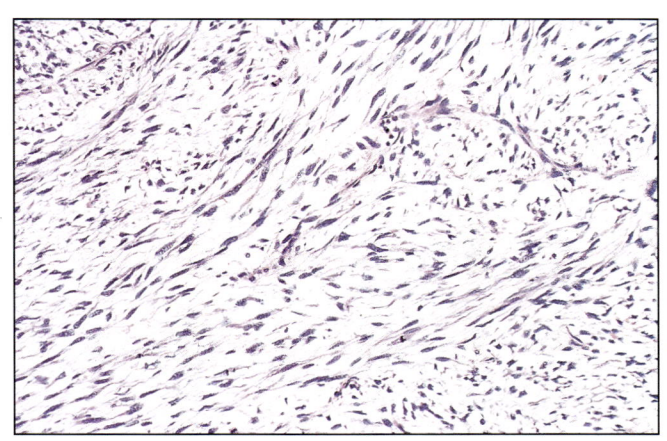

图24.85 黏液性平滑肌肉瘤。对于与神经鞘肿瘤的鉴别，免疫组化或电镜是必要的。

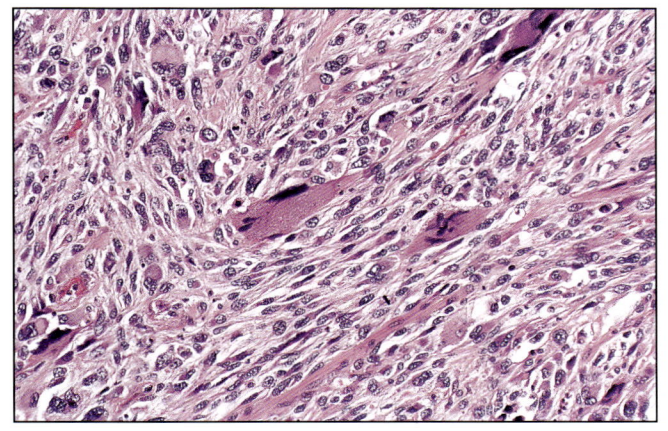

图24.84 多形性平滑肌肉瘤。显著多形性可类似于所谓的"MFH"，但背景中的嗜酸性梭形细胞提示肌源性分化。

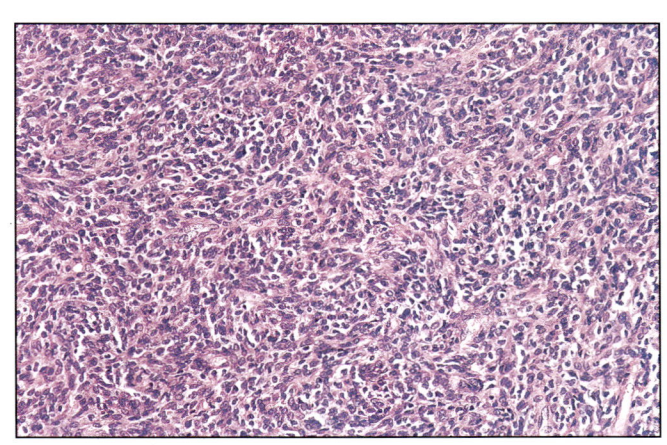

图24.86 炎性平滑肌肉瘤。肿瘤性平滑肌细胞淹没于大量淋巴细胞中。

性[394,395]；可呈局灶、点状或弥漫性，见于多数常用抗体。其他辅助诊断包括三色法染色呈嗜品红性以及固定良好的病例中胞浆内糖原PAS呈阳性。一个偶见的特征是出现透明的核旁空泡，尽管过去曾经高估了这一点，因为非肌源性KIT阳性的胃肠道间质瘤时常也出现这一特征表现；5%～10%的病例出现明显的细胞核栅栏状表现。

许多病例中除了以明显嗜酸性束状成分为主要特征之外，其他特征变化不定，包括明显（MFH样）多形性（图24.84）[339,396]、广泛玻璃样变性、不同程度黏液变性（图24.85）[397]、混以多量破骨细胞性巨细胞（见图24.78）[349]以及混合数量不等的炎细胞，包括淋巴细胞和黄瘤细胞（图24.86）[398]。这些亚型在行为上与普通型平滑肌肉瘤没有明显差别；特别是软组织黏液性平滑肌肉瘤并不具有与前面提到的子宫病变一样的侵袭性。尽管资料有限，但是炎性平滑肌肉瘤（具有特殊的核型）[399]的预后似乎相对较好[398]。极少数特殊的病例出现明显的颗粒细胞改变[400]或上皮样细胞形态学表现[401]；后者容易被误诊为黑色素瘤，尤其是在浅表软组织。一般来说，非内脏部位的上皮样平滑肌肿瘤极少见。细胞遗传学方面，平滑肌肉瘤一般具有非常复杂的核型[402]，出现与以前诊断为所谓的MFH的重叠等位基因失衡或许并不令人惊奇[403]。

最后一点有关定义问题。毋庸置疑，存在一组数量少但具有重要意义的梭形细胞肉瘤，其肌动蛋白呈阳性，结蛋白呈阴性，形态学上并非完全典型的平滑肌肉瘤（图24.87），或因为胞浆染色较淡，或因为细胞核较细长和轻度波浪状。对于这些肿瘤如何分类有着不同的观点，但似乎许多此类病例都出现肌纤维母细胞分化，如果能够达成一致的定义，最好将其分类为肌纤维肉瘤[288,289]。形态学上此类病变的低级别亚型

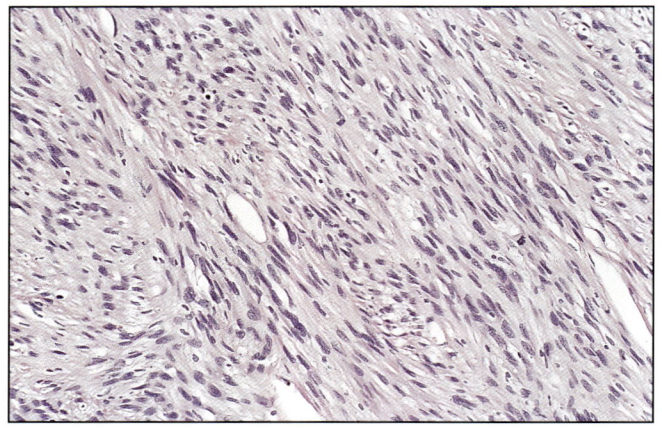

图24.87 平滑肌肉瘤或黏液纤维肉瘤？伴有胞浆淡染、胞核细长的肌动蛋白阳性的梭形细胞的本质还有争议。

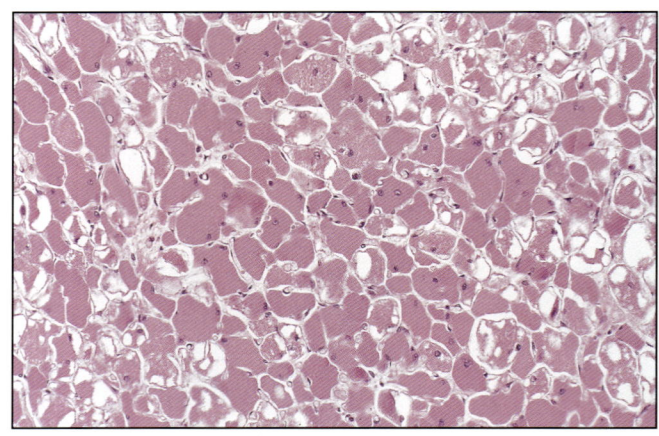

图24.88 成人横纹肌瘤。典型的大多角形嗜酸性细胞，伴有局灶空泡。

已经这样定义[287]（见1554页）。

骨骼肌肿瘤　Skeletal muscle tumors

在整体名称当中，肿瘤出现骨骼肌分化并不常见。它们重要性在于：横纹肌肉瘤在孤立性儿童恶性肿瘤中具有重要地位。心脏横纹肌瘤在第2章描述。

间叶性横纹肌瘤样错构瘤 Rhabdomyomatous mesenchymal hamartoma

间叶性横纹肌瘤样错构瘤[404,405]是一种极其少见的先天性病变，通常发生于新生儿或婴儿，表现为头颈部的一个或多个皮肤小息肉。组织学上，其特征是网状真皮内出现分布不规则的成熟骨骼肌纤维成分。

成人横纹肌瘤 Adult rhabdomyoma

横纹肌瘤整体上罕见，其中以成人型最常见。成人横纹肌瘤[406-408]几乎都发生于中年人头颈部（尤其是口咽部）；有明显男性倾向。整体上发病年龄范围和解剖学分布十分广泛，尽管四肢病例还未曾描述过。高达10%的病例为多发性的，个别病例局部切除后可复发。多数病例病变小于5cm，有被膜，由大多角形嗜酸性细胞构成，胞浆呈颗粒状，胞核小，位于周边（图24.88）。PTAH染色不仅常可见到横纹结构，也可见到杂乱的结晶状或丝状包涵体，与线状体肌病所见相同。如果需要与颗粒细胞瘤或冬眠瘤鉴别，可依据免疫染色结蛋白和肌红蛋白呈强阳性。

胎儿横纹肌瘤 Fetal rhabdomyoma

胎儿横纹肌瘤[406,407,409,410]可发生于任何年龄，但以儿童为主，最常见于头颈部，尤其是耳后。与成人型一样，病变生长缓慢，通常小于5cm。这些病变似乎从没有过多发，局部复发极为少见[410,411]。组织学上，除了缺乏细胞核非典型性以及核分裂象极少以外，病变与胚胎性横纹肌肉瘤极为类似（图24.89）。病变具有带状分布表现，较成熟的嗜酸性横纹肌母细胞位于周边，伴有不成熟骨骼肌细胞成分的原始间叶细胞分布于黏液性基质当中，位于病变中央。个别细胞更为丰富、甚至呈束状的病变已被命名为富于细胞的胎儿横纹肌瘤[412]，但这一诊断概念的有效性令人质疑，而且有些病例实际上为横纹肌肉瘤[413]。

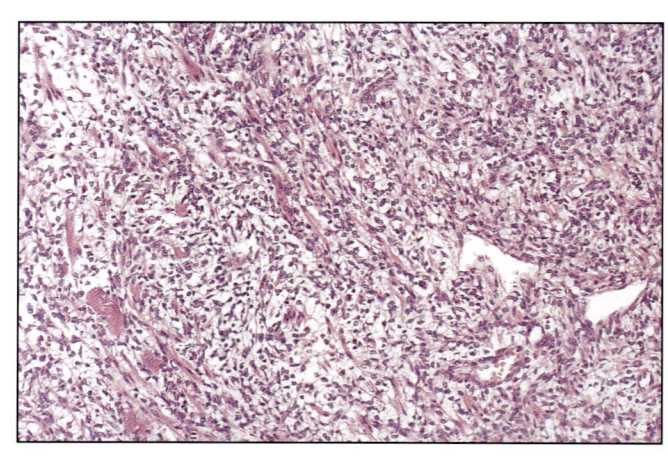

图24.89 胎儿横纹肌瘤。注意缺乏非典型性，并且向左下角方向呈进行性分化。

生殖器横纹肌瘤
Gentinal rhabdomyoma

生殖器横纹肌瘤[406,414]发生在中年女性的外阴、阴道或宫颈，呈孤立性息肉样病变。多数病例的病变小于3cm，没有局部复发倾向。组织学上，黏膜下出现细长、梭形或带状嗜酸性横纹肌母细胞增生，细胞核呈卵圆或细长（图24.90）。一般容易见到横纹，结蛋白和肌红蛋白呈强阳性。与葡萄状横纹肌肉瘤的区别在于：患者年龄、缺乏生发层和细胞核非典型性以及核分裂象。

横纹肌肉瘤　　Rhabdomyosarcoma

横纹肌肉瘤分类中所包含的恶性肿瘤出现原始骨骼肌分化的形态学、免疫组化、超微结构或分子遗传学表现，一般缺乏任何其他分化形式。出现异源性横纹肌肉瘤分化的肿瘤[415]在其各自章节中描述，以恶性müller混合瘤、恶性Triton肿瘤以及肾母细胞瘤为代表。

临床特征

依据目前定义，横纹肌肉瘤主要分为三大类：胚胎性、腺泡状和多形性，一般来说，前两者主要发生于儿童，而单纯的多形性病变几乎完全发生在成人。儿童横纹肌肉瘤[416-420]主要发生在10岁以前，高峰在4岁以前，男性有中度好发倾向。最常见部位是头颈部（包括眼眶和脑膜），其次是生殖道、四肢及躯干。一般情况下，胚胎性病变所累及的患者比腺泡性病变所累及的患者稍年轻，后者多见于青少年；四肢肿瘤中，腺泡性比胚胎性更常见。其他两种虽不常见但较特殊的临床特性为女性患者容易发生乳腺转移[421]，以及由于广泛骨髓受累而出现非常少见的、与白血病十分类似的表现，没有明确的原发病变[422]。病变的后一种表现代表了骨髓间叶性干细胞的恶性转化（"横纹肌母细胞血症"）。由于其解剖学上令人棘手的好发部位，使得多数儿童病例的病变不能完全切除，因此在过去的25年中进行了有效的放疗和化疗。将用于肿瘤切除以及肿瘤扩散程度的临床分类IRS系统考虑在内[417,420,423]，总体5年生存率现已达到70%，在所有儿童横纹肌肉瘤病例中，现在据说几乎50%可以治愈，这是25年来所取得的明显进步。葡萄状和梭形细胞性胚胎性横纹肌肉瘤（见下文）有极好的预后，5年生存率超过90%，但即使出现局灶的腺泡状结构，存活率也会降低。儿童横纹肌肉瘤治疗后复发也是预后不良的标志[424]。

与之相比，成人横纹肌肉瘤[342,343,425-428]主要发生在四肢，不论组织学类型如何，化疗敏感性似乎稍差，5年生存率仅为20%左右。此年龄组中，多形性亚型的数量明显超过胚胎性和腺泡性病变的数量，尽管后两者也可发生。从总体比例上，成人病例不超过10%。

组织学特征

胚胎性横纹肌肉瘤大约占儿童病例的60%，其经典型由小圆形或梭形未分化（嗜碱性）细胞构成，在黏液性间质中混有数量不等的圆形、带状或蝌蚪状嗜酸性横纹肌母细胞（图24.91）。不超过20%～30%的病例具有胞浆内横纹，但即使在几乎没有可识别的横纹肌母细胞的肿瘤当中，95%以上的病例结蛋白和肌肉肌动蛋白免疫染色呈阳性[429,430]（图24.92），因此这是常规诊断最为可靠的方法。另外，特殊肌源性细胞核转录因子蛋白产物的特异性抗体，即MyoD1和肌细胞生成素(myf4)[431-433]极为有用，尽管肌细胞生成素(myf4)染色常常更为清晰和可靠，但与腺泡型相比，阳性肿瘤细胞所占比例较小。个别病例（胚胎型多于腺泡型）出现明显的胞浆分化，化疗后出现更为显著的横纹肌母细胞性表现[434,435]。

葡萄状横纹肌肉瘤只是代表胚胎性肿瘤的一个解剖学亚型，发生在黏膜表面下方，呈外生性葡萄样生长方式。这些肿瘤的特征是50%或更多的病例存在于

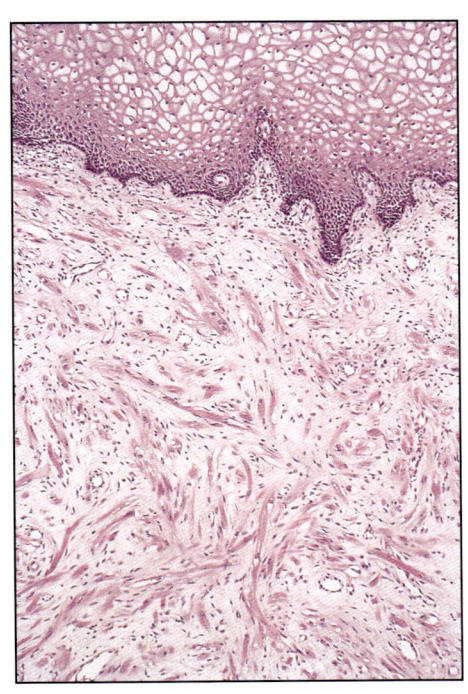

图24.90　生殖器横纹肌瘤。此阴道病变中，细长横纹肌母细胞成分较明显。

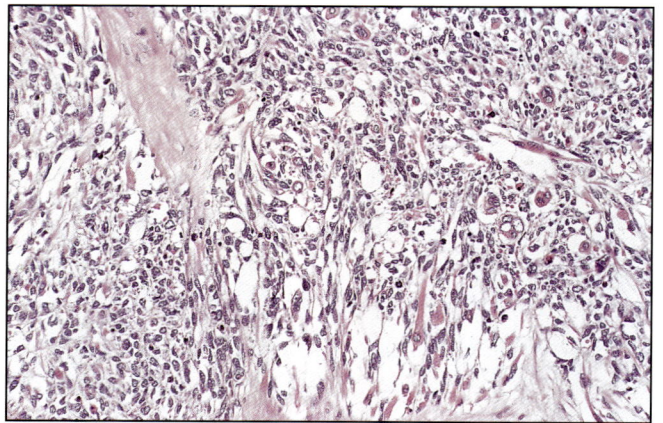

图24.91 胚胎性横纹肌肉瘤。此例中嗜酸性横纹肌母细胞容易识别。

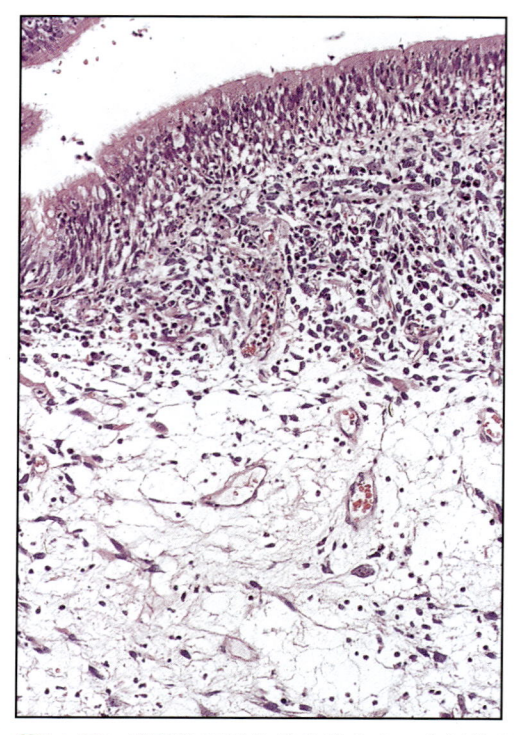

图24.93 葡萄状胚胎性横纹肌肉瘤。此例幼儿息肉样鼻腔肿瘤出现独特的黏膜下富于细胞区（生发层）。

上皮下生发层，由密集的相对未分化的肿瘤细胞构成（图24.93）。

间变性横纹肌肉瘤[436]目前更多用于儿童多形性病例，胶原性间质中至少局部存在片状奇异性细胞，伴有巨大细胞核和非典型核分裂象；此类病例常常也可见到胚胎性或少数腺泡性病灶，预后相对较差。也存在伴有胞浆内玻璃样（"横纹肌样"）包涵体的横纹肌肉瘤[437]；需要与所谓的"横纹肌样"肿瘤鉴别，其预后与普通型横纹肌肉瘤相同，比"横纹肌样"肿瘤好得多（见1581页）。

腺泡状横纹肌肉瘤[430,438,439]：一般特征为较大、较圆的未分化细胞，细胞核比胚胎型的大，混以数量不等的嗜酸性横纹肌母细胞以及多核巨细胞的细胞核位于周边（环状）（图24.94）；这些细胞大多排列成腺泡状结构，使其沿胶原间隔呈线性排列或覆盖胶原间隔，并且容易失去黏附"脱落"进入腺泡腔中央。只有不超过10%的病例可见横纹。早已明确，伴有明显腺泡状结构的肿瘤具有侵袭性行为，然而，重要的是也已明确[440,441]，当肿瘤出现实性胚胎样生长结构时（图24.95），其细胞（和细胞核）大于胚胎型的，原有腺泡状结构可通过网织纤维染色来证实，有预后明显降低的作用，即所谓的"实性型"腺泡状横纹肌肉瘤。尽管不常见，腺泡状病例也可出现间变特征或横纹肌样包涵体，与上面胚胎性肿瘤中所述相同。个别病例也可出现容易令人误解的透明细胞表现[442,443]。免疫组化方面，腺泡状横纹肌肉瘤

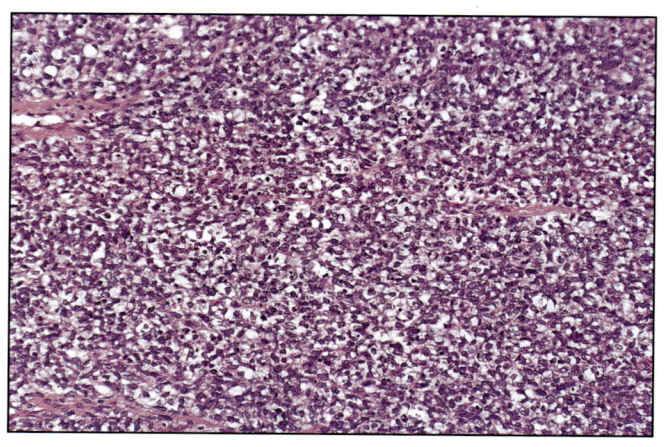

A

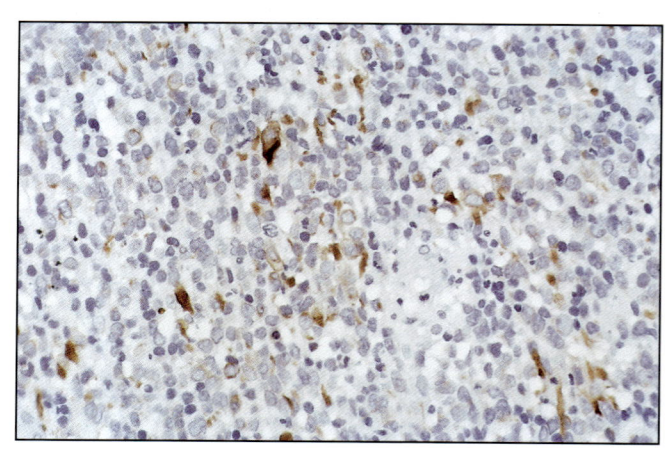

B

图24.92 胚胎性横纹肌肉瘤。此例分化较差（A），结蛋白仍然呈强阳性（B），后者具有辅助诊断意义。ABC法。

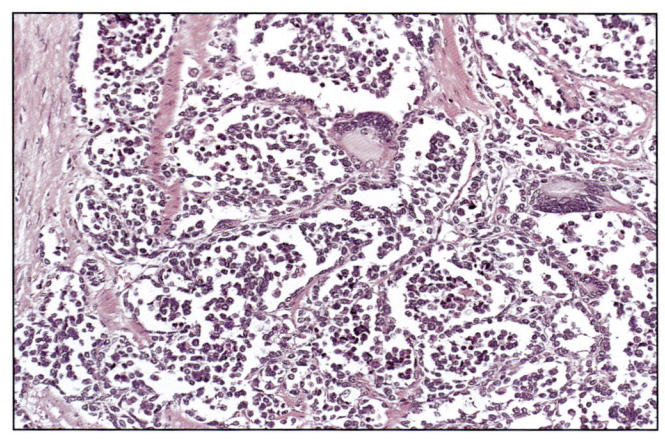

图24.94 腺泡状横纹肌肉瘤。经典病例出现典型纤维间隔和花环样多核细胞。

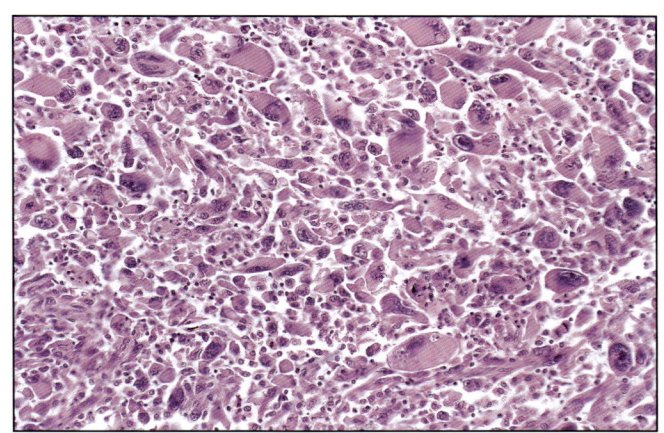

图24.96 多形性胚胎性横纹肌肉瘤。病变无结构排列，由大的奇异形横纹肌母细胞构成。

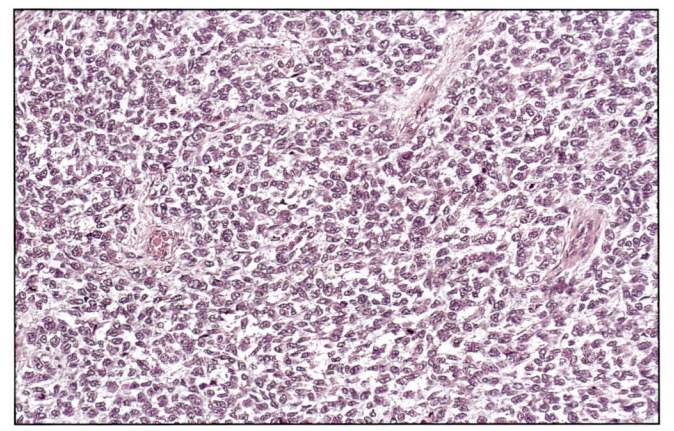

图24.95 实性型腺泡状横纹肌肉瘤。注意其细胞大于胚胎性病变的。也有轻度纤维分隔。

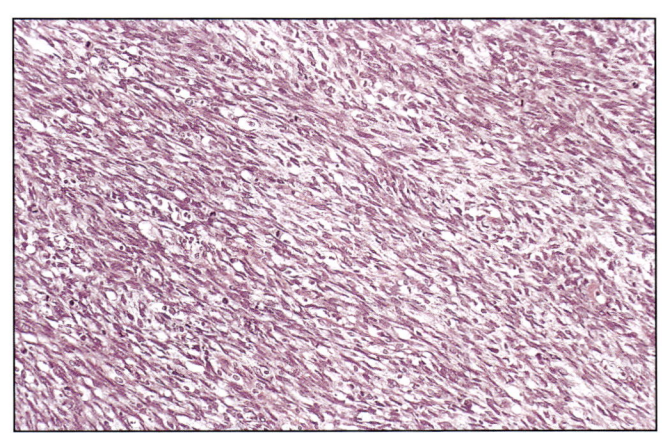

图24.97 梭形细胞横纹肌肉瘤。此附睾肿瘤可被误认为是纤维肉瘤或神经鞘肿瘤。

的多数肿瘤细胞常常表现为肌细胞生成素(myf4)呈弥漫强阳性[432,433]。

多形性横纹肌肉瘤[342,343,444] 依据目前定义，为高级别多形性肉瘤，主要由无排列结构的奇异形大多角或梭形横纹肌母细胞构成，背景为数量不等的胶原性间质（图24.96）。有些肿瘤呈明显的席纹状，与所谓的多形性MFH极为类似。完全见不到横纹。儿童病例中，在其他区域几乎总能见到至少为小灶状的胚胎性或（少数）腺泡状肿瘤成分，"间变性"一词多指此类肿瘤（见上文），极少数纯粹多形性肿瘤病例也在这个年龄组[445]。确诊最好依据结蛋白、fast myosin和(或)肌细胞生成素(myf4)免疫染色，适当结合电镜。

梭形细胞横纹肌肉瘤[446,447] 传统上被认为是胚胎型的一个亚型，但没有明确的遗传学资料将这一亚型与胚胎性或腺泡状病变联系起来。此型主要发生在附睾区，头颈部不常见，其主要特征为嗜酸性梭形细胞排列成束状（图24.97）或席纹状结构，至少在儿童，5年生存率超过90%。这些病变可极其类似于其他类型的束状梭形细胞肉瘤，包括恶性外周神经鞘瘤。类似病变可见于成人[448]，主要位于头颈部区域，在此年龄组似乎并不具有预后优势。

硬化性横纹肌肉瘤[449-451] 是新近识别的一种特殊亚型，准确的疾病学分类还不清楚，因为在遗传学上与胚胎性或腺泡状亚型无关。这些肿瘤可发生在成人或儿童，四肢和头颈部最常见。这些肿瘤主要由原始样梭形、卵圆形或圆形细胞构成，常常有假血管裂隙，背景是显著玻璃样的胶原性间质。可以见到小灶明显的横纹肌母细胞分化。作者已经见到过一些病例，具有这些与梭形细胞横纹肌肉瘤无法区别的区域，这两种少见类型似乎极有可能具有相关性。

用以证实和精确横纹肌肉瘤诊断的分子遗传学方法近来已取得了巨大进展，尤其是在儿童肿瘤中心，并已成为标准化服务[441,452-455]。这里简单概括一下，从细胞遗传学角度，腺泡状横纹肌肉瘤携带（在多数病例中）可复制的肿瘤特殊染色质易位，即 t(2;13)(q35;q14)，导致 PAX3-FOXO1 融合；少数病例出现变异性易位，即 t(1;13)(q36;q14)，导致 PAX7-FOXO1 融合（见表 24.1）。这些异常在核型上与胚胎性横纹肌肉瘤中常见的 11 号染色体断臂缺失差别很大。可通过经典核型、RT-PCR 或原位杂交荧光等方法将这些差异应用于诊断。此外，携带 PAX7-FOXO1 融合基因的肿瘤，即使有转移，其预后也好于携带 PAX3-FOXO1 融合基因的病例[456]。总体上，年轻人的小圆细胞肿瘤的诊断在过去 20 年间已发生了转变。此时，免疫组织化学和更新的分子遗传学在很大程度上取代了 HE 形态学，因为一般来说，这些方法的结果判定更加一致，在治疗方案存在明显不同的情况下很必要。

软骨-骨肿瘤 Chondro-osseous tumors

软组织软骨瘤、间叶性软骨肉瘤（骨组织比软组织更常见）、骨化性肌炎以及进展性骨化性纤维结构不良等都在第 25 章描述。现在认为，骨外黏液样软骨肉瘤为不明分化系，与软骨无关，在 1580 页讨论。

动脉瘤样骨囊肿 Aneurysmal bone cyst

病变与骨的动脉瘤样骨囊肿基本相同（见第 25 章），目前认为偶尔可发生在软组织[457,458]。主要发生于肢端深部软组织，一般见于成人，特征是外层一圈成熟骨组织围绕出血囊腔，间隔以细胞数量不等的纤维性间隔，其中含有破骨性巨细胞，局灶可见编织骨。与骨的相应病变相同，目前认为这些病变为克隆性肿瘤，多数病例具有特征性的 17p13 染色体 USP6 基因重排[459]，此遗传学事件在继发性动脉瘤样骨囊肿中从未见到。

皮肤骨瘤 Osteoma cutis

皮肤的骨性结节绝大多数为先前病变继发性骨化的结果，尤其是毛母质瘤和黑色素细胞痣[460]。确有极少数病人出现组织学上由成熟骨构成的皮肤多发性结节，发病机制不清[461,462]，尽管有些病例与长期寻常型痤疮或假性甲状腺功能不全有关；脸部是最常见的部位[463]。尽管骨化生常见于多种软组织肿瘤，但深部软组织没有发现原发性骨瘤。

骨外骨肉瘤 Extraskeletal osteosarcoma

临床特征

原发于软组织的骨肉瘤[464-468]大约占所有骨肉瘤的 5%，主要累及 51～80 岁的成年人，男性稍多见。大部分病例发生在四肢，尤其是股部，但其解剖学分布广泛。大约 15% 的病例发生在先前受伤或受照射的部位。多数病例具有侵袭和转移的临床过程，整体 5 年死亡率为 60%～70%，尽管治疗上应用与年轻骨病患者相同的化疗方案有效[469]。然而，老年人常常不能耐受这样的强化治疗方案，可能会减少有效治疗的机会。

病理学特征

骨肉瘤的形态学特征在第 25 章有详细描述。在软组织病变中，最常见的类型为 MFH 样，少数为骨母细胞性。软组织中软骨母细胞性骨肉瘤相对不常见[466]，毛细血管扩张型也不常见[466,470]。如果识别确切的骨样基质存在问题，有些作者已经发现碱性磷酸酶染色[468]（与普通骨肿瘤同样）或免疫组织化学染色显示鲑鱼降钙素[471]可有帮助。富于巨细胞的病变亚型先前认为是巨细胞 MFH（见 1561 页），从逻辑上可能被划归为骨肉瘤，具有与其他类型骨肉瘤相类似的临床病理学特征。

其他良性病变 Miscellaneous benign lesions

黏液瘤 Myxoma

"黏液瘤"一词不应该宽泛地用于描述几乎所有良性、细胞稀少的胶样肿瘤。多数此类病变可重复再分类，以便更为可靠地预测临床行为[472]。不精心的"非特殊型黏液瘤"诊断其主要危险在于对低级别恶性病变的识别，尤其是低级别黏液纤维肉瘤或黏液样脂肪肉瘤。

肌内黏液瘤[473-477]或许是这个组别中最好定义的病变。主要累及 30～70 岁成人，女性中等程度好发。多数病例表现为生长缓慢的无痛性肿物，位于股部肌肉或下肢肢带。不常累及上肢；个别病例可发生在其他部位。大约 5% 的病人出现多发性病变，病变下方骨组织通常伴有纤维结构不良[474,478]，被称为 Mazabraud 综合征。孤立散发性病变患者也可出现放射性骨异常[479]。局部单纯切除后，极少复发，复发病例不足 5%。组织学上识别这些病变常常依据细胞稀少和轻度富于血管（图 24.98）。肿瘤细胞小，良性，梭形或星形，细胞核小而深染，细胞浆不甚明显。常可见极少数含有黏液或（少数）

脂质的微泡状细胞。没有多形性或核分裂象。这些细胞均匀分布于透明质酸背景当中，周边局灶性伸入肌纤维之间。肿瘤区域可含有少量呈疏松束状排列的胶原。实际上多数病例缺乏血管成分，可以排除黏液样脂肪肉瘤和黏液纤维肉瘤，缺乏多形性也有助于除外后者。S-100蛋白呈阴性有助于排除黏液样神经纤维瘤或低级别恶性外周神经鞘瘤。**富于细胞性黏液瘤**[480]一词是指该病变比"经典"肌内黏液瘤具有更为丰富的细胞和血管成分（图24.99）[477,480]，尽管它们代表了形态学连续性改变的关键点。这一亚型有时可位于皮下。此类肿瘤中没有低级别黏液纤维肉瘤的细胞核非典型性和深染。尽管这些细胞较丰富的病变以前被称为"伴有复发潜能的低级别黏液性肿瘤"，但局部复发似乎非常少见[480]。从生物学方面来看，值得注意的是，肌内黏液瘤隐含 *GNAS1* 突变[481]，与纤维结构不良所见相似。

关节旁黏液瘤[482]一词用于描述一组不常见的发生于大关节附近的胶样病变，尤其是膝部。此类病变主要累及中年男性，与肌内黏液瘤相比，常有局部复发。组织学方面，病变类似于富于细胞的黏液瘤（见上文），尽管值得注意的是这些病变缺乏 *GNAS1* 突变[483]。有些病例最初被描述为与低级别黏液纤维肉瘤有重叠。有限的资料表明，这些病变也为克隆性（肿瘤性）病变[484]。

指（趾）部纤维黏液瘤也称为浅表性肢端纤维黏液瘤[72,485]，病变不常见，表现为指（趾）部小结节，一般见于成人手或足，男性稍多。甲周最多见。病变为边界不清的真皮内病变，由无结构排列的增生性良性纤维母细胞构成，背景是数量不等的胶原或黏液样基质（图24.100）。过去称为指（趾）部黏液样或黏液性囊肿的病变，代表了同种病变的特殊黏液类型。非破坏性的局部复发十分常见。

浅表性血管黏液瘤[486-488]主要累及成人，大多见于头颈部、躯干或外阴阴道区域，表现为浅表性生长缓慢的结节，直径一般小于3～4cm。局部复发常见，并可反复复发，除非切除病变且切缘干净。最常累及真皮和皮下，组织学上由多结节、境界不清的黏液性肿物构成，其中可见散在的肥胖梭形和星形纤维母细胞，有大量薄壁血管以及炎细胞成分，具有特征性的中性粒细胞，不伴有坏死和溃疡（图24.101）。可见个别核分裂象，但缺乏多形性，尽管个别病例可出现细胞核轻度深染，但其有可能是退行性的。高达1/3的病例含有陷入的、多有增生的上皮性成分，原发或复发性病变均可出现，大多包含表皮样囊肿、纤细的鳞状细胞条索或小团基底样细胞出芽。这被认为是反映了陷入附属器结构的诱导性结果。任何部位的多发浅表性血管黏液瘤或外耳[489]或乳

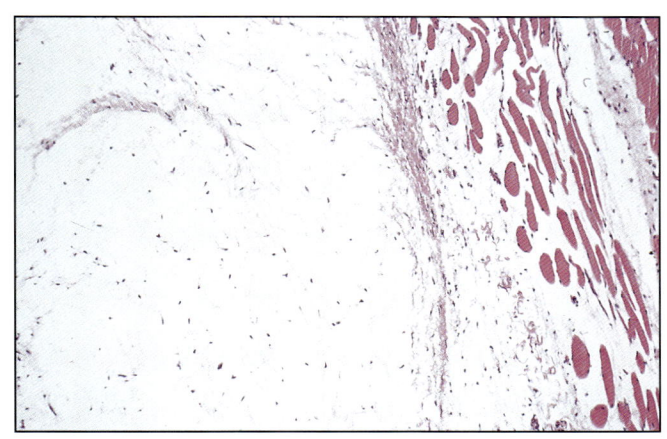

图24.98　肌内黏液瘤。注意事实上缺乏血管，细胞核没有异型。

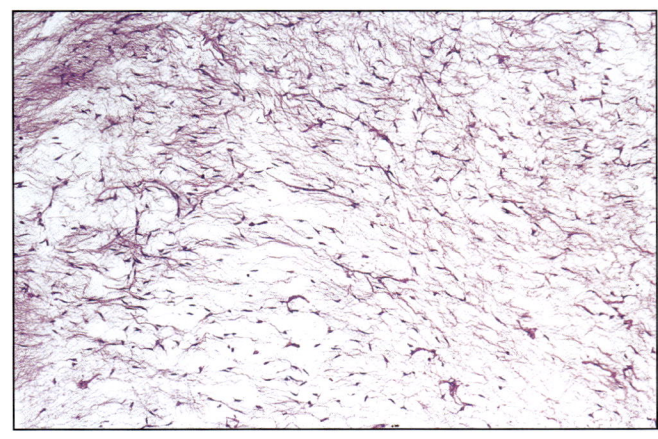

图24.99　富于细胞性黏液瘤。细胞学良性的病变比肌内黏液瘤具有更丰富的细胞和血管成分。

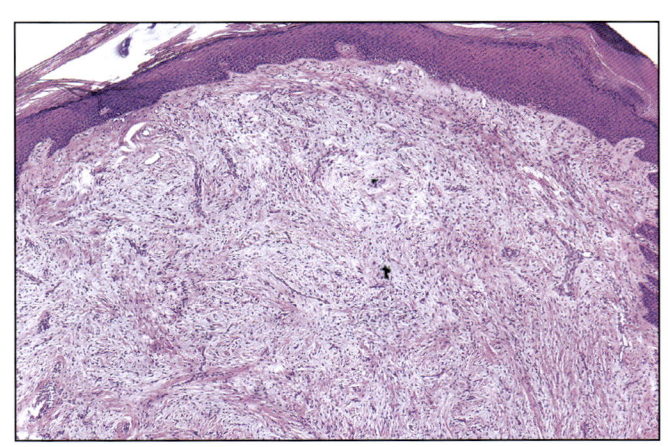

图24.100　指（趾）部纤维黏液瘤。无结构排列的纤维母细胞增生，伴有数量不等的黏液或胶原性基质。

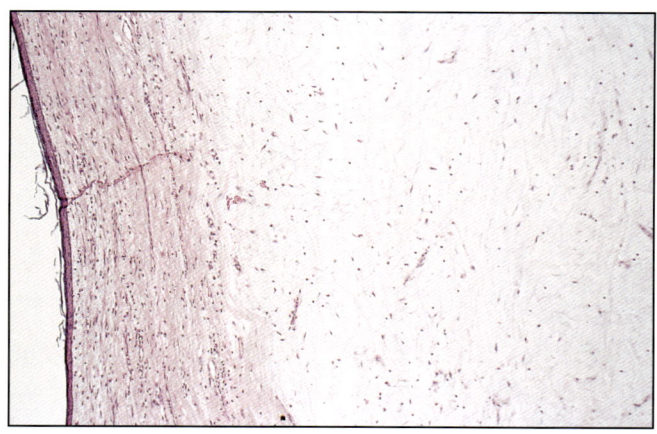
图24.101　浅表性血管黏液瘤。典型的细胞稀少的真皮病变，其中可见一个表皮样囊肿（左）。

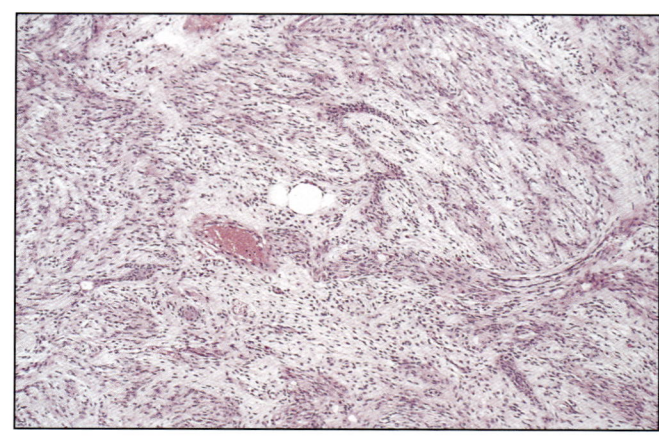
图24.102　异位性错构瘤性胸腺瘤。上皮性索条和散在的脂肪细胞与显著的均一性梭形细胞成分关系密切。

腺[490]发生的组织学上类似的孤立性病变，均与Carney综合征关系密切，可能处于较危险的病变之前，其中以心脏黏液瘤最为重要。

侵袭性血管黏液瘤[200,491,492]最常发生在成年女性的外阴或盆腔，往往很大，大概30%的病例有局部复发，虽然一般不会再次复发。第13章对此有比较详细的描述，但重要的是，极少数类似病变也会发生在男性盆腔[493,494]。不论性别如何，个别病例可出现与血管肌纤维母细胞瘤重叠的特征。

异位性错构瘤性胸腺瘤
Ectopic hamartomatous thymoma

异位性错构瘤性胸腺瘤[495-497]放在这里而不是胸腺章节是因为：病变发生在软组织，常与滑膜肉瘤或神经鞘瘤混淆。这种病变通常被认为是发生错位的鳃囊衍生物（正常发生在胸腺组织），尽管有些作者提出了鳃裂始基肌上皮性分化[497]。病变发生在成人，男性为主，表现为胸骨上或锁骨上区生长缓慢的筋膜下隆起。不易复发。

多数病例的病变为5cm或更小，界限清楚。组织学方面，由不同比例的良性梭形细胞构成，胞浆淡染，细胞核两端细长，排列成束状，混有成熟脂肪组织岛和第三种上皮性成分（图24.102）。后者由索条状、管状或腺体构成，上皮成分为非角化鳞状上皮，立方性或明显腺性。所有三种成分在细胞学上均为良性，通常缺乏核分裂象。梭形细胞成分角蛋白广泛呈强阳性。角蛋白染色程度远远超过滑膜肉瘤中所见，也可与神经鞘瘤区别开。

尿磷酸盐增多性的间叶性肿瘤
Phosphaturic mesenchymal tumor

尿磷酸盐增多性的间叶性肿瘤是一个临床病理病变，多数通过其伴有的由磷酸盐尿所致的肿瘤源性骨质软化而容易确诊[498,499]，然而，后者并非恒定不变，形态学相同的病变可以没有任何生化异常。多数受累患者为长期骨质软化的成人（没有性别差异），出现软组织肿瘤或少数骨肿瘤。病变分布广泛，四肢最常见。病变切除后，磷酸盐尿可以治愈，多数病例为良性过程，仅有个别病例复发。极个别可以发生转移。

组织学上，许多病例有些类似于肌纤维瘤/肌血管外皮细胞瘤，常有分枝状薄壁血管，而其他特点是几乎都存在蓝色无定形或颗粒状钙化，常见破骨巨细胞反应。此外，可见局灶软骨分化和编织骨形成。间质出血常见，但坏死并非常见特征，核分裂象稀少。具有磷酸盐尿属性的纤维母细胞生长因子-23（FGF23），在多数肿瘤中有表达[499]。

含铁血黄素性纤维脂肪瘤性肿瘤
Hemosiderotic fibrolipomatous tumor

含铁血黄素性纤维脂肪瘤性肿瘤也被称为含铁血黄素性纤维组织细胞脂肪瘤性病变，是一种不明细胞系的少见肿瘤，几乎都表现为成人踝/足部肿物[500,501]。儿童病例极少见。这些病变有时复发，但不具有破坏性。有些作者提出这种肿瘤为多形性玻璃样变性血管扩张性肿瘤的前期病变（见下文）[502]，但还有争议。

组织学上，病变由不同比例的成熟脂肪细胞和均一的纤维母细胞性梭形细胞混合而成，后者在脂肪中呈束状、旋涡状或蜂窝状结构，伴有明显的含铁血黄素沉积。

梭形细胞成分可伴有散在的破骨性巨细胞。极少数病例可出现局灶细胞核非典型和多形性，其生物学意义目前还不明确。免疫组化对诊断没有帮助。

中间性生物学潜能的其他病变
Miscellaneous lesions of intermediate biologic potential

骨化性纤维黏液样肿瘤
Ossifying fibromyxoid tumor

临床特征

骨化性纤维黏液样肿瘤[503-507]是一个相对较新、具有特征性的肿瘤，尽管总体的部位和年龄分布广泛，但主要表现为中老年人（男性为主）的四肢皮下结节。病变的一种亚型部位较深。切除不完全可有局部复发。有些病例伴有明确的系统性扩散[507,508]，但这些病变有微小的组织学差异（见下文）。

病理学特征

这些病变界限清楚，多结节性，常有厚的纤维被膜，直径通常小于5cm。肿瘤由分叶状圆形细胞构成，胞浆淡染或嗜酸，单一形态的圆形或卵圆形泡状细胞核，在含有多量薄壁血管的黏液样基质中呈条索或花边样带状排列（图24.103）。通常缺乏核分裂象。小叶结构被纤维间隔分隔。在纤维性被膜内，有时也在间隔内，至少有75%的病例中存在成熟的板层骨壳（图24.104）。这种骨成分有时只在广泛取材后方可发现，其周围常常围有薄层的良性骨母细胞。还不清楚对于明显缺乏骨的病例这是代表真正的非骨化类型还是由于取材误差所

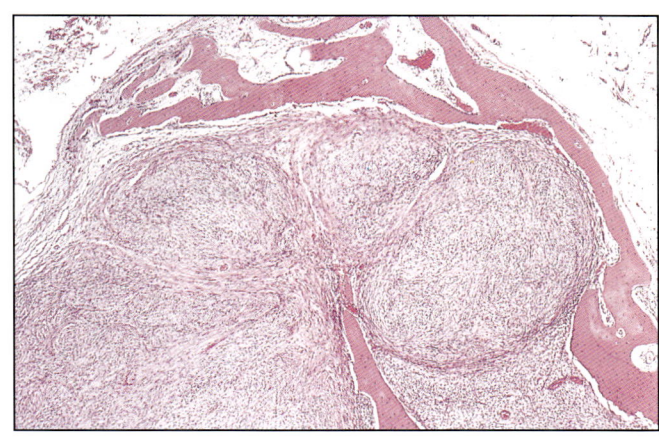

图24.104　骨化性纤维黏液样肿瘤。注意特殊的板层骨圈。

致。免疫组化[505-507]显示，大约80%的病例S-100蛋白呈阳性，50%～60%的病例结蛋白呈阳性，同时大约50%的病例SMA呈阳性。电镜出现特殊的随机分布的中间丝、短的细胞突起以及一般较厚、常有重叠但不连续的外板。精确的分化系还不清楚，但肌上皮分化似乎有可能[509]。

有少数病例尽管具有典型结构和细胞学特征，但骨性成分的分布更为不规则，并且显然置于肿瘤细胞下方[508]。其他病例也可出现细胞丰富程度、细胞核异型以及核分裂活性的增加[506,508]。由于其免疫表型和超微结构与普通病例相同，因此这些病变被称为"非典型"或"恶性"骨化性纤维黏液样肿瘤，其中有些病例出现反复复发和肺转移更加支持这一观点。

软组织肌上皮瘤/混合瘤
Soft tissue myoepithelima / mixed tumor

发生在非皮肤软组织的肌上皮病变最近才得以明确[510,512]，可能是因为陈旧的组织发生概念已基本上排除了这种可能性。实际上，这些病变似乎并不罕见（但以前被误认为是黏液样软骨肉瘤或是隐性转移），在1997年初一项相对小量的病例研究报告发表之后，作者目前已经见过另外150例以上的病例，提示病理医生很愿意做出这种诊断。这些肿瘤可累及所有年龄组，但最常见于50岁之前；一个重要亚型（大约10%）发生在幼儿。四肢（包括手和足）是最常见部位，尽管多数病例的病变位于皮下，但高达35%的病例病变位于肌内或筋膜下。与涎腺的相应肿瘤相同，大约15%～20%的病例有局部复发，经验表明，有10%～15%的病例最终出现转移，虽然多数病变具有非典型细胞学特征（见下文）。

组织学上，软组织的肌上皮病变（图24.105）出现与涎腺同样宽泛的谱系（见第7章）。混合瘤和肌上

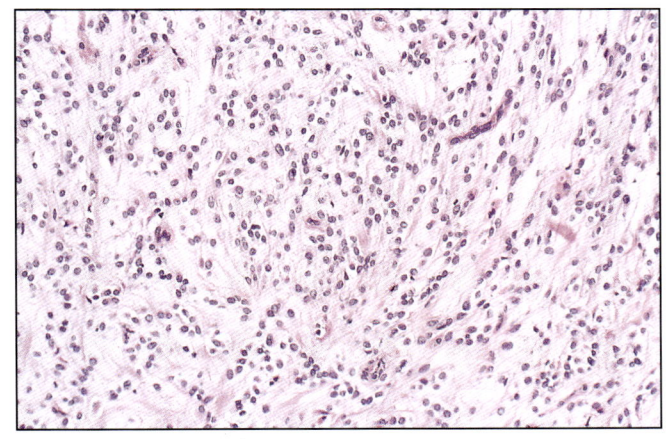

图24.103　骨化性纤维黏液样肿瘤。典型的均一性圆形细胞呈线性排列，分布于纤维黏液样间质内。

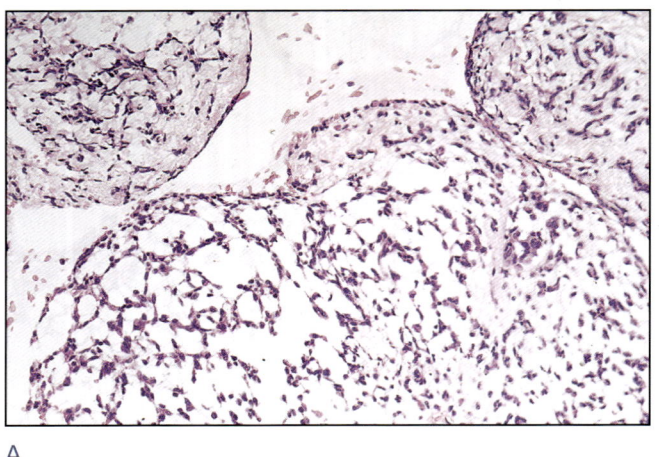 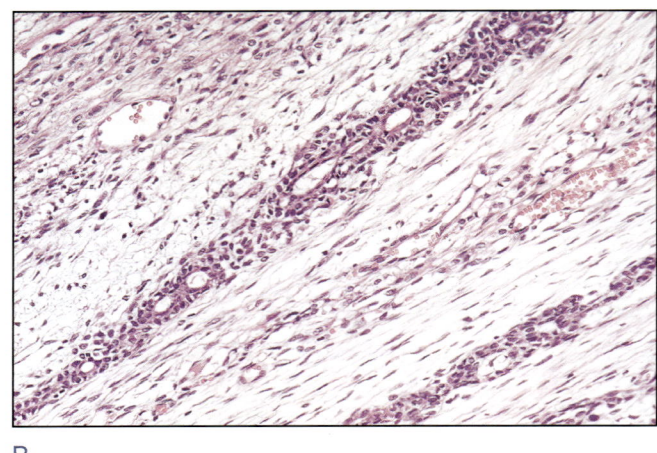

图24.105 肌上皮瘤/混合瘤。许多病例与骨外黏液样软骨肉瘤极为类似（A）。如果出现导管/结构（B），是有用的鉴别特征。

皮瘤之间的唯一（其有效性存在疑问）区别是存在导管成分，见于15%~20%的病例。黏液样/软骨黏液样组织和上皮性/肌上皮性成分的相对比例变化很大：大约10%~15%的病例出现明显的软骨-分化，极少数病例出现脂肪细胞分化。个别病例与涎腺病变一样，具有明显的癌或肉瘤转化，但侵袭性潜能比较常见的线索是：细胞核异型或明显的核仁。核分裂象和边缘的特征并不能判断预后。免疫组织化学方面，多数（但并非全部）病例角蛋白呈阳性，几乎90%的病例S-100蛋白呈阳性，大约45%的病例GFAP呈阳性[512]。多数病例calponin染色呈阳性，而EMA为60%着色，SMA仅有20%~25%呈阳性。S-100的一致阳性得以与多数转移癌（除了可能的乳腺肿瘤）鉴别，黏液样软骨肉瘤角蛋白呈阳性，常见上皮样细胞形态学表现，以及有些病变存在导管成分。

副脊索瘤[513-515]是一种令人难以理解的肿瘤，还没有被确认是一种"疾病"。尽管其部分形态学表现与脊索瘤重叠，但它与后者之间在局部解剖、临床以及免疫组化方面存在重要差异。相比之下，它与肌上皮瘤/混合瘤基本上不能鉴别，除了肿瘤细胞胞浆多为明显空泡状以外[512]，目前WHO分类[215]也认为其是肌上皮瘤的一个亚型。

外胚间质软骨黏液样肿瘤[516]在第7章有比较全面的描述。这个病变最常见于舌部，但也可以发生在口腔的其他部位，也被认为是肌上皮瘤的一个亚型。

血管瘤样MFH（所谓的）
Angiomatoid MFH (so-called)

毋庸置疑，血管瘤样MFH是一种特殊的明确病变，与其家族中其他成员的明显区别在于：它所累及的年龄组较小[517]。然而，这些病变的分化系还不清楚。

临床上，所谓的血管瘤样MFH最常见于儿童或青少年，没有性别差异，常常发生在浅表软组织，四肢比躯干更常见[517-520]，然而，总体年龄范围广，少部分病例位置较深。一小部分但重要的患者伴发系统性特征，如发热、贫血、体重减轻或异常蛋白血症，这些症状在肿瘤切除后可以消失。多数病例位于皮下，通常小于3~4cm。切除后，局部复发率是10%~15%，但不超过1%~2%的患者发生淋巴结或系统转移，肿瘤相关性死亡极为少见。鉴于此原因，在目前WHO分类中，这个肿瘤被认为是"中间性，很少转移"[215]。

病理学方面，病变为界限清楚、多结节状囊性肿物，常有广泛出血。组织学上[517-520]，肿瘤由多结节和成片的良性、嗜酸性、卵圆形到梭形的细胞构成，伴有一致的泡状、有些梭形的细胞核，核分裂象不常见（图24.106）。除了个别病例之外，细胞核轻度多形性，巨细胞少见。这些结节分布于胶原性间质中，常有显著的含铁血黄素沉着以及明显的淋巴浆细胞浸润，可类似于

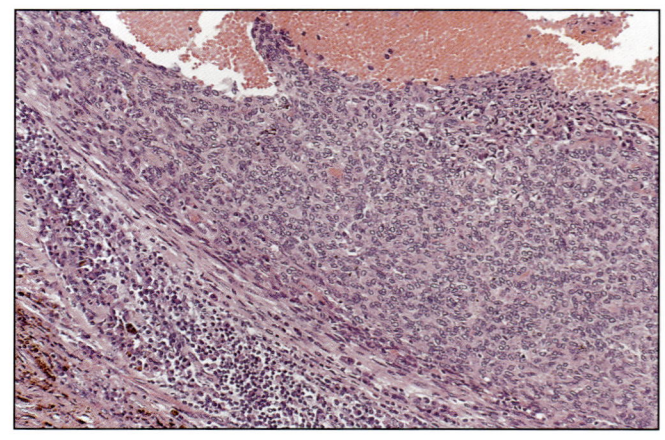

图24.106 血管瘤样"MFH"。良性嗜酸性细胞伴有出血和淋巴浆细胞浸润。

淋巴结。这种结构可以发生变化，在有些病例中，炎症或充满血液的腔隙可不明显甚或缺乏；偶尔腔隙中缺乏内皮被覆，只含有嗜酸性蛋白液。免疫组化方面[520-522]，100例以上的个人经验提示，大约40%～50%的嗜酸性肿瘤细胞结蛋白呈阳性（图24.107），EMA和肌肉肌动蛋白（HHF-35）（而非SMA）许多为阳性；CD68一般为阳性，尽管其特异性值得怀疑。在许多病例报告中，电镜检查显示了相互矛盾和不确定性结果。目前，这些病变从本质上最有可能是黏液性的，从形态学和临床特征方面，肿瘤细胞极有可能向所谓的"纤维母细胞性网织细胞"和正常情况下可见于淋巴结的黏液样细胞分化。一个值得注意的新进展已经明确，这些病变的特征为具有一致性的 *ATF1* 基因重排[523,524]，大多伴有（12;16）易位。鉴别诊断主要包括动脉瘤样良性纤维组织细胞瘤，该肿瘤通常更为表浅，细胞学更具多形性，且结蛋白呈阴性（见第23章）。个别病例可与梭形细胞血管内皮瘤或结节性Kaposi肉瘤混淆，但应该容易区分（见第3章）。

多形性玻璃样血管扩张性肿瘤
Pleomorphic hyalinizing angiectatic tumor

多形性玻璃样血管扩张性肿瘤（PHAT）是一种少见而有些争议的肿瘤[502,525]，主要发生在成人下肢的皮下组织。临床上可类似血肿或血管肿瘤。尽管其组织学形态令人担忧，但到目前为止，已经发布的病例表明，某仅有局部复发趋势，没有转移的报道。组织学上，肿瘤境界表现不一，或为浸润性病变，由成团的扩张薄壁血管构成，管壁有明显的纤维蛋白样变性（有时为玻璃样变性），常常伴有血栓形成。所涉及的间质组织含有数量不等的梭形和奇异性多角形或多核细胞（图24.108），出现明显细胞核多形性和深染，常伴

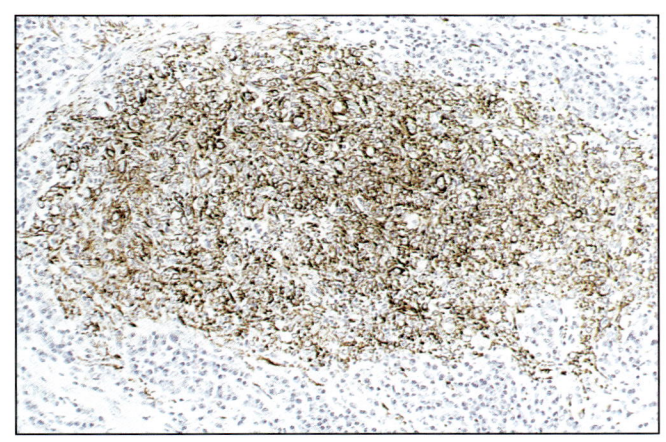

图24.107　血管瘤样"MFH"。多数病例出现明确结蛋白阳性。ABC法。

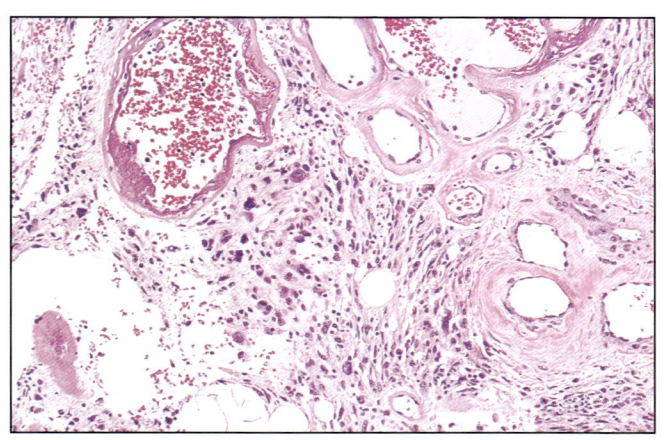

图24.108　多形性玻璃样血管扩张性肿瘤。注意纤维蛋白样及玻璃样变血管之间的奇异形肿瘤细胞。

有胞核内的假包涵体。通常缺乏核分裂象，发现核分裂象应及时重新评估诊断。在有些病例中，这些奇异形细胞CD34呈阳性，但更具特异性分化的标记物为阴性，如S-100蛋白。S-100蛋白呈阴性和多形性程度有助于排除古老的Schwann细胞瘤。所谓的"共质性"（symplastic）血管瘤[526]也需要进行鉴别诊断，但是通常具有更为经典的血管瘤性表现，其多形性程度比较有限。另一个重要的关注点在于，类似的纤维蛋白样血管改变在几乎所有肉瘤中都可以偶尔见到，尤其是下肢远端，这些病变容易误诊为PHAT。最后，作者已经见到过几个病例呈"典型"PHAT表现，后来复发为明确的黏液纤维肉瘤，其他作者也报道了同样的现象[527]。迄今为止，PHAT的精确疾病分类和生物学潜能还没有完全明确。

血管周围上皮样细胞肿瘤　PEComa

血管周围上皮样细胞肿瘤现在称为PEComa，代表一个肿瘤家族，最初是由Bonetti和Pea提出[528]，其特征是免疫组化染色具有肌黑色素细胞双重分化表现[215,529]。在一般分类中，病变包括血管肌脂肪瘤（和其上皮样的亚型）（见第12章）、透明细胞（"糖"）肿瘤（见第5章）以及淋巴管平滑肌瘤病（见第13章）。近年来已经明确，组织学上类似的病变可发生在许多部位[529,530]，包括腹内和躯体软组织以及多种器官，最主要为子宫和胃肠道。多数病例发生在成人，有非常显著的女性倾向。多数病例似乎具有良性过程（尽管迄今为止资料相对有限），也有少数亚型的形态学令人烦恼（见下文），可发生转移。

组织学上，除了上文提到的明确类型外，PEComa具有相当广泛的形态学表现，最常见的是巢状和上皮样（图24.109），但有时以梭形为主，个别极具多形性。

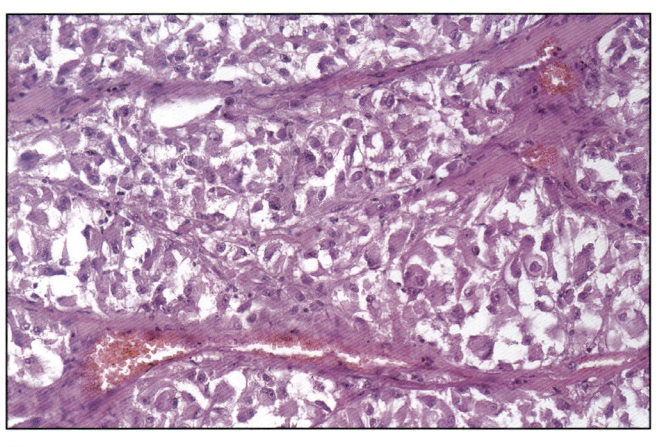 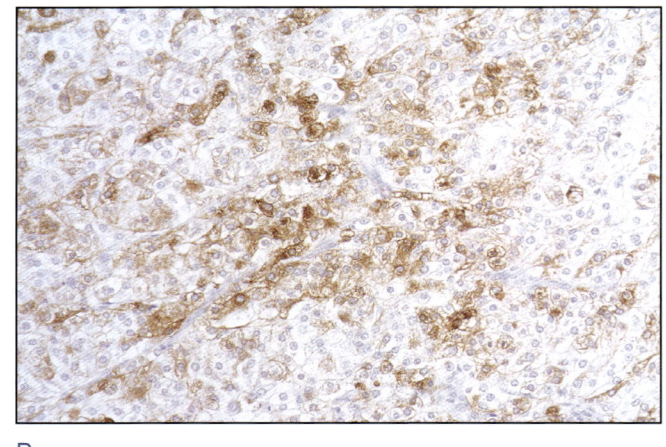

图24.109　PEComa。多数病例具有巢状上皮样形态学表现，伴有颗粒状胞浆（A）。黑色素小体相关抗原阳性为一致性表现，如HMB45。

肿瘤细胞通常具有颗粒状嗜酸性或透明胞浆，泡状细胞核，有时伴有明显的核仁。通常可见明显的薄壁分枝状血管结构，至少局灶性的肿瘤细胞围绕这些血管呈向心性排列方式，有些病例，尤其是腹膜后的病例，可以出现明显的间质玻璃样变性。少数出现明显异型或多形性，容易见到核分裂象，或坏死的病例具有恶性行为潜能。

免疫组织化学在这些病变的诊断中具有重要作用[529,530]，尤其是这些肿瘤几乎总是同时表达SMA和HMB-45，50%以上的病例Melan-A呈阳性（有时缺乏HMB-45），大约25%呈结蛋白呈阳性。有些病例S-100蛋白（可能与黑色素瘤相混淆）和TFE3也可着色。

其他恶性病变
Miscellaneous malignant lesions

在此标题下描述了多种分化系（或"组织发生"）的尚不明确的软组织肉瘤。读者可以参考第27章的骨外Ewing肉瘤/PNET和透明细胞肉瘤（软组织黑色素瘤）、第15章的腹内促结缔组织增生性小细胞肿瘤和第21章的结外型滤泡性树突细胞肉瘤。应该记住的是，即使在转诊中心，高达5%的软组织肉瘤仍然不能分类（因此生物学上常常不可预测）。

滑膜肉瘤
Synovial sarcoma

临床特征

滑膜肉瘤[531-536]可发生在任何年龄，但发病高峰在10～35岁之间；男性略多。解剖分布广泛，但60%以上的病例在下肢，尤其是股部。少数但重要的病例发生在躯干，尤其是腹壁[537]、颈部[538]、头部[539]（包括眼眶）[540]、纵隔[541]、甚至腹腔[542]。现已明确，肿瘤可原发于内脏许多部位，包括肺/胸膜（见第5章）、肾和胃肠道，在其他部位中，过去许多此类病例常被误诊为纤维肉瘤或血管外皮细胞瘤。极个别病例据报道可发生于血管内[543]、神经[544]或关节[545]，尽管许多病变发生于大关节结构附近，但已不再认为这些病变来源于（或与之真正相关）滑膜[546]。多数病变部位较深，大小差异较大。特殊的是，许多患者表现为长期疼痛，常常发生在能够触及肿物之前；即使在无疼痛的病例，许多患者术前也存在长期病史，长至10年或更长。放射学检查常常发现病变有钙化。总体5年生存可能性大约为60%～65%，但10年降到仅为30%左右。通常，肿瘤小（<5cm）、临床分期早、发病年龄小（<10岁）以及组织学分级较低（通过核分裂象和坏死来确定）是预后好的指标[547-549]。

组织学特征

滑膜肉瘤分为两大组：双相性和单相性梭形细胞。后者更为常见，依赖于取材。两种类型都具有梭形细胞成分，排列呈束状，细胞核均一，纺锤状，胞浆淡染，界限不清，背景是数量不等的胶原性间质，常常呈丝状或玻璃样表现（图24.110）。这些梭形细胞一般呈单一形态，具有数量不等的核分裂象，常伴有间质肥大细胞和分枝状血管外皮细胞瘤样血管结构（图24.111）。典型的双相病变含有数量不等的腺样结构，内衬高分化立方性或柱状上皮（图24.112）。其他双相病例更加隐蔽（"隐匿"），但可以通过存在较肥胖和

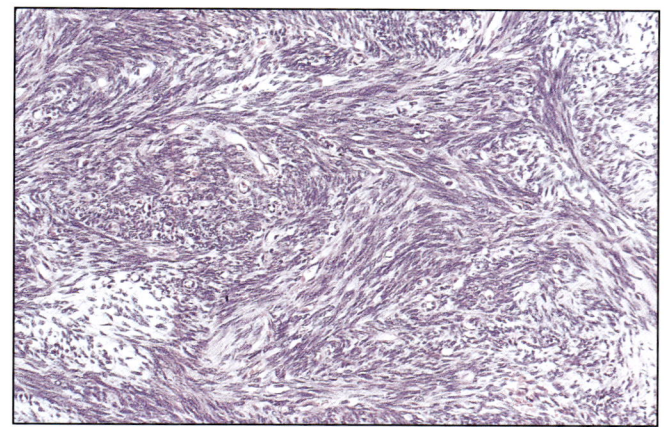

图24.110 单相型滑膜肉瘤。除了粉色胶原性间质，束状梭形细胞肿瘤类似于神经鞘肉瘤（恶性神经鞘瘤）。注意还有肥大细胞。

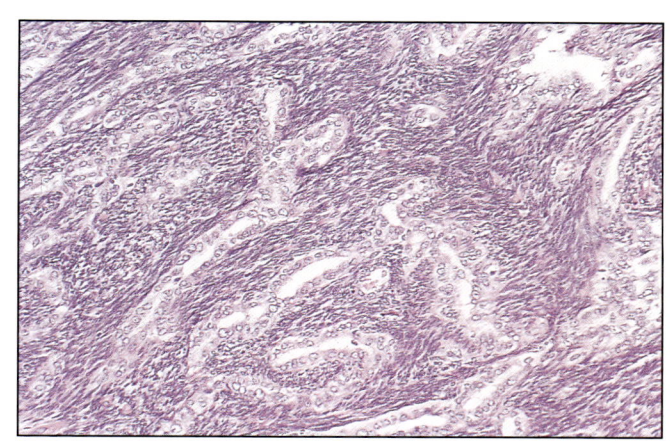

图24.112 双相型滑膜肉瘤。此经典类型容易诊断。

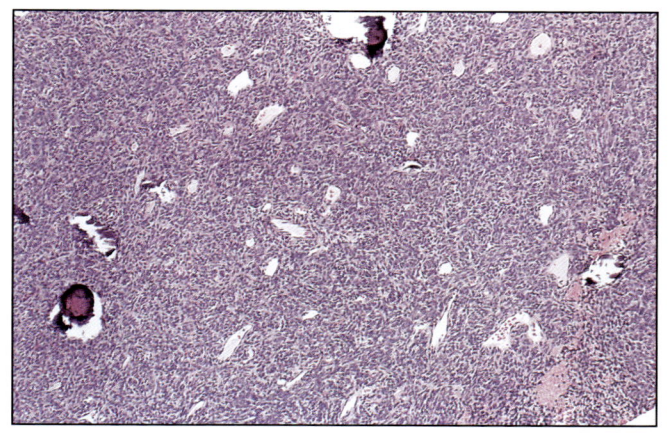

图24.111 单相型滑膜肉瘤。分枝状外皮细胞瘤样血管结构常见。注意还有钙化。

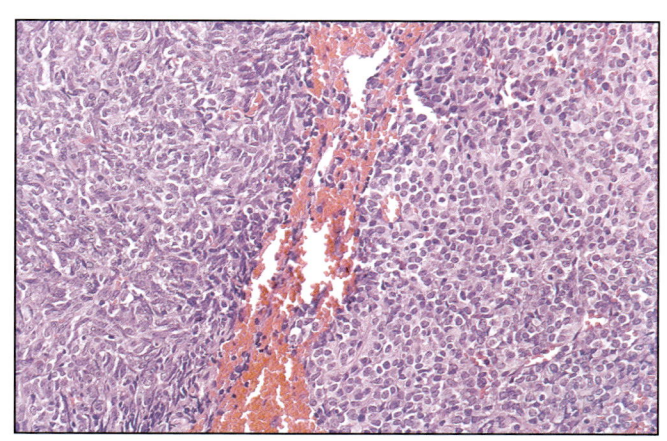

图24.113 分化较差的滑膜肉瘤。注意明显的圆形细胞形态表现。

较圆的细胞团来确认，这些细胞被网织纤维包裹，分布于其他梭形细胞病变中。大约5%~10%的病例出现低分化表现[534,536,550,551]，最常见的特征为未分化圆形细胞形态，类似Ewing肉瘤（图24.113）。低分化肿瘤在老年性滑膜肉瘤病人中更常见[552]。其他病例具有非特异性纤维肉瘤样结构，小部分具有大细胞性上皮样或显著多形性表现。伴有圆形细胞形态学表现的肿瘤有时出现嗜酸性横纹肌样胞浆内包涵体。尽管单相型和双相型之间没有明确的预后差异，但低分化形态学表现的病变明显预后较差[534,549,551]。极少数的滑膜肉瘤几乎均为单相上皮性结构[553]，但是所报道的病例不足以明确临床相关意义。所有滑膜肉瘤类型中的一个常见表现是小灶间质（或有时为腺体内）钙化或骨化。这些改变可以广泛，据说可以改善预后[554,555]。

免疫组织化学方面[536,556,557]，除了明显上皮性成分的染色阳性之外，几乎所有病例的梭形细胞成分至少出现局灶的EMA和角蛋白阳性；此表现与形态学线索结合，通常是区别单相型病变与恶性外周神经鞘瘤（MPNST）或纤维肉瘤的最好方法（图24.114）。一般说来，EMA比角蛋白更敏感，染色细胞更多[557,558]。大约30%的滑膜肉瘤病例S-100蛋白呈阳性[557,558]，这可能存在潜在的误导，尽管EMA着色在MPNST中并不常见。同样，至少2/3的滑膜肉瘤病例CD99染色呈阳性[557,559]，此抗体无助于与Ewing肉瘤的鉴别。细胞角蛋白亚型有助于区分形态学有重叠的滑膜肉瘤和MPNST病例，因为CK7和CK19阳性在前者更常见[560]。多数病例CD34呈阴性[557]，有助于与孤立性纤维性肿瘤的进一步鉴别。超微结构上，双相型和单相型病变通常

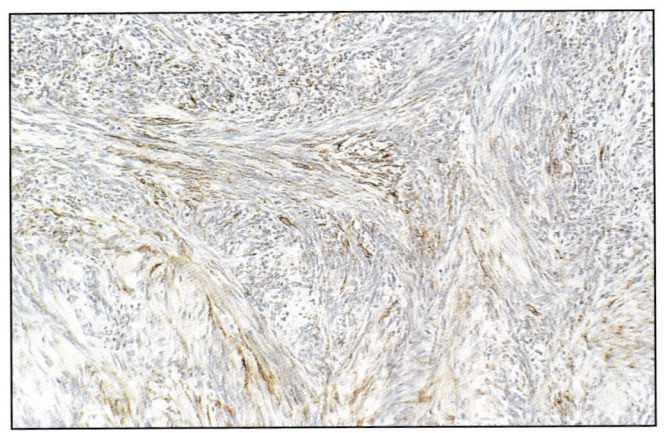

图24.114 单相型滑膜肉瘤。EMA至少局部呈阳性，具有诊断意义。ABC法。

都具有明确的上皮分化证据，后者存在明显的桥粒样连接和微绒毛。细胞遗传学上，双相型和单相型（以及低分化病变）具有重复性肿瘤特异染色体易位，即 t (X;18)(p11.2;q11.2)[9,561,562]，导致两个主要融合基因 *SYT-SSX1* 和 *SYT-SSX2*[562-564] 中的某一个产生（见表24.1）。就形态学关系而言，几乎所有出现 *SYT-SSX1* 融合的肿瘤均为双向型的[565,566]。尽管伴有 *SYT-SSX1* 的病例据说预后较差[565-567]，但还存有争议，有待证实[549]。在几年前的个案报道中，*SYT-SSX* 转录也见于恶性外周神经鞘瘤，但在其他许多研究中没有被证实，总体上不可信。

上皮样肉瘤　Epithelioid sarcoma

临床特征

上皮样肉瘤[568-572]有明显的青少年和年轻人倾向，以男性为主。多数病例发生在肢体远端，尤其是手和腕部周围。但总体上年龄范围和解剖学分布广泛。多数患者表现为浅表性或腱膜的结节及斑块，生长缓慢。常有疼痛和溃疡。个别病例病变部位较深。这些肿瘤具有的局部亚临床扩散能力很独特且令人震惊：病变沿筋膜或神经血管结构呈进行性扩散，常形成卫星结节，局部出现源自原发部位的可达30cm或更大的病变。这是这些病例的特征性反复局部复发和根治性手术至关重要的主要原因。淋巴结转移常常扩散至肺。5年生存率达到50%～60%或更高，总体最终死亡率（经10～20年随访）可能接近80%。转移性头皮受累尤为常见。在某种程度上，生存率与肿瘤大小有关，病变如小于5cm,则预后较好[571,573]。位于较近端的病变，尤其是盆腔、会阴和外阴，其形态学表现稍有不同（见下文），尤其具有侵袭性[574-577]，较早发生转移。

病理学特征

上皮样肉瘤常常是界限不清的灰白质硬肿物，伴有质软的棕色（坏死）病灶。大小不等，但最初多数肿瘤小于5cm。组织学上，多结节和弥漫性病变由明显单一形态的嗜酸性细胞构成，细胞呈圆形、上皮样或梭形不等，背景是致密的胶原性间质。有轻度多形性，但可见核仁，多少不等的核分裂象（图24.115）。玻璃样胞浆（横纹肌样）包涵体可见于许多病例。经典的是，肿瘤细胞围绕地图样坏死或黏液玻璃样变性区域排列（图24.116）。肿瘤细胞以不规则的、常常是单个细胞的方式浸润，往往围绕各种大小的血管和神经。大约30%的病例至少局灶可见胞浆空泡；这一特征加上常常容易形成假血管裂隙，可导致与上皮样内皮细胞肿瘤混淆。个别病例出现骨化生或极少数软骨化生。极少数病例具有

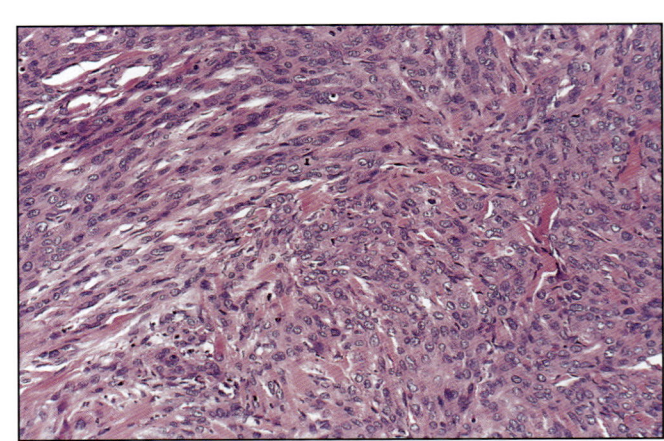

图24.115 上皮样肉瘤。多数病例出现明显单一形态的细胞学表现。

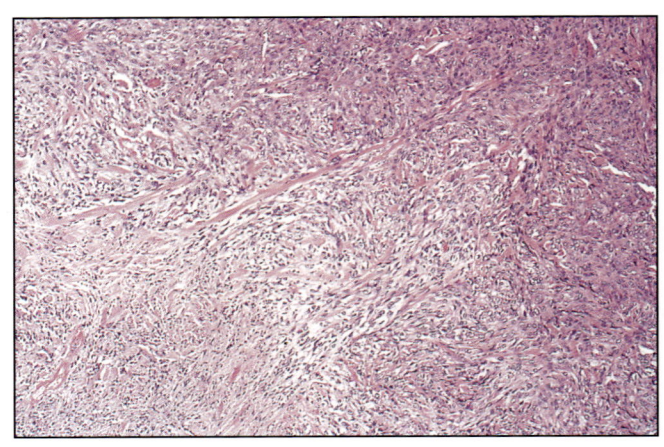

图24.116 上皮样肉瘤。所谓"地图样"（区域样）坏死可见于大约50%的病例。

梭形细胞性、几乎假肌源性形态学表现[578,579]。"近端"型上皮样肉瘤[575,576]过去常与肾外横纹肌样肿瘤（见下文）和未分化癌混淆，往往出现更为成片的生长结构，大且明显为上皮样表现的肿瘤细胞（图24.117）常常具有较大的泡状核以及横纹肌样胞浆包涵体。这个类型中通常见不到肉芽肿样坏死。极个别病例具有普通型和近端型混合性形态学特征，说明了这些病变的相关性。

免疫组织化学方面，这些肿瘤角蛋白（图24.118）、波形蛋白和EMA均为阳性，有助于与所有渐进坏死或肉芽肿性病变区别。缺乏表皮受累可与原发性鳞状细胞癌鉴别，上皮性转移常常容易出现显著多形性。与上皮样恶性血管肿瘤（见第3章）的不同点在于：后者的细胞和细胞核一般较大，且此类肿瘤几乎都表达特异性内皮标记物（如CD31和von Willebrand因子）及角蛋白。然而，重要的是要注意，大约50%的上皮样肉瘤CD34呈阳性[575,579]；因此该抗原在与血管性肿瘤的鉴别中没有帮助。然而，其在与癌的鉴别中有作用，癌组织中CD34免疫染色极其不常见。上皮样肉瘤的超微结构表现稍有不同，但往往出现未分化、肌纤维母细胞性或原始上皮性特征。细胞遗传学上，已发表的病例报告出现多种核型异常，但分子学研究显示，普通型和近端性病变均存在22q异常[580,581]。

腺泡状软组织肉瘤
Alveolar soft part sarcoma

腺泡状软组织肉瘤尽管已被熟知且研究较多，但仍是尚未明确的肿瘤，其分化系尚不清楚。十多年前发现，这些病变可出现骨骼肌分化[582]，但并未得到证实，近来这些肿瘤已经通过基因工程得以明确[583]。

临床特征

腺泡状软组织肉瘤[584-587]极为少见，但一般见于青少年或年轻成人，女性稍多见，表现为深在性肿物，主要见于下肢或肢带周围。在儿童，主要累及头颈部区域。总体上，发病年龄范围及分布广泛，极少见的部位包括纵隔[588]、女性生殖道（尤其是宫颈或子宫）[589]，甚至骨[590]。常常具有较长的缓慢生长病史。一经诊断，病变呈惰性表现，但大多为致死性肿瘤，2年生存率为87%，随访20年减少至18%[586]。多数病人最终死于转移，尤其是肺转移；发病年龄较大、肿瘤大于10cm似乎预后较差，儿童病例一般预后较好[591,592]。

组织学特征

腺泡状软组织肉瘤的形态极为特殊。由境界清楚的细胞巢构成，细胞较大，呈圆形或卵圆形，嗜酸性，常常出现中央性解离，因而成腺泡状结构（图24.119）。细胞巢周围围以纤维性间隔，其中常常含有明显的血管成分。肿瘤细胞自身具有丰富的、有些颗粒状的胞浆，偏心的圆形细胞核具有明显的核仁。在不超过50%的病例中，淀粉酶消化PAS染色显示细胞浆内颗粒和棒状结晶，此为病变的诊断性标志（图24.120）。超微结构上，这些成分对应于细胞膜结合性的结晶体或丝状物质，似乎与高尔基体关系密切，常常形成明显的几何形状[593]（见第31章）。已经表明，这些成分主要是由单羧酸转运蛋白1和CD147混合而成[594]。尽管坏死和出血可以很明显，但细胞核多形性通常有限，并且局灶，核分裂象也如此。少见病例具有副节瘤样、甚至假腺样表现，其他出现沙粒体性钙化[595]（图24.121）。一个见于多数病例的常见表现是：肿瘤周边有明显的血管浸润，尤其是扩张的静脉。

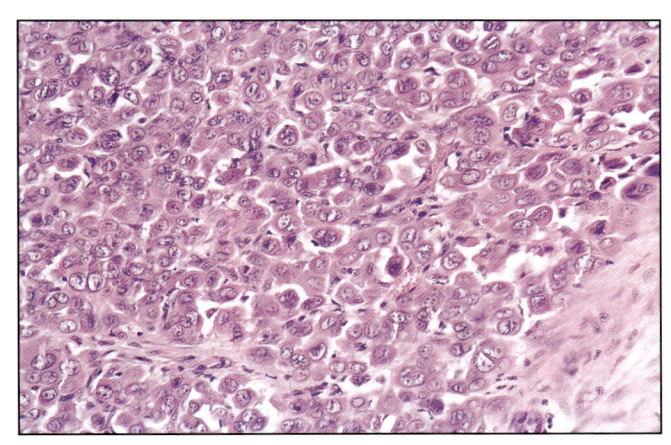

图24.117　近端型上皮样肉瘤。注意较大肿瘤细胞的形态表现为癌样。

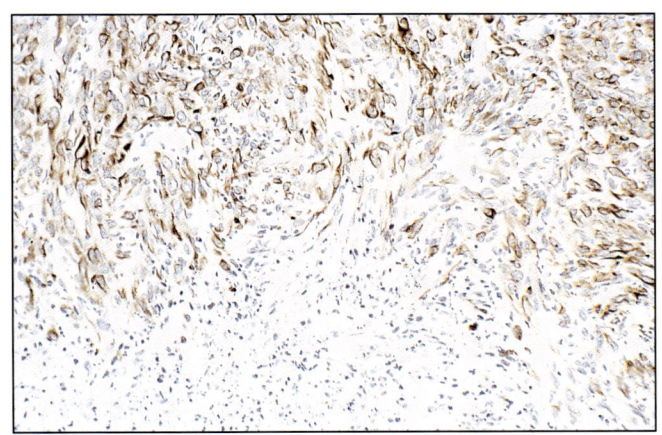

图24.118　上皮样肉瘤。基本上所有病例角蛋白（如此处）和EMA均为阳性。ABC法。

其他恶性病变

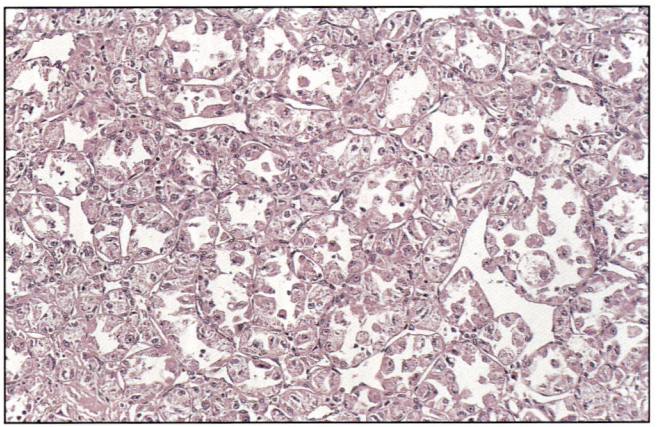

图24.119　腺泡状软组织肉瘤。经典的腺泡状生长结构，伴有插入的血管成分。

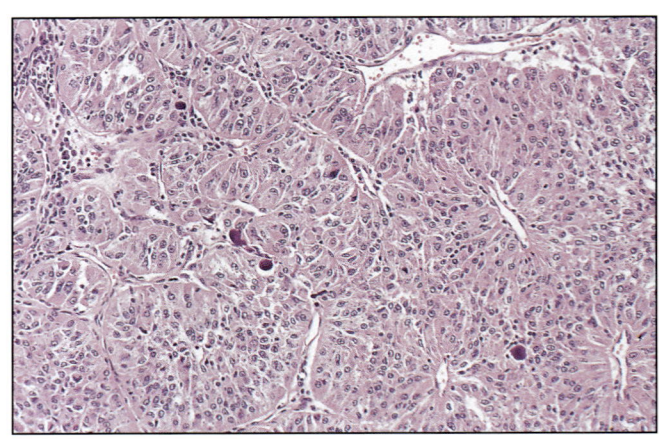

图24.121　腺泡状软组织肉瘤。这种不常见的病例具有明显副节瘤样表现，也可见沙粒体性钙化。

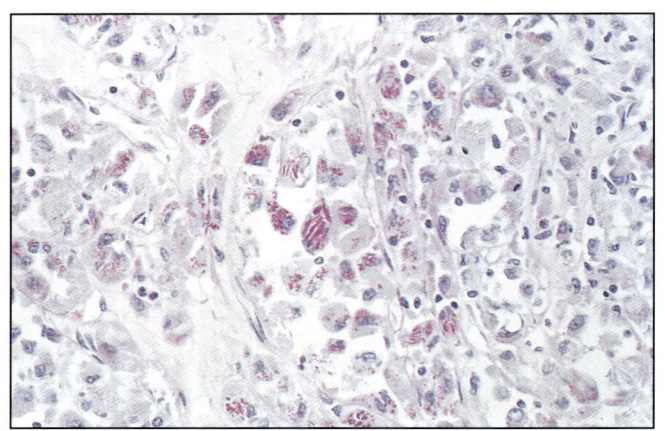

图24.120　腺泡状软组织肉瘤。多数病例中，通过淀粉酶消化的PAS染色可以显示特征性的结晶样包涵体。

在过去20年中，有关这些病变免疫表型的辩论和争议一直存在[582]。许多病例似乎结蛋白、肌肉肌动蛋白、肌节肌动蛋白和β-enolase染色均为阳性，尽管必须使用冰冻切片。相当一部分病例NSE和S-100蛋白也有染色，但是这两者在正常骨骼肌中通常呈阳性，这些结果并不能否认肌源性假说。当4病变中出现令人信服的MyoD1表达时，支持了病变为横纹肌母细胞性这一理念[596]，并且与腺泡状软组织肉瘤类似的特殊结晶体结构在骨骼肌梭形细胞器中也可见到[597]。然而，随后的更为广泛的研究并没有提供令人信服的横纹肌母细胞分化证据，尤其是肌浆调节蛋白MyoD1和肌细胞生成素的表达并没有可重复性特征[598,599]。从遗传学角度，17q25重排是独特的[600,601]（见表24.1），一种特征性的失衡（x;17）易位随后已被克隆，表现为 *TFE3-ASPL* 融合基因[582]。这种融合可导致细胞核过度表达TFE3蛋白，该成分随后被证实为腺泡状软组织肉瘤和其他伴有 *TFE3* 融合肿瘤（主要是儿童肾细胞癌）的有价值和特殊的免疫组化标记物[602]。多数病例不存在鉴别诊断问题：唯一真正类似这种表现的肿瘤是转移性肾细胞癌以及少数转移性黑色素瘤。然而，后两者往往更具多形性，依据免疫组化也容易鉴别。

骨外黏液样软骨肉瘤（所谓的）Extraskeletal myxoid chondrosarcoma (so-called)

不管其名称如何，现已逐渐认识到，这个肿瘤并不具有令人确信的软骨分化的证据，这种命名可能最终不得已而更改。与腺泡状软组织肉瘤一样，这些病变的分化系还不明确，但是这些病变的确是一种具有特殊遗传性的病变（见下文）。

临床特征

骨外黏液样软骨肉瘤[603-607]有时也被称为脊索瘤，主要发生在31～60岁，男性稍多见。个别病例发生在幼儿[608]。病变为无痛性、生长缓慢的筋膜下或深在性皮下肿物，大多位于肢体近端部分，少数发生于躯干。罕见病例发生在其他部位，如颈部、腹膜后或纵隔[609]。现在已认识到，这一特殊类型的软骨肉瘤可以发生在骨[610]，因此需要与骨的普通黏液样软骨肉瘤鉴别。肿瘤多数为分叶状，界限清楚，最大直径在5～15cm之间。传统上认为它是容易复发的低级别肿瘤，但5年转移率大约仅为10%～15%。然而，现在认为，至少40%～50%的此类病例最终会发生转移并导致患者死亡，常常是诊断后10年或更长时间[605,606]。

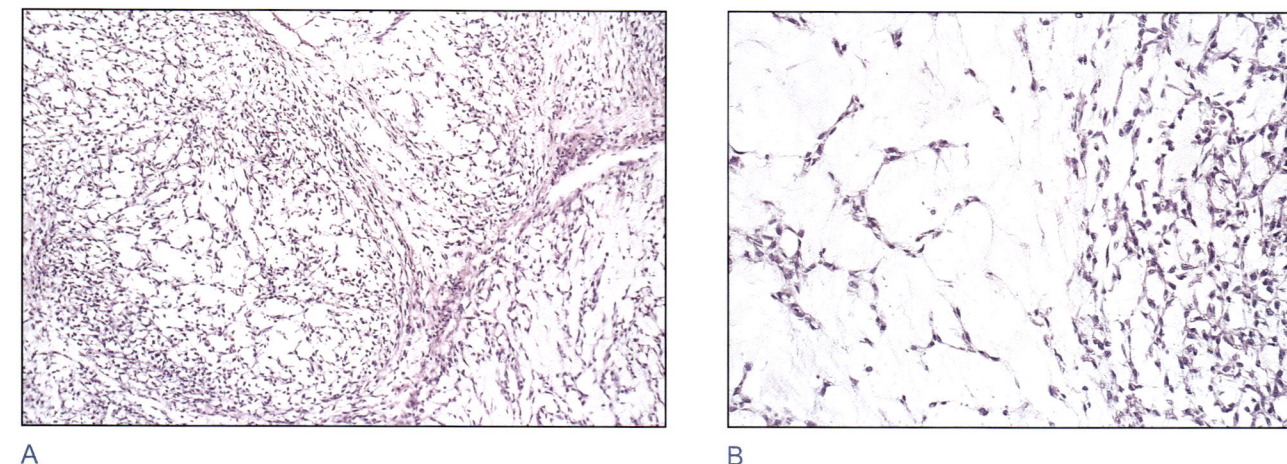

图24.122　骨外黏液样软骨肉瘤。分叶状生长结构具有特征性（A），小叶周边常常细胞较丰富，中心区有梁状结构（B）。

组织学特征

黏液样软骨肉瘤一般具有多结节生长方式，是由均一性的、以卵圆形为主的小的细胞条索或细带构成，有极少量的嗜酸性胞浆，细胞核圆形，背景为丰富的黏液样基质，主要由硫酸黏多糖构成[606,611]（图24.122）。小叶周边细胞常常较丰富，而中心部位的细胞具有胞浆空泡，并形成软骨母细胞样陷窝。显著的软骨样分化极为少见，过去描述的具有这种特征的病例多数可能为肌上皮性肿瘤，那时还没有认识到。大约10%的病例至少局灶含有明显嗜酸的、伴有胞浆内玻璃样（横纹肌样）包涵体的细胞[612]（图24.123）。在有些病例中，肿瘤细胞是较为梭形的，具有轻度多形性，但核分裂象大多比较散在。现已明确，有些病例明显富于细胞，梭形细胞更为弥漫，甚至以上皮样为主[606,613]，这些形态学上高级别的病变在小活检或缺乏典型区域情况下很难识别并更具侵袭性。

在多数病例中，特殊染色可以显示丰富的细胞浆内糖原，但与早先的报告相比[611]，显然大约不超过20%的病例出现明确的S-100蛋白免疫染色阳性[614]，个别病例EMA也呈阳性。超微结构检查显示，至少在30%的病例中，粗面内质网内可见明显的微管聚集[615,616]（见第13章）。值得注意的是，近来免疫组织化学资料[607,616]显示，这些肿瘤出现神经内分泌分化（NSE和Syn显著呈阳性），并已从基因表达谱中获得额外支持[617]。然而，这些表现的意义还不明确。黏液样软骨肉瘤也是具有一致性核型异常的肉瘤之一，与Ewing肉瘤、透明细胞癌和促纤维组织增生性小细胞肿瘤一样，通常导致22号染色体*EWSRI*基因重排（见表24.1）。尤其是，多数病例出现t(9;22)(q22;q12)相互易位[618,619]。个别病例出现t(9;17)(q22;q11)变异易位[620]，导致*NR4A3-RBP56*融合。主要的鉴别诊断为软组织（见1573页）或皮肤附属器来源的混合瘤/肌上皮瘤，病变出现明显的上皮（通常是导管）分化灶，除了S-100蛋白一致呈阳性、GFAP常常阳性以外，角蛋白和肌动蛋白通常也呈阳性。

肾外横纹肌样肿瘤
Extrarenal rhabdoid tumor

自肾外病变首次[621]被报道之后，所谓的"横纹肌样肿瘤"几乎在每一个可以想到的部位都有描述[622]，尽管多数病例发生在幼儿，但据说总体上年龄范围广泛。位于软组织的病例报道[622-627]具有广泛的解剖分布，容易出现极具侵袭性的临床过程，多数在2年内死亡。所有这些病变唯一一致的组织学特征是：出现透明小球样胞浆包涵体，并且在泡状核内有较大的核仁（图

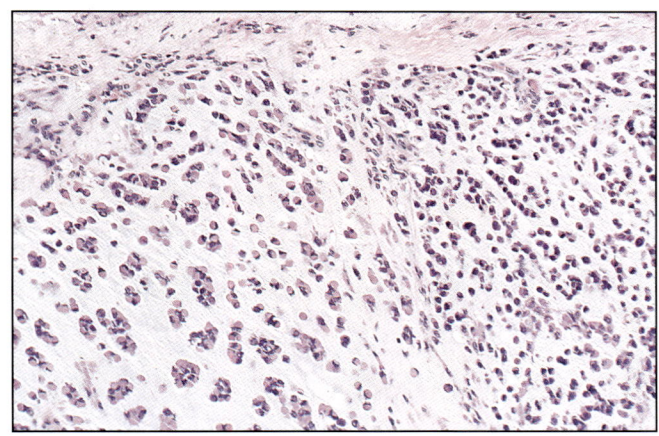

图24.123　骨外黏液样软骨肉瘤。横纹肌样胞浆内包涵体极为常见，同样也见于上皮样肉瘤。

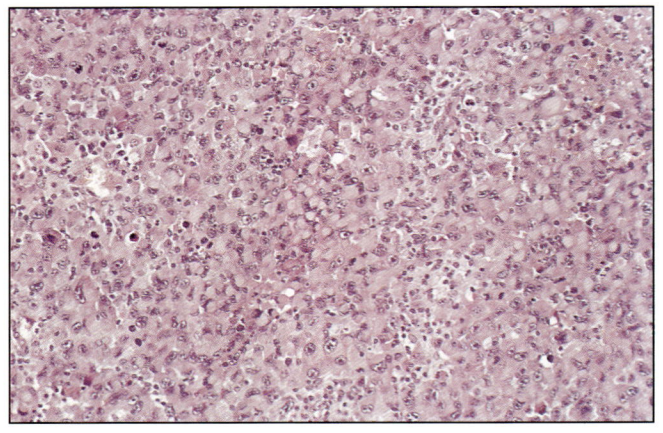

图24.124 所谓的"肾外横纹肌样肿瘤"。注意特殊的胞浆包涵体和大核仁。这个病例被证实为转移性黑色素瘤。

24.124)。尽管肿瘤细胞一般为圆形和有些上皮样,但从细胞形态学和生长方式表现上很少会使人怀疑这是一组异源性肿瘤而并非一个独立疾病[215,622,628],其他许多特殊肿瘤中出现"横纹肌样"包涵体进一步支持了这一点。另外,尽管多数肿瘤出现角蛋白、EMA 和波形蛋白一致阳性,但它们也常常表达其他多种不同抗原[622,627],

使得将它们定义为相互关联的一组肿瘤几乎是不可能的,除非是婴儿病例亚型。超微结构上,包涵体对应于聚集于核旁的中间丝成分。与肾和中枢神经系统对应的肿瘤常常出现 22q11 核型重排不同,软组织病例极少有这种特征,通常仅见于幼儿。这种染色体异常导致 hSNF5/INI1 基因缺失或突变,因此在真正的肾和(更少见的)肾外横纹肌样肿瘤中表达缺失[629]。

恶性间叶瘤
Malignant mesenchymoma

恶性间叶瘤[630-632]定义为出现两种或更多特殊类型间叶分化的软组织肉瘤,不同于任何未分化的、"纤维肉瘤样"、MFH 样或血管外皮细胞瘤样成分。任何出现去分化的特殊肉瘤以及异源性分化的恶性神经鞘瘤传统上不包括在这个分类中。在精确定义情况下,这些肿瘤目前被认为极其罕见[215],但似乎主要发生在成人的四肢。过去描述的多数腹膜后病例现在被认为是伴有异源成分的去分化脂肪肉瘤(见1536页)。真正的恶性间质瘤的分化系不一致,没有真正的特殊组合。临床过程似乎具有侵袭性。

参考文献

1. Nielsen T O, West R B, Linn S C et al. 2002 Molecular characterisation of soft tissue tumours: a gene expression study. Lancet 359: 1301–1307
2. Segal N H, Pavlidis P, Antonescu C R et al. 2003 Classification and subtype prediction of adult soft tissue sarcoma by functional genomics. Am J Pathol 163: 691–700
3. West R B, Corless C L, Chen X et al. 2004 The novel marker, DOG1, is expressed ubiquitously in gastrointestinal stromal tumors irrespective of KIT or PDGFRA mutation status. Am J Pathol 165: 107–113
4. Hess J L 1998 Chromosomal translocations in benign tumors. The HMGI proteins. Am J Clin Pathol 109: 251–261
5. Tallini G, Dal Cin P 1999 HMGI(Y) and HMGI-C dysregulation: a common occurrence in human tumors. Adv Anat Pathol 6: 237–246
6. Hahn H P, Fletcher C D M 2005 The role of cytogenetics and molecular genetics in soft tissue tumour diagnosis – a realistic appraisal. Curr Diagn Pathol 11: 361–370
7. Antonescu C R 2006 The role of genetic testing in soft tissue sarcoma. Histopathology 48: 13–21
8. Mertens F, Fletcher C D M, Dal Cin P et al. 1998 Cytogenetic analysis of 46 pleomorphic soft tissue sarcomas and correlation with morphologic and clinical features. A report of the CHAMP study group. Genes Chromos Cancer 22: 16–25
9. Fletcher C D M, Dal Cin P, De Wever I et al. 1999 Correlation between clinicopathological features and karyotype in spindle cell sarcomas: a report of 130 cases from the CHAMP study group. Am J Pathol 154: 1841–1847
10. Costa J, Wesley R A, Glatstein E, Rosenberg S A 1984 The grading of soft tissue sarcomas. Results of a clinicohistopathologic correlation in a series of 163 cases. Cancer 53: 530–541
11. Trojani M, Contesso G, Coindre J-M et al. 1984 Soft tissue sarcomas of adults: study of pathologic prognostic variables and definition of a histopathological grading system. Int J Cancer 33: 37–42
12. Coindre J-M, Terrier P, Bui N B et al. 1996 Prognostic factors in adult patients with locally controlled soft tissue sarcoma: a study on 546 patients from the French Federation of Cancer Centers Sarcoma Group. J Clin Oncol 14: 869–877
13. Association of Directors of Anatomic and Surgical Pathology 1998 Recommendations for the reporting of soft tissue sarcomas. Mod Pathol 11: 1257–1261
14. Brown F M, Fletcher C D M 2000 Problems in grading soft tissue sarcomas. Am J Clin Pathol 114 (Suppl): S82–S89
14a. Gustafson P, Akerman M, Alvegard T A et al. 2003 Prognostic information in soft tissue sarcoma using tumour size, vascular invasion and microscopic tumour necrosis – the SIN system. Eur J Cancer 39: 1568–1576
15. Rubin B P, Dal Cin P 2001. The genetics of lipomatous tumours. Semin Diagn Pathol 18: 286–293
16. Adair F E, Pack G T, Farrior J H 1932 Lipomas. Am J Cancer 16: 1104–1120
17. Bick E M 1936 Lipoma of the extremities. Ann Surg 104: 139–143
18. Rydholm A, Berg N O 1983 Size, site and clinical incidence of lipoma. Factors in the differential diagnosis of lipoma and sarcoma. Acta Orthop Scand 54: 929–934
19. Truhan A P, Garden J M, Caro W A et al. 1985 Facial and scalp lipomas: case reports and study of prevalence. J Dermatol Surg Oncol 11: 981–984
20. Dorfman H D, Levin S, Robbins H 1980 Cartilage-containing benign mesenchymomas of soft tissue. Report of two cases. J Bone Joint Surg 62A: 472–475
21. Milchgrub S, McMurry S K, Vuitch F, Dorfman H D 1990 Chondrolipoangioma. A cartilage-containing benign mesenchymoma of soft tissue. Cancer 66: 2636–2641
22. Sreekantaiah C, Leong S P L, Karakousis C P et al. 1991 Cytogenetic profile of 109 lipomas. Cancer Res 51: 422–433
23. Willen H, Akerman M, Dal Cin P et al. 1998 Comparison of chromosomal patterns with clinical features in 165 lipomas: a report of the CHAMP study group. Cancer Genet Cytogenet 102: 46–49
24. Wilson Jones E, Marks R, Pongeshirun D 1975 Naevus lipomatosus superficialis. A clinicopathological report of twenty cases. Br J Dermatol 93: 121–133
25. Fergin P E, MacDonald D M 1980 Naevus lipomatosus superficialis. Clin Exp Dermatol 5: 365–367
26. Placeo T, Tassi D 1953 Considerazioni cliniche su 62 osservazioni di lipoma arborescente posttraumatico del ginocchio come entit patologica a se sante ed associata a lesione meniscale. Minerva Chir 8: 316–322
27. Enzinger F M 1977 Benign lipomatous tumors simulating a sarcoma. In: Martin R G, Ayala A G (eds) Management of primary bone and soft tissue tumors. Year Book Medical Publishers, Chicago, p 11–24

28. Kindblom L–G, Angervall L, Stener B et al. 1974 Intermuscular and intramuscular lipomas and hibernomas. A clinical, roentgenologic, histologic and prognostic study of 46 cases. Cancer 33: 754–762
29. Fletcher C D M, Martin-Bates E 1988 Intramuscular and intermuscular lipoma: neglected diagnoses. Histopathology 12: 275–287
30. Dickmann O, Bilde T, Damgaard K 1987 Pelvic lipomatosis. Br J Urol 59: 591
31. Enzi G, Busetto L, Ceschin E et al. 2002. Multiple symmetric lipomatosis: clinical aspects and outcome in a long-term longitudinal study. Int J Obes Relat Metab Disord 26: 253–261
32. Enzi G, Digito M, Enzi G B et al. 1985 Asymmetrical lipomatosis: report of two cases. Postgrad Med J 61: 797–800
33. Enzi G, Digito M, Marin R et al. 1984 Mediastino-abdominal lipomatosis: deep accumulation of fat mimicking a respiratory disease and ascites. Clinical aspects and metabolic studies in vitro. J Med 22: 453–463
34. Enzi G, Inelmen E M, Baritussio A et al. 1977 Multiple symmetric lipomatosis. A defect in adrenergic-stimulated lipolysis. J Clin Invest 60: 1221–1229
35. Klein F A, Smith M J, Kasenetz I 1988 Pelvic lipomatosis: 35-year experience. J Urol 139: 998–1001
36. Chung E B, Enzinger F M 1973 Benign lipoblastomatosis. Cancer 32: 482–492
37. Mentzel T, Calonje E, Fletcher C D M 1993 Lipoblastoma and lipoblastomatosis: a clinicopathological study of 14 cases. Histopathology 23: 527–533
38. Collins M H, Chatten J 1997 Lipoblastoma/lipoblastomatosis: a clinicopathologic study of 25 tumors. Am J Surg Pathol 21: 1131–1137
39. Gisselsson D, Hibbard M K, Dal Cin P et al. 2001. PLAG1 alterations in lipoblastoma: involvement in varied mesenchymal cell types and evidence for alternative oncogenic mechanisms. Am J Pathol 159: 955–962
40. Howard W R, Helwig E B 1960 Angiolipoma. Arch Dermatol 82: 924–931
41. Dixon A Y, McGregor D H, Lee S H 1981 Angiolipomas: an ultrastructural and clinicopathological study. Hum Pathol 12: 739–747
42. Hunt S J, Santa Cruz D J, Barr R J 1990 Cellular angiolipoma. Am J Surg Pathol 14: 75–81
43. Stimpson N 1971 Infiltrating angiolipomata of skeletal muscle. Br J Surg 58: 464–466
44. Meis J M, Enzinger F M 1991 Myolipoma of soft tissue. Am J Surg Pathol 15: 121–125
45. Meis J M, Enzinger F M 1993 Chondroid lipoma. A unique tumor simulating liposarcoma and myxoid chondrosarcoma. Am J Surg Pathol 17: 1103–1112
46. Kindblom L-G, Meis-Kindblom J M 1995 Chondroid lipoma: an ultrastructural and immunohistochemical analysis with further observations regarding its differentiation. Am J Surg Pathol 26: 706–715
47. Gisselsson D, Domanski H A, Hoglund M et al. 1999 Unique cytological features and chromosome aberrations in chondroid lipoma. Am J Surg Pathol 23: 1300–1304
48. Hruban R H, Bhagavan B S, Epstein J I 1989 Massive retroperitoneal angiomyolipoma. A lesion that may be confused with well-differentiated liposarcoma. Am J Clin Pathol 92: 805–808
49. Chan J K C, Tsang W Y W, Pau M Y et al. 1993 Lymphangiomyomatosis and angiomyolipoma: closely related entities characterized by hamartomatous proliferation of HMB-45 positive smooth muscle. Histopathology 22: 445–455
50. Pea M, Bonetti F, Martignoni G et al. 1998 Apparent renal cell carcinomas in tuberous sclerosis are heterogeneous. The identification of malignant epithelioid angiomyolipoma. Am J Surg Pathol 22: 180–187
51. Grignon D J, Shkrum M J, Smout M S 1989 Extra-adrenal myelolipoma. Arch Pathol Lab Med 113: 52–54
52. Hunter S B, Schemankewitz E H, Patterson C et al. 1992 Extra-adrenal myelolipoma. A report of two cases. Am J Clin Pathol 97: 402–404
53. Amin M B, Tickoo S Z, Schultz D 1999 Myelolipoma of the renal sinus. An unusual site for a rare extra-adrenal lesion. Arch Pathol Lab Med 123: 631–634
54. Enzinger F, Harvey D A 1975 Spindle cell lipoma. Cancer 36: 1852–1859
55. Shmookler B M, Enzinger F M 1981 Pleomorphic lipoma: a benign tumor simulating liposarcoma. A clinicopathologic analysis of 48 cases. Cancer 47: 126–133
56. Azzopardi J G, Iocco J, Salm R 1973 Pleomorphic lipoma: a tumour simulating liposarcoma. Histopathology 7: 511–523
57. Fletcher C D M, Martin-Bates E 1987 Spindle cell lipoma: a clinicopathological study with some original observations. Histopathology 11: 803–817
58. Billings S D, Henley J D, Summerlin DJ et al. 2006 Spindle cell lipoma of the oral cavity. Am J Dermatopathol 28: 28–31
59. Bartley R B, Yeatts R P, Garrity J A et al. 1985 Spindle cell lipoma of the orbit. Am J Ophthalmol 100: 605–609
60. French C A, Mentzel T, Kutzner H, Fletcher C D M 2000 Intradermal spindle cell/pleomorphic lipoma: a distinct subset. Am J Dermatopathol 22: 496–502
61. Fanburg-Smith J C, Devaney K O, Miettinen M, Weiss S W 1998 Multiple spindle cell lipomas: a report of 7 familial and 11 nonfamilial cases. Am J Surg Pathol 22: 40–48
62. Suster S, Fisher C, Moran C A 1998 Dendritic fibromyxolipoma: a clinicopathologic study of a distinctive benign soft tissue lesion that may be mistaken for a sarcoma. Ann Diagn Pathol 2: 111–120
63. Hawley I C, Krausz T, Evans D J et al. 1994 Spindle cell lipoma a pseudoangiomatous variant. Histopathology 24: 565–569
64. Dal Cin P, Sciot R, Polito P et al. 1997 Lesions of 13q may occur independently of deletion of 16q in spindle cell/pleomorphic lipomas. Histopathology 31: 222–225
65. Furlong M A, Fanburg-Smith J C, Miettinen M 2001 The morphologic spectrum of hibernoma: a clinicopathologic study of 170 cases. Am J Surg Pathol 25: 809–814
66. Gaffney E F, Hargreaves H K, Semple E et al. 1983 Hibernoma: distinctive light and electron microscopic features and relationship to brown adipose tissue. Hum Pathol 14: 677–687
67. Rigor V V, Goldstone S E, Jones J et al. 1986 Hibernoma. A case report and discussion of a rare tumor. Cancer 57: 2207–2211
68. Gisselsson D, Hoglund M, Mertens F et al. 1999 Hibernomas are characterized by homozygous deletions in the multiple endocrine neoplasia type I region. Am J Pathol 155: 61–66
69. Shmookler B M, Enzinger F M 1983 Liposarcoma occurring in children. An analysis of 17 cases and review of the literature. Cancer 52: 567–574
70. Enzinger F M, Winslow D J 1962 Liposarcoma. A study of 103 cases. Virchow's Arch [A] 335: 367–388
71. Kindblom L-G, Angervall L, Svendsen P 1975 Liposarcoma. A clinicopathologic, radiographic and prognostic study. Acta Pathol Microbiol Scand Sect A Suppl 253: 1–71
72. Azumi N, Curtis J, Kempson R L et al. 1987 Atypical and malignant neoplasms showing lipomatous differentiation. A study of 111 cases. Am J Surg Pathol 11: 161–183
73. Evans H L 1988 Liposarcomas and atypical lipomatous tumors: a study of 66 cases followed for a minimum of 10 years. Surg Pathol 1: 41–54
74. Weiss S W, Rao V K 1992 Well-differentiated liposarcoma (atypical lipoma) of deep soft tissue of the extremities, retroperitoneum and miscellaneous sites. A follow-up study of 92 cases with analysis of the incidence of 'dedifferentiation.' Am J Surg Pathol 16: 1051–1058
75. Evans H L, Soule E H, Winkelmann R K 1979 Atypical lipoma, atypical intramuscular lipoma and well differentiated retroperitoneal liposarcoma. A reappraisal of 30 cases formerly classified as well differentiated liposarcoma. Cancer 43: 574–584
76. Laurino L, Furlanetto A, Orvieto E, Dei Tos A P 2001 Well differentiated liposarcoma (atypical lipomatous tumor). Semin Diagn Pathol 18: 258–262
77. Evans H L 1990 Smooth muscle in atypical lipomatous tumors. A report of three cases. Am J Surg Pathol 14: 714–718
78. Folpe A L, Weiss S W 2002 Lipoleiomyosarcoma (well differentiated liposarcoma with leiomyosarcomatous differentiation): a clinicopathologic study of nine cases including one with dedifferentiation. Am J Surg Pathol 26: 742–749
79. Kraus M D, Guillou L, Fletcher C D M 1997 Well-differentiated inflammatory liposarcoma: an uncommon and easily overlooked variant of a common sarcoma. Am J Surg Pathol 21: 518–527
80. Argani P, Facchetti F, Inghirani G, Rosai J 1997 Lymphocyte-rich well differentiated liposarcoma: report of nine cases. Am J Surg Pathol 21: 884–895
81. Dei Tos A P, Mentzel T, Newman P L et al. 1994 Spindle cell liposarcoma: a hitherto unrecognised variant of liposarcoma: analysis of six cases. Am J Surg Pathol 18: 913–921
82. Nascimento A F, Fletcher C D M 2005 Spindle cell liposarcoma/atypical lipomatous tumor: a clinicopathologic study of 120 cases. Mod Pathol 18: 19A (abstract).
83. Dal Cin P, Kools P, Sciot R et al. 1993 Cytogenetic and fluorescence in situ hybridization investigation of ring chromosomes characterizing a specific pathologic subgroup of adipose tissue tumors. Cancer Genet Cytogenet 68: 85–90
84. Rosai J, Akerman M, Dal Cin P et al. 1996 Morphologic-karyotypic study of 59 atypical lipomatous tumors: evaluation of their relationship and differential diagnosis with other adipose tissue tumors. Am J Surg Pathol 20: 1182–1189
85. Binh M B, Sastre-Garau X, Guillou L et al. 2005 MDM2 and CDK4 immunostainings are useful adjuncts in diagnosing well differentiated and dedifferentiated liposarcoma subtypes: a comparative analysis of 559 soft tissue neoplasms with genetic data. Am J Surg Pathol 29: 1340–1347
86. McCormick D, Mentzel T, Beham A et al. 1994 Dedifferentiated liposarcoma: clinicopathological analysis of 32 cases suggesting a better prognostic subgroup among the pleomorphic sarcomas. Am J Surg Pathol 18: 1213–1223
87. Henricks W H, Chu Y C, Goldblum J R, Weiss S W 1997 Dedifferentiated liposarcoma: a clinicopathological analysis of 155 cases with a proposal for an expanded definition of dedifferentiation. Am J Surg Pathol 21: 271–281
88. Coindre J M, Hostein I, Maire G et al. 2004 Inflammatory malignant fibrous histiocytomas and dedifferentiated liposarcomas: histological review, genomic profile and MDM2 and CDK4 status favour a single entity. J Pathol 203: 820–830
89. Tallini G, Erlandson R A, Brennan M F et al. 1993 Divergent myosarcomatous differentiation in retroperitoneal liposarcoma. Am J Surg Pathol 17: 546–556
90. Evans H L, Khurana K K, Kemp B L, Ayala G 1994 Heterologous elements in the dedifferentiated component of dedifferentiated liposarcoma. Am J Surg Pathol 18: 1150–1157
91. Nascimento A G, Kurtin P J, Guillou L, Fletcher C D M 1998 Dedifferentiated liposarcoma: a report of nine cases showing a peculiar neural-like (whorling) pattern associated with metaplastic bone formation. Am J Surg Pathol 22: 945–955
92. Fanburg-Smith J C, Miettinen M 1998 Liposarcoma with meningothelial-like whorls: study of 17 cases of a distinctive histological pattern associated with dedifferentiated liposarcoma. Histopathology 33: 414–424

93. Aman P, Ron D, Mandahl N et al. 1992 Rearrangement of the transcription factor gene CHOP in myxoid liposarcomas with t(12;16)(q13;p11). Genes Chromos Cancer 5: 278–285
94. Knight J, Renwick P J, Dal Cin P, van den Berghe H, Fletcher C D M 1995 Translocation t(12;16)(q13;p11) in myxoid liposarcoma and round cell liposarcoma: molecular and cytogenetic analysis. Cancer Res 55: 24–27
95. Antonescu C R, Elahi A, Humphrey M et al. 2000 Specificity of TLS-CHOP rearrangement for classic myxoid/round cell liposarcoma: absence in predominantly myxoid well differentiated liposarcomas. J Mol Diagn 2: 132–138
96. Hosaka T, Nakashima Y, Kusuzaki K et al. 2002 A novel type of EWS-CHOP fusion gene in two cases of myxoid liposarcoma. J Mol Diagn 4: 164–171
97. Kilpatrick S E, Doyon J, Choong P F, Sim F, Nascimento A G 1996 The clinicopathologic spectrum of myxoid and round cell liposarcoma. A study of 95 cases. Cancer 77: 1450–1458
98. Fletcher C D M 1997 Will we ever reliably predict prognosis in a patient with myxoid and round cell liposarcoma? Adv Anat Pathol 4: 108–113
99. Dei Tos A P, Wadden C, Fletcher C D M 1996 S-100 protein staining in liposarcoma: its diagnostic utility in the high grade myxoid (round cell) variant. Appl Immunohistochem 4: 95–101
100. Gebhard S, Coindre J M, Michels J J et al. 2002 Pleomorphic liposarcoma: clinicopathologic, immunohistochemical and follow-up analysis of 63 cases: a study from the French Federation of Cancer Centers Sarcoma Group. Am J Surg Pathol 26: 601–616
101. Hornick J L, Bosenberg M W, Mentzel T et al. 2004 Pleomorphic liposarcoma: clinicopathologic analysis of 57 cases. Am J Surg Pathol 28: 1257–1267
102. Miettinen M, Enzinger F M 1999 Epithelioid variant of pleomorphic liposarcoma: a study of 12 cases of a distinctive variant of high grade liposarcoma. Mod Pathol 12: 722–728
103. Mentzel T, Fletcher C D M 1997 Dedifferentiated myxoid liposarcoma: a clinicopathological study suggesting a closer relationship between myxoid and well-differentiated liposarcoma. Histopathology 30: 457–463
104. Garb J, Stone M J 1942 Keloids. Review of the literature and a report of 80 cases. Am J Surg 58: 315–335
105. Lee J Y, Yang C C, Chao S C, Wong T W 2004 Histopathological differential diagnosis of keloid and hypertrophic scar. Am J Dermatopathol 26: 379–384
106. Lee C P 1982 Keloids – their epidemiology and treatment. Int J Dermatol 21: 504–505
107. Ehrlich H P, Desmouliere A, Diegelmann R F et al. 1994 Morphological and immunochemical differences between keloid and hypertrophic scar. Am J Pathol 145: 105–113
108. Konwaler B E, Keasbey L, Kaplan L 1955 Subcutaneous pseudosarcomatous fibromatosis (fasciitis). Am J Clin Pathol 25: 241–252
109. Allen P W 1972 Nodular fasciitis. Pathology 4: 9–26
110. Bernstein K E, Lattes R 1982 Nodular (pseudosarcomatous) fasciitis, a non-recurrent lesion: clinicopathologic study of 134 cases. Cancer 49: 1668–1678
111. Shimizu S, Hashimoto H, Enjoji M 1984 Nodular fasciitis: an analysis of 250 patients. Pathology 16: 161–166
112. Sarangarajan R, Dehner L P 1999 Cranial and extracranial fasciitis of childhood: a clinicopathologic and immunohistochemical study. Hum Pathol 30: 87–92
113. Hutter R V P, Foote F W, Francis K C et al. 1962 Parosteal fasciitis. A self-limited benign process that simulates a malignant neoplasm. Am J Surg 104: 800–807
114. Goodlad J R, Fletcher C D M 1990 Intradermal variant of nodular fasciitis. Histopathology 17: 569–571
115. Price S K, Kahn L B, Saxe N 1993 Dermal and intravascular fasciitis. Unusual variants of nodular fasciitis. Am J Dermatopathol 15: 539–543
116. Lauer D H, Enzinger F M 1980 Cranial fasciitis of childhood. Cancer 45: 401–406
117. Patchefsky A S, Enzinger F M 1981 Intravascular fasciitis. A report of 17 cases. Am J Surg Pathol 5: 29–36
118. Montgomery E A, Meis J M 1991 Nodular fasciitis. Its morphologic spectrum and immunohistochemical profile. Am J Surg Pathol 15: 942–948
119. Kwittken J, Branche M 1969 Fasciitis ossificans. Am J Clin Pathol 51: 251–255
120. Chung E B, Enzinger F M 1975 Proliferative fasciitis. Cancer 36: 1450–1458
121. Kitano M, Iwasaki H, Enjoji M 1997 Proliferative fasciitis. A variant of nodular fasciitis. Acta Pathol Jpn 27: 485–493
122. Meis J M, Enzinger F M 1992 Proliferative fasciitis and myositis of childhood. Am J Surg Pathol 16: 364–372
123. Enzinger F M, Dulcey F 1967 Proliferative myositis. Report of thirty three cases. Cancer 20: 2213–2223
124. Dupree W B, Enzinger F M 1986 Fibro-osseous pseudotumor of the digits. Cancer 58: 2103–2109
125. Spjut H J, Dorfman H D 1981 Florid reactive periostitis of the tubular bones of the hands and feet. A benign lesion which may simulate osteosarcoma. Am J Surg Pathol 5: 423–433
126. Wilson J D, Montague C J, Salcuni P et al. 1999 Heterotopic mesenteric ossification ('intraabdominal myositis ossificans'). Report of five cases. Am J Surg Pathol 23: 1464–1470
127. Perosio P M, Weiss S W 1993 Ischemic fasciitis: a juxta-skeletal fibroblastic proliferation with a predilection for elderly patients. Mod Pathol 6: 69–72
128. Montgomery E A, Meis J M, Mitchell M S et al. 1992 Atypical decubital fibroplasia. A distinctive fibroblastic pseudotumor occurring in debilitated patients. Am J Surg Pathol 16: 708–715
129. Proppe K H, Scully R E, Rosai J 1984 Postoperative spindle cell nodules of genitourinary tract resembling sarcomas. A report of eight cases. Am J Surg Pathol 8: 101–108
130. Young R H, Scully R E 1987 Pseudosarcomatous lesions of the urinary bladder, prostate gland and urethra. Arch Pathol Lab Med 111: 354–358
131. Hirsch M S, Dal Cin P, Fletcher C D M 2006 ALK expression in pseudosarcomatous myofibroblastic proliferations of the genitourinary tract. Histopathology 48: 569–578
132. Hollowood K, Fletcher C D M 1992 Pseudosarcomatous myofibroblastic proliferations of the spermatic cord ('proliferative funiculitis'). Am J Surg Pathol 16: 448–454
133. Barr J R 1966 Elastofibroma. Am J Clin Pathol 45: 679–683
134. Jarvi O H, Saxen A E, Hopsu-Havu V K et al. 1969 Elastofibroma – a degenerative pseudotumor. Cancer 23: 42–63
135. Renshaw T S, Simon M A 1973 Elastofibroma. J Bone Joint Surg 55A: 409–412
136. Nagamine N, Nohara Y, Ito E 1982 Elastofibroma in Okinawa. A clinicopathologic study of 170 cases. Cancer 50: 1794–1805
137. McComb E N, Feely M G, Neff J R et al. 2001 Cytogenetic instability, predominantly involving chromosome 1, is characteristic of elastofibroma. Cancer Genet Cytogenet 126: 68–72
138. Hisaoka M, Hashimoto H 2006 Elastofibroma: clonal fibrous proliferation with predominant CD34-positive cells. Virchows Arch 448: 195–199
139. Kumaratilake J S, Krishnan R, Lomax-Smith J et al. 1991 Elastofibroma: disturbed elastic fibrillogenesis by periosteal-derived cells? An immunoelectron microscopic and in situ hybridization study. Hum Pathol 22: 1017–1029
140. Enjoji M, Sumiyoshi K, Sueyoshi K 1985 Elastofibromatous lesion of the stomach in a patient with elastofibroma dorsi. Am J Surg Pathol 9: 233–237
141. Enzinger F M 1965 Fibrous hamartoma of infancy. Cancer 18: 241–248
142. Paller A S, Gonzalez-Crussi F, Sherman J O 1989 Fibrous hamartoma of infancy. Eight additional cases and a review of the literature. Arch Dermatol 125: 88–91
143. Maung R, Lindsay R, Trevenen C et al. 1987 Fibrous hamartoma of infancy. Hum Pathol 18: 652–653
144. Efem S E E, Ekpo M D 1993 Clinicopathological features of untreated fibrous hamartoma of infancy. J Clin Pathol 46: 522–524
145. Fletcher C D M, Powell G, van Noorden S et al. 1988 Fibrous hamartoma of infancy: a histochemical and immunohistochemical study. Histopathology 12: 65–74
146. Michal M, Mukensnabl P, Chlumska A et al. 1992 Fibrous hamartoma of infancy. A study of eight cases with immunohistochemical and electron microscopical findings. Pathol Res Pract 188: 1049–1053
147. Granter S R, Badizadegan K, Fletcher C D M 1998 Myofibromatosis in adults, glomangiopericytoma and myopericytoma: a spectrum of tumors showing perivascular myoid differentiation. Am J Surg Pathol 22: 513–525
148. Chung E B, Enzinger F M 1981 Infantile myofibromatosis. Cancer 48: 1807–1818
149. Briselli M F, Soule E H, Gilchrist G S 1980 Congenital fibromatosis. Report of 18 cases of solitary and 4 cases of multiple tumors. Mayo Clin Proc 55: 554–562
150. Fletcher C D M, Achu P, van Noorden S et al. 1987 Infantile myofibromatosis: a light microscopic, histochemical and immunohistochemical study suggesting true smooth muscle differentiation. Histopathology 11: 245–258
151. Inwards C Y, Unni K K, Beabout J W et al. 1991 Solitary congenital fibromatosis (infantile myofibromatosis) of bone. Am J Surg Pathol 15: 935–941
152. Bracko M, Cindro L, Golouh R 1992 Familial occurrence of infantile myofibromatosis. Cancer 69: 1294–1299
153. Zand D J, Huff D, Everman D et al. 2004 Autosomal dominant inheritance of infantile myofibromatosis. Am J Med Genet A 126: 261–266
154. Mentzel T, Calonje E, Nascimento A G et al. 1994 Infantile hemangiopericytoma versus infantile myofibromatosis: study of a series suggesting a continuous spectrum of infantile myofibroblastic lesions. Am J Surg Pathol 18: 922–930
155. Lidge R T, Bechtol R C, Lambert C N 1957 Congenital muscular torticollis. Etiology and pathology. J Bone Joint Surg 39A: 1165–1182
156. Coventry M B, Harris L E 1959 Congenital muscular torticollis in infancy. Some observations regarding treatment. J Bone Joint Surg 41A: 815–822
157. MacDonald D 1969 Sternomastoid tumour and muscular torticollis. J Bone Joint Surg 51B: 432–443
158. Drescher E, Woyke S, Markiewicz C et al. 1967 Juvenile fibromatosis in siblings (fibromatosis hyalinica multiplex juvenilis). J Pediatr Surg 2: 427–430
159. Remberger K, Krieg T, Kunze D et al. 1985 Fibromatosis hyalinica multiplex (juvenile hyaline fibromatosis). Light microscopic, electron microscopic, immunohistochemical and biochemical findings. Cancer 56: 614–624
160. Breier F, Fang-Kircher S, Wolff K, Jurecka W 1997 Juvenile hyaline fibromatosis: impaired collagen metabolism in human skin fibroblasts. Arch Dis Child 77: 436–440
161. Hanks S, Adams S, Douglas J et al. 2003 Mutations in the gene encoding capillary morphogenesis protein 2 cause juvenile hyaline fibromatosis and infantile systemic hyalinosis. Am J Hum Genet 73: 791–800
162. Chung E B, Enzinger F M 1979 Fibroma of tendon sheath. Cancer 44: 1945–1954
163. Hashimoto H, Tsuneyoshi M, Daimaru Y et al. 1985 Fibroma of tendon sheath: a tumor of myofibroblasts. A clinicopathologic study of 18 cases. Acta Pathol Jpn 35: 1099–1107
164. Pulitzer D R, Martin P C, Reed R J 1989 Fibroma of tendon sheath. A clinicopathologic study of 32 cases. Am J Surg Pathol 13: 472–479

165. Satti M B 1992 Tendon sheath tumours: a pathological study of the relationship between giant cell tumour and fibroma of tendon sheath. Histopathology 20: 213–220
166. Dal Cin P, Sciot R, Desmet L, Van den Berghe H 1998 Translocation 2;11 in a fibroma of tendon sheath. Histopathology 32: 433–435
167. Evans H L 1995 Desmoplastic fibroblastoma. A report of seven cases. Am J Surg Pathol 19: 1077–1081
168. Nielsen G P, O'Connell J X, Dickersin G R, Rosenberg A E 1996 Collagenous fibroma (desmoplastic fibroblastoma): a report of seven cases. Mod Pathol 9: 781–785
169. Miettinen M, Fetsch J F 1998 Collagenous fibroma (desmoplastic fibroblastoma): a clinicopathological analysis of 63 cases of a distinctive soft tissue lesion with stellate-shaped fibroblasts. Hum Pathol 29: 676–682
170. Bernal K, Nelson M, Neff J R et al. 2004 Translocation (2;11)(q31;q12) is recurrent in collagenous fibroma (desmoplastic fibroblastoma). Cancer Genet Cytogenet 149: 161–163.
171. Rapini R P, Golitz L E 1989 Sclerotic fibromas of the skin. J Am Acad Dermatol 20: 266–271
172. Metcalf J S, Maize J C, LeBoit P E 1991 Circumscribed storiform collagenoma (sclerosing fibroma). Am J Dermatopathol 13: 122–129
173. High W A, Stewart D, Essary L D et al. 2004 Sclerotic fibroma-like change in various neoplastic and inflammatory skin lesions: is sclerotic fibroma a distinct entity? J Cutan Pathol 31: 373–378
174. Hugel H 1991 Die plaqueformige dermale Fibromatose. Hautarzt 42: 223–226
175. Kamino H, Reddy V B, Gero M et al. 1992 Dermatomyofibroma. A benign cutaneous plaque-like proliferation of fibroblasts and myofibroblasts in young adults. J Cutan Pathol 19: 85–93
176. Mentzel T, Calonje E, Fletcher C D M 1993 Dermatomyofibroma – additional observations of a distinctive cutaneous myofibroblastic tumour with emphasis on differential diagnosis. Br J Dermatol 129: 69–73
177. Mentzel T, Kutzner H. 2003 Haemorrhagic dermatomyofibroma (plaque-like dermal fibromatosis): clinicopathological and immunohistochemical analysis of three cases resembling plaque-stage Kaposi sarcoma. Histopathology 42: 594–598
178. Smith K J, Skelton H G, Barrett T L et al. 1989 Cutaneous myofibroma. Mod Pathol 2: 603–609
179. Daimaru Y, Hashimoto H, Enjoji M 1989 Myofibromatosis in adults (adult counterpart of infantile myofibromatosis). Am J Surg Pathol 13: 859–865
180. Beham A, Badve S, Suster S et al. 1993 Solitary myofibroma in adults: clinicopathological analysis of a series. Histopathology 22: 335–341
181. Foss R D, Ellis G L. 2000 Myofibromas and myofibromatosis of the oral region: a clinicopathologic analysis of 79 cases. Oral Surg Oral Med Oral Pathol Oral Radiol Endod 89: 57–65
182. Balachandran K, Allen R W, MacCormac L B 1995 Nuchal fibroma. A clinicopathological study of nine cases. Am J Surg Pathol 19: 313–317
183. Michal M, Fetsch J F, Hes O, Miettinen M 1999 Nuchal-type fibroma: a clinicopathologic study of 52 cases. Cancer 85: 156–163
184. Wehrli B M, Weiss S W, Yandow S, Coffin C M 2001 Gardner-associated fibromas in young patients: a distinct fibrous lesion that identifies unsuspected Gardner syndrome and risk for fibromatosis. Am J Surg Pathol 25: 645–651
185. Coffin C M, Hornick J L, Zhou H, Fletcher C D M 2006 Gardner fibroma: a clinicopathologic and immunohistochemical study of 45 patients with 57 fibromas. Am J Surg Pathol – in press.
186. Diwan A H, Graves E D, King J A, Horenstein M G 2000 Nuchal–type fibroma in two related patients with Gardner's syndrome. Am J Surg Pathol 24: 1563–1567
187. Reye R D K 1965 Recurring digital fibrous tumors of childhood. Arch Pathol 80: 228–231
188. Allen P W 1972 Recurring digital fibrous tumours of childhood. Pathology 4: 215–223
189. Sarma D P, Hoffman E O 1980 Infantile digital fibroma-like tumor in an adult. Arch Dermatol 116: 578–579
190. Viale G, Doglioni C, Iuzzolino P et al. 1988 Infantile digital fibromatosis-like tumour (inclusion body fibromatosis) of adulthood: report of two cases with ultrastructural and immunocytochemical findings. Histopathology 12: 415–424
191. Purdy L J, Colby T V 1984 Infantile digital fibromatosis occurring outside the digit. Am J Surg Pathol 8: 787–790
192. Pettinato G, Manivel J C, Gould E W, Albores-Saavedra J 1994 Inclusion body fibromatosis of the breast. Two cases with immunohistochemical and ultrastructural findings. Am J Clin Pathol 101: 714–718
193. Iwasaki H, Kikuchi M, Ohtsuki I et al. 1983 Infantile digital fibromatosis. Identification of actin filaments in cytoplasmic inclusions by heavy meromyosin binding. Cancer 52: 1653–1661
194. Bittesini L, Dei Tos A P, Doglioni C et al. 1994 Fibroepithelial tumor of the breast with digital fibroma-like inclusions in the stromal component. Am J Surg Pathol 18: 296–301
195. Fletcher C D M, Tsang W Y W, Fisher C et al. 1992 Angiomyofibroblastoma of the vulva. A benign neoplasm distinct from aggressive angiomyxoma. Am J Surg Pathol 16: 373–382
196. Nielsen G P, Rosenberg A E, Young R H et al. 1996 Angiomyofibroblastoma of the vulva and vagina. Mod Pathol 9: 284–291
197. Laskin W B, Fetsch J F, Tavassoli F A 1997 Angiomyofibroblastoma of the female genital tract: analysis of 17 cases including a lipomatous variant. Hum Pathol 28: 1046–1055
198. Cao D, Srodon M, Montgomery E A, Kurman R J 2005 Lipomatous variant of angiomyofibroblastoma: report of two cases and review of the literature. Int J Gynecol Pathol 24: 196–200
199. Nielsen G P, Young R H, Dickersin G R, Rosenberg A E 1997 Angiomyofibroblastoma of the vulva with sarcomatous transformation ('angiomyofibrosarcoma'). Am J Surg Pathol 21: 1104–1108
200. Granter S R, Nucci M R, Fletcher C D M 1997 Aggressive angiomyxoma: reappraisal of its relationship to angiomyofibroblastoma in a series of 16 cases. Histopathology 30: 3–10
201. Nucci M R, Granter S R, Fletcher C D M 1997 Cellular angiofibroma: a benign neoplasm distinct from angiomyofibroblastoma and spindle cell lipoma. Am J Surg Pathol 21: 636–644
202. Iwasa Y, Fletcher C D M 2004 Cellular angiofibroma: clinicopathologic and immunohistochemical analysis of 51 cases. Am J Surg Pathol 28: 1426–1435
203. Laskin W B, Fetsch J F, Mostofi F K 1998 Angiomyofibroblastoma-like tumor of the male genital tract. Analysis of 11 cases with comparison to female angiomyofibroblastoma. Am J Surg Pathol 22: 6–16
204. Dei Tos A P, Seregard S, Calonje E, Chan J K C, Fletcher C D M 1995 Giant cell angiofibroma. A distinctive orbital tumor in adults. Am J Surg Pathol 19: 1286–1293
205. Guillou L, Gebhard S, Coindre J M 2000 Orbital and extraorbital giant cell angiofibroma: a giant cell-rich variant of solitary fibrous tumor? Clinicopathologic and immunohistochemical analysis of a series in favor of a unifying concept. Am J Surg Pathol 24: 971–979
206. Fetsch J F, Miettinen M 1998 Calcifying aponeurotic fibroma: a clinicopathologic study of 22 cases arising in uncommon sites. Hum Pathol 29: 1504–1510
207. Keasbey L E 1953 Juvenile aponeurotic fibroma (calcifying fibroma). A distinctive tumor arising in the palms and soles of young children. Cancer 6: 338–346
208. Allen P W, Enzinger F M 1970 Juvenile aponeurotic fibroma. Cancer 26: 857–867
209. Fetsch J F, Montgomery E A, Meis J M 1993 Calcifying fibrous pseudotumor. Am J Surg Pathol 17: 502–508
210. Pinkard N B, Wilson R W, Lawless N et al. 1996 Calcifying fibrous pseudotumor of pleura. A report of three cases of a newly described entity involving the pleura. Am J Clin Pathol 105; 189–194
211. Nascimento A F, Ruiz R, Hornick J L, Fletcher C D M 2002 Calcifying fibrous 'pseudotumor': clinicopathologic study of 15 cases and analysis of its relationship to inflammatory myofibroblastic tumor. Int J Surg Pathol 10: 189–196
212. Chen K T 2003 Familial peritoneal multifocal calcifying fibrous tumor. Am J Clin Pathol 119; 811–815
213. Van Dorpe J, Ectors N, Geboes K et al. 1999 Is calcifying fibrous pseudotumor a late sclerosing stage of inflammatory myofibroblastic tumor? Am J Surg Pathol 23: 329–335
214. Hill K A, Gonzalez-Crussi F, Chou P M 2001 Calcifying fibrous pseudotumor versus inflammatory myofibroblastic tumor: a histological and immunohistochemical comparison. Mod Pathol 14: 784–790
215. Fletcher C D M, Unni K K, Mertens F (eds) 2002 World Health Organization Classification of Tumours. Pathology and Genetics of Tumours of Soft tissue and Bone. IARC Press, Lyon
216. Gengler C, Guillou L. 2006. Solitary fibrous tumour and haemangiopericytoma: evolution of a concept. Histopathology 48: 63–74
217. Goodlad J R, Fletcher C D M 1991 Solitary fibrous tumour arising at unusual sites: analysis of a series. Histopathology 19: 515–522
218. Young R H, Clement P B, McCaughey W T E 1990 Solitary fibrous tumors ('fibrous mesotheliomas') of the peritoneum. A report of three cases and a review of the literature. Arch Pathol Lab Med 114: 493–495
219. Witkin G B, Rosai J 1989 Solitary fibrous tumor of the mediastinum. A report of 14 cases. Am J Surg Pathol 13: 547–557
220. Witkin G B, Rosai J 1991 Solitary fibrous tumor of the upper respiratory tract. A report of six cases. Am J Surg Pathol 15: 842–848
221. Dorfman D M, To K, Dickersin G R et al. 1994 Solitary fibrous tumor of the orbit. Am J Surg Pathol 18: 281–287
222. Suster S, Nascimento A G, Miettinen M et al. 1995 Solitary fibrous tumor of soft tissue. A clinicopathologic and immunohistochemical study of 12 cases. Am J Surg Pathol 19: 1257–1266
223. Hasegawa T, Hirose T, Seki K, Yang P, Sano T 1996 Solitary fibrous tumour of the soft tissue. An immunohistochemical and ultrastructural study. Am J Clin Pathol 106: 325–331
224. Nielsen G P, O'Connell J X, Dickersin G R, Rosenberg A E 1997 Solitary fibrous tumor of soft tissue: a report of 15 cases, including 5 malignant examples with light microscopic, immunohistochemical and ultrastructural data. Mod Pathol 10: 1028–1037
225. Brunnemann R B, Ro J Y, Ordonez N G et al. 1999 Extrapleural solitary fibrous tumor: a clinicopathologic study of 24 cases. Mod Pathol 12: 1034–1042
226. Alawi F, Stratton D, Freedman P D 2001 Solitary fibrous tumor of the oral soft tissues: a clinicopathologic and immunohistochemical study of 16 cases. Am J Surg Pathol 25: 900–910
227. Chan J K C 1997 Solitary fibrous tumour – everywhere and a diagnosis in vogue. Histopathology 31: 568–576
228. Vallat–Decouvelaere A, Dry S M, Fletcher C D M 1998 Atypical and malignant solitary fibrous tumors in extrathoracic locations: evidence of their comparability to intrathoracic tumors. Am J Surg Pathol 22: 1501–1511

229. Gold J S, Antonescu C R, Hajdu C et al. 2002 Clinicopathologic correlates of solitary fibrous tumors. Cancer 94: 1057–1068
230. De Saint Aubain Somerhausen N, Rubin B P, Fletcher C D M 1999 Myxoid solitary fibrous tumor: a study of seven cases with emphasis on differential diagnosis. Mod Pathol 12: 463–471
231. Ng T L, Gown A M, Barry T S et al. 2005 Nuclear beta catenin in mesenchymal tumors. Mod Pathol 18: 68–74
232. Nielsen G P, Dickersin G R, Provenzal J M, Rosenberg A E 1995 Lipomatous hemangiopericytoma. A histologic, ultrastructural and immunohistochemical study of a unique variant of hemangiopericytoma. Am J Surg Pathol 19: 748–756
233. Folpe A L, Devaney K, Weiss S W 1999 Lipomatous hemangiopericytoma. A rare variant of hemangiopericytoma that may be confused with liposarcoma. Am J Surg Pathol 23: 1201–1207
234. Guillou L, Gebhard S, Coindre J M 2000 Lipomatous hemangiopericytoma: a fat-containing variant of solitary fibrous tumor? Clinicopathologic, immunohistochemical and ultrastructural analysis of a series in favor of a unifying concept. Hum Pathol 31: 1108–1115
235. Allen P W 1977 The fibromatoses: a clinicopathologic classification based on 140 cases. Part I. Am J Surg Pathol 1: 255–270
236. Hasegawa S, Fletcher C D M 1996 Fibromatosis in the adult. Adv Pathol Lab Med 9: 259–275
237. Yost J, Winters T, Fett H C 1955 Dupuytren's contracture. A statistical study. Am J Surg 90: 568–571
238. Early P F 1962 Population studies in Dupuytren's contracture. J Bone Joint Surg 44B: 602–613
239. Chiu H F, McFarlane R M 1978 Pathogenesis of Dupuytren's contracture: a correlative clinical–pathological study. J Hand Surg 3: 1–10
240. Ushijima M, Tsuneyoshi M, Enjoji M 1984 Dupuytren type fibromatosis. A clinicopathologic study of 62 cases. Acta Pathol Jpn 34: 991–1001
241. Rombouts J J, Noel H, Legrain Y, Munting E 1989 Prediction of recurrence in the treatment of Dupuytren's disease: evaluation of a histologic classification. J Hand Surg (Am) 14: 644–652
242. Dal Cin P, De Smet L, Sciot R, van Damme B, van den Berghe H 1999 Trisomy 7 and trisomy 8 in dividing and non-dividing tumor cells in Dupuytren's disease. Cancer Genet Cytogenet 108: 137–140
243. Montgomery E, Lee J H, Abraham S C, Wu T T 2001 Superficial fibromatoses are genetically distinct from deep fibromatoses. Mod Pathol 14: 695–701
244. Aviles E, Arlen M, Miller T 1971 Plantar fibromatosis. Surgery 69: 117–120
245. Evans H L 2002 Multinucleated giant cells in plantar fibromatosis. Am J Surg Pathol 26: 244–248
246. Breiner J A, Nelson M, Bredthauer B D, Neff J R, Bridge J A 1999 Trisomy 8 and trisomy 14 in plantar fibromatosis. Cancer Genet Cytogenet 108: 176–177
247. Allison J R, Allison J R 1966 Knuckle pads. Arch Dermatol 93: 311–316
248. McRoberts J W 1969 Peyronie's disease. Surg Gynecol Obstet 129: 1291–1294
249. Billig R, Baker R, Immergut M et al. 1975 Peyronie's disease. Urology 6: 409–418
250. Guerneri S, Stioui S, Mantovani F et al. 1991 Multiple clonal chromosomal abnormalities in Peyronie's disease. Cancer Genet Cytogenet 52: 181–185
251. Ballo M T, Zagars G K, Pollack A, Pisters P W, Pollack R A 1999 Desmoid tumor: prognostic factors and outcome after surgery, radiation therapy, or combined surgery and radiation therapy. J Clin Oncol 17: 158–167
252. Lewis J J, Boland P J, Leung D H, Woodruff J M, Brennen M F 1999 The enigma of desmoid tumors. Ann Surg 229: 866–872
253. Merchant N B, Lewis J J, Woodruff J M, Leung D H Y, Brennan M F 1999 Extremity and trunk desmoid tumors. A multifactorial analysis of outcome. Cancer 86: 2045–2052
254. Heinrich M C, McArthur G A, Demetri G D et al. 2006 Clinical and molecular studies of the effect of imatinib on advanced aggressive fibromatosis (desmoid tumor). J Clin Oncol 24: 1195–1203
255. Das Gupta T K, Brasfield R D, O'Hara J 1969 Extra-abdominal desmoids: a clinicopathologic study. Ann Surg 170: 109–121
256. Rock M G, Pritchard D J, Reiman H M et al. 1984 Extra-abdominal desmoid tumors. J Bone Joint Surg 66A: 1369–1374
257. Jones I T, Jagelman D J, Fazio V W et al. 1986 Desmoid tumors in familial polyposis coli. Ann Surg 204: 94–97
258. Burke A P, Sobin L H, Shekitka K M 1990 Mesenteric fibromatosis. A follow-up study. Arch Pathol Lab Med 114: 832–835
259. Burke A P, Sobin L H, Shekitka K M et al. 1990 Intra-abdominal fibromatosis. A pathologic analysis of 130 tumors with comparison of clinical subgroups. Am J Surg Pathol 14: 335–341
260. Watanabe K, Ogura G, Tajino T, Suzuki T 2002 Extra-abdominal desmoid fibromatosis: two familial cases with synchronous and metachronous multicentric hyalinizing nodules. Histopathology 41: 118–121
261. Miyaki M, Konishi M, Kikuchi-Yanoshita R et al. 1993 Coexistence of somatic and germ line mutations of the APC gene in desmoid tumors from patients with familial adenomatous polyposis. Cancer Res 53: 5079–5082
262. Nugent K P, Philips R K, Hodgson S V et al. 1994 Phenotypic expression in familial adenomatous polyposis: partial prediction by mutation analysis. Gut 35: 1622–1623
263. Eccles D M, van der Luijt R, Breukel C et al. 1996 Hereditary desmoid disease due to a frameshift mutation at codon 1924 of the APC gene. Am J Hum Genet 59: 1193–1201
264. Caspari R, Oschwang S, Friedl W et al. 1995 Familial adenomatous polyposis: desmoid tumours and lack of ophthalmic lesions (CHRPE) associated with APC mutations beyond codon 1444. Hum Mol Genet 4: 337–340
265. Lynch H T 1996 Desmoid tumors: genotype–phenotype differences in familial adenomatous polyposis – a nosological dilemma. Am J Hum Genet 59: 1184–1185
266. Brasfield R D, Das Gupta T K 1969 Desmoid tumors of the anterior abdominal wall. Surgery 65: 241–246
267. Hayry P, Reitamo J J, Totterman S et al. 1982 The desmoid tumor II. Analysis of factors possibly contributing to the etiology and growth behavior. Am J Clin Pathol 77: 674–680
268. Deyrup A T, Tretiakova M, Montag A G 2006 Estrogen receptor-beta expression in extra-abdominal fibromatoses: an analysis of 40 cases. Cancer 106: 208–213
269. Ayala A G, Ro J Y, Goepfert H et al. 1986 Desmoid fibromatosis: a clinicopathologic study of 25 children. Semin Diagn Pathol 3: 138–150
270. Yokoyama R, Tsuneyoshi M, Enjoji M et al. 1989 Extra-abdominal desmoid tumors: correlations between histological features and biologic behavior. Surg Pathol 2: 29–42
271. Schmidt D, Klinge P, Leuschner I et al. 1991 Infantile desmoid-type fibromatosis: morphological features correlate with biological behaviour. J Pathol 164: 315–319
272. Lucas D R, al-Abbadi M, Tabaczka P et al. 2003 c-kit expression in desmoid fibromatosis. Comparative immunohistochemical evaluation of two commercial antibodies. Am J Clin Pathol 119: 339–345
273. Fletcher J A, Naeem R, Xiao S et al. 1995 Chromosome aberrations in desmoid tumors: trisomy 8 may be a predictor of recurrence. Cancer Genet Cytogenet 79: 139–143
274. Li M, Cordon-Cardo C, Gerald W L, Rosai J 1996 Desmoid fibromatosis is a clonal process. Hum Pathol 27: 939–943
275. Li C, Bapat B, Alman B A 1998 Adenomatous polyposis coli gene mutation alters proliferation through its beta-catenin-regulatory function in aggressive fibromatosis (desmoid tumor). Am J Pathol 153: 709–714
276. Bhattacharya B, Dilworth H P, Iacobuzio-Donahue C et al. 2005. Nuclear beta-catenin expression distinguishes deep fibromatosis from other benign and malignant fibroblastic and myofibroblastic lesions. Am J Surg Pathol 29:653–659
277. De Wever I, Dal Cin P, Fletcher C D M et al. 2000 Cytogenetic, clinical and morphologic correlations in 78 cases of fibromatoses: a report from the CHAMP Study Group. Mod Pathol 13: 1080–1085
278. Schofield D E, Fletcher J A, Grier H E et al. 1994 Fibrosarcoma in infants and children. Application of new techniques. Am J Surg Pathol 18: 14–24
279. Fetsch J F, Miettinen M, Laskin W B et al. 2000 A clinicopathologic study of 45 pediatric soft tissue tumors with an admixture of adipose tissue and fibroblastic elements and a proposal for classification as lipofibromatosis. Am J Surg Pathol 24: 1491–1500
280. Coffin C M, Dehner L P, Meis-Kindblom J M 1998 Inflammatory myofibroblastic tumor, inflammatory fibrosarcoma and related lesions: an historical overview with differential diagnostic considerations. Semin Diagn Pathol 15: 102–110
281. Coffin C M, Watterson J, Priest J, Dehner L P 1995 Extrapulmonary inflammatory myofibroblastic tumor: a clinicopathologic and immunohistochemical study of 84 cases. Am J Surg Pathol 19: 859–872
282. Meis J M, Enzinger F M 1991 Inflammatory fibrosarcoma of the mesentery and retroperitoneum. A tumor closely simulating inflammatory pseudotumor. Am J Surg Pathol 15: 1146–1156
283. Lawrence B, Perez-Atayde A, Hibbard M K et al. 2000 TPM3-ALK and TPM4-ALK oncogenes in inflammatory myofibroblastic tumors. Am J Pathol 157: 377–384
284. Debelenko L, Arthur D C, Pack S D et al. 2003 Identification of CARS-ALK fusion in primary and metastatic lesions in inflammatory myofibroblastic tumor. Lab Invest 83: 1255–1265
285. Cessna M H, Zhou H, Sanger W G et al. 2002 Expression of ALK1 and p80 in inflammatory myofibroblastic tumor and its mesenchymal mimics: a study of 135 cases. Mod Pathol 15: 931–938
286. Coffin C M, Hornick J L, Fletcher C D M 2006 Inflammatory myofibroblastic tumor: comparison of clinicopathologic, histologic, immunohistochemical features and ALK expression in atypical and aggressive cases. Am J Surg Pathol – in press
287. Mentzel T, Dry S M, Katenkamp D, Fletcher C D M 1998 Low grade myofibroblastic sarcoma. Analysis of 18 cases in the spectrum of myofibroblastic tumors. Am J Surg Pathol 22: 1228–1238
288. Montgomery E, Goldblum J R, Fisher C 2001 Myofibrosarcoma: a clinicopathologic study. Am J Surg Pathol 25: 219–228
289. Fisher C 2004 Myofibrosarcoma. Virchows Arch 445: 215–223
290. Pritchard D J, Sim F H, Ivins J C et al. 1977 Fibrosarcoma of the bone and soft tissues of the trunk and extremities. Orthop Clin North Am 8: 869–881
291. Iwasaki H, Enjoji M 1979 Infantile and adult fibrosarcomas of the soft tissues. Acta Pathol Jpn 29: 377–388
292. Scott S M, Reiman H M, Pritchard D J et al. 1989 Soft tissue fibrosarcoma. A clinicopathologic study of 132 cases. Cancer 64: 925–931
293. Chung E B, Enzinger F M 1976 Infantile fibrosarcoma. Cancer 38: 729–739
294. Soule E H, Pritchard D J 1977 Fibrosarcoma in infants and children. A review of 110 cases. Cancer 40: 1711–1721
295. Coffin C M, Jaszcz W, O'Shea P A, Dehner L P 1994 So-called congenital infantile fibrosarcoma: does it exist and what is it? Pediatr Pathol 14: 133–150
296. Variend S, Bax N M, van Gorp J 1995 Are infantile myofibromatosis, congenital fibrosarcoma and congenital haemangiopericytoma histogenetically related? Histopathology 26: 57–62

297. Bourgeois J M, Knezevich S R, Mathers J A, Sorenson P H 2000 Molecular detection of the *ETV6-NTRK3* gene fusion differentiates congenital fibrosarcoma from other childhood spindle cell tumors. Am J Surg Pathol 24: 937–946
298. Sandberg A A, Bridge J A 2002 Updates on the cytogenetics and molecular genetics of bone and soft tissue tumors: congenital (infantile) fibrosarcoma and mesoblastic nephroma. Cancer Genet Cytogenet 132: 1–13
299. Merck C, Angervall L, Kindblom L-G et al. 1983 Myxofibrosarcoma. A malignant soft tissue tumour of fibroblastic-histiocytic origin. A clinicopathologic and prognostic study of 110 cases using multivariate analysis. Acta Pathol Microbiol Immunol Scand Sect A 91 (suppl 282): 1–40
300. Weiss S W, Enzinger F M 1977 Myxoid variant of malignant fibrous histiocytoma. Cancer 39: 1672–1685
301. Mentzel T, Calonje E, Wadden C et al. 1996 Myxofibrosarcoma: clinicopathologic analysis of 75 cases with emphasis on the low grade variant. Am J Surg Pathol 20: 391–405
302. Huang H Y, Lal P, Qin J et al. 2004 Low grade myxofibrosarcoma: a clinicopathological analysis of 49 cases treated at a single institution with simultaneous assessment of the efficacy of a 3-tier or 4-tier grading system. Hum Pathol 35: 612–621
302a. Nascimento A F, Fletcher C D M. 2006 Epithelioid variant of myxofibrosarcoma: expanding the clinicopathologic spectrum of myxofibrosarcoma in a series of 17 cases. Am J Surg Pathol – in press
303. Kindblom L-G, Merck C, Angervall L 1979 The ultrastructure of myxofibrosarcoma. A study of 11 cases. Virchow's Arch [A] 381: 121–139
304. Hirose T, Sano T, Hizawa K 1988 Ultrastructural study of the myxoid area of malignant fibrous histiocytomas. Ultrastruct Pathol 12: 621–630
305. Willems S M, Debiec-Rychter M, Szukai K et al. 2006 Local recurrence of myxofibrosarcoma is associated with increase in tumor grade and cytogenetic aberrations, suggesting a multistep tumor progression model. Mod Pathol 19: 407–416
306. Evans H L 1987 Low-grade fibromyxoid sarcoma. A report of two metastasizing neoplasms having a deceptively benign appearance. Am J Clin Pathol 88: 615–619
307. Evans H L 1993 Low grade fibromyxoid sarcoma. A report of 12 cases. Am J Surg Pathol 17: 595–600
308. Goodlad J R, Mentzel T, Fletcher C D M 1995 Low grade fibromyxoid sarcoma. Clinicopathological analysis of eleven new cases in support of a distinct entity. Histopathology 26: 229–237
309. Folpe A L, Lane K L, Paull G W, Weiss S W 2000 Low grade fibromyxoid sarcoma and hyalinizing spindle cell tumor with giant rosettes: a clinicopathologic study of 73 cases supporting their identity and assessing the impact of high grade areas. Am J Surg Pathol 24: 1353–1360
310. Billings S D, Giblen G, Fanburg-Smith J C 2005 Superficial low grade fibromyxoid sarcoma (Evans tumor): a clinicopathologic analysis of 19 cases with a unique observation in the pediatric population. Am J Surg Pathol 29: 204–210
311. Mertens F, Fletcher C D M, Antonescu C R et al. 2005 Clinicopathologic and molecular genetic characterization of low grade fibromyxoid sarcoma and cloning of a novel FUS/CREB3L1 fusion gene. Lab Invest 85: 408–415
312. Reid R, de Silva M V, Paterson L et al. 2003 Low grade fibromyxoid sarcoma and hyalinizing spindle cell tumor with giant rosettes share a common t(7;16)(q34;p11) translocation. Am J Surg Pathol 27: 1229–1236
313. Lane K L, Shannon R J, Weiss S W 1997 Hyalinizing spindle cell tumor with giant rosettes. A distinctive tumor closely resembling low grade fibromyxoid sarcoma. Am J Surg Pathol 21: 1481–1488
314. Meis-Kindblom J M, Kindblom L-G, Enzinger F M 1995 Sclerosing epithelioid fibrosarcoma. A variant of fibrosarcoma simulating carcinoma. Am J Surg Pathol 19: 979–993
315. Eyden B P, Marson C, Banerjee S S, Roberts I S, Harris M 1998 Sclerosing epithelioid fibrosarcoma: a study of five cases emphasizing diagnostic criteria. Histopathology 33: 354–360
316. Antonescu C R, Rosenblum M K, Pereira P et al. 2001 Sclerosing epithelioid fibrosarcoma: a study of 16 cases and confirmation of a clinicopathologically distinct tumor. Am J Surg Pathol 25: 699–709
317. Meis-Kindblom J M, Kindblom L-G 1998 Acral myxoinflammatory fibroblastic sarcoma. A low grade tumor of the hands and feet. Am J Surg Pathol 22: 911–924
318. Montgomery E A, Devaney K O, Giordano T J, Weiss S W 1998 Inflammatory myxohyaline tumor of distal extremities with virocyte or Reed–Sternberg-like cells: a distinctive lesion with features simulating inflammatory conditions, Hodgkin's disease and various sarcomas. Mod Pathol 11: 384–391
319. Myers B W, Masi A T, Feigenbaum S L 1980 Pigmented villonodular synovitis and tenosynovitis: a clinical epidemiologic study of 166 cases and literature review. Medicine 59: 223–238
320. Ushijima M, Hashimoto H, Tsuneyoshi M et al. 1986 Giant cell tumor of the tendon sheath (nodular tenosynovitis). A study of 207 cases to compare the large joint group with the common digit group. Cancer 57: 875–884
321. Monaghan H, Salter D M, Al-Nafussi A. 2001. Giant cell tumour of tendon sheath (localised nodular tenosynovitis): clinicopathological features of 71 cases. J Clin Pathol 54: 404–407
322. Bertoni F, Unni K K, Beabout J W, Sim F H 1997 Malignant giant cell tumor of the tendon sheaths and joints (malignant pigmented villonodular synovitis). Am J Surg Pathol 21: 153–163
323. Somerhausen N S, Fletcher C D M 2000 Diffuse-type giant cell tumor: clinicopathological and immunohistochemical analysis of 50 cases with extra-articular disease. Am J Surg Pathol 24: 479–492
324. Darling J M, Goldring S R, Harada Y et al. 1997 Multinucleated giant cells in pigmented villonodular synovitis and giant cell tumor of tendon sheath express features of osteoclasts. Am J Pathol 150: 1383–1393
325. Alguacil-Garcia A, Unni K K, Goellner J R 1978 Giant cell tumor of tendon sheath and pigmented villonodular synovitis. An ultrastructural study. Am J Clin Pathol 69: 6–17
326. O'Connell J X, Fanburg J C, Rosenberg A E 1995 Giant cell tumor of tendon sheath and pigmented villonodular synovitis: immunophenotype suggests a synovial cell origin. Hum Pathol 26: 771–775
327. Folpe A L, Weiss S W, Fletcher C D M, Gown A M 1998 Tenosynovial giant cell tumors: evidence for a desmin-positive dendritic cell subpopulation. Mod Pathol 11: 939–944
328. Sciot R, Rosai J, Dal Clin P et al. 1999 Analysis of 35 cases of localized and diffuse tenosynovial giant cell tumor: a report from the Chromosomes and Morphology (CHAMP) study group. Mod Pathol 12: 576–579
329. Vogrincic G S, O'Connell J X, Gilks C B 1997 Giant cell tumor of tendon sheath is a polyclonal cellular proliferation. Hum Pathol 28: 815–819
330. West R B, Rubin B P, Miller M A et al. 2006 A landscape effect in tenosynovial giant cell tumor from activation of CSF1 expression by a translocation in a minority of tumor cells. Proc Natl Acad Sci USA 103: 690–695
331. Fletcher C D M 1990 Benign fibrous histiocytoma of subcutaneous and deep soft tissue: a clinicopathologic analysis of 21 cases. Am J Surg Pathol 14: 801–809
332. Enzinger F M, Zhang R Y 1988 Plexiform fibrohistiocytic tumor presenting in children and young adults. An analysis of 65 cases. Am J Surg Pathol 12: 818–826
333. Hollowood K, Holley M P, Fletcher C D M 1991 Plexiform fibrohistiocytic tumour: clinicopathological, immunohistochemical and ultrastructural analysis in favour of a myofibroblastic lesion. Histopathology 19: 503–513
334. Remstein E D, Arndt C A, Nascimento A G 1999 Plexiform fibrohistiocytic tumor: clinicopathologic analysis of 22 cases. Am J Surg Pathol 23: 662–670
335. Folpe A L, Morris R J, Weiss S W 1999 Soft tissue giant cell tumor of low malignant potential: a proposal for the reclassification of malignant giant cell tumor of soft parts. Mod Pathol 12: 894–902
336. Oliveira A M, Dei Tos A P, Fletcher C D M, Nascimento A G 2000 Primary giant cell tumor of soft tissues: a study of 22 cases. Am J Surg Pathol 24: 248–256
337. O'Connell J X, Wehrli B M, Nielsen G P, Rosenberg A E 2000 Giant cell tumors of soft tissue: a clinicopathologic study of 18 benign and malignant tumors. Am J Surg Pathol 24: 386–395
338. Salm R, Sissons H A 1972 Giant cell tumours of soft tissues. J Pathol 107:27–39
339. Fletcher C D M 1992 Pleomorphic malignant fibrous histiocytoma: fact or fiction? A critical reappraisal based on 159 tumors diagnosed as pleomorphic sarcoma. Am J Surg Pathol 16: 213–228
340. Hollowood K, Fletcher C D M 1995 Malignant fibrous histiocytoma: morphologic pattern or pathologic entity? Semin Diagn Pathol 12: 210–220
341. Akerman M 1997 Malignant fibrous histiocytoma – the commonest soft tissue sarcoma or a nonexistent entity? Acta Orthop Scand 68 (suppl 273): 41–46
342. Gaffney E F, Dervan P A, Fletcher C D M 1993 Pleomorphic rhabdomyosarcoma in adulthood: analysis of 11 cases with definition of diagnostic criteria. Am J Surg Pathol 17: 601–609
343. Schurch W, Begin L R, Seemayer T A et al. 1996 Pleomorphic soft tissue myogenic sarcomas of adulthood. A reappraisal in the mid-1990s. Am J Surg Pathol 20: 131–147
344. Fletcher C D M, Gustafson P, Rydholm A, Willen H, Akerman M 2001 Clinicopathologic re-evaluation of 100 malignant fibrous histiocytomas: prognostic relevance of subclassification. J Clin Oncol 19: 3045–3050
345. Deyrup A T, Haydon R C, Huo D et al. 2003 Myoid differentiation and prognosis in adult pleomorphic sarcomas of the extremity: an analysis of 92 cases. Cancer 98: 805–813
346. Massi D, Beltrami G, Capanna R, Franchi A 2004 Histopathological reclassification of extremity pleomorphic soft tissue sarcoma has clinical relevance. Eur J Surg Oncol 30: 1131–1136
347. Guccion J G, Enzinger F M 1972 Malignant giant cell tumor of soft parts. An analysis of 32 cases. Cancer 29: 1518–1529
348. Angervall L, Hagmar B, Kindblom L-G et al. 1981 Malignant giant cell tumor of soft tissues: a clinicopathologic, cytologic, ultrastructural, angiographic and microangiographic study. Cancer 47: 736–747
349. Mentzel T, Calonje E, Fletcher C D M 1994 Leiomyosarcoma with prominent osteoclast-like giant cells: analysis of eight cases closely mimicking the so-called giant cell variant of 'MFH.' Am J Surg Pathol 18: 258–265
350. Mentzel T, Fletcher C D M 1994 Malignant mesenchymomas of soft tissue associated with numerous osteoclast-like giant cells mimicking the so-called giant cell variant of 'MFH.' Virchows Arch 424: 539–545
351. Kyriakos M, Kempson R L 1976 Inflammatory fibrous histiocytoma. An aggressive and lethal lesion. Cancer 37: 1584–1606
352. Roques A W W, Horton L W L, Leslie J et al. 1979 Inflammatory fibrous histiocytoma in the left upper abdomen with a leukemoid blood picture. Cancer 43: 1800–1804
353. Berger T G, Levin M W 1984 Congenital smooth muscle hamartoma. J Am Acad Dermatol 11: 709–712

354. Johnson M D, Jacobs A H 1989 Congenital smooth muscle hamartoma. A report of six cases and a review of the literature. Arch Dermatol 125: 820–822
355. Gran-Massanes M, Rainier S, Colomme-Grimmer M et al. 1996 Congenital smooth muscle hamartoma presenting as a linear atrophic plaque: case report and review of the literature. Pediatr Dermatol 13: 222–225
356. Stout A P 1937 Solitary cutaneous and subcutaneous leiomyoma. Am J Cancer 29: 435–469
357. Fisher W C, Helwig E B 1963 Leiomyomas of the skin. Arch Dermatol 88: 510–520
358. Raj S, Calonje E, Kraus M et al. 1997 Cutaneous pilar leiomyoma: clinicopathologic analysis of 53 lesions in 45 patients. Am J Dermatopathol 19: 2–9
359. Jolliffe D S 1978 Multiple cutaneous leiomyomata. Clin Exp Dermatol 3: 89–92
360. Alam N A, Olpin S, Leigh I M. 2005. Fumarate hydratase mutations and predisposition to cutaneous leiomyomas, uterine leiomyomas and renal cancer. Br J Dermatol 153: 11–17
361. Newman P L, Fletcher C D M 1991 Smooth muscle tumours of the external genitalia: clinicopathological analysis of a series. Histopathology 18: 523–529
362. Templeton A C 1972 Subcutaneous leiomyoma – a neglected tumour. East Afr Med J 49: 521–525
363. Hachisuga T, Hashimoto H, Enjoji M 1984 Angioleiomyoma. A clinicopathologic reappraisal of 562 cases. Cancer 54: 126–130
364. Fox S B, Heryet A, Khong T Y 1990 Angioleiomyomas: an immunohistological study. Histopathology 16: 495–496
365. Kilpatrick S E, Mentzel T, Fletcher C D M 1994 Leiomyoma of deep soft tissue. Clinicopathologic analysis of a series. Am J Surg Pathol 18: 576–582
366. Billings S D, Folpe A L, Weiss S W 2001 Do leiomyomas of deep soft tissue exist? An analysis of highly differentiated smooth muscle tumors of deep soft tissue supporting two distinct subtypes. Am J Surg Pathol 25: 1134–1142
367. Paal E, Miettinen M 2001 Retroperitoneal leiomyomas: a clinicopathologic and immunohistochemical study of 56 cases with a comparison to retroperitoneal leiomyosarcomas. Am J Surg Pathol 25: 1355–1363
368. Hornick J L, Fletcher C D M 2003 Criteria for malignancy in nonvisceral smooth muscle tumors. Ann Diagn Pathol 7: 60–66
369. Miettinen M, Fetsch J F 2006 Evaluation of biologic potential of smooth muscle tumours. Histopathology 48: 97–105
370. Nielsen G P, Rosenberg A E, Koerner F C et al. 1996 Smooth muscle tumors of the vulva. A clinicopathological study of 25 cases and review of the literature. Am J Surg Pathol 20: 779–793
371. Slone S, O'Connor D 1998 Scrotal leiomyomas with bizarre nuclei: a report of three cases. Mod Pathol 11: 282–287
372. Quinn T R, Young R H 1997 Smooth muscle hamartoma of the tunica dartos of the scrotum: report of a case. J Cutan Pathol 24: 322–326
373. Van Kooten E O, Hage J J, Meinhardt W et al. 2004 Acquired smooth muscle hamartoma of the scrotum: a histological simulator? Cutis 31: 388–392
374. Wile A G, Evans H L, Romsdahl M M 1981 Leiomyosarcoma of soft tissue: a clinicopathologic study. Cancer 48: 1022–1032
375. Shmookler B M, Lauer D H 1983 Retroperitoneal leiomyosarcoma. A clinicopathologic analysis of 36 cases. Am J Surg Pathol 7: 269–280
376. Hashimoto H, Tsuneyoshi M, Enjoji M 1985 Malignant smooth muscle tumors of the retroperitoneum and mesentery: a clinicopathologic analysis of 44 cases. J Surg Oncol 28: 177–186
377. Farshid G, Pradhan M, Goldblum J, Weiss S W 2002 Leiomyosarcoma of somatic soft tissues: a tumor of vascular origin with multivariate analysis of outcome in 42 cases. Am J Surg Pathol 26: 14–24
378. Fields J P, Helwig E B 1981 Leiomyosarcoma of the skin and subcutaneous tissue. Cancer 47: 156–169
379. Hashimoto H, Daimaru Y, Tsuneyoshi M et al. 1986 Leiomyosarcoma of the external soft tissues. A clinicopathologic, immunohistochemical and electron microscopic study. Cancer 57: 2077–2088
380. Gustafson P, Willen H, Baldertorp B et al. 1992 Soft tissue leiomyosarcoma. A population-based epidemiologic and prognostic study of 48 patients, including cellular DNA content. Cancer 70: 114–119
381. Dahl I, Angervall L 1974 Cutaneous and subcutaneous leiomyosarcoma. A clinicopathologic study of 47 patients. Pathol Eur 9: 307–315
382. Kaddu S, Beham A, Cerroni L et al. 1997 Cutaneous leiomyosarcoma. Am J Surg Pathol 21: 979–987
383. Kevorkian J, Cento D P 1973 Leiomyosarcoma of large arteries and veins. Surgery 73: 390–400
384. Varela-Duran J, Oliva H, Rosai J 1979 Vascular leiomyosarcoma. The malignant counterpart of vascular leiomyoma. Cancer 44: 1684–1691
385. Berlin O, Stener B, Kindblom L-G et al. 1984 Leiomyosarcomas of venous origin in the extremities. A correlated clinical, roentgenologic and morphologic study with diagnostic and surgical implications. Cancer 54: 2147–2159
386. Lack E E 1986 Leiomyosarcomas in childhood: a clinical and pathological study of 10 cases. Pediatr Pathol 6: 181–197
387. Swanson P E, Wick M R, Dehner L P 1991 Leiomyosarcoma of somatic soft tissues in childhood: an immunohistochemical analysis of six cases with ultrastructural correlation. Hum Pathol 22: 569–577
388. De Saint Aubain Somerhausen N, Fletcher C D M 1999 Leiomyosarcoma of soft tissue in children: clinicopathologic analysis of 20 cases. Am J Surg Pathol 23: 755–763
389. Jenson H B, Leach C T, McClain K L et al. 1997 Benign and malignant smooth muscle tumors containing Epstein–Barr virus in children with AIDS. Leuk Lymphoma 27: 303–314
390. Granovsky M O, Mueller B U, Nicholson H S et al. 1998 Cancer in human immunodeficiency virus-infected children: a case series from the Children's Cancer Group and the National Cancer Institute. J Clin Oncol 16: 1729–1735
391. Deyrup A T, Lee V K, Hill C E et al. 2006. Epstein–Barr virus-associated smooth muscle tumors are distinctive mesenchymal tumors reflecting multiple infection events: a clinicopathologic and molecular analysis of 29 tumors from 19 patients. Am J Surg Pathol 30: 75–82
392. Schurch W, Skalli O, Seemayer T A et al. 1987 Intermediate filament proteins and actin isoforms as markers for soft tissue tumor differentiation and origin. I. Smooth muscle tumors. Am J Pathol 128: 91–103
393. Lundgren L, Seidal T, Kindblom L-G et al. 1989 Intermediate and fine filaments of vascular leiomyomas (angiomyoma), leiomyoma and leiomyosarcomas of large veins. APMIS 97: 637–645
394. Lundgren L, Kindblom L-G, Seidal T et al. 1991 Intermediate and fine filaments in cutaneous and subcutaneous leiomyosarcomas. APMIS 99: 820–828
395. Iwata J, Fletcher C D M 2000 Immunohistochemical detection of cytokeratin and epithelial membrane antigen in leiomyosarcoma: a systematic study of 100 cases. Pathol Int 50: 7–14
396. Oda Y, Miyajima K, Kawaguchi K et al. 2001 Pleomorphic leiomyosarcoma: clinicopathologic and immunohistochemical study with special emphasis on its distinction from ordinary leiomyosarcoma and malignant fibrous histiocytoma. Am J Surg Pathol 25: 1030–1038
397. Rubin B P, Fletcher C D M 2000 Myxoid leiomyosarcoma of soft tissue: an underrecognized variant. Am J Surg Pathol 24: 927–936
398. Merchant W, Calonje E, Fletcher C D M 1995 Inflammatory leiomyosarcoma: a morphological subgroup within the heterogeneous family of so-called inflammatory 'MFH.' Histopathology 27: 525–532
399. Dal Cin P, Sciot R, Fletcher C D M et al. 1998 Inflammatory leiomyosarcoma may be characterised by specific near-haploid chromosome changes. J Pathol 185: 112–115
400. Mentzel T, Wadden C, Fletcher C D M 1994 Granular cell change in smooth muscle tumours of skin and soft tissue. Histopathology 24: 223–231
401. Suster S 1994 Epithelioid leiomyosarcoma of the skin and subcutaneous tissue. Clinicopathologic, immunohistochemical and ultrastructural study of five cases. Am J Surg Pathol 18: 232–240
402. Mandahl N, Fletcher C D M, Dal Cin P et al. 2000 Comparative cytogenetic study of spindle cell and pleomorphic leiomyosarcomas of soft tissues: a report from the CHAMP Study Group. Cancer Genet Cytogenet 116: 66–73
403. Derre J, Lagace R, Nicolas A et al. 2001 Leiomyosarcomas and most malignant fibrous histiocytomas share very similar comparative genomic hybridization imbalances: an analysis of a series of 27 leiomyosarcomas. Lab Invest 81:211–215
404. Sahn E E, Garen P D, Pai G S et al. 1990 Multiple rhabdomyomatous mesenchymal hamartomas of skin. Am J Dermatopathol 12: 485–491
405. Rosenberg A S, Kirk J, Morgan M B 2002 Rhabdomyomatous mesenchymal hamartoma: an unusual dermal entity with a report of two cases and a review of the literature. J Cutan Pathol 29: 238–243
406. Willis J, Abdul-Karim F W, Di Sant' Agnese P A 1994 Extracardiac rhabdomyoma. Semin Diagn Pathol 11: 15–25
407. Eusebi V, Ceccarelli C, Daniele E et al. 1988 Extracardiac rhabdomyoma: an immunocytochemical study and a review of the literature. Appl Pathol 6:197–207
408. Hansen T, Katenkamp D 2005 Rhabdomyoma of the head and neck: morphology and differential diagnosis. Virchows Arch 447: 849–854
409. Dehner L P, Enzinger F M, Font R L 1972 Fetal rhabdomyoma. An analysis of nine cases. Cancer 30: 160–166
410. Kapadia S B, Meis J M, Frisman D M et al. 1993 Fetal rhabdomyoma of the head and neck. A clinicopathologic and immunophenotypic study of 24 cases. Hum Pathol 24: 754–765
411. Smith N M, Thornton C M 1996 Fetal rhabdomyoma: two instances of recurrence. Pediatr Pathol Lab Med 16: 673–680
412. Di Sant' Agnese P A, Knowles D M 1980 Extracardiac rhabdomyoma: a clinicopathologic study and review of the literature. Cancer 46: 780–789
413. Kodet R, Fajstavr J, Kabelka Z et al. 1991 Is fetal cellular rhabdomyoma an entity or a differentiated rhabdomyosarcoma? A study of patients with rhabdomyoma of the tongue and sarcoma of the tongue enrolled in the Intergroup Rhabdomyosarcoma Studies I, II and III. Cancer 67: 2907–2913
414. Chabrel C M, Beilby J W 1980 Vaginal rhabdomyoma. Histopathology 4: 645–651
415. Woodruff J M, Perino G 1994 Non-germ-cell or teratomatous malignant tumors showing additional rhabdomyoblastic differentiation, with emphasis on the malignant Triton tumor. Semin Diagn Pathol 11: 69–81
416. Bale P M, Parsons R E, Stevens M M 1983 Diagnosis and behaviour of juvenile rhabdomyosarcoma. Hum Pathol 14: 596–611
417. Maurer H M, Beltangady M, Gehan E A et al. 1988 The Intergroup Rhabdomyosarcoma Study I. A final report. Cancer 61: 209–220
418. Crist W M, Garnsey L, Beltangady M S et al. 1990 Prognosis in children with rhabdomyosarcoma: a report of the Intergroup Rhabdomyosarcoma Studies I and II. J Clin Oncol 8: 443–452
419. Maurer H M, Gehan E A, Beltangady M et al. 1993 The Intergroup Rhabdomyosarcoma Study II. Cancer 71: 1904–1922
420. Newton W A, Soule E H, Hamoudi A B et al. 1988 Histopathology of childhood sarcomas, Intergroup Rhabdomyosarcoma Studies I, II and III. Clinicopathologic correlation. J Clin Oncol 6: 67–75

421. Hays D M, Donaldson S S, Shimada H et al. 1997 Primary and metastatic rhabdomyosarcoma in the breast: neoplasms of adolescent females. A report from the Intergroup Rhabdomyosarcoma Study. Med Pediatr Oncol 29: 181–189
422. Douglass E C, Shapiro D N, Valentine M et al. 1993 Alveolar rhabdomyosarcomas with the t(2;13): cytogenetic findings and clinicopathologic correlations. Med Pediatr Oncol 21: 83–87
423. Crist W M, Anderson J R, Meza J L et al. 2001 Intergroup rhabdomyosarcoma study – IV: results for patients with non-metastatic disease. J Clin Oncol 19: 3091–3102
424. Pappo A S, Anderson J R, Crist W M et al. 1999 Survival after relapse in children and adolescents with rhabdomyosarcoma: a report from the Intergroup Rhabdomyosarcoma Study Group. J Clin Oncol 17: 3487–3493
425. Lloyd R V, Hajdu S I, Knapper W H 1983 Embryonal rhabdomyosarcoma in adults. Cancer 51: 557–565
426. Seidal T, Kindblom L-G, Angervall L 1989 Rhabdomyosarcoma in middle-aged and elderly individuals. APMIS 97: 236–248
427. Hawkins W G, Hoos A, Antonescu C R et al. 2001 Clinicopathologic analysis of patients with adult rhabdomyosarcoma. Cancer 91: 794–803
428. La Quaglia M P, Heller G, Ghavimi F et al. 1994 The effect of age at diagnosis on outcome in rhabdomyosarcoma. Cancer 73: 109–117
429. Parham D M, Webber B, Holt H et al. 1991 Immunohistochemical study of childhood rhabdomyosarcomas and related neoplasms. Cancer 67: 3072–3080
430. Tsokos M 1994 The diagnosis and classification of childhood rhabdomyosarcoma. Semin Diagn Pathol 11: 26–38
431. Wang N P, Marx J, McNutt M A, Rutledge J C, Gown A M 1995 Expression of myogenic regulatory proteins (myogenin and MyoD1) in small blue round cell tumors of childhood. Am J Pathol 147: 1799–1810
432. Dias P, Chen B, Dilday B et al. 2000 Strong immunostaining for myogenin in rhabdomyosarcoma is significantly associated with tumors of the alveolar subclass. Am J Pathol 156: 399–408
433. Kumar S, Perlman E, Harris C A et al. 2000 Myogenin is a specific marker for rhabdomyosarcoma: an immunohistochemical study in paraffin-embedded tissues. Mod Pathol 13: 988–993
434. D'Amore E S G, Tollot M, Stracca-Pansa V et al. 1994 Therapy-associated differentiation in rhabdomyosarcoma. Mod Pathol 7: 69–75
435. Coffin C M, Rulon J, Smith L, Bruggers C, White F V 1997 Pathologic features of rhabdomyosarcoma before and after treatment: a clinicopathologic and immunohistochemical analysis. Mod Pathol 10: 1175–1187
436. Kodet R, Newton W A, Hamoudi A B et al. 1993 Childhood rhabdomyosarcoma with anaplastic (pleomorphic) features. A report of the Intergroup Rhabdomyosarcoma Study. Am J Surg Pathol 17: 443–453
437. Kodet R, Newton W A, Hamoudi A B et al. 1991 Rhabdomyosarcoma with intermediate filament inclusions and features of rhabdoid tumors. Light microscopic and immunohistochemical study. Am J Surg Pathol 15: 257–267
438. Enterline H T, Horn R C 1958 Alveolar rhabdomyosarcoma. A distinctive tumor type. Am J Surg Pathol 29: 356–366
439. Enzinger F M, Shiraki M 1969 Alveolar rhabdomyosarcoma. An analysis of 110 cases. Cancer 24: 18–31
440. Tsokos M, Webber B L, Parham D M et al. 1992 Rhabdomyosarcoma. A new classification scheme related to prognosis. Arch Pathol Lab Med 116: 847–855
441. Qualman S J, Coffin C M, Newton W A et al. 1998 Intergroup Rhabdomyosarcoma Study: update for pathologists. Pediatr Dev Pathol 1: 550–561
442. Chan J K C, Ng H–K, Wan K Y et al. 1989 Clear cell rhabdomyosarcoma of the nasal cavity and paranasal sinuses. Histopathology 14: 391–399
443. Begin L R, Schurch W, LaCoste J, Hiscott J, Melnychuk D A 1994 Glycogen-rich clear cell rhabdomyosarcoma of the mediastinum. Potential diagnostic pitfall. Am J Surg Pathol 18: 302–308
444. Furlong MA, Mentzel T, Fanburg-Smith JC 2001 Pleomorphic rhabdomyosarcoma in adults: a clinicopathologic study of 38 cases with emphasis on morphologic variants and recent skeletal muscle-specific markers. Hum Pathol 14: 595–603
445. Furlong M A, Fanburg-Smith J C. 2001. Pleomorphic rhabdomyosarcoma in children: four cases in the pediatric age group. Ann Diagn Pathol 5: 199–206
446. Cavazzana A O, Schmidt D, Ninfo V et al. 1992 Spindle cell rhabdomyosarcoma. A prognostically favorable variant of rhabdomyosarcoma. Am J Surg Pathol 16: 229–235
447. Leuschner I, Newton W A, Schmidt D et al. 1993 Spindle cell variants of embryonal rhabdomyosarcoma in the paratesticular region. A report of the Intergroup Rhabdomyosarcoma Study. Am J Surg Pathol 17: 221–230
448. Nascimento A F, Fletcher C D M 2005 Spindle cell rhabdomyosarcoma in adults. Am J Surg Pathol 29: 1106–1113
449. Mentzel T, Katenkamp D 2000 Sclerosing pseudovascular rhabdomyosarcoma in adults. Clinicopathologic and immunohistochemical analysis of three cases. Virchows Arch 436: 305–311
450. Folpe A L, McKenney J K, Bridge J A, Weiss S W 2002 Sclerosing rhabdomyosarcoma in adults: report of four cases of a hyalinizing, matrix-rich variant of rhabdomyosarcoma that may be confused with osteosarcoma, chondrosarcoma or angiosarcoma. Am J Surg Pathol 26: 1175–1183
451. Chiles M C, Parham D M, Qualman S J et al. 2004 Sclerosing rhabdomyosarcomas in children and adolescents: a clinicopathologic review of 13 cases from the Intergroup Rhabdomyosarcoma Study Group and Children's Oncology Group. Pediatr Dev Pathol 7: 583–594
452. Scrable H, Witte D, Shimada H et al. 1989 Molecular differential pathology of rhabdomyosarcoma. Genes Chromosomes Cancer 1: 23–35
453. Kushner B H, LaQuaglia M P, Cheung N K et al. 1999 Clinically critical impact of molecular genetic studies in pediatric solid tumors. Med Pediatr Oncol 33: 530–535
454. Anderson J, Gordon A, Pritchard-Jones K, Shipley J 1999 Genes, chromosomes and rhabdomyosarcoma. Genes Chromos Cancer 26: 275–285
455. Hostein I, Andraud-Fregeville M, Guillou L et al. 2004 Rhabdomyosarcoma: value of myogenin expression analysis and molecular testing in diagnosing the alveolar subtype: an analysis of 109 paraffin-embedded specimens. Cancer 101: 2817–2824
456. Sorenson P H, Lynch J C, Qualman S J et al. 2002 PAX3-FKHR and PAX7-FKHR gene fusions are prognostic indicators in alveolar rhabdomyosarcoma: a report from the Children's Oncology Group. J Clin Oncol 20: 2672–2679
457. Rodriquez-Peralto J L, Lopez-Barea F, Sanchez-Herrara S, Atienza M 1994 Primary aneurysmal cyst of soft tissues. Am J Surg Pathol 18: 632–636
458. Nielsen G P, Fletcher C D M, Smith M A et al. 2002 Soft tissue aneurysmal bone cyst: a clinicopathologic study of five cases. Am J Surg Pathol 26: 64–69
459. Oliveira A M, Perez-Atayde A R, Inwards C Y et al. 2004 USP6 and CDH11 oncogenes identify the neoplastic cell in primary aneurysmal bone cysts and are absent in so-called secondary aneurysmal bone cysts. Am J Pathol 165: 1773–1780
460. Roth S I, Stowell R E, Helwig E B 1963 Cutaneous ossification. Report of 120 cases and review of the literature. Arch Pathol 76: 56–66
461. Donaldson E M, Summerly R 1962 Primary osteoma cutis and diaphyseal aclasis. Arch Dermatol 85: 141–145
462. Peterson W C, Mandel S L 1963 Primary osteomas of the skin. Arch Dermatol 87: 132–138
463. Bergonse F N, Nico M M, Kavamura M I, Sotto M N 2002 Miliary osteoma of the face: a report of 4 cases and review of the literature. Cutis 69: 383–386
464. Allan C J, Soule E H 1971 Osteogenic sarcoma of the somatic soft tissues. Clinicopathologic study of 26 cases and review of the literature. Cancer 27: 1121–1133
465. Sordillo P P, Hajdu S I, Magill G B et al. 1983 Extraosseous osteogenic sarcoma. A review of 48 patients. Cancer 51: 727–734
466. Chung E B, Enzinger F M 1987 Extraskeletal osteosarcoma. Cancer 60: 1132–1142
467. Lee J S, Fetsch J F, Wasdahl D A et al. 1995 A review of 40 patients with extraskeletal osteosarcoma. Cancer 76: 2253–3259
468. Lidang Jensen M, Schumacher B, Myhre Jensen O et al. 1998 Extraskeletal osteosarcomas: a clinicopathologic study of 25 cases. Am J Surg Pathol 22: 588–594
469. Goldstein-Jackson S Y, Gosheger G, Delling G et al. 2005 Extraskeletal osteosarcoma has a favourable prognosis when treated like conventional osteosarcoma. J Cancer Res Clin Oncol 131:520–526
470. Mirra J M, Fain J S, Ward W G et al. 1993 Extraskeletal telangiectatic osteosarcoma. Cancer 71: 3014–3019
471. Fanburg-Smith J C, Bratthauer G L, Miettinen M 1999 Osteocalcin and osteonectin immunoreactivity in extraskeletal osteosarcoma: a study of 28 cases. Hum Pathol 30: 32–38
472. Van Roggen J F G, Hogendoorn P C W, Fletcher C D M 1999 Myxoid tumours of soft tissue. Histopathology 35: 291–312
473. Enzinger F M 1965 Intramuscular myxoma. A review and follow-up study of 34 cases. Am J Clin Pathol 43: 104–113
474. Ireland D C R, Soule E H, Ivins J C 1973 Myxoma of somatic soft tissues. A report of 58 patients, 3 with multiple tumors and fibrous dysplasia of bone. Mayo Clin Proc 48: 401–410
475. Kindblom L-G, Stener B, Angervall L 1974 Intramuscular myxoma. Cancer 34: 1737–1744
476. Hashimoto H, Tsuneyoshi M, Daimaru Y et al. 1986 Intramuscular myxoma. A clinicopathologic, immunohistochemical and electron microscopic study. Cancer 58: 740–747
477. Nielsen G P, O'Connell J X, Rosenberg A E 1998 Intramuscular myxoma: a clinicopathologic study of 51 cases with emphasis on hypercellular and hypervascular variants. Am J Surg Pathol 22: 1222–1227
478. Wirth W A, Leavitt D, Enzinger F M 1971 Multiple intramuscular myxomas. Another extraskeletal manifestation of fibrous dysplasia. Cancer 27: 1167–1173
479. Miettinen M, Hockerstedt K, Reitamo J et al. 1985 Intramuscular myxoma – a clinicopathologic study of twenty three cases. Am J Clin Pathol 84: 265–272
480. Van Roggen J F, McMenamin M E, Fletcher C D M. 2001. Cellular myxoma of soft tissue: a clinicopathologic study of 38 cases confirming indolent clinical behaviour. Histopathology 39: 287–297
481. Okamoto S, Hisaoka M, Ushijima M et al. 2000 Activating Gs(alpha) mutations in intramuscular myxomas with and without fibrous dysplasia of bone. Virchows Arch 437: 133–137
482. Meis J M, Enzinger F M 1992 Juxta-articular myxoma. A clinical and pathologic study of 65 cases. Hum Pathol 23: 639–646
483. Okamoto S, Hisaoka M, Meis-Kindblom J M et al. 2002 Juxta-articular myxoma and intramuscular myxoma are two distinct entities. Activating Gs(alpha) mutation at Arg 201 codon does not occur in juxta-articular myxoma. Virchows Arch 440: 12–15
484. Sciot R, Dal Cin P, Samson I et al. 1999 Clonal chromosomal changes in juxta-articular myxoma. Virchow's Arch 434: 177–180
485. Fetsch J F, Laskin W B, Miettinen M 2001 Superficial acral fibromyxoma: a clinicopathologic and immunohistochemical analysis of 37 cases of a distinctive soft tissue tumor with a predilection for the fingers and toes. Hum Pathol 32: 704–714

486. Allen P W, Dymock R B, MacCormac W B 1988 Superficial angiomyxomas with and without epithelial components. Report of 30 tumors in 28 patients. Am J Surg Pathol 12: 519–530
487. Fetsch J F, Laskin W B, Tavossoli F A 1997 Superficial angiomyxoma (cutaneous myxoma): a clinicopathologic study of 17 cases arising in the genital region. Int J Gynecol Pathol 16: 325–334
488. Calonje E, Guerin D, McCormick D, Fletcher C D M 1999 Superficial angiomyxoma: clinicopathologic analysis of a series of distinctive but poorly recognized cutaneous tumors with a tendency for recurrence. Am J Surg Pathol 23: 910–917
489. Ferreiro J A, Carney J A 1994 Myxomas of the external ear and their significance. Am J Surg Pathol 18: 274–280
490. Carney J A, Toorkey B C 1991 Myxoid fibroadenoma and allied conditions (myxomatosis) of the breast. A heritable disorder with special associations including cardiac and cutaneous myxomas. Am J Surg Pathol 15: 713–721
491. Steeper T A, Rosai J 1983 Aggressive angiomyxoma of the female pelvis and perineum. Report of nine cases of a distinctive type of gynecologic soft tissue neoplasm. Am J Surg Pathol 7: 463–475
492. Fetsch J F, Laskin W B, Lefkowitz M et al. 1996 Aggressive angiomyxoma. A clinicopathologic study of 29 female patients. Cancer 78: 79–90
493. Tsang W Y W, Chan J K C, Lee K C et al. 1992 Aggressive angiomyxoma. A report of four cases occurring in men. Am J Surg Pathol 16: 1059–1065
494. Iezzoni J C, Fechner R E, Wong L S, Rosai J 1995 Aggressive angiomyxoma in males: a report of four cases. Am J Clin Pathol 104: 391–396
495. Rosai J, Limas C, Husband E M 1984 Ectopic hamartomatous thymoma: a distinctive benign lesion of the lower neck. Am J Surg Pathol 8: 501–513
496. Chan J K C, Rosai J 1991 Tumors of the neck showing thymic or related branchial pouch differentiation: a unifying concept. Hum Pathol 22: 349–367
497. Fetsch J F, Laskin W B, Michal M et al. 2004 Ectopic hamartomatous thymoma: a clinicopathologic and immunohistochemical analysis of 21 cases with data supporting reclassification as a branchial anlage mixed tumor. Am J Surg Pathol 28: 1360–1370
498. Weidner N, Santa Cruz D 1987 Phosphaturic mesenchymal tumors. A polymorphous group causing osteomalacia or rickets. Cancer 59: 1442–1454
499. Folpe A L, Fanburg-Smith J C, Billings S D et al. 2004 Most osteomalacia-associated mesenchymal tumors are a single histopathologic entity: an analysis of 32 cases and a comprehensive review of the literature. Am J Surg Pathol 28: 1–30
500. Marshall-Taylor C, Fanburg-Smith J C 2000 Hemosiderotic fibrohistiocytic lipomatous lesion: ten cases of a previously undescribed fatty lesion of the foot/ankle. Mod Pathol 13: 1192–1199
501. Browne T J, Fletcher C D M 2006 Haemosiderotic fibrolipomatous tumour (so-called haemosiderotic fibrohistiocytic lipomatous tumour): analysis of 13 new cases in support of a distinct entity. Histopathology 48: 453–461
502. Folpe A L, Weiss S W 2004 Pleomorphic hyalinizing angiectatic tumor: analysis of 41 cases supporting evolution from a distinctive precursor lesion. Am J Surg Pathol 28: 1417–1425
503. Enzinger F M, Weiss S W, Liang C Y 1989 Ossifying fibromyxoid tumor of soft parts. A clinicopathologic analysis of 59 cases. Am J Surg Pathol 13: 817–827
504. Miettinen M 1991 Ossifying fibromyxoid tumor of soft parts. Additional observations of a distinctive soft tissue tumor. Am J Surg Pathol 95: 142–149
505. Schofield J B, Krausz T, Stamp G W H et al. 1993 Ossifying fibromyxoid tumour of soft parts – immunohistochemical and ultrastructural analysis of a series. Histopathology 22: 101–112
506. Zamecnik M, Michal M, Simpson R H et al. 1997 Ossifying fibromyxoid tumor of soft parts: a report of 17 cases with emphasis on unusual histological features. Ann Diagn Pathol 1: 73–81
507. Folpe A L, Weiss S W 2003 Ossifying fibromyxoid tumor of soft parts: a clinicopathologic study of 70 cases with emphasis on atypical and malignant variants. Am J Surg Pathol 27: 421–431
508. Kilpatrick S E, Ward W G, Mozes M et al. 1995 Atypical and malignant variants of ossifying fibromyxoid tumor. Clinicopathologic analysis of six cases. Am J Surg Pathol 19: 1039–1046
509. Min K W, Seo I S, Pitha J 2005 Ossifying fibromyxoid tumor: modified myoepithelial cell tumor? Report of three cases with immunohistochemical and electron microscopic studies. Ultrastruct Pathol 29: 535–548
510. Kilpatrick S E, Hitchcock M G, Kraus M D, Calonje E, Fletcher C D M 1997 Mixed tumors and myoepitheliomas of soft tissue: a clinicopathologic study of 19 cases with a unifying concept. Am J Surg Pathol 21: 13–22
511. Michal M, Miettinen M 1999 Myoepitheliomas of the skin and soft tissues. Report of 12 cases. Virchow's Arch 434: 393–400
512. Hornick J L, Fletcher C D M 2003 Myoepithelial tumors of soft tissue: a clinicopathologic and immunohistochemical study of 101 cases with evaluation of prognostic parameters. Am J Surg Pathol 27: 1183–1198
513. Dabska M 1977 Parachordoma. A new clinicopathologic entity. Cancer 40: 1586–1592
514. Fisher C, Miettinen M 1997 Parachordoma: a clinicopathologic and immunohistochemical study of four cases of an unusual soft tissue neoplasm. Ann Diagn Pathol 1: 3–10
515. Folpe A L, Agoff S N, Willis J, Weiss S W 1999 Parachordoma is immunohistochemically and cytogenetically distinct from axial chordoma and extraskeletal myxoid chondrosarcoma. Am J Surg Pathol 23: 1059–1067
516. Smith B C, Ellis G L, Meis-Kindblom J M, Williams S B 1995 Ectomesenchymal chondromyxoid tumor of the anterior tongue. Nineteen cases of a new clinicopathologic entity. Am J Surg Pathol 19: 519–530

517. Enzinger F M 1979 Angiomatoid malignant fibrous histiocytoma. A distinct fibrohistiocytic tumor of children and young adults simulating a vascular neoplasm. Cancer 44: 2147–2157
518. Costa M J, Weiss S W 1990 Angiomatoid malignant fibrous histiocytoma. A follow-up study of 108 cases with evaluation of possible histologic predictors of outcome. Am J Surg Pathol 14: 1126–1132
519. Pettinato G, Manivel J C, De Rosa G et al. 1990 Angiomatoid malignant fibrous histiocytoma: cytologic, immunohistochemical, ultrastructural and flow cytometric study of 20 cases. Mod Pathol 3: 479–487
520. Fanburg-Smith J C, Miettinen M 1999 Angiomatoid 'malignant' fibrous histiocytoma: a clinicopathologic study of 158 cases and further exploration of the myoid phenotype. Hum Pathol 30: 1336–1343
521. Fletcher C D M 1991 Angiomatoid 'malignant fibrous histiocytoma': an immunohistochemical study indicative of myoid differentiation. Hum Pathol 22: 563–568
522. Smith M E F, Costa M J, Weiss S W 1991 Evaluation of CD68 and other histiocytic antigens in angiomatoid malignant fibrous histiocytoma. Am J Surg Pathol 15: 757–763
523. Waters B L, Panagopoulos I, Allen E F 2000 Genetic characterization of angiomatoid fibrous histiocytoma identifies fusion of the FUS and ATF-1 genes induced by a chromosomal translocation involving bands 12q13 and 16p11. Cancer Genet Cytogenet 121: 109–116
524. Hallor K H, Mertens F, Jin Y et al. 2005 Fusion of the EWSR1 and ATF1 genes without expression of MITF-M transcript in angiomatoid fibrous histiocytoma. Genes Chromos Cancer 44: 97–102
525. Smith M E F, Fisher C, Weiss S W 1996 Pleomorphic hyalinizing angiectatic tumor of soft parts. A low grade neoplasm resembling neurilemoma. Am J Surg Pathol 20: 21–29
526. Tsang W Y W, Chan J K C, Fletcher C D M, Rosai J 1993 Symplastic hemangioma: a distinctive vascular neoplasm featuring bizarre stromal cells. Int J Surg Pathol 1: 202 (abstract)
527. Mitsuhashi T, Barr R J, Machtinger L A, Cassarino DS 2005 Primary cutaneous myxofibrosarcoma mimicking pleomorphic hyalinizing angiectatic tumor (PHAT): a potential diagnostic pitfall. Am J Dermatopathol 27: 322–326
528. Bonetti F, Pea M, Martignoni G et al. 1992 PEC and sugar. Am J Surg Pathol 16: 307–308 (letter)
529. Hornick J L, Fletcher C D M 2006 PEComa: what do we know so far? Histopathology 48: 75–82
530. Folpe A L, Mentzel T, Lehr H A et al. 2005 Perivascular epithelioid cell neoplasms of soft tissue and gynecologic origin: a clinicopathologic study of 26 cases and review of the literature. Am J Surg Pathol 29: 1558–1575
531. Cadman N L, Soule E H, Kelly P J 1965 Synovial sarcoma. An analysis of 134 tumors. Cancer 18: 613–627
532. Wright P H, Sim F H, Soule E H et al. 1982 Synovial sarcoma. J Bone Joint Surg 64A: 112–122
533. Schmidt D, Thun P, Med C et al. 1991 Synovial sarcoma in children and adolescents. A report from the Kiel Pediatric Tumor Registry. Cancer 67: 1667–1672
534. Bergh P, Meis-Kindblom J M, Gherlinzoni F et al. 1999 Synovial sarcoma: identification of low and high risk groups. Cancer 85: 2596–2607
535. Skytting B, Bauer H C F, Perfekt R et al. 1999 Clinical course in synovial sarcoma. A Scandinavian Sarcoma Group study of 104 patients. Acta Orthop Scand 70: 536–542
536. Fisher C 1998 Synovial sarcoma. Ann Diagn Pathol 2: 401–421
537. Fetsch J F, Meis J M 1993 Synovial sarcoma of the abdominal wall. Cancer 72: 469–477
538. Roth J A, Enzinger F M, Tannenbaum M 1975 Synovial sarcoma of the neck: a follow-up study of 24 cases. Cancer 35: 1243–1253
539. Shmookler B M, Enzinger F M, Brannon R B 1982 Orofacial synovial sarcoma. A clinicopathologic study of 11 new cases and review of the literature. Cancer 50: 269–276
540. Ratnatunga N, Goodlad J R, Sankarakumaran N et al. 1992 Primary biphasic synovial sarcoma of the orbit. J Clin Pathol 45: 265–267
541. Suster S, Moran C 2005 Primary synovial sarcomas of the mediastinum: a clinicopathologic, immunohistochemical and ultrastructural study of 15 cases. Am J Surg Pathol 29: 569–578
542. Fisher C, Folpe A L, Hashimoto H, Weiss SW 2004 Intra-abdominal synovial sarcoma: a clinicopathological study. Histopathology 45: 245–253
543. Miettinen M, Santavirta S, Slatis P 1987 Intravascular synovial sarcoma. Hum Pathol 18: 1075–1079
544. O'Connell J X, Browne W L, Gropper P T, Berean K W 1996 Intraneural biphasic synovial sarcoma: an alternative 'glandular' tumor of peripheral nerve. Mod Pathol 9: 738–741
545. McKinney C D, Mills S E, Fechner R E 1992 Intraarticular synovial sarcoma. Am J Surg Pathol 16: 1017–1020
546. Miettinen M, Virtanen I 1984 Synovial sarcoma – a misnomer. Am J Pathol 117: 18–25
547. Lewis J J, Antonescu C R, Leung D H et al. 2000 Synovial sarcoma: a multivariate analysis of prognostic factors in 112 patients with primary localized tumors of the extremity. J Clin Oncol 18: 2087–2094
548. Trassard M, Le Doussal V, Hacene K et al. 2001 Prognostic factors in localized primary synovial sarcoma: a multicenter study of 128 adult patients. J Clin Oncol 19: 525–534
549. Guillou L, Benhattar J, Bonichon F et al. 2004 Histologic grade, but not SYT–SSX fusion type, is an important prognostic factor in patients with synovial sarcoma: a multicenter retrospective analysis. J Clin Oncol 22: 4040–4050

550. Folpe A L, Schmidt R A, Chapman D, Gown A M 1998 Poorly differentiated synovial sarcoma: immunohistochemical distinction from primitive neuroectodermal tumors and high grade malignant peripheral nerve sheath tumors. Am J Surg Pathol 22: 673–682
551. Van de Rijn M, Barr F G, Xiong Q B et al. 1999 Poorly differentiated synovial sarcoma: an analysis of clinical, pathologic and molecular genetic features. Am J Surg Pathol 23: 106–112
552. Chan J A, McMenamin M E, Fletcher C D M 2003 Synovial sarcoma in older patients: clinicopathological analysis of 32 cases with emphasis on unusual histological features. Histopathology 43: 72–83
553. Majeste R M, Beckman E N 1988 Synovial sarcoma with an overwhelming epithelial component. Cancer 61: 2527–2531
554. Varela Duran J, Enzinger F M 1982 Calcifying synovial sarcoma. Cancer 50: 345–352
555. Milchgrub S, Ghandur-Mnaymneh L, Dorfman H D et al. 1993 Synovial sarcoma with extensive osteoid and bone formation. Am J Surg Pathol 17: 357–363
556. Ordonez N G, Mahfouz S M, Mackay B 1990 Synovial sarcoma: an immunohistochemical and ultrastructural study. Hum Pathol 21: 733–749
557. Pelmus M, Guillou L, Hostein I et al. 2002 Monophasic fibrous and poorly differentiated synovial sarcoma: immunohistochemical reassessment of 60 t(x;18)(SYT–SSX)-positive cases. Am J Surg Pathol 26: 1434–1440
558. Guillou L, Wadden C, Kraus M D, Dei Tos A P, Fletcher C D M 1996 S-100 protein reactivity in synovial sarcomas – a potentially frequent diagnostic pitfall. Immunohistochemical analysis of 100 cases. Appl Immunohistochem 4: 167–175
559. Dei Tos A P, Wadden C, Calonje E et al. 1995 Immunohistochemical demonstration of glycoprotein p30/32^{MIC2} (CD99) in synovial sarcoma. A potential cause of diagnostic confusion. Appl Immunohistochem 3: 168–173
560. Smith T A, Machen S K, Fisher C, Goldblum J R 1999 Usefulness of cytokeratin subsets for distinguishing monophasic synovial sarcoma from malignant peripheral nerve sheath tumor. Am J Clin Pathol 112: 641–648
561. Dal Cin P, Rao U, Jani-Sait S et al. 1992 Chromosomes in the diagnosis of soft tissue tumors. I. Synovial sarcoma. Mod Pathol 5: 357–362
562. Sandberg A A, Bridge J A 2002 Updates on the cytogenetics and molecular genetics of bone and soft tissue tumors. Synovial sarcoma. Cancer Genet Cytogenet 133: 1–23
563. Clark J, Rocques P J, Crew A J et al. 1994 Identification of novel genes, SYT and SSX, involved in the t(X;18)(p11.2;q11.2) translocation found in human synovial sarcoma. Nature Genet 7: 502–508
564. Crew A J, Clark J, Fisher C et al. 1995 Fusion of SYT to two genes, SSX1 and SSX2, encoding proteins with homology to the Kruppel-associated box in synovial sarcoma. EMBO J 14: 2333–2340
565. Kawai A, Woodruff J, Healey J H et al. 1998 SYT–SSX gene fusion as a determinant of morphology and prognosis in synovial sarcoma. N Engl J Med 338: 153–160
566. Ladanyi M, Antonescu CR, Leung D H et al. 2002 Impact of SYT-SSX fusion type on the clinical behavior of synovial sarcoma: a multi-institutional retrospective study of 243 patients. Cancer Res 62: 135–140
567. Nilsson G, Skytting B, Xie Y et al. 1999 The SYT–SSX1 variant of synovial sarcoma is associated with a high rate of tumor cell proliferation and poor clinical outcome. Cancer Res 59: 3180–3184
568. Enzinger F M 1970 Epithelioid sarcoma. A sarcoma simulating a granuloma or a carcinoma. Cancer 26: 1029–1041
569. Dabska M, Koszarowski T 1982 Clinical and pathologic study of aponeurotic (epithelioid) sarcoma. Pathol Annu 17: 129–153
570. Chase D R, Enzinger F M 1985 Epithelioid sarcoma. Diagnosis, prognostic indicators and treatment. Am J Surg Pathol 9: 241–263
571. Evans H L, Baer S C 1993 Epithelioid sarcoma: a clinicopathologic and prognostic study of 26 cases. Semin Diagn Pathol 10: 286–291
572. Halling A C, Wollan P C, Pritchard D J, Vlasak R, Nascimento A G 1996 Epithelioid sarcoma: a clinicopathologic review of 55 cases. Mayo Clin Proc 71: 636–642
573. El-Naggar A K, Garcia G M 1992 Epithelioid sarcoma. Flow cytometric study of DNA content and regional DNA heterogeneity. Cancer 69: 1721–1728
574. Ulbright T M, Brokaw S A, Stehman F B et al. 1983 Epithelioid sarcoma of the vulva. Evidence suggesting a more aggressive behaviour than extragenital epithelioid sarcoma. Cancer 52: 1462–1469
575. Guillou L, Wadden C, Coindre J M, Krausz T, Fletcher C D M 1997 'Proximal-type' epithelioid sarcoma, a distinctive aggressive neoplasm showing rhabdoid features. Clinicopathologic, immunohistochemical and ultrastructural study of a series. Am J Surg Pathol 21: 130–146
576. Hasegawa T, Matsuno Y, Shimoda T et al. 2001 Proximal-type epithelioid sarcoma: a clinicopathologic study of 20 cases. Mod Pathol 14: 655–663
577. Casanova M, Ferrari A, Collini P et al. 2006 Epithelioid sarcoma in children and adolescents: a report from the Italian Soft Tissue Sarcoma Committee. Cancer 106: 708–717
578. Mirra J M, Kessler S, Bhuta S et al. 1992 The fibroma-like variant of epithelioid sarcoma. A fibrohistiocytic/myoid cell lesion often confused with benign and malignant spindle cell tumors. Cancer 69: 1382–1395
579. Miettinen M, Fanburg-Smith J C, Virolainen M, Shmookler B M, Fetsch J F 1999 Epithelioid sarcoma: an immunohistochemical analysis of 112 classical and variant cases and a discussion of the differential diagnosis. Hum Pathol 30: 934–942
580. Quezado M M, Middleton L P, Bryant B et al. 1998 Allelic loss on chromosome 22q in epithelioid sarcomas. Hum Pathol 29: 604–608
581. Lualdi E, Modena P, Debiec-Rychter M et al. 2004 Molecular cytogenetic characterization of proximal-ype epithelioid sarcoma. Genes Chromos Cancer 41: 283–390
582. Foschini M P, Eusebi V 1994 Alveolar soft-art sarcoma: a new type of rhabdomyosarcoma? Semin Diagn Pathol 11: 58–68
583. Ladanyi M, Lui M Y, Antonescu C R et al. 2001 The der(17)t(x;17)(p11;q25) of human alveolar soft part sarcoma fuses the TFE3 transcription factor gene to ASPL, a novel gene at 17q25. Oncogene 20: 48–57
584. Christopherson W M, Foote F W, Stewart F W 1952 Alveolar soft-art sarcomas: structurally characteristic tumors of uncertain histogenesis. Cancer 5: 100–111
585. Auerbach H E, Brooks J J 1987 Alveolar soft part sarcoma. A clinicopathologic and immunohistochemical study. Cancer 60: 66–73
586. Lieberman P H, Brennan M F, Kimmel M et al. 1989 Alveolar soft-part sarcoma. A clinicopathologic study of half a century. Cancer 63: 1–13
587. Portera C A, Ho X, Patel S R et al. 2001 Alveolar soft part sarcoma: clinical course and patterns of metastasis in 70 patients treated at a single institution. Cancer 91: 585–591
588. Flieder D B, Moran C A, Suster S 1997 Primary alveolar soft-part sarcoma of the mediastinum: a clinicopathological and immunohistochemical study of two cases. Histopathology 31: 469–473
589. Nielsen G P, Oliva E, Young R H et al. 1995 Alveolar soft-part sarcoma of the female genital tract: a report of nine cases and review of the literature. Int J Gynecol Pathol 14: 283–292
590. Park Y K, Unni K K, Kim Y W et al. 1999 Primary alveolar soft part sarcoma of bone. Histopathology 35: 411–417
591. Pappo A S, Parham D M, Cain A et al. 1996 Alveolar soft part sarcoma in children and adolescents: clinical features and outcome of 11 patients. Med Pediatr Oncol 26: 81–84
592. Kayton M L, Meyers P, Wexler L H et al. 2006 Clinical presentation, treatment and outcome of alveolar soft part sarcoma in children, adolescents and young adults. J Pediatr Surg 41: 187–193
593. Ordonez N G, Ro J Y, Mackay B 1989 Alveolar soft part sarcoma. An ultrastructural and immunocytochemical investigation of its histogenesis. Cancer 63: 1721–1736
594. Ladanyi M. Antonescu C R, Drobnjak M et al. 2002 The precrystalline cytoplasmic granules of alveolar soft part sarcoma contain monocarboxylate transporter 1 and CD147. Am J Pathol 160: 1215–1221
595. Persson S, Willems J S, Kindblom L-G et al. 1988 Alveolar soft part sarcoma. An immunohistochemical, cytologic and electron microscopic study and a quantitative DNA analysis. Virchow's Arch [A] 412: 499–513
596. Rosai J, Dias P, Parham D M et al. 1991 MyoD1 protein expression in alveolar soft part sarcoma as confirmatory evidence of its skeletal muscle nature. Am J Surg Pathol 15: 974–981
597. Carstens P H B 1990 Membrane-bound cytoplasmic crystals, similar to those in alveolar soft part sarcoma, in a human muscle spindle. Ultrastruct Pathol 14: 423–428
598. Cullinane C, Thorner P S, Greenberg M L et al. 1992 Molecular, genetic, cytogenetic and immunohistochemical characterization of alveolar soft part sarcoma. Implications for cell of origin. Cancer 70: 2444–2450
599. Wang N P, Bacchi C E, Jiang J J, McNutt M A, Gown A M 1996 Does alveolar soft-part sarcoma exhibit skeletal muscle differentiation? An immunocytochemical and biochemical study of myogenic regulatory protein expression. Mod Pathol 9: 496–506
600. van Echten J, van den Berg E, van Baarlen J et al. 1995 An important role for chromosome 17, band q25, in the histogenesis of alveolar soft-part sarcoma. Cancer Genet Cytogenet 82: 57–61
601. Joyama S, Ueda T, Shimizu K et al. 1999 Chromosome rearrangement at 17q25 and Xp11.2 in alveolar soft-part sarcoma: a case report and review of the literature. Cancer 86: 1246–1250
602. Argani P, Lal P, Hutchinson B et al. 2003 Aberrant nuclear immunoreactivity for TFE3 in neoplasms with TFE3 gene fusions: a sensitive and specific immunohistochemical assay. Am J Surg Pathol 27: 750–761
603. Enzinger F M, Shiraki M 1972 Extraskeletal myxoid chondrosarcoma. An analysis of 34 cases. Hum Pathol 3: 421–435
604. Tsuneyoshi M, Enjoji M, Iwasaki H et al. 1981 Extraskeletal myxoid chondrosarcoma. A clinicopathologic and electron microscopic study. Acta Pathol Jpn 31: 439–447
605. Saleh G, Evans H L, Ro J Y et al. 1992 Extraskeletal myxoid chondrosarcoma. A clinicopathologic study of ten patients with long-term follow-up. Cancer 70: 2827–2830
606. Meis-Kindblom J M, Bergh P, Gunterberg B, Kindblom L G 1999 Extraskeletal myxoid chondrosarcoma: a reappraisal of its morphologic spectrum and prognostic factors based on 117 cases. Am J Surg Pathol 23: 636–650
607. Okamoto S, Hisaoka M, Ishida T et al. 2001 Extraskeletal myxoid chondrosarcoma: a clinicopathologic, immunohistochemical and molecular analysis of 18 cases. Hum Pathol 32: 116–1124
608. Hachitanda Y, Tsuneyoshi M, Daimaru Y et al. 1988 Extraskeletal myxoid chondrosarcoma in young children. Cancer 61: 2521–2526
609. Suster S, Moran C A 1997 Malignant cartilaginous tumors of the mediastinum: clinicopathological study of six cases presenting as extraskeletal soft tissue masses. Hum Pathol 28: 588–594
610. Kilpatrick S E, Inwards C Y, Fletcher C D M, Smith M A, Gitelis S 1997 Myxoid chondrosarcoma (chordoid sarcoma) of bone: a report of two cases and review of the literature. Cancer 79: 1903–1910

611. Fletcher C D M, Powell G, McKee P H 1986 Extraskeletal myxoid chondrosarcoma: a histochemical and immunohistochemical study. Histopathology 10: 489–499
612. Tsuneyoshi M, Daimaru Y, Hashimoto H et al. 1987 The existence of rhabdoid cells in specified soft tissue sarcomas. Histopathological, ultrastructural and immunohistochemical evidence. Virchow's Arch [A] 411: 509–514
613. Lucas D R, Fletcher C D M, Adsay N V, Zalupski M M 1999 High-grade extraskeletal myxoid chondrosarcoma: a high-grade epithelioid malignancy. Histopathology 35: 201–208
614. Dei Tos A P, Wadden C, Fletcher C D M 1997 Extraskeletal myxoid chondrosarcoma: an immunohistochemical reappraisal of 39 cases. Appl Immunohistochem 5: 73–77
615. DeBlois G, Wang S, Kay S 1986 Microtubular aggregates within rough endoplasmic reticulum: an unusual ultrastructural feature of extraskeletal myxoid chondrosarcoma. Hum Pathol 17: 469–475
616. Goh Y W, Spagnolo D V, Platten M et al. 2001 Extraskeletal myxoid chondrosarcoma: a light microscopic, immunohistochemical, ultrastructural and immunoultrastructural study indicating neuroendocrine differentiation. Histopathology 39: 514–524
617. Subramanian S, West R B, Marinelli R J et al. 2005 The gene expression profile of extraskeletal myxoid chondrosarcoma. J Pathol 206: 433–444
618. Labelle Y, Zucman J, Stenman G et al. 1995 Oncogenic conversion of a novel orphan nuclear receptor by chromosome translocation. Hum Mol Genet 4: 2219–2226
619. Sciot R, Dal Cin P, Fletcher C D M et al. 1995 t(9;22)(q22–31;q11–12) is a consistent marker of extraskeletal myxoid chondrosarcoma: evaluation of three cases. Mod Pathol 8: 765–768
620. Sjogren H, Meis-Kindblom J, Kindblom L G, Aman P, Stenman G 1999 Fusion of the EWS-related gene TAF2N to TEC in extraskeletal myxoid chondrosarcoma. Cancer Res 59: 5064–5067
621. Lynch H T, Shurin S B, Dahms B B et al. 1983 Paravertebral malignant rhabdoid tumor in infancy. In vitro studies of a familial tumor. Cancer 52: 290–296
622. Parham D M, Weeks D A, Beckwith J B 1994 The clinicopathologic spectrum of putative extrarenal rhabdoid tumors. An analysis of 42 cases studied with immunohistochemistry and/or electron microscopy. Am J Surg Pathol 18: 1010–1029
623. Tsuneyoshi M, Daimaru Y, Hashimoto H et al. 1985 Malignant soft tissue neoplasms with the histologic features of renal rhabdoid tumors: an ultrastructural and immunohistochemical study. Hum Pathol 16: 1235–1242
624. Sotelo-Avila C, Gonzalez-Crussi F, deMello D et al. 1986 Renal and extrarenal rhabdoid tumors in children: a clinicopathologic study of 14 patients. Semin Diagn Pathol 3: 151–163
625. Schmidt D, Leuschner I, Harms D et al. 1989 Malignant rhabdoid tumor. A morphological and flow cytometric study. Pathol Res Pract 184: 202–210
626. Kodet R, Newton W A, Sachs N et al. 1991 Rhabdoid tumors of soft tissue: a clinicopathologic study of 26 cases enrolled on the Intergroup Rhabdomyosarcoma Study. Hum Pathol 22: 674–681
627. Fanburg-Smith J C, Hengge M, Hengge U R, Smith S, Miettinen M 1998 Extrarenal rhabdoid tumors of soft tissue: a clinicopathologic and immunohistochemical study of 18 cases. Ann Diagn Pathol 2: 351–362
628. Weeks D A, Beckwith J B, Mierau G W 1989 Rhabdoid tumor. An entity or a phenotype? Arch Pathol Lab Med 113: 113–114
629. Hoot A C, Russo P, Judkins A R et al. 2004 Immunohistochemical analysis of hSNF5/INI1 distinguishes renal and extrarenal malignant rhabdoid tumors from other pediatric soft tissue tumors. Am J Surg Pathol 28: 1485–1491
630. Stout A P 1948 Mesenchymoma, the mixed tumor of mesenchymal derivatives. Ann Surg 127: 278–290
631. Newman P L, Fletcher C D M 1991 Malignant mesenchymoma. Clinicopathologic analysis of a series with evidence of low-grade behavior. Am J Surg Pathol 15: 607–614
632. Brady M S, Perino G, Tallini G, Russo P, Woodruff J M 1996 Malignant mesenchymoma. Cancer 77: 467–473

骨关节系统肿瘤
Tumors of the osteoarticular system

25

K. Krishnan Unni 和 Carrie Y. Inwards 著

鲍冬梅 译　　沈丹华 校

引言	1593
分类	1594
活检方法	1595
小细胞肿瘤	1597
软骨肿瘤	1602
成骨性肿瘤	1613
来源不明的肿瘤	1623
血管肿瘤	1627
纤维组织细胞肿瘤	1630
纤维源性肿瘤	1631
脊索肿瘤	1632
神经源性肿瘤	1634
脂肪源性瘤	1634
类似于原发性骨肿瘤的病变	1634
骨的囊性病变	1634
纤维性病变	1636
伴有反应性新骨形成的病变	1639
其他各类疾病	1641
关节肿瘤	1644

引言

骨肿瘤是相对少见的肿瘤。在美国，据估计每年新增骨肉瘤病例为2440例，而新增的肺癌病例为93 000例，新增的乳腺癌病例则为88 000例。因此，骨肿瘤从数量上讲相对不重要。然而恶性骨肿瘤好发于幼儿，治疗涉及范围广，有时要应用威胁生命的化疗和截肢手术。预后通常仍很差。故而对骨肿瘤的诊断总是有很多的担忧。由于骨肿瘤较少见，大部分医疗中心在处理骨肿瘤上并没有丰富的经验。因此，大部分外科病理医生不熟悉骨肿瘤。这就导致了诊断的不确定性，即使是对非常典型的病例，也是如此。

骨肿瘤患者的处理需要一个团队来进行。1958年，Jaffe[1]就曾指出在骨组织病变诊断中外科医生、放射科医生和病理科医生合作的重要性。一个病理医生在不了解临床特征和放射影像表现时就试图进行骨肿瘤的诊断，会使自己处于十分不利的地位。

骨肿瘤的临床症状常常是非特异性的。多数患者表现疼痛、肿胀或两者均有。偶尔，患者表现为病理性骨折。这些特征均不能提示特殊诊断。然而，一些骨组织病变却伴有特异性症状。骨样骨瘤患者伴有强烈的疼痛，这种疼痛使用阿司匹林可以迅速缓解。另一方面，临床症状可能会误导诊断。骨Ewing肉瘤患者可能出现发热和血沉加快，提示骨髓炎的诊断。这可能导致不当的治疗并延误诊断。

虽然症状对诊断的价值有限，但是患者的年龄和肿瘤生长的确切部位非常重要。大部分高度恶性的肉瘤，如Ewing肉瘤和骨肉瘤，发生在儿童。低级别肉瘤，如软骨肉瘤，通常发生在成人。因此，当外科病理医生遇到一个儿童的恶性软骨肿瘤时，一定要考虑软骨母细胞型骨肉瘤。病变部位和范围非常重要。巨细胞瘤通常发生在骨端（骨骺）。而发生在干骺端和骨干的含有大量巨细胞的病变提示其他一些疾病的可能性，如甲状旁腺功能亢进、骨肉瘤或动脉瘤样骨囊肿。病变在骨的确切位置非常重要。发生在手和足的小骨的软骨肿瘤最有可能是软骨瘤。但发生在胸骨的相同组织学表现的软骨肿瘤是软骨肉瘤。病变是孤立的还是多发的也非常重要。大多数梭形细胞肉瘤是孤立的。然而血管肉瘤、恶性淋巴瘤、多发性骨髓瘤、转移癌倾向于表现为多灶性病变。如果多发性病变有局限于一侧肢体的倾向，则提示恶性血管瘤。

放射学影像表现非常重要，而且放射学影像是病变定位的最好方法。如一位年轻女性出现一个累及桡骨远端的单纯性溶骨性病变，几乎可以肯定是一个良性的巨细胞瘤。一些放射学影像特征有助于良性病变与恶性病变的鉴别。良性病变倾向于边界清楚，而且可以有硬化的边缘。恶性肿瘤则界限不清。梭形细胞肉瘤多表现为地图样破坏，地图样破坏是指一个骨中的巨大空洞。小细胞恶性肿瘤，如 Ewing 肉瘤，表现为穿透性的破坏过程；这是一种虫蚀表现，是指在骨中有多灶的小洞，其间掺杂着残留骨。骨旁反应的特征非常重要。良性病变，如 Langerhans 组织细胞增生症，刺激厚的、规则的骨旁新骨形成。恶性肿瘤，如 Ewing 肉瘤，倾向于在骨周围形成组织结构不清的多层的新生骨。虽然外科病理医生熟悉不同骨肿瘤的放射影像学特征非常重要，但是得到有经验的放射科医生的帮助更为重要。

同样重要的是要认识到，影像检查也可能导致误诊。很显然，临床医生更容易接受与影像学一致的组织学诊断；但是，如果病理医生能够确定其组织学表现，应该不管其他特征而做出明确诊断。

骨的影像学检查有很多进展；但是，平片是对诊断最有帮助的辅助检查。计算机断层扫描（CT）和核磁共振成像（MRI）在解剖学复杂的区域有优势；它们也有助于病变的分期。

分类

骨肿瘤既要基于细胞学特征也要基于肿瘤细胞所产生的基质来进行分类。Mayo Clinic 应用的分类是由 Lichtenstein[2] 首次推荐的分类标准修改的版本，与世界卫生组织的分类[3] 相似。肿瘤被分为良性和恶性。虽然这是一个便于记住不同疾病的方法，但是不应该理解为：恶性肿瘤是经由良性肿瘤转化而来。这种情况极为罕见。表 25.1 显示的分类是在 Mayo Clinic[4] 以前版本的基础上修改的版本。小细胞恶性肿瘤（包括造血系统肿瘤）是骨肿瘤中最大的一组肿瘤。然而，骨髓瘤作为

表25.1	骨肿瘤分类[a]				
		良性肿瘤		恶性肿瘤	
组织学类型	病例总数	类型	病例数	类型	病例数
造血性	1974	–	–	骨髓瘤 恶性淋巴瘤	1069[b] 905[b]
软骨源性	3129	骨软骨瘤 软骨瘤 软骨母细胞瘤 软骨黏液纤维瘤	1024 490 147 50	原发性软骨肉瘤 继发性软骨肉瘤 去分化软骨肉瘤 间叶性软骨肉瘤	1073 154 145 46
骨源性	2521	骨样骨瘤 骨母细胞瘤	396 108	骨肉瘤 骨旁骨肉瘤	1942 75
不明来源	1365	巨细胞瘤	671	巨细胞瘤中的恶性病变 釉质瘤 Ewing肿瘤	39 44 611
组织细胞源性	107	纤维组织细胞瘤	9	恶性（纤维）组织细胞瘤	98
纤维源性	301	–	–	纤维组织增生性纤维瘤 纤维肉瘤	16 285
脊索	437	–	–	脊索瘤	437
血管	273	血管瘤	149	血管肉瘤 血管周围细胞瘤	109 15
脂肪源性	13	脂肪瘤	11	脂肪肉瘤	2
神经源性	23	神经纤维瘤	23	–	
总数	10143		3078		7065

[a] 病例来自Mayo Clinic，截止到2004年1月。
[b] 此表中仅包括外科活检诊断的骨髓瘤病例。以前的版本包括骨髓活检诊断的病例。
After Unni 1996,[4] with the permission of Mayo Foundation for Medical Education and Research.

最常见的骨肿瘤，其中的大部分病例是通过骨髓穿刺标本而不是骨活检标本诊断的。在外科系统中，骨恶性肿瘤的数量多于良性肿瘤的，比例为3:1。然而，这并不能反映良性和恶性骨肿瘤的真实发病率，因为很多良性骨肿瘤是没有症状的。因此，外科系统会偏重于恶性肿瘤的诊断和治疗。

除骨肿瘤外，一些骨的非肿瘤性病变也可能类似于原发骨肿瘤。为避免误诊，认识这些病变是非常重要的。

分级和分期

肿瘤分期的提出是肿瘤学领域的一个非常重要的进展。肿瘤学家对上皮性肿瘤进行分期已经有很多年。这个分期系统是熟知的肿瘤、淋巴结以及转移（TNM）系统。直到最近，仍没有满意的骨和软组织肿瘤的分期系统。用TNM系统对肉瘤进行分期并不适合，因为在肉瘤中淋巴结受累并不常见。

由Enneking及其同事[5]在1980年首先提出的分期系统已经在全世界或多或少地被接受了。这个分期系统为那些对肉瘤感兴趣的临床医生在世界范围内交流提供了共同的语言。它也提供了预后的重要信息和影响治疗的决定因素。

这个分期系统基于肿瘤的两个特征：肿瘤的分级和解剖学位置。肉瘤有数个分级系统。一个系统[6]是根据坏死的数量对软组织肉瘤进行分级。肉瘤中坏死的数量与预后成反比。我们认为高级别肉瘤倾向于有更多的坏死。然而，我们并不认为坏死应该作为肿瘤分级的标准。

我们最初对肿瘤的分级是根据由Broders[7]首次提出的概念进行的，Broders在唇的鳞状细胞癌的治疗中认识到：肿瘤高分化以至类似于正常鳞状上皮时，预后要比低分化癌好得多。Broders设计了数量分级系统，1级肿瘤分化最好，而4级肿瘤分化最差。他证实了预后与这种分级系统有非常好的相关性。我们最初对肉瘤的分级系统也是根据肿瘤的细胞学特征制定的。

第二个分期标准是肿瘤的解剖学位置。骨和软组织肿瘤可以被认为是由很多部位组成的。如仅局限在股骨的骨肉瘤应该被认为仅累及一个部位。然而，如果肿瘤已经突破骨皮质累及软组织，就应该认为肿瘤累及两个部分。通过应用肿瘤分级和累及部位的数量，肉瘤被分为两期。

所有低级别肉瘤是Ⅰ期。所有高级别肉瘤是Ⅱ期。对于肉瘤，无论级别，如果有远处转移的证据，则为Ⅲ期。这三期再根据部位分为A和B两期。如果肿瘤局限于一个部位，归为A期，而超过一个部位受累，则为B期。这个分期系统也考虑到外科手术的切缘。当一个肉瘤生长时，它会挤压周围组织，以至于形成假包膜。围绕着假包膜的通常是一个血管增生带，称为反应带。外科切缘的确定如下所示：

1. 病变内切缘（intralesional margin）。如果外科医生切除肿瘤并没有试图得到干净边缘，这种边缘被认为是病变内切缘。这可能适合于治疗骨的一些良性和非肿瘤性病变的方法。
2. 边缘性切缘（marginal margin）。如果病变包括假包膜被完整切除，这种边缘称作边缘性切缘。这种治疗适合于良性和稍有局灶侵袭的病变，如骨巨细胞瘤。
3. 宽泛切缘（wide margin）。如果病变包括假包膜和周围的反应带完全被切除，以至于整个病变由正常的组织覆盖，这种边缘称作宽泛切缘。这种切缘通常适合于大多数肉瘤。
4. 根治性切缘（radical margin）。如果含有肿瘤的整个部位被切除，这种边缘称作根治性切缘。如股骨远端的骨肉瘤仅仅当整个股骨被切除时，通常通过臀部的关节远端，才能获得根治性切缘。虽然这种治疗可能看上去很理想，但是很少有好的效果。一些研究显示，保留肢体的外科手术并不会对预后产生不利影响[8]。

活检方法

当怀疑为骨肿瘤时，有数种方法来获得肿瘤组织用于确诊。

细针针吸活检
Fine-needle aspiration biopsy

细针针吸活检这种用于诊断不同器官肿瘤的方法已受到越来越多的欢迎。一个恶性肿瘤的穿刺结果呈阳性，可能免除切开活检的必要。现在一些主要的医疗中心首选细针针吸活检作为骨肿瘤的诊断方法。我们认为细针针吸活检非常适用于确诊转移的恶性病变，而对于原发性骨肿瘤的诊断并不理想。尽管如此，细针针吸活检对于诊断小细胞恶性肿瘤可能是足够了，如骨髓瘤、淋巴瘤和Ewing肉瘤。如果针吸标本足够，有可能对骨肉瘤的病例作出诊断。然而，我们认为不可能根据细针针吸所获得的材料进一步细分骨肉瘤的类型。不过，大多数患者如果在术前确诊为恶性肿瘤，则会进行术前化疗。我们还认为，细针针吸活检不适合于软骨肿瘤的诊断。细针针吸活检对骨的良性和假肿瘤性病变的诊断作用更小。

活检方法

细针针吸活检的一些优点：

1. 可以避免开放性的外科活检，降低费用，避免常规麻醉的风险。
2. 正常组织的污染少于切开活检，因此可以行保肢手术。
3. 可行多次活检并获得组织，进一步可以用于特殊检查，如免疫过氧化物酶染色和细胞遗传学研究。

细针针吸活检也有它的缺点：

1. 获得的组织可能不够，甚至可能造成误诊，这样可能需要切开活检，增加费用。
2. 当为了特殊检查而获取组织时，并不能确保获取的是具有代表性的材料或获得材料足够充分。
3. 在具有多种形态的肿瘤中，如去分化软骨肉瘤，获取的组织可能不会提供完整的病变情况。在去分化的骨旁骨肉瘤病例中，CT引导针吸穿刺活检有助于从不同病变区域成功取材。然而，这在去分化软骨肉瘤的诊断中可能就受到限制，因为在25%的病例中，放射学不能提示诊断。

在 Mayo Clinic，用于骨肿瘤诊断的细针针吸活检的数量逐渐增加。细针针吸活检是由放射医生在 CT 引导下用 14-18 号针进行的。采用一种快速 Papanicolaou 试验，放射科医生通常能在 30 分钟内确认是否取到了具有诊断意义的材料。通过针吸我们几乎总能得到一小块组织。如果细胞标本呈阴性结果，我们常常将组织块行冰冻切片。如果两者都不能诊断，放射科医生可能选择再次活检。如果细胞学标本结果是阳性，我们将组织块仅做永久（石蜡）切片。大约所有细针针吸活检中一半是用于明确有无转移癌存在的。我们认为，细针针吸活检在骨科肿瘤学实际工作中可能是非常有用的。尽管如此，细胞学材料应该结合病变的临床和影像特征的所有知识进行解释。

穿刺活检　　Needle biopsy

一些文章[9,10]肯定了穿刺活检在骨病变诊断中的作用。穿刺活检可以由放射科医生或外科医生在荧光镜的引导下实施。可以应用不同大小的针。穿刺活检优于细针针吸活检是由于它通常可以提供更为理想的组织材料。缺点是获得的组织可能并不具有病变的代表性。随着细针针吸活检不断推广，骨病变的穿刺活检数量已经下降。

开放活检　　Open biopsy

绝大部分骨肿瘤的诊断仍依赖于开放活检。开放活检可以是切开或是切除的。切开活检设计非常重要，以便活检通道与肿瘤能被完整切除。如果外科医生确信病变是良性的或是局部侵袭性的，可以行切除活检。

在 Mayo Clinic，我们常规对几乎所有的外科标本制备冰冻切片。骨肿瘤也不例外。骨肿瘤几乎总是有质软的区域，应该可以制备冰冻切片。然而重要的是，病理医生要检查大体标本并能将质软的部分从骨成分中分离出来。我们仅有几个标本因为组织太硬不能行冰冻切片。我们认为，几乎所有的骨肿瘤和肿瘤样病变都可以通过冰冻切片进行诊断。当然，对于病理医生来说，最为重要的是在检查组织之前查看影像图片，了解临床表现。我们认为并不需要对所有的病例都做出肯定的冰冻切片诊断。然而，在创面关闭之前至少能根据冰冻切片确定活检材料的性质是至关重要的。冰冻切片能够识别感染，以便获得合适的标本用于培养。冰冻切片检查手术切缘也非常有用。

在 Mayo Clinic，我们使用冷冻切片机制备冰冻切片。有经验的技术员几秒钟就能切出好的切片。我们用亚甲基蓝对切片染色。整个过程通常用 30～45 秒。

如果不需要立即诊断，在 24 小时内还可能做出诊断。全部活检标本，包括碎骨片，不应送去脱钙。如果将皮质骨碎片仔细与肿瘤分离，标本应该能够像其他活检标本那样处理。

许多活检标本需要脱钙，有数种不同的方法。在 Mayo Clinic，常规用 20% 的甲酸和 10% 的甲醛溶液。如果骨被制成薄片，则脱钙不应该超过 24 小时。定时检查标本非常重要，以确保不过度脱钙。绝大多数恶性骨肿瘤常规行切除治疗，而不进行截肢。不论是手术切除的标本还是截肢的标本，处理方式是相同的。我们通常通过活检部位切开来确定病变部位。一旦病变明确，病变周围的所有软组织和骨都要与之分离剔除。留下完整的带有骨的肿瘤组织。我们认为不可能在伴有软组织包块的巨大骨肿瘤标本中检查软组织边界，因此，我们不标记这样的标本。但是，可以将那些外科医生可能特别关注的区域（如神经血管束）制成切片。我们也会检查骨段的骨髓切缘。我们用条锯锯断骨。剖开骨之后，应该在流动冷水下用刷子彻底清理干净。这样可以减少骨尘的数量，否则它可能进入骨的缝隙间，掩盖组织学的细微结构。

绝大多数骨肉瘤患者常规行术前化疗。通过检查外科标本评估化疗效果非常重要。我们常规从带有肿瘤的整个骨取一薄片。整个薄片进行脱钙。由于标本含有皮质骨，脱钙可能需要几天时间。一旦标本充分脱钙，标本就可以分成多块完全包埋。组织块要编号，以便整个标本可以重现。评估化疗后标本坏死百分率的详细情况将在骨肉瘤部分讨论（见1619页）。

小细胞肿瘤　Small cell tumors

常规应用的分类方案已经稍有改动，以便Ewing肿瘤与其他小细胞恶性肿瘤可以一起讨论。这样显得更为合理，因为Ewing肉瘤的鉴别诊断包括其他小细胞恶性肿瘤，特别是恶性淋巴瘤。小细胞恶性肿瘤组成了骨肿瘤中最大的一组病变。

骨髓瘤　Myeloma

骨髓瘤（也见第22章）是最常见的骨肿瘤。在Mayo Clinic的档案中，骨髓瘤占所有骨肿瘤的1/3，几乎占所有恶性骨肿瘤的一半。绝大多数骨髓瘤的患者是通过髂骨骨髓针吸和活检标本诊断的（表25.1提供的数据不包括这些病例）。仅有很少数病例是经外科开放取活检的。

骨痛是骨髓瘤最常见的症状。患者可能出现病理性骨折；脊椎受累患者常出现脊髓压迫。骨髓瘤患者常常有全身症状和体征，如体重减轻和疲劳。许多骨髓瘤患者有高钙血症，并且一些患者可以出现高血钙危象。实验室检查通常显示贫血，在外周血涂片中，红细胞呈卷轴样，红细胞沉降率增高。几乎所有的骨髓瘤患者的血浆和（或）尿中都可以识别到单克隆蛋白质。

放射学的典型表现为骨的多发性、穿凿样、单纯溶骨性病变（图25.1）。骨髓瘤极少伴有任何硬化性改变。有小部分骨髓瘤呈现弥漫性骨密度降低的影像。

多发性骨髓瘤的大体表现通常被描述为类似于红浆果果冻。病变质软色红。尽管如此，许多骨髓瘤显示恶性淋巴瘤的典型的鱼肉样外观。

组织学上，骨髓瘤由成片的浆细胞组成（图25.2）。在几乎所有的骨髓瘤病例中，肿瘤的浆细胞特性很明显，至少在局灶区域如此。细胞有丰富的蓝染或粉染的胞浆和偏位的细胞核。偶尔胞浆还含有结晶包涵体。细胞核呈圆形，染色质呈集块状。常见双核细胞。浆细胞常常显示细胞学的非典型性。尽管如此，我们认为，这些不能用来诊断骨髓瘤。巨核细胞也经常可见。偶尔，细胞核多形性非常显著，以至于肿瘤的浆细胞特性可能被掩盖（图25.3）。在这种情况下，通常要与恶性淋巴瘤进行鉴别。

骨髓瘤血管通常十分丰富。偶尔，这种血管构成呈窦隙状，可能类似于内分泌肿瘤，如类癌的表现。大约10%～15%的骨髓瘤含有淀粉样沉积物。淀粉样物可

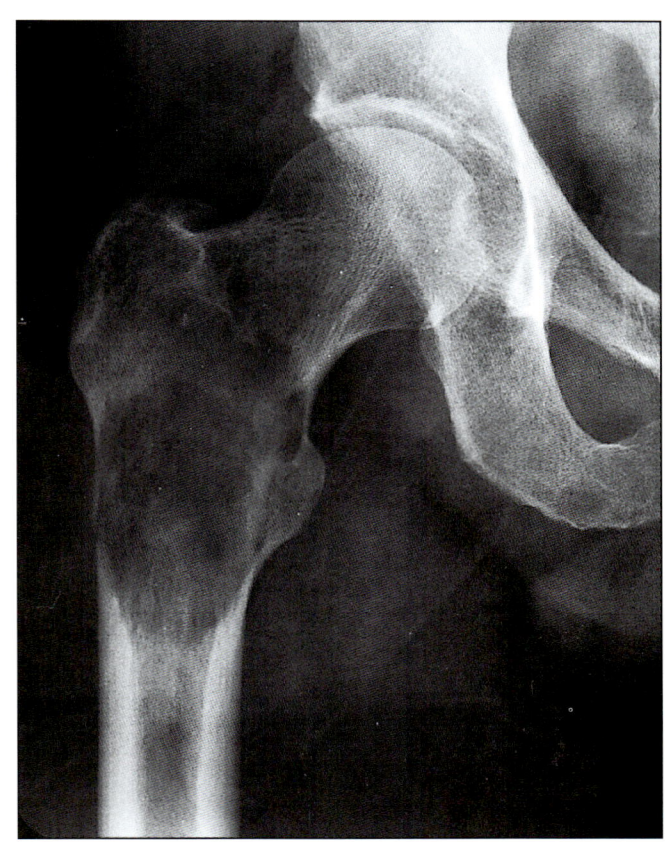

图25.1　右侧股骨远端的多发性骨髓瘤。显示界限清晰的、破坏性单纯溶骨性病变。

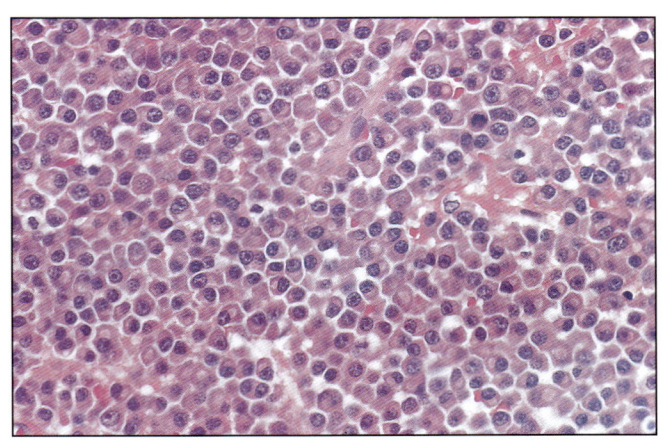

图25.2　骨髓瘤由相对成熟的浆细胞组成，细胞核偏位，胞浆嗜酸性，核周透亮。

以沉积在血管壁，或可能在肿瘤细胞间形成团块状沉积。当淀粉样物形成呈团块状时，可能引起巨细胞反应。在少见的情况下，淀粉样物和巨细胞反应非常明显，可能使背景中增生的浆细胞被忽视。在我们的经验中，几乎所有的骨淀粉样沉积都与骨髓瘤有关，罕见的例外可能

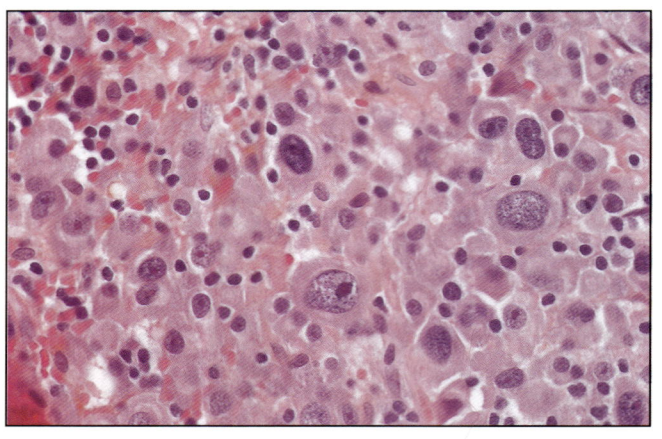

图25.3 间变性骨髓瘤含有几个大的非典型性浆细胞，可能类似于在恶性淋巴瘤中见到的免疫母细胞。

只有长期接受血液透析的患者出现的骨淀粉样沉积[11]。

骨髓瘤细胞产生单克隆免疫球蛋白，因此细胞或 κ 或 λ 轻链染色呈阳性。肿瘤细胞常常表达 CD56，但不表达 CD20 或 CD45。在这种特定的情况下，CD138 被认为是浆细胞的特异标记物。

绝大多数患者表现为多发性骨髓瘤。然而，小部分为孤立性浆细胞瘤（图 25.4）。骨髓瘤患者在诊断孤立性骨髓瘤之前需要进行广泛检查。孤立性骨髓瘤患者比多发性骨髓瘤患者要年轻一些，他们中的很多患者有漫长的临床病程[12,13]，最终发展成多发性骨髓瘤。虽然在影像学上，骨髓瘤常表现为单纯的溶骨性病变，但是有小部分病变也可以伴有骨的硬化，这种变型被称为骨硬化性骨髓瘤（osteosclerotic myeloma）[14,15]。这些患者常常有特征性的临床和实验室表现，包括多发性神经病、浆细胞恶病质、器官肿大症、内分泌疾病、皮肤改变、单克隆血清蛋白。多发性神经病通常随着骨髓瘤的治疗而消退。硬化性骨髓瘤的组织学特征除了有非常显著的骨硬化外，与典型的骨髓瘤没有差别。活检标本在诊断前可能需要脱钙。孤立性和骨硬化性骨髓瘤患者可能有很长的临床病程，甚至一些多发性骨髓瘤患者可能也有这样的病程[16]。

鉴别诊断通常要考虑慢性骨髓炎。一定情况下，慢性骨髓炎也伴有浆细胞的显著增生；然而，慢性骨髓炎几乎总是伴有散在的其他细胞，如淋巴细胞和中性粒细胞。骨髓瘤仅会显示浆细胞的增生。慢性骨髓炎也有间质毛细血管增生，类似于肉芽组织的表现。在有些情况下，有必要采用免疫过氧化物酶染色确定骨髓瘤的单克隆性。偶尔，骨髓瘤也可呈簇状生长，类似转移癌的表现。浆细胞的上皮膜抗原染色经常呈阳性反应。然而，角蛋白染色是阴性的，少数情况下，有必要用免疫组化染色鉴别转移癌和骨髓瘤。

淋巴瘤　Lymphoma

骨的恶性淋巴瘤可以是孤立性病变也可以是全身性病变的一部分。原发性和继发性淋巴瘤的影像学和组织学特征是一致的。两者的区别纯粹是基于分期的结果。在 Mayo Clinic 的资料中，恶性淋巴瘤大约占恶性骨肿瘤的 8%。男性稍多，骨的淋巴瘤通常累及年轻成人或

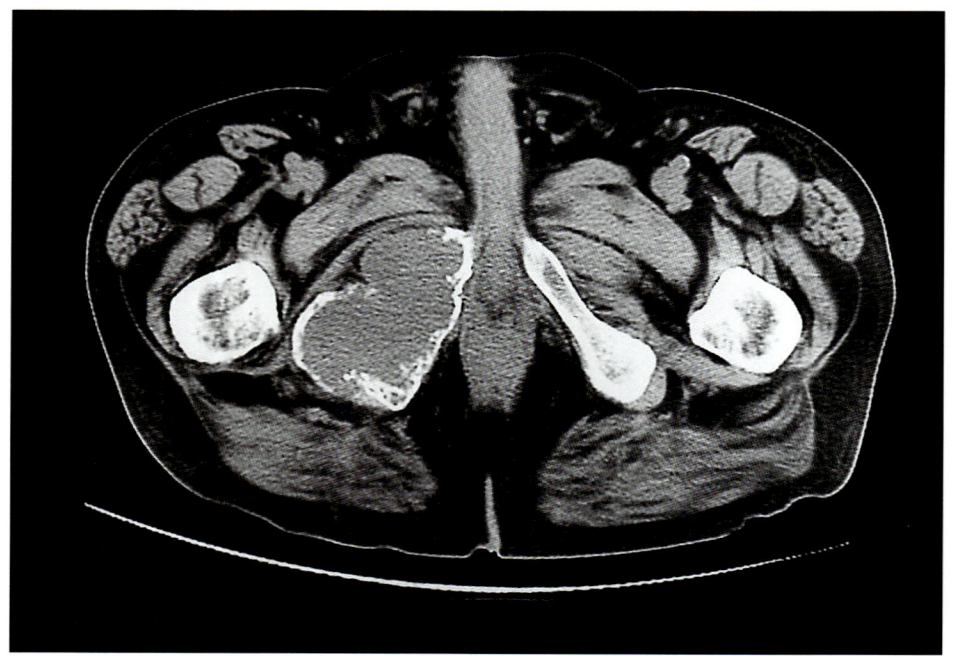

图25.4 计算机断层扫描（CT）显示右侧坐骨发生的孤立性浆细胞瘤的巨大膨胀性病变。

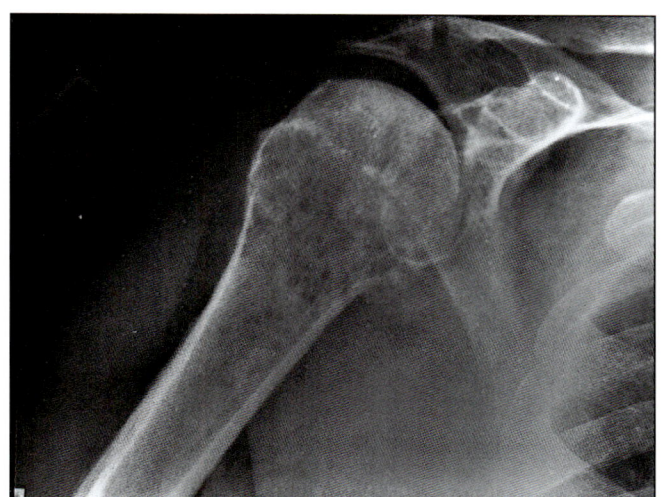

图25.5 肱骨近段干骺端淋巴瘤，形成界限不清的、溶骨性、破坏性病变。

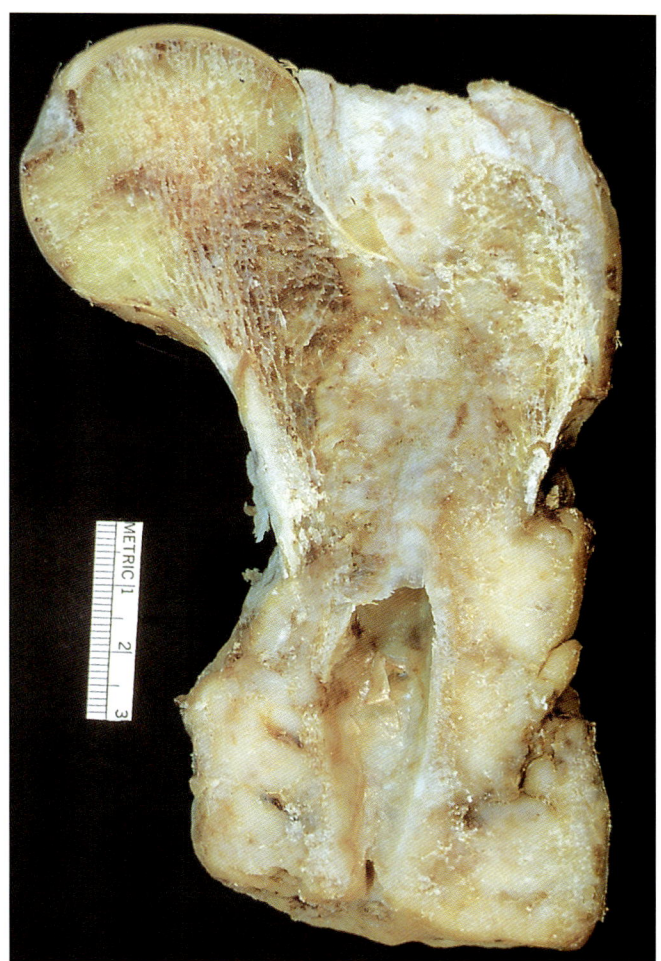

图25.6 恶性淋巴瘤的大体表现。灰白色（鱼肉样）肿瘤侵透骨皮质至周围软组织。

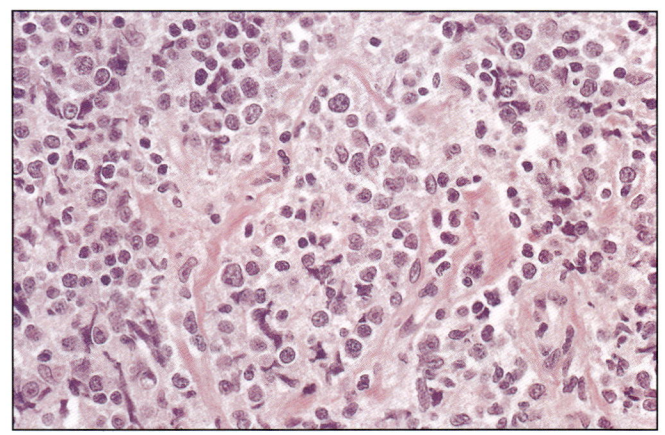

图25.7 骨的恶性淋巴瘤。显示恶性淋巴瘤细胞在细胞学上的多样性，细胞核轮廓不规则。肿瘤细胞间还可见到纤细的编织样纤维。

老年人。然而，淋巴瘤也可累及儿童，但比这一年龄组的 Ewing 肉瘤少见得多[17]。骨的任何部分都可受累，但是倾向于累及在成年期仍然含有骨髓的骨。

患者常常表现为骨痛或病理性骨折。可能出现全身性症状，如发热、体重减轻。累及脊椎的患者常常出现脊髓压迫。放射影像通常显示骨组织广泛累及，并伴有浸润性破坏性病变。骨干常常受累，影像学表现就像在骨中有多个小洞，其间穿插着正常骨。淋巴瘤患者影像学上也可呈溶骨性和硬化性的混合表现（图25.5）。大多数恶性淋巴瘤在诊断时已经蔓延到软组织。然而，骨膜反应性新骨形成并不常见。骨扫描具有特征性的阳性表现。平片表现可能呈阴性，甚至当骨髓广泛受累时也没什么变化。骨扫描呈阳性，或放射平片表现正常，而 MRI 上可以看到病变，提示骨的恶性淋巴瘤。

大约 20% 的骨淋巴瘤患者显示骨骼多区域受累。因此，当遇到多骨部位受累的患者，鉴别诊断应该考虑恶性淋巴瘤。

骨淋巴瘤的大体表现与其他部位的淋巴瘤相似（如鱼肉样外观；图25.6）。一些骨淋巴瘤可以有非常明显的反应性硬化。从这样的肿瘤取得的活检标本可能需要广泛的脱钙。由此可导致细胞形态丢失并使诊断变得困难。

骨恶性淋巴瘤的镜下表现差异很大。在低倍镜下，可见病变位于正常骨小梁间和骨髓脂肪中。骨小梁可能显示一些硬化。结节状生长方式在骨淋巴瘤中十分少见。在肿瘤细胞间纤维可能十分明显。大多数骨淋巴瘤显示多样性浸润（图25.7）。细胞核的大小及形状不一致。这种不一致的表现有助于骨淋巴瘤与 Ewing 肉瘤鉴别。

肿瘤细胞的细胞学特征与身体其他部位的淋巴瘤细胞相似。原发性骨淋巴瘤绝大多数是大 B 细胞系淋巴瘤，较少部分表现为间变大细胞（Ki-1 阳性）淋巴瘤[18-23]。

骨恶性淋巴瘤可能显示一些不常见的组织学特征。因为肿瘤细胞间的纤维化，细胞表现为梭形。偶尔，细胞甚至可能出现编席状生长，可能导致误诊为所谓的恶性纤维组织细胞瘤。重要的是要注意肿瘤细胞的细胞学特征和细胞核的多形性，以便得到正确的诊断。此外，细胞也有呈簇状生长的情况，这提示可能是转移癌。

关于骨淋巴瘤的准确组织学分类是否具有重要的预后意义，尚有争议[24,25]。以我们的经验，疾病的临床分期对于预测预后更为重要。当诊断为骨淋巴瘤时，可能表现为四种临床状况：

1. 据骨活检诊断淋巴瘤。广泛检查，包括骨骼体检、骨扫描、骨髓检查以及胸腹部CT，显示无其他部位受累，应该考虑骨的原发性淋巴瘤，预后好。
2. 患者表现为累及骨的淋巴瘤。骨骼检查和骨扫描显示骨骼多部位受累。然而，没有其他器官受累，如肝、脾或淋巴结。尽管有如此广泛的骨骼受累，根据其他临床状况，这些患者可能仍有好的预后。
3. 患者表现为骨淋巴瘤，检查显示多发的结外部位受累。这些患者预后不会很好。
4. 患者有一些部位有淋巴瘤，接受化疗。在治疗过程中，确定在骨上有新的病变，并确诊为淋巴瘤。同淋巴瘤化疗不敏感的其他患者一样，这种情况预后很差。

恶性淋巴瘤的鉴别诊断包括这样几种病变：肉瘤、转移癌、白血病浸润和慢性骨髓炎。一些研究显示，淋巴瘤可能有肉瘤样表现[26]。间变大细胞（Ki-1）淋巴瘤是一个高度多形性肿瘤的例子，偶尔可以累及骨[21,27]。如果患者有骨多发受累，组织学特征提示肉瘤，应该慎重考虑恶性淋巴瘤的诊断。免疫过氧化物酶染色，如CD45（白细胞共同抗原）、CD30以及T和B细胞相关标记物检查，对鉴别都会有很大帮助。转移癌可能有类似于恶性淋巴瘤的表现。两者都可能表现为多处骨受累。如果簇状肿瘤细胞周围纤维化，则更多提示为转移癌。在恶性淋巴瘤中，纤维化更弥漫，通常没有与转移癌相关的促纤维结缔组织增生表现。角蛋白和血液细胞标记物免疫过氧化物酶染色应该有助于鉴别诊断。多形性细胞浸润可能导致误诊为慢性骨髓炎。注意临床病史和细胞核的细胞学改变应该有助于避免误诊。

白血病细胞浸润，尤其是髓性白血病，表现可能像骨肿瘤[28,29]。除非发现有明确的嗜酸性粒细胞和中性粒细胞前体，否则仅以HE染色切片诊断粒细胞肉瘤可能很困难。在所有怀疑粒细胞肉瘤的病例，都应该进行髓过氧化物酶和CD43染色[30,31]。一些粒细胞肉瘤患者在确认白血病之前可能存活数年。

在极少见情况下，Hodgkin淋巴瘤患者可以有骨骼症状。Hodgkin淋巴瘤晚期骨骼受累可能并不少见。尽管如此，Hodgkin淋巴瘤在发现时以骨骼病变为表现者并不常见。当病变累及骨骼时，脊椎最易受累，因此，当脊椎活检显示淋巴瘤样病变并伴有散在的多形性细胞核时，应该怀疑Hodgkin淋巴瘤。CD15（Leu-M1）和CD30（Ber-H2）染色对于确定Hodgkin淋巴瘤的诊断是非常必要的。以我们的经验，骨的Hodgkin淋巴瘤几乎总是伴有淋巴结受累，尤其是大动脉旁区域的淋巴结。

Ewing肉瘤　Ewing sarcoma

Ewing肉瘤在骨的原发性肿瘤中较为罕见，在Mayo Clinic的资料中，Ewing肉瘤约占整个恶性骨肿瘤的6%。Ewing肉瘤发病男性略多于女性。大多数患者（Mayo Clinic超过一半的患者）在11～20岁发病。小于5岁的Ewing肉瘤患者很少见（仅占Mayo Clinic患者的2%）。同样，仅有略多于3%的患者发病年龄在50岁左右。骨骼任何部位都可受累，但是超过一半的肿瘤累及长骨，通常发生在骨干。扁骨也可以受累，尤其是髂骨和肋骨（骨外病变在第27章讨论）。患者通常表现为局部疼痛或肿胀。病理性骨折也可出现。一些Ewing肉瘤患者表现为全身性症状，如发热和体重减轻。实验室检查可显示贫血和红细胞沉积率上升。所有这些结果可能导致误诊为骨髓炎，从而延误治疗。

影像学通常显示病变范围广泛，有时累及整个骨骼（图25.8）。典型病变累及骨干，表现为浸润性破坏，类似于恶性淋巴瘤。然而，一些病变表现为大片的地图样破坏。Ewing肉瘤的典型表现是引起明显的新膜化骨形成。新骨形成多层，产生洋葱皮样表现。

大体标本上，Ewing肉瘤常为白色，鱼肉样伴有坏死（图25.9）。病变可能质地非常软，以至于类似于脓液。活检时外科医生可能误将肿瘤组织当做脓液，而将所有材料送去做微生物培养。

典型的Ewing肉瘤由一致的小圆细胞组成（图25.10）。细胞核呈圆形，核仁不清。细胞核有点像烟熏样表现。细胞浆边界不清，以至于几个细胞的胞浆似乎形成合体状，细胞核陷入其中。只要有轮廓鲜明的梭形

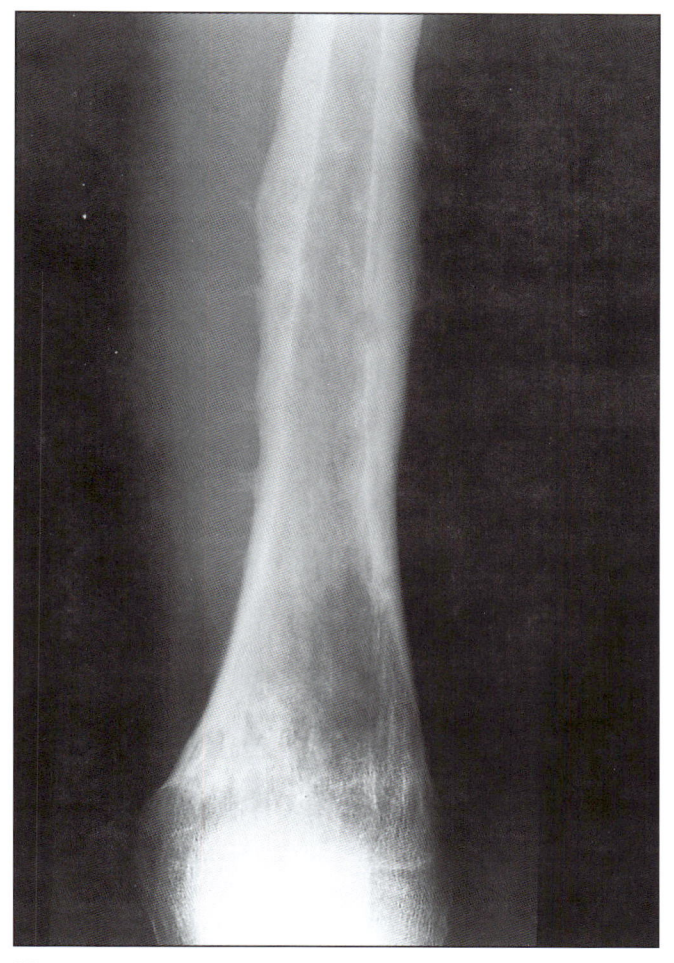

图25.8 X光片显示Ewing肉瘤广泛累及股骨的骨干和远端。溶骨性破坏及新骨膜化骨形成。

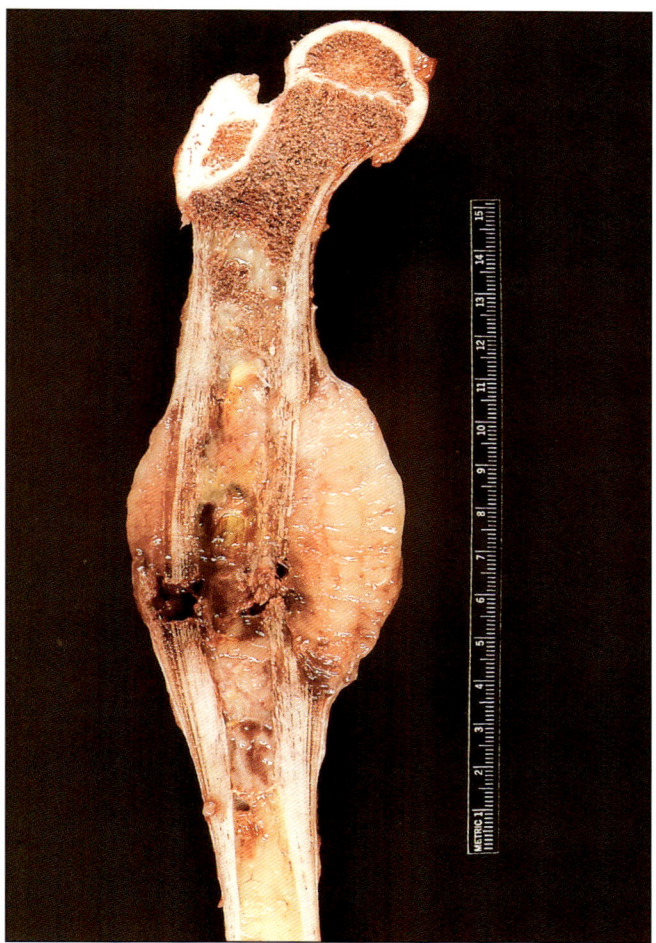

图25.9 Ewing肉瘤的大体标本显示病理性骨折，灰白质软的肿块延伸至软组织。

核就应该除外 Ewing 肉瘤的诊断。但是，必须确定这种梭形核不是活检标本周围的人工假象。在典型的 Ewing 肉瘤中，核分裂活动通常不明显。在高达 70% 的 Ewing 肉瘤中，特殊染色和电镜常常可以显示胞浆糖原[32]。

Ewing 肉瘤和周围神经外胚层肿瘤（peripheral neuroectodermal tumor）强烈表达 p30/32^{MIC} 抗原，它是一种由假性-常染色体 *MIC2* 基因编码的糖蛋白，集合成簇成为 CD99 抗原[33]。在高达 90% 的 Ewing 肉瘤中，包括 O13、HBA-71 和 12E7 在内的单克隆抗体可以识别这一抗原[34]。虽然它们是敏感的标记物，但是并不特异。诸如淋巴母细胞淋巴瘤、急性淋巴细胞白血病、滑膜肉瘤、神经内分泌癌、间叶性软骨肉瘤、横纹肌肉瘤等也可能呈阳性[35-42]。因此，CD99 阳性应该考虑支持此诊断，但不是诊断 Ewing 肉瘤的证据。

细胞遗传学和分子遗传学在诊断 Ewing 肉瘤中可以起作用（也见第 27 章）。t(11;22)(q24;q12) 的相互易位在大约 90% 的 Ewing 肉瘤中都能见到。其他少见的易

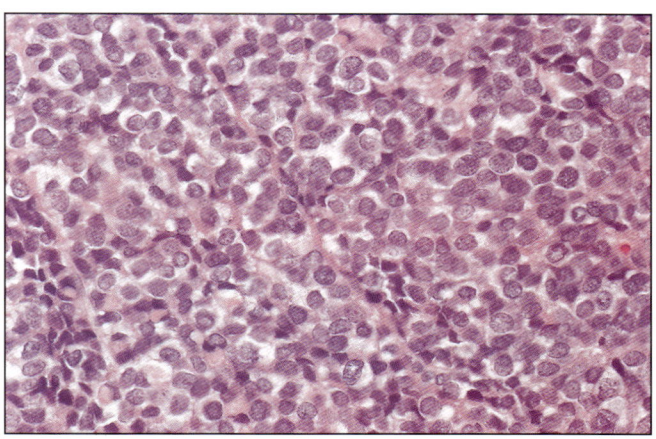

图25.10 Ewing肉瘤显示一致的细胞群，细胞核呈圆形到卵圆形，染色质呈细小颗粒状。

位，如 t(21;22)(q22;q12)，大约在 10% 的肿瘤中可见[43]。已经显示这些易位的断点克隆涉及 22 号染色体的 *EWS* 基因、11 号染色体的 *FLI-1* 基因以及 21 号染色体的 *ERG* 基因[43]。这可导致 EWS-FLI-1 和 EWS-ERG 杂

交转录物的形成，后者可通过反转录 PCR 检测到[44-46]。融合基因转录的类型（不同外显子组合的结果）可能对预后有重要意义[47]。

大约 5% 的 Ewing 肉瘤显示更大、更多形性的细胞核。这些细胞中有些有明显的核仁，核分裂活动通常比典型的 Ewing 肉瘤更明显。有些作者将这一类型的 Ewing 肉瘤命名为非典型性 Ewing 肉瘤或大细胞 Ewing 肉瘤[48]。以我们的经验，它们的预后与典型的 Ewing 肉瘤相似。一些研究试图研究 Ewing 肉瘤组织学特征与预后的相关性。已经有报告：丝状生长方式[49]、非典型的组织学特征[50]和坏死[51]与不良预后有关。鉴别诊断包括其他小细胞肿瘤，尤其是转移性神经母细胞瘤和恶性淋巴瘤。转移性神经母细胞瘤患者通常发生在 2 岁之前，原发病灶通常容易找到。神经母细胞瘤通常显示清楚的玫瑰花结，并且出现神经纤维性基质。然而，一些神经母细胞瘤分化很差，鉴别诊断可能很困难。患者的临床检查以及确定与神经母细胞瘤相关的血清标记物可能有所帮助。恶性淋巴瘤通常有多形性细胞浸润，而 Ewing 肉瘤的细胞形态更为一致。尽管如此，在一些情况下，特别是送检的材料有限时，鉴别诊断可能非常困难。Ewing 肉瘤通常在儿童发病，而恶性淋巴瘤并不常见于儿童。白细胞共同抗原染色阳性可以排除 Ewing 肉瘤的诊断。

一些年前，Askin 等[52]描述了一种儿童胸肺来源的小细胞肿瘤。由于具有少见的组织学特征，他们把这种病变与 Ewing 肉瘤区别开来，并且认为它来源于神经系统。在他们的研究中，这种肿瘤的预后比 Ewing 肉瘤的更差。Contesso 等[53]将 Askin 肿瘤与其他部位的经典的 Ewing 肉瘤做了比较，他们发现，Askin 肿瘤与经典的 Ewing 肉瘤在免疫组化谱系上没有明显的差异。出现在 Ewing 肉瘤中的特征性染色体易位（11;22），在 Askin 肿瘤、外周神经外胚叶肿瘤和触觉神经母细胞瘤（esthesioneuroblastoma）中也有记述，但在脑的原始神经外胚叶肿瘤中没有[43,54]。

一些电子显微镜、组织培养和免疫组化研究已经支持 Ewing 肉瘤可能是神经外胚叶肿瘤中的一种的观点[55,56]。

Tsuneyoshi 等[57]将骨的小细胞肿瘤分为四个不同的组：(1) 经典的 Ewing 肉瘤；(2) 骨的神经外胚叶肿瘤；(3) 具有神经外胚叶肿瘤和 Ewing 肉瘤特征的中间型肿瘤；以及 (4) 局灶形成玫瑰花结的梭形细胞肿瘤。他们提出，只有在整个病变中出现弥漫的玫瑰花结时，才应该做出神经外胚叶肿瘤的诊断（图 25.11）。应用这个标准他们发现，神经外胚叶肿瘤神经标记物染色呈阳性，而仅有少数典型的 Ewing 肉瘤显示这种标记物呈阳性。研究并没有提及这种区分是否在预后上有何不同。

Ushigome 等[56]将可出现明确的 Homer Wright 玫

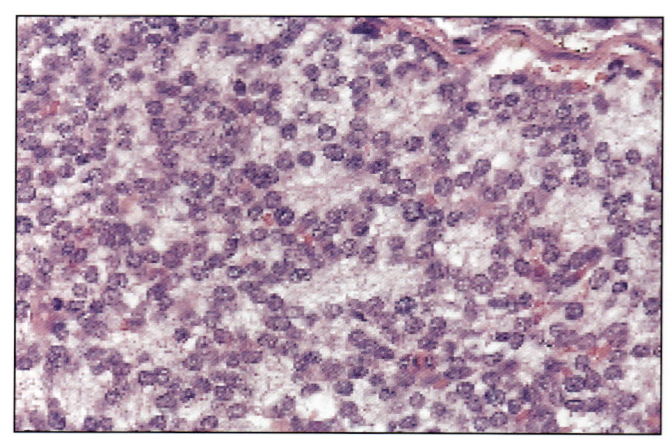

图 25.11　原始神经外胚叶肿瘤。显示明显的玫瑰花结结构。

瑰花结或局灶神经节分化（或两者均有）的肿瘤分类为原始神经外胚叶肿瘤。在大部分病例中，神经标记物呈阳性。在这组病例中，3 例肿瘤在最初的部位是典型的 Ewing 肉瘤，在转移部位显示出明确的 Homer Wright 玫瑰花结结构。这些作者也提出，Ewing 肉瘤和原始神经外胚叶肿瘤是相关联的病变。Ewing 肉瘤可能代表原始神经外胚叶肿瘤一种未分化的形式。

仅有一项研究[58]提示，原始神经外胚叶肿瘤的预后比 Ewing 肉瘤的差。内科肿瘤医生采用相同的方案治疗 Ewing 肉瘤和原始神经外胚叶肿瘤。因此，至少到目前为止，Ewing 肉瘤和原始神经外胚叶肿瘤间的差别只是一种学术上的问题，还没有显示出任何实用的价值。

在现代治疗模式——如放疗和化疗——取得进展之前，Ewing 肉瘤被认为是所有骨肿瘤中最致命的。5 年生存率在 5% ~ 10% 之间。然而，采用现代治疗方案后，5 年生存率提高到 50% ~ 60%。一些研究表明，化疗后肿瘤的坏死范围与预后有关[59]。虽然放疗和化疗一直是主要的治疗方式，但外科切除骨的受累部分也是一种重要的辅助治疗[60,61]。

软骨肿瘤　Chondroid tumors

软骨分化的相关肿瘤构成了第二大类骨肿瘤。

良性软骨肿瘤　Benign cartilage tumors

骨软骨瘤　Osteochondroma

骨软骨瘤是最常见的良性骨肿瘤。骨软骨瘤一直被认为并非真性肿瘤，而是错位了的骺板。然而，最近的遗传学资料显示，它是真正的肿瘤性病变[62]。当骨软骨瘤很小时，是没有症状的，因此无法知道真实的发病率。

骨软骨瘤产生症状则是由于它们的大小（破坏了邻近结构，如神经），或穿过肿瘤的骨柄部骨折引起了疼痛。大多数骨软骨瘤的年轻患者是在外科检查时发现的。以男性为主。骨骼的任何部位都可受累，但最好发于长骨的干骺端。累及手足小骨的真正骨软骨瘤非常少见。发生在这些部位的类似于骨软骨瘤的病变是反应性改变，如奇异型骨旁骨软骨瘤样增生和指（趾）下骨疣[63,64]。我们从未见过发生在颅骨和颌骨的骨软骨瘤。

影像学检查具有特征性，显示从骨表面开始的一个突出性病变（图25.12）。病变可能是广基底的或有蒂的。无论哪种病变，下方的骨皮质与骨软骨瘤的皮质都是连续的；同样，下方的骨松质与骨软骨瘤的松质也是连续的。当病变累及长骨的干骺端时，典型的生长方式是从最近的关节向远端生长。有蒂的骨软骨瘤是由骨柄和软骨帽构成蘑菇状外壳组成。表面的帽光滑而规则。

在大体标本上，骨软骨瘤有薄而光滑的软骨帽，下方为骨柄（图25.13）。骨梁间可见骨髓的造血成分和脂肪组织。显微镜下，骨软骨瘤的软骨帽中显示软骨细胞位于陷窝中。软骨帽的细胞从基底向上呈柱状排列，类似于骺板的表现。在骺板的基底，软骨经历软骨内骨化到形成骨小梁。在骨柄中，成分之间常常可以看到残留的软骨岛。骨小梁间的空隙既可含有脂肪也可含有骨髓造血成分（图25.14）。小部分患者有遗传性多发外生性骨疣。后者为常染色体显性遗传[65]，是由于*EXT1*或*EXT2*基因突变造成的[66]。这些患者还有其他的骨骼异常，如生长迟缓[67]。这些骨软骨瘤的放射学、大体解剖和镜下特征与孤立的外生性骨疣相似。然而，其放射学显示通常缺乏骨的管腔结构，如在股骨颈。一些骨软骨瘤发生在滑囊之上；这在临床检查和影像学表现上会给人以一个肿块的印象，可能导致误诊为继发性软骨肉瘤。

鉴别诊断包括奇异型骨旁骨软骨瘤样增生（bizarre parosteal osteochondromatous proliferation）和指（趾）下骨疣（subungual exostosis）。奇异型骨旁骨软骨瘤样增生通常累及手的小骨，足骨较少见。但是，大约20%的病变累及长骨。病变类似于骨软骨瘤，由增生的软骨和逐渐成熟的梁状骨组成。软骨常常很丰富，而且细胞也很多。在骨梁间可以看到梭形细胞增生。软骨有特征性的蓝染性质，尤其是在软骨内骨化的位置[63]。这些病变可以复发，但是它们的临床病程一定

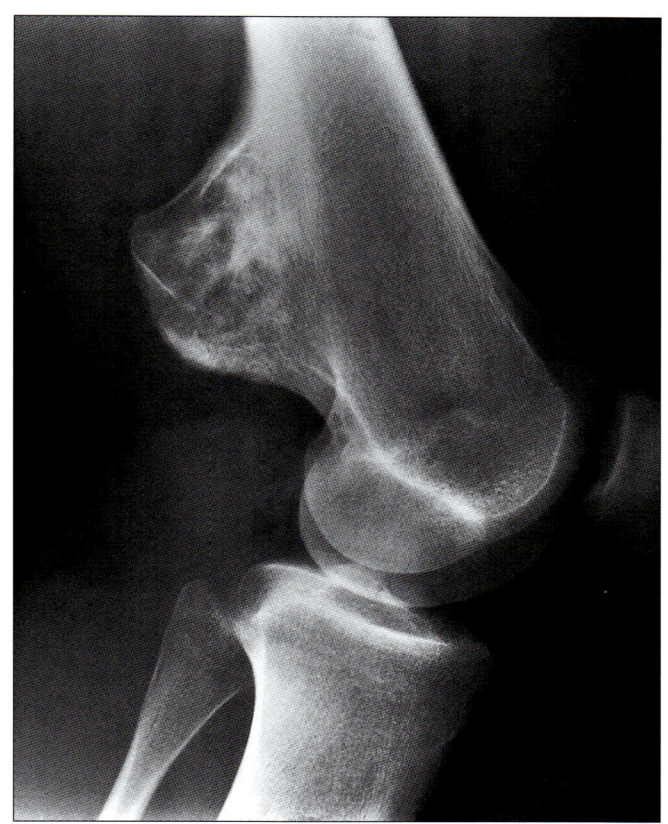

图25.12　X光片显示突出于股骨干骺端的骨软骨瘤。注意下方的股骨与病变的皮质和松质相连续。

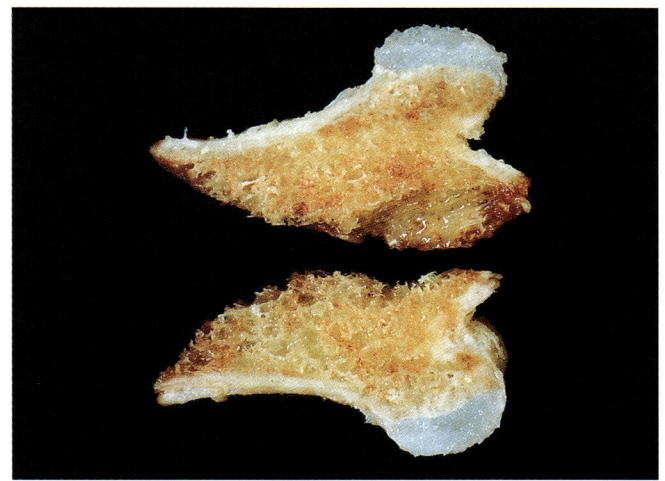

图25.13　骨软骨瘤的大体标本，松质骨上方有软骨帽。

是良性的。指（趾）下骨疣（见1640页），如病名所示，发生在甲床下，尤其是大拇趾[64]。影像学显示为起自骨表面的钙化性病变。大体上，病变类似于骨软骨瘤的表现，有软骨帽和其下的骨柄。然而，它不像骨软骨瘤，不具有梭形细胞增生成熟为软骨，再成熟为骨

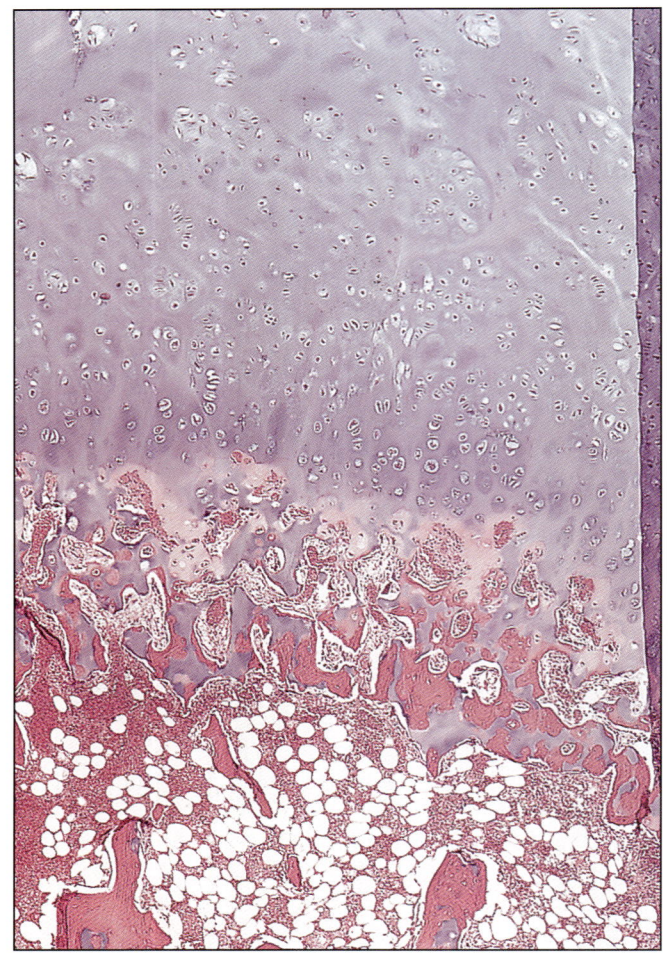

图25.14 骨软骨瘤的镜下照片，有增厚的透明软骨帽，由软骨内钙化成熟转化为骨小梁，骨小梁周边为骨髓的脂肪和造血组织。

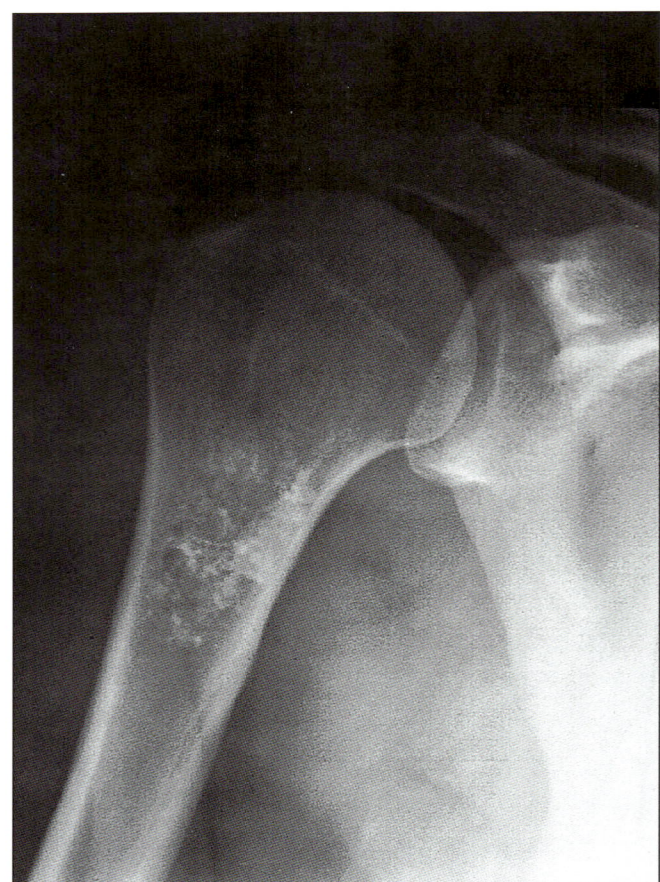

图25.15 右侧肱骨近端X光片显示骨髓腔内软骨肿瘤，伴有典型的内生性软骨瘤的特征。

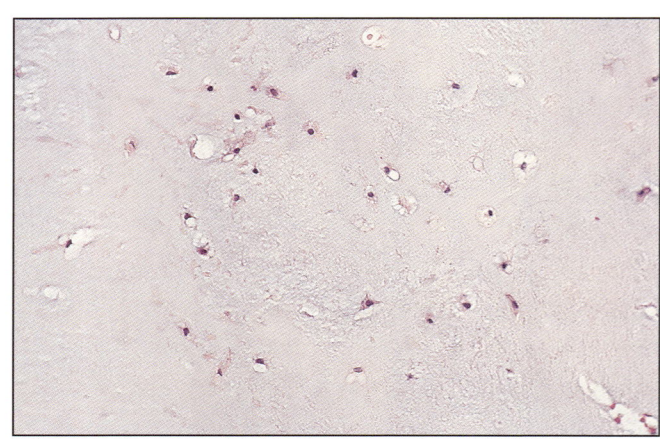

图25.16 股骨近端内生性软骨瘤。显示细胞稀疏，细胞核小而规则，不伴有细胞非典型性，以及一致的蓝灰色基质。

小梁的过程。

软骨瘤 Chondroma

软骨瘤一词是指良性软骨肿瘤。这些肿瘤中一些可能不是真正的肿瘤，而有可能是发育异常。病变可能出现在骨内，这样的病例被命名为内生性软骨瘤；而骨表面发生的病例则被命名为骨膜软骨瘤；在软组织中发生的病例命名为软组织软骨瘤。

内生性软骨瘤（enchondroma）是无症状的病变；因此不清楚它的真正发病率。此病无性别和年龄发病倾向。在外科病例中，大部分内生性软骨瘤是由累及手足小骨的病变组成。发生在较大骨骼的内生性软骨瘤可能是在影像学检查中的偶然发现。内生性软骨瘤在骨扫描中可呈阳性表现，并且有可能在为除外转移癌进行扫描时被检测到。影像学显示内生性软骨瘤是界限清楚的局限于髓腔内的病变。肿瘤不侵犯骨皮质内面。大部分内生性软骨瘤病变内有分布均匀一致的钙化（图25.15）。在大体标本上，内生性软骨瘤具有特征性的淡蓝色软骨表现。可见（石灰）白色钙化斑点。显微镜下，内生性软骨瘤呈分叶状，病变细胞稀少，软骨细胞排列成簇状，伴有丰富的细胞间基质（图25.16）。小叶周围常常有一薄的骨边。基质是实性的，没有广泛的黏液样变性或囊性变。

软骨细胞总是在陷窝中,一个陷窝有几个软骨细胞。细胞核小、呈圆形、不明显。双核细胞罕见。内生性软骨瘤呈膨胀性生长,破坏骨髓,因此不会浸润到骨小梁之间。

手和足小骨的内生性软骨瘤具有不同的特征。它们常常因为发生病理性骨折而引起疼痛。影像学检查显示骨皮质变薄。这种特征在较大的骨的软骨肿瘤中则提示恶性。然而,在小骨,除非肿瘤穿透骨侵犯软组织,否则不能诊断软骨肉瘤。在大体标本上,软骨瘤常常充满整个骨腔,表面覆盖的骨皮质可以薄如纸。镜下,小骨的内生性软骨瘤细胞十分丰富(图25.17)。常常见到双核细胞,甚至可以有黏液变性。然而病变不穿透骨皮质进入软组织。

在骨肿瘤病理中,较难解决的问题之一是鉴别软骨瘤与高分化软骨肉瘤。我们已经指出:小骨与大骨的病变有不同的评价规则。当评估大骨的软骨肿瘤时,我们认为有必要由有经验的放射科医生查看X片。软骨肿瘤广泛破坏骨皮质一定要考虑恶性的可能。大体检查时,基质的黏液变性或囊性变应作为恶性的证据。显微镜下,我们认为是否穿透周围结构可能是鉴别低级别软骨肉瘤与内生性软骨瘤的一个最好标准。

骨膜软骨瘤(periosteal chondromas)非常罕见,是发生在骨表面的良性软骨肿瘤[68,69]。这些病变通常累及肱骨近端和股骨远端。罕见情况下可累及手和足的小骨。影像学显示骨表面界限清楚的病变,伴有下方皮质的碟形凹陷。在大体标本上,病变呈现软骨肿瘤的典型表现,没有侵犯周围组织的倾向。组织学上,骨膜软骨瘤的细胞非常丰富。细胞核深染,常见双核细胞。如不结合其他情况,所有这些特征支持1级或甚至2级软骨肉瘤的诊断。然而,如果病变小,边界清楚,这些细胞的改变可以忽略。

大部分**软组织软骨瘤**(soft tissue chondromas)发生在手和足[70,71]。以我们的经验,在身体的其他任何部位,软组织的良性玻璃样软骨肿瘤都非常少见。软组织软骨瘤呈分叶状,可以有多个结节。组织学上,软骨细胞呈簇排列,但是可以显示轻到中度的细胞非典型性。组织学特征与滑膜软骨瘤病非常相似(见1646页)[70,71]。无论细胞学特征多么让人不放心,软组织软骨瘤的临床病程总是良性的。局部复发并不少见,肿瘤恶变极罕见。

少数患者可出现多发性软骨病变,可能是发育异常而不是真正的肿瘤。Ollier病患者表现为软骨肿块,通常累及长骨末端和扁骨。其病变可累及单一肢体或一侧肢体,也可为两侧病变。此病发生在儿童时,影像学表现非常有特点。此病发生在长骨干骺端-骨干部分则表现为膨胀以及纵向条纹状钙化(图25.18)。发生在

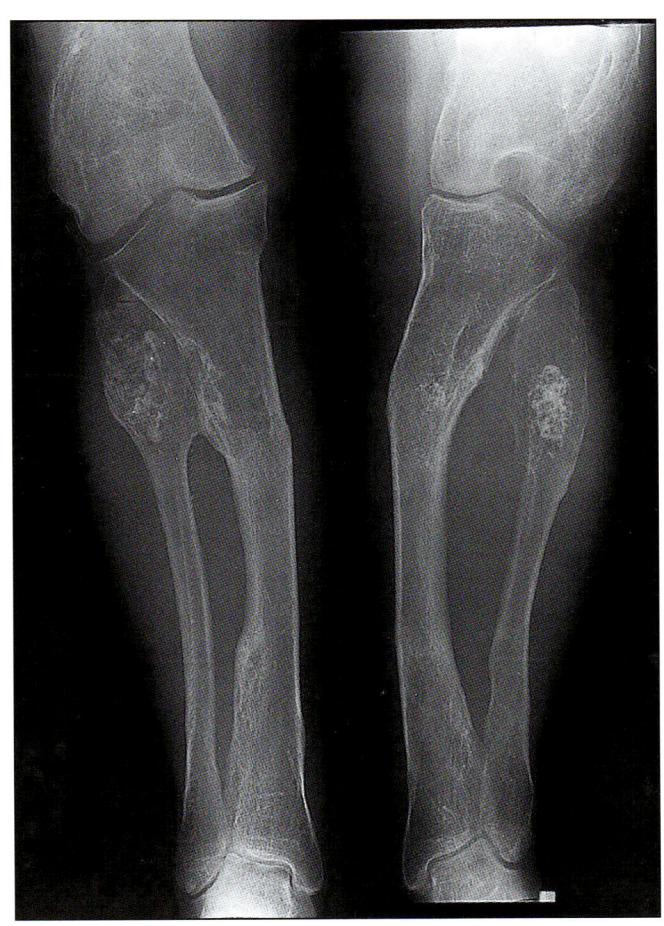

图25.18 X光片显示双下肢长骨干骺区域的Ollier病的典型发育异常改变,伴有弓形畸形。有多发性软骨病变,与多发性内生性软骨瘤相同。

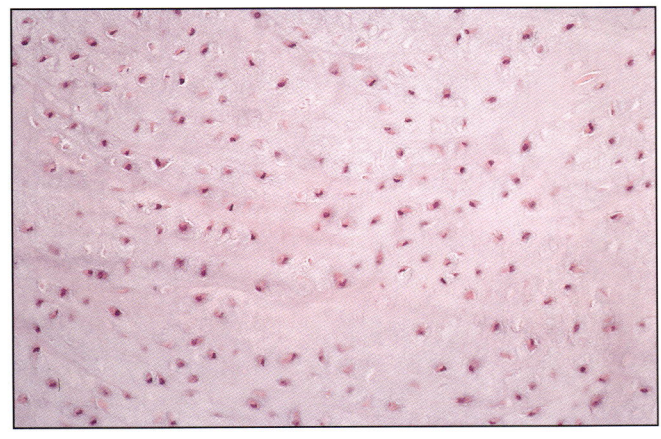

图25.17 发生在手指骨的内生性软骨瘤。此病变比发生在长骨内的内生性软骨瘤细胞丰富。

Ollier病的软骨发育异常可以有高分化软骨肉瘤的表现。其病变常常细胞十分丰富，有双核细胞，细胞核增大深染。然而，如果影像学表现为Ollier病，则这些组织学特征就不是恶性特征。当骨骼成熟时，病变逐渐呈退行性改变。起自Ollier病的患者很少发生软骨肉瘤。区别Ollier病软骨发育异常与软骨肉瘤可能很困难。放射学上显示破坏和浸润改变。我们发现，比较怀疑恶性变的区域和良性发育异常区域的组织学特征是很有用的。基质的明显黏液变性和周围组织的浸润应该考虑为恶性表现[72]。

更罕见的疾病称作Maffucci综合征。除了骨骼软骨发育异常外，Maffucci综合征患者还有软组织血管瘤。Maffucci综合征患者有较高的恶变几率。事实上，该综合征可能是某些恶性肿瘤的标志，或是骨骼或是内脏[73]。伴发血管瘤的大多数病例显示梭形细胞血管瘤的特征（见第3章）[74]。

软骨母细胞瘤 Chondroblastoma

软骨母细胞瘤是一种良性肿瘤，好发年龄为11～20岁。男性稍多。临床表现完全不具特异性。骨骼的任何部位都可能受累，但是主要发生于长骨末端，延伸至关节软骨。累及颅骨的患者年龄比累及长骨的患者年龄更大[75]。软骨母细胞瘤主要发生于骺端，但偶尔也有典型的软骨母细胞瘤发生在干骺端[75-80]。影像学表现非常有特征。病变边界清晰，可以有硬化的边缘。病变的中心几乎都在骺端[81]。此病一半以上的病变累及骺端，但也可通过开放的骺板扩展到干骺端。这种表现几乎可以够得上诊断软骨母细胞瘤了。

大约15%的肿瘤累及骨的突起部分，即股骨的大转子或肱骨的结节（图25.19）。大约1/3的软骨母细胞瘤影像学上显示有矿化。

在大体标本上，软骨母细胞瘤通常呈白色，质韧。少数情况下，病变可以呈囊性。显微镜下，软骨母细胞瘤由单核细胞和巨细胞组成。其巨细胞数量通常不像在典型的巨细胞瘤中见到的那么多。单核细胞的细胞核呈卵圆形，伴有纵行的核沟，类似于Langerhans组织细胞增生症的细胞。细胞浆轮廓常常很清晰，胞浆淡染或透明。我们认为，软骨母细胞瘤的细胞学特征十分典型。但是，诊断软骨母细胞瘤要有明确的软骨样分化或肿瘤细胞间的钙化（图25.20）。软骨岛通常粉染，紧邻单核细胞增生的典型区域。单个肿瘤细胞间形成纤细的线样钙化。Kurt等[75]的研究显示，95%的病例可见到软骨分化，而仅有35%的病例可以见到钙化。在单核细胞中常可找到核分裂象。但是，细胞并没有非典型性。

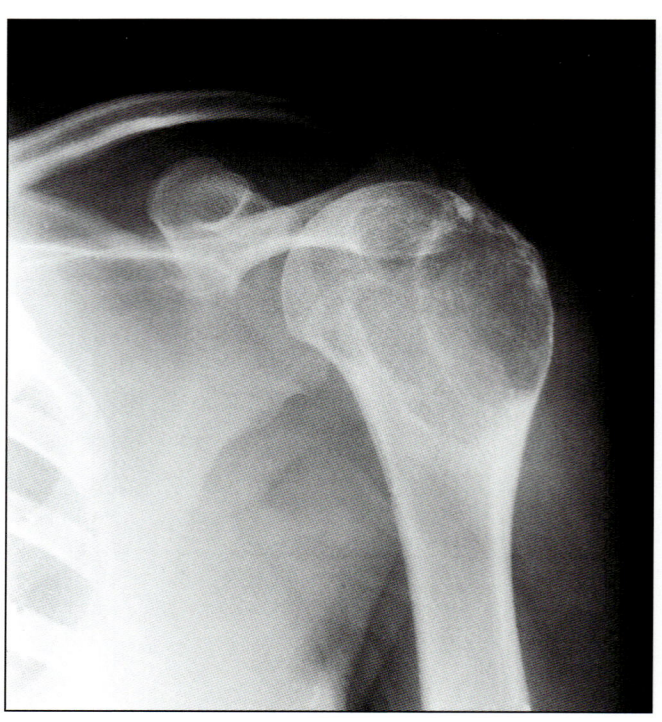

图25.19 肱骨骨突发生的软骨母细胞瘤的X-线表现，呈现一种膨胀性表现，周围伴有硬化。

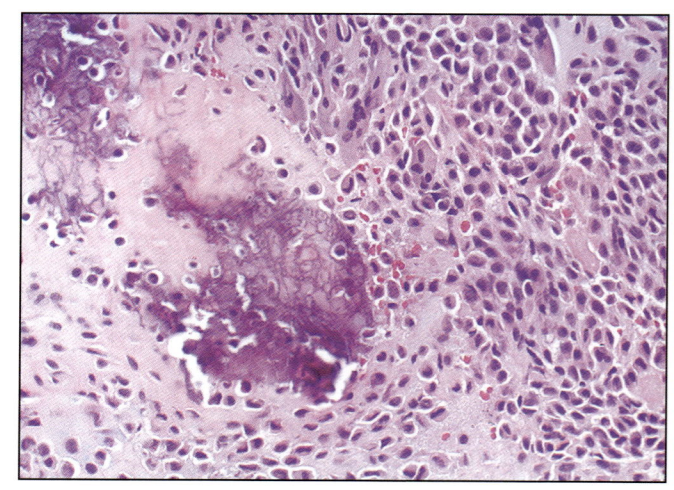

图25.20 典型的软骨母细胞瘤表现嗜酸性软骨样基质伴有钙盐沉积。单核细胞含有圆形到卵圆形的细胞核，周围为淡染的胞浆。

大约1/3的软骨母细胞瘤显示有继发性动脉瘤样骨囊肿形成的区域。这可能是局灶的表现，也可能是主要特征。这种组织学特征不影响预后。软骨母细胞瘤是良性病变，但可能会局部复发。软骨母细胞瘤甚至可能种植到软组织中。据文献记载：组织学良性的软骨母细胞瘤可出现肺转移[82,83]。这些转移性病变多数在肺内形成孤立病灶，外科切除可以治愈。然而，极少数情况下，转移病变为弥漫性的，可导致患者死亡[84]。软骨母细胞瘤远处转移非常罕见，在 Mayo Clinic 的档案记录中，495 例中仅有 7 例出现转移[75]。

鉴别诊断包括软骨黏液样纤维瘤和软骨肉瘤，尤其是透明细胞软骨肉瘤。软骨黏液样纤维瘤发生在干骺端，而软骨母细胞瘤发生在骺端。两种肿瘤组织学上有一些相似之处（见下文）。透明细胞软骨肉瘤也出现在长骨末端。然而，透明细胞软骨肉瘤细胞的核是圆形的，可以有明显的核仁。

软骨黏液样纤维瘤　Chondromyxoid fibroma

软骨黏液样纤维瘤十分少见，发生率仅为软骨母细胞瘤的一半。直到 1982 年，Mayo Clinic 的资料中仅有 48 例，而到 1983 年，Rizzoli 研究所也仅有 27 例[85]。最近的 Mayo Clinic 的一次研究包括会诊病例在内，积累了 278 例[86]。患者发病常在 11～30 岁之间。软骨黏液样纤维瘤通常累及长骨的干骺端。此病也常常累及足部的小骨。放射学显示病变界限非常清晰，干骺端单纯溶骨性破坏。病变通常有硬化性边缘，可以呈波浪状或扇贝样外观（图 25.21）。

在大体标本上，软骨黏液样纤维瘤常常为灰白色分叶状。病变边界清楚，常突出于骨周围。

显微镜下，软骨黏液样纤维瘤是分叶状病变。小叶可小可大。典型者，小叶中心细胞稀少，小叶周边部细胞丰富（图 25.22）。因此，在小叶融合的区域，细胞可以呈片状。背景呈淡蓝色，但液化性黏液变性不常见。在软骨黏液样纤维瘤中，界限清晰的玻璃样软骨分化并不常见。细胞呈梭形或星芒状。肿瘤细胞可以增大深染，提示恶变的可能。可以见到动脉瘤样骨囊肿样变，但是不像在软骨母细胞瘤中那样常见。细胞较丰富的区域可能有类似于软骨母细胞瘤的细胞。细胞遗传学分析显示，这些病变常常有染色体 6q13 的重排[87]。

软骨黏液样纤维瘤是良性病变，单纯切除可以治愈。然而，有 15%～20% 的病例可能复发，甚至可能出现软组织种植。

鉴别诊断包括软骨母细胞瘤、软骨肉瘤和黏液样纤维异常增生。软骨肉瘤倾向于呈分叶状，高级别软骨肉瘤可能有与软骨黏液样纤维瘤细胞相似的细胞。软骨肉瘤在影像学中总是呈侵袭性表现，而软骨黏液样纤维瘤总是呈良性放射学表现。所有分叶状肿瘤的周边部细胞都很丰富。软骨肉瘤即使在小叶中心区，细胞也相当丰富，而软骨黏液样纤维瘤小叶中心区细

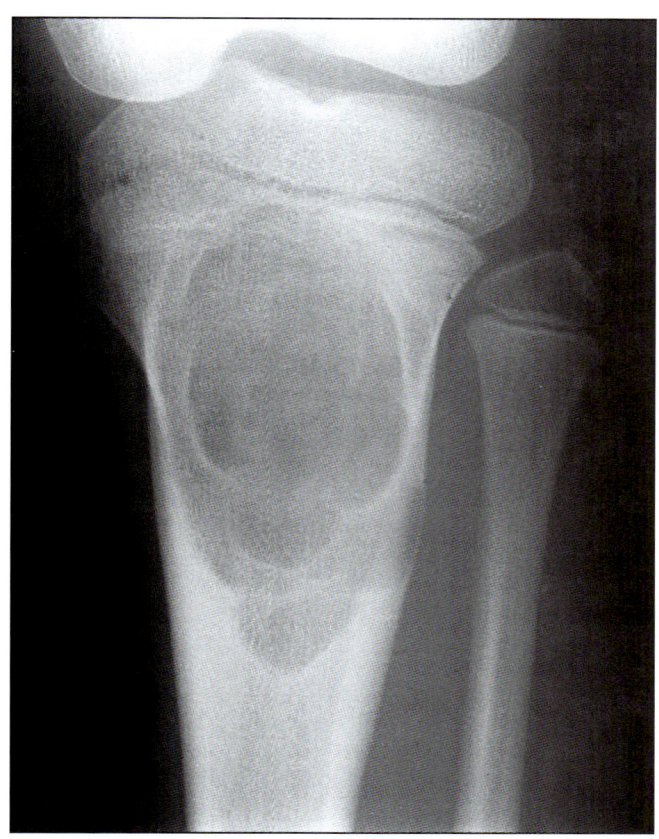

图 25.21　发生在胫骨近端干骺端的软骨黏液样纤维瘤的影像学表现。病变有硬化和扇贝样边缘，这是典型的软骨黏液样纤维瘤的表现。(Courtesy of Dr. M. Miller, Middlemore Hospital, Auckland, New Zealand.)

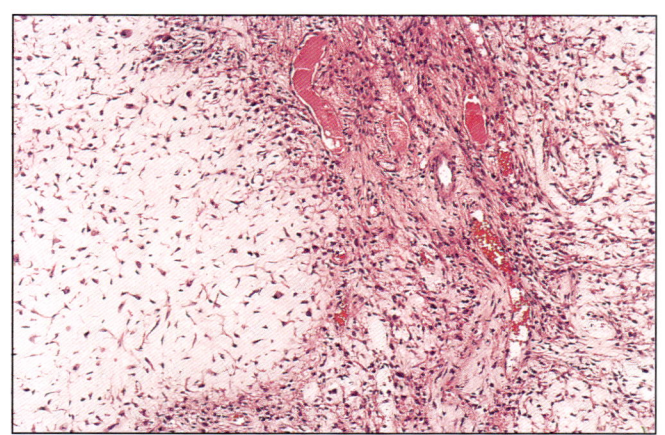

图 25.22　软骨黏液样纤维瘤的显微照片，显示分叶状生长。在小叶的周边有富于梭形或星芒状细胞区。

胞稀少。软骨母细胞瘤通常没有像软骨黏液样纤维瘤那样明确的分叶结构。然而，在一些病例中，两者几乎不能区别。在这种情况下，我们常常依据病变的位置来区别两者。纤维异常增生可以出现明显的黏液变性，类似于软骨黏液样纤维瘤。但是，纤维异常增生没有分叶结构。

恶性软骨肿瘤　Malignant cartilage tumors

软骨肉瘤　Chondrosarcoma

软骨肉瘤在骨的最常见恶性肿瘤中列第三位，发病率仅次于骨髓瘤和骨肉瘤。骨的软骨肉瘤根据临床、影像学和组织学特征可以分为几个不同的亚型[88]，如普通型软骨肉瘤、小骨的软骨肉瘤、继发性软骨肉瘤、骨旁软骨肉瘤、透明细胞软骨肉瘤、去分化软骨肉瘤和间叶性软骨肉瘤。

最大的一组累及成人的长骨和扁骨，是由恶性玻璃样软骨组成的肿瘤。这组可以命名为普通型软骨肉瘤。虽然骨骼的任何部位都可以发生，但肩胛和骨盆区是最常见的部位。大部分软骨肉瘤患者的年龄在31～60岁。临床症状不特异，患者常常主诉疼痛，可能为长期持续性疼痛。病理性骨折不常见。

软骨肉瘤的影像学表现是具有诊断意义的。虽然仅在1/5的病例中出现骨膨胀和皮质增厚的联合表现，但这是软骨肉瘤具有确诊意义的表现。肿瘤通常显示为钙化影（图25.23）。在良性软骨肿瘤中，钙化影常常均匀分布于病变中。当一个软骨肿瘤显示有透光区和钙化区时，应该考虑软骨肉瘤。肿瘤最终突破骨皮质而形成软组织包块。一些软骨肉瘤并不出现骨皮质增厚，而是显示骨内皮质部分的溶骨性破坏，形成圆齿样表现。

软骨肉瘤通常有特征性大体表现。软骨为淡蓝色或珍珠白色（图25.24）。钙化灶可以形成白色沙砾样区域。一个给人以黏液般感觉的软骨肿瘤应该高度怀疑为软骨肉瘤。当软骨肉瘤黏液样变明显时，肿瘤切开时基质可能是液态的并可流出。这可能引起病变内出现囊性变。

软骨肉瘤镜下表现多种多样，依据肿瘤分级而不同。低级别软骨肉瘤与内生性软骨瘤鉴别很困难。低倍镜下，软骨肉瘤侵犯已存在的骨，将骨小梁包裹在内（图25.25）。肿瘤往往充满骨髓腔。广泛的黏液样变使得基质呈颗粒状、黏稠丝状或泡沫样外观。软骨细胞在陷窝中，通常不是梭形的。内生性软骨瘤的软骨细胞的细胞

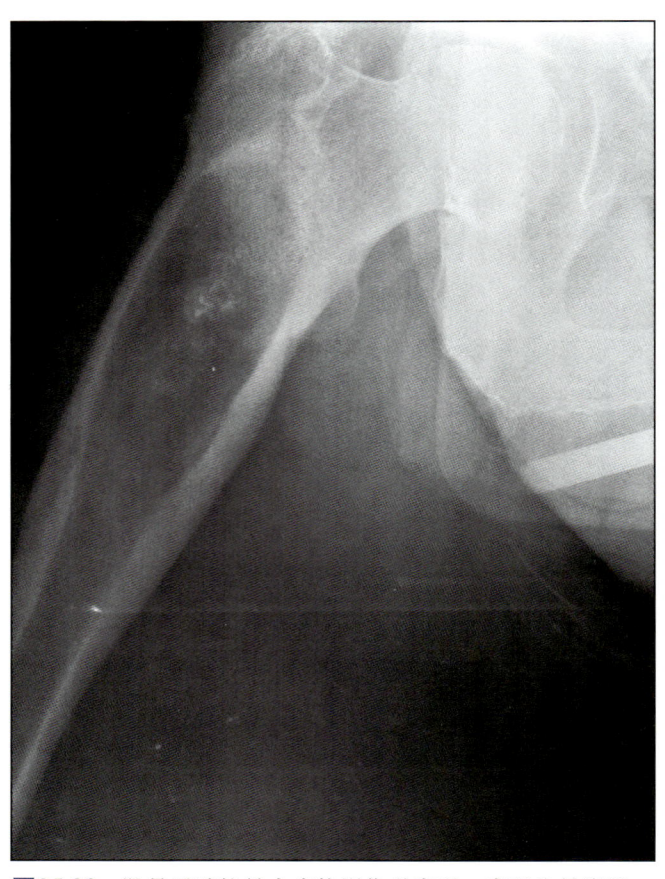

图25.23　股骨近端软骨肉瘤的影像学表现。表现为骨膨胀，皮质增厚，以及散在的钙化影。

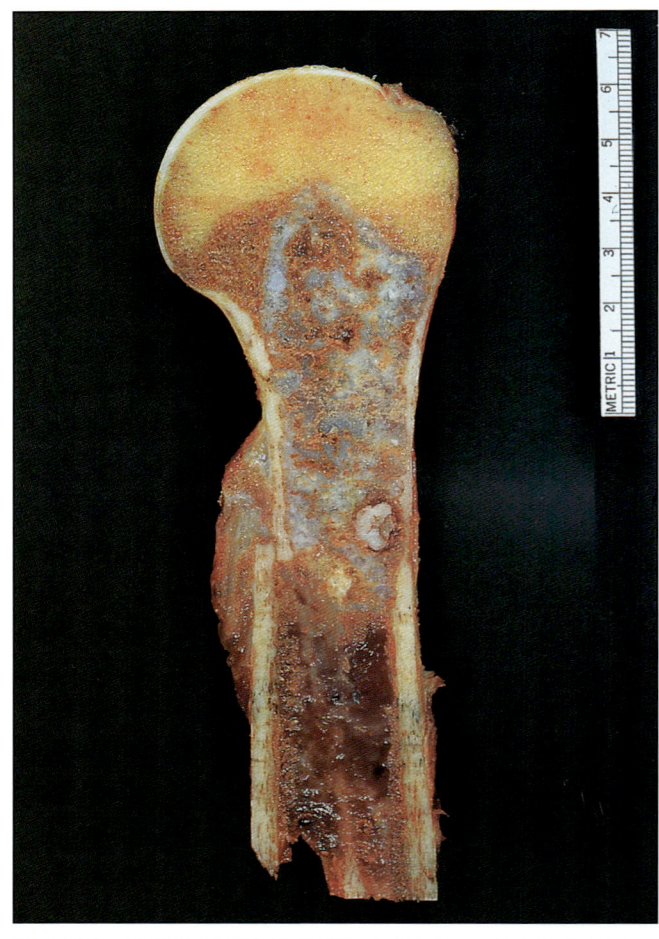

图25.24　软骨肉瘤病理性骨折的大体标本。肿瘤呈蓝灰色，侵透骨皮质形成软组织包块。

核小、呈圆形、规则。恶性软骨肿瘤中细胞核增大，实际上染色可能比良性细胞的浅。可以见到双核细胞。

和前面一样，软骨肉瘤的分级与疾病预后密切相关[89-93]。已经提出了几种不同的软骨肉瘤分级系统[90,92]。软骨肉瘤一般并不显示核分裂活性，因此，我们不能使用这一指标对软骨肉瘤进行分级。我们根据病变中的细胞密集程度和软骨细胞核的改变来对软骨肉瘤进行分级。1级，软骨肉瘤显示的细胞密度较内生性软骨瘤高。软骨细胞增大且更不规则（图25.26）。2级软骨肉瘤的细胞比1级软骨肉瘤的细胞更丰富，细胞核的改变更为明显（图25.27）。3级软骨肉瘤显示细胞非常丰富，细胞核的多形性很显著，小叶周边部有一些梭形细胞（图25.28）。以我们的经验，任何广泛的梭形细胞表现，除非是去分化软骨肉瘤（见下文），否则可以排除软骨肉瘤的诊断。这种分级系统有判断预后的意义[92]。

软骨肉瘤通常是局部侵袭性肿瘤，远处转移的潜能较低。一项来自Mayo Clinic的研究[94]发现，虽然不断有患者有局部复发，甚至在长达20年以后出现远处转移，但其5年存活率仍能达到77%。1级肿瘤的远处转移风险是4%，而高级别肿瘤则为30%。在这项研究中，66%的肿瘤为1级，31%为2级，仅有3%是3级。

许多作者指出，鉴别低级别软骨肉瘤和内生性软骨瘤非常困难[95]。细胞学改变、基质的黏液变性和浸润的特征都非常重要。我们主要依赖影像学表现来进行解释。位于中轴骨的、大的、疼痛性病变很可能是软骨肉瘤，而累及手和足的小骨的病变可能是良性病变。

虽然大部分手和足的小骨的软骨病变是良性的，但是确有累及小骨的软骨肉瘤。用于诊断小骨的软骨肉瘤的标准与大骨的并不相同[96-98]。

正如先前提到的那样，小骨的内生性软骨瘤常常使皮质变薄。肿瘤清晰的皮质穿透进入软组织，支持小骨软骨肉瘤的诊断。在这个位置上的肿瘤细胞学改变不足

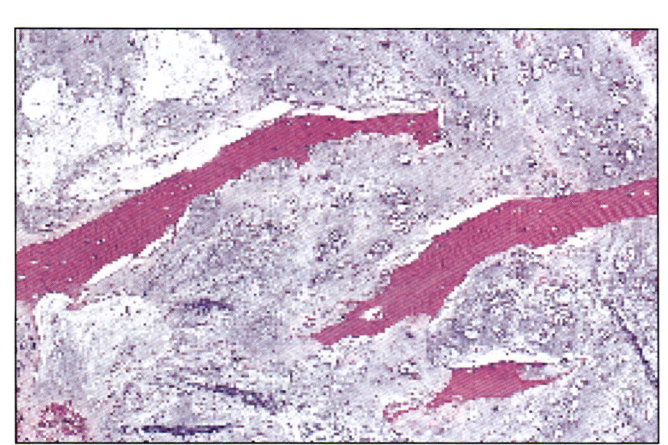

图25.25　1级软骨肉瘤侵犯周围已存在的骨小梁。

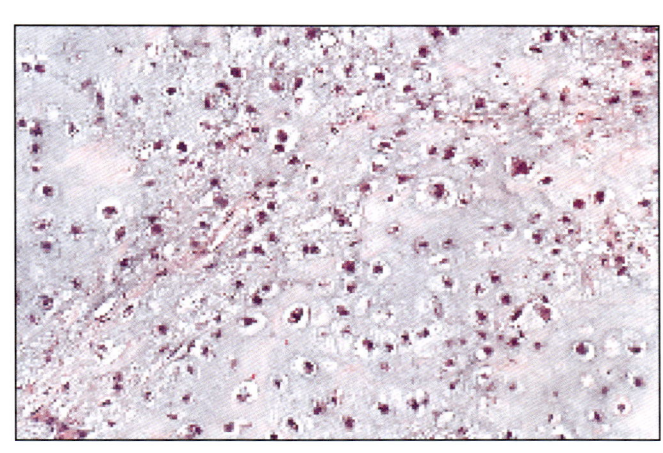

图25.27　与1级软骨肉瘤相比，2级软骨肉瘤的细胞核非典型性更加明显，细胞更加丰富。

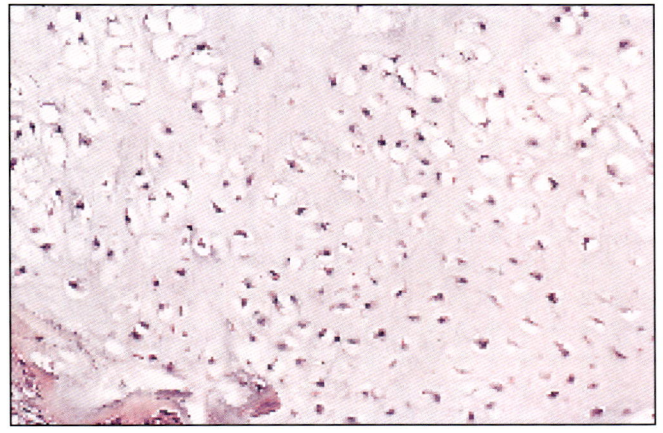

图25.26　股骨远端的1级软骨肉瘤的细胞比同一位置的内生性软骨瘤的细胞更丰富。

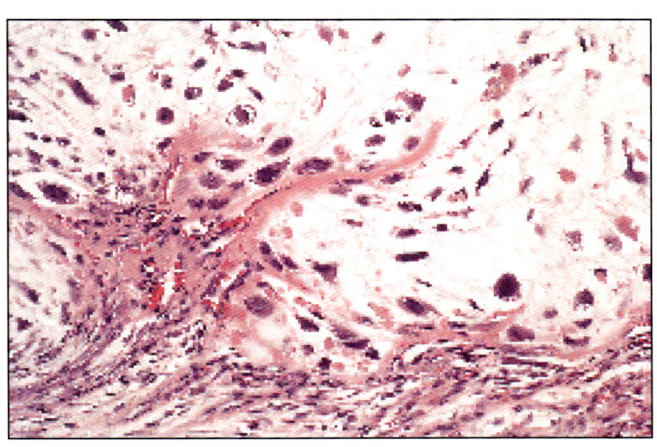

图25.28　3级软骨肉瘤显示细胞核明显深染和多形性。

以将内生性软骨瘤和软骨肉瘤区别开来。间质的明显黏液变性应该引起关注。虽然这些肿瘤患者的预后常常较好，但是转移确实可能发生[96-98]。

继发性软骨肉瘤
Secondary chondrosarcoma

绝大部分软骨肉瘤发生在原先正常的骨。然而，有一小部分是发生在先前骨骼有病变的部位。在 Mayo Clinic 的资料中，大约 14% 的软骨肉瘤是继发性的。这些病例可能起自单发或多发的外生性骨疣，或来自软骨发育异常。大部分来自骨软骨瘤的软骨肉瘤分化非常好，因此在组织学上鉴别非常困难。静止的骨软骨瘤在患者成年后开始生长，应该高度怀疑软骨肉瘤。从骨软骨瘤进展为软骨肉瘤可能与甲状旁腺激素相关性肽及 bcl-2 的上调有关[99]。

影像学特征非常重要。骨软骨瘤有薄而规则的软骨帽。当继发软骨肉瘤时，软骨帽会变得厚而不规则，边界不清。随着现代影像学技术的进步，如 CT 和 MRI，影像学医生能准确地测量软骨帽的厚度。大体标本的表现也非常重要。绝大部分骨软骨瘤软骨帽光滑，通常不超过 1cm 厚。而一个厚的、有圆形突起的软骨帽，特别是显示有黏液样改变时，则提示可能是软骨肉瘤（图 25.29）。大部分继发性软骨肉瘤是低级别肿瘤。肿瘤向周围组织侵犯应该考虑为恶性的指征。继发性软骨肉瘤的预后一般较好[100]。我们已经指出，在软骨异常增生的背景中发生的软骨肉瘤其诊断非常困难。在孤立的软骨瘤中很难或不可能确定是否是恶性的。

继发性软骨肉瘤患者通常比普通型软骨肉瘤患者大约年轻 10 岁。

个别普通型软骨肉瘤患者可在 16 岁之前就发病。一项 Mayo Clinic 研究[101]显示，这些患者的预后与成年患者相同。无论什么时候在儿童发现软骨肿瘤，都应该小心除外软骨母细胞骨肉瘤，后者的可能性要大得多。

骨旁软骨肉瘤　Periosteal chondrosarcoma

发生在骨表面的软骨肉瘤非常少见。大部分发生在皮质的软骨肿瘤是良性的。少数情况下，软骨肉瘤可以发生在骨表面。这些病变往往很大，通常最大直径可超过 5cm。影像学显示肿块的界限不清，伴有不均匀的钙化。组织学上，肿瘤往往侵犯周围软组织。虽然转移很少见，但肿瘤确实能转移到肺[68]。

透明细胞软骨肉瘤
Clear cell chondrosarcoma

透明细胞软骨肉瘤是少见的软骨肿瘤。病变常常发生在长骨末端，与软骨母细胞瘤和骨巨细胞瘤相似（图 25.30）。影像学表现可能类似于软骨母细胞瘤，病变通常界限清晰，甚至可以有硬化性边缘。在影像学表现提

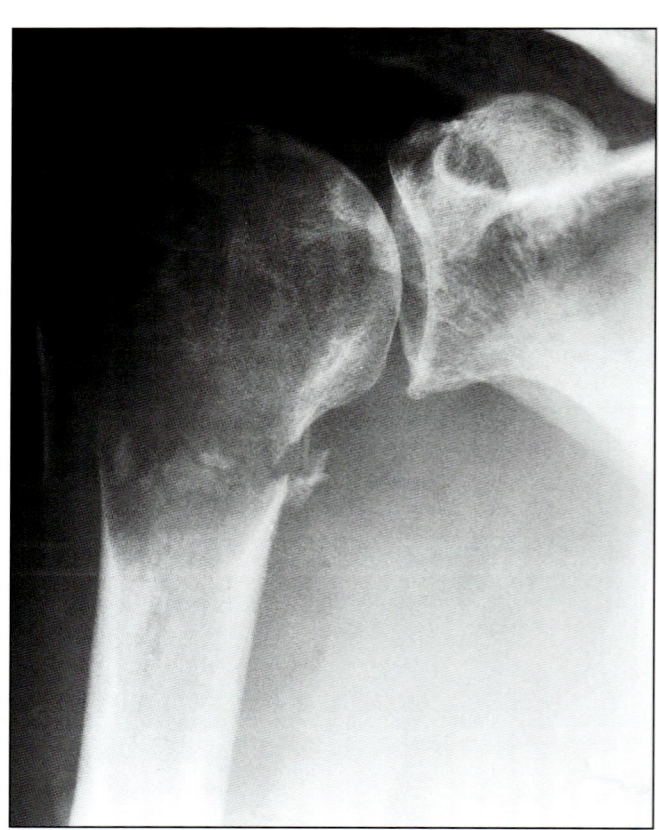

图25.30　肱骨近段的透明细胞软骨肉瘤。有向骨端延伸的膨胀性病变。

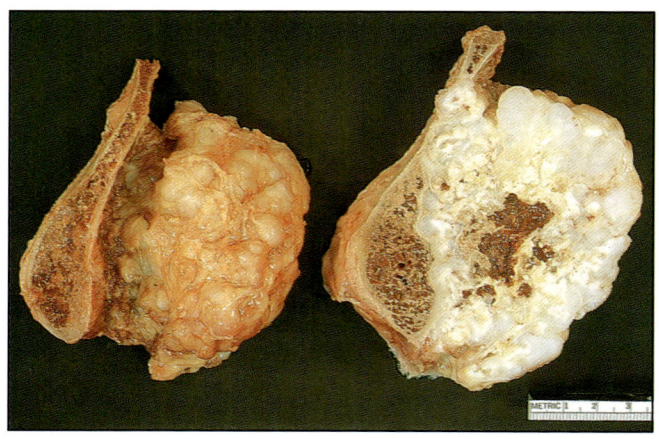

图25.29　发生于骨软骨瘤基础上的软骨肉瘤，其大体标本显示软骨帽厚，中心有退行性变。

示恶性之前，病变可能会经历几年时间。在大体标本上（图 25.31），透明细胞软骨肉瘤显示玻璃样软骨区和表现为灰白鱼肉样的区域。常可找到囊性变。显微镜下，透明细胞软骨肉瘤是分叶状肿瘤。小叶的边缘通常可见良性巨细胞（这在普通型软骨肉瘤中少见）。小叶的中心通常显示骨样或骨形成。肿瘤细胞有边界清楚的胞浆和位于中心的圆形细胞核（图 25.32）。有时核仁很明显。大约 50% 的透明细胞软骨肉瘤显示和普通型软骨肉瘤一样的区域。在透明细胞软骨肉瘤中常常可以发现动脉瘤样骨囊肿样改变。以我们的经验，继发性动脉瘤样骨囊肿伴有恶性骨肿瘤非常少见。有时动脉瘤样骨囊肿样改变非常明显，以至于肿瘤可能仅仅是一个附壁结节。

透明细胞软骨肉瘤的临床行为与一个低级别的软骨肉瘤相同[102]。

去分化软骨肉瘤
Dedifferentiated chondrosarcoma

去分化软骨肉瘤最先是在 1971 年作为一个独特的临床病理疾病来描述的[103]。去分化软骨肉瘤发生在年龄较大的成人，通常比普通型软骨肉瘤的患者大 10 岁。累及的部位与普通型软骨肉瘤相同。患者可能主诉症状已出现几年，随后有症状数量突然增加或程度突然加重。影像学检查显示软骨肉瘤的经典特征，但是，与之并存的是更具破坏性表现的区域（图 25.33）。在所有的去分化软骨肉瘤中，大约 1/3 具有普通型软骨肉瘤的影像学表现。在大体标本上，我们能找到低级别软骨肉瘤才有的淡蓝染软骨样基质的典型表现。同时存在的还有质软的鱼肉样肉瘤样肿瘤（图 25.34）。显微镜下，低级别软骨肉瘤与高级别梭形细胞肉瘤并存（图 25.35）。软骨肉瘤并不与梭形细胞肉瘤融合。首次描述时，软骨肉瘤被认为总为 1 级。然而，随后的研究[104]发现，大约 1/4 的去分化软骨肉瘤是 2 级软骨肉瘤。梭形细胞恶性程度总是高级别的，可以具有纤维肉瘤、平滑肌肉瘤或未分类的多形性肉瘤的特征。少数情况下，可能显示横纹肌母细胞分化[105,106]。一些研究[107,108a]已经证实我们最初的经验，即这种肿瘤的患者预后非常差。一些作者质疑

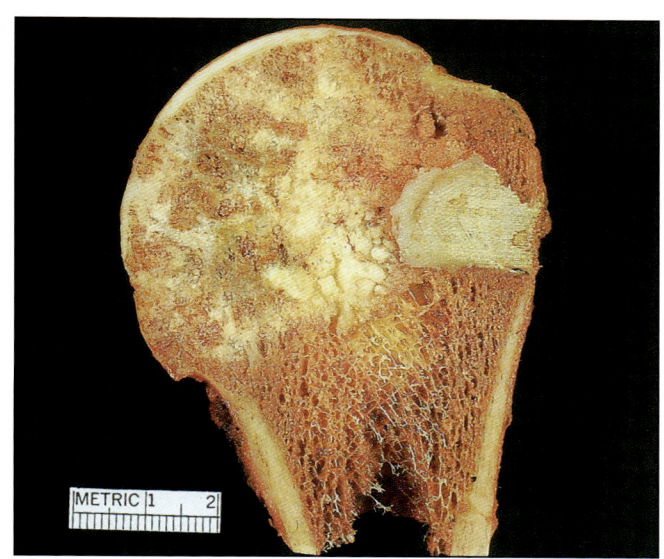

图25.31 透明细胞软骨肉瘤的大体标本，钙化非常明显，向骨端延伸。

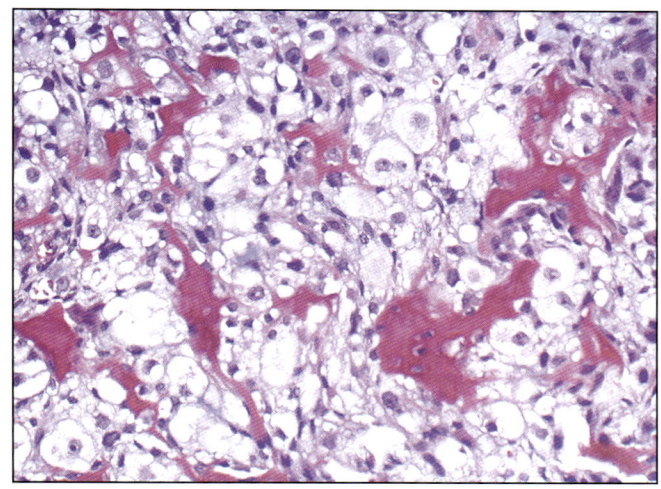

图25.32 透明细胞软骨肉瘤在镜下表现为编织骨，细胞界限非常清晰，胞浆丰富透明，散在明显的核仁。

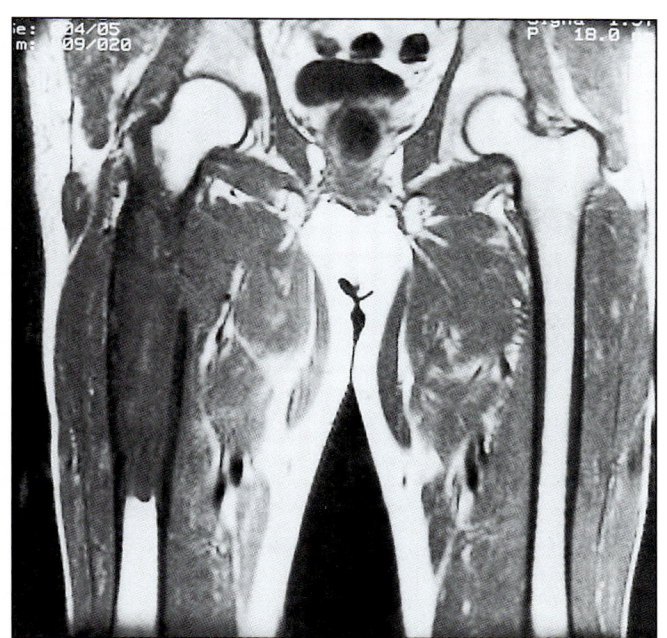

图25.33 发生在股骨内的去分化软骨肉瘤的核磁共振影像。病变位于整个干骺端，肿瘤广泛破坏皮质，并向软组织扩展。

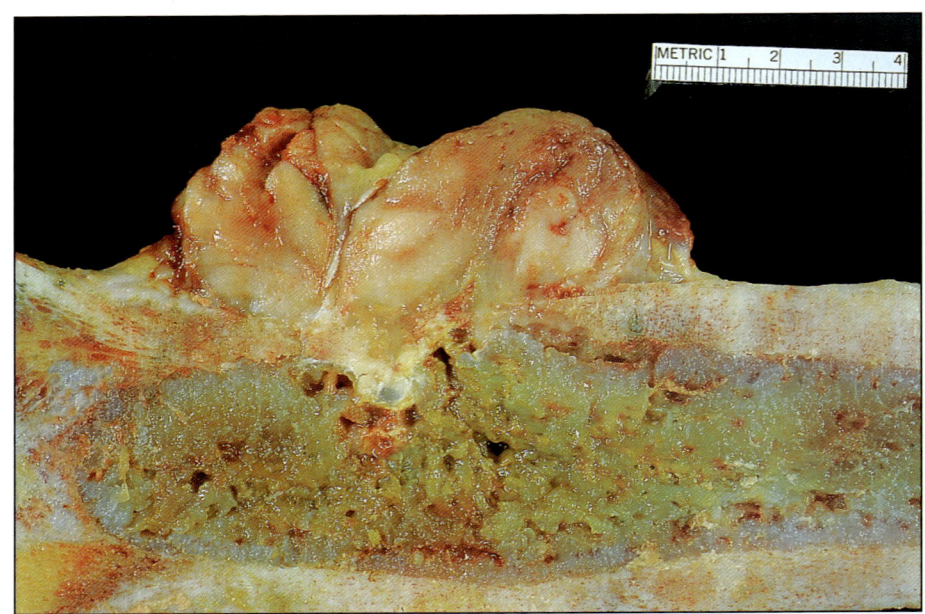

图25.34 去分化软骨肉瘤的大体标本，与图25.33显示的是同一个病例。骨髓部分显示具有特征性的分叶状、蓝-灰色玻璃样软骨肿瘤；然而，软组织包块表现为质软、棕褐色的高级别肉瘤。

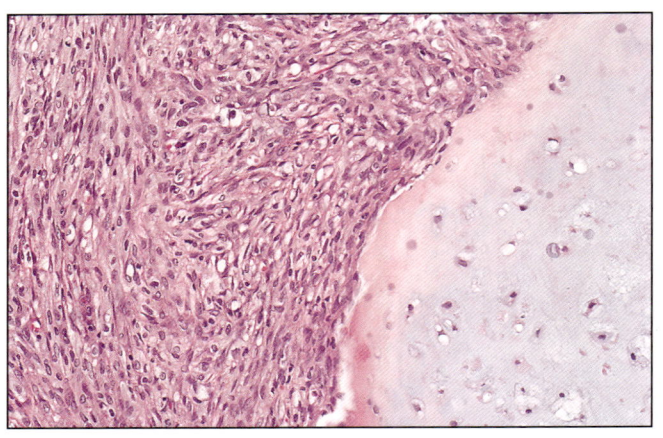

图25.35 去分化软骨肉瘤显示肿瘤的玻璃样软骨成分，具有低级别软骨肉瘤的特征，同时并存高级别的梭形细胞肉瘤（左）。

去分化软骨肉瘤这个诊断，他们更喜欢用伴有额外间叶成分的软骨肉瘤这个术语。无论去分化软骨肉瘤的名词从科学上讲是否准确，在文献中这个名词已经得到公认。去分化软骨肉瘤可能来源于与其相关的、位于下方的骨软骨瘤。这些肿瘤的预后也较差[109,110]。

去分化软骨肉瘤一定要与软骨母细胞骨肉瘤鉴别。软骨母细胞骨肉瘤通常累及青少年，而去分化软骨肉瘤累及老年人。在软骨母细胞骨肉瘤中，软骨细胞看上去是恶性的，而且与梭形细胞肉瘤融合。而在去分化软骨肉瘤中，软骨分化好，恶性梭形细胞成分与其并存，但相互不融合。这种鉴别非常重要，因为去分化软骨肉瘤的预后比软骨母细胞骨肉瘤更差。

间叶性软骨肉瘤
Mesenchymal chondrosarcoma

1959年，间叶性软骨肉瘤首次被提出[111]。它主要好发于青少年和青年人，无性别差异。大约1/3的间叶性软骨肉瘤发生在软组织或脑膜。它们的组织学和临床特征与发生在骨的间叶性软骨肉瘤相似。间叶性软骨肉瘤常常累及下颌骨和肋骨。影像学表现缺乏特异性。X线通常提示其为恶性肿瘤，可伴有或不伴有钙化（图25.36）。在大体标本上，病变常常呈粉红色鱼肉样，但可显示局灶钙化。

间叶性软骨肉瘤的显微镜下表现是特征性的。分化好的软骨和恶性的小细胞混合存在。在最初的描述中，软骨总被认为是良性的。然而，随着经验的积累，我们已经了解到，软骨可能显示高分化软骨肉瘤的表现。软骨和小细胞恶性肿瘤的比例变化相当大。一些肿瘤显示大片的软骨岛与大片的恶性小细胞岛并存（图25.37）。在另一些病例，肿瘤以软骨成分为主，仅在软骨样小叶间有小的不明显的恶性细胞灶。小细胞通常显示细胞核深染，细胞通常呈圆形或卵圆形。然而，在间叶性软骨肉瘤可以找到明显的梭形（纺锤形）区域。特征性的表现是：小细胞围绕大小不等的、裂开的或裂隙样鹿角形血管间隙排列，很像血管周围细胞瘤的表现（图25.38）。

间叶性软骨肉瘤的预后很难预测[112]。一些患者出现广泛转移，并在几个月内死亡。而其他患者在转移发生之前可能存活很长一段时间。间叶性软骨肉瘤长期预后不好。组织学特征不能预测预后。

鉴别诊断包括其他小细胞恶性肿瘤，如Ewing肉瘤

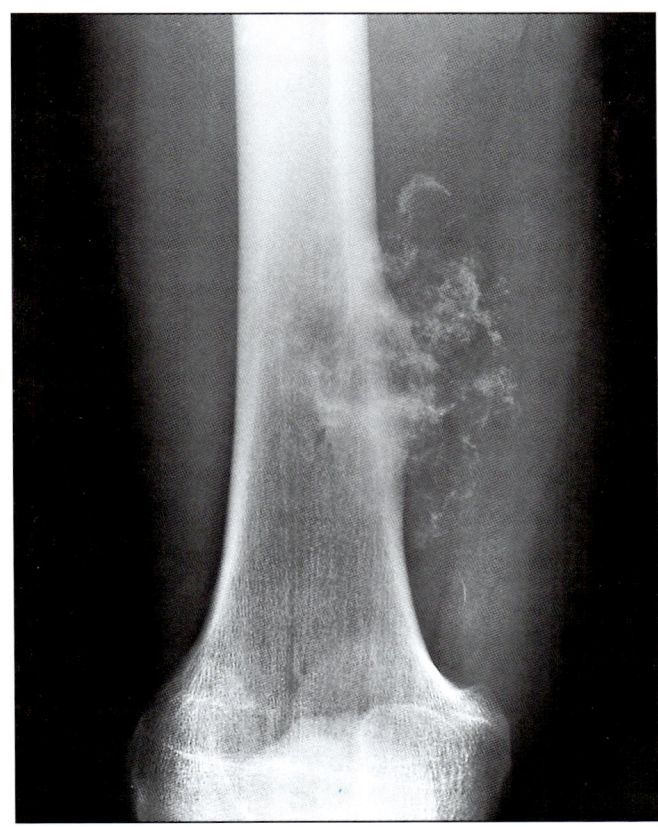

图25.36 间叶性软骨肉瘤的X光片，显示股骨干骺区钙化性病变，伴有巨大软组织包块。

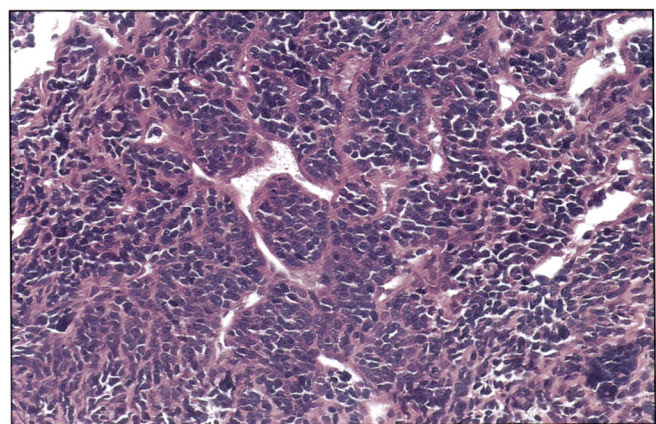

图25.38 间叶性软骨肉瘤中显示血管周围细胞瘤样生长方式，表现为圆形或卵圆形小细胞围绕鹿角样血管间隙分布。

很好的软骨岛。

成骨性肿瘤 Osteogenic tumors

成骨性肿瘤是以肿瘤细胞产生骨或骨样基质来命名的，它们构成了骨肿瘤的第三大部分。这类肿瘤可以进一步分为良性和恶性两类。

良性成骨性肿瘤
Benign osteogenic tumors

骨样骨瘤 Osteoid osteoma

骨样骨瘤是非常罕见的根据患者临床表现即可诊断的骨病变。骨样骨瘤是否是真正的肿瘤尚有争议。毫无疑问的是，这种病变的生长具有自限性。

在 Mayo Clinic 的资料中，骨样骨瘤大约占所有良性骨肿瘤的12%。男性好发。绝大多数患者为11～20岁。骨骼的任何部分都可受累，但是大部分肿瘤发生在长骨的干骺端和骨干。病变常常累及皮质而不是髓腔。

骨样骨瘤总是引起疼痛。疼痛可能十分严重，并且在夜间加重。服用阿司匹林能明显缓解疼痛。脊柱受累可以导致脊柱侧弯。

骨样骨瘤的影像学表现很典型。病变通常伴有广泛的硬化区域。硬化可以很广泛，以至于掩盖了引起硬化的基础病变。瘤巢是具有硬化边缘的放射透亮区。广泛硬化可能使病变的定位非常困难。骨样骨瘤放射核素骨扫描总呈阳性，并且可能对病变定位有帮助。CT 扫描图像也有助于病变定位（图 25.39）。

骨样骨瘤的大体表现很典型。病变界限非常清楚，表现为红色颗粒状（图 25.40）。如果进行骨段切除，可

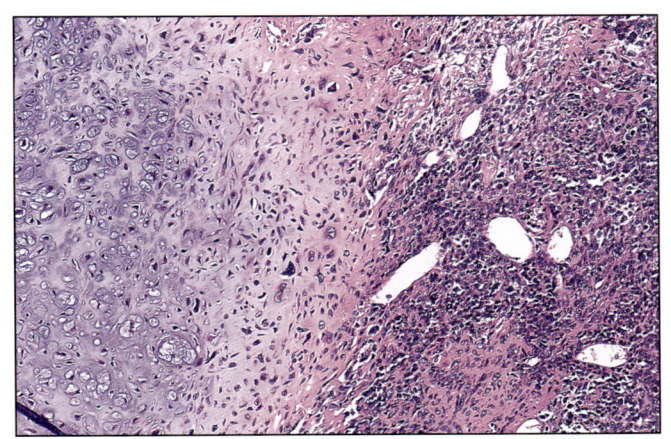

图25.37 间叶性软骨肉瘤，显示恶性软骨结节与小细胞构成的富细胞区相互融合。

和恶性淋巴瘤。间叶性软骨肉瘤也表现 CD99 阳性，这一事实使得其与 Ewing 肉瘤更容易混淆[113]。在肿瘤中出现软骨岛应该除外 Ewing 肉瘤和恶性淋巴瘤。与间叶性软骨肉瘤的细胞相比，血管周围细胞瘤的细胞通常很少有恶性表现。在血管周围细胞瘤中应该找不到软骨岛。小细胞骨肉瘤可以有软骨样分化和血管周围细胞瘤样结构。然而，在小细胞骨肉瘤中很难看到发育

成骨性肿瘤

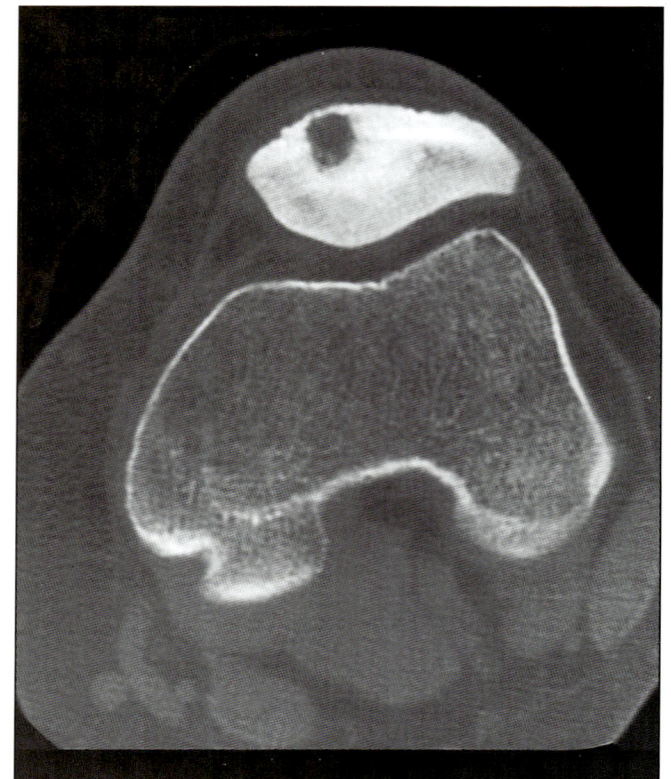

图25.39　计算机断层扫描确定的膝部皮质骨样骨瘤。

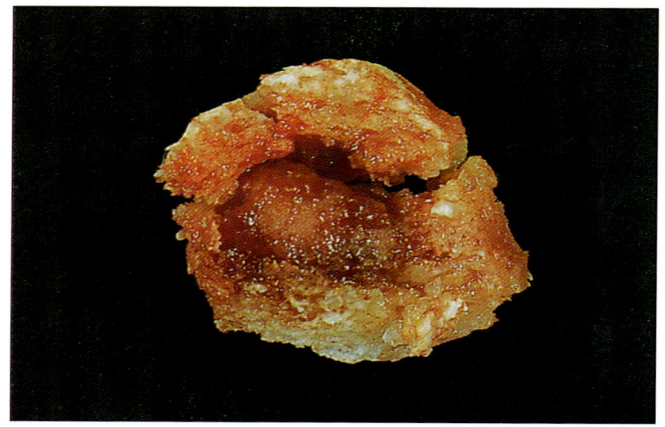

图25.40　大体上，骨样骨瘤的核心呈红色颗粒状，围以致密的硬化骨。

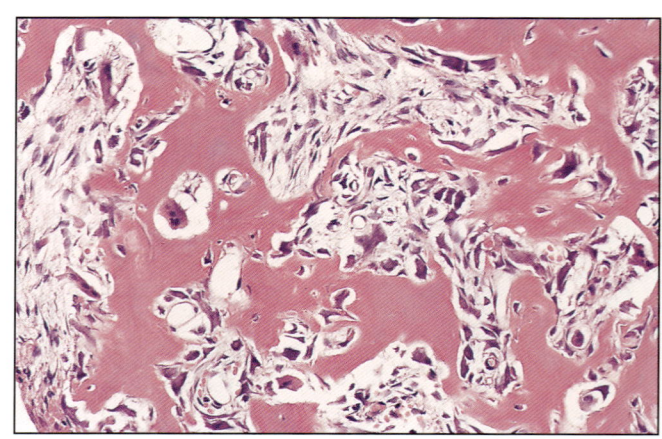

图25.41　骨样骨瘤，显示在细胞稀少的纤维血管结缔组织间质中，有骨母细胞镶边的相互吻合的不规则骨小梁。

见病变有致密硬化的骨围绕。病理医生检查大体标本非常重要，尤其是对于那些外科医生已经进行过治疗的可疑区域。如果整个病变一起脱钙，瘤巢可能会丢失。检查大体标本之后，可确认瘤巢，并分别进行处理。骨样骨瘤的瘤巢由骨样小梁相互交织成网状，有不同程度的钙化。骨小梁纤细，显示明显的骨母细胞镶边的表现。小梁间间隙由没有明显恶性表现的梭形细胞和毛细血管填充（图25.41）。

骨样骨瘤的特征之一是病变界限非常清楚。病变不穿透周围组织。一些作者已确认，在少见情况下，靠近瘤巢存在有明显的神经纤维，这或许是引起疼痛的原因[114]。骨样骨瘤的常规治疗是外科切除。手术前确定瘤巢的位置非常困难，有可能需要实施多次外科手术进行治疗[115]。

我们已经发现，手术前四环素标记或CT引导定位对肿瘤的定位有帮助[116,117]。对一些患者只进行随访，而不进行外科干预，服用阿司匹林可控制疼痛。许多患者可在CT引导下进行热消融治疗[118]。

骨样骨瘤的鉴别诊断包括骨髓炎和骨母细胞瘤。骨髓炎可能形成局限性脓肿，称为Brodie脓肿，影像学表现可能类似于骨样骨瘤。然而，组织学上，Brodie脓肿显示炎症表现，没有瘤巢。骨母细胞瘤在组织学上与骨样骨瘤无法区别。人为地规定，病变小于1.5cm考虑为骨样骨瘤，病变大于1.5cm考虑为骨母细胞瘤。

骨母细胞瘤　Osteoblastoma

1954年，Dahlin和Johnson[119]指出了骨母细胞瘤与骨样骨瘤的相似性。当时他们用巨大骨样骨瘤一词来命名这一病变。然而，Jaffe[120]提出用良性骨母细胞瘤来命名这一肿瘤，并且已被人们普遍接受。骨母细胞瘤仅占骨样骨瘤的1/4，男性好发。与骨样骨瘤不同，骨母细胞瘤可能会累及脊柱；脊柱后部常常受累（图25.42）。临床特征也不像骨样骨瘤那样具有特征性。病变可有疼痛，这可能与病变周围的结构受累有关，如当病变累及脊柱而神经根受累时可引起疼痛。

骨母细胞瘤的影像学表现也没什么特异性。少数病例伴有硬化的瘤巢（就像在骨样骨瘤中见到的那样）；但是，骨母细胞瘤的瘤巢较大。在所有骨母细胞瘤中，大约1/4出现侵袭性，影像学提示恶性诊断[121,122]。

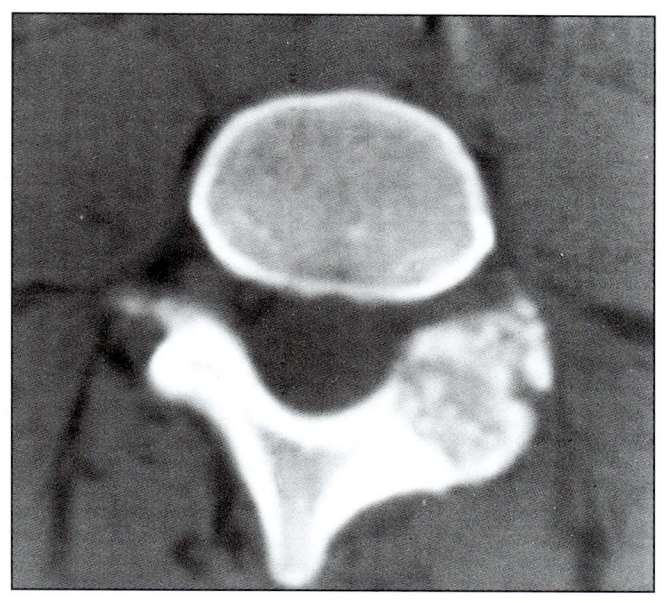

图25.42 发生在腰椎后部的骨母细胞瘤的CT扫描图像，呈膨胀和钙化表现。(Courtesy of Dr. R. Jeffrey, St. Mary's Hospital, San Francisco, CA.)

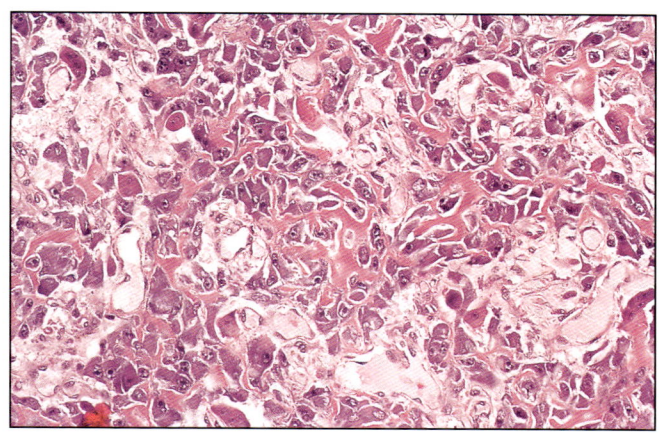

图25.43 骨母细胞瘤显微镜下图像，显示明显的上皮样表现。

骨母细胞瘤的大体表现常常为红色颗粒状的肿瘤。病变缺乏肉瘤所常见的鱼肉样外观。如果切除病变，可见病变界限非常清楚，可能有硬化骨包绕在周围。

显微镜下，骨母细胞瘤类似于骨样骨瘤。相互吻合的骨小梁边缘有单层的骨母细胞被覆。骨小梁间隙排列疏松，偶尔含有梭形细胞和毛细血管。肿瘤可能形成带状结构，在中心骨样粘合线没有钙化，而在周边骨样粘合线，钙化明显，并且与周围的原有骨组织融合。病变边缘总是非常清楚，没有向原有骨小梁之间侵犯的倾向。在骨母细胞瘤中可以看到继发性动脉瘤状骨囊肿样改变。一些骨母细胞瘤显示多发的小的瘤巢。

有关骨母细胞瘤的文献非常混乱。Dorfman和Weiss已经着重强调了这些问题[123]。1976年，Schajowicz和Lemos引入了恶性骨母细胞瘤这一名词[124]。这些作者描述了有骨母细胞瘤组织学表现的病变，但病变中细胞更丰富，并伴有大量良性巨细胞和许多针状蓝染的骨。他们发现，这些病变具有局灶侵袭性，但不发生远处转移。Dorfman和Weiss[123]使用侵袭性骨母细胞瘤一词来命名那些出现上皮样骨母细胞、具有小梁状或片状骨样组织和骨硬化再吸收特征的肿瘤。然而，他们没有提及是否所有的肿瘤细胞都必须有上皮样表现。他们也认为，侵袭性骨母细胞瘤仅仅是局部侵袭性疾病，往往不出现远处转移。Bertoni等[125]认为，如果肿瘤细胞全部具有上皮样表现，则应命名为侵袭性骨母细胞瘤（图25.43）。他们也发现，这些病变具有更高的复发率。Della Rocca和Huvos[126]发现，组织学特征和疾病的预后没有相关性。我们不完全相信侵袭性骨母细胞瘤是一种真正的病变。由于出现假恶性骨母细胞瘤这一名称[127]，这个问题变得更加复杂，在假恶性骨母细胞瘤中，肿瘤细胞有增大深染的细胞核。然而，细胞核有假恶性细胞的模糊不清的表现。

骨母细胞瘤的治疗是保守性的：完整外科切除。复发不常见，鉴别诊断包括骨样骨瘤（鉴别完全根据大小）和骨肉瘤。在有些病例中骨肉瘤和骨母细胞瘤之间的鉴别非常困难。支持骨肉瘤诊断的两个特征是：没有基质产生的成片细胞和对原有骨的侵犯。

骨瘤 Osteoma

骨瘤是少见的骨的良性过度生长，通常发生在鼻窦或下颌骨表面。骨瘤可能与Gardner综合征有关[128]。在少数情况下，骨瘤可以长在长骨表面。颅骨骨瘤可能是对其下方的脑膜瘤的一种反应。

恶性成骨性肿瘤
Malignant osteogenic tumors

骨肉瘤可以被简单的定义为那些肿瘤细胞产生骨样或骨基质的恶性肿瘤。骨肉瘤大致可分为两组：占多数的一类发生在骨内，而占少数的一类发生在骨表面。这两大类可以根据临床、影像学和组织学特征进一步划分[129]（表25.2）。

发生在骨内的骨肉瘤
Osteosarcomas arising within bone

绝大多数骨肉瘤起源于骨内，即使它们中的一些有明显的骨外成分，也是如此。这种骨肉瘤可以进一步分为几类。

表25.2　骨肉瘤分类

骨内骨肉瘤
　　普通型骨肉瘤
　　　　骨母细胞型
　　　　软骨母细胞型
　　　　纤维母细胞型
　　小细胞骨肉瘤
　　血管扩张型骨肉瘤
　　低级别中心型骨肉瘤
　　发生在Paget病中的骨肉瘤
　　放疗后骨肉瘤
　　发生在其他良性病变基础上的骨肉瘤

表面骨肉瘤
　　骨旁骨肉瘤
　　骨膜骨肉瘤
　　高级别表面骨肉瘤

普通型骨肉瘤　Conventional osteosarcoma

普通型骨肉瘤是好发于儿童长骨干骺端的高级别恶性肿瘤。大多数骨肉瘤发生在青少年和年轻成人。小于5岁或大于50岁的骨肉瘤患者非常少见，除非是在易感情况下。男性好发。绝大多数普通型骨肉瘤的中心发生在长骨干骺端。大约10%发生在骨干上。

有一小部分骨肉瘤发生在扁骨，如骨盆骨和肩胛。这些病变可能与以前进行过放疗或存在疾病（如Paget病）有关。发生在手足骨者更加少见。虽然在Mayo Clinic的资料中有少数几例发生在腕骨和跗骨的病例，但是没有发生在指（趾）骨的骨肉瘤。然而，我们在会诊的过程中，偶尔看到过发生在指（趾）骨的骨肉瘤[130]。发生在骶部的骨肉瘤很少见。临床症状没有特异性。患者主诉疼痛或肿胀，或两者都有，持续时间长短不一，可从数天到数月不等。病理性骨折也可以是首发症状。

骨肉瘤的影像学特征多种多样。肿瘤常常引起大片区域的骨破坏，并延伸到软组织中（图25.44）。病变中出现钙化的数量不等，与骨肉瘤的类型有一定的关系（图25.45）。当肿瘤破坏皮质时会掀起骨膜。这将导致在抬起的骨膜与其下的皮质之间的连接处有反应性新骨形成。这就是所谓的Codman三角。在少数情况下，骨肉瘤很小并有非常清楚的界限，提示是一个良性病变。

骨肉瘤大体表现也多种多样。大部分具有肉瘤的鱼肉样外观（图25.46）。一些病变钙化很明显，因此非常硬。一些病变有非常明显的大片蓝色软骨区域。

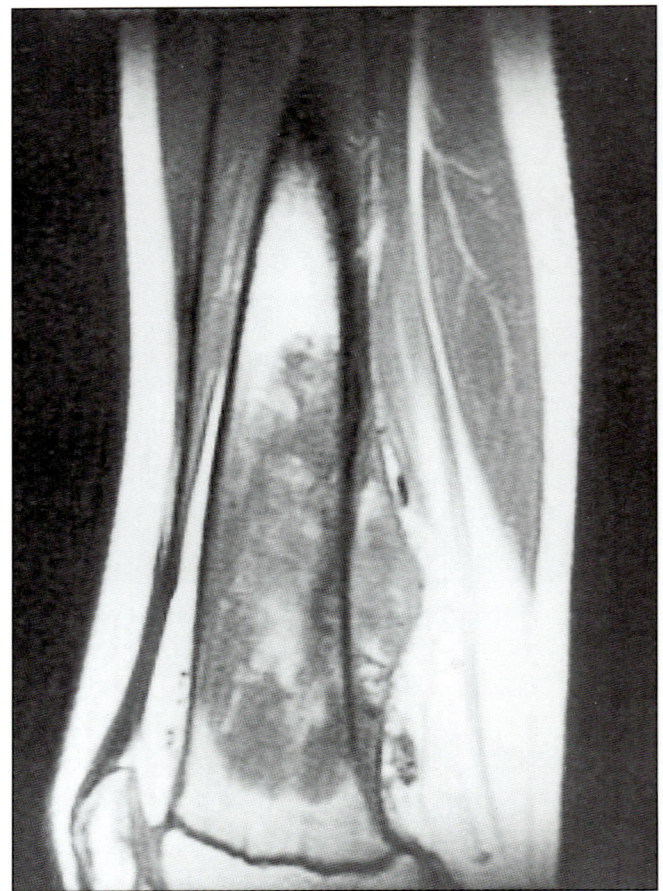

图25.44　这张核磁图像显示了普通型骨肉瘤向软组织的扩展。

显微镜下，大部分骨肉瘤是高度恶性的肿瘤；肿瘤的梭形细胞有多形性非常明显的细胞核。普通型骨肉瘤根据主要的基质成分可进一步分为骨母细胞型、软骨母细胞型和纤维母细胞型。

骨母细胞型骨肉瘤大约占整个骨肉瘤的一半。其特征是：每个肿瘤细胞之间产生纤细网状基质。基质可以是非钙化的骨样基质，也可以是钙化的骨小梁。一些骨肉瘤有大量的团块状基质，肿瘤细胞核不明显。偶尔，骨肉瘤的诊断纯粹是根据浸润至原有骨小梁之间的骨基质确定的（图25.47）。

大约25%的骨肉瘤显示有明显的软骨分化。软骨形成小叶，陷窝中的细胞显示明显的多形性。小叶周围肿瘤细胞变得丰富，小叶周围的细胞呈梭形（图25.48）。在梭形细胞之间或软骨小叶中心可以见到骨样基质。在小的活检标本中，在梭形细胞之间可能看不到骨样基质。然而，我们认为，如果软骨看上去像是恶性的，并伴有成片的梭形细胞，应该诊断为软骨母细胞型骨肉瘤。

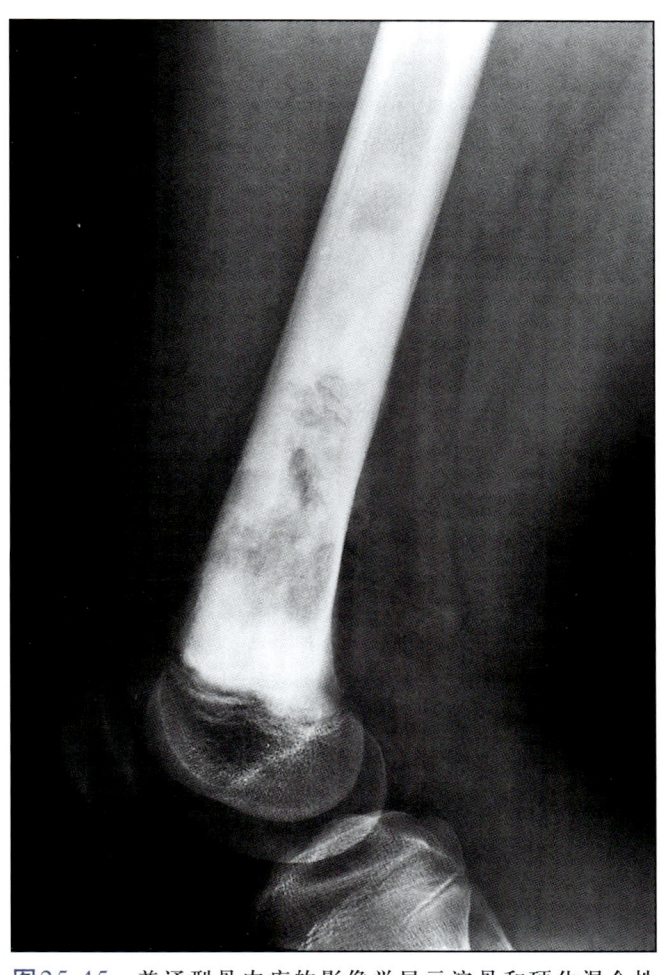

图25.45 普通型骨肉瘤的影像学显示溶骨和硬化混合性表现。

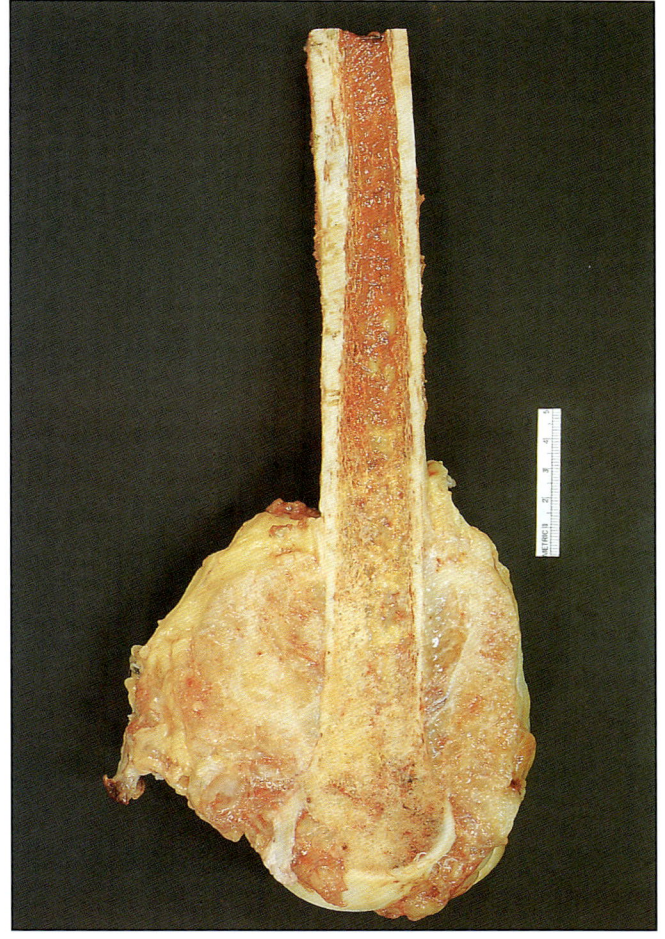

图25.46 普通型骨肉瘤的大体标本显示，股骨远端被大量的鱼肉样软组织包块包绕。

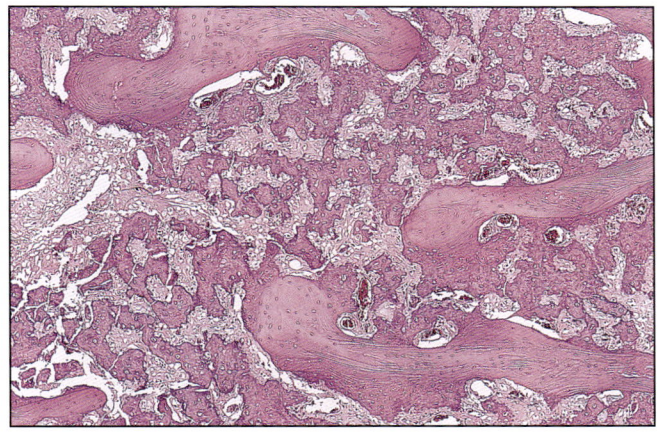

图25.47 显微镜下显示恶性基质和骨母细胞型骨肉瘤的间质弥漫浸润到已存在的大的骨小梁中。

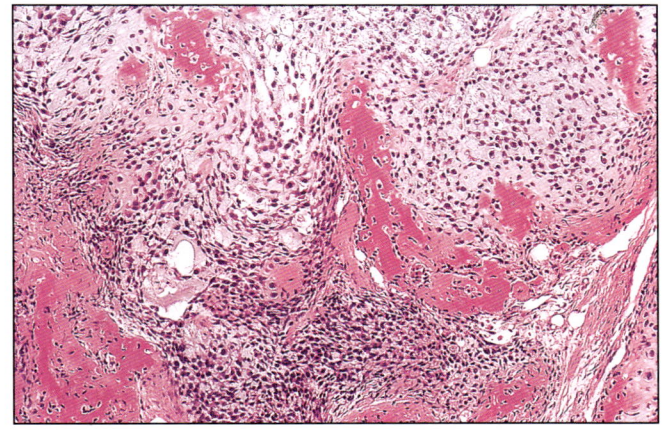

图25.48 软骨母细胞型骨肉瘤伴有恶性软骨小叶。小叶的周边有梭形细胞以及骨样基质形成。

大约25%的骨肉瘤中梭形细胞结构占优势，仅产生很少的骨样基质。这类骨肉瘤被称为纤维母细胞型骨肉瘤。大部分骨肉瘤混合有不同的成分，所以根据活检进行进一步分类有些武断。几乎可以肯定的是：这种组织学的进一步分类并没有预测预后的意义。

除了上述亚型外，普通型骨肉瘤还可能出现几种不常见的组织学结构。一些纤维母细胞骨肉瘤有明显的血管结构，使人联想起所谓的血管周围细胞瘤。大约1/4

的骨肉瘤病变中含有良性巨细胞。一个罕见的病例有大量的巨细胞，以至我们考虑应诊断为良性巨细胞瘤。单核细胞的非典型性可能非常轻微。当一个发生在年轻患者的骺端病变有巨细胞瘤的组织学表现时，应该考虑诊断为富巨细胞的骨肉瘤。一些骨肉瘤有上皮样表现。甚至有伴有腺体形成的骨肉瘤报道。但是这并不常见；最常见的情况是：这些细胞仅仅具有明显核仁和丰富淡粉色胞浆的上皮样表现。如果年轻患者的骨活检标本中有癌的表现，应该疑为骨肉瘤。一些骨肉瘤有明显的分化好的骨小梁和骨母样细胞，让人联想起骨母细胞瘤。这种病变可诊断为骨母细胞瘤样的骨肉瘤[131]。骨母细胞瘤样骨肉瘤与骨母细胞瘤的鉴别可能非常困难。在这种情况下，向周围组织浸润可能是最可靠的恶性特征。

骨肉瘤通常可转移至肺，但少数情况下，淋巴结和其他骨也可能受累。过去该病的5年生存率被认为约为20%[132]。现代化疗的应用改善了骨肉瘤的预后，5年生存率可达50%~60%[133]。然而，一些研究提示，骨肉瘤甚至不进行化疗其生存率本身也可有所提高[134]。

现在几乎所有研究机构对骨肉瘤患者的治疗方式都是进行术前化疗。这使骨肉瘤的截肢率明显下降。大多数骨肉瘤患者接受的是受累骨段的切除术。一些研究显示，骨肉瘤的预后与化疗后标本坏死的数量有关；因此，对手术标本化疗效果的评估非常重要[135]。我们取一片有骨和整个肿瘤全貌的切片。切片应该很薄以便能很快脱钙。将整个标本编号包埋成块，以便被重现。化疗的结果可能表现为：肿瘤被硬化骨、具有良性表现的纤维组织、肉芽组织样物质或真正坏死的碎屑所替代。有时候异型细胞很难评价。尽管有这样的缺点，但研究显示，肿瘤化疗效果（"坏死"）至少为95%的患者其预后要比对化疗没有反应的患者好。有研究提示，肿瘤细胞P-糖蛋白（一种多药耐药基因产物）染色阳性可能与预后不良有关，因为此种肿瘤对化疗不敏感[136]。

放疗后肉瘤　Postirradiation sarcoma

在受过放疗的骨可能生长肉瘤[137]。放疗后肉瘤的准确发病率尚不清楚，但是危险性较小。在肉瘤出现之前通常有一个很长的潜伏期。在Mayo Clinic的资料中，潜伏期大约有14年，但是患者可能永远处于发生肉瘤的危险中。肿瘤可以发生在原发肿瘤接受放疗的区域，或可以发生在与肿瘤无关的放疗区域内。肿瘤通常是高级别的，可以是骨肉瘤，纤维肉瘤或是未分类多形性肉瘤（恶性纤维组织细胞瘤）。这种肉瘤的预后与骨肉瘤的总体预后大致相同[138]。

Paget肉瘤　Paget sarcoma

Paget病患者发生肉瘤的危险较小。Paget肉瘤患者多是老年人。患者通常主诉疼痛加剧，或可能出现病理性骨折。影像学显示典型的Paget病特征，伴有皮质增厚和髓腔内的骨化。从外观上看，肉瘤看上去通常像骨内溶骨。在大体标本上，肿瘤常常是破坏性的，伴有鱼肉样质软的肿瘤成分（图25.49）。组织学上，肉瘤为高级别肿瘤，可以是纤维肉瘤、骨肉瘤或恶性纤维组织细胞瘤（图25.50）。几项研究[139,140]证实，Paget肉瘤预后差。

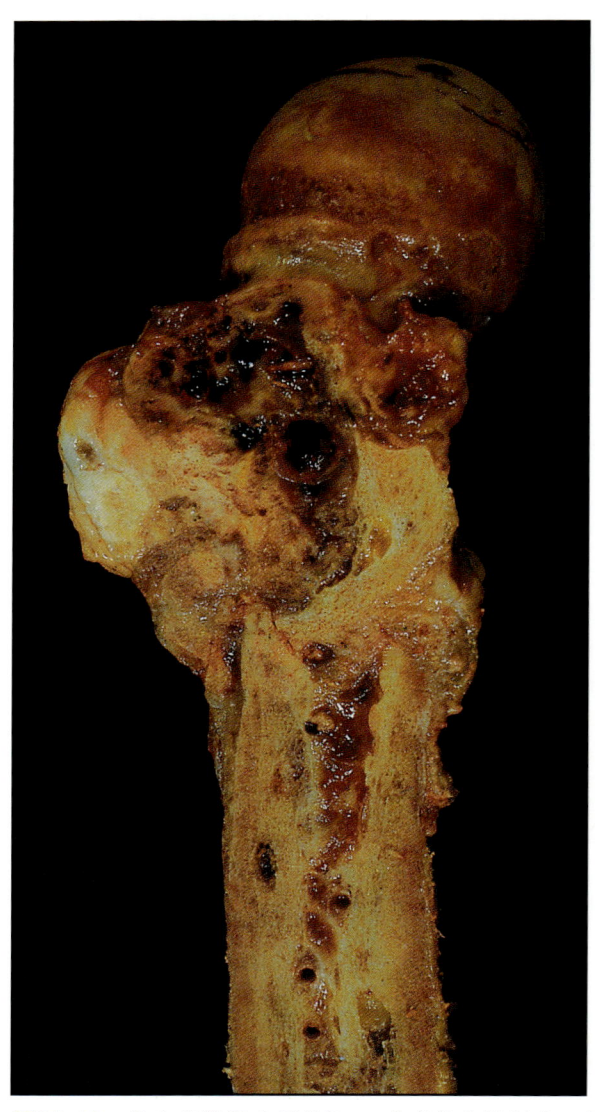

图25.49　发生在股骨末端的Paget肉瘤的大体标本，显示在Paget病基础上，皮质增厚，髓腔内骨化，以及巨大的出血性的棕褐色-白色肉瘤样肿瘤突破皮质。

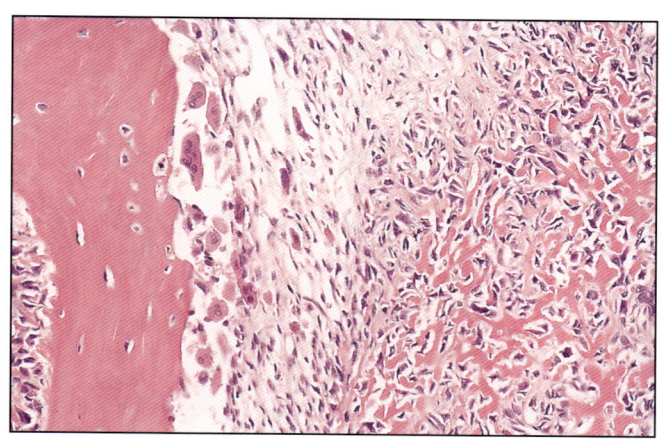

图25.50 Paget肉瘤。显示在Paget病（左）中有高级别骨肉瘤（右）侵犯Paget病中见到的异常骨，这些骨增厚并衬有破骨细胞。

毛细血管扩张型骨肉瘤
Telangiectatic osteosarcoma

在 Mayo Clinic 的资料中，毛细血管扩张性骨肉瘤大约占所有骨肉瘤的4%。在文献中，有关毛细血管扩张型骨肉瘤与普通型骨肉瘤的鉴别的重要性是有争议的。产生这种争议的部分原因是因为：不同的医疗中心采用的诊断标准不同。我们应用的标准如下：

1. 影像学显示单纯的溶骨破坏性病变，通常发生在年轻患者的长骨干骺端（图25.51）。
2. 大体标本显示：空腔被间隔分开，或空腔内含有凝血块（图25.52）。
3. 显微镜下，由间隔分隔出空隙，类似于动脉瘤样骨囊肿的表现。然而，内衬的细胞呈多形性（图25.53）。肿瘤细胞产生的骨非常少。

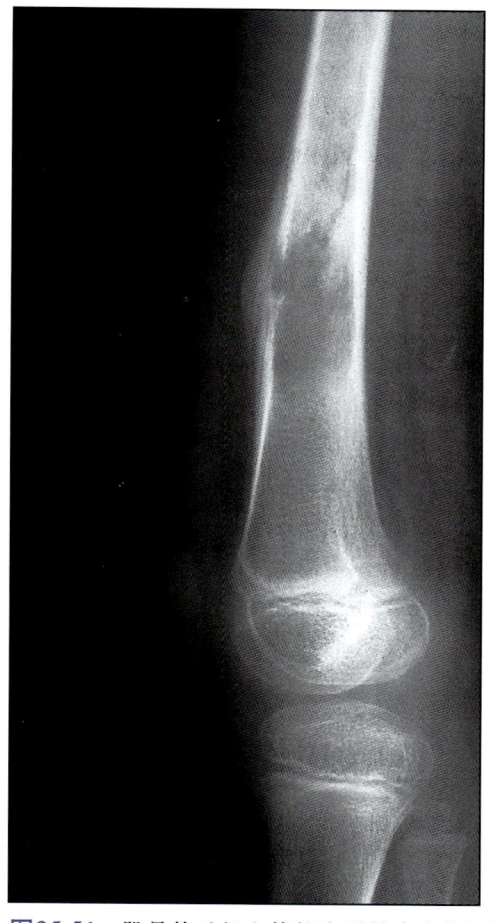

图25.51 股骨的毛细血管扩张型骨肉瘤的X线片。病变为溶骨性的，边缘不清，显示为皮质骨的破坏。

在这组病变中，我们不将部分呈毛细血管扩张表现的骨肉瘤包括在内。Mayo Clinic[141]的最初研究认为，毛细血管扩张型骨肉瘤的预后非常差。然而，Memorial 医院的一项病例研究[142]提示，毛细血管扩张型骨肉瘤的预后与普通型骨肉瘤的相同。Mayo

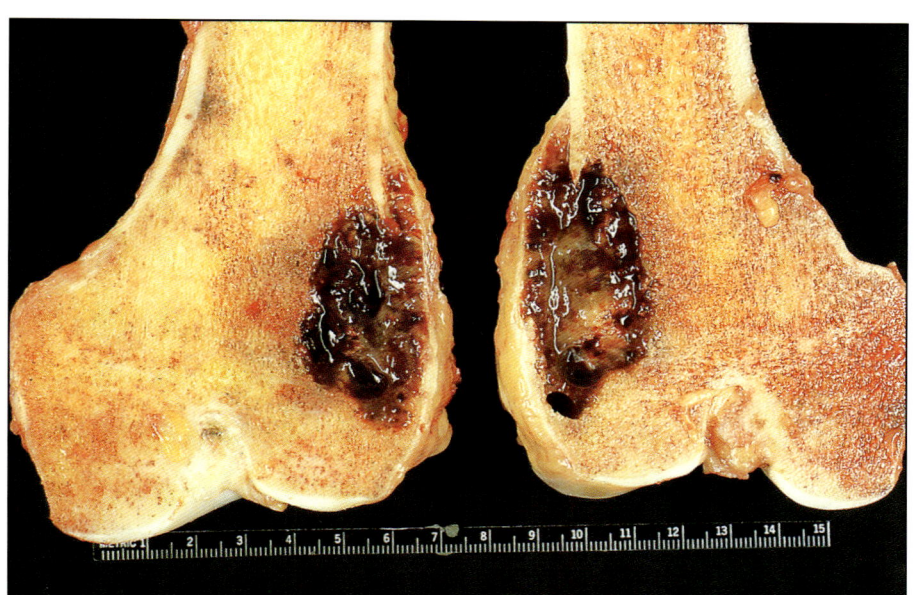

图25.52 发生在股骨末端的毛细血管扩张型骨肉瘤的大体标本。肿瘤有出血的红褐色表现，类似于血凝块。

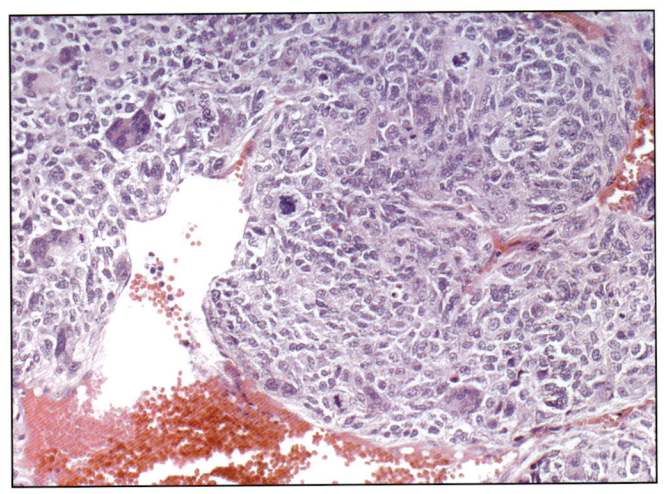

图25.53　毛细血管扩张型骨肉瘤的镜下图像，显示在邻近囊腔的实性间隔中有丰富的间质细胞，具有明显的多形性。出现大量非典型核分裂象。

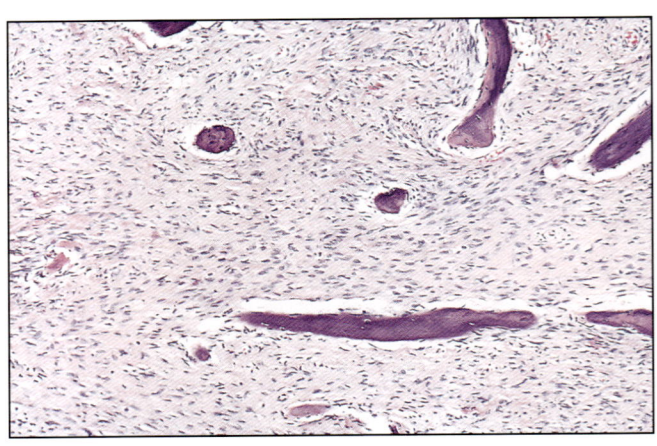

图25.54　中心型低级别骨肉瘤，显示骨小梁周围围绕细胞稀少的梭形细胞间质，表现出轻微的细胞非典型性。

Clinic 的后期研究[143]发现，最近的毛细血管扩张型骨肉瘤患者的预后与普通型骨肉瘤相同。这似乎与化疗的应用无关；但是，以我们的经验，毛细血管扩张型骨肉瘤对化疗非常敏感。

我们认为，毛细血管扩张型骨肉瘤应该作为一种单独的疾病存在，因为它的大体标本和镜下表现具有独特性。更为重要的是，这有助于提醒我们：诊断动脉瘤样骨囊肿时，有毛细血管扩张型骨肉瘤的可能性。动脉瘤样骨囊肿和毛细血管扩张型骨肉瘤在包括影像学、大体标本和低倍镜下表现的许多方面具有相似的特征。唯一的不同是：在毛细血管扩张型骨肉瘤的间隔中可能出现明显的非典型细胞。

中心型低级别骨肉瘤
Central low-grade osteosarcoma

绝大部分骨肉瘤都是高度恶性的，因此，细胞学表现很明显。然而，有一小部分骨肉瘤分化非常好，可能被误诊为良性病变，如纤维发育不良[144,145]。低级别骨肉瘤是非常少见的疾病；在 Mayo Clinic 的资料中仅有20例。患者年龄常常比普通型骨肉瘤患者的要大。症状一般持续时间长。病变常常累及长骨末端。

影像学表现通常没有诊断意义。一些病变有良性表现，然而，大部分病例显示至少有局部的皮质破坏。长期存在的病变可能会向骨外扩展。

在大体标本上，中心型低级别骨肉瘤有质韧、纤维性外观。此病缺乏高级别骨肉瘤的质软、鱼肉样表现。组织学上，肿瘤细胞稀少，由增生的梭形细胞构成。骨基质形成很好的骨小梁。梭形细胞显示轻微的非典型性（图25.54）。核分裂象稀少。肿瘤常常侵犯骨髓的脂肪和周围骨小梁。这是这种低级别肿瘤最可靠的恶性特征。

低级别骨肉瘤的预后很好。病变可能局部复发，但是转移的能力有限。然而，高达15%的病例可能继续发展成去分化成高级别骨肉瘤[145]。

小细胞骨肉瘤　Small cell osteosarcoma

在少数情况下，骨肉瘤有类似于 Ewing 肉瘤或恶性淋巴瘤表现的小细胞。然而，肿瘤细胞至少可在局灶区域产生骨样或骨基质。Ewing 肉瘤，尤其是大细胞 Ewing 肉瘤，与小细胞骨肉瘤之间的鉴别非常困难。一些 Ewing 肉瘤在肿瘤细胞之间显示一些纤维素样沉积。因此，我们认为在做出明确的小细胞骨肉瘤诊断之前一定要看到钙化的基质。小细胞骨肉瘤是一种预后很差的非常少见的肿瘤[146,147]。

以上所有的肿瘤都发生在髓腔内。在少数情况下，骨肉瘤起源于骨皮质内[148]。

除组织学类型之外，骨肉瘤累及的部位对预测预后也有重要意义；如颚骨骨肉瘤患者的预后要比普通型骨肉瘤好得多[149]。然而，颅骨骨肉瘤患者的预后非常差[150]。

骨表面的骨肉瘤
Osteosarcomas of the surface of bone

发生在骨表面的任何类型的骨肉瘤都非常少见。这些肿瘤可以被分为三个不同的组：骨旁、骨膜或高级别表面骨肉瘤。

骨旁骨肉瘤　Parosteal osteosarcoma

骨旁骨肉瘤是发生在骨表面的低级别骨肉瘤。之所以使用骨旁骨瘤这一名称来命名这一病变[151]，是因为其可突现出肿瘤的高分化属性。此病女性好发，患者年龄常常比普通型骨肉瘤患者大10岁左右。在所有骨旁骨肉瘤中，大约有3/4发生在股骨末端后方。

患者通常由于腘窝出现肿物而表现为膝部弯曲受限。影像学显示为具有宽基底的、附着于骨皮质的明显骨化的肿块（图25.55和25.56）。当病变增大时，基底并不相应地增大，因此，在肿瘤与其下方的皮质之间形成空隙。骨旁骨肉瘤有包绕受累骨的倾向。在大体标本上，骨旁骨肉瘤外观为实性质硬的包块，并不出现鱼肉样的区域（图25.57）。病变周围钙化较少，在这些区域病变侵犯周围的骨骼肌。表面可能覆有帽状软骨。

显微镜下，骨旁骨肉瘤是分化很好的骨肉瘤。肿瘤细胞稀少，由增生的梭形细胞组成（图25.58）。梭形细胞缺少细胞非典型性。肿瘤细胞之间有大量的胶原。骨由形成很好的骨小梁构成。骨旁骨肉瘤中看不到缎带样骨样组织。细胞核显示出轻微的非典型性，核分裂象少见。越往病变的周边，梭形细胞增生越明显，将骨骼肌纤维包裹在内。在骨旁骨肉瘤中可见多少不等的软骨成分。有时候可看到软骨帽形成，类似于骨软骨瘤的表现。然而，与骨软骨瘤不同的是，此病骨小梁之间充满增生的梭形细胞。在所有骨旁骨肉瘤中，大约有1/4在大体标本或镜下有髓腔受累的迹象。

大约15%的骨旁骨肉瘤伴有高级别骨肉瘤，为一种去分化形式[152,153]。这种去分化可以发生在最初发病时，而更为常见的是发生在复发肿瘤中。骨旁骨肉瘤的

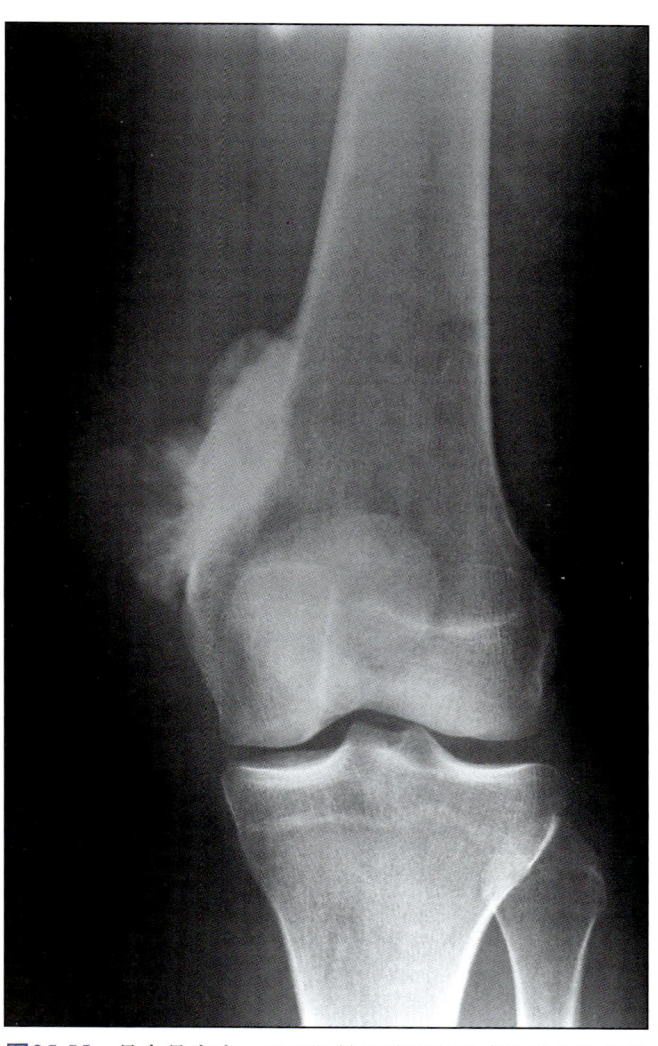

图25.55 骨旁骨肉瘤，显示股骨远端干骺端表面发生的骨性肿块。

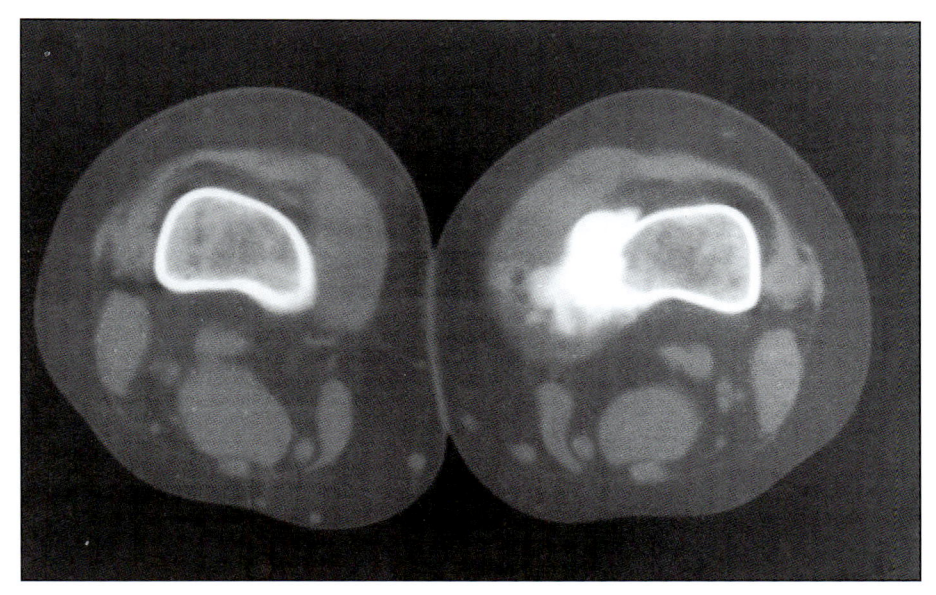

图25.56 骨旁骨肉瘤的CT扫描图像，显示病变广泛附着于骨表面，缺乏髓腔受累。

预后非常好。远处转移不常见。然而，当出现去分化时，预后与普通型骨肉瘤相同。

鉴别诊断包括骨软骨瘤和骨化性肌炎。在骨软骨瘤中，影像学显示骨和骨软骨瘤之间是连续性的。骨旁骨肉瘤的影像学表现则没有这种连续性。在骨软骨瘤中，骨小梁之间的空隙有脂肪或造血成分填充，而骨旁骨肉瘤空隙中含有梭形细胞成分。骨化性肌炎不累及骨皮质，而是一个软组织肿块。骨化性肌炎比骨旁骨肉瘤的细胞更加丰富（见1639页）。

骨膜骨肉瘤 Periosteal osteosarcoma

1976年，骨膜骨肉瘤被描述为一种独立的疾病[154]。这种肿瘤也被描述为近皮质的软骨肉瘤[155]。骨膜骨肉瘤患者通常为11～20岁，女性略多见。长骨干，尤其是胫骨和股骨，容易受累。患者常常主述短暂的疼痛。影像学显示为附着于下方皮质的透光性病变，在皮质上形成一个碟形缺损。病变延伸至软组织，并与之融合（图25.59）。

通常在软组织中的扩散病灶中可以看到平行排列的钙化，形成一种日光放射的表现。在大体标本上，骨膜骨肉瘤有软骨样表现（图25.60）。显微镜下，骨膜骨

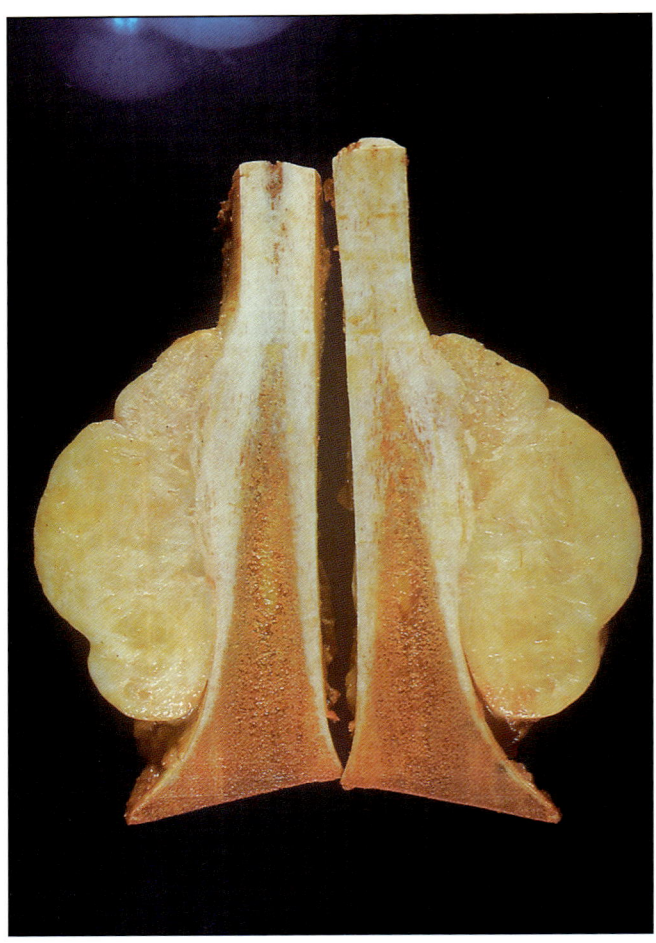

图25.57 骨旁骨肉瘤的大体标本，显示实性分叶状棕褐-白色的肿物，仅累及骨表面。

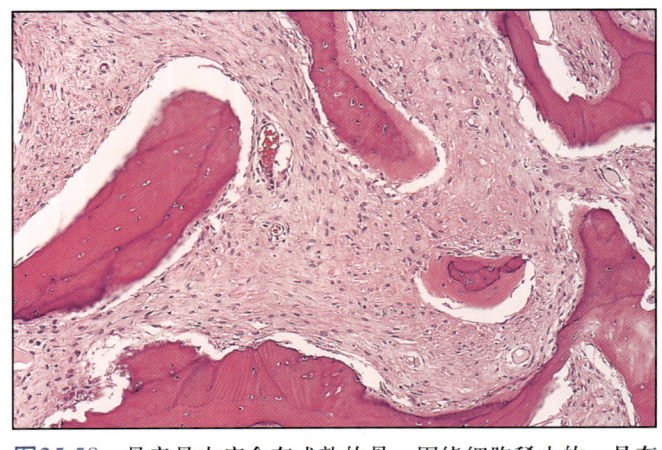

图25.58 骨旁骨肉瘤含有成熟的骨，围绕细胞稀少的、具有轻度细胞非典型性的纤维母细胞间质。

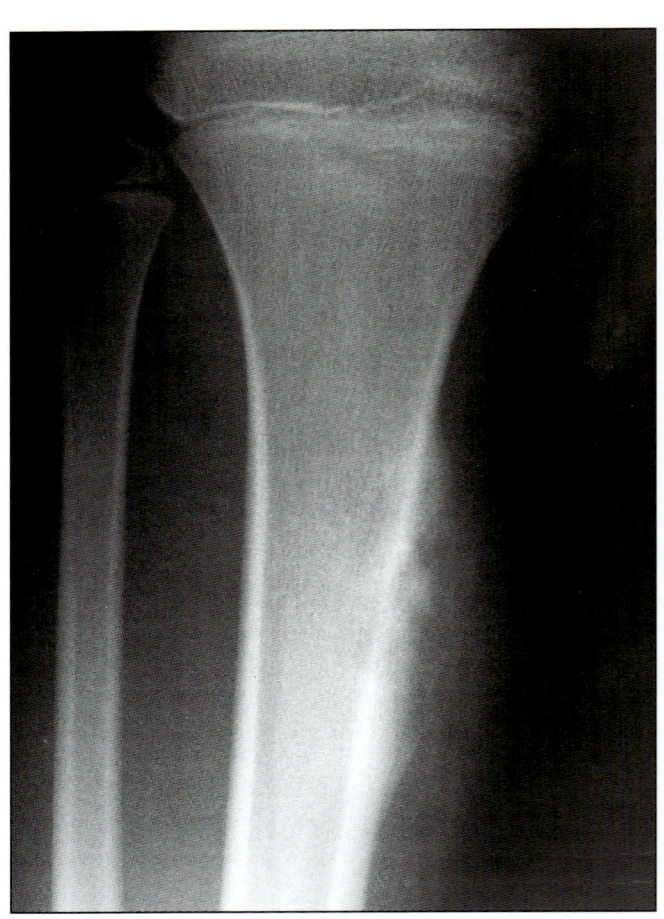

图25.59 位于胫骨表面的骨膜骨肉瘤的影像学图像，显示部分骨化，皮质增厚。(Courtesy of Dr. D. S. Dyke, Geisinger Medical Center, Danville, PA.)

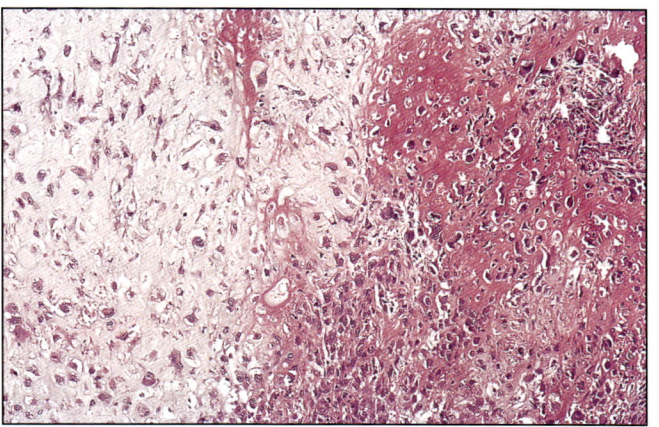

图25.61 骨膜骨肉瘤，显示恶性软骨样基质与骨样组织和非典型梭形细胞混合。

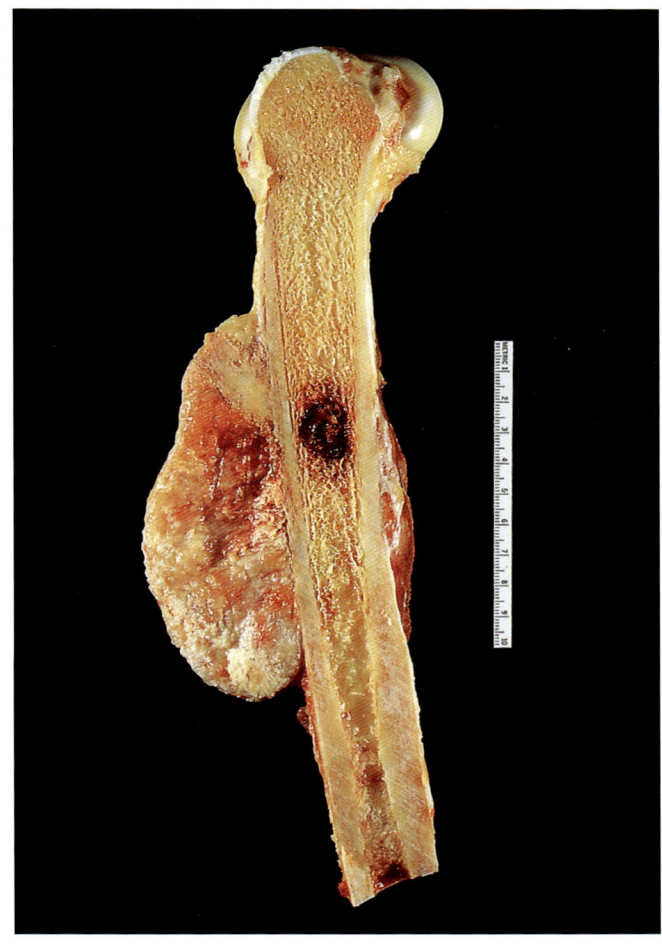

图25.60 大体标本显示位于骨干的典型的骨膜骨肉瘤，未累及其下的髓腔。肿瘤有混合性的外观，白色的针状骨区域与透明软骨的蓝灰色肿块相混合。邻近肿瘤处显示活检部位的髓内出血。

维母细胞性或软骨母细胞性的。预后与普通型骨肉瘤相似。鉴别诊断通常包括骨膜骨肉瘤。任何高级别骨肉瘤，如这种病变，不应包括在骨膜骨肉瘤中。

上文所提到的进一步分类可能看上去比较详细和繁琐。这些类型中有一些并不具有指导预后的意义。但是，知道这些病变有助于正确诊断。一些肿瘤仍被归为来源不明的肿瘤。这些肿瘤能够进一步分为良性和恶性肿瘤。

肉瘤是具有中等分化程度的软骨母细胞型骨肉瘤（图25.61）。肿瘤排列成小叶状，软骨母细胞具有中等程度的非典型性。在周围病变有梭形结构存在，梭形细胞可产生骨样基质。软骨样小叶的中心也显示有骨形成。

骨膜骨肉瘤的预后很好。我们认为，出现任何髓腔的浸润就应排除骨膜骨肉瘤的诊断。骨膜骨肉瘤的组织学特征是典型的，但是不具有特异性。如果伴有髓腔受累的骨肉瘤被归为骨膜骨肉瘤，则我们认为对这种疾病的认识将会慢慢消失。

高级别骨表面骨肉瘤
High-grade surface osteosarcoma

在少数情况下，主要发生在骨表面的骨肉瘤具有所有高级别普通型骨肉瘤的所有组织学特征[156,157]。影像学显示为恶性肿瘤，但是没有特异性。此病可能有轻微的髓内受累；然而，肿瘤的主要部分在骨表面。组织学上，肿瘤通常是间变性的，并且可能是骨母细胞性、纤

来源不明的肿瘤
Tumors of unknown origin

来源不明的良性肿瘤
Benign tumors of unknown origin

良性巨细胞肿瘤　Benign giant cell tumors

虽然几乎所有的骨肿瘤都可能含有巨细胞，但巨细胞肿瘤只显示良性巨细胞明显增生。此病好发于女性。患者通常是骨骼已经成熟的年轻成人。绝大部分患者年龄在21～40岁之间。巨细胞瘤很少发生在年龄很小和年龄很老的人身上。

骨骼的任何部位都可以受累，但是，绝大部分巨细胞瘤发生在长骨末端。最常受累的部位按顺序依次为：股骨远端、胫骨近端、桡骨远端和骶骨。虽然骶骨是发生巨细胞瘤相对常见的部位，但骶骨以上的椎骨受累却不常见。病变总是会扩展到骨的末端。如果在长骨的干骺端或骨干部看到一个含有巨细胞的病变，几乎可以肯定不是巨细胞瘤，而是富于巨细胞的骨肉瘤或是动脉瘤样骨囊肿。具有巨细胞瘤组织学特征的病变出现在不常见的部位，如扁骨，应该考虑其他情况，如甲状旁腺功

能亢进。当然，偶尔真正的巨细胞瘤也可以发生在不常见的部位，如在肩胛骨和颅骨[158]。发生在手和足小骨的含有巨细胞的病变更有可能是反应性病变，如动脉瘤样骨囊肿，而不是巨细胞瘤；但是，手和足的小骨的确可发生真正的巨细胞瘤。它们也可延伸至骨末端。一些报道显示，这些发生在小骨的病变的临床病程更具有侵袭性[159]。

影像学显示，此病为扩展到骨末端的纯溶骨性破坏性病变（图25.62）。骺板通常已经闭合。然而，当一个真正的巨细胞瘤发生在干骺端时，患者的骨骼通常是不成熟的。影像学通常显示界限不清的病变。病变内的钙化非常少见。肿瘤可以破坏皮质并扩展到软组织。虽然发生在骨末端的单纯溶骨性病变应该提示巨细胞瘤的可能性，但是在很多情况下，根据影像学表现不能除外恶性肿瘤的可能。

巨细胞瘤的大体表现可以非常明显。病变质软，典型者为深褐色（图25.63）。然而，巨细胞瘤中的继发性改变很常见。最常见的继发性改变之一是出现囊性区。代表泡沫细胞出现的黄变区域也常常见到。

显微镜下，巨细胞瘤有两种细胞群增生。单核细胞呈圆形或卵圆形，通常均匀地分布在整个病变中（图25.64）。巨细胞的细胞核类似于单核细胞的细胞核。在单核细胞中常见核分裂活动，但是在巨细胞中却看不到。然而，在典型的巨细胞瘤中不应该见到非典型性核分裂。不应该有细胞学的非典型性。

在巨细胞瘤中可见泡沫细胞聚集，有时，这种表现可能成为主要的组织学表现。单核细胞可能是梭形的，甚至可能有席纹状结构。如果梭形结构非常明

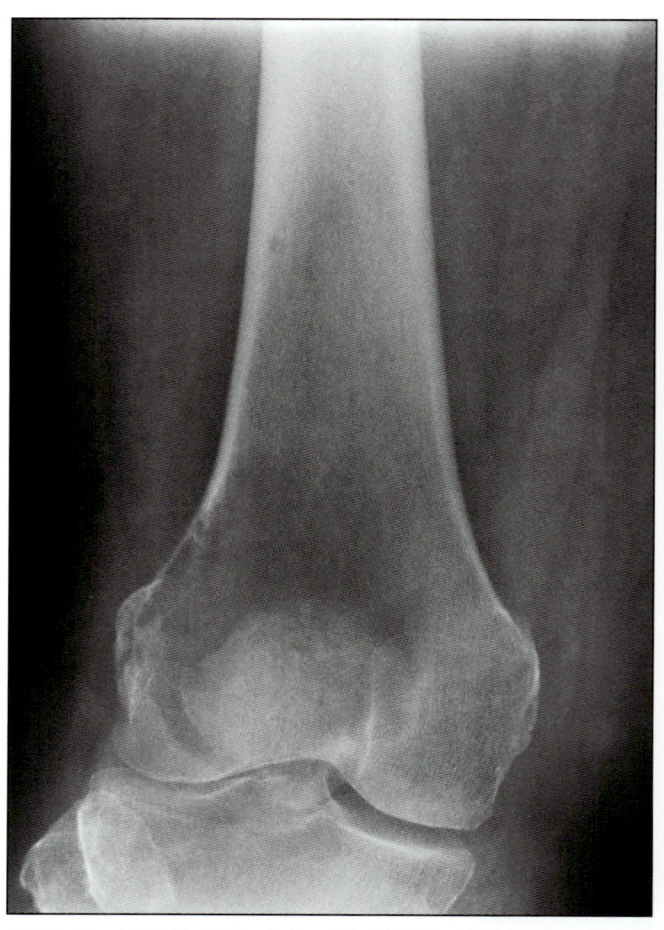

图25.62 巨细胞瘤的X光片，显示股骨远端的单纯溶骨性病变延伸至骨末端。

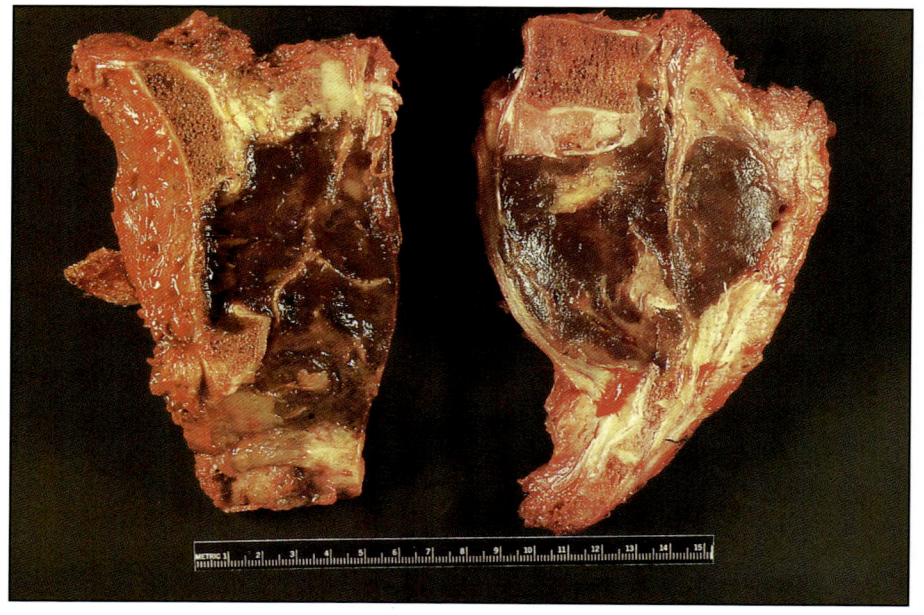

图25.63 巨大骶骨巨细胞瘤的大体标本，显示侵犯周围软组织，病变为红褐色，是典型的巨细胞瘤的表现。

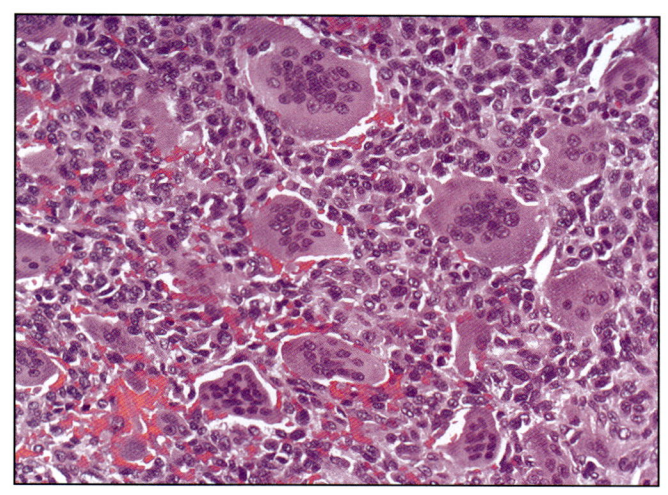

图25.64 巨细胞瘤由均匀分布的巨细胞组成，巨细胞周围围绕着圆形或卵圆形单核细胞，后者没有非典型性。

显，则有可能导致误诊为纤维组织细胞瘤，既可以是良性的也可以是非典型性的。我们认为，一个具有巨细胞瘤所有临床特征的病变，即使组织学上以纤维组织细胞瘤的结构为主，而仅有小灶状的典型巨细胞瘤表现，也应该做出巨细胞瘤的诊断。在经典的巨细胞瘤中经常可以见到与继发性动脉瘤样骨囊肿相似的改变。如果是一个扩展至骨末端并有动脉瘤样骨囊肿表现的病变，那么就应该彻底寻找哪怕是很小的巨细胞瘤病灶。

在巨细胞瘤中很少见到新骨形成。然而，在肿瘤与软组织交界的边缘处常常会形成骨壳。当软组织中的病变复发时，病变会出现特征性的骨壳包裹，这在X线平片上很明显[160]。少数情况下，巨细胞瘤中可以显示在肿瘤实质内有新骨形成。骨组织通常呈现一种反应性病变的形态，就像在动脉瘤样骨囊肿中见到的那样。骨小梁有明显的骨母细胞镶边。这种表现可能导致误诊为骨母细胞瘤甚至骨肉瘤。

我们发现，巨细胞瘤的组织学分级并没有意义。我们认为，巨细胞瘤的局部侵袭性决定于肿瘤局部侵犯的能力以及外科切除的完整性。少数情况下，良性的巨细胞瘤可能转移到远处部位，通常是肺。甚至有报道显示，淋巴结也可以被良性表现的转移性巨细胞瘤累及[161-164]。转移灶通常是孤立的，而且如果病变被切除，患者可以痊愈。然而，在非常少见的情况下，更加弥漫的转移可能导致患者死亡。我们还没有找到可靠的方法来预测有良性表现的巨细胞瘤发生转移的可能性。我们还看到过弥漫转移的病灶出现自发性消退以及发生转移后长期存活的报道。

大多数早期报道强调，良性巨细胞瘤具有较高的局部复发率。然而，随着现代外科技术的应用，复发率已明显降低了。治疗上常常采用外科切除，放疗的作用有限。在诸如脊椎和骶骨部位发生的巨细胞瘤，可能必须采用放疗缩小肿瘤，以便于能进行外科切除。巨细胞瘤的鉴别诊断包括很多可能含有巨细胞的病变。伴有骨骼棕色瘤产生的甲状旁腺功能亢进通常不再是一个鉴别难题。影像学特征经常显示其他甲状旁腺功能亢进的证据，如骨膜下的骨吸收。

动脉瘤样骨囊肿发生在更为年轻的患者的干骺端。

软骨母细胞瘤与巨细胞瘤有很多相似之处，包括部位和一些组织学特征。然而，大多数软骨母细胞瘤患者的骨骼未成熟，而巨细胞瘤患者的骨骼是成熟的。诊断软骨母细胞瘤一定要找到软骨分化或钙化灶。

来源不明的恶性肿瘤
Malignant tumors of unknown origin

巨细胞瘤中的恶性肿瘤
Malignancy in giant cell tumor

正如前面提到的，虽然没有恶性组织学证据的巨细胞瘤可以转移，但并不认为这是恶性骨巨细胞瘤的证据。巨细胞瘤中的恶性肿瘤这一名词要好于恶性巨细胞瘤。许多诊断为恶性巨细胞瘤的肿瘤可能是骨肉瘤以及所谓的恶性纤维组织细胞瘤。

巨细胞瘤中恶性肿瘤的发生可能有三种不同的形式。首先，患者有典型部位的巨细胞瘤。作为治疗的一部分，病变接受了放疗。几年后，相同的部位出现了高级别肉瘤。当然，这可以被认为是巨细胞瘤中的恶性肿瘤或是放疗后的肉瘤。在确定巨细胞瘤中的恶性肿瘤时，这是最常见的情况。

另一个少见的情况是：巨细胞瘤患者仅仅进行了外科治疗。几年后在相同部位发生了肉瘤。

较为常见的情况是：在经典的巨细胞瘤中发生了明显的肉瘤。这种类型才被称为原发性恶性巨细胞瘤[165]。

长骨的釉质瘤 Adamantinoma of long bones

釉质瘤是一种非常罕见的肿瘤，几乎总是累及胫骨。命名为釉质瘤是由于其组织学类似于颌骨的成釉细胞瘤。虽然胫骨好发，但其他骨也可以发生。在一项Mayo Clinic的研究中，Keeney等[166]发现，在此病85例中，70例发生在胫骨。然而，在这70例中，11例也累及同侧腓骨。一些釉质瘤可能开始于腓骨病变，继而累及同侧胫骨。在这项研究中，受累的其他骨是股骨、尺骨、肱骨和桡骨。其中一例肿瘤明显发生在胫前软组织，而其下的骨没有受累。男性和女性的发病率几乎相等，大多数是年轻成人。症状常为疼痛和肿胀。症状可能持续相当长的时间：在Mayo Clinic的病例中，有1/4的患者症状持续时间长达5年以上。

釉质瘤的X线表现具有诊断意义。病变倾向于累及胫骨皮质。病变常常累及胫骨中部，并且骨组织广泛受累（图25.65）。典型的表现是：在皮质中出现周围有硬化的透光区。通常透光区会很大，破坏性表现很明显。

在大体标本上，釉质瘤常常发生在长骨，主要累及皮质。然而，病变也常常累及髓腔（图25.66）。肿瘤呈白色和纤维状，并且插入骨的硬化区。少数情况下，釉质瘤肉眼可见囊性变。

显微镜下，釉质瘤为由纤维间质包绕的上皮细胞簇。细胞为柱状，特征性地显示外周栅栏样结构。中心类似于星网状结构，与成釉细胞瘤相似。上皮岛大小不等，一些上皮岛不明显。角蛋白免疫染色可以突出上皮细胞[167]。肿瘤细胞不显示间变状态。鳞状分化不常见；而角化形成更不常见。一些釉质瘤显示纯粹的梭形结构，以至于活检标本可能被误诊为纤维肉瘤。在胫骨皮质出现的梭形细胞病变，几乎都可诊断为釉质瘤。此外，肿瘤细胞缺乏明显的间变状态，但是病变细胞比低级别纤维肉瘤更加丰富。即使肿瘤细胞呈梭形时，它们也常常显示一种簇状排列，周围围绕着缺乏细胞的纤维性间质。一些釉质瘤有腺体形成，肿瘤细胞排列成滤泡状。在一些釉质瘤中也可见到明显的血管结构。血管样腔隙内衬圆胖细胞，这些细胞与上皮岛融合。过去，这种明显的结构导致一些作者认为：釉质瘤是血管源性肿瘤[168]。已有比较少见的去分化釉质瘤病例的报道[169]，肿瘤伴有高级别多形性形态学表现。

在釉质瘤中可能出现不良纤维结构样改变[170-172]。纤维结构不良区域可能是局灶的，伴有细胞稀疏的梭形细胞增生和化生骨形成。这些区域可能是肿瘤的主要成分，以至于仅有小的上皮细胞岛出现（图25.67）。也有人提出，纤维发育不良样改变是骨纤维发育不良的一种形式[173]。的确，釉质瘤的影像学表现经常在骨的不良纤维结构中见到。一些作者认为，伴有骨纤维发育不良特征的病例其骨纤维发育不良，至少在一些情况下既可能是退化的釉质瘤的一种形式[174]，也可能是釉质瘤形态学谱系的一部分[17,176]。电镜和过氧化物酶染色已经证实：在年轻患者中，其他方面都典型的骨纤维发育不良病例也有上皮分化[177]。这一证据提示，它们是"分化型"釉质瘤。然而，这些患者的临床随访结果提示，病变没有进展。

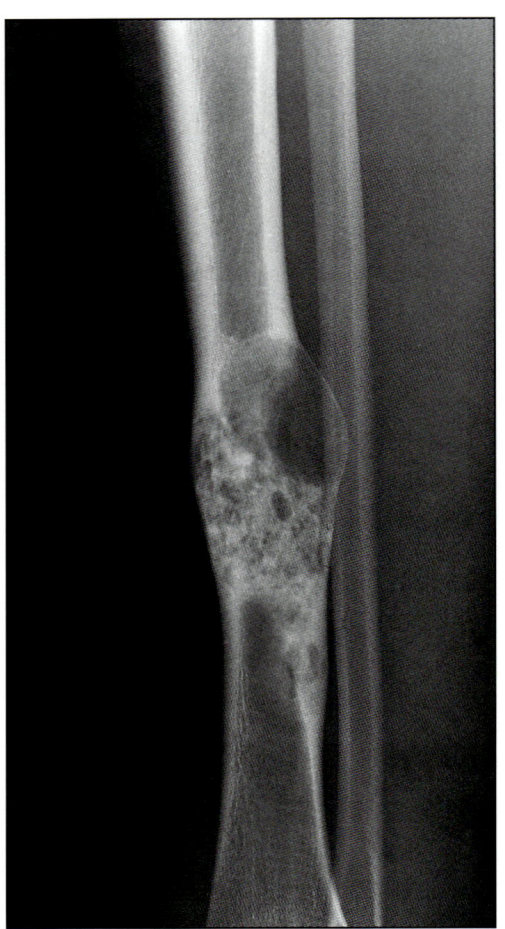

图25.65 胫骨中段釉质瘤的X光片，显示骨膨胀和多中心的病变。

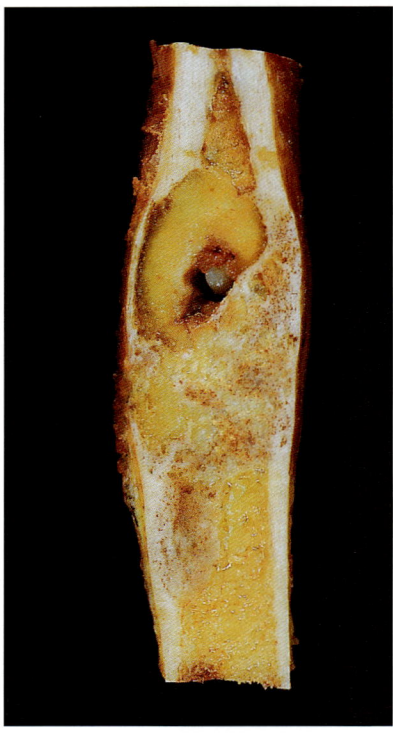

图25.66 釉质瘤的大体标本，呈灰白色，伴有骨硬化区，与图25.65为同一病例。肿瘤累及骨皮质及髓腔。可见中心活检部位出血。

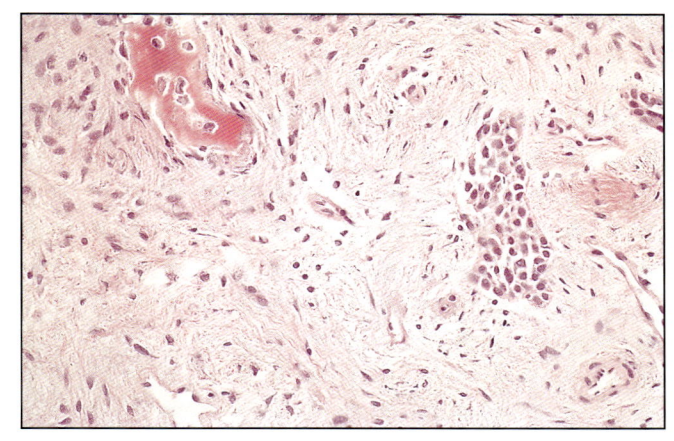

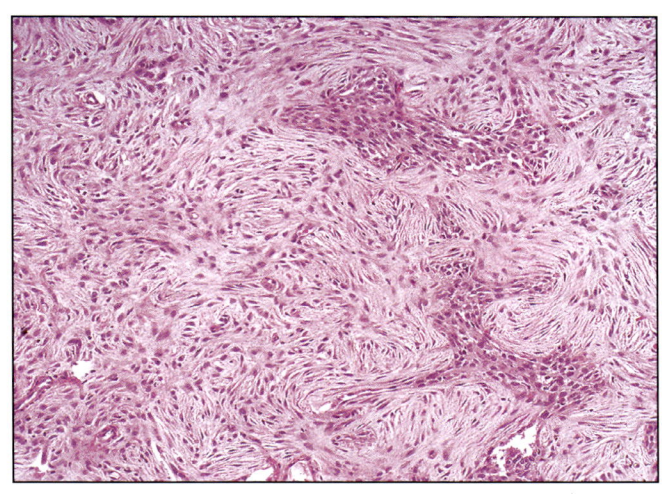

图25.67 （A）这是釉质瘤的主要组织学表现：类似于纤维发育不良；然而，在整个细胞稀少的梭形细胞间质中散在分布着不规则的小的上皮细胞岛。（B）釉质瘤含有不规则的上皮巢，周围围绕着质硬的纤维间质，没有骨组织生成。

我们认为，在釉质瘤中可以见到骨纤维发育不良或纤维发育不良样区域。两者之间是否有某种联系则存在疑问。但毫无疑问的是，有些釉质瘤病例，在先前的活检标本中仅有纤维发育不良表现；现在看来这可能仅仅是取材有误。有关发生在儿童的典型的骨纤维发育不良发生在成年人就是"分化型"釉质瘤的观点，我们认为是没有根据的。已有报道称，大部分骨纤维发育不良病例免疫过氧化物酶染色发现有角蛋白阳性的细胞[178]，在一些釉质瘤中也有相似的核型[179]。我们仍不能确信这些可以作为骨纤维发育不良是釉质瘤的一种形式的证据。大多数骨纤维发育不良患者的预后非常好，将这些发育异常诊断为肿瘤可能是不正确的。虽然几项研究证实，釉质瘤有上皮分化[180-182]，但是其组织来源一直不清楚。即使病变是上皮来源的，也无法解释为什么它会出现在胫骨的皮质中。

釉质瘤的预后通常很好。在Keeney等[166]的研究中，11例患者死于本病，7例发生转移后仍存活。41例患者在治疗后无病生存1个月到47年。然而，此病可能发生转移，甚至是在首次治疗后20年之久才出现。大多数转移至肺，但是，大约7%的患者也可以累及淋巴结。主要的治疗方式是手术切除。

此病的鉴别诊断包括转移癌和纤维肉瘤。转移癌常出现在老年人，而釉质瘤常常发生在较年轻的成人。临床上很少见胫骨转移癌。此外，大多数转移癌的细胞学表现要比釉质瘤有更加显著的间变性。单纯的梭形釉质瘤可能会被误诊为纤维肉瘤。然而，即使釉质瘤细胞非常丰富，也不会表现出细胞学非典型性。大多数低级别纤维肉瘤在肿瘤细胞间有胶原形成。纤维肉瘤常常发生在髓腔，而釉质瘤则累及骨皮质。

血管肿瘤 Vascular tumors

良性血管肿瘤 Benign vascular tumors
血管瘤 Hemangiomas

骨的良性血管肿瘤非常少见。有症状的血管肿瘤更为少见。许多在尸体解剖时描述为椎体血管瘤的病变其实是血管畸形。在外科病例中，血管瘤女性好发。

绝大多数血管瘤没有症状，是在影像学检查中偶然发现的。它们通常是在对与其无关的症状（如头痛）进行颅骨X光检查时发现的。椎体的血管瘤可能引起压缩性骨折，并可延伸到软组织，导致脊髓压迫。骨骼的任何部位都可受累，但在外科病例中，绝大部分血管瘤位于颅骨、椎骨和颌骨。

影像学表现可能具有诊断意义，尤其是在颅骨和脊柱。在脊柱，平片显示锥体密度减低的区域，残留有骨的梁状结构。在交叉断面CT中，显示特征性的圆点花布样表现（图25.68）。在颅骨，病变显示为一个透亮区。病变可以有骨梁结构穿过。然而，当从一侧观察时，骨梁结构呈现特征性的日光放射表现。在长骨，表现无特异性；病变表现为透光区。

血管瘤的大体表现是伴有囊性区域的红色或蓝色病变。新骨形成可能很明显。显微镜下，血管瘤显示多发性小管腔，也可以有更大的管腔。常常可以见到两者混合出现的病变。

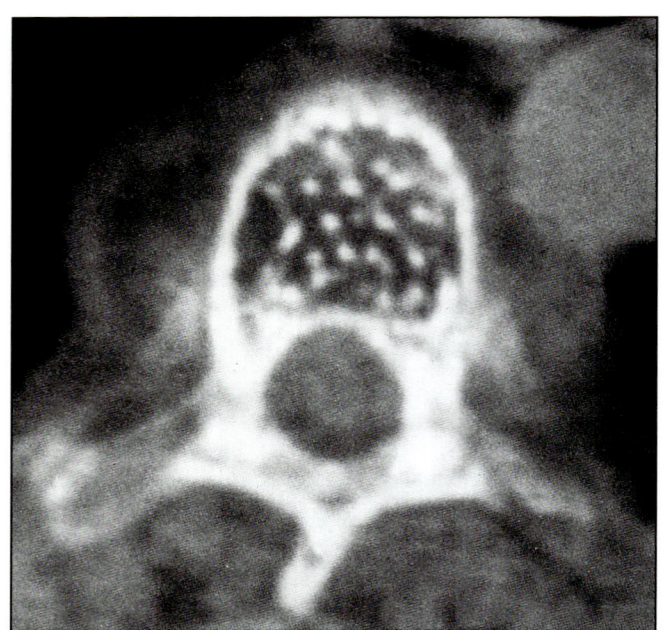

图25.68 CT扫描显示累及椎体的血管瘤呈现典型的圆点小花布样表现。

在少数情况下，血管瘤的内皮细胞相当明显，但是不会看到乳头状形式。文献对骨的上皮样血管瘤也有记载[183]。这些病变常常有分化好的血管腔隙，内衬单层内皮细胞，伴有嗜酸性胞浆和明显的稍显立方的细胞核。血管腔相互并不吻合，基质可出现黏液变。可能会出现炎细胞，尤其是嗜酸性粒细胞（也见第3章）。此外，有一组特有的病变，主要侵犯手足小骨，命名为上皮样和梭形细胞血管瘤[184]。

血管瘤是良性病变，并不会进展。只有在少数情况下发生在椎体的血管瘤，因为脊髓压迫可能会出现问题。在少数情况下，患者可能发生多发血管瘤。然而，良性肿瘤的这种多中心性病变要比恶性血管肿瘤少得多（见下文）。一些患者出现弥漫性血管瘤，可累及全部肢体，包括骨和软组织。这可能引起临床症状，如出血倾向，这是由血小板捕获所致。

大块溶骨性病变，或Gorham病，是一种不常见的骨破坏性病变，可能与血管瘤有关[185]。患者多是青少年或年轻成人。这种疾病常常累及身体的一部分。这些病变可以跨关节扩散，骨似乎消失了。这种消失显然是从外开始向内延伸，所以，早期影像学表现像吮吸的糖果。活检材料可能表现为非特异性的纤维化或血管增生。

一些患者伴有软组织淋巴管瘤，这种病变实际上由于乳糜液外渗可能引起死亡。这种疾病常常是自限性的。伴有脊椎和肋骨受累的患者可能会并发感染而死亡。

原发于骨的血管球肿瘤非常罕见[186]。此病通常见于指（趾）骨。放射学显示界限清楚的透光区。组织学上为典型的血管球细胞瘤的表现，可见小圆形细胞排列在不明显的血管腔隙周围。

恶性血管肿瘤　Malignant vascular tumors

血管肉瘤　Angiosarcoma

恶性血管肿瘤的命名一直有些混乱。作者们曾使用血管内皮瘤（hemangioendothelioma）、血管内皮肉瘤（hemangioendothelial sarcoma）、血管肉瘤（angiosarcoma）来命名，或作为同义词使用，或意指不同的肿瘤。一些作者使用血管内皮瘤来命名低级别的血管肿瘤，而使用血管肉瘤来命名高级别的血管肿瘤。血管肉瘤这个命名已经被世界卫生组织（World Health Organization）采用[3]。

血管肉瘤是非常少见的骨肿瘤；到2004年为止，在Mayo Clinic的资料中仅有109例。男性好发。血管肉瘤可发生于不同年龄段，多少不一。骨骼的任何位置都可受累，没有一个特殊的好发部位。在所有的血管肉瘤中，大约1/3的患者为多中心性病变。多中心病变中大约又有一半是倾向于集中在一个解剖部位；如血管肉瘤可能累及一条腿的所有骨。影像学上这种表现应该具有诊断意义。但是，血管肉瘤可能广泛累及不同区域，如双手的骨骼。

除了出现单一肢体多骨受累的病例外，血管肉瘤的影像学表现并不具有特异性（图25.69）。病变常常表现为单纯的透光区。低级别病变的界限比高级别病变的更清楚。反应性新骨形成非常少见。

在大体标本上，病变常常质软，出血。血管肉瘤显示出相互吻合的血管腔，内衬具有非典型性的血管内皮细胞（图25.70）。一般情况下，血管肉瘤没有促结缔组织反应。在骨的血管肉瘤中，内皮细胞形成乳头状簇并不常见。较高级别的血管肉瘤可能显示肿瘤细胞呈梭形，伴有明显的多形性。这可能会导致误诊为梭形细胞肉瘤。常常可见良性巨细胞，有时可能非常明显，甚至掩盖了真正的病变。病灶中常常可以见到炎症细胞，尤其是嗜酸性粒细胞，特别是在低级别病变中。反应性新骨形成也经常可以见到，骨小梁显示明显的骨母细胞活性。新骨形成可能很多，以至于病变被误诊为骨样肿瘤，尤其是骨母细胞瘤。

我们发现，骨的血管肉瘤分级很有用。分级系统几乎完全是根据肿瘤细胞的细胞学特征进行的。我们仅将血管肉瘤分为1～3级。1级血管肉瘤患者有非常好的预后，而3级血管肉瘤患者的预后非常差[187,188]。然而，有一些研究[189]表明，血管肉瘤的预后是无法预知的。

一些恶性的血管肿瘤有上皮样表现（也见第3章）。这些肿瘤曾经用过上皮样血管内皮瘤和上皮样血管肉瘤的名称[190-193]。**上皮样血管内皮瘤**（epithelioid

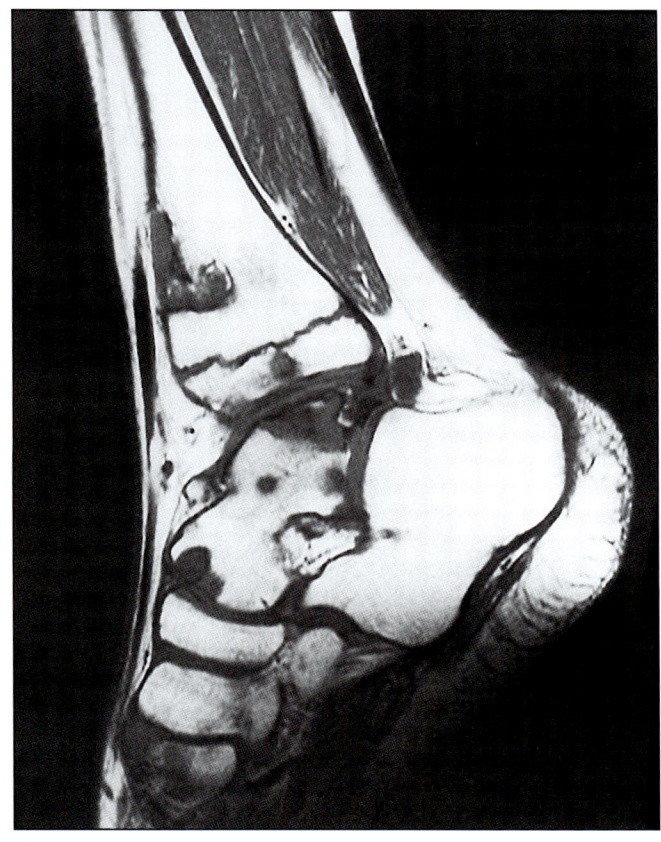

图25.69 核磁共振图像显示累及足和远端胫骨的多处骨的多中心血管内皮细胞瘤。

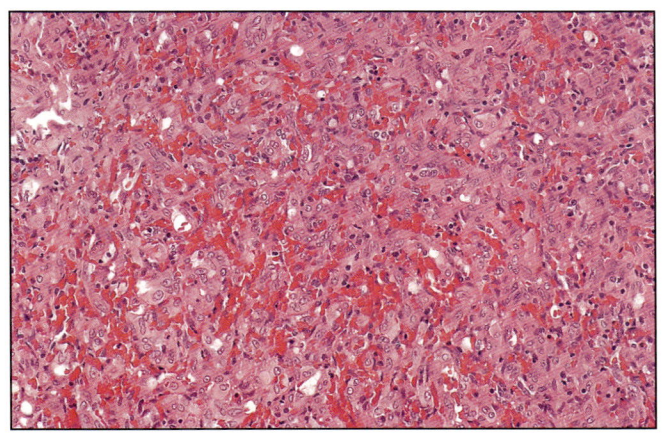

图25.70 2级血管内皮细胞瘤，显示一个成熟血管性肿瘤，具有相互吻合的血管腔，内衬肥胖的内皮细胞。

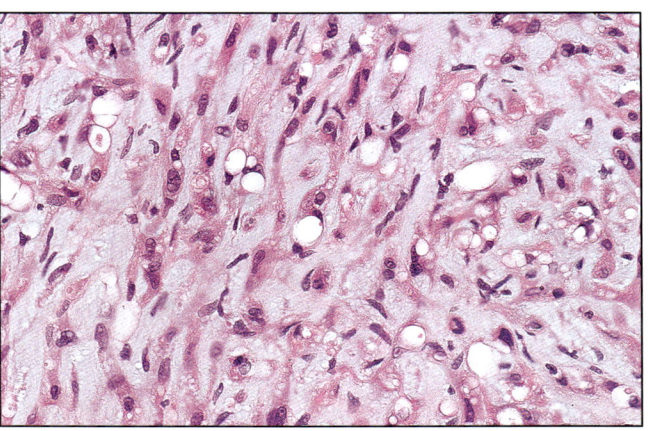

图25.71 上皮样血管内皮瘤，在略嗜碱性的背景中，有细胞条索和胞浆空泡。

hemangioendothelioma）被认为是低级别肿瘤，经常是多灶性的，显示为明显的分叶状生长，背景中具有软骨样或玻璃样变基质。肿瘤细胞常常有丰富的粉染胞浆，出现上皮样表现。通常情况下，胞浆有空泡，显然是代表血管腔。可以见到细胞埋于间质中并常常形成条索（图25.71）。

上皮样血管肉瘤（epithelioid angiosarcoma）：背景中常常没有基质，而是更多的成片结构。然而，肿瘤细胞有大的泡状细胞核，具有明显的核仁和粉染的胞浆。这种细胞常常让人联想起肝细胞。继发性改变，如炎细胞出现，尤其是嗜酸性粒细胞，就像在普通型的血管内皮瘤中看到的一样，在上皮样血管内皮瘤中也可以看到。肿瘤常常累及多处骨组织。黏液样血管母细胞瘤病（myxoid angioblastomatosis）的名称有时被用于描述这种病变[194]。

治疗常常采取外科切除。至今为止，化疗对血管肉瘤无效。然而，有些病变对放疗有非常好的反应。

低级别血管肉瘤的鉴别诊断是良性血管瘤。这种区别仅仅是以细胞学为基础的。高级别血管肉瘤可能被误诊为梭形细胞肉瘤或转移癌。血管内皮瘤的腔隙表现为相互吻合，而这在转移癌中是非常少见的。血管肿瘤中角蛋白染色可能是阳性的；此外，CD31和CD34在血管肿瘤中呈典型的阳性，而在癌中是阴性的。与其他梭形细胞肿瘤的鉴别只能通过充分取材、找到血管形成的区域。一些转移癌，尤其是肾细胞癌，常常血管非常丰富，因此会被误诊为血管肉瘤。

血管外皮细胞瘤 Hemangiopericytoma

骨的原发性血管外皮细胞瘤非常罕见[195,196]。截止到2004年，在Mayo Clinic的资料中仅有15例。许多骨的梭形细胞肿瘤都在局灶区域有血管外皮细胞瘤的结构；因此，在诊断之前，病变要充分取材，以确保这个病变有一致的血管外皮细胞瘤的形态。现在有一些专家更愿意将这类病变命名为孤立性纤维瘤。血管外皮细胞瘤在低倍镜下很有特点，小圆形或卵圆形细胞排列在变形的血管腔周围。血管腔被周围增生的细胞挤压，形成典型的鹿角样形态。在血管外皮细胞瘤中通常看不到巨细胞。细胞核并没有明显的多形性。

虽然在软组织的血管外皮细胞瘤（孤立性纤维瘤），恶性通常表现为核分裂活性、坏死和核非典型性，但我们认为，大多数的骨血管外皮细胞瘤都是恶性的。即使细胞稀少，而且没有恶性组织学证据，病变的生物学行为常常也是恶性的，但临床过程可能是迟缓的。

一些作者还将脑膜血管外皮细胞瘤（也见第3章和第26章）看成是孤立纤维性肿瘤，具有转移到骨的特殊倾向；在诊断骨的原发性血管外皮细胞瘤之前，应该排除这种可能。

纤维组织细胞肿瘤
Fibrohistiocytic tumors

良性纤维组织细胞肿瘤
Benign fibrohistiocytic tumors

良性纤维组织细胞瘤
Benign fibrous histiocytoma

骨的良性纤维组织细胞瘤非常罕见。其组织学特征表现是：伴有席纹状结构的梭形细胞肿瘤。整个病变常常可见散在分布的良性巨细胞。泡沫细胞常见。组织学表现可见纤维干骺缺损（见1638页）。事实上，一些作者提出，纤维干骺缺损就是纤维组织细胞瘤。当有这种组织学表现的病变发生在不常见的位置或发生在不常见的年龄段时，而且有症状出现，则诊断为良性纤维组织细胞瘤是合适的。有纤维干骺缺损的患者其年龄通常小于20岁，而良性纤维组织细胞瘤则发生在成人。良性纤维组织细胞瘤发生的部位也不是纤维干骺缺损好发的部位，如骨盆骨。疼痛的出现可能提示这种病变是真正的肿瘤，而不只是纤维性缺损。临床病程符合良性肿瘤的表现[197,198]。

恶性纤维组织细胞肿瘤
Malignant fibrohistiocytic tumors

恶性纤维组织细胞瘤（所谓的）
Malignant fibrous histiocytoma (so-called)

直到最近，恶性纤维组织细胞瘤可能仍是软组织肉瘤中最常诊断的肿瘤（见第24章）。多形性恶性肿瘤，尤其是伴有席纹状结构者，常常考虑为恶性纤维组织细胞瘤。根据是否出现黏液性间质或炎细胞浸润，可以将这些病变再分为几种亚型。恶性纤维组织细胞瘤常常含有破骨样巨细胞。甚至软组织的恶性纤维组织细胞瘤也可以出现骨和软骨形成。然而，免疫过氧化物酶染色和电子显微镜研究对这种恶性纤维组织细胞瘤的观点提出

了挑战[199]。这些研究表明，许多多形性软组织肉瘤实际上是多形性恶性肿瘤或其他特殊肉瘤的某种类型。我们认为，在多形性肉瘤中只要有基质产生就要排除恶性纤维组织细胞瘤的诊断。许多骨肉瘤有大片病灶，与恶性纤维组织细胞瘤无法区别。因此，如果取材充分，骨的恶性纤维组织细胞瘤的诊断将会减少。如果有任何怀疑，我们宁愿倾向于诊断骨肉瘤，因为肿瘤学家已经注意到，恶性纤维组织细胞瘤不像骨肉瘤那样对化疗比较敏感。

当病变有席纹状排列或肿瘤细胞呈现上皮样或组织细胞样表现时，我们诊断为恶性纤维组织细胞瘤（或未分类多形性肉瘤）。应该没有任何其他方向分化的证据——换句话说，这是一种排除性诊断。应用这些标准，到2004年为止，我们仅发现了98例骨原发性恶性纤维组织细胞瘤。相比之下，我们在同一时期诊断了1941例骨肉瘤以及271例纤维肉瘤。男性发病略多。任何年龄的患者均可发病，且恶性纤维组织细胞瘤似乎并没有像骨肉瘤那样显示明显好发于青少年的特点。此病常见的症状是疼痛和肿胀。

这些多形性肉瘤的影像学表现没有特异性。病变显示溶骨性破坏区。在病变内应该没有钙化。肿瘤往往边缘不清，提示为恶性。在大体标本上，病变可能是纤维性或鱼肉样。常常可见黄色斑点。

组织学上，所谓的恶性纤维组织细胞瘤总是多形性肿瘤。梭形细胞经常显示席纹状结构。肿瘤内常常可见破骨样巨细胞、Touton巨细胞和泡沫细胞。一些细胞有泡状细胞核，有丰富的粉染胞浆，呈现组织细胞的表现。以我们的经验，所有骨的恶性纤维组织细胞瘤都是高级别肿瘤。一些作者按照在软组织中应用的亚分类进一步细分骨的恶性纤维组织细胞瘤[200]。在骨病变中进行这样的分类是否有预测预后的意义，尚不清楚。

恶性纤维组织细胞瘤中大约有25%是继发于先前存在的病变，如Paget病、早期放疗或骨折[201,202]。

一些研究证实，发生在骨的恶性纤维组织细胞瘤的预后与高级别纤维肉瘤和骨肉瘤相同[203-207]。

鉴别诊断涉及几种疾病。恶性纤维组织细胞瘤必须与纤维肉瘤和骨肉瘤鉴别。任何基质的产生都可排除恶性纤维组织细胞瘤。多形性非常显著的肿瘤通常不考虑是纤维肉瘤。这些鉴别可能仅具有理论意义。然而重要的是，要将恶性纤维组织细胞瘤与恶性淋巴瘤和转移癌区别开。一些恶性淋巴瘤有梭形细胞，可能类似于恶性纤维组织细胞瘤。如果病变累及骨骼多个部位，则更可能是恶性淋巴瘤而不是恶性纤维组织细胞瘤。

如果病变是恶性淋巴瘤，大的多形细胞应该会被造血系统的免疫过氧化物酶染色着色。肉瘤样癌也可以非常类似于恶性纤维组织细胞瘤。针对角蛋白的免疫过氧

化物酶染色可能会对鉴别有帮助。我们认为，仔细的临床检查，包括适当的影像学检查，是区别转移性肉瘤样癌与骨原发肉瘤的最好方法。

纤维源性肿瘤　Fibrogenic tumors

骨没有良性纤维源性肿瘤。我们认为，非骨化性纤维瘤或骨干骺纤维缺损是一种非肿瘤性病变（见1638页）。

交界性纤维源性肿瘤
Borderline fibrogenic tumors

纤维组织增生性纤维瘤
Desmoplastic fibroma

命名为"交界性"就意味着这一肿瘤通常具有局部侵袭性，但缺乏远处转移的潜能。Jaffe[1]首先将纤维组织增生性纤维瘤作为一种疾病详细描述。然而，他将其放在纤维肉瘤的章节中，并指出其与纤维肉瘤相似。

纤维组织增生性纤维瘤是非常罕见的肿瘤。至2004年为止，在Mayo Clinic的资料中仅有16例。在Mayo Clinic对包括会诊病例在内所有患者的研究中[208]，男性明显好发。虽然患者发病年龄从2岁到60岁都有，但27个患者中有20例发生在21～30岁之间。骨盆骨、长骨和颌骨是最常发生的部位。疼痛和膨胀分别是最常见的症状和体征。5个患者出现病理性骨折。

影像学显示累及长骨的干骺端或骨干的单纯透光性病变。在骺板闭合后，病变常常延伸至骨端。受累的骨有轻度或中度的膨胀。边缘呈分叶状，但界限清楚（图25.72）。

在大体标本上，纤维组织增生性纤维瘤常常有质韧、纤维性漩涡状表现。显微镜下，纤维组织增生性纤维瘤是发生在骨内的、与韧带样瘤相似的病变。病变细胞稀少，由呈束状增生的梭形细胞组成，缺乏细胞学非典型性（图25.73）。肿瘤细胞可以显示β-catenin免疫染色呈阳性[208a]。

在肿瘤细胞之间有丰富的间质胶原。核分裂象非常少见。肿瘤内可能出现直径较大的血管腔，与在一些韧带样瘤中见到的相似。

病变具有局部侵袭性。切除不充分一定会引起复发；然而，广泛切除通常能确保治愈。直到最近，我们还没有见过在纤维组织增生性纤维瘤基础上发生的高级别肉瘤。而现在我们已见到一例这样的病例，是患病很长时间后发生转变的。

鉴别诊断包括纤维发育不良、低级别纤维肉瘤和骨肉瘤。纤维发育不良有化生骨形成，后者在纤维组织增

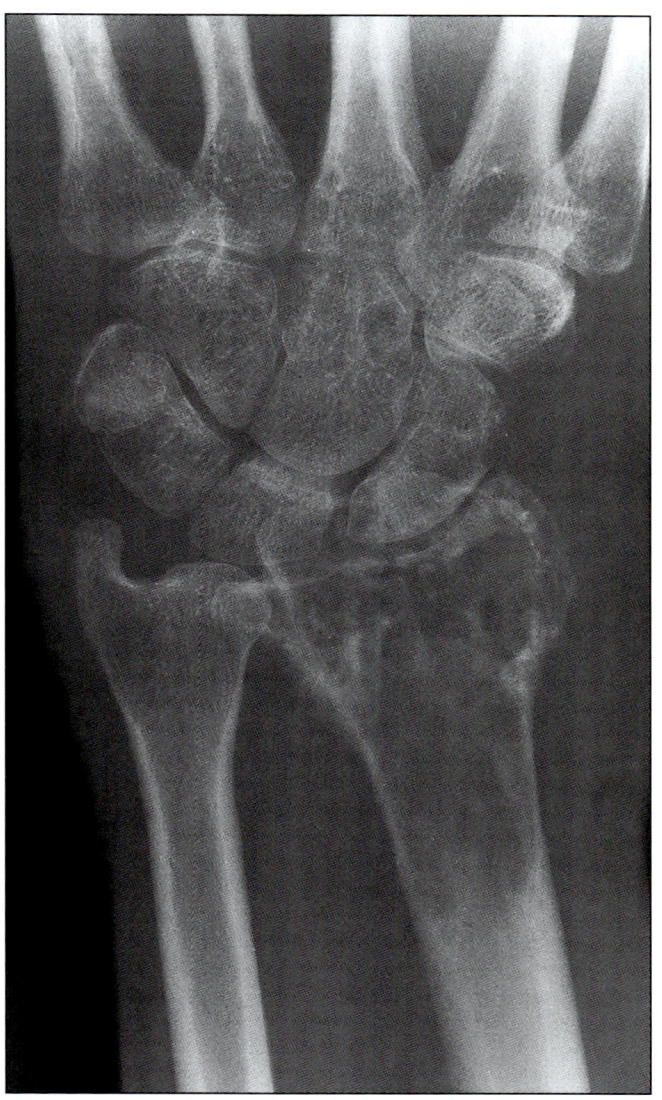

图25.72　纤维组织增生性纤维瘤的X光片，显示溶骨性病变，骨伴有分叶状膨胀。

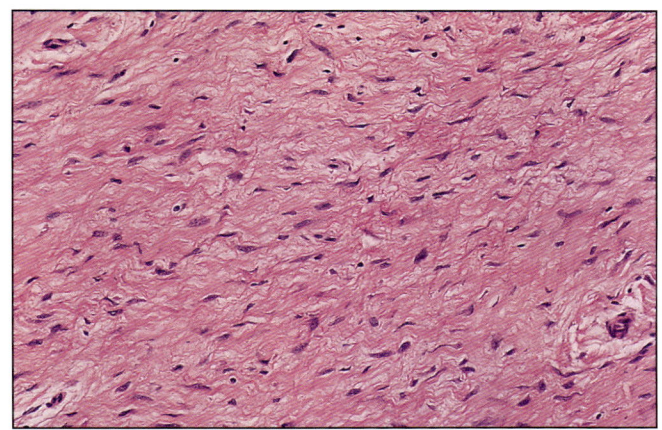

图25.73　骨的纤维组织增生性纤维瘤，显示病变细胞稀少，由一致的拉长的梭形细胞组成，伴有波浪状胶原纤维。

生性纤维瘤中是不会出现的。一些低级别纤维肉瘤有类似于纤维组织增生性纤维瘤的区域。然而有骨形成可排除纤维组织增生性纤维瘤的诊断。低级别纤维肉瘤与纤维组织增生性纤维瘤的表现有些许的相似性（见下文）。

恶性纤维源性肿瘤
Malignant fibrogenic tumors

纤维肉瘤　Fibrosarcoma

纤维肉瘤是骨的唯一恶性纤维源性肿瘤。在 Mayo Clinic 的资料中，此病发病率大约是骨肉瘤的 1/6。大约有 1/4 的病例继发于先前存在的病变，如 Paget 病、早期放疗或骨折。男女受累比例大致相当。此病不像骨肉瘤那样以年轻患者为主。年龄分布没有规律，在 10～80 岁之间都有发生。骨骼的任何部位都可以受累，但是解剖部位分布类似于骨肉瘤。大多数病变发生在长骨干骺端。症状没有特异性。

此病的影像学表现也没有特异性。就像提到的那样，病变通常是长骨干骺端的破坏性区域。边界常不清晰。在少数情况下，纤维肉瘤有明确的边界，可能有类似于良性病变的表现。

纤维肉瘤的大体表现根据肿瘤的分级而有所不同。低级别纤维肉瘤常常质韧、白色并呈纤维性。高级别肉瘤呈鱼肉样，可能出现出血和坏死区域。

显微镜下，纤维肉瘤表现为具有不同程度的非典型性的梭形细胞排列成束状，这种束状结构常常相互交错，出现一种鱼骨样结构（图 25.74）。胶原分布于肿瘤细胞之间。在肿瘤中出现的胶原的数量与肿瘤的分级成反比。低级别纤维肉瘤常常细胞稀少，细胞仅有轻微非典型性和稀少的核分裂活动。高级别纤维肉瘤细胞非常丰富，显示明显的细胞学非典型性，但是几乎没有多形性，核分裂活性明显并有坏死区域。良性巨细胞的出现通常不是纤维肉瘤的特征。恶性度分级与预后密切相关[209]。

一些纤维肉瘤细胞非常小，类似于 Ewing 肉瘤的表现。即使出现非常小的梭形区域和鱼骨样结构，也支持纤维肉瘤的诊断。一些纤维肉瘤常常显示广泛的黏液变性；在这些病变中，细胞可能出现虚假的良性表现。

治疗方式是外科切除。对于化疗尚没有足够的经验来了解是否有效。

鉴别诊断包括纤维组织增生性纤维瘤和骨肉瘤。低级别纤维肉瘤与纤维组织增生性纤维瘤相似，但是通常至少有一些细胞核的非典型性。高级别纤维肉瘤与纤维母细胞型骨肉瘤难以区别，区别可能是人为的，并且完全是由取材决定的。

目前仅有几个骨的平滑肌肉瘤（leiomyosarcoma）的报道[210-212]。这些病变与软组织相对应的病变相似，显示出平滑肌分化的免疫组化染色特点。预后可能与纤维肉瘤相同。然而，如果骨的梭形细胞肿瘤有肌源性肿瘤的表现，应该仔细考虑除外是否肿瘤是从诸如女性生殖道或后腹膜等部位转移而来的。

我们没有骨的原发性神经纤维肉瘤病例。Mayo Clinic 的资料中有 3 例梭形细胞肉瘤的病例，伴有神经纤维瘤病[213]。尽管如此，这些肿瘤的组织学特征表现为纤维肉瘤而不是神经纤维肉瘤。

脊索肿瘤　Notochordal tumors

仅在最近才认识到有罕见的良性脊索病变，它在疾病分类学中的准确位置仍在考虑中（见 1634 页）。已有报道称发现了异位脊索残件的团块——被称为颅内脊索瘤[214]。这些病变没有症状，是在尸检时偶然发现的。

脊索瘤　Chordoma

脊索瘤是唯一起源于脊索成分的恶性肿瘤。其之所以被认为是真正的脊索来源，是由于其表达鼠短尾突变体表型，这可能是一个有用的诊断标记[214a]。它们总是发生在中线。然而，组织学上类似于脊索瘤但发生在其他部位的肿瘤，如软组织的肿瘤，实际上主要是黏液性软骨肉瘤或混合（肌上皮）瘤（见第 24 章）。

男性脊索瘤发病率是女性的两倍，常常发生在脊柱的两端。在 Mayo Clinic 的资料中，大约一半的脊索瘤发生在骶骨，而 37% 累及大脑底部。累及椎骨的病变则主要累及颈椎。胸椎则极少受累。大多数脊索瘤发生在成年人，而少见的涉及儿童的脊索瘤最常发生在颅底[214b]。

脊索瘤的临床症状根据解剖部位的不同而不同。患者可能出现症状月至数年。疼痛最为常见。骶骨的脊

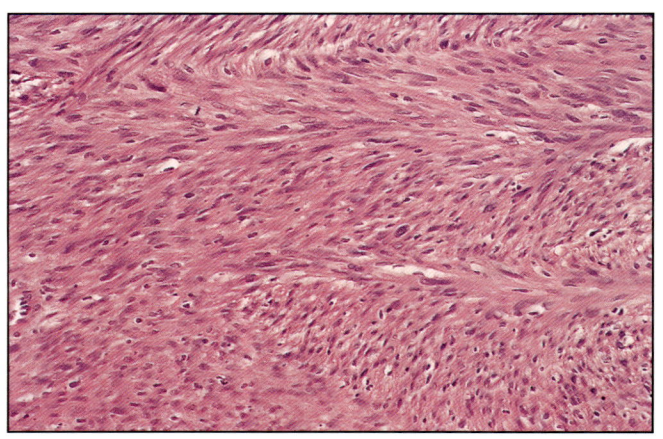

图 25.74　骨的纤维肉瘤显示细胞丰富，由非典型梭形细胞构成，细胞排列成束状并形成鱼骨样结构。

索瘤患者常常因为神经损伤而出现便秘。大多数尾骨脊索瘤患者出现前方的包块，但是少数情况下也可以出现后方的包块。蝶-枕部脊索瘤可出现颅神经受累症状。肿瘤可能破坏垂体腺并产生垂体功能障碍症状。脊索瘤可能表现为小脑脑桥角肿瘤，或可能向下扩散，在鼻或在鼻咽部形成肿块。

影像学上，脊索瘤显示地图样破坏区。可见残留的骨梁和钙化成分。由于骶骨的脊索瘤与阴影重叠，可能会被放射科医生忽略。在CT和MRI上能更好地观察病变。颅底的脊索瘤总是显示累及斜坡。

在大体标本上，脊索瘤常常质软，呈分叶状胶冻样外观（图25.75）。少数情况下，脊索瘤可能显示囊性变。

脊索瘤总是分叶状病变；如果获得了足够的材料，则肿瘤可显示被纤维间隔分成小叶状。小叶由在黏液样基质中的肿瘤细胞组成。肿瘤细胞常常排列成条索。病变细胞核通常较小，胞浆丰富。胞浆可能有多泡状表现，这样的细胞被称作空泡细胞。虽然空泡细胞被认为是脊索瘤的典型表现，但我们发现，分叶状结构和细胞条索对于诊断脊索瘤更有帮助（图25.76）。

脊索瘤细胞可能显示一些不寻常的表现。细胞经常出现上皮样表现，非常类似于转移癌。细胞有时呈梭形。一些脊索瘤显示奇异的细胞学改变。然而，这些都与预后无关。

1973年，Heffelfinger等[215]描述了颅底的脊索瘤显示明显的软骨样分化。这些软骨样脊索瘤的预后要比普通型脊索瘤好得多。以我们的经验，累及颅底的普通型脊索瘤并不常见。如果从颅底取材的活检标本显示单纯的软骨样分化，且放射科医生向我们保证这个病变确实累及斜坡，则我们认为应该诊断为软骨样脊索瘤。

文献中关于软骨样脊索瘤的真正本质是有争论的。一些作者[216]认为，软骨样脊索瘤实际上是软骨肉瘤，因为在软骨样脊索瘤中缺乏上皮标记物的染色。然而，其他研究反对这一观点[217]。上皮标记物在普通型脊索瘤中呈典型的阳性[217,218]。电子显微镜研究支持软骨样脊索瘤的观点[219]。这些少见的病变是真正的脊索瘤还是软骨肉瘤，由于临床的原因需要辨认，因为它们通常临床病程较长。

已经有经过[220,221]或未经过[222]放疗的脊索瘤转变成高级别梭形细胞肉瘤（去分化）的报道。

直到最近，脊索瘤的预后还是很差。以我们的经验，脊索瘤是一种可局部复发、转移潜能有限的疾病；然而，也有一些作者[223,224]报告：脊索瘤有高的转移率。患者常常长期存活，但是因为有神经系统问题，患者可能会有较严重的临床表现。现代手术技术使此病的预后有了相当大程度的改善[225-227]，但是局部控制以及因此有了

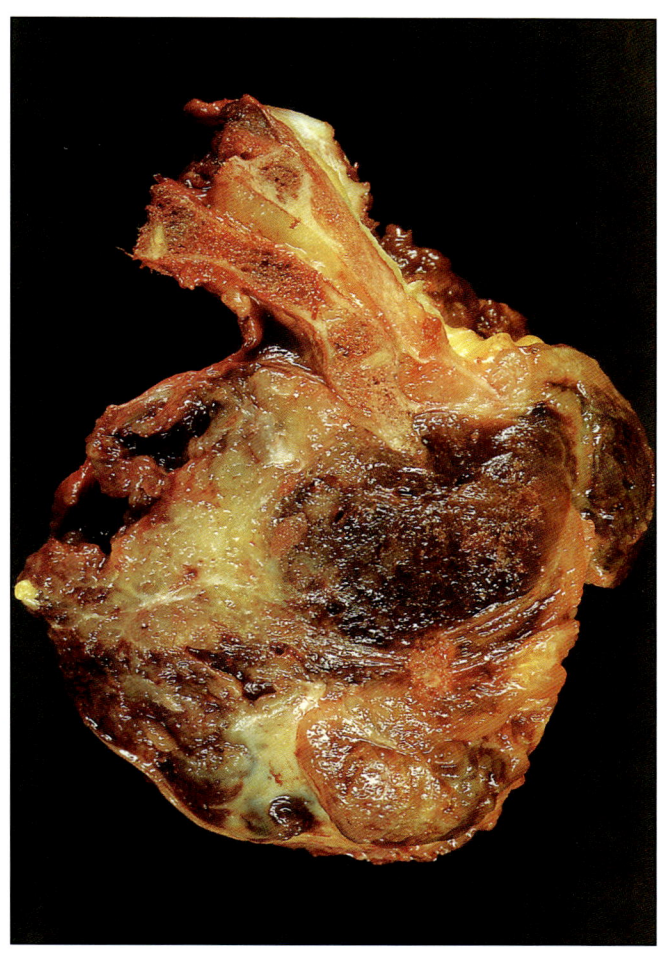

图25.75 具有破坏性的脊索瘤的大体标本，显示分叶状胶冻样肿块。

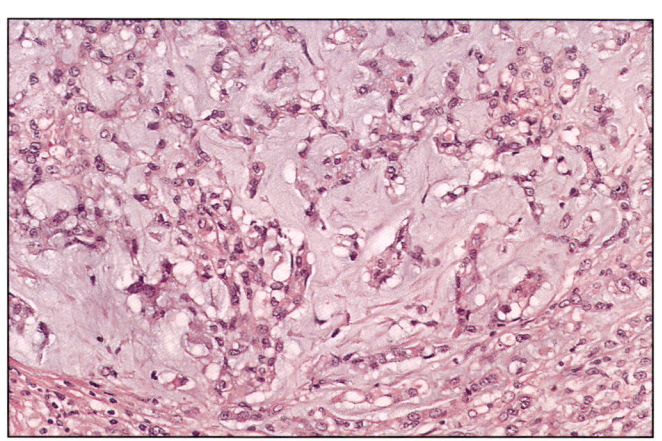

图25.76 脊索瘤显示肿瘤细胞排列成条索，周围为黏液样基质。

更长的生存时间反而导致远期转移率更高了。

鉴别诊断主要包括软骨肉瘤、转移癌和黏液性乳头状室管膜瘤。转移癌和脊索瘤的上皮标记物染色都可出现阳性表现。但是，除此之外，脊索瘤S-100蛋白呈阳性。以我们的经验，在转移癌中很少见到伴有纤维间隔的明确的分叶状生长。软骨肉瘤常常呈分叶状，但是并没有纤维间隔。软骨肉瘤上皮标记物呈阴性。黏液性乳头状

骨的囊性病变

室管膜瘤上皮标记物也为阴性[228]。

良性脊索细胞肿瘤（benign notochordal cell tumor）[229,230]或错构瘤（hamartoma）是一种相对新近才命名的疾病，且此病偶尔可能发展成脊索瘤[230]。这种病变可以完全取代椎体，在 X 光片上可以表现为硬化。许多病例是在尸检时发现的。低倍镜下，肿瘤具有浸润性，充满髓腔。肿瘤细胞呈空泡状，可能提示是一个脂肪性肿瘤。肿瘤细胞不排列成条索，缺乏黏液性基质，与在脊索瘤中所见的典型排列不同。

神经源性肿瘤　Neural tumors

在骨中，神经起源的肿瘤非常少见。在 Mayo Clinic 的资料中，我们没有神经纤维瘤和神经纤维肉瘤的病例，即使在神经纤维瘤病的患者中也没有发现此病。

神经鞘瘤　Neurilemmoma

神经鞘瘤在骨也不常见。许多巨大神经鞘瘤位于骶骨周围而累及骨。然而，在这些病例中，很难知道病变最初是始于骨内，还是骨是继发受累部位。截止到 2004 年，在 Mayo Clinic 的资料中仅有 23 例骨的神经鞘瘤。最常见的发病部位是下颌骨；但是其他部位的骨也可能受累[231,232]。影像学总是显示界限非常清晰的、具有良性表现的病变。如果影像学显示边界不清，神经鞘瘤的诊断是不能成立的。

显微镜下，这些神经鞘瘤与其他部位的神经鞘瘤相似（见第 27 章），显示梭形细胞局灶呈栅栏样排列。可见玻璃样变的厚壁血管。治疗方式应该选择保守切除，预后很好。

脂肪源性肿瘤　Lipogenic tumors

良性脂肪源性肿瘤　Benign lipogenic tumors
脂肪瘤　Lipoma

发生在骨的脂肪源性肿瘤非常少见。在 Mayo Clinic 的资料中仅有 8 例骨内脂肪瘤。文献报道了一组大型病例研究[233]。虽然骨的任何部位都可能受累，但是跟骨是最好发部位[234,235]。X 光片显示为境界清晰的透光区，伴有中心钙化区。中心钙化区与在骨梗死中所见的钙化相似。CT 显示缺损处只含有脂肪。

组织学上，我们可以看到正常骨小梁被脂肪组织替代。中心常常有钙化灶。有报道可发生恶变[236]。

恶性脂肪源性肿瘤　Malignant lipogenic tumors
脂肪肉瘤　Liposarcoma

发生在骨的脂肪肉瘤极为少见。大多数骨的脂肪肉瘤既可以是从其他软组织转移而来（通常为黏液性/小圆细胞型），也可以是软组织脂肪肉瘤的直接侵犯所致。在 Mayo Clinic 的资料中仅有 2 例真正的骨的原发性脂肪肉瘤。

类似于原发性骨肿瘤的病变　Conditions that simulate primary neoplasms of bone

几种病变可能类似于原发性骨肿瘤。最近的一些资料[237,238]表明，至少有一些传统上认为是非肿瘤的病变事实上可能是肿瘤。不过，为了实用的目的，以及因为还有另外一些不确定的资料和这些病变的临床特点，或许仍然可以将它们认为是类似于肿瘤的病变。这些病变中一些很常见，而另一些非常少见。重要的是要知道这些病变以避免误诊。转移癌可能是骨中最常见的恶性肿瘤。通常转移发生在原发性肿瘤诊断之前，来自骨病变的活检通常并不会出现误诊。骨转移可能是隐匿性原发性肿瘤出现的体征。即使在这些病变中，转移癌的组织学特征也是特征性的，诊断并不会出问题。但在少数情况下，转移癌可能类似于原发性梭形细胞肉瘤的表现。以我们的经验，最常见的类似于骨的梭形细胞肉瘤的原发肿瘤是肉瘤样肾细胞癌。当在一个老年人的骨骼中出现明显的梭形细胞肉瘤时，应该牢记肉瘤样癌的可能性。

下列疾病是骨骼系统中很有特点的疾病，常常引起诊断上的困难。

骨的囊性病变　Cystic lesions of bone

动脉瘤样骨囊肿　Aneurysmal bone cyst

动脉瘤样骨囊肿是略有局部侵袭性的骨病变，虽然最近的研究显示，在这些病变中有克隆性染色体异常[237]，但至少，传统上一直认为它是非肿瘤性病变。绝大多数病变发生在 20 岁之前。女性略好发。绝大多数病变发生在长骨干骺端。大约 15% 累及椎骨；当病变累及椎骨时，它的常见部位在脊侧。

动脉瘤样骨囊肿的影像学表现具有明显的特征。病变是纯溶骨性的，累及长骨的干骺端，偏心性，显示一种爆炸样表现，并向软组织扩展。边界可以很清晰，也

1634

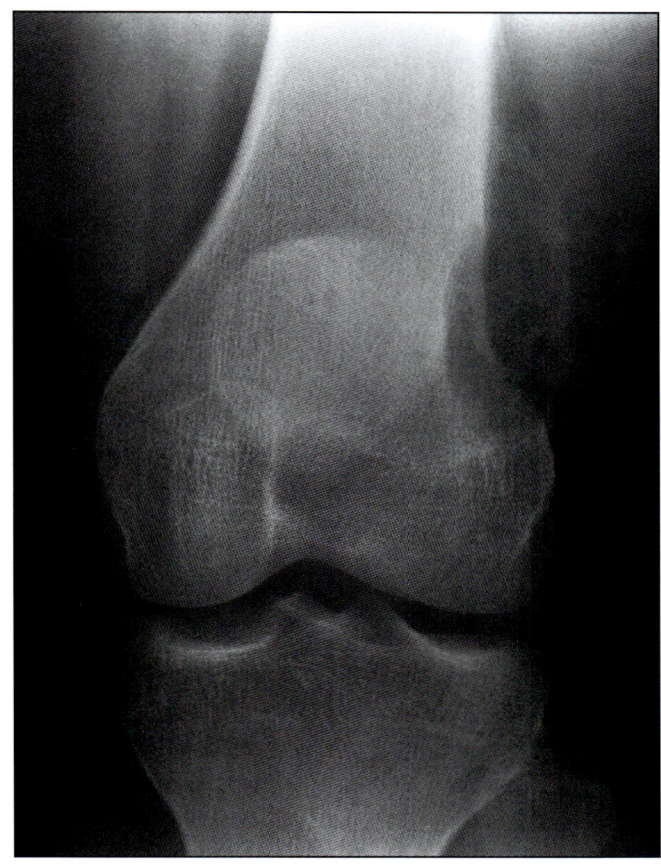

图25.77 动脉瘤样骨囊肿，在股骨干骺端形成偏心性包块。病变膨胀，周围有薄的新生骨壳。

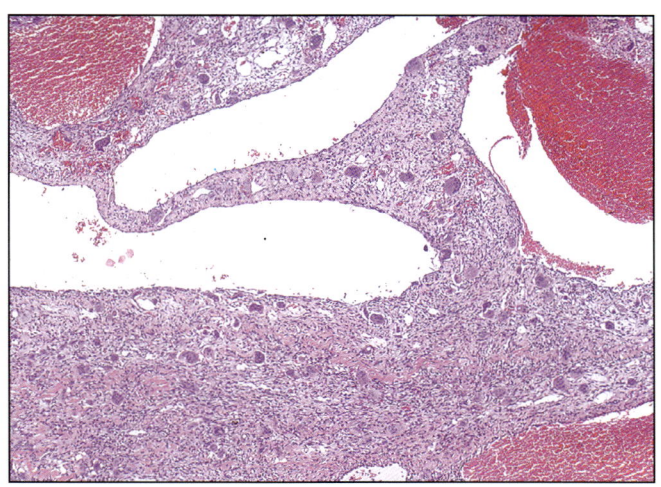

图25.78 动脉瘤样骨囊肿，显示囊腔是由不具有非典型性的梭形细胞和散在的多核巨细胞构成的间隔围绕而成。

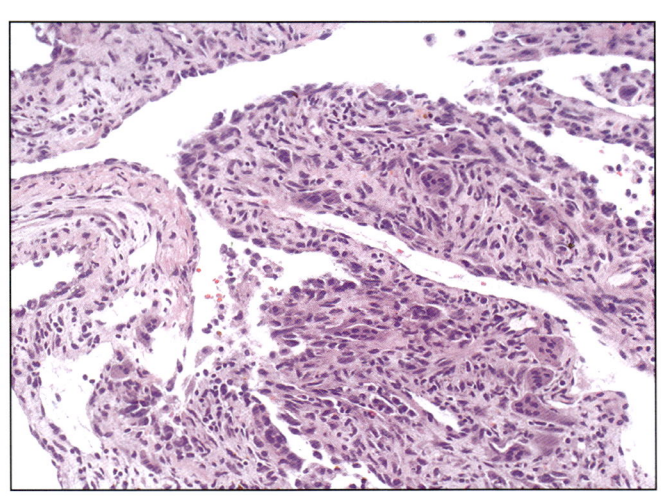

图25.79 动脉瘤样骨囊肿的纤维间隔由梭形的纤维母细胞和散在的多核巨细胞构成。

可以表现为浸润性生长。

　　软组织扩展通常受新骨形成的骨壳限制（图25.77）。CT 和 MRI 显示有液平，这是有益于诊断的特征[239]。然而，毛细血管扩张型骨肉瘤也可以显示有液平。在大体标本上，病变显示由间隔分成腔隙。腔隙通常含有血液或浆液。获得的病理标本的数量与 X 光片提示的尺寸相比通常要小得多。这是因为当病变刮除后腔隙被破坏所致。

　　显微镜下，低倍镜显示动脉瘤样骨囊肿被间隔分成大小不等的囊腔。囊腔可能含有血液或浆液。间隔由疏松排列的梭形细胞和良性巨细胞组成（图25.78）。腔隙内衬立方细胞。间隔有毛细血管增生。梭形细胞显示核分裂活跃，但是没有细胞学非典型性。典型的表现是：在立方细胞下层有薄层骨形成，称为纤维骨样组织。区域内可见相对实性的细胞增生区域，在后者通常能发现相当数量的反应性新骨形成。新生骨可以在梭形细胞间形成缎带样基质，通常逐渐形成更多成熟的骨小梁。骨小梁衬覆肥胖的、具有良性表现的骨母细胞。纤细的钙化基质出现也是特征性的，这对动脉瘤样骨囊肿具有诊断意义（图25.79）[240]。动脉瘤样骨囊肿可以继发于一种基础病变，后者几乎总是良性的[241,242]。以我们的经验，最常见的病变是软骨母细胞瘤、巨细胞瘤和纤维发育不良。

　　如上文提到的，一些动脉瘤样骨囊肿显示或多或少的实性区域。由此产生了一些动脉瘤样骨囊肿是完全实性的观点[243]。这些病变显示梭形细胞增生，伴有活跃的核分裂，但是没有细胞学非典型性。但是，梭形细胞排列疏松，不像在肿瘤中那样致密。梭形细胞没有明显的生长方式。在典型的病变，新骨形成向其周边部逐渐成熟，类似于在异位骨化中见到的表现。一些作者不同意实性动脉瘤样骨囊肿这一名称。他们将这种病变与已熟知的巨细胞反应或手或足的小骨的巨细胞修复性肉芽肿进行了对比，倾向于使用巨细胞修复性肉芽肿（giant cell reparative granuloma）这一名称[244-246]。无论使用什么名称，重要的是要认识到，这种病变不是肉瘤。动脉瘤样骨囊肿是良性病变，单纯刮除通常可以治愈。但是，病变可能复发，而且可以非常迅速地长到很大。治疗应该保守些，但是要完整切除。

鉴别诊断应该包括巨细胞瘤和骨肉瘤。动脉瘤样骨囊肿中常常出现良性巨细胞。大多数情况下，它们呈簇状排列。然而，在一些罕见的情况下，肿瘤可以有非常丰富的巨细胞，这种表现可能提示是巨细胞瘤。然而，肿瘤背景显示纤维化，细胞为梭形而不是像巨细胞瘤中那样呈卵圆形。巨细胞瘤发生在成人的骨端，而动脉瘤样骨囊肿发生在年轻患者的干骺端。巨细胞瘤发生在脊椎，累及椎体，而动脉瘤样骨囊肿累及脊侧椎骨。需与实性动脉瘤样骨囊肿鉴别的是骨肉瘤；但是低级别骨肉瘤比动脉瘤样骨囊肿细胞要少得多。高级别骨肉瘤表现出显著的多形性。

单纯性囊肿　Simple cyst

骨的单纯性囊肿发生在年幼儿童的肱骨近端和股骨近端。男孩受累比女孩明显多见，常见的症状是病理性骨折。X光片显示位于骨中心的单纯性透亮缺损，向上延伸至骺板（图25.80）。受累骨通常不膨胀。

在大体标本上，标本显示囊性，伴有薄层的纤维衬覆，含有清亮的黄色液体。显微镜下，可见薄的纤维间隔，

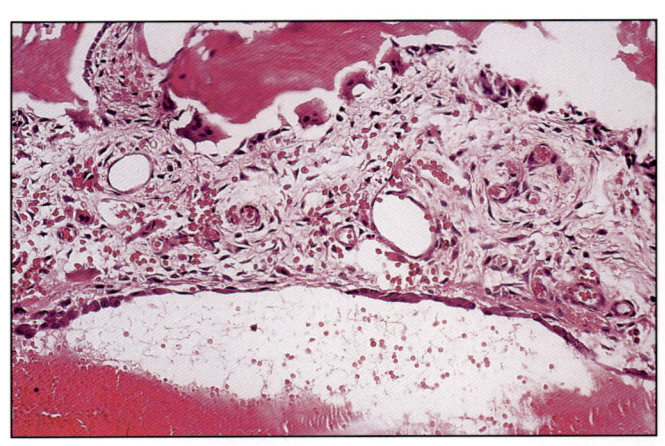

图25.81　单纯性骨囊肿的纤维间隔含有疏松的纤维母细胞间质，并有散在的炎细胞和良性巨细胞。

偶尔可见巨细胞（图25.81）。一些单纯性囊肿有与牙骨质相似的独特的钙化性间质。当出现这种物质时，就可以明确诊断为单纯性骨囊肿了。

单纯性囊肿的现代治疗是将液体吸出，注入醋酸甲泼尼龙[247]。因此，大多数单纯性囊肿并不取活检。注射醋酸甲泼尼龙失败后复发的病变可采用手术治疗。

腱鞘囊肿　Ganglion cyst

腱鞘囊肿是少见的骨内病变，总是发生在骨末端。此病可能与邻近的关节相连。

X光片显示单纯性的透亮缺损，偶尔伴有硬化的边缘（图25.82）。大体标本上和显微镜下，表现与更为常见的软组织腱鞘囊肿相似，有纤维性衬覆和黏液性物质[248]。

纤维性病变　Fibrous lesions

骨的几种纤维性病变可能类似于肿瘤。

纤维发育不良　Fibrous dysplasia

纤维发育不良可能代表一种骨化缺陷，然而新近的资料显示（主要来自遗传性病例），GNAS1中的突变可能是重要的发病机制。纤维发育不良可能为骨的单发病灶，也可能累及多骨。多骨性纤维发育不良患者可能伴有皮肤色素沉着和青春期性早熟，尤其是在女孩，这种改变称作Albright综合征[249]。已经有报道称一些Albright综合征患者伴有佝偻病[250]。

大多数纤维发育不良患者是青少年或年轻成人。病变常常累及近端股骨、肋骨、颌骨和颅骨。纤维发育不

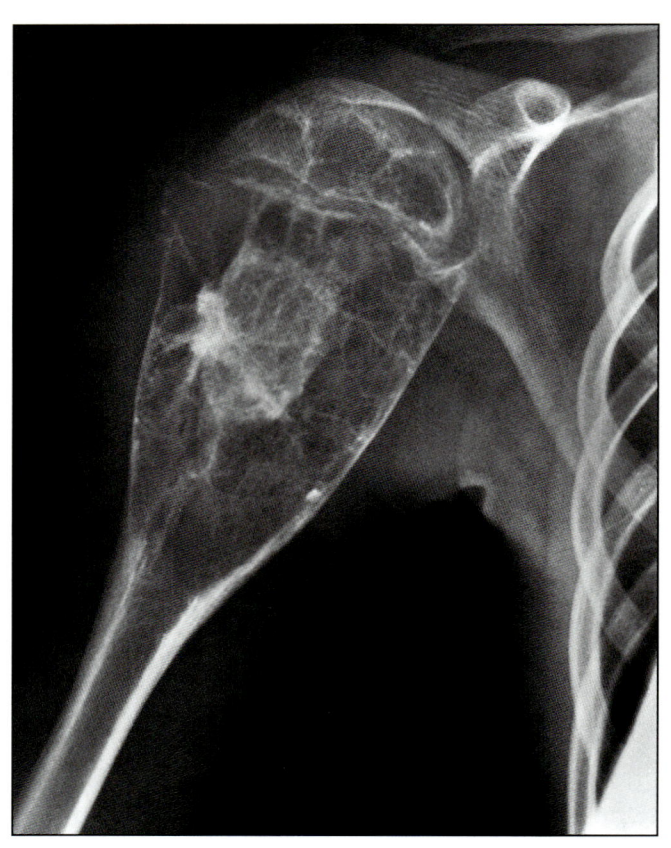

图25.80　肱骨近端单纯性囊肿的X光片，显示穿过溶骨性病变的病理性骨折，病变扩展到骨末端。

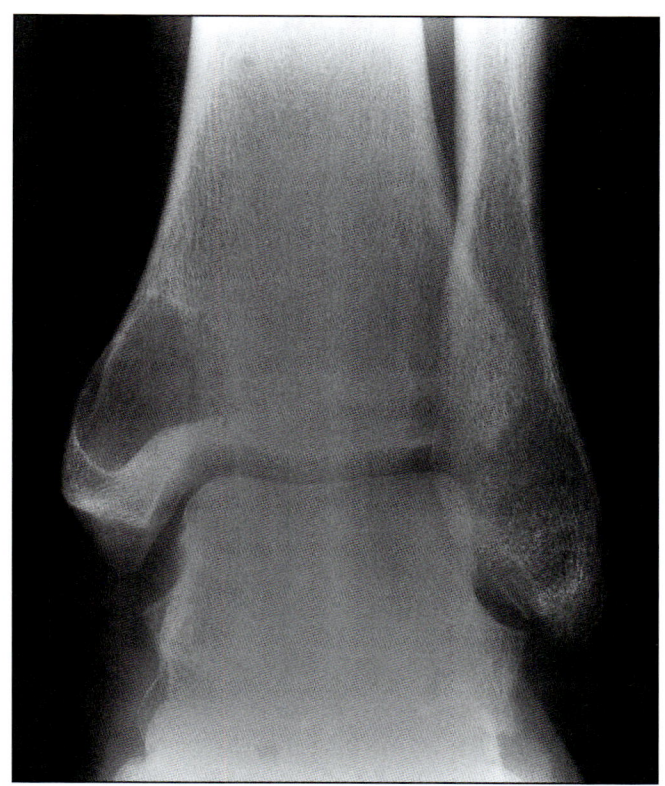

图25.82 骨内腱鞘囊肿的X光片，显示溶骨性表现，周围有硬化。

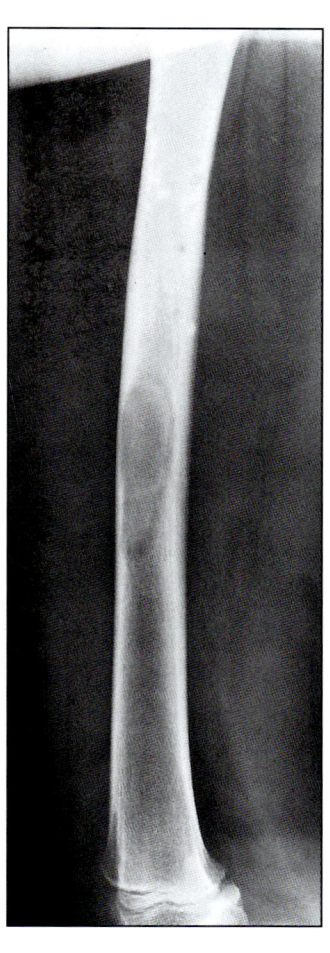

图25.83 纤维发育不良的X光片，显示股骨的骨干有一边界清晰的透光性病变。

良通常没有什么症状。颌骨的纤维发育不良患者可能有面部轮廓的不对称。累及眼眶周围区域的可以引起眼球突出。累及股骨颈的患者可能出现病理性骨折。

纤维发育不良的影像学表现通常十分典型。病变为边界清晰的、伴有硬化边缘的透亮区（图25.83）。病变可能会有些模糊不清；这种表现被描述为毛玻璃样表现。

在大体标本上，纤维发育不良质韧并具呈纤维状。由于出现化生性骨化，当切开时可能有砂砾感。显微镜下，纤维发育不良显示梭形细胞增生。病变细胞相当稀少，有丰富的胶原形成。梭形细胞通常较短，不像真正的梭形细胞肉瘤的那样拉长。细胞生长没有结构；但是偶尔可能见到席纹状排列的区域。纤维发育不良的特征性表现是产生化生骨。这种骨是由看似被梭形细胞分割的小梁构成，特征明显（图25.84）。梭形细胞表现为直接成骨，不伴有骨母细胞形成；然而，骨的边缘出现骨母细胞并不能排除纤维发育不良的诊断。

以上描述是纤维发育不良的常见表现，一些少见的特征也可以看到。一些纤维发育不良伴有大量的泡沫细胞。一些纤维发育不良，尤其是在股骨颈部，含有大量的软骨岛[251]。这可能导致误诊为软骨肿瘤。纤维发育不良常常显示黏液样变，这可能提示黏液瘤或软骨黏液

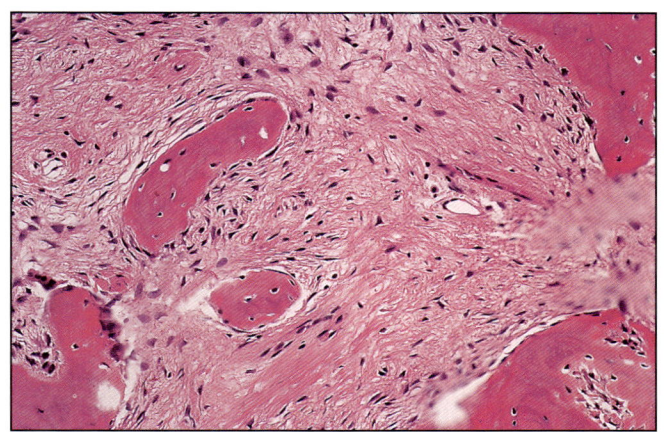

图25.84 纤维发育不良，显示不规则的骨小梁穿过细胞稀疏的增生的梭形细胞，无细胞学非典型性。

样纤维瘤的诊断。纤维发育不良常常显示出圆形沙粒体样骨形成，类似脑膜瘤的表现。也可能见到继发性动脉瘤样骨囊肿，并且可能出现快速生长，提示肉瘤样[252,253]。纤维发育不良的恶变不常见。一些有肉瘤

变的患者常有放疗病史。尽管如此，一些文献也报道了纤维发育不良自发转变为软骨肉瘤或梭形细胞肉瘤的病例[254-256]。

骨纤维发育不良　Osteofibrous dysplasia

我们认为，骨纤维发育不良是一种纤维发育不良的变型[257-260]。这种病变最初被描述为骨化纤维瘤[261]。病变主要累及幼儿的胫骨，偶尔累及腓骨。一些患者可能是先天性的。X 光片显示骨皮质受累，为溶骨和硬化混合性病变（图 25.85）。这种表现类似于釉质瘤的影像学表现。显微镜下，骨纤维发育不良显示梭形细胞增生和骨形成。骨形成常常有活跃的骨母细胞镶边。这与在纤维发育不良中看到的表现十分不同。骨纤维发育不良是一种自限性病变，如果对有骨折的患者施以保守性治疗，病变常常可以退化。如上文所提到的（见 1626 页），有现象表明，釉质瘤和骨纤维发育不良可能有关联。

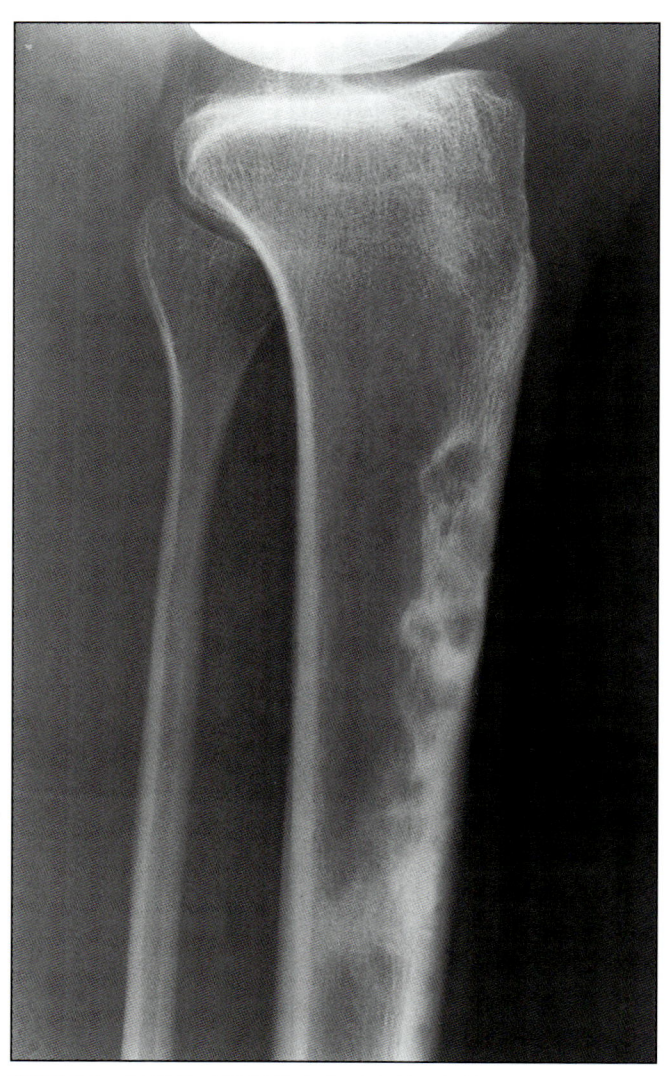

图 25.85　胫骨骨干的纤维发育不良的 X 光片，显示累及皮质的多处透亮区，间隔处有明显的硬化。

干骺纤维缺损　Metaphyseal fibrous defect

纤维瘤、非骨化性纤维瘤和纤维皮质缺损这些名称都曾被用于描述这种病变。我们更愿意使用干骺纤维缺损这一名称，因为它描述了病变的位置，而且提示了这种病变并非真正的肿瘤。病变通常是在小于 20 岁的年轻患者进行 X 光片检查时偶然发现的。在骨骼成熟后，干骺纤维缺损非常少见。患者可能出现病理性骨折。X 光片显示位于长骨干骺端的单纯性透亮性缺损。病变有硬化、波浪形边缘，形成扇贝样表现。在少数情况下，具有所有干骺纤维缺损特征表现的病变可能出现在少见的位置，如锁骨和髂骨。

在大体标本上，组织呈颗粒状，为褐色和黄色。组织学上，干骺纤维缺损显示梭形细胞增生，细胞排列疏松并有特征性的席纹状结构（图 25.86）。良性巨细胞常常散在分布。总是出现泡沫细胞和含铁血黄素沉积。常见核分裂象，但是缺乏细胞学非典型性。

干骺纤维缺损常是偶然发现的，除非即将发生病理性骨折，否则不需要治疗[262]。在少数情况下，患者可出现多发性干骺纤维缺损（图 25.87）。这可能导致骨骼畸形。其中一些患者可能有皮肤色素沉着、智力发育迟缓和内分泌异常[263,264]。

两种其他病变可能与干骺纤维缺损有关。一些干骺纤维缺损含有明显的泡沫细胞成分，包括胆固醇结晶沉积。在少数情况下，病变只含有胆固醇结晶和泡沫细胞。这些病变被命名为黄色瘤。它们可能是干骺纤维缺损这类病变的终末阶段。

1951 年，Kimmelstiel 和 Rapp[265] 描述了累及年幼儿童股骨远端的病变，采用了骨膜纤维组织增生性纤维

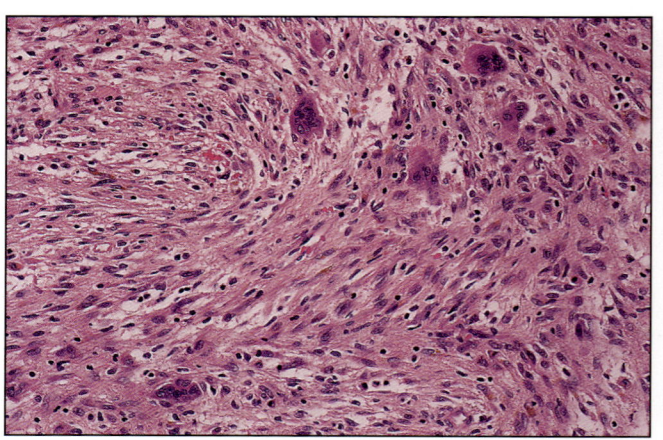

图 25.86　干骺纤维缺损，显示无细胞学非典型性的梭形细胞排列成席纹状结构，散在慢性炎细胞和良性巨细胞。

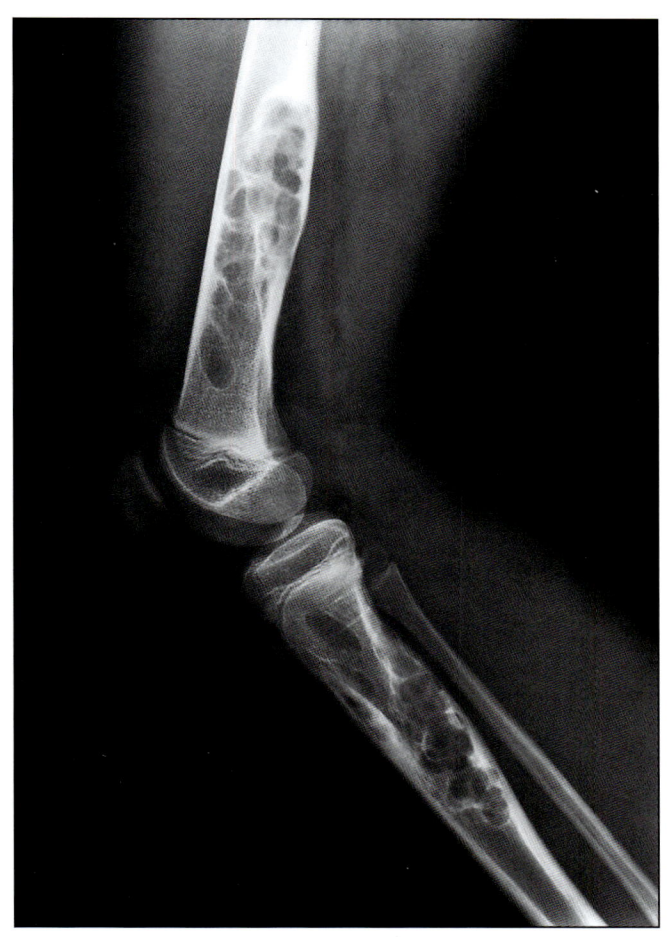

图25.87 干骺纤维缺损的X光片，显示在股骨末端骨干的多发病变以及胫骨近端骨干透亮的多房性表现。

状增生。病变常常有黏液样或软骨样背景。其特征性表现是：在血管腔隙周围排列着更多的梭形细胞区域，类似于血管外皮细胞瘤的表现。这种表现在骨骼病变中非常罕见。更常见的是有扩张的血管腔。这些梭形细胞有肥胖的细胞核和嗜酸性胞浆，与肌纤维母细胞一致。病变可自行消退，预后很好。

伴有反应性新骨形成的病变
Conditions with reactive new bone formation

骨痂　Fracture callus

骨痂通常不会引起诊断问题。受累患者通常有创伤史，X线显示骨折并伴有新骨形成。然而，当检查骨痂切片时，X线表现必须与单纯骨痂形成的诊断符合。重要的是，我们不要漏掉可能引起病理性骨折的潜在的肿瘤性病变。组织学表现为软骨增生，并逐渐成熟变为骨组织。这种表现可能导致误诊为软骨肉瘤。然而，在软骨肉瘤中，没有从软骨形成小梁状骨的证据。

压缩性骨折常常引起诊断困难。创伤很轻微，X线可能显示不出骨折线。此时常常有弥漫的新骨膜化骨形成，可能类似于小细胞恶性肿瘤的表现，如 Ewing 肉瘤的表现。骨折也可能是在骨质疏松基础上新增加的病变，典型的病变发生在绝经后妇女，累及骨盆骨，尤其是耻骨支和骶骨翼。这些病变被称为不完全性骨折[269]。患者可能先前有恶性肿瘤病史。患者常常主诉骨盆区疼痛。骨扫描通常显示在骶骨和耻骨的多灶浓聚点。平片可能仅仅显示反应性新骨形成；然而，CT通常可显示骨折线。了解这种病变非常重要，可以避免进行不必要的活检。

瘤来命名。这不是一个合适的名称，因为其提示这是一种侵袭性病变。然而，其仅仅是远端皮质纤维的不规则病变，可能与肌腱和韧带的插入有关。如果影像学可以识别，那么不必对这些皮质的不规则病变进行活检[266]。

婴儿肌纤维瘤病
Infantile myofibromatosis

婴儿肌纤维瘤病是相对罕见的病变（也见第24章）。它常发生在婴儿，主要累及软组织。这种病变可以是孤立性的也可是多发性的。病变也可以累及骨骼，通常在受累的长骨干骺端形成双侧对称的透光性病变。即使骨骼多处受累，预后也很好。病变常常自行退化。仅仅当病变累及内脏器官时，如肝和胃肠道，才会出现严重的临床问题。

婴儿肌纤维瘤病可能表现为孤立性的骨骼病变[267,268]。在 Mayo Clinic 的资料中[268]，发病年龄范围从6个月到16岁，中位年龄为15.5个月。X线一般表现为边界清楚的透光区。

组织学上，婴儿肌纤维瘤病表现为梭形细胞的结节

骨化性肌炎　Myositis ossification

骨化性肌炎或异位骨化（heterotopic ossification）并不累及骨。很少能看到异位骨化附着于其下的骨组织。患者一般为年轻成人，可能或不能回忆起曾有外伤史。病变增长速度很快。影像学显示界限清楚的病变，周围伴有钙化，中心为透亮区（图25.88）。这种分带在CT上可以显示得更加清楚。在大体标本上，病变界限非常清晰，中心显示为水肿样外观的骨骼肌。病变周围为钙化灶（图25.89）。组织学上，中心区域显示疏松排列的梭形细胞增生，使人想起结节性筋膜炎。虽然核分裂象很明显，但没有细胞学非典型性。病变越接近周边越趋于成熟，产生骨样层，这层钙化逐渐形成小梁状骨（图25.90）。这种分带的表现，正如 Ackerman[270] 描述的那

伴有反应性新骨形成的病变

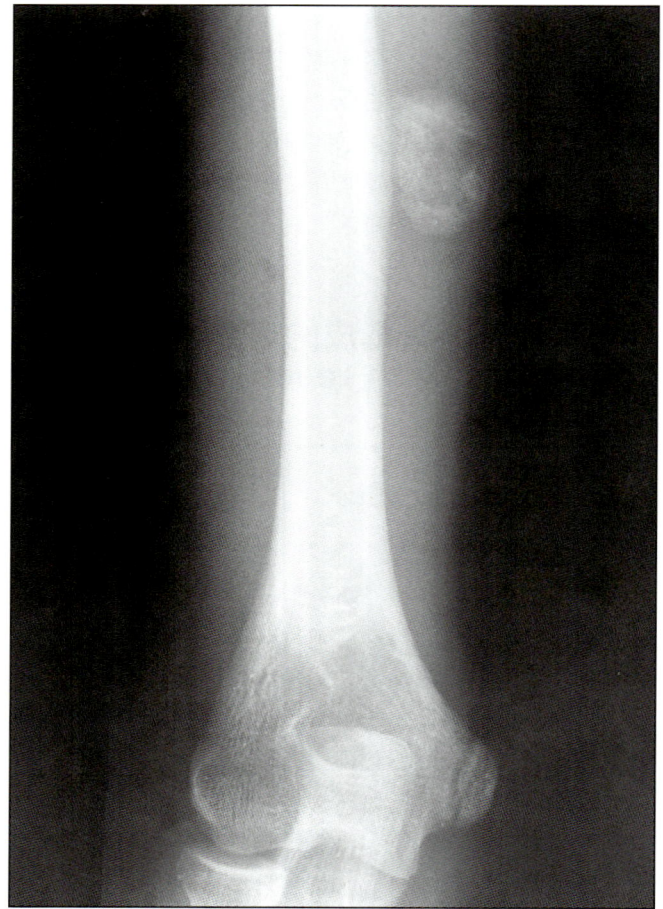

图25.88　骨化性肌炎。有界限清楚、部分骨化的影像学表现。(Courtesy of Dr. B. Khan, Thorek Medical Center, Chicago, IL.)

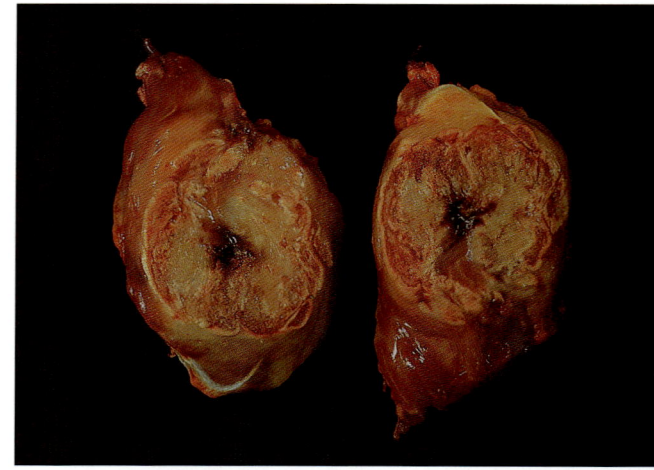

图25.89　骨化性肌炎的大体标本，显示为界限清楚的病变，伴有中心出血，周围为质地较硬的灰黄色组织，外周为骨壳。

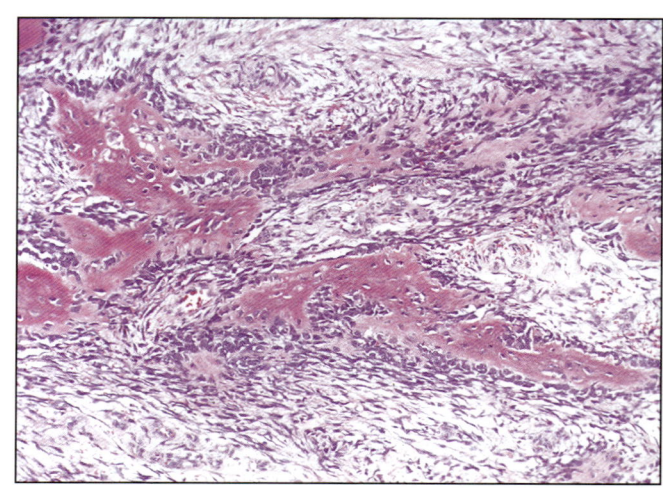

图25.90　在这例骨化性肌炎中，可见分带表现，含有增生活跃的纤维母细胞区域，逐渐成熟形成完好的骨小梁。

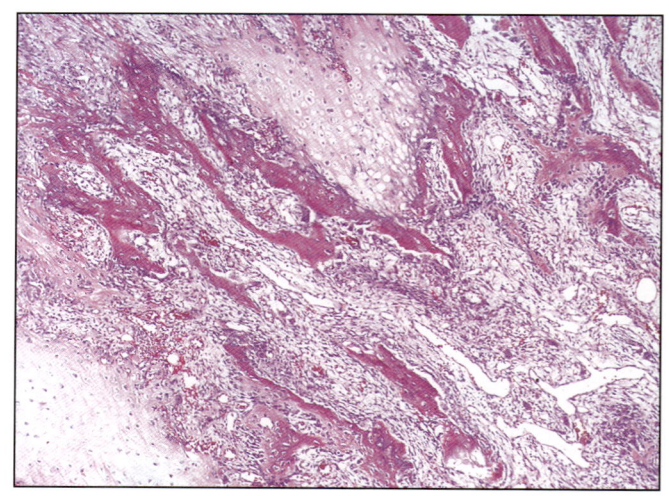

图25.91　甲下外生性骨疣的软骨组织侵入编织骨的骨小梁中，小梁周围为疏松纤维血管结缔组织。

样，一直是鉴别异位骨化和骨外骨肉瘤的最好的标准。在少数情况下，患者表现为多中心的骨化性肌炎，也称为进行性骨化性肌炎（或纤维发育不良）[myositis (or fibrodysplasia) ossification progressive]。这些患者也伴有骨骼的异常，长期预后不良[271]。虽然，异位骨化如果不予治疗最终会消融，但是有报道说，偶尔有病例可以在此基础上发生骨肉瘤[272]。

指（趾）甲下外生性骨疣
Subungual exostosis

指（趾）甲下外生性骨疣是很少见的病变，仅发生在甲床下。这种病变出现独有的染色体异常，t (X;6)，提示其发病机制是肿瘤性的而非反应性的[273]。病变明显好发于大拇趾。患者年龄通常为11～20岁[274]。病变处可感疼痛，可能掀起趾甲，并引起溃疡。整个病变可能看起来是黑色的，临床上可能与甲下黑色素瘤混淆。影像学显示为附着于脚趾趾骨末端的钙化性病变，但是并不与其相连续，就像在真正的骨软骨瘤中见到的那样[64]。大体表现可能与骨软骨瘤一样，具有厚的不规则的软骨帽和骨柄。组织学上，软骨呈增生表现，细胞数量增加，常常有双核细胞；但是有规则性地逐渐成熟，变为小梁样骨（图 25.91）。小梁间隙含有增生的梭形细胞。这种骨、软骨和梭形细胞的联合增生可能导致误诊为骨肉瘤。然而，典型的部位和良性的影像学表现可为正确诊断做出提示。某种形式的甲下黑色素瘤可产生化生骨及软骨，可能误诊为甲下外生性骨疣[275]。

奇异性骨旁骨软骨瘤样增生
Bizarre parosteal osteochondromatous proliferation

奇异性骨旁骨软骨瘤样增生是 1983 年由 Nora 等[61]最先描述的，它是一种少见的累及小骨的反应性病变，手比足常见。然而最近确定，这些病变易复发，并且有特异性的 t(1;17) 易位[276]，提示这可能是一种克隆性肿瘤性病变。一项来自 Mayo Clinic[277] 的综述描述了 65 例患者；其中 1/4 累及长骨。女性稍好发，病变可以发生在任何年龄段。影像学显示非常明显的钙化包块以宽基底附着于其下的皮质（图 25.92）。组织学上，低倍镜下，病变类似于骨软骨瘤。大量软骨可以排列成帽状或小叶状结构。典型的表现是：软骨发生软骨内骨化，成熟变为骨组织。这种成骨会有特征性的深蓝色质地，尤其是在软骨界面上更是如此（图 25.93）。骨小梁间隙含有增生的梭形细胞，这些细胞缺乏细胞学非典型性。

软骨增生的性质和骨小梁间梭形细胞的出现常常会导致误诊为软骨肉瘤或骨肉瘤。尽管如此，典型的影像学表现和软骨逐渐成熟为少见的蓝色的骨，有助于做出正确的诊断。复发很常见，但是还没有报告发生恶变的病例。这种病变在组织学上与指（趾）活跃的反应性骨膜炎[278]和纤维骨样假瘤[279]不同（见第 24 章）。

其他各类疾病
Miscellaneous conditions

骨髓炎　Osteomyelitis

骨髓炎有特征性的临床表现，包括疼痛、发热和红细胞沉降率升高，因此不会出现诊断困难。然而，骨髓炎可能类似于肿瘤[280]。急性骨髓炎在临床和影像学上都可以类似于恶性淋巴瘤或 Ewing 肉瘤。慢性骨髓炎或 Brodie 脓肿可能会提示骨样骨瘤的诊断。

大多数骨髓炎是由金黄色葡萄球菌引起的，显示由炎性细胞构成的渗出物（图 25.94）。然而，骨髓炎也可以由真菌和结核杆菌引起，表现为肉芽肿。在骨骼中，骨髓炎几乎总是表现为单发病变（图 25.95）。但是，在少数情况下，患者表现为多灶性骨髓炎。

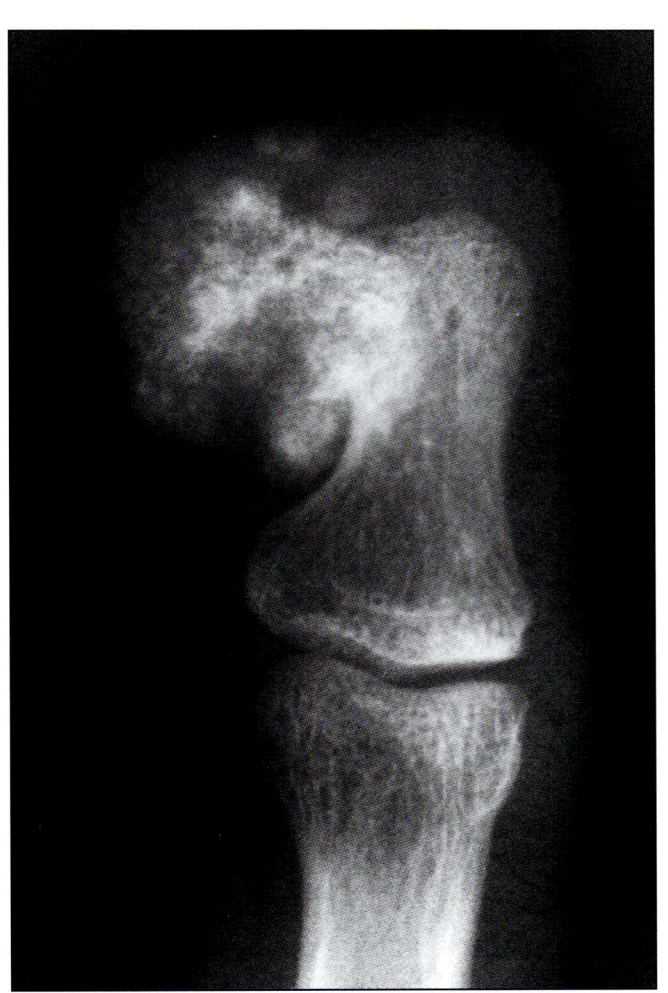

图25.92 奇异性骨旁骨软骨瘤样增生的影像学，显示钙化包块附着于指（趾）骨的末端的表面。（Courtesy of Dr. I. M. M. Taylor, Medlab Tauranga, Tauranga, New Zealand.）

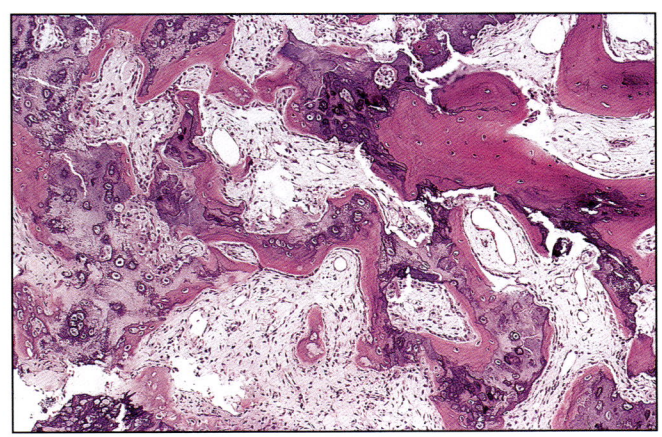

图25.93 奇异性骨旁骨软骨瘤样增生。显示软骨成熟化骨，周围有纤维母细胞增生，不伴有细胞学非典型性。注意图中具有特征性的深蓝色软骨，它逐渐成熟为骨。

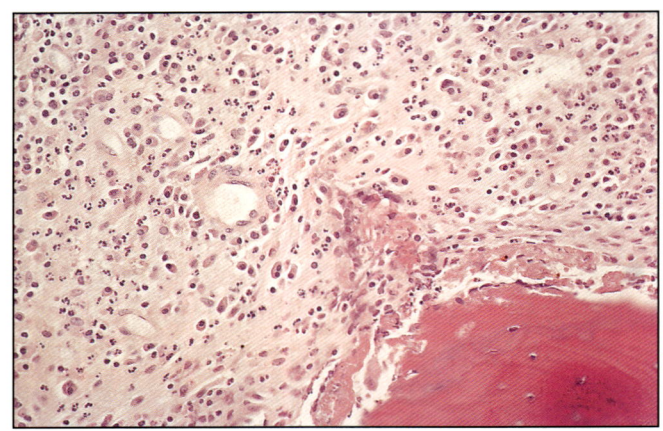

图25.94 急性骨髓炎。显示毛细血管增生，骨小梁周围有大量中性粒细胞、浆细胞和淋巴细胞。

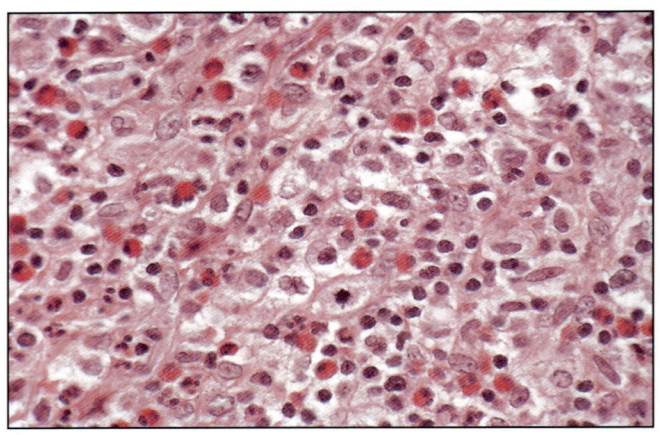

图25.96 Langerhans细胞组织细胞增生症的X线片，显示一种多形性病变，由具有折叠或沟纹状细胞核的Langerhans细胞、中性粒细胞、嗜酸性粒细胞、淋巴细胞和浆细胞组成。

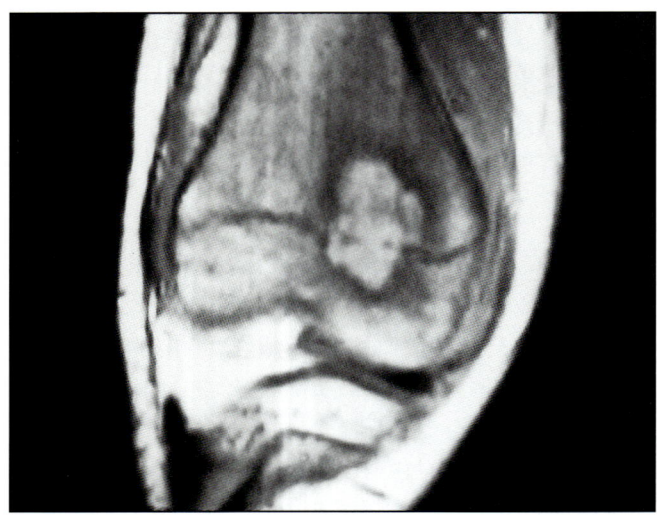

图25.95 10岁女孩的股骨远端的跨过骺板的骨髓炎的核磁共振影像。（Courtesy of Dr. D. S. Forth, The Permanente Medical Group, Walnut Creek, CA.）

一些患者有迁延不愈的骨髓炎，可能伴有引流的窦道。在一些长期伴有窦道的骨髓炎患者，其窦道可以发生恶变，恶变几乎总是分化非常好的鳞状细胞癌。癌通常分化得非常好，以至于单独根据细胞学无法作出诊断。然而，在一个有窦道的骨内出现鳞状上皮，就可以诊断鳞状细胞癌。由于在大多数病例中，癌分化非常好，故其预后也很好。治疗通常采用截肢术。在少数情况下，可出现高级别癌[281]。更为罕见的是慢性骨髓炎的窦道可以伴发肉瘤[282]。

Langerhans细胞组织细胞增生症
Langerhans cell histiocytosis

1953年，Lichtenstein[283]提出，嗜酸性肉芽肿、Hand-Schüller-Christian病和Letterer-Siwe病具有共同的病理学特征。他采用组织细胞增生症X这个名称来提示这是一种原因不清的疾病[283]。这种一病论的假说受到Lieberman等[284]的挑战，后者提出，Letterer-Siwe病不是一种特异的组织学病变，而是一种伴有不同病理学过程的临床综合征，就像白血病。然而，至少有一些Letterer-Siwe病例的临床综合征显示出Langerhans细胞组织细胞增生症的组织学特征[285]。因为所有类型的Langerhans细胞组织细胞增生症的患者都被发现有克隆性组织细胞，故现在认为，Langerhans细胞组织细胞增生症是一种克隆增生性疾病（见第21章）[286]。

Langerhans细胞组织细胞增生症患者的临床表现与其受累的范围有关。单一病灶（所谓的嗜酸性肉芽肿）可能是影像学检查发现，也可能有疼痛症状。呈慢性播散性表现的患者可能表现为眼球突出症或糖尿病尿崩症。

骨的影像学表现通常比较典型。在长骨，病变常常累及骨干，显示出边界清楚的透光区，伴有增厚的、具有良性表现的新骨膜化骨形成。在颅骨的表现被比作洞中有洞，这是由于两片颅骨的破坏几率不同。

组织学上，Langerhans细胞组织细胞增生症由增生的所谓Langerhans细胞构成。这些细胞有卵圆形细胞核和粉染或透亮的胞浆（图25.96）。细胞核有特征性的纵形沟纹，呈咖啡豆样外观。嗜酸性粒细胞通常很多（图25.97），甚至可能形成嗜酸性脓肿。良性巨细胞可能出现，并且可能很显著。其他炎细胞也可以见到，如浆细胞、淋巴细胞和多形核白细胞。在骨的Langerhans细胞组织细胞增生症中，广泛的坏死并不少见。

鉴别诊断包括骨髓炎和恶性淋巴瘤。仅有一些少见的形成肉芽肿的骨髓炎要考虑与Langerhans细胞组织细胞增生症鉴别。Langerhans细胞组织细胞增生症的细胞S-100蛋白呈阳性，但是CD1a是最特异性的标记物[287]。

恶性淋巴瘤显示成片的肿瘤细胞，而在Langerhans细胞组织细胞增生症，细胞常常成簇。此外，Langerhans

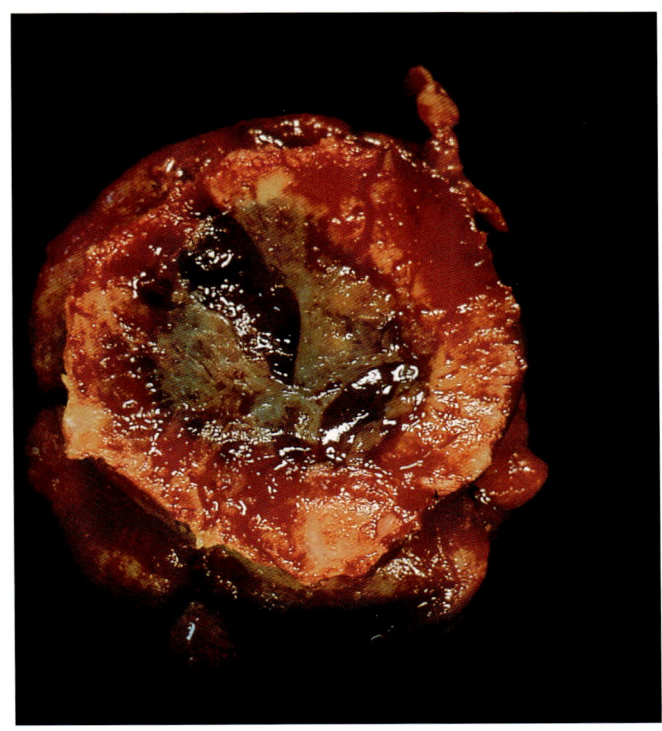

图25.97 组织细胞增生症X的颅骨大体标本，由于病变组织中有大量嗜酸性粒细胞，所以标本呈棕绿色。

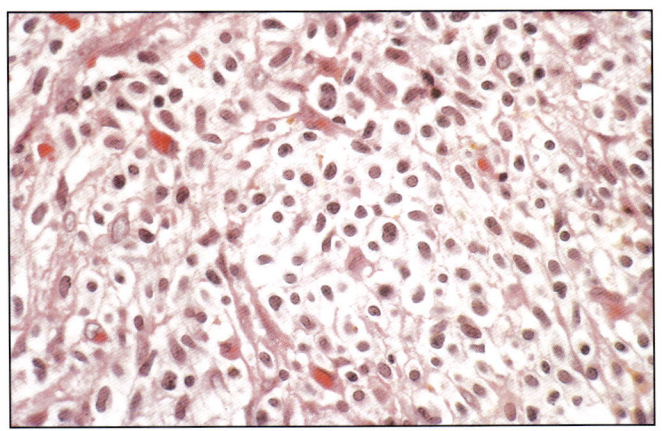

图25.98 累及股骨头的系统性肥大细胞疾病。显示肥大细胞聚集，特征为细胞核呈圆形或卵圆形，胞浆透亮，胞界清晰。

细胞组织细胞增生症的细胞并不显示细胞学非典型性，而且常用的造血系统免疫标记物，如CD45、CD20盒CD3，呈阴性。

一些较早的研究[288-289]提示，Langerhans细胞组织细胞增生症的预后可以根据组织学特征预测。另一些研究提出，若患者诊断时年龄小、肝脾大、血小板减少和多骨受累，则预后可能不良[290]。

肥大细胞增多症 Mastocytosis

目前认为，肥大细胞增多症可能表现为皮肤疾病，这样的病例命名为色素性荨麻疹，也可以表现为系统性疾病伴有或不伴有皮肤受累（见第22章）。皮肤受累的患者预后好，而系统性肥大细胞疾病的预后无法预测。患有系统性肥大细胞疾病的患者可能伴有其他导致死亡的恶性疾病[291]。

大约1/4的系统性肥大细胞疾病患者出现骨骼的症状，如骨骼疏松症或病理性骨折[292]；然而，60%显示有骨骼受累的影像学表现。影像学可能显示出弥漫的骨质疏松或出现伴有硬化的多发性溶骨性区域。后者的表现通常会导致误诊为转移癌。

组织学上，肥大细胞疾病患者通常有骨髓的局灶性病变。肥大细胞趋向于聚集于骨小梁附近，骨小梁可能增厚。肥大细胞呈圆形或卵圆形，有非常清晰的细胞边界（图25.98）。细胞常常形成结节，出现肉芽肿表现，并且经常伴有嗜酸性粒细胞。免疫组化能检测到类胰蛋白酶（tryptase），后者出现在肥大细胞的分泌颗粒中，是一种能在石蜡切片中进行检测的又敏感又特异的标记物[293]。

虽然肥大细胞疾病的预后无法预测，但它极少会引起死亡[294]。

伴有巨大淋巴结病的窦组织细胞增生症 Sinus histiocytosis with massive lymphadenopathy

伴有巨大淋巴结病的窦组织细胞增生症（Rosai-Dorfman病）最先是作为一种累及淋巴结的不明病因的疾病进行描述的[295]，但是不久就认识到，这种疾病过程可以累及其他器官。在对伴有巨大淋巴结病的窦组织细胞增生症进行全面回顾中，我们发现，骨骼是这种疾病第五最常累及的部位[296]。累及骨的窦组织细胞增生症的影像学表现不是很明显。我们见过累及骨的单一部位的病例以及累及多部位的病例。一些患者的病程会不断进展。组织学表现与在淋巴结中的表现相似。增生的组织细胞有透明或粉染的胞浆。组织细胞的胞浆中含有淋巴细胞和浆细胞（细胞吞噬作用）。浆细胞散布在组织细胞之间，有纤维化的背景。组织细胞S-100蛋白呈强阳性。虽然大多数病例的预后似乎很好，但是对于这种罕见的病变，还没有足够的信息来预测其长期的预后。

胸壁错构瘤 Chest wall hamartoma

胸壁错构瘤是一种非常罕见的良性病变，累及新生儿的肋骨。此病的首次介绍是作为胸廓内的间叶性肿瘤来描述的[297]。从那时起，我们已经认识到病变的良性性质，并命名为错构瘤[298,299]。

患者是新生儿或婴儿，表现为累及胸壁的多分叶的

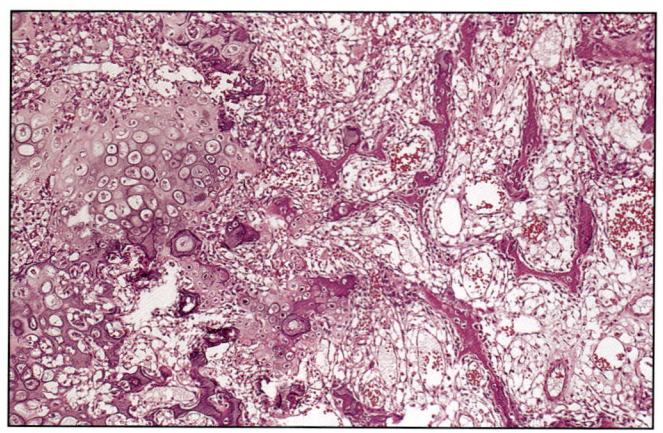

图25.99 胸壁错构瘤。显示一种混合性表现，不规则的软骨结节逐渐成熟为骨小梁。骨小梁周围有细胞丰富的纤维母细胞增生。

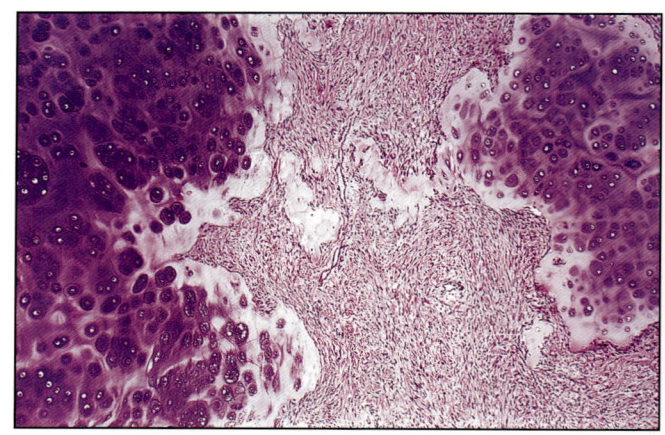

图25.100 具有透明软骨结节状包块的纤维软骨间叶瘤，显示软骨内骨化区域，周围围绕着富于细胞的梭形细胞间质。

包块。病变可能影响正常分娩。影像学显示累及多个肋骨的畸形和软组织包块。在新生儿中，影像学表现为累及多处肋骨的边界清楚的包块，可诊断为胸壁错构瘤。显微镜下，病变由软骨、骨和增生的梭形细胞构成（图25.99）。囊性空隙常常提示动脉瘤样骨囊肿的诊断。梭形细胞排列成疏松的束状结构。软骨形成软骨板，并逐渐成熟为骨小梁，类似于骺板的表现。

胸壁错构瘤的预后非常好，如果已经认识到是这种病变，不必要施行外科手术。病变应能够自行消退。

纤维软骨间叶瘤
Fibrocartilaginous mesenchymoma

1984年，Dahlin等[300]报告了一种罕见的以前未见过的骨肿瘤。他们所描述的病变显示为软骨和梭形细胞增生。这些病例是从Mayo Clinic诊断为纤维发育不良的会诊记录中重新检索到的。由于一些病例局部复发，有作者采用具有低度恶性的纤维软骨间质瘤来命名它。12例该病病例的后续研究显示，先前的低度恶性的印象并不正确[301]。长期随访，肿瘤没有出现侵袭行为。

这种病变可以累及骨骼的任何部位；但是绝大多数发生在长骨的干骺端。影像学显示以透光性病变为主，但伴有钙化，提示软骨源性。显微镜下，病变显示梭形细胞增生、骨形成以及软骨岛形成。梭形细胞排列成束状，没有非典型性。在增生的梭形细胞中出现化生骨，类似于在纤维发育不良中见到的。病变中软骨岛很常见。这些软骨岛可以表现为梭形细胞间质中的结节，但更为常见的是软骨内骨化的软骨板（图25.100）。这些软骨板中的细胞常常呈现柱状排列，伴有软骨内骨化，类似于骺板的表现。

鉴别诊断有纤维发育不良。在纤维软骨间叶瘤中，细胞增生比纤维发育不良中的更加密集，胶原常常在单个肿瘤细胞间充填。虽然在纤维发育不良中可以看到软骨结节，但是很少见到骺板样结构。

关节肿瘤 Tumors of joints

关节的肿瘤性病变非常少见。关节的恶性肿瘤就更为少见了。偶尔有发生在关节内的滑膜肉瘤的报道。我们在Mayo Clinic的资料中仅见到少数这样的病例。骨的其他肿瘤，如累及骨末端的骨肉瘤，偶尔会累及关节。我们甚至见过股骨末端的骨肉瘤侵入滑膜，在低倍镜下观察，显示类似于色素性绒毛结节状滑膜炎的表现。

Coventry等[302]回顾了1945—1964年Mayo Clinic所做的4000例膝部关节切开术，发现95例滑膜的肿瘤样病变：27例滑膜软骨瘤病，27例色素性绒毛结节状滑膜炎，19例局限性色素性绒毛结节状滑膜炎，11例血管瘤，8例滑膜脂肪瘤，丛状神经瘤、血管肌瘤和黏液瘤各一例。在这组病例中没有一例为恶性肿瘤。

色素性绒毛结节状滑膜炎（同义名：弥漫型巨细胞瘤）
Pigmented villonodular synovitis (synonym: diffuse-type giant cell tumor)

色素性绒毛结节状滑膜炎是由Jaffe等[303]在1941年提出的名称，Jaffe等将累及关节、肌腱和滑膜囊的滑膜增生性病变统一起来。在大关节中，病变趋于弥漫，但是当病变累及肌腱时，则趋于局限，称为腱鞘巨细胞瘤（见24章）。女性略好发，患者通常为年轻成人。患者主诉疼痛、肿胀或活动受限。症状长期持续存在，通常为5年或更长时间。体检通常显示受累关节肿胀、发热。疾病总是累及单关节，且常常累及大关节。在 Mayo Clinic 的一项研究中[304]，有 99 例患者：75 例显示膝部受累，20 例为髋部，2 例为肩部，2 例为肘部。然而，其他关节也可以受累，包括脊柱的关节[305-307]。脊柱的色素性绒毛结节状滑膜炎可能发生在关节面。病变延伸至关节外软组织也十分常见，一些色素性绒毛结节状滑膜炎病例甚至完全发生在关节之外（见第 24 章）[308]。

色素性绒毛结节状滑膜炎的影像学表现通常没有诊断意义。影像学常常显示受累关节弥漫肿胀。MRI 可能检测到病变中的铁色素（图 25.101）。病变中钙化十分少见。一些病例显示两侧关节的骨都有侵蚀[309]。文献有报道，严重的浸润可造成大段的骨破坏[310]。

色素性绒毛结节状滑膜炎的大体表现具有典型性。滑膜增厚非常明显，表面显示出绒毛状结构。如果将标本浸入水中，则能更好地观察绒毛结构。滑膜呈褐色，部分区域有黄色斑点（图 25.102）。

显微镜下，低倍镜观察，滑膜显示绒毛肥大。由于滑膜的组织细胞样细胞增生，绒毛非常明显（图 25.103）。增生的细胞小，呈圆形到卵圆形，有咖啡豆样细胞核。核分裂象常见到，但是没有细胞学非典型性。良性的巨细胞散布在整个病变中。病变中总会找到泡沫细胞聚集和含铁血黄素沉积，但可能是局灶性的。病变中可以看到玻璃样变区域，甚至类似于骨样基质的病变也可找到。肿瘤细胞常常形成假滑膜样裂隙。

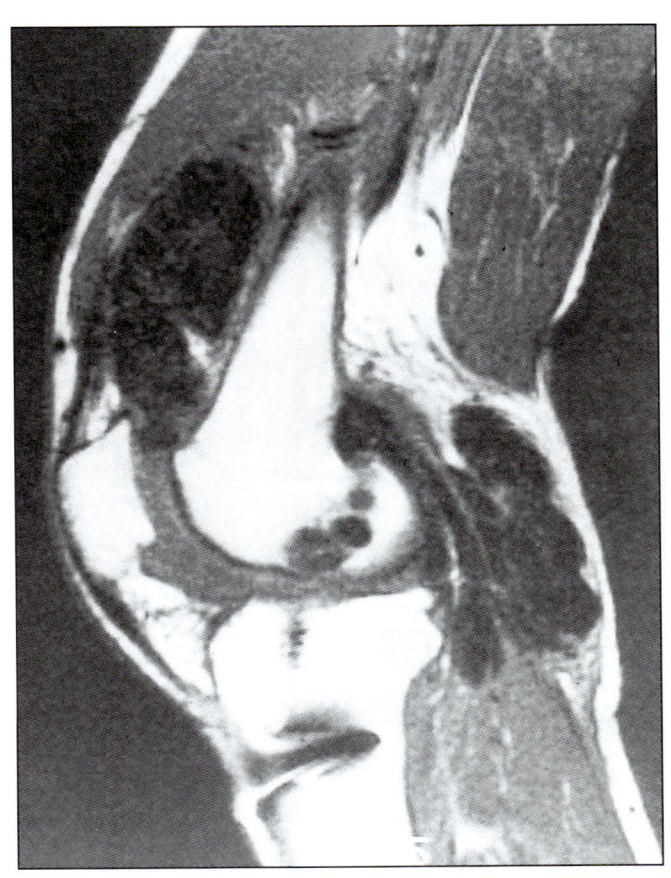

图 25.101　T2 强化的核磁共振影像矢状面，显示膝关节内的大的低信号包块。这种低信号（黑色）是色素性绒毛结节状滑膜炎的特征。大多数肿瘤显示高信号（白色）。

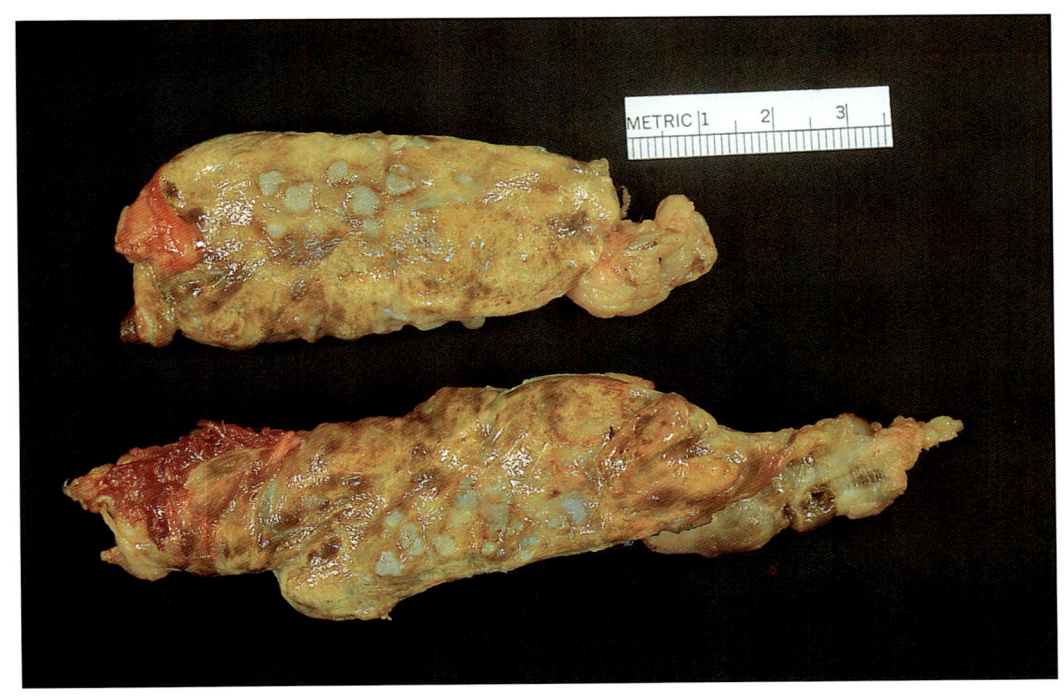

图 25.102　色素性绒毛结节状滑膜炎的大体标本，显示金-黄-褐色和灰色的结节状病变。

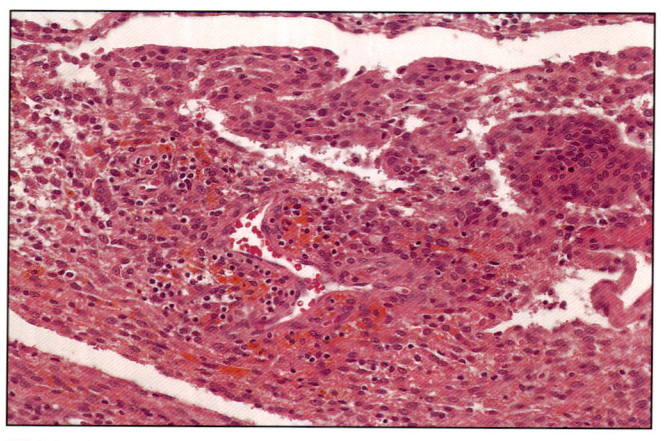

图25.103 色素性绒毛结节状滑膜炎。显示增生的绒毛含有成片的圆形滑膜样细胞、慢性炎性细胞和吞噬含铁血黄素的巨噬细胞。

我们已见到有非常罕见的色素性绒毛结节状滑膜炎发生恶变。后者有结节状浸润性生长方式，并伴有坏死带。细胞变大，呈圆形或卵圆形，伴有明显的核仁[311]。我们至少见过一例发生在关节的肉瘤病例，患者先前有色素性绒毛结节状滑膜炎，并且进行过放疗。真正的恶性肿瘤可以发生在关节，它们与色素性绒毛结节状滑膜炎可能有关，也可能无关[312]。

滑膜软骨瘤病　Synovial chondromatosis

滑膜软骨瘤病是一种罕见的疾病，在关节滑膜中形成软骨结节。同色素性绒毛结节状滑膜炎一样，该病总是单关节发病[313]。膝关节最常受累。男性明显好发，且通常为年轻成人。患者常主诉活动受限、疼痛或肿胀。影像学可显示关节弥漫肿胀（图25.104）。但是，病变中可以见到特征性的软骨型钙化体，使病变易于在术前确诊。

在大体标本上，滑膜明显增厚。蓝白色软骨结节被包埋在增厚的滑膜中（图25.105）。在关节腔内也可以见到漂浮的游离软骨结节。

在滑膜内出现软骨必须诊断滑膜软骨瘤病。在制备良好的切片中，在软骨结节表面可以看到一层扁平的滑膜细胞。软骨是以结节的形式出现的，在结节中的细胞常常成簇排列（图25.106）。这种簇状生长方式具有典型性，但对于滑膜软骨瘤病来说并不具有诊断意义。然而，如果怀疑滑膜软骨瘤病的诊断，并且细胞不显示为簇状生长方式，那么就不能诊断滑膜软骨瘤病。软骨细胞通常显示出中度到显著的非典型性。细胞簇中的细胞可能非常丰富，而且有大量的双核细胞。在特定的情况下，这些表现并不是恶性表现。虽然大部分滑膜软骨瘤病都累及大关节，但是也有累及

鉴别诊断包括患者的滑膜病变。所有类型的滑膜病变中都可以见到绒毛状增生，包括退行性关节炎和类风湿性关节炎的滑膜组织。病变中也可以见到巨细胞，尤其是在类风湿性关节炎中。但是在这些病变中，增生的滑膜不伴有滑膜细胞的增生。用于关节成形术的材料引起的异物反应可能类似于色素性绒毛结节状滑膜炎的表现；甚至可以见到褐色的斑点。然而，在这些病变中可以很清楚地见到异物的碎片，尤其是在巨细胞中。

绝大多数累及大关节的色素性绒毛结节状滑膜炎呈弥漫的生长方式。但是有少数病变显示为局限型色素性绒毛结节状滑膜炎。病变表现为褐色结节，通过一个蒂与滑膜相连。

色素性绒毛结节状滑膜炎的长期预后非常好。然而，弥漫性病变需行全滑膜切除术。预计大约有1/4的患者可能复发。但是在局限型病变，复发极其少见。

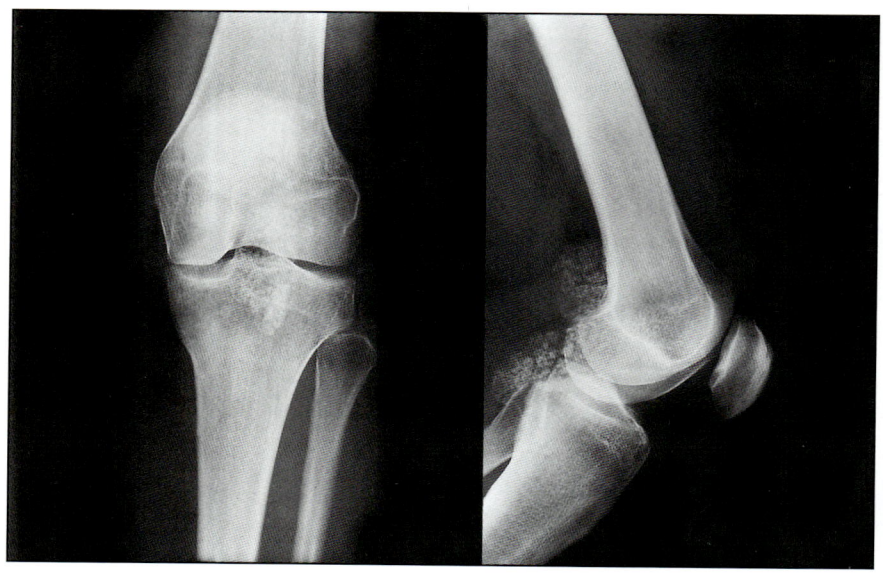

图25.104 滑膜软骨瘤病的影像学，显示关节腔增大，含有多量小的钙化性聚集体。

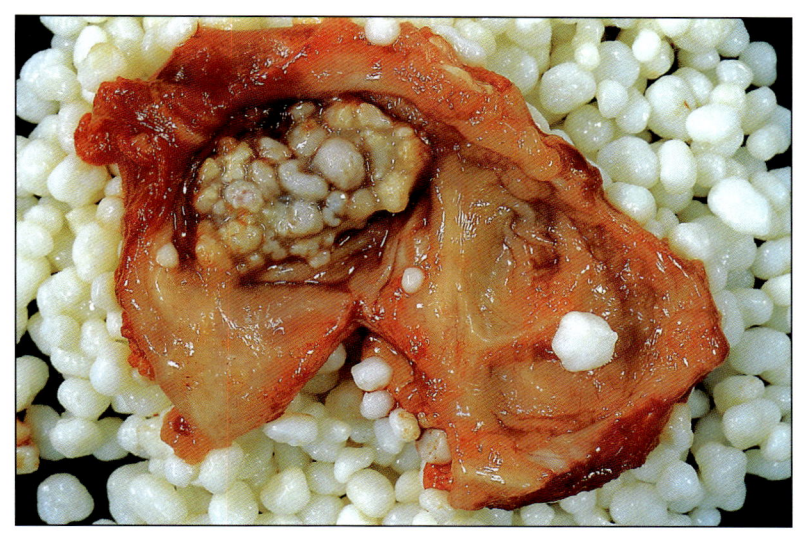

图 25.105 滑膜软骨瘤病的大体标本显示红褐色滑囊组织，伴有大量小的、圆形、白色的软骨性结节。

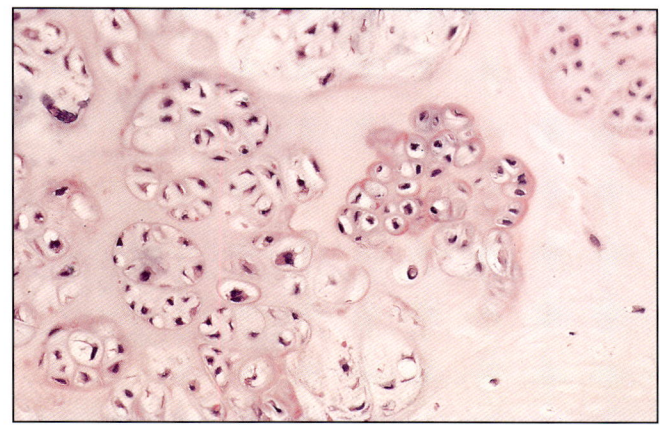

图 25.106 滑膜软骨瘤病由具有大而深染细胞核的软骨细胞组成，细胞常常保持结节状排列。

小关节的报道，如颞下颌关节[314,315]。我们也见过累及脊柱关节面的滑膜软骨瘤病。最近的资料显示，滑膜软骨瘤病有恒定的克隆性细胞遗传学异常，支持将其命名为一种肿瘤病变[316]。鉴别诊断包括骨软骨性的游离小体，后者伴有其下方的原发性关节病变，如退行性关节病。这些游离体通常较小且在关节腔内自由漂浮，当然，它们也可以包埋在滑膜内。它们可能数量很多，并且体积可以变得很大。影像学上，与滑膜软骨瘤病的鉴别可能很困难。

组织学上，滑膜软骨瘤病看上去与游离小体不同。游离小体显示为非肿瘤性软骨，有层状表现。软骨细胞没有在滑膜软骨瘤病中所见的典型的簇状生长方式。它也没有任何细胞学非典型性。滑膜软骨瘤病与游离小体的鉴别很重要。前者的治疗是行完全的滑膜切除术，而后者则需治疗基础疾病。

来自滑膜的**软骨肉瘤**（chondrosarcoma）已有报道。在 Mayo Clinic 报告[317]的 10 例滑膜软骨肉瘤中，仅有 2 例考虑是原发性病变。其余病例考虑是继发于滑膜软骨瘤病。已经发现，能区别滑膜软骨瘤病和软骨肉瘤的有用特征是黏液样基质、坏死和成片的细胞；这些特征在滑膜软骨瘤病中见不到。滑膜的软骨肉瘤是真正的恶性病变，10 例中有 4 例是死于转移性软骨肉瘤。然而，更为要紧的问题是滑膜软骨瘤病被过度诊断为软骨肉瘤，而不是罕见的滑膜软骨肉瘤被降低诊断。

滑膜血管瘤
Hemangioma of the synovium

发生在滑膜的血管瘤是非常少见的。自 1959 年以来，Mayo Clinc 的资料中仅记载有 11 例[318]。这些病变通常发生在青少年或年轻的成人。膝部常常受累。疼痛是主要症状。滑膜的大体表现为增厚，呈褐色或红色斑点样。

组织学上，血管瘤可以是毛细血管或海绵状血管，或可能两种结构混合存在。

滑膜脂肪瘤　Lipoma of the synovium

脂肪瘤发生在滑膜中很少见。滑膜呈沼泽样、分叶状表现。显微镜下，滑膜组织充满脂肪。大多数滑膜弥漫性脂肪肥大的原因可能是反应性的，有时可能被认为是树枝状脂肪瘤。

参考文献

1. Jaffe H L 1958 Tumors and tumorous conditions of the bones and joints. Lea & Febiger, Philadelphia
2. Lichtenstein L 1951 Classification of primary tumors of bone. Cancer 4: 335-341
3. Fletcher C D M, Unni K K, Mertens F 2002 Pathology and genetics of tumours of soft tissue and bone. IARC Press, Lyon
4. Unni K K 1996 Dahlin's bone tumors: general aspects and data on 11 087 cases, 5th edn. Lippincott-Raven, Philadelphia
5. Enneking W F, Spanier S S, Goodman M A 1980 The surgical staging of musculoskeletal sarcoma. J Bone Joint Surg [Am] 62: 1027-1030
6. Costa J, Wesley R A, Glatstein E et al. 1984 The grading of soft tissue sarcomas: results of a clinicohistopathologic correlation in a series of 163 cases. Cancer 53: 530-541
7. Broders A C 1920 Squamous cell epithelioma of the lip: a study of 537 cases. JAMA 74: 656-664
8. Simon M A, Aschliman M A, Thomas N et al. 1986 Limb-salvage treatment versus amputation for osteosarcoma of the distal end of the femur. J Bone Joint Surg [Am] 68: 1331-1337
9. DeSantos L A, Murray J A, Ayala A G 1979 The value of percutaneous needle biopsy in the management of primary bone tumors. Cancer 43: 735-744
10. Moore T M, Meyers M H, Patzakis M J et al. 1979 Closed biopsy of musculoskeletal lesions. J Bone Joint Surg [Am] 61: 375-380
11. Casey T T, Stone W J, DiRaimondo C R et al. 1986 Tumoral amyloidosis of bone of beta$_2$-microglobulin origin in association with long-term hemodialysis: a new type of amyloid disease. Hum Pathol 17: 731-738
12. Bataille R, Sany J 1981 Solitary myeloma: clinical and prognostic features of a review of 114 cases. Cancer 48: 845-851
13. Frassica D A, Frassica F J, Schray M F et al. 1989 Solitary plasmacytoma of bone: Mayo Clinic experience. Int J Radiat Oncol Biol Phys 16: 43-48
14. Resnick D, Greenway G D, Bardwick P A et al. 1981 Plasma-cell dyscrasia with polyneuropathy, organomegaly, endocrinopathy, M-protein, and skin changes: the POEMS syndrome. Distinctive radiographic abnormalities. Radiology 140: 17-22
15. Kelly J J Jr, Kyle R A, Miles J M et al. 1983 Osteosclerotic myeloma and a peripheral neuropathy. Neurology 33: 202-210
16. Kyle R A 1983 Long-term survival in multiple myeloma. N Engl J Med 308: 314-316
17. Howat A J, Thomas H, Waters K D et al. 1987 Malignant lymphoma of bone in children. Cancer 59: 335-339
18. Fairbanks R K, Bonner J A, Inwards C Y et al. 1994 Treatment of stage IE primary lymphoma of bone. Int J Radiat Oncol Biol Phys 28: 363-372
19. Pettit C K, Zukerberg L R, Gray M H et al. 1990 Primary lymphoma of bone: a B-cell neoplasm with a high frequency of multilobulated cells. Am J Surg Pathol 14: 329-334
20. Clayton F, Butler J J, Ayala A G et al. 1987 Non-Hodgkin's lymphoma in bone: pathologic and radiologic features with clinical correlates. Cancer 60: 2494-2501
21. Jones D, Kraus M D, Dorfman D M 1999 Lymphoma presenting as a solitary bone lesion. Am J Clin Pathol 111: 171-178
22. Nagasaka T, Nakamura S, Medeiros L J et al. 2000 Anaplastic large cell lymphomas presented as bone lesions: a clinicopathologic study of six cases and review of the literature. Mod Pathol 13: 1143-1149
23. de Leval L, Braaten K M, Ancukiewicz M et al. 2003 Diffuse large B-cell lymphoma of bone: an analysis of differentiation-associated antigens with clinical correlation. Am J Surg Pathol 27: 1269-1277
24. Dosoretz D E, Raymond A K, Murphy G F et al. 1982 Primary lymphoma of bone: the relationship of morphologic diversity to clinical behavior. Cancer 50: 1009-1014
25. Ostrowski M L, Unni K K, Banks P M et al. 1986 Malignant lymphoma of bone. Cancer 58: 2646-2655
26. Kluin P M, Slootweg P J, Schuurman H J et al. 1984 Primary B-cell malignant lymphoma of the maxilla with a sarcomatous pattern and multilobulated nuclei. Cancer 54: 1598-1605
27. Chan J K C, Ng C-S, Hui P-K et al. 1991 Anaplastic large cell Ki-1 lymphoma of bone. Cancer 68: 2186-2191
28. Meis J M, Butler J J, Osborne B M et al. 1986 Granulocytic sarcoma in nonleukemic patients. Cancer 58: 2697-2709
29. Welch P, Grossi C, Carrol A et al. 1986 Granulocytic sarcoma with an indolent course and destructive skeletal disease: tumor characterization with immunologic markers, electron microscopy, cytochemistry, and cytogenetic studies. Cancer 57: 1005-1010
30. Goldstein N S, Ritter J H, Argenyi Z B et al. 1995 Granulocytic sarcoma: potential diagnostic clues from immunostaining patterns seen with anti-lymphoid antibodies. Int J Surg Pathol 2: 177-186
31. Traweek S T, Arber D A, Rappaport H et al. 1993 Extramedullary myeloid cell tumors: an immunohistochemical and morphologic study of 28 cases. Am J Surg Pathol 17: 1011-1019
32. Schajowicz F 1959 Ewing's sarcoma and reticulum-cell sarcoma of bone: with special reference to the histochemical demonstration of glycogen as an aid to differential diagnosis. J Bone Joint Surg [Am] 41: 349-356
33. Weidner N, Tjoe J 1994 Immunohistochemical profile of monoclonal antibody O13: antibody that recognises glycoprotein p30/32^{MIC2} and is useful in diagnosing Ewing's sarcoma and peripheral neuroepithelioma. Am J Surg Pathol 18: 486-494
34. Perlman E J, Dickman P S, Askin F B et al. 1994 Ewing's sarcoma - routine diagnostic utilization of MIC2 analysis: a Pediatric Oncology Group/Children's Cancer Group Intergroup Study. Hum Pathol 25: 304-307
35. Stevenson A J, Chatten J, Bertoni F et al. 1994 CD99 (p30/32^{MIC2}) neuroectodermal/Ewing's sarcoma antigen as an immunohistochemical marker: review of more than 600 tumors and the literature experience. Appl Immunohistochem 2: 231-240
36. Lumadue J A, Askin F B, Perlman E J 1994 MIC2 analysis of small cell carcinoma. Am J Clin Pathol 102: 692-694
37. Dei Tos A P, Wadden C, Calonje E et al. 1995 Immunohistochemical demonstration of glycoprotein p30/32^{MIC2} (CD99) in synovial sarcoma: a potential cause of diagnostic confusion. Appl Immunohistochem 3: 168-173
38. Riopel M, Dickman P S, Link M P et al. 1994 MIC2 analysis in pediatric lymphomas and leukemias. Hum Pathol 25: 396-399
39. Vartanian R K, Sudilovsky D, Weidner N 1996 Immunostaining of monoclonal antibody O13 [anti-MIC2 gene product (CD99)] in lymphomas: impact of heat-induced epitope retrieval. Appl Immunohistochem 4: 43-55
40. Dorfman D M, Pinkus G S 1996 CD99 (p30/32^{MIC2}) immunoreactivity in the diagnosis of thymic neoplasms and mediastinal lymphoproliferative disorders: a study of paraffin sections using monoclonal antibody O13. Appl Immunohistochem 4: 34-42
41. Soslow R A, Bhargava V, Warnke R A 1997 MIC2, TdT, bcl-2, and CD34 expression in paraffin-embedded high-grade lymphoma/acute lymphoblastic leukemia distinguishes between distinct clinicopathologic entities. Hum Pathol 28: 1158-1165
42. Hess E, Cohen C, DeRose P B et al. 1997 Nonspecificity of p30/32^{MIC2} immunolocalization with the O13 monoclonal antibody in the diagnosis of Ewing's sarcoma: application of an algorithmic immunohistochemical analysis. Appl Immunohistochem 5: 94-103
43. Stephenson C F, Bridge J A, Sandberg A A 1992 Cytogenetic and pathologic aspects of Ewing's sarcoma and neuroectodermal tumors. Hum Pathol 23: 1270-1277
44. Delattre O, Zucman J, Melot T et al. 1994 The Ewing family of tumors - a subgroup of small-round-cell tumors defined by specific chimeric transcripts. N Engl J Med 331: 294-299
45. Downing J R, Head D R, Parham D M et al. 1993 Detection of the (11;22)(q24;q12) translocation of Ewing's sarcoma and peripheral neuroectodermal tumor by reverse transcription polymerase chain reaction. Am J Pathol 143: 1294-1300
46. Scotlandi K, Serra M, Manara M C et al. 1996 Immunostaining of the p30/32^{MIC2} antigen and molecular detection of EWS rearrangements for the diagnosis of Ewing's sarcoma and peripheral neuroectodermal tumor. Hum Pathol 27: 408-416
47. de Alava E, Kawai A, Healey J H et al. 1998 EWS-FLI1 fusion transcript structure is an independent determinant of prognosis in Ewing's sarcoma. J Clin Oncol 16: 1248-1255
48. Nascimento A G, Unni K K, Pritchard D J et al. 1980 A clinicopathologic study of 20 cases of large-cell (atypical) Ewing's sarcoma of bone. Am J Surg Pathol 4: 29-36
49. Kissane J M, Askin F B, Foulkes M et al. 1983 Ewing's sarcoma of bone: clinicopathologic aspects of 303 cases from the Intergroup Ewing's Sarcoma Study. Hum Pathol 14: 773-779
50. Hartman K R, Triche T J, Kinsella T J et al. 1991 Prognostic value of histopathology in Ewing's sarcoma: long-term follow-up of distal extremity primary tumors. Cancer 67: 163-171
51. Llombart-Bosch A, Contesso G, Henry-Amar M et al. 1986 Histopathological predictive factors in Ewing's sarcoma of bone and clinicopathological correlations: a retrospective study of 261 cases. Virchows Arch [A] 409: 627-640
52. Askin F B, Rosai J, Sibley R K et al. 1979 Malignant small cell tumor of the thoracopulmonary region in childhood: a distinctive clinicopathologic entity of uncertain histogenesis. Cancer 43: 2438-2451
53. Contesso G, Llombart-Bosch A, Terrier P et al. 1992 Does malignant small round cell tumor of the thoracopulmonary region (Askin tumor) constitute a clinicopathologic entity? An analysis of 30 cases with immunohistochemical and electron-microscopic support treated at the Institut Gustave Roussy. Cancer 69: 1012-1020
54. Davison E V, Pearson A D J, Emslie J et al. 1989 Chromosome 22 abnormalities in Ewing's sarcoma. J Clin Pathol 42: 797-799
55. Lizard-Nacol S, Lizard G, Justrabo E et al. 1989 Immunologic characterization of Ewing's sarcoma using mesenchymal and neural markers. Am J Pathol 135: 847-855
56. Ushigome S, Shimoda T, Nikaido T et al. 1992 Primitive neuroectodermal tumors of bone and soft tissue: with reference to histologic differentiation in primary or metastatic foci. Acta Pathol Jpn 42: 483-493
57. Tsuneyoshi M, Yokoyama R, Hashimoto H et al. 1989 Comparative study of neuroectodermal tumor and Ewing's sarcoma of the bone: histopathologic,

57. immunohistochemical and ultrastructural features. Acta Pathol Jpn 39: 573-581
58. Schmidt D, Herrmann C, Jürgens H et al. 1991 Malignant peripheral neuroectodermal tumor and its necessary distinction from Ewing's sarcoma: a report from the Kiel Pediatric Tumor Registry. Cancer 68: 2251-2259
59. Picci P, Rougraff B T, Bacci G et al. 1993 Prognostic significance of histopathologic response to chemotherapy in nonmetastatic Ewing's sarcoma of the extremities. J Clin Oncol 11: 1763-1769
60. Pritchard D J, Dahlin D C, Dauphine R T et al. 1975 Ewing's sarcoma: a clinicopathological and statistical analysis of patients surviving five years or longer. J Bone Joint Surg [Am] 57: 10-16
61. Wilkins RM, Pritchard DJ, Burgert EO Jr et al. 1986 Ewing's sarcoma of bone: experience with 140 patients. Cancer 58: 2551-2555
62. Bovée J V M G, Cleton-Jansen A-M, Wuyts W et al. 1999 EXT-mutation analysis and loss of heterozygosity in sporadic and hereditary osteochondromas and secondary chondrosarcomas. Am J Hum Genet 65: 689-698
63. Nora F E, Dahlin D C, Beabout J W 1983 Bizarre parosteal osteochondromatous proliferations of the hands and feet. Am J Surg Pathol 7: 245-250
64. Landon G C, Johnson K A, Dahlin D C 1979 Subungual exostoses. J Bone Joint Surg [Am] 61: 256-259
65. Peterson H A 1989 Multiple hereditary osteochondromata. Clin Orthop 239: 222-230
66. Wuyts W, Van Hul W, De Boulle K et al. 1998 Mutations in the EXT1 and EXT2 genes in hereditary multiple exostoses. Am J Hum Genet 62: 346-354
67. Shapiro F, Simon S, Glimcher M J 1979 Hereditary multiple exostoses: anthropometric, roentgenographic, and clinical aspects. J Bone Joint Surg [Am] 61: 815-824
68. Nojima T, Unni K K, McLeod R A et al. 1985 Periosteal chondroma and periosteal chondrosarcoma. Am J Surg Pathol 9: 666-677
69. Bauer T W, Dorfman H D, Latham J T Jr. 1982 Periosteal chondroma: a clinicopathologic study of 23 cases. Am J Surg Pathol 6: 631-637
70. Dahlin D C, Salvador A H 1974 Cartilaginous tumors of the soft tissues of the hands and feet. Mayo Clin Proc 49: 721-726
71. Chung E B, Enzinger F M 1978 Chondroma of soft parts. Cancer 41: 1414-1424
72. Liu J, Hudkins P G, Swee R G et al. 1987 Bone sarcomas associated with Ollier's disease. Cancer 59: 1376-1385
73. Lewis R J, Ketcham A S 1973 Maffucci's syndrome: functional and neoplastic significance: case report and review of the literature. J Bone Joint Surg [Am] 55: 1465-1479
74. Fanburg J C, Meis-Kindblom J M, Rosenberg A E 1995 Multiple enchondromas associated with spindle-cell hemangioendotheliomas: an overlooked variant of Maffucci's syndrome. Am J Surg Pathol 19: 1029-1038
75. Kurt A M, Unni K K, Sim F H et al. 1989 Chondroblastoma of bone. Hum Pathol 20: 965-976
76. Schajowicz F, Gallardo H 1970 Epiphysial chondroblastoma of bone: a clinico-pathological study of sixty-nine cases. J Bone Joint Surg [Br] 52: 205-226
77. Springfield D S, Capanna R, Gherlinzoni F et al. 1985 Chondroblastoma: a review of seventy cases. J Bone Joint Surg [Am] 67: 748-755
78. Huvos A G, Marcove R C 1973 Chondroblastoma of bone: a critical review. Clin Orthop 95: 300-312
79. Dahlin D C, Ivins J C 1972 Benign chondroblastoma: a study of 125 cases. Cancer 30: 401-413
80. Turcotte R E, Kurt A M, Sim F H et al. 1993 Chondroblastoma. Hum Pathol 24: 944-949
81. McLeod R A, Beabout J W 1973 The roentgenographic features of chondroblastoma. AJR Am J Roentgenol 118: 464-471
82. Kahn L P, Wood S M, Ackerman L V 1969 Malignant chondroblastoma: report of two cases and review of the literature. Arch Pathol Lab Med 88: 371-376
83. Green P, Whittaker R P 1975 Benign chondroblastoma: case report with pulmonary metastasis. J Bone Joint Surg [Am] 57: 418-420
84. Kyriakos M, Land V J, Penning H L et al. 1985 Metastatic chondroblastoma: report of a fatal case with a review of the literature on atypical, aggressive, and malignant chondroblastoma. Cancer 55: 1770-1789
85. Gherlinzoni F, Rock M, Picci P 1983 Chondromyxoid fibroma: the experience at the Istituto Ortopedico Rizzoli. J Bone Joint Surg [Am] 65: 198-204
86. Wu C T, Inwards C Y, O'Laughlin S et al. 1998 Chondromyxoid fibroma of bone: a clinicopathologic review of 278 cases. Hum Pathol 29: 438-446
87. Granter S R, Renshaw A A, Kozakewich H P et al. 1998 The pericentromeric inversion, inv (6)(p25q13), is a novel diagnostic marker in chondromyxoid fibroma. Mod Pathol 11: 1071-1074
88. Dahlin D C 1976 Chondrosarcoma and its "variants." Monogr Pathol 17: 300-311
89. Meachim G 1979 Histological grading of chondrosarcomata [editorial]. J Bone Joint Surg [Br] 61: 393-394
90. Evans H L, Ayala A G, Romsdahl M M 1977 Prognostic factors in chondrosarcoma of bone: a clinicopathologic analysis with emphasis on histologic grading. Cancer 40: 818-831
91. Gitelis S, Bertoni F, Picci P et al. 1981 Chondrosarcoma of bone: the experience of the Istituto Ortopedico Rizzoli. J Bone Joint Surg [Am] 63: 1248-1257
92. Pritchard D J, Lunke R J, Taylor W F et al. 1980 Chondrosarcoma: a clinicopathological and statistical analysis. Cancer 45: 149-157
93. Henderson E D, Dahlin D C 1963 Chondrosarcoma of bone - a study of two hundred and eighty-eight cases. J Bone Joint Surg [Am] 45: 1450-1458
94. Björnsson J, McLeod R A, Unni K K et al. 1998 Primary chondrosarcoma of long bones and limb girdles. Cancer 83: 2105-2119
95. Mirra J M, Gold R, Downs J et al. 1985 A new histologic approach to the differentiation of enchondroma and chondrosarcoma of the bones: a clinicopathologic analysis of 51 cases. Clin Orthop 201: 214-237
96. Dahlin D C, Salvador A H 1974 Chondrosarcomas of bones of the hands and feet - a study of 30 cases. Cancer 34: 755-760
97. Ogose A, Unni K K, Swee R G et al. 1997 Chondrosarcoma of small bones of the hands and feet. Cancer 80: 50-59
98. Bovee J V, van der Heul R O, Taminiau A H et al. 1999 Chondrosarcoma of the phalanx: a locally aggressive lesion with minimal metastatic potential: a report or 35 cases and a review of the literature. Cancer 86: 1724-1732
99. Bovee J V, van den Broek L J, Cleton-Jansen A M, Hogendoorn P C W 2000 Upregulation of PTHrP and Bcl-2 expression characterizes the progression of osteochondroma towards peripheral chondrosarcoma and is a late event in central chondrosarcoma. Lab Invest 80: 1925-1934
100. Garrison R C, Unni K K, McLeod R A et al. 1982 Chondrosarcoma arising in osteochondroma. Cancer 49: 1890-1897
101. Young C L, Sim F H, Unni K K et al. 1990 Chondrosarcoma of bone in children. Cancer 66: 1641-1648
102. Björnsson J, Unni K K, Dahlin D C et al. 1984 Clear cell chondrosarcoma of bone: observations in 47 cases. Am J Surg Pathol 8: 223-230
103. Dahlin D C, Beabout J W 1971 Dedifferentiation of low-grade chondrosarcomas. Cancer 28: 461-466
104. Frassica F J, Unni K K, Beabout J W et al. 1986 Dedifferentiated chondrosarcoma: a report of the clinicopathological features and treatment of seventy-eight cases. J Bone Joint Surg [Am] 68: 1197-1205
105. Tetu B, Ordonez N G, Ayala A G et al. 1986 Chondrosarcoma with additional mesenchymal component (dedifferentiated chondrosarcoma). II. An immunohistochemical and electron microscopic study. Cancer 58: 287-298
106. Reith J D, Bauer T W, Fischler D F et al. 1996 Dedifferentiated chondrosarcoma with rhabdomyosarcomatous differentiation. Am J Surg Pathol 20: 293-298
107. Capanna R, Bertoni F, Bettelli G et al. 1988 Dedifferentiated chondrosarcoma. J Bone Joint Surg [Am] 70: 60-69
108. Johnson S, Têtu B, Ayala A G et al. 1986 Chondrosarcoma with additional mesenchymal component (dedifferentiated chondrosarcoma): 1. A clinicopathologic study of 26 cases. Cancer 58: 278-286
108a. Staals E L, Bacchini P, Bertoni F 2006 Dedifferentiated central chondrosarcoma. Cancer 106: 2682-2691
109. Matsuno T, Ichioka Y, Yagi T et al. 1988 Spindle-cell sarcoma in patients who have osteochondromatosis: a report of two cases. J Bone Joint Surg [Am] 70: 137-141
110. Bertoni F, Present D, Bacchini P et al. 1989 Dedifferentiated peripheral chondrosarcomas: a report of seven cases. Cancer 63: 2054-2059
111. Lichtenstein L, Bernstein D 1959 Unusual benign and malignant chondroid tumors of bone: a survey of some mesenchymal cartilage tumors and malignant chondroblastic tumors, including a few multicentric ones, as well as many atypical benign chondroblastomas and chondromyxoid fibromas. Cancer 12: 1142-1157
112. Nakashima Y, Unni K K, Shives T C et al. 1986 Mesenchymal chondrosarcoma of bone and soft tissue: a review of 111 cases. Cancer 57: 2444-2453
113. Granter S R, Renshaw A A, Fletcher C D et al. 1996 CD99 reactivity in mesenchymal chondrosarcoma. Hum Pathol 27: 1273-1276
114. O'Connell J X, Nanthakumar S S, Nielsen G P et al. 1998 Osteoid osteoma: the uniquely innervated bone tumor. Mod Pathol 11: 175-180
115. Sim F H, Dahlin D C, Beabout J W 1975 Osteoid osteoma: diagnostic problems. J Bone Joint Surg [Am] 57: 154-159
116. Ayala A G, Murray J A, Erling M A et al. 1986 Osteoid osteoma: intraoperative tetracycline-fluorescence demonstration of the nidus. J Bone Joint Surg [Am] 68: 747-751
117. Marcove R C, Heelan R T, Huvos A G et al. 1991 Osteoid osteoma: diagnosis, localization, and treatment. Clin Orthop 267: 197-201
118. Rosenthal D I, Springfield D S, Gebhardt M C et al. 1995 Osteoid osteoma: percutaneous radio-frequency ablation. Radiology 197: 451-454
119. Dahlin D C, Johnson E W Jr 1954 Giant osteoid osteoma. J Bone Joint Surg [Am] 36: 559-572
120. Jaffe H L 1956 Benign osteoblastoma. Bull Hosp Jt Dis 17: 141-151
121. Lucas D R, Unni K K, McLeod R A et al. 1994 Osteoblastoma: clinicopathologic study of 306 cases. Hum Pathol 25: 117-134
122. McLeod R A, Dahlin D C, Beabout J W 1976 The spectrum of osteoblastoma. AJR Am J Roentgenol 126: 321-335
123. Dorfman H D, Weiss S W 1984 Borderline osteoblastic tumors: problems in the differential diagnosis of aggressive osteoblastoma and low-grade osteosarcoma. Semin Diagn Pathol 1: 215-234
124. Schajowicz F, Lemos C 1976 Malignant osteoblastoma. J Bone Joint Surg [Br] 58: 202-211
125. Bertoni F, Donati D, Bacchini P et al. 1992 The morphologic spectrum of osteoblastoma (OBL): is its aggressive nature predictable? Lab Invest 66: 3A

(abstract)
126. Della Rocca C, Huvos A G 1996 Osteoblastoma: varied histological presentations with a benign clinical course: an analysis of 55 cases. Am J Surg Pathol 20: 841-850
127. Mirra J M, Kendrick R A, Kendrick R E 1976 Pseudomalignant osteoblastoma versus arrested osteosarcoma: a case report. Cancer 37: 2005-2014
128. Haggitt R C, Reid B J 1986 Hereditary gastrointestinal polyposis syndrome. Am J Surg Pathol 10: 871-887
129. Dahlin D C, Unni K K 1977 Osteosarcoma of bone and its important recognizable varieties. Am J Surg Pathol 1: 61-72
130. Okada K, Wold L E, Beabout J W et al. 1993 Osteosarcoma of the hand: a clinicopathologic study of 12 cases. Cancer 72: 719-725
131. Bertoni F, Unni K K, McLeod R A et al. 1985 Osteosarcoma resembling osteoblastoma. Cancer 55: 416-426
132. Dahlin D C, Coventry M B 1967 Osteogenic sarcoma: a study of six hundred cases. J Bone Joint Surg [Am] 49: 101-110
133. Rosen G, Marcove R C, Caparros B et al. 1979 Primary osteogenic sarcoma: the rationale for preoperative chemotherapy and delayed surgery. Cancer 43: 2163-2177
134. Taylor W F, Ivins J C, Unni K K et al. 1989 Prognostic variables in osteosarcoma: a multi-institutional study. J Natl Cancer Inst 81: 21-30
135. Raymond A K, Ayala A G 1988 Specimen management after osteosarcoma chemotherapy. Contemp Issues Surg Pathol 11: 157-181
136. Baldini N, Scotlandi K, Barbanti-Bròdano G et al. 1995 Expression of P-glycoprotein in high-grade osteosarcoma in relation to clinical outcome. N Engl J Med 333: 1380-1385
137. Cahan W G, Woodard H Q, Higinbotham N L et al. 1948 Sarcoma arising in irradiated bone: report of eleven cases. Cancer 1: 3-29
138. Weatherby R P, Dahlin D C, Ivins J C 1981 Postradiation sarcoma of bone: review of 78 Mayo Clinic cases. Mayo Clin Proc 56: 294-306
139. Wick M R, Siegal G P, Unni K K et al. 1981 Sarcomas of bone complicating osteitis deformans (Paget's disease): fifty years' experience. Am J Surg Pathol 5: 47-59
140. Huvos A G, Butler A, Bretsky S S 1983 Osteogenic sarcoma associated with Paget's disease of bone: a clinicopathologic study of 65 patients. Cancer 52: 1489-1495
141. Matsuno T, Unni K K, McLeod R A et al. 1976 Telangiectatic osteogenic sarcoma. Cancer 38: 2538-2547
142. Huvos A G, Rosen G, Bretsky S S et al. 1982 Telangiectatic osteogenic sarcoma: a clinicopathologic study of 124 patients. Cancer 49: 1679-1689
143. Mervak T R, Unni K K, Pritchard D J et al. 1991 Telangiectatic osteosarcoma. Clin Orthop 270: 135-139
144. Unni K K, Dahlin D C, McLeod R A et al. 1977 Intraosseous well-differentiated osteosarcoma. Cancer 40: 1337-1347
145. Kurt A-M, Unni K K, McLeod R A et al. 1990 Low-grade intraosseous osteosarcoma. Cancer 65: 1418-1428
146. Sim F H, Unni K K, Beabout J W et al. 1979 Osteosarcoma with small cells simulating Ewing's tumor. J Bone Joint Surg [Am] 61: 207-215
147. Nakajima H, Sim F H, Bond J R et al. 1997 Small cell osteosarcoma of bone: review of 72 cases. Cancer 79: 2095-2106
148. Kyriakos M 1980 Intracortical osteosarcoma. Cancer 46: 2525-2533
149. Clark J L, Unni K K, Dahlin D C et al. 1983 Osteosarcoma of the jaw. Cancer 51: 2311-2316
150. Nora F E, Unni K K, Pritchard D J et al. 1983 Osteosarcoma of extragnathic craniofacial bones. Mayo Clin Proc 58: 268-272
151. Geschickter C F, Copeland M M 1951 Parosteal osteoma of bone: a new entity. Ann Surg 133: 790-806
152. Wold L E, Unni K K, Beabout J W et al. 1984 Dedifferentiated parosteal osteosarcoma. J Bone Joint Surg [Am] 66: 53-59
153. Okada K, Frassica F J, Sim F H et al. 1994 Parosteal osteosarcoma: a clinicopathological study. J Bone Joint Surg [Am] 76: 366-378
154. Unni K K, Dahlin D C, Beabout J W 1976 Periosteal osteogenic sarcoma. Cancer 37: 2476-2485
155. Schajowicz F 1977 Juxtacortical chondrosarcoma. J Bone Joint Surg [Br] 59: 473-480
156. Wold L E, Unni K K, Beabout J W et al. 1984 High-grade surface osteosarcomas. Am J Surg Pathol 8: 181-186
157. Okada K, Unni K K, Swee R G et al. 1999 High grade surface osteosarcoma: a clinicopathologic study of 46 cases. Cancer 85: 1044-1054
158. Wolfe J T III, Scheithauer B W, Dahlin D C 1983 Giant-cell tumor of the sphenoid bone: review of 10 cases. J Neurosurg 59: 322-327
159. Biscaglia R, Bacchini P, Bertoni F 2000 Giant cell tumor of the bones of the hand and foot. Cancer 88: 2022-2032
160. Cooper K L, Beabout J W, Dahlin D C 1984 Giant cell tumor: ossification in soft-tissue implants. Radiology 153: 597-602
161. Bertoni F, Present D A, Sudanese A et al. 1988 Giant-cell tumor of bone with pulmonary metastases: six case reports and a review of the literature. Clin Orthop 237: 275-285
162. Present D A, Bertoni F, Springfield D et al. 1986 Giant cell tumor of bone with pulmonary and lymph node metastases: a case report. Clin Orthop 209: 286-291
163. Bertoni F, Present D, Enneking W F 1985 Giant-cell tumor of bone with pulmonary metastases. J Bone Joint Surg [Am] 67: 890-900
164. Rock M G, Pritchard D J, Unni K K 1984 Metastases from histologically benign giant-cell tumor of bone. J Bone Joint Surg [Am] 66: 269-274

165. Nascimento A G, Huvos A G, Marcove R C 1979 Primary malignant giant cell tumor of bone: a study of eight cases and review of the literature. Cancer 44: 1393-1402
166. Keeney G L, Unni K K, Beabout J W et al. 1989 Adamantinoma of long bones: a clinicopathologic study of 85 cases. Cancer 64: 730-737
167. Hazelbag H M, Fleuren G J, v d Broek L J C M et al. 1993 Adamantinoma of the long bones: keratin subclass immunoreactivity pattern with reference to its histogenesis. Am J Surg Pathol 17: 1225-1233
168. Huvos A G, Marcove R C 1975 Adamantinoma of long bones: a clinicopathological study of fourteen cases with vascular origin suggested. J Bone Joint Surg [Am] 57: 148-154
169. Hazelbag H M, Laforga J B, Roels H J et al. 2003 Dedifferentiated adamantinoma with revertant mesenchymal phenotype. Am J Surg Pathol 27: 1530-1537
170. Dockerty M B, Meyerding H W 1942 Adamantinoma of the tibia: report of two new cases. JAMA 119: 932-937
171. Cohen D M, Dahlin D C, Pugh D G 1962 Fibrous dysplasia associated with adamantinoma of the long bones. Cancer 15: 515-521
172. Weiss S W, Dorfman H D 1977 Adamantinoma of long bone: an analysis of nine new cases with emphasis on metastasizing lesions and fibrous dysplasia-like changes. Hum Pathol 8: 141-153
173. Alguacil-Garcia A, Alonso A, Pettigrew N M 1984 Osteofibrous dysplasia (ossifying fibroma) of the tibia and fibula and adamantinoma: a case report. Am J Clin Pathol 82: 470-474
174. Czerniak B, Rojas-Corona R R, Dorfman H D 1989 Morphologic diversity of long bone adamantinoma: the concept of differentiated (regressing) adamantinoma and its relationship to osteofibrous dysplasia. Cancer 64: 2319-2334
175. Kuruvilla G, Steiner G C 1998 Osteofibrous dysplasia-like adamantinoma of bone: a report of five cases with immunohistochemical and ultrastructural studies. Hum Pathol 29: 809-814
176. Hazelbag H M, Taminiau A H, Fleuren G J et al. 1994 Adamantinoma of the long bones. A clinicopathological study of thirty-two patients with emphasis on histological subtype, precursor lesion, and biological behavior. J Bone Joint Surg Am 76: 1482-1499
177. Kuruvilla G, Steiner G C 1993 Adamantinoma of the tibia in children and adolescents simulating osteofibrous dysplasia of bone [abstract]. Lab Invest 68: 7A
178. Sweet D E, Vinh T N, Devaney K 1992 Cortical osteofibrous dysplasia of long bone and its relationship to adamantinoma: a clinicopathologic study of 30 cases. Am J Surg Pathol 16: 282-290
179. Hazelbag H M, Wessels J W, Mollevangers P et al. 1997 Cytogenetic analysis of adamantinoma of long bones: further indications for a common histogenesis with osteofibrous dysplasia. Cancer Genet Cytogenet 97: 5-11
180. Rosai J 1969 Adamantinoma of the tibia: electron microscopic evidence of its epithelial origin. Am J Clin Pathol 51: 786-792
181. Rosai J, Pinkus G S 1982 Immunohistochemical demonstration of epithelial differentiation in adamantinoma of the tibia. Am J Surg Pathol 6: 427-434
182. Mori H, Yamamoto S, Hiramatsu K et al. 1984 Adamantinoma of the tibia: ultrastructural and immunohistochemical study with reference to histogenesis. Clin Orthop 190: 299-310
183. O'Connell J X, Kattapuram S V, Mankin H J et al. 1993 Epithelioid hemangioma of bone: a tumor often mistaken for low-grade angiosarcoma or malignant hemangioendothelioma. Am J Surg Pathol 17: 610-617
184. Keel S B, Rosenberg A E 1999 Hemorrhagic epithelioid and spindle cell hemangioma: a newly recognized, unique vascular tumor of bone. Cancer 85: 1966-1972
185. Gorham L W, Stout A P 1955 Massive osteolysis (acute spontaneous absorption of bone, phantom bone, disappearing bone): its relation to hemangiomatosis. J Bone Joint Surg [Am] 37: 985-1004
186. Sugiura I 1976 Intra-osseous glomus tumour. J Bone Joint Surg [Br] 58: 245-247
187. Wold L E, Unni K K, Beabout J W et al. 1982 Hemangioendothelial sarcoma of bone. Am J Surg Pathol 6: 59-70
188. Campanacci M, Boriani S, Giunti A 1980 Hemangioendothelioma of bone: a study of 29 cases. Cancer 46: 804-814
189. Volpe R, Mazabraud A 1982 Hemangioendothelioma (angiosarcoma) of bone: a distinct pathologic entity with an unpredictable course? Cancer 49: 727-736
190. Weiss S W, Enzinger F M 1982 Epithelioid hemangioendothelioma: a vascular tumor often mistaken for a carcinoma. Cancer 50: 970-981
191. Maruyama N, Kumagai Y, Ishida Y et al. 1985 Epithelioid haemangioendothelioma of the bone tissue. Virchows Arch [A] 407: 159-165
192. Tsuneyoshi M, Dorfman H D, Bauer T W 1986 Epithelioid hemangioendothelioma of bone: a clinicopathologic, ultrastructural, and immunohistochemical study. Am J Surg Pathol 10: 754-764
193. Kleer C G, Unni K K, McLeod R A 1996 Epithelioid hemangioendothelioma of bone. Am J Surg Pathol 20: 1301-1311
194. Mirra J M, Kameda N 1986 Case report 366. Skeletal Radiol 15: 323-326
195. Wold L E, Unni K K, Cooper K L et al. 1982 Hemangiopericytoma of bone. Am J Surg Pathol 6: 53-58
196. Tang J S H, Gold R H, Mirra J M et al. 1988 Hemangiopericytoma of bone. Cancer 62: 848-859
197. Bertoni F, Calderoni P, Bacchini P et al. 1986 Benign fibrous histiocytoma of

198. Clark B E, Xipell J M, Thomas D P 1985 Benign fibrous histiocytoma of bone. Am J Surg Pathol 9: 806-815
199. Fletcher C D M 1992 Pleomorphic malignant fibrous histiocytoma: fact or fiction? A critical reappraisal based on 159 tumors diagnosed as pleomorphic sarcoma. Am J Surg Pathol 16: 213-228
200. Huvos A G, Heilweil M, Bretsky S S 1985 The pathology of malignant fibrous histiocytoma of bone: a study of 130 patients. Am J Surg Pathol 9: 853-871
201. Mirra J M, Gold R H, Marafiote R 1977 Malignant (fibrous) histiocytoma arising in association with a bone infarct in sickle-cell disease: coincidence or cause-and-effect? Cancer 39: 186-194
202. Huvos A G, Woodard H Q, Heilweil M 1986 Postradiation malignant fibrous histiocytoma of bone: a clinicopathologic study of 20 patients. Am J Surg Pathol 10: 9-18
203. Taconis W K, van Rijssel T G 1985 Fibrosarcoma of long bones: a study of the significance of areas of malignant fibrous histiocytoma. J Bone Joint Surg [Br] 67: 111-116
204. Nakashima Y, Morishita S, Kotoura Y et al. 1985 Malignant fibrous histiocytoma of bone: a review of 13 cases and an ultrastructural study. Cancer 55: 2804-2811
205. Ghandur-Mnaymneh L, Zych G, Mnaymneh W 1982 Primary malignant fibrous histiocytoma of bone: report of six cases with ultrastructural study and analysis of the literature. Cancer 49: 698-707
206. Capanna R, Bertoni F, Bacchini P et al. 1984 Malignant fibrous histiocytoma of bone: the experience at the Rizzoli Institute: report of 90 cases. Cancer 54: 177-187
207. Nishida J, Sim F H, Wenger D E et al. 1997 Malignant fibrous histiocytoma of bone: a clinicopathologic study of 81 patients. Cancer 79: 482-493
208. Inwards C Y, Unni K K, Beabout J W et al. 1991 Desmoplastic fibroma of bone. Cancer 68: 1978-1983
208a. Hauben E I, Jundt G, Cleton-Jansen A M et al. 2005 Desmoplastic fibroma of bone: an immunohistochemical study including beta-catenin expression and mutational analysis for beta-catenin. Hum Pathol 36: 1025-1030
209. Jeffree G M, Price C H G 1976 Metastatic spread of fibrosarcoma of bone: a report on forty-nine cases, and a comparison with osteosarcoma. J Bone Joint Surg [Br] 58: 418-425
210. Myers B L, Arocho A, Bernreuter W et al. 1991 Leiomyosarcoma of bone: a clinicopathologic, immunohistochemical, and ultrastructural study of five cases. Cancer 67: 1051-1056
211. Angervall L, Berlin Ö, Kindblom L-G et al. 1980 Primary leiomyosarcoma of bone: a study of five cases. Cancer 46: 1270-1279
212. Antonescu C R, Erlandson R A, Huvos A G 1997 Primary leiomyosarcoma of bone: a clinicopathologic, immunohistochemical, and ultrastructural study of 33 patients and a literature review. Am J Surg Pathol 21: 1281-1294
213. Ducatman B S, Scheithauer B W, Dahlin D C 1983 Malignant bone tumors associated with neurofibromatosis. Mayo Clin Proc 58: 578-582
214. Ulich T R, Mirra J M 1982 Ecchordosis physaliphora vertebralis. Clin Orthop 163: 282-289
214a. Vujovic S, Henderson S, Presneau N et al. 2006 Brachyury, a crucial regulator of notochordal development, is a novel biomarker for chordomas. J Pathol 209: 157-165
214b. Hoch B L, Nielson G P, Leibsch N J, Rosenberg A E 2006 Base of skull chordomas in children and adolescents: a clinicopathologic study of 73 cases. Am J Surg Pathol 30:811-818
215. Heffelfinger M J, Dahlin D C, MacCarty C S et al. 1973 Chordomas and cartilaginous tumors at the skull base. Cancer 32: 410-420
216. Brooks J J, LiVolsi V A, Trojanowski J Q 1987 Does chondroid chordoma exist? Acta Neuropathol (Berl) 72: 229-235
217. Rosenberg A E, Brown G A, Bahn A K et al. 1994 Chondroid chordoma - a variant of chordoma: a morphologic and immunohistochemical study. Am J Clin Pathol 101: 36-41
218. Salisbury J R 1987 Demonstration of cytokeratins and an epithelial membrane antigen in chondroid chordoma. J Pathol 153: 37-40
219. Mierau G W, Weeks D A 1987 Chondroid chordoma. Ultrastruct Pathol 11: 731-737
220. Belza M G, Urich H 1986 Chordoma and malignant fibrous histiocytoma: evidence for transformation. Cancer 58: 1082-1087
221. Miettinen M, Letho V-P, Virtanen I 1984 Malignant fibrous histiocytoma within a recurrent chordoma: a light microscopic, electron microscopic, and immunohistochemical study. Am J Clin Pathol 82: 738-743
222. Makek M, Leu H J 1982 Malignant fibrous histiocytoma arising in a recurrent chordoma: case report and electron microscopic findings. Virchows Arch [A] 397: 241-250
223. Chambers P W, Schwinn C P 1979 Chordoma: a clinicopathologic study of metastasis. Am J Clin Pathol 72: 765-776
224. Volpe R, Mazabraud A 1983 A clinicopathologic review of 25 cases of chordoma (a pleomorphic and metastasizing neoplasm). Am J Surg Pathol 7: 161-170
225. O'Connell J X, Renard L G, Liebsch N J et al. 1994 Base of skull chordoma: a correlative study of histologic and clinical features of 62 cases. Cancer 74: 2261-2267
226. Kaiser T E, Pritchard D J, Unni K K 1984 Clinicopathologic study of sacrococcygeal chordoma. Cancer 53: 2574-2578
227. Björnsson J, Wold L E, Ebersold M J et al. 1993 Chordoma of the mobile spine: a clinicopathologic analysis of 40 patients. Cancer 71: 735-740
228. Miettinen M 1984 Chordoma: antibodies to epithelial membrane antigen and carcinoembryonic antigen in differential diagnosis. Arch Pathol Lab Med 108: 891-892
229. Mirra J M, Brien E W 2001 Giant notochordal hamartoma of intraosseous origin: a newly reported benign entity to be distinguished from chordoma. Report of two cases. Skeletal Radiol 30: 698-709
230. Yamaguchi T, Suzuki S, Ishikawa H et al. 2004 Benign notochordal cell tumors: a comparative histological study of benign notochordal cell tumors, classic chordomas, and notochordal vestiges of fetal intervertebral discs. Am J Surg Pathol 28: 756-761
231. Divertie M B, Dahlin D C 1963 Neurilemmoma of rib: report of a case. Dis Chest 44: 635-637
232. Gordon E J 1976 Solitary intraosseous neurilemmoma of the tibia: review of intraosseous neurilemmoma and neurofibroma. Clin Orthop 117: 271-282
233. Milgram J W 1988 Intraosseous lipomas: a clinicopathologic study of 66 cases. Clin Orthop 231: 277-302
234. Gunterberg B, Kindblom L-G 1978 Intraosseous lipoma: a report of two cases. Acta Orthop Scand 49: 95-97
235. Chow L T-C, Lee K-C 1992 Intraosseous lipoma: a clinicopathologic study of nine cases. Am J Surg Pathol 16: 401-410
236. Milgram J W 1990 Malignant transformation in bone lipomas. Skeletal Radiol 19: 347-352
237. Oliveira A M, Hsi B L, Weremowicz S et al. 2004 USP6 (Tre2) fusion oncogenes in aneurysmal bone cyst. Cancer Res 64: 1920-1923
238. Zambrano E, Nose V, Perez-Atayde A R et al. 2004 Distinct chromosomal rearrangements in subungual (Dupuytren) exostosis and bizarre parosteal osteochondromatous proliferation (Nora lesion). Am J Surg Pathol 28: 1033-1039
239. Hudson T M 1984 Fluid levels in aneurysmal bone cysts: a CT feature. Am J Roentgenol 142: 1001-1004
240. Gold R H, Mirra J M 1983 Case report 234. Skeletal Radiol 10: 57-60
241. Levy W M, Miller A S, Bonakdarpour A et al. 1975 Aneurysmal bone cyst secondary to other osseous lesions: report of 57 cases. Am J Clin Pathol 63: 1-8
242. Martinez V, Sissons H A 1988 Aneurysmal bone cyst: a review of 123 cases including primary lesions and those secondary to other bone pathology. Cancer 61: 2291-2304
243. Sanerkin N G, Mott M G, Roylance J 1983 An unusual intraosseous lesion with fibroblastic, osteoclastic, osteoblastic, aneurysmal and fibromyxoid elements: "solid" variant of aneurysmal bone cyst. Cancer 51: 2278-2286
244. Lorenzo J C, Dorfman H D 1980 Giant-cell reparative granuloma of short tubular bones of the hands and feet. Am J Surg Pathol 4: 551-563
245. Wold L E, Dobyns J H, Swee R G et al. 1986 Giant cell reaction (giant cell reparative granuloma) of the small bones of the hands and feet. Am J Surg Pathol 10: 491-496
246. Ratner V, Dorfman H D 1990 Giant-cell reparative granuloma of the hand and foot bones. Clin Orthop 260: 251-258
247. Scaglietti O, Marchetti P G, Bartolozzi P 1979 The effects of methylprednisolone acetate in the treatment of bone cysts: results of three years follow-up. J Bone Joint Surg [Br] 61: 200-204
248. Bauer T W, Dorfman H D 1982 Intraosseous ganglion: a clinicopathologic study of 11 cases. Am J Surg Pathol 6: 207-213
249. Dockerty M B, Ghormley R K, Kennedy R L J et al. 1945 Albright's syndrome (polyostotic fibrous dysplasia with cutaneous pigmentation in both sexes and gonadal dysfunction in females). Arch Intern Med 75: 357-375
250. McArthur R G, Hayles A B, Lambert P W 1979 Albright's syndrome with rickets. Mayo Clin Proc 54: 313-320
251. Ishida T, Dorfman H D 1993 Massive chondroid differentiation in fibrous dysplasia of bone (fibrocartilaginous dysplasia). Am J Surg Pathol 17: 924-930
252. Simpson A H R W, Creasy T S, Williamson D M et al. 1989 Cystic degeneration of fibrous dysplasia masquerading as sarcoma. J Bone Joint Surg [Br] 71: 434-436
253. Diercks R L, Sauter A J M, Mallens W M C 1986 Aneurysmal bone cyst in association with fibrous dysplasia: a case report. J Bone Joint Surg [Br] 68: 144-146
254. Ruggieri P, Sim F H, Bond J R et al. 1994 Malignancies in fibrous dysplasia. Cancer 73: 1411-1424
255. Feintuch T A 1973 Chondrosarcoma arising in a cartilaginous area of previously irradiated fibrous dysplasia. Cancer 31: 877-881
256. Huvos A G, Higinbotham N L, Miller T R 1972 Bone sarcomas arising in fibrous dysplasia. J Bone Joint Surg [Am] 54: 1047-1056
257. Campanacci M, Laus M 1981 Osteofibrous dysplasia of the tibia and fibula. J Bone Joint Surg [Am] 63: 367-375
258. Nakashima Y, Yamamuro T, Fujiwara Y et al. 1983 Osteofibrous dysplasia (ossifying fibroma of long bones): a study of 12 cases. Cancer 52: 909-914
259. Blackwell J B, McCarthy S W, Xipell J M et al. 1988 Osteofibrous dysplasia of the tibia and fibula. Pathology 20: 227-233
260. Park Y-K, Unni K K, McLeod R A et al. 1993 Osteofibrous dysplasia: clinicopathologic study of 80 cases. Hum Pathol 24: 1339-1347
261. Kempson R L 1966 Ossifying fibroma of the long bones: a light and electron microscopic study. Arch Pathol 82: 218-233
262. Arata M A, Peterson H A, Dahlin D C 1981 Pathological fractures through non-ossifying fibromas: review of the Mayo Clinic experience. J Bone Joint Surg [Am] 63: 980-988

263. Campanacci M, Laus M, Boriani S 1983 Multiple non-ossifying fibromata with extraskeletal anomalies: a new syndrome? J Bone Joint Surg [Br] 65: 627-632
264. Mirra J M, Gold R H, Rand F 1982 Disseminated nonossifying fibromas in association with café-au-lait spots (Jaffe-Campanacci syndrome). Clin Orthop 168: 192-205
265. Kimmelstiel P, Rapp I 1951 Cortical defect due to periosteal desmoids. Bull Hosp Jt Dis 12: 286-297
266. Barnes G R Jr, Gwinn J L 1974 Distal irregularities of the femur simulating malignancy. AJR Am J Roentgenol 122: 180-185
267. Kindblom L-G, Angervall L 1978 Congenital solitary fibromatosis of the skeleton: case report of a variant of congenital generalized fibromatosis. Cancer 41: 636-640
268. Inwards C Y, Unni K K, Beabout J W et al. 1991 Solitary congenital fibromatosis (infantile myofibromatosis) of bone. Am J Surg Pathol 15: 935-941
269. Cooper K L, Beabout J W, Swee R G 1985 Insufficiency fractures of the sacrum. Radiology 156: 15-20
270. Ackerman L V 1958 Extra-osseous localized non-neoplastic bone and cartilage formation (so-called myositis ossificans): clinical and pathological confusion with malignant neoplasms. J Bone Joint Surg [Am] 40: 279-298
271. Smith R, Russell R G G, Woods C G 1976 Myositis ossificans progressiva: clinical features of eight patients and their response to treatment. J Bone Joint Surg [Br] 58: 48-57
272. Eckardt J J, Ivins J C, Perry H O et al. 1981 Osteosarcoma arising in heterotopic ossification of dermatomyositis: case report and review of the literature. Cancer 48: 1256-1261
273. Zambrano E, Nose V, Perez-Atayde A R et al. 2004 Distinct chromosomal rearrangements in subungual (Dupuytren) exostosis and bizarre parosteal osteochondromatous proliferation (Nora lesion). Am J Surg Pathol 28: 1033-1039
274. Miller-Breslow A, Dorfman H D 1988 Dupuytren's (subungual) exostosis. Am J Surg Pathol 12: 368-378
275. Lucas D R, Tazelaar H D, Unni K K et al. 1993 Osteogenic melanoma: a rare variant of malignant melanoma. Am J Surg Pathol 17: 400-409
276. Nilsson M, Domanski H A, Mertens F et al. 2004 Molecular cytogenetic characterization of recurrent translocation breakpoints in bizarre parosteal osteochondromatous proliferation (Nora's lesion). Am J Surg Pathol 35: 1063-1069
277. Meneses M F, Unni K K, Swee R G 1993 Bizarre parosteal osteochondromatous proliferation of bone (Nora's lesion). Am J Surg Pathol 17: 691-697
278. Spjut H J, Dorfman H D 1981 Florid reactive periostitis of the tubular bones of the hands and feet: a benign lesion which may simulate osteosarcoma. Am J Surg Pathol 5: 423-433
279. Dupree W B, Enzinger F M 1986 Fibro-osseous pseudotumor of the digits. Cancer 58: 2103-2109
280. Cabanela M E, Sim F H, Beabout J W et al. 1974 Osteomyelitis appearing as neoplasms: a diagnostic problem. Arch Surg 109: 68-72
281. Fitzgerald R H Jr, Brewer N S, Dahlin D C 1976 Squamous-cell carcinoma complicating chronic osteomyelitis. J Bone Joint Surg [Am] 58: 1146-1148
282. Akbarnia B A, Wirth C R, Colman N 1976 Fibrosarcoma arising from chronic osteomyelitis: case report and review of the literature. J Bone Joint Surg [Am] 58: 123-125
283. Lichtenstein L 1953 Histiocytosis X: integration of eosinophilic granuloma of bone, "Letterer-Siwe disease," and "Schuller-Christian disease" as related manifestations of a single nosologic entity. Arch Pathol 56: 84-102
284. Lieberman P H, Jones C R, Dargeon H W K et al. 1969 A reappraisal of eosinophilic granuloma of bone, Hand-Schüller-Christian syndrome and Letterer-Siwe syndrome. Medicine (Baltimore) 48: 375-400
285. Simmons P S, Wold L E, Elveback L R et al. 1981 Prognostic factors and management of histiocytosis X [abstract]. J Pediatr 98: 1023
286. Willman C L, Busque L, Griffith B B et al. 1994 Langerhans'-cell histiocytosis (histiocytosis X) - a clonal proliferative disease. N Engl J Med 331: 154-160
287. Emile J F, Wechsler J, Brousse N et al. 1995 Langerhans' cell histiocytosis: definitive diagnosis with the use of monoclonal antibody O10 on routine paraffin-embedded samples. Am J Surg Pathol 19: 636-641
288. Newton W A Jr, Hamoudi A B 1973 Histiocytosis: a histologic classification with clinical correlation. Perspect Pediatr Pathol 1: 251-283
289. Nezelof C, Frileux-Herbet F, Cronier-Sachot J 1979 Disseminated histiocytosis X: analysis of prognostic factors based on a retrospective study of 50 cases. Cancer 44: 1824-1838
290. Kilpatrick S E, Wenger D E, Gilchrist G S et al. 1995 Langerhans' cell histiocytosis (histiocytosis X) of bone: a clinicopathologic analysis of 263 pediatric and adult cases. Cancer 76: 2471-2484
291. Travis W D, Li C-Y, Bergstralh E J 1989 Solid and hematologic malignancies in 60 patients with systemic mast cell disease. Arch Pathol Lab Med 113: 365-368
292. Travis W D, Li C-Y, Bergstralh E J et al. 1988 Systemic mast cell disease: analysis of 58 cases and literature review. Medicine (Baltimore) 67: 345-368
293. Hughes D M, Kurtin P J, Hanson C A et al. 1995 Identification of normal and neoplastic mast cells by immunohistochemical demonstration of tryptase in paraffin sections. J Surg Pathol 1: 87-96
294. Webb T A, Li C-Y, Yam L T 1982 Systemic mast cell disease: a clinical and hematopathologic study of 26 cases. Cancer 49: 927-938
295. Rosai J, Dorfman R F 1969 Sinus histiocytosis with massive lymphadenopathy: a newly recognized benign clinicopathological entity. Arch Pathol 87: 63-70
296. Foucar E, Rosai J, Dorfman R 1990 Sinus histiocytosis with massive lymphadenopathy (Rosai-Dorfman disease): review of the entity. Semin Diagn Pathol 7: 19-73
297. Blumenthal B I, Capitanio M A, Queloz J M et al. 1972 Intrathoracic mesenchymoma: observations in two infants. Radiology 104: 107-109
298. McLeod R A, Dahlin D C 1979 Hamartoma (mesenchymoma) of the chest wall in infancy. Radiology 131: 657-661
299. Odell J M, Benjamin D R 1986 Mesenchymal hamartoma of chest wall in infancy: natural history of two cases. Pediatr Pathol 5: 135-146
300. Dahlin D C, Bertoni F, Beabout J W et al. 1984 Fibrocartilaginous mesenchymoma with low-grade malignancy. Skeletal Radiol 12: 263-269
301. Bulychova I V, Unni K K, Bertoni F et al. 1993 Fibrocartilaginous mesenchymoma of bone. Am J Surg Pathol 17: 830-836
302. Coventry M B, Harrison E G Jr, Martin J F 1966 Benign synovial tumors of the knee: a diagnostic problem. J Bone Joint Surg [Am] 48: 1350-1358
303. Jaffe H L, Lichtenstein L, Sutro C J 1941 Pigmented villonodular synovitis, bursitis and tenosynovitis: a discussion of the synovial and bursal equivalents of the tenosynovial lesion commonly denoted as xanthoma, xanthogranuloma, giant cell tumor or myeloplaxoma of the tendon sheath, with some consideration of this tendon sheath lesion itself. Arch Pathol 31: 731-765
304. Schwartz H S, Unni K K, Pritchard D J 1989 Pigmented villonodular synovitis: a retrospective review of affected large joints. Clin Orthop 247: 243-255
305. Pulitzer D R, Reed R J 1984 Localized pigmented villonodular synovitis of the vertebral column. Arch Pathol Lab Med 108: 228-230
306. Giannini C, Scheithauer B W, Wenger D E et al. 1996 Pigmented villonodular synovitis of the spine: a clinical, radiological, and morphological study of 12 cases. J Neurosurg 84: 592-597
307. Weidner N, Challa V R, Bonsib S M et al. 1986 Giant cell tumors of synovium (pigmented villonodular synovitis) involving the vertebral column. Cancer 57: 2030-2036
308. Somerhausen N S, Fletcher C D 2000 Diffuse-type giant cell tumor: clinicopathologic and immunohistochemical analysis of 50 cases with extraarticular disease. Am J Surg Pathol 24: 479-492
309. Dorwart R H, Genant H K, Johnston W H et al. 1984 Pigmented villonodular synovitis of synovial joints: clinical, pathologic, and radiologic features. Am J Roentgenol 143: 877-885
310. Kindblom L-G, Gunterberg B 1978 Pigmented villonodular synovitis involving bone: case report. J Bone Joint Surg [Am] 60: 830-832
311. Bertoni F, Unni K K, Beabout J W et al. 1997 Malignant giant cell tumor of the tendon sheaths and joints (malignant pigmented villonodular synovitis). Am J Surg Pathol 21: 153-163
312. Nielsen A L, Klaer T 1989 Malignant giant cell tumor of synovium and locally destructive pigmented villonodular tenosynovitis: ultrastructural and immunohistochemical study and review of the literature. Hum Pathol 20: 765-771
313. Murphy F P, Dahlin D C, Sullivan C R 1962 Articular synovial chondromatosis. J Bone Joint Surg [Am] 44: 77-86
314. Ronald J B, Keller E E, Weiland L H 1978 Synovial chondromatosis of the temporomandibular joint. J Oral Surg 36: 13-19
315. Blankestijn J, Panders A K, Vermey A et al. 1985 Synovial chondromatosis of the temporo-mandibular joint: report of three cases and a review of the literature. Cancer 55: 479-485
316. Buddingh E P, Krallman P, Neff J R et al. 2003 Chromosome 6 abnormalities are recurrent in synovial chondromatosis. Cancer Genet Cytogenet 140: 18-22
317. Bertoni F, Unni K K, Beabout J W et al. 1991 Chondrosarcomas of the synovium. Cancer 67: 155-162
318. Lewis R C Jr, Coventry M B, Soule E H 1959 Hemangioma of the synovial membrane. J Bone Joint Surg [Am] 41: 264-271

中枢神经系统肿瘤
Tumors of the central nervous system

M. Beatriz S. Lopes 和 Scott R.VandenBerg 著

孙昆昆 译　钱利华 校

引言	1653	起源未定的神经上皮肿瘤	1686
术中诊断技术	1653	神经元和混合性神经元-胶质肿瘤	1688
组织处理	1654	松果体实质肿瘤	1697
特殊染色和免疫组织化学	1654	胚胎性肿瘤	1700
神经上皮性肿瘤	1655	脑膜肿瘤	1707
星形细胞瘤	1655	组织发生未定的肿瘤	1714
少突胶质细胞肿瘤和混合性胶质瘤	1673	生殖细胞肿瘤	1717
室管膜肿瘤	1678	非神经上皮性肿瘤和囊肿	1720
脉络丛肿瘤	1684		

引言

在过去的十年，外科神经病理学的一个重点在于：以特殊组织病理学和免疫组织化学特征为依据来进行肿瘤的精确分类。对于有些病例，将这些特征与临床资料和细胞遗传学数据相结合已经成为确定临床病理病变的基础。在今后的十年，临床神经-肿瘤学的进展将包括新的用药模式：应用直接作用于多种组织病理肿瘤类型的特定生物靶向药物。这些药物将包括细胞受体和可调控增殖[1]、肿瘤浸润和（或）血管形成[2]的信号通路，后者在不同肿瘤细胞种群中有不同的表达。外科神经病理学需要通过结合常规技术和免疫组化技术以及分子形态学方法来确定和识别这些靶点。分子形态学方法包括分子细胞遗传学技术、活化蛋白质的磷酸化抗原决定簇的检测以及表达谱的确定（结合激光捕获显微分离），通过特殊的基因扩增和（或）信号通路活化来识别肿瘤细胞亚群。这些基因和蛋白方法当与现代组织病理学框架融合时，可以使神经-肿瘤学家能够更准确地预测生物学行为和确定治疗靶点[3]。脑肿瘤的分子遗传学评估，尤其是星形细胞瘤和少突胶质细胞瘤，已经增强了我们对组织病理学相同或不同的胶质瘤亚型肿瘤的发生和进展的认识。最后，重点需要强调的是，所有组织病理学资料都应该与临床和神经影像学资料相结合，以便对CNS肿瘤进行最佳的评估。

术中诊断技术

目前神经-影像引导技术的进展以使医生能够对肿瘤进行精确的定位，并可对异质性肿瘤进行多部位的准确取材。但是，这些技术通常还需要对小标本样本进行病理学评估。术中对全部小标本样本进行冰冻切片处理常常会使随后的石蜡标本的免疫组织化学和分子形态学技术达不到最佳效果。组织涂片技术既可对小的活检标本进行选择性的多处检查，又可保留多数组织进行快速和有效的保存和处理，以便进行最佳的免疫组织化学检查。涂片可以避免小的、不可替代的标本进行术中冰冻切片，这样可以防止重要的诊断材料扭曲或丢失的危险出现。作为一种术中CNS活检评估的准确和有效方法，涂片技术[4-6]在许多神经肿瘤中心已确立和应用。其结果与冰冻切片的诊断准确率相当[5,6]。从涂片中获得的细胞学信息足以进行术中诊断，并且常常可为石蜡包埋组织切片提供补充信息。这种组织处理方法也适用于进行组织化学、免疫组织化学和荧光原位杂交（FISH）研究，即可直接也可在Morris染色之后应用[7,8]。FISH可用于室温下经100%的甲醇固定/脱水几分钟后储存在-25℃无水甲醇的涂片。对于细胞脆性极大且间质极其致密或质硬的肿瘤，印片[9]也可有助于提供额外的细胞学信息（如硬膜或硬膜外组织的浆细胞瘤）。涂片作为对组织病理切片的一种常规补充方法其特点在本章全章都有讨论。

组织处理

在外科病理学中，甲醛溶液仍然优于大多数常规使用的固定剂。最好的结果通常可通过使用轻度酸化加 $ZnSO_4$ 的甲醛溶液或 10% 的甲醛缓冲液来获得。对分子形态学研究的更多重视也使 methacarn[10] 或乙醇[11-13]、标准石蜡包埋得以使用，即作为用甲醛溶液固定的替代方法，以便对同一个标本进行蛋白质组分析 [免疫组化和（或）用于 2D 凝胶电泳 / 质谱分析的蛋白萃取]、表达谱（RNA）和基因组研究（DNA）。低温熔点包埋介质的应用，如聚酯蜡[14]，其包埋组织可以更好地保存温度敏感成分，包括纤细的嗜银性突起。近来，组织经甲醇和聚乙二醇混合固定，随后用微波加强固定以及脱水和石蜡包埋，已经用于常规免疫组化和分子形态学研究的组织处理[15,16]。抗原修复技术常常需要对非甲醛溶液固定技术进行改进。需要着重强调的是，无论采用何种固定技术，减少标本从切除到固定的热缺血时间都是获得最佳分子形态学的关键。

特殊染色和免疫组织化学

目前神经病理学的常用方法包括特殊技术，尤其是免疫组织化学和少数组化银染色以及超微结构免疫细胞化学。银染色技术，尤其是改良的 Bielschowsky 染色，仍然是检测神经突起的重要手段，尤其是对来源于神经母细胞和不成熟神经元的纤细突起。然而，固定和包埋过程可显著地影响这些技术的成功应用。尽管改良的 Bielschowsky 染色可以用于常规的甲醛溶液固定、石蜡包埋的组织，但是根据我们的经验，为了使大多数纤细不成熟的细胞突起获得最佳染色，应该采用甲醛溶液固定、低熔点聚酯蜡（37℃）包埋，或者采用甲醛溶液固定的冰冻切片。Bouin 固定液和乙醇不适合银染色。经 10% 的甲醛缓冲液处理的脱蜡组织切片可明显增强神经的嗜银性，无论最初固定如何。

过去十年间，大量多克隆和单克隆抗体已经作为常规组织技术的补充手段应用于脑肿瘤的诊断分类。不同程度的细胞分化可以通过与细胞骨架和表面膜蛋白抗原决定簇产生反应的抗体来检测。肿瘤性神经母细胞和神经元细胞可以通过与神经丝蛋白抗原决定簇（尤其是 NF-M/H，但不是 NF-L 抗原决定簇）[17]、微管和微管相关蛋白（MAP-2 和 MAP-Tau）[18,19]、突触素[20]、突触蛋白 I[21]、Neu-N[22] 和 α-synuclein[23,24] 产生反应的抗体来识别。肿瘤的胶质分化可以通过中间丝蛋白来评估，如胶质纤维酸性蛋白（GFAP）、波形蛋白和 nestin 以及细胞表面或细胞膜相关蛋白，如 Leu-7（CD57）、髓鞘碱性蛋白（MBP）、髓鞘相关糖蛋白（MAG）和胞浆蛋白（S-100 和谷氨酰胺合成酶）[18,25]。肿瘤性脑膜上皮细胞可以通过若干上皮和间叶细胞相关蛋白来识别，如上皮膜抗原（EMA）、细胞角蛋白、S-100 蛋白和波形蛋白[26-29]。

组织经过固定处理后的抗原保留以及它们在石蜡处理和储存过程中的稳定性是影响免疫组织化学技术成功运用的主要因素。这些因素对于神经元细胞骨架蛋白和突触素的研究尤为关键。对于这些抗原决定簇，Bouin 固定液一般最为理想，但是添加 $ZnSO_4$ 的甲醛固定液也可以得到满意的结果。总的来说，短暂的固定结合低熔点石蜡可以更好地检测许多细胞骨架和细胞膜相关蛋白。如突触素，如果甲醛溶液或 Bouin 固定的时间不超过 2～4 小时，其免疫反应最佳[30]。相比之下，理想的乙醇固定通常不是时间依赖型的[30]，神经丝蛋白表型经乙醇处理后不溶解[31]；但是，乙醇固定的组织经过石蜡包埋和储存后其抗原性减少[30]。在常规处理过程中，乙醇固定非常不适于微管抗原决定簇的保留[31]。至于其他中间丝蛋白表型，如 GFAP、波形蛋白和角蛋白以及其他抗原，后者如 S-100 蛋白、Leu-7（CD57）和 EMA，非常适于缓冲液或 $ZnSO_4$- 甲醛溶液短暂固定。

大多数常规甲醛溶液固定和石蜡包埋的组织在对照条件下，采用蛋白酶或加热进行脱蜡组织的预处理可使免疫组化分析效果明显增强。读者可以参阅有关加强"抗原修复"的各种蛋白水解、热修复和缓冲系统的优秀综述[32-36]。对于特殊的表型，采用蛋白水解酶（蛋白酶 XXV、蛋白酶 E、胃蛋白酶或蛋白酶 K）来处理脱蜡组织切片，可以提高免疫反应的敏感性而不改变抗体的选择；但是，对每一种表型而言，最佳的酶处理明显不同。这对于长时间在甲醛溶液中固定的标本尤其有用[31]。敏感性明显增加，而特异性不变，已可通过在 GFAP、角蛋白和 S-100 蛋白（0.4% 的胃蛋白酶于 0.01N HCl 中）得以实现。但是必须慎重，因为波形蛋白、微管 - 相关蛋白和许多神经丝蛋白表型会选择性地受到某些蛋白酶处理的显著影响。在不同的螯合条件下，热处理可能是最常用的预处理形式。微波和高压锅，无论有无额外的温度控制和湿度饱和装置，都很有效[34,37]。该过程的优点是加强了选择性的免疫组化反应，而不产生明显新的人工免疫反应位点，也不增加非特异性背景水平。尤其易于受此影响的抗原大多数是中间丝蛋白，包括波形蛋白和神经丝蛋白表型，微管相关蛋白，包括Tau、NeuN、胞核和胞膜受体[38]。最重要的是，微波处理技术可使许多先前只能用于冰冻组织的抗体能够用于甲醛溶液固定、石蜡包埋的组织。非常重要的例子是单克隆抗体MIB-1，直接抗Ki-67抗原的重组部分[39]（见下文），它们只有经过微波热处理后才能成功应用于石蜡包埋组织[40,41]。这种方法也使免疫组化技术可用于氧化脱黑色素或EDTA脱钙之后[41]。

一个最常见的对常规组织病理学的补充方法是：运用特殊技术来评估细胞周期相关核蛋白，以更好地勾画出增殖性细胞部分。这些方法尤其适用于胶质和脑膜肿瘤以及特异性蛋白，包括Ki-67蛋白、增殖细胞核抗原（PCNA）以及新近的拓扑异构酶Ⅱα。涉及这些表型的免疫组化最好采用甲醛溶液固定的组织而非酒精或Bouin固定的组织。

在三种核蛋白中，Ki-67蛋白的免疫染色，即单克隆抗体MIB-1，已被用于多数CNS肿瘤的研究，它是日常工作中最实用的增殖性标记物。Ki-67蛋白是一种细胞核非组蛋白，是维持细胞周期所必需，表达于细胞周期G1、S、G2、M期，但是G0期不表达[39,42,43]。与PCNA相比（见下文），Ki-67在G1中晚期有少量表达，在整个S期明显聚集。很多项研究已证实了Ki-67免疫组化作为一种评估生长潜能方法的重要性。而且，MIB-1标记指数与弥漫性星形细胞瘤[44]和脑膜瘤[45]的WHO分级具有很好的相关性。

PCNA/cyclin（大约为36KDa）是DNA聚合酶δ的辅助因子，在S期早期合成率稍高[46,47]，而当细胞进入非周期状态时相对减少。但是，采用常规免疫组化来检测这些改变很有争议[47-49]，而且依特殊的细胞类型、组织处理类型、特异性抗体以及阳性免疫反应的染色阈值而有所不同[50,51]。因此，对于PCNA免疫反应"阳性"的简单解释应慎重，除了分批组织处理外，应考虑到每一种抗体的细致规范化和总体免疫反应强度。尽管在研究的大多数胶质瘤中，一般来说间变性增加与PCNA-标记细胞核增加之间具有相关性[50-52]，但多数试验室目前在日常工作中并不常规运用该抗体。

大多数Ⅱ型拓扑异构酶的催化活性是清除DNA复制后残留的拓扑复合体。α-异构体，为细胞生存所必需，是已定性哺乳类动物的拓扑异构酶Ⅱ的异构体。拓扑异构酶Ⅱα（TopoⅡα）在染色体的构型上也具有作用，在间期和有丝分裂期间，可形成染色体环与蛋白框架之间的黏附[53]。在胶质瘤和非胶质瘤性脑肿瘤的谱系中，通过反转录聚合酶链反应（RT-PCR）分析[54]，免疫反应性TopoⅡα表达与TopoⅡα mRNA表达密切相关。应用TopoⅡα免疫反应来检测增殖细胞最初是用于室管膜瘤[55,56]。在一大组肿瘤研究中，TopoⅡα免疫反应与MIB-1免疫反应具有很好的相关性；但是，TopoⅡα免疫反应细胞的标记指数大约为25%~54%，低于MIB-1指数。这种绝对误差是由TopoⅡα活性所致，后者在S晚期，以复制依赖的方式，集中在异染色质的复制，在G2和M期，集中在中心性异染色质[53]，而MIB-1表型聚集在大部分增殖细胞周期。

核仁组成区（NOR）的银染色（AgNOR）已经成功地用于常规处理的组织，与Ki-67的免疫组化具有相关性[7,57,59]。核糖体DNA环在调节细胞蛋白合成中起到不可缺少的作用[60]，除了在一些组织中受增殖活性的影响外，核仁组成区还受细胞生理状态的影响。因此，AgNOR与增殖活性的相关性应该在每种细胞类型进行验证。应该注意到，采用AgNOR技术来区分反应性星形细胞增生和星形细胞瘤的潜在可行性[61]。

神经上皮性肿瘤
Tumors of neuroepithelial tissue

星形细胞瘤　Astrocytic tumors

目前，星形细胞瘤[44]的WHO分类定义了六种主要肿瘤类型（表26.1），通常被归为两大类。这些是依据浸润邻近脑和脊髓组织的能力来定义的，后者表现为病变边缘的弥漫性细胞浸润以及CNS内的远处细胞播散。除了能弥漫浸润邻近的神经毡或白质及远处播散外，弥漫型星形细胞瘤具有随时间推移向具有更为恶性的生物学行为发展的显著潜能。前三种肿瘤类型（星形细胞瘤、间变性星形细胞瘤以及多形性胶质母细胞瘤）及其变型组成弥漫性星形细胞瘤。对于弥漫性星形细胞瘤而言，细胞浸润局部神经元的程度以及肿瘤细胞远处播散的能力随分级的升高而均有增加[62-64]。同样，肿瘤内异质性也增加。胶质母细胞瘤作为最高级别的弥漫性星形细胞瘤，最具浸润性生长和广泛转移的能力。相反，第二大类中的星形细胞瘤，如毛细胞性星形细胞瘤、多形性黄色瘤性星形细胞瘤及室管膜下巨细胞性星形细胞瘤恶性进展能力有限，很少出现浸润邻近神经毡的侵袭性生长。

星形细胞肿瘤和神经干细胞的多样性（diversity of astrocytic tumors and neural stem cells）：星形细胞瘤的生物学行为谱系部分源于靶细胞的异质性，一旦发生转化，就会表达不同的星形细胞表型。实验室研究表明，这些成人脑组织中的靶点包括神经干细胞和前体细胞以及更加分化的细胞群[65,66]。这些靶点对于外源性微环境因子

表26.1　神经上皮性肿瘤

星形细胞瘤
1. 星形细胞瘤
   变型：纤维、原浆、肥胖或混合型
2. 间变性（恶性）星形细胞瘤
3. 胶质母细胞瘤
   变型：巨细胞胶质母细胞瘤、胶质肉瘤
4. 毛细胞型星形细胞瘤
5. 多形性黄色瘤型星形细胞瘤
6. 室管膜下巨细胞型星形细胞瘤（常伴有结节性硬化）

少突胶质细胞肿瘤
1. 少突胶质细胞瘤
2. 间变性（恶性）少突胶质细胞瘤

混合性胶质瘤
1. 混合性少突星形细胞瘤
2. 间变性（恶性）少突星形细胞瘤
3. 其他

室管膜肿瘤
1. 室管膜瘤
   变型：富于细胞型、乳头型、上皮型、透明细胞型、伸展细胞型
2. 间变性（恶性）室管膜瘤
3. 黏液乳头型室管膜瘤
4. 室管膜下瘤

脉络丛肿瘤
1. 脉络丛乳头状瘤
2. 脉络丛癌

起源未定的神经上皮肿瘤
1. 第三脑室脊索样胶质瘤
2. 星形母细胞瘤
3. 大脑胶质瘤病

神经元和混合性神经元-胶质肿瘤
1. 节细胞瘤
2. 小脑发育不良性节细胞瘤（Lhermitte-Duclos）
3. 促纤维增生性婴儿型星形细胞瘤和节细胞胶质瘤
4. 胚胎发育不良性神经上皮性肿瘤
5. 节细胞胶质瘤
6. 间变性（恶性）节细胞胶质瘤
7. 中枢神经细胞瘤

松果体肿瘤
1. 松果体瘤
2. 松果体母细胞瘤
3. 中分化松果体实质肿瘤

胚胎性肿瘤
1. 髓母细胞瘤
   经典型髓母细胞瘤
   促纤维增生型/结节型髓母细胞瘤
   大细胞髓母细胞瘤
   髓肌母细胞瘤
   黑色素型髓母细胞瘤
2. 幕上原始神经外胚层肿瘤
3. 髓上皮瘤
4. 室管膜母细胞瘤
5. 大脑神经母细胞瘤
   变型：节细胞神经母细胞瘤
6. 视网膜母细胞瘤
7. 非典型畸胎样/横纹肌样瘤

以及肿瘤转化和肿瘤形成过程中的特殊基因和后生事件具有不同的易感性。神经干和前体细胞具有特殊的区域性分布和生成胶质和神经元细胞系的不同的潜能[67]。神经干细胞可自我更新，能够针对复杂的环境活化迁移和（或）分化，由特殊的环境提示来介导，包括细胞连接、一系列生长因子以及细胞外基质中的信号分子。尽管这些细胞已经从不同的哺乳动物脑组织的脑室下区域、侧脑室内层、海马齿状回和皮层下白质区中分离出来，但在人类，这些生发区域中最大的似乎是脑室下区，其具有双相潜能，伴有星形细胞特性（GFAP$^+$）的放射状胶质样细胞似乎行使着神经干细胞功能[66,68]。能够自我更新的前体细胞具有产生星形细胞和少突胶质细胞的潜能，也可以位于整个神经轴，包括皮质、胼胝体、脑室周围的白质、脑室下区以及齿状回。

成人神经干和前体细胞明确位于CNS中提示，局部适宜的微环境对维持干细胞池自我更新、增殖以及形成星形和少突胶质细胞系特异性胶质前体细胞的正常调节是必需的。Notch受体信号在此调节中可能起关键作用[66,69,70]。Hedgehog-Gli通路是调节神经干细胞增殖的另一个关键通路，也可以调节脑室下区后来形成的前体细胞的增殖。这些通路的异常刺激似乎与弥漫性胶质瘤的形成有关[71]。放射状胶质细胞的分化残留体，如Bergmann胶质和下丘脑的伸展细胞[66]，可以是细胞靶点，如果出现转化，会形成特殊类型的胶质瘤。小脑和下丘脑的毛细胞型星形细胞瘤也可以源自放射状胶质残留体的衍生物。有关CD133表型的试验研究为某些胶质瘤起源中有干细胞存在提供了额外的证据。小脑毛细胞型星形细胞瘤和胶质母细胞瘤均含有不同干细胞片段，可以通过CD133免疫反应识别，从胶质母细胞瘤中纯化的CD133阳性细胞群可以产生类似于原发肿瘤的高效异种移植物[72,73]。

试验小鼠模型提示，原始胶质和神经前体细胞以及更加分化的胶质细胞系对肿瘤性转化具有不同的易感性，在相同基因病变的诱导下，可形成不同的胶质瘤表型，包括*PDGF-β*、*Ras*和*Akt*相关信号通路的活化[74-76]。不同神经细胞靶点中的一个基因病变如何形成生物行为显著不同的非典型性或增殖性病变的另外一个令人困惑的例子是小脑发育不良性节细胞瘤（也见于神经元肿瘤部分）。它是惰性的、细胞增生性病变，伴有*PTEN*功能丧失，原因是种系突变（Cowden病）和体细胞*PTEN*突变。出现小脑神经母细胞群异位性扩展，可能是正常发育性凋亡的减少或丢失、迁移缺陷以及体积增加所致。增殖性星形细胞病变则缺乏。这与胶质细胞中*PTEN*功能如何缺失和磷酸肌醇-3激酶（PI3K）调节通路活化具有高度恶性的生物学行为（见下文）形成对比。与发

育中的脑组织的对应部分相比，成人神经前体细胞的令人困惑的致癌作用尚有待于进一步确定。有关原始前体细胞和分化细胞群作为致癌靶点对肿瘤转化和随后的肿瘤形成过程中的特定基因和后期事件具有不同易感性的概念，将进一步影响胶质瘤的分类。

弥漫性星形细胞肿瘤分级（grading diffuse astrocytic tumors）：在WHO分类中，目前确诊弥漫性星形细胞肿瘤主要依赖组织病理学特征，免疫组化可作为补充[44,77,78]。弥漫性星形细胞肿瘤对应于三级系统的三种主要类型：星形细胞瘤（WHO Ⅱ级）、间变性星形细胞瘤（WHO Ⅲ级）和多形性胶质母细胞瘤（GBM）及其变型、巨细胞型胶质母细胞瘤和胶质肉瘤（星形细胞瘤，WHO Ⅳ级）。尽管过去应用过多种组织病理学分级系统[79-81]，但WHO分类目前仍被广泛使用（图26.2）。

因此，仅有细胞核非典型性的肿瘤被认为是Ⅱ级，命名为星形细胞瘤；那些除了细胞核非典型性以外还具有核分裂活性的肿瘤被认为是Ⅲ级，命名为间变性星形细胞瘤；肿瘤出现非典型性、核分裂象、微血管增生（"内皮细胞增生"）和（或）坏死者被认为是Ⅳ级，命名为胶质母细胞瘤。肿瘤取材适当时，这种简化的系统一般适于进行肿瘤分级。随着肿瘤分级的增加，其组织病理学的异质性增加，对于有限的肿瘤标本，可能难以精确分级。在这种病例中，非典型性的出现，结合内皮/外皮细胞增生（微血管增生），即使没有看到核分裂象或坏死，也提示胶质母细胞瘤。对于有限的或立体定位活检病例，多处组织位点应当与神经影像学参数结合。这些有利于在细胞丰富和微血管增生明显增多的肿瘤区域取材[82-84]。

由于出现核分裂象细胞对鉴别WHO Ⅱ级和WHO Ⅲ级星形细胞瘤是关键特征，免疫组化技术一直被用来进行更为精确的增殖细胞群计数。Ki-67蛋白免疫染色，如用单克隆抗体MIB-1，是目前最好的"增殖"细胞标记物。对于一个取自弥漫性星形细胞瘤的特定组织标本，尽管单一Ki-67免疫反应还不足以进行明确分级，但对于弥漫性星形细胞瘤，MIB-1标记指数与WHO分级之间具有很好的相关性[85]。但是，采用小分子抑制剂治疗的复发性肿瘤可干扰细胞周期G1期和G1-S的过渡，因此评判Ki-67标记指数需要谨慎，因为有可能导致Ki-67抗原指数反常增加，尽管是低增殖分数[86]。

具有显著"肾小球样"微血管增生表现的异常血管增生是将弥漫性星形细胞肿瘤分级为胶质母细胞瘤的关键性组织病理学特征。其基础生物学在一定程度上与肿瘤细胞中血管内皮生长因子（VEGF）表达和肿瘤微血管细胞中VEGF受体（flt-1；flk-1/KDR）的非均匀性上调有关[87,88]。有关胶质母细胞瘤中的明显"肾小球样"增生以及缺氧诱导因子（HIF-1α）和VEGF表达的微血管结构研究提示，微血管结构可能与原发性胶质母细胞瘤的临床预后相关[89]。此外，有证据表明，依据VEGF免疫组化反应类型进行肿瘤分类具有重要的预后价值[90]，并且放射性治疗可以诱导VEGF表达增加[91]。

胶质母细胞瘤进展时出现的血管生成也涉及微血管细胞成分（内皮细胞和外皮细胞）与若干生长因子和间质细胞外环境多种成分的相互作用[92]，包括与肿瘤细胞浸润有关的基质蛋白酶（MMP-2）的活化[93]。

要在星形细胞瘤诊断方面取得进展，其挑战在于除了评估增殖活性以外，需要更为精确地评估特殊肿瘤的侵袭潜能。用来确定弥漫性星形细胞瘤恶性潜能的组织学特征评估过程，是将异质性和动态生长过程赋予静态

表26.2	胶质瘤和WHO分级
肿瘤命名	WHO分级
弥漫性浸润型星形细胞瘤	
星形细胞瘤	Ⅱ
间变性星形细胞瘤	Ⅲ
多形性胶质母细胞瘤	Ⅳ
星形细胞瘤的特殊类型	
毛细胞型星形细胞瘤	Ⅰ
多形性黄色瘤型星形细胞瘤	Ⅱ~Ⅲ
室管膜下巨细胞型星形细胞瘤	Ⅰ
少突胶质细胞肿瘤	
少突胶质细胞瘤	Ⅱ
间变性少突胶质细胞瘤	Ⅲ
混合性少突星形细胞瘤	Ⅱ
间变性少突星形细胞瘤	Ⅲ
室管膜肿瘤	
室管膜瘤	Ⅱ
间变性室管膜瘤	Ⅲ
黏液乳头型室管膜瘤	Ⅰ
室管膜下瘤	Ⅰ
脉络丛肿瘤	
脉络丛乳头状瘤	Ⅰ
脉络丛癌	Ⅲ

和相关性的组织病理学命名。因此，星形细胞瘤分级理当明确哪一种组织病理学和分子形态学特征可以预测：(1) 快速生长的潜能（增殖、细胞死亡和血管形成）；(2) 肿瘤-脑交界处相互间的（协同）生物学行为；(3) 肿瘤细胞浸润脑组织和中枢神经轴远处播散的能力。最近一项有关41例胶质母细胞瘤患者生存率与基因表达水平和基因标记的相关性研究强烈提示：评估星形细胞瘤浸润性具有重要意义。三种细胞迁移相关基因（即doublecortin、骨连接素、信号素3B）一致高表达，患者存活期较短[94]。

肿瘤浸润（tumor invasiveness）：弥漫性星形细胞肿瘤浸润邻近脑组织、软脑膜以及沿脑脊液通路播散的能力已有报道[95-97]。一项伴有CSF播散的有14例胶质母细胞瘤的研究[95]提示了令人费解的可能性，即根据表型分化，特殊肿瘤细胞亚群的一种特征为远处转移，并且浸润邻近结构为其另外一个特征。星形细胞瘤浸润是一个复杂表现，涉及粘附性、细胞外基质修饰和细胞活动，并且与这些属性在间变进程中的不同调节相关。粘附分子研究方面已经产生了最终会有助于诊断的数据。至于细胞表面粘附分子，整合素（integrin）表达的改变伴有星形胶质细胞的转化。特别是，αv和β1整合素在星形细胞瘤浸润中已经被提及[98]；β4在星形细胞瘤中上调[99]；两种玻璃粘连蛋白受体，即αvβ3和αvβ5，在部分星形细胞恶性表型中上调[100,101]。胶质母细胞瘤的细胞与肿瘤间质和浸润性肿瘤边缘的反应性星形胞都可以分泌一定量的似乎利于肿瘤细胞浸润的基质分子。后者包括透明质烷[102,103]、NG2[104,105]、黏蛋白、tenascin[106-109]和层粘连蛋白[110,111]，尤其是含有α4、β1和β2链（层粘连蛋白8和9）的成分。胶质母细胞瘤细胞的透明质烷（HA）受体可介导细胞迁移[112,113]和对邻近脑组织的浸润[114]。HA受体（CD44）的表达水平似乎与肿瘤对他莫昔芬/卡铂的化疗反应相关[114]。运用功能蛋白组筛查检测有助于发现另外的膜表面受体，后者参与介导胶质母细胞瘤浸润性生长过程中肿瘤细胞的活动[115,116]。肿瘤转化和恶性进展后，星形胶质细胞分泌的细胞外基质（ECM）分子也可有改变，可以调节肿瘤浸润[98,101,117,118]。层粘连蛋白在肿瘤细胞浸润、血管生成和肿瘤内炎细胞相互作用中起作用[110,111,119]。最近的资料表明，层粘连蛋白8在肿瘤浸润、进展和复发过程中起重要作用。结合层粘连蛋白的巨噬细胞可上调尿激酶型纤溶酶原激活物（uPA）和基质金属蛋白酶9（MMP-9）的分泌，两者在肿瘤浸润中起关键作用。综合脑组织区域性ECM变化、这种ECM的肿瘤性胶质改变以及肿瘤细胞粘附分子的进行性变化，对于活检或切除标本来说，究竟何种浸润"标志"能够预测体内特殊肿瘤的生物学潜能，给我们的诊断提出了挑战。

肿瘤性星形细胞表达和分泌一定量的丝氨酸蛋白酶和金属蛋白酶[120]，以及几种蛋白酶抑制剂（包括纤溶酶原激活物-1和蛋白酶连接蛋白Ⅰ和Ⅱ）[121]。若干种蛋白酶和蛋白酶膜受体在胶质母细胞瘤浸润和血管生成过程中作用已被论及[64,122]。恶性转化后，与正常脑组织或低级别胶质瘤相比[123,124]，尿激酶型纤溶酶原激活物（uPA）明显上调，uPA活性在恶性星形细胞瘤中较高，尤其是在胶质母细胞瘤。uPA直接和间接介导浸润性迁移，即通过直接与其膜受体——uPAR的相互作用以及间接活化基质金属蛋白酶2（MMP-2）[125-127]。与低级别星形细胞瘤相对比，胶质母细胞瘤的uPAR表达水平也有增加[128,129]。胶质母细胞瘤细胞的uPAR过表达也被视为免疫毒素治疗的潜在靶点[130]。MMP-2和MMP-9的表达/活化与肿瘤细胞和肿瘤间质细胞表达血管形成和浸润因子VEGF、ang-2和uPA相关[91,126,131,132]。

弥漫性星形细胞瘤的间变性进展和分子病理学（anaplastic progression and molecular pathology of diffuse astrocytomas）：星形细胞肿瘤的所有类型都有间变性进展的潜能；但只有弥漫性星形细胞瘤随时间进展至间变性或高级别肿瘤的几率较高。间变性改变的过程大不相同，增加了预测个体病例的难度。在一组79例复发性低级别星形细胞瘤病例中，50%的病例发生进展[133]。在一项有231例患者的低级别肿瘤研究中，依据手术前后的肿瘤体积，肿瘤进展至较高组织学分级的占复发肿瘤的大约4%～46%[134]。除了这一显著倾向以外，能够预测个体病例迅速间变性进展为有侵袭性生物学行为的明确的诊断性特征还有待今后明确。有关星形细胞瘤肿瘤发生的关键步骤在于，在增加增殖刺激情况下，细胞周期调节进行性缺失。转化最早阶段涉及自体分泌（也可能是旁分泌）增殖性刺激以及G1检测点（*TP53*突变/17p丢失）异常调控的形成。在细胞周期中，G1-S过渡的异常进展，伴有未修复的DNA损伤的危险增加和凋亡减少，可能伴有增殖性增加。这一状态可能与WHO Ⅱ级星形细胞瘤相对应。

分子学方法，尤其是基因异常的独特类型和时机选择，可以补充现有系统，从而更好地定义低级别星形细胞瘤亚型，预测个体肿瘤的生物学潜能[135]。基因组杂交的对比综合分析资料显示，复制异常的平均数、受累 GTG- 带获得和丢失的平均数量与弥漫型星形细胞瘤的 WHO 分级之间具有相关性[136]。至于特殊的基因位点，$p14^{ARF}$ 或 $p16^{INK4a}$ 的甲基化，不伴其他基因缺失，均可发生于低级别星形细胞瘤。如此基因功能的后生衰减可伴有阻滞性复制衰老，以维系有丝分裂生长因子刺激和高水平的 ras 活性[137-139]。尽管 TP53 基因突变、血小板源性生长因子（PDGF）以及胰岛素样生长因子（IGF-1）的表达增加似乎发生于弥漫型星形细胞瘤肿瘤发生的早期阶段[140,141]，这些分子特征并非Ⅱ级肿瘤所特有。关于肿瘤发生和增殖刺激早期阶段生长因子的作用方面，一些不同的因子，包括细胞因子[142]，也起作用。在星形细胞瘤中，生长因子活性可以发生改变[70]，或者为配体改变，或者为受体表达改变，包括 PDGF[143]、bFGF、TGFα、TGFβ 和 IGF-1[140]。异常自分泌环作为这些生长因子/受体体系的可能性也已提出[140]，PDGF/R 在刺激增殖中的致病作用则已得到有力的证实[143]。

尽管细胞核多形性和核分裂活性伴有细胞密度增加等重要特征常常被广泛应用于 WHO Ⅱ级肿瘤与非肿瘤、反应性病变的区分或与 WHO Ⅲ级肿瘤的区分，但是现有的组织病理学分类过于简化了该肿瘤谱系的生物学复杂性。重叠的形态学表型妨碍了 WHO Ⅱ～Ⅲ级谱系中个体肿瘤生物学行为的精确预测。WHO Ⅱ级星形细胞瘤间变性进展至 WHO Ⅲ级间变性星形细胞瘤通常伴有 19q 染色体的基因丢失、CDK4 过表达/放大、Rb 基因通路改变、13q 染色体杂合性缺失（LOH）以及 11p 染色体缺失[144]。随着细胞周期调节变得更加失控，细胞非典型性和肿瘤细胞数量都会有显著增加，伴有在 G1-S 期过渡的调节过程中获得的其他病变。近10%～17%的间变性星形细胞瘤有 EGFR 基因扩增[145,146]，后者是原发性胶质母细胞瘤的一个常见基因改变（见下文），并且这些病例中大约20%～75%表达 EGFRvⅢ 突变型[146,147]。间变性星形细胞瘤中，EGFR 扩增和 EGFRvⅢ 表达似乎与老年人发生的肿瘤和预后较差有关。大约18%的间变性星形细胞瘤具有 PTEN 点突变，这些肿瘤的预后也较差[145]。

WHO Ⅳ级星形细胞瘤（GBM）的恶性细胞表型是一个存在差异的生物学变化谱系，伴有侵袭性增加、异常血管生成、多个间变性克隆形成以及不受调节的异常增殖，加上凋亡控制的缺失，共同促使肿瘤形成。结合临床参数与分子遗传学改变，已经提出两种胶质母细胞瘤亚型[148]。原发性胶质母细胞瘤发生于老年患者（平均62岁），病程相对较短（月），没有前期低级别病变，而继发性胶质母细胞瘤发生于较年轻的患者（平均45岁），具有低级别胶质瘤病史。但是，继发性胶质母细胞瘤的发病率明显低于前期的低级别病变，大约占所有胶质瘤的5%。提示很大比例的低级别星形细胞瘤患者没有存活至胶质母细胞瘤形成[149]。

作为一种亚型，原发性与继发性 GBM 具有相同的组织病理特征表现，但似乎发生自不同的分子遗传学改变。对于从低级别肿瘤进展而来的继发性胶质母细胞瘤，最常见的遗传学病变在于 TP53 基因（65%）；而原发性胶质母细胞瘤，MDM2 基因扩增对 p53/MDM/p21 调节通路似乎有相似（但未被证实）的影响[150,151]。另外一种细胞周期调节通路为 p16/p15-CDK4/6-Rb，其中的基因病变是在弥漫性星形细胞瘤间变性进展过程中逐步形成。p16（CDKN2a）基因的缺失见于原发性胶质母细胞瘤（31%），通常伴发 EGFR 基因扩增，后者发生于大约40%～60%的肿瘤[145,151]。PTEN 突变（45%）也是原发性胶质母细胞瘤重要的基因改变。与成人原发性胶质母细胞瘤相比，EGFR 扩增在儿童肿瘤中并不常见[152,153]。在继发性胶质母细胞瘤中，p16（CDKN2a）基因缺失、EGFR 扩增和 PTEN 突变的发生率较低，分别为19%、8%和4%。在两类胶质母细胞瘤中，10q 的杂合性丢失（LOH）是最常见的基因病变，发生于70%的原发性和63%的继发性胶质母细胞瘤病例[148]。鉴于在胶质母细胞瘤的肿瘤发生过程中 PTEN 功能缺失的重要性，以及随后 PI3 调节下游通路的活化[154]，继发性胶质母细胞瘤低比例的 PTEN 突变提示可能发生了非活化的后生机制。PTEN 启动子位点的过度甲基化是低级别星形细胞瘤恶性进展的机制（Stokoe, D，未发表的资料），并且常见于胶质母细胞瘤[155]。

星形细胞瘤 Astrocytomas

星形细胞瘤、间变性星形细胞瘤和胶质母细胞瘤占所有胶质瘤的60%～80%左右，大约占所有成人 CNS 肿瘤的30%[149,156]。尽管所有年龄均可受累，但对于临床症状明显的肿瘤，分级增高，年龄也较大。年轻人（20～34岁）中，所有级别的弥漫型星形细胞瘤大约占胶质瘤的20%，大约占胶质母细胞的6%。胶质母细胞瘤是45岁以上人群第二位常见的脑肿瘤，大约占所有胶质瘤的21%，发病率为3～3.55人/10万人。与之相比，15岁以下人群中，胶质母细胞瘤仅占胶质瘤的3%～4%。

星形细胞瘤（WHO Ⅱ级）一般发生于31～40岁左右（平均为40岁），然而间变性星形胶质细胞瘤和肥胖细胞星形细胞瘤多见于41～50岁的患者[133,157,158]。一般来说，男性比女性更容易受累（男：女为1.18～1.0）[44]，肿瘤可发生于 CNS 的任何部位。多数大脑半球的肿瘤为实性肿瘤，尽管由于退变可形成小囊。

所有弥漫性星形细胞瘤患者的生存率具有显著的年

龄相关性，对于任何组织病理学分级，生存率与年龄呈负相关。总之，基于人群的生存期，在星形细胞瘤、间变性星形细胞瘤和胶质母细胞瘤中分别是 5.6、1.6 和 0.4 年。对于 0～19 岁人群，间变性星形细胞瘤和胶质母细胞瘤的 5 年生存率分别在 52% 和 19% 左右[149,156]。

星形细胞瘤的计算机成像（CT）研究显示，不论何种组织学类型，与脑组织相比均为低密度，没有对比增强。核磁共振成像（MRI）显示，星形细胞瘤相对周围脑组织显示 T2-加权像高密度信号，T1-加权序列低信号[159]。CT 对比增强和 MRI 非均匀密度提示其间变性进展。根据 MRI 的七个特征（即中线的交叉、水肿、异质性、出血、边界情况、囊性变/坏死及占位效应），可以将肿瘤分为星形细胞瘤、间变性星形细胞瘤或胶质母细胞瘤，总体准确率是 94.4%[160]。

构成星形细胞瘤的肿瘤性星形细胞可部分类似于正常和反应性脑组织中通过经典形态学技术识别的基本星形胶质细胞类型，即纤维、原浆和肥胖细胞。以其中一种类型为主的肿瘤分别称为纤维型、原浆型和肥胖型，然而这些细胞类型在同一肿瘤中通常混合存在，没有任何特殊的预后意义。但是含有肥胖型星形细胞的星形细胞肿瘤例外（见下文）。然而，基于这些细胞学特征的星形细胞瘤亚型有很大局限性。这些特征并不能确切反映可能的生理性差异，原因在于局部组织发生以及局部细胞间相互作用或其他肿瘤因子不同可导致异质性（见上文）。因此，肿瘤性星形细胞的复杂的功能多样性可进一步混淆特殊细胞学特征与肿瘤生物学行为之间的相关性。

星形细胞瘤术中涂片可以显示这些肿瘤的典型纤维性特征。肿瘤组织的质地取决于肿瘤的优势成分。多数纤维型星形细胞瘤比原浆和肥胖细胞型硬很多。由多数胞浆突起形成的富于纤维性基质在纤维型星形细胞瘤中容易识别（图 26.1 和 26.2）。细胞含有一种胞浆几何构型，从境界不清的少量核周轮圈至伴有拉长细胞核的纺锤形结构。"原浆型"星形细胞群更具星状结构，细胞突起短而细。基质纤维性不明显，依据肿瘤中纤维性星形细胞的丰富程度而有差异。肥胖细胞型星形细胞瘤涂片的特征为细胞含有大量嗜酸性、圆形至轻度成角的胞浆和偏心性细胞核（图 26.5）。与多发性硬化或慢性脓肿周边区域伴发的反应性肥胖细胞的明显突起相比，肿瘤细胞仅仅出现短而不明显的突起。

没有一种细胞骨架蛋白对肿瘤性星形细胞完全特异。GFAP 作为星形胶质细胞中间丝的主要组成成分，相对选择性地可见于成人脑组织的正常（纤维性）和反应性星形细胞，但是不成熟的少突胶质细胞、反应性室管膜和脉络丛上皮也出现 GFAP 免疫反应性。在脑发育

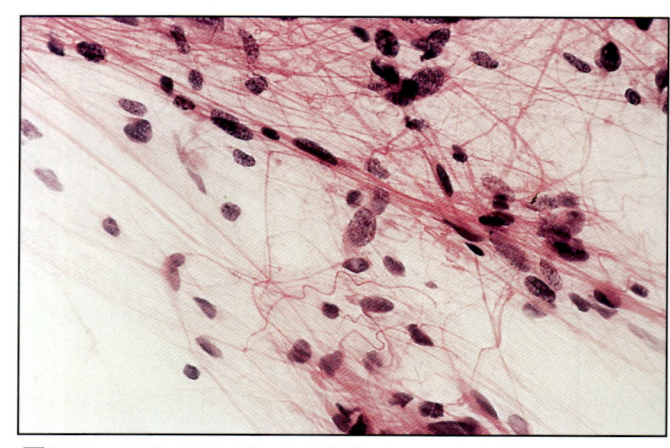

图 26.1 纤维型星形细胞瘤涂片显示，肿瘤性星形细胞的细胞核拉长，染色质粗。注意胞浆稀少、境界不清的单个肿瘤细胞分布于由纤细突起构成的网中。Morris 染色。

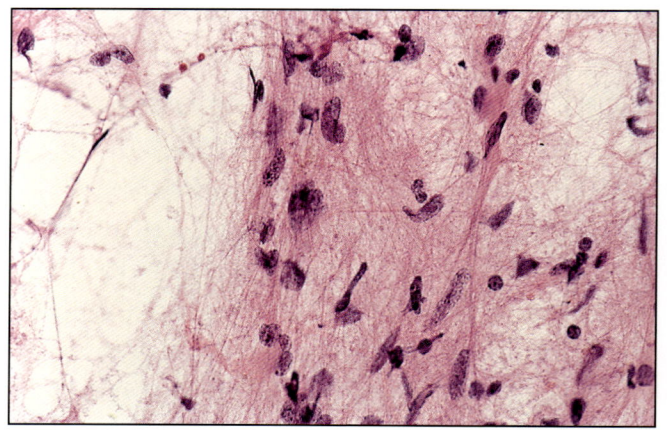

图 26.2 纤维型星形细胞瘤涂片。单个细胞的突起在纤细的纤维性背景中不明显，但细胞核呈典型分化好的肿瘤性星形细胞表现。Morris 染色。

和细胞反应中的表达多样化，对于应用 GFAP 免疫组化来确定肿瘤星形胶质分化具有重要意义。大多数星形细胞瘤 GFAP 免疫染色阳性，但原浆型星形细胞瘤例外，其免疫反应呈低表达或缺少表达[161,162]。在间变性星形细胞瘤和多形性胶质母细胞中，GFAP 免疫反应呈阳性的细胞的分布比较局灶，且数量减少，原因是分化程度比较有限。波形蛋白是一种中间丝蛋白，细胞分布相对广泛，包括正常的和肿瘤性的间叶性衍生物，在早期神经形态发生过程中有短暂表达。它们常常表达于星形细胞肿瘤，与 GFAP 的分布相似，但较不明显[163]。事实上，所有间变性星形细胞瘤和胶质母细胞都含有波形蛋白阳性的细胞群。星形细胞性的肿瘤细胞也表达 S-100 蛋白

（位于胞核及胞浆突起）和神经元特异烯醇化酶[161]。但是，这些表型在鉴别星形细胞和其他神经上皮性肿瘤中的诊断价值有限。

纤维型星形细胞瘤（fibrillary astrocytoma）：纤维型星形细胞瘤是最常见的变型，累及成人大脑半球和儿童及青少年的脑干。术中涂片显示纤维性基质，与背景中反应性星形细胞增生相比，其境界不清（图26.1和26.2）。与反应性星形细胞相比，肿瘤细胞的细胞核稍大，更为不规则、浓染、染色质粗。胞浆形态从境界不清、比较稀少的核周轮廓至比较明显的星状结构（图26.3和26.4）。总之，分化好的星形细胞瘤与反应性星形细胞增生相比，细胞结构改变较少。但是，随着肿瘤非典型性的增加，差异变大。丰富的纤维性基质通过磷钨酸苏木素（PTAH）染色和GFAP免疫反应可更为明显。

肥胖型星形细胞瘤（gemistocytic astrocytoma）：肥胖型星形细胞瘤为第二位常见类型，占星形细胞瘤的比例不足20%[166]。在人群相关性研究中，这些肿瘤患者比纤维型星形细胞瘤患者稍年长（平均50岁）[149]。除了这种特殊的组织学亚型（即肿瘤的每个高倍视野中，60%以上为肥胖细胞）以外，具有肥胖细胞特征的细胞也可见于纤维型（图26.3）和间变性星形细胞瘤。肥胖细胞型星形细胞瘤常见于幕上，表现为大体境界清楚的肿物，可有囊性变。肥胖细胞型星形细胞瘤的涂片和组织学切片可显示特殊细胞成分，较多的嗜酸性、肥胖至轻度成角的胞浆，以及偏位的细胞核（图26.5）。肿瘤细胞可有短而纤细的胶质突起，使肿瘤基质呈轻度纤维性结构（图26.6）。多核细胞并不少见，但与肥胖细胞型肿瘤细胞相比，具有核分裂活性的小胶质细胞成分差异较大。肥胖细胞和小细胞成分均出现细胞核p53免

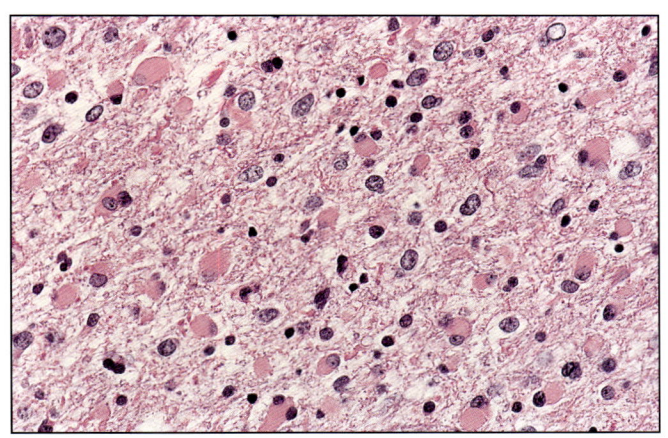

图26.3　星形细胞瘤中的肥胖型细胞常常混以纤维性肿瘤细胞。

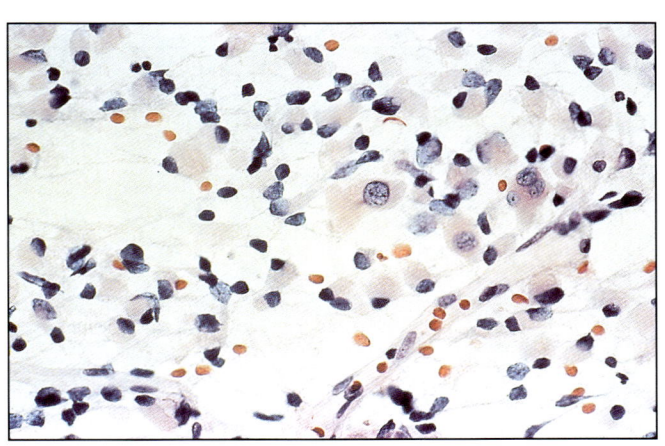

图26.5　肥胖型星形细胞瘤涂片显示典型的多角形细胞，伴有较多的致密嗜酸性胞浆，核偏位，浓染。尽管基质的纤维性不甚明显，但是短的胶质突起容易见到。Morris染色。

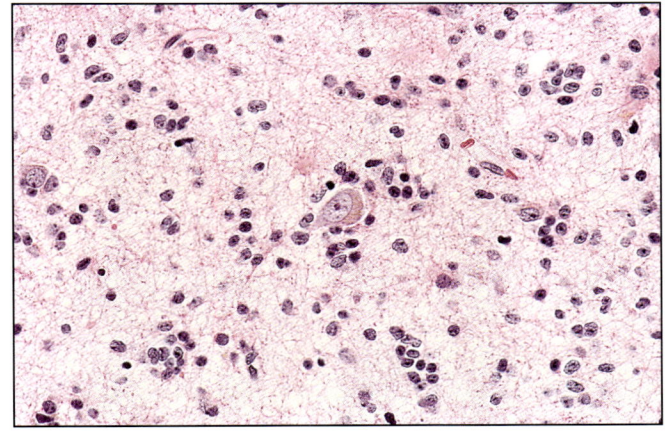

图26.4　靠近图26.3肿瘤的皮质成分，显示星形细胞瘤的浸润特征，表现为正常神经元的卫星现象。

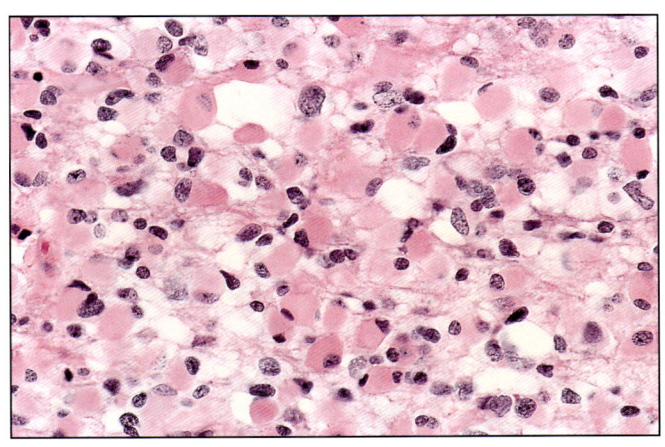

图26.6　肥胖型星形细胞瘤的高倍观，显示肿瘤细胞的星形胶质特征，即纤细的胞浆突起，不同程度的纤维性背景。

疫反应阳性。相比之下，肥胖细胞是唯一具有 bcl-2 免疫反应性的细胞群[165]。肥胖细胞 GFAP 免疫反应较强，与超微结构出现大量胞浆纤维束相符合[162]。血管周围淋巴细胞浸润在此型比在其他星形细胞瘤更为常见。肥胖型星形细胞瘤常常具有侵袭性行为[164]，大约 80% 的肿瘤进展为胶质母细胞瘤[162]。对一组 28 例肥胖型细胞星形细胞瘤病例进行的分子遗传学分析显示，*TP53* 突变是此类型的遗传学标志，而 *PTEN* 突变在低级别肥胖型星形细胞瘤中缺乏，在间变性肥胖型星形细胞瘤中极少见[166]。

原浆型星形细胞瘤（protoplasmic astrocytoma）：该少见变型所占比例不足星形细胞瘤的 1%[162]，大多位于儿童和年轻成人的大脑。肿瘤常常位于表浅皮层，表现为胶样肿物伴不同程度囊腔形成。镜下，原浆型星形细胞瘤由相对一致的小星形细胞构成，具有极少数短而纤细的胞浆突起，分布于丰富的嗜酸性基质当中（图26.7）。PTAH 阳性胶质纤维和 GFAP 免疫反应少见或缺乏。常常可见微囊变性。这些少见肿瘤的组织学发生尚不清楚，尽管具有这些特征的细胞构成了相对较多的毛细胞型星形细胞瘤成分（见下文）。取材不当可使毛细胞型星形细胞瘤被误诊为原浆型星形细胞瘤。

间变性星形细胞瘤（图26.8和26.9）
Anaplastic astrocytoma

所有星形细胞瘤都具有不同程度的、向间变性星形细胞瘤进展的能力，一般来说，可见于 50%～75% 的复发肿瘤[162]。但是，间变性星形细胞瘤可以是原发的，不经过低级别肿瘤的恶性转化。WHO 分类确定的间变性星形细胞瘤的诊断标准包括：局灶或弥漫性细胞密度增加、细胞核非典型性以及核分裂活性（图 26.8 和 26.9）。不应当出现内皮细胞增生和坏死。一般来说，间变性肿瘤的纤维性基质比分化好的星形细胞瘤的更为稀少。这种组织质地较软，在涂片准备过程中能够感觉到。

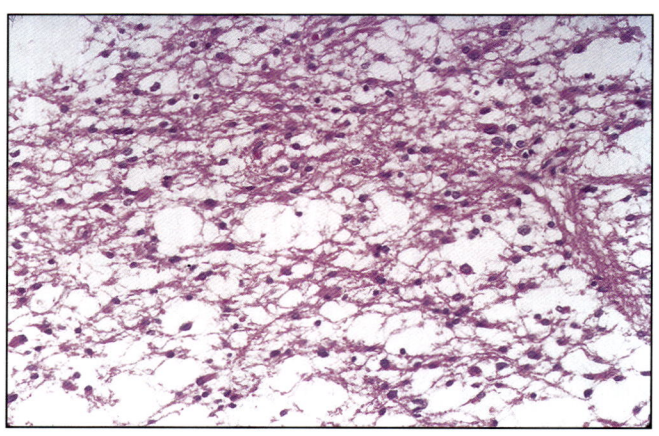

图26.7　原浆型星形细胞瘤具有星状细胞标志性特征，即短而纤细的突起，形成微囊性网架。

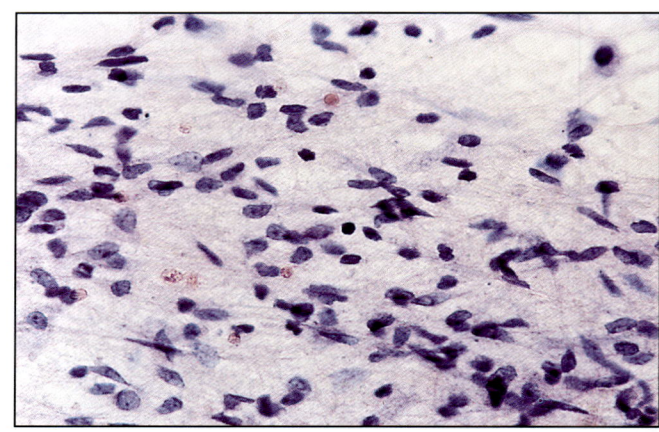

图26.8　中等细胞密度、细胞多形性及核染色质增多是间变性星形细胞瘤的细胞学特征，这在涂片中易于见到。注意纤维性基质。

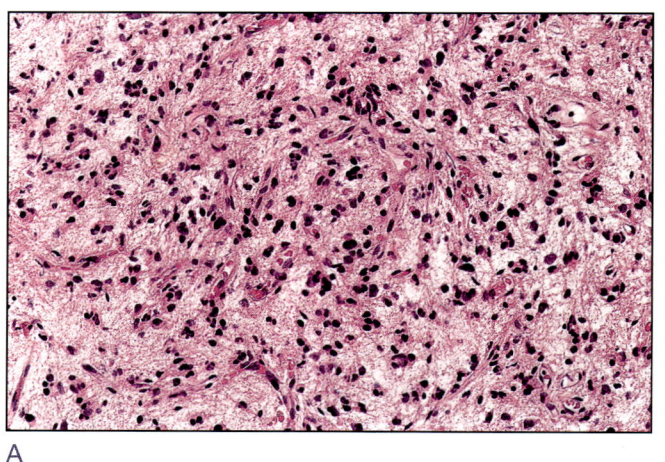

A

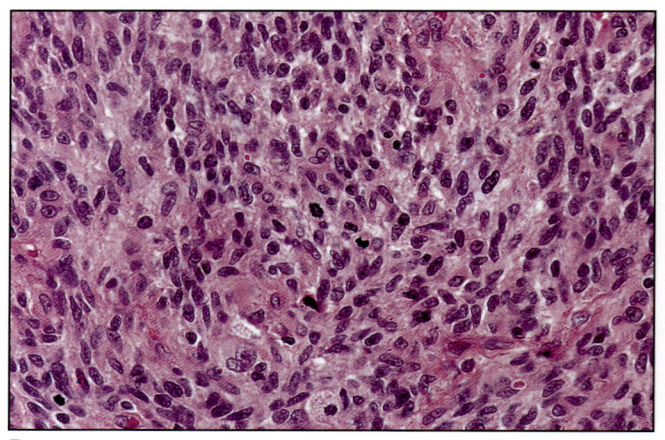

B

图26.9　间变性星形细胞瘤的组织学切片显示中度到显著的细胞多形性。仔细检查肿瘤的多个视野，没有见到血管内皮细胞/外皮细胞增生或坏死。注意纤细的血管和多个核分裂象。

神经影像学研究显示，信号不均匀，边界欠清，占位效应增加，血管源性水肿。可见局灶对比增强，与胶质母细胞瘤所见不同，不是一个恒定特征。

在间变性星形细胞瘤的组织病理学谱系中，有一种变型称为小细胞星形细胞瘤[167]。这种肿瘤有以下特征：（1）类似于少突胶质细胞肿瘤的常见的一系列组织病理学特征；（2）采用常规染色，小星形细胞具有相对良性特征，伴有轻度多形性；（3）细胞密度和MIB-1指数较高（平均为24%，17%～61%）；以及（4）有与间变性星形细胞瘤和胶质母细胞瘤相关的分子病理学特征[EGFR扩增（58%）、EGFR VIII突变（50%）、10q缺失（83%）]。其组织病理学与少突胶质细胞肿瘤的相似性包括：细胞核的一致性、微小钙化、鸡笼样毛细血管、核周透明空晕及神经元周围卫星现象。尽管神经影像学检查仅有轻度或无对比增强（大约40%病例），但这些肿瘤具有侵袭性生物学行为，存活率为3～19个月不等（平均6个月）。在绝大多数肿瘤中，对比增强更为显著对应于胶质母细胞瘤标志性特征的出现（见下文），其中10q缺失和EGFR扩增分别占到100%和72%。

多形性胶质母细胞瘤（图26.10至26.23）
Glioblastoma multiforme

在成人，胶质母细胞瘤好发于大脑半球，尽管它们可以发生于任何部位。胶质母细胞瘤也可以发生于新生儿和儿童[168]，其中小脑和脑干是最常见部位[169-171]。胶质母细胞瘤的大体表现反映了肿瘤的侵袭性生长方式。胶质母细胞瘤的CT和MR影像学极为不同。一种最常见的表现是：境界相对清楚的膨胀性（"推挤性"）肿瘤边界。此外，特征性的"环形强化"，通过钆造影剂尤其可以很好地显示，对应的是显著微小新生血管形成和高细胞密度区域。肿瘤内信号（T2加权影像）不均匀对应的是细胞丰富和坏死混合区域伴以低细胞密度区。常见弥漫性浸润超出肿瘤的大体边界。有关胶质母细胞瘤的详细定位研究显示，肿瘤细胞的浸润范围差异较大，从几毫米至几厘米[172]。在坏死与细胞丰富的环状强化区域之间进行立体定向活检最有可能获得典型胶质母细胞瘤的组织学特征，而其他区域对于诊断和分级可能疑问较多。因此，多部位影像学立体定位活检可增加活检诊断的准确性，六个部位为最佳[173]。

原始肿瘤细胞沿深部纤维束的远处播散也可以很广泛，可以跨越连合浸润对侧半球（"蝴蝶"样式）。目前的神经影像学分析采用了先进的MR技术，增加了检出这种播散的敏感性，包括弥散加权成像、灌注加权以及多回波序列T2-加权MRI[83,84]，这些技术对于细胞密度、血-脑屏障改变以及水肿更加敏感。在此背景下，肿瘤定位分析将胶质母细胞瘤分成几类，包括"多灶"型，即在细胞不丰富的区域内含有多处细胞丰富和坏死区[172]。依据影像技术的分辨率，这些肿瘤表现为多发、孤立性病变。

胶质母细胞瘤在涂片和组织切片上均显示明显的胞浆和胞核多形性，从紧密排列的小细胞，胞浆稀少、圆形到卵圆形浓染细胞核，到奇异形多核巨细胞（图26.10、26.11、26.14和26.15）。然而，多数肿瘤含有呈明显星形细胞特征（即纤细纤维性突起）的成分，正如PTAH和GFAP阳性所示（图26.13）。也可出现胞浆脂质[174]以及更为少见的、伴有鳞状或腺性特征[175]的上皮性结构（图26.16）。此时，细胞角蛋白（CK）表达（图26.16）并非少见[175]。核分裂象常见，包括非典型核分裂象，但肿瘤内不同部分差别很大，MIB-1增殖指数一般较高（图26.17）。

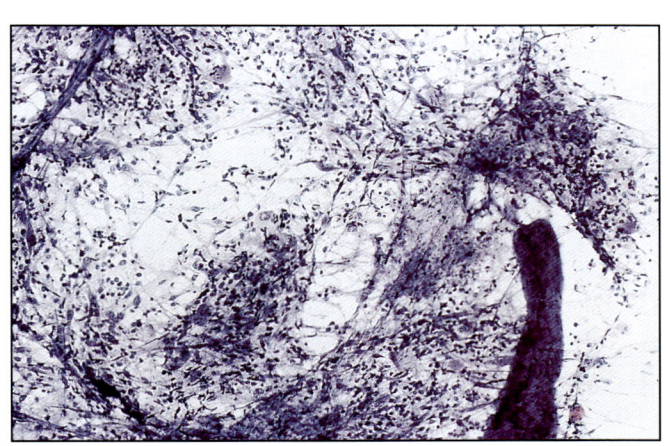

图26.10 多形性胶质母细胞瘤涂片显示广泛胞浆和胞核多形性。注意片状坏死，致密内皮细胞增生。局灶纤维性背景显示肿瘤的星形细胞特征。Morris染色。

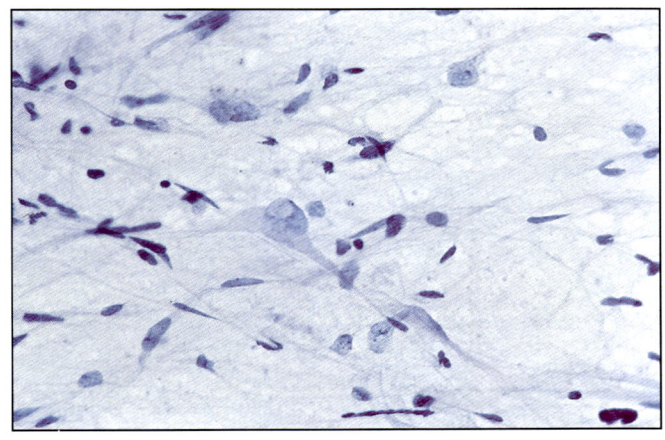

图26.11 多形性胶质母细胞瘤。大细胞伴有奇异形、多形性细胞核，混杂有明显纤维性但极具非典型性的星形细胞。Morris染色。

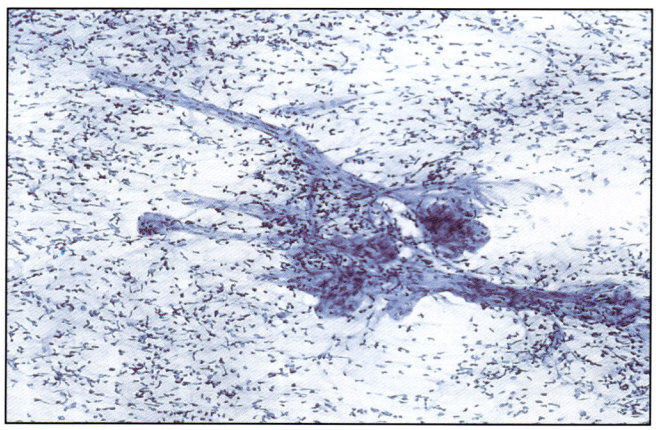

图26.12 多形性胶质母细胞瘤。在涂片中也可见到内皮细胞/外皮细胞增生，伴有肾小球样血管形成，散在分布于致密肿瘤细胞之间。Morris染色。

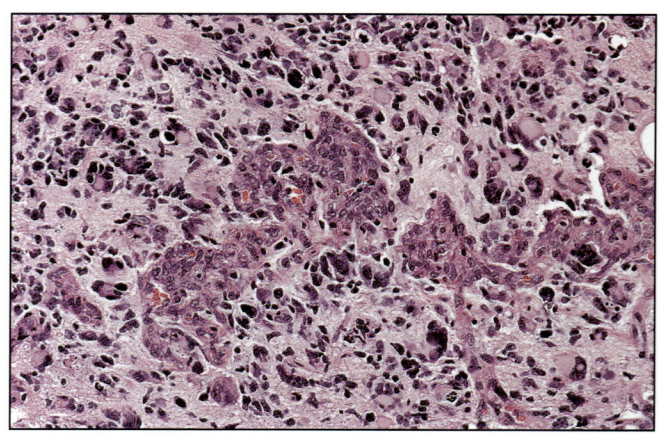

图26.15 图26.14肿瘤的其他区域，显示奇异形星形细胞及巨细胞。注意肾小球样血管增生（中央）。

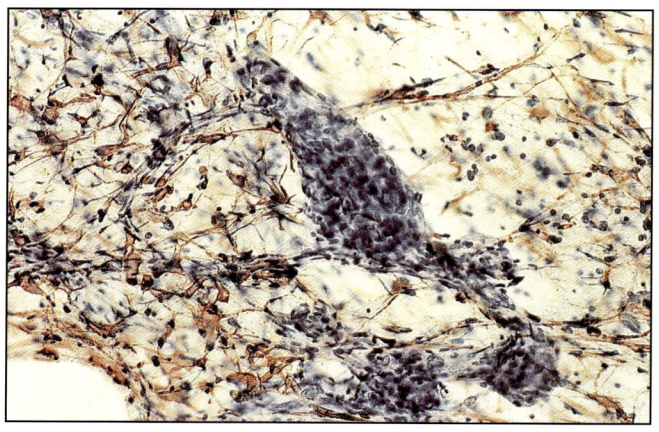

图26.13 多形性胶质母细胞瘤。涂片胶质纤维酸性蛋白（GFAP）免疫组织化学染色可以突出内皮细胞增生和致密多形性星形细胞团。GFAP-ABC免疫过氧化物酶-苏木素双重染色。

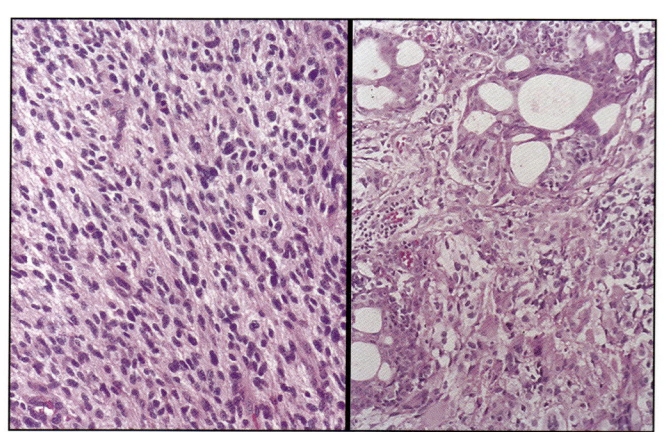

图26.16 胶质母细胞的多种组织学结构。（A）左：胶质母细胞瘤浸润髓鞘通路时，小的肿瘤细胞常常表现为单一形态特征的梭形细胞束。右：胶质母细胞瘤偶尔可见上皮化生，伴有腺腔形成。（B）该胶质母细胞瘤的腺体结构通过CK免疫组化染色更为突出（左），而胶质肿瘤细胞GFAP呈强阳性（右）。GFAP和CK为ABC免疫过氧化物酶，苏木素双重染色。

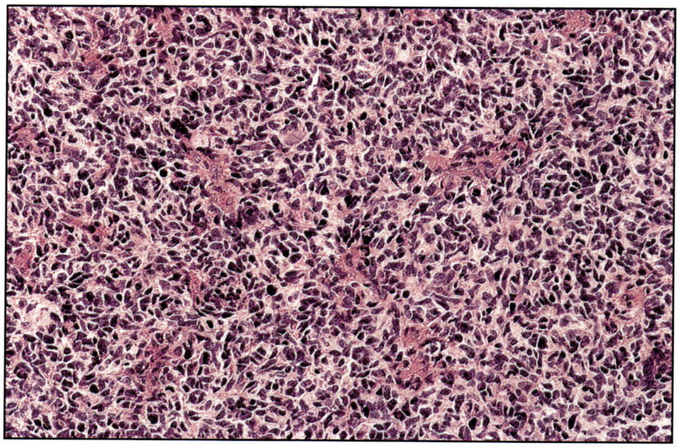

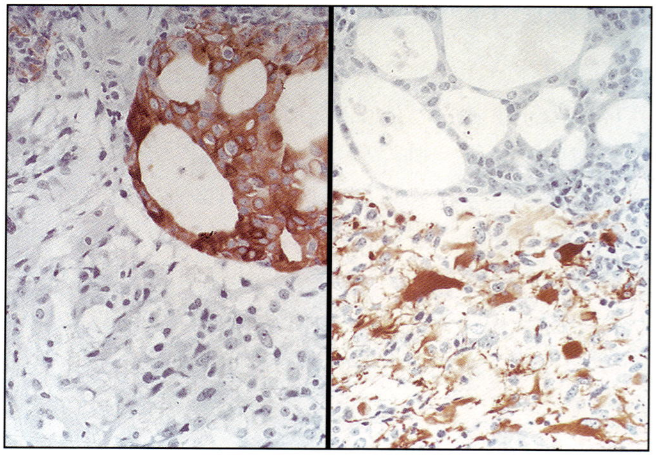

图26.14 胶质母细胞瘤的一个视野显示细胞密集，细胞境界不清。胞浆及胞核明显多形性，染色极深。注意大量核分裂象。

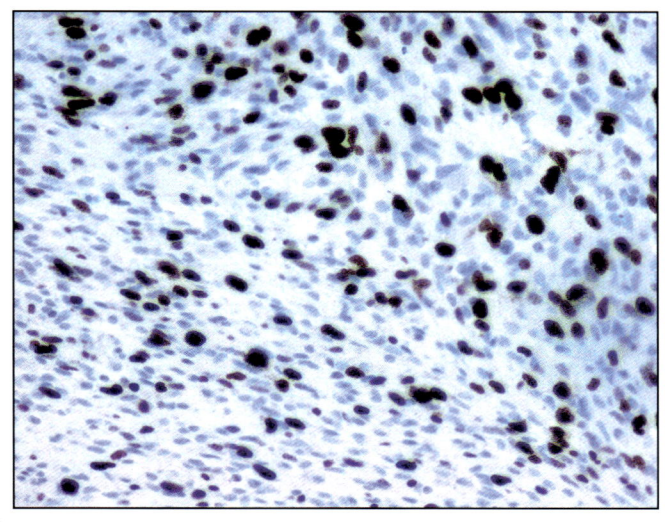

图26.17 Ki-67免疫组化染色（MIB-1单克隆）显示这种肿瘤的高度增殖活性。ABC免疫过氧化物酶法，苏木素双重染色。

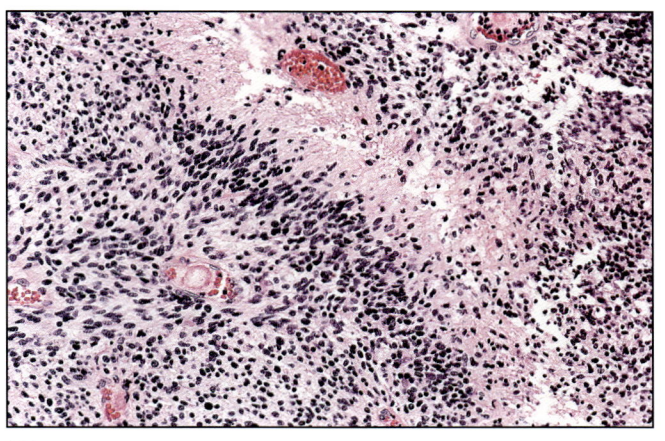

图26.18 围绕中心坏死区的假栅栏状排列是胶质母细胞瘤的诊断特征。

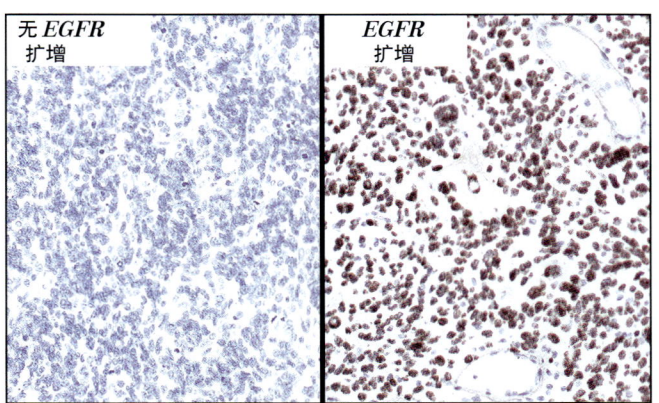

图26.19 胶质母细胞瘤的原位杂交显色是识别EGFR扩增的可靠方法。

内皮［和（或）外皮细胞］增生和坏死相结合是胶质母细胞瘤的诊断特征，在涂片和切片中，这些特征都可将它们与间变性星形细胞瘤鉴别开（图26.12和26.13）。微小坏死常见，多呈"地图样"结构，坏死周围是栅栏状排列的分化差的梭形细胞成分（"假栅栏样"）（图26.18）。内皮增生常常出现在紧邻的脑组织中，与肿瘤性星形细胞散布的血管生长因子的出现一致。在此边缘进行立体定位活检，常常可以见到这些"肾小球样"血管，而没有肿瘤细胞。此外，胶质母细胞瘤可以引起大量纤维结缔组织增生，伴有软脑膜和硬脑膜的浸润，不应与胶质肉瘤相混淆（见下文）。

如上所述，大约40%的胶质母细胞瘤和10%~20%的间变性星形细胞瘤有 EGFR 扩增（图26.19），而后者在星形细胞瘤（WHO Ⅱ）中从未出现。在小活检中，在出现高MIB-1指数但没有其他明确的间变性组织病理特征情况下，EGFR 扩增应当考虑为高级别病变的指征。

胶质母细胞瘤的诊断性分子学分析（diagnostic molecular analyses of glioblastomas）：有关组织提取物基因组和表型的分子形态学和分子生物学技术可为常规组织病理特征提供有益的补充，以便更好地确定传统治疗可以增加生存率以及对新型靶向治疗有效的胶质母细胞瘤亚型。在一项有97例病例的连续性GBM研究中，TP53 突变和 LOH 10q 的出现分别为预后较好和差的因素。在胶质母细胞瘤中，1p 和 19q 联合缺失的患者生存率较好[176]。一项有50例胶质母细胞瘤的芯片比较基因组杂交（CGH）研究显示有三种主要亚型：肿瘤出现7号染色体增加和10号染色体丢失；肿瘤出现10号染色体丢失，但无7号染色体增加；以及肿瘤没有7号或10号染色体复制数改变[177]。基因表达谱 EGFR 过表达也可以确定胶质母细胞瘤的分子亚型；位于12q13-15[178]染色体的基因上调结合 EGFR 过表达与特殊的总体基因表达类型有关[179,180]。基因表达谱也显示了预后相关基因[179,180]。芯片 CGH 结合芯片表达谱也被用于识别不同分子亚型的生存率[181]。

近来分析活化信号通路和生长因子受体表达/扩增的研究，结合临床试验的有关预后数据，提出一个新的新型靶向治疗有效患者的诊断模式。有关小分子抑制剂靶向 EGFR 和下游信号通路表型的临床试验显示，具有高水平 EGFR 表达或扩增以及低水平蛋白激酶 B/Akt 活性（使用磷酸 Akt 免疫组化）的胶质母细胞瘤治疗效果较好[181a]。这些特征都可以通过甲醛溶液固定和石蜡包埋组织的免疫组化和分子形态学技术来检测。重要的是要注意，此时，EGFR 基因扩增伴有免疫组化 EGFR 染色过表达（约96%的病例）。组织的 EGFR 扩增可以通过荧光原位杂交[182,183]或显色原位杂交技术检测[184]（图

26.19）。此外，EGFR vIII 和 PTEN 的共同表达似乎预示对 EGFR 激酶抑制剂的反应性[184a]。

巨细胞胶质母细胞瘤（giant cell glioblastoma）：依据临床病理和遗传学数据，巨细胞胶质母细胞瘤似乎为特殊病变[185]。在短暂临床病史后，肿瘤临床上可较为明显，同原发性胶质母细胞瘤一样，但患者较年轻。这组肿瘤的生存期通常超过报道的经典胶质母细胞瘤的中位生存期[162,186]。有一组病例提示，颞叶稍微多见[186]。肿瘤通常境界清楚，神经影像学显示非均质性增强表现，没有常见的周围强化。尽管放射学上和大体上境界清楚，但肿瘤通常浸润邻近脑组织和软脑膜。一般坏死较多，通常形成大的囊腔。组织学特征以大的奇异型多核巨细胞为主，含有丰富的嗜酸性胞浆和大的空泡状核（图 26.20）。在术中涂片中，这些细胞是令人印象最为深刻的成分，通常分布于广泛坏死的背景下。仔细检查更具纤维性的细胞，可以证实这些肿瘤的星形细胞本质。其他特征有血管内皮增生较少，网织纤维增加与血管关系密切，以及大片坏死。巨细胞 GFAP 免疫反应呈阳性，尽管 GFAP 通常在梭形细胞中更明显。非典型核分裂象常见，细胞可重度脂质化。

巨细胞性胶质母细胞瘤具有特殊的"杂合性"分子遗传学表型，介于原发性及继发性胶质母细胞瘤之间，它们通常：（1）没有 CDK（4/6）抑制剂（*CDKN2a* 基因）缺失；（2）缺乏 *EGFR* 或 *CDK4* 基因扩增；（3）具有 30% 的 *PTEN* 突变率；以及（4）出现高 *TP53* 突变率[185,187-189]。这些表现不同于其他 GBM 亚型，临床预后相对较好，包括浸润脑组织能力明显减低。

胶质肉瘤（gliosarcoma）：尽管微血管（内皮/外皮细胞）增生是所有胶质母细胞瘤的显著特征，但胶质肉瘤出现明显间叶表型的肿瘤性细胞成分。胶质母细胞瘤中，这种肉瘤表型的发生率为 2%～8% 不等[190-192]。胶质和肉瘤成分比例不同，但组织学上常常可以区分两种细胞群体（图 26.21 和 26.22）。肉瘤成分可以超过胶质肿瘤细胞，因而可能会使诊断复杂化，但通过网织纤维染色可使其更为明显。有必要对适当的组织标本进行 GFAP 免疫组化（图 26.23）和 PTAH 染色来证实肿瘤性胶质成分。恶性的间叶性表型可有不同，从类似于未分化多形性肉瘤（所谓的恶性纤维组织细胞瘤）到纤维肉瘤结构。也可见到骨和软骨化生以及横纹肌肉瘤成

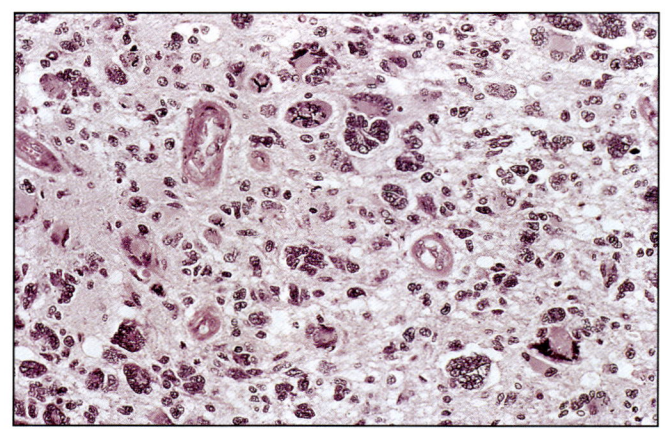

图 26.20 巨细胞型胶质母细胞瘤的组织切片显示相似的细胞混合。有些肿瘤几乎完全由巨大多核细胞和多角形细胞组成，有必要仔细检查以识别细胞的星形细胞本质。

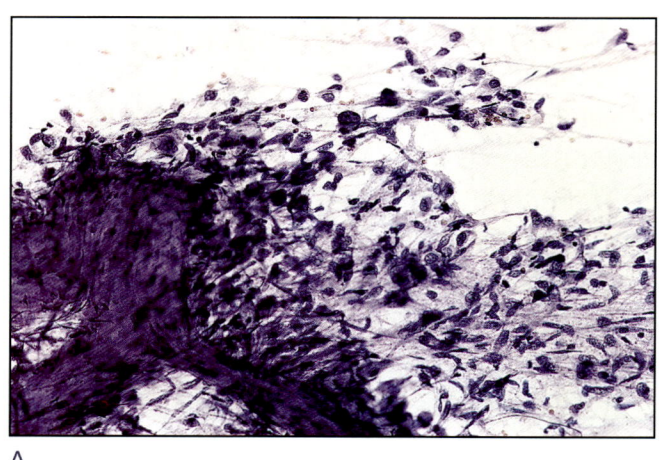

A

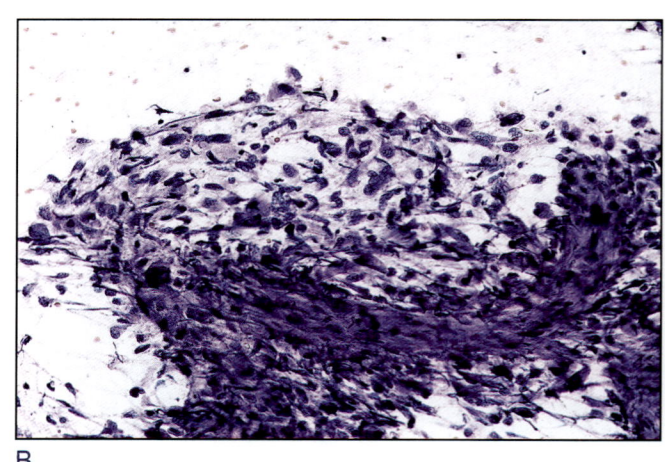

B

图 26.21 胶质肉瘤的涂片显示双重细胞成分。（A）胶质细胞成分可通过细胞致密聚集边缘的纤维性胞浆突起来识别。（B）与胶质细胞成分相比，梭形肉瘤细胞成分源自增生明显的血管。注意细胞境界清楚，缺乏纤维性背景。Morris 染色。

分[190]。免疫组化和超微结构研究表明，肉瘤成分可能源自与血管外膜有关的未分化间叶细胞，它不同于内皮细胞、平滑肌和外皮细胞[190]。但是，由于肿瘤性星形胶质细胞具有产生基底膜和间叶分化相关性细胞外基质的能力，所以"肉瘤"成分肯定来源于非胶质细胞的假设很可能过于简单化了。事实上，分子遗传学分析显示，胶质肉瘤的胶质和间叶成分具有类似的遗传学异常[190,192-195]。相同的 TP53 和 PTEN 基因突变可见于胶质瘤及肉瘤成分中[193,195]，提示肉瘤区域为胶质细胞的一种表型改变。

毛细胞型星形细胞瘤（图26.24至26.32）
Pilocytic astrocytoma

毛细胞型星形细胞瘤是生长缓慢的肿瘤，大约占所有胶质瘤的5%～6%[156]，总的发病率是每年0.37/10万人[149]。肿瘤最常见于20岁以内，没有性别倾向。在5～19岁，它是最常见的脑肿瘤，年龄校正后的发病率（每10万人/年）在0～19岁是0.8。在成人，这些肿瘤一般较低级别弥漫浸润性大脑星形细胞瘤早10年（平均年龄为22岁）[196]。毛细胞型星形细胞瘤特征性地位于中线结构（如小脑、第三脑室区、视神经交叉和脑干）。这些肿瘤不常见于大脑半球，但是如果出现的话，则以颞叶或颞叶顶部和丘脑稍多见[196,197]。与其他部位相比，在脊髓，这些肿瘤容易发生在年长的患者，在一些病例研究中，占脊髓星形细胞肿瘤的重要部分（58%）[198]。

与弥漫型星形细胞肿瘤相比，毛细胞型星形细胞瘤、多形性黄色瘤型星形细胞瘤和室管膜下巨细胞型星形细胞瘤由特殊的肿瘤性星形细胞组成，境界具有清楚的生长方式。毛细胞型星形细胞瘤并不弥漫性浸润周围的神经毡，仅有极少数出现恶性进展。但肿瘤细胞活性可有选择性地增加，表现为经常浸润邻近的软脑膜和白质束，尤其是脑干、视神经和视交叉。软脑膜浸润可能在极少数没有间变特征的播散型中起一定作用[199]。

神经放射影像学证实，这些显著囊性变的病变边界清楚，在 MR 的 T1- 和 T2- 加权像上，弛豫时间增加[159]。常见对比强化，这是由于肿瘤内血管增生所致。

镜下，毛细胞型星形细胞瘤通常是双相肿瘤（图26.24至26.28）。双极纤维样伸展的（毛样）细胞与含有短突起的类似于原浆型星形细胞的星状细胞区域混合存在（图26.27和26.28）。毛样细胞易于呈束状排列，

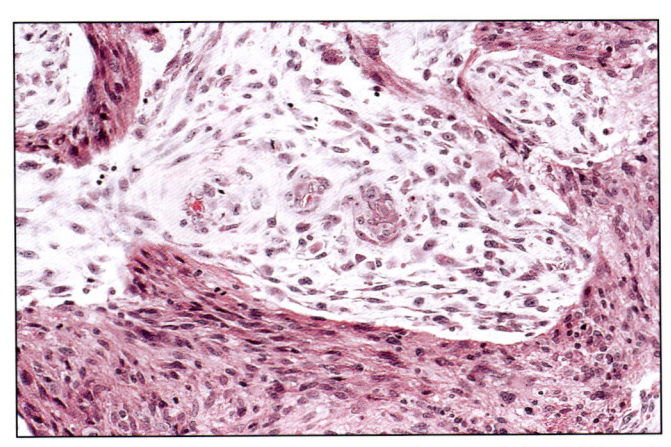

图26.22 胶质肉瘤的组织切片明确显示两种不同的细胞群，并且通常境界清楚。一种为不甚致密的肉瘤成分，另一种为比较致密的纤维性胶质成分。注意两种成分中有众多核分裂象。

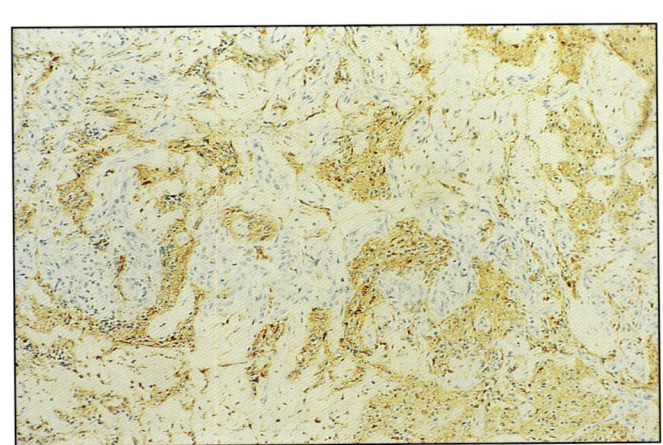

图26.23 胶质纤维酸性蛋白（GFAP）免疫组化染色显示肿瘤性星形胶质成分，与GFAP阴性的肉瘤成分交错分布。GFAP-ABC免疫过氧化物酶法，苏木素双重染色。

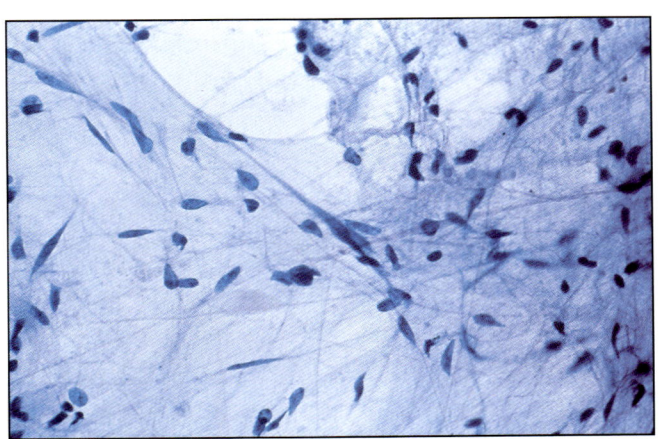

图26.24 毛细胞型星形细胞瘤。涂片中显示星形细胞的毛细胞特征。注意明显嗜酸的丝状细胞突起和相当于Rosenthal纤维的局灶膨胀。Morris染色。

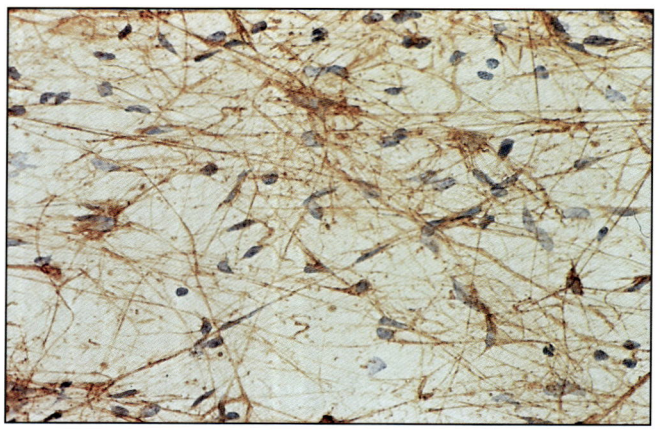

图26.25 毛细胞型星形细胞瘤涂片中，胶质纤维酸性蛋白（GFAP）免疫组化染色显示众多的双极纤维性突起。GFAP-ABC过氧化物酶法，苏木素双重染色。

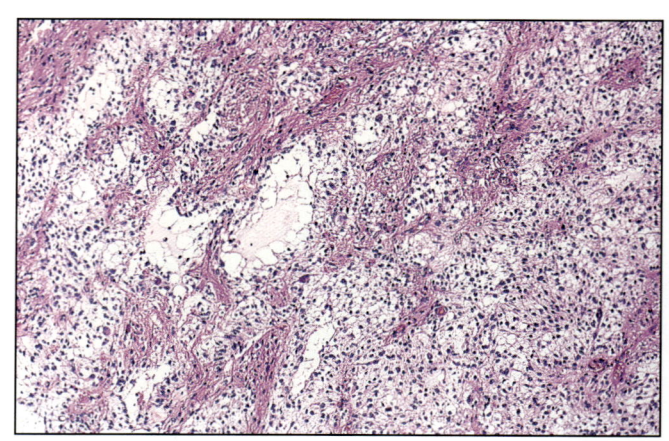

图26.27 毛细胞型星形细胞瘤的双向结构常可见于组织切片。毛样和较为星状的星形细胞（伴有微囊改变）在整个肿瘤中以不同比例混合。伴有血管间质的纤维性成分聚集常见。

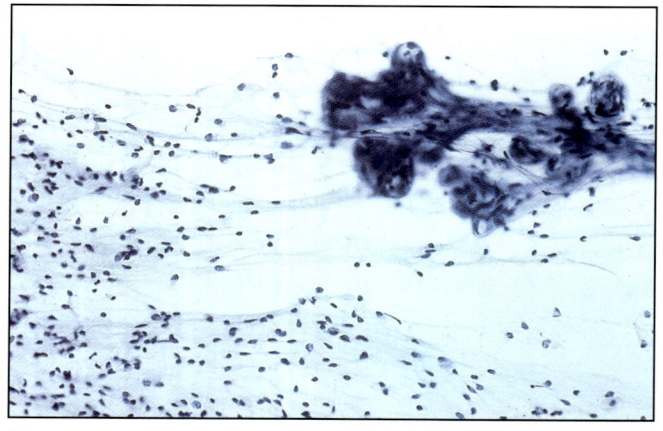

图26.26 伴有肾小球样血管的内皮增生在毛细胞型星形细胞瘤涂片中容易见到，应当小心，不要误诊为是胶质母细胞瘤成分。Morris染色。

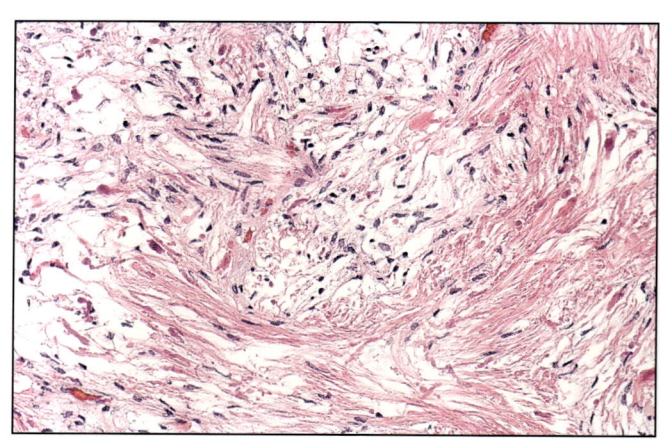

图26.28 毛细胞型星形细胞瘤。在有些肿瘤中，毛样细胞交错分布于致密束状和疏松网状结构之间。

常常在血管周围分布明显。星状细胞出现明显丝带样结构，常伴有微囊变。Rosenthal 纤维、颗粒状玻璃样变小体和嗜酸性、胞浆内小体是特征性结构，为退行性改变（图 26.28 至 26.30）。极具纤维性的毛细胞 GFAP 免疫反应呈阳性，而微囊区域的星状细胞 GFAP 仅为弱阳性。细胞突起波形蛋白明显呈阳性。

肾小球样毛细血管和内皮细胞增生常见（图 26.26），但不像间变性星形细胞瘤那样意味着恶性转化。同样，细胞核非典型性和伴有多核细胞多形性出现，也没有任何恶性含意（图 26.31 和 26.32）。局灶软脑膜浸润而无脑脊髓通路播散并非少见，但不意味着恶性。因此，与弥漫浸润的星形细胞瘤相比，仅有细胞非典型性和微血管增生并不提示恶性转化。但是，与细胞核非典型性、坏死和核分裂活性增加结合以后，应该怀疑间变性进展，这在该肿瘤并不常见[199,200]。核分裂比例一般较低，报道的范围是 0~4 个/10HPF，MIB-1 标记指数为 0%~4%（平均 1.1%）[85]。少数情况下，间变性进展也可以发生于较长间隔之后。在 Virginia 大学的病例报告中，间变性进展的特征可见于最初肿瘤切除后近乎 40 年、临床相对静止的小脑病变活检样本。在 107 例小脑毛细胞型星形细胞瘤中，原发性间变性进展仅发生于 0.9% 的病例，这些病变具有较高 S- 期分值（5%~11%），相当于流式细胞术的 3.19（± 0.237 SEM）[201]。只有与微血管增生和（或）坏死相结合，活跃的核分裂活性才是间变性进展最可靠的提示。

一种组织学变型，即单相型毛细胞黏液样型星形细胞瘤，需要特别注意[202]。该变型发生于婴儿和幼儿的下丘脑/视交叉部位。与经典的毛细胞型星形细胞瘤相比，这些肿瘤出现更为单一形态的组织学结构、明显黏液样基质和 Rosenthal 纤维，嗜酸性颗粒状小体不明显

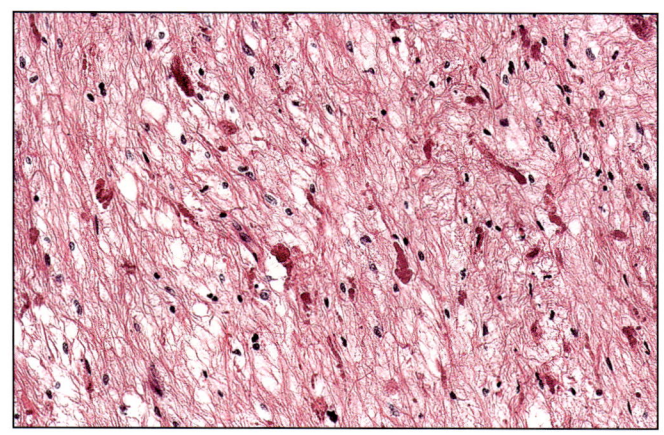

图26.29 毛细胞型星形细胞瘤。高倍放大显示纤维束中有大量的Rosenthal纤维。

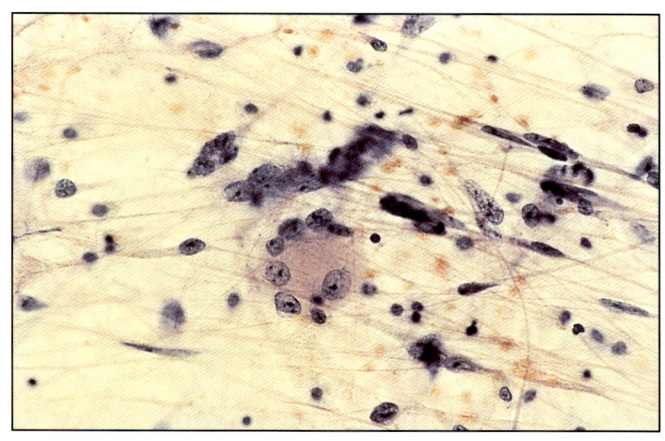

图26.31 毛细胞型星形细胞瘤常有退变表现，不应当认为是间变性改变。在此颞叶肿瘤中，高倍放大显示，在极为纤维性的基质中，多核细胞与毛细胞型星形细胞的典型的并列分布。Morris染色。

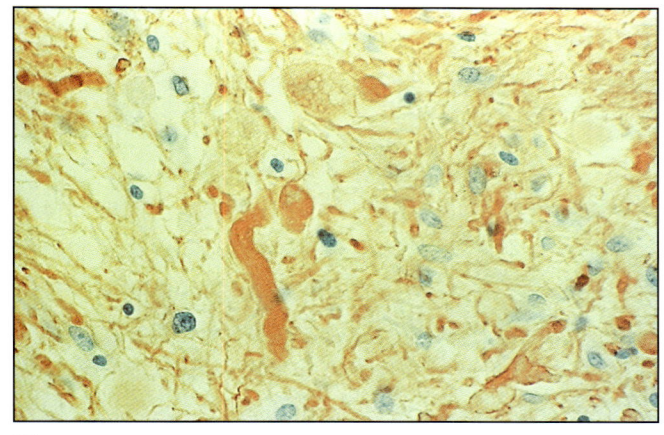

图26.30 毛细胞型星形细胞瘤。Rosenthal纤维和颗粒状嗜酸性小体显示不同程度的胶质纤维酸性蛋白（GFAP）免疫反应。该视野中，强阳性的Rosenthal纤维包埋于致密纤维性星形细胞基质当中。GFAP-ABC免疫过氧化酶法，苏木素双重染色。

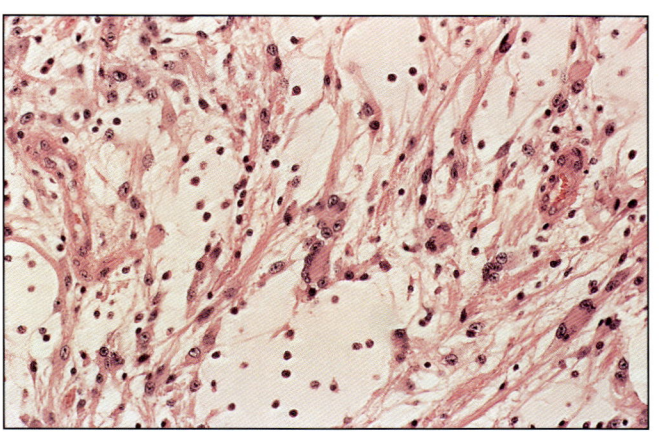

图26.32 毛细胞型星形细胞瘤。图26.31涂片所用组织的组织学切片，显示退变的多核细胞，伴有微囊变和大量毛细胞型星形细胞。

或缺乏。这些肿瘤的复发率明显较高，1年时无进展生存率仅为经典毛细胞型星形细胞瘤的56%。

毛细胞型星形细胞瘤的分子细胞遗传学（molecular cytogenetics of pilocytic astrocytomas）：毛细胞型星形细胞瘤的分子生物学表现同其组织病理学特征一样，明显不同于弥漫型星形细胞瘤。TP53突变以及血小板源性生长因子受体α（PDGF-α）和PDGF-R表达增加常见，可能是弥漫型星形细胞瘤形成的早期事件，但TP53突变或异常PDGF信号在毛细胞型星形细胞瘤的发生中不起作用[203,204]。有关散发性星形细胞瘤的基因表达的对比分析显示，这些肿瘤不同于非肿瘤性白质和其他低级别胶质瘤，与胎儿星形细胞更为相似[205]。然而，毛细胞型星形细胞瘤也表达少突胶质细胞谱系的基因（PEN5、PLP、PMP-22、MBP、少突胶质细胞髓鞘糖蛋白）[203,205]。大约30%的毛细胞型星形细胞瘤发生于患有神经纤维瘤病Ⅰ型（NF1）的患者，并且这些肿瘤的发生年龄通常较早（诊断时平均年龄为4.5岁）[203]。在这一肿瘤亚群中，NF1基因表达的减少或丢失为肿瘤发生的初级事件，而在散发性肿瘤中，NF1基因甚至有过表达[206,208]。NF1相关性与散发性毛细胞型星形细胞瘤除了NF1基因表达不同以外，EF-1α2基因仅在散发性肿瘤中出现表达增加。因此，NF-1相关型与散发性毛细胞型星形细胞瘤尽管具有相同的组织学特征，但其发生和发展经历了不同的遗传学改变，结果是出现类似的组织学表型。

毛细胞型星形细胞瘤的特殊组织学特征和好发部位提示这些肿瘤来源于特殊的、与放射状胶质细胞或前体细胞（类似于O-2A）有关的胶质细胞群增生，它们很可能存在于儿童和年轻人的神经系统中[209,210]。这些肿瘤常见的GFAP免疫反应双相性及其区域性好发倾向与这一假说相一致。正常O-2A起源的星形细胞缺乏EGF反应性，在单层培养中出现低的核分裂活性[211]，类似于毛细胞型星形细胞瘤的通常的惰性生长。毛细胞型星形细胞瘤的纤维突起GFAP和波形蛋白呈强阳性，胎儿放射状胶质出现同样特征[163,212,213]。

多形性黄色瘤型星形细胞瘤 （图26.33至26.36）
Pleomorphic xanthoastrocytoma

多形性黄色瘤型星形细胞瘤（PXA）是发生于CNS的相对不常见的胶质瘤，在大多数病例研究中占星形细胞肿瘤的比例不足1%。此星形细胞瘤的特殊临床病理学特征最初报道于1979年[214]，迄今已报道了大约100例。这些肿瘤常常发生于有长期癫痫病史的儿童和年轻人，没有性别倾向。临床出现肿瘤时的平均年龄通常在1～20岁，但病例范围为1～30岁。发生于31～40岁以后年长病人的肿瘤极少见[215,216]。

肿瘤大多发生于幕上，好发于颞叶及其被覆的软脑膜。但硬脑膜受累极其少见[214,217-219]。伴有多形性黄色瘤型星形细胞瘤特征的肿瘤也可以见于CNS的其他部位，包括小脑和脊髓[215,220]。在9例小脑病例中，除1例婴儿病例以外，平均年龄是40岁，多数病变为实性病变，40%以上的肿瘤具有节细胞成分。尽管有些病例具有间变特征，但其生物学在总体上相对呈惰性；然而，发生在非颞叶部位的肿瘤过少，难以得出普遍性结论。重点强调的是，发生在其他部位的肿瘤其生物学行为有可能不同于幕上的肿瘤[215]。

颞叶部位的肿瘤通常呈囊性，也可以表现为附壁结节。尽管大体上与下部脑组织通常有明确的界限，但镜下常可见局灶浸润。肿瘤较邻近脑组织稍硬，但其明显的粘附性在进行术中涂片时容易感觉到。肿瘤的粘附性增加，部分是由于丰富的网织纤维阳性间质，后者常常为显著特征。它们包裹细胞束，并且程度不同地分布于单个肿瘤细胞之间（图26.35）。尽管此间质在肿瘤中所占比例多少不等，但它们在伴有软脑膜受累和显著微血管成分的肿瘤中最为显著。超微结构研究可显示细胞间的基底膜成分[221,222]，该特征为肿瘤性星形细胞和软脑膜下星形细胞所共有[162]。但也报道了一些病例，没有明显的网状间质，而伴有PXA的其他典型特征[219,223]。

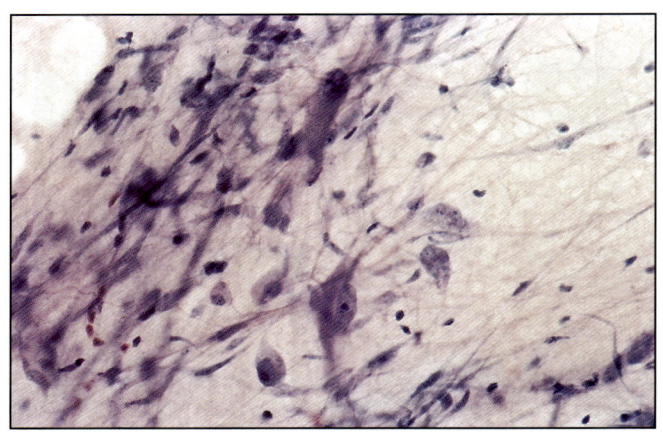

图26.33 多形性黄色瘤型星形细胞瘤的涂片，以显著多形性为特征。注意多角形、细长及纤维性的星形细胞。组织的显著粘附性在涂片过程中很明显。Morris染色。

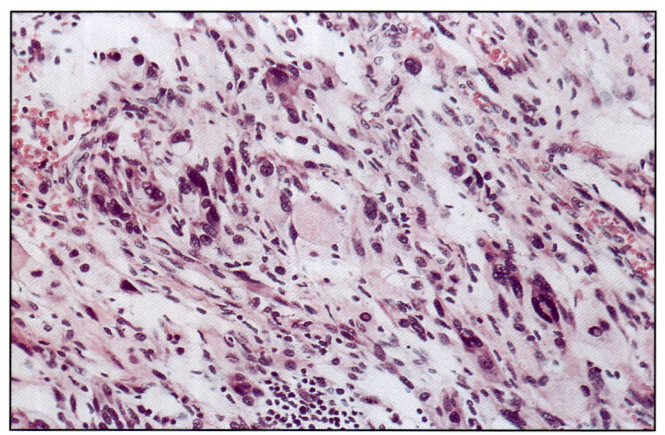

A　　　　　　　　　　　　　　　　　　B

图26.34 多形性黄色瘤型星形细胞瘤具有明显不同的肿瘤细胞构型，从排列成束状的梭形细胞到具有非典型细胞核的明显球状的嗜酸性细胞（A）。脂性细胞常见，但必须除外脂性胶质母细胞瘤（B）。

异质性的星形胶质肿瘤细胞可通过 GFAP 免疫组化染色显示（图 26.36），从没有突起的肥胖性多角形细胞到呈束状交错排列、分布于多少不等的纤维性间质中的较梭形的细胞（图 26.33,26.34）。一般细胞密度中等，但可有局灶增加。多形性细胞核通常深染，多核巨细胞易见（图 26.34）。核分裂象可以见到，但不多，与免疫荧光流式细胞术分析的 S- 期细胞比例极低一致[224]，一般 MIB-1 指数较低[223]。细胞浆的脂质化，尤其是在多角及巨细胞中，可以很明显。该特征差异较大，与肿瘤持续时间以及周围神经毡的相对退变数量有关。在 PXA 中，血管周围不同程度的淋巴细胞浸润并不少见，但没有特殊意义。

少数病例出现非典型节细胞与其他典型 PXA 混合[225-228]。神经元和胶质细胞成分的比例和类型不同，从可能为陷入的神经元成分到 PXA 内、代表节细胞胶质瘤中胶质部分的肿瘤[228]。关于这些少见病例与其他促结缔组织增生性胶质神经元肿瘤之间的组织遗传学相关性，目前尚不清楚。

尽管最初关于 PXA 类型的临床数据提示这些肿瘤应为低级别[214]，但 PXA 的生物学行为及其间变性进展的潜能仍然不清楚。有些病例有复发，并表现为间变性进展[221-223]，但与弥漫浸润性星形细胞瘤相比，此行为明显少见。尽管如此，与其他境界更清楚、预后较好的星形细胞瘤（即毛细胞性和室管膜下巨细胞型星形细胞瘤）相比，应将 PXA 视为一种具有显著侵袭性生物行为潜能的肿瘤。因此，将这些肿瘤确定为 WHO 分类 II 级或 III 级[229]。浸润性边界的组织病理学特征是复发和间变性进展潜能的重要线索[221,222]。这在增殖能力增加的情况下尤其重要，因为核分裂象罕见，MIB-1 指数常常是 2%[223]。可以见到 Virchow-Robin 间隙浸润，但其本身并不提示预后更差。肿瘤的星形胶质特征在原始和复发肿瘤中也有不同。在一例 7 岁男性病例中，第一次和第二次肿瘤切除之间经历了 20 年的时间间隔，在两次样本中，网织纤维阳性间质和纤维性星形细胞成分存在明显不同。复发并不伴有胶质细胞间变特征强调，有些 PXA 病例复发可有或无间变进展。

多形性黄色瘤型星形细胞瘤的分子细胞遗传学（molecular cytogenetics of pleomorphic xanthoastrocytomas）：目前没有确切的资料表明有分子事件在 PXA 的发病机制上起作用。PXA 有限的分子分析证实，它不同于弥漫型星形细胞瘤。同样，关于肿瘤发生和从 WHO II 级进

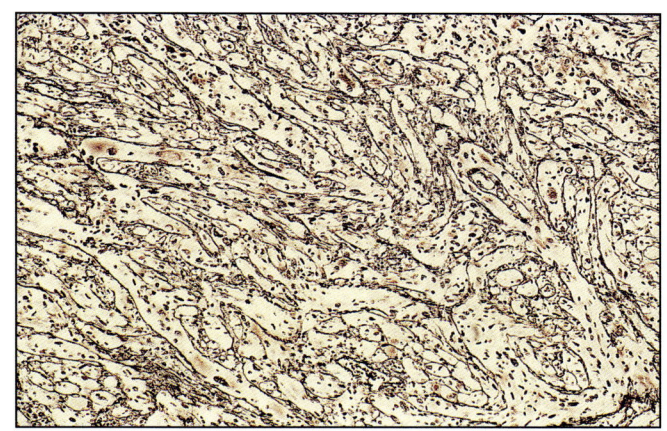

图 26.35 多形性黄色瘤型星形细胞瘤。单个细胞和不规则的细胞簇被沉积的网状纤维所包围。这和电镜下看到的包裹性基底膜相对应。网织纤维染色。

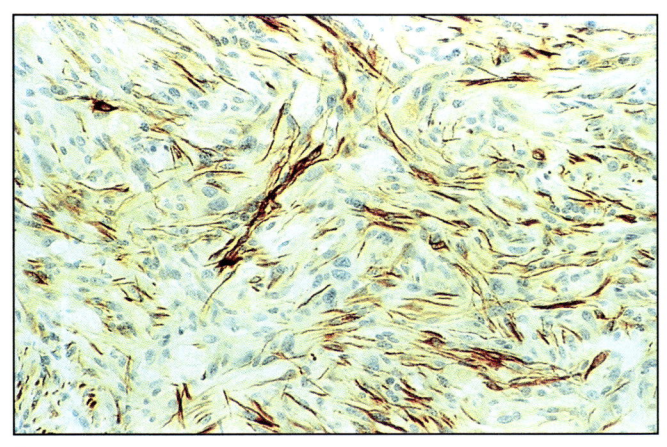 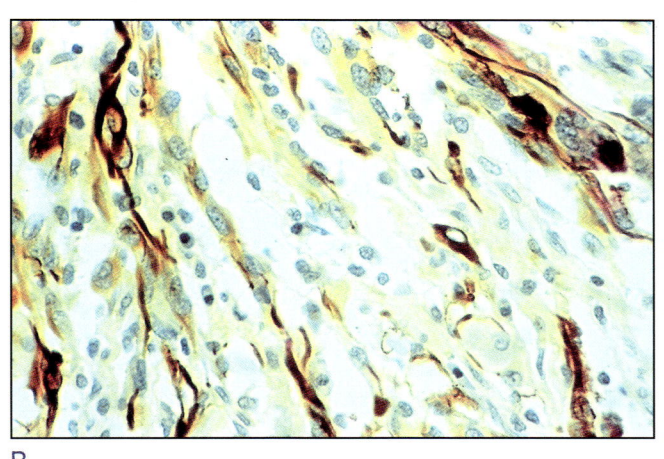

图 26.36 多形性黄色瘤型星形细胞瘤。胶质纤维酸性蛋白（GFAP）免疫染色证实了多形性细胞的胶质本质，并且常常可以突出较为梭形的细胞成分（A）。注意黄色瘤样细胞GFAP-免疫反应的胞浆环（B）。GFAP-ABC免疫过氧化物酶法，苏木素双重染色。

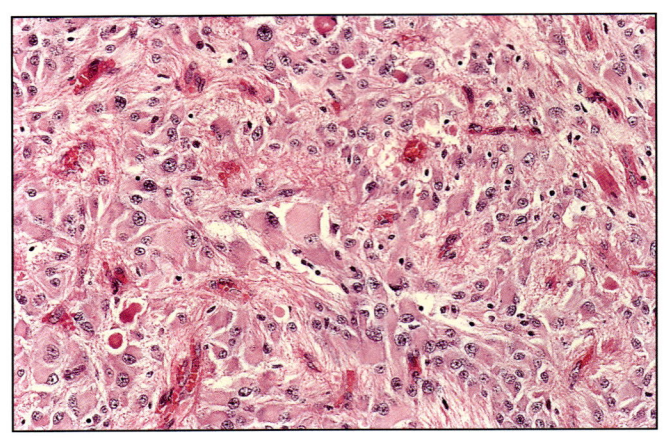
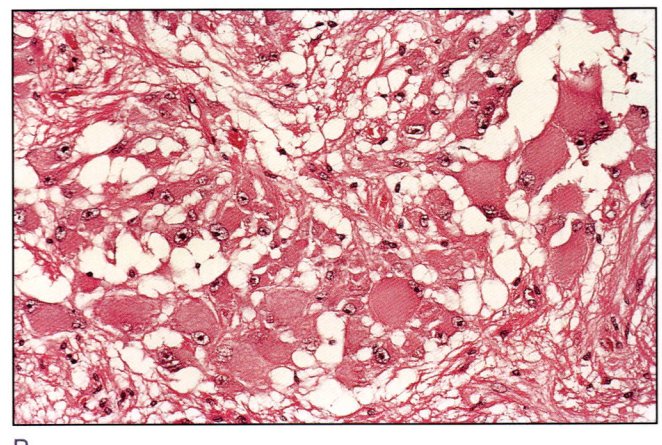

图26.37 室管膜下巨细胞型星形细胞瘤典型的细胞异质性。大的锥体样细胞与梭形和较小的纤维性星形细胞混合（A）。注意节细胞样细胞，有时为双核，核仁明显（B）。

展到WHO Ⅲ级的特殊机制方面也没有明确的资料。遗传性病变通常可见于弥漫型星形细胞瘤，*TP53*突变和*EGFR*基因扩增在PXA的发病机制中比较少见，但在弥漫型星形细胞瘤中不常见的遗传性缺失（8p染色体）可起到更重要的作用[229,230]。

室管膜下巨细胞型星形细胞瘤（图26.37和26.38）
Subependymal giant cell astrocytoma

室管膜下巨细胞型星形细胞瘤（SEGA）通常发生于1~20岁，有结节性硬化背景，但也可以是原发性表现。这些肿瘤也可发生于随后没有斑痣性错构瘤病的患者。SEGA境界清楚、常常为结节状及多囊状，伴有钙化[231]。大多位于基底节水平的侧脑室壁，少数邻近第三脑室。症状一般与室间孔阻塞有关。

SEGA的肿瘤细胞群出现宽泛的星形胶质细胞表型。典型表现由含有丰富毛玻璃样胞浆的多角形细胞到随机分布的、更为细长的小细胞构成，分布于多少不等的纤维型基质中（图26.37和26.38）。细胞核具有细颗粒状染色体结构，核仁明显（图26.37B）。具有"节细胞样"表现的巨大锥体细胞并不少见。肿瘤细胞大多表现为不同程度的GFAP（图26.38）和S-100蛋白阳性，证实了该肿瘤的星形胶质细胞本质。然而，有些肿瘤表现为胶质和神经元相关表型，如class Ⅲ β-微管蛋白、NF-H/M和神经递质[231-233]。

肿瘤也可以出现提示神经元分化的超微结构特征，包括微管、极个别致密核心颗粒和极少数突触形成。这些特征可令人联想起结节性硬化中的错构瘤性皮层病变。细胞核显著多形性、数量不等的核分裂象以及个别多核细胞的出现并不意味着间变。在一个有20例

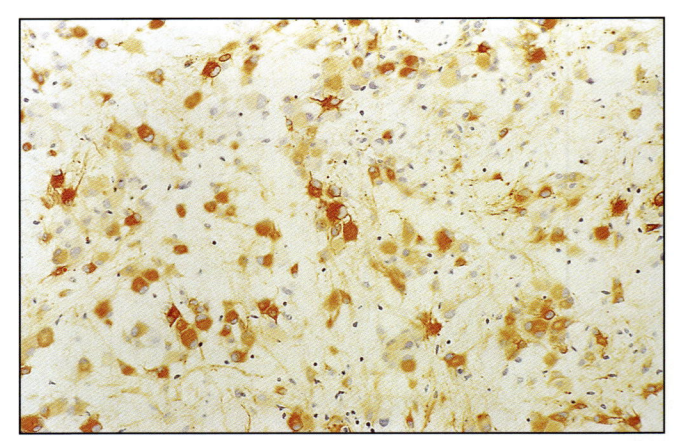

图26.38 胶质纤维酸性蛋白（GFAP）免疫反应也不同程度地见于室管膜下巨细胞型星形细胞瘤，常常突出了多角形细胞和梭形细胞。GFAP-ABC免疫过氧化物酶法，苏木素双重染色。

SEGA病例的研究中[234]，内皮增生、坏死、核分裂象增加以及出现显著的细胞多形性与不良的临床过程或生存时间减少并不相关。这种相关性的缺乏与弥漫性浸润性星形细胞肿瘤形成对比，说明识别室管膜下巨细胞型星形细胞瘤的重要性。极少数复发性肿瘤并不出现恶性转化[235]。

室管膜下巨细胞型星形细胞瘤的分子细胞遗传学：室管膜下巨细胞型星形细胞瘤的分子遗传学显示：*TSC2*基因（16p13）杂合性丢失以及*TSC2*基因产物、tuberin、一个Rap 1同系物和公认的肿瘤抑制因子丢失[236,237]。在鼠*TSC2*突变模型中，TSC（+/-）杂合的星形胶质细胞$p27^{kip1}$表达减少，提示在这些肿瘤性病变的形成过程中，星形细胞增殖的调节异常（单层细胞培养中出现接触抑制减少）[238]。

少突胶质细胞肿瘤和混合性胶质瘤
Oligodendroglial tumors and mixed gliomas

少突胶质细胞肿瘤的组织病理学分类包括两个普通类别中的四种主要肿瘤类型（见表26.1）。少突胶质细胞瘤（WHO Ⅱ级）和间变性少突胶质细胞瘤（WHO Ⅲ级）为第一种较为同质性的组织病理学分类。其次，更为多相性的分类包括少突星形细胞瘤（WHO Ⅱ级）和间变性少突星形细胞瘤（WHO Ⅲ级）被划归为"混合型"胶质瘤，具有少突胶质细胞和星形细胞表型。在美国和欧洲的大型病例研究中，少突胶质细胞瘤大约占所有 CNS 原发性脑肿瘤的 4%，占成人胶质瘤的 9.5%，校正后的整体发病率为每年 0.27/10 万人～0.37/10 万人[149,156]。年轻人（20～34 岁）中，少突胶质细胞瘤占所有原发性脑肿瘤的 9.4%，而高峰发生率在 35～44 岁（每年 0.66/10 万人）。儿童阶段极其少见，大约占原发性 CNS 肿瘤的 2%。在大多数病例研究中，少突胶质细胞瘤男性与女性的比例为 0.92～1.75；但在最大的病例研究中，只有轻微的男性倾向。

神经轴的任何区域均可受累，但额颞区和基底节是常见部位。低级别与高级别少突胶质瘤（WHO Ⅱ级：Ⅲ级）的比率为 2.1～4.5，在少突胶质细胞肿瘤的一般分类中（包括少突星形胶质细胞瘤），少突胶质细胞瘤占 WHO Ⅱ级肿瘤的 71%～79%（见表 26.2）。间变性少突胶质细胞瘤和间变性少突星形细胞瘤在 WHO Ⅲ级肿瘤中大约占有同等比例。对于少突胶质细胞瘤，最初手术时的平均年龄为 40～42.5 岁[149,239,240]；但在年龄上额叶肿瘤患者比非额叶肿瘤患者稍微年轻[240]。有些病例研究中，年龄超过 40 岁可短期内出现进展，总体生存时间减少[241]。

少突胶质瘤（图26.39至26.44） Oligodendroglioma

少突胶质细胞瘤大体上一般质软，呈胶样，伴有微小钙化。涂片中，肿瘤细胞的胞浆境界不清，疏松粘附于境界不清的嗜酸性基质中（图 26.39）。与星形细胞瘤相比，其细胞核呈特征性的圆形，稍有分叶，具有较纤细的染色质结构。尽管其核仁较星形细胞瘤易见，但多个染色质结节更为常见。缺乏星形细胞瘤的明显的纤维性基质以及出现大量纤细的微血管结构等其他特征有助于在涂片中识别少突胶质细胞瘤。微小矿化也易于识别。

在经过固定、石蜡包埋的组织切片中，少突胶质细胞瘤的细胞学特征和组织学结构变化较大（图 26.40 至 26.43）。部分是由于不同程度的人工假象所致的核周胞浆透明，形成所谓的"煎蛋"样外观（图 26.40）。细胞

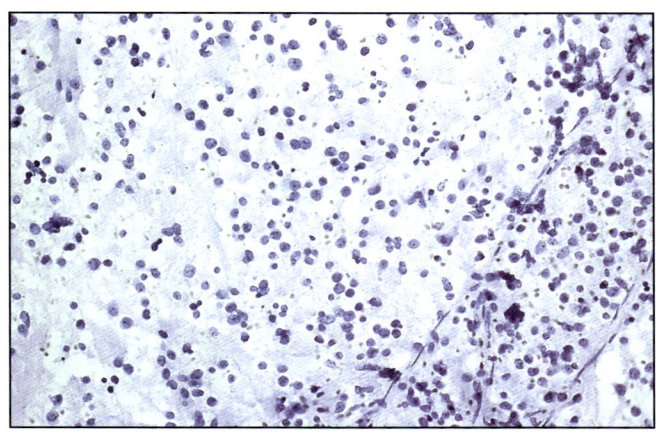

图26.39 少突胶质细胞瘤涂片，在纤细的纤维性基质中出现粘附较差的细胞具有诊断性。细胞核相对一致，但常有分叶，胞浆界限不清。Morris染色。

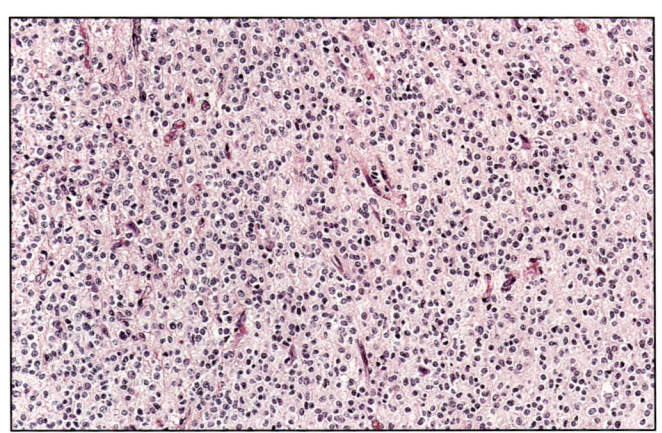

图26.40 少突胶质细胞瘤。组织切片显示均匀一致的细胞结构，纤细血管的数量增加。

核从均质圆形至稍呈梭形（图 26.41）。细胞核分叶不如在涂片中易见。通常胞浆突起稀少，发育不良，与星形细胞相比，其细胞间基质的纤维性特征不甚明显。大量血管性间质形成了纤细薄壁血管构成的几何性网状结构，类似于"鸡笼样结构"以及不完全分隔的肿瘤细胞簇（图 26.41）。其他细胞分布包括平行排列的细胞行，形成栅栏样结构，血管周围的假玫瑰花结或明显球形细胞乳头状结构。少数情况下，球形细胞呈空泡状，类似于印戒细胞。少数情况下，细胞间基质可出现黏液或囊性变。反应性星形细胞常常散在分布于肿瘤当中，常常靠近血管（图 26.42）。细胞密度从低度至中度，以致细胞核分散，相互不接触。细胞增殖活性在少突胶质细胞瘤中较低。核分裂象罕见，总体 MIB-1 标记指数（LI）较低。一项有关少突胶质细胞瘤中的 Ki-67 研究显示，平均 MIB-1 标记指数在少突胶质细胞瘤（低级别）中小

于 2，MIB-1 标记指数大于 5 的肿瘤生存期较短[242]。毛细血管可以比较明显，但真正的微血管增生一般只限于间变性少突胶质细胞瘤。

对于固定过的石蜡包埋组织，肿瘤性少突胶质细胞没有特异的免疫细胞化学标记物。尽管 bHLH 转录因子（OLIG1 和 OLIG2）与少突胶质细胞系和发育过程中的分化相关，但在胶质细胞肿瘤中，两者似乎都不是仅特异性地表达于少突胶质细胞瘤中[243-245]。

少突胶质细胞瘤大多不表达中间丝蛋白 GFAP 和波形蛋白。小肥胖细胞型少突胶质细胞瘤，即所谓的"胶质纤维型少突胶质细胞"[246,247]，出现 GFAP 强阳性（图26.44），见于大约 50% 的少突胶质细胞瘤[246,248]。对于小肥胖细胞型少突胶质细胞的 GFAP 免疫反应检测，不应该解释为提示星形细胞成分。仔细分析 PTAH 组织化学和波形蛋白免疫组化，应当区分开肿瘤性少突胶质瘤的 GFAP 免疫反应与多数肿瘤中反应性胶质血管基质内的星形细胞或少突星形细胞瘤中具有星形胶质细胞表型的肿瘤细胞（见下文）。在肿瘤性少突胶质瘤中，GFAP 免疫反应类似于不成熟的少突细胞瘤的先前正常髓鞘形成过程中的短暂 GFAP 表达[249]。这在分化较差的少突胶质细胞瘤中比较明显[250]。这些肿瘤中的 GFAP 免疫阳性细胞比例在伴有间变性进展时有增加的趋势，更加类似于经典肥胖细胞型星形细胞，而不是"胶质原纤维少突胶质细胞"或"小肥胖细胞"[246]。但这些 GFAP 阳性细胞的组织发生尚不清楚。

少突胶质细胞瘤出现 Leu-7 抗原[251]、半乳糖脑苷脂[252]及 S-100 蛋白阳性；但是，这些标记物不能特异性的判定少突胶质细胞瘤。

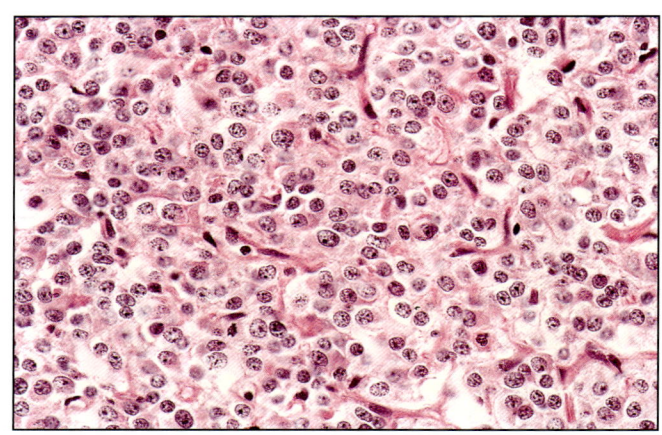

图26.41　少突胶质细胞瘤。高倍放大显示不规则性细胞核分叶，染色质粗，不同程度胞浆收缩，细胞境界不清。注意细胞间基质境界不清，缺乏星形细胞瘤常见的纤维性。

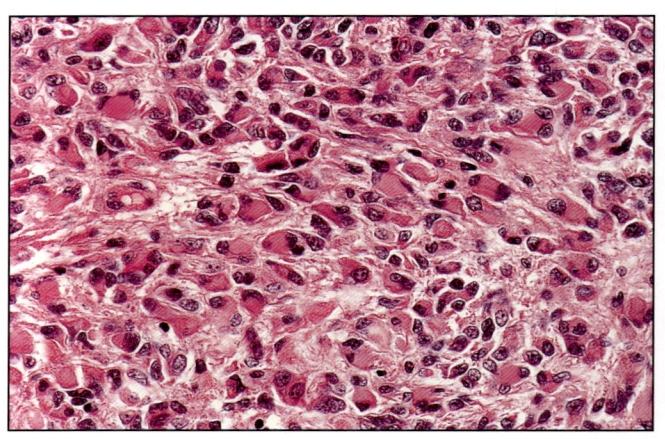

图26.43　少突胶质细胞瘤的非典型性增加，胞浆体积和多形性加大，通常为嗜酸性胞浆和偏位的细胞核。

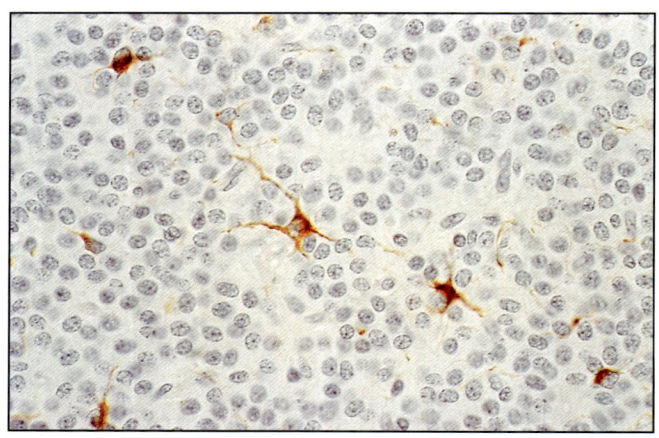

图26.42　少突胶质细胞瘤中出现典型的反应性星形细胞常见。GFAP-PAP免疫过氧化物酶法，苏木素双重染色。

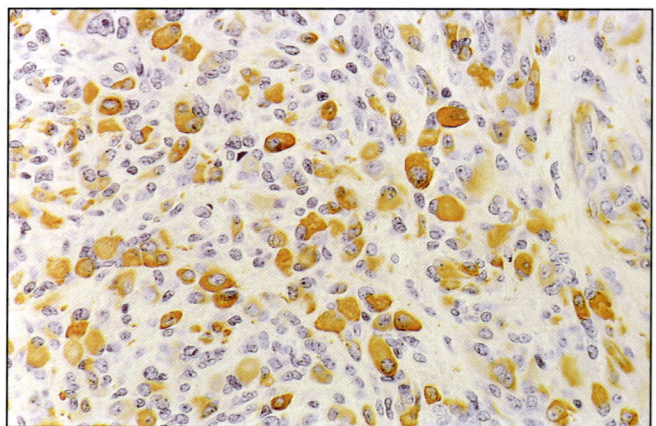

图26.44　胶质纤维酸性蛋白（GFAP）免疫反应细胞，伴有典型少突胶质细胞特征（"胶质原纤维少突胶质细胞"），见于大约50%的少突胶质细胞瘤；但是，这些GFAP免疫反应细胞的数量在间变性肿瘤中常有增加。GFAP-ABC免疫过氧化物酶法。

间变性少突胶质细胞瘤（图26.45至26.51）
Anaplastic oligodendroglioma

间变性少突胶质细胞瘤为少数的少突胶质细胞肿瘤，占新发生恶性胶质瘤的比例不到5%[253]。间变性少突胶质细胞瘤可由低级别少突胶质细胞瘤间变转化而来，或者为原发性的。识别间变性少突胶质细胞瘤及其与其他间变性胶质瘤的鉴别具有临床和预后意义，因为它们具有独特的化疗敏感性[253,254]。

间变性少突胶质细胞瘤不但具有低级别少突胶质细胞瘤的组织学特征，还出现间变转化特征，类似于弥漫性星形细胞瘤伴发间变，包括高度富于细胞、核分裂活性较高、细胞核多形性增加、地图样坏死以及微血管增生（图26.45至26.51）[255-257]。日常诊断中采用与弥漫性星形细胞瘤同样的标准。

间变性少突胶质细胞瘤的组织病理特征在预测肿瘤行为方面是否具有预后意义，有关报道结果不一。有些研究者发现，经典参数（如核分裂活性和坏死）是最重

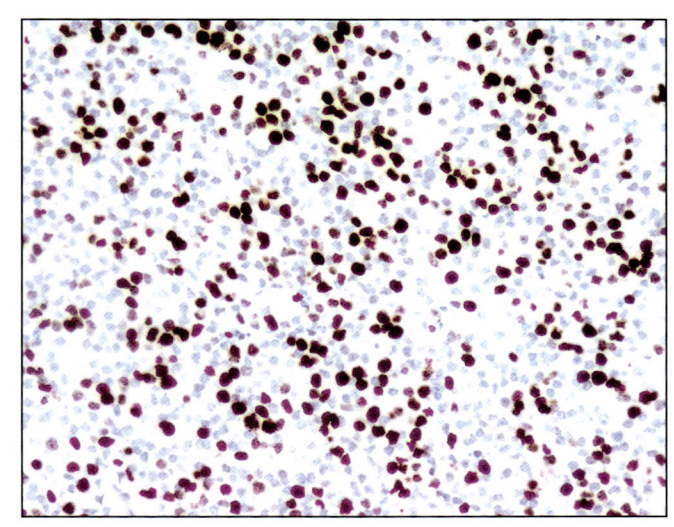

图26.47　间变性少突胶质细胞瘤中，Ki-67（MIB1单克隆）免疫组化染色显示较高的标记指数。ABC免疫过氧化物酶法，苏木素双重染色。

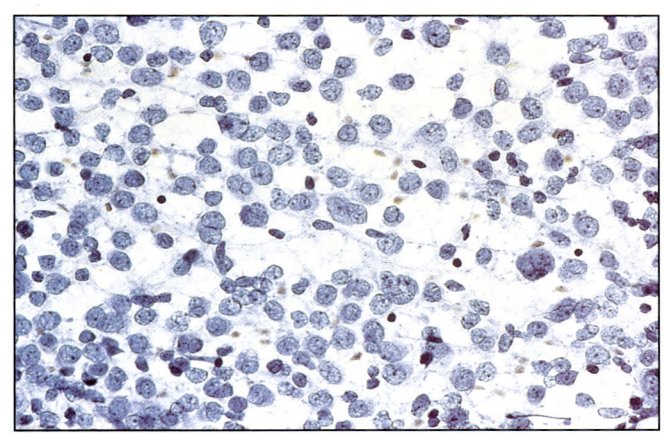

图26.45　细胞多形性显著增加、明显细胞核分叶以及浓染细胞核是间变性少突胶质细胞瘤涂片中的典型特征。常见有多核。Morris染色。

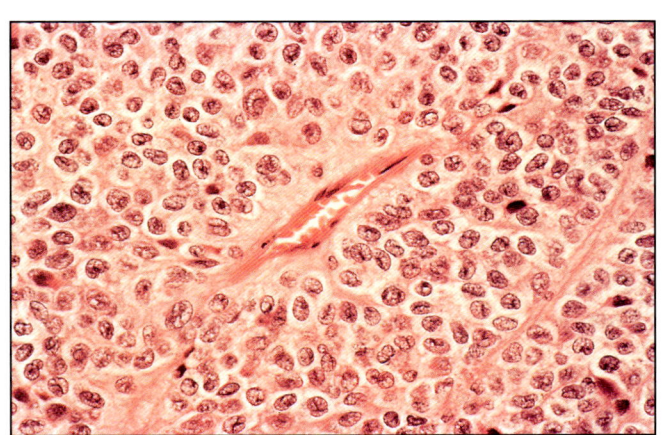

图26.48　间变性少突胶质细胞瘤。更高倍放大，显示同样含有粗大染色质的分叶状核，在涂片中易于识别。注意血管周围的细胞缺乏清楚的突起。

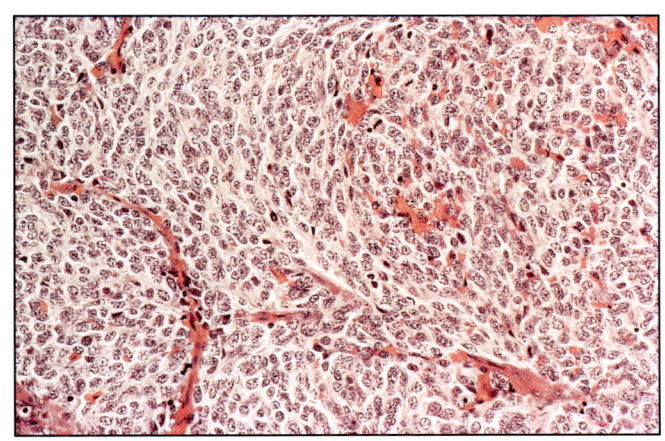

图26.46　此间变性少突胶质细胞瘤视野中出现丰富的细胞和众多的核分裂象。

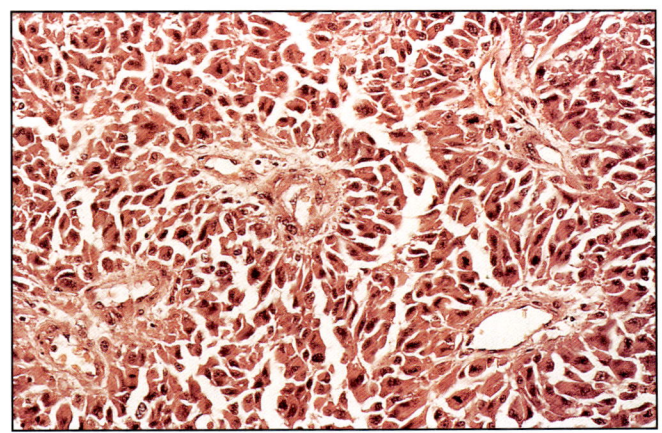

图26.49　间变性肿瘤细胞排列在血管周围，可以形成乳头状结构，如在同此间变性少突胶质细胞瘤中。

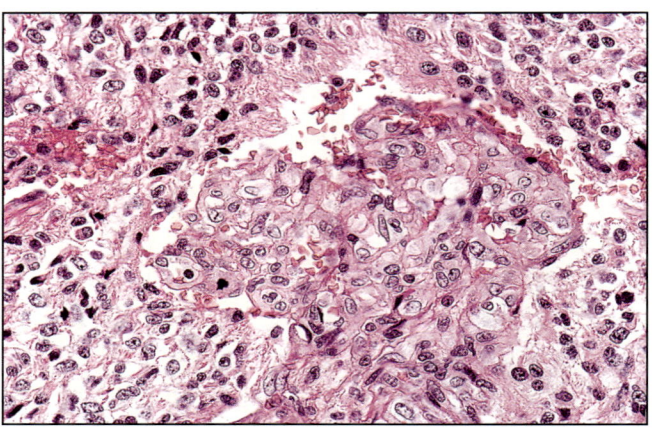

图26.50 呈肾小球样结构的显著内皮细胞/外皮细胞增生是少突胶质细胞瘤间变转化的重要指标。

要的预后指标[257]。其他人则认为，采用 Ki-67（MIB-1）评估增殖活性与患者生存率的关系更为密切[242,258]。少突胶质细胞肿瘤的精确分级系统尚未完全形成或验证。进展为胶质母细胞瘤被认为是少突胶质细胞瘤和间变性少突胶质细胞瘤中极为少见的已被认可的事件。

混合性少突星形细胞肿瘤
Mixed oligoastrocytic tumors

Bailey 和 Bucy[259] 早在 3/4 个世纪以前就注意到，胶质细胞的异质性是少突胶质细胞肿瘤的属性。他们除了描述了主要的少突胶质肿瘤细胞外，还描述了出现多少不等的多形性星形细胞瘤以及介于"真正的"星形细胞和更为原始的胶质样细胞之间的"所有阶段的转化"。这些肿瘤的组织学发生尚不清楚；然而，与同级别星形细胞瘤相比，少突星形细胞瘤病人的存活率要好得多。

最近，有关干细胞的研究提供的数据支持成人脑内存在多潜能和双相潜能胶质细胞祖细胞[66,260]。实验工作已经证实了胶质祖细胞系的真正的祖细胞活性，即产生分化后代和维持稳定的祖细胞池[261,262]。这些祖细胞群的存在，作为成人神经系统肿瘤转化的关键点，是理解少突胶质细胞瘤和混合性少突星形细胞瘤组织学发生的关键所在[263]。

大多数基于人群的研究没有特别报告混合性少突星形细胞瘤。在有数据的病例研究中，混合性少突星形细胞瘤大约占少突胶质细胞瘤的 35%，WHO Ⅱ 级肿瘤大约占 20%（每年发生率为 0.1/10 万人）[149,239]。对于"混合性胶质瘤"[156]，诊断时的平均年龄为 42 岁，发病率是每年 0.15/10 万人，尽管高峰发病率位于下一个 10 年。

少突星形细胞瘤（图26.52和26.53）
Oligoastrocytoma

少突星形细胞瘤（WHO Ⅱ 级）由少突胶质细胞和相当比例的肿瘤性星形细胞组成。少突星形细胞瘤原发于大脑半球，额叶最常受累，其次是颞叶[264]。与低级别少突胶质细胞瘤类似，患者常常具有长期癫痫病史。

目前没有诊断混合性少突星形细胞瘤的明确组织学标准。少突胶质细胞瘤和少突星形细胞瘤的鉴别有困难，因为肿瘤内两种细胞成分的组成差异较大，并且缺乏明确的鉴别参数。这两种胶质性肿瘤的细胞成分可呈局灶或弥漫性分布（图 26.52）。这些病例的涂片可以大大方便识别这两种不同细胞成分的细胞形态学特征（图 26.53）。有些研究者认为，混合性胶质瘤至少应在 1 个 100 倍视野里见到第二种次要胶质成分[265]。与低级别少突胶质细胞瘤一样，混合性少突星形细胞瘤出现轻度多形性，很少有核分裂象。缺乏内皮增生和坏死。

新近一项平均随访 40.3 个月的报告强调，应用 MIB-1 评估 WHO Ⅱ 级少突星形细胞瘤的增殖细胞[266]。相对于低增殖活性的 WHO Ⅱ 级肿瘤，MIB-1 标记指数大于等于 10% 的肿瘤出现肿瘤进展的时间较短，总体预后更差。

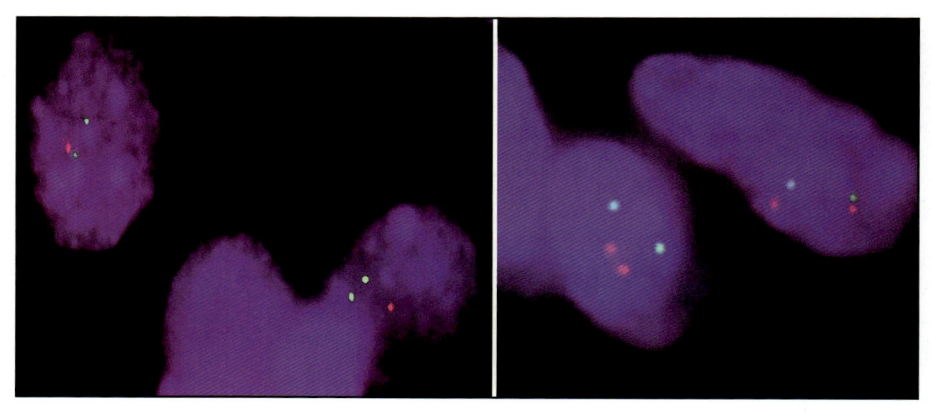

图26.51 荧光原位杂交（FISH）分析间变性少突胶质细胞瘤的1和19号染色体。（A）间变性少突胶质细胞瘤出现1p缺失（每个核一个红点，与之对比，2个绿点标记1q）。（B）同一肿瘤显示完整19q（每个核2个红点，与之对比，2个绿点标记19p）。[（A）1号染色体：1p = 罗丹明（红色），1q = FITC（绿色）；（B）19号染色体：19p = FIFC（绿色）；19q = 罗丹明（红色）。]

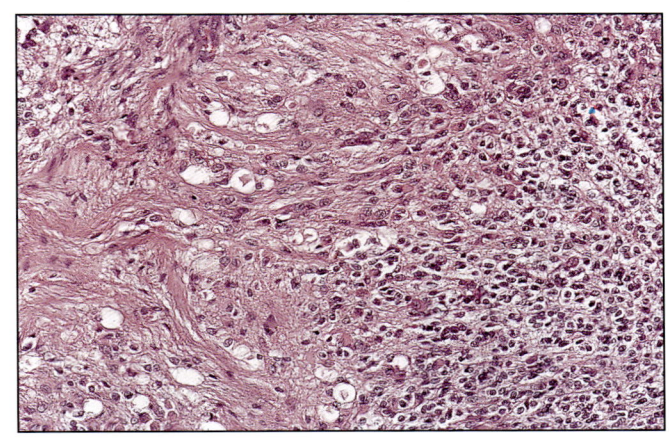

图26.52 混合性少突星形细胞瘤的组织切片,两种成分的组织学结构或者紧密混合,或者并列分布,此处显示纤维性星形细胞瘤(左)和少突胶质细胞瘤(右)。

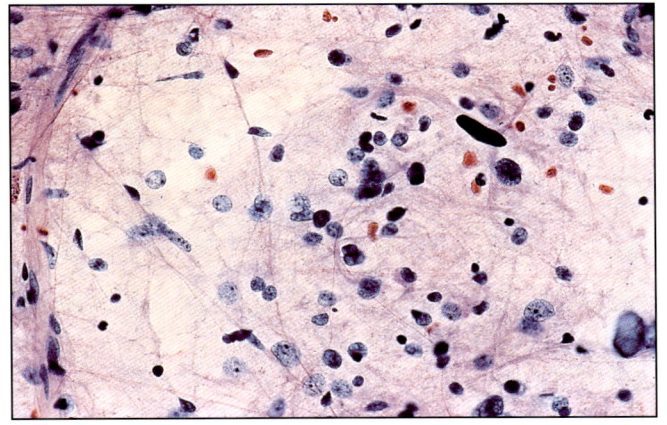

图26.53 混合性少突星形细胞瘤。涂片有助于区别肿瘤性星形细胞和少突胶质细胞的混合成分。Morris染色。

间变性少突星形细胞瘤
Anaplastic oligoastrocytoma

少突星形胶质细胞瘤的确切的间变性进展发生率尚不清楚。间变性少突星形胶质细胞瘤(WHO Ⅲ级)是混合性胶质瘤,伴有间变性组织学特征,包括细胞密度增加、细胞核非典型性和高度核分裂活性。血管内皮细胞增生和局灶坏死常见。在大多数病例中,间变性改变在少突胶质细胞和星形细胞成分中均可见到。然而,星形细胞成分更易于出现间变进展。

由于这些混合性胶质瘤的潜在的化疗敏感性,间变性少突星形细胞瘤与间变性星形细胞瘤或多形性胶质母细胞瘤的鉴别具有临床意义。尽管这些间变性少突星形细胞瘤的预后尚在监测中,但其平均生存期比胶质母细胞瘤患者的好得多[267]。

少突胶质细胞肿瘤的分子细胞遗传学:分子遗传学分析结合化疗后治疗效果和生存率数据,已极大地增加了少突胶质细胞瘤的WHO组织病理学定义的复杂性[268]。此外,这些分析显示了其与弥漫性星形细胞瘤的相对明确的分子遗传学差异。符合"经典"少突胶质细胞瘤组织病理学定义的肿瘤至少有两种不同的临床基因组。第一组,一般在成人少突胶质细胞瘤中占大多数(60%～92%),但在儿童组为罕见肿瘤[239,269],具有 1p(1p34.2-p36.1;1p36.22-p36.31、1p36.3-pter)和 19q(19q13.3)(34-37,1,3)遗传缺失(见图26.51)。伴有1p遗传缺失的肿瘤的神经影像学特征包括:T1-加权像境界不清,T1和T2-加权像混合信号密度[270,271]。对于具有该特征的特定肿瘤是否具有特殊好发部位,存在一些分歧[272];但是,起源于颞叶的少突胶质细胞瘤通常没有1p/19q缺失,与发生于其他部位的肿瘤的发生率相同[273]。尽管项研究表明,同低级别星形细胞瘤一样,少突胶质细胞瘤有p14ARF和CDKN2A(p16INK4a)遗传位点的过度甲基化,但这些位点在少突胶质细胞瘤中的过度甲基化更为常见。同样,多个遗传位点的5'-CpG岛过度甲基化可能是一种重要后生遗传机制,调节伴有1p和19q缺失肿瘤的多位点基因表达[274]。因此,1p和1p/19q缺失可以确定少突胶质细胞瘤的特殊亚型,具有特殊的基因表达谱[275]。

*EGF*和*PDGF*受体通路的过表达可以发生于少突胶质细胞瘤;同样,功能性*GRO1-PDGF*通路[*PDGFA*、*PDGFαR*、*GRO1*细胞因子及受体(*CXCR2*)]的所有成分也表达于多数少突胶质细胞瘤(WHO Ⅱ～Ⅲ级),与弥漫型星形细胞瘤(WHO Ⅱ～Ⅲ级)相比[276]。在伴有1p丢失的少突胶质细胞瘤中,*EGFR*或*PDGFR*基因扩增以及*PTEN*丢失罕见,即使是在间变性少突胶质细胞瘤中[277-279]。伴有混合LOH1p/19q的少突胶质细胞瘤倾向有较长的进展间期和总体生存期,但对于当前的治疗方法并没有显著差异[241,280]。

第二位和较小一组的少突胶质细胞瘤最初定义为具有完整1p染色体和*TP53*突变。与第一组相比,这些肿瘤在T1-加权像上也具有比较离散的界限[271]。野生型*EGFR*可有过表达,没有高级别弥漫性星形细胞瘤的基因扩增或常见的突变(*EGFR* vⅢ)[142,281]。与第一组少突胶质细胞瘤1p染色体丢失相比,*TP53*突变状况似乎明显预示着少突胶质细胞瘤有一个较短的生存间期,并且极易出现一个较短的无进展存活间期[280]。

少突胶质细胞瘤的间变性肿瘤进展可伴有细胞周期调节基因改变增加、显著缺失性突变,以及影响*CDKN2A/B/p14ARF*的9p21位点甲基化[277,279]。血管形成生长因子、血管内皮生长因子(VEGF)的过表达也可见于恶性进展。与少突胶质细胞瘤稍有些类似的是,间变性少突胶质细胞瘤的定义以分子遗传学改变的等级为依据：(1) 肿瘤伴有 1p 和 19q 丢失，没有其他可以检测的遗传性病变；(2) 肿瘤伴有 1p 丢失和其他遗传学改变，没有 19q 丢失；以及 (3) 肿瘤伴有完整 1p 染色体，伴有或者不伴有 TP53 突变。这些肿瘤亚型回顾起来似乎在发病年龄、常见受累部位、临床反应以及生存时间上存在差异[279]。同少突胶质细胞瘤一样，TP53 突变可使其预后较差[280]。将间变性少突胶质细胞瘤单独分组考虑时，位于 1p 和 19q 的 LOH 与肿瘤进展间期较长和总体生存期较长有关。具有 1p/19q 丢失的间变性少突胶质细胞瘤其 5 年生存率是 63%，相比之下，无此基因标志的是 19%[241]。部分是由于具有 1p/19q 丢失的间变性少突胶质细胞瘤对化疗药物有效所致。含有 9p21q 染色体改变的间变性少突胶质细胞瘤无论 1p/19q 染色体状况如何，容易出现无进展生存期较短和总体预后较差，生存期短[280]。

分子遗传学研究显示，混合性少突星形细胞瘤是基因异质性的一组肿瘤[282,283]。肿瘤的一个亚群具有少突胶质细胞瘤常见的遗传学病变，另一个亚群显示弥漫浸润性星形细胞瘤的分子遗传学特征。大约 30%~70% 的少突星形胶质细胞瘤其特征为少突胶质细胞和星形细胞成分均出现 1p 和 19q 染色体等位基因丢失[284-286]。另外 30% 的肿瘤具有弥漫性星形细胞瘤常见的遗传学改变，包括 TP53 基因突变和（或）17p 丢失[284,285]。具有 1p 和 19q 丢失的少突星形胶质细胞瘤亚群多为少突胶质细胞瘤占优的肿瘤，而具有 TP53 基因突变和（或）17p 丢失的肿瘤多为星形细胞瘤为主[284]。此时，9p21 染色体改变在少突星形细胞瘤比少突胶质细胞瘤更常见[280]。

室管膜肿瘤　Ependymal tumors

室管膜肿瘤的 WHO 分类包括四组：室管膜瘤及其变型（WHO Ⅱ级）、间变性室管膜瘤（WHO Ⅲ级）、黏液乳头状室管膜瘤（WHO Ⅰ级）以及室管膜下瘤（WHO Ⅰ级）（见表 26.1 和 26.2）。这些肿瘤绝大多数起源于脑室及脊髓中央管有关的室管膜神经上皮。其他来源可能源自妊娠后半期侧脑室扩张的[287]发育性皱缩的室管膜细胞巢残件以及马尾终室（ventriculus terminalis）和室管膜残件[288,289]。关于侧脑室的脑室下区中移位的室管膜细胞的作用尚不清楚[290]。

室管膜瘤整体上大约占所有原发性 CNS 肿瘤的 2.3% 及胶质瘤的 5.5%，但出现明显的双峰年龄分布，第 1 个高峰是幼儿期，后一个高峰是 31~50 岁[156,291]。1~4 岁期间，室管膜肿瘤约占神经上皮肿瘤的 11%，特定年龄比例是每年 0.44 人 /10 万人。在随后的两个 10 年里，发病率下降，20~34 岁时，肿瘤约占原发性脑肿瘤的 4.7%，发病率为每年 0.19/10 万人。31~50 岁时，发病率再次上升至每年 0.35/10 万人。所有儿童和成人的室管膜肿瘤均出现程度不一的男性优势（1.3:1~1.5），包括髓内的脊髓肿瘤[292-294]。在马尾和终丝内，黏液乳头状室管膜瘤具有更为明显的男性倾向（1.7:1）[295]。

室管膜肿瘤随着年龄出现不同的解剖学分布。多数儿童室管膜肿瘤位于颅内，起源于幕下后颅窝[294]。较大比例的成人病例起源于脊髓，约占脊髓胶质瘤的 60%[296]。颈部是常见的髓内部位，但大约 40% 的硬膜内脊髓肿瘤起源于终丝[297]。幕上肿瘤成人较儿童常见，至少一半的肿瘤发生于大脑半球，与脑室系统没有任何明确的空间关系[298-300]。多发性脊髓室管膜瘤常常伴有神经纤维瘤病 2 型。

室管膜瘤（图26.54至26.59）
Ependymoma

室管膜瘤是相对境界清楚的肿瘤，相对于其他胶质瘤，其大体上呈"推挤性边缘"。大体上，室管膜瘤具有比星形细胞瘤更为多样的表现。脑室内肿瘤一般较软，呈乳头状，而脑实质发生的肿瘤出现更为一致的颗粒状改变。囊性变和钙化常见。尽管室管膜瘤相对境界清楚，但脑室内肿瘤常常扩展至脑室系统以外，累及蛛网膜下腔。不论其部位如何，室管膜瘤在 CT 和 MR 影像上常常显示类似的特征。这些肿瘤高度富于血管特征，使其静脉对比有不同程度的加强。MR 影像上，这些肿瘤 T1 像一般呈低密度，T2 像密度稍高。

室管膜瘤涂片显示，肿瘤细胞的胞浆境界清楚，通常含有细的突起。它们可形成小"玫瑰花结"样细胞巢或附着于薄壁血管上（图 26.54）。细胞核染色质通常分布不规则，形成纤细小结节，产生"椒盐"或"开放"结构。与星形细胞瘤和少突胶质细胞瘤的相对粗大的染色质形成对比。核仁相对不明显。肿瘤之间纤维性细胞间基质差异较大，但与脉络膜特征相比，病变的胶质本质容易识别（图 26.56）。

室管膜瘤组织切片的结构特征是呈极性排列的肿瘤细胞围绕血管形成"假玫瑰花结"结构（图 26.55 和 26.57）。真正室管膜玫瑰花结和衬有上皮成分的小管结构并不常见（图 26.58）。HE 染色中见到的细胞突起，或者形成细长的纤维性突起，或者形成致密纤维网络（图 26.56）。纤细的、相对细长的突起可经 PTAH 染色和波形蛋白染色以及不同程度的 GFAP 免疫组织化学而更加突出（图 26.57）。除了玫瑰花结和上皮性结构外，肿瘤中等细胞密度，细胞排列紧密，伴有不同程度的纤维性基质。可以见到核分裂象、细胞核非典型性甚至小灶坏死，这些

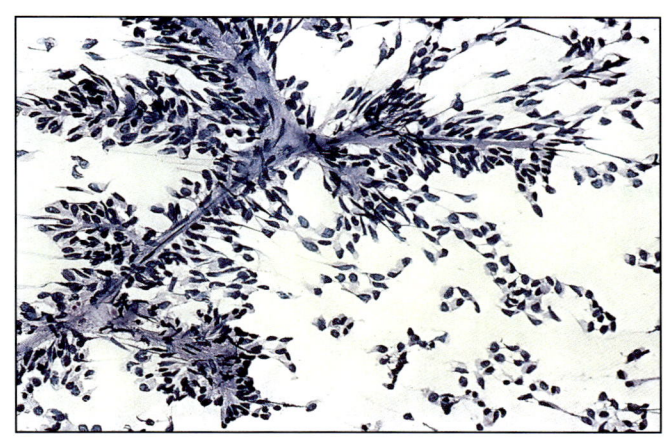

图26.54 血管周围的假玫瑰花结结构常常是室管膜瘤涂片的显著特征。除了血管周围极性分布的细胞形成叶状结构外，显著的细胞学特征包括境界相对清楚的伸长胞浆，伴有数量不等的纤细突起。细胞间基质为纤维性。Morris染色。

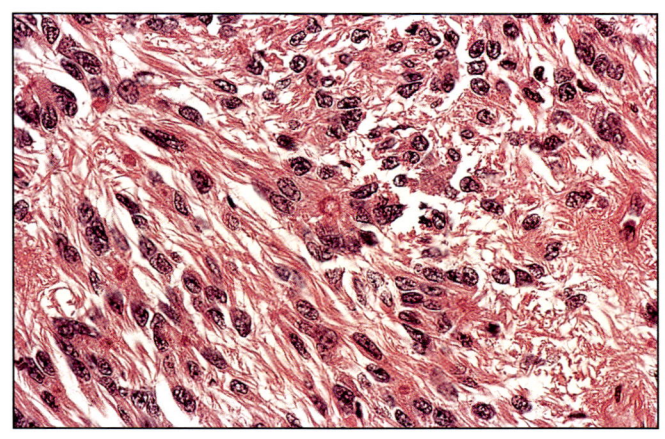

图26.56 室管膜瘤的细胞间基质可为致密纤维性的，正如此肿瘤中所见（来自一个17岁患有神经纤维瘤病的女性）。

并不提示间变性改变（见下文）。

WHO分类中有四种类型的室管膜瘤：**细胞型、乳头型、透明细胞型**以及**伸展型**[292]。肿瘤较少出现这些组织病理学亚型混合。这些变型基本上具有相同的临床行为，重要的是确认其为室管膜瘤，而不与间变性星形细胞瘤、脑膜瘤和脉络膜肿瘤以及少突胶质细胞瘤混淆。**细胞型室管膜瘤**，细胞较致密，玫瑰花结结构不甚明显，类似弥漫性胶质瘤。**乳头型室管膜瘤**，肿瘤细胞形成明显的乳头状和管状结构。因为伴有上皮样结构的室管膜瘤可以类似转移癌，重要的是它们不同程度地表达EMA和CAM5.2[300]。肿瘤的室管膜属性可通过细胞核染色质结构以及细胞突起的纤维特征来证实，GFAP和波形蛋白免疫反应可使其更为明显。对于脊髓肿瘤，EMA和CAM5.2结合通常具有鉴别脊髓髓内室管膜瘤与星形细胞瘤的意义。**透明细胞室管膜瘤**[302]（图26.59）可通过明显的PTAH阳性纤维和波形蛋白免疫反应与少突胶质细胞瘤鉴别。至少一半的透明细胞室管膜瘤起源于幕上，而多数幕下肿瘤位于小脑，而不是第四脑室。**透明细胞型**在儿童阶段比较少见[303,304]，相对更具侵袭性。**伸展型室管膜瘤**罕见，一般发生于脊髓，尽管有几例报道发生于侧脑室和第三脑室[305]。多数伸展型室管膜瘤仅显示境界不清的血管周围假玫瑰花结，真正的室管膜玫瑰花结极其少见。显著的组织病理学特征是相对一致的分化较好的肿瘤细胞，具有伸长纤细的突起，通过GFAP免疫反应可使其更为明显。细胞突起常常形成紧密排列的纤维网，可随机分布或呈

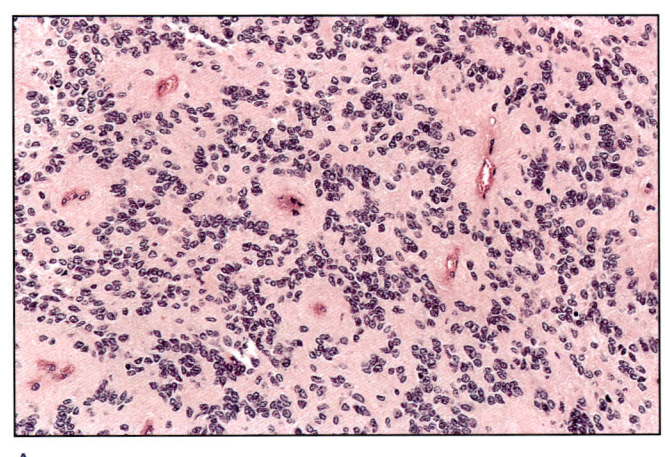

A

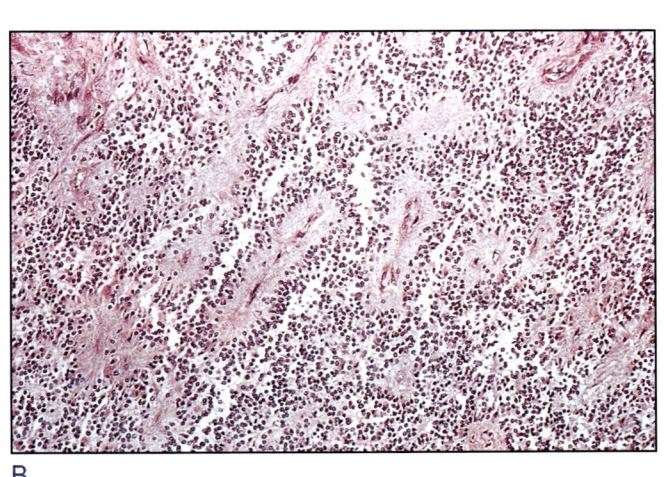

B

图26.55 室管膜瘤中，血管周围假玫瑰花结单个突起的显著程度差异较大。注意一致性的圆形细胞核和显著的细胞极性，伴有突起的纤维性基质延伸至血管壁。

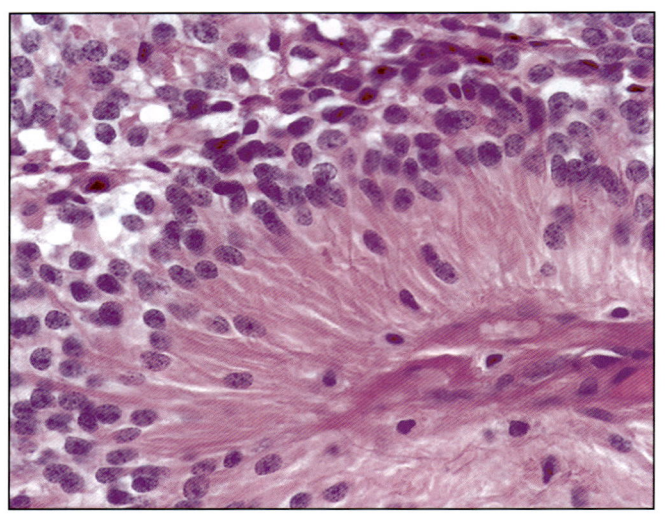
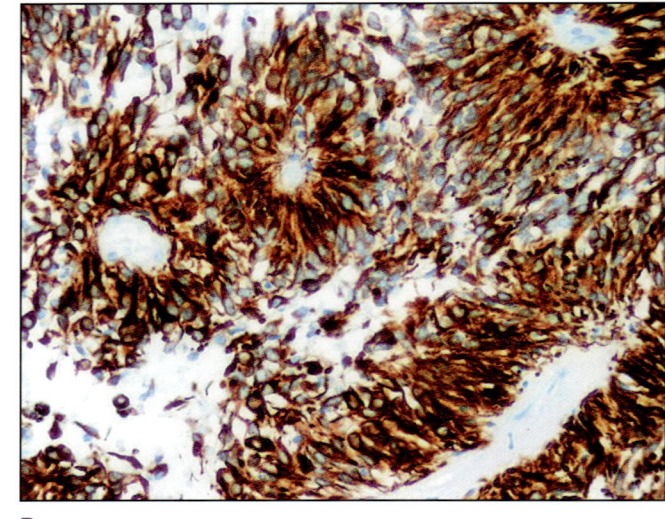

图26.57 室管膜瘤。（A）室管膜瘤的高倍放大观，显示一致性细胞核，染色质分布均匀。血管周围假玫瑰花结纤细的纤维性突起也可见到。（B）胶质纤维酸性蛋白（GFAP）免疫反应在这些血管周围结构中常常最为致密。（A）HE染色；（B）GFAP-PAP免疫过氧化物酶法，苏木素双重染色。

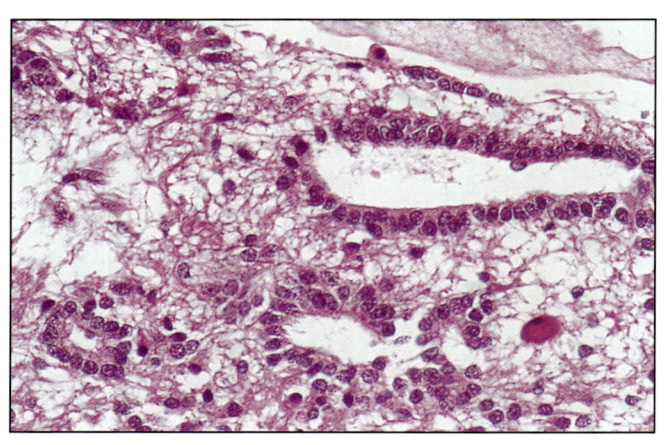
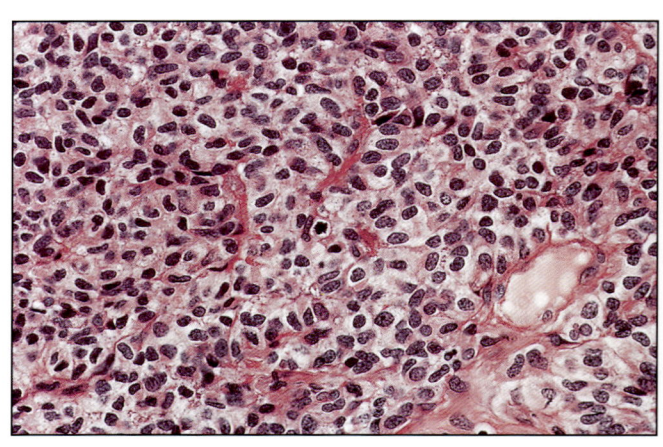

图26.58 对于室管膜瘤来说，真正的室管膜玫瑰花结尽管罕见，但是诊断性的。注意细小结节状染色质一般分布不规则，形成"开放"结构，不同于其他胶质瘤的粗大染色质。

图26.59 室管膜瘤的透明细胞变型类似于少突胶质细胞瘤。胶质纤维酸性蛋白（GFAP）和波形蛋白免疫反应有助于鉴别这两种类型的肿瘤。

流水状结构。

间变性室管膜瘤（图26.60）
Anaplastic ependymoma

间变性室管膜瘤可以发生于室管膜瘤的所有发生部位。然而在幕上区比在脊髓更为常见[292]。总体上，室管膜瘤（WHO Ⅱ级）比间变性室管膜瘤（WHO Ⅲ级）常见得多。低级别肿瘤随时间推移出现间变进展的发生率远低于星形细胞肿瘤，进展性基因异常也同样[306]。对于哪些特征可以精确定义间变还没有达成共识，儿童和成人室管膜瘤的经典组织病理学评估受制于生物学行为的判定。然而，室管膜瘤的间变通常结合以下几点来确定：(1) 细胞密度增加，伴有细胞核多形性；(2) 显著核分裂；以及 (3) 明显微血管增生，由于复杂的多层细胞成分而较为明显（图26.60）。可以出现镜下或地图样坏死，但仅有坏死并不是有力的鉴别特征，因为这种特征可不同程度地见于其他不起眼的低级别室管膜瘤中。间变性肿瘤可呈细胞致密的片状生长结构，但常常保留假玫瑰花结结构，特别是结合有微血管增生时。幕上病变中特别重要的预后因子是核分裂指数[307]，MIB-1标记指数是最有力的预后因素，不论组织病理学分级如何[308-314]。多项研究表明，高标记指数与组织学分级和早期肿瘤复发呈正相关。拓扑异构酶Ⅱα（TOPOⅡα）免疫组织化学也可以定量增生细胞[56,315]。

11%～14%的病例最终出现远处播散。幕上脑室肿瘤和脊髓肿瘤更可能发生软脑膜播散种植。对于幕下肿瘤，脊髓播散比幕上肿瘤更常见，此种远处播散可能没有局部复发[330]。出现肿瘤播散的平均年龄要小十岁，临床出现症状时就有肿瘤远处播散者预后极差，不论其组织病理学分级如何。组织病理学分级（见表26.2）影响CSF播散潜能，所以，WHO Ⅲ级病变的远处播散比例是WHO Ⅱ级病变的6倍[331]。至于硬膜外腰骶部的脊髓肿瘤病例，局部播散可以发生，并且常有疑问，尤其是伴有骶骨前肿物时[332]。

室管膜瘤沿脑室系统和中央管分布的好发部位会妨碍根治性手术切除，这是在第一次切除后的3～5年内，肿瘤总体复发可能性为50%的部分因素[333]。仅在原发部位复发者较在远处播散者更常见，见于大约14%～24%的病例[331]。儿童WHO Ⅱ级肿瘤中，局部复发是最常见的复发形式[294]。除了切除不完全外，与早期复发和总体预后较差相关的其他因素为：年龄小（小于3岁）[294,334]和间变组织学表现。至于总体生存率，位于脑室外幕上的间变性肿瘤预后较差，其5年肿瘤相关性死亡率为100%。

成人发生于第四脑室的肿瘤通常是WHO Ⅱ级，10年生存率高达90%，而侧脑室和第三脑室肿瘤的生存率下降，10年生存率分别为60%和35%[298]。在儿童，预后一般较差，平均存活约为4.3年，5年和7年的整体生存率分别为57%和46%。此生物学行为与婴幼儿WHO Ⅲ级颅内肿瘤的百分比较高一致[335]。

室管膜肿瘤的分子病理学（Molecular pathology of ependymal tumors） 与其他星形细胞或少突胶质细胞肿瘤相比，对室管膜瘤的分子病理学知之甚少。但新出现了几个重要的基本观念。首先，与其他胶质瘤相比，室管膜肿瘤具有不同的分子生物学病变位点[306,336]。与弥漫性星形细胞瘤相比，其TP53、Rb、p16以及PTEN的突变或缺失罕见，同10q染色体上任何基因丢失一样；同样，与少突胶质细胞瘤相比，1p和19q丢失也少见。

22q染色体的遗传丢失是最常见的异常表现，22单体见于大约1/3的肿瘤。6q染色体丢失和1q增加也可出现，尤其是间变性室管膜瘤。通过显色原位杂交（CISH）可以检测到7号染色体的多倍体，见于大约2/3的成人室管膜瘤中[337]，但EGFR和CDK4扩增在室管膜瘤中不常见。与高级别星形细胞瘤的EGFR过表达相比，儿童室管膜瘤表现为ERBB2和ERBB4高表达，在体外培养中，它们可以调节室管膜瘤细胞增殖[293]。与星形细胞肿瘤相似，肿瘤抑制基因RASSF1A甲基化[338]。在室管膜瘤中，RASSF1A中CpG位点的甲基化较为广泛，有些肿瘤显示100%的甲基化[339]。

第二个有关室管膜肿瘤分子病理学的基本观念在于，与其他胶质瘤类似，儿童室管膜瘤出现不同于成人肿瘤的分子遗传学标记。与成人肿瘤相比，22q染色体的遗传丢失在低级别散发性儿童肿瘤中极为少见[340]。导致这种差异的原因之一是：伴有22q丢失的肿瘤具有区域倾向，脊髓的发生率最高[306,341]，而脊髓肿瘤在儿童少见。17p染色体的遗传丢失是散发性儿童肿瘤最常见的遗传病变[340]，但7号多倍体不如成人肿瘤常见（25%对66%）[337]。应用CGH，儿童室管膜瘤更多出现平衡表型[306,342]。CDKN2A、CDKN2B和p141ARF的启动子位点甲基化在儿童比在成人少[343]。相比之下，肿瘤抑制基因HIC-1（染色体17p13.3）甲基化常见于10岁以内的肿瘤[344]。

室管膜瘤的第三个分子病理学特征是：发生于不同解剖部位的肿瘤也具有特殊的分子病理学。这在黏液乳头型肿瘤特别如此，黏液乳头型室管膜瘤显示13和14q/14染色体丢失[306,345]。同时常见9号和18号染色体增加，并且10q/10丢失在黏液乳头型肿瘤中极其多见。相比之下，1q和9号的增加以及6q丢失是后颅窝起源室管膜瘤的特殊特征，此处的间变性肿瘤常见1q增加[306,342]。幕上肿瘤显示9号染色体丢失。

除了遗传失衡外，基因甲基化和表达类型在不同部位之间也有差异。对于9号染色体基因而言，依据部位和分级的不同，CDKN2A、CDKN2B和p141ARF甲基化程度也有不同[343]。总体上，WHO Ⅱ级肿瘤较WHO Ⅲ级肿瘤的甲基化发生率低，CDKN2A例外，两者没有差异。对于CDKN2A来说，甲基化在后颅窝WHO Ⅱ级室管膜瘤中最少见，在幕上WHO Ⅱ级室管膜瘤中最常见。CDKN2B和p14/ARF启动子甲基化见于大约21%～32%的肿瘤。对于CDKN2B而言，颅外室管膜癌较颅内室管膜瘤更常见甲基化。P14/ARF甲基化比较常见于WHO Ⅱ级肿瘤中，但在黏液乳头型室管膜瘤中比较罕见。

对于基因表达，一组21个基因似乎可对39例中的34例的肿瘤分布（脊髓与颅内）进行精确分类[335]。脊髓室管膜瘤，包括100%的黏液乳头型室管膜瘤，高度表达HOXB5、PLA2G5、ITIH2。在一组26个基因中，幕上分布和分级也似乎不同，6例儿童幕上Ⅲ级室管膜瘤的特征为高度表达GPX3、STAM、COL6A1、PYCRI、HSPB1以及ARHGD。此外，NF2基因在颅内和脊髓肿瘤中表达不同。

脉络丛肿瘤 Choroid plexus tumors

脉络丛肿瘤罕见，占所有颅内胶质瘤的 2.0%，大约占所有脑肿瘤的 0.5%[346,347]。与癌相比，脉络丛乳头状瘤更为多见，比例是 5:1[347]。这些肿瘤起源于任何正常可以见到脉络丛的部位，如脑室，但多数限于侧脑室和第四脑室，仅有少数病例见于第三脑室[346,348]。多数乳头状瘤起源于儿童的侧脑室[348,349]，尽管成人也有发生。脉络丛肿瘤大约占 15 岁以下儿童肿瘤的 2%~3%[347]。大约 80% 的癌发生于儿童，他们中大多数不到 2 岁。据报道，癌的平均患病年龄约为 26~32 个月[348,350,351]。尽管发生于侧脑室的病例没有性别倾向，但第四脑室肿瘤更多见于男性，与女性的比例是 3:2[346]。临床症状常常是由颅内压升高所致，继发于 CSF 通路梗阻或 CSF 生成增加。

脉络丛肿瘤为一个肿瘤谱系，从高分化乳头状瘤（WHO Ⅰ 级）到高度侵袭性的脉络丛癌（WHO Ⅲ 级），极少数的中间型称为"非典型脉络丛乳头状瘤"，其生物学行为仍有待确定[346]。

脉络丛乳头状瘤（图 26.66 至 26.69） Choroid plexus papilloma

这些境界清楚、常有钙化的肿瘤比较特殊，因为其表面呈乳头状，类似于正常脉络丛。镜下表现为良性乳头状肿瘤，由单层或多层立方或柱状上皮组成，具有纤细的纤维血管轴心（图 26.66 和 26.67）。这些特征在涂片中易于识别（图 26.66）。可见黄色瘤性和嗜酸性变，没有任何临床意义[352,353]。出现核分裂象增加、坏死和（或）浸润邻近脑实质，提示恶变为癌（见下文），并且复发和播散潜能也增加[354,355]。报道的脉络丛乳头状瘤平均 Ki-67（MIB-1）标记指数是 1.9%，脉络丛乳头状癌为 13.8%[356]。

脉络丛乳头状瘤可表达 GFAP，与其常常起源自脑室神经上皮一致[357-361]。然而，大量病例中，GFAP 表达可为局灶性甚或缺乏。波形蛋白、S-100 蛋白和细胞角蛋白在绝大多数病例中为阳性[346]。Transthyretin（前-白蛋白）在脉络丛乳头状瘤中有一致性表达[362]，尽管此标记对于脉络丛肿瘤并不特异[363]。应用芯片方法，近来报道了新的脉络丛肿瘤特异性诊断标记物，包括 stanniocalcin-1（一种糖蛋白，正常表达于人脉络丛，可参与调节 CSF 的钙水平）和 Kir7.1（一种钾内向整流通道家族成员，在跨上皮运转钾的过程中起作用，其表达见于脉络丛上皮细胞膜顶端）[364]。

室管膜瘤乳头状变型在脑室内乳头状肿瘤的鉴别诊断中必须考虑到。此诊断常常在常规切片中可以排

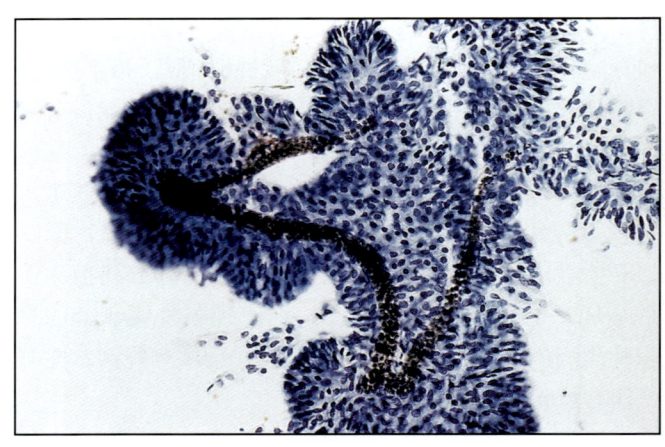

图 26.66　脉络丛乳头状瘤涂片，显示典型的围绕血管周围排列的良性矮柱状上皮成分。仔细检查，乳头状排列的上皮成分均可见纤细的纤维血管轴心，不同于室管膜瘤。Morris 染色。

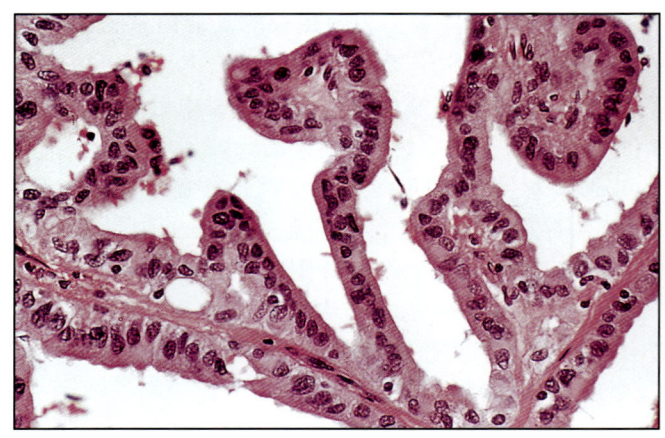

图 26.67　脉络丛乳头状瘤的组织切片类似于正常脉络丛的，具有单层、部分假复层的柱状上皮，被覆于纤维血管轴心之上。

除，因为室管膜瘤缺乏脉络丛乳头状瘤的特征性纤维血管轴心，并且常常具有更明显的纤维神经胶质细胞结构。GFAP 免疫组化对鉴别这两种肿瘤并不可靠，因为它们对此中间丝都有反应。乳头状瘤的角蛋白、EMA 和 transthyretin 免疫反应对鉴别有帮助（图 26.68 和 26.69）[359,360]，然而，这些蛋白偶尔也可见于单纯室管膜肿瘤，尤其是乳头状和上皮性变型。超微结构特征在这方面有帮助，因为与正常脉络丛一样，乳头状瘤具有仅限于紧密连接的顶端连接复合体。这些不同于室管膜瘤内极其广泛的连接带。

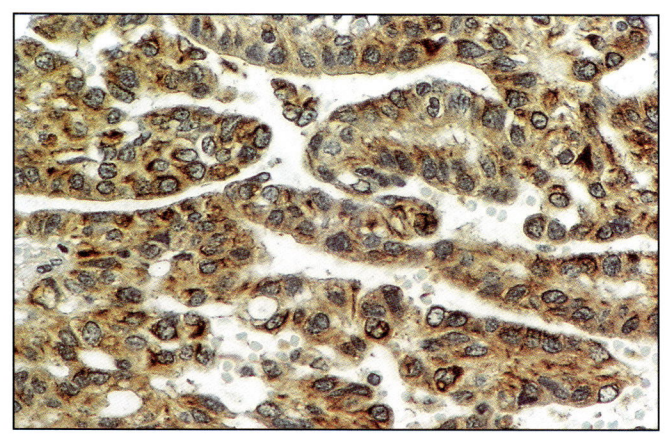

图26.68 细胞角蛋白表型在大多数脉络丛乳头状瘤中容易检测。细胞角蛋白PAP免疫过氧化物酶法。

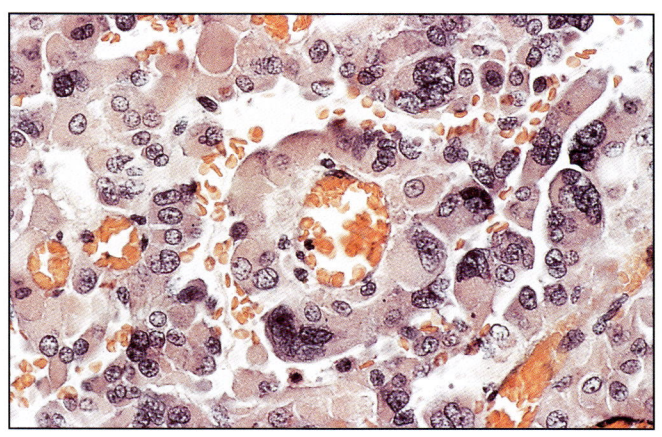

图26.70 细胞/细胞核多形性伴有明显的非典型性、多核细胞,以及缺乏分化好的乳头状结构为脉络丛癌的组织病理学特征。

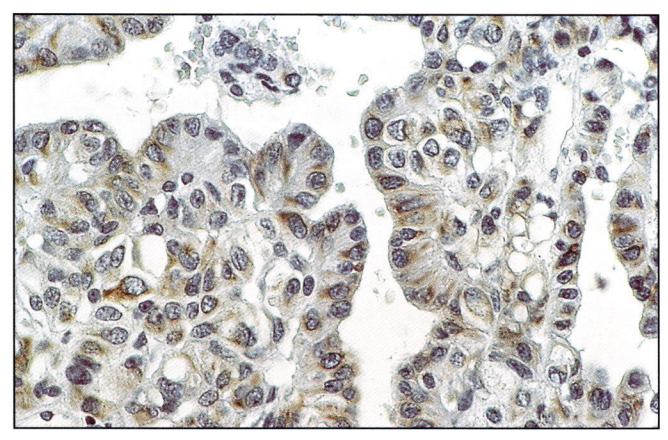

图26.69 转甲状腺蛋白(TTR)免疫反应有助于鉴别脉络丛乳头状瘤与乳头状室管膜瘤。TTR-PAP免疫过氧化物酶法。

脉络丛癌(图26.70) Choroid plexus carcinoma

脉络丛癌多数是原发性恶性肿瘤,对应于WHO Ⅲ级。脉络丛乳头状瘤恶性转化见于不到20%的病例[349],CSF播散和蛛网膜下腔播散常见,极个别病例报告有CNS以外转移[365]。

组织学上,癌容易出现不明显的乳头状结构,细胞排列密集,生长结构成型较差。可出现弥漫或局灶间变[如奇异形细胞和(或)细胞核非典型性]、核分裂象增加和坏死(图26.70)。

必须除外转移性腺癌的可能,尤其是在累及成人的病例。常用的诊断标记物,如transthyretin、GFAP、EMA或细胞角蛋白,大多并不可靠,因为缺乏特异性,并且在脉络丛肿瘤中的表达也不一致。如上所述,尽管transthyretin免疫反应可以将脉络丛肿瘤与其他上皮性肿瘤鉴别开,但腺癌中的transthyretin免疫反应也有报道[363]。由于脉络丛癌多数发生于儿童,因此,与其他儿童恶性肿瘤的鉴别具有重要意义,如生殖细胞肿瘤(恶性畸胎瘤、胚胎癌和绒癌)和非典型畸胎样/横纹肌样肿瘤(AT/RT)。即使出现22q11.2染色体上的 *hSNF5/INI-1* 基因失活突变被认为是AT/RT的标志(见胚胎性肿瘤),但近来有极少数的脉络丛肿瘤病例已被描述具有类似的突变[366]。这两种肿瘤之间的发病机制的相关性尚未完全清楚[366]。

脉络丛肿瘤的生物学行为:脉络丛乳头状瘤多数可以手术治愈,5年存活率高达100%[367]。另一方面,脉络丛癌是极具侵袭性的、生长迅速的肿瘤,预后不良,5年生存率为40%[367]。然而脉络丛癌可沿CSF通路发生显著转移,甚至良性脉络丛乳头状瘤也可以在CSF内种植细胞[368,369]。一项52例患者的临床病理研究显示,预后差表现为复发和(或)致死性后果,与核分裂活性增加、坏死、脑浸润、缺乏transthyretin免疫反应以及S-100蛋白表达减少有关[355]。

脉络丛肿瘤的分子细胞遗传学:脉络丛肿瘤的发病机制大多不清楚。在一些肿瘤中已检测到SV40乳多泡病毒的DNA序列,提示后者在这些肿瘤的演化过程中可能起作用[346]。脉络丛乳头状瘤的分子学分析显示超二倍体,尤其是7、9、12、15、17和18号染色体增加,而一例脉络丛癌出现7p11-12、9q11-12、15q22和19q13.4染色体重排[347]。正如先前提到的,*hSNF5/INI-1* 失活对脉络丛肿瘤的生物学行为可能有作用。脉络丛乳头状瘤和癌偶尔也可发生于Li-Fraumeni综合征[370]。

起源未定的神经上皮肿瘤（见表26.1）
Neuroepithelial tumors of uncertain origin

有三种肿瘤性病变，尽管具有与各种胶质表型相关的特殊组织学特征，但仍没有明确组织学发生，阻碍了它们进一步分类。它们是第三脑室脊索样胶质瘤、星形母细胞瘤以及大脑胶质瘤病。鉴于这些罕见肿瘤的最初描述，现在越来越多的证据表明，脊索样胶质瘤和星形母细胞瘤的确为不同的临床病理性病变，而大脑胶质瘤病仍然是一种描述性经验性定义的肿瘤性病变。

第三脑室脊索样胶质瘤（图26.71）
Chordoid glioma of the third ventricle

在起源未定的神经上皮性肿瘤类别中，第三脑室脊索样胶质瘤是最近才被认识和定义的临床病理性病变，目前文献中有超过30例的报道[371-375]。这些肿瘤通常发生于成人，女性好发（1.5:1），平均年龄为44岁。个别病例发生于30岁以下[376]，仅有一例儿童病例报道，见于一位12岁男孩[377]。神经影像学特征包括境界清楚的、以实性为主的肿物，伴有囊性区域，在T1、T2和FLAIR序列为等密度，加强（注射钆）后，T1像均匀强化。肿瘤可以很大，最大直径为1.6～4cm。尽管这些肿瘤有些呈惰性生长，但相对较高的发病率和死亡率与就诊时肿瘤大小以及常常不能安全地完全切除有关。复发可见于次全切除的病例。

尽管可以出现不同的组织病理学类型，但最常见、通常也是最明显的生长方式为密集的上皮样肿瘤细胞排列呈条索状、细长簇状或分叶状结构，被纤细的胶原、网织纤维阳性的网络分隔。具有大量空泡状黏液丰富的PAS阳性基质；黏液样间质改变可较为局灶。肿瘤细胞通常具有境界清楚的多角形外观，伴有明显的胞浆，卵圆形至圆形的细胞核，核仁不明显（图26.71）。其他不常见的结构有：形成腺泡及乳头状结构，肿瘤细胞衬于假腺样腔隙，遍布纤细的纤维血管轴心，或者宽大的波浪状胞浆突起直接连至血管，形成假花环结构。肿瘤与周围脑组织境界清楚，在反应性脑组织界面，可引起明显的星形细胞增生，Rosenthal 纤维形成，常有明显的淋巴及浆细胞浸润，可见 Russell 小体。此外，慢性炎症细胞团散在分布于整个肿瘤基质。缺乏间变特征，如坏死和微血管增生，特征性的是，核分裂象稀少或缺乏。与低核分裂活性一致的是 MIB-1 标记指数较低，从 0.5% 以下到不足 2%[374,375]。

多数肿瘤细胞显示 GFAP（图26.71）和波形蛋白弥漫强阳性，可以突显更局灶的纤维突起。此外，绝大多数肿瘤出现局灶但通常较强的细胞角蛋白（包括 AE1/AE3）、CD34（突出细胞界限）和 S-100 蛋白免疫反应，另外，EMA 呈弱阳性。超微结构特征明确提示胶质以及更特异的室管膜样表型，圆形至梭形细胞中含有中等量的微管，聚集有丰富的 10nm 胞浆中间丝、微绒毛、中间连接（带状连接）以及局灶基底膜形成。众多微绒毛样突起包裹管状空隙，但一般见不到真正的含有细胞的微小管腔。没有明确的纤毛，但极少数异常胞浆内有纤毛已有报道。细胞及胞浆突起常常排列成马赛克结构，胞浆突起相对短且单一[374,375]。

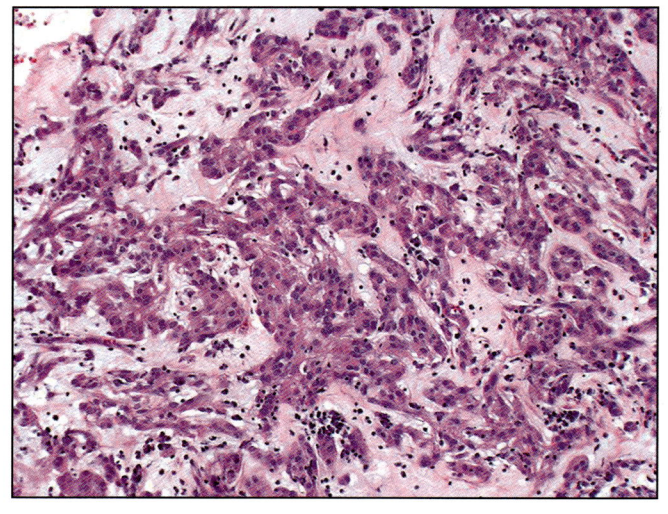 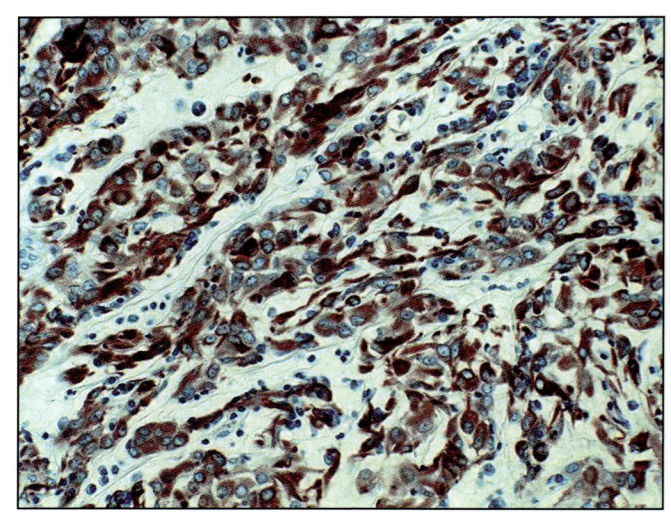

图26.71 第三脑室脊索样胶质瘤的典型上皮样细胞条索散布于黏液样基质中（A）。在这些胶质瘤中，胶质纤维酸性蛋白（GFAP）免疫反应较强（B）。GFAP-ABC免疫过氧化物酶法，苏木素双重染色。

星形母细胞瘤（图26.72至26.73） Astroblastoma

星形母细胞瘤是罕见的胶质瘤类型，占所有胶质瘤的比例不足3%[378]。这些肿瘤境界清楚，较大，常为多囊性，大多发生于年轻人的幕上部位。临床就诊时的平均年龄在15～20岁。在2个最大的病例研究中，患者年龄为3～58岁不等[379,380]，女性好发（2.3:1）。尽管肿瘤偶尔发生于幼儿，但只有2例先天性星形母细胞瘤的报道[378]。肿瘤可以发生在大脑半球深部和中脑，但脑室内生长或与脑室系统有明确关系者极为罕见。神经影像学研究显示特征性分叶表现，具有实性和囊性成分以及轻度血管源性水肿。T2像显示信号不均匀，整体上与灰质等密度。加强（注射钆）后，T1像一般出现实性部分不均匀强化，伴有囊性区域周围边缘强化[381]。

该胶质瘤的标志性组织病理学结构为大量相互交织的细胞团呈特殊的血管周围排列方式，粘附性较差。细胞结构不一，在血管周围玫瑰花结中，可见具有粗大波浪状或宽大突起的细胞，延伸至血管壁（图26.72），以及疏松成片的、更具多角形的细胞，具有稀少而境界不清的突起。血管周围玻璃样变和局部玻璃样物质沉积很常见，并可出现微小钙化。与室管膜瘤相比，胶质细胞通常没有PTAH阳性纤维，除了血管周围的极少数细胞。星形母细胞瘤的明显的血管中心性分布不同于星形细胞瘤、少突胶质细胞瘤和混合性少突星形细胞瘤偶尔出现的血管周围排列。体外研究提示，这些肿瘤来源于伸展细胞[382]，然而，CGH提示染色体异常类型与室管膜瘤和弥漫型星形细胞瘤不同[380]。

多数星形母细胞瘤显示GFAP、S-100蛋白和波形

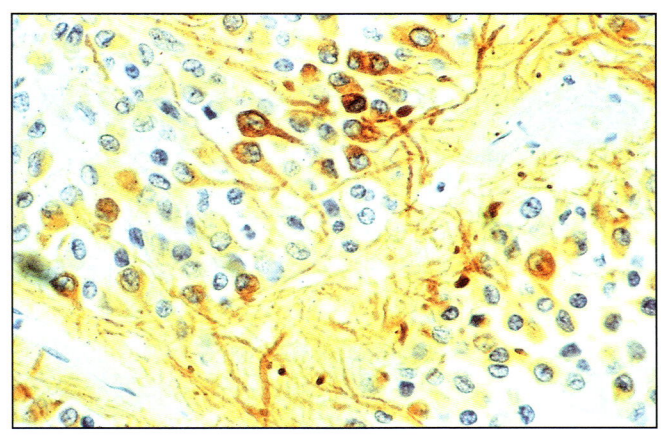

图26.73 星形母细胞瘤。与一般缺乏磷钨酸苏木素（PTAH）染色的纤维不同，血管周围细胞的粗大细胞突起呈胶质纤维酸性蛋白（GFAP）强阳性。GFAP-PAP免疫过氧化物酶法。

蛋白免疫反应，但是GFAP在单个肿瘤细胞中的表达不同，在血管周围玫瑰花结内尤为明显（图26.73）。与室管膜瘤类似，有时也可有EMA免疫反应[380]。星形母细胞瘤可依据是否出现胶质细胞间变的组织病理结构进行分类，包括有假栅栏状坏死和微血管增生。这些较为间变的星形母细胞瘤其平均MIB-1标记指数高于分化好的没有间变特征的肿瘤（15.5%对3.2%），尽管MIB-1的标记范围有重叠[380]。

虽然高分化病变具有复发率减低的倾向，但胶质细胞间变特征与随后的临床行为相关性并不一致；总体上该系列肿瘤的生物学行为比其组织病理学所表现的要好[379]。

大脑胶质瘤病 Gliomatosis cerebri

大脑胶质瘤病极少见[383,384]，特征为弥漫性、常常相互连续的神经轴肿瘤性浸润，缺乏独立的肿瘤。这种病变可以累及多个脑叶、整个大脑半球、幕下区域和（或）脊髓。这种肿瘤性增殖的唯一的大体表现是受累结构弥漫性增大，MR影像学显示T2像高信号区域[385]。

显微镜下大脑胶质瘤病的标志性表现为中度多形性的胶质细胞浸润原有结构，并不伴有明显的结构破坏。这些细胞结构不一，从梭形到细胞核浓染的卵圆形表现。细胞可表现为星形细胞，显示不同程度的GFAP免疫反应，但更具少突胶质细胞样表现的肿瘤细胞相对少见[386]。由于受累结构（包括软脑膜下）中肿瘤细胞数量差异较大，在有限的或非定位的活检组织，确诊的可能性极小。因此，在考虑大脑胶质瘤病的诊断之前，应当仔细区分多中心性胶质瘤和源自不明胶质

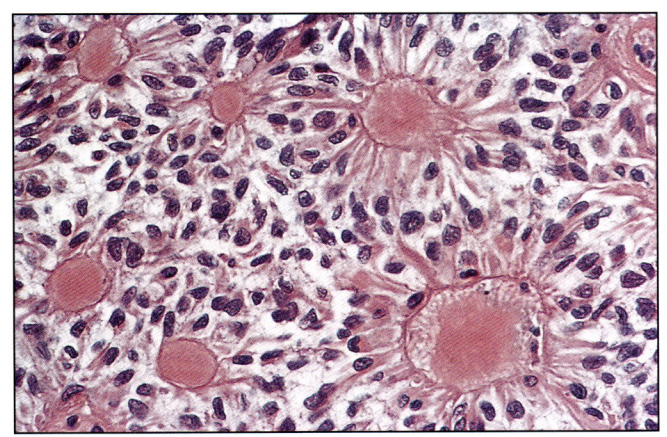

图26.72 星形母细胞瘤。该视野中，有明显伸展突起的细胞形成的典型的假玫瑰花结结构。

瘤的转移性播散。

神经元和混合性神经元-胶质肿瘤（见表26.1至26.3）
Neuronal and mixed neuronal-glial tumors

节细胞瘤　Gangliocytomas

此类神经上皮肿瘤的细胞成分显示节细胞特征，没有真正肿瘤性胶质成分。尽管事实上有些作者认为这些肿瘤中有些为发育不良性（错构瘤性）病变，但WHO视其为真正的肿瘤[387]。这些病变具有良性临床行为，被认为是WHO I级肿瘤[387]。

节细胞瘤为罕见肿瘤，由成熟节细胞神经元组成。肿瘤一般境界清楚，最常发生于颞叶和脊髓颈胸段[388,389]。其他部位包括下丘脑和垂体区，以及极少数的松果体[388,390,391]。多数病变在30岁以内出现临床症状。尽管颞叶肿瘤可以伴发癫痫，但是其他部位的节细胞瘤可出现特异性症状，如垂体区发生的肿瘤伴有内分泌异常[391]，下丘脑的节细胞瘤可出现性早熟[392]。

节细胞瘤的特征是细胞成分稀少的胶质-间叶性基质中有肿瘤性节细胞增生。节细胞不规则性分布，出现显著细胞多形性，包括奇异形和双核表现。异常节细胞和神经突起可以通过银染色（如改良的Bielschowsky）和神经元相关性标记物免疫组化染色来显示。由于病变的胶质成分本质上不是肿瘤成分，因此这些肿瘤没有间变进展潜能[387,388]。

小脑发育不良性节细胞瘤（图26.74至26.76）
Dysplastic gangliocytoma of the cerebellum

小脑发育不良性节细胞瘤，也称为Lhermitte-Duclos病，是限于小脑的罕见节细胞瘤类型。病变常常在31～40岁时出现明显的临床症状，尽管患者早年出现症状已有报道，主要是由于巨脑和颅内高血压所致[393]。在最近的一项有31例Lhermitte-Duclos病的病例报道中，患者平均就诊年龄为34.8岁，为13～63岁不等[394]。尽管早期综述表明，男性受累多于女性[393]，但好像没有明显的性别倾向[394]。病变出现典型的神经影像学表现，T2像为条状或层状表现，可见多灶、狭窄的高信号带与等密度条带交替出现[394]。

病变的组织学特征是异常的节细胞和神经元细胞增生所致的小脑肥厚，占据正常颗粒层和Purkinje细胞层（图26.74至26.76）。过度髓鞘化的纤维和增大的神经突起可替代正常分子层，导致整叶扩大。邻近颗粒层减少和皮层白质脱髓鞘常见。免疫组化研究，这些神经节细胞表达Purkinje细胞突触蛋白和表面膜蛋白，提示可能为Purkinje细胞系[393,395-397]。然而，其他实验室也提出

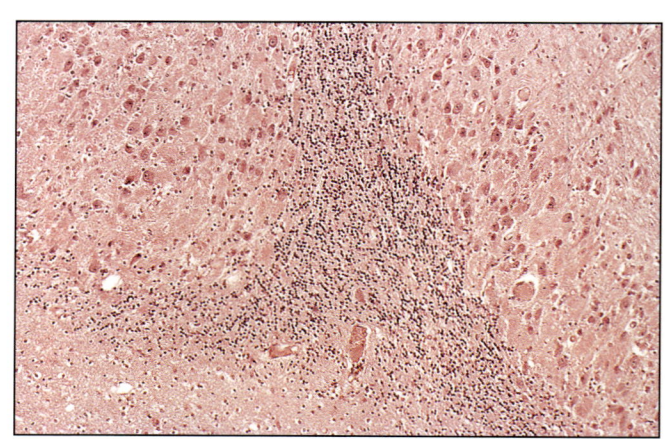

图26.74　小脑发育不良性节细胞瘤。显示大且异常的节细胞替代颗粒层，大体上对应于增厚的脑叶。

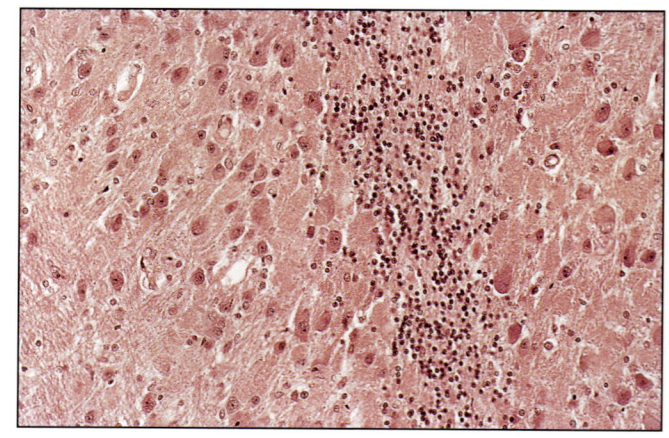

图26.75　小脑发育不良性节细胞瘤。高倍放大，与图26.74为同一病例，显示节细胞类似于Purkinje细胞。

表26.3	神经元和混合性神经元-胶质肿瘤以及WHO分级
肿瘤命名	WHO分级
神经元肿瘤	
节细胞瘤	I
小脑发育不良性节细胞瘤	I
中枢神经细胞瘤及变型	II
混合性神经元-胶质肿瘤	
节细胞胶质瘤	I～II
间变性节细胞胶质瘤	II～IV
婴儿促结缔组织增生性节细胞胶质瘤	I
胚胎发育不良性神经上皮性肿瘤	I

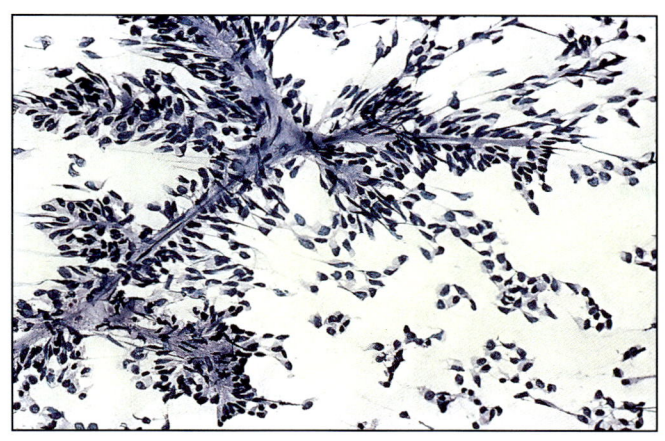

图26.54 血管周围的假玫瑰花结结构常常是室管膜瘤涂片的显著特征。除了血管周围极性分布的细胞形成叶状结构外，显著的细胞学特征包括境界相对清楚的伸长胞浆，伴有数量不等的纤细突起。细胞间基质为纤维性。Morris染色。

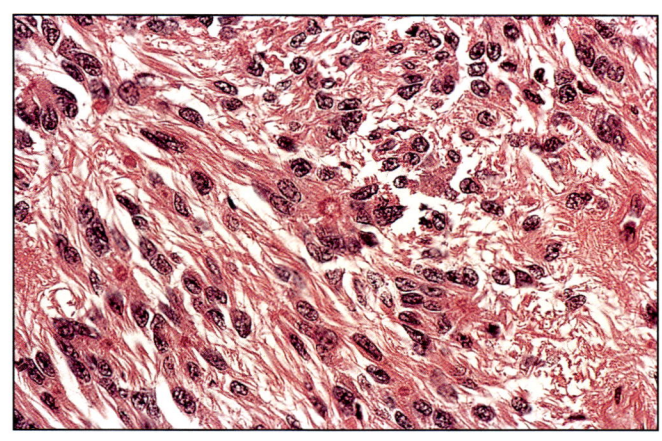

图26.56 室管膜瘤的细胞间基质可为致密纤维性的，正如此肿瘤中所见（来自一个17岁患有神经纤维瘤病的女性）。

并不提示间变性改变（见下文）。

WHO 分类中有四种类型的室管膜瘤：**细胞型、乳头型、透明细胞型**以及**伸展型**[292]。肿瘤较少出现这些组织病理学亚型混合。这些变型基本上具有相同的临床行为，重要的是确认其为室管膜瘤，而不与间变性星形细胞瘤、脑膜瘤和脉络膜肿瘤以及少突胶质细胞瘤混淆。**细胞型室管膜瘤**，细胞较致密，玫瑰花结结构不甚明显，类似弥漫性胶质瘤。**乳头型室管膜瘤**，肿瘤细胞形成明显的乳头状和管状结构。因为伴有上皮样结构的室管膜瘤可以类似转移癌，重要的是它们不同程度地表达 EMA 和 CAM5.2[300]。肿瘤的室管膜属性可通过细胞核染色质结构以及细胞突起的纤维特征来证实，GFAP 和波形蛋白免疫反应可使其更为明显。对于脊髓肿瘤，EMA 和 CAM5.2 结合通常具有鉴别脊髓髓内室管膜瘤与星形细胞瘤的意义。**透明细胞室管膜瘤**[302]（图26.59）可通过明显的 PTAH 阳性纤维和波形蛋白免疫反应与少突胶质细胞瘤鉴别。至少一半的透明细胞室管膜瘤起源于幕上，而多数幕下肿瘤位于小脑，而不是第四脑室。**透明细胞型**在儿童阶段比较少见[303,304]，相对更具侵袭性。**伸展型室管膜瘤**罕见，一般发生于脊髓，尽管有几例报道发生于侧脑室和第三脑室[305]。多数伸展型室管膜瘤仅显示境界不清的血管周围假玫瑰花结，真正的室管膜玫瑰花结极其少见。显著的组织病理学特征是相对一致的分化较好的肿瘤细胞，具有伸长纤细的突起，通过 GFAP 免疫反应可使其更为明显。细胞突起常常形成紧密排列的纤维网，可随机分布或呈

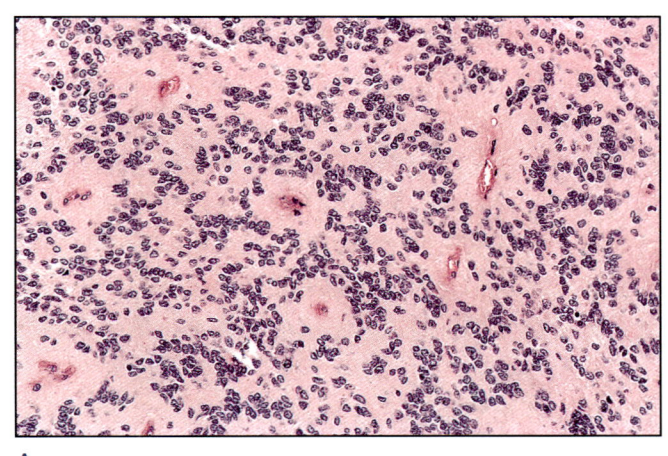

A

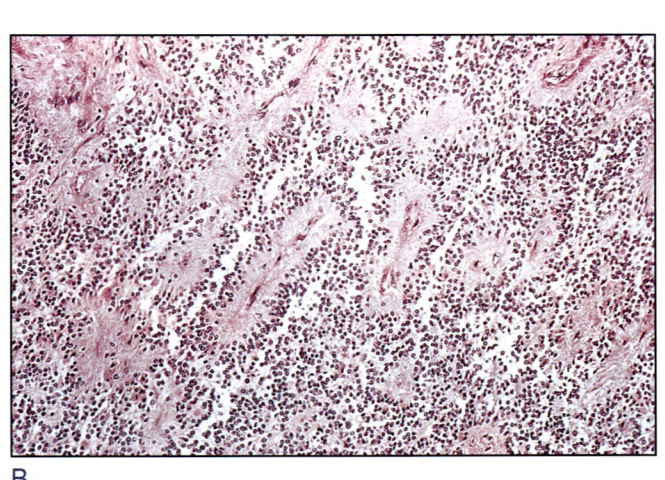

B

图26.55 室管膜瘤中，血管周围假玫瑰花结单个突起的显著程度差异较大。注意一致性的圆形细胞核和显著的细胞极性，伴有突起的纤维性基质延伸至血管壁。

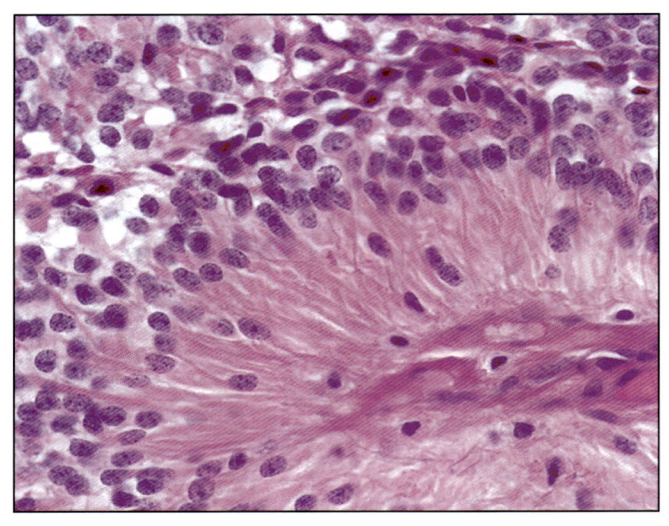
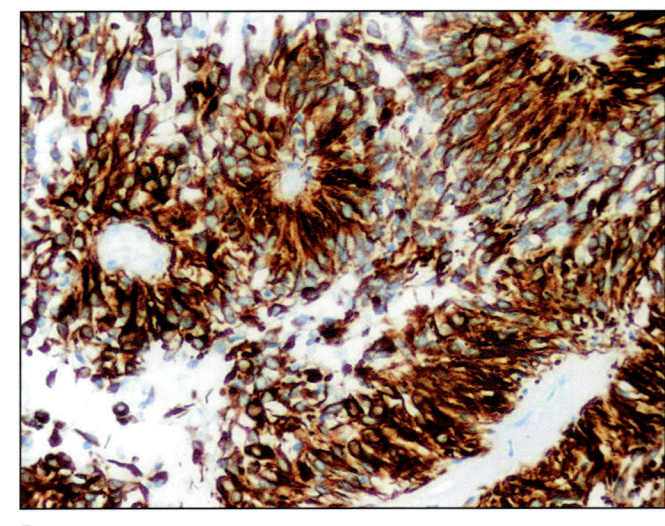

图26.57 室管膜瘤。（A）室管膜瘤的高倍放大观，显示一致性细胞核，染色质分布均匀。血管周围假玫瑰花结纤细的纤维性突起也可见到。（B）胶质纤维酸性蛋白（GFAP）免疫反应在这些血管周围结构中常常最为致密。（A）HE染色；（B）GFAP-PAP免疫过氧化物酶法，苏木素双重染色。

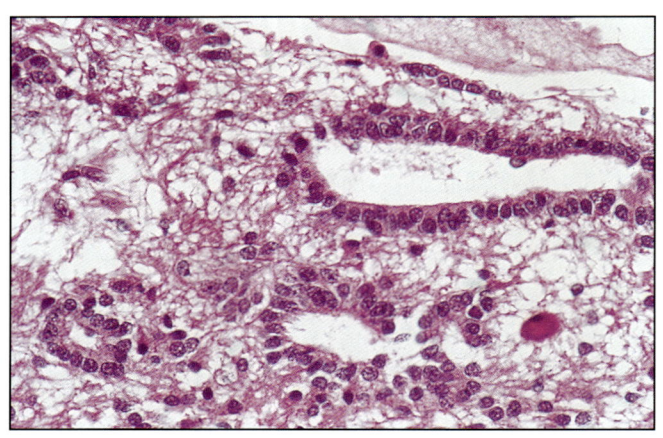
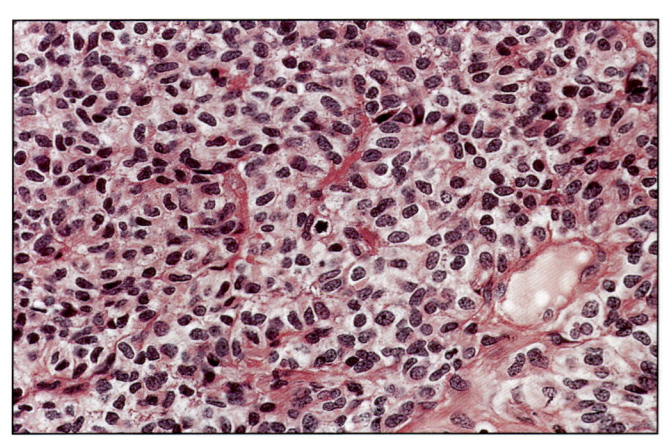

图26.58 对于室管膜瘤来说，真正的室管膜玫瑰花结尽管罕见，但是诊断性的。注意细小结节状染色质一般分布不规则，形成"开放"结构，不同于其他胶质瘤的粗大染色质。

图26.59 室管膜瘤的透明细胞变型类似于少突胶质细胞瘤。胶质纤维酸性蛋白（GFAP）和波形蛋白免疫反应有助于鉴别这两种类型的肿瘤。

流水状结构。

间变性室管膜瘤（图26.60）
Anaplastic ependymoma

间变性室管膜瘤可以发生于室管膜瘤的所有发生部位。然而在幕上区比在脊髓更为常见[292]。总体上，室管膜瘤（WHO Ⅱ级）比间变性室管膜瘤（WHO Ⅲ级）常见得多。低级别肿瘤随时间推移出现间变进展的发生率远低于星形细胞肿瘤，进展性基因异常也同样[306]。对于哪些特征可以精确定义间变还没有达成共识，儿童和成人室管膜瘤的经典组织病理学评估受制于生物学行为的判定。然而，室管膜瘤的间变通常结合以下几点来确定：(1) 细胞密度增加，伴有细胞核多形性；(2) 显著核分裂；以及 (3) 明显微血管增生，由于复杂的多层细胞成分而较为明显（图 26.60）。可以出现镜下或地图样坏死，但仅有坏死并不是有力的鉴别特征，因为这种特征可不同程度地见于其他不起眼的低级别室管膜瘤中。间变性肿瘤可呈细胞致密的片状生长结构，但常常保留假玫瑰花结结构，特别是结合有微血管增生时。幕上病变中特别重要的预后因子是核分裂指数[307]，MIB-1标记指数是最有力的预后因素，不论组织病理学分级如何[308-314]。多项研究表明，高标记指数与组织学分级和早期肿瘤复发呈正相关。拓扑异构酶Ⅱα（TOPOⅡα）免疫组织化学也可以定量增生细胞[56,315]。

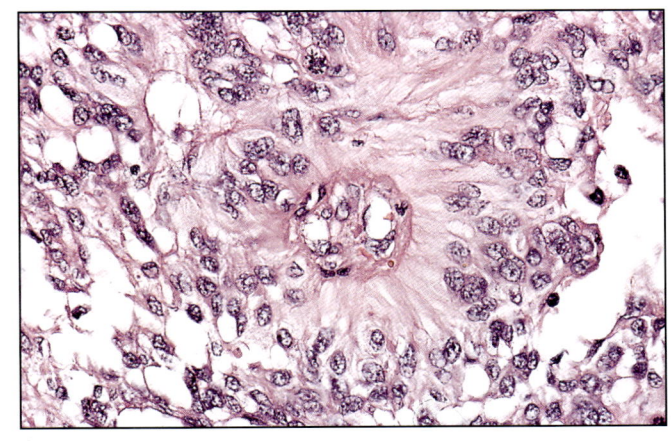

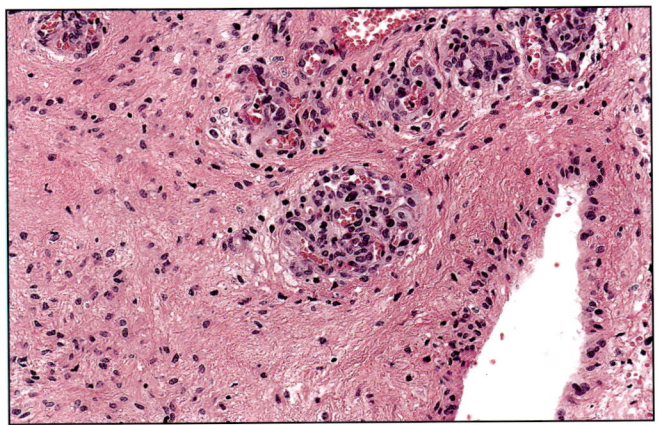

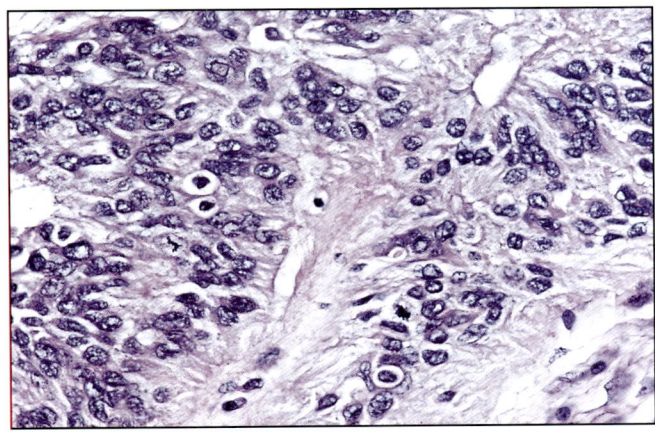

图26.60 在间变性室管膜瘤中，血管周围假玫瑰花结的血管成分常常显示内皮/外皮细胞增殖（A）。注意后颅窝肿瘤浸润性边缘的这些丰富的肾小球样结构（B）。不完全性室管膜小管不常见。细胞核显著多形性和众多核分裂象伴细胞密度增加是室管膜肿瘤的间变特征（C）。

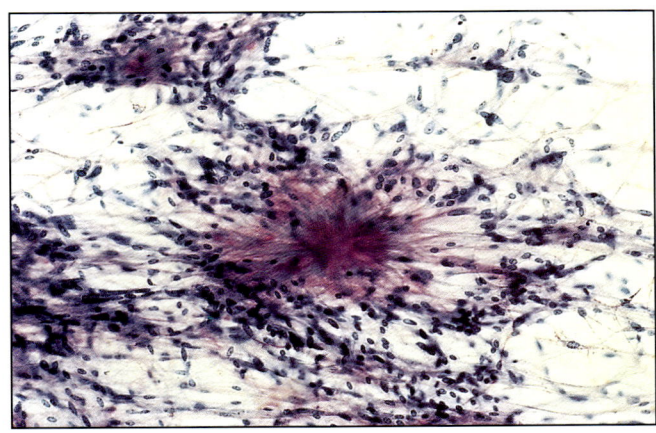

图26.61 黏液乳头状室管膜瘤涂片通常显示丰富黏液性基质中的细胞具有纤维性突起。Morris染色。

期较短的间变性肿瘤[314,316]。尽管复杂微血管增生被认为是间变的前哨性组织病理学标志，作为一个独立性特征，它与预后的相关性较低[317,318]。

区分间变性室管膜瘤与室管膜母细胞瘤很重要，因为后者是高度恶性的胚胎性肿瘤，大多累及婴儿和5岁以下的儿童。与室管膜瘤相比，室管膜母细胞瘤容易弥漫性侵袭邻近结构，特别容易出现脑脊髓种植（见胚胎性肿瘤）。

黏液乳头状室管膜瘤（图26.61至26.63）
Myxopapillary ependymoma

黏液乳头状室管膜瘤绝大多数发生于马尾和终丝，但少数也可以发生于颅内，但保留与脊髓肿瘤相同的生物行为[249,319]（也见第27章软组织的相应部分）。

肿瘤常为分散的腊肠形肿块，含有混合性纤维和上皮样细胞成分，伴有丰富的细胞外基质，黏液染色阳性（图26.61和26.62）。细长纤维细胞的乳头状排列是这些肿瘤最为典型的结构，细胞的纤细突起常常延伸至玻璃样变性的血管（图26.62和26.63）。胶质原纤维可通过GFAP免疫组织化学来证实，可将这一肿瘤与该区域的副神经节细胞瘤和神经鞘瘤区分开。电镜可以证实该肿瘤的室管膜属性[320,321]。但超微结构特征，即大量基底膜、纤毛相对稀少和众多致密细胞突起，仅限于黏液乳头状室管膜瘤。在这些WHO I级肿瘤中，MIB-1标记通常很低[322]，MIB-1标记指数在预测黏液乳头状肿瘤复发上没有作用[323]。

室管膜下瘤（图26.64和26.65）
Subependymoma

除了评估增生细胞以外，其他研究也不同程度地表明，结合p27/kip1低表达、p53高表达、p14/ARF低表达以及生存素（survivin）表达升高可以确定无进展生存

室管膜下瘤是境界清楚的无症状结节，位于相关的脑室壁内。大多在尸检时偶然发现，但由于CSF流

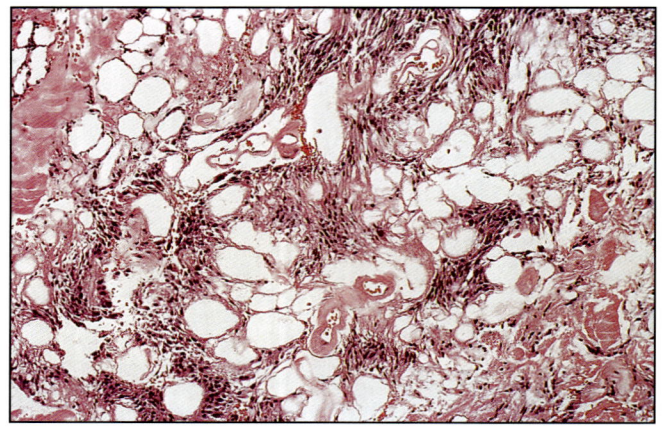

图26.62 栅栏状排列的梭形细胞与黏液沉积区域混合出现是黏液乳头型室管膜瘤的特征。注意在这些肿瘤中常见玻璃样变血管。

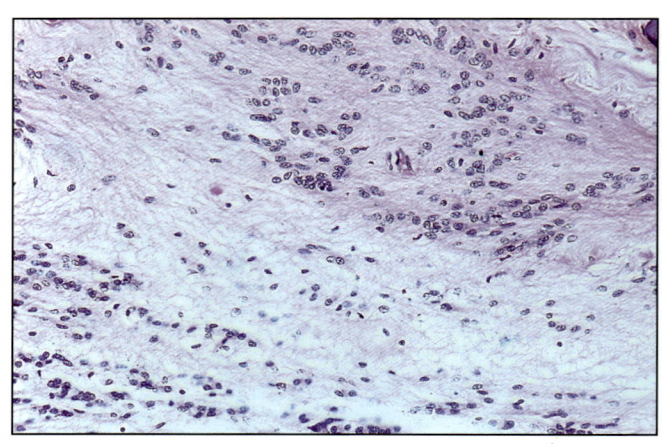

图26.64 位于无核纤维基质内的小的细胞团构成了室管膜下瘤的典型特征。尽管肿瘤细胞常常显示室管膜细胞特征，但见不到特殊的细胞极向。在同一肿瘤中，更具星形细胞特征的肿瘤细胞可与细胞团并列存在。

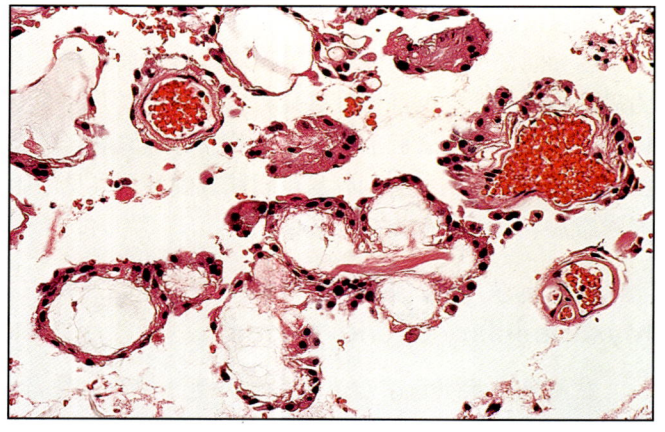

图26.63 黏液乳头型室管膜瘤。除了肿瘤的胶质细胞特征外，在这些肿瘤中常可见围绕血管的乳头状排列。

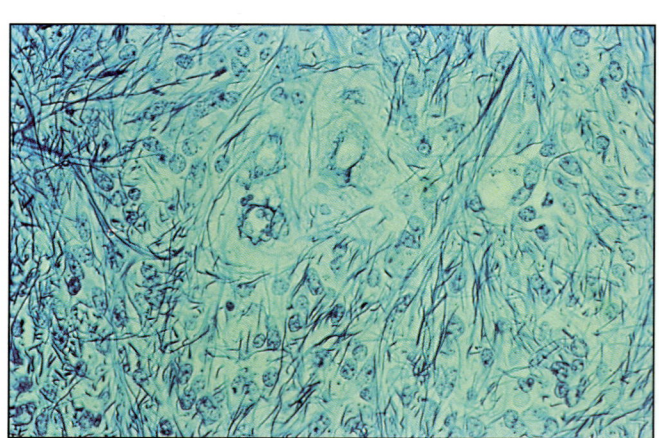

图26.65 室管膜下瘤的致密纤维性基质可通过磷钨酸苏木素（PTAH）染色来显示。

出受阻或肿瘤内出血，临床上会出现颅内压升高症状。50%～70%的室管膜下瘤通常发生于成人(23～81岁)，表现为无症状性肿瘤，与第四脑室有关。最常见的幕上部位是侧脑室和透明隔周围，随后是第三脑室。与其他室管膜肿瘤相比，脊髓的室管膜下瘤极为少见[323-327]，大约仅占所有室管膜瘤的2%。不同于一般41～60岁发病的无症状的室管膜下瘤，有症状的肿瘤发生于较年轻的成人（平均44岁）以及10岁以内的儿童，其肿瘤常常出现细胞型室管膜瘤和室管膜下瘤的混合性特征。

室管膜下瘤出现室管膜和星形细胞混合性特征。与纤维性星形细胞成分相比，确切的"室管膜瘤"区域通常很稀少且发育较差。肿瘤细胞通常排列成簇状，致密纤维与细胞稀少区域交替出现。基质的纤维性属性即使在富于细胞的区域也可以见到（图26.64和26.65）。混合性星形细胞和室管膜特征已经通过电镜和组织培养得到证实[328,329]。也常可见微囊变性和微小钙化。尽管偶尔出现非典型性和细胞核分裂活性增加，但肿瘤部位和成功完全切除是最重要的预后因素[325]。此病变的组织学发生尚未确定，但与室管膜瘤的鉴别很重要，可以避免不必要的辅助治疗。

室管膜肿瘤的生物学行为：室管膜肿瘤的生物学行为（不包括室管膜下瘤）除了局部生长以外，还具有显著的远处转移潜能。室管膜肿瘤靠近脑室系统及蛛网膜下腔，易于沿神经轴向远处播散。但与所有胶质瘤一样，神经轴以外转移罕见。在大型病例研究中，大约了其源于颗粒细胞神经元的假设[398,399]。

小脑发育不良性节细胞瘤与一种常染色体显性遗传以及导致多发性错构瘤及肿瘤形成的系统性综合征有关，后者被称为Cowden病[400-407]。这两种疾病都与10号染色体磷酸酶和张力蛋白同源（PTEN）基因的种系突变有关[407-410]。Cowden病具有标志性的皮肤黏膜表现，包括外毛根鞘瘤、相关毛囊畸形和特殊类型的玻璃样变性黏液纤维瘤，此外，Cowden病还有肢端角化病和口腔乳头状瘤[411]。很大一部分患者也有甲状腺腺瘤或多结节性甲状腺肿、乳腺纤维囊性病和（或）腺癌、胃肠道息肉（结肠、胃和食管）以及卵巢囊肿和息肉[412,413]。尽管这些相关性已有很多报道，但是，Lhermitte-Duclos病、Cowden病和PTEN种系突变之间的确切关系尚未完全清楚，因为并非所有Lhermitte-Duclos病患者都有Cowden病的临床表现，而且有些Lhermitte-Duclos病患者缺乏PTEN种系突变[409]。此外，不是所有具有PTEN种系突变的患者均出现Cowden病[414]。最近的遗传学分析提示，儿童发生的Lhermitte-Duclos病可以通过缺乏PTEN种系突变和缺少Cowden病表型来与那些成人病变鉴别[409]。近来Abel等[394]的研究表明，Lhermitte-Duclos病的发病机制与磷脂酰肌醇3-激酶（PI3K）通路（PTEN基因的下游通路）的PTEN抑制作用丢失有关，后者可对神经元迁移和细胞大小调节产生有害影响。这些作者认为，病变为发育异常基础上的肥厚表现。

无论其组织发生如何，这些进展性小脑病变最终需要外科切除，手术后复发并不少见[415-421]。在Abel等的最新研究中[394]，有31%的长期随访患者至少进行过一次复发肿瘤切除。

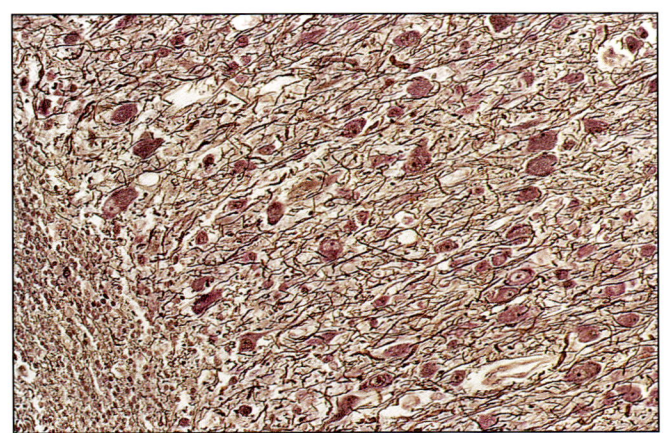

图26.76 小脑发育不良性节细胞瘤。镀银染色显示源自这些肿瘤性神经元的形态和分布异常的神经突起。Bodian。

婴儿促纤维增生型节细胞胶质瘤和促纤维增生型大脑星形细胞瘤（图26.77至26.80）
Desmoplastic infantile ganglioglioma and desmoplastic cerebral astrocytoma of infancy

此类肿瘤罕见，文献中收集的病例大约有60例，在一些病例研究中，约占颅内肿瘤的0.4%～1.25%[422-424]。

婴儿促纤维增生型节细胞胶质瘤通常在2～24个月出现临床症状（平均6个月，中位年龄为4个月），男女比为1.7:1[423,424]。大约有10例非婴儿患者的肿瘤具有与婴儿促纤维增生型节细胞胶质瘤相同的临床放射及病理学特征，年龄为5～25岁[425,426]。

该肿瘤位于幕上，相对较大，超过60%的病例不止一个脑叶受累，额顶区最常受累，但肿瘤也可源于半球的其他部位；连合处发生极其常见。枕叶例外，通常不受累（<15%），但发生多叶性肿瘤时受累程度较大[423]。尽管最初出现临床症状时肿瘤相对很大，但没有双侧肿瘤的报道。浅表软脑膜受累以及不同程度的硬膜粘连很常见。限于深部结构或与脑室系统相通极为少见，只有极个别病例报告[427-429]。多数患者最初表现为头围迅速增大，伴有急性且差异较大的局部体征出现，包括麻痹和癫痫。

婴儿促纤维增生性大脑星形细胞瘤：与婴儿促纤维增生性节细胞胶质瘤有很多相同的临床病理特征；但这些肿瘤之间的组织遗传学关系尚不清楚[424]。在一个病例研究中，这些肿瘤具有类似的人口统计学特征，年龄在1.5～14个月（平均为6.8个月；中位年龄为6个月），男女比例为0.8:1[422]。生长结构方面，该肿瘤境界相对清楚，一般发生于额顶叶的浅表部分。除了缺乏具有神经元表型的肿瘤性成分外，其组织病理学和超微结构特征与婴儿促纤维结缔组织增生性节细胞胶质瘤极其类似。平均术后随访2年以上（11个月至5.5年），这些肿瘤经过适当外科切除后，预后相对较好[422]。一项有2例病例的分子遗传学研究显示，与弥漫性星形细胞瘤相比较，婴儿促纤维组织增生性大脑星形细胞瘤没有任何17p或10号染色体的等位基因丢失[430]。

两种类型的肿瘤的神经影像学特征极其类似[423,424,431]。CT神经影像学显示这些大肿瘤有显著的囊性成分。实性部分为等密度或稍高密度，应用血管造影剂后有显著强化，尤其是脑膜表面的区域。MRI方面，囊性部分在T1加权像上一般为低密度，而实性皮质成分通常与灰质等密度。在T2加权像上，囊性部分通常信号密度增加，而实性成分通常不均匀，密度不等。CT影像上，相当一部分的实性成分常有显著血管强化。肿瘤周围水肿差异较大。

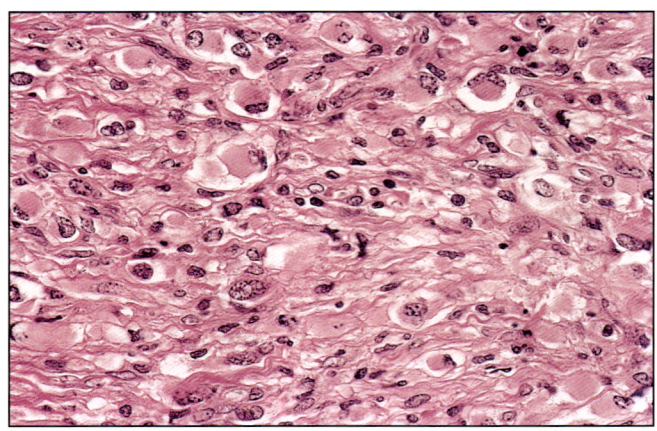

图26.77 婴儿促纤维增生性节细胞胶质瘤由异质性胶质和球状神经元混合而成，分布于有不同程度胶原沉积的显著间质当中。

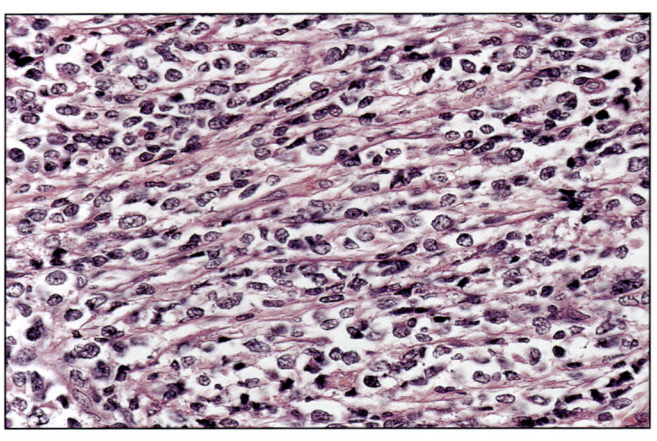

图26.78 婴儿促纤维增生性节细胞胶质瘤。显著的间质内可见更为原始的神经元细胞。

这些肿瘤的标志性组织病理学特征是有大量的致密结缔组织增生，使这些肿瘤具有特征性的硬度。这在与硬脑膜的交界处尤其明显，与胶原沉积有关。镜下，增生结缔组织具有明显的致密基质沉积，混合有神经上皮和纤维母细胞成分。特殊染色可显示波浪状网织纤维阳性的致密间质沉积，胶原纤维包绕两种细胞成分。细胞外基质的密度以及明显的纤维母细胞成分在每个肿瘤中差异极大。范围从神经细胞数量相对较少，被丰富的结缔组织反应包裹，到含有大量肿瘤性神经细胞的细胞丰富区与不甚明显的细胞外基质松散交织。

在节细胞胶质瘤中，肿瘤的神经上皮成分由不同比例的星形胶质细胞和神经元细胞组成（图26.77至26.80），在星形细胞瘤中仅有胶质细胞成分。此外，常可见更为原始的细胞成分（图26.78和26.79D），在某些区域偶尔可成为最显著的部分[424]。在每个肿瘤内，星形细胞和神经元成分的分布一般不均匀，部分与间质密度有关。总体上，星形细胞为最显著的神经成分，尤其是在结缔组织增生最丰富的区域。神经元成分最具异质性，从非典型节细胞样到更常见的小多角形细胞表现。银浸染和免疫组化[神经微丝表型、NF-H/M和（或）突触素]可很方便地识别神经元细胞。双重免疫组化标记明确显示，代表胶质细胞和神经元分化的细胞骨架表型在单个细胞内并不共存。

在两种类型的肿瘤中，可以见到分化较差的细胞聚集。尽管这些比较原始的细胞在HE染色中分化较差，但是，数量不等的这些细胞的免疫组化染色显示神经元或胶质细胞的细胞骨架标记物。在两种类型的肿瘤中，如果出现核分裂象和微小坏死灶，那么最常见于原始细胞群（图26.78和26.29D）。据报道，婴儿促结缔组织增生性节细胞胶质瘤的Ki-67标记指数从不到0.5%到15%[432]，而在婴儿促结缔组织增生性星形细胞瘤中是5%（平均3.5%）[424]。

大体上全部或近乎全部切除后预后较好，这是婴儿促结缔组织增生性节细胞胶质瘤和星形细胞瘤的重要临床特征[424]，见于多个报道。在这些病例中，临床随访超过8年，肿瘤无复发，提示出现明显原始细胞成分并非特别提示间变或更为侵袭性行为的潜能增加。但是，据报道，少数病例出现更为侵袭性的行为。一例进展病例首诊6年后死亡，尸检时可见显著软脑膜播散[428]。在另外2例，最初切除几个月后肿瘤出现复发，伴有软脑膜和室管膜转移性播散[433]。在此3例，由于在最初治疗时有包括下丘脑、中脑和脑干在内的深部结构受累，大体上无法完全切除，这可能对更为侵袭性的临床过程产生了影响。

胚胎发育不良性神经上皮肿瘤（图26.81和26.82）
Dysembryoplastic neuroepithelial tumor

胚胎发育不良性神经上皮肿瘤（DNT）是一种特殊类型的混合性神经元-胶质肿瘤，发生于有长期复杂部分性癫痫的儿童和年轻成人[435,436]。胚胎发育不良性神经上皮肿瘤罕见，占所有脑肿瘤的比例不足1%[435]。然而在专业癫痫外科中心，其发生率可较高。

DNT为特征性多结节皮质内肿瘤，好发于颞叶[435]。但少数也可发生于皮质的其他部位，包括额叶、顶叶和枕叶[437]。少数病例累及其他部位也有报道，包括尾状核、小脑和脑干[436,438,439]。偶尔出现多病灶性病变[440]。

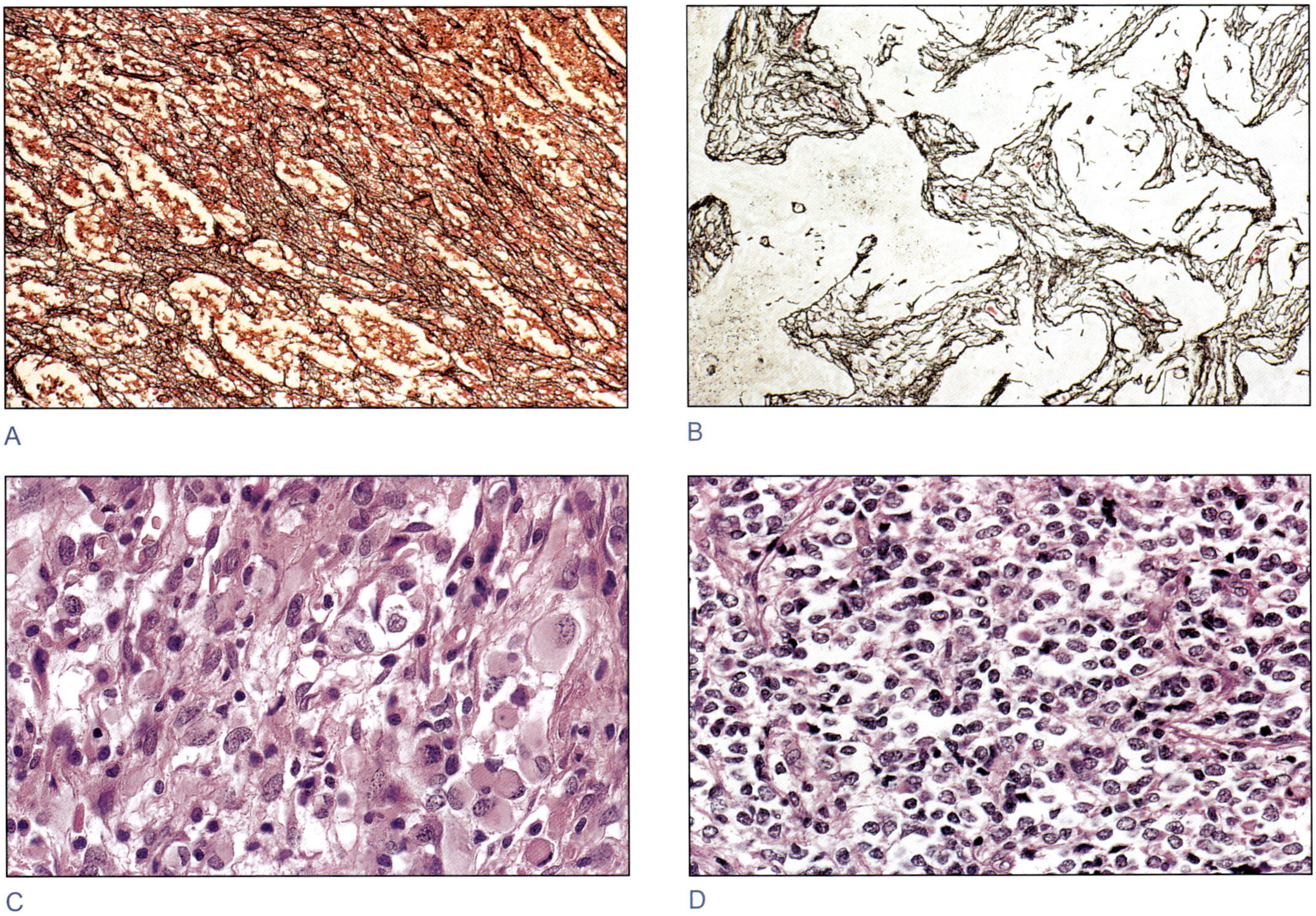

图26.79 婴儿促纤维增生型节细胞胶质瘤。网织纤维沉积是这些肿瘤的显著特征,部分与肿瘤性星形细胞产生的基底膜相对应。网织纤维的密度不一,从弥漫性聚集(A)到紧凑的岛状(B)散在分布于较密集的细胞当中,混有不同细胞成分(C)或原始神经细胞(D)。(A,B)网织纤维染色。

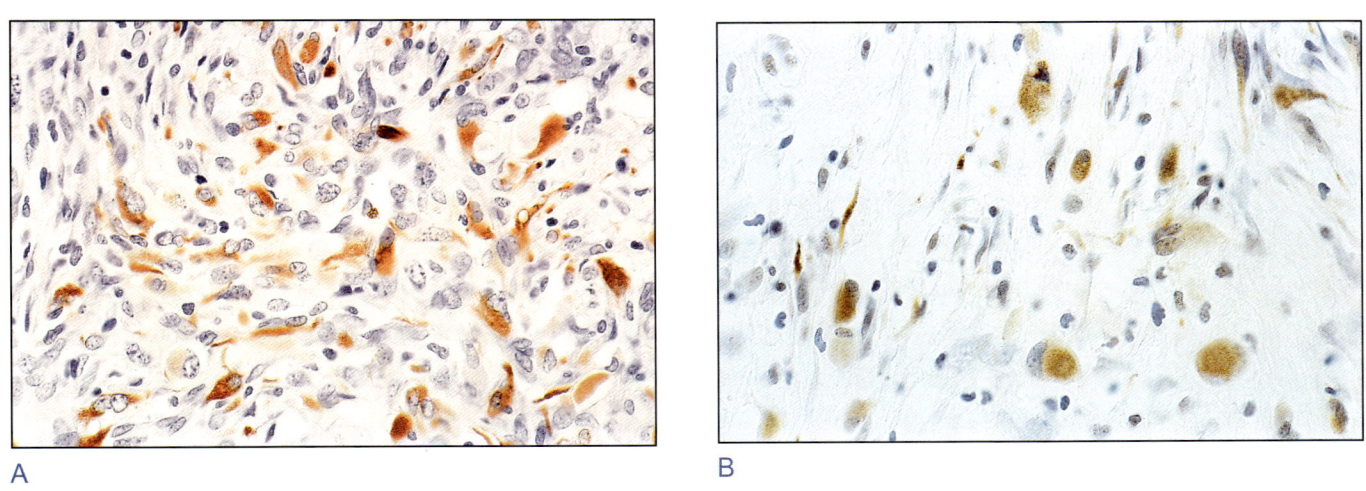

图26.80 婴儿促纤维增生型节细胞胶质瘤。胶质和神经元细胞骨架蛋白免疫组织化学显示异质性神经上皮细胞的分化不同。大量肿瘤性星形细胞具有胶质纤维酸性蛋白(GFAP)免疫反应(A)。神经元细胞具有神经微丝(NF-H/M)表型免疫反应(B)。(A)GFAP-PAP免疫过氧化物酶法,苏木素双重染色;(B)SMI33-PAP免疫过氧化物酶法,苏木素双重染色。

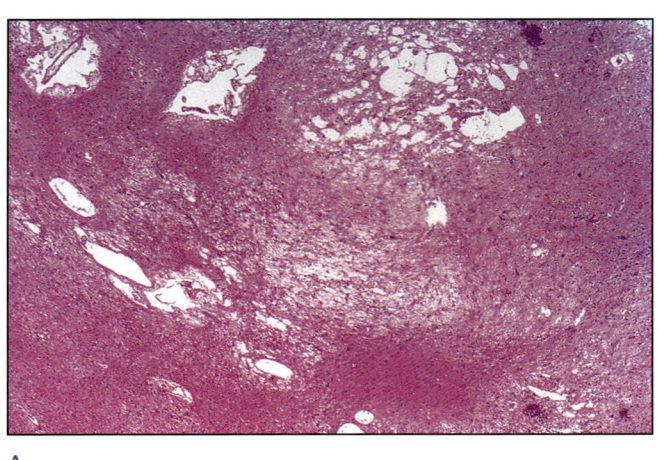
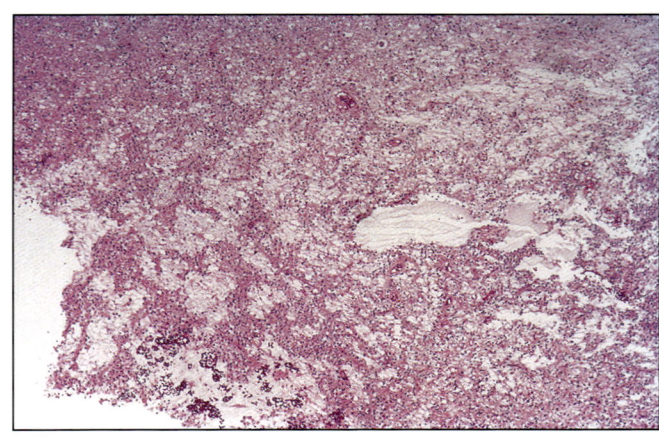

图26.81 2例经典型胚胎发育不良性神经上皮性肿瘤，低倍显示肿瘤轻度富于细胞，浅表皮质内有微囊改变（A和B）。

神经影像学常常出现多囊性表现[441]。这些肿瘤通常位于皮质内，没有占位效应，没有肿瘤周围水肿。DNT 在 CT 上多为低密度，MR 影像上，T1 加权像为低信号，T2 加权像为高信号[442]。普通放射影像学征象为被覆颅骨变形，提示是一个长期病变。

DNT 的组织学标志是多结节肿瘤结构，低倍镜下最易观察。结节由"少突胶质细胞样细胞"、星形细胞和神经元细胞混合而成，包裹于黏液和微囊性基质中。神经元成分大多由漂浮于黏液样基质中的大细胞组成。通常，DNT 周围皮质显示不同程度的皮层发育不良（图 26.81 和 26.82）；高达 80% 的病例伴发皮层发育不良[443]。细胞非典型性不是 DNT 的典型特征，但是可以出现核分裂活性，Ki-67（MIB-1）增生指数一般较低（小于 1%）[444,445]。

免疫组化研究已经证实了这些病变的胶质神经元属性。不仅成熟的、个别发育不良的神经元为必要成分，而且，DNT 免疫组化和超微结构研究表明，少突胶质细胞样细胞为早期胶质及神经元分化细胞的混合[446]。神经元相关标记物（突触素、神经微丝蛋白、Ⅲ型 β-微管蛋白、NeuN）证实了特殊神经元成分，而 GFAP、波形蛋白和 S-100 蛋白印证了胶质成分[22,446]。

考虑到这些病变的不同的形态学表现，有些方面最好在低倍镜下观察，取材恰当对诊断非常重要。最常见的是，不具代表性的或微小的标本可类似于混合性少突星形细胞瘤。区分 DNT 和低级别胶质瘤对于准确评估预后和治疗非常重要。即使是次全切除，DNT 也有非常好的预后[436,447]；放疗和化疗对 DNT 没有意义。肿瘤复发仅见于最初未完全切除的病例[437,445]，仅有一例恶性转化的报道[448]。

DNT 样病变发生于其他部位而非半球皮层已有报

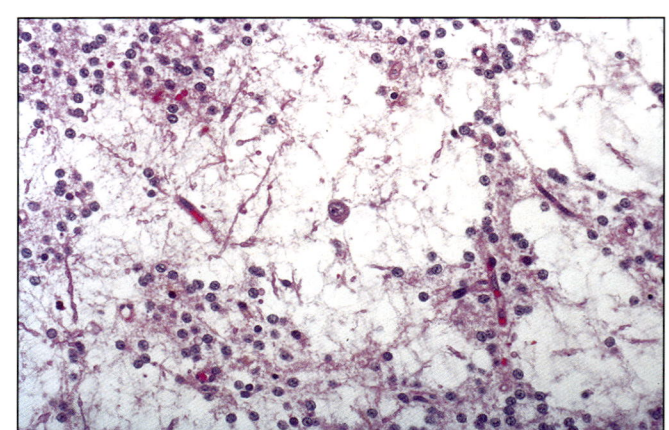

图26.82 胚胎发育不良性神经上皮性肿瘤。混合性细胞成分由少突胶质细胞、星形细胞和神经元以不同比例组合而成；但少突细胞成分最为明显。

道。一例 DNT 样肿瘤发生于透明隔和尾状核部位是其中之一，已被广泛报道[449,450]。与皮层 DNT 类似，这些病变的特征是富于黏液的基质以及少突胶质细胞样细胞、漂浮的神经元和特殊胶质神经元成分。区分这些病变与更具侵袭性的胶质瘤很必要，因为这些肿瘤与经典皮层 DNT 一样，其行为更为良性。

节细胞胶质瘤（图26.83至26.88）
Ganglioglioma

节细胞胶质瘤大约仅占所有脑组织的 1%[451]，大约占所有儿童 CNS 肿瘤的 1%～4%[452]。节细胞胶质瘤是最常见的混合性神经元-胶质肿瘤，主要发生于 1～30 岁[453,454]。肿瘤可伴有癫痫，尤其是复杂部分性癫痫[453]。

节细胞胶质瘤大多位于颞叶，其次是顶叶和额

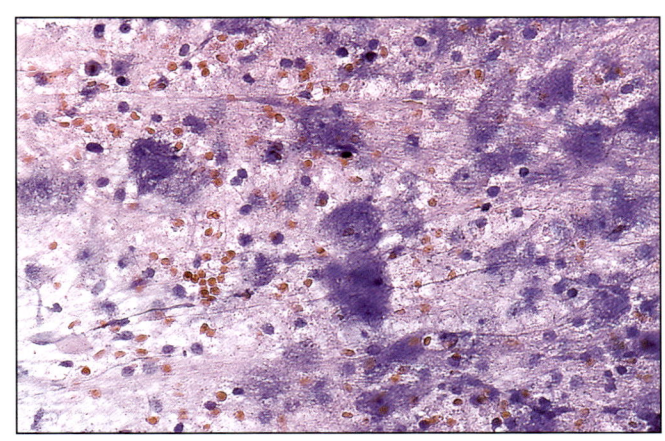

图26.83 节细胞胶质瘤涂片大多显示纤维性间质内的混合性星形细胞和节细胞成分。Morris染色。

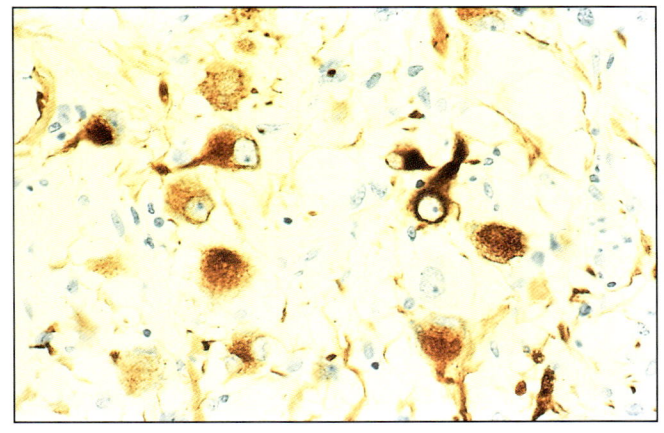

图26.85 该节细胞胶质瘤的肿瘤性胶质细胞成分显示非磷酸化依赖性神经丝蛋白（NF-H/M）表型免疫反应性。SMI33-ABC免疫过氧化物酶及苏木素双重染色。

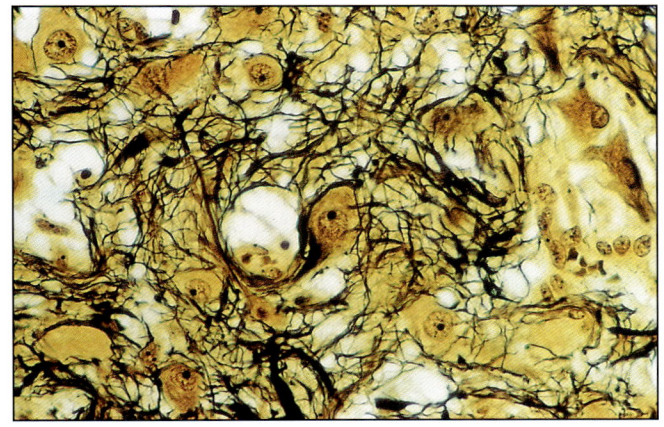

图26.84 节细胞胶质瘤。Bielschowsky镀银染色常常出现发自节细胞的排列及形状异常的神经突起。Bielschowsky染色。

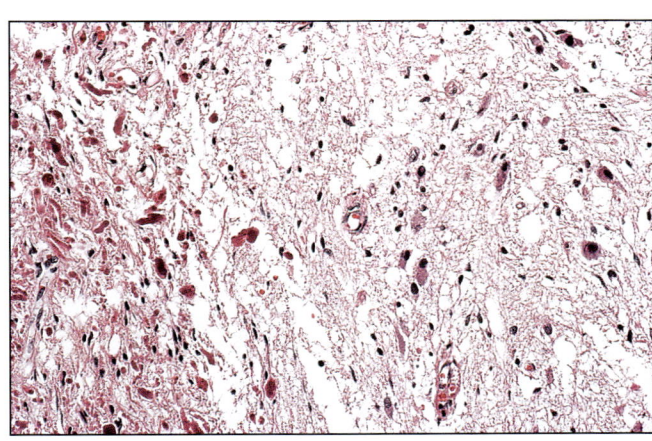

图26.86 此颞叶节细胞胶质瘤中，星形细胞成分类似于毛细胞型星形细胞瘤。注意大量Rosenthal纤维与肿瘤性节细胞相邻。

叶[451-455]。神经影像学研究显示，肿瘤境界相对清楚，常常出现囊性变和钙化成分。在一些病例中，肿瘤周围皮层可出现皮层发育不良[451,455]。可以见到肿瘤累及软脑膜。

节细胞胶质瘤组织学上由肿瘤性节细胞和胶质细胞混合而成（图26.83）。节细胞形态异常，大小和密度差异较大。可以见到奇异形和双核表现，但后者在某些肿瘤中罕见。胶质成分大多由纤维和毛细胞型星形细胞组成；少突胶质细胞成分相当少见[455]。胶质成分可出现特殊区域或细胞类型的典型胶质瘤表型，如毛细胞型星形细胞瘤（图26.86）。嗜酸性颗粒或玻璃小体常混杂于胶质成分中。其他特征包括微囊变性和钙化。细胞脂质化也可以见于胶质细胞，仔细检查肿瘤性神经元，以除外多形性黄色瘤性星形细胞瘤（PXA）诊断[456]。在此背景下，一些复合性节细胞瘤/PXA瘤已有报道[225-228]。

神经元相关蛋白的免疫组化，包括神经微丝蛋白、突触素以及NeuN[451,453]、镀银染色技术、尼氏体物质染色，通常有助于证实肿瘤性神经元细胞（图26.84和26.85）。突触、致密核心囊泡和突起内微管等超微结构常见[457]。胶质成分通常是星形细胞，通过GFAP、波形蛋白和S-100蛋白来显现。有趣的是，较高比例的节细胞瘤CD34呈阳性。

节细胞胶质瘤的一个显著特征是：出现丰富的纤维性间质，常常伴有淋巴细胞浸润。间质成分有差异，从纤细的纤维血管成分混以大量胶质成分，到相对致密的促结缔组织反应，几乎掩盖了胶质性基质（图26.87和26.88）。不同程度的血管瘤病可出现纤维血管增生。血

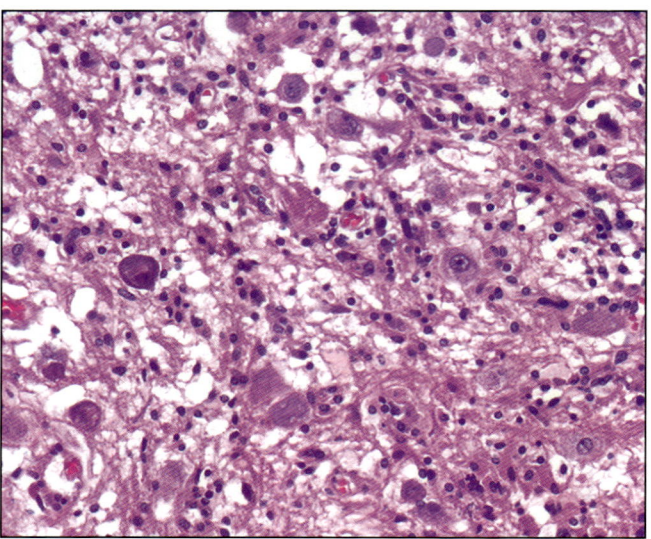

图26.87 节细胞胶质瘤。组织切片中，混合性的肿瘤性星形细胞瘤和异常节细胞成分通常包埋于纤维血管性间质当中。注意淋巴细胞浸润与血管并存。

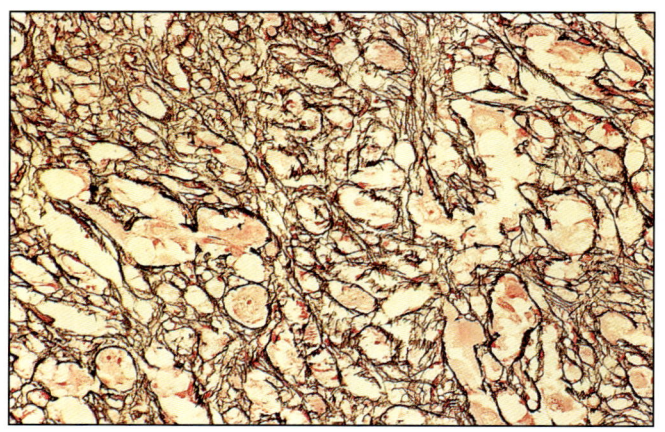

图26.88 节细胞胶质瘤。网织纤维阳性的间质在节细胞胶质瘤中可极其丰富。网织纤维染色。

管周围淋巴细胞浸润不应误认为是神经母细胞。

节细胞胶质瘤根据胶质成分分为Ⅰ级或Ⅱ级[458]。胶质成分常常使这些混合性神经元-胶质肿瘤具有复发和间变进展潜能[458,459]。尽管绝大部分节细胞胶质瘤的Ki-67标记指数较低，但Ki-67染色似乎局限于胶质成分[451,453]。高标记指数的重要性在于行为更具侵袭性[453]。除了有间变转化的病例外，预后相对较好[460]（见下文）。

间变性（恶性）节细胞胶质瘤
Anaplastic (malignant) ganglioglioma

据报道，节细胞胶质瘤的恶性转化大约发生于10%的病例[451,453,455,459,460]。临床上，对于慢性癫痫活动近期有加剧、T2信号密度增加以及神经影像学对比增强的患者，应该怀疑有间变性转化。间变性进展（图26.89）不同程度地发生于胶质成分，最终导致与多形性胶质母细胞瘤难以区别的组织学图像。在高度富于细胞的胶质成分为主的情况下，神经元和胶质标记物免疫组化染色有助于识别不同的细胞成分。

混合性神经元-胶质肿瘤的新变型（new variants of mixed neuronal-glial tumors）：最近几年，有些报道描述了具有特殊形态学表现的混合性神经元-胶质肿瘤。这些病变主要是低级别肿瘤，识别它们很重要，可以避免误认为是普通胶质瘤，防止不必要的辅助治疗。

乳头状胶质神经元肿瘤（papillary glioneuronal tumor）：这种不常见肿瘤的特征为：单层假复层状小立方性胶质细胞围绕玻璃样变的血管形成假乳头状结构。在假乳头状结构之间，可见片状或局灶神经元细胞聚集，从神经细胞到小的节细胞。这些肿瘤最常发生于深部白

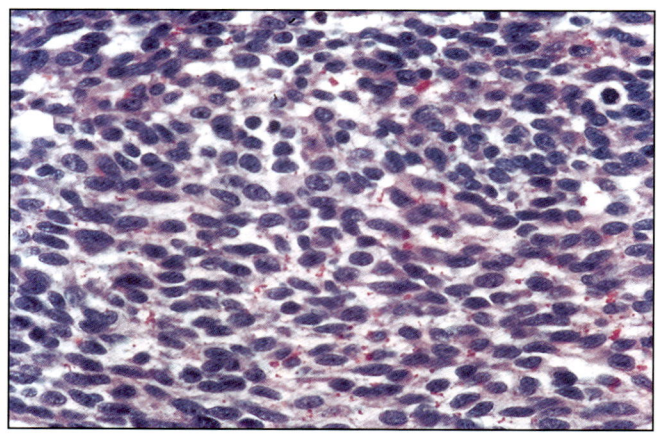

A

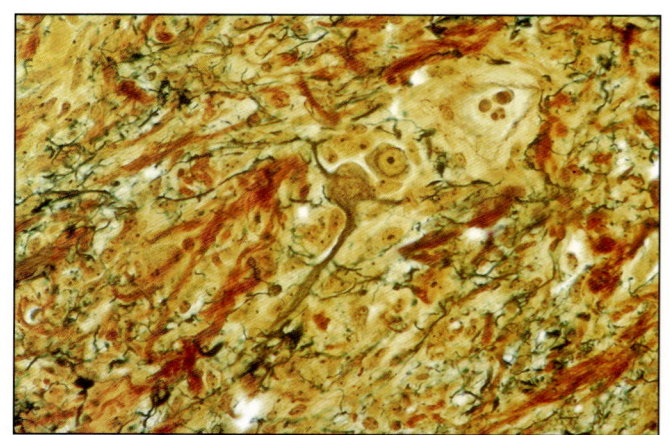

B

图26.89 间变性节细胞胶质瘤。（A）此间变性节细胞胶质瘤的胶质成分由小细胞组成，胶质性胞浆稀少，细胞核深染。（B）同一肿瘤，节细胞通过镀银染色易于识别。

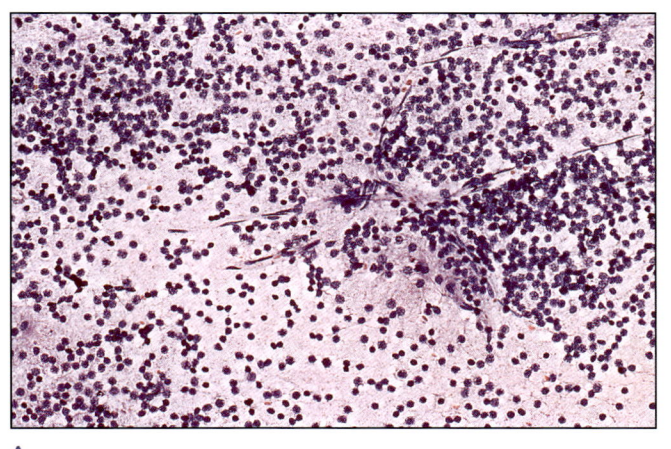
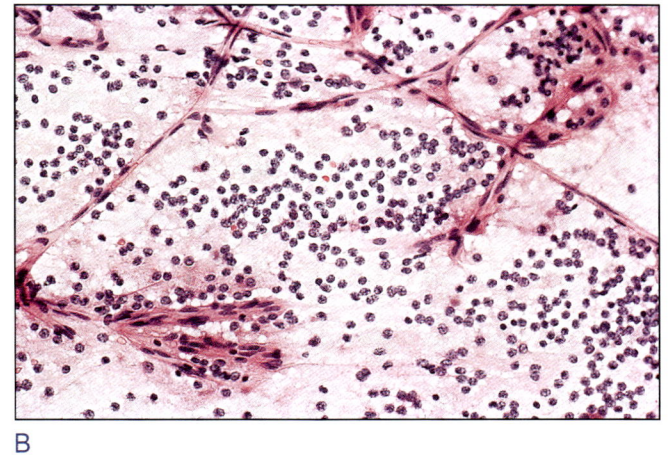

图26.90 （A，B）中枢神经细胞瘤涂片显示一致性的细胞，具有圆形核和纤细分散的染色质。胞浆境界不清，嗜酸性基质呈中等程度的纤维性。血管成分纤细程度不等。Morris染色。

质，呈脑室旁分布，放射学上表现为对比增强的囊性肿物。肿瘤可发生于不同年龄的患者，没有性别倾向。与节细胞胶质瘤类似，该肿瘤核分裂活性低，Ki-67标记指数低。尽管迄今为止仅有几例报道，但随访资料提示，在6个月至7年之间，没有肿瘤复发证据[461-465]。

第四脑室形成玫瑰花结结构的胶质神经元肿瘤（rosette-forming glioneuronal tumor of the fourth ventricle）：此第四脑室的罕见病变以双相结构为特征，由小神经细胞排列成小玫瑰花结结构和具有毛细胞特征的第二种星形细胞成分混合而成[466,467]。也可出现节细胞。胶质成分偶尔可出现Rosenthal纤维、颗粒或透明样小体以及微小钙化，类似于毛细胞型星形细胞瘤。神经影像学上，肿瘤位于中线，占据脑室系统。累及小脑蚓部、中脑、脑桥和丘脑的多中心性病变已有报道[466,467]。与其他混合性神经元-胶质肿瘤相似，这些肿瘤呈惰性病程。报道的Ki-67标记指数较低。

近来，小型病例研究报道的胶质神经元肿瘤的其他变型包括：胶质神经元肿瘤，伴有神经毡样岛状结构，以及少突胶质细胞瘤，伴有神经细胞分化[468-471]。

中枢神经细胞瘤 （图26.90至26.95）
Central neurocytoma

中枢神经细胞瘤是脑室内的神经元肿瘤，外科切除后预后良好[472,473]。这些肿瘤罕见，在大型外科病例研究中，其发病率占所有颅内肿瘤的0.25%～0.5%[473,474]。大多见于年轻成人，无性别差异。在Virginia大学的10例病例研究中，手术时患者年龄6～52岁（平均24岁）[475]，与其他研究报道的一致。

肿瘤境界清楚，部分有钙化，发生于侧脑室和（或）第三脑室，常常位于室间孔区。巨大肿瘤累及侧脑室和第三脑室也可出现。近来，Schmidt等将中枢神经细胞瘤的典型神经影像表现进行了回顾分析[476]。

中枢神经细胞瘤的组织学结构典型且相对一致。肿瘤由一致性的细胞成分组成，细胞核呈圆形至稍有分叶，染色质细斑状，位于明显纤维性基质中（图26.90至26.92）。纤细的微血管成分形成分枝状网状结构，有些类似于少突胶质细胞瘤。一致的细胞、纤细的基质以及典型的微血管在涂片中易于识别（图26.90），容易除外少突胶质细胞瘤和松果体肿瘤。这些肿瘤的一个一致性及特征性结构是致密纤维性基质构成的无核岛（图26.92）。极少数情况下，可以出现局灶性坏死。核分裂活性和Ki-67（MIB-1）标记指数一般较低[477]。没有内皮增生（见下文）。在极少数报道中，成熟节细胞可见

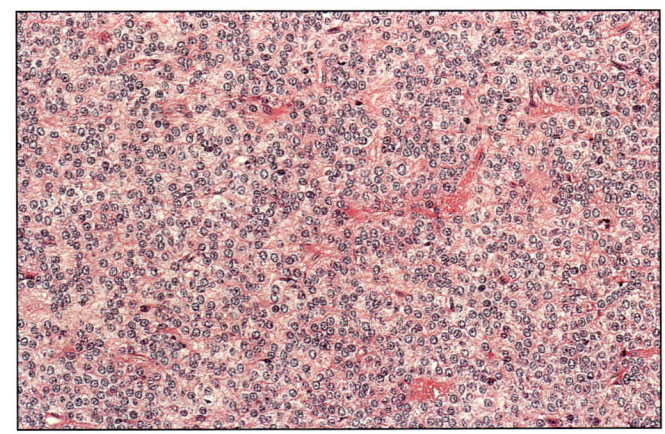

图26.91 组织切片中，中枢神经细胞瘤通常由均匀一致的细胞组成，一定程度上可被纤细血管间质的轻度增殖勾画出来。

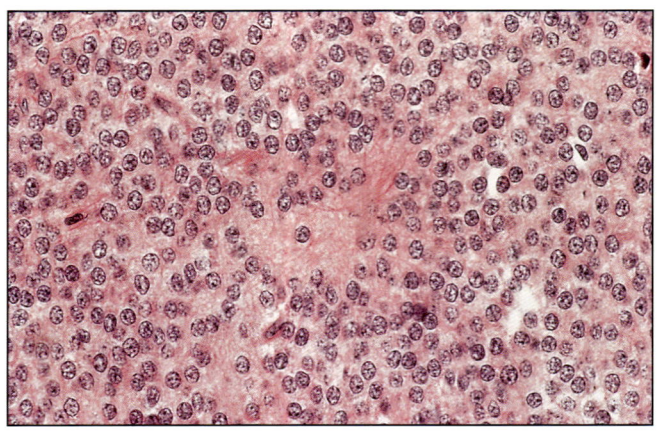

图26.92 中枢神经细胞瘤常规制片的高倍表现，显示一致的圆形细胞核中弥散而纤细的染色质结构。致密纤维性细胞突起的无核区很常见。

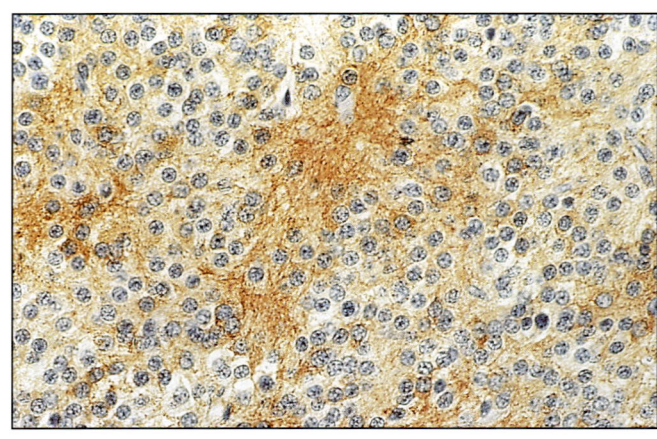

图26.93 中枢神经细胞瘤。突触素免疫反应，与肿瘤的神经细胞本质相一致，弥漫分布于肿瘤内，但在无核区更为明显。SY38-ABC免疫过氧化物酶苏木素双重染色。

于中枢神经细胞瘤[472]。

肿瘤的神经元分化可通过突触素和其他神经元细胞骨架蛋白的免疫组化来证实，包括神经微丝蛋白和Neu-N[472,473,475]（图26.93和26.94）。GFAP免疫反应在少数病例报告中有报道[472]，但在大多数病例中，其仅限于间质的反应性星形细胞[475]（图26.95）。超微结构特征可明确地证实诊断，包括透明及致密核心囊泡、充满平行排列的微管的细胞突起和突触[473]。

中枢神经细胞瘤是良性病变，多数肿瘤的行为表现为WHO Ⅱ级肿瘤。但也有肿瘤复发的报道[477-480]，主要是次全切除的病例。有些肿瘤复发时也出现脑室和蛛网膜下腔播散[479,481]。在几个报告中，该肿瘤具有中度核分裂活性、血管增生以及局灶性坏死[473]。中枢神经细胞瘤的增生潜能与其临床行为具有相关性[482,483]。在1982年以来发表的大量研究分析中，Rades等提出，MIB-1指数大于3%与局部病变复发和总体生存期较差相关[483]。其他作者提出，肿瘤出现血管内皮增生和高Ki-67（MIB-1）标记指数，应当称为"非典型中枢神经细胞瘤"[482]。

多数中枢神经细胞瘤可通过单独外科治疗。然而，对于不完全或次全切除的病例，常规体外放射治疗或聚焦放射外科治疗也已运用[476]。

其他与中枢神经细胞瘤组织结构类似的肿瘤也可见于脑室外部位，称为"脑室外神经细胞瘤"。这些肿瘤与中枢神经细胞瘤出现相同的组织学特征，但在细胞密度和增生比例方面，出现更为宽泛的形态学谱系。此外，多数脑室外的神经细胞瘤出现程度不同的节细胞

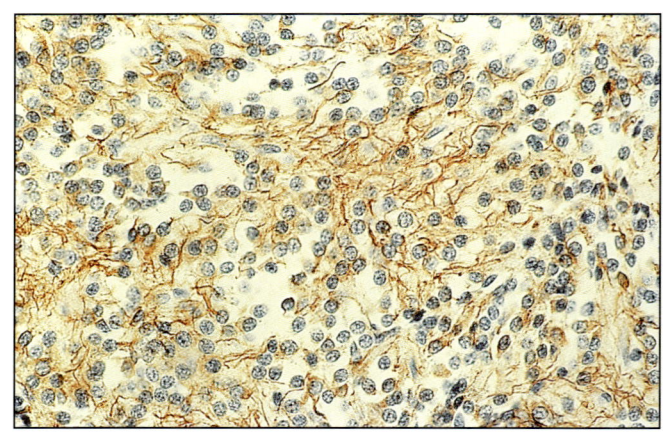

图26.94 中枢神经细胞瘤。微管相关蛋白（MAP-2）免疫组织化学显示，致密包裹的神经突起呈强阳性。AP18-ABC免疫过氧化物酶苏木素双重染色。

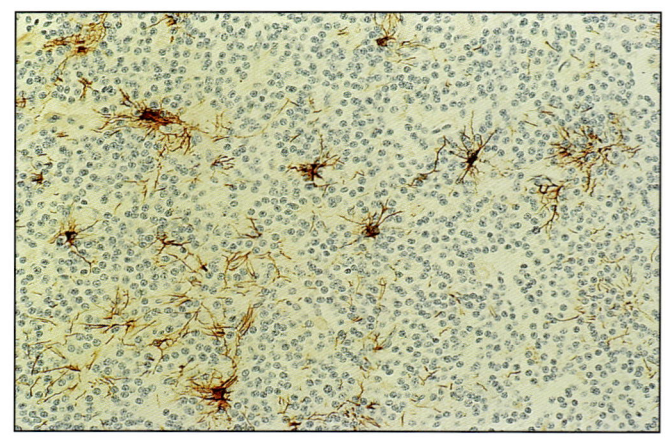

图26.95 中枢神经细胞瘤。被认为是反应性的星形细胞通常散在分布于肿瘤当中。它们主要与血管间质相关，可通过胶质纤维酸性蛋白（GFAP）免疫组织化学染色来显示。注意高分化的星形细胞的典型星状结构。GFAP-ABC免疫过氧化物酶苏木素双重染色。

分化[484]。这些肿瘤与典型的中枢神经细胞瘤的确切关系尚不清楚。

小脑脂肪神经细胞瘤
Cerebellar liponeurocytoma

小脑脂肪神经细胞瘤是极其少见的肿瘤，发生于成人小脑，组织学特征为神经元/神经细胞分化，可见脂化病灶[485]。最初定义为髓母细胞瘤的一个变型（所谓的脂肪瘤性髓母细胞瘤），这些肿瘤在 2000 年 WHO 分类中被重新分类为小脑脂肪神经细胞瘤，原因是肿瘤内在的低增殖潜能和临床预后较好，这两个重要因子不同于更具侵袭性的髓母细胞瘤。此外，该名称也强调了这些肿瘤在进一步神经元分化方面与中枢神经细胞瘤类似。

与中枢神经细胞瘤相比，小脑脂肪神经细胞瘤发生于较年长的人群，即 41~60 岁，平均发病年龄为 51 岁[485]。肿瘤境界大多清楚，位于两侧小脑半球和小脑蚓部。CT 上，病变与脑实质相比呈低密度或等密度，显示中度不均匀对比增强[486]。MR 影像上，T1-加权序列在整体低密度肿瘤中出现高信号密度灶，与肿瘤内脂肪的出现相一致。可见不同程度的肿瘤周围水肿[486,487]。肿瘤大体上出现明显的片状黄色区域，与典型的质软灰红组织混合[486,487]。

这些肿瘤的组织学标志是双相结构：相对一致的圆形细胞、胞浆稀少、圆形或卵圆形浓染细胞核与数量不等的脂化细胞相混合。前一种细胞会使人联想起神经细胞瘤或神经母细胞瘤的组织学特征。核分裂象的数量较少，坏死和微血管增生不明显或缺乏。

神经元免疫反应标记物可以检测小细胞和脂肪细胞成分，如突触素和 MAP-2。GFAP、S-100 以及波形蛋白可呈局灶免疫反应阳性，但在范围及分布上差异较大[485,488]。超微结构也显示神经元分化证据，包括含有微管束的突起、致密核心囊泡和极少数的突触连接。可以见到充满中间丝的星形细胞突起，但并不明显。肿瘤细胞含有细胞浆内脂质，可以聚成巨大脂滴[488]。

这些肿瘤总体上增殖活性相对较低，MIB-1 标记指数为 1%~6%，平均约为 3%[485]。尽管病例数太少，无法确定有意义的预后标准，但相当数量的患者无复发生存率大于 5 年[486,489]。小脑脂肪神经细胞瘤 WHO 分级为 I 或 II 级[485]。

小脑脂肪神经细胞瘤的发病机制以及与其他神经元和神经元-胶质肿瘤的关系尚不清楚。近来分子遗传学研究显示，这些肿瘤在遗传学方面不同于髓母细胞瘤[490]。与髓母细胞瘤不同，这些肿瘤缺乏常见的 17q 等位染色体，大约 20% 的病例出现 TP53 错义突变，该百分比明显高于髓母细胞瘤或中枢神经细胞瘤。小脑脂肪神经细胞瘤可能是一种病理学和遗传学特殊的神经元/胶质神经元肿瘤。

松果体实质肿瘤
Pineal parenchymal tumors

松果体实质肿瘤（PPT）占所有颅内肿瘤的比例不足 0.1%[491,492]，大约占儿童松果体区肿瘤的 11%~28%[493,494]。目前 WHO 分类将这些松果体自身肿瘤分成三个亚型——松果体母细胞瘤、松果体瘤、中分化 PPT（见表 26.1）。这些亚型代表连续性的肿瘤特征谱系，从原始松果体母细胞瘤到相对高分化的松果体细胞瘤。两个极端之间是中分化肿瘤，出现松果体母细胞和松果体细胞瘤结构。

从临床角度来看，PPT 的三个亚型也有不同。松果体细胞瘤常常发生于年长患者，多为境界比较清楚的病变，没有脑脊液（CSF）种植倾向。松果体细胞瘤在 WHO 分类中被分为 II 级肿瘤[491]，生存时间长于松果体母细胞瘤（5 年生存率为 67%）[495]。相比之下，松果体母细胞瘤的临床行为与 CNS 其他原始神经外胚层肿瘤相似（见胚胎性肿瘤），即一般发生于儿童和年轻成人，是高度侵袭性肿瘤，具有经 CSF 通路播散的潜能。一般来说，这些肿瘤表现为 IV 级恶性肿瘤。松果体母细胞瘤患者的总体生存时间较短（16 个月）[496]，5 年无进展生存率较低（在一个病例研究中为 38%）[497]。中间型 PPT 病例可出现过渡性行为表现，依据是否出现较多的松果体母细胞瘤成分[491,495]。中间型 PPT 在 WHO 分类中为 II~III 级[491]。局部浸润和 CSF 播散潜能显著，其临床行为比松果体细胞瘤更具侵袭性[495]。

松果体细胞瘤 （图 26.96 至 26.98）
Pineocytoma

松果体细胞瘤大约占 PPT 的 7%~30%。这些肿瘤可发生于任何年龄，但常见于年轻成人（平均年龄为 35~47 岁），具有相同的性别分布[491,495,496]。松果体细胞瘤一般表现为境界清楚的肿物，神经影像学上与邻近脑组织结构界限清楚[498]，这与它们有限的局部浸润倾向相一致。这些肿瘤质软，切面呈颗粒状，常常伴有囊性变。可以出现局灶坏死。

松果体细胞瘤是中度富于细胞的肿瘤（图 26.96），特征为相对一致的细胞围绕纤维性无核区，称为"松果体细胞瘤性玫瑰花结"（图 26.97 和 26.98）。这些玫瑰花结类似 Homer Wright 玫瑰花结，但较大。它们在肿瘤中可极为广泛，但通常相互连接，分散的结构不易见到。玫瑰花结的出现以前被当做"神经元"分化的证据，但

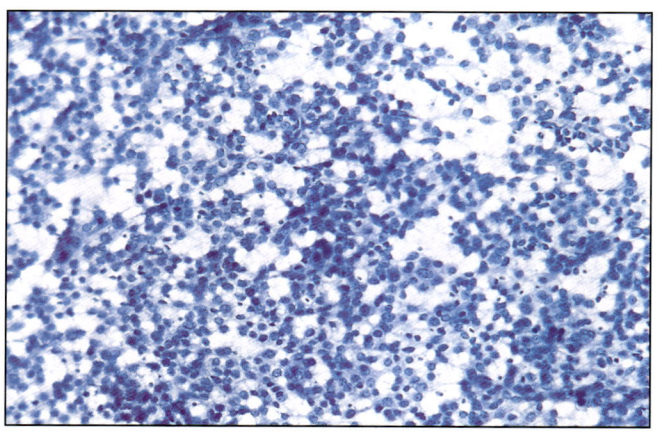

图26.96 松果体细胞瘤的涂片显示,细胞的胞浆境界清楚,核呈轻度多形性。注意细胞间基质稀少,与中枢神经细胞瘤涂片中的花边基质形成对比。Morris染色。

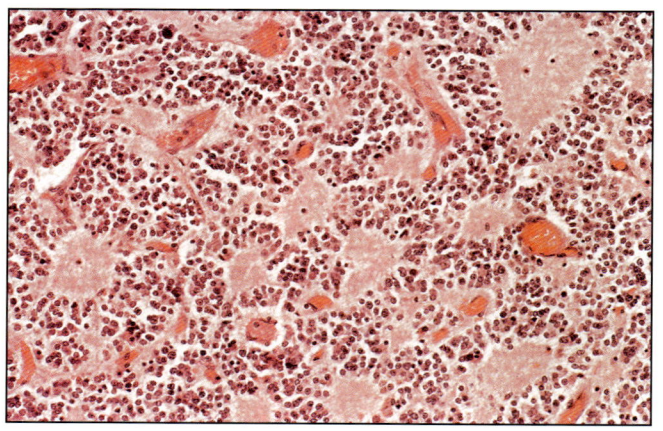

图26.97 松果体细胞瘤。"松果体细胞瘤性"玫瑰花结显示纤维性无核中央区,周围有细胞围绕,细胞核小且一致。这些玫瑰花结代表松果体细胞的成熟。注意玫瑰花结之间更为密集的细胞区。

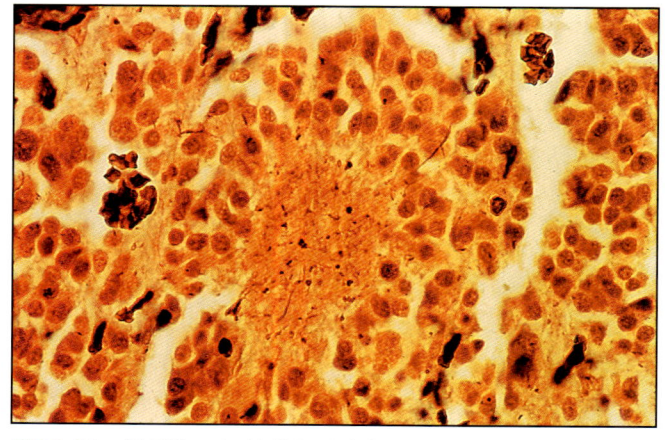

图26.98 银浸染,松果体细胞瘤性玫瑰花结的中央区内显示纤细的神经突起。注意小的终末膨大。Bielschowsky染色。

更为恰当的解释是:肿瘤性松果体细胞的成熟化。它们的出现伴有更为良性的临床过程[499]。在松果体细胞瘤中,显著细胞多形性不常见,但可见个别巨细胞。核分裂象可以见到,但不与临床行为直接相关。大体成功切除后,预后通常较好。

神经元-相关蛋白(NF-H/M和突触素)和光感标记物(视网膜S抗原)在松果体母细胞瘤中均有表达[500-502]。此种表达与松果体细胞的成熟化相一致。极少数肿瘤也可出现节细胞分化,并伴有(或不伴有)肿瘤性星形细胞成分[499]。这些少见肿瘤应被认为是松果体的节细胞瘤和节细胞胶质瘤。这些混合性神经元-胶质肿瘤与CNS内其他部位的同种肿瘤具有相同的行为。

电镜显示,出现9+0神经感觉纤毛、中心粒形成、含有致密核心及透明囊泡的突起、微管鞘、成束的中间丝以及发育良好的环形片层[503],与正常松果体细胞和(或)神经感觉分化的超微结构类似。

松果体母细胞瘤 (图26.99和26.100)
Pineoblastoma

松果体母细胞瘤是最原始的PPT,大约占儿童松果体区肿瘤的3%~17%[491,493,494]。它们好发于1~10岁[491],尽管最初诊断时的年龄极为不同,从新生儿早期至60岁[496,504]。松果体母细胞瘤的男女比为2:1。神经影像学显示多叶状肿物、不均匀对比增强及与邻近结构边界不清[498]。局灶浸润性生长,常常伴有水肿。松果体母细胞瘤是极具侵袭性的肿瘤,容易经CSF通路播散。少数病例出现手术后神经系统外转移[505,506]。

大体上,肿瘤境界不清,切面呈胶样及出血。坏死常见,钙化的出现差异较大。松果体母细胞瘤的镜下所见类似于CNS的原始神经外胚层肿瘤。松果体细胞瘤高度富于细胞,由小而多形的细胞组成,含有圆形或卵圆形的细胞核,具有粗大、浓染的染色质。细胞一般呈无结构片状排列,但可形成Homer Wright玫瑰花结(图26.99)。碳酸银浸染可以显示钝性的细胞突起。极少数可见伴有Flexner-Wintersteiner玫瑰花结的视网膜母细胞瘤样分化和花环样结构[507],反映了人松果体早期光感器个体发育[508,509]。在有些病例中,这种光感器分化也可通过视网膜S抗原免疫组织化学反应来显示[501](图26.100)。节细胞性神经元分化已有报道[510]。这些肿瘤极少数也可有间叶性分化,包括横纹肌和软骨以及黑色素[511,512]。

超微结构特征与分化差的神经上皮性肿瘤一致。然

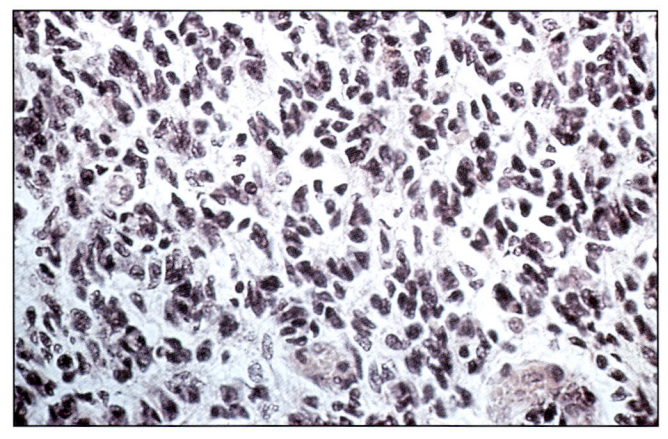

图26.99 松果体母细胞瘤。注意富于密集细胞的排列紧密的原始细胞，界限不清，类似于髓母细胞瘤的原始玫瑰花结（中心）。

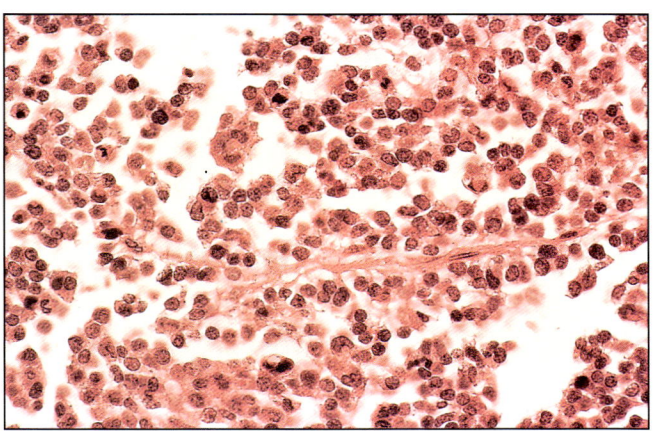

图26.101 中间型松果体实质肿瘤。这些少见的混合性肿瘤的组织学表现从类似于松果体母细胞瘤的高度富于细胞区域到分化更好的区域。一个与早期松果体细胞分化相关的特征是：形成由纤维血管间质分隔的部分叶状结构。注意细胞伸向血管壁的胖胖突起。这种与纤维血管间质的关系可以夸张成更为乳头状的结构，可见于临床更具侵袭性的松果体肿瘤。

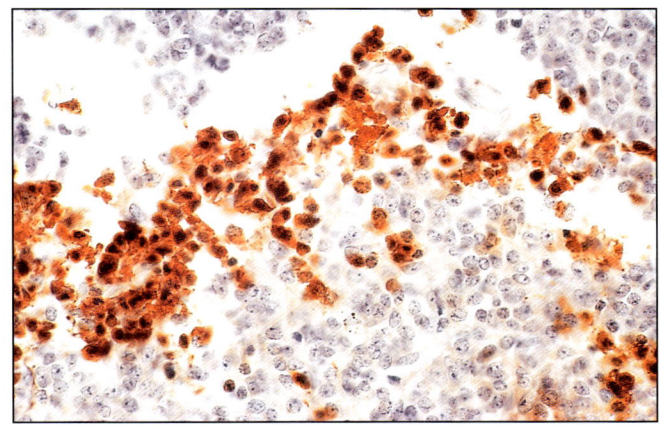

图26.100 松果体母细胞瘤可以显示视网膜S抗原免疫反应性，与肿瘤细胞的光感器谱系一致。S-Ag-PAP免疫过氧化物酶-苏木素双重染色。

而，可以见到早期光感器表型的表达，特征为胞浆细胞器极化、9+0纤毛、环形片层以及发育良好的滑面内质网[503]。

中分化松果体实质肿瘤（图26.101）
Pineal parenchymal tumor intermediate differentiation

相当数量的PPT不能准确地归入松果体母细胞瘤和松果体细胞瘤，可出现介于这两种肿瘤之间的特征。根据新的WHO分类指南[496]，在新近一组病例研究中，中分化PPT占病例的56%。该组包括组织学特征介于松果体细胞瘤和松果体母细胞瘤之间的肿瘤，或者是具有松果体细胞瘤和松果体母细胞瘤混合区域的肿瘤。中分化PPT比松果体细胞瘤更具侵袭性，常常出现局部浸润和远处

CSF播散。

其形态学特征介于松果体细胞瘤和松果体母细胞瘤之间，尤其容易出现单极性肿瘤细胞分叶状分布，被纤细的血管间质整齐勾画出来（图26.101）。当出现分叶状结构而缺乏松果体细胞瘤性玫瑰花结结构时，这些肿瘤常常伴有局部浸润以及沿CSF通路的播散。细胞多形性、坏死和核分裂象也是常见特征。松果体细胞瘤性玫瑰花结极为少见。

松果体实质肿瘤的鉴别诊断：松果体实质肿瘤的稀少强化了区分这些肿瘤与侵犯松果体区的其他神经上皮性肿瘤的重要性，后者包括中枢神经细胞瘤、室管膜瘤以及少突胶质细胞瘤。因此，必须特别注意，对于松果体区的肿瘤应当保留标本进行免疫组化和超微结构分析。相对于中枢神经细胞瘤而言，松果体细胞瘤和中间性肿瘤显示细胞的胞浆境界清楚，细胞多形性更为显著。其细胞间基质不明显，细胞与纤维血管间质的关系更为明显。两种肿瘤中，神经元相关蛋白免疫组化染色均为阳性，因此在鉴别这些肿瘤中帮助不大。中枢神经细胞瘤的超微结构特征因神经细胞分化而具有诊断性，包括众多含有微管排列的突起、致密核心及透明囊泡和突触。与松果体细胞瘤不同，中枢神经细胞瘤并没有粘附带型的细胞间连接。室管膜和少突胶质细胞肿瘤则由于它们的胶质分化而更易于识别。分析光感器的基因表达，尤其是光感受器间维甲酸类结合蛋白（IRBP）和视网膜S抗原，是鉴别松果体肿瘤和此处发生的其他神经上皮性

松果体实质肿瘤的分子细胞遗传学：松果体实质肿瘤的发生机制尚不清楚。有关这些肿瘤的分子和细胞遗传学资料很少，可能归因于病例稀有。然而，单个病例的细胞遗传学研究已经发现这些肿瘤中的极少数特殊染色体异常。松果体细胞瘤出现 11 和 22 号染色体丢失，12q 远端缺失；而松果体母细胞瘤表现为 11q 染色体缺失[504,515-517]。近来，有关 CGH 的报道见于一组 9 例 PPT 中[518]。尽管松果体细胞瘤中没有染色体的增加或丢失，但松果体母细胞瘤和中等分化 PPT 最常见的 DNA 复制数量改变是：12q、4q、5p 和 5q 的增加，以及 22、9q 和 16q 的丢失。然而，迄今为止，由于分析的肿瘤病例数量过少，有关这些染色体异常在肿瘤发病机制中的作用，不难有定论。在 PPT 中，TP53 肿瘤抑制基因分析显示，其既没有 TP53 基因突变，也没有免疫组化 p53 蛋白过表达，提示 TP53 基因通路没有参与这些肿瘤的形成[519]。

胚胎性肿瘤　Embryonal tumors

胚胎性肿瘤（见表 26.1）是原始性的临床侵袭性肿瘤，通常发生于 1 ～ 10 岁。与间变性肿瘤不同，后者常常发生于成人，尽管两者的组织病理学特征相同。有大量证据表明，致癌基因转化事件和胚胎性或原始神经上皮性肿瘤的靶细胞分子学基础上不同于恶性转化或间变性胶质瘤进展[520-523]。所有胚胎性肿瘤，无论其组织发生如何，具有共同的特征，包括细胞丰富、众多核分裂象以及至少局灶性坏死。通常容易出现软脑膜浸润和随后的沿 CSF 通路转移。所有这些特征反映了胚胎性肿瘤的临床侵袭性行为，WHO 分类将其确定为 IV 级肿瘤。

尽管这些胚胎性肿瘤具有共有的特性，但有些肿瘤依据其特殊的组织学特征和假定的组织发生而被划分出来。目前 WHO 分类认为，大脑神经母细胞瘤 / 大脑节细胞神经母细胞瘤和室管膜母细胞瘤为胚胎性肿瘤，分别显示神经元和室管膜分化。髓上皮瘤是一种极为罕见的胚胎性肿瘤，具有特征性的形态学表现，也是 WHO 分类中的一种独立病变。非典型畸胎样 / 横纹肌样肿瘤也归入该类，原因在于其特殊的临床、病理和遗传学特征。最常见的胚胎性肿瘤是髓母细胞瘤，发生于小脑。与髓母细胞瘤无法区别的、位于神经轴其他部位的胚胎性肿瘤为幕上原始神经外胚叶肿瘤（sPNET）。

髓上皮瘤（图 26.102 和 26.103）
Medulloepithelioma

髓上皮瘤是 CNS 最为罕见的胚胎性肿瘤。这种肿瘤临床上见于 0 ～ 5 岁（平均年龄为 29 个月；中位年龄为 22 个月）[524,525]，没有性别倾向[524-527]。在颅内肿瘤患者中，颅内压升高的症状和体征很常见。多数患者在诊断后 1 年内死亡[528]；但是，据报道，极少数病例存活期长达 12 年[524,527,529]。

这种肿瘤多数发生于大脑半球，与侧脑室相关。其他部位也可受累，包括小脑、脑干、第 3 脑室区、中脑和脊髓。脑脊液种植或广泛播散超出原发部位可见于大约 10% 的病例。髓上皮瘤也可位于眼内，源自睫状体，继而浸润视网膜和视神经（见第 29 章）[530]。但多数眼内肿瘤具有良性病程。

髓上皮瘤的组织学标志是核分裂活跃、假复层柱状上皮常常排列成管状或乳头状玫瑰花结，内有多少不等的纤细间质成分（图 26.102）。这些结构再现了神经管原始上皮。大约 50% 的病例出现多系分化，包括神经元、胶质和间叶，或者与神经管混合密切，或者出现境界明显的区域[525]。

免疫组织化学研究显示，原始上皮弥漫表达 nestin[531] 和波形蛋白[525]（图 26.103）。相比之下，神经母细胞和胶质细胞骨架蛋白在上皮结构中仅有极少数散在表达，而这些蛋白在更为分化的细胞成分中表达常见。胰岛素样生长因子 I 以及碱性成纤维生长因子也可见于这种肿瘤[532]。这些病变中的原始神经上皮的超微结构研究显示，胞浆内细胞器稀少、发育中等的腔旁粘附带以及明显缺乏顶部分化[533,534]。

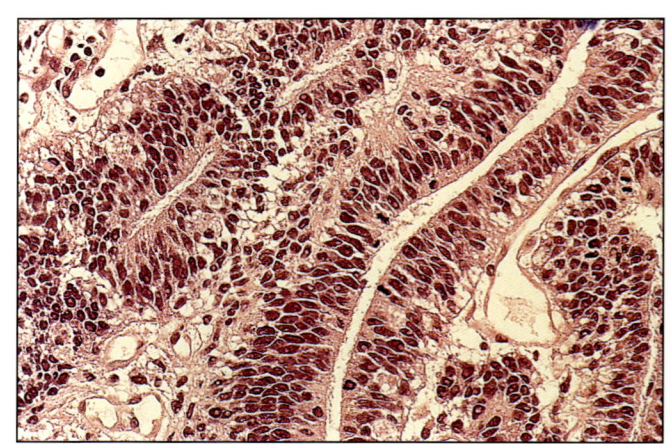

图 26.102　髓上皮瘤的标志性特征是假复层柱状上皮排列成乳头和管状结构。注意上皮的内外界膜。注意与胚胎性神经管的原始神经上皮类似。

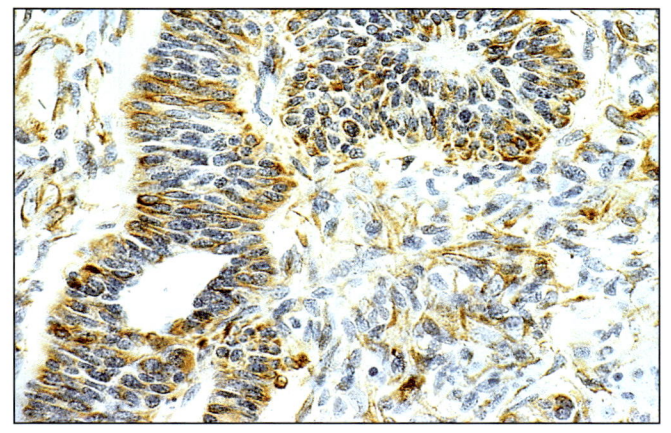

图26.103 髓上皮瘤。波形蛋白免疫反应显示原始神经上皮细胞的细胞突起。波形蛋白-ABC，免疫过氧化物酶-苏木素双重染色。

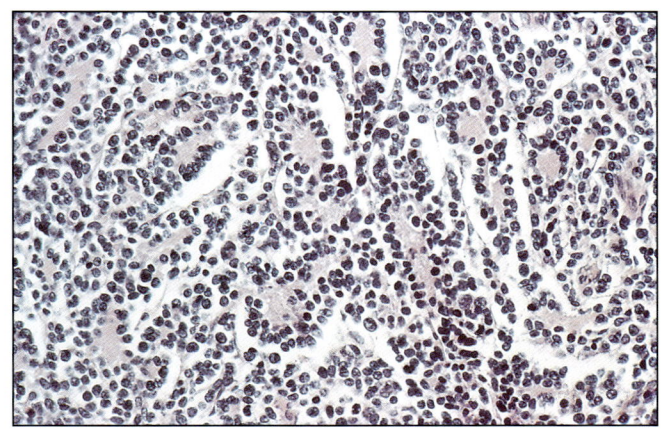

图26.104 神经母细胞瘤的低倍观，常常显示小细胞排列成密集的细胞巢，不同程度勾勒出Homer Wright（神经母细胞）玫瑰花结。

大脑神经母细胞瘤（图26.104至26.107）
Cerebral neuroblastoma

大脑神经母细胞瘤是一种罕见的胚胎性肿瘤，可显示特殊的神经元分化。这肿瘤通常见于10岁以内的较小儿童。尽管肿瘤可发生于整个CNS，包括脑桥、脊髓和马尾，但大多是幕上的、大且多囊性的肿瘤[535-537]。数量不等的结缔组织基质可使这些大体分散的肿瘤质地较硬且部分呈分叶状表现。

在胚胎性肿瘤类型中，大脑神经母细胞瘤是一种特殊的病理学改变，尽管在临床、放射学，甚至形态学方面很难与幕上PNET鉴别[538]。

肿瘤高度富于细胞，由分化较差、但显示不同阶段神经元分化的细胞组成。细胞学特征极为不同，但胞浆境界不清、胞核呈圆形或卵圆形浓染的小细胞最为常见（图26.104）。也可以出现较大的细胞，极性突起清晰，细胞核呈泡状。轻度纤维性基质被纤细的神经突起贯穿为其特征（图26.105）。散在神经母细胞性（Homer Wright）玫瑰花结表现差异较大（图26.104）。可以出现平行排列的细胞成分，细胞核排成规律的栅栏状，类似于髓母细胞瘤[539,540]。节细胞分化，或者是孤立细胞，或者是细胞巢，均可见于中等比例的病例当中[537]（图26.106和26.107），此时，诊断为大脑节细胞神经母细胞瘤[538]。

银浸染和神经元相关细胞骨架蛋白免疫组化染色可以更为特异性地识别神经母细胞性细胞和神经突起。不同于PNET（见下文），大脑神经母细胞瘤和节细胞神经母细胞瘤不出现不同的胶质和神经元分化。因此，GFAP免疫组化可以证实这些原始肿瘤缺乏肿瘤性胶质成分。

超微结构分析证实了这些肿瘤的神经母细胞本质，显示神经元成熟，表现为细胞器密度增加和突触连接分化。

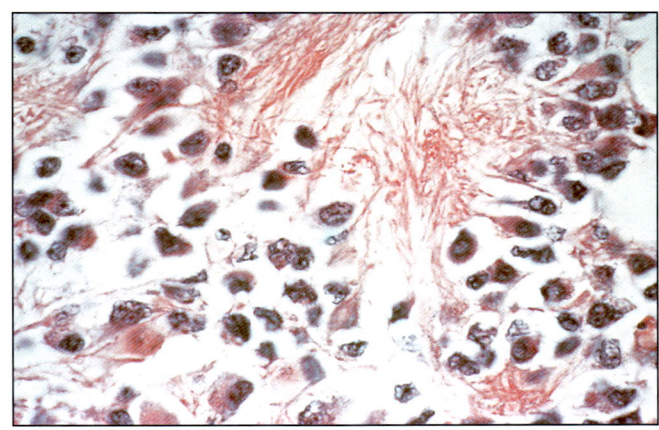

图26.105 5岁男孩右眼的大脑神经母细胞瘤，源自极性细胞的纤细神经突起形成不完全的玫瑰花结。

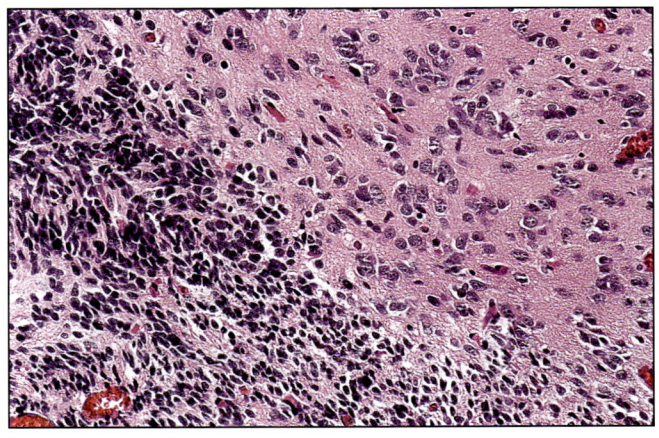

图26.106 在此分化性神经母细胞瘤中，致密的小原始细胞区与神经元分化增多部分相邻。

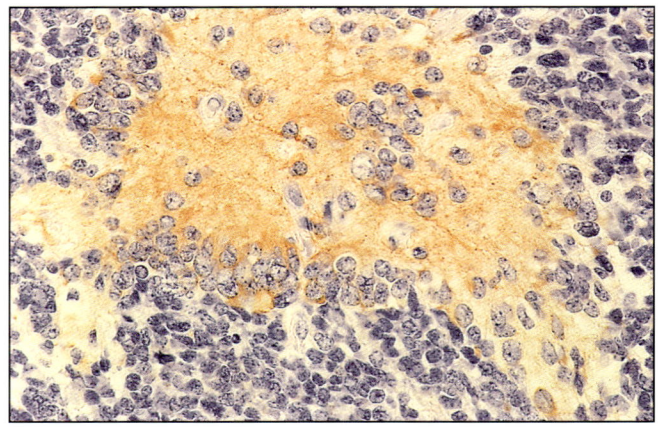

图26.107 神经母细胞瘤。这些细胞成分不甚密集的区域（如图26.106）为Ⅲ型β-微管蛋白表型的免疫反应，与早期神经元分化相一致。TUJ1-ABC免疫过氧化物酶-苏木素双重染色。

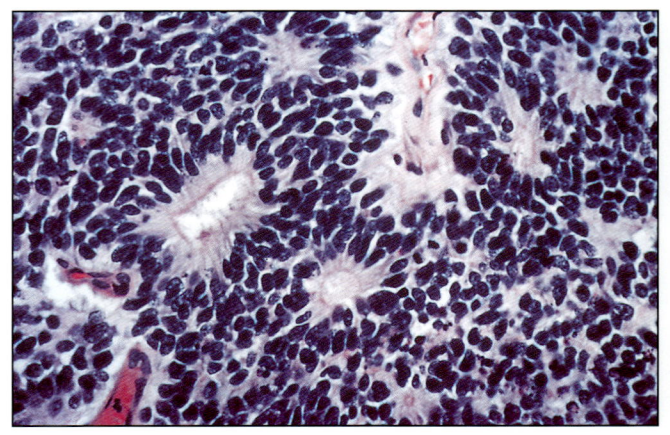

图26.108 此区域显示室管膜母细胞瘤的典型特征，具有实性排列的浓染原始细胞，形成复层的复杂室管膜母细胞玫瑰花结和室管膜管。不同于间变性室管膜瘤，这些肿瘤由相对一致的、分化差的细胞组成，没有明显多形性，缺乏内皮/外皮细胞增生。

室管膜母细胞瘤（图26.108和26.109）
Ependymoblastoma

室管膜母细胞瘤是一种罕见的胚胎性肿瘤，通常见于新生儿和幼儿（平均年龄为 2 岁）[542,543]。所有报道的病例均为颅内肿瘤，尤其是在幕上。尽管这些肿瘤大体上孤立存在，但常常浸润周围脑实质。由于病变常常较大，与脑室的关系难以判定。软脑膜播散和神经以外转移已有报道[544]。

室管膜母细胞瘤的镜下特征包括：高度富于细胞的、分化较差的小细胞呈不定型排列，以及细胞核分裂活性较高，类似于其他胚胎性肿瘤；然而，这种肿瘤的标志是出现特征性的多层玫瑰花结及小管，即所谓的"室管膜母细胞瘤性玫瑰花结"（图26.108）。与室管膜瘤不同，这些玫瑰花结为假复层，常有腔旁核分裂象。此外，常见于室管膜瘤的分化好的血管周围玫瑰花结在室管膜母细胞瘤中极为少见。

GFAP 免疫组化[545,546]可进一步明确肿瘤细胞的原始细胞突起，在血管周围尤其明显（图26.109）。GFAP 免疫反应也可不同程度地见于无定型原始细胞成分以及室管膜玫瑰花结和小管内的个别细胞。也可见到波形蛋白和 S-100 蛋白免疫反应。

超微结构特征可以证实室管膜母细胞瘤的室管膜来源[547]。在玫瑰花结当中，细胞具有腔面胞浆特化，包括微绒毛和 9+2 纤毛。可见腔旁粘附带。在玫瑰花结以外的细胞排列中，胞浆极化形成内衬基底膜的迷路结构。

依据几个镜下特征可将这些肿瘤与间变性室管膜瘤区分开。室管膜母细胞瘤没有分化好的假玫瑰花结，极

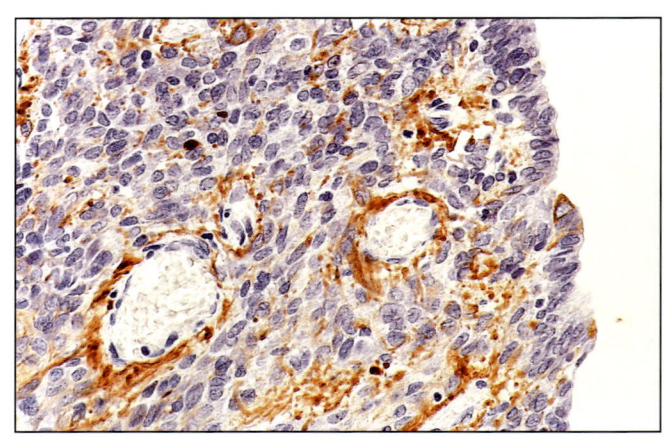

图26.109 室管膜母细胞瘤。胶质纤维酸性蛋白（GFAP）免疫反应细胞散在分布于整个致密排列的细胞密集区。在血管周围区，常常有显著的GFAP免疫反应聚集，即使没有血管周围玫瑰花结形成。GFAP-ABC免疫过氧化物酶-苏木素双重染色。

少见到间变性室管膜瘤的特征性胞浆和胞核多形性。很少或没有微血管内皮细胞增生，但后者在间变性室管膜瘤中常见甚或显著。两种肿瘤均可见坏死，尽管地图样和假栅栏样坏死仅见于间变性室管膜瘤。邻近脑实质的镜下浸润见于两类肿瘤。

视网膜母细胞瘤（图26.110和26.111）
Retinoblastoma

视网膜母细胞瘤（也见第 29 章）是儿童最常见的眼内肿瘤，并且是唯一已知肿瘤性转化遗传性基础的胚胎性肿瘤。这些转化事件发生于不成熟视网膜，在单个细胞内，RB-1 肿瘤抑制基因的两个等位基因失活[548]。

这种肿瘤主要由无定形片状分化差的小细胞组成，但多数视网膜母细胞瘤至少局部出现数量不等的 Flexner-Wintersteiner 和 Homer Wright 玫瑰花结（图 26.110）。偶尔可见分化较好的光感器结构（"菊形团"，"fluerettes"）。神经元/光感器-相关蛋白的表达，如神经微丝亚型、神经元相关性Ⅲ型β-微管蛋白[549]、视网膜 S 抗原[549]、IRBP（图 26.111）以及杆状/锥状视蛋白[513]，也可通过免疫组化或 cDNA 探针来检测，但玫瑰花结或 fluerettes 没有好发部位。GFAP 可标记反应性"间质"星形细胞[513]，这些细胞与血管相关，如在正常视网膜中[550]，位于视网膜与浸润性肿瘤交界处。

研究显示，视网膜母细胞瘤含有多种细胞类型，提示它们来源于多潜能细胞。我们实验室对于原位视网膜母细胞瘤的研究表明，这些肿瘤组织具有类似于不成熟视网膜神经上皮的组织发生潜能，但限于光感器（锥状和杆状）和 Müller 细胞系[513]。

髓母细胞瘤（图 26.112 至 26.116）
Medulloblastoma

髓母细胞瘤是最常见的胚胎性肿瘤，是儿童最常见的恶性 CNS 肿瘤[551]。在儿童，大约占所有颅内肿瘤的 1/4，多数发生于 1～10 岁，高峰年龄是 7 岁，具有轻度男性倾向[551]。

这些肿瘤多数位于小脑中线，尽管也发生于小脑半球侧面。大体上，为质软、易碎的肿块。坏死为其一致性特征，可弥漫分布，表现为点状或更广泛的带状病灶，有时形成中央空洞。与该部位的毛细胞型星形细胞瘤相比，囊肿形成极为少见。促纤维增生型或结节型（见下文）更多见于小脑半球侧面，境界清楚，质地较硬。

髓母细胞瘤细胞丰富，由相对较小的细胞组成，胞浆稀少，细胞境界不清（图 26.112）。胞核深染，具有特征性的不规则胞膜，成角或呈卵圆形（图 26.112）。这些特征使其在术中涂片中与正常颗粒细胞易于区别。细胞通常排列成片状，尽管局部可形成规律的栅栏状细胞核。肿瘤细胞弥漫浸润小脑皮质，颗粒层和分子层消失。核分裂象易见。凋亡和坏死常见，但微血管内皮细胞增生罕见。

尽管常规光镜下肿瘤分化较差，但是大约 1/3 的髓母细胞瘤具有神经母细胞分化，表现为出现神经母细胞（Homer Wright）玫瑰花结、明显的细胞间纤维性基质以及大的泡状核细胞增生[552]；具有神经母细胞分化的少数肿瘤也含有肿瘤性节细胞成分。神经元相关标记物呈阳性，包括Ⅲ型β-微管蛋白同型、神经微丝表型，并且突触素常常见于细胞及其细胞突起（图 26.113 和 26.114）。星形细胞分化，可通过 GFAP 反应性来显示，见于近乎 10% 的病例[551,553]。然而，反应性间质星形细胞与真正肿瘤性星形细胞很难鉴别。

髓母细胞瘤的几种变型已经明确，不仅因为其组织学特征，还因为其自身重要的预后意义。它们是：（1）经典型，由片状未分化细胞组成，伴有数量不等的上述神经母细胞玫瑰花结和栅栏状结构；（2）促结缔组织增生或结节型髓母细胞瘤；（3）大细胞或间变性髓母细胞瘤；（4）髓肌母细胞瘤；以及（5）黑色素型髓母细胞瘤。

促结缔组织增生或结节型髓母细胞瘤大约占肿瘤的大约 10%～12%[552,554]。这些肿瘤因其质地较硬且含有较多量的结缔组织而引人注意，因其双相结构及伴有结

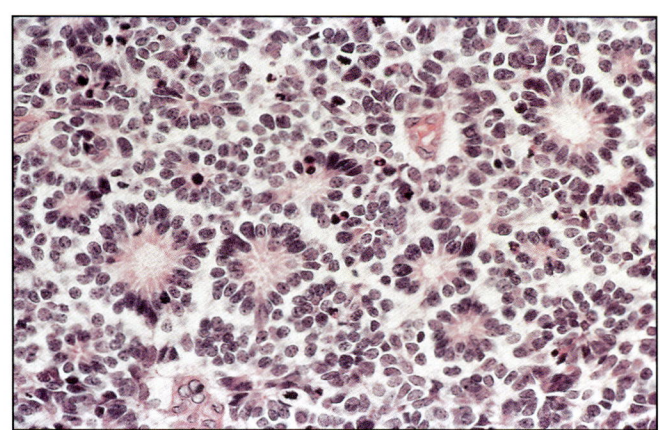

26.110　Flexner-Wintersteiner玫瑰花结，如果出现，为视网膜母细胞瘤的诊断性组织病理学特征之一。

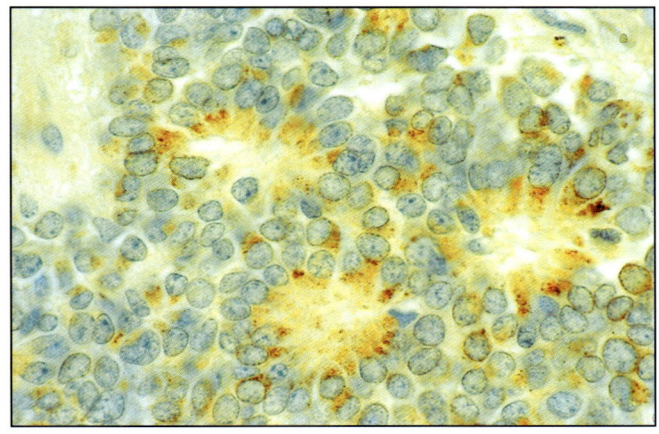

26.111　视网膜母细胞。玫瑰花结和单个肿瘤细胞出现光感器间视网膜结合蛋白（IRRP）免疫反应，与视网膜母细胞瘤的光感器分化一致。注意细胞极性分布，形成玫瑰花结。IRBP-ABC免疫过氧化物酶-苏木素双重染色。

胚胎性肿瘤

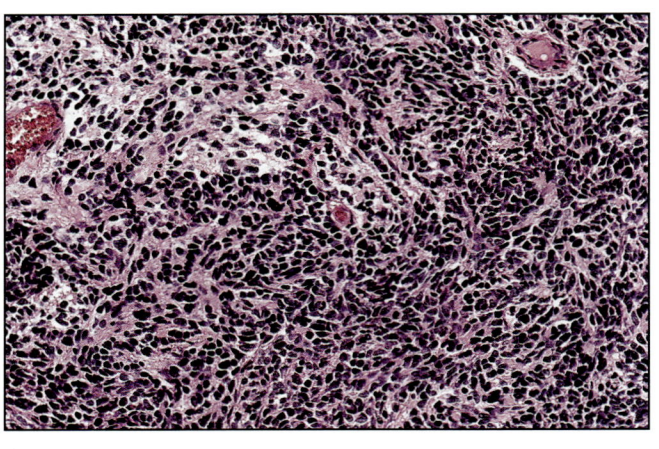
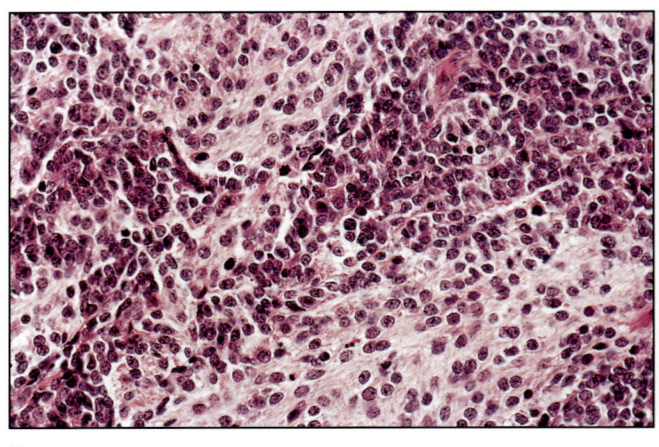

A　　　　　　　　　　　　　　　　　　　　　B

图26.112　髓母细胞瘤是细胞丰富的肿瘤，由紧密排列的原始细胞组成（A）。高度富于细胞的区域常常与细胞较少、出现细丝状细胞间基质的区域混合出现（B）。

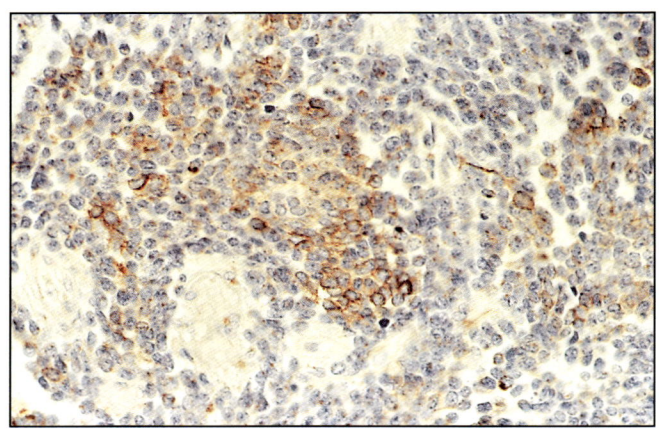
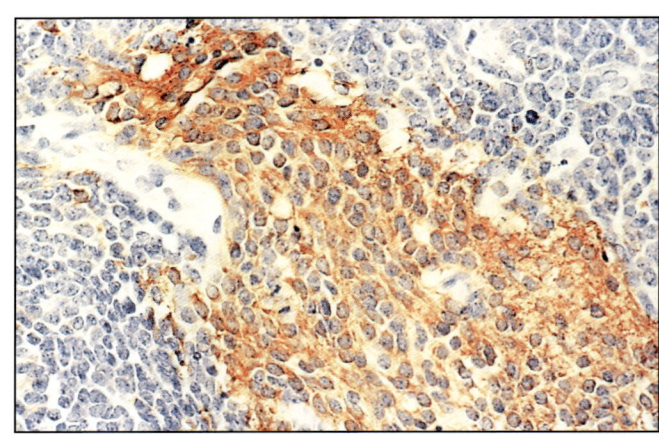

26.113　髓母细胞瘤。非磷酸化依赖性神经微丝（NF-H/M）表型的免疫反应常常显示肿瘤细胞较少区域的神经母细胞/神经元分化。SMI 33-ABC免疫过氧化物酶-苏木素双重染色。

26.114　髓母细胞瘤。神经元相关Ⅲ型β-微管蛋白免疫组化（与图26.113为同一病例）显示，Ⅲ型β-微管蛋白免疫反应与神经微丝标记的分布相似。TUJ1-ABC免疫过氧化物酶-苏木素双重染色。

节状排列的肿瘤细胞而与众不同（图 26.115）。结节的特征是：细胞不甚丰富，与细胞丰富的结节间区交替出现。形成结节的细胞稍大，具有较大的常染色质细胞核，呈神经细胞样表现，包埋在细丝状的神经毡样背景之中。这些神经元样分化特征也可以通过神经元相关标记物的免疫反应来显示[551,555,556]。相比之下，细胞丰富区域由原始性表现的小细胞组成，核分裂活性和增殖标记指数增加。这种独特的双相结构通过网织染色表现最为明显，网织纤维阴性的结节与富于细胞的网织纤维丰富的区域形成对比。这种髓母细胞瘤亚型的临床行为好于经典型的，因此识别这些肿瘤成为治疗髓母细胞瘤的重要一步（见下文）。

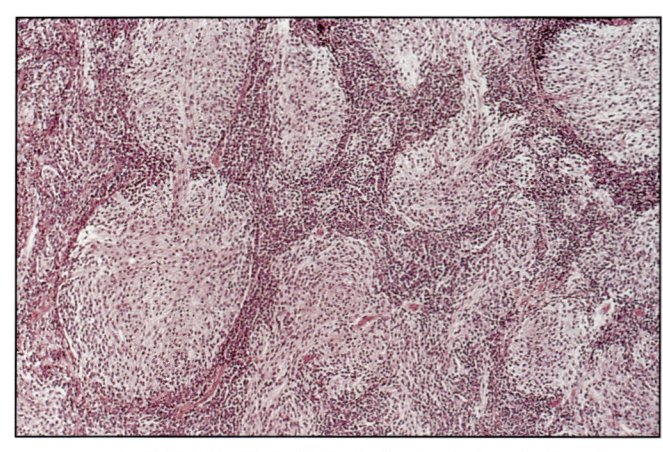

26.115　促结缔组织增生/结节型髓母细胞瘤。低倍放大，可使促结缔组织增生型髓母细胞瘤的结节状外观更为明显。在细胞不丰富区域，没有网织纤维，而神经微丝和Ⅲ型β-微管蛋白表型呈强阳性。

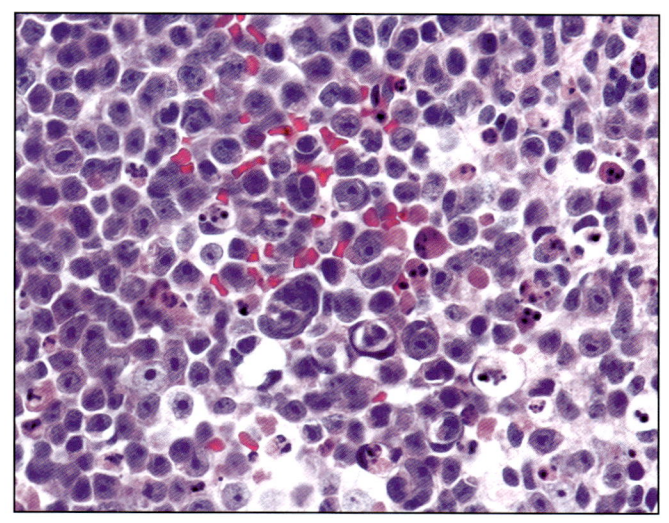

26.116 间变性/大细胞髓母细胞瘤。细胞核较大,众多核分裂象及核型是此型髓母细胞瘤的特征性结构。注意大量凋亡表现。

髓母细胞瘤的一个不常见变型是**大细胞**或**间变性髓母细胞瘤**[551,557]。这些肿瘤大约占髓母细胞瘤的4%,极具侵袭性生物行为。组织学上,它们以多角形细胞为特征,细胞核较大,多形性,核仁明显,与较为经典的肿瘤相比,其胞浆更丰富(图26.116)。核型典型。肿瘤出现高核分裂活性、凋亡以及明显坏死区。

髓母细胞瘤的其他罕见变型包括**髓肌母细胞瘤和黑色素型髓母细胞瘤**,前者显示横纹肌细胞分化,具有与横纹肌肉瘤类似的更为原始的细胞成分[558];后者具有色素性乳头状结构。这些变型与普通类型的髓母细胞瘤的关系尚不清楚。

近来,大量临床研究显示,髓母细胞瘤是异质性肿瘤,具有不同的临床预后以及治疗效果,与其组织学特征和分子表型有关[551,559]。组织学谱系中两个极端是前面提到的促结缔组织增生型/结节型髓母细胞瘤和大细胞/间变性髓母细胞瘤。尽管髓母细胞瘤的官方分级系统还没有被广泛接受,但建议根据肿瘤的分化程度或间变性进行分级[559,560]。间变性髓母细胞瘤的特征是:核增大、有明显的细胞学间变、核分裂及凋亡比例增加,具有侵袭性临床行为[560,561]。另一方面,肿瘤显示神经元分化特征包括:广泛结节状表现,在统计学上比经典髓母细胞瘤具有更长的存活期[559,561]。组织病理学上,随着时间进展,从分化较好的结节状髓母细胞瘤发展到间变性类型已有报道。此外,最新的研究表明,髓母细胞瘤的组织学分类与分子表型相结合是将来对这些肿瘤进行更为精确的预后分级的基础[562-564]。

髓母细胞瘤的分子细胞遗传学:细胞遗传学研究显示,17q等位染色体[i(17q)]是髓母细胞瘤最常见的异常表现,见于大约1/3的肿瘤[551]。分子研究已经证实,常常出现17p染色体的杂合性丢失(LOH)[565]。尽管这是一个含有*TP53*基因位点的区域,但是该基因突变很少见于髓母细胞瘤[565,567]。

其他多种细胞遗传学改变已有报道,包括1q、10q、11p/11q、16q和9q染色体缺失。在后者当中,位于9q22(*PTCH*)的基底细胞癌细胞综合征位点分布于此处。具有*PTCH*基因种系突变的患者(Gorlin综合征)容易发生髓母细胞瘤,尤其是促结缔组织增生型/结节型变型[568]。此基因突变也见于散发性髓母细胞瘤[569]。具有*PTCH1*基因突变的髓母细胞瘤其下游DNA结合蛋白(如Gli1)表达发生改变,是新型治疗的潜在分子靶点。因此,识别这种具有*PTCH1*信号改变的髓母细胞瘤亚型具有预后和治疗意义[570,571]。结肠腺瘤性息肉基因(*APC*)突变及其相应的2型Turcot综合征(*APC*体系突变)相关性Wnt信号通路,也与髓母细胞瘤的发生有关;然而,仅有少数散发性髓母细胞瘤具有Wnt/APC通路突变[572]。

在几项研究中,*myc*癌基因扩增与恶性行为有关[559],*c-myc* mRNA表达增加被认为是预后不良的指标[573,574]。*c-myc*癌基因改变与大细胞/间变型髓母细胞瘤亚型密切相关[559]。或者,*N-myc*下调和神经营养因子受体TrkC表达较高与生存期较长有关[565,575,576]。此外,最新资料表明,*ERBB2*表达与预后较差有关,无论其组织学亚型如何[577]。

非典型畸胎样/横纹肌样肿瘤 (图26.117)
Atypical teratoid/rhabdoid tumor

非典型畸胎样/横纹肌样肿瘤(AT/RhT)是一组罕见的儿童脑肿瘤,因具有特殊的"横纹肌样"细胞而与众不同。这些肿瘤大多发生于后颅窝,幕上肿瘤和累及多部位的肿瘤并不少见[578-580]。75%的患为3岁或更小儿童,男性相对好发。

大体上,肿瘤一般较大、质软,出现局灶性坏死和出血区。1/3的肿瘤在诊断时已经沿CSF通路播散,颅神经受累很常见。组织学上,肿瘤以大多角形细胞为特征,细胞核偏位,核仁明显,嗜酸性胞浆含有球状纤维性胞浆内包涵体(图26.117)。横纹肌样细胞成簇排列,或者与原始神经上皮细胞混杂,可产生具有髓母细胞瘤、间叶性梭形细胞成分以及多种上皮成分特征的混合性肿瘤印象。

尽管标志性细胞称为"横纹肌样",但它们缺乏真正的肌肉分化,结蛋白免疫染色呈阴性。细胞波形蛋白

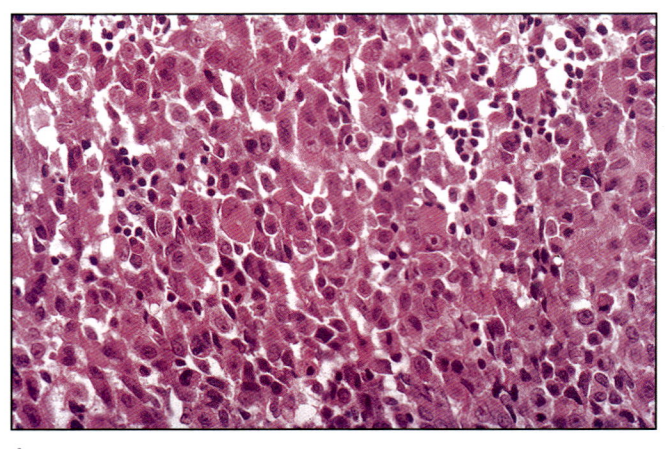
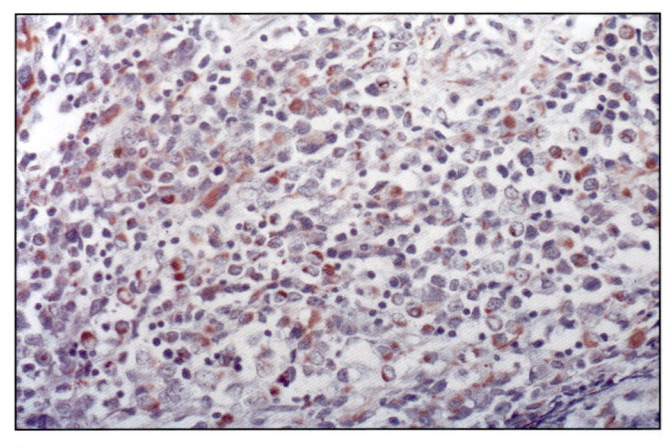

26.117 非典型畸胎样/横纹肌样肿瘤。（A）许多肿瘤细胞有丰富的嗜酸性胞浆，使该胚胎性肿瘤呈横纹肌样表现。（B）波形蛋白免疫组化反应在大多数肿瘤细胞呈强阳性，包涵体更加明显。ABC免疫过氧化物酶-苏木素双重染色。

呈强阳性（图26.117B），上皮膜抗原（EMA）和平滑肌肌动蛋白（SMA）呈不同程度免疫染色阳性；与GFAP、细胞角蛋白和神经微丝蛋白偶尔也有反应[580]。生殖细胞标记物多数呈阴性，包括PLAP、AFP和β-HCG[581]。

AT/RhT遗传学分析对于将此独立性病变从胚胎性肿瘤中鉴别出来是必不可少的。细胞遗传学分析显示特殊的22染色体异常，或者是单体，或者是22q11.2部分性缺失，可以区分这些肿瘤和髓母细胞瘤[582,583]。此区域含有INI1/hSNF5基因，该基因编码SW1/SNF染色体重构复合体成分[366, 584]。

非典型畸胎样/横纹肌样肿瘤是极具侵袭性的肿瘤。报道的平均生存期是6个月，随访2年时，总体生存率不足20%[580,582]。肿瘤预后极差，部分原因可能是容易脑脊髓种植[585]。

幕上原始神经外胚叶肿瘤
Supratentorial primitive neuroectodermal tumors

原始神经外胚叶肿瘤（PNET）的定义包含一个概念，即这些肿瘤源自遍布于整个神经轴的原始神经上皮的前体细胞。因此，这些肿瘤具有相似的组织病理学特征和生物学行为。这一概念提示，未分化的神经上皮细胞转化后，PNET中可出现多潜能表型分化[586]。也就是说，胚胎性肿瘤出现肿瘤转化之前即确定了稳定而有限的基因型特征。

目前，将幕上PNET用于诊断分类还只限于组织学上与小脑髓母细胞瘤无法区别但位于大脑或鞍上区域的肿瘤；对于这些肿瘤的推荐术语是幕上PNET[538]。

幕上PNET极其少见。在由美国国家癌症研究所流行病学监测和最终结果项目（SEER）进行的最新调查中，诊断为髓母细胞瘤或PNET（M/PNET）的肿瘤发生率是每年4.9/100万人，男性好发[587]。在同一调查中，有768例患者诊断为M/PNET，只有53例(7%)为幕上肿瘤。

幕上PNET的组织病理学特征与髓母细胞瘤相似（见下文）。肿瘤细胞丰富，由原始未分化细胞构成，无排列结构。相对纤维性的背景。诸如Homer Wright玫瑰花结的特殊排列也可以见到。核分裂活性较高，常见有凋亡现象。单个细胞坏死以及大片融合性坏死也可出现。与髓母细胞瘤类似，通过神经元和胶质细胞相关标记物的免疫组化表达，幕上PNET可出现多种分化证据[538]。

与髓母细胞瘤相比，有关幕上PNET的遗传学异常知之甚少。目前有关资料表明，幕上PNET的染色体和遗传学异常与髓母细胞瘤常见的那些不同。17q等位染色体可例外地见于幕上PNET[588]，而幕上PNET不出现LOH 17p[589,590]。这些肿瘤的基因表达谱系显示缺乏集群以及分子异质性，可能反映了此类肿瘤的多种谱系[588]。

区分幕上PNET和外周PNET很重要。除了这两类PNET的起源和自然病程外，这两类胚胎性肿瘤的病理生理学和分子生物学完全不同。外周PNET源于软组织、骨及周围神经，与骨外和骨内的Ewing肉瘤关系密切（见第25章和第27章）。Ewing家族的这些小蓝细胞肿瘤绝大多数以常见的t（11;22)(q24;q12)染色体易位和EWS/FLI-1融合基因为特征[591]。可以识别MIC2基因产物的CD99免疫反应是外周PNET肿瘤的特征[591]。然而，重要的是要强调，幕上PNET不具有这种遗传学表型，因此不表达CD99。然而，原发性硬膜内外周 PNET 也有报道，源自颅内和脊髓内硬膜的周围神经部分[592,593]。

脑膜肿瘤（表26.4）
Tumors of the meninges

脑膜上皮细胞肿瘤（表26.4和26.5）
Tumors of meningothelial cells

脑膜瘤（图26.118至26.125） Meningioma

脑膜瘤是源于蛛网膜细胞的肿瘤，蛛网膜细胞见于蛛网膜绒毛和颗粒以及血管旁间隙和脉络膜丛的间质内[594]。脑膜瘤大约占所有原发性 CNS 肿瘤的28%[156]，颅内肿瘤的15%，脊髓内肿瘤的25%[595]。脑膜瘤出现临床症状多在中年，极少数见于儿童。在成人有明显的女性倾向（3:1），尤其是硬膜内肿瘤。硬膜外肿瘤常见于儿童病例[594]，其中男性好发[596]。多发性脑膜瘤发生于近8%的病例[597]，尤其是伴有神经纤维瘤病2型（NF2）的病例[594]。这种相关性在儿童更高，近40%的患有脑膜瘤的儿童伴有 NF2[596]。极少数家族性非-NF2 相关的脑膜瘤也有发生[595]。

表26.4　脑膜肿瘤

脑膜上皮细胞肿瘤

1. 脑膜瘤
   变型：脑膜上皮（合体）型，过渡型，纤维（纤维母细胞）型，沙粒体型，血管瘤型，微囊型，分泌型，富于淋巴浆细胞型，化生型，透明细胞型，脊索瘤样型，嗜酸细胞型
2. 非典型脑膜瘤
3. 乳头状脑膜瘤
4. 横纹肌样脑膜瘤
5. 间变性脑膜瘤

非脑膜上皮脑膜肿瘤

1. **良性肿瘤**
   骨软骨瘤
   脂肪瘤
   纤维组织细胞瘤
   孤立性纤维性肿瘤
2. **恶性肿瘤**
   血管外皮细胞瘤
   软骨肉瘤
   间叶性软骨肉瘤
   横纹肌肉瘤
   脑膜肉瘤病
   黑色素瘤

表26.5　脑膜瘤和WHO分级

脑膜瘤变型	WHO分级
脑膜上皮型	I
纤维（纤维母细胞）型	
过渡（混合）型	
沙粒体型	
血管瘤样型	
微囊型	
分泌型	
富于淋巴浆细胞型	
化生型	
脊索样型	II
透明细胞型	
非典型*	
横纹肌样	III
乳头状	
间变性（恶性）*	

*任何亚型的脑膜瘤均可分为非典型或间变性。

脑膜瘤可发生于具有脑膜上皮细胞的任何神经轴部位。然而，有些部位比较好发。颅内最常见于大脑镰部、大脑凸面、嗅沟、蝶骨嵴、鞍结节和蝶鞍旁区。脑室内的脑膜瘤可能源自脉络组织或脉络丛间质内的蛛网膜细胞，左边侧脑室是最常见的部位，虽然15%源于第三脑室[598]。脑膜瘤也可以位于松果体区。脑膜瘤占眼眶膨胀性病变的3%，也可见于颞骨（岩骨内）[599]。在后颅窝，岩骨上方的小脑脑桥角是常见部位[600]。在椎管，脑膜瘤见于胸、颈及腰部，发生率依次降低。与成人相比，儿童脑膜瘤好发于不常见部位，包括脑室、后颅窝和硬脊膜区[596]。这些肿瘤的各种其他颅外和异位部位也有报道[594,601]。

神经影像学分析是脑膜瘤组织病理学诊断的重要补充，尤其是对形态学表现不同寻常的病例。血管造影常常可显示特征性的肿瘤红色，表明这些肿瘤高度富于血管，同样，CT 和 MRI 显示弥漫性对比增强。MRI 对于区分该肿瘤的优势组织学结构也有些帮助，尤其是 T2 加权像，与纤维母细胞成分比较，合体细胞和血管瘤样成分的密度较高[602]。MRI 也可以区分肿瘤-大脑的相互关系不同类型，包括良好的胶原性包膜、CSF 间隙或脑粘附及浸润，因而有助于对脑与肿瘤交界处进行直接细致的评估。

多数脑膜瘤为大体上境界清楚的、具有薄层包膜的球形肿块；但也有例外，表现为斑块、扁平、地毯状肿瘤，常常见于蝶骨嵴上方。肿瘤生长缓慢，压迫脑组织，侵蚀邻近结构。常见有硬膜侵犯和骨组织受累，后者可引

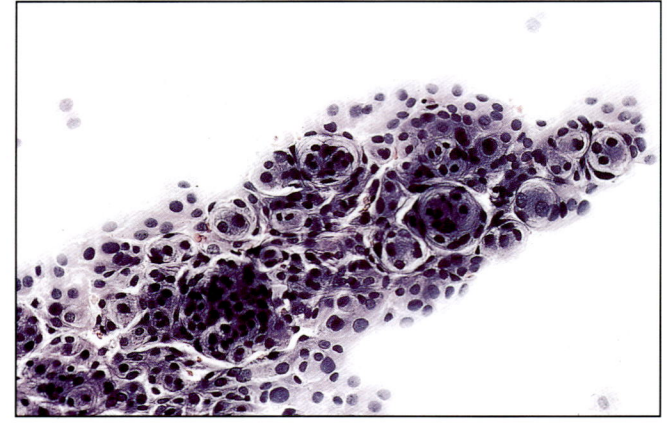

图26.118 脑膜瘤。涂片显示典型脑膜上皮细胞，胞浆境界不清。细胞核染色质淡染，粉末状，伴有明显的染色质结节。此例中漩涡状结构明显。Morris染色。

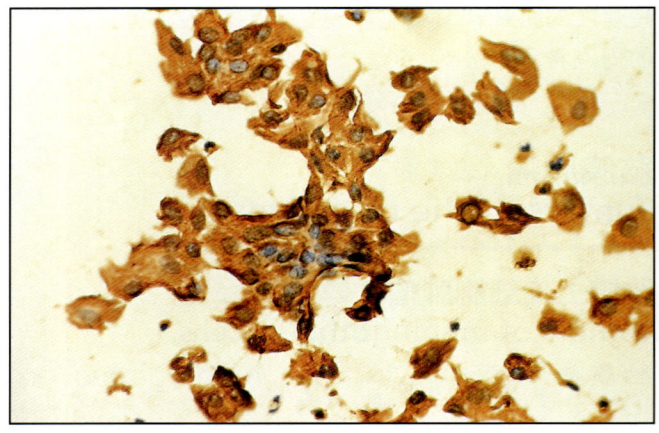

图26.120 在术中活检涂片中，波形蛋白免疫染色见于大多数脑膜瘤，如图所示。波形蛋白-ABC免疫过氧化物酶-苏木素双重染色。

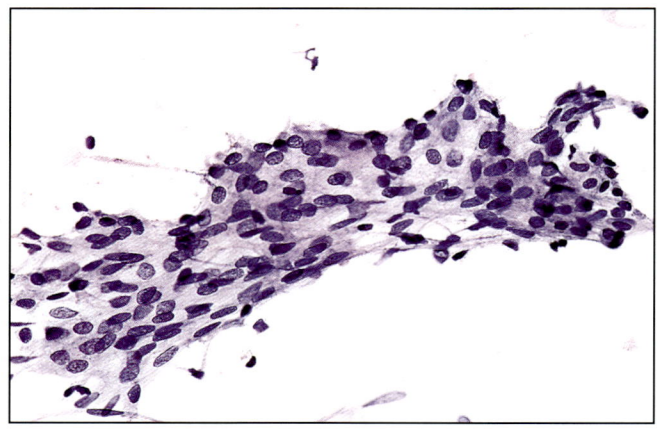

图26.119 高倍放大后易见脑膜瘤的特征性纤细染色质结构。Morris染色。

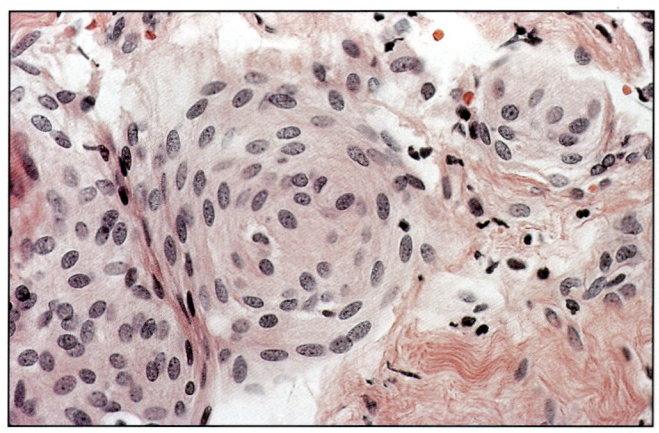

图26.121 过渡型脑膜瘤的组织学切片中，其典型的脑膜上皮漩涡状结构与图26.118中的结构很类似。注意其显示与图26.119相同的染色质特征。

起不同程度的骨质增生。切面特征差异极大，常常可反映优势组织学亚型，如质地坚韧，伴有大量沙粒体，或者质地为更为脂性的分泌型。

组织学表型：众多脑膜瘤变型已有报道[595]，表明有蛛网膜细胞间叶和上皮性组织发生潜能（见表26.4）。尽管这些变型中的绝大多数出现类似的生物学行为，但有些伴发系统性疾病，如脊索样变型伴有Castleman病[595]、富于淋巴浆细胞型肿瘤伴有多克隆丙种球蛋白病[595]。最为重要的是，四种脑膜瘤变型（透明细胞型、脊索样型、乳头型和横纹肌样型）具有较高的侵袭性行为潜能。

脑膜细胞型（合体性）和**过渡型**脑膜瘤可以出现这些肿瘤中最为典型的"脑膜上皮"表现，特征是境界不清的细胞团围绕血管或间质成分形成漩涡状结构（图26.118和26.121）以及出现沙粒体。细胞核染色质均匀分布，核仁不明显（图26.119和26.121）。核内的胞浆包涵体常常被描述为核"空泡"或核"假包涵体"，在这些变型中常见。

蛛网膜细胞的间叶和上皮表型在其他类型的脑膜瘤中也有很好的反映。纤维型（纤维母细胞性）、血管瘤型（图26.125）以及化生型组成"间叶性"变型。它们含有不同程度的网织纤维且富于胶原；也可以见到细胞外基质蛋白，如层粘连蛋白[603]、纤维结合素以及Ⅳ型和Ⅴ型胶原。化生性病变可出现软骨-骨分化甚或明显的脂化[604]。脑膜瘤"上皮"表型的表达可见于微囊型（图26.122）、分泌型（图26.123）、透明细胞型（图26.124）（富于糖原）、脊索样型以及乳头型（图26.130）变型。PAS-阳性包涵体多见于分泌型，胞浆腔缘被覆微绒毛[605]。透明细胞型和脊索样型更具侵袭性生长方式，类似于非典型脑膜瘤。这两种类型的脑膜瘤被认为是WHO Ⅱ级

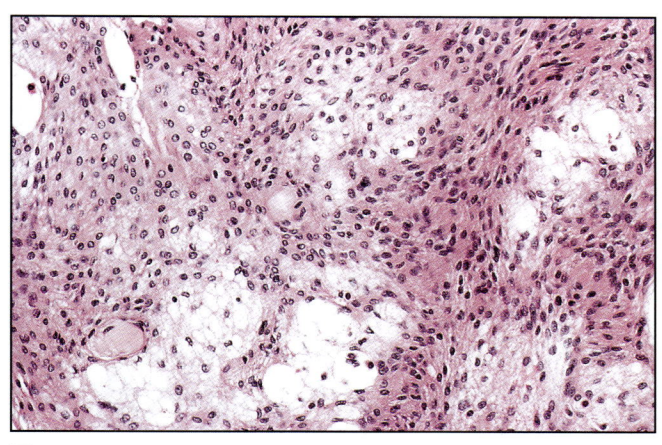

图26.122 微囊型脑膜瘤由合体/脑膜上皮细胞型混合而成，伴有微囊区域。

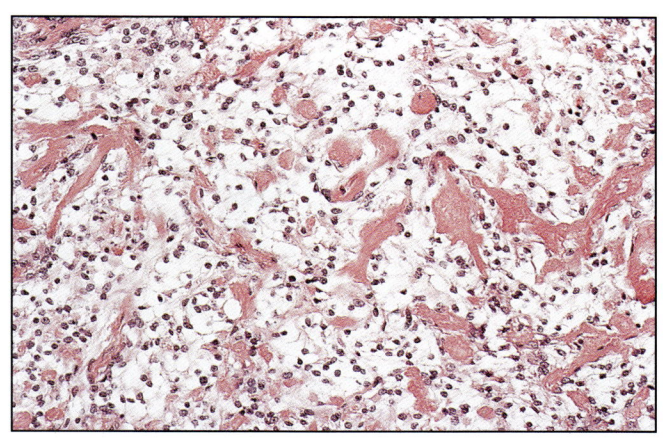

图26.124 透明细胞型脑膜瘤由充满大量糖原的细胞构成。注意特征性的脑膜上皮染色质结构。

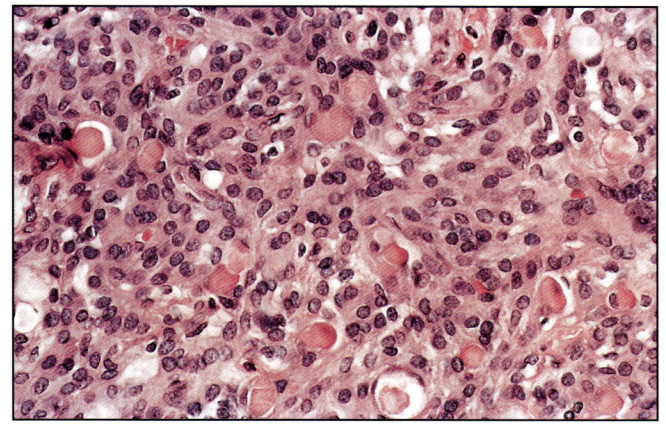

图26.123 多角形细胞，胞浆境界清楚，含有嗜酸性包涵体，一般为分泌型脑膜瘤。

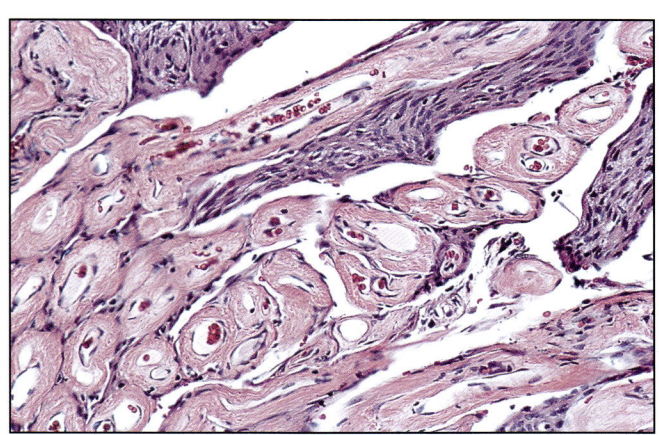

图26.125 血管瘤型脑膜瘤中，玻璃样变血管与小巢合体性排列的脑膜上皮细胞相混合。对于此变型，有必要仔细检查，以证明这些肿瘤的脑膜上皮属性。

肿瘤（见下文）。透明细胞脑膜瘤含有丰富的糖原，常常位于后颅窝或脊柱，具有侵袭性生长方式，包括复发率较高和脊髓播散[606]。脊索样型脑膜瘤可出现特殊的核型[607]，含有类似脊索瘤组织学结构区域，即在黏液样基质中，可见带状排列的嗜酸性空泡状细胞。

    脑膜瘤的免疫组化特征与前体细胞间叶及上皮双相属性一致。主要的中间纤维丝是波形蛋白，见于几乎100%的病例[27,594]（图26.120），支持其为间叶性本质。然而，CK 表型和 EMA 可出现不同程度的局灶或弥漫性分布。CK 免疫反应阳性率在整个脑膜瘤中大约为20%，但在上皮性亚型中接近40%[27,29]。CEA 免疫染色见于分泌型[595]。S-100 蛋白免疫反应不一，见于大约50%的病例，主要位于纤维母细胞区域[26,27]。GFAP 均为阴性。最近，一种紧密连接相关蛋白，即 claudin-1，被认为对鉴别诊断有益，尽管只有大约50%的脑膜瘤为阳性[607a]。

    脑膜瘤的分级：脑膜瘤依据组织学间变和侵袭性行为潜能进行分级（见表26.5）。这里依据间变组织学特征列出了三种主要类别，即脑膜瘤（WHO Ⅰ级）、非典型脑膜瘤（WHO Ⅱ级）以及间变性（恶性）脑膜瘤（WHO Ⅲ级）。此外，特殊变型的脑膜瘤由于其特殊的侵袭性行为潜能也予以强调。包括透明细胞和脊索样脑膜瘤（WHO Ⅱ级）以及乳头型和横纹肌样脑膜瘤（WHO Ⅲ级）。WHO Ⅰ级脑膜瘤是良性肿瘤，增殖指数低，报道的平均 Ki-67（MIB-1）标记指数约为4%[608]。

非典型脑膜瘤——WHO Ⅱ级（图26.126和26.127）
Atypical meningioma-WHO grade Ⅱ

非典型脑膜瘤是体现复发潜能相关组织学特征的肿瘤[595]。尽管这些肿瘤缺乏明确的与恶性相关的组织学特征，但它们更容易出现复发及局部侵袭性行为[609,610]。这些肿瘤与**脊索样型**和**透明细胞型**一起被认为是WHO Ⅱ级肿瘤。

WHO分类认为，非典型脑膜瘤具有高的核分裂指数 [≥ 4/10 高倍视野（HPF）]；或者出现下列五种组织学特征中的至少三个：片状结构、大核仁、小细胞形成、细胞密集以及坏死。这些特征可见于任何组织学变型。通常，这些组织学特征在整个肿瘤中的分布并不一致，说明了细致检查多张组织学切片对于评估脑膜瘤的必要性。Ki-67（MIB-1）标记指数与肿瘤分级增加相关[610-612]。

非典型脑膜瘤Ki-67标记指数平均约为7%[608]。

脑组织浸润：脑组织浸润（图26.128）表现为脑实质浸润和融合，强烈提示侵袭性临床行为[596]。具有这一特征的肿瘤，不论其间变程度如何，均容易复发。有些作者认为，脑膜瘤出现脑浸润至少应当为WHO Ⅱ级[596]。然而，WHO分类对于本身有脑浸润的肿瘤并没有一个分级标准[595]。仔细检查经GFAP免疫组化染色的肿瘤与脑组织交界处，有助于识别脑浸润和融合情况（图26.128B）。此标准仅限于评估首次切除标本，因为在复发标本中，脑组织与肿瘤交界处可能由于先前的外科操作而出现明显改变。

间变性（恶性）脑膜瘤（图26.129）
Anaplastic (malignant) meningioma

非典型与间变性脑膜瘤的不同在于程度，它们具有相同的组织病理学特征；因此，间变性脑膜瘤出现显著细胞核及细胞多形性、核分裂活性高以及坏死（图26.129）。核分裂活性为此类肿瘤分类的重要部分，指数可高达20个/10HPF以上[595]。

两种特殊的脑膜瘤变型为Ⅲ级脑膜瘤，类似于间变性脑膜瘤，即**乳头型**和**横纹肌样脑膜瘤**。

乳头型脑膜瘤，极少见的恶性变型，较多见于儿童和年轻成人，极易浸润和复发，常常出现远处转移[596,613]。因此，该变型被确定为WHO Ⅲ级[595]。组织学上，这种肿瘤高度富于细胞，由上皮样细胞组成，呈立方性/

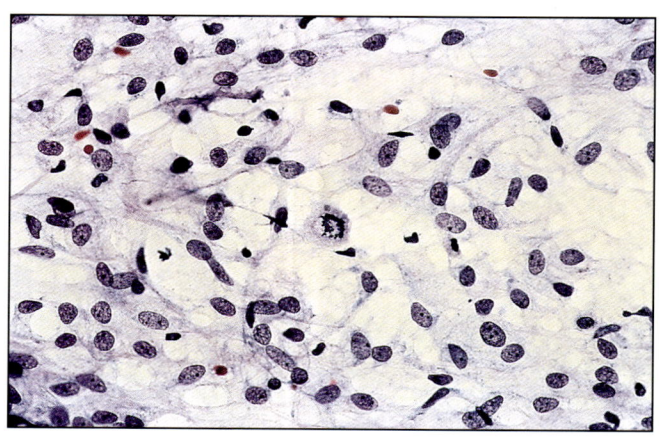

图26.126　非典型脑膜瘤涂片，显示脑膜瘤的特征性脑膜上皮染色质结构。注意核分裂象和细胞多形性增加。Morris染色。

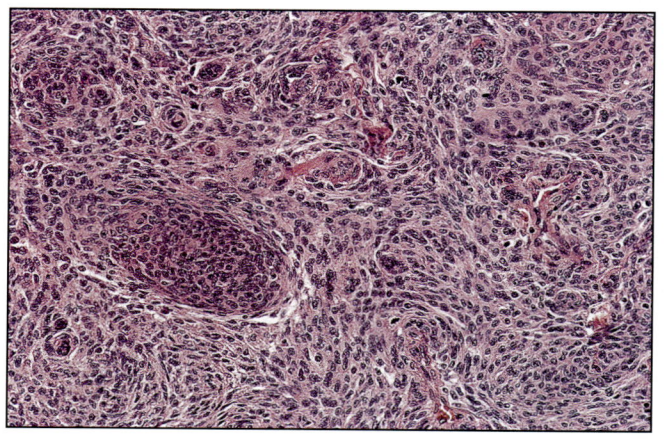

A

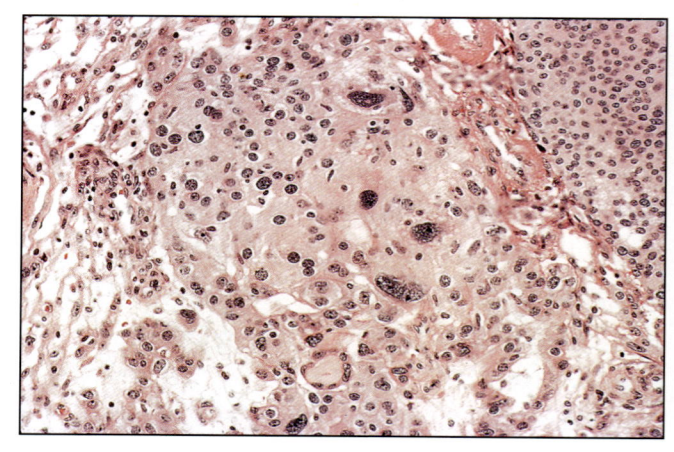

B

图26.127　细胞密度增加伴有细胞结构模式丢失、多形性核伴有明显核仁以及微小坏死是非典型脑膜瘤的组织病理学特征。注意，此细胞密集区仅保留部分合体细胞结构（A）。仅有奇异形的细胞核多形性并不提示间变，但它是间变性脑膜瘤的一个常见表现（B）。

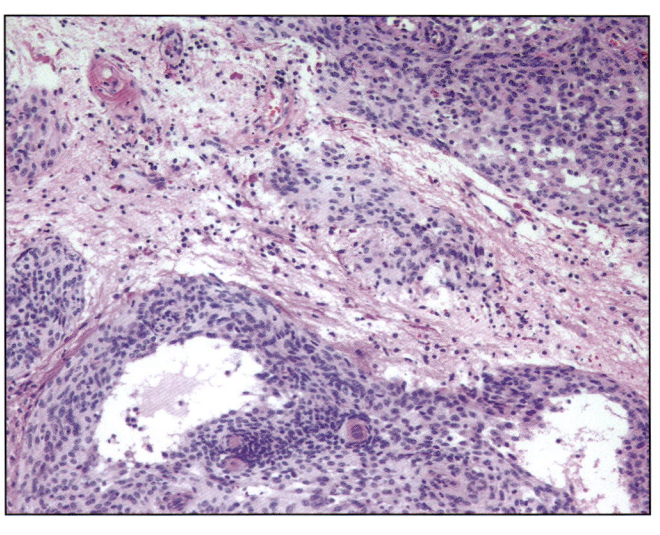
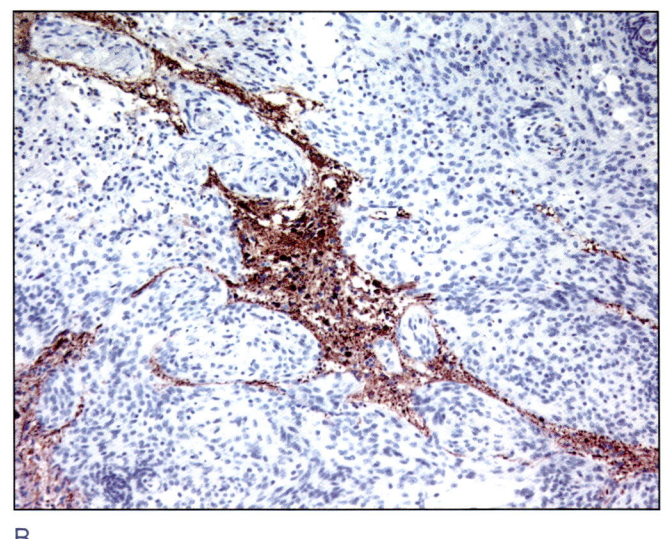

图26.128 脑组织浸润强烈提示侵袭性脑膜瘤，与组织病理学类型或间变程度无关（A）。胶质纤维酸性蛋白（GFAP）免疫组化染色可显示具有脑组织侵犯的恶性脑膜瘤中的反应性脑组织融合（B）。（B）GFAP-ABC免疫过氧化物酶-苏木素双重染色。

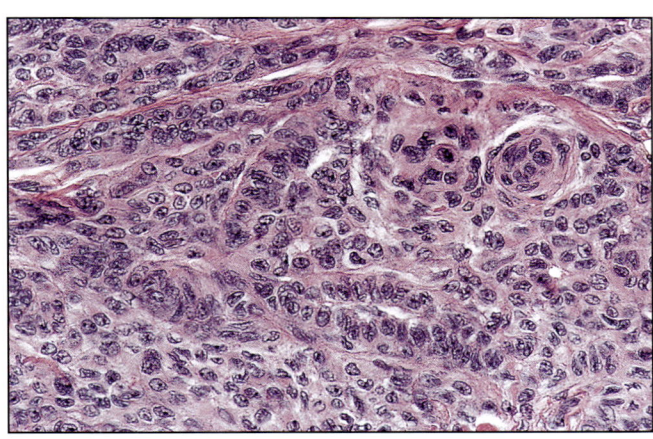

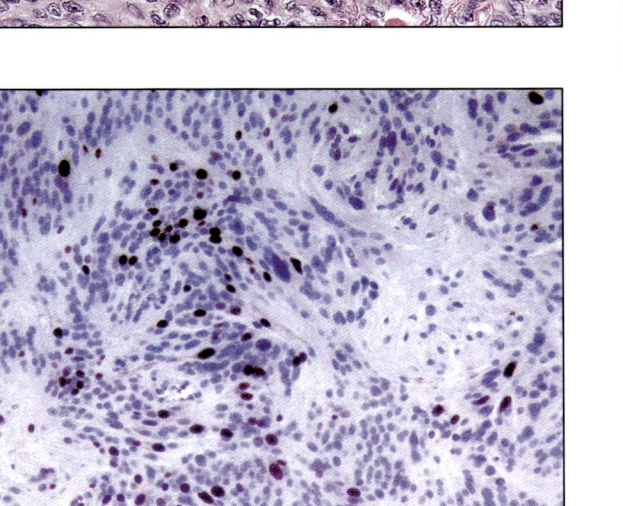

图26.129 间变性脑膜瘤中致密细胞区的局灶乳头状结构（A）。间变性脑膜瘤出现中等至较高的Ki-67增殖指数（B）。MIB-1-ABC免疫过氧化物酶-苏木素双重染色。

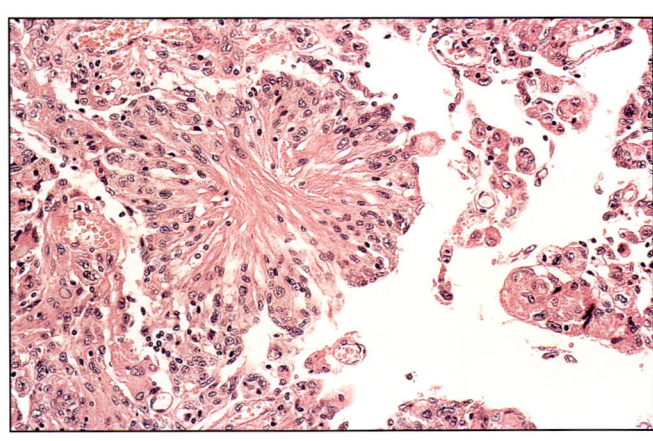

图26.130 乳头状脑膜瘤显示立方至柱状细胞排列成假乳头状结构。此型脑膜瘤都应被视为恶性。

柱状，胞浆境界清楚（图26.130）。肿瘤细胞常常围绕血管排列成乳头状结构，或者排列成"上皮"带，后者可融合成没有明显结构的片状，类似于转移性腺癌[614]。高度富于细胞和分裂活性，脑组织浸润常见。尽管乳头状结构可能明显，但仔细查找，常常可以见到比较经典的脑膜上皮表现。甚至，出现局灶乳头状结构常常伴有复发的可能性增加[611]。

横纹肌样脑膜瘤：脑膜瘤含有显著横纹肌样形态的细胞成分并不常见[595,615,616]，但是这种肿瘤以其侵袭性生物学行为类似于间变或恶性脑膜瘤而引人注意。因此，这种肿瘤与间变性和乳头型变型一起被定义为WHO Ⅲ级。横纹肌样细胞呈相对松散的片状排列，或者呈斑片状。细胞学形态类似于其他部位的横纹肌肿瘤细胞，表现为圆形,具有泡状核,巨型核仁,明显嗜酸性胞浆,其中含有透明核旁包涵体。这些包涵体的超微结构是呈明显漩涡状的中间丝,常常包含有其他细胞器。脑膜上皮细胞的细胞学特征在这种肿瘤中可以见到,但多少不一。只有局灶横纹肌样结构而没有其他恶性表现,可能并不一定代表侵袭性生物学行为。

脑膜瘤分子遗传:脑膜瘤最常见的细胞遗传学异常是 22q 等位基因丢失[595]。此染色体也是神经纤维瘤病基因 *NF2* 所在的位置,这一发现与此家族性病变中脑膜瘤的高发生率相一致。然而,*NF2* 基因突变不只限于 *NF2* 患者发生的肿瘤。在散发性脑膜瘤中,*NF2* 突变的发生率高达 60%[595]。脑膜瘤的肿瘤发生中也涉及其他几种基因[595,617]。

间叶性、非脑膜上皮肿瘤(见表26.4)
Mesenchymal, non-meningothelial tumors

许多间叶性肿瘤偶尔也可发生于脑膜。一般来说,这些肿瘤与 CNS 以外的相应肿瘤具有相似的特征。此类中较常见的良性肿瘤包括孤立性纤维性肿瘤、软骨瘤、骨软骨瘤、骨瘤及脂肪瘤。最常见的肉瘤包括所谓的血管外皮细胞瘤、软骨肉瘤、未分化多形性肉瘤(所谓的"恶性纤维组织细胞瘤")以及横纹肌肉瘤。尤其要注意地是,血管外皮细胞瘤是非脑膜上皮性的间叶性肿瘤,并不是血管母细胞型脑膜瘤的变型。在此仅详细讨论血管外皮细胞瘤和孤立性纤维性肿瘤。

脑膜血管外皮细胞瘤(所谓的)(图26.131和26.132)
Meningeal hemangiopericytoma(so-called)

所谓的脑膜血管外皮细胞瘤,大约占所有脑膜肿瘤的 1%~7%,是极具侵袭性的肿瘤,复发和远处转移的发生率很高[618,619]。肿瘤大多发生于成人,男性比女性稍多见,年龄范围(30~50岁)常常比脑膜瘤稍年轻[620]。这些肿瘤的组织发生是神经病理学家长期争议的话题。曾经被认为是脑膜瘤的特殊血管(血管母细胞性)变型,目前已划归为一种独立性疾病,与软组织病理学中较有争议性的疾病之一——孤立性纤维性肿瘤的关系密切(见第3章和第24章)[621]。

脑膜血管外皮细胞瘤发生于硬膜,常常位于幕内或其周围,可以压迫甚至侵犯下方的脑组织。可以导致被覆颅骨的溶骨性病变,与脑膜瘤不同,不会引起骨的肥厚性病变。大体上,血管外皮细胞瘤通常呈球形,质硬,高度富于血管,外科切除困难。

肿瘤组织学上富于细胞,由片状卵圆形至梭形肿瘤细胞组成,胞浆境界不清,核为卵圆形、细长,核仁明显(图 26.131)。裂隙状的纤细血管网呈典型"鹿角"状分支,可通过网织纤维染色勾勒出来。不常见的是,单个肿瘤细胞也可围以网织纤维染色阳性的间质成分。核分裂象可以见到,但即使在同一肿瘤内,数量上也有较大差异。尽管命名变更一般较慢,但愈加明确的是,目前还不具备有意义的方法将这些病变从细胞型孤立性纤维性肿瘤中分离出来(见下文)。肿瘤细胞的免疫反应见于波形蛋白和 CD34[620] 的反应(图 26.132B)。与

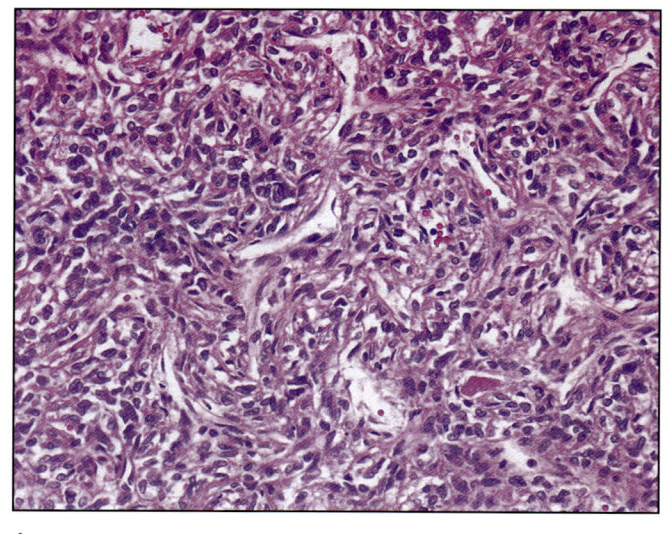

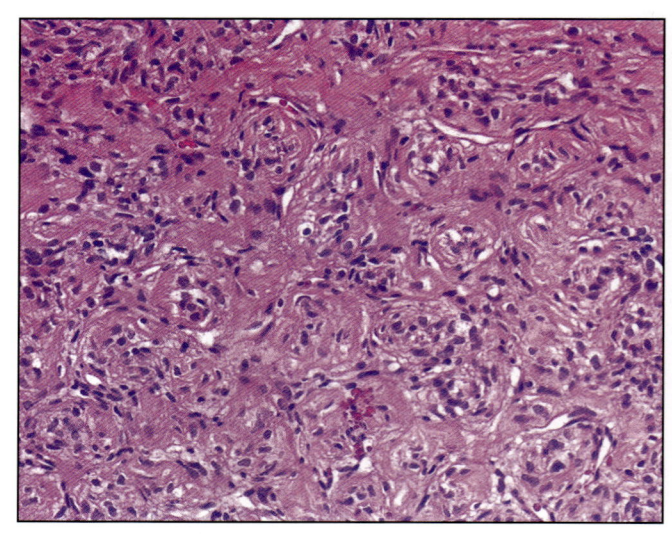

A B

图26.131 血管外皮细胞瘤的组织学切片显示细胞密集和丰富的纤细血管网(A)。在同一肿瘤的其他区域,致密胶原性间质与细胞较丰富的区域交织出现(B)。

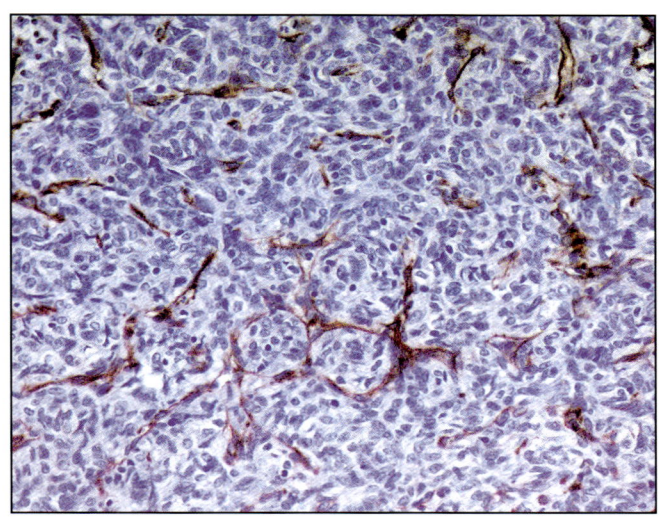 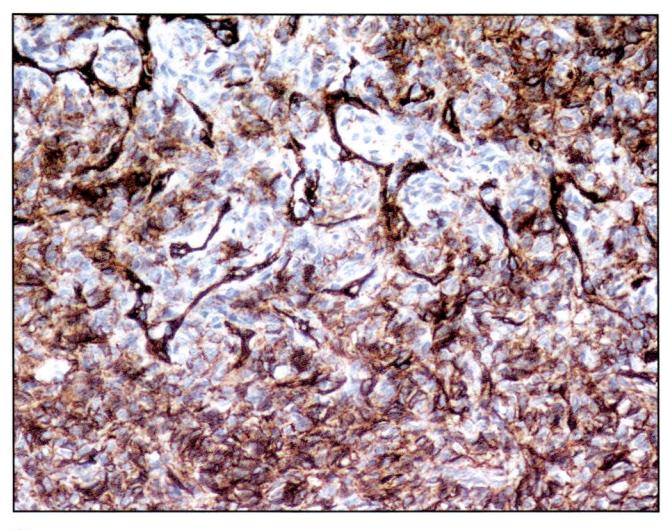

图26.132 与26.131为同一肿瘤的波形蛋白免疫组化染色，突出了血管外皮细胞瘤的血管网（A）。血管和细胞成分CD34明显呈阳性（B）。CD34-ABC免疫过氧化物酶-苏木素双重染色。

脑膜瘤不同，EMA和其他上皮标记物为阴性[621,622]。重要的是，没有外皮细胞分化的表型证据。

Ki-67（MIB-1）标记指数不一，但平均为10%[620]。核分裂比例高（≥5～6/10HPF），并且出现核多形性和肿瘤性坏死，与生存率减低有关[619]。脑膜的血管外皮细胞瘤为低级别肉瘤，原因在于其高复发率（即使外科明确完全切除）以及易于CNS外转移通常是在间隔很长时间之后。15年复发的危险高达90%[622]。

孤立性纤维性肿瘤（图26.133）
Solitary fibrous tumor

孤立性纤维性肿瘤（SFT）是相对不常见的间叶性肿瘤，大多累及神经系统以外的不同部位（见第24章）。尽管多见于胸膜和腹膜，但SFT发生在其他许多组织已有报道，包括深部软组织、乳腺、甲状腺、涎腺、上呼吸道、鼻腔以及眼眶[624,625]。过去的十年间已报道了数个CNS内病例[626-630]。诊断时年龄为11～73岁不等，平均大约为46岁，具有男性倾向（M:F为1.8:1～2.0:1）。大约75%的肿瘤位于颅内，部位包括大脑凸面及矢状窦、侧脑室、脑幕、小脑脑桥角以及鞍上池。脊髓肿瘤大多见于胸腰部，几乎均为髓外，一般以硬膜为基底，大体上与软脑膜明显附着。神经影像学显示境界清楚、常常非均质性的肿物，注射对比剂后，出现弥漫性相对显著的血管强化。肿瘤周围水肿不常见。

尽管这些肿瘤没有包膜，但它们与邻近脑组织或脊

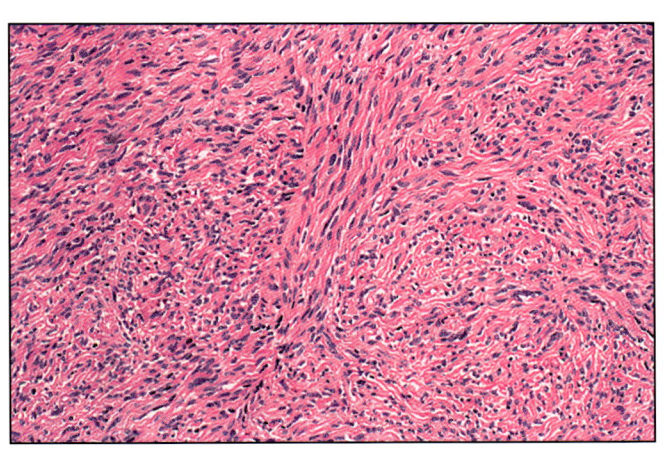 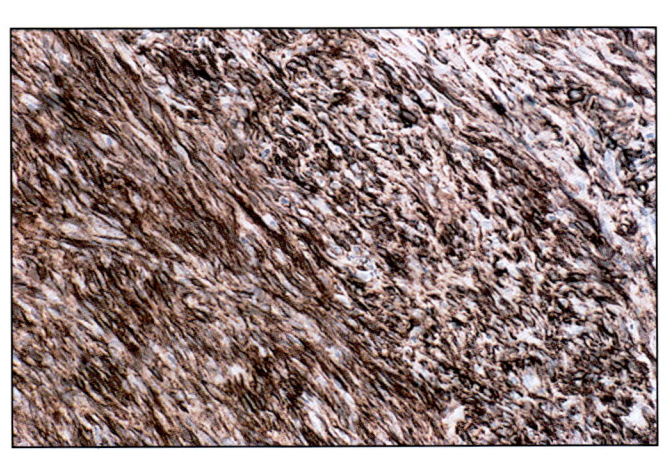

图26.133 孤立性纤维性肿瘤。（A）梭形细胞排列成不明显的束状结构，混合有致密胶原带。（B）肿瘤细胞CD34呈强阳性。CD34-ABC免疫过氧化物酶法-苏木素双重染色。

髓之间呈明显"膨胀性"界面。不常见的是，可出现邻近结构的局灶微小浸润，这一点并不提示任何生物学潜能改变。与在其他解剖部位一样，孤立性纤维性肿瘤的典型组织学表现为：中度富于细胞，波浪状的梭形细胞形态一致，无排列结构，或者呈不明显的束状结构，伴有大量带状玻璃样胶原纤维沉积（图26.133A），血管成分显著。血管常有分支，呈血管外皮细胞瘤样。血管玻璃样变并不是明显特征；然而一旦出现，可为局灶性。细胞核一般呈卵圆形至细长，染色质纤细，核仁不明显，没有假包涵体或核周晕。最近报道了一例小脑脑桥角发生的SFT病例，与异位涎腺有关[630]。

主要的鉴别诊断是纤维母细胞型脑膜瘤和（有争议的）血管外皮细胞瘤。与纤维母细胞型脑膜瘤相比，SFT既没有脑膜上皮或合体漩涡的典型细胞结构，也没有沙粒体；细胞间胶原一般较明显，分布均匀。局部胶原基质可如此量大，以致成为其显著特征，表现为致密瘢痕疙瘩样的束带。可以出现局灶黏液变性，但是与CNS外的肿瘤一样[631]，以黏液变性为主的肿瘤尚无报道。免疫组化分析在与脑膜瘤的鉴别方面可提供诊断性帮助。CD34免疫反应通常呈弥漫强阳性（图26.133B），相比之下，在纤维性脑膜瘤和血管外皮细胞瘤中，肿瘤细胞着色呈现较为局灶、不均匀的弱阳性[621,632]。波形蛋白表达显著，而结蛋白和肌肉特异性肌动蛋白免疫反应不常见且不弥漫。没有发现S-100蛋白或上皮性标记物免疫反应，如细胞角蛋白或EMA。然而，如上所述，SFT与血管外皮细胞瘤的鉴别更成问题[621]，因为这些病变可能代表了单一病变的形态学连续统一体。

软脑膜孤立性纤维性肿瘤的转移潜能较低，但是没有完全切除时，肿瘤常有复发。据报道，核分裂指数为1～5（平均为1.5）/10HPF，Ki-67标记指数为0.2%～18.3%（平均为4.5%）[632]。与CNS以外的肿瘤不同，CNS的恶性SFT的标准还没有确立。高度富于细胞、核分裂指数较高、显著细胞多形性以及坏死[633]联合起来高度提示恶性潜能，但事实上，后一种亚型的病变表现常常被认为是（没有理由）脑膜血管外皮细胞瘤。

组织发生未定的肿瘤
Tumors of uncertain histogenesis

血管母细胞瘤（图26.134至26.137）
Hemangioblastoma

毛细血管性血管母细胞瘤占所有颅内肿瘤的比例不足2.5%，可为散发或与Hippel-Lindau（VHL）病伴发[634]。其经典部位是小脑，但肿瘤累及延髓和脊髓者并不少见，尤其是VHL患者[635]。幕上和视网膜的血管母细胞瘤极为少见，大多伴有VHL病[594,635,636]。此外，多发性病变具有诊断性。CNS以外的血管母细胞瘤病例也有极少数报道，大多与外周神经有关[637,638]。

VHL病患者出现CNS血管母细胞瘤一般较散发病例患者年轻[635,636]，出现临床症状时两者的平均年龄分别为36岁和45岁[635]。

血管母细胞瘤为境界清楚的囊性病变，含有一个或多个附壁结节。该肿瘤的特征是纤细的血管成分相互吻合成网状，分隔大多角形细胞团，这些细胞常常含有脂质性胞浆和浓染的胞核（图26.135）。这些非血管成分被认为是"间质细胞"（图26.135和26.137）。各种内皮细胞、血管外皮细胞和间质细胞在涂片中容易识别（图26.134）。肿瘤容易推挤邻近的实质，明显浸润不常见。然而，周围实质中常可见大量星形胶质细胞增生，伴有Rosenthal纤维形成，这在小活检和术中涂片时容易产生误导。

间质细胞出现广泛的免疫组化标记物表达，包括波形蛋白和神经元特异性烯醇化酶（NSE）（图26.137）呈强阳性，S-100蛋白、transthyretin、孕激素受体、Leu7和GFAP呈不同程度阳性[634]。但是，NSE、S-100和GFAP的出现并不提示细胞的神经上皮性组织发生。内皮细胞出现典型的内皮细胞标记物免疫反应，间质细胞缺乏这些标记物表达，包括CD34、CD31[634]。研究显示，血管母细胞瘤的所有间质细胞均表达缺氧诱导因子（HIF）-家族蛋白和VEGF[639-641]。这些发现已成为新近应用针对VEGF信号的血管母细胞瘤特异性抗血管生成治疗的依据[642]。此外最近报道，间质细胞出现水通道蛋白1（aquaporin 1）表达[643]，这一发现意义不明。

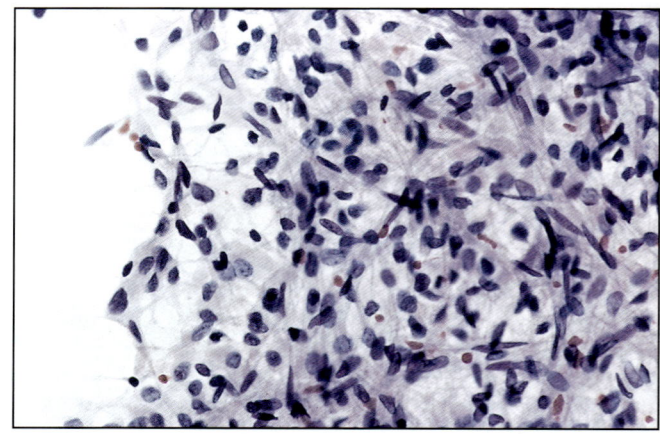

图26.134　涂片显示构成血管外皮细胞瘤的两种不同的细胞成分。较肥胖、常有脂化的间质细胞，细胞核呈圆形，与较为梭形的内皮细胞混合存在。Morris染色。

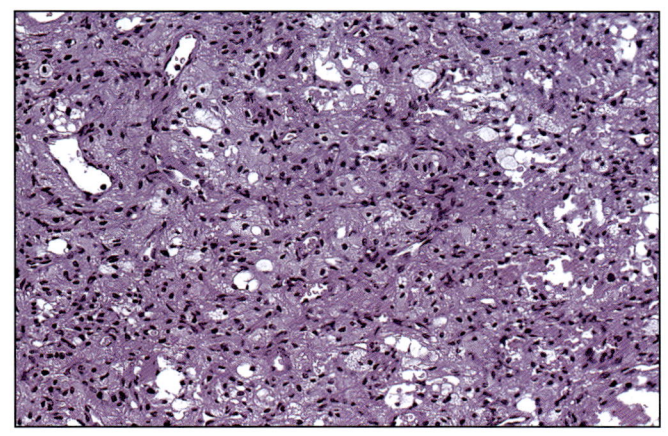

图26.135 血管母细胞瘤。组织学切片常常显示被多数血管分隔的间质细胞团。

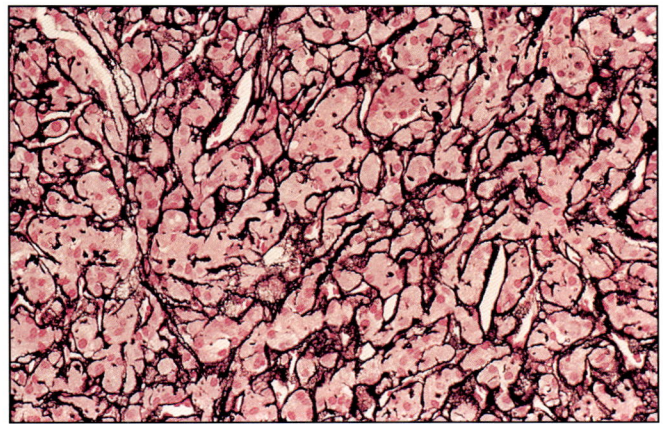

图26.136 网织纤维染色勾勒出血管母细胞瘤的复杂的毛细血管网。网织纤维染色。

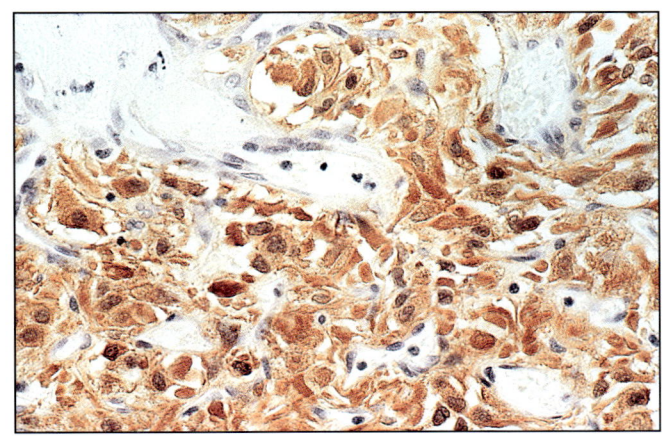

图26.137 血管母细胞瘤。神经特异性烯醇化酶（NSE）染色，间质细胞明显呈阳性。NSE-PAP免疫过氧化物酶-苏木素双重染色。

间质细胞上皮标记物为阴性，包括细胞角蛋白和EMA，这是与转移性肾细胞癌鉴别的有用工具[644]。最近的研究显示，在大多数散发以及VHL相关性血管母细胞瘤中，间质细胞表达抑制素α亚单位（抑制素A），并且显著高于肾细胞癌[645,646]。因此，上皮标记和抑制素A的联合应用对鉴别血管母细胞瘤和转移性肾细胞癌有益。

CNS原发性淋巴瘤（图26.138）
Primary lymphomas of the CNS

原发性CNS淋巴瘤（PCNSL）为结外非Hodgkin淋巴瘤，发生于CNS，并且神经系统以外缺乏明确的淋巴瘤。该肿瘤稀发的历史（先前约占CNS肿瘤的1%）在近十年来出现了稳步性转变，在有些病例研究中，其发生率约占所有原发性CNS肿瘤的7%[647]。尽管这种增加多数是由于免疫功能低下患者的发病率增加所致，尤其是与AIDS和器官移植相关；但也有明确证据表明，CNS淋巴瘤在所有年龄组均有增加，没有性别差异，无论人群的免疫状况如何[648-650]。在一般人群，PCNSL大多见于51～70岁的男性。但在免疫功能低下人群中较为年轻，平均为30～40岁[651]。PCNSL一般是高级别肿瘤，5年生存率极差，尤其是AIDS患者[652]。

PCNSL一般发生于幕上大脑半球的深部白质。其他部位包括颅后窝和基底节，常常累及脑室周围地区。与多数原发性CNS髓内肿瘤不同，这些肿瘤常为多发及多灶，类似于转移性肿瘤。多发性病变在AIDS和移植后人群中尤为多见。

CT影像显示，PCNSL通常为高信号密度，血管造影呈相对均匀强化。MR影像上，病变在T1像上通常为等密度至稍低密度，在T2像扫描上为等密度至高密度。对比增强后，免疫活性患者的多数病变出现显著的均匀强化。AIDS中的病变较不均匀，伴有出血和坏死灶，以及环状强化[654,655]。由于PCNSL弥漫浸润脑实质，病变可以境界不清，类似于炎症性病变[655]。

大体检查上，CNS淋巴瘤通常为苍白色，质软，边界不清。治疗后，肿瘤常有坏死、出血，边界模糊。

PCNSL最常见的镜下表现为弥漫大细胞淋巴瘤（图26.138）：大细胞的细胞核呈圆形或分叶状，染色质呈泡状，核仁明显，常常混有数量不等的反应性淋巴细胞、组织细胞、小胶质细胞和星形细胞。细胞涂片常常可反映病变的高级别属性，淋巴瘤细胞散在分布于这些混合性细胞成分中，背景为颗粒状的崩解神经毡（图

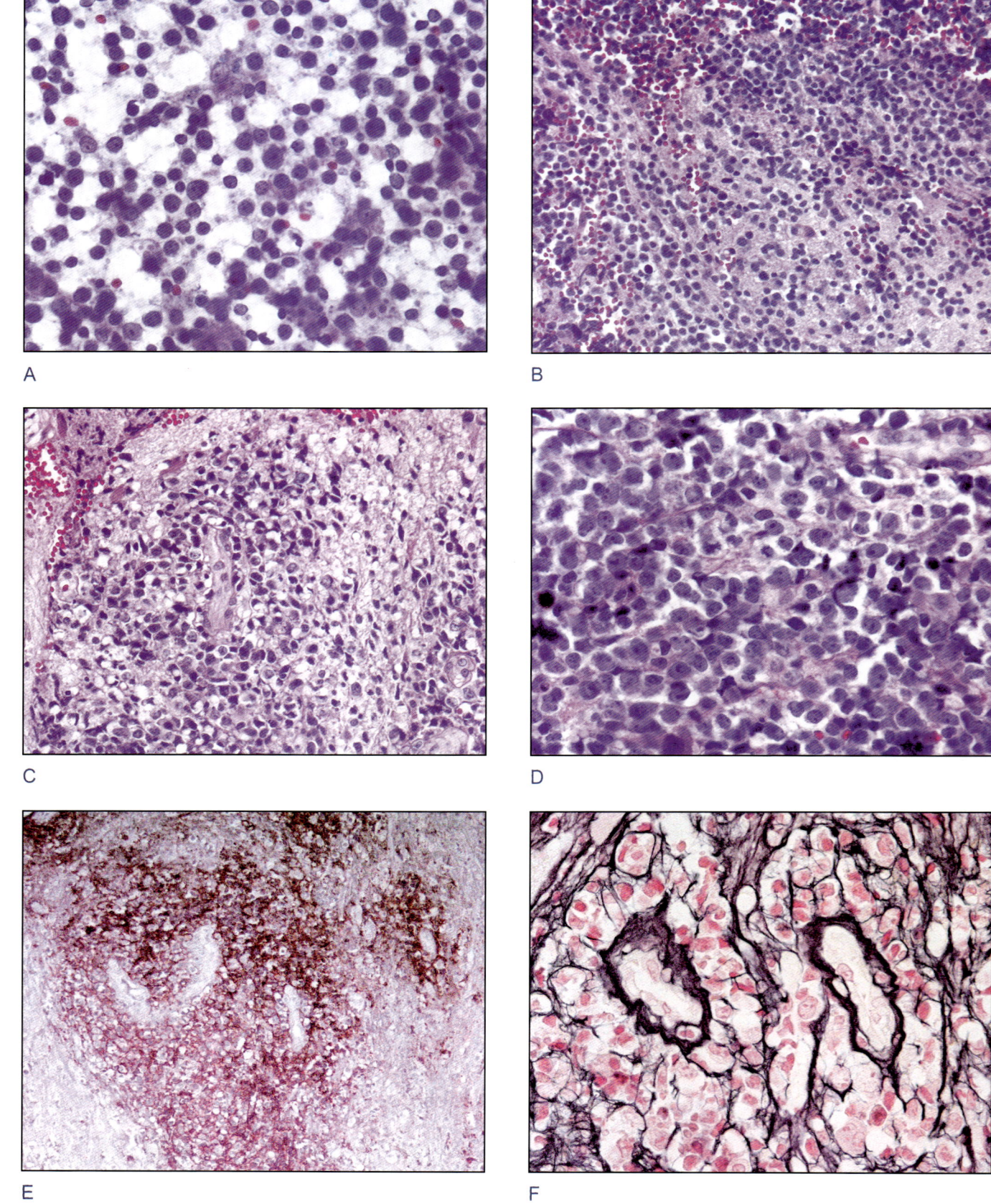

图26.138 原发性CNS恶性淋巴瘤。（A）原发性CNS淋巴瘤（PCNSL）涂片。显示颗粒状和"污秽"背景中的多形性大淋巴细胞。（B）大细胞淋巴瘤弥漫浸润脑组织。（C）注意，肿瘤细胞周围血管聚集是PCNSL的典型特征。（D）多数PCNSL为高级别病变，肿瘤细胞出现单个坏死和高核分裂活性。（E）CD20免疫染色可突出肿瘤细胞的典型血管中心性分布。（F）血管壁浸润伴网织纤维网膨胀是PCNSL的特征。

26.138A 和 26.138D）。这些涂片中常可见反应性的肥大星形细胞（图 26.138B）。多数淋巴瘤浸润境界不清，呈片状分布，以血管为中心，包括血管周围浸润和血管浸润（图 26.138C、26.138E 和 26.138F）。肥大的反应性星形细胞常可见到，并在病变中度富于细胞的区域比较明显。致密反应性星形细胞增多也可见于浸润区。有必要进行补充性的免疫组织化学染色，以确定免疫表型和除外胶质瘤和癌，尤其是在立体定向穿刺的有限活检标本。

绝大多数的 PCNSL 为 B 细胞系，T 细胞 PCNSL 仅占病例的比例不足 5%[651]。组织遗传学方面，多数 B 细胞 PCNSL 源于生发中心 B 细胞，表现为 bcl-6 蛋白表达[656]。少数 B 细胞 PCNSL 为低级别病变，大多在边缘区型，通常表现为以硬脑膜为基底的肿物[657]。T 细胞 PCNSL，一般为外周 T 细胞型，常常累及软脑膜，最常见于免疫活性个体[658]。尽管 T 细胞 PCNSL 在西方国家仅有少数病例，但文献报道，亚洲人群发病率较高，与那些地区 T 细胞淋巴瘤发病率较高相一致[659]。极其少见的是间变性淋巴瘤（Ki-1，通常为 T 细胞亚型）[660]以及 Hodgkin 淋巴瘤[651]。然而，播散性 Hodgkin 性淋巴瘤可累及 CNS[651]。

PCNSL 的分子遗传学：B 细胞 PCNSL 的分子研究已经证实了典型的 B 细胞淋巴瘤基因重排，即免疫球蛋白 H（*IgH*）和 *BCL6* 基因位点的经常性异位[651]。这些肿瘤中的其他几种体细胞突变也有报道，包括肿瘤抑制基因 *CD95* 和原癌基因 *c-MYC*、*PAX5*、*RhoH/TTF* 和 *PIM1*[661]。绝大多数发生于 AIDS 患者的 B 细胞 PCNSL 病例可以检测到 EB 病毒，但在有免疫活性的淋巴瘤患者中 EBV 不常见[662]。其他病毒，如 HHV-6、HHV-8 和 SV40 已被除外，是该人群淋巴瘤发病机制的相关辅助因子[663]。对 PCNSL（B 细胞和 T 细胞淋巴瘤）免疫活性个体的遗传学研究显示，常见 *CDKN2A* 基因失活，只有极少数有 *TP53* 或 *BCL2* 基因改变[664]。

生殖细胞肿瘤（表26.6；图26.139至26.141）
Germ cell tumors

原发性颅内生殖细胞肿瘤极少见，主要发生于儿童和青少年。与性腺外的生殖细胞肿瘤一样，几乎都发生于中线结构，包括松果体和蝶鞍区、第三脑室和下丘脑，脊髓罕见[665]。生殖细胞肿瘤是松果体区的最大一组肿瘤，在累及该区域的肿瘤中所占比例接近 50%[666-668]。然而，其发生率依地理位置不同而有差异，亚洲病例数最多。多数颅内肿瘤发生于 20 岁以内，绝大多数患者在 11～20 岁之间确诊[669]。有明确的性别倾向，无论生殖细胞肿瘤的类型如何，在一个病例研究中，男女比例为 11:1[669]。

CNS 生殖细胞肿瘤的组织发生和分化与其性腺内和性腺外的相应病变一致（表 26.6），被认为是起源于原始生殖细胞的肿瘤性转化。有假说认为，在胚胎发育过程中，多数原始生殖细胞迁移至泌尿生殖嵴，从而产生了性腺。然而，原始细胞也可以异常散布于其他组织，尤其是中线结构沿线，包括纵隔和胸腺以及 CNS 的间脑-松果体区[670]。

有关性腺外原始生殖细胞恶性转化的机制尚不清楚。据说神经内分泌因子在颅内细胞的肿瘤性转化中起一定作用，主要是由于原始性腺细胞靠近间脑促性腺激素调节中心。此外，绝大多数生殖细胞肿瘤的临床表现与青春期该区域的改变类似[671,672]。

所有类型的生殖细胞肿瘤在 CNS 都有报道，包括生殖细胞瘤、胚胎癌、绒毛膜癌、内胚窦（卵黄囊）瘤和畸胎瘤[671]。混合性生殖细胞肿瘤，即肿瘤具有两种或更多的组织学类型，也有较高的百分比[495]。生殖细胞肿瘤的组织学类型是有关患者生存期的最重要的预后因素。单纯生殖细胞瘤与其他生殖细胞肿瘤相比，生存期最长，复发率最低[673,674]。单纯生殖细胞瘤的 5 年生存率为 90%～95%，而 10 年生存率可达 91%[673,674]。恶性肿瘤包括绒毛膜癌、胚胎癌、卵黄囊瘤和混合性生殖细胞肿瘤，5 年生存率最低，大约 44%[671]。畸胎瘤的生存率依分化程度而不同。成熟性畸胎瘤的 5 年生存率高达 93%，未成熟畸胎瘤和伴有恶性转化的畸胎瘤的 5 年生存率低至 75%[674]。

表26.6	生殖细胞肿瘤

1. 生殖细胞瘤
2. 胚胎癌
3. 卵黄囊瘤（内胚窦瘤）
4. 绒毛膜癌
5. 畸胎瘤
   变型：成熟，未成熟，恶性
6. 混合性生殖细胞肿瘤

生殖细胞瘤（图26.139） Germinoma

生殖细胞瘤是发生于神经轴的最常见的生殖细胞肿瘤[665,667]。绝大多数病例发生于松果体和蝶鞍区。在松果体区，生殖细胞瘤占生殖细胞肿瘤的50%～80%[675]。男性明显好发。生殖细胞瘤通常为境界清楚的实性肿瘤，肿瘤与正常组织之间有明显的界面。然而，有些病例可以侵犯周围脑组织。大体上，肿瘤质软、易碎，伴有不同程度的囊性成分。常可见钙化。坏死和出血区不常见。

组织学特征类似于性腺相应病变（见第14章）。生殖细胞瘤由均匀一致的大多角形细胞组成，因为含有大量糖原，胞浆淡染或透明。细胞中央可见大的泡状核，通常含有一个或多个明显的核仁（图26.139）。肿瘤细胞呈较大的分叶状排列，间隔以纤细的纤维血管间隔。后者含有淋巴或淋巴浆细胞浸润，其中有大量的T淋巴细胞和活化的巨噬细胞[676]。可以出现伴有上皮样组织细胞聚集的肉芽肿性反应[677]。

生殖细胞瘤的免疫组织化学反应显示：胎盘碱性磷酸酶（PLAP）呈阳性[677-679]，是临床随访肿瘤复发的一种有用标记物[679]。人绒毛膜促性腺激素（β-hCG）在典型肿瘤细胞中呈散在阳性[678]，然而，β-hCG着色也可以提示肿瘤内具有合体滋养叶细胞样细胞[680]。生殖细胞瘤伴有合体滋养叶细胞成分在行为上与普通型生殖细胞瘤不同。据报道，产生β-hCG的生殖细胞瘤与单纯生殖细胞瘤相比，具有较高的复发率[673]和较短的生存期[674]。软脑膜和（或）CSF播散并不少见。生殖细胞瘤对放疗极其敏感，因而生殖细胞瘤的预后好于其他恶性生殖细胞肿瘤。

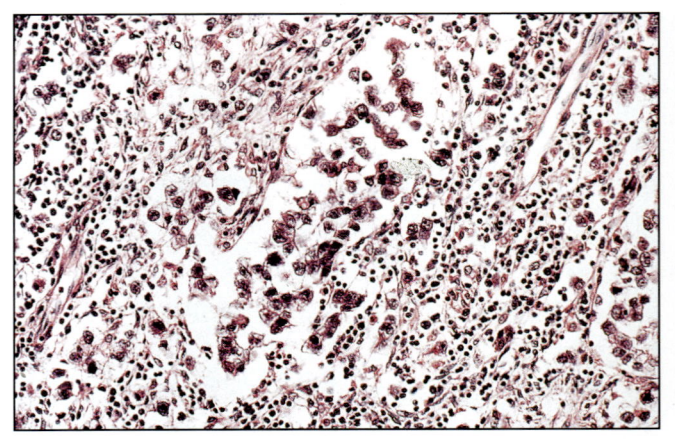

图26.139 颅内生殖细胞瘤出现与性腺内和性腺外相应病变相同的组织病理学特征。具有明显的泡状核的大细胞被富于淋巴细胞的间质分隔成团。

胚胎癌（图26.140） Embryonal carcinoma

胚胎癌是极为原始的生殖细胞肿瘤，仅次于生殖细胞瘤。在CNS内，极少数为单一性肿瘤，大约仅占所有颅内生殖细胞肿瘤的5%[681]。更为常见的是，胚胎癌为混合性肿瘤的一种成分，最常与未成熟畸胎瘤和绒毛膜癌伴发。

胚胎癌通常为巨大肿瘤，质硬为纤维性质地。肿瘤血供丰富，容易包绕其周围的大血管，因而完整切除更为复杂[675]。组织学上，肿瘤由大多角形细胞组成，呈密集巢状或片状增生。细胞含有大的泡状核，核仁明显。肿瘤细胞也可排列成上皮样结构，包括乳头状及腺样结构。高核分裂活性和广泛坏死常可见到。

胚胎癌的免疫组织化学表型是细胞角蛋白呈显著弥漫阳性，可将其与生殖细胞瘤鉴别开。PLAP见于绝大多数肿瘤细胞，甲胎蛋白（AFP）和β-hCG见于数量不等的病例[680,682]。

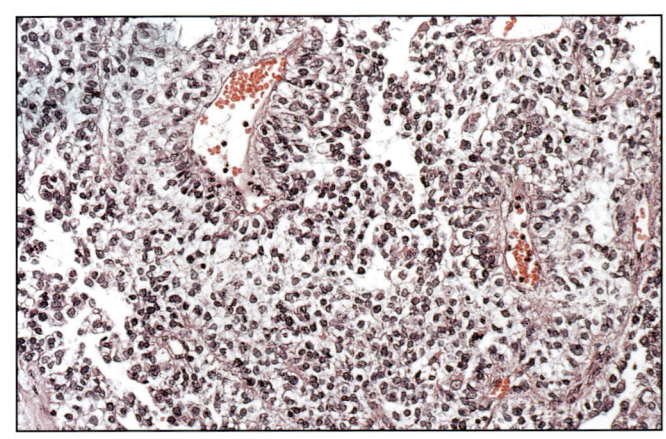

图26.140 松果体区胚胎癌的低倍放大图像，显示典型的乳头状/小管状结构，混有较多的网织纤维。

内胚窦瘤（卵黄囊瘤） Endodermal sinus tumor (yolk sac tumor)

内胚窦瘤是高度恶性的生殖细胞肿瘤。多数病例生存期不超过14个月[683]。这些肿瘤约占颅内生殖细胞肿瘤的7%[670,681]，好发于松果体区[677,683]。然而，大约50%的松果体病例实际上是混合性肿瘤，含有不同比例的内胚窦瘤和其他生殖细胞成分[683]。

内胚窦瘤的特征是出现假腺样结构，由黏液样基质中的内胚层细胞排列而成[678,684]。肿瘤细胞一般为透明的立方至柱状上皮样细胞，排列成片状、条索状，并且有不同程度的小管形成或有真正乳头状结构。经典的Schiller-Duval小体和PAS阳性小体常可见到[680]。内胚窦瘤有特征性的甲胎蛋白（AFP）免疫反应，上皮细成分以及玻璃样小体均为阳性。CSF和（或）单独血中AFP升高强烈提示内胚窦瘤[685]。

绒毛膜癌　Choriocarcinoma

单纯绒毛膜癌在神经轴中极其少见，但可作为混合性生殖细胞肿瘤的一种成分存在[686,687]。松果体区是这些肿瘤的好发部位。绒毛膜癌一般伴有性早熟，以及β-hCG和（或）促黄体激素水平升高[681]。

绒毛膜癌的境界清楚，常有出血。镜下，它们由合体滋养叶细胞和细胞滋养叶细胞呈双层结构排列而成，绒毛膜癌一般为出血性肿瘤，具有丰富的窦状血管结构。合体滋养叶细胞呈β-hCG强阳性[678,687]。PLAP和细胞角蛋白在多数肿瘤中也呈阳性[677,682]。

畸胎瘤（图26.141）　Teratoma

畸胎瘤是由源于三个胚胎生发层的组织混合组成的。因此，其被认为是胚胎组织对应的肿瘤性病变。畸胎瘤大约占所有颅内肿瘤的0.5%，松果体区是最常见部位，占松果体生殖细胞肿瘤的比例近乎15%[495,675,688]。与生殖细胞瘤相比，畸胎瘤通常发生于较年轻的患者，就诊时平均年龄为11岁[688]。与生殖细胞瘤一样，有明显的男性倾向。

畸胎瘤一般为较大的境界清楚的肿物，与邻近脑实质结构紧密附着。肿瘤一般呈多囊性，由可识别的成熟成分混合而成，包括角珠、毛发、软骨和骨组织。未成熟成分不明显，但常常伴有坏死和出血。畸胎瘤的组织学表现依这些未成熟成分及其分化程度而有不同。与性腺内和性腺外病例相同，有三种变型：**成熟、未成熟和恶性**。

在CNS中，**成熟畸胎瘤**比未成熟畸胎瘤相对少见。绝大多数为囊性，由于有不同组织和成分出现，其大体上呈多样性表现。组织学上，病变由高度分化的"成人型"外胚层、中胚层和内胚层成分组成。常常排列成类似成人组织的有序结构，如含有附属器的皮肤、软骨及骨、脂肪组织、横纹肌和平滑肌束、伴有脉络膜的胶质神经元组织、伴有色素性眼部上皮的视网膜成分等。

未成熟畸胎瘤在颅内畸胎瘤中最常见[665,669]。在未成熟畸胎瘤中，任何或者全部三个生发层的组织由类似于未成熟胚胎组织的较为原始的成分组成。未成熟成分的主要部分一般为神经上皮，包括胚胎髓质上皮、原始性玫瑰花结或更为特殊的结构，如Flexner-Wintersteiner和Homer Wright玫瑰花结以及类似于胚胎性肿瘤的结构，包括髓上皮瘤、神经母细胞瘤、视网膜母细胞瘤或室管膜母细胞瘤（图26.141）。源于其他生发层的未成熟成分不常见。未成熟畸胎瘤的临床过程较成熟性畸胎

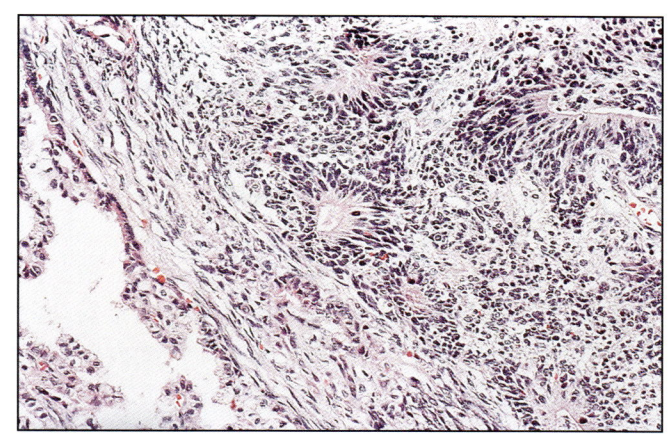

图26.141　在未成熟畸胎瘤中，室管膜母细胞瘤型玫瑰花结是极为常见的神经上皮分化表现。

瘤差[689]。肿瘤更容易沿CSF通路播散[665,690,691]，复发和死亡率高于成熟性畸胎瘤[665,689]。然而，出现未成熟成分并不代表畸胎瘤的恶性转化（见下文）。未成熟成分的成熟化极少见于残留或复发性肿瘤[692]。

恶性畸胎瘤表现为三种成人组织出现一种或多种恶性转化，与其他器官和组织常见的一样，如癌和肉瘤，混以常见的成熟或未成熟畸胎瘤成分。横纹肌肉瘤或未分化肉瘤最为常见[671]。这些肿瘤较先前的畸胎瘤类型少见。应当采用畸胎瘤伴腺癌或畸胎瘤伴横纹肌肉瘤来替代笼统的恶性畸胎瘤名称。

成熟和未成熟畸胎瘤中常常伴有恶性生殖细胞成分，尤其是生殖细胞瘤和胚胎性癌[671]。据估计，生殖细胞瘤与畸胎瘤伴发的病例约占畸胎瘤的1/5[693]。在这些病例中，命名为畸胎瘤伴有生殖细胞瘤或畸胎瘤伴有胚胎癌，较以前的畸胎癌更为恰当。

生殖细胞肿瘤的分子细胞遗传学：有关颅内生殖细胞肿瘤的细胞遗传学分析已有个别报道，但从这些研究中并没有得出明确的细胞遗传学表型。所分析的病例中绝大多数可见多数或复杂的结构性染色体异常[694-698]。性腺生殖细胞肿瘤最常见的核型异常即12p等位染色体[i(12p)][699]，在有些病例中也可出现[696,698-701]，表明在性腺及颅内生殖细胞肿瘤形成过程中具有相似的遗传途径。

非神经上皮性肿瘤和囊肿
Non-neuroepithelial neoplasms and cysts

颅咽管瘤（图26.142和26.143）
Craniopharyngioma

颅咽管瘤是组织学良性的肿瘤，起源于"鳞状细胞残留"（从垂体腺的灰结节，沿着不完整且复杂的垂体-咽管路径分布）。颅咽管瘤大约占颅内肿瘤的1%～4%[702]，较常见于儿童和青少年，为该组人群最常见的非胶质细胞脑肿瘤，大约占所有颅内肿瘤的5%～10%[702]。在儿童，发病高峰在5～14岁；第二个小高峰在41～60之间[702]。

颅咽管瘤绝大多数（80%）位于鞍上，尽管近乎一半的肿瘤有蝶鞍内成分。20%的颅咽管瘤源于蝶鞍区，导致蝶鞍区扩大，类似于垂体腺瘤[703]。极少数颅咽管瘤全部位于第三脑室内，在视交叉、蝶骨、小脑脑桥角和松果体区已有报道[704]。目前WHO分类分为两型：**造釉细胞型**和**乳头型**颅咽管瘤[702]。造釉细胞型颅咽管瘤最常见于青少年，而乳头型颅咽管瘤多常见于成人[705]。尽管有些肿瘤可含有不同比例的两种组织学类型，但对这两种类型分别进行讨论。

大体上，所有颅咽管瘤中大约50%为囊性，15%为实性，其余由囊性和实性成分组成。**造釉细胞型**大多为囊性，而**乳头型**一般为实性。大体切面，肿瘤的囊性成分含有闪亮双折光胆固醇结晶和钙化性脱落碎屑的黏性混合物，使得内容物呈现"机油"表现。实性成分质地较韧，可含有钙盐甚或骨灶。

造釉细胞型颅咽管瘤组织学特征是复层上皮，基底细胞呈栅栏状排列，其中混有实性和囊性结节状上皮条索（图26.143）。常见有退变表现，可见细胞解离和微小囊肿形成。囊性成分被覆单层鳞状上皮，以胶原性基底膜为依托。这些继发变性改变也可导致层状角化物质形成，常有融合并出现钙化。结节状角化物也称为"湿性角化"，对颅咽管瘤具有特殊诊断意义。钙化区域可有板层骨沉积。除了上皮成分以外，广泛纤维化、慢性炎症和胆固醇裂隙伴有巨细胞反应也很明显。

乳头型颅咽管瘤比较散在孤立，缺乏造釉细胞型肿瘤典型的钙化和"机油"囊肿成分。组织学方面，肿瘤由被覆高分化鳞状上皮的乳头状结构组成，中间可见明显的纤维血管间质轴心。鳞状细胞样上皮成分缺乏真正的角化和角质透明颗粒，因此不同于表皮样及皮样囊肿（见下文）。肿瘤没有柱状栅栏结构、微囊变性、钙化、角质结节和胆固醇性裂隙，这些均为造釉细胞型的特征。

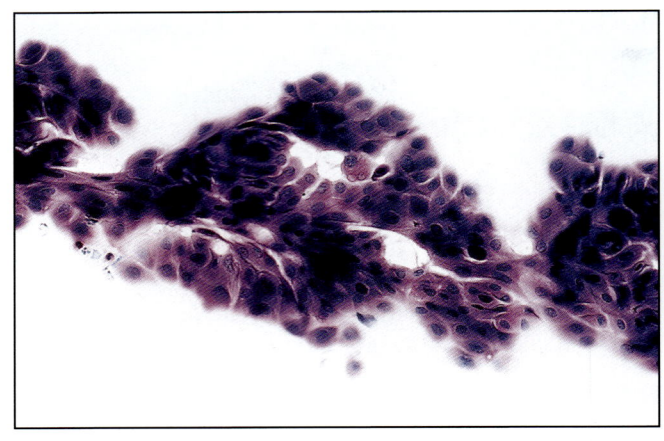

图26.142 颅咽管瘤。涂片显示由小乳头结构组成的特征性上皮结构。小心不要与脑膜瘤的上皮漩涡状结构混淆。Morris染色。

尽管颅咽管瘤一般境界清楚，但它们没有包膜，常常与相邻结构粘连。颅咽管瘤的这一特征可使其潜入周围重要结构，导致难以根治性切除以及潜在的极度危险。应该强调的是，肿瘤与脑组织交界处脑实质丰富的胶质属性。相邻脑组织出现丰富星形细胞增生，伴有Rosenthal纤维形成（图26.143），在小标本和不具代表性的活检中可被误诊为毛细胞型星形细胞瘤。

颅咽管瘤从病理角度基本为良性，但是如上所述，它们容易浸润周围结构。除了局部浸润以外，核分裂象和其他组织学侵袭特征极为少见。MIB-1标记指数显示的肿瘤增殖潜能较低，具有预后意义[706]。

颅咽管瘤，特别是那些**造釉细胞型**，即便是根治性切除的肿瘤，因其术后复发率较高而声名狼藉。据报道，复发率是25%或更高[707]。最初研究报告，乳头型与造釉细胞型相比，更容易完全切除，因此，不容易术后复发[705]。然而，多数最新报道显示，这两种颅咽管瘤类型的总体生存率没有显著差异[708]。复发和总体生存率与肿瘤切除范围和术后治疗具有更为直接的关系[709,710]。

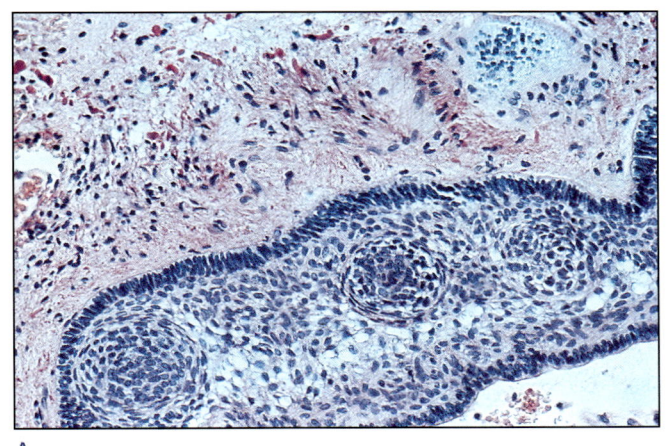
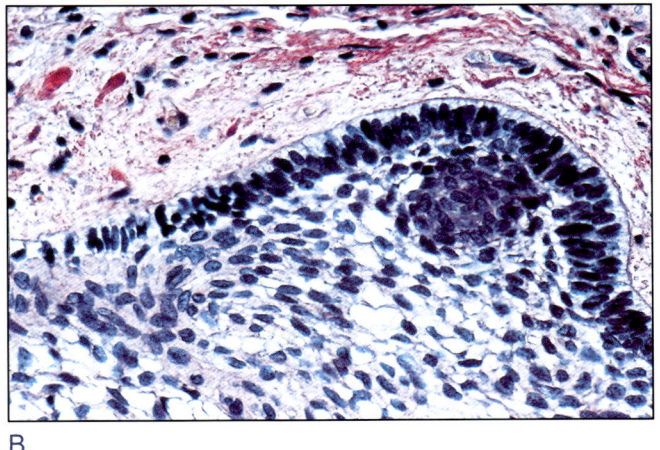

A

B

图26.143 颅咽管瘤。组织学切片通常显示类似于"造釉细胞瘤型"的区域，以及比较致密的基底样细胞栅栏，形成不规则的巢状和梁状结构（A）。这些区域可见疏松附着的鳞状细胞基质。注意相邻脑实质内反应性胶质细胞增生伴有Rosenthal纤维成分（左上）（B）。

表皮样和皮样囊肿（图26.144）
Epidermoid and dermoid cysts

表皮样和皮样囊肿可以发生于神经轴的任何部分，但最多见于小脑脑桥角、脑桥前池、蝶鞍区和脑室系统[711]。这些病变大约占颅内肿瘤的1%，表皮样囊肿比皮样囊肿的发病率高。表皮样囊肿出现较薄的复层上皮伴有角化，而皮样囊肿还具有附属器结构，如毛囊和腺体成分（图26.144）。这些囊肿，尤其是表皮样囊肿，可以破裂导致周围实质大量炎症反应。手术切除不完全可有复发[711]。

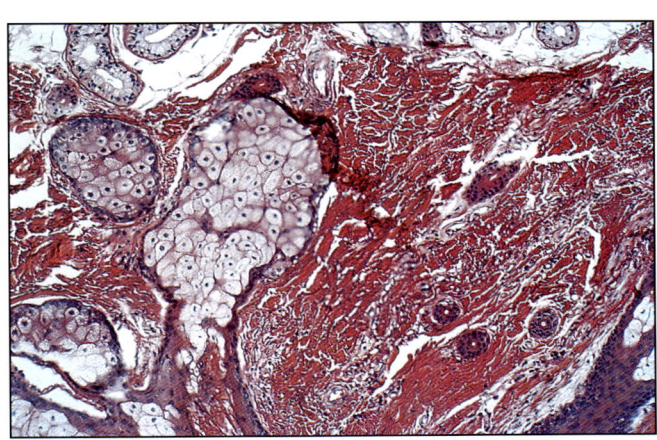

图26.144 枕叶的皮样囊肿，显示皮脂腺和汗腺成分。

参考文献

1. Choe G, Horvath S, Cloughesy T F et al. 2003 Analysis of the phosphatidylinositol 3′-kinase signaling pathway in glioblastoma patients in vivo. Cancer Res 63: 2742–2746
2. Gagner J-P, Law M, Fischer I et al. 2005 Angiogenesis in gliomas: imaging and experimental therapeutics. Brain Pathol 15: 342–363
3. Mellinghoff I K, Wang M Y, Vivanco I et al. 2005 Molecular determinants of the response of glioblastomas to EGFR kinase inhibitors. N Engl J Med 353: 2012–2024
4. Adams J H, Graham D I, Doyle D 1981 Brain biopsy: the smear technique for neurosurgical biopsies. J B Lippincott, Philadelphia
5. Burger P C 1985 Use of cytological preparations in the frozen section diagnosis of central nervous system neoplasia. Am J Surg Pathol 5: 344–354
6. Chandrasoma P T, Apuzzo M L J 1989 Stereotactic brain biopsy. Igaku-Shoin, New York
7. Plate K H, Rüschoff J, Mennel H D 1991 Cell proliferation in intracranial tumours: selective silver staining of nucleolar organizer regions (AgNORs). Application to surgical and experimental neuro-oncology. Neuropathol Appl Neurobiol 17: 121–132
8. Perentes E, Rubinstein L J 1987 Recent applications of immunoperoxidase histochemistry in human neurooncology. Arch Pathol Lab Med 111: 796–812
9. Martinez A J, Pollack I, Hall W A et al. 1988 Touch preparations in the rapid intraoperative diagnosis of central nervous system lesions. A comparison with frozen sections and paraffin-embedded sections. Mod Pathol 1: 378–384
10. Uneyama C, Shibutani M, Masutomi N et al. 2002 Fixation for genomic DNA analysis in microdissected paraffin-embedded tissue specimens. J Histochem Cytochem 50: 1237–1245
11. Kabbarah O, Pinto K, Mutch D G et al. 2003 Expression profiling of mouse endometrial cancers microdissected from ethanol-fixed paraffin-embedded tissues. Am J Pathol 162:755–762
12. Ahram M, Flaig M J, Gillespie J W et al. 2003 Evaluation of ethanol-fixed paraffin-embedded tissues for proteomic applications. Proteomics 3: 413–421
13. Perlmutter M A, Best C J M, Gillespie J W et al. 2004 Comparison of snap freezing versus ethanol fixation for gene expression profiling of tissue specimens. J Mol Diagn 6: 371–377
14. Steedman H F 1957 Polyester wax; a new ribboning embedding medium for histology. Nature 179: 1345
15. Morales A R, Essenfeld H, Essenfeld E et al. 2002 Continuous-specimen-flow high-throughput 1-hour tissue processing. A system for rapid diagnostic tissue preparation. Arch Pathol Lab Med 126: 583–590
16. Morales A R, Nassiri M, Kanhoush R et al. 2004 Experience with an automated microwave-assisted rapid tissue processing method validation of histologic quality and impact on the timeliness of diagnostic surgical pathology. Am J Clin Pathol 121: 528–536
17. Tohyama T, Lee V M-Y, Trojanowski J Q 1993 Co-expression of low molecular weight neurofilament protein and glial fibrillary acidic protein in established human glioma cell lines. Am J Pathol 142: 883–892
18. Rubinstein L J 1988 Diagnostic markers in human neurooncology. Ann NY Acad Sci 540: 78–90

19. VandenBerg S R 1991 Desmoplastic infantile ganglioglioma: a clinicopathologic review of sixteen cases. Brain Tumor Pathol 8: 25–31
20. Miller D C, Koslow M, Budzilovich G N et al. 1990 Synaptophysin: a sensitive and specific marker for ganglion cells in central nervous system neoplasms. Hum Pathol 21: 93–98
21. Smith T W, Nikulasson S, De Girolami U et al. 1993 Immunohistochemistry of synapsin and synaptophysin in human nervous system and neuroendocrine tumors. Applications in diagnostic neuro-oncology. Clin Neuropathol 12: 335–342
22. Wolf H K, Buslei R, Schmidt-Kastner R et al. 1996 NeuN: a useful neuronal marker for diagnostic histopathology. J Histochem Cytochem 44: 1167–1171
23. Kawashima M, Suzuki S O, Doh-ura K 2000 Alpha-synuclein is expressed in a variety of brain tumors showing neuronal differentiation. Acta Neuropathol 99: 154–160
24. Raghavan R, White C L III, Rogers B, et al. 2000 Alpha-synuclein expression in central nervous system tumors showing neuronal or mixed neuronal/glial differentiation. J Neuropathol Exp Neurol 59: 490–494
25. Dahlstrand J, Collins V P, Lendahl U 1992 Expression of the class VI intermediate filament nestin in human central nervous system tumors. Cancer Res 52: 5334–5341
26. Artlich A, Schmidt D 1990 Immunohistochemical profile of meningiomas and their histological subtypes. Hum Pathol 21: 843–849
27. Schnitt S J, Vogel H 1986 Meningiomas: diagnostic value of immunoperoxidase staining for epithelial membrane antigen. Am J Surg Pathol 10: 640–649
28. Meis J M, Ordóñez N G, Bruner J M 1986 Meningiomas: an immunohistochemical study of 50 cases. Arch Pathol Lab Med 110: 934–937
29. Theaker J M, Gatter K C, Esiri M M et al. 1986 Epithelial membrane antigen and cytokeratin expression by meningiomas: an immunohistological study. J Clin Pathol 39: 435–439
30. Hoog A, Gould V E, Grimelius L et al. 1998 Tissue fixation methods alter the immunohistochemical demonstrability of synaptophysin. Ultrastruct Pathol 12: 673–678
31. Riederer B M, Porchet R, Marugg R A et al. 1993 Solubility of cytoskeletal proteins in immunohistochemistry and the influence of fixation. J Histochem Cytochem 41: 609–616
32. Kim S H, Kook M C, Shin Y K et al. 2004 Evaluation of antigen retrieval buffer systems. J Mol Histol 35: 409–416
33. MacIntyre N 2001 Unmasking antigens for immunohistochemistry. Br J Biomed Sci 58: 190–196
34. Shi S R, Cote R J, Taylor C R 2001 Antigen retrieval techniques: current perspectives. J Histochem Cytochem 49: 931–937
35. Boon M E, Kok L P 1994 Microwaves for immunohistochemistry. Micron 25: 151–170
36. Ezaki T 2000 Antigen retrieval on formaldehyde-fixed paraffin sections: its potential drawbacks and optimization for double immunostaining. Micron 31: 639–649
37. Shin R-W, Iwaki T, Kitamoto T et al. 1992 Massive accumulation of modified tau and severe depletion of normal tau characterize the cerebral cortex and white matter of Alzheimer's disease. Am J Pathol 140: 937–945
38. Shi S R, Key M E, Kalra K 1991 Antigen retrieval in formalin-fixed, paraffin-embedded tissues: an enhancement method for immunohistochemical staining based on microwave oven heating of tissue sections. J Histochem Cytochem 39: 741–748
39. Gerdes J, Ki L, Schlüter C et al. 1991 Cell cycle analysis of a cell proliferation-associated human nuclear antigen that is defined by monoclonal antibody Ki-67. Am J Pathol 138: 867–873
40. Gerdes J, Becker M H G, Key G et al. 1992 Immunohistochemical detection of tumour growth fraction (Ki-67 antigen) in formalin-fixed and routinely processed tissues. J Pathol 168: 85–87
41. Cattoretti G, Becker M H G, Key G et al. 1992 Monoclonal antibodies against recombinant parts of the Ki-67 antigen (MIB 1 and MIB 3) detect proliferating cells in microwave-processed formalin-fixed paraffin sections. J Pathol 168: 357–363
42. Sawhney N, Hall P A 1992 Ki67 – structure function and new antibodies (editorial). J Pathol 168: 161–162
43. Duchrow M, Gerdes J, Schluter C 1994 The proliferation-associated Ki-67 protein: definition in molecular terms. Cell Prolif 27: 235–242
44. Kleihues P, Davis R L, Ohgaki H et al. 2000 Diffuse astrocytoma. In: Kleihues P, Cavenee WK (eds) World Health Organization classification of tumours. Pathology and genetics of tumours of the nervous system. IARC, Lyon, p 22–26
45. Roser F, Samii M, Ostertag H et al. 2004 The Ki-67 proliferation antigen in meningiomas, Experience in 600 cases. Acta Neurochir (Wien) 146: 37–44
46. Bravo R, Frank R, Blundell P A et al. 1987 Cyclin/PCNA is the auxiliary protein of DNA polymerase-d. Nature 326: 515–517
47. Morris G F, Mathews M B 1989 Regulation of proliferating cell nuclear antigen during the cell cycle. J Biol Chem 264: 13856–3864
48. Van Dierendonck J H, Wijsman J H, Keijzer R et al. 1991 Cell-cycle-related staining patterns of anti-proliferating cell nuclear antigen monoclonal antibodies, Comparison with BrdUrd labeling and Ki-67 staining. Am J Pathol 138: 1165–1172
49. McCormick D, Hall P A 1992 The complexities of proliferating cell nuclear antigen. Histopathology 21: 591–594
50. Allegranza A, Girlando S, Arrigoni G L et al. 1991 Proliferating cell nuclear antigen expression in central nervous system neoplasms. Virchow's Arch [A] 419: 417–423
51. Schiffer D, Chiỳ A, Giordana M T et al. 1993 Proliferating cell nuclear antigen expression in brain tumors and its prognostic role in ependymomas: an immunohistochemical study. Acta Neuropathol 85: 495–502
52. Revesz T, Alsanjari N, Darling J L et al. 1993 Proliferating cell nuclear antigen (PCNA): expression in samples of human astrocytic gliomas. Neuropathol Appl Neurobiol 19: 152–158
53. Agostinho M, Rino J, Braga J et al. 2004 Human topoisomerase II alpha: targeting to subchromosomal sites of activity during interphase and mitosis. Mol Biol Cell 15: 2388–2400
54. Oda M, Arakawa Y, Kano H et al. 2005 Quantitative analysis of topoisomerase IIa to rapidly evaluate cell proliferation in brain tumors. Biochem Biophys Res Commun 331: 971–976
55. Korshunov A, Golanov A, Timirgaz V 2000 Immunohistochemical markers for intracranial ependymoma recurrence. An analysis of 88 cases. J Neurol Sci 177: 72–82
56. Wolfsberger S, Fischer I, Höftberger R et al. 2004 Ki-67 immunolabeling index is an accurate predictor of outcome in patients with intracranial ependymoma. Am J Surg Pathol 28: 914–920
57. Shiraishi T, Tabuchi K, Mineta T et al. 1991 Nucleolar organizer regions in various human brain tumors. J Neurosurg 74: 979–984
58. Hara A, Hirayama H, Sakai N et al. 1990 Correlation between nucleolar organizer region staining and Ki-67 immunostaining in human gliomas. Surg Neurol 33: 320–324
59. Kajiwara K, Orita T, Nishizaki T et al. 1992 Glial fibrillary acidic protein (GFAP) expression and nucleolar organizer regions (NORs) in human gliomas. Brain Res 572: 314–318
60. Smith P J, Skilbeck N, Harrison A et al. 1988 The effect of a series of fixatives on the AgNOR technique. J Pathol 155: 109–112
61. Louis D N, Meehan S M, Ferrante R J et al. 1992 Use of the silver nucleolar organizer region (AgNOR) technique in the differential diagnosis of central nervous system neoplasia. J Neuropathol Exp Neurol 51: 150–157
62. Loeffler P M B J 1997 Cancer of the nervous system. Blackwell, Oxford
63. Silbergeld D L, Chicoine M R 1997 Isolation and characterization of human malignant glioma cells from histologically normal brain. J Neurosurg 86: 525–531
64. Tysnes B, Mahesparan R 2001 Biological mechanisms of glioma invasion and potential therapeutic targets. J Neurooncol 53: 129–147
65. Sanai N, Alvarez-Buylla A, Berger M S 2005 Neural stem cells and the origin of gliomas. N Engl J Med 353: 811–822
66. Rakic P 2003 Developmental and evolutionary adaptations of cortical radial glia. Cerebral Cortex 13: 541–549
67. Temple S, Alvarez-Buylla A 1999 Stem cells in the adult mammalian central nervous system. Curr Opin Neurobiol 9: 135–141
68. Tramontin A D, García-Verdugo J M, Lim D A et al. 2003 Postnatal development of radial glia and the ventricular zone (VZ): a continuum of the neural stem cell compartment. Cerebral Cortex 13: 580–587
69. Ma D K, Ming G-L, Song H 2005 Glial influences on neural stem cell development: cellular niches for adult neurogenesis. Curr Opinion Neurobiol 15: 514–520
70. Hu Q D, Cui X Y, Ng Y K et al. 2004 Axoglial interaction via the notch receptor in oligodendrocyte differentiation. Ann Acad Med Singapore 33(5): 581–588
71. Stecca B, Ruiz I, Altaba A 2005 Brain as a paradigm of organ growth: Hedgehog-Gli signaling in neural stem cells and brain tumors. J Neurobiol 64: 476–490
72. Singh S K, Clarke I D, Terasaki M et al. 2003 Identification of a cancer stem cell in human brain tumours. Cancer Res 63: 5821–5828
73. Singh S K, Clarke I D, Hide T et al. 2004 Cancer stem cells in nervous system tumors. Oncogene 23: 7267–7273
74. Dai C, Celestino J C, Okada Y et al. 2001 PDGF autocrine stimulation dedifferentiates cultured astrocytes and induces oligodendrogliomas and oligoastrocytomas from neural progenitors and astrocytes in vivo. Genes Dev 15: 1913–1925
75. Holland E C 2001 Progenitor cells and glioma formation. Curr Opin Neurol 14: 683–688
76. Holland E C 2001 Gliomagenesis: genetic alterations and mouse models. Nat Rev Genet 2: 120–129
77. Kleihues P, Davis R L, Coons S W et al. 2000 Anaplastic astocytoma. In: Kleihues P, Cavenee WK (eds) WHO Classification of tumors, pathology and genetics: tumours of the nervous system. IARC Press, Lyon, p 27–28
78. Kleihues P, Burger P C, Collins V P et al. Glioblastoma. In: Kleihues P, Cavenee WK (eds) WHO Classification of tumors, pathology and genetics: tumours of the nervous system. IARC Press, Lyon, p 29–39
79. Daumas-Duport C, Scheithauer B W, O'Fallon J et al. 1988 Grading of astrocytomas. A simple and reproducible method. Cancer 62: 2152–2165
80. VandenBerg S R 1992 Current diagnostic concepts of astrocytic tumors. J Neuropathol Exp Neurol 51: 644–657
81. Kleihues P, Burger P C, Scheithauer B W 1993 The new WHO classification of brain tumours. Brain Pathol 3: 255–268
82. Gagner J-P, Law M, Fischer I et al. 2005 Angiogenesis in gliomas: imaging and experimental therapeutics. Brain Pathol 15: 342–363
83. Nelson S J, Cha S 2003 Imaging glioblastoma multiforme. Cancer J 9: 134–145
84. Cha S 2005 Update on brain tumor imaging. Curr Neurol Neurosci Rep 5(3): 169–177
85. Giannini C, Scheithauer B W, Burger P C et al. 1999 Cellular proliferation in pilocytic and diffuse astrocytomas. J Neuropathol Exp Neurol 58: 46–53

86. Couldwell W T, Weiss M H, Law R E et al. 1995 Paradoxical elevation of Ki-67 labeling with protein kinase inhibition in malignant gliomas. J Neurosurg 82: 461–468
87. Plate K H, Risau W 1995 Angiogenesis in malignant gliomas. Glia 15: 339–347
88. Stratmann A, Machein M R, Plate K H 1995 Anti-angiogenic gene therapy of malignant glioma. Acta Neurochir Suppl 68: 105–110
89. Birner P, Piribauer M, Fischer I et al. 2003 Vascular patterns in glioblastoma influence clinical outcome and associate with variable expression of angiogenic proteins: evidence for distinct angiogenic subtypes. Brain Pathol 13: 133–143
90. Yao Y, Kubota T, Sato K et al. 2001 Prognostic value of vascular endothelial growth factor and its receptors Flt-1 and Flk-1 in astrocytic tumours. Acta Neurochir (Wien) 143: 159–16
91. Steiner H H, Karcher S, Mueller M M 2004 Autocrine pathways of the vascular endothelial growth factor (VEGF) in glioblastoma multiforme: clinical relevance of radiation-induced increase of VEGF levels. J Neurooncol 66: 129–138
92. Wang D, Anderson J C, Gladson C L 2005 The role of the extracellular matrix in angiogenesis in malignant glioma tumors. Brain Pathol 15: 318–326
93. Hu B, Guo P, Fang Q et al. 2003 Angiopoietin-2 induces human glioma invasion through the activation of matrix metalloprotease-2. Proc Natl Acad Sci USA 100: 8904–8909
94. Rich J N, Hans C, Jones B et al. 2005 Gene expression profiling and genetic markers in glioblastoma survival. Cancer Res 65: 4051–4058
95. Onda K, Tanaka R, Takahashi H et al. 1989 Cerebral glioblastoma with cerebrospinal fluid dissemination: a clinicopathological study of 14 cases examined by complete autopsy. Neurosurgery 25: 533–540
96. Onda K, Tanaka R, Takahashi H et al. 1990 Symptomatic cerebrospinal fluid dissemination of cerebral glioblastoma. Computed tomographic findings in 11 cases. Neuroradiology 32: 146–150
97. Grabb P A, Albright A L, Pang D 1992 Dissemination of supratentorial malignant gliomas via the cerebrospinal fluid in children. Neurosurgery 30: 64–71
98. Zagzag D, Friedlander D R, Dosik J et al. 1996 Tenascin-C expression by angiogenic vessels in human astrocytomas and by human brain endothelial cells in vitro. Cancer Res 56: 182–189
99. Previtali S, Quattrini A, Nemni R et al. 1996 αvβ4 and αvβ1 integrins in astrocytomas and other CNS tumors. J Neuropathol Exp Neurol 55: 456–465
100. Gladson C L, Cheresh D A 1991 Glioblastoma expression of vitronectin and the alpha v beta 3 integrin. Adhesion mechanism for transformed glial cells. J Clin Invest 88: 1924–1932
101. Gladson C L, Wilcox J N, Sanders L et al. 1995 Cerebral microenvironment influences expression of the vitronectin gene in astrocytic tumors. J Cell Sci 108: 947–956
102. Hayen W, Goebeler M, Kumar S et al. 1999 Hyaluronan stimulates tumor cell migration by modulating the fibrin fiber architecture. J Cell Sci 112 (Pt 13): 2241–2251
103. Junker N, Latini S, Petersen L N et al. 2003 Expression and regulation patterns of hyaluronidases in small cell lung cancer and glioma lines. Oncol Rep 10: 609–616
104. Chekenya M, Rooprai H K, Davies D et al. 1999 The NG2 chondroitin sulfate proteoglycan: role in malignant progression of human brain tumours. Int J Dev Neurosci 17: 421–435
105. Tang X, Davies J E, Davies S J 2003 Changes in distribution, cell associations, and protein expression levels of NG2, neurocan, phosphacan, brevican, versican V2, and tenascin-C during acute to chronic maturation of spinal cord scar tissue. J Neurosci Res 71: 427–444
106. Hausmann R, Betz P 2001 Course of glial immunoreactivity for vimentin, tenascin and alpha1-antichymotrypsin after traumatic injury to human brain. Int J Legal Med 114: 338–342
107. Brenneke F, Schachner M, Elger C E et al. 2004 Up-regulation of the extracellular matrix glycoprotein tenascin-R during axonal reorganization and astrogliosis in the adult rat hippocampus. Eur J Neurosci 58: 133–143
108. Swindle C S, Tran K T, Johnson T D et al. 2001 Epidermal growth factor (EGF)-like repeats of human tenascin-C as ligands for EGF receptor. J Cell Biol 154: 459–468
109. Ventimiglia R, Wikstrand C J, Ostrowski L E et al. 1992 Tenascin expression in human glioma cell lines and normal tissues. J Neuroimmunol 36: 41–55
110. Ljubimova J Y, Fugita M, Khazenzon N M et al. 2004 Association between laminin-8 and glial tumor grade, recurrence, and patient survival. Cancer 101: 604–612
111. Ljubimova J Y, Lakhter A J, Loksh A et al. 2001 Overexpression of alpha4 chain-containing laminins in human glial tumors identified by gene microarray analysis. Cancer Res 61: 5601–5610
112. Okada H, Yoshida J, Sokabe M et al. 1996 Suppression of CD44 expression decreases migration and invasion of human glioma cells. Int J Cancer 66: 255–260
113. Akiyama Y, Jung S, Salhia B et al. 2001 Hyaluronate receptors mediating glioma cell migration and proliferation. J Neurooncol 53: 115–127
114. Hagel C, Park S H, Puchner M J et al. 2004 CD44 expression and tumour cell density correlate with response to tamoxifen/carboplatin chemotherapy in glioblastomas. J Neurooncol 66: 139–146
115. Sloan K E, Eustace B K, Stewart J K et al. 2004 D155/PVR plays a key role in cell motility during tumor cell invasion and migration. BMC Cancer 4: 7386
116. Sloan K E, Stewart J K, Treloar A F et al. 2005 CD155/PVR enhances glioma cell dispersal by regulating adhesion signaling and focal adhesion dynamics. Cancer Res 65: 10930–10937
117. Giese A, Loo M A, Norman S A et al. 1996 Contrasting migratory response of astrocytoma cells to tenascin mediated by different integrins. J Cell Sci 109: 2161–2168
118. Chintala S K, Gokaslan Z L, Go Y et al. 1996 Role of extracellular matrix proteins in regulation of human glioma cell invasion in vitro. Clin Exp Metastasis 14: 358–366
119. Khan K M, Falcone D J 1997 Role of laminin in matrix induction of macrophage urokinase-type plasminogen activator and 92-kDa metalloproteinase expression. J Biol Chem 272: 8270–8275
120. Rao J S, Steck P A, Tofilon P et al. 1994 Role of plasminogen activator and of 92 kDa type IV collagenase in glioblastoma invasion using an in vitro matrigel model. J Neurooncol 18: 129–138
121. Keohane M E, Hall S W, VandenBerg S R et al. 1990 Glioblastoma multiforme in primary culture synthesizes and secretes α2-macroglobulin α2-antitrypsin and plasminogen activator inhibitor-1. J Neurosurg 73: 234–241
122. Bu X, Khankaldyyan V, Gonzales-Gomez I et al. 2004 Species-specific urokinase receptor ligands reduce glioma cell growth and increase survival primarily by an antiangiogenesis mechanism. Lab Invest 84: 667–678
123. Landau B K, Kwaan H C, Verrusio E N et al. 1994 Elevated levels of urokinase-type plasminogen activator and plasminogen activator inhibitor type-1 in malignant human brain tumors. Cancer Res 54: 1105–1108
124. Yamamoto M, Sawaya R, Mohanam S et al. 1994 Activities, localizations, and roles of serine proteases and their inhibitors in human brain tumor progression. J Neurooncol 22: 139–151
125. Chandrasekar N, Mohanam S, Gujrati M et al. 2003 Downregulation of uPA inhibits migration and PI3k/Akt signaling in glioblastoma cells. Oncogene 22: 392–400
126. Le D M, Besson A, Fogg D K et al. 2003 Exploitation of astrocytes by glioma cells to facilitate invasiveness: a mechanism involving matrix metalloproteinase-2 and the urokinase-type plasminogen activator-plasmin cascade. J Neurosci 23: 4034–4043
127. Yu J, Bian D, Mahanivong C et al. 2004 p38 Mitogen-activated protein kinase regulation of endothelial cell migration depends on urokinase plasminogen activator expression. J Biol Chem 279: 50446–50454
128. Yamamoto M, Sawaya R, Mohanam S et al. 1994 Expression and localization of urokinase-type plasminogen activator in human astrocytomas in vivo. Cancer Res 54: 3656–3661
129. Gladson C L, Pijuan-Thompson V, Olman M A et al. 1995 Up-regulation of urokinase and urokinase receptor genes in malignant astrocytoma. Am J Pathol 146: 1150–1160
130. Rustamzadeh E, Li C, Doumbia S et al. 2003 Targeting the over-expressed urokinase-type plasminogen activator receptor on glioblastoma multiforme. J Neurooncol 65: 63–75
131. Munaut C, Noel A, Hougrand O et al. 2003 Vascular endothelial growth factor expression correlates with matrix metalloproteinases MT1-MMP, MMP-2 and MMP-9 in human glioblastomas. Int J Cancer 106: 848–855
132. Kyrkanides S, Moore A H, Olschowka J A et al. 2002 Cyclooxygenase-2 modulates brain inflammation-related gene expression in central nervous system radiation injury. Brain Res Mol Brain Res 104: 159–169
133. Laws E R Jr, Taylor W F, Clifton M E et al. 1984 Neurosurgical management of low-grade astrocytoma of the cerebral hemispheres. J Neurosurg 61: 665–673
134. Berger M S, Deliganis A V, Dobbins J et al. 1994 The effect of extent of resection on recurrence in patients with low grade cerebral hemisphere gliomas. Cancer 74: 1784–1791
135. Louis D N, Holland E C, Cairncross J G 2001 Glioma classification. Am J Pathol 159: 779–786
136. Koschny R, Koschny T, Froster U G et al. 2002 Comparative genomic hybridization in glioma: a meta-analysis of 509 cases. Cancer Genet Cytogene; 135: 147–149
137. Besson A, Wee Yong V 2001 Mitogenic signaling and the relationship to cell cycle regulation in astrocytomas. J Neurooncol 51: 245–264
138. Ivanchuk S M, Mondal S, Dirks P B et al. 2001 The INK4A/ARF locus: role in cell cycle control and apoptosis and implications for glioma growth. J Neurooncol 51: 219–229
139. Parkinson E K, Munro J, Steeghs K et al. 2000 Replicative senescence as a barrier to human cancer. Biochem Soc Trans 28(2): 226–233
140. Hirano H, Lopes M B S, Carpenter J et al. 1999 The IGF-I content and pattern of expression correlates with histopathologic grade in diffusely infiltrating astrocytomas. Neuro-Oncology 1: 109–119
141. Louis D N 1997 A molecular genetic model of astrocytoma histopathology. Brain Pathol 7: 755–764
142. Van Meir E G 1995 Cytokines and tumors of the central nervous system. Glia 15: 264–288
143. Westermark B, Heldin C H, Nister M 1995 Platelet-derived growth factor in human glioma. Glia 15: 257–263
144. Kitange G J, Templeton K L, Jenkins R B 2003 Recent advances in the molecular genetics of primary gliomas. Curr Opin Oncol 15: 197–203
145. Smith J S, Tachibana I, Passe S M et al. 2001 PTEN mutation, EGFR amplification, and outcome in patients with anaplastic astrocytoma and glioblastoma multiforme. J Natl Cancer Inst 93: 1246–1256
146. Liu L, Backlund L M, Nilsson B R et al. 2005 Clinical significance of EGFR amplification and the aberrant EGFR vIII transcript in conventionally treated astrocytic gliomas. J Mol Med 83: 917–926
147. Aldape K D, Ballman K, Furth A et al. 2004 Immunohistochemical detection of EGFRvIII in high malignancy grade astrocytomas and evaluation of prognostic significance. J Neuropathol Exp Neurol 63: 700–707

148. Kleihues P, Ohgaki H 1999 Primary and secondary glioblastoma: from concept to clinical diagnosis. Neuro-Oncology 1: 44–445
149. Ohgaki H, Kleihues P 2005 Population-based studies on incidence, survival rates, and genetic alterations in astrocytic and oligodendroglial gliomas. J Neuropathol Exp Neurol 64: 479–489
150. Bögler O, Su Huang H-J, Kleihues P et al. 1995 The p53 gene and its role in human brain tumors. Glia 15: 308–327
151. Collins V P 1995 Gene amplification in human gliomas. Glia 15: 289–296
152. Sung T, Miller D C, Hayes R L et al. 2000 Preferential inactivation of the p53 tumor suppressor pathway and lack of EGFR amplification distinguish de novo high grade pediatric astrocytomas from de novo adult astrocytomas. Brain Pathol 10: 249–259
153. Sure U, Ruedi D, Tachibana O et al. 1997 Determination of p53 mutations, EGFR over expression, and loss of p16 expression in pediatric glioblastomas. J Neuropathol Exp Neurol 56: 782–789
154. Choe G, Horvath S, Cloughesy T F et al. 2003 Analysis of the phosphatidylinositol 3′-kinase signaling pathway in glioblastoma patients in vivo. Cancer Res 63: 2742–2746
155. Baeza N, Weller M, Yonekawa Y et al. 2003 PTEN methylation and expression in glioblastomas. Acta Neuropathol (Berl) 106: 479–485
156. CBTRUS (2005) Statistical Report: Primary Brain Tumors in the United States, 1998–2002. Published by the Central Brain Tumor Registry of the United States.
157. Kim T S, Halliday A L, Hedley-Whyte E T et al. 1991 Correlates of survival and the Daumas-Duport grading system for astrocytomas. J Neurosurg 74: 27–37
158. Müller W, Afra D, Schroder R 1997 Supratentorial recurrences of gliomas: morphological studies in relation to time intervals with 544 astrocytomas. Acta Neurochir 37: 75–91
159. Huk W J, Gademann G, Friedmann G 1990 MRI of the central nervous system diseases.: Springer-Verlag, Berlin
160. Dean B L, Drayer B P, Bird C R et al. 1990 Gliomas: classification with MR imaging. Radiology 174: 411–415
161. Perentes E, Rubinstein L J 1987 Recent applications of immunoperoxidase histochemistry in human neurooncology. Arch Pathol Lab Med 111: 796–812
162. Russell D S, Rubinstein L J 1989 Astrocytic group. In: Pathology of tumours of the nervous system, 5th edn. Edward Arnold, London, p 95–112
163. Schiffer D, Giordana M T, Mauro A et al. I. 1986 Immunohistochemical demonstration of vimentin in human cerebral tumors. Acta Neuropathol 70: 209–219
164. Krouwer H G J, Davis R L, Silver R et al. 1991 Gemistocytic astrocytomas: a reappraisal. J Neurosurg 74: 399–406
165. Watanabe K, Tachibana O, Yonekawa Y et al. 1997 Role of gemistocytes in astrocytoma progression. Lab Invest 76: 277–284
166. Watanabe K, Peraud A, Gratas C et al. 1998 TI-p53 and PTEN gene mutations in gemistocytic astrocytomas. Acta Neuropathol 95: 559–564
167. Perry A, Aldape K D, George D H et al. 2004 Small cell astrocytoma: an aggressive variant that is clinicopathologically and genetically distinct from anaplastic oligodendroglioma. Cancer 101: 2318–2326
168. Itoh Y, Kowada M, Mineura K et al. 1987 Congenital glioblastoma of the cerebellum with cytofluorometric deoxyribonucleic acid analysis. Surg Neurol 27: 163–167
169. Chin H W, Maruyama Y, Tibbs P et al. 1984 Cerebellar glioblastoma in childhood. J Neurooncol 2: 79–84
170. Dohrmann G J, Farwell J R, Flannery J T 1976 Glioblastoma multiforme in children. J Neurosurg 44: 442–448
171. Georges P M, Noterman J, Flament-Durand J 1983 Glioblastoma in childhood. J Neurooncol 1: 275–278
172. Burger P C, Kleihues P 1989 Cytologic composition of the untreated glioblastoma with implications for evaluation of needle biopsies. Cancer 63: 2014–2023
173. Daumas-Duport C 1992 Histological grading of gliomas. Curr Opin Neurol Neurosurg 5: 924–931
174. Kepes J J, Rubinstein L J 1981 Malignant gliomas with heavily lipidized (foamy) tumor cells: a report of three cases with immunoperoxidase study. Cancer 47: 2451–2459
175. Mørk S J, Rubinstein L J, Kepes J J 1988 Patterns of epithelial metaplasia in malignant gliomas. I. Papillary formations mimicking medulloepithelioma. J Neuropathol Exp Neurol 47: 93–100
176. Schmidt M C, Antweiler S, Urban N et al. 2002 Impact of genotype and morphology on the prognosis of glioblastoma. J Neuropathol Exp Neurol 61: 321–328
177. Misra A, Pellarin M, Nigro J et al. 2005 Array comparative genomic hybridization identifies genetic subgroups in grade 4 human astrocytoma. Clin Cancer Res 11: 2907–2918
178. Mischel P S, Shai R, Shi T et al. 2003 Identification of molecular subtypes of glioblastoma by gene expression profiling. Oncogene 22: 2361–2373
179. Freije W A, Castro-Vargas F E, Fang Z et al. 2004 Gene expression profiling of gliomas strongly predicts survival. Cancer Res 64: 6503–6510
180. Rich J N, Hans C, Jones B et al. 2005 Gene expression profiling and genetic markers in glioblastoma survival. Cancer Res 65: 4051–4058
181. Nigro J M, Misra A, Zhang L et al. 2005 Integrated array-comparative genomic hybridization and expression array profiles identify clinically relevant molecular subtypes of glioblastoma. Cancer Res 65: 1678–1686
181a. Haas-Kogan D A, Prados M D, Tihan T et al. 2005 Epidermal growth factor receptor, protein kinase B/Akt and glioma response to erlotinib. J Natl Cancer Inst 97: 880–887
182. Fuller C E, Perry A 2002 Fluorescence in situ hybridization (FISH) in diagnostic and investigative neuropathology. Brain Pathol 12: 67–86
183. Petersen B L, Sorensen M C, Pedersen S et al. 2004 Fluorescence in situ hybridization on formalin-fixed and paraffin-embedded tissue: optimizing the method. Appl Immunohistochem Mol Morphol 12: 259–265
184. Quezado M, Ronchetti R, Rapkiewicz A et al. 2005 Chromogenic in situ hybridization accurately identifies EGFR amplification in small cell glioblastoma multiforme, a common subtype of primary GBM. Clin Neuropathol 24: 163–169
184a. Mellinghoff I K, Wang M Y, Vivanco I et al. 2005 Molecular determinants of the response of glioblastomas to EGFR kinase inhibitors. N Engl J Med 353: 2012–2024
185. Peraud A, Watanabe K, Schwechheimer K et al. 1999 Genetic profile of the giant cell glioblastoma. Lab Invest 79: 123–129
186. Margetts J C, Kalyan-Raman U P 1989 Giant-celled glioblastoma of brain: a clinicopathological and radiological study of ten cases (including immunohistochemistry and ultrastructure). Cancer 63: 524–531
187. Meyer-Puttlitz B, Haayashi Y, Whah A et al. 1997 Molecular genetic analysis of giant cell glioblastomas. Am J Pathol 151: 853–857
188. Peraud A, Watanabe K, Plate K H et al. 1997 p53 mutations versus EGF receptor expression in giant cell glioblastomas. J Neuropathol Exp Neurol 56: 1236–1241
189. Ohgaki H, Peraud A, Nakazato Y et al. 2000 Giant cell glioblastoma. In: Kleihues P, Cavenee WK (eds) WHO classification of tumors, pathology and genetics: tumours of the nervous sytem. IARC Press, Lyon, p 40–41
190. Ohgaki H, Biernat W, Reis R et al. 2000 Gliosarcoma. In: Kleihues P, Cavenee WK (eds) WHO classification of tumors, pathology and genetics: tumours of the nervous sytem. IARC Press, Lyon, p 42–44
191. Meis J M, Martz K L, Nelson J S 1991 Mixed glioblastoma multiforme and sarcoma. A clinicopathologic study of 26 radiation therapy oncology group cases. Cancer 67: 2342–2349
192. Albrecht S, Connelly J H, Bruner J M 1993 Distribution of p53 protein expression in gliosarcomas: an immunohistochemical study. Acta Neuropathol 85: 222–226
193. Biernat W, Aguzzi A, Sure U et al. 1995 Identical mutations of the p53 tumor suppressor gene in the glial and sarcomatous part of gliosarcomas suggest a common origin from glial cells. J Neuropathol Exp Neurol 54: 651–655
194. Boerman R H, Anderl K, Herath J et al. 1996 The glial and mesenchymal elements of gliosarcoma share similar genetic alterations. J Neuropathol Exp Neurol 55: 973–981
195. Reis R M, Konu-Lebleblicioglu D, Lopes J M et al. 2000 Genetic profile of gliosarcomas. Am J Pathol 156: 425–431
196. Garcia J D M, Fulling K H 1985 Juvenile pilocytic astrocytoma of the cerebrum in adults. A distinctive neoplasm with favorable prognosis. J Neurosurg 63: 382–386
197. Burger P C, Scheithauer B W, Vogel F S 2002 Pilocytic astocytoma. In: Surgical pathology of the nervous system and its coverings, 4th edn. Churchill Livingstone, New York, p 203–215
198. Minehan K J, Shaw E G, Scheithauer B W et al. 1995 Spinal cord astrocytoma: pathological and treatment considerations. J Neurosurg 83: 590–595
199. Schwartz A N, Ghatak N R 1990 Malignant transformation of benign cerebellar astrocytoma. Cancer 56: 333–336
200. Dirks P B, Jay V, Becker L E et al. 1994 Development of anaplastic changes in low grade astrocytomas of childhood. Neurosurgery 34: 68–78
201. Tomlinson F H, Scheithauer B W, Hayostek C H et al. 1994 The significance of atypia and histologic malignancy in pilocytic astrocytoma of the cerebellum: a clinicopathologic and flow cytometric study. J Child Neurol 9: 301–310
202. Tihan T, Fisher P G, Kepner J L et al. 1999 Pediatric astrocytomas with monomorphous pilomyxoid features and a less favorable outcome. J Neuropathol Exp Neurol 58: 1061–1068
203. Li J, Perry A, James C D et al. 2001 Cancer-related gene expression profiles in NF1-associated pilocytic astrocytomas. Neurology 56: 885–890
204. Ohgaki H, Eibl R H, Schwab M et al. 1993 Mutations of the p53 tumor suppressor gene in neoplasms of the human nervous system. Mol Carcinog 8: 74–80
205. Gutmann D H, Medrick N M, Li J et al. 2002 Comparative gene expression profile analysis of neurofibromatosis 1-associated and sporadic pilocytic astrocytomas. Cancer Res 2: 2085–2091
206. Kluwe L, Hagel C, Tatagiba M et al. 2001 Loss of NF1 alleles distinguish sporadic from NF1-associated pilocytic astrocytomas. J Neuropathol Exp Neurol 60: 917–920
207. Platten M, Giordano M J, Dirven C M et al. 1996 Up-regulation of specific NF 1 gene transcripts in sporadic pilocytic astrocytomas. Am J Pathol 149: 621–627
208. Wimmer K, Eckart M, Meyer-Puttlitz B et al. 2002 Mutational and expression analysis of the NF1 gene argues against a role as tumor suppressor in sporadic pilocytic astrocytomas. J Neuropathol Exp Neurol 61: 896–902
209. French-Constant C, Raff M C 1996 Proliferating bipotential glial progenitor cells in adult rat optic nerve. Nature 319: 499–502
210. Norton W T, Farooq M 1989 Astrocytes cultured from mature brain derive from glial precursor cells. J Neurosci 9: 769–775
211. Raff M C, Miller R H, Noble M 1983 A glial progenitor cell that develops in vitro into an astrocyte or an oligodendrocyte depending on culture medium. Nature 303: 390–396

212. Pixley S K R, De Vellis J 1984 Transition between immature radial glia and mature astrocytes studied with a monoclonal antibody to vimentin. Dev Brain Res 15: 201–209
213. Wilkinson M, Hume R, Stragne R et al. 1990 Glial and neuronal differentiation in the human fetal brain 9-23 weeks of gestation. Neuropathol Appl Neurobiol 16: 193–204
214. Kepes J J, Rubinstein L J, Eng L F 1979 Pleomorphic xanthoastrocyoma: a distinctive meningocerebral glioma of young subjects with relatively favorable prognosis. a study of 12 cases. Cancer 44: 1839–1852
215. Herpers M J, Freling G, Beuls E A 1994 Pleomorphic xanthoastrocytoma in the spinal cord. Case report. J Neurosurg 80: 564–569
216. MacKenzie J M 1987 Pleomorphic xanthoastrocytoma in a 62-year-old male. Neuropathol Appl Neurobiol 13: 481–487
217. Strom E H, Skullerud K 1983 Pleomorphic xanthoastrocytoma: report of 5 cases. Clin Neuropathol 2: 188–191
218. Pasquier B, Kojder I, Labat F et al. 1985 Le xanthoastrocytome du sujet jeune. Ann Pathol 5: 29–43
219. Kawano N 1991 Pleomorphic xanthoastrocytoma (PXA) in Japan: its clinico-pathologic features and diagnostic clues. Brain Tumor Pathol 8: 5–10
220. Gil-Gouveia R, Cristino N, Farias J P et al. 2004 Pleomorphic xanthoastrocytoma of the cerebellum: illustrated review. Acta Neurochir (Wien) 146: 1241–1244
221. Weldon-Linne G M, Victor T A, Groothuis D R et al. 1983 Pleomorphic xanthoastrocytoma: ultrastructural and immunohistochemical study of a case with a rapidly fatal outcome following surgery. Cancer 52: 2055–2063
222. Kepes J J, Rubinstein L J, Ansbacher L et al. 1989 Histopathological features of recurrent pleomorphic xanthoastrocytomas: further corroboration of the glial nature of this neoplasm. Acta Neuropathol 78: 585–593
223. Giannini C, Scheithauer B W, Burger P C et al. 1999 Pleomorphic xanthoastrocytoma. What do we really know about it? Cancer 85: 2033–2045
224. Hosokawa Y, Tsuchihashi Y, Okabe H et al. 1991 Pleomorphic xanthoastrocytoma. Ultrastructural, immunohistochemical, and DNA cytofluorometric study of a case. Cancer 68: 853–859
225. Furuta A, Takahashi H, Ikuta F et al. 1992 Temporal lobe tumor demonstrating ganglioglioma and pleomorphic xanthoastrocytoma components. Case report. J Neurosurg 77: 143–147
226. Lindboe C, Cappelen J, Kepes J 1992 Pleomorphic xanthoastrocytoma as a component of a cerebellar ganglioglioma: case report. Neurosurgery 31: 353–355
227. Kordek R, Biernat W, Sapieja W et al. 1995 Pleomorphic xanthoastrocytoma with gangliomatous component: an immunohistochemical and ultrastructural study. Acta Neuropathol 89: 194–197
228. Perry A, Giannini C, Scheithauer B W et al. 1997 Composite pleomorphic xanthoastrocytoma and ganglioglioma: report of four cases and review of the literature. Am J Surg Pathol 21: 763–771
229. Kepes J J, Louis D N, Giannini C et al. 2000 Pleomorphic xanthoastrocytoma. In: Kleihues P, Cavenee WK (eds) WHO classification of tumors, pathology and genetics: tumours of the nervous sytem. IARC Press, Lyon, p 52–54
230. Yin X L, Hui A B, Liong E C et al. 2002 Genetic imbalances in pleomorphic xanthoastrocytoma detected by comparative genomic hybridization and literature review. Cancer Genet Cytogenet 132: 14–19
231. Wiestler O D, Lopes M B S, Green A J et al. 2000 Tuberous sclerosis complex and subependymal giant cell astrocytoma. In: Kleihues P, Cavenee WK (eds) WHO classification of tumors, pathology and genetics: tumours of the nervous system. IARC Press, Lyon, p 227–230
232. Hirose T, Scheithauer B W, Lopes M B et al. 1995 Tuber and subependymal giant cell astrocytoma associated with tuberous sclerosis: an immunohistochemical, ultrastructural, and immunoelectron and microscopic study. Acta Neuropathol 90: 387–399
233. Lopes M B S, Altermatt H T, Scheithauer B W et al. 1996 Immunohistochemical characterization of subependymal giant cell astrocytomas. Acta Neuropathol 91: 368–375
234. Shepherd C W, Scheithauer B W, Gomez M R et al. 1991 Subependymal giant cell astrocytoma: a clinical, pathological, and flow cytometric study. Neurosurgery 28: 864–868
235. Halmagyi G M, Bignold L P, Allsop J L 1979 Recurrent subependymal giant-cell astrocytoma in the absence of tuberous sclerosis. J Neurosurg 50: 106–109
236. Henske E P, Wessner L L, Golden J et al. 1997 Loss of tuberin in both subependymal giant cell astrocytomas and angiomyolipomas supports a two-hit model for the pathogenesis of tuberous sclerosis tumors. Am J Pathol 151: 1639–1647
237. Mizuguchi M, Kato M, Yamanouchi H et al. 1996 Loss of tuberin from cerebral tissues with tuberous sclerosis and astrocytomas. Ann Neurol 40: 941–944
238. Uhlmann E J, Apicelli A J, Baldwin R L et al. 2002 Heterozygosity for the tuberous sclerosis complex (TSC) gene products results in increased astrocyte numbers and decreased p27-Kip1 expression in TSC2± cells. Oncogene 21: 4050–4059
239. Kim S H, Kim H, Kim T S 2005 Clinical, histological, and immunohistochemical features predicting 1p/19q loss of heterozygosity in oligodendroglial tumors. Acta Neuropathol 110: 27–38
240. Kros J M, Pieterman H, van Eden C G et al. 1994 Oligodendroglioma: The Rotterdam-Dijzigt experience. Neurosurgery 34: 959–966
241. Felsberg J, Erkwoh A, Sabel M C et al. 2004 Oligodendroglial tumors: refinement of candidate regions on chromosome arm 1p and correlation of 1p/19q status with survival. Brain Pathol 14: 121–130
242. Coons S W, Johnson P C, Pearl D K 1997 The prognostic significance of Ki-67 labeling indices for oligodendrogliomas. Neurosurgery 41: 878–884
243. Ligon K L, Alberta J A, Kho A T et al. 2004 The oligodendroglial lineage marker OLIG2 is universally expressed in diffuse gliomas. J Neuropathol Exp Neurol 63: 499–509
244. Bouvier C, Bartoli C, Aguirre-Cruz L et al. 2003 Shared oligodendrocyte lineage gene expression in gliomas and oligodendrocyte progenitor cells. J Neurosurg 99:344–350
245. Ohnishi A, Sawa H, Tsuda M et al. 2003 Expression of the oligodendroglial lineage-associated markers Olig1 and Olig2 in different types of human gliomas. J Neuropathol Exp Neurol 62: 1052–1059
246. Herpers M J H M, Budka H 1994 Glial fibrillary acidic protein (GFAP) in oligodendroglial tumors: gliofibrillary oligodendroglioma and transitional oligoastrocytoma as subtypes of oligodendroglioma. Acta Neuropathol 64: 265-272
247. Wondrusch E, Huemer M, Budka H 1991 Production of glial fibrillary acidic protein (GFAP) by neoplastic oligodendrocytes: gliofibrillary oligodendroglioma and transitional oligoastrocytoma revisited. Brain Tumor Pathol 8: 11–15
248. Nakagawa Y, Perentes E, Rubinstein L J 1986 Immunohistochemical characterization of oligodendrogliomas: an analysis of multiple markers. Acta Neuropathol 72: 15–22
249. Choi B H, Kim R C 1985 Expressions of glial fibrillary acidic protein by immature oligodendroglia and its implications. J Neuroimmunol 8: 215–235
250. Kros J M, van Eden C G, Stefanko S Z et al. 1990 Prognostic implications of glial fibrillary acidic protein containing cell types in oligodendrogliomas. Cancer 66: 1204–1212
251. Perentes E, Rubinstein L 1986 Immunohistochemical recognition of human neuroepithelial tumors by anti-Leu 7 (HNK-1) monoclonal antibody. Acta Neuropathol 69: 227–233
252. De La Monte S M 1989 Uniform lineage of oligodendrogliomas. Am J Pathol 135: 529–540
253. Cairncross J G, Macdonald D R, Ramsay D A 1992 Aggressive oligodendroglioma. A chemosensitive tumor. Neurosurgery 31: 78–82
254. Cairncross J G, Ueki K, Zlatescu M C et al. 1998 Specific genetic predictors of chemotherapeutic response and survival in patients with anaplastic oligodendrogliomas. J Natl Cancer Inst 90: 1473–1479
255. Mørk S J, Lindegaad K-F, Halvorsen T B et al. 1985 Oligodendroglioma: incidence and biological behavior in a defined population. J Neurosurg 63: 881–889
256. Smith M T, Ludwig C L, Godfrey A D et al. 1983 Grading of oligodendrogliomas. Cancer 52: 2107–2114
257. Burger P C 1989 The grading of astrocytomas and oligodendrogliomas. In: Fields WS (ed) Primary brain tumors. A review of histologic classification. Springer-Verlag, New York, p 171–180
258. Schiffer D, Dutto A, Cavalla P et al. 1997 Prognostic factors in oligodendrogliomas. Can J Neurol Sci 24: 313–319
259. Bailey P, Bucy P C 1929 Oligodendrogliomas of the brain. J Pathol Bacteriol 32: 735–751
260. Tramontin A D, Garcia-Verdugo J M, Lim D A et al. 2003 Postnatal development of radial glia and the ventricular zone (VZ): a continuum of the neural stem cell compartment. Cereb Cortex 3: 580–587
261. Wren D, Wolwijk G, Noble M 1992 In vitro analysis of the origin and maintenance of 0-2A adult progenitor cells. J Cell Biol 116: 167–176
262. Nishiyama A, Chang A, Trapp B D 1999 NG2+ glial cells: A novel glial cell population in the adult brain. J Neuropathol Exp Neurol 58: 1113–1124
263. Lillien L E, Raff M C 1990 Differentiation signals in the CNS: type-2 astrocyte development in vitro as a model system. Neuron 5: 111–119
264. Reifenberger G, Kros J M, Burger P C et al. 2000 Oligoastrocytoma. In: Kleihues P, Cavenee WK (eds) Pathology and genetics of tumours of the nervous system. IARC, Lyon, p 65–67
265. Coons S W, Johnson P C, Scheithauer B W et al. 1997 Improving diagnostic accuracy and interobserver concordance in the classification and grading of primary gliomas. Cancer 79: 1381–1393
266. Shaffrey M E, Farace E, Schiff D et al. 2005 The Ki-67 labeling index as a prognostic factor in Grade II oligoastrocytomas. J Neurosurg 102: 1033–1039
267. Reifenberger G, Kros J M, Burger P C et al. 2000 Anaplastic oligoastrocytoma. In: Kleihues P, Cavenee WK (eds) Pathology and genetics of tumours of the nervous system. IARC, Lyon, p 68–69
268. Hartmann C, Mueller W, Lass U et al. 2005 Molecular genetic analysis of oligodendroglial tumors. J Neuropathol Exp Neurol 64: 10–14
269. Kreiger P A, Okada Y, Simon S et al. 2005 Losses of chromosomes 1p and 19q are rare in pediatric oligodendrogliomas. Acta Neuropathol (Berl) 109: 387–392
270. Van den Bent M J 2004 Advances in the biology and treatment of oligodendrogliomas. Curr Opin Neurol 17: 675–680
271. Megyesi J F, Kachur E, Lee D H et al. 2004 Imaging correlates of molecular signatures in oligodendrogliomas. Clin Cancer Res 10: 4303–4306
272. Zlatescu M C, Tehrani Yazdi A, Sasaki H et al. 2001 Tumor location and growth pattern correlate with genetic signature in oligodendroglial neoplasms. Cancer Res 61: 6713–6715
273. Mueller W, Hartmann C, Hoffmann A et al. 2002 Genetic signature of oligoastrocytomas correlates with tumor location and denotes distinct molecular subsets. Am J Pathol 161: 313–319

274. Wolter M, Reifenberger J, Blaschke B et al. 2001 Oligodendroglial tumors frequently demonstrate hypermethylation of the CDKN2A (MTS1, p16INK4a, and 14ARF, and CDKN2B (MTS2,p15INK4b) tumor suppressor genes. J Neuropathol Exp Neurol 60: 1170–1180
275. Mukasa A, Ueki K, Matsumoto S et al. 2002 Distinction in gene expression profiles of oligodendrogliomas with and without allelic loss of 1p. Oncogene 21: 3961–3968
276. Robinson S, Cohen M, Prayson R et al. 2001 Constitutive expression of growth-related oncogene and its receptor in oligodendrogliomas. Neurosurgery 48: 864–873
277. Engelhard H H, Stelea A, Cochran E J 2002 Oligodendroglioma: pathology and molecular biology. Surg Neurol 58: 111–117
278. Hoang-Xuan K, He J, Huguet S et al. 2001 Molecular heterogeneity of oligodendrogliomas suggests alternative pathways in tumor progression. Neurology 57: 1278–1281
279. Reifenberger G, Louis D N 2003 Oligodendroglioma: toward molecular definitions in diagnostic neuro-oncology. J Neuropathol Exp Neurol 62: 111–126
280. McLendon R E, Herndon J E 2nd, West B et al. 2005 Survival analysis of presumptive prognostic markers among oligodendrogliomas. Cancer 104: 1693–1699
281. McLendon R E, Wikstrand C J, Matthews M R et al. 2000 Glioma associated antigen expression in oligodendroglial neoplasms: Tenascin and epidermal growth factor receptor. J Histochem Cytochem 48: 1103–1110
282. Bigner S H, Raheed A, Wiltshire R et al. 1999 Morphologic and molecular genetic aspects of oligodendroglial neoplasms. Neuro-Oncology 1: 52–60
283. Bigner S H, Matthews M R, Rasheed B K et al. 1999 Molecular genetic aspects of oligodendrogliomas including analysis by comparative genomic hybridization. Am J Pathol 155: 375–386
284. Reifenberger J, Reifenberger G, Liu L et al. 1994 Molecular genetic analysis of oligodendroglial tumors shows preferential allelic deletions on 19q and 1p. Am J Pathol 145: 175–1190
285. Kraus J A, Koopmann J, Kaskel P et al. 1995 Shared allelic losses on chromosomes 1p and 19q suggest a common origin of oligodendroglioma and oligo-astrocytoma. J Neuropathol Exp Neurol 54: 91–95
286. Kros J M, Lie S-T, Stefanko S Z 1994 Familial occurrence of polymorphous oligodendroglioma. Neurosurgery 34: 732–736
287. Gilles F H, Gomez I G 2005 Developmental neuropathology of the second half of gestation. Early Hum Dev 81: 245–253
288. Morantz R A, Kepes J J, Batnitzky S et al. 1979 Extraspinal ependymomas: report of three cases. J Neurosurg 51: 383–391
289. Pulitzer D R, Martin P C, Collins P C et al. 1988 Subcutaneous sacrococcygeal ("myxopapillary") ependymal rests. Am J Surg Pathol 12: 672–677
290. Quinones-Hinojosa A, Sanai N, Soriano-Navarro M et al. 2006 Cellular composition and cytoarchitecture of the adult human subventricular zone: a niche of neural stem cells. J Comp Neurol 494: 415–434
291. Preusser M, Wolfsberger S, Haberler C et al. 2005 Vascularization and expression of hypoxia-related tissue factors in intracranial ependymoma and their impact on patient survival. Acta Neuropathol 109: 211–216
292. Wiestler O D, Schiffer D, Coons S W et al. 2000 Ependymoma. In: Kleihues P, Cavenee WK (eds) World Health Organization classification of tumours. Pathology and genetics of tumours of the nervous system. IARC, Lyon, p 72–77
293. Gilbertson R J, Bentley L, Hernan R et al. 2002 ERBB receptor signaling promotes ependymoma cell proliferation and represents a potential novel therapeutic target for this disease. Clin Cancer Res 8: 3054–3064
294. Horn B, Heideman R, Geyer R et al. 1999 A multi-institutional retrospective study of intracranial ependymoma in children: identification of risk factors. J Ped Hematol/Oncol 21: 203–211
295. Sonneland P R, Scheithauer B W, Onofrio B M 1985 Myxopapillary ependymoma: a clinicopathologic and immunocytochemical study of 77 cases. Cancer 56: 883–893
296. Sloof J L, Kernohan J W, MacCarty C S 1964 Primary intramedullary tumors of the spinal cord and filum terminale. WB Saunders, Philadelphia
297. McCormick P C, Stein B M 1990 Intramedullary tumors in adults. Neurosurg Clin N Am 1: 609–630
298. Guyotat J, Signorelli F, Desme S et al. 2002 Intracranial ependymomas in adult patients: analyses of prognostic factors. Neuro-Oncol 60: 255–268
299. Korshunov A, Golanov A, Sycheva R 2004 The histologic grade is a main prognostic factor for patients with intracranial ependymomas treated in the microneurosurgical era: an analysis of 258 patients. Cancer 100: 1230–1237
300. Roncaroli F, Consales A, Fioravanti A 2005 Supratentorial cortical ependymoma: report of three cases. Neurosurgery 57: 192
301. Takeuchi H, Kubota T, Sato K et al. 2002 Epithelial differentiation and proliferative potential in spinal ependymomas. J Neuro-Oncol 58: 13–19
302. Min K-W, Scheithauer B W 1997 Clear cell ependymoma: a mimic of oligodendroglioma: clinicopathologic and ultrastructural considerations. Am J Surg Pathol 21: 820–826
303. Katoh M, Satoh T, Nishiya M et al. 2004 Clear cell ependymoma of the fourth ventricle. Neuropathology 24: 330–335
304. Fouladi M, Helton K, Dalton J et al. 2003 Clear cell ependymoma: a clinicopathologic and radiographic analysis of 10 patients. Cancer 98: 2232–2244
305. Ragel B T, Townsend J J, Arthur A S et al. 2005 Intraventricular tanycytic ependymoma: case report and review of the literature. J Neuro-Oncol 71: 189–193
306. Carter M, Nicholson J, Ross F et al. 2002 Genetic abnormalities detected in ependymomas by comparative genomic hybridization. Br J Cancer 86: 929–939
307. Schiffer D, Chio A, Giordana M T et al. 1991 Histologic prognostic factors in ependymoma. Childs Nerv Syst 7: 177–182
308. Schröder R, Ploner C, Ernestus R I 1993 The growth potential of ependymomas with varying grades of malignancy measured by the Ki-67 labelling index and mitotic index. Neurosurg Rev 16: 145–150
309. Rezai A R, Woo H H, Lee M et al. 1996 Disseminated ependymomas of the central nervous system. J Neurosurg 85: 618–624
310. Rushing E J, Yashima K, Brown D F et al. 1997 Expression of telomerase RNA component correlates with the MIB-1 proliferation index in ependymomas. J Neuropathol Exp Neurol 56: 1142–1146
311. Rushing E J, Brown D F, Hladik C L et al. 1998 Correlation of bcl-2, p53, and MIB-1 expression with ependymoma grade and subtype. Mod Pathol 11: 464–470
312. Prayson R A 1999 Clinicopathologic study of 61 patients with ependymoma including MIB-1 immunohistochemistry. Ann Diagn Pathol 3: 11–18
313. Bennetto L, Foreman N, Harding B et al. 1998 Ki-67 immunolabelling index is a prognostic indicator in childhood posterior fossa ependymomas. Neuropathol Appl Neurobiol 24: 434–440
314. Preusser M, Wolfsberger S, Czech T et al. 2005 Survivin expression in intracranial ependymomas and its correlation with tumor cell proliferation and patient outcome. Am J Clin Pathol 124: 543–549
315. Korshunov A, Golanov A, Timirgaz V 2001 p14ARF protein (FL-132) immunoreactivity in intracranial ependymomas and its prognostic significance: an analysis of 103 cases. Acta Neuropathol (Berl) 102: 271–277
316. Korshunov A, Golanov A, Timirgaz V 2000 Immunohistochemical markers for intracranial ependymoma recurrence. An analysis of 88 cases. J Neurol Sci 177: 72–82
317. Ross G W, Rubinstein L J 1989 Lack of histopathological correlation of malignant ependymomas with postoperative survival. J Neurosurg 70: 31–36
318. Schiffer D, Chio A, Cravioto H et al. 1991 Ependymoma: internal correlations among pathological signs: the anaplastic variant. Neurosurgery 29: 206–210
319. Tzerakis N, Georgakoulias N, Kontogeorgos G et al. 2004 Intraparenchymal myxopapillary ependymoma: case report. Neurosurgery 55: 981–985
320. Rawlinson D G, Herman M M, Rubinstein L J 1973 The fine structure of a myxopapillary ependymoma of the filum terminale. Acta Neuropathol 25: 1–13
321. Specht C S, Smith T W, DeGirolami U et al. 1986 Myxo-papillary ependymoma of the filum terminale: a light and electron microscopic study. Cancer 58: 310–317
322. Prayson R A, Suh J H 1999 Subependymomas: clinicopathologic study of 14 tumors, including comparative MIB-1 immunohistochemical analysis with other ependymal neoplasms. Arch Pathol Lab Med 123: 306–309
323. Prayson R A 1997 Myxopapillary ependymoma: a clinicopathologic study of 14 cases including MIB-1 and p53 immunoreactivity. Mod Pathol 10: 304–310
324. Scheithauer B W 1978 Symptomatic subependymoma: report of 21 cases with review of the literature. J Neurosurg 49: 689–696
325. Lombardi D, Scheithauer B W, Meyer F B et al. 1991 Symptomatic subependymoma: a clinical, pathological and flow cytometric study. J Neurosurg 75: 583–588
326. Chiechi M V, Smirniotopoulos J G, Jones R V 1995 Intracranial subependymomas: CT and MR imaging features in 24 cases. Am J Roentgenol 165: 1245–1250
327. Kim H-C, Kima I-O, Kimb C J et al. 2004 Subependymoma in the third ventricle in a child. J Clin Imag 28: 381–384
328. Fu Y-S, Chen A T L, Kay S et al. 1974 Is subependymoma (subependymal glomerate astrocytoma) an astrocytoma or ependymoma? A comparative ultrastructural and tissue culture study. Cancer 34: 1992–2008
329. Azzarelli B, Rekate H L, Roessman U 1997 Subependymoma: a case report with ultrastructural study. Acta Neuropathol 40: 279–282
330. Nakasu S, Ohashi M, Suzuki F et al. 2001 Late dissemination of fourth ventricle ependymoma: a case report. J Neuro-Oncol 55: 117–120
331. Kawabata Y, Takahashi J A, Arakawa Y et al. 2005 Long-term outcome in patients harboring intracranial ependymoma. J Neurosurg 103: 31–37
332. Fassett D R, Schmidt M H 2003 Lumbosacral ependymomas: a review of the management of intradural and extradural tumors. Neurosurg Focus 15: E13
333. Chen C-J, Tseng Y-C, Hsu H-L et al. 2004 Imaging predictors of intracranial ependymomas. J Comput Assist Tomogr 28: 407–413
334. Agaoglu F Y, Ayan I, Dizdar Y et al. 2005 Ependymal tumors in childhood. Pediatr Blood Cancer 45: 298–303
335. Korshunov A, Neben K, Wrobel G et al. 2003 Gene expression patterns in ependymomas correlate with tumor location, grade, and patient age. Am J Pathol 163: 1721–1727
336. Goussia A C, Kyritsis A P, Mitlianga P et al. 2001 Genetic abnormalities in oligodendroglial and ependymal tumours. J Neurol 248: 1030–1035
337. Santi M, Quezado, M, Ronchetti R et al. 2005 Analysis of chromosome 7 in adult and pediatric ependymomas using chromogenic in situ hybridization. J Neurooncol 72: 25–28
338. Yu J, Zhang H, Gu J et al. 2004 Methylation profiles of thirty four promoter-CpG islands and concordant methylation behaviours of sixteen genes that may contribute to carcinogenesis of astrocytoma. BMC Cancer 4: 65–79
339. Hamilton D W, Lusher M E, Lindsey J C et al. 2005 Epigenetic inactivation of the RASSF1A tumour suppressor gene in ependymoma. Cancer Lett 227: 75–81

340. Von Haken MS, White EC, Daneshvar-Shyesther L et al. 1996 Molecular genetic analysis of chromosome arm 17p and chromosome arm 22q DNA sequences in sporadic pediatric ependymomas. Genes Chromos Cancer 17: 37–44
341. Ebert C, von Haken M, Meyer-Puttlitz B et al. 1999 Molecular genetic analysis of ependymal tumors. NF2 mutations and chromosome 22q loss occur preferentially in intramedullary spinal ependymomas. Am J Pathol 155: 627–632
342. Jeuken J W M, Sprenger S H E, Gilhuis J et al. 2002 Correlation between localization, age, and chromosomal imbalances in ependymal tumours as detected by CGH. J Pathol 197: 238–244
343. Rousseau E, Ruchoux M-M, Scaravilli F et al. 2003 CDKN2A, CDKN2B and p14^{ARF} are frequently and differentially methylated in ependymal tumours. Neuropathol Appl Neurobiol 29: 574-583
344. Waha A, Koch A, Hartmann W et al. 2004 Analysis of HIC-1 methylation and transcription in human ependymomas. Int J Cancer 110: 542–549
345. Mahler-Araujo M B, Sanoudou D, Tingby O et al. 2003 Structural genomic abnormalities of chromosomes 9 and 18 in myxopapillary ependymomas. J Neuropathol Exp Neurol 62: 927–935
346. Aguzzi A, Brandner S, Paulus W 2000 Choroid plexus tumours. In: Kleihues P, Cavenee WK (eds) World Health Organization classification of tumours. Pathology and genetics of tumours of the nervous system. IARC, Lyon, p 84–86
347. Rickert C H, Paulus W 2001 Tumors of the choroid plexus. Microsc Res Tech 52: 104–111
348. Russell D S, Rubinstein L J 1989 Papillomas and carcinomas of the choroid plexus. In: Pathology of tumours of the nervous system, 5th edn. Edward Arnold, London, p 394–404
349. Laurence K M 1979 The biology of choroid plexus papilloma in infancy and childhood. Acta Neurochir 50: 79–90
350. Packer R J, Perilongo G, Johnson D et al. 1992 Choroid plexus carcinoma of childhood. Cancer 69: 580–585
351. Pierga J Y, Kalifa C, Terrier-Lacombe M J et al. 1993 Carcinoma of the choroid plexus: a pediatric experience. Med Pediat Oncol 21: 480–487
352. Kepes J J 1983 Oncocytic transformation of choroid plexus epithelium. Acta Neuropathol 62: 145–148
353. Bonnin J M, Colon L E, Morawetz R B 1987 Focal glial differentiation and oncocytic transformation in choroid plexus papilloma. Acta Neuropathol 72: 277–280
354. Masuzawa T, Shimabukuro H, Yoshimuzu N et al. 1981 Ultrastructure of disseminated choroid plexus papilloma. Acta Neuropathol 54: 321–324
355. Paulus W, Jänisch W 1990 Clinicopathologic correlations in epithelial choroid plexus neoplasms: a study of 52 cases. Acta Neuropathol 80: 635–641
356. Vajtai I, Varga Z, Aguzzi A 1996 MIB-1 immunoreactivity reveals different labelling in low-grade and in malignant epithelial neoplasms of the choroid plexus. Histopathology 29: 147–151
357. Rubinstein L J, Brucher J M 1981 Ependymal differentiation in choroid plexus papillomas. Acta Neuropathol 53: 29–33
358. Taratuto A L, Molina H, Monges J 1983 Choroid plexus tumors in infancy and childhood. Focal ependymal differentiation. An immunoperoxidase study. Acta Neuropathol 59: 304–308
359. Miettinen M, Clark R, Virtanen I 1986 Intermediate filament proteins in choroid plexus and ependyma and their tumors. Am J Pathol 123: 231–240
360. Lopes M B S, Rosenberg S, de Almeida P C et al. 1989 Glial fibrillary acidic protein and cytokeratin in choroid plexus neoplasms: an immunohistochemical study. Pathol Res Pract 185: 339–341
361. Doglioni C, Dell'Orto P, Coggi G et al. 1987 Choroid plexus tumors. An immunocytochemical study with particular reference to the coexpression of intermediate filament proteins. Am J Pathol 127: 519–529
362. Herbert J, Cavallaro T, Dwork A J 1990 A marker for primary choroid plexus neoplasms. Am J Pathol 136: 1317–1325
363. Albrecht S, Rouah E, Becker L E et al. 1991 Transthyretin immunoreactivity in choroid plexus neoplasms and brain metastases. Mod Pathol 4: 610–614
364. Hasselblatt M, Bohm C, Tatenhorst L et al. 2006 Identification of novel diagnostic markers for choroid plexus tumors: a microarray-based approach. Am J Surg Pathol 30: 66–74
365. Vraa-Jensen G 1950 Papilloma of the choroid plexus with pulmonary metastases. Acta Psychiatr Neurol 25: 299–306
366. Gessi M, Giangaspero F, Pietsch T 2003 Atypical teratoid/rhabdoid tumors and choroid plexus tumors: when genetics "surprise" pathology. Brain Pathol 13: 409–414
367. Pencalet P, Sainte-Rose C, Lellouch-Tubiana A et al. 1998 Papillomas and carcinomas of the choroid plexus in children. J Neurosurg 88: 521–528
368. Wolfson W L, Brown W J 1997 Disseminated choroid plexus papilloma: an ultrastructural study. Arch Pathol Lab Med 101: 366–368
369. McGirr S J, Ebersold M J, Scheithauer B W 1988 Choroid plexus papillomas: long term follow-up of a surgically treated series. J Neurosurg 69: 843–849
370. Oghaki H, Vital A, Kleihues P et al. 2000 Li-Fraumeni syndrome and *TP53* germline mutations. In: Kleihues P, Cavenee WK (eds) World Health Organization classification of tumours. Pathology and genetics of tumours of the nervous system. IARC, Lyon, p 231–234
371. Wanschitz J, Schmidbauer M, Maier H et al. 1995 Suprasellar meningioma with expression of glial fibrillary acidic protein: a peculiar variant. Acta Neuropathol 90: 539–544
372. Brat D J, Scheithauer B W, Staugaitis S M et al. 1998 Third ventricular chordoid glioma: a distinct clinicopathologic entity. J Neuropathol Exp Neurol 57: 283–290
373. Vajtai I, Varga Z X, Scheithauer B W et al. 1999 Chordoid glioma of the third ventricle: confirmatory report of a new entity. Hum Pathol 30: 723–726
374. Pasquier B, Péoc'h M, Morrison A L et al. 2002 Chordoid glioma of the third ventricle: a report of two new cases, with further evidence supporting an ependymal differentiation, and review of the literature. Am J Surg Pathol 26: 1330–1342
375. Raizer J J, Shetty T, Gutin P H et al. 2003 Chordoid glioma: report of a case with unusual histologic features, ultrastructural study and review of the literature. J Neurooncol 63: 39–47
376. Oda M, Sasajima T, Kinouchi H et al. 2002 Third ventricular chordoid glioma: report of a surgical case. No Shinkei Geka 30: 973–979
377. Castellano-Sanchez A A, Schemankewitz E, Mazewski C et al. 2001 Pediatric chordoid glioma, with chondroid metaplasia. Pediatr Dev Pathol 4: 564–567
378. Pizer B L, Moss T, Oakhill A et al. 1995 Congenital astroblastoma: an immunohistochemical study. Case report. J Neurosurg 83: 550–555
379. Bonnin J M, Rubinstein L J 1989 Astroblastomas: a pathological study of 23 tumors, with a postoperative follow-up in 13 patients. Neurosurgery 25: 6–13
380. Brat D J, Hirose Y, Cohen K J et al. 2000 Astroblastoma: clinicopathologic features and chromosomal abnormalities defined by comparative genomic hybridization. Brain Pathol 10: 342–352
381. Port J D, Brat D J, Burger P C et al. 2003 Astroblastoma: radiologic-pathologic correlation and distinction from ependymoma. Am J Neuroradiol 23: 243–247
382. Rubinstein L J, Herman M M 1989 The astroblastoma and its possible cytogenetic relationship to the tancyte. Acta Neuropathol 78: 472–483
383. Artigas J, Cervos-Navarro J, Iglesias J R et al. 1985 Gliomatosis cerebri: clinical and histological findings. Clin Neuropathol 4: 135–148
384. Kandler R H, Smith C M, Broome J C et al. 1991 Gliomatosis cerebri: a clinical, radiological and pathological report of four cases. Br J Neurosurg 5: 187–193
385. Rust P, Ashkan K, Ball C et al. 2001 Gliomatosis cerebri: pitfalls in diagnosis. J Clin Neurosci 8: 361–363
386. Vates G E, Chang S, Lamborn K R et al. 2003 Gliomatosis cerebri: a review of 22 cases. Neurosurgery 53: 261–271
387. Nelson J S, Bruner J M, Wiestler O D et al. 2000 Ganglioglioma and gangliocytoma. In: Kleihues P, Cavenee WK (eds) World Health Organization classification of tumours. Pathology and genetics: tumours of the nervous system. IARC Press, Lyon, p 96–98
388. Russell D C, Rubinstein L J 1989 Pathology of tumours of the nervous system, 5th edn. Edward Arnold, London, p 289–306
389. Russo C P, Katz D S, Corona R J et al. 1995 Gangliocytoma of the cervicothoracic spinal cord. Am J Neuroradiol 16: 889–891
390. Beal M F, Kleinman G M, Pjemann R G et al. 1981 Gangliocytoma of third ventricle. Hyperphagia, somnolence, and dementia. Neurology 31: 1224–1228
391. Towfighi J, Salam M M, McLendon R E et al. 1996 Ganglion cell-containing tumors of the pituitary gland. Arch Pathol Lab Med 120: 369–377
392. Boyko O B, Curnes J T, Oakes W J et al. 1991 Hamartomas of the tuber cinereum. CT, MR, and pathologic findings. Am J Neuroradiol 12: 309–314
393. Tuli S, Provias J P, Bernstein M 1997 Lhermitte-Duclos disease. Literature review and novel treatment strategy. Can J Neurol Sci 24: 155–160
394. Abel T W, Baker S J, Fraser M M et al. 2005 Lhermitte-Duclos disease: a report of 31 cases with immunohistochemical analysis of the PTEN/AKT/mTOR pathway. J Neuropathol Exp Neurol 64: 341–349
395. Shiruba R A, Gessaga E C, Eng L F et al. 1998 Lhermitte-Duclos disease: an immunohistochemical study of the cerebellar cortex. Acta Neuropathol 75: 474–480
396. Faillot T, Sichez J-P, Brault J-L et al. 1990 Lhermitte-Duclos disease (dysplastic gangliocytoma of the cerebellum). Report of a case and review of the literature. Acta Neurochir 105: 44–49
397. Hair L S, Symmans F, Powers J M et al. 1992 Immunohistochemistry and proliferative activity in Lhermitte-Duclos disease. Acta Neuropathol 84: 570–573
398. Reznik M, Schoenen J 1983 Lhermitte-Duclos disease. Acta Neuropathol 59: 88–94
399. Yachnis A T, Trojanowski J Q, Memmo M et al. 1988 Expression of neurofilament proteins in the hypertrophic granule cells of Lhermitte-Duclos disease: an explanation for the mass effect and the myelination of parallel fibers in the disease state. J Neuropathol Exp Neurol 47: 206–216
400. Vinchon M, Blond S, Lejeune J P et al. 1994 Association of Lhermitte-Duclos and Cowden disease: report of a new case and review of the literature. J Neurol Neurosurg Psych 57: 699–704
401. Albrecht S, Haber R M, Goodman J C et al. 1992 Cowden syndrome and Lhermitte-Duclos disease. Cancer 70: 869–876
402. Eng C, Murday V, Seal S et al. 1994 Cowden syndrome and Lhermitte-Duclos disease in a family: a single genetic syndrome with pleiotropy. J Med Genet 31: 458–461
403. Rimbau J, Isamat F 1994 Dysplastic gangliocytoma of the cerebellum (Lhermitte-Duclos disease) and its relation to the multiple hamartoma syndrome (Cowden's disease). J Neurooncol 18: 191–197
404. Vital A, Vital C, Martin-Negrier M L et al. 1994 Lhermitte-Duclos type cerebellum hamartoma and Cowden disease. Clin Neuropathol 13: 229–231
405. Wells G B, Lasner T M, Yousem D M et al. 1994 Lhermitte-Duclos disease and Cowden's syndrome in an adolescent patient. J Neurosurg 81: 133–136
406. Robinson S, Cohen A R 2000 Cowden's disease and Lhermitte-Duclos disease: characterization of a new phakomatosis. Neurosurgery 46: 371–383

407. Padberg G W, Schot J D, Vielvoye G J et al. 1991 Lhermitte-Duclos disease and Cowden disease: a single phakomatosis. Ann Neurol 29: 517–523
408. Nelen M R, Padberg G W, Peeters E A et al. 1996 Localization of the gene for Cowden disease to chromosome 10q22-23. Nat Genet 13: 114–116
409. Zhou X P, Marsh D J, Morrison C D et al. 2003 Germline inactivation of PTEN and dysregulation of the phosphoinositol-3-kinase/Akt pathway cause human Lhermitte-Duclos disease in adults. Am J Hum Genet 73: 1191–1198
410. Liaw D, Marsh D J, Li J et al. 1997 Germline mutations of the PTEN gene in Cowden disease, an inherited breast and thyroid cancer syndrome. Nat Genet 16: 64–67
411. Starink T M, Meijer C J L M, Brownstein M H 1985 The cutaneous pathology of Cowden's disease: new findings. J Cutan Pathol 12: 83–93
412. Carlson G J, Nivatvong S, Snover D C 1984 Colorectal polyps in Cowden's disease (multiple hamartoma syndrome). Am J Surg Pathol 8: 763–770
413. Williard W, Borgen P, Bol R et al. 1992 Cowden's disease. A case report with analyses at the molecular level. Cancer 69: 2969–2974
414. Staal F J, van der Luijt R B, Baert M R et al. 2002 A novel germline mutation of PTEN associated with brain tumors of multiple lineages. Br J Cancer 86: 1586–1591
415. Banerjee A K, Gleadhill C A 1979 Lhermitte-Duclos disease (diffuse cerebellar hypertrophy): prolonged postoperative survival. Ir J Med Sci 148: 97–99
416. Marano S R, John P C, Spetzler R F 1988 Recurrent Lhermitte-Duclos disease in a child. J Neurosurg 69 599–603
417. Reeder R F, Saunders R L, Fratkin J D et al. 1988 Magnetic resonance imaging in the diagnosis and treatment of Lhermitte-Duclos disease. Neurosurgery 23: 140–245
418. Hair L S, Symmans F, Powers J M et al. 1992 Immunohistochemistry and proliferative activity in Lhermitte-Duclos disease. Acta Neuropathol 84: 570–573
419. Stapleton S R, Wilkins P R, Bell B A 1992 Recurrent dysplastic cerebellar gangliocytoma (Lhermitte-Duclos disease) presenting with subarachnoid haemorrhage. Br J Neurosurg 6: 153–156
420. Williams D W, Elster A D, Ginsberg L E et al. 1992 Recurrent Lhermitte-Duclos disease: report of two cases and association with Cowden's disease. Am J Neuroradiol 13: 287–290
421. Hashimoto H, Iida J, Masui K et al. 1997 Recurrent Lhermitte-Duclos disease: case report. Neurol Med Chir (Tokyo) 37: 692–696
422. Taratuto A L, Monges J, Lylyk P et al. 1984 Superficial cerebral astrocytoma attached to dura. Report of six cases in infants. Cancer 54: 2505–2512
423. VandenBerg S R 1993 Desmoplastic infantile ganglioglioma and desmoplastic cerebral astrocytoma of infancy. Brain Pathol 3: 275–281
424. Taratuto A L, VandenBerg S R, Rorke L B 2000 Desmoplastic infantile astrocytoma and ganglioglioma. In: Kleihues P, Cavenee WK (eds) World Health Organization classification of tumours. Pathology and genetics: tumours of the nervous system. IARC Press, Lyon, p 99–102
425. Onguru O, Celasun B, Gunhan O 2005 Desmoplastic non-infantile ganglioglioma. Neuropathology 25: 150–152
426. Pommepuy I, Delage-Corre M, Moreau J et al. 2005 A report of a desmoplastic ganglioglioma in a 12-year-old girl with review of the literature. J Neurooncol Sep 9 (Epub ahead of print)
427. Duffner P K, Burger P C, Cohen M E et al. 1994 Desmoplastic infantile gangliogliomas: an approach to therapy. Neurosurgery 34: 583–589
428. Komori T, Scheithauer B W, Parisi J E et al. 2001 Mixed conventional and desmoplastic infantile ganglioglioma: an autopsied case with 6-year follow-up. Mod Pathol 14: 720–726
429. Setty S N, Miller D C, Camras L et al. 1997 Desmoplastic infantile astrocytoma with metastases at presentation. Mod Pathol 10: 945–951
430. Louis D N, von Deimling A, Dickersin G R et al. 1992 Desmoplastic cerebral astrocytomas of infancy: A histopathologic, immunohistochemical, ultrastructural, and molecular genetic study. Hum Pathol 23: 402–409
431. Trehan G, Bruge H, Vinchon M et al. 2004 MR Imaging in the diagnosis of desmoplastic infantile tumor: retrospective study of six cases. Am J Neuroradiol 25: 1028–1033
432. Tamburrini G, Colosimo C, Giangaspero F et al. 2003 Desmoplastic infantile ganglioglioma. Childs Nerv Syst 19: 292–297
433. Fan X, Larson T C, Jennings M T et al. 2001 December 2000: 6 month old boy with 2 week history of progressive lethargy. Brain Pathol 11: 265–266
434. De Munnynck K, Van Gool S, Van Calenbergh F et al. 2002 Desmoplastic infantile ganglioglioma: a potentially malignant tumor? Am J Surg Pathol 26: 1515–1522
435. Daumas-Duport C 1993 Dysembryoplastic neuroepithelial tumours. Brain Pathol 3: 283–295
436. Daumas-Duport C, Pietsch T, Lantos P L 2000 Dysembryoplastic neuroepithelial tumour. In: Kleihues P, Cavenee WK (eds) World Health Organization classification of tumours. Pathology and genetics: tumours of the nervous system. IARC Press, Lyon, p 103–106
437. Nolan M A, Sakuta R, Chuang N et al. 2004 Dysembryoplastic neuroepithelial tumors in childhood. Long-term outcome and prognostic features. Neurology 62: 2270–2276
438. Kuchelmeister K, Demirel T, Schlorer E et al. 1995 Dysembryoplastic neuroepithelial tumour of the cerebellum. Acta Neuropathol 89: 385–390
439. Fijumoto K, Ohnishi H, Tsujimoto M et al. 2000 Dysembryoplastic neuroepithelial tumor of the cerebellum and brainstem. Case report. J Neurosurg 93: 487–489
440. Leung S Y, Gwi E, Ng H K et al. 1994 Dysembryoplastic neuroepithelial tumor. A tumor with small neuronal cells resembling oligodendroglioma. Am J Surg Pathol 18: 604–614
441. Ostertun B, Wolf H K, Campos M G et al. 1996 Dysembryoplastic neuroepithelial tumors. MR and CT evaluation. Am J Neuroradiol 17: 419–430
442. Stanescu Cosson R, Varlet P, Beuvon F et al. 2001 Dysembryoplastic neuroepithelial tumors: CT, MR findings and imaging follow-up: a study of 53 cases. J Neuroradiol 28: 230–240
443. Takahashi A, Hong S-C, Seo D W et al. 2005 Frequent association of cortical dysplasia in dysembryoplastic neuroepithelial tumor treated by epilepsy surgery. Surg Neurol 64: 419–427
444. Taratuto A L, Pomata H, Sevlever G et al. 1995 Dysembryoplastic neuroepithelial tumor: morphological, immunocytochemical, and deoxyribonucleic acid analyses in a pediatric series. Neurosurgery 36: 474–481
445. Prayson R A, Morris H H, Estes M L et al. 1996 Dysembryoplastic neuroepithelial tumor: a clinicopathologic and immunohistochemical study of 11 tumors including MIB-1 immunoreactivity. Clin Neuropathol 15: 47–53
446. Hirose T, Scheithauer B W, Lopes M B S et al. 1994 Dysembryoplastic neuroepithelial tumor (DNT): an immunohistochemical and ultrastructural study. J Neuropathol Exp Neurol 53: 184–195
447. Daumas-Duport C, Scheithauer B W, Chodkiewicz J-P et al. 1988 Dysembryoplastic neuroepithelial tumor: a surgically curable tumor of young patients with intractable partial seizures: report of thirty-nine cases. Neurosurgery 23: 545–556
448. Hammond R R, Duggal N, Woulfe J M et al. 2000 Malignant transformation of a dysembryoplastic neuroepithelial tumor. Case report. J Neurosurg 92: 722–725
449. Cervera-Pierot P, Varlet P, Chodkiewicz J P et al. 1997 Dysembryoplastic neuroepithelial tumors located in the caudate nucleus area: report of four cases. Neurosurgery 40: 1065–1070
450. Baisden B L, Brat D J, Melhem E R et al. 2001 Dysembryoplastic neuroepithelial tumor-like neoplasm of the septum pellucidum: a lesion often misdiagnosed as glioma. Report of 10 cases. Am J Surg Pathol 25: 494–499
451. Wolf H K, Muller M B, Spanle M et al. 1994 Ganglioglioma. A detailed histopathological and immunohistochemical analysis of 61 cases. Acta Neuropathol 88: 166–173
452. Johnson J H Jr, Hariharan S, Berman J et al. 1997 Clinical outcome of pediatric gangliogliomas. Ninety-nine cases over 20 years. Pediatr Neurosurg 27: 203–207
453. Hirose T, Scheithauer B W, Lopes M B et al. 1997 Ganglioglioma. An ultrastructural and immunohistochemical study. Cancer 79: 989–1003
454. Blumcke I, Wiestler O D 2002 Gangliogliomas: an intriguing tumor entity associated with focal epilepsies. J Neuropathol Exp Neurol 61: 575–584
455. Prayson R A, Khajavi K, Comair Y G 1995 Cortical architectural abnormalities and MIB1 immunoreactivity in gangliogliomas. A study of 60 patients with intracranial tumors. J Neuropathol Exp Neurol 54: 513–520
456. Giannini C, Scheithauer B W, Lopes M B et al. 2002 Immunophenotype of pleomorphic xanthoastrocytoma. Am J Surg Pathol 26: 479–485
457. Takahashi H, Ikuta F, Tsuchida T et al. 1987 Ultrastructural alterations of neuronal cells in a brain stem ganglioglioma. Acta Neuropathol 74: 307–312
458. Luyken C, Blumcke I, Fimmers R et al. 2004 Supratentorial gangliogliomas: histopathologic grading and tumor recurrence in 184 patients with a median follow-up of 8 years. Cancer 101: 146–155
459. Kalyan-Raman U P, Olivero W C 1987 Ganglioglioma: a correlative clinicopathological and radiological study of ten surgically treated cases with follow-up. Neurosurgery 20: 428–433
460. Hakim R, Loeffler J S, Anthony D C et al. 1997 Gangliogliomas in adults. Cancer 79: 127–131
461. Komori T, Scheithuaer B W, Anthony D C et al. 1998 Papillary glioneuronal tumor: a new variant of mixed neuronal-glial neoplasm. Am J Surg Pathol 22: 1171–1183
462. Prayson R A 2000 Papillary glioneuronal tumor. Arch Pathol Lab Med 20: 558–563
463. Bouvier-Labit C, Daniel L, Dufour H et al. 2000 Papillary glioneuronal tumour: clinicopathological and biochemical study of one case with 7-year follow-up. Acta Neuropathol 99: 321–326
464. Tsukayama C, Arakawa Y 2002 A papillary glioneuronal tumor arising in an elderly woman: a case report. Brain Tumor Pathol 19: 35–39
465. Broholm H, Madsen F F, Wagner A A et al. 2002 Papillary glioneuronal tumor – a new tumor entity. Clin Neuropathol 21: 1–4
466. Komori T, Scheithauer B W, Hirose T 2002 A rosette-forming glioneuronal tumor of the fourth ventricle. Infratentorial form of dysembryoplastic neuropeithelial tumor? Am J Surg Pathol 26: 582–591
467. Preusser M, Dietrich W, Czech T et al. 2003 Rosette-forming glioneuronal tumor of the fourth ventricle. Acta Neuropathol 106: 506–508
468. Teo J G C, Gultekin S H, Bilsky M et al. 1999 A distinctive glioneuronal tumor of adult cerebrum with neuropil-like (including "rosetted") islands. Report of 4 cases. Am J Surg Pathol 23: 502–510
469. Prayson R A, Abramovick C M 2000 Glioneuronal tumor with neuropil-like islands. Hum Pathol 31: 1435–1438
470. Keyvani K, Rickert C H, von Wild K et al. 2001 Rosetted glioneuronal tumor: a case with proliferating neuronal nodules. Acta Neuropathol 101: 525–528
471. Perry A, Scheithauer B W, Macaulay R J B et al. 2002 Oligodendrogliomas with neurocytic differentiation. A report of 4 cases with diagnostic and histogenesis implications. J Neuropathol Exp Neurol 61: 947–955
472. Von Deimling A, Janzer R, Kleihues P et al. 1990 Patterns of differentiation in central neurocytoma: an immunohistochemical study of eleven biopsies. Acta Neuropathol 79: 473–479

602. Elster A D, Challa V R, Gilbert T H et al. 1989 Meningiomas: MR and histopathologic features. Radiology 170: 857–862
603. McComb R D, Bigner D D 1985 Immunolocalization of laminin in neoplasms of the central and peripheral nervous systems. J Neuropathol Exp Neurol 44: 242–253
604. Roncaroli F, Scheithauer B W, Laeng R H et al. 2001 Lipomatous meningioma. A clinicopathologic study of 18 cases with special reference to the issue of metaplasia. Am J Surg Pathol 25: 769–775
605. Radley M G, Di Sant'Agnese P A, Eskin T A et al. 1989 Epithelial differentiation in meningiomas. An immunohistochemical, histochemical and ultrastructural study – with review of literature. Am J Clin Pathol 92: 266–272
606. Zorludemir S, Scheithauer B W, Hirose T et al. 1995 Clear cell meningioma. A clinicopathologic study of a potentially aggressive variant of meningioma. Am J Surg Pathol 19: 493–505
607. Steilen-Gimbel H, Niedermayer I, Feiden W et al. 1999 Unbalanced translocation t(1;3)(p12-13;q11) in meningiomas as the unique feature of chordoid differentiation. Genes Chromos Cancer 26: 270–272
607a. Hahn H P, Bundock E A, Hornick J L 2006 Immunohistochemical staining for Claudin-1 can help distinguish meningiomas from histologic mimics. Am J Clin Pathol 125: 203–208
608. Perry A, Stafford S L, Scheithauer B W et al. 1998 The prognostic role of MIB-1, p53 and DNA flow cytometry in completely resected primary meningiomas. Cancer 82: 2262–2269
609. Perry A, Stafford S L, Scheithauer B W et al. 1997 Meningioma grading. An analysis of histologic parameters. Am J Surg Pathol 21: 1455–1465
610. Perry A, Scheithauer B W, Stafford S L et al. 1999 "Malignancy" in meningiomas. A clinicopathologic study of 116 patients, with grading implications. Cancer 85: 2046–2056
611. Chen W Y, Liu H C 1990 Atypical (anaplastic) meningioma: relationship between histologic features and recurrence – a clinicopathologic study. Clin Neuropathol 9: 74–81
612. Maier H, Wanschitz J, Sedivy R et al. 1997 Proliferation and DNA fragmentation in meningioma subtypes. Neuropathol Appl Neurobiol 23: 496–506
613. Ludwin S K, Rubinstein L J, Russell D S 1975 Papillary meningiomas: a malignant variant of meningioma. Cancer 36: 1363–1373
614. Kepes J J, Goldware S, Leoni R 1983 Meningioma with pseudoglandular pattern. J Neuropathol Exp Neurol 42: 61–68
615. Kepes J J, Moral L A, Wilinson S B et al. 1998 Rhabdoid transformation of tumor cells in meningiomas: a histologic indication of increased proliferative activity: report of four cases. Am J Surg Pathol 22: 231–238
616. Perry A, Scheithauer B W, Stafford S L et al. 1998 "Rhabdoid" meningioma: an aggressive variant. Am J Surg Pathol 22: 1482–1490
617. Perry A, Gutmann D H, Reifenberger G 2004 Molecular pathogenesis of meningiomas. J Neuro-Oncol 70: 183–202
618. Jellinger K, Paulus W 1991 Mesenchymal, non-meningothelial tumors of the central nervous system. Brain Pathol 1: 79–87
619. Mena H, Ribas J L, Pezeshkpur G H et al. 1991 Hemangiopericytoma of the central nervous system: a review of 94 cases. Hum Pathol 22: 84–91
620. Jääskeläinen J, Louis D N, Paulus W et al. 2000 Haemangiopericytoma. In: Kleihues P, Cavenee WK (eds) World Health Organization classification of tumours. Pathology and genetics: tumours of the nervous system. IARC Press, Lyon, p 190–192
621. Guillou L, Fletcher J A, Fletcher C D M et al. 2002 Extrapleural solitary fibrous tumour and haemangiopericytoma. In: Fletcher CDM, Unni KK, Mertens F (eds) World Health Organization classification of tumours. Pathology and genetics of tumours of soft tissue and bone. IARC, Lyon, p 86–90
622. Winek R R, Scheithauer B W, Wick M R 1989 Meningioma, meningeal hemangiopericytoma (angioblastic meningioma), peripheral hemangiopericytoma and acoustic schwannoma. A comparative immunohistochemical study. Am J Surg Pathol 13: 251–261
623. Vuorinen V, Salinen P, Haapasalo H et al. 1996 Outcome of 31 intracranial hemangiopericytomas. Poor predictive value of cell proliferation indices. Acta Neurochir 138: 1399–1408
624. Nascimento A G 1996 Solitary fibrous tumor: a ubiquitous neoplasm of mesenchymal differentiation. Adv Anat Pathol 3: 388–395
625. Chan J K C. 1997 Solitary fibrous tumor: everywhere, and a diagnosis in vogue. Histopathology 31: 568–576
626. Carneiro S S, Scheithauer B W, Nascimento A G et al. 1996 Solitary fibrous tumors of the meninges: a lesion distinct from fibrous meningioma. A clinicopathologic and immunohistochemical study. Am J Clin Pathol 106: 217–224
627. Nikas D C, Girolami U D, Fokeerth R D et al. 1999 Parasagittal solitary fibrous tumor of the meninges. Case report and review of the literature. Acta Neurochir 141: 307–313
628. Kanahara T, Hirokawa M, Shimizu M et al. 1999 Solitary fibrous tumor of the spinal cord: Report of a case with scrape cytology. Acta Cytol 43: 425–428
629. Brunori A, Cerasoli S, Donati R et al. 1999 Solitary fibrous tumor of the meninges: Two new cases and review of the literature. Surg Neurol 51: 636–640
630. Rodriguez F, Scheithauer B W, Ockner D M et al. 2004 Solitary fibrous tumor of the cerebellopontine angle with salivary gland heterotopia: a unique presentation. Am J Surg Pathol 28: 139–142
631. Somerhausen N de S A, Rubin B P, Fletcher C D M 1999 Myxoid solitary fibrous tumor: a study of seven cases with emphasis on differential diagnosis. Mod Pathol 12: 463–471
632. Perry A, Scheithauer B W, Nascimento A G 1997 The immunophenotypic spectrum of meningeal hemangiopericytoma: a comparison with fibrous meningioma and solitary fibrous tumor of meninges. Am J Surg Pathol 21: 1354–1360
633. Vallat-Decouvelaere A-V, Dry S, Fletcher C D M 1998 Atypical and malignant solitary fibrous tumors in extrathoracic locations: evidence of their comparability to intrathoracic tumors. Am J Surg Pathol 22: 1501–1511
634. Böhling T, Plate K H, Haltia M J et al. 2000 von Hippel-Lindau disease and capillary haemangioblastoma. In: Kleihues P, Cavenee WK (eds) World Health Organization classification of tumours. Pathology and genetics: tumours of the nervous system. IARC Press, Lyon, p 223–226
635. Conway J E, Chou D, Clatterbuck R E et al. 2001 Hemangioblastomas of the central nervous system in von Hippel-Lindau syndrome and sporadic disease. Neurosurgery 48: 55–63
636. Neumann H P H, Lips C J M, Hsia Y E et al. 1995 Von Hippel-Lindau syndrome. Brain Pathol 5: 181–193
637. Giannini C, Scheithauer B W, Hellbusch L C et al. 1998 Peripheral nerve hemangioblastoma. Mod Pathol 11: 999–1004
638. Patton K T, Satcher R L, Laskin W B 2005 Capillary hemangioblastoma of soft tissue: report of a case and review of the literature. Hum Pathol 36: 1135–1139
639. Krieg M, Marti H H, Plate K H 1998 Coexpression of erythropoietin and vascular endothelial growth factor in nervous system tumors associated with von Hippel-Lindau tumor suppressor gene loss of function. Blood 92: 3388–3393
640. Zagzag D, Zhong H, Scalzitti J M et al. 2000 Expression of hypoxia-inducible factor 1 alpha in brain tumors: Association with angiogenesis, invasion, and progression. Cancer 88: 2606–2618
641. Krieg M, Haas R, Brauch H et al. 2000 Up-regulation of hypoxia-inducible factors HIF-1 alpha and HIF-2 alpha under normoxic conditions in renal cell carcinoma cells by von Hippel-Lindau suppressor gene loss of function. Oncogene 19: 5435–5443
642. Madhusudan S, Deplanque G, Braybrooke J P et al. 2004 Antiangiogenic therapy for von Hippel-Lindau disease. J Am Med Assoc 291: 943–944
643. Longatti P, Basaldella L, Orvieto E et al. 2006 Aquaporin 1 expression in cystic hemangioblastomas. Neurosci Lett 392: 178–180
644. Mills S E, Ross G W, Perentes E et al. 1990 Cerebellar hemangioblastoma: immunohistochemical distinction from metastatic renal cell carcinoma. Surg Pathol 3: 121–132
645. Hoang M P, Amirkan R H 2003 Inhibin alpha distinguishes hemangioblastoma from clear cell renal cell carcinoma. Am J Surg Pathol 27: 1152–1156
646. Jung S M, Kuo T T 2005 Immunoreactivity of CD10 and inhibin alpha in differentiating hemangioblastoma of central nervous system from metastatic clear cell renal cell carcinoma. Mod Pathol 18: 788–794
647. Miller D C, Hochberg F H, Harris N L 1994 Pathology with clinical correlations of primary central nervous system non-Hodgkin's lymphoma. Cancer 74: 1383–1397
648. Eby N L, Grufferman S, Flannelly C M et al. 1988 Increasing incidence of primary brain lymphomas in the US. Cancer 62: 2461–2465
649. Hao D, DiFrancesco L M, Brasher P M et al. 1999 Is primary CNS lymphoma really becoming more common? A population-based study of incidence, clinicopathological features and outcome in Alberta from 1975 to 1996. Ann Oncol 10: 65–70
650. Olson J E, Janney C A, Rao R D et al. 2002 The continuing increase in the incidence of primary central nervous system non-Hodgkin lymphoma. Cancer 95: 1504–1510
651. Paulus W, Jellinger K, Morgello S et al. 2000 Malignant lymphomas. In: Kleihues P, Cavenee WK (eds) World Health Organization classification of tumours. Pathology and genetics: tumours of the nervous system. IARC Press, Lyon, p 198–203
652. Tomlinson F H, Kurtin P J, Suman V J et al. 1995 Primary intracerebral malignant lymphoma: a clinicopathological study of 89 patients. J Neurosurg 82: 558–566
653. Roman-Goldstein S M, Goldman D L, Howieson J et al. 1992 MR in primary CNS lymphoma in immunologically normal patients. Am J Neuroradiol 13: 1207–1213
654. Ruiz A, Post M J, Bundschia C et al. 1997 Primary central nervous system lymphoma in patients with AIDS. Neuroimaging Clin North Am 7: 281–296
655. Brecher K, Hochberg F H, Louis D N et al. 1998 Case report of unusual leukoencephalopathy preceding primary CNS lymphoma. J Neurol Neurosurg Psychiatr 65: 917–920
656. Montesinos-Rongen M, Küppers R, Schlüter D et al. 1999 Primary central nervous system lymphomas are derived from germinal-center B cells and show a preferential usage of the V4-34 gene segment. Am J Pathol 155: 2077–2086
657. Tu P-H, Giannini C, Judkins A R et al. 2005 Clinicopathologic and genetic profile of intracranial marginal zone lymphoma: a primary low grade CNS lymphoma that mimics meningioma. J Clin Oncol 23: 5718–5727
658. Shenkier T N, Blay J-Y, O'Neill B P et al. 2005 Primary CNS lymphoma of T cell origin: a descriptive analysis from the International Primary CNS Lymphoma Collaborative Group. J Clin Oncol 23: 2233–2239
659. Choi J S, Nam D-H, Ko Y H et al. 2003 Primary central nervous system lymphomas in Korea: comparison of B- and T-cell lymphoma. Am J Surg Pathol 27: 919–928
660. Paulus W, Ott M M, Strik H et al. 1994 Large cell anaplastic (Ki-1) brain lymphoma of T-cell genotype. Hum Pathol 25: 1253–1256
661. Montesinos-Rongen M, Roost D V, Schaller C et al. 2004 Primary diffuse large B-cell lymphomas of the central nervous system are targeted by aberrant somatic hypermutation. Blood 103: 1869–1875

662. Morgello S 1995 Pathogenesis and classification of primary central nervous system lymphoma: an update. Brain Pathol 5: 383–393
663. Montesinos-Rongen M, Besleaga R, Heinsohn S et al. 2004 Absence of simian virus 40 DNA sequences in primary central nervous system lymphoma in HIV-negative patients. Virchow's Arch 444: 436–438
664. Cobbers J M, Wolter M, Reifenberger J et al. 1998 Frequent inactivation of CDKN2A and rare mutation of TP53 in PCNSL. Brain Pathol 8: 263–276
665. Bjornsson J, Scheithauer B W, Okazaki H et al. 1985 Intracranial germ cell tumors: pathobiological and immunohistochemical aspects of 70 cases. J Neuropathol Exp Neurol 44: 32–46
666. Bruce J N, Stein B M 1990 Pineal tumors. Neurosurg Clin North Am 1: 123–138
667. Hoffman H J, Otsubo H, Hendrick E B et al. 1991 Intracranial germ-cell tumors in children. J Neurosurg 74: 545–551
668. Fauchon F, Jouvet A, Paquis P et al. 2000 Parenchymal pineal tumors: a clinicopathological study of 76 cases. Int J Radiat Oncol Biol Phys 46: 959–968
669. Hoffman H J, Yoshida M, Becker L E et al. 1994 Pineal region tumors in childhood. Pediatr Neurosurg 21: 91–104
670. Gonzalez-Crussi F (ed) 1982 Extragonadal teratomas. Atlas of tumor pathology, series 2, fascicle 18. Armed Forces Institute of Pathology, Washington, DC
671. Rosenblum M K, Matsutani M, Van Meir E G 2000 Germ cell tumours. In: Kleihues P, Cavenee WK (eds) World Health Organization classification of tumours. Pathology and genetics: tumours of the nervous system. IARC Press, Lyon, p 207–214
672. Glenn O A, Barkovich A J 1996 Intracranial germ cell tumors: A comprehensive review of proposed embryologic derivation. Pediatr Neurosurg 24: 242–251
673. Sawamura Y, Ikeda J, Shirato H et al. 1998 Germ cell tumours of the central nervous system: treatment consideration based on 111 cases and their long-term clinical outcomes. Eur J Cancer 34: 104–110
674. Sano K 1995 So-called intracranial germ cell tumours: are they really of germ cell origin? Br J Neurosurg 9: 391–401
675. Bruce D A, Schut L, Sutton L N 1989 Pineal region tumors. In: McLaurin RL, Schut L, Venes JL et al. (eds) Pediatric neurosurgery: surgery of the developing nervous system. WB Saunders, Philadelphia, p 409–416
676. Wei Y-Q, Hang Z-B, Liu K-F 1992 In situ observation of inflammatory cell-tumor cell interaction in human seminomas (germinomas): light, electron microscopic, and immunohistochemical study. Hum Pathol 23: 421–428
677. Ho D M, Liu H-C 1992 Primary intracranial germ cell tumor. Pathologic study of 51 patients. Cancer 70: 1577–1584
678. Felix I, Becker L E 1990 Intracranial germ cell tumors in children: an immunohistochemical and electron microscopic study. Pediatr Neurosurg 16: 156–162
679. Shinoda J, Yamada H, Sakai N et al. 1988 Placental alkaline phosphatase as a tumor marker for primary intracranial germinoma. J Neurosurg 68: 710–720
680. Yamagami T, Handa H, Yamashita J et al. 1987 An immunohistochemical study of intracranial germ cell tumors. Acta Neurochir 86: 33–41
681. Jennings M T, Gelman R, Hochberg F 1985 Intracranial germ-cell tumors: natural history and pathogenesis. J Neurosurg 63: 155–167
682. Niehans G A, Manivel C, Copland G T et al. 1988 Immunohistochemistry of germ cell and trophoblastic neoplasms. Cancer 62: 1113–1123
683. Kirkove C S, Brown A P, Symon L 1991 Successful treatment of a pineal endodermal sinus tumor. J Neurosurg 74: 832–836
684. Masuzawa T, Shimabukuro H, Nakahara N et al. 1986 Germ cell tumors (germinoma and yolk sac tumor) in unusual sites in the brain. Clin Neuropathol 5: 190–202
685. Edwards M B S, Baumgartner J E 1994 Pineal region tumors. In: Cheek WR, Marlin AE, McLone DG et al. (eds) Pediatric neurosurgery 3rd edn. WB Saunders, Philadelphia, p 429–436
686. Shinoda J, Sakai N, Yano H et al. 2004 Prognostic factors and therapeutic problems of primary intracranial choriocarcinoma/germ-cell tumors with high levels of HCG. J Neurooncol 66: 225–240
687. Hoffman H J, Otsubo H, Hendrick B et al. 1991 Intracranial germ-cell tumors in children. J Neurosurg 74: 545–551
688. Dearnaley D P, A'Hern R P, Whittaker S et al. 1990 Pineal and CNS germ cell tumors: Royal Marsden Hospital experience 1962–1987. Int J Rad Oncol Biol Phys 18: 773–781
689. Sano K, Matsutani M, Seto T 1989 So-called intracranial germ cell tumours: personal experiences and a theory of their pathogenesis. Neurol Res 11: 118–126
690. Kamiya M, Tateyama H, Fujiyoshi Y et al. 1991 Cerebrospinal fluid cytology in immature teratoma of the central nervous system: A case report. Acta Cytol 35: 757–760
691. Smirniotopoulus J G, Rushing E J, Mena H 1992 Pineal region masses: differential diagnosis. RadioGraphics 12: 577–596
692. Shaffrey M E, Lanzino G, Lopes M B S et al. 1996 Maturation of intracranial immature teratoma – report of two cases. J Neurosurg 85: 672–676
693. Dayan A D, Marshall A H E, Miller A A et al. 1966 Atypical teratomas of the pineal and hypothalamus. J Pathol Bacteriol 92: 1–28
694. Shen V, Chaparro M, Choi B H et al. 1990 Absence of isochromosome 12p in a pineal region malignant germ cell tumor. Cancer Genet Cytogenet 50: 153–160
695. Albrecht S, Armstrong D, Mahoney D H et al. 1993 Cytogenetic demonstration of gene amplification in a primary intracranial germ cell tumor. Genes Chromos Cancer 6: 61–63
696. De Bruin T W A, Slater R M, Defferrari R et al. 1994 Isochromosome 12p-positive pineal germ cell tumor. Cancer Res 54: 1542–1544
697. Yu I T, Griffin C A, Phillips P C et al. 1995 Numerical sex chromosomal abnormalities in pineal teratomas by cytogenetic analysis and fluorescence in situ hybridization. Lab Invest 72: 419–423
698. Losi L, Polito P, Hagemeijer A et al. 1998 Intracranial germ cell tumour (embryonal carcinoma with teratoma) with complex karyotype including isochromosome 12p. Virchow's Arch 433: 571–574
699. Atkin N B, Baker M C 1983 I(12p): specific chromosomal marker in seminoma and malignant teratoma of the testis. Cancer Genet Cytogenet 10: 199–204
700. Dal Cin P, Dei Tos A P, Qi H et al. 1998 Immature teratoma of the pineal gland with isochromosome 12p. Acta Neuropathol 95: 107–110
701. Suijkerbuijk R F, Looijenga L, de Jong B et al. 1992 Verification of isochromosome 12p and identification of other chromosome 12 aberrations in gonadal and extragonadal human germ cell tumors by bicolor double fluorescence in situ hybridization. Cancer Genet Cytogenet 63: 8–16
702. Janzer R C, Burger P C, Giangaspero F 2000 Craniopharyngioma. In: Kleihues P, Cavenee WK (eds) World Health Organization classification of tumours. Pathology and genetics: tumours of the nervous system. IARC Press, Lyon, p 244–246
703. Laws E R Jr, Thapar K 1994 The diagnosis and management of craniopharyngioma. Growth, Genet Hormones 10: 6–11
704. Burger P C, Scheithauer B W, Vogel F S 2002 Craniopharyngiomas. In: Surgical pathology of the nervous system and its coverings, 4th edn. Churchill Livingstone, New York, p 475–483
705. Crotty T B, Scheithauer B W, Young W F Jr et al. 1995 Papillary craniopharyngioma: a clinicopathological study of 48 cases. J Neurosurg 83: 206–214
706. Duo D, Gasverde S, Benech F et al. 2003 MIB-1 immunoreactivity in craniopharyngiomas: a clinico-pathological analysis. Clin Neuropathol 22: 229–234
707. Coffey R J, Lunsford L D 1990 The role of stereotactic techniques in the management of craniopharyngiomas. Neurosurg Clin N Am 1: 161–172
708. Duff J M, Meyer F B, Ilstrup D M et al. 2000 Long-term outcomes for surgically resected craniopharyngiomas. Neurosurgery 46: 291–305
709. Van Effenterre R, Boch A L 2002 Craniopharyngioma in adults and children: a study of 122 surgical cases. J Neurosurg 97: 3–11
710. Karavitaki N, Brufani C, Warner J T et al. 2005 Craniopharyngiomas in children and adults: systematic analysis of 121 cases with long-term follow-up. Clin Endocrinol 62: 397–409
711. Gormley W B, Tomecek F J, Qureshi N et al. 1994 Craniocerebral epidermoid and dermoid tumors: a review of 32 cases. Acta Neurochir (Wien) 128: 115–121

周围神经外胚层肿瘤
Peripheral neuroectodermal tumors

27

Christopher D. M. Fletcher 著

王莉芬 译

引言	1733	良性肿瘤	1735
反应性病变	1733	恶性肿瘤	1747
错构瘤性病变	1734	其他软组织神经外胚层肿瘤	1753

引言

传统上，与本章内容类似的章节标题应该是"周围神经系统肿瘤"或"周围神经鞘肿瘤"。本书弃用这些名称是为了回避现在越来越难以站得住脚的组织发生学问题，同时也可以更加合乎逻辑地将那些显示神经外胚层分化特性、但没有起源于周围神经的证据或可能性的软组织肿瘤包括在内；属于后一类的肿瘤包括诸如异位的脑膜上皮病变和软组织恶性黑色素瘤（透明细胞肉瘤）。

真正显示某种形式的神经鞘分化的病变，乃是一组非常异质性和复杂的病变，具有不同的明确的诊断标准。这反映了周围神经的错综复杂的结构。周围神经由有髓或无髓神经轴突构成，后者被包裹在由神经鞘细胞和纤维母细胞组成的神经内膜基质中，其外围绕一层神经束膜细胞；这种神经"束"与被称为神经外膜的纤维母细胞结缔组织结合在一起形成周围神经。因此，当所谓的"神经鞘肿瘤"发生或分化时其结构和细胞类型相当广泛。

反应性病变　Reactive lesions

创伤性神经瘤（断肢性神经瘤）
Traumatic neuroma（amputation neuroma）

创伤性神经瘤[1]，顾名思义，可发生在周围神经被切断而未能正常愈合的任何部位。创伤性神经瘤的两个主要发病原因是创伤——包括撕裂伤或穿透伤——和手术，尤其是截肢术。前者好发于年轻人，而后者最常见于老年人，与因周围血管病变所致的肢体局部缺血的发病率一致。不管由何种原因引起，这种病变通常表现为发生在浅表软组织的伴有疼痛的小结节。临床上在外科患者中有一独特的亚群，表现为胆囊切除术后出现右上腹痛甚至黄疸[2]。如果手术中注意处理好被切断的神经断端，则任何部位的术后创伤性神经瘤都可以减少发生。

组织学上，创伤性神经瘤是由神经束所有正常成分构成的赘疣组成，这些成分包括纤维母细胞、神经鞘细胞、神经束膜细胞以及许多小的神经纤维。赘疣界限不清，排列紊乱（图27.1）。这种增生通常发生在胶原纤维组织中；有时胶原纤维组织可以发生炎症或黏液样变，这取决于病变是否受到外界因素（如反复创伤或伤口感染）的影响。

Morton神经瘤（Morton跖骨痛）
Morton's neuroma（Morton's metatarsalgia）

Morton神经瘤在有关肿瘤的书籍内描述仅仅是因为其在临床上可能表现为局灶性肿胀。Morton神经瘤[3]表现为足底的严重的撕裂样疼痛，通常在跖骨头或跖趾

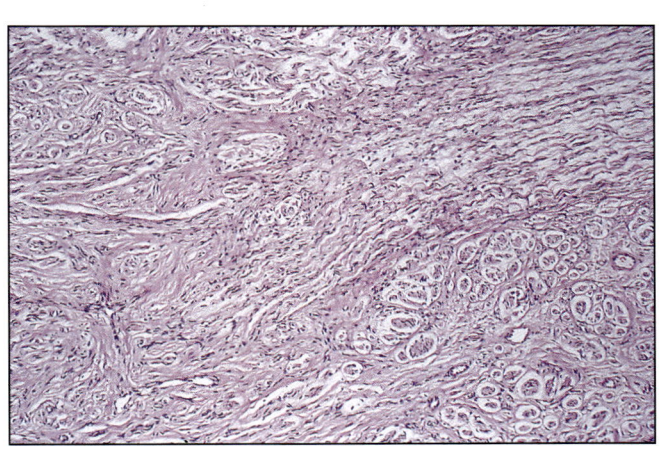

图27.1　创伤性神经瘤。注意神经纤维和纤维组织的杂乱混合。右上角是明显水肿的受损神经末梢。

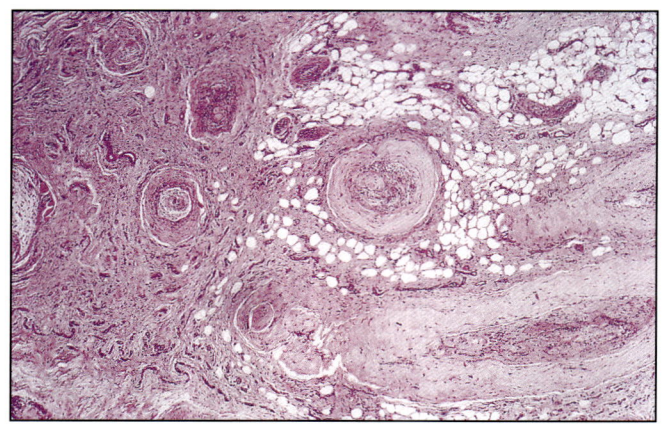

图27.2 Morton跖骨痛。注意神经束膜和神经内膜明显纤维化。

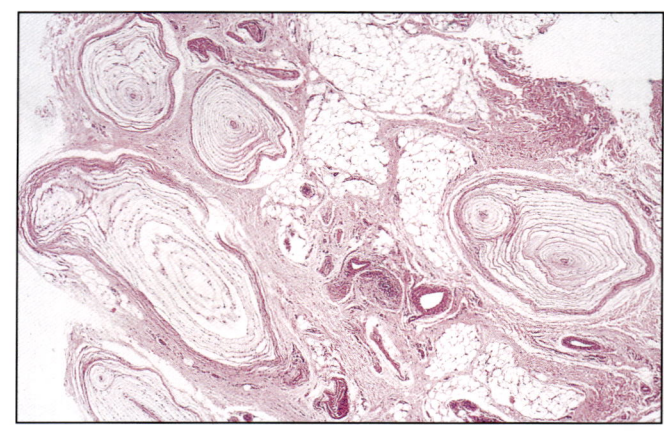

图27.3 手指Pacini神经瘤。注意典型的增生性环层小体。

关节区。疼痛在行走时加剧，休息时缓解。这种病变局限于成人，女性明显多见。穿鞋袜可迫使脚的跖趾关节延伸，如穿高跟鞋，可能导致此病发生。手术时可见一支或多支趾跖神经变粗或梭形肿胀，常常伴有邻近腱鞘组织增厚。手术切除即可治愈。

组织学上，Morton 神经瘤以明显的神经内膜、神经束膜和神经外膜纤维化和透明变性为特征，伴有轴突消失[4]（图 27.2）。此外，一般还有邻近血管壁纤维化和增厚以及脂肪组织内纤维化。纤维内膜明显增厚，甚至可导致较小的动脉闭塞。

Pacini神经瘤　Pacinian neuroma

Pacini 神经瘤是环层小体的一种少见而又独特的肿瘤，通常发生在成年人受过损伤的手指[5]。病变表现为一个小而十分疼痛的结节，切除后无复发倾向。因为几乎所有报道的病例都发生在局部创伤之后，所以这些神经瘤被认为是反应性病变而非肿瘤性病变。组织学上相似的病变偶尔也可发生在腹膜后。

组织学上，手指 Pacini 神经瘤 （digital pacinian neuroma） 完全由增生的正常大小的环层小体集聚而成，没有包膜（图 27.3），在周围的纤维组织中可见许多小神经。本病与 Pacini 神经鞘瘤 （pacinian schwannoma） 在形态学上没有相似之处 （见 1740 页）。

错构瘤性病变　Hamartomatous lesions

在错构瘤性病变这一部分，我们描述从发病年龄或形态学结构上看好像是某种发育异常的病变。尽管如此，必须承认，这类病变与良性肿瘤的区别常常模糊不清或不太一致。

神经脂肪瘤病（纤维脂肪瘤性错构瘤；神经纤维脂肪瘤）
Lipomatosis of nerve (fibrolipomatous hamartoma; neural fibrolipoma)

神经脂肪瘤病是一种罕见的病变，尽管有许多个案报道，但只有一项大型病例研究对此有适当的描述[6]。本病的特征是：缓慢生长的梭形肿物，最常发生在正中神经（少数情况下发生于尺神经），伴有与腕管综合征（carpal tunnel syndrome）相似的压迫性神经病（compression neuropathy）的症状。通常在儿童早期发病，刚成年即就诊。男女发病率相同，25% 的患者伴有由于脂肪肥大而引起的巨指（趾）症（macrodactyly）。少数病例可发生在手腕/前臂以外区域，通常在近端的部位[7]。除了取活检和试图手术解压以外，没有其他有效的治疗方法。粗略地(或试图)切除梭形肿物会导致明显的神经缺损。

组织学上，有大量的境界不清的成熟纤维脂肪组织使受累神经外膜膨大（图 27.4）。神经束本身结构保存，仅见神经束膜纤维化。组织学上明显的轴突变性很少见。

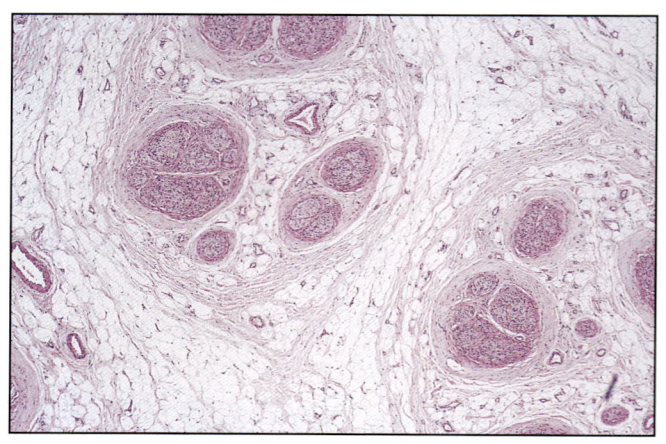

图27.4 神经的纤维脂肪瘤性错构瘤。纤维脂肪组织使神经外膜膨大。

黏膜神经瘤　Mucosal neuroma

黏膜神经瘤几乎总是多发性的，并参与构成IIb型（Gorlin）多发性内分泌肿瘤综合征的一部分特征性病变[8,9]。本病十分罕见，多成簇分布在黏膜皮肤交界附近区域，尤其是口腔，但也有少数病例可在其他部位的皮肤发生。本病伴有肠肌神经丛肥大或有时伴有神经节瘤病。临床上，这种常染色体显性遗传综合征的最重要的组成部分是甲状腺髓样癌（见第18章）。

组织学上，每一处病变在真皮层或黏膜下层可见由增生的神经纤维组成的境界不清的肿块，神经纤维排列紊乱，并有不规则的分支（图27.5）。某些病例表面上可能与创伤性神经瘤相似，但黏膜神经瘤只是单纯的神经内膜增生而无纤维化。增生的神经束常常被神经束膜包裹，神经束膜上皮膜抗原（EMA）染色呈阳性。

神经肌肉错构瘤（良性蝾螈瘤）　Neuromuscular hamartoma (benign Triton tumor)

神经肌肉错构瘤是发生在婴儿的一种十分罕见的病变，其特征是发生于大神经的先天性肿块，如在臂丛或坐骨神经[10,11]。病变由正常骨骼肌和许多小的神经纤维交织混合而成，神经纤维常常位于肌束膜鞘内。随着幼儿生长，病变似乎可以消失，但不可能完全消退。

其他错构瘤　Miscellaneous hamartomata

还有各种各样的稀奇的错构瘤散发病例报道，主要发生在皮肤，有些是先天性的，其特征通常是完全由增生的神经纤维或神经鞘细胞组成[12-15]。也有十分罕见的先天性病变，由增生的环层小体组成，有时伴有神经管缺失[16,17]。

良性肿瘤　Benign tumors

这里用"肿瘤"（tumor）一词而不是用新生物（neoplasm）一词是因为：这些病变的真正生物学本质仍不肯定并存在争议，如孤立的局限性神经瘤，甚至常见的神经纤维瘤（及其变型）。在20世纪60年代后期和70年代早期，人们将神经鞘瘤、神经纤维瘤以及孤立的局限性神经瘤（solitary circumscribed neuroma）不加以区别地归为"良性神经鞘肿瘤"，但这种普遍的倾向已被制止，因为这样掩盖了它们之间的显著的临床病理差异，尤其是有并发神经纤维瘤病或恶变的危险性。

孤立的局限性神经瘤（栅栏状包裹性神经瘤）　Solitary circumscribed neuroma (palisaded encapsulated neuroma)

临床特征

孤立的局限性神经瘤（由Reed等[18]于1972年首先描述）是一种非常常见但又经常不被临床医生和病理医生充分重视的疾病。此病通常表现为孤立的无痛性皮肤结节，直径小于1cm，好发于面部的"口鼻"或"蝶形"区[18-20]，但少数病例也可累及其他黏膜皮肤部位，包括口腔和龟头。发病高峰年龄在30～60岁之间，无性别差异。此病不伴有任何神经性分泌性病变（neurocristopathy），临床病程完全表现为良性。多数病例最初被误诊为皮内黑色素细胞痣。极少数患者表现为多发性病变[21]。

组织学特征

多数病例表现为真皮内境界清楚的小结节，但也有些病变呈棒状。当外科或病理医生切开病变时，结节有时可从周围组织"爆出"。在大多数情况下，结节侧面和底部有不完全的包膜，但表面与真皮层界限不清（图27.6）；邻近底部常可见起源的神经。病变本身由温和的嗜酸性梭形细胞构成，细胞界限不清，细胞核小，呈波浪形，深染。细胞在胶原间质中呈束状排列，常被人工裂隙分开（图27.7）；血管数量很少。真正的呈栅栏状排列的核少见，没有Antoni A区和Antoni B区。许多病例可见被覆上皮棘层轻度增厚，少数病例伴有假上皮瘤样增生[19,22]。个别病例的肿瘤细胞核显示非典型性退行性（"陈旧性"）改变，并且已有局灶性上皮样形态的描

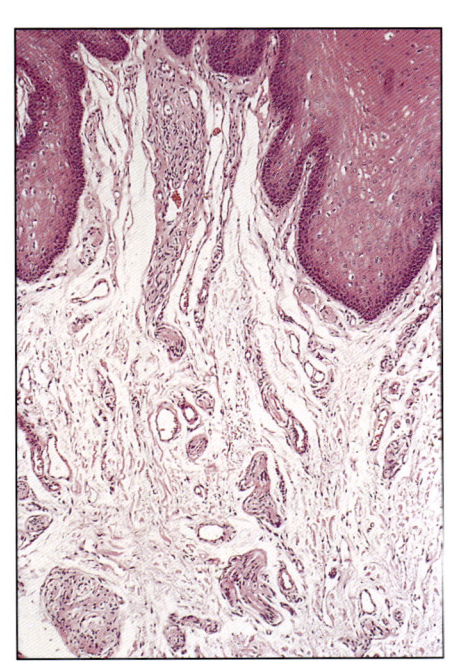

图27.5　黏膜神经瘤。黏膜下层有许多大小不同的神经纤维。

良性肿瘤

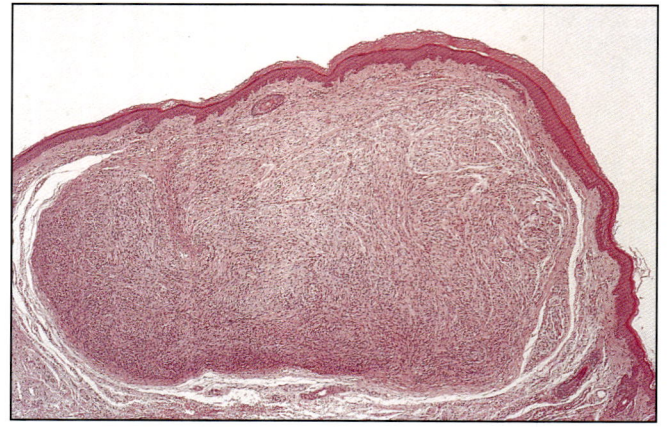

图27.6 孤立的局限性神经瘤。注意表面缺少包膜，右下角为起源的神经。

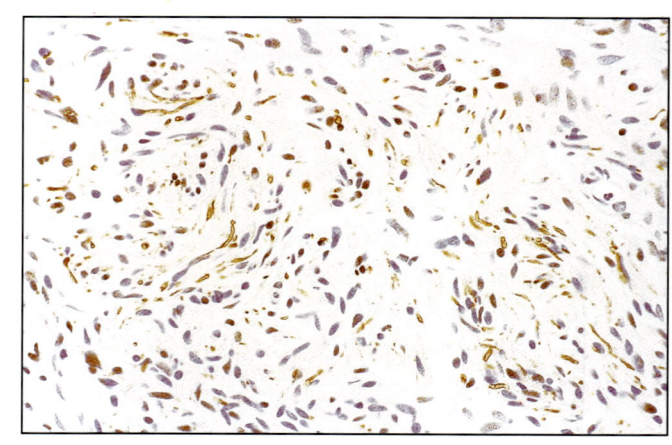

图27.8 孤立的局限性神经瘤。注意神经细丝染色证实有无数小的轴突。ABC方法。

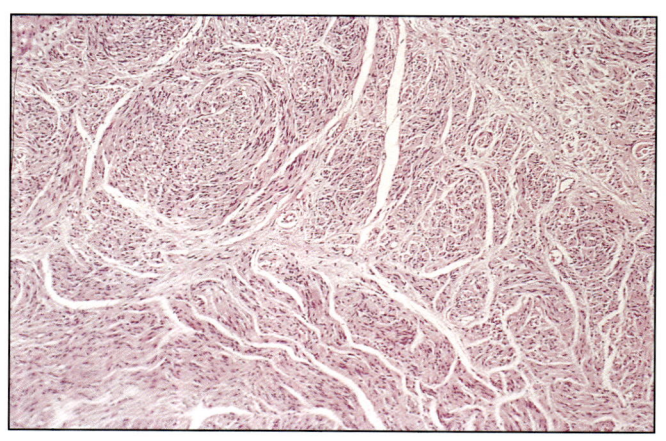

图27.7 孤立的局限性神经瘤。良性的神经鞘细胞束被人工裂隙分开。

述[23]。应用特殊染色[18]或比较简单的免疫组织化学染色[19,24]可证明，病变神经鞘细胞 S-100 呈阳性，混合有许多细小的轴突（神经细丝阳性，图27.8），这些轴突在 HE 染色切片上并不明显，因此被命名为"神经瘤"（neuroma）。包膜细胞 EMA 几乎全部呈阳性，证明其属于神经束膜。本病病变相对局限，加之有明显的轴突成分，易与神经瘤或神经纤维瘤鉴别开来。

神经鞘瘤　Schwannoma（neurilemmoma）

临床特征

典型的神经鞘瘤是一种良性非复发性肿瘤，发生于成年人，没有性别差异[25,26]。病变的解剖学分布十分广泛，包括诸如颅神经[27]、骨[28]或胃肠道，尤其是胃[29,30]等不同部位，但是绝大多数发生在皮下组织，肌肉少见，

略好发于肢体远端或头颈部。双侧听神经鞘瘤是 2 型神经纤维瘤病（NF2）的主要（或能确定诊断的）特征病变[31]。肢体病变最常发生在屈侧。手术时这些起源于神经的肿瘤通常易于分离而不遗留神经损伤。极少数患者可发生多发性周围局限性神经鞘瘤，但是除非同时存在前庭神经鞘瘤，否则这些病变一般与神经纤维瘤病无关[32,33]。多数孤立性神经鞘瘤没有症状，肿瘤直径大多小于 5 cm。确定的良性神经鞘瘤恶变的病例报道十分罕见[34,35]。

组织学特征

典型的神经鞘瘤是有包膜的肿瘤，有两种成分，称为 Antoni A 和 Antoni B 组织，以不同比例组成（图27.9）。Antoni A 区细胞丰富，由形态单一的梭形神经鞘细胞组成，包含有混杂的嗜酸性胞浆，细胞核明显嗜碱性染色，间质为数量不等的胶原纤维（图27.10）。这些细胞的细胞核常呈栅栏状，并与间插的嗜酸性胞浆（突起）平行排列，后者称为 Verocay 小体（图27.11）。Antoni B 区也是由神经鞘细胞组成的，但其胞浆不明显，

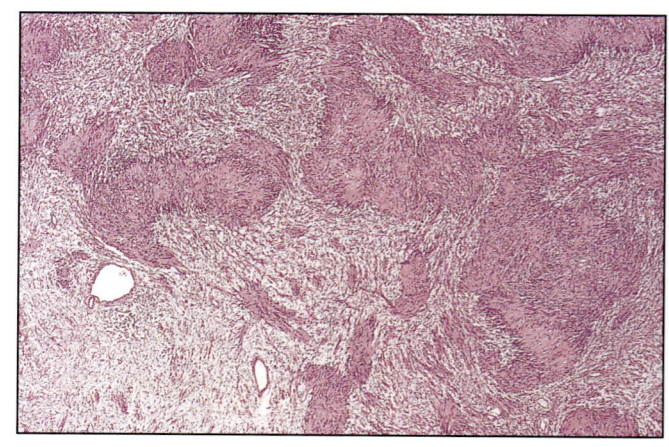

图27.9 良性神经鞘瘤。本例有典型的双相表现。

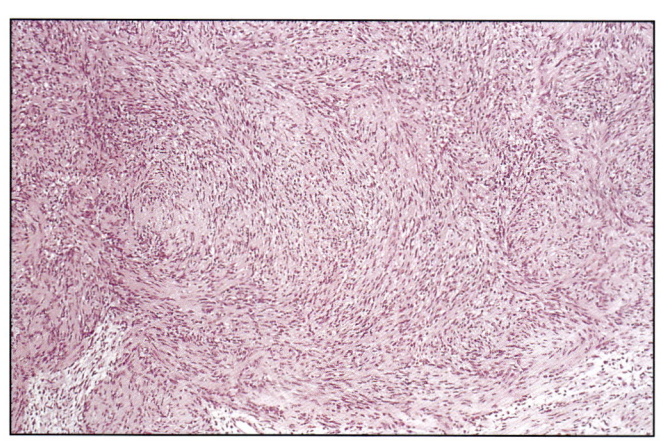

图27.10 良性神经鞘瘤。Antoni A区细胞丰富，核呈栅栏状排列。

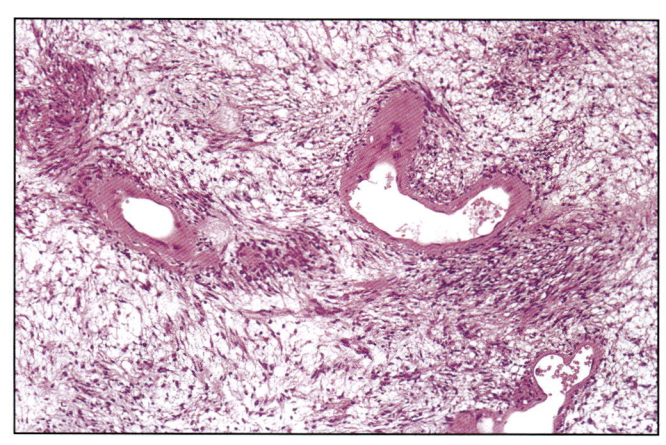

图27.12 良性神经鞘瘤。注意Antoni B区黏液性基质和透明样变的血管壁。

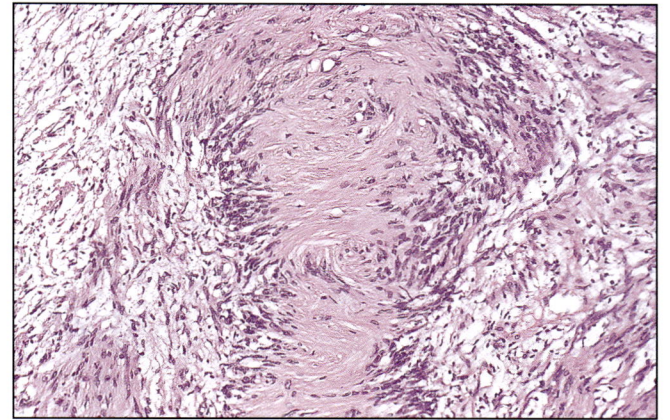

图27.11 良性神经鞘瘤。典型的Verocay小体。

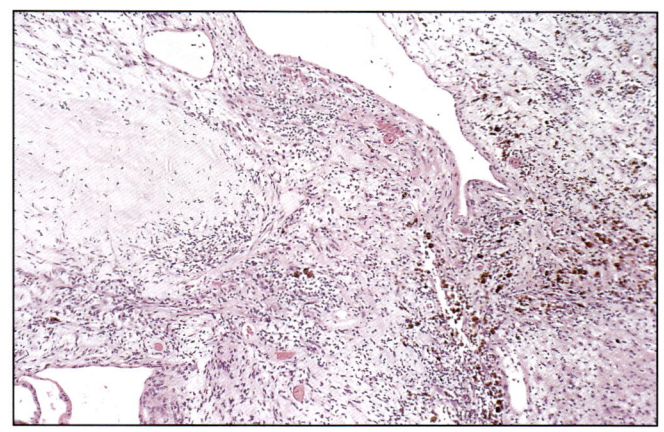

图27.13 退变的神经鞘瘤。注意透明化，含铁血黄素沉积和囊性变。

细胞核似乎悬浮在透明的黏液样基质中，常常形成微囊。这些区域可能发生了变性。Antoni B区常见的最明显的特征是：出现管壁透明变性的厚壁血管（图27.12）。值得注意的是，发生于胃肠道或上呼吸道的神经鞘瘤的特点是没有包膜。良性神经鞘瘤常见正常核分裂象，尤其在 Antoni A 区，但是核分裂象很少超过 5 个 /10HPF。虽然在包膜处偶尔可见明显被牵拉的起源神经，但良性神经鞘瘤通常没有轴突或神经存在。然而，与NF2 有关的神经鞘瘤病（schwannomatosis）可能含有散在的轴突[36]。也有十分罕见的神经鞘瘤和典型的(常常是丛状)神经纤维瘤混合存在的病变（见下文）；在这样的病变中，神经纤维瘤成分确实含有神经，有时伴有神经纤维瘤病[37]。神经鞘瘤常见进行性退变，这常常反应了肿瘤存在时间较长或发生在经常受伤的部位。这些变化最初是局灶性的，包括透明变性、间质出血、囊性变和钙化（图27.13）。此种肿瘤被归为"陈旧性神经鞘瘤"（ancient schwannoma），但诊断标准并不确切（见下文）。

神经鞘瘤恶变十分罕见[33,34]，最常见表现为高级别的上皮样恶性外周神经鞘肿瘤（malignant peripheral nerve sheath tumor，MPNST）或具有特征的上皮样血管肉瘤（图 27.14）。个别病例可能具有小圆细胞的形态学

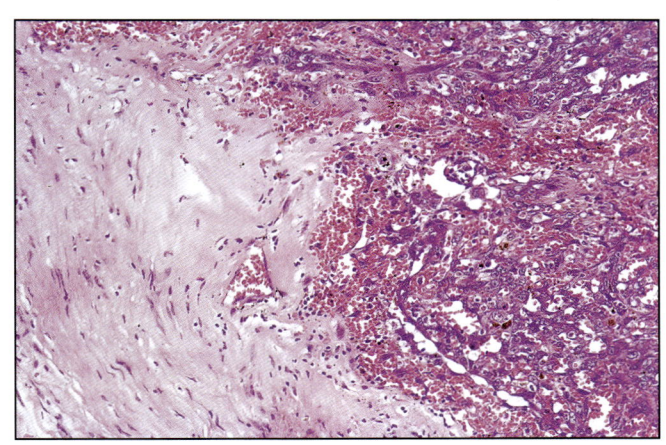

图27.14 发生在良性神经鞘瘤基础上的上皮样血管肉瘤。注意两种成分之间的突变。

结构[33]。偶尔，神经鞘瘤可以显示原位上皮样恶性改变（in-situ epithelioid malignant change），其特征是单个散在分布的大的上皮样神经鞘细胞，细胞核呈空泡状，核仁明显[34]。迄今为止，随访显示这些病例的临床经过均呈良性，最好将其称为伴有上皮样细胞的非典型性神经鞘瘤（atypical schwannoma with epithelioid cells）。

免疫组织化学染色，神经鞘瘤 S-100 蛋白呈弥漫性强阳性。位于胃肠道的神经鞘瘤还常常显示胶质原纤维酸性蛋白（GFAP）阳性，而位于腹膜后和纵隔的神经鞘瘤角蛋白阳性十分常见。神经鞘瘤的神经束膜性包膜 EMA 呈阳性。超微结构检查显示，组成良性神经鞘瘤（包括其变型）的细胞胞体小，有被覆完整外板的细长的犬牙交错的细胞突起，外板常常是双层的。这些胞浆突常常由桥粒样结构连接。细胞器相对较少且无特异性。间质内常常可见长间隙的胶原纤维束（称为 Luse 小体）。细胞遗传学分析显示，多数神经鞘瘤伴有 22 号染色体单体或 22 号染色体短臂缺失[38]，与 NF2 等位基因缺失一致。有趣的是，其他类型的良性神经鞘瘤以及脑脊膜瘤也有这种染色体突变表现（见第 26 章）。

良性神经鞘瘤亚型
Variants of benign schwannoma

陈旧性神经鞘瘤（ancient schwannoma）[39]：这种类型基本上是良性神经鞘瘤，其中有严重的退行性变。如前所述，诊断这种病变没有严格的标准，但是这个作者倾向于保留这种诊断，用于那些有明显的非典型核或核多形性的病例（图 27.15），以及（Antoni A）细胞成分不明显或呈局灶性以至不通过 S-100 染色（图 27.16）就难以做出神经鞘瘤诊断的病例。非典型退变细胞核的特征是：细胞核显著深染，染色质呈粗块状；核仁不明显或缺失，通常找不到核分裂象。这种类型的神经鞘瘤可以发生在任何部位，但通常位于深部。没有复发倾向。

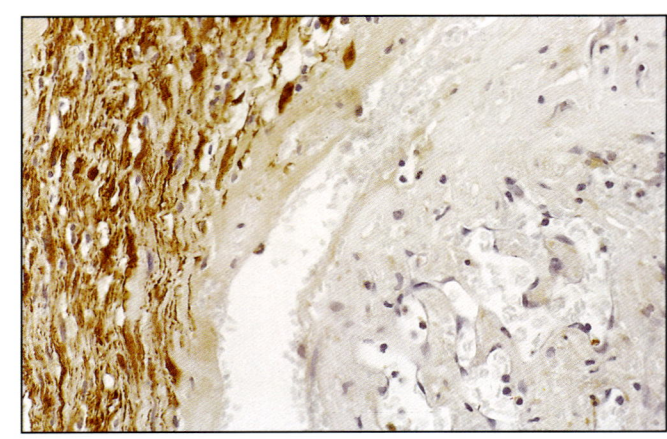

图 27.16 陈旧性神经鞘瘤。高度透明变性的假血管区域只有小灶状 S-100 阳性的残留的神经鞘细胞。ABC 法。

富细胞性神经鞘瘤（cellular schwannoma）[40-43]最先报道于 1981 年，这种类型的神经鞘瘤的高达 30% 的病例被误诊为肉瘤（至少在过去是这样）。典型的富细胞性神经鞘瘤是大而深在的肿瘤，好发于腹膜后或纵隔，并且常常起源于大神经。女性稍多见，少数病例伴有神经纤维瘤病。虽然肿瘤通常有包膜，但是某些病例可能有局部浸润并侵蚀或侵犯骨组织。如果切除不完全，有时可能局部复发。

组织学上，这些病变不同于普通的神经鞘瘤，整个肿瘤细胞丰富（Antoni B 成分不明显或仅仅为局灶性），细胞呈明显束状（图 27.17）或漩涡状生长，细胞核很少呈栅栏状排列。核分裂象可达 10 个/10HPF，也可见多形细胞核；后者本质上是一种退行性（固缩性）改变，并且常常与分裂核不在同一部位。其他常见的特征包括：被覆一个厚的纤维包膜，其中可见致密的淋巴细胞浸润，肿瘤组织内可见很多泡沫样（黄瘤）细胞（图 27.18）。偶尔可见局灶性坏死。

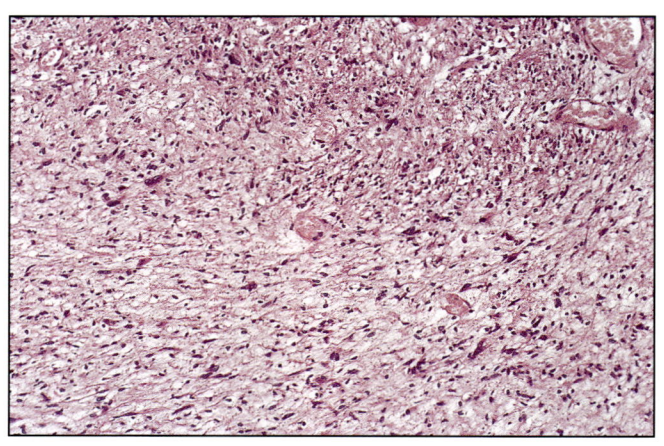

图 27.15 陈旧性神经鞘瘤。注意细胞核的非典型性。

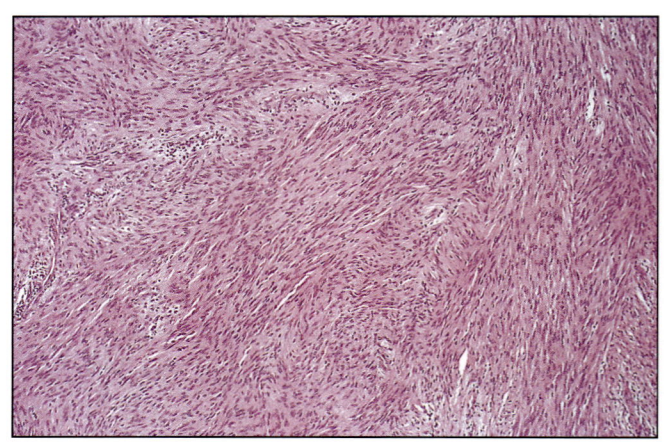

图 27.17 富细胞性神经鞘瘤。注意均匀一致的嗜酸性束状生长方式。

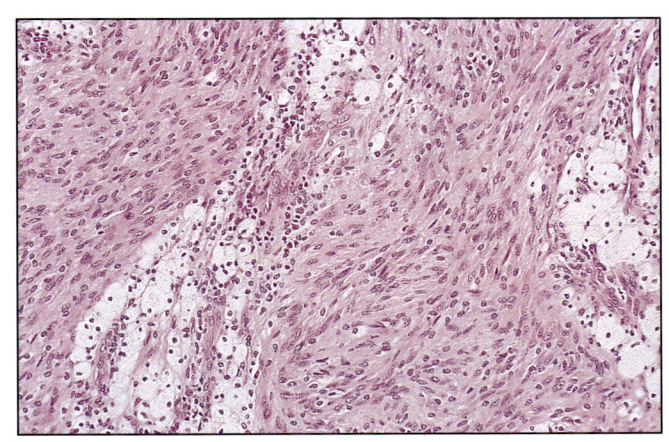

图27.18 富细胞性神经鞘瘤。许多病例存在泡沫样组织细胞聚集。

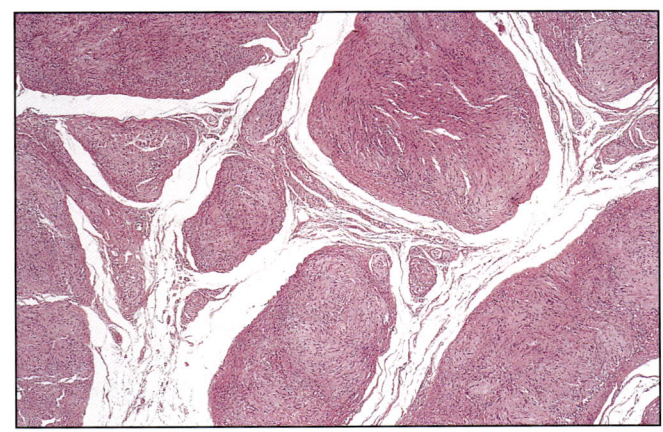

图27.19 丛状神经鞘瘤。明显的多发性结节,每个结节均由Antoni A区组织组成。

肿瘤境界清楚,有管壁玻璃样变性的血管和小灶状Antoni B区,神经纤维瘤样区域相对缺乏,结合其他临床病理特征和免疫组化染色 S-100 蛋白弥漫强阳性,几乎所有病例都可与低度恶性的 MPNST 很好地鉴别开。其 S-100 蛋白免疫染色阳性和结蛋白阴性可避免被误诊为平滑肌肉瘤,后者是排列成束的嗜酸性梭形细胞肿瘤,核分裂象较常见,一般容易做出诊断。

值得重视的是,极少数富细胞性神经鞘瘤可呈明显的丛状结构[44]。这样的病变在过去曾被误认为是恶性的[45],最常发生在婴儿的四肢,局部复发十分常见。

丛状神经鞘瘤(plexiform schwannoma)[46-48]:这种类型的肿瘤少见,累及的患者常比普通神经鞘瘤患者年轻。丛状神经鞘瘤略好发于躯干部位。值得注意的是,至少 2/3 的患者病变起源于真皮。深在的病变十分少见[49]。除了极少数病例外,一般不伴有神经纤维瘤病,因此,与丛状神经纤维瘤的鉴别十分重要。肿瘤直径通常小于 3 cm,有时有疼痛,组织学上表现为主要由 Antoni A 型组织构成的多发性孤立性结节(图 27.19)。与普通神经鞘瘤一样,每个结节都有包膜,可见核分裂。局部复发十分少见,尚无恶变的报道。

黑色素性神经鞘瘤(melanotic schwannoma)[50-52]:这是一种罕见的神经鞘瘤亚型,通常发生于中年人,好发于脊髓神经根,但其他部位也有个案报道。其组织学特征是神经鞘细胞常常呈上皮样,存在核沟,大多数肿瘤细胞含有明显的 Fontama 染色阳性的黑色素,但不是全部(图 27.20)。超微结构上,肿瘤细胞具有典型的神经鞘细胞的特征,还含有黑色素小体。有包膜的病变缺乏核分裂象,临床病程是良性的。相当数量的病例含有

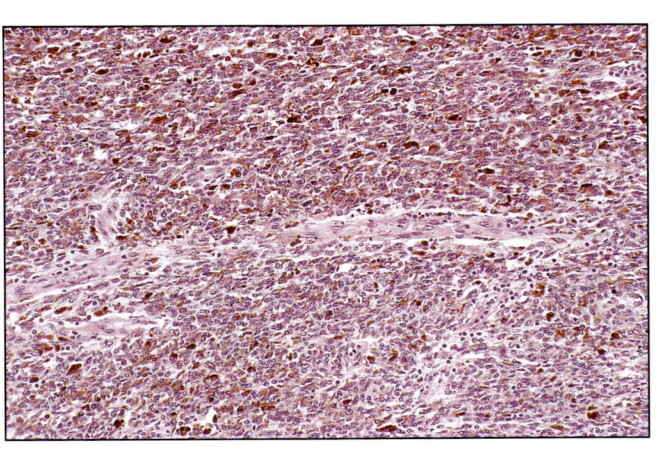

A

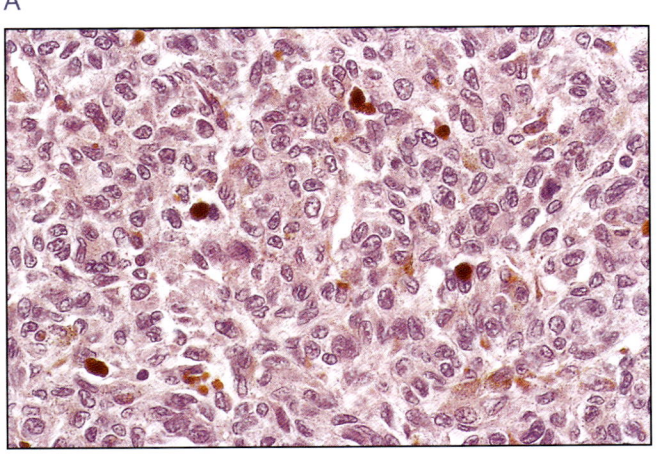

B

图27.20 黑色素性神经鞘瘤。注意典型的重度色素沉积(A),肿瘤细胞核具有明显的空泡状有核沟的细胞核(B)。

数量不等的层状钙化小球(沙粒体性黑色素性神经鞘瘤,psammomatous melanotic schwannoma),这类患者至少 50% 伴有 Carney 综合征(黏液瘤、色素斑、内分泌异常)[53]。

一定比例的黑色素性神经鞘瘤（不管是不是沙粒体型）在临床上表现为恶性，具有转移的生物学行为[53-56]。这类病变最常发生于交感神经链或非中轴部位，肿瘤细胞常显示明显的核仁，核分裂象十分常见。有些病例与转移性黑色素瘤的鉴别十分困难。然而，在其他一些病例，原发性肿瘤的组织学特征可能出现假良性。

上皮样神经鞘瘤（epithelioid schwannoma）[57,58]：良性上皮样神经鞘瘤直到最近几年才受到关注。它主要发生于成年人肢体的真皮深层或皮下组织。典型病变有包膜，但缺乏普通神经鞘瘤的 Antoni A/B 分区或玻璃样变的血管，是由呈巢或小梁状排列的嗜酸性上皮样细胞组成，间质常常表现为黏液样变（图27.21）。它们可能与肌上皮瘤十分相似，但是 S-100 蛋白呈强阳性，角蛋白和 EMA 呈阴性。

混合性神经鞘瘤/神经束膜瘤（hybrid schwannoma/perineurioma）：有一小部分良性神经鞘肿瘤主要由 Antoni A 型组织构成，有的区域呈明显的漩涡状生长方式。这些病变显示明显的 S-100 蛋白和 EMA 混合染色阳性。它们似乎与任何的神经性分泌病（neurocristopathy）均无关系。

腺样神经鞘瘤（glandular schwannoma）[59,60]：这是一个有争议的概念。多数显示局灶性腺样分化的神经鞘瘤为恶性肿瘤（见下文，恶性外周神经鞘肿瘤一节）。然而，确实存在极其罕见的对应的良性肿瘤，但在大多数（如果不是所有）这样的病例，腺样成分可能是陷入的正常结构，这些结构已经发生了某种形式改变。

Pacini 神经鞘瘤（Pacinian schwannoma）：这是一种非常罕见的良性神经鞘肿瘤，含有类似于环层小体的漩涡状结构。尽管它们以前被命名为 Pacini 神经纤维瘤，但肿瘤一般有包膜，具有神经鞘瘤而不是神经纤维瘤的结构[5]。

淋巴结神经鞘瘤（lymph node schwannoma）：这一名称过去是指那些现在认为是淋巴结内肌纤维母细胞瘤（intranodal myofibroblastoma）的病变（见第21章）。然而，确实存在十分罕见的真正发生在淋巴结内的良性神经鞘瘤病例[61]。

孤立性神经纤维瘤　Solitary neurofibroma

临床特征

大多数神经纤维瘤[62,63]是孤立的局限性病变，其中大多数表现为成人皮肤的息肉样或结节状病变，没有特异的临床特征。这种发生在皮肤的孤立性病变通常不伴有 NF1，在解剖学上分布非常广泛。极少数情况下，孤立的神经纤维瘤可发生在深部软组织，多见于身体的中轴部位。深部病变常伴有 NF1，而值得注意的是，这一部位的肿瘤具有较小的恶变危险，但这种风险似乎没有显著性差异。孤立性的小皮肤病变似乎没有这种恶变潜能，如果有，也极其罕见。与神经鞘瘤不同，神经纤维瘤似乎起源于神经内膜，事实上，少数神经纤维瘤亚型完全位于神经内。在 NF1 患者中，这种病变常常是恶变的前兆[64]。如果可以辨认起源的神经，那么这个神经不可避免地会陷到肿瘤团块中，因此，手术切除大而深在的病变有可能导致严重的功能损害。局限的神经纤维瘤似乎没有局部复发倾向；事实上，其混合性细胞成分（见下文）和明显神经内膜起源均提示：它可能不是肿瘤性病变，或许将其看成是错构瘤性病变更好。这个问题可能直到肿瘤定义统一时（见第1章）才能得到解决，因为尽管有多种类型细胞成分的形态学证据，但神经纤维瘤已证明是克隆性生长的[65,66]。

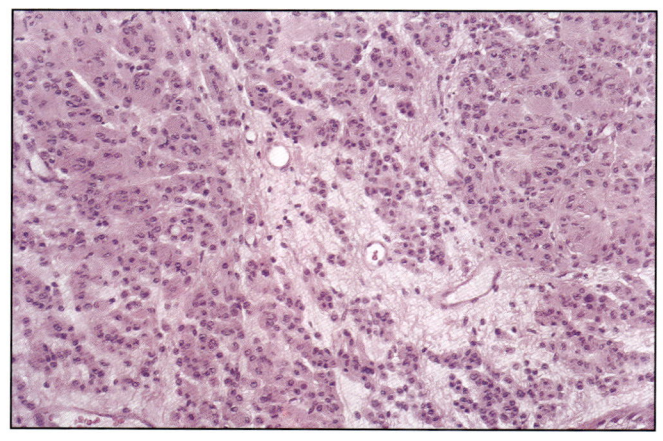

图27.21　上皮样神经鞘瘤。上皮样细胞巢状分布在黏液性基质中。

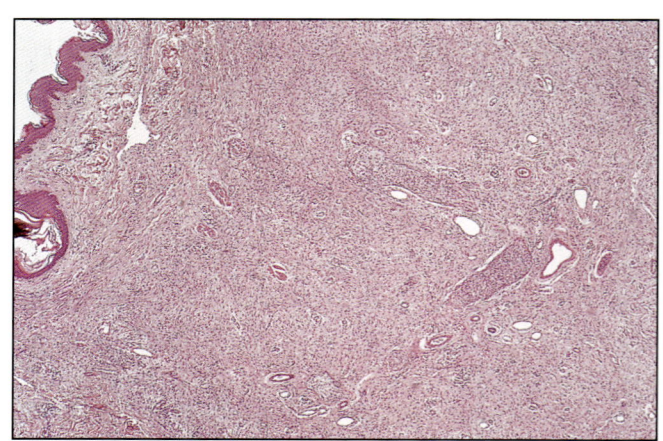

图27.22　神经纤维瘤。典型的皮肤病变，中央可见增生的神经。

组织学特征

局限性神经纤维瘤（图 27.22）是一个界限清楚但没有包膜的病变。肿瘤边界并不十分清楚。组织学形态多种多样，但大多数病例由界线不清的长梭形细胞组成，细胞浆淡嗜酸性，细胞核两端变细，波浪状或弯曲，混有一些种类不明确的短梭形细胞、许多小的神经纤维以及肥大细胞（图 27.23）。这些混合性成分多位于数量不等的纤维黏液样基质中；有些病例黏液沉积可非常明显，应该诊断为黏液样神经纤维瘤（myxoid neurofibroma）（图 27.24）。在较少见的情况下，肿瘤间质可有明显的玻璃样变，或肿瘤细胞与粗大的胶原纤维束混合分布在黏液样间质中（胶原性神经纤维瘤，collagenous neurofibroma；图 27.25）。在少数病例，肿瘤像陈旧性神经鞘瘤一样，细胞核呈现染色过深和退变性多形性改变（奇异性或非典型性神经纤维瘤，bizarre or atypical neurofibroma；图 27.26）。同样的变化如果出现在 NF1 患者中，应高度警惕恶变的可能性，要仔细寻找核分裂象。有些作者认为[67]，神经纤维瘤性病变只要有任何核分裂活性，通常伴有细胞核的非典型性或细胞数量增多，都应该认为是恶性的证据（真皮神经纤维瘤中可见个别核分裂象除外），本人个人经验也支持上述看法；这与良性神经鞘瘤明显不同，后者可以出现一些核分裂象。已有报道在十分罕见的情况下，良性神经纤维瘤可出现横纹肌母细胞分化[68]。超微结构上[69]，神经纤维瘤由神经鞘、神经束膜细胞以及纤维母细胞多种细胞成分混合组成。因此，在神经纤维瘤中，通常仅有 30%～50% 的细胞显示 S-100 蛋白阳性，而良性神经鞘瘤几乎 100% 的细胞 S-100 阳性。

多发神经纤维瘤　Multiple neurofibromas

对于出现少数几个皮肤神经纤维瘤而缺乏任何其他诸如咖啡牛乳色斑或虹膜 Lisch 结节特征的患者，不应机械地认为是 NF1。NFI 的诊断需要综合多种特征[70,71]。目前，还没有普遍接受的诊断 NF1 的严格标准，但一般认为出现 5 个以上咖啡牛乳色斑、大的咖啡牛乳色斑、Lisch 结节或丛状神经纤维瘤（见下文）对本病具有诊断意义。

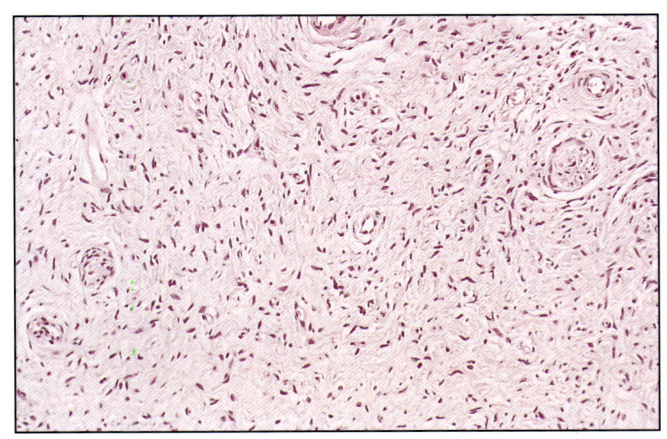

图 27.23　神经纤维瘤。病变显示典型的深染而弯曲的细胞核和几个小的神经纤维。

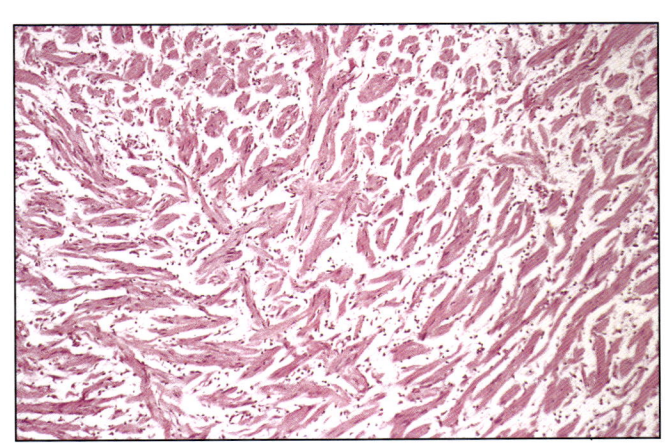

图 27.25　胶原性神经纤维瘤。在一些区域，肿瘤细胞分布在纵行排列的胶原束间或胶原束内。

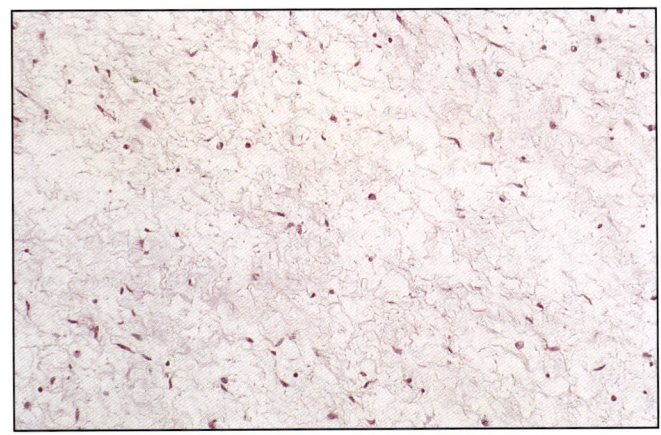

图 27.24　黏液样神经纤维瘤。这种疾病与黏液瘤的鉴别可能需要 S-100 免疫染色。

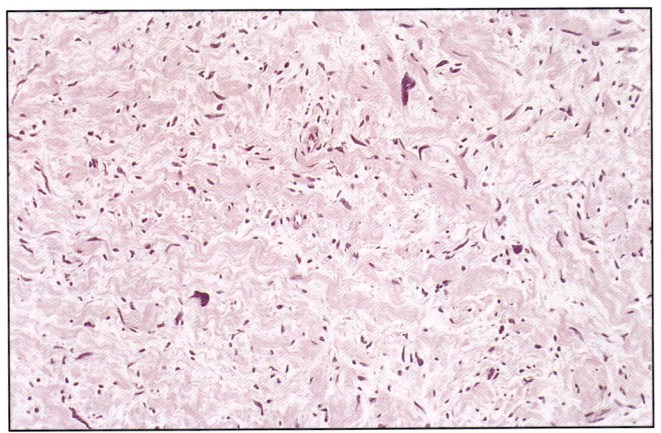

图 27.26　奇异性神经纤维瘤。注意退变细胞核的非典型性。

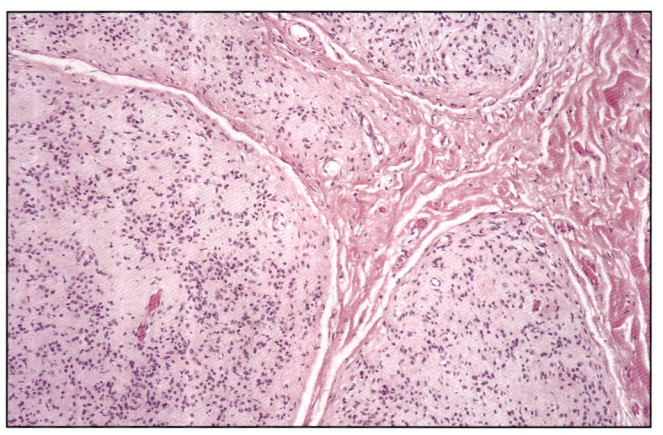

图27.27 树突状细胞神经纤维瘤。小的嗜碱性细胞围绕较大而淡染的细胞排列成玫瑰花结样。

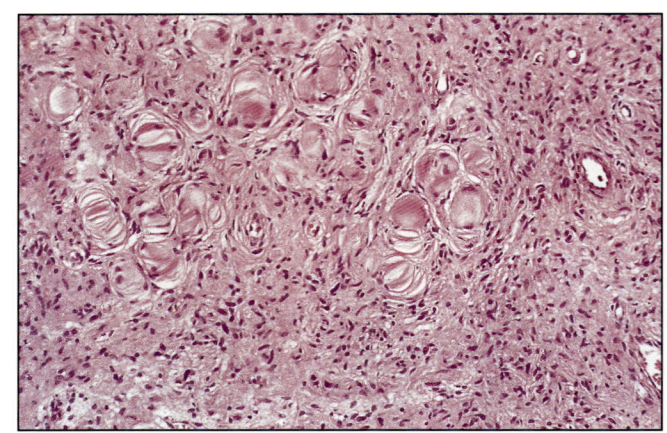

图27.28 弥漫性神经纤维瘤。触觉小体分化是一种常见而突出的表现。

局限性神经纤维瘤亚型 Variants of localized neurofibroma

确定的局限性神经纤维瘤亚型很少见。它们包括：上皮样神经纤维瘤（epithelioid neurofibroma），部分肿瘤细胞呈圆形，伴有嗜酸性胞浆；颗粒细胞神经纤维瘤（granular cell neurofibroma），许多肿瘤细胞含有明显的细颗粒状、耐淀粉酶消化 PAS 染色阳性的嗜酸性胞浆；以及色素神经纤维瘤（pigmented neurofibroma），肿瘤中散在一些含有黑色素的肿瘤细胞。最近描述的树突状细胞神经纤维瘤（dendritic cell neurofibroma）[72]其疾病分类仍有一些争议。本病一般是小的皮肤病变，发生在成年人，组织学特征是由圆形-梭形细胞组成的微小分叶状或玫瑰花结样生长，围绕着体积较大的胞浆淡嗜酸性的细胞排列，有些像神经节样细胞（图 27.27）。所谓的 Pacini 神经纤维瘤，同前面提到的一样，最好是将其看成是神经鞘瘤的变型。典型的皮肤神经鞘黏液瘤（见 1744 页）过去也被误认为是 Pacini 神经纤维瘤[73]。

弥漫性神经纤维瘤 Diffuse neurofibroma

临床特征

弥漫性神经纤维瘤表现为皮下增厚所形成的境界不清的斑块样区域，发病年龄最常为 10～30 岁，无性别差异。根据作者的经验，最常受累的部位是躯干，其次为头颈部，然后为四肢；大约 10% 的病例伴有 NF1。这些病变常常较大，并且毁损外形，可能需要较大的整形外科手术加以适当地控制。尽管肿瘤较大，但它们似乎没有恶变的倾向，或者至少是恶变的发生极其罕见。

组织学特征

弥漫性神经纤维瘤的特征是：真皮和皮下组织被弥漫性增生的神经纤维瘤性组织取代，非常类似于局限性神经纤维瘤。唯一的差别是：几乎所有的弥漫性神经纤维瘤均可见局灶性触觉小体（meissnerian）分化（图 27.28）；此外，组成的神经（或神经纤维）常常呈现明显肥大和水肿。在这些肿瘤中，发现含有黑色素的树突状细胞并不少见[74]。偶尔可见起源不明的多核巨细胞。肿瘤弥漫性浸润浅层皮下脂肪组织，可能被误认为是皮肤纤维肉瘤，后者有较明显的席纹状排列方式，CD34 阳性，S-100 阴性，容易与弥漫性神经纤维瘤区别。

丛状神经纤维瘤 Plexiform neurofibroma

临床特征

丛状神经纤维瘤最常见于儿童，发病没有性别差异，少数可发生在年轻成人。即使在就诊时其他特征不明显，但它通常仍被认为是 NF1 的特殊表现。病变解剖分布和深度变异很大，但以头颈部最为常见，并且浅表软组织比深部组织更常受累。这种类型的神经纤维瘤常常伴有皮肤色素的不同程度增加，形成粗大冗赘的皱襞，邻近软组织普遍增厚，骨骼肥大，可导致明显畸形。丛状神经纤维瘤具有恶变的危险性，尤其是体积较大的和发生在深部组织的病变，但恶变的发生率似乎较低[64,75]。

组织学特征

丛状神经纤维瘤是由膨胀的神经或神经纤维组成的，这些神经纤维大部分被类似于局限性神经纤维瘤的神经纤维瘤性组织取代（图 27.29）。这些膨胀的神经形成肉眼可见的粗大扭曲的条索和结节。大多数肿瘤有明显的黏液样变，此外，具有与弥漫性神经纤维瘤类似特征的肿瘤常常见于邻近的软组织。兼有丛状神经纤维瘤和弥漫性神经纤维瘤二者临床病理学特征的混合性病变并不少见。需要重申的是，在这一类型肿瘤中见到任何

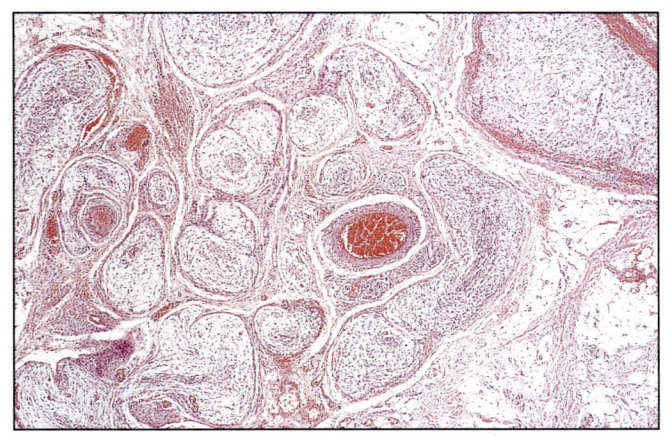

图27.29　丛状神经纤维瘤。典型的表现为黏液样神经纤维瘤小叶，其中央为神经束。

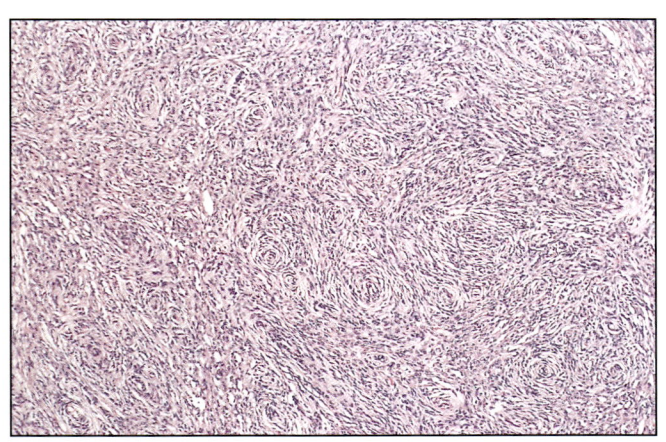

图27.30　软组织神经束膜瘤。注意细胞呈不同程度的席纹状或漩涡状排列。

的核分裂活动均代表发生恶变，一般还伴有细胞密度增加或细胞核的非典型性。

神经束膜瘤　Perineurioma

临床特征

目前已知神经束膜瘤的发生有三种主要形式：软组织（神经外）、神经内和硬化性神经束膜瘤。软组织神经束膜瘤（过去称为席纹状神经束膜纤维瘤）直到近年来才被认识到是神经鞘肿瘤的特殊类型[76-80]。此病最常见于中年人的肢体或躯干；女性多发。大多数患者表现为皮下无痛性肿块，肿块直径一般小于 5 cm；原发于皮肤的大约占10%。此病不伴有神经纤维瘤病，临床病程几乎都是良性的，局部复发极其少见[80]。组织形态相似的病变也可发生在肠壁[81]。神经内神经束膜瘤[82]，从前称为局限性肥大性神经病（localized hypertrophic neuropathy）[83,84]，现在认为是一种主要发生在年轻人的良性肿瘤，临床特征是主干神经梭形肿胀，伴有运动（感觉少见）神经功能障碍。硬化性神经束膜瘤[85]是一种良性非复发性肿瘤，表现为孤立性小结节，典型病变发生在手指或手掌皮肤，主要见于年轻人。

组织学特征

软组织神经束膜瘤（soft tissue perineurioma）是一种境界清楚但无包膜的肿瘤，其特征是细胞数量不等并呈明显的漩涡状或席纹状排列（图 27.30）。它至少在表面上类似于颅内脑膜瘤；鉴于神经束膜和软脑膜在胚胎学和解剖学上关系密切，这种现象就不足为奇了。肿瘤细胞呈梭形，双极，胞浆淡嗜酸性，细胞核尖细或圆胖不一，取决于切面的位置（图 27.31）。此病常见间质局灶性玻璃样变，有些病例可见明显的黏液样变性。极少数的病例具有明显的网状生长方式（图 27.32）[86]。核

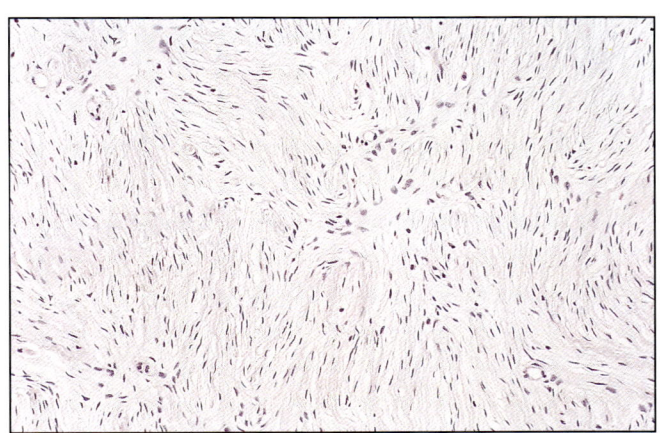

图27.31　软组织神经束膜瘤。本例细胞稀少，显示双极梭形细胞，伴有局灶圆胖型细胞核。

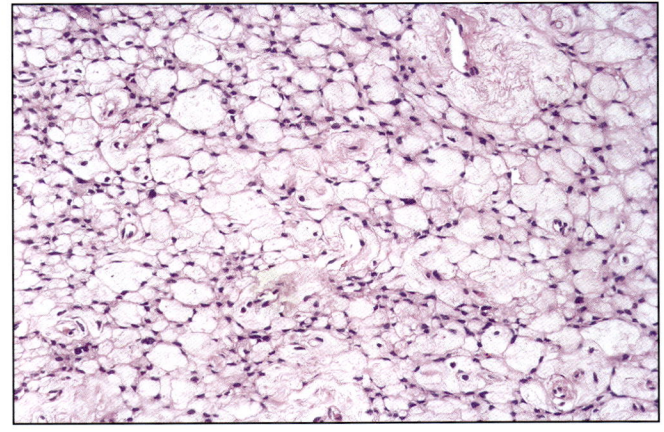

图27.32　网状神经束膜瘤。长的肿瘤细胞围绕基质排列成网状结构。

分裂象罕见，但少数病例可显示非典型性灶状变性的细胞核，类似于陈旧性神经鞘瘤[80]。肿瘤细胞 EMA 免疫组化染色几乎总是阳性，支持其神经束膜的性质（图27.33）。Claudin-1 可能也是一个有用的标记物[87]，但是仅有 20%～25% 病例呈阳性[80]。超微结构观察可以进

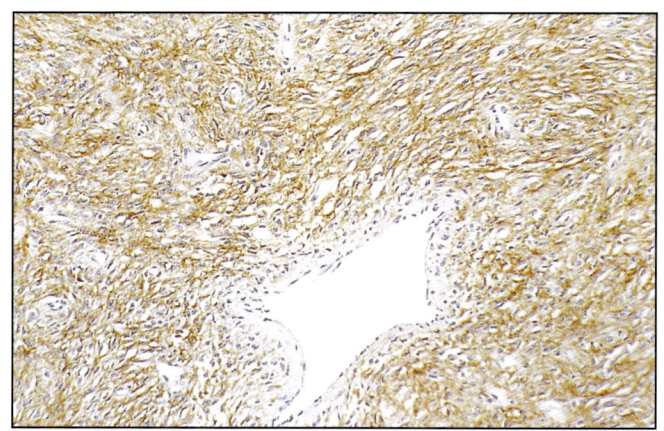

图27.33 软组织神经束膜瘤。注意上皮膜抗原（EMA）染色呈强阳性。ABC法。

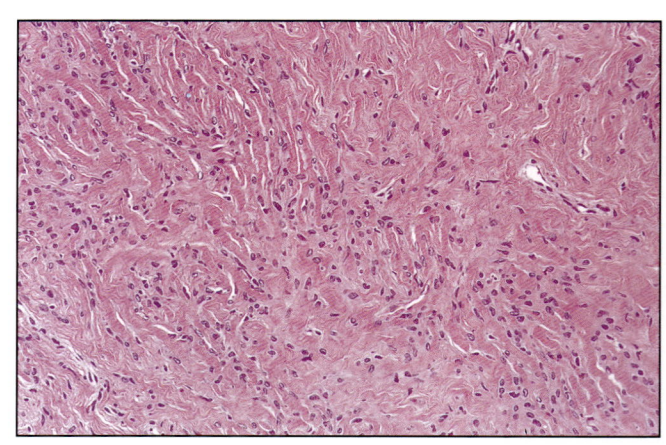

图27.35 硬化性神经束膜瘤。这个手指病变是由小的上皮样细胞组成的，位于玻璃样的胶原间质中。

一步证实神经束膜分化，诸如具有细长的细胞突起，伴有不完全的外板，常见吞饮小泡。胞浆突起非常纤细，尤其在细胞数量较少的病例更是如此，使 EMA 染色容易被忽略。大约50%的病例CD34呈阳性，少数病例S-100蛋白可呈局灶性阳性。

神经内神经束膜瘤（intraneural perineurioma）：可引起神经圆柱状膨大，最常见于肢体的不同部位。其特征是形态温和的梭形神经束膜细胞围绕单个轴突增生：纵切面上这些细胞在神经外鞘（epineural scheath）内呈束状排列，而横切面则呈同心圆的"洋葱头样"结构（图 27.34）。此病几乎没有细胞非典型性。EMA 免疫染色阳性是一个重要的诊断标志。

硬化性神经束膜瘤（sclerosing perineurioma）形成界限相对清楚但没有包膜的胶原性结节，通常位于真皮，其中可见小的上皮样细胞或圆胖的梭形细胞，呈条索状、漩涡状和相互吻合的丝条状分布，细胞核轻度深染（图27.35）。细胞数量多少不一，胞浆淡染而不明显，很难辨认双极胞浆突起。同其他类型的神经束膜瘤一样，肿瘤细胞 EMA 阳性。有时也可见到肌动蛋白或角蛋白灶状阳性 [85]。

虽然分析的病例数目不多，但是所有这三种类型的神经束膜瘤均出现22号染色体重排，最常见的是染色体缺失 [38,79,82]。

皮肤神经鞘黏液瘤（神经鞘黏液瘤）
Dermal nerve sheath myxoma (neurothekeoma)

临床特征

皮肤神经鞘黏液瘤最常表现为上肢或头颈部的浅表孤立性无痛性肿块，好发于青少年或年轻人。女性多见 [88,89]；尽管如此，总的发病年龄和部位变化非常大。多数肿物最大直径不超过3 cm，且皮肤的临床表现没有特殊性。不伴有神经纤维瘤病。此病可出现局部复发，但并没有破坏性 [89a]。发生在椎管的组织学上与之类似的病变极少见，但已有报道 [90]，作者也见过发生在脊柱旁软组织和乳房皮肤的病例。

组织学特征

这种皮肤肿瘤的特征是：膨胀性的、典型的分叶状或多结节状生长方式，有明显的黏液样基质（图27.36）。肿瘤细胞大多为梭形，少数有时也可以是上皮样，甚至出现多核细胞（图27.37）；它们在黏液样间质中呈束状或漩涡状排列。少数病变可累及皮下脂肪组织。细胞核多呈空泡状，局部可见多形性；很容易找到核分裂象，但通常为正常核分裂象。少数病例显示灶状软骨化生。典型的黏液样神经鞘黏液瘤 S-100 蛋白反应都呈阳性。

近年来我们已经注意到一些个案报道，肿瘤中有些细胞比较丰富的小叶状结构 [89,91,92]，但是，只要肿瘤主要呈黏液样改变，S-100保持阳性，就支持可能具有神经鞘分化。有限的超微结构资料也支持这种解释 [93]。这样的

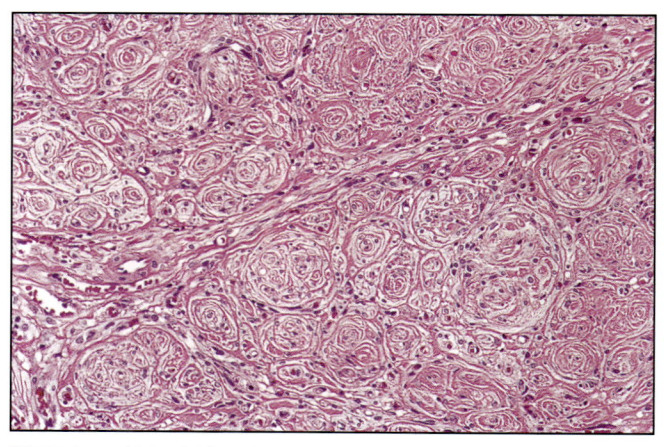

图27.34 神经内神经束膜瘤。这是膨胀的坐骨神经的部分横切面。注意神经束膜细胞呈同心圆的漩涡状排列。

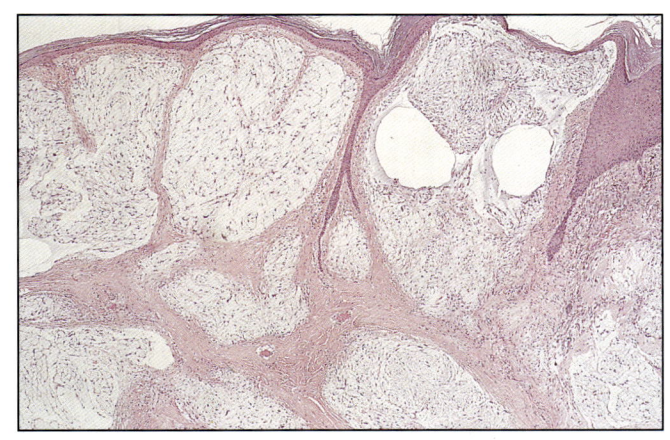

图27.36 皮肤神经鞘黏液瘤。真皮胶原可见典型的分叶状结构，病变中细胞稀少。

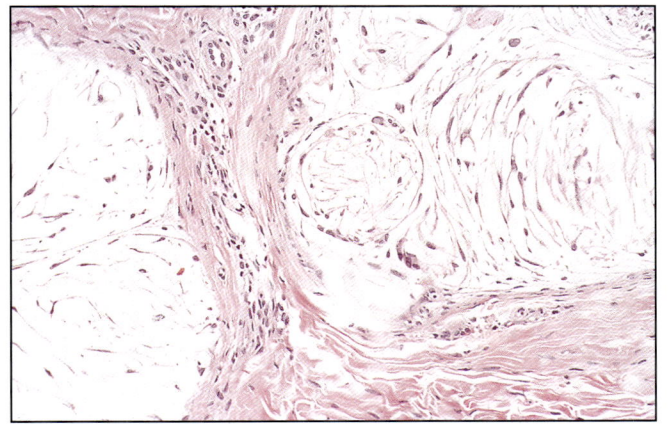

图27.37 皮肤神经鞘黏液瘤。细胞大多数为梭形，有些细胞呈圆形和上皮样，这个视野还有多核细胞。

病例最初被描述为"富细胞性神经鞘黏液瘤"（cellular neurothekeoma）[91]，但事实上，这些病变似乎不同于之后文献中命名的肿瘤类型（见下文）。S-100阴性的富细胞病变最好被看成是所谓的富细胞性神经鞘黏液瘤黏液样变的实例，其本质可能是非神经性的。

富细胞性神经鞘黏液瘤
Cellular "neurothekeoma"

现在已经普遍接受的观点是：被描述为富细胞性神经鞘黏液瘤的疾病[94,95]本质上不属于神经外胚层，与皮肤神经鞘黏液瘤无关。这一病变在23章有详细的讨论。

颗粒细胞瘤（以前称之为颗粒细胞肌母细胞瘤，Abrikossof瘤）
Granular cell tumor (formerly granular cell myoblastoma, Abrikossof tumor)

有关颗粒细胞瘤是代谢性、退行性还是肿瘤性病变的争论已经持续多年[96-98]，现在这个问题似乎已经得到解决，多数人支持它是肿瘤性病变。然而，应当注意的是，虽然多数颗粒细胞肿瘤本质上可能是神经外胚层来源[99]，但是其免疫表型及其与神经的密切关系说明，显示颗粒性胞浆形态学改变的所有病变决不都是颗粒细胞瘤。由于次级溶酶体积聚引起的胞浆颗粒性改变可以见于各种类型的肿瘤，包括平滑肌肿瘤[100]、其他结缔组织肿瘤、神经胶质肿瘤，甚至基底细胞癌（见Mentzel等[100]的综述）。根据这个作者的经验，显示颗粒细胞改变的所有类型的肿瘤都有共同的免疫组织化学染色特征，即神经元特异性烯醇化酶（NSE）和NKI-C3染色阳性[101]，CD68也常常呈阳性。因此，当诊断任何一种颗粒细胞肿瘤时，重要的是应当寻找可排除一系列可能的鉴别诊断的线索。以下描述的特征与大多数显示神经外胚层分化的病变相关。

临床特征

大多数颗粒细胞瘤发生于中年人的皮肤或皮下组织，女性稍多见[102,103]。然而，总的来说，发病年龄范围广泛。此病在任何解剖部位都可发生，但躯干（包括女性外阴部）和舌也许是最常见的部位。发生在乳房[104]、胆管分支（biliary tree）[105]、喉（见第4章）以及其他内脏部位的病例均有很多报道；但是发生在骨骼肌内的颗粒细胞瘤相对少见。高达10%的颗粒细胞瘤患者为多发性病变[103,106,107]，这种现象似乎更常见于黑人。多数情况下肿瘤生长缓慢，很少有触痛，最大直径通常小于3 cm。良性颗粒细胞瘤的局部复发率<5%，通常是由于切除不彻底所致。

组织学特征

颗粒细胞瘤无论发生在什么部位均具有明显均匀一致的形态。肿瘤境界变化不一，多达50%的肿瘤境界不清或呈浸润性边界。肿瘤细胞排列成巢状或小梁状（图

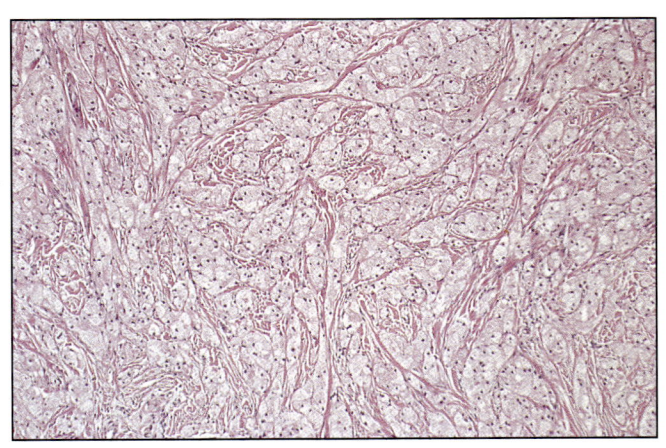

图27.38 颗粒细胞瘤。颗粒细胞呈巢状和条索状分布，被薄的纤维性间隔分开。

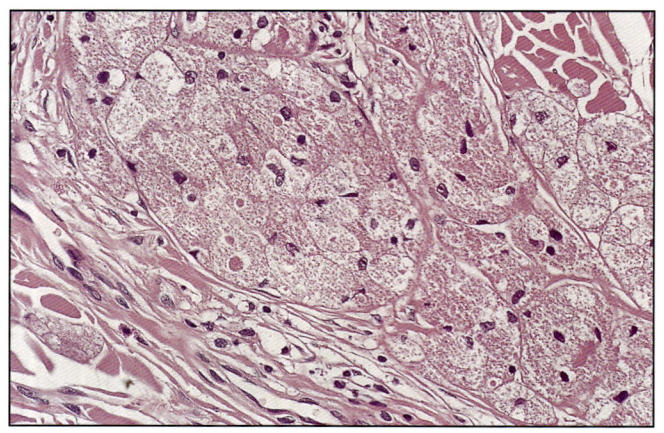

图27.39 颗粒细胞瘤。注意典型的小而深染的细胞核和细颗粒状胞浆，其内偶有嗜酸性小滴。

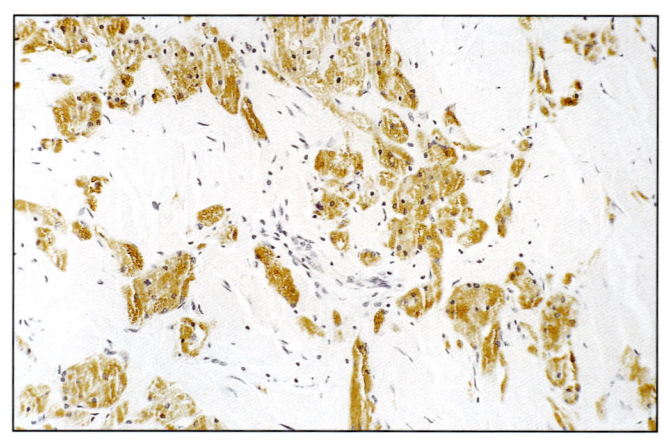

图27.41 颗粒细胞瘤。在这个浸润性较为明显的病例中，S-100蛋白免疫染色显示肿瘤细胞阳性。

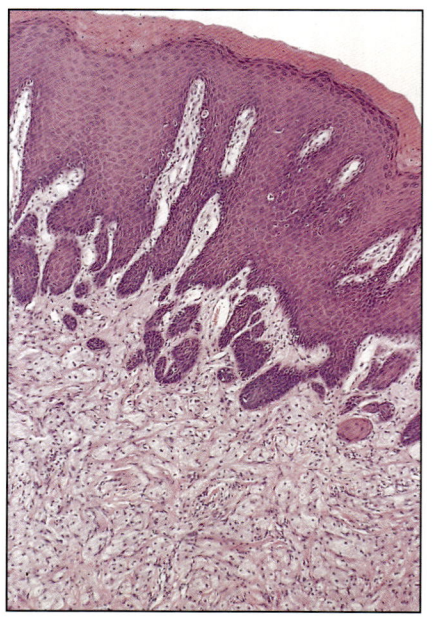

图27.40 颗粒细胞瘤。表面上皮或黏膜增生，常呈不同程度的假上皮瘤性增生，尤其在口腔。

27.38）。细胞体积较大，呈圆形或多边形，具有明显的细颗粒状嗜酸性胞浆（图27.39）；有时可见较大的嗜酸性小滴或颗粒。肿瘤细胞核小，居中，常常呈固缩状或深染，但也有些核呈空泡状。有些病变有散在核分裂象或轻度核非典型性，后者常常是退变性的。传统观点认为，颗粒细胞呈一致性耐淀粉酶消化的 PAS 阳性染色，但作者的经验认为，只有不超过 1/3 的病例如此。肿瘤细胞巢常常围绕或邻近小的神经，常位于神经外膜内。浅表部位的病变常常伴有被覆的鳞状上皮棘层增厚或假上皮瘤性增生（图27.40），在表浅活检时（尤其在口腔或喉）不小心可能被误认为鳞状细胞癌。

免疫组化染色，除了 NSE 和 NK1-C3 阳性外（见上文），常见的神经外胚层型颗粒细胞瘤在几乎所有病例 S-100 蛋白均呈阳性[99,108,109]（图 27.41）。有趣的是，几乎所有的病变抑制素（inhibin）和钙视网膜蛋白（calretinin）也呈阳性反应[110]。其他标记物几乎没有类似的应用价值。20 世纪 80 年代中期，一些短篇报道描述，颗粒细胞瘤对癌胚抗原（CEA）表达呈阳性，其实只不过是应用了（现在已经废弃的）交叉反应抗体。超微结构特征如前所述，颗粒细胞有许多含有明显髓鞘样结构的次级溶酶体。此外，肿瘤细胞具有不同程度的完整的外板和多数胞浆突起。大多数病例的鉴别诊断并不困难，但应考虑到上面提到的显示颗粒细胞改变的其他类型的肿瘤的可能性。有些肿瘤可能需要与成人横纹肌瘤、组织细胞样癌（如来自乳腺）或罕见的既往创伤或炎症合并的反应性病变鉴别[111]。

颗粒细胞瘤的亚型 Variants of granular cell tumor

新生儿牙龈颗粒细胞瘤（gingival granular cell tumor of newborn infants）[112]也称为先天性牙龈瘤，是一种十分少见的肿瘤，呈息肉样肿胀，最常位于牙槽嵴外侧，尤其是上颌。90% 以上的病例为女性，几乎全都见于出生时或出生后不久。随后病变似乎不再长大。少数患者有多发性病变[112,113]。随着时间的推移，病变倾向于逐渐缩小，且切除后似乎不再复发。组织学上它们是由与成人神经外胚层型颗粒细胞瘤相同的细胞组成的（图27.42），伴有明显的丛网状毛细血管，散在的炎细胞，偶尔可见陷入其中的牙源性上皮巢（图27.43）。免疫组化染色[114]，肿瘤细胞 S-100 蛋白呈阴性，而且没有任何特异性分化证据；电镜观察[114,115]，细胞无外板，显示部分组织细胞特征。这些病变的本质极有可能是反应性的。

原始息肉样颗粒细胞瘤（primitive polyploid granular cell tumor）[116,117]：LeBoit 等最先应用这一术语描述一种罕见的颗粒细胞瘤亚型，表现为皮肤外生性肿物，可发生在不同部位和任何年龄。肿瘤细胞丰富，呈梭形，

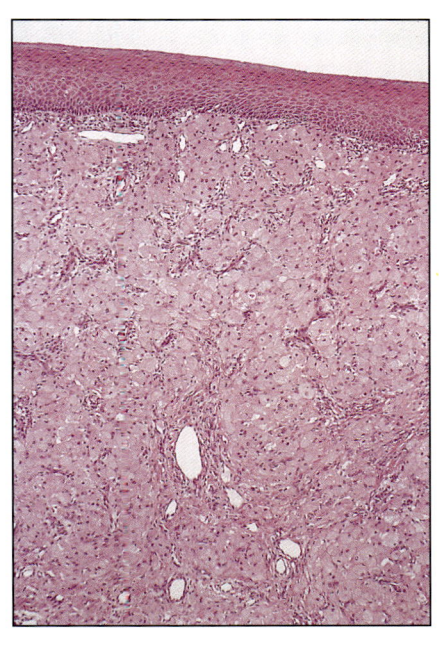

图27.42 牙龈颗粒细胞瘤。病变来自新生儿，显示血管和炎症细胞比成人颗粒细胞瘤病例常见到的丰富。

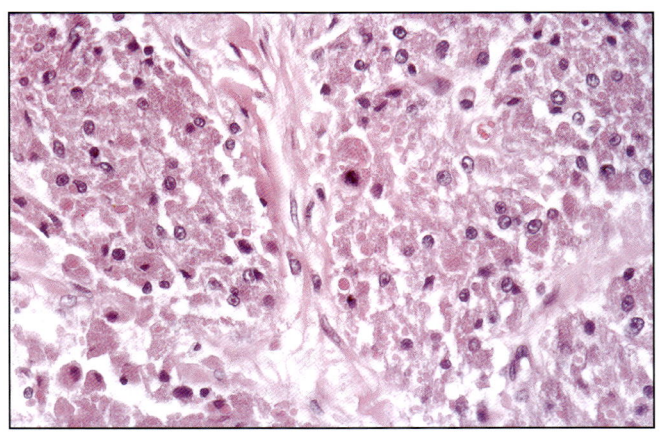

图27.44 恶性颗粒细胞瘤。大的腹膜后肿块伴有骨转移，显示核的非典型性，核分裂象多见。

恶性肿瘤　Malignant tumors

在这一标题下描述恶性外周神经鞘肿瘤（MPNST）和外周（骨外）原始神经外胚层肿瘤（PNET）。发生在软组织的其他具有神经外胚层分化的恶性肿瘤，包括透明细胞肉瘤，将在其他神经外胚层肿瘤的章节中讨论。

恶性外周神经鞘瘤（恶性神经鞘瘤，神经纤维肉瘤）
Malignant peripheral nerve sheath tumor（malignant schwannoma, neurofibrosarcoma）

喜欢用恶性外周神经鞘瘤（MPNST）这一术语来描述神经鞘型肉瘤是因为：其构成细胞具有异质性，而且与普通良性神经鞘瘤或神经纤维瘤完全不同或少有相似性。从前认为诊断 MPNST 必须证实肿瘤：（1）起源于神经或起源于先前存在的良性神经鞘瘤；（2）超微结构显示神经鞘细胞分化的证据；或（3）NF1 患者出现梭形细胞肉瘤，但是随着时间的推移，已经明确，很多 MPNST 病例都具有可重复的形态学特征（见下文），足以能够做出 MPNST 诊断，尤其是在缺乏上述诊断标准的情况下，如果能够得到免疫组化的支持，则更加确定[122]。

临床特征

MPNST 主要以两种形式出现：散发或 30%～50% 的患者伴有 NF1 特征或 NF1 家族史[123-127]。NF1 患者终生发生 MPNST 的危险估计为 2%[128]。发病年龄范围较广，但主要发生在成年人。在散发病例中，发病性别相同，发病高峰为 40～50 岁，而在 NF1 患者中，发病高峰要年轻 10～15 岁，而且男性多见。病变解剖部位很广泛，肢体比躯干（包括腹膜后）更常见，头部和颈部

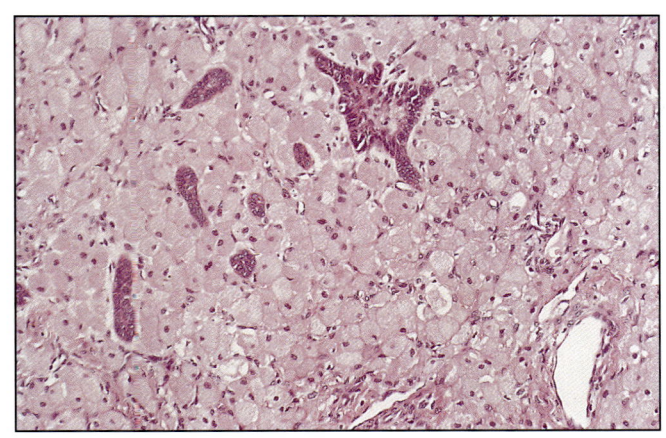

图27.43 牙龈颗粒细胞瘤。常见陷入的非肿瘤牙源性上皮巢。

常见细胞核的多形性，核分裂象非常常见。免疫表型基本阴性，且这种少见病变的分化路径尚不清楚。临床经过一般为良性，但有一例淋巴结转移的病例报告[117]。

恶性颗粒细胞瘤(malignant granular cell tumor)[102,103,118-121] 发病率不超过所有颗粒细胞瘤的 2%～3%，似乎主要发生在成人的深部软组织。在所报道的病例中，50% 以上发生转移或有致死性临床过程。诊断标准很难确定，因为有些病变在组织学上呈明显的良性和单形性改变。当肿瘤体积异常增大或位于深部且伴有浸润性生长或坏死时，其细胞多形性或核仁明显以及核分裂象非常常见，应该怀疑为恶性（图 27.44）。

恶性肿瘤

发生的很少见。与 NF1 相关的肿瘤，肿瘤通常起源于神经或原有的神经纤维瘤。

如前所述，极少数病例起源于良性神经鞘瘤[34,35]，其他一些可起源于神经节瘤，或新发或继发于神经母细胞瘤放疗后[129,130]。多达 10% 的 MPNST 病例似乎是放射诱导所致[131,132]，放疗后的潜伏期一般超过 10 年。少数病例为儿童[133,134]，其中伴有 NF1 的病例比成人更常见。由于 MPNST 以高分化病变为主，因此 MPNST 的 5 年生存率在散发病例中大约为 50%，在 NF1 患者中为 20%～25%，而在放疗后的病例中不超过 10%～15%。与 NF1 相关的 MPNST 更具侵袭性，可能与其通常发生在中心部位和肿瘤体积较大有关。大多数患者死于肺转移。

病理学特征

除非有明显的神经系统症状（通常罕见），大多数 MPNST 患者在就诊时肿瘤的最大直径已超过 10 cm，这反映了肿瘤位置通常很深。发生在大神经的病变常表现为邻近神经的梭形肿大，而先前存在的良性肿瘤病变在显微镜下可见分区现象，但这种改变常不明显。

组织学上，多数病例表现为梭形细胞呈束状分布；提示神经分化的显著特征是：富细胞区和黏液样区之间的突然转变（图 27.45），以及血管周围肿瘤细胞较密集或呈漩涡状排列（图 27.46），有时肿瘤细胞直接蔓延到血管壁导致血栓形成。在其他病例，整个肿瘤的细胞均匀一致，呈束状分布，在 HE 染色切片上，与单相型滑膜肉瘤和纤维肉瘤几乎无法区别（图 27.47）。高达 10% 的病例整个肿瘤组织有丰富的黏液样间质（黏液性 MPNST；图 27.48）。在细胞水平有助于诊断的线索是：细胞浆淡染，细胞界线不清，细胞核窄，两端逐渐变细，在一些区域常呈波浪状或弯曲状（图 27.49）；后一特征并不像在神经纤维瘤中那样常见。核倾向于深染，至少

呈局灶多形性，核仁不明显。细胞核栅栏状排列不常见（实际上，可能还不如在平滑肌肉瘤和滑膜肉瘤常见），而且触觉小体分化也很罕见。除了不常见的富细胞性或非典型性神经纤维瘤外，核分裂象在 MPNST 中一般容

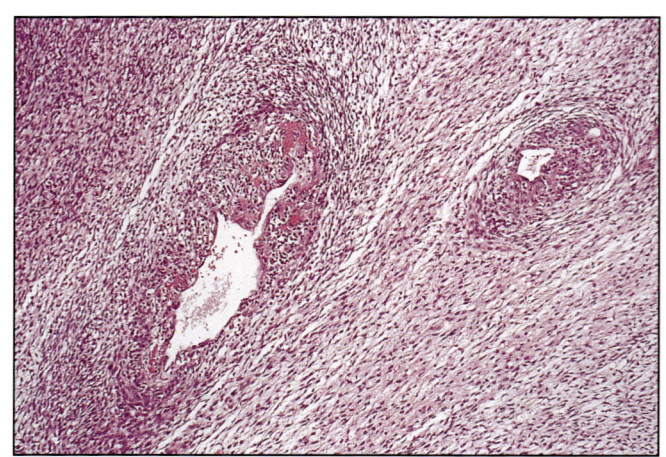

图27.46　恶性外周神经鞘瘤。常见的特征是肿瘤细胞聚集在血管周围并浸润血管壁。

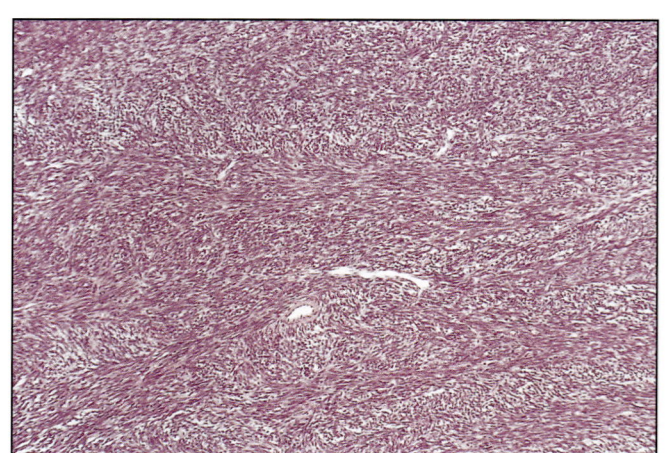

图27.47　恶性外周神经鞘肿瘤。这种束状排列方式使其与其他梭形细胞肿瘤很难鉴别。

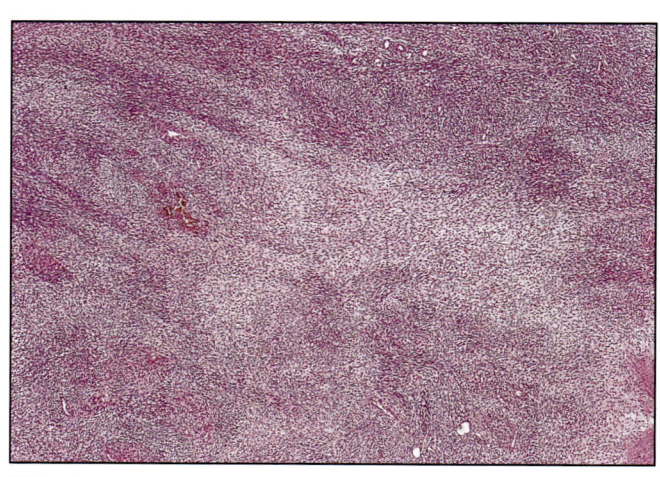

图27.45　恶性外周神经鞘瘤。注意细胞多少不一并有较明显的黏液样区域。

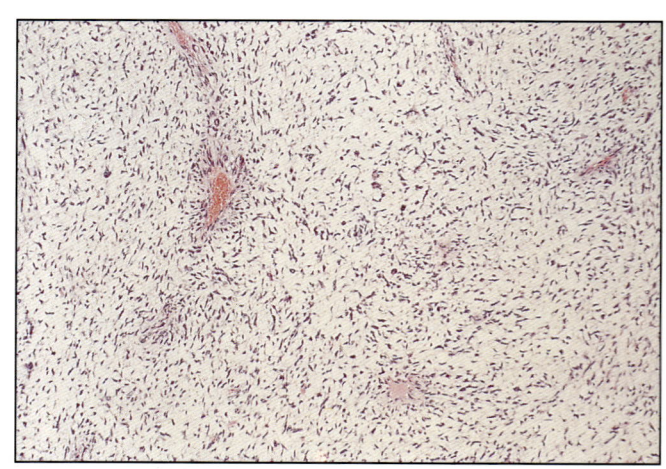

图27.48　黏液性恶性外周神经鞘肿瘤。注意肿瘤细胞明显聚集在血管周围。

易找到。在伴有NF1的患者中，区别良性和恶性通常完全依靠是否出现核分裂象，但核分裂象很少见（图27.50）。少数MPNST被认为是神经束膜型的[135]，其病变倾向于呈非常明显的旋涡状生长（图27.51），而且预后被认为较好，但目前资料有限。极少数MPNST病例在HE染色上难以与所谓的"多形性恶性纤维组织细胞瘤"（见第24章）鉴别，确诊需要辅助技术（通常是电镜检查）。

大约10%~15%的MPNST患者，尤其是发生于NF1的患者，其显著特征是出现异源性分化[136]。其中最常见的是出现横纹肌肉瘤成分[137-139]，形成所谓的恶性蝾螈瘤（malignant Triton tumor 图27.52），其预后尤为不佳。骨肉瘤（图27.53）和软骨肉瘤分化的区域也较常见，后者显示不同程度的恶性细胞学特征。血管肉瘤分化罕见。一般不将这些肿瘤称为恶性间叶瘤。极少见的病例可出现上皮分化，主要是腺上皮分化[59,136]，有时需要与滑膜肉瘤鉴别[140]。

在免疫组化方面，不超过50%的MPNST病例呈S-100阳性[141,142]（图27.54）。这似乎暗合了在超微水

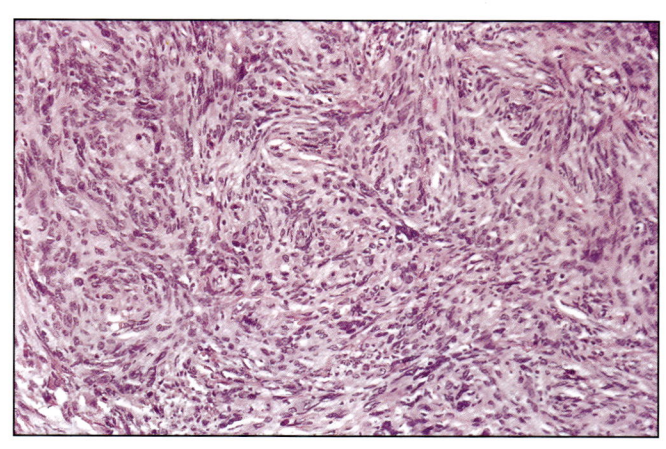

图27.51　恶性外周神经鞘瘤。注意漩涡状的生长方式和细胞的非典型性。

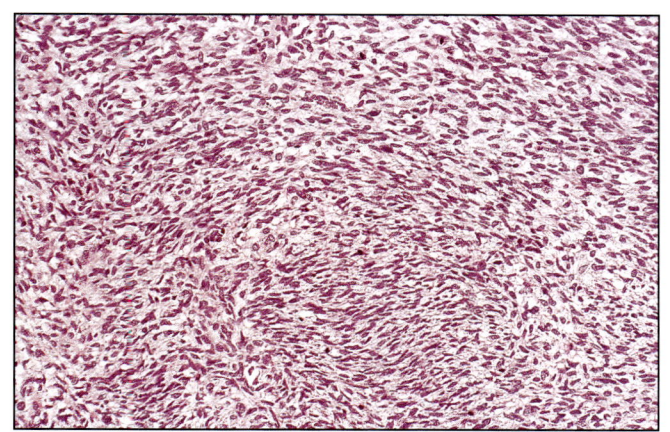

图27.49　恶性外周神经鞘瘤。注意细胞核两端变细，局部弯曲或呈波浪状的形态。

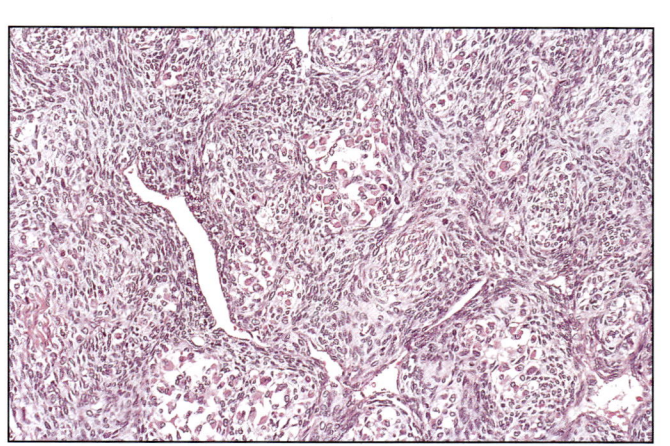

图27.52　恶性蝾螈瘤。注意本例恶性外周神经鞘瘤中有圆胖的横纹肌母细胞。

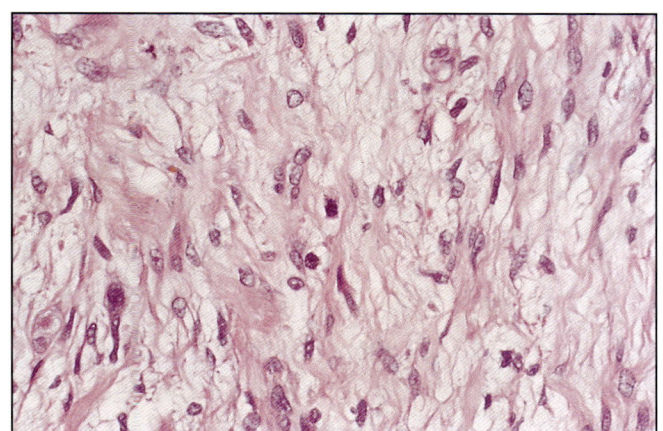

图27.50　恶性外周神经鞘瘤。这个病变来自伴有NF1的患者，除了有轻度核的非典型性和罕见的核分裂象以外，与神经纤维瘤非常相似，这种低级别的形态学所见并非总是与缓慢的临床病程相关。

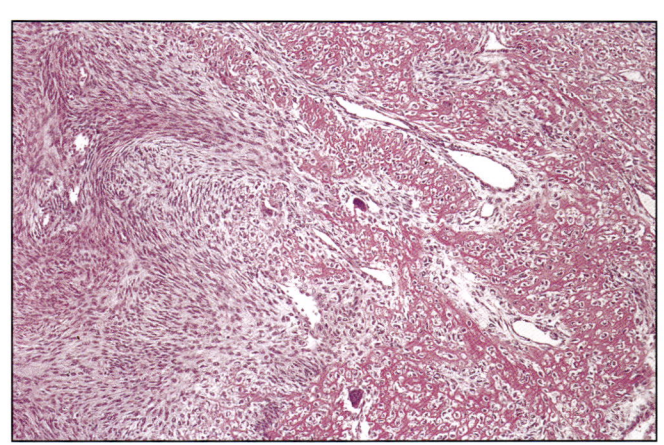

图27.53　恶性外周神经鞘瘤。本例显示有异源性骨肉瘤分化区域。

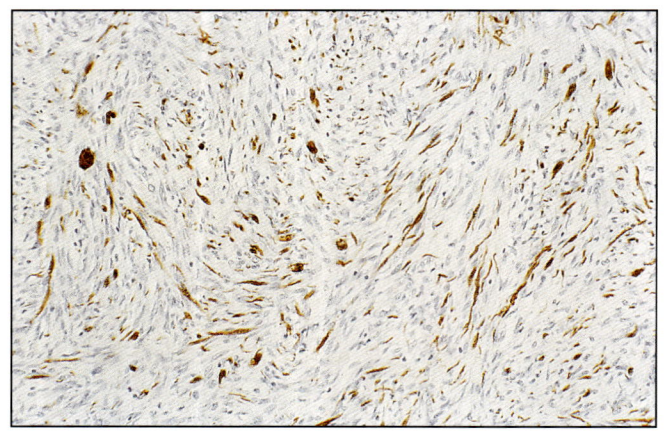

图27.54 恶性外周神经鞘瘤。大约50%的病例S-100阳性，一般不超过50%。ABC法。

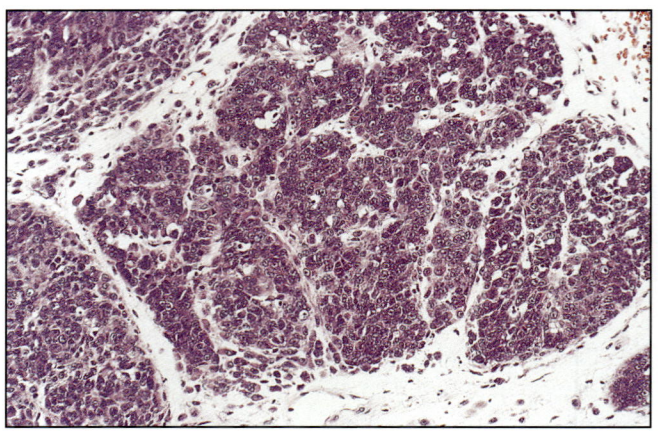

图27.55 上皮样恶性外周神经鞘瘤。注意与无色素性黑色素瘤相似。

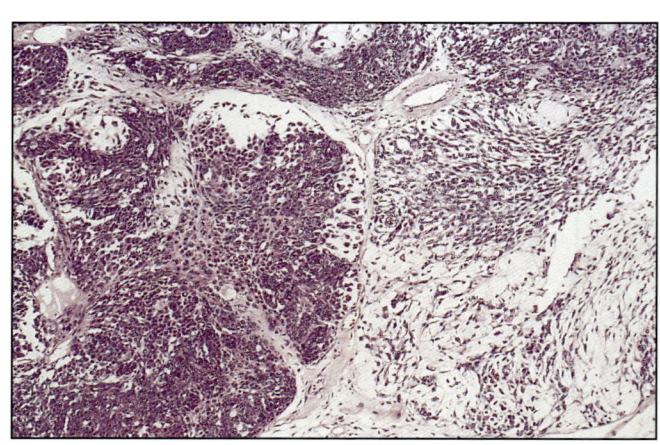

图27.56 上皮样恶性外周神经鞘瘤。证明至少有局灶性的比较典型的梭形细胞区域有利于诊断。

平上仅有不超过50%的病例显示广泛而发育良好的神经鞘分化，而其他病例显示纤维母细胞、神经束膜或不同程度的混合性分化特征[142-144]。即使在阳性的病例，S-100阳性细胞的比例也常常小于20%～30%。在出现神经束膜分化的病例，EMA阳性并具有特征性的超微结构特征[135,145]（见1774页）。研究证实，其他神经标记物，如Leu-7和髓磷脂碱蛋白（myelin basic protein），对于常规诊断MPNST是不足以信赖或欠敏感的，但根据作者个人的经验，GFAP作为诊断MPNST的"二线"标记物有时具有价值，20%～30%的病例可能呈阳性。通过免疫组化染色易于证实异源性横纹肌母细胞或上皮样分化的存在。从预后的角度观察，拓扑异构酶-II-α（topoisomerase-II-alpha）的表达似乎与高级别和侵袭性高的肿瘤相关[146,147]，而在染色体17q同一区域的其他基因在这一方面可能也很重要[147a]。在细胞遗传学上，MPNST通常具有复杂而非特异性的细胞核型，不具有特征性[38]。有人提出，同滑膜肉瘤一样，这些病变可能具有（X;18）染色体易位，现在认为这种说法是错误的，这可能与PCR的污染有关。然而在分子水平上，无论是散发的病例还是与NF1相关的病例都常常显示NF1基因缺失[148]。

MPNST的亚型 Variants of MPNST

上皮样MPNST：大约占所有MPNST的5%，其除了高达50%的病例发生在真皮深层和皮下组织外，临床上没有特征性表现，而发生在浅表部位的肿瘤的预后似乎明显较好[151]。很少有病例发生于以前存在的神经鞘瘤[35]。组织学上，上皮样MPNST大多呈多叶状结构，由数量不等的巢状和条索状排列的上皮样细胞组成；细胞呈圆形，胞浆嗜酸性或嗜双染性，细胞核空泡状，核仁明显，有时类似于无色素性恶性黑色素瘤（图27.55）。许多病例出现普通MPNST的典型的梭形细胞区域（图27.56），且免疫组化检查黑色素瘤抗原（如HMB-45）阴性，必要时结合电镜观察可与转移性黑色素瘤区别。与普通的MPNST不同，上皮样MPNST通常S-100阳性，而且阳性细胞比例常常很高。MPNST与癌（原发的或转移的）的鉴别通过免疫组化染色很容易进行。

色素性（黑色素性）MPNST：在黑色素性神经鞘瘤中已经讨论过（见1739页）。除了通常发生于交感神经链的具有特征性的恶性病变之外，据报道，极少数普通MPNST病例也会出现局灶性黑色素性色素沉积[152]。

外周原始神经外胚层肿瘤（外周神经上皮瘤、Askin瘤、骨外Ewing肉瘤） Peripheral primitive neuroectodermal tumor (peripheral neuroepithelioma, Askin tumor, extraosseous Ewing's sarcoma)

外周PNET[153-155]这一概念一直存在着争议，近20年来发展迅速，现在这些病变已被命名为Ewing

肉瘤/PNET，在本质上这些病变都是同一家族内互相连续的肿瘤，它们具有不同程度（通常很少）的神经分化和单一的 *EWS* 基因重排[156]，后者常常是 t(11;22)(q24;q12) 染色体交互易位的结果[157]。来自大量病例的经验表明，除了 11 号染色体外，还有其他几种染色体易位可导致 22 号染色体 *EWS* 基因重排。其中最常见的是 t(21;22)(q22;q12)，产生 *ERG-EWS* 融合基因，大约 5% 的病例如此，而其他类型的易位则并不常见[158]。这些断裂点上的细微差别可能具有提示预后的意义（见下文）。通过反转录 PCR 可证实这些易位的克隆性融合基因产物的存在[159]，可在分子水平上做出准确的诊断。应用荧光原位杂交探针可以证实 *EWS* 基因重排，在石蜡包埋组织也可以做[160]。将 Ewing 肉瘤和 PNET 区分开是否有临床意义仍存在争议，目前得到的大量证据显示，这种做法没有实际意义，而且神经外胚层分化的程度和预后之间没有相关性。骨 Ewing 肉瘤/PNET 见骨和关节一章（见第 25 章），本节仅探讨骨外软组织病变。

临床特征

骨外 Ewing 肉瘤/PNET 发病年龄范围很广，但好发于 10～30 岁，无性别差异[161-166]。大多发生在深部软组织，特别是躯干（以脊柱旁多见）或下肢。少数病例发生于可识别的神经，就像 1918 年 Arthur Purdy Stout 描述的最早认识的一例病例那样[167]。Askin 瘤这一术语用于描述发生在胸壁的临床病变，后者常常累及肋骨、胸膜和肺[168,169]。经现代诊断技术证实，目前公认的 Ewing 肉瘤/PNET 也可以原发于皮肤[160,170]和各种内脏[171-173]。PNET 患者通常表现为快速生长的肿块，常伴疼痛，位于身体中轴和深部的肿瘤常常不易外科切除。但是这类肿瘤对化疗敏感，大多数病例反应较好，至少初治阶段如此。但即使是这样，作者发现，目前在大多数医疗中心，被确诊为骨外 Ewing 肉瘤/PNET 的患者其 5 年生存率也不超过 20%～30%，但这常常是较大的非儿科年龄组患者的生存率，因为这类患者对于大剂量化疗相对不能耐受。

病理学特征

在化疗之前，这些病变通常只是经过活检而没有被切除。手术切除的肿瘤体积较大，灰白色，质软，伴有广泛的坏死。在身体中轴部位的肿瘤常常累及骨，无法判断肿瘤是原发于骨还是原发于软组织。

组织学上，有一系列的表现反映了神经外胚层分化程度。各种表现都具有显著的分叶状、有时呈小梁状生长（图 27.57），伴有显著的分枝状毛细血管网。一般来说，几乎没有间质成分（虽然个别的也有透明间质成

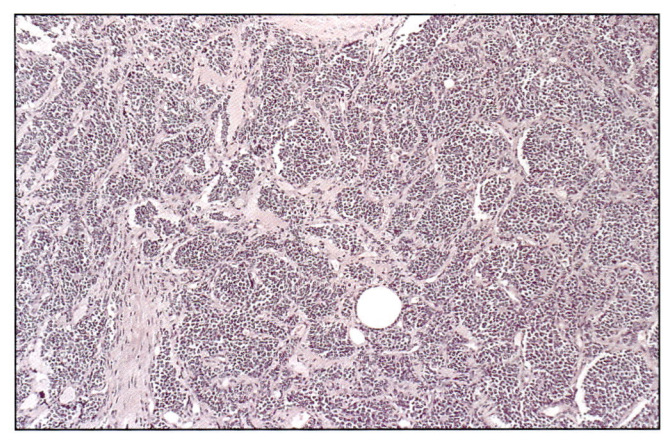

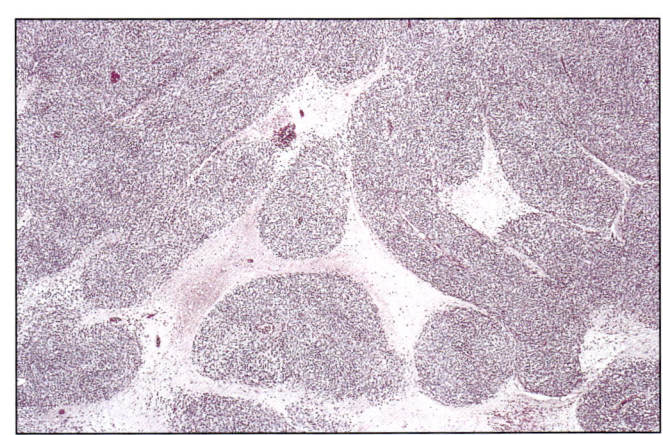

图 27.57 恶性外周神经外胚层肿瘤。这些病变典型表现为小叶状（A）或有些小梁状（B）的生长方式。注意（A）中有显著的纤维血管间隔。

分），常见融合性或条带状坏死。形态谱系一端为低分化（Ewing）的肿瘤细胞，胞浆稀少，淡染，细胞核呈圆形或卵圆形，空泡状，染色质细腻（"粉末状"）（图 27.58），可见小核仁。相反，某些病例由较大的细胞组成，常常伴有看得出来的透明的胞浆，但如出现梭形细胞，则要排除这一诊断。在谱系的另一端（所谓的神经上皮瘤），细胞可能有弱嗜酸性胞浆，染色质可能粗糙，常见核仁。重要的是，在这一形态谱系中分化较好的一端（图 27.59），可见多量玫瑰花结，通常所谓的 Homer Wright 型玫瑰花结，以及血管周围假玫瑰花结。这一谱系是连续的，没有明确的分界点，这就可以用来解释多年来为什么在典型的 Ewing 肉瘤病例中总可见少数菊形团结构。PAS 阳性证明细胞内存在糖原，这种现象可见于任何病变，但较常见于未分化肿瘤，而伴有菊形团结构的肿瘤中大约有 40% 的病例 PAS 阳性。由于多种其他类型的圆形细胞肿瘤都可以出现 PAS 阳性，所以，这项技术用于鉴别诊断价值有限。

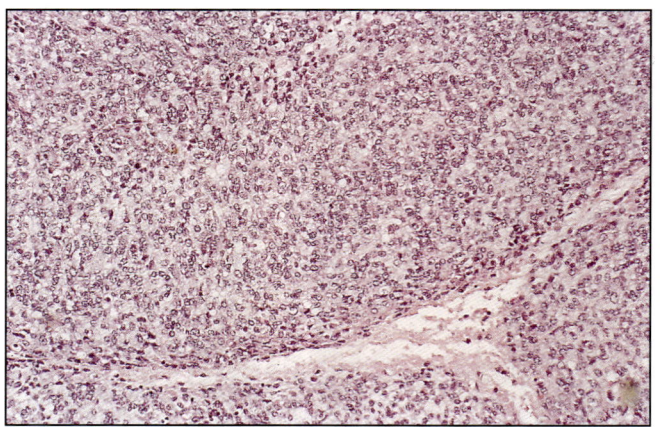

图27.58 恶性外周神经外胚层肿瘤。本例显示未分化的细胞形态改变，是以前公认的Ewing肉瘤。

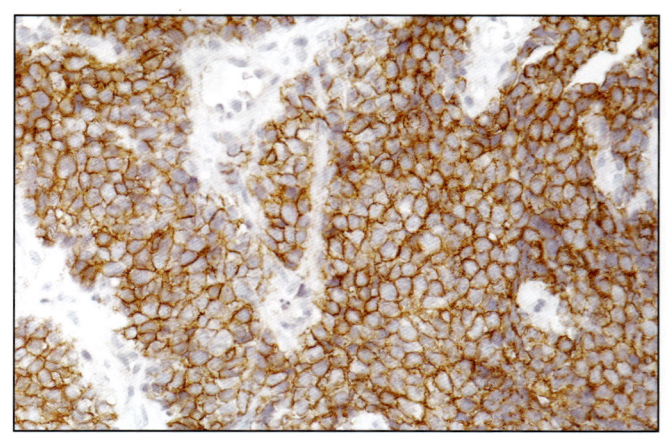

图27.60 恶性外周神经外胚层肿瘤。大部分病例不管分化程度如何，细胞膜CD99均呈弥漫阳性。ABC法。

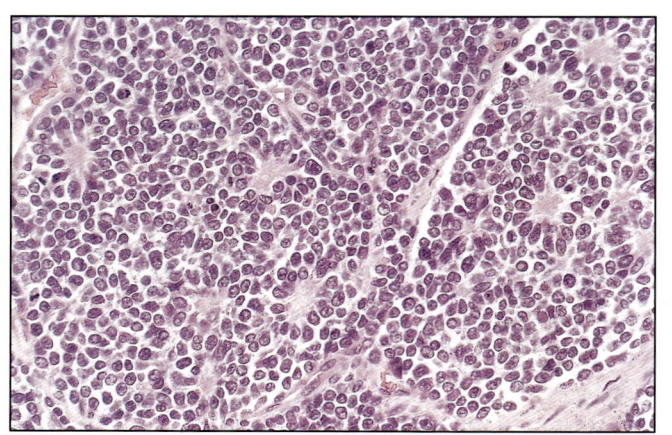

图27.59 恶性外周神经外胚层肿瘤。这个分化较好的病例发生于胸壁，常见菊形团结构，可能被归类于外周神经上皮瘤。

在免疫组化方面，这一形态学谱系中的所有肿瘤都表达CD99抗原，后者是X染色体上 *MIC2* 基因编码的产物，可用O-13、MIC-2或HBA-71抗体染色证实[174-177]；大多数病例β2-微球蛋白（β2-microglobulin）也呈阳性[165,175]。抗CD99的抗体对于证实Ewing/PNET诊断特别有用，但是这种抗原不是特异性的，必须根据病变本质严格加以解释；在小圆细胞肿瘤、T-淋巴母细胞淋巴瘤、低分化滑膜肉瘤、一些神经内分泌癌以及少数横纹肌肉瘤（通常是腺泡状横纹肌肉瘤）病例中，CD99可能呈阳性。在真正的Ewing/PNET病例，CD99呈散在阳性，在细胞膜表面甚为明显（图27.60）。此外，PNET谱系中的很多肿瘤在免疫组化上都显示不同程度的神经外胚层分化，表现为NSE、蛋白基因产物（protein gene product）9.5（PGP9.5）、神经细丝、Leu-7和突触素阳性。值得注意的是，在PNET谱系中，20%~30%的病例角蛋白常呈点状阳性[178]。在超微结构方面，正如所预期的那样，这种肿瘤有一个类似的连续分化的谱系，分化范围从传统的细胞器稀少和糖原丰富的"Ewing"一端，经过微管和神经分泌颗粒数目增多，到形成发育良好的神经突起的所谓的"神经上皮瘤"的另外一端。

还有小部分肿瘤无论是形态学上还是免疫组化方面都显示多种表型的分化。此外，那些特殊的形成菊形团的PNET病例还显示神经胶质、神经节、甚至上皮样分化[179-181]，这可能表明神经嵴有多向分化潜能。关于包括角蛋白阳性在内的异常或有复杂中间丝表达的比较原始的肿瘤的性质，尚有争议[182-184]。这可能也反映了神经嵴的可塑性，但是以前已报道的病例中至少部分可能是纤维组织增生性小圆细胞肿瘤（见第24章）。不论这些病例是什么，其中一些可能是真正的"母细胞瘤"（blastoma）。

尽管PNET的预后与神经分化程度的关系尚有争议[185,186]，但目前基本上已被摒弃。资料显示，EWS嵌合融合基因转录子类型与预后明显相关；至少一些研究发现，伴有I型融合转录子（涉及 *EWS* 的7号外显子和 *FLI1* 的6号轴突）的患者其无瘤生存期明显延长[187,188]。

外胚层间叶瘤 Ectomesenchymoma

外胚层间叶（ectomesenchyme）是用于神经嵴组织的一个术语，在胚胎发生中，神经嵴显示间叶分化。神经嵴肿瘤的异向分化是一种公认的现象，因此，尽管它有横纹肌母细胞成分，但外胚层间叶瘤在本章中讨论较为合乎逻辑。外胚层间叶瘤[189-192]是一种非常罕见的肿瘤，令人信服的病例报道只有不到30例。几乎所有肿瘤都发生在幼婴，男性优势明显。肿瘤通常位于腹膜后、盆腔和睾丸旁。组织学上，此病的特点是胚胎性横纹肌肉瘤与神经节瘤、神经母细胞瘤或MPNST混合存在；其他各种混合性间叶或神经外胚层成分在一些个案报告中也有描述（见Kawamoto等[191]的综述）。随访发现，大约50%的病例临床预后为死亡。随着分子病理研究的进展，外胚层间叶瘤这一术语也被某些人用于描述与横纹肌肉瘤相似但有 t(11;22) 染色体易位、通常与 PNET 相关的肿瘤[193]。

自主神经瘤（神经丛肉瘤、胃肠自主神经瘤）Autonomic nerve tumor (plexosarcoma, gastrointestinal autonomic nerve tumor)

过去认为自主神经瘤是一组特殊的腹腔内肿瘤，认为其发生于胃肠道肠肌神经丛，由其超微结构特征所确定[194]。然而，现在认为它们是胃肠间质瘤（GIST）的一种形态学亚型，没有特殊的临床意义。它们与普通的 GIST[195]（见第9章）相同，均表现为 CD117（KIT）免疫组化染色阳性和 c-kit 基因突变，现在已不再认为它们是独立的病变。

其他软组织神经外胚层肿瘤 Misccellaneous neuroectodermal tumors presenting in soft tissue

异位脑膜病变 Heterotopic meningeal lesions

Lopez 等[196]于1974年提出了实用的皮肤（或颅外）脑膜病变的分类。这些病变基本上分为三类，尽管前两类的区分有些模糊。

第一类病变称为异位脑膜上皮错构瘤（ectopic meningothelial hamartoma）[197]或隔离性脑膜膨出（sequestrated meningocele）[198,199]，它们实际上是发生在头皮（尤其是枕部）或整个脊柱的错构瘤。可能所有的病例都是先天性的，大多数在儿童期发病，表现为没有特征的皮肤肿块或囊肿，或表现为皮肤发育不全或斑秃。这些病例没有真正的颅骨或脊柱缺损。组织学上，其特征为真皮和皮下组织异常的不同程度狭窄或扩张的分枝状间隙，伴有异常表现的胶原（图27.61）和许多血管。小圆形上皮样脑膜上皮细胞衬覆于间隙内或在其旁成簇分布（图27.62），其性质可通过 EMA 染色阳性得到证实（图27.63）。这些细胞可以围绕在玻璃样变的胶原纤维束周围，随后似乎可以钙化，有时形成沙粒体性钙化小球。还可见散在分布的多核细胞。低倍镜下这些病变容易被误认为某种类型的淋巴管瘤（见图27.61）或假血管肉瘤性病变。此病变切除后无复发倾向。

第二类病变通常称为皮肤脑膜瘤（cutaneous meningioma）[196,200]，较少见，主要发生在成人，最常见于头部。此类病变与第一类病变的根本不同之处只是：这种病变表现为由脑膜上皮细胞组成的散在结节（或肿块），有时也可伴有沙粒体。临床病程为良性病程。

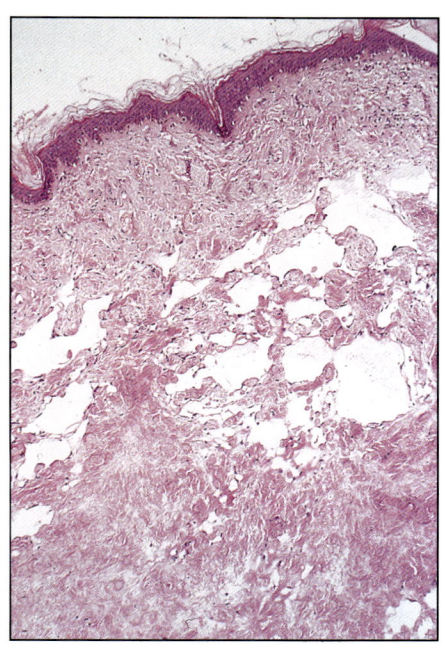

图27.61 异位脑膜上皮错构瘤。注意假血管间隙和异常致密的真皮胶原。

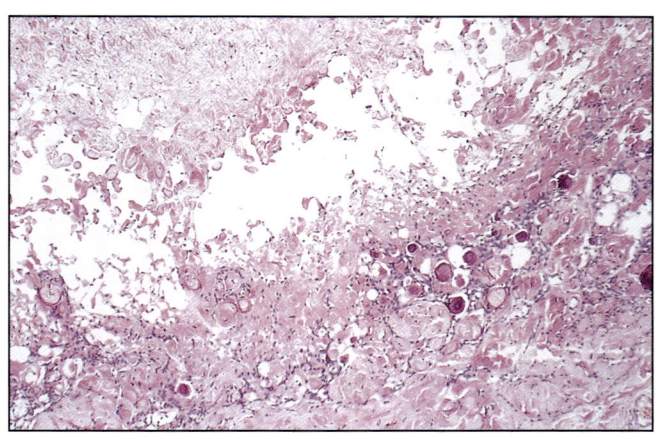

图27.62 异位脑膜上皮错构瘤。本例假血管间隙旁可见簇状分布的脑膜上皮细胞和大量沙粒体。

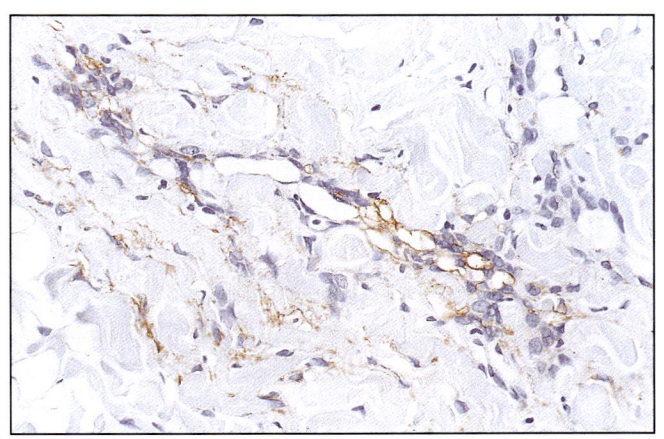

图27.63 异位脑膜上皮错构瘤。内衬间隙的细胞呈纤细的 EMA 膜阳性。ABC 法。

Lopez 等人提出的第三类病变称为 III 型，是中枢神经系统脑膜瘤在原来手术部位或通过颅骨缝播散到被覆皮肤和皮下组织而形成的[196]。

异位胶质结节　Heterotopic glial nodules

异位胶质结节[201-204]由于最常发生在鼻部，故通常被称为鼻神经胶质瘤（nasal gliomas）。这种先天性病变被认为是神经胶质组织异位发展而来，发生在鼻附近的皮下组织或鼻内。少数情况下可发生在口腔或鼻咽部。病变经常在出生后即被发现，偶尔也会在成人期才发现。多达 15% 的病例通过骨的缺损可能仍与额叶相连，或通过残留的纤维条索相连，或表现为真正的脑膨出。如果是这样，就有形成脑脊液鼻漏或脑膜炎的危险，尤其是在轻率的手术后更易发生。切除不完全的患者可能出现局部复发。极其罕见的移位胶质病变已有报道，可发生于很难用神经管闭合缺损来解释的部位[205,206]。

组织学上，大多数病变界限清晰，但没有包膜，为具有原纤维背景的成熟神经胶质组成的多叶状肿块（图 27.64）。一般缺乏神经元成分。一些病例可有囊性变，而时间较长的病变间质常常明显硬化。神经胶质组织 GFAP 阳性可为诊断提供强有力的证据。有趣的是，形态学和免疫组织化学证明，这些异位胶质结节没有脑膜覆盖[203]；这一点提示我们，将这些病变看成是隔离性脑膨出（sequestrated encephaloceles）的观点可能过于简单。除了少数成人病例可能需要与通过骨质侵入的星形细胞瘤鉴别以外，的确没有其他需要鉴别诊断的疾病[207]。

软组织室管膜病变　Soft tissue ependymal lesions

软组织室管膜病变是由室管膜细胞组成的，主要分为两组：异位室管膜残余（heterotopic ependymal rsts）[208]和更为常见的皮下黏液乳头状室管膜瘤（subcutaneous myxopapillary ependymomas）[209,210]。两者均发生在骶尾部皮下组织。良性异位病变通常发生在婴儿早期，而肿瘤性病变则主要发生在 21～40 岁的成年人（虽然这不是绝对的）。实际上，软组织室管膜瘤可能起源于临床上隐性的异位室管膜细胞残余。这种罕见的异位在临床上表现为尾骨表面皮肤小孔（无明显肿块），而室管膜瘤表现为缓慢生长的肿物，有时伴有神经功能缺损；多达 20% 的肿瘤性病变可发生转移，通常发生在多年以后。

组织学上，发生在婴幼儿的异位性病变由排列成巢或小梁状的室管膜细胞组成，细胞为立方形或多边形，核小，嗜碱性，胞浆呈不同程度嗜酸性或透明状。这些细胞分布在淡染的黏液样基质中，偶尔形成假腺腔结构。肿瘤性病变的组织学表现与之相似，但肿瘤体积更大，呈分叶状，通常有局部浸润。此外，肿瘤通常形成具有

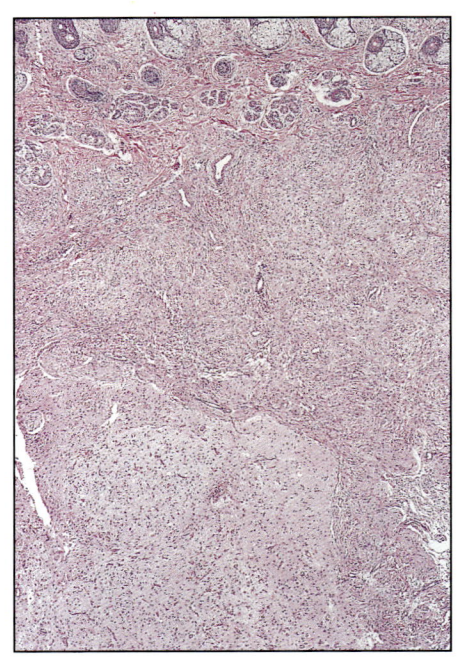

A

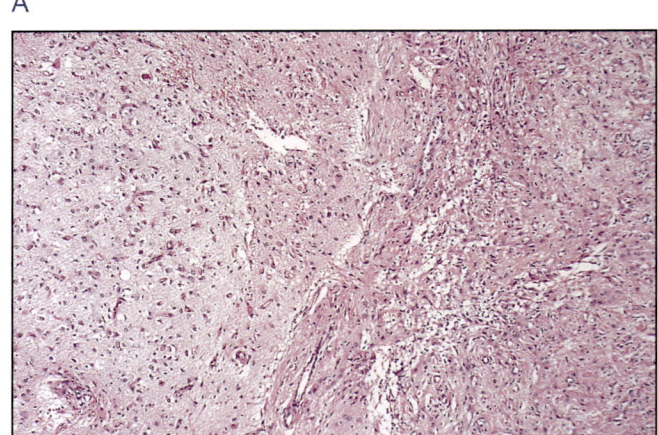

B

图 27.64　鼻神经胶质瘤。本例发生于鼻梁，真皮深层（A）被分叶状的原纤维神经胶质组织取代（B）。

纤维血管轴心的乳头状结构（图 27.65），同发生在脊髓终丝的室管膜瘤一样（见第 26 章），核分裂活跃。细胞多形性通常不是它的特征。这两类病变 GFAP 均呈阳性反应（图 27.66），可与脊索瘤、软骨肉瘤或转移癌鉴别。极少数发生在纵隔的不同类型的室管膜也有报道，它们也可能起源于室管膜残余[211]。

婴儿黑色素性神经外胚层肿瘤（视网膜原基瘤、黑色素性突变瘤）
Melanotic neuroectodermal tumor of infancy (retinal anlage tumor, melanotic progonoma)

婴儿黑色素性神经外胚层肿瘤是一种令人迷惑和难以理解的肿瘤，过去 30 多年间本病引起了相当大的关

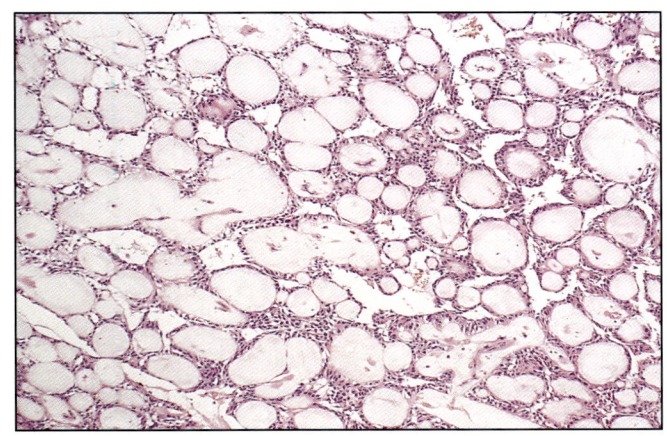

图27.65 皮下室管膜瘤。本例为从骶骨表面切除的肿瘤，具有典型的黏液乳头状结构。

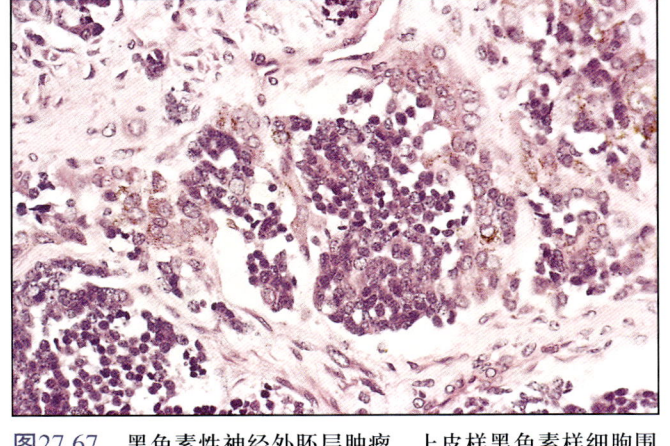

图27.67 黑色素性神经外胚层肿瘤。上皮样黑色素样细胞围绕成簇的较原始的神经母细胞样细胞排列。

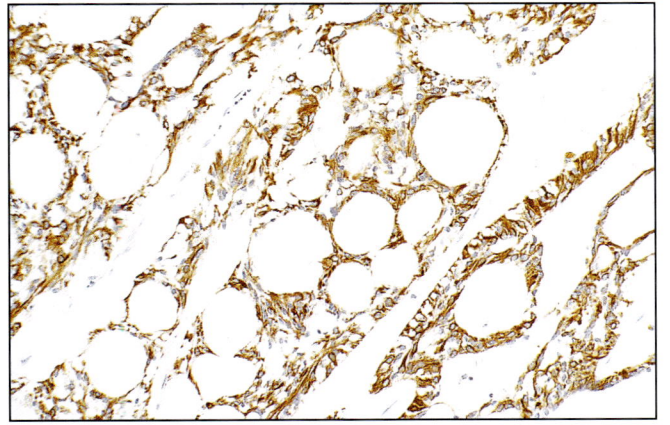

图27.66 皮下室管膜瘤。GFAP强阳性即可确诊。ABC法。

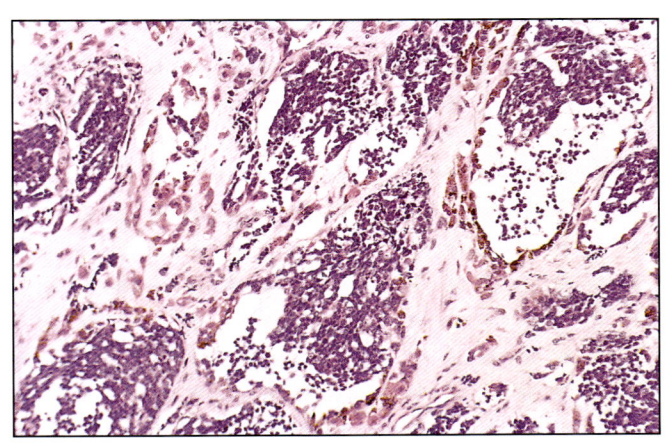

图27.68 黑色素性神经外胚层肿瘤。注意肿瘤细胞在纤维性间质中呈典型的腺泡状生长方式。

注，有大量的病例报道[212]，主要是关于其组织发生或分化方式的研究。错误认识有许多来源，而最近的资料提示，这种病变重现了视网膜上皮的早期发育阶段[213]。

临床特征：90%以上的婴儿黑色素性神经外胚层肿瘤病例发生在头颈部，尤其是上颌骨；其他部位少见，但在附睾和颅外骨组织中也可见到[212-216]。绝大多数病例发生在1岁以内，男性略多；普遍认为发生在成人的极少数病例报道是误诊。尽管此病常缺乏组织学上的恶性表现，但是高达5%的病例可出现转移，而且有时呈致死性的临床经过[212-214,217]。少数病例伴有尿液香草扁桃酸（anillylmandelic acid）水平升高[217,218]，提示与其他类型神经母细胞肿瘤密切相关。

组织学特征：这种肿瘤具有一种非常特征性和可重复性的表现，特征是具有两种主要细胞成分：一种是小的嗜碱性神经母细胞样细胞，常常位于原纤维性基质中；另一种是较大的嗜酸性上皮样细胞，细胞核呈空泡状，胞浆内含有数量不等的黑色素（黑色素细胞样细胞；图27.67）。产生黑色素的细胞常常排列成腺泡状或假腺管样结构，位于致密的纤维母细胞性间质中（图27.68）。发生在上颌骨的肿瘤不规则地向周围骨组织浸润。核分裂数多少不一，通常既没有细胞多形性也没有明显坏死。

在免疫组化方面[213,215,216,219]，两种类型细胞NSE和突触素染色均呈阳性，但是有些奇怪的是，S-100呈阴性；此外，大细胞还一致表达细胞角蛋白（图27.69）和HMB-45，与色素性视网膜上皮的表现平行。GFAP和Leu-7染色不同程度呈阳性。超微结构检查证实，肿瘤细胞具有神经母细胞和黑色素细胞的特征。此外，在黑色素细胞样细胞中还可见到桥粒、张力丝和神经内分泌颗粒[213]。这种免疫表型和电镜特征，结合肿瘤通常是先天性的，支持婴儿黑色素性神经外胚层肿瘤是一种胚胎发育不良性肿瘤，重现了视网膜发育的早期阶段[213]。

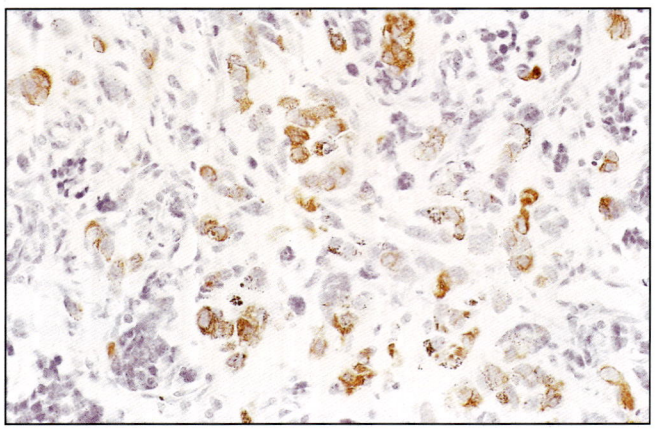

图27.69 黑色素性神经外胚层肿瘤。圆胖的黑色素细胞样细胞角蛋白呈阳性，但S-100蛋白染色呈阴性。ABC法。

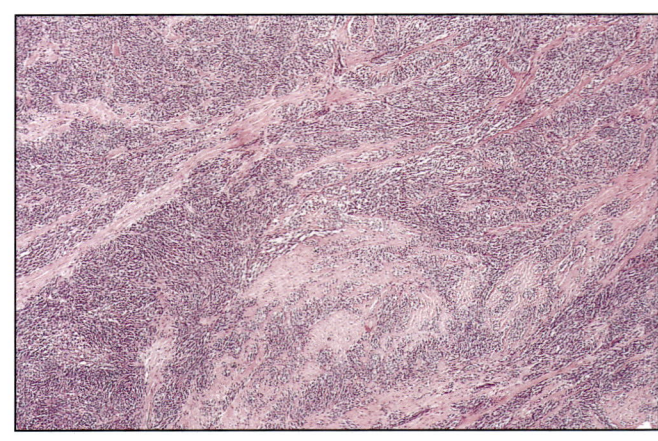

图27.70 软组织恶性黑色素瘤。注意典型的部分呈巢状，部分呈束状浸润肌腱组织。

软组织恶性黑色素瘤（透明细胞肉瘤）
Malignant melanoma of soft tissues (clear cell sarcoma)

软组织恶性黑色素瘤，又称为肌腱和腱膜透明细胞肉瘤[220]，显示单一的黑色素细胞分化的证据[221]，因此将其归在显示神经外胚层分化的肿瘤一章中阐述似乎最合乎逻辑。基因表达谱也支持这种肿瘤与普通黑色素瘤密切相关，虽然它们并非同一肿瘤[222]。

临床特征

软组织恶性黑色素瘤[221,223,224]多发于青少年或年轻成人，女性略多见，肿物生长缓慢，表现为伴有显著疼痛的结节，好发于四肢远端，特别是足踝部位。但实际上，发病年龄范围和解剖部位都很广泛。多数肿瘤直径小于5cm，与筋膜或腱膜关系密切；常波及皮下甚至真皮层。极少见的病例可发生在内脏[225,228]，最常见于小肠。它们的解剖部位常使其只能行伴有宽切缘的非根治性手术，故病变常常在局部反复复发，除非截肢。50%以上的患者最后发生转移，最常转移到淋巴结、肺或骨，但转移常常发生在多年以后。5年存活率可能超过60%，以本作者经验来看，20年存活率不会高于20%。辅助性放化疗的效果尚有待确定。

组织学特征

尽管此病原来被称为透明细胞肉瘤，但并非所有肿瘤或所有肿瘤细胞胞质均具有透明的胞浆。低倍镜下，肿瘤表现为无包膜的肿瘤细胞巢或细胞束，不规则地浸润纤维腱膜（图27.70）、皮下或深层真皮组织。网状纤维染色可很好地显示瘤细胞的巢状生长（图27.71）。肿瘤细胞小叶由大的多边形透明细胞组成，或由胞浆淡嗜

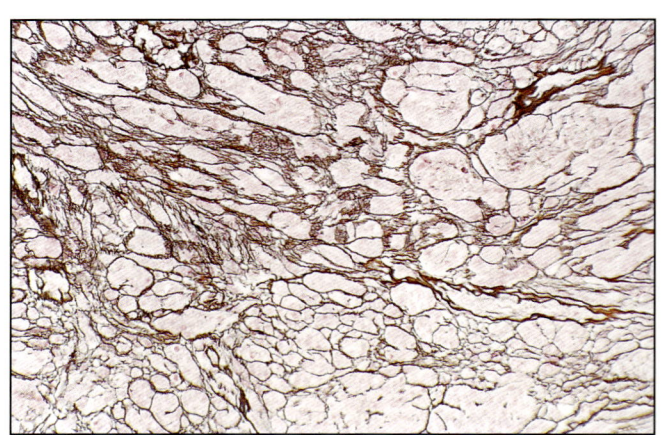

图27.71 软组织恶性黑色素瘤。网状纤维染色显示明显的巢状或束状结构。

酸性的梭形细胞组成（图27.72）；两种类型的细胞均有空泡状的细胞核和明显的核仁，与皮肤黏膜组织的黑色素瘤相似（图27.73）。50%以上的病例含有多核巨细胞，细胞核一般位于周边部（花冠型巨细胞）（图27.74）。大约2/3的肿瘤含有数量不等的黑色素，通过HE染色或特殊染色可以证实。一些位置比较表浅的病例缺乏与正常组织的交界，这是与皮肤黑色素瘤鉴别的关键；其他有鉴别意义的特性还有：透明细胞肉瘤具有一致性的巢状生长方式，而且一般缺乏多形性。

在免疫组化方面，此病与皮肤原发性或转移性黑色素瘤无法区分，因为这些病变S-100、NSE和HMB-45均呈相同的阳性反应。然而，HMB-45阳性有助于此病与某些上皮样MPNST病例的鉴别（图27.75）。另外，其HMB-45阳性表达常常比转移性黑色素瘤更加广泛。电镜观察发现[229-231]，在一些病例中，肿瘤细胞显示典型的黑色素细胞分化和部分神经鞘细胞的特征。肿瘤大

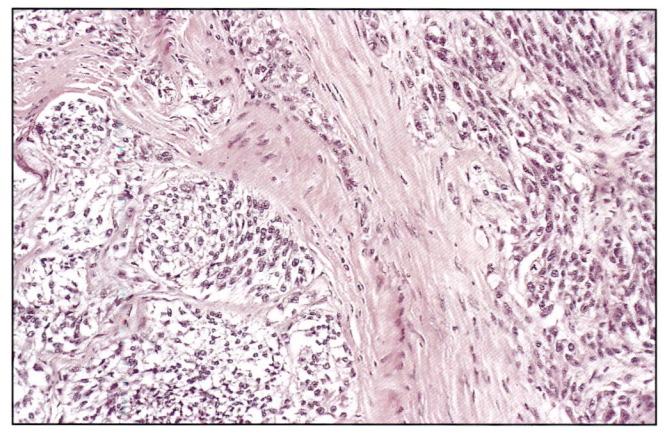

图27.72 软组织恶性黑色素瘤。注意这个视野透明细胞巢向梭形细胞的转化。

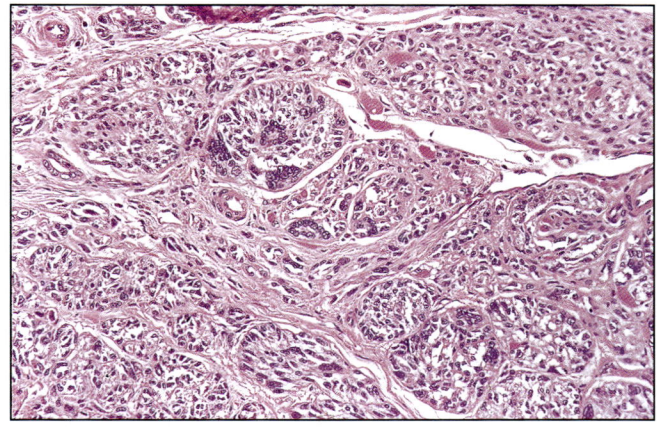

图27.74 软组织恶性黑色素瘤。独特的花冠样巨细胞伴有典型的巢状生长。

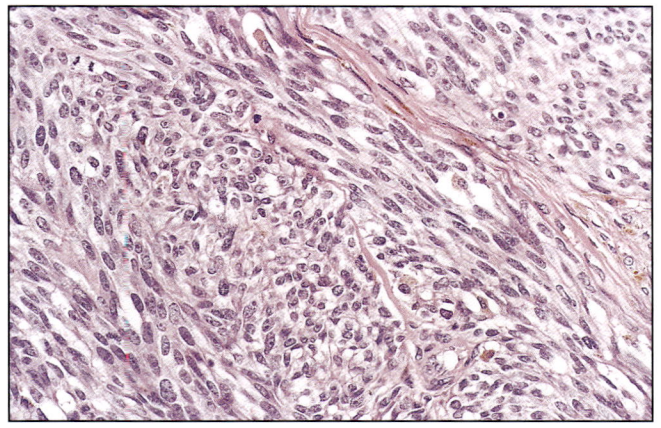

图27.73 软组织恶性黑色素瘤。注意常见的黑色素瘤样细胞核的形态学和小的黑色素颗粒沉积。

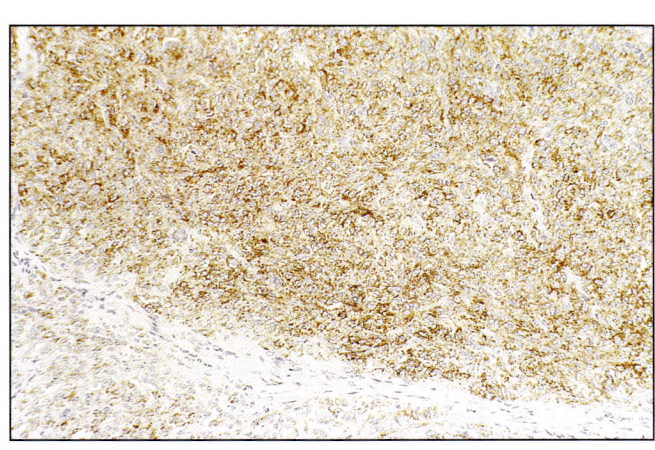

图27.75 软组织恶性黑色素瘤。黑色素瘤抗原HMB-45呈阳性,有助于排除上皮样恶性外周神经鞘肿瘤。ABC法。

于5 cm和出现坏死是判定预后的决定性因素[223,224,232],这一点与损害的结果有关;一个小样本研究提示,肿瘤细胞二倍体DNA似乎与改善生存率相关[233]。同样有趣的是,也有人认为这种类型的肿瘤是另外的肉瘤(见第24章、第32章),其特征是具有可复制性的染色体易位,特别是t(12;22)(q13;q13)[234,235],其融合基因产物涉及22号染色体上的 *EWS* 基因[236,237],在石蜡包埋和冷冻的新鲜组织中,可以很容易地检测到具有诊断意义的基因重排。证实 *EWS-ATF1* 融合基因可以用于与转移性黑色素瘤的鉴别诊断[238]。

参考文献

1. Cieslak A K, Stout A P 1946 Traumatic and amputation neuromas. Arch Surg 53: 646–651
2. Tancino B, Petras B, Gerken K et al. 1985 Traumatic "neuromas" of the biliary tract: a clinicopathologic study of eight cases. Am J Clin Pathol 84: 562 (abstract)
3. Meachim G, Abberton M J 1971 Histological findings in Morton's metatarsalgia. J Pathol 103: 209–217
4. Lassmann G, Lassmann H, Stockinger L 1976 Morton's metatarsalgia. Light and electron microscopic observations and their relation to entrapment neuropathies. Virchow's Arch [A] 370: 307–321
5. Fletcher C D M, Theaker J M 1989 Digital Pacinian neuroma: a distinctive hyperplastic lesion. Histopathology 15: 249–256
6. Silverman T A, Enzinger F M 1985 Fibrolipomatous hamartoma of nerve. A clinicopathologic analysis of 26 cases. Am J Surg Pathol 9: 7–14
7. Price A J, Compson J P, Calonje E 1995 Fibrolipomatous hamartoma of nerve arising in the brachial plexus. J Hand Surg [Br] 20: 16–18
8. Williams E D, Pollock D J 1966 Multiple mucosal neuromata with endocrine tumours: a syndrome allied to von Recklinghausen's disease. J Pathol Bacteriol 91: 71–80
9. Gorlin R J, Sedano H O, Vickers R A et al. 1968 Multiple mucosal neuromas, pheochromocytoma and medullary carcinoma of the thyroid – a syndrome. Cancer 22: 293–299
10. Louhimo I, Rapola J 1972 Intraneural muscular hamartoma: report of two cases in small children. J Pediatr Surg 7: 696–699
11. Markel S F, Enzinger F M 1982 Neuromuscular hamartoma – a benign "Triton tumor" composed of mature neural and striated muscle elements. Cancer 49: 140–144
12. Argenyi Z B, Goodenberger M E, Strauss J S 1990 Congenital neural hamartoma ("fascicular schwannoma"). Am J Dermatopathol 12: 283–293
13. Dupre A, Christol B, Bonafé J L et al. 1974 Neurome cutané a tumeur unique avec importantes alterations des cellules schwanniennes. Ann Dermatol Syphilog 101: 271–276

14. Guillet G, Gauthier Y, Tamisier J M et al. 1987 Linear cutaneous neuromas (dermatoneurie en stries). J Cutan Pathol 14: 43–48
15. Shames B, Fretzin D 1989 Cutaneous nerve hamartoma – a new entity. J Cutan Pathol 16: 325 (abstract)
16. Bale P M 1980 Sacrococcygeal paciniomas. Pathology 12: 231–235
17. McCormack K, Kaplan D, Murray J C et al. 1988 Multiple hairy pacinian neurofibromas (nerve sheath myxomas). J Am Acad Dermatol 18: 416–419
18. Reed R J, Fine R M, Meltzer H D 1972 Palisaded, encapsulated neuromas of the skin. Arch Dermatol 106: 865–870
19. Fletcher C D M 1989 Solitary circumscribed neuroma of the skin (so-called palisaded, encapsulated neuroma). A clinicopathologic and immunohistochemical study. Am J Surg Pathol 13: 574–580
20. Dover J S, From L, Lewis A 1989 Palisaded encapsulated neuromas. A clinicopathologic study. Arch Dermatol 125: 386–389
21. Holm T W, Prawer S E, Sahl W J et al. 1973 Multiple cutaneous neuromas. Arch Dermatol 107: 608–610
22. Alexander J, Theaker J M 1991 An unusual solitary circumscribed neuroma (palisaded encapsulated neuroma) of the skin – with observations on the nature of pseudoepitheliomatous hyperplasia. Histopathology 18: 175–177
23. Tsang W Y W, Chan J K C 1992 Epithelioid variant of solitary circumscribed neuroma of the skin. Histopathology 20: 439–441
24. Albrecht S, Kahn H J, From L 1989 Palisaded encapsulated neuroma: an immunohistochemical study. Mod Pathol 2: 403–406
25. Stout A P 1935 The peripheral manifestations of the specific nerve sheath tumor (neurilemmoma). Am J Cancer 24: 751–796
26. Hennessee M T, Walter M H, Wallace G et al. 1985 Benign schwannoma. Clinical and histopathologic findings. J Am Podiatr Med Assoc 75: 310–314
27. Shuangshoti S, Panyathanya R 1983 Nerve sheath tumors of neuraxis: study of 181 cases. J Med Assoc Thai 66: 397–409
28. De La Monte S M, Dorfman H D, Chandra R et al. 1984 Intraosseous schwannoma: histological features, ultrastructure and review of the literature. Hum Pathol 15: 551–558
29. Daimaru Y, Kido H, Hashimoto H et al. 1988 Benign schwannoma of the gastrointestinal tract: a clinicopathologic and immunohistochemical study. Hum Pathol 19: 257–264
30. Sarlomo-Rikala M, Miettinen M 1995 Gastric schwannoma. A clinicopathological analysis of six cases. Histopathology 27: 355–260
31. Martuza R L, Eldridge R 1988 Neurofibromatosis 2 (bilateral acoustic neurofibromatosis). N Engl J Med 318: 684–688
32. MacCollin M, Woodfin W, Kronn D et al. 1996 Schwannomatosis: a clinical and pathologic study. Neurology 46: 1072–1079
33. Seppala M T, Sainio M A, Haltia M J et al. 1998 Multiple schwannomas: schwannomatosis or neurofibromatosis type 2? J Neurosurg 89: 36–41
34. Woodruff J M, Selig A M, Crowley K et al. 1994 Schwannoma (neurilemoma) with malignant transformation. A rare, distinctive peripheral nerve tumor. Am J Surg Pathol 18: 882–895
35. McMenamin M E, Fletcher C D M 2001 Expanding the spectrum of malignant change in schwannomas: epithelioid malignant change, epithelioid malignant peripheral nerve sheath tumor and epithelioid angiosarcoma: a study of 17 cases. Am J Surg Pathol 25: 13–25
36. Wechsler J, Lantieri L, Zeller J et al. 2003 Aberrant axon neurofilaments in schwannomas associated with phacomatoses. Virchows Arch 443: 768–773
37. Feany M B, Anthony D C, Fletcher C D M 1998 Nerve sheath tumours with hybrid features of neurofibroma and schwannoma: a conceptual challenge. Histopathology 32: 405–410
38. Mertens F, Dal Cin P, De Wever I et al. 2000 Cytogenetic characterization of peripheral nerve sheath tumors. A report of the CHAMP study group. J Pathol 190: 31–38
39. Dahl I 1977 Ancient neurilemmoma (schwannoma). Acta Pathol Microbiol Scand A 85: 812–818
40. Woodruff J M, Godwin T A, Erlandson R A et al. 1981 Cellular schwannoma. A variety of schwannoma sometimes mistaken for a malignant tumor. Am J Surg Pathol 5: 733–744
41. Fletcher C D M, Davies S E, McKee P H 1987 Cellular schwannoma: a distinct pseudosarcomatous entity. Histopathology 11: 21–35
42. White W M, Shiu M F H, Rosenblum M K et al. 1990 Cellular schwannoma. A clinicopathologic study of 57 patients and 58 tumors. Cancer 66: 1266–1275
43. Casadei G P, Scheithauer B W, Hirose T et al. 1995 Cellular schwannoma. A clinicopathologic, DNA flow cytometric and proliferation marker study of 70 patients. Cancer 75: 1109–1119
44. Woodruff J M, Scheithauer B W, Kurtkaya-Yapicier O et al. 2003 Congenital and childhood plexiform (multinodular) cellular schwannoma: a troublesome mimic of malignant peripheral nerve sheath tumor. Am J Surg Pathol 27: 1321–1329
45. Meis-Kindblom J M, Enzinger F M 1994 Plexiform malignant peripheral nerve sheath tumor of infancy and childhood. Am J Surg Pathol 18: 479–485
46. Fletcher C D M, Davies S E 1986 Benign plexiform (multinodular) schwannoma: a rare tumour unassociated with neurofibromatosis. Histopathology 10: 971–980
47. Iwashita T, Enjoji M 1987 Plexiform neurilemmoma: a clinicopathological and immunohistochemical analysis of 23 tumours from 20 patients. Virchow's Arch [A] 411: 305–309
48. Kao G F, Laskin W B, Olson T G 1989 Solitary cutaneous plexiform neurilemmoma (schwannoma): a clinicopathologic, immunohistochemical and ultrastructural study of 11 cases. Mod Pathol 2: 20–26
49. Agaram N P, Prakash S, Antonescu C R 2005 Deep-seated plexiform schwannoma. A pathologic study of 16 cases and comparative analysis with the superficial variety. Am J Surg Pathol 29 1042–1048
50. Mennemeyer R P, Hammar S P, Tytus J S et al. 1979 Melanocytic schwannoma. Clinical and ultrastructural studies of three cases with evidence of intracellular melanin synthesis. Am J Surg Pathol 3: 3–10
51. Font R L, Truong L D 1984 Melanotic schwannoma of soft tissues. Electron microscopic observations and review of the literature. Am J Surg Pathol 8: 129–138
52. Killeen R M, Davy C L, Bayserman S C 1988 Melanocytic schwannoma. Cancer 62: 174–183
53. Carney J A 1990 Psammomatous melanotic schwannoma. A distinctive heritable tumor with special associations including cardiac myxoma and the Cushing syndrome. Am J Surg Pathol 14: 206–222
54. Fu Y-S, Kaye G I, Lattes R 1975 Primary malignant melanocytic tumors of the sympathetic ganglia, with an ultrastructural study of one. Cancer 36: 2029–2041
55. Krausz T, Azzopardi J G, Pearse E 1984 Malignant melanoma of the sympathetic chain with a consideration of pigmented nerve sheath tumours. Histopathology 8: 881–894
56. Rowlands D, Edwards C, Collins F 1987 Malignant melanotic schwannoma of the bronchus. J Clin Pathol 40: 1449–1455
57. Kindbom L-G, Meis-Kindblom J M, Haver G et al. 1998 Benign epithelioid schwannoma. Am J Surg Pathol 22: 762–770
58. Laskin W B, Fetsch J F, Lasota J et al. 2005 Benign epithelioid peripheral nerve sheath tumors of the soft tissues: clinicopathologic spectrum of 33 cases. Am J Surg Pathol 29: 39–51
59. Woodruff J M, Christensen W M 1993 Glandular peripheral nerve sheath tumors. Cancer 72: 3618–3628
60. Fletcher C D M, Madziwa D, Heyderman E et al. 1986 Benign dermal schwannoma with glandular elements: true heterology or a local organiser effect? Clin Exp Dermatol 11: 475–485
61. Griffiths A P, Ironside J W, Gray C 1991 True neurilemmoma arising in a lymph node in infancy. Histopathology 18: 180–183
62. Geschickter C F 1935 Tumors of the peripheral nerves. Am J Cancer 25: 377–410
63. Reed R J 1977 Cutaneous manifestations of neural crest disorders (neurocristopathies). Int J Dermatol 16: 807–826
64. Woodruff J M 1999 Pathology of tumors of the peripheral nerve sheath in type I neurofibromatosis. Am J Med Genet 89: 23–30
65. Colman D S, Williams C A, Wallace M R 1995 Benign neurofibromas in type I neurofibromatosis (NF1) show somatic deletions of the NF1 gene. Nat Genet 11: 90–92
66. Daschner K, Assum G, Eisenbarth I et al. 1997 Clonal origin of tumor cells in a plexiform neurofibroma with LOH in NF1 intron 38 and in dermal neurofibromas without LOH of the NF1 gene. Biochem Biophys Res Commun 234: 346–350
67. Lin B T, Weiss L M, Medeiros L J 1997 Neurofibroma and cellular neurofibroma with atypia: a report of 14 tumors. Am J Surg Pathol 21: 1443–1449
68. Azzopardi J G, Eusebi V, Tison V et al. 1983 Neurofibroma with rhabdomyomatous differentiation: benign "Triton" tumour of the vagina. Histopathology 7: 561–572
69. Erlandson R A 1985 Peripheral nerve sheath tumors. Ultrastruct Pathol 9: 113–122
70. Riccardi V M 1981 Von Recklinghausen's neurofibromatosis. N Engl J Med 305: 1617–1627
71. Riccardi V M 1989 Neurofibromatosis update. Neurofibromatosis 2: 284–291
72. Michal M, Fanburg-Smith J, Mentzel T et al. 2001 Dendritic cell neurofibroma with pseudorosettes: a report of 18 cases of a distinct and hitherto unrecognized neurofibroma variant. Am J Surg Pathol 25: 587–594
73. MacDonald D M, Wilson Jones E 1977 Pacinian neurofibroma. Histopathology 1: 247–255
74. Fetsch J F, Michal M, Miettinen M 2000 Pigmented (melanotic) neurofibroma: a clinicopathologic and immunohistochemical analysis of 19 lesions from 17 patients. Am J Surg Pathol 24: 331–343
75. Williams G D, Hoffman S, Schwartz I S 1984 Malignant transformation in a plexiform neurofibroma of the median nerve. J Hand Surg 9A: 583–587
76. Lazarus S S, Trombetta L D 1978 Ultrastructural identification of a benign perineurial cell tumor. Cancer 41: 1823–1829
77. Tsang W Y W, Chan J K C, Chow L T C et al. 1992 Perineurioma: an uncommon soft tissue neoplasm distinct from localised hypertrophic neuropathy and neurofibroma. Am J Surg Pathol 16: 756–763
78. Mentzel T, Dei Tos A P, Fletcher C D M 1994 Perineurioma (storiform perineurial fibroma): clinicopathological analysis of four cases. Histopathology 25: 261–267
79. Giannini C, Scheithauer B W, Jenkins R B et al. 1997 Soft-tissue perineurioma. Evidence for an abnormality of chromosome 22, criteria for diagnosis and review of the literature. Am J Surg Pathol 21: 164–173
80. Hornick J L, Fletcher C D M 2005 Soft tissue perineurioma: clinicopathologic analysis of 81 cases including those with atypical histologic features. Am J Surg Pathol 29: 845–858
81. Hornick J L, Fletcher C D M 2005 Intestinal perineuriomas: clinicopathologic definition of a new anatomic subset in a series of 10 cases. Am J Surg Pathol 29: 859–865

82. Emory T S, Scheithauer B W, Hirose T et al. 1995 Intraneural perineurioma. A clonal neoplasm associated with abnormalities of chromosome 22. Am J Clin Pathol 103: 696–704
83. Bilbao J M, Khoury N J S, Hudson A R et al. 1984 Perineurioma (localized hypertrophic neuropathy). Arch Pathol Lab Med 108: 557–560
84. Johnson P C, Kline D G 1989 Localized hypertrophic neuropathy: possible focal perineurial barrier defect. Acta Neuropathol 77: 514–518
85. Fetsch J F, Miettinen M 1997 Sclerosing perineurioma. A clinicopathologic study of 19 cases of a distinctive soft tissue lesion with a predilection for the fingers and palms of young adults. Am J Surg Pathol 21: 1433–1442
86. Van Roggen J F G, McMenamin M E, Belchis D A et al. 2001 Reticular perineurioma: a distinctive variant of soft tissue perineurioma. Am J Surg Pathol 25: 485–493
87. Folpe A L, Billings S D, McKenney J K et al. 2002 Expression of claudin-1, a recently described tight junction-associated protein, distinguishes soft tissue perineurioma from potential mimics. Am J Surg Pathol 26: 1620–1626
88. Gallager R L, Helwig E B 1980 Neurothekeoma – a benign cutaneous tumor of neural origin. Am J Clin Pathol 74: 759–764
89. Pulitzer D R, Reed R J 1985 Nerve sheath myxoma (perineurial myxoma). Am J Dermatopathol 7: 409–421
89a. Fetsch J F, Laskin W B, Miettinen M 2005 Nerve sheath myxoma: a clinicopathologic and immunohistochemical analysis of 57 morphologically distinctive, S-100 protein- and GFAP-positive, myxoid peripheral nerve sheath tumors with a predilection for the extremities and a high local recurrence rate. Am J Surg Pathol 29: 1615–1624
90. Paulus W, Jellinger K, Perneczy G 1991 Intraspinal neurothekeoma (nerve sheath myxoma). A report of two cases. Am J Clin Pathol 95: 511–516
91. Rosati L A, Fratamico C M, Eusebi V 1986 Cellular neurothekeoma. Appl Pathol 4: 186–191
92. Argenyi Z B, LeBoit P E, Santa Cruz D et al. 1993 Nerve sheath myxoma (neurothekeoma) of the skin: light microscopic and immunohistochemical reappraisal of the cellular variant. J Cutan Pathol 20: 294–303
93. Argenyi Z B, Kutzner H, Seaba M M 1995 Ultrastructural spectrum of cutaneous nerve sheath myxoma/cellular neurothekeoma. J Cutan Pathol 22: 137–145
94. Barnhill R L, Mihm M C 1990 Cellular neurothekeoma. A distinctive variant of neurothekeoma mimicking nevomelanocytic tumors. Am J Surg Pathol 14: 113–120
95. Hornick J L, Fletcher C D M 2006 Cellular neurothekeoma: detailed characterization in a series of 133 cases. Am J Surg Pathol: in press
96. Azzopardi J G 1956 Histogenesis of the granular cell "myoblastoma." J Pathol Bacteriol 71: 85–94
97. Fisher E R, Wechsler H 1962 Granular cell myoblastoma – a misnomer. Electron microscopic and histological evidence concerning its Schwann cell derivation and nature (granular cell schwannoma). Cancer 15: 936–954
98. Ordonez N G, Mackay B 1999 Granular cell tumor: a review of the pathology and histogenesis. Ultrastruct Pathol 23: 207–222
99. Buley I D, Gatter K C, Kelly P M A et al. 1988 Granular cell tumours revisited. An immunohistochemical and ultrastructural study. Histopathology 12: 263–274
100. Mentzel T, Wadden C, Fletcher C D M 1994 Granular cell change in smooth muscle tumours of skin and soft tissue. Histopathology 24: 223–231
101. Vennegoor C, Calafat J, Hageman P et al. 1985 Biochemical characterization and cellular localization of a formalin-resistant melanoma-associated antigen reacting with antibody NK1/C3. Int J Cancer 35: 287–295
102. Strong E W, McDivitt R W, Brasfield R D 1970 Granular cell myoblastoma. Cancer 25: 415–422
103. Khansur T, Balducci L, Tavassoli M 1987 Granular cell tumor. Clinical spectrum of the benign and malignant entity. Cancer 60: 220–222
104. Adeniran A, Al-Abmadie H, Mahoney M C et al. 2004 Granular cell tumor of the breast: a series of 17 cases and review of the literature. Breast J 10: 528–531
105. Eisen R N, Kirby W M, O'Quinn J L 1991 Granular cell tumor of the biliary tree. A report of two cases and a review of the literature. Am J Surg Pathol 15: 460–465
106. Moscovic E A, Azar H A 1967 Multiple granular cell tumors ("myoblastomas"). Case report with electron microscopic observations and review of the literature. Cancer 20: 2032–2047
107. Papageorgiou S, Litt J Z, Pomeranz J R 1967 Multiple granular cell myoblastomas in children. Arch Dermatol 96: 168–171
108. Nathrath W B J, Remberger K 1986 Immunohistochemical study of granular cell tumours. Demonstration of neuron specific enolase, S-100 protein, laminin and alpha-1-antichymotrypsin. Virchow's Arch [A] 408: 421–434
109. Mazur M T, Shultz J J, Myers J L 1990 Granular cell tumor. Immunohistochemical analysis of 21 benign tumors and one malignant tumor. Arch Pathol Lab Med 114: 692–696
110. Fine S W, Li M 2003 Expression of calretinin and the alpha-subunit of inhibin in granular cell tumors. Am J Clin Pathol 119: 259–264
111. Sobel J H, Churg J 1964 Granular cells and granular cell lesions. Arch Pathol 77: 132–141
112. Lack E E, Worsham G F, Callihan M D et al. 1981 Gingival granular cell tumors of the newborn (congenital "epulis"). A clinical and pathologic study of 21 patients. Am J Surg Pathol 5: 37–46
113. Park S H, Kim T J, Chi J G 1991 Congenital granular cell tumor with systemic involvement. Immunohistochemical and ultrastructural study. Arch Pathol Lab Med 115: 934–938
114. Tucker M C, Rusnock E J, Azumi N et al. 1990 Gingival granular cell tumors of the newborn. An ultrastructural and immunohistochemical study. Arch Pathol Lab Med 114: 895–898
115. Lack E E, Perez-Atayde A R, McGill T J et al. 1982 Gingival granular cell tumor of the newborn (congenital "epulis"): ultrastructural observations relating to histogenesis. Hum Pathol 13: 686–689
116. LeBoit P E, Barr R J, Burall S et al. 1991 Primitive polypoid granular cell tumor and other cutaneous granular cell neoplasms of apparent non-neural origin. Am J Surg Pathol 15: 48–58
117. Lazar A J F, Fletcher C D M 2005 Primitive non-neural granular cell tumors of skin: clinicopathologic analysis of 13 cases. Am J Surg Pathol 29: 927–934
118. Tamaoki N, Osamura Y, Ueyama Y et al. 1984 Malignant granular cell tumor of the right sciatic nerve. Cancer 53: 524–529
119. O'Donovan D G, Kell P 1989 Malignant granular cell tumor with intraperitoneal dissemination. Histopathology 14: 417–419
120. Thunold S, von Eyben F E, Maehle B 1989 Malignant granular cell tumor of the neck: immunohistochemical and ultrastructural studies of a case. Histopathology 14: 655–657
121. Fanburg-Smith J C, Meis-Kindblom J M, Fante R et al. 1998 Malignant granular cell tumor of soft tissue. Diagnostic criteria and clinicopathologic correlation. Am J Surg Pathol 22: 779–794
122. Fletcher C D M 1994 Malignant peripheral nerve sheath tumours. In: Harms D, Schmidt D (eds) Current topics in pathology: soft tissue tumours, vol 89. Springer-Verlag, Heidelberg, p 333–354
123. Ghosh B C, Ghosh L, Huvos A G et al. 1973 Malignant schwannoma. A clinicopathologic study. Cancer 31: 184–190
124. Guccion J G, Enzinger 1979 Malignant schwannoma associated with von Recklinghausen's neurofibromatosis. Virchow's Arch [A] 383: 43–57
125. Sordillo P P, Helson L, Hajdu S I et al. 1981 Malignant schwannoma – clinical characteristics, survival and response to therapy. Cancer 47: 2503–2509
126. Ducatman B S, Scheithauer B W, Piepgras D G et al. 1986 Malignant peripheral nerve sheath tumors. A clinicopathologic study of 120 cases. Cancer 57: 2006–2021
127. Hruban R H, Shiu M H, Senie R T et al. 1990 Malignant peripheral nerve sheath tumors of the buttock and lower extremity. Cancer 66: 1253–1265
128. King A A, Debaun M R, Riccardi V M, Gutmann D H 2000 Malignant peripheral nerve sheath tumors in neurofibromatosis 1. Am J Med Genet 93: 388–392
129. Fletcher C D M, Fernando I N, Braimbridge M V et al. 1988 Malignant nerve sheath tumour arising in a ganglioneuroma. Histopathology 12: 445–448
130. Ghali V S, Gold J E, Vincent R A et al. 1992 Malignant peripheral nerve sheath tumor arising spontaneously from a retroperitoneal ganglioneuroma: a case report, review of the literature and immunohistochemical study. Hum Pathol 23: 72–75
131. Foley K M, Woodruff J M, Ellis F T et al. 1980 Radiation-induced malignant and atypical peripheral nerve sheath tumors. Ann Neurol 7: 311–318
132. Ducatman B S, Scheithauer B W 1983 Postirradiation neurofibrosarcoma. Cancer 51: 1028–1033
133. Ducatman B S, Scheithauer B W, Piepgras D G et al. 1984 Malignant peripheral nerve sheath tumors in childhood. J Neurooncol 2: 241–248
134. Meis J M, Enzinger F M, Martz K L et al. 1992 Malignant peripheral nerve sheath tumors (malignant schwannomas) in children. Am J Surg Pathol 16: 694–707
135. Hirose T, Scheithauer B W, Saio T 1998 Perineurial malignant peripheral nerve sheath tumor (MPNST). A clinicopathologic, immunohistochemical and ultrastructural study of seven cases. Am J Surg Pathol 22: 1368–1378
136. Ducatman B S, Scheithauer B W 1984 Malignant peripheral nerve sheath tumors showing divergent differentiation. Cancer 54: 1049–1057
137. Daimaru Y, Hashimoto H, Enjoji M 1984 Malignant "Triton" tumors: a clinicopathologic and immunohistochemical study of nine cases. Hum Pathol 15: 768–778
138. Brooks J S J, Freeman M, Enterline H T 1985 Malignant "Triton" tumors. Natural history and immunohistochemistry of nine new cases with literature review. Cancer 55: 2543–2549
139. Woodruff J M, Perino G 1994 Non-germ cell or teratomatous malignant tumors showing additional rhabdomyoblastic differentiation, with emphasis on the malignant Triton tumor. Semin Diagn Pathol 11: 69–81
140. Christensen W N, Strong E W, Bains M S et al. 1988 Neuroendocrine differentiation in the glandular peripheral nerve sheath tumor. Pathologic distinction from the biphasic synovial sarcoma with glands. Am J Surg Pathol 12: 417–426
141. Wick M R, Swanson P E, Scheithauer B W et al. 1987 Malignant peripheral nerve sheath tumor. An immunohistochemical study of 62 cases. Am J Clin Pathol 87: 425–433
142. Johnson T L, Lee M W, Meis J M et al. 1991 Immunohistochemical characterization of malignant peripheral nerve sheath tumors. Surg Pathol 4: 121–135
143. Fisher C, Carter R L, Ramachandra S et al. 1992 Peripheral nerve sheath differentiation in malignant soft tissue tumours: an ultrastructural and immunohistochemical study. Histopathology 20: 115–125
144. Hirose T, Hasegawa T, Kudo E et al. 1992 Malignant peripheral nerve sheath tumors: an immunohistochemical study in relation to ultrastructural features. Hum Pathol 23: 865–870

145. Hirose T, Sumimoto M, Kudo E et al. 1989 Malignant peripheral nerve sheath tumor (MPNST) showing perineurial cell differentiation. Am J Surg Pathol 13: 613–620
146. Zhou H, Coffin C M, Perkins S L et al. 2003 Malignant peripheral nerve sheath tumor: a comparison of grade, immunophenotype and cell cycle/growth activation marker expression in sporadic and NF-1 related lesions. Am J Surg Pathol 27: 1337–1345
147. Skotheim R I, Kallioniemi A, Bjerkehagen B et al. 2003 Topoisomerase-II-alpha is upregulated in malignant peripheral nerve sheath tumors and associated with clinical outcome. J Clin Oncol 21: 4586–4591
147a. Storlazzi C, Brekke H, Mandahl N et al. 2006 Identification of a novel amplicon at distal 17q containing the BIRC5/SURVIVIN gene in malignant peripheral nerve sheath tumors. J Pathol 209: 492–500
148. Perry A, Roth K A, Banerjee R et al. 2001 NF1 deletions in S100 protein-positive and negative cells of sporadic and NF1-associated plexiform neurofibromas and malignant peripheral nerve sheath tumors. Am J Pathol 159: 57–61
149. Lodding P, Kindblom L-G, Angervall L 1986 Epithelioid malignant schwannoma. A study of 14 cases. Virchow's Arch [A] 409: 433–451
150. DiCarlo E F, Woodruff J M, Bansal M et al. 1986 The purely epithelioid malignant peripheral nerve sheath tumor. Am J Surg Pathol 10: 478–490
151. Laskin W B, Weiss S W, Bratthauer G L 1991 Epithelioid variant of malignant peripheral nerve sheath tumor (malignant epithelioid schwannoma). Am J Surg Pathol 15: 1136–1145
152. Janzer R C, Makek M 1983 Intraoral malignant melanotic schwannoma. Ultrastructural evidence for melanogenesis by Schwann's cells. Arch Pathol Lab Med 107: 298–301
153. Dehner L P 1986 Peripheral and central primitive neuroectodermal tumors. A nosologic concept seeking a consensus. Arch Pathol Lab Med 110: 997–1005
154. Dehner L P 1990 Whence the primitive neuroectodermal tumor? (editorial). Arch Pathol Lab Med 114: 16–17
155. Dehner L P 1993 Primitive neuroectodermal tumor and Ewing's sarcoma. Am J Surg Pathol 17: 1–13
156. Delattre O, Zucman J, Melot T et al. 1994 The Ewing family of tumors – a subgroup of small round cell tumors defined by specific chimeric transcripts. N Engl J Med 331: 294–299
157. Turc-Carel C, Aurias A, Mugneret F et al. 1988 Chromosomes in Ewing's sarcoma. I. An evaluation of 85 cases and remarkable consistency of t(11;22)(q24;q12). Cancer Genet Cytogenet 32: 229–238
158. Sandberg A A, Bridge J A 2000 Updates on cytogenetics and molecular genetics of bone and soft tissue tumors: Ewing sarcoma and peripheral primitive neuroectodermal tumors. Cancer Genet Cytogenet 123: 1–26
159. Downing J R, Head D R, Parham D M et al. 1993 Detection of the (11;22)(q24;q12) translocation of Ewing's sarcoma and peripheral neuroectodermal tumor by reverse transcription polymerase chain reaction. Am J Pathol 143: 1294–1300
160. Hasegawa S, Davison J M, Rutten A et al. 1998 Primary cutaneous Ewing's sarcoma. Immunophenotypic and molecular cytogenetic evaluation of five cases. Am J Surg Pathol 22: 310–318
161. Angervall L, Enzinger F M 1975 Extraskeletal neoplasm resembling Ewing's sarcoma. Cancer 36: 240–251
162. Shimada H, Newton W A, Soule E H et al. 1988 Pathologic features of extraosseous Ewing's sarcoma: a report from the Intergroup Rhabdomyosarcoma study. Hum Pathol 19: 442–453
163. Jurgens H, Bier V, Harms D et al. 1988 Malignant peripheral neuroectodermal tumors. A retrospective analysis of 42 patients. Cancer 61: 349–357
164. Rud N F, Reiman H M, Pritchard D J et al. 1989 Extraosseous Ewing's sarcoma. A study of 42 cases. Cancer 64: 1548–1553
165. Cavazzana A O, Ninfo V, Roberts J et al. 1992 Peripheral neuroepithelioma: a light microscopic, immunocytochemical and ultrastructural study. Mod Pathol 5: 71–78
166. Shishikura A, Ushigome S, Shimoda T 1993 Primitive neuroectodermal tumors of bone and soft tissue: histological subclassification and clinicopathologic correlations. Acta Pathol Jpn 43: 176–186
167. Stout A P 1918 A tumor of the ulnar nerve. Proc NY Pathol Soc 18: 2–12
168. Askin F B, Rosai J, Sibley R K et al. 1979 Malignant small cell tumor of the thoracopulmonary region in childhood. A distinctive clinicopathologic entity of uncertain histogenesis. Cancer 43: 2438–2451
169. Contesso G, Llombart-Bosch A, Terrier P et al. 1992 Does malignant small round cell tumor of the thoracopulmonary region (Askin tumor) constitute a clinicopathologic entity? An analysis of 30 cases with immunohistochemical and electron-microscopic support treated at the Institut Gustave Roussy. Cancer 69: 1012–1020
170. Banerjee S S, Agbamu D A, Eyden B P et al. 1997 Clinicopathological characteristics of peripheral primitive neuroectodermal tumour of skin and subcutaneous tissue. Histopathology 31: 355–366
171. O'Sullivan M J, Perlman E J, Furman J et al. 2001 Visceral primitive peripheral neuroectodermal tumors: a clinicopathologic and molecular study. Hum Pathol 32: 1109–1115
172. Jimenez R E, Folpe A L, Lapham R L et al. 2002 Primary Ewing's sarcoma/primitive neuroectodermal tumor of the kidney: a clinicopathologic and immunohistochemical analysis of 11 cases. Am J Surg Pathol 26: 320–327
173. Movahedi-Lankarani S, Hruban R H, Westra W H et al. 2002 Primitive neuroectodermal tumors of the pancreas: a report of seven cases of a rare neoplasm. Am J Surg Pathol 26: 1040–1047
174. Ambros I M, Ambros P F, Strehl S et al. 1991 MIC2 is a specific marker for Ewing's sarcoma and peripheral primitive neuroectodermal tumors. Cancer 67: 1886–1893
175. Pappo A S, Douglass E C, Meyer W H et al. 1993 Use of HBA-71 and anti-beta-2-microglobulin to distinguish peripheral neuroepithelioma from neuroblastoma. Hum Pathol 24: 880–885
176. Weidner N, Tjoe J 1994 Immunohistochemical profile of monoclonal antibody O13: Antibody that recognizes glycoprotein p30/32^{MIC2} and is useful in diagnosing Ewing's sarcoma and peripheral neuroepithelioma. Am J Surg Pathol 18: 486–494
177. Stevenson A J, Chatten J, Bertoni F et al. 1994 CD99 (p30/32^{MIC2}) neuroectodermal/Ewing's sarcoma antigen as an immunohistochemical marker. Review of more than 600 tumors and the literature experience. Appl Immunohistochem 2: 231–240
178. Folpe A L, Goldblum J R, Rubin B P et al. 2005 Morphologic and immunophenotypic diversity in Ewing family tumors: a study of 66 genetically confirmed cases. Am J Surg Pathol 29: 1025–1033
179. Hachitanda Y, Tsuneyoshi M, Enjoji M et al. 1990 Congenital primitive neuroectodermal tumor with epithelial and glial differentiation. An ultrastructural and immunohistochemical study. Arch Pathol Lab Med 114: 101–105
180. Parham D M, Thompson E, Fletcher B et al. 1991 Metastatic small cell tumor of bone with "true" rosettes and glial fibrillary acidic protein positivity. Am J Clin Pathol 95: 166–171
181. Ushigome S, Shimoda T, Nikaido T et al. 1992 Primitive neuroectodermal tumors of bone and soft tissue with reference to histologic differentiation in primary or metastatic foci. Acta Pathol Jpn 42: 483–493
182. Moll R, Lee I, Gould V E et al. 1987 Immunocytochemical analysis of Ewing's tumors. Patterns of expression of intermediate filaments and desmosomal proteins indicate cell type heterogeneity and pluripotential differentiation. Am J Pathol 127: 288–304
183. Swanson P E, Dehner L P, Wick M R 1988 Polyphenotypic small cell tumors of childhood. Lab Invest 58: 9P (abstract)
184. Parham D M, Dias P, Kelly D R et al. 1992 Desmin positivity in primitive neuroectodermal tumors. Am J Surg Pathol 16: 483–493
185. Schmidt D, Herrmann C, Jurgens H et al. 1991 Malignant peripheral neuroectodermal tumor and its necessary distinction from Ewing's sarcoma. A report from the Kiel Pediatric Tumor Registry. Cancer 68: 2251–2259
186. Terrier P, Henry-Amar M, Triche T J et al. 1995 Is neuroectodermal differentiation of Ewing's sarcoma of bone associated with an unfavourable prognosis? Eur J Cancer 31: 307–314
187. Zoubek A, Dockhorn-Dworniczak B, Delatrre O et al. 1996 Does expression of different EWS chimeric transcripts define clinically distinct risk groups of Ewing tumor patients? J Clin Oncol 14: 1245–1251
188. de Alava E, Kawai A, Healey J H et al. 1998 EWS-FLI1 fusion transcript structure is an independent determinant of prognosis in Ewing's sarcoma. J Clin Oncol 16: 1248–1255
189. Karcioglu Z, Someren A, Mathes S J 1977 Ectomesenchymoma. Cancer 39: 2486–2496
190. Kodet R, Kasthuri N, Marsden H B et al. 1986 Gangliorhabdomyosarcoma: a histopathological and immunohistochemical study of three cases. Histopathology 10: 187–193
191. Kawamoto E H, Weidner N, Agostini R M et al. 1987 Malignant ectomesenchymoma of soft tissue. Report of two cases and review of the literature. Cancer 59: 1791–1802
192. Oppenheimer O, Athanasian E, Meyers P et al. 2005 Malignant ectomesenchymoma in the wrist of a child: case report and review of the literature. Int J Surg Pathol 13: 113–116
193. Sorensen P H, Shimada H, Liu X F et al. 1995 Biphenotypic sarcomas with myogenic and neural differentiation express the Ewing's sarcoma EWS/FLI1 fusion gene. Cancer Res 55: 1385–1392
194. Lauwers G Y, Erlandson R A, Casper E S et al. 1993 Gastrointestinal autonomic nerve tumors. A clinicopathological, immunohistochemical and ultrastructural study of 12 cases. Am J Surg Pathol 17: 887–897
195. Lee J R, Joshi V, Griffin J W Jr et al. 2001 Gastrointestinal autonomic nerve tumor: immunohistochemical and molecular identity with gastrointestinal stromal tumor. Am J Surg Pathol 25: 979–987
196. Lopez D A, Silvers D N, Helwig E B 1974 Cutaneous meningiomas – a clinicopathologic study. Cancer 34: 728–744
197. Suster S, Rosai J 1990 Hamartoma of the scalp with ectopic meningothelial elements. A distinctive benign soft tissue lesion that may simulate angiosarcoma. Am J Surg Pathol 14: 1–11
198. Bale P M, Hughes L, De Silva M 1990 Sequestrated meningoceles of scalp: extracranial meningeal hamartoma. Hum Pathol 21: 1156–1163
199. Sibley D A, Cooper P H 1989 Rudimentary meningocele: a variant of "primary cutaneous meningioma." J Cutan Pathol 16: 72–80
200. Theaker J M, Fletcher C D M, Tudway A J 1990 Cutaneous heterotopic meningeal nodules. Histopathology 16: 475–479
201. Bradley P J, Singh S D 1985 Nasal glioma. J Laryngol Otol 99: 247–252
202. Fletcher C D M, Carpenter G, McKee P H 1986 Nasal glioma – a rarity. Am J Dermatopathol 8: 341–346
203. Theaker J M, Fletcher C D M 1991 Heterotopic glial nodules: a light microscopic and immunohistochemical study. Histopathology 18: 255–260
204. Penner C R, Thompson L 2003 Nasal glial heterotopia: a clinicopathologic and immunophenotypic analysis of 10 cases with a review of the literature. Ann Diagn Pathol 7: 354–359

205. Shepherd N A, Coates P A, Brown A A 1987 Soft tissue gliomatosis – heterotopic glial tissue in the subcutis: a case report. Histopathology 11: 655–660
206. McDermott M B, Glasner S D, Nielsen P L et al. 1996 Soft tissue gliomatosis. Morphologic unity and histogenetic diversity. Am J Surg Pathol 20: 148–155
207. Chan J K C, Lau W-H 1989 Nasal astrocytoma or nasal glial heterotopia? Arch Pathol Lab Med 113: 943–945
208. Pulitzer D R, Martin P C, Collins P C et al. 1988 Subcutaneous sacrococcygeal ("myxopapillary") ependymal rests. Am J Surg Pathol 12: 672–677
209. Anderson M S 1966 Myxopapillary ependymomas presenting in the soft tissue over the sacrococcygeal region. Cancer 19: 585–590
210. King P, Cooper P N, Malcolm A J 1993 Soft tissue ependymoma: a report of three cases. Histopathology 22: 394–396
211. Wilson R W, Moran C A 1998 Primary ependymoma of the mediastinum: a clinicopathologic study of three cases. Ann Diagn Pathol 2: 293–300
212. Young S, Gonzalez-Crussi F 1985 Melanotic neuroectodermal tumor of the foot. Report of a case with multicentric origin. Am J Clin Pathol 84: 371–378
213. Pettinato G, Manivel J C, d'Amore E S G et al. 1991 Melanotic neuroectodermal tumor of infancy. A reexamination of a histogenetic problem based on immunohistochemical, flow cytometric and ultrastructural study of 10 cases. Am J Surg Pathol 15: 233–245
214. Johnson R E, Scheithauer B W, Dahlin D C 1983 Melanotic neuroectodermal tumor of infancy. A review of seven cases. Cancer 52: 661–666
215. Stirling R W, Powell G, Fletcher C D M 1988 Pigmented neuroectodermal tumour of infancy: an immunohistochemical study. Histopathology 12: 425–435
216. Barrett A W, Morgan M, Ramsay A D et al. 2002 A clinicopathologic and immunohistochemical analysis of melanotic neuroectodermal tumor of infancy. Oral Surg Oral Med Oral Pathol Oral Radiol Endod 93: 688–698
217. Dehner L P, Sibley R K, Sauk J J et al. 1979 Malignant melanotic neuroectodermal tumor of infancy. A clinical, pathologic, ultrastructural and tissue culture study. Cancer 43: 1389–1410
218. Borello E D, Gorlin R J 1966 Melanotic neuroectodermal tumor of infancy – a neoplasm of neural crest origin. Report of a case with high urinary excretion of vanilmandelic acid. Cancer 19: 196–206
219. Raju U, Zarbo R J, Regezi J A et al. 1993 Melanotic neuroectodermal tumors of infancy: intermediate filament, neuroendocrine and melanoma-associated antigen profiles. Appl Immunohistochem 1: 69–76
220. Enzinger F M 1965 Clear cell sarcoma of tendons and aponeuroses. An analysis of 21 cases. Cancer 18: 1163–1174
221. Chung E B, Enzinger F M 1983 Malignant melanoma of soft parts. A reassessment of clear cell sarcoma. Am J Surg Pathol 7: 405–413
222. Segal N H, Pavlidis P, Noble W S et al. 2003 Classification of clear cell sarcoma as a subtype of melanoma by genomic profiling. J Clin Oncol 21: 1775–1781
223. Lucas D R, Nascimento A G, Sim F H 1992 Clear cell sarcoma of soft tissues. Mayo Clinic experience with 35 cases. Am J Surg Pathol 16: 1197–1204
224. Montgomery E A, Meis J M, Ramos A G et al. 1993 Clear cell sarcoma of tendons and aponeuroses. A clinicopathologic study of 58 cases with analysis of prognostic factors. Int J Surg Pathol 1: 89–100
225. Donner L R, Trompler R A, Dobin S 1998 Clear cell sarcoma of the ileum: the crucial role of cytogenetics for the diagnosis. Am J Surg Pathol 22: 121–124
226. Rubin B P, Fletcher J A, Renshaw A A 1999 Clear cell sarcoma of soft parts. Report of a case primary in the kidney with cytogenetic confirmation. Am J Surg Pathol 23: 589–594
227. Zambrano E, Reyes-Mugica M, Franchi A et al. 2003 An osteoclast-rich tumor of the gastrointestinal tract with features resembling clear cell sarcoma of soft parts: report of 6 cases of a GIST simulator. Int J Surg Pathol 11: 75–81
228. Covinsky M, Gong S, Rajaram V et al. 2005 EWS-AFT1 fusion transcripts in gastrointestinal tumors previously diagnosed as malignant melanoma. Hum Pathol 36: 74–81
229. Kindblom L-G, Lodding P, Angervall L 1983 Clear cell sarcoma of tendons and aponeuroses. An immunohistochemical and electron microscopic analysis indicating neural crest origin. Virchow's Arch [A] 401: 109–128
230. Benson J D, Kraemer B, Mackay B 1985 Malignant melanoma of soft parts: an ultrastructural study of four cases. Ultrastruct Pathol 8: 57–70
231. Hasegawa T, Hirose T, Kudo E et al. 1989 Clear cell sarcoma. An immunohistochemical and ultrastructural study. Acta Pathol Jpn 39: 321–327
232. Sara A S, Evans H L, Benjamin R S 1990 Malignant melanoma of soft parts (clear cell sarcoma). A study of 17 cases with emphasis on prognostic factors. Cancer 65: 367–374
233. El-Naggar A K, Ordonez N G, Sara A et al. 1991 Clear cell sarcomas and metastatic soft tissue melanomas. A flow cytometric comparison and prognostic implications. Cancer 67: 2173–2179
234. Bridge J A, Sreekantaiah C, Neff J R et al. 1991 Cytogenetic findings in clear cell sarcoma of tendons and aponeuroses. Malignant melanoma of soft parts. Cancer Genet Cytogenet 52: 101–106
235. Reeves B R, Fletcher C D M, Gusterson B A 1992 Translocation t(12;22)(q13;q13) is a non random rearrangement in clear cell sarcoma. Cancer Genet Cytogenet 64: 101–103
236. Zucman J, Delattre O, Desmaze C et al. 1993 EWS and ATF-1 gene fusion induced by t(12;22) translocation in malignant melanoma of soft part. Nat Genet 4: 341–345
237. Speleman F, Delattre O, Peter M et al. 1997 Malignant melanoma of the soft parts (clear cell sarcoma): confirmation of EWS and ATF-1 gene fusion caused by a t(12;22) translocation. Mod Pathol 10: 496–499

自主神经系统（包括副神经节）肿瘤
Tumors of the autonomic nervous system (including paraganglia)

28

Ernest E. Lack 著

回允中 李莹杰 译

肾上腺外副神经节	1763
头颈部副神经节瘤	1764
交感肾上腺神经内分泌系统的肾上腺外副神经节瘤	1769
神经节细胞副神经节瘤	1770
神经母细胞瘤和相关肿瘤	1771
神经节细胞瘤	1777

肾上腺外副神经节
Extra-adrenal paraganglia

肾上腺外副神经节大致对称地向心性分布于中线的两侧，并从中耳部位和颅底向盆底延伸。交感肾上腺神经内分泌系统是由交感神经系统组成的复合体，伴有节后神经元通过神经递质去甲肾上腺素介导的效应器反应，而肾上腺髓质合成并分泌肾上腺素和少量去甲肾上腺素[1]。这些副神经节通过神经元（节后交感神经元释放去甲肾上腺素）和激素作用迅速调节以适应环境的改变，而激素作用依赖于肾上腺髓质分泌的儿茶酚胺（主要是肾上腺素）。头颈部副神经节的部位很关键，它们与副交感神经系统的排列比较接近，使其能够发挥化学感受器的作用，在动脉血成分改变时，呼吸和心血管系统功能发生反射性变化[1]。

头颈部副神经节
Paraganglia of the head and neck region

头颈部副神经节的排列接近副交感神经系统，常常与鳃弓中胚层衍生物并列（图28.1）。最大而又最致密的副神经节集合是颈动脉体，它位于两侧颈动脉分叉的内侧（图28.2）。成人颈动脉体的总重量平均为稍大于12 mg[1]。每一个颈动脉体都是由许多小叶组成的，低倍镜下（图28.3A），小叶排列紧密，高倍镜下（图28.3B），小叶含有主细胞（或叫I型血管球）和支持（或叫II型血管球）细胞。嗜铬素（chromogranin）A免疫染色可清楚地显示主细胞（chief cells）呈小簇或短条索状分布（图28.3C）。S-100蛋白染色可勾画出主细胞条索和小簇周围的支持细胞（sustentacular cells）（图28.3D），但是主动脉体和其他副神经节内的神经鞘细胞也呈阳性反应。

其他副神经节位于颅底（如中耳岬、颈静脉球外膜、面神经管）、与神经节小结密切相关的迷走神经突、喉以及与大血管有关的心脏底部。这些副神经节在显微镜下才能看到，相当于颈动脉体小叶的大小或较小的亚单

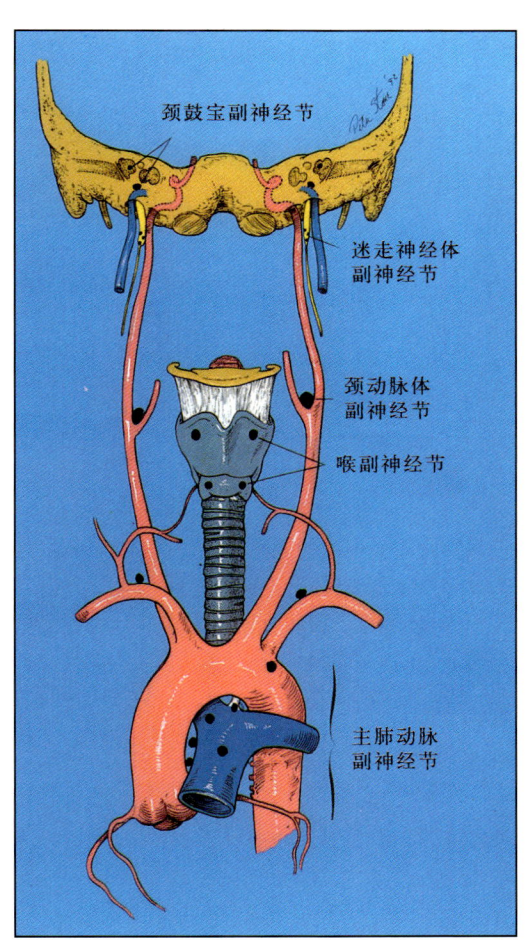

图28.1 头颈部副神经节的解剖学分布，它们的排列紧贴副交感神经系统。

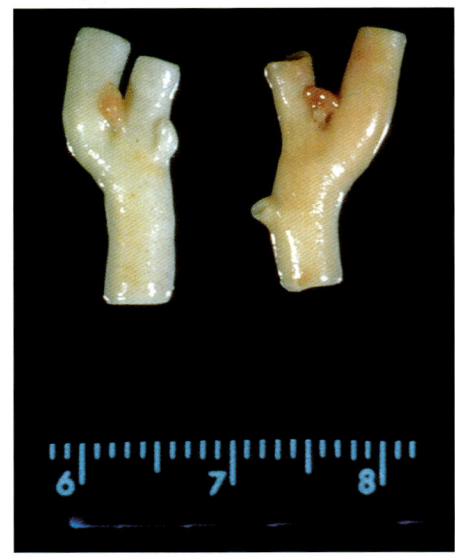

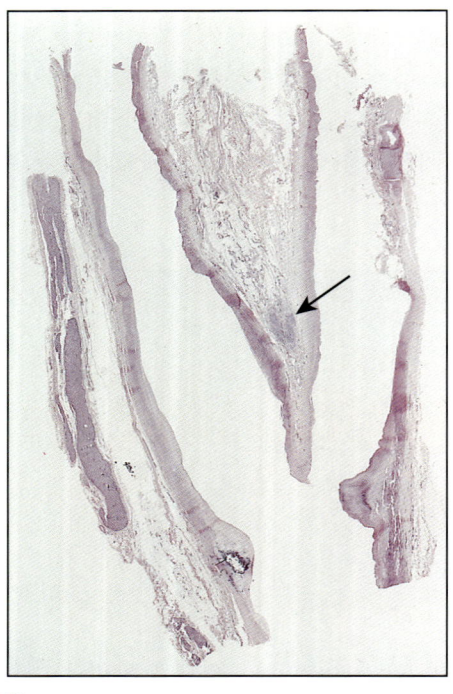

图28.2 （A）5周大女孩的颈动脉体，位于两侧颈总动脉分叉的内侧，表现为卵圆形的粉红色结构，其总重量为1.9 mg。（B）切片来自成人尸检，通过颈总动脉以及内侧（左）和外侧（右）颈动脉分支切开。颈动脉体是颈动脉分叉处外膜软组织内的一个明显的小的卵圆形结构（箭头所示）。

位。动物实验研究证实，颈动脉体和心底附近的副神经节具有化学感受器的作用。

生活在高原的人[2]以及在低于正常气压情况下的某些慢性血氧过低的病人[3,4]，其颈动脉体肥大和增生已有报道。类似的改变在其他部位也见到过，如迷走神经和主动脉与肺动脉之间的副神经节[1]。

头颈部副神经节瘤
Paragangliomas of the head and neck region

颈动脉体副神经节瘤
Carotid body paragangliomas

颈动脉体副神经节瘤（CBP）通常累及成人，年龄常见于41～50岁，在大多数报道中，男女的发病率几乎相等，但某些报道显示女性病人略多。CBP也叫"化学感受器瘤"（chemodectoma）（尽管没有证据表明这些肿瘤具有化学感受器的功能），通常表现为靠近下颌角的一个无痛性缓慢生长的肿块[1,5-10]。这是这种类型肿瘤在头颈部最常见的部位。依据它们的解剖学部位进行鉴别诊断可能存在严重的问题。据报道，在高原地区，CBP的发生率有所增加[11]。

来自Memorial医院的一项研究显示，CBP的平均直径是3.8 cm（1.8～8.5 cm）[6,7]。血管造影可用于证实肿瘤血管供应以及探索CBP和其他头颈部副神经节瘤的精确位置（图28.4）。肿瘤一般表现为孤立的，单侧，褐色到"肉色"，切面呈棕红色（图28.5）。有些肿瘤可有明显的出血，当肿瘤较大时，可能出现伴有纤维化和一些囊性改变的退行性区域。

镜下的特征性表现是腺泡状，伴有"细胞球"（Zellballen）或细胞巢结构（图28.6A），这种结构可以通过网织纤维染色显示（图28.6B）。肿瘤细胞的这种排列方式部分类似于正常头颈部副神经节主细胞的器官样结构（图28.3B和C）。在有些肿瘤，肿瘤性主细胞簇可能较大，伴有中心退行性改变（图28.7）。由于组织取样小或没有代表性，或有挤压假象，准确诊断可能比较困难。在一些肿瘤，核的多形性可能是一个显著特征，可见类似于嗜铬细胞瘤的细胞核的"假包涵体"（图28.8）。核的多形性和核深染对于诊断恶性并不是可靠的证据。一般缺乏核分裂象。只有少数肿瘤应用DNA流式细胞分析进行了研究[1,10,12,13]，但是DNA倍体状态好像不是一个可靠的恶性指征[14]。下面将讨论恶性标准。

由于充血，巢状或腺泡状结构可能更加明显，伴有肿瘤细胞巢分离（图28.9）。肿瘤可出现各种间质改变，如陈旧或新鲜出血、纤维化以及血管硬化（图28.10）。在一些病例，间质变化可能造成诊断困难，如突出的硬化[14a]，但是肿瘤的其他部分通常有保存完好的器官样结构。

少数肿瘤的肿瘤细胞具有显著的嗜酸细胞特征，伴有丰富的强嗜酸性胞浆；"细胞拥抱"（cell-embracing）现象也有报道，伴有细胞突起犬牙交错，这在正常副神经节也可以见到（图28.11）。少数情况下可能有梭形细

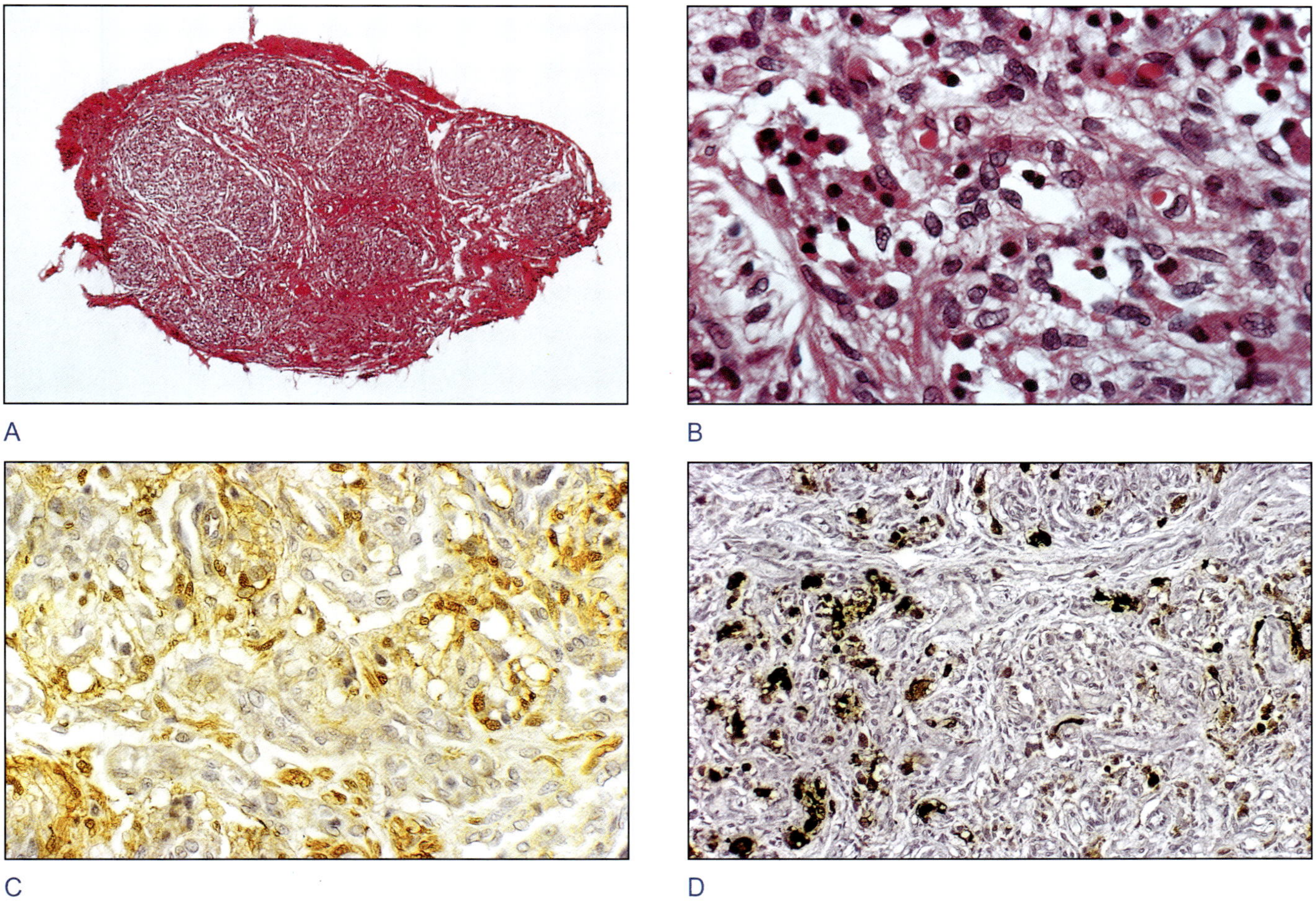

图28.3 （A）来自一个幼儿的正常颈动脉体的横切面。注意分叶状结构，伴有交叉的纤维血管结缔组织带。（B）正常颈动脉体小叶。主细胞排列成短条索和细胞簇（细胞球），具有颗粒状粉染的胞浆。支持细胞具有扁豆状淡染的细胞核，出现在主细胞簇的周围。（C）正常主动脉体嗜铬素A免疫染色显示特征性的主细胞巢。（D）正常颈动脉体的支持细胞S-100蛋白染色显示核和胞浆。有些细胞可能是神经鞘细胞，因为颈动脉体神经支配丰富。

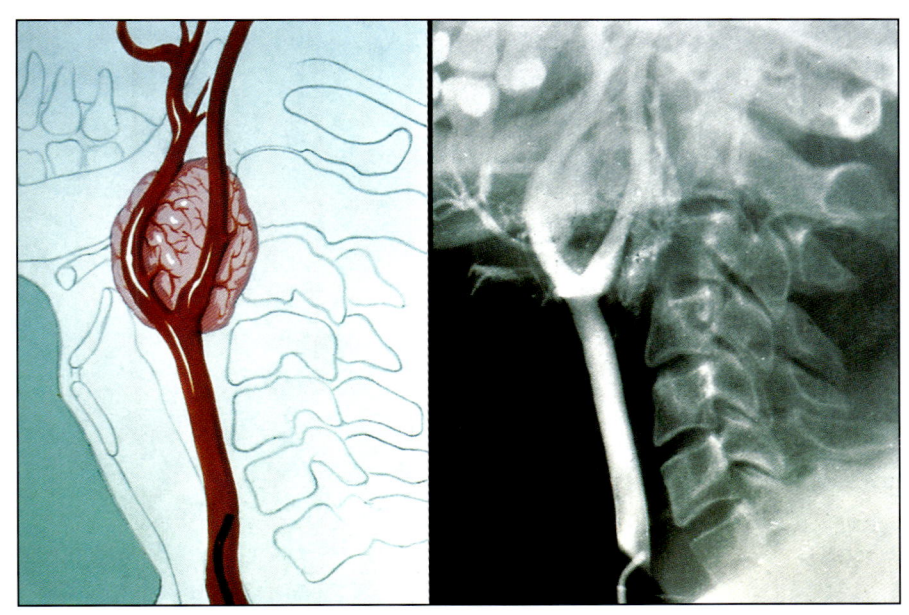

图28.4 选择性动脉造影。显示颈动脉体副神经节瘤引起颈动脉分叉增宽，具有独特的肿瘤红染。(Reproduced with permission from Lack E E, Cubilla A L, Woodruff J M 1979 Paragangliomas of the head and neck region: a pathologic study of tumors from 71 patients. Hum Pathol 10: 191-218.)

头颈部副神经节瘤

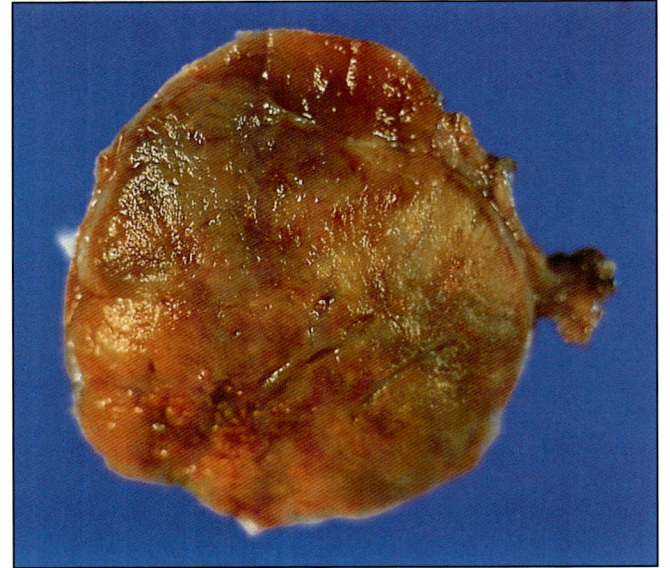

图28.5　从一位40岁女性患者体内切除的颈动脉体副神经节瘤。患者对侧切除了一个类似的肿瘤，有颈动脉体副神经节瘤家族史。由于手术切除之前进行了肿瘤栓塞，所以有缺血性坏死区域。

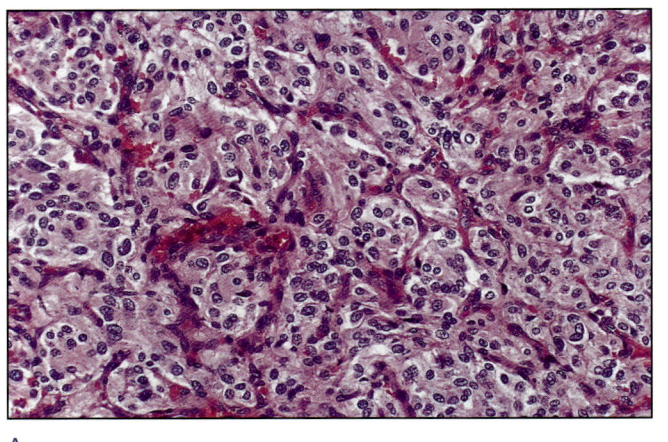

A

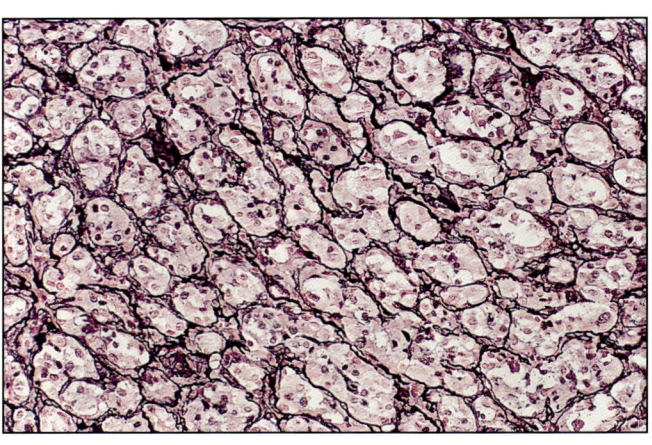

B

图28.6　颈动脉体副神经节瘤。（A）注意肿瘤细胞呈器官样排列，伴有粉红色颗粒状胞浆。（B）网织纤维染色，突显了腺泡状巢状结构。

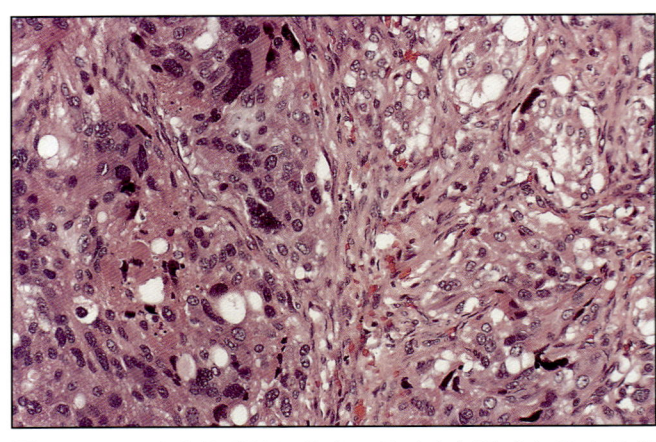

图28.7　颈动脉体副神经节瘤。显示左侧肿瘤细胞大片集聚，伴有中心退变区域。注意杂乱分布的透明空泡，可能是由于固定造成的人工假象。8年来患者生存良好。

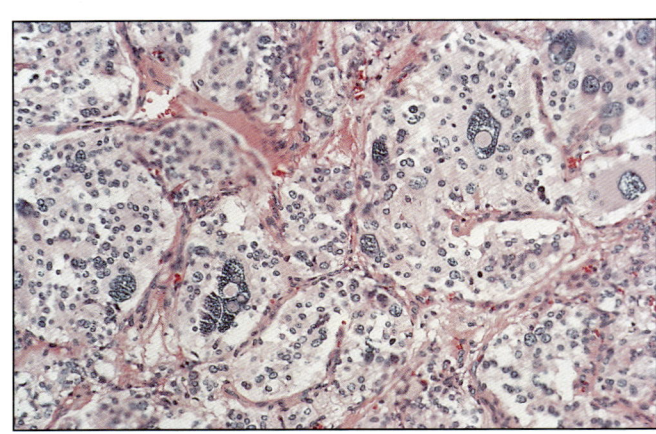

图28.8　颈动脉体副神经节瘤。显示核的多形性和核深染的区域，少数细胞核可见"假包涵体"。

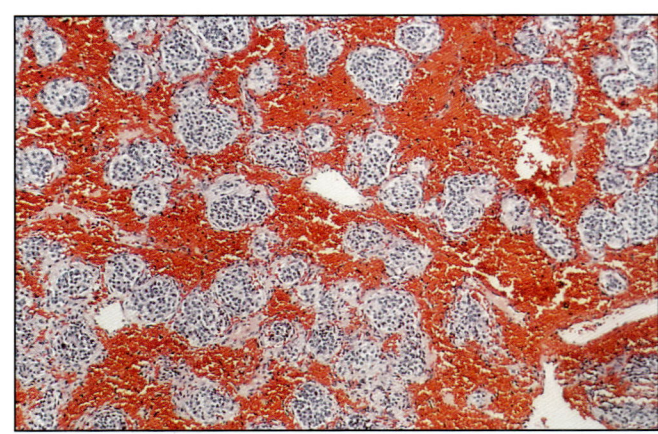

图28.9　颈动脉体副神经节瘤。显示显著出血和充血，伴有分散的肿瘤细胞巢。其他部位具有更典型的组织学表现。

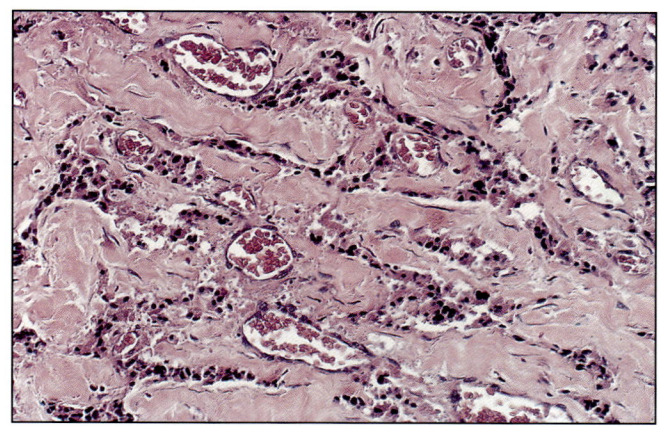

图28.10 迷走神经副神经节瘤。明显硬化的部位为肿瘤细胞受压形成的条索；其他部位显示大量的含铁血黄素沉积。

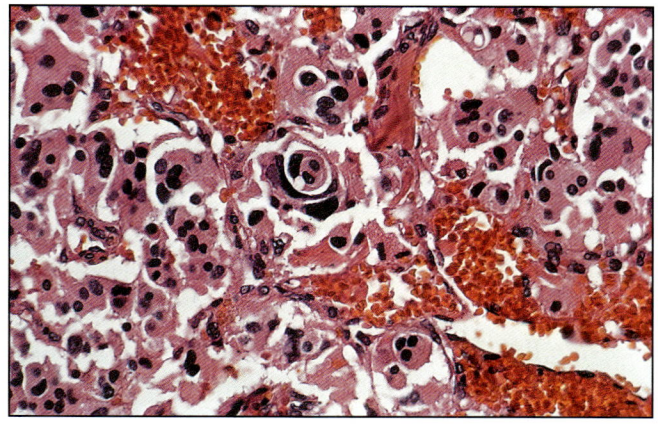

图28.11 颈动脉体副神经节瘤由嗜酸瘤细胞组成，含有丰富的深染的强嗜酸性细颗粒状胞浆。靠近视野的中心，肿瘤细胞胞浆突起相互交织，呈同心圆性排列。

胞结构，但是通常存在其他更具有诊断意义的区域[1,10]。

迷走神经和其他副神经节瘤
Vagal and other paragangliomas

副神经节瘤根据它们的大小和解剖学部位可以引起各种不同的症状和体征，但是它们的形态学表现本身却与颈动脉体副神经节瘤没有明显不同。如迷走神经副神经节瘤从上颈部的小的副神经节发生，接近或位于迷走神经节小结的较下部分。即使解剖学上它们在镜下是散在的结构，这些副神经节又叫迷走神经体副神经节（vagal body paraganglia）。迷走神经副神经节瘤和颈静脉鼓室副神经节瘤好发于女性。这些肿瘤很少累及颈动脉分叉（图28.12）。迷走神经副神经节瘤可以不规则地向迷走神经头侧延伸并累及颅底。其他常见的部位是中耳（颈静脉鼓室副神经节瘤，jugulotympanic paragangliomas）、

喉[15,16]、鼻咽[1]、眶[17]和心底[1]。

家族性副神经节瘤　Familial paragangliomas

编码线粒体呼吸链复合体Ⅱ亚单位D（SDHD）的丁二酸脱氢酶的基因种系突变是头颈部遗传性副神经节瘤的遗传性因素之一[18]。遗传方式是常染色体显性遗传，而且两侧颈动脉体副神经节瘤和头颈部其他部位多灶性肿瘤的发生率可能会有所增加[19,20]。在明显是散发的单个肿瘤患者，SDHD种系突变比较罕见[20a]。

副神经节瘤的特殊染色、免疫组织化学和超微结构

副神经节瘤一般是非嗜铬性副神经节瘤，且其被认为与副交感神经系统密切相关；但也有例外，甚至在功能活跃的肿瘤，也有儿茶酚胺分泌过多的报道[1,10]。

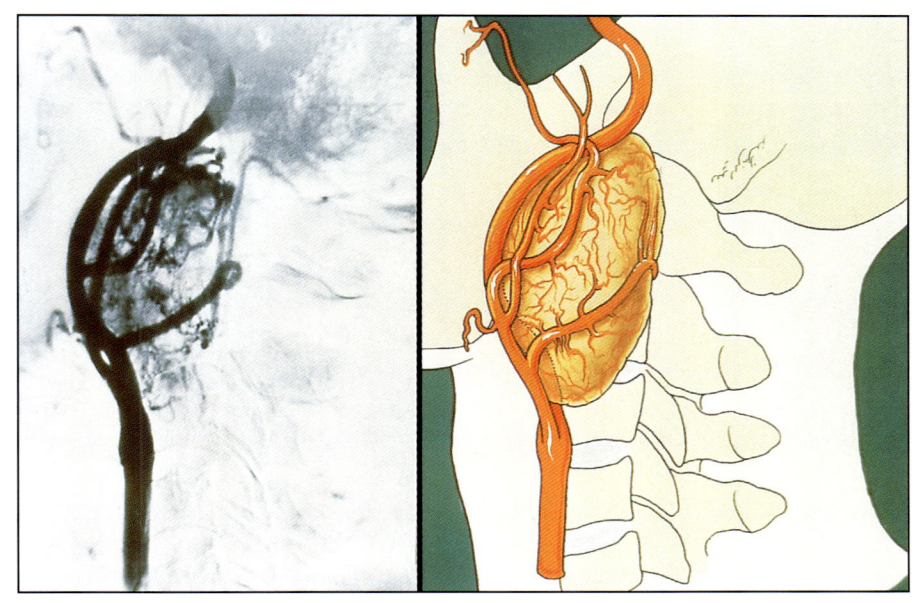

图28.12 迷走神经副神经节瘤。没有累及颈动脉分叉。肿瘤取代颈动脉分支前部，并延伸至颅底。

以往，对确定诊断最有帮助的染色之一是嗜银染色，可显示胞浆内有针尖大的颗粒（图28.13）。神经内分泌免疫组化标记物能够提供更加特异和敏感的诊断信息。主细胞表现为NSE染色和其他更特异的神经内分泌分化标记物呈阳性，如嗜铬素（chromogranin）呈阳性[1, 10, 21, 22]（图28.14）。在这种肿瘤，各种激素物质免疫染色也可呈阳性，包括5-羟色胺（serotonin）、血管活性肠多肽（vasoactive intestinal polypeptide）、胃泌素（gastrin）、P物质（substance P）、生长抑素（somatostatin）和铃蟾肽（bombesin）。S-100蛋白的特征性的染色形态可以证实支持细胞的存在，这有助于这种肿瘤与其他肿瘤的鉴别诊断，如与甲状腺髓样癌和喉神经内分泌癌[1]。据报道，GFAP免疫染色也能突出支持细胞（图28.15）[23]，但是S-100蛋白可能更可靠。在有些副神经节瘤，细胞角蛋白免疫染色阳性比较罕见，这可能是免疫组化诊断的一个缺陷[22]。

超微结构研究显示，主细胞含有不同数量的致密轴心神经内分泌颗粒，直径通常在120～250 nm[1, 7, 24]；通常是规则圆形，伴有均匀一致的空晕（图28.16）。有些细胞有发育良好的细胞连接，但是真正的桥粒连接并不是它的特征。可能有"暗"细胞和"亮"细胞，取决于细胞浆的总的电子透明的差异，但是这并没有显著性差异[24]。支持细胞也可见到，但是并不恒定，S-100蛋白（或有时用GFAP）免疫染色能够最好地显示出这种细胞。

恶性副神经节瘤
Malignant paragangliomas

与恶性行为有关的形态学特征尚没有明确的界定；一项研究就这种肿瘤的核分裂象、坏死和血管浸润进行了分析，但是也没有得出结论[7]。非典型性的组织学特征表现（如核分裂象和坏死）与S期和（或）G2/M期细胞分裂或非整倍体细胞群的出现大致相关[12]。在一项

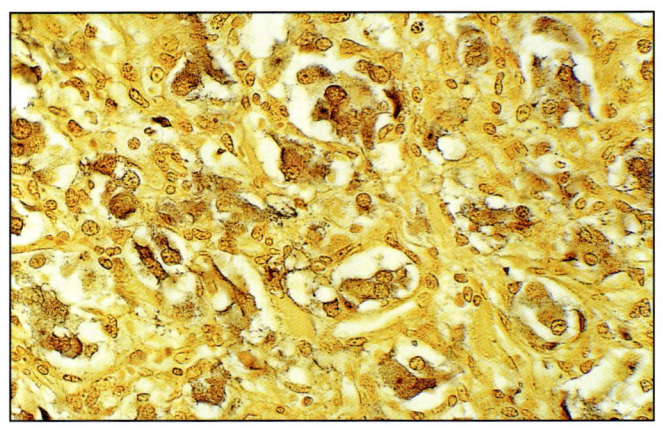

图28.13 一位年轻妇女的喉副神经节瘤。患者伴有进行性声音嘶哑。肿瘤细胞具有散在的巢状结构，多数细胞具有独特的胞浆嗜银颗粒。Grimelius 染色。

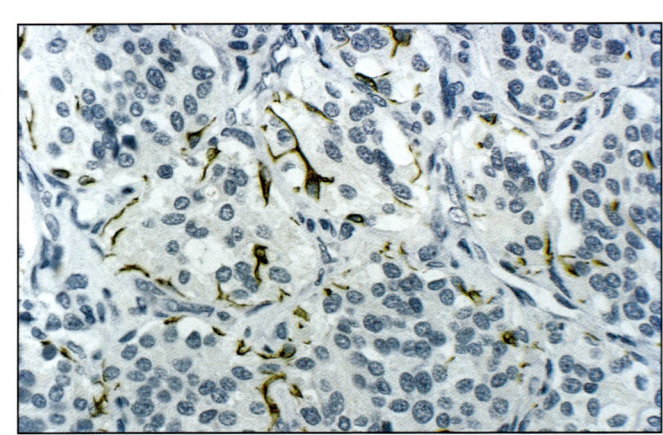

图28.15 颈动脉体副神经节瘤。GFAP染色显示支持细胞核和胞浆呈阳性反应。大多数支持细胞在成簇的肿瘤主细胞周围。过氧化物酶-抗过氧化物酶反应。

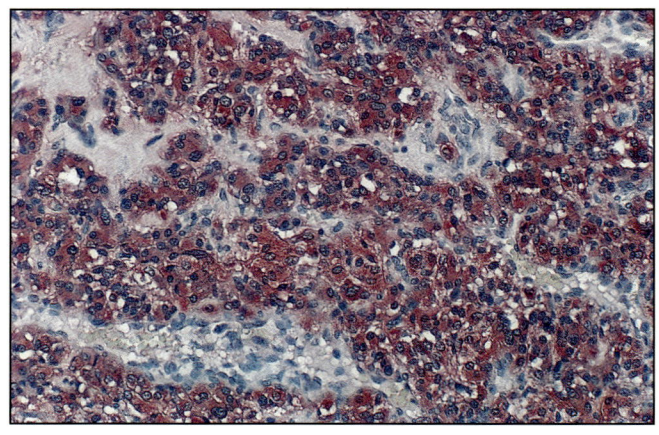

图28.14 颈动脉体副神经节瘤。显示嗜铬素染色呈阳性。抗生物素蛋白链菌素碱性磷酸酶反应。

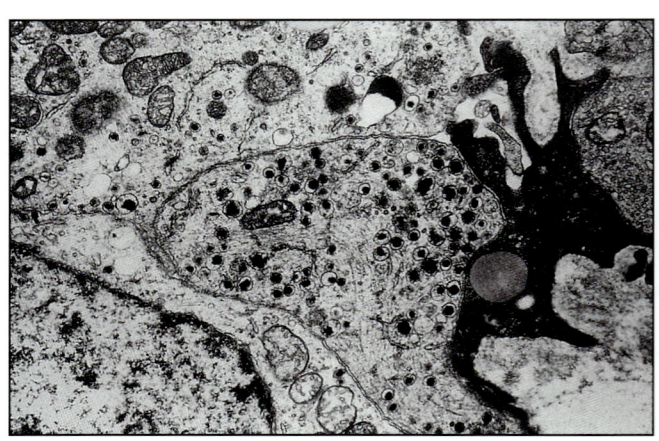

图28.16 相互交织的细胞突起伴有相对一致的致密轴心神经内分泌颗粒。界膜内的一些颗粒呈偏心性分布。

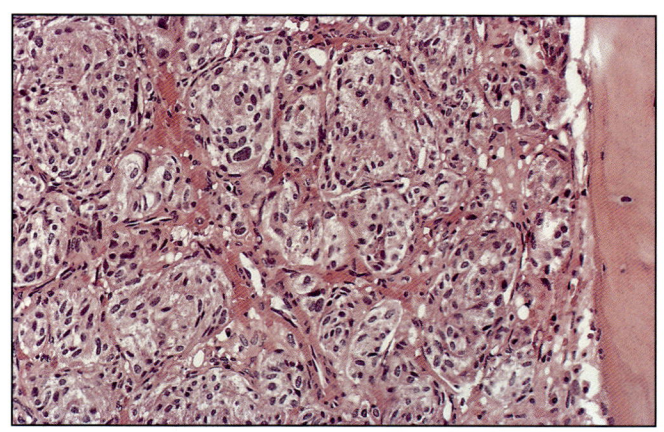

图28.17 临床上主动脉与肺动脉间的恶性副神经节瘤发生于心底附近。骨转移的肿瘤细胞具有明显的器官样排列，同原发性肿瘤一样。

研究中，多数侵袭性或转移性副神经节瘤缺乏支持细胞[23]。肿瘤转移少见[25]，一旦出现，则最常累及局部淋巴结、肺、肝和骨骼[1]（图28.17）。

交感肾上腺神经内分泌系统的肾上腺外副神经节
Extra-adrenal paraganglia of the sympathoadrenal neuroendocrine system

这个系统的肾上腺外副神经节沿着脊柱旁和主动脉干旁分布，从颈部向下延伸到骨盆，紧靠交感神经系统排列[1,10]。出生之后，肾上腺髓质最终将变成最大最致密的副神经节，但是在胎儿发育和新生儿中，肾上腺外副神经节最为明显，特别是在腹主动脉的两侧。Zuckerkandl描述，这些副神经节85%是多发的（图28.18），并将其称为"主动脉小体"（aortic bodies）[26]。这些副神经节（也叫Zuckerkandl器）在10岁之前就退化了，但在任何年龄的成人均可见到遗迹，表现为非常类似于肾上腺髓质的细胞的小的结构（图28.19）。去甲肾上腺素是肾上腺外嗜铬细胞分泌的主要儿茶酚胺，因为这是一个强有力的加压剂，所以有人提出，在子宫内，Zuckerkandl器可以帮助维持血管张力[1]。

交感肾上腺神经内分泌系统的肾上腺外副神经节瘤
Extra-adrenal paragangliomas of the sympathoadrenal neuroendocrine system

这些副神经节瘤的分布平行于交感神经系统的肿瘤，它们可以发生于从盆底（如膀胱）到颈部的任何

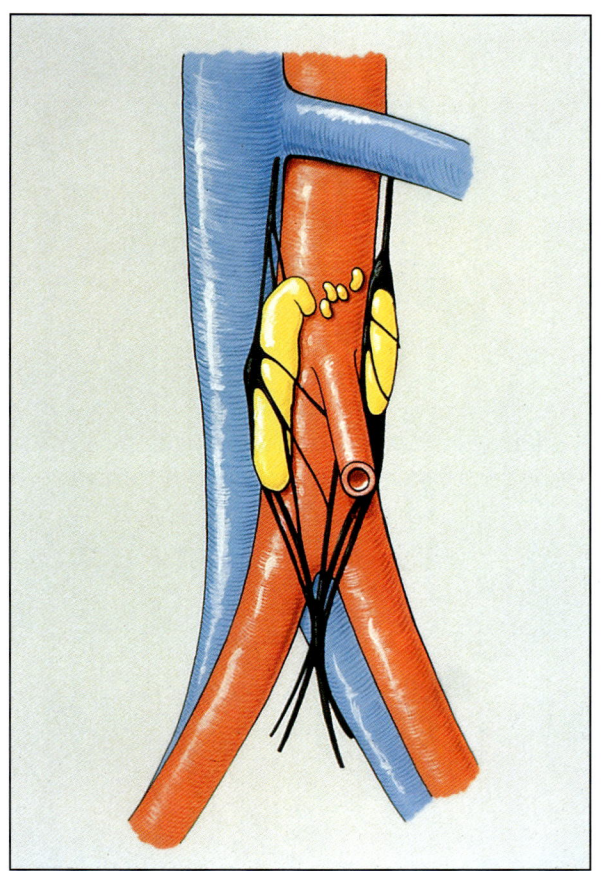

图28.18 根据1901年最初做的研究，Zuckerkandl器的分布[26]。在15%的新生儿，嗜铬组织是通过肠系膜动脉正上方的主动脉前面的一个岬延续并连接。

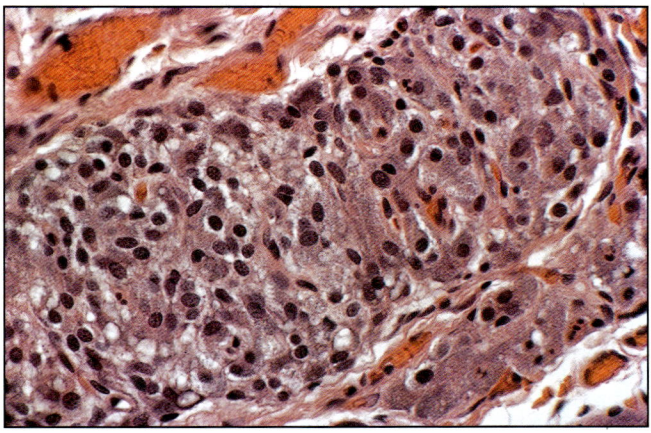

图28.19 腹膜后小的副神经节，含有与肾上腺髓质嗜铬细胞一样的内分泌细胞。

部位[1,10,27-29]。椎管，包括马尾的部位，比较少见[30,31]。在腹部，肿瘤可能起源于Zuckerkandl器的遗迹（图28.18），其组织学表现与肾上腺髓质的嗜铬细胞相同（见上文）。腹部肾上腺外副神经节瘤的大小从6～20 cm不等，切面可能显示有坏死和囊性退变的区域[29]（图28.20）。虽然这些肿瘤组织学上可以类似于伴有细胞小巢（腺泡状结构或"细胞球"）的头颈部副神经节瘤，

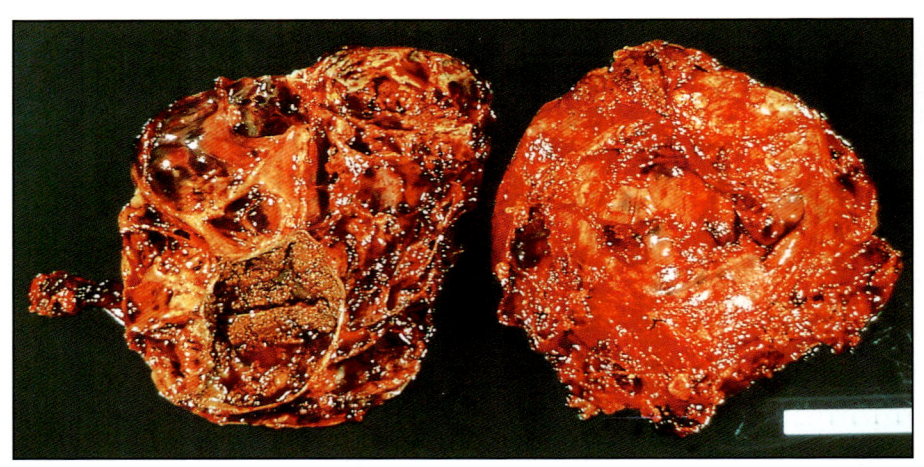

图28.20 肾上腺外副神经节瘤。切面显示囊性变（左侧），伴有出血区。右侧为肿瘤外表面。肿瘤直径为20 cm。

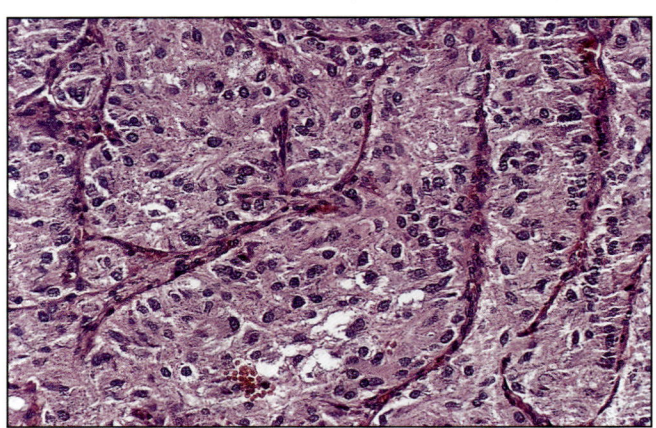

图28.21 吻合的小梁状或盘绕的细胞索是肾上腺外副神经节瘤相对常见的病变形态。胞浆为嗜酸性颗粒状，边界不清。有些细胞核可能增大和深染。

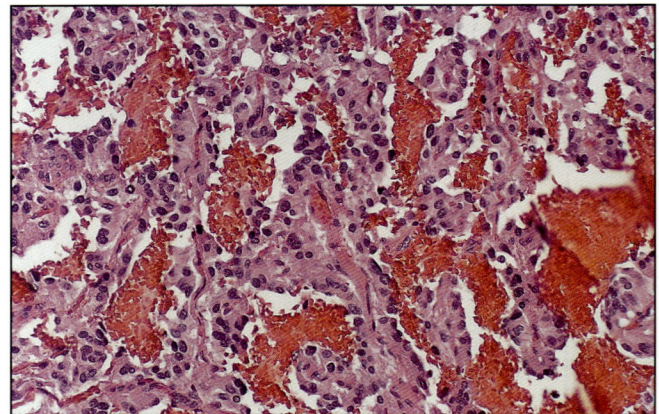

图28.22 胸部肾上腺外副神经节瘤。肿瘤细胞呈假乳头状排列，伴有显著的充血。肿瘤发生在椎旁沟，临床表现为恶性，伴有骨转移。

但是广泛吻合的或小梁状结构表现更具有特征性（图28.21）。肿瘤内出血或充血可能将肿瘤细胞分离呈细小梁状，形成血管周围假玫瑰花结（图28.22）。复杂的血管网被称为"内分泌样结构"，因为多数肿瘤细胞位于内衬内皮细胞的血管腔的附近。在一些病例，小梁状或巢状结构并不显著，肿瘤细胞具有弥漫性或实性生长方式，少数情况下可能为梭形细胞状。有些情况下可见胞浆内玻璃样小体，像嗜铬细胞瘤（肾上腺髓质副神经节瘤）一样。极少见的病例含有大量的色素，有一例好像是神经黑色素（neuromelanin）[32]。

膀胱副神经节瘤是一种少见而又特殊的肿瘤[33]（见第12章）。显微镜下，切面似乎有膀胱壁固有肌层浸润（图28.23A），但是仅仅根据这一点不能认为其是恶性的；其他部位可显示吻合的或盘绕的细胞条索结构，这是见于这些肿瘤的一种典型病变（图28.23B）。

胃间质肉瘤（最常见伴有上皮样结构）、肺软骨瘤和肾上腺外副神经节瘤三联征（Carney 三联征）已有人报道[34]。我们已经认识到，这样的患者还有肾上腺皮质肿瘤，有些病例是家族性的，但遗传方式尚未明确[34]。

肾上腺外副神经节瘤的免疫组化所见在几项研究中也有过描述[35-37]。初步结果提示，同嗜铬细胞瘤一样[37]，缺乏支持细胞与侵袭性行为相关[36]。虽然支持细胞稀少或缺乏可以发生在临床上表现为恶性的肿瘤，但这并不是恶性的绝对可靠的指征，因为这也可以见于一些随访证实是良性的肿瘤[38]。

神经节细胞副神经节瘤
Gangliocytic paraganglioma

神经节细胞副神经节瘤是一种罕见的良性肿瘤（也叫十二指肠非嗜铬副神经节瘤）[39]，它是由上皮样细胞组成的，具有内分泌样的生长方式，伴有梭形细胞和神经节细胞[40-44]（图28.24）。这些病变主要累及中年成人，表现为黏膜下结节，最常见于十二指肠的第二部分。上皮样细胞排列成巢或小梁状，伴有类似于副神经节瘤和（或）类癌/胰岛细胞瘤的形态学结构。梭形细胞和神经节细胞成分可能酷似神经节细胞瘤（ganglioneuroma）。肿瘤可能在平滑肌内浸润性生长，但这并不是恶性表现；尽管有几个患者有局部淋巴结受累，但实际上，

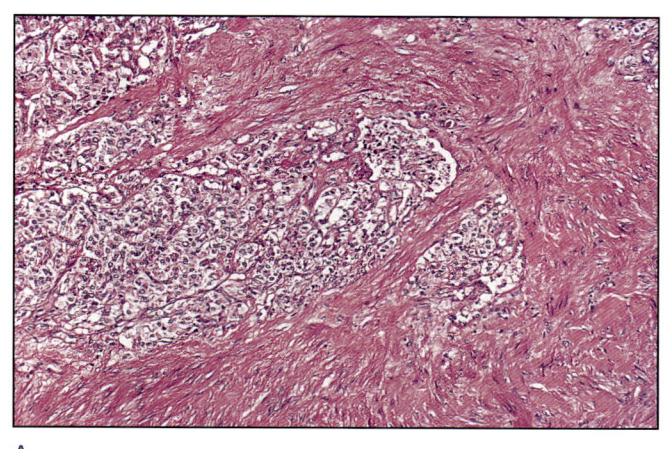
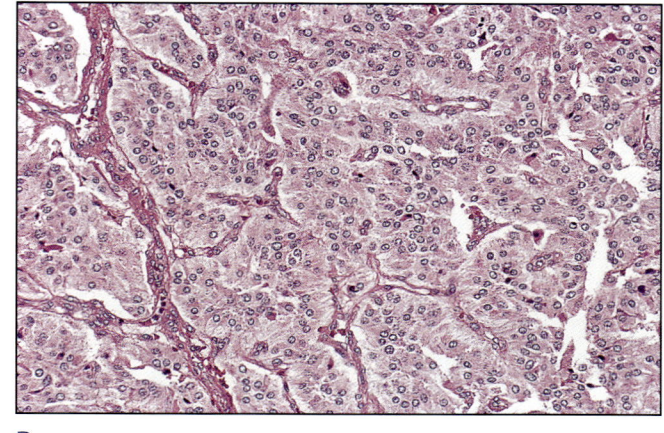

图28.23 膀胱副神经节瘤。（A）注意肿瘤侵及膀胱壁肌层。（B）为（A）所示同一膀胱副神经节瘤的另外一个部位，具有吻合性小梁状结构，伴有相互连接的细胞索和突出的微血管结构。

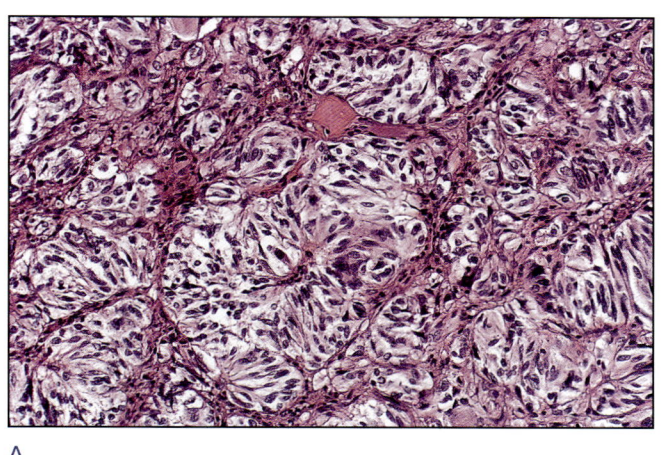
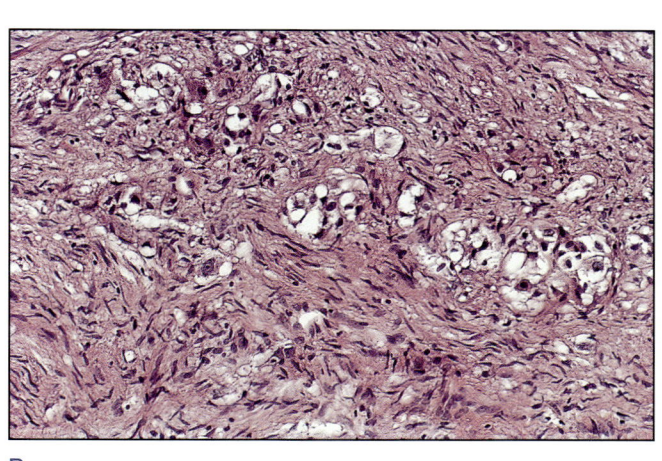

图28.24 神经节细胞副神经节瘤。（A）注意上皮样细胞呈小梁状排列，伴有突出的微血管结构，酷似副神经节瘤。（B）梭形细胞增生，偶尔出现神经节样细胞，酷似神经节细胞瘤。

随访发现是良性的[44]。有人认为，这种肿瘤是错构瘤／迷芽瘤，包含异位的胚胎性胰腺组织。虽然这种肿瘤具有神经内分泌病变的结构和免疫组化特征，但还是应与肾上腺外副神经节瘤鉴别，后者通常缺乏神经节样细胞和梭形细胞。

神经母细胞瘤和相关肿瘤
Neuroblastoma and related tumors

原位神经母细胞瘤　In-situ neuroblastoma

根据1963年最初描述的概念[45]，原位神经母细胞瘤是指小的肾上腺肿瘤（通常为0.7～9.5 mm），与典型的儿童期神经母细胞瘤一样，但是大体或显微镜下，在身体其他部位没有发现肿瘤的证据。在3个月以下的婴儿的尸检中，大约每200例可发现1例原位神经母细胞瘤[45]。这远远超出了临床上神经母细胞瘤的发病率，

如果假定这些病变是真性肿瘤，那么绝大多数必定是经历了自发性退化（或成熟）。图28.25显示了一个原位神经母细胞瘤病例。在尝试鉴别神经母细胞结节和原位神经母细胞瘤时出现了问题；前者是肾上腺正常发育的组成部分，且可能存留直到出生或新生儿早期。

神经母细胞瘤和神经节母细胞瘤
Neuroblastoma and ganglioneuroblastoma

大约85%的神经母细胞瘤和神经节母细胞瘤发生在4岁之前，中位年龄大约为21个月；发病率没有性别差异[1,10,46,47]。不到10%的神经母细胞瘤和神经节母细胞瘤发生在10岁以上；在青春期和成年患者，这种肿瘤表现出不同的生物学特征和更长的临床病程，但是不管年龄如何，最终预后都不好[48]。大约70%的病例病变发生在肾上腺或腹腔内的交感神经链，而至少20%的病例病变发生在胸腔（包括胸腺）[49]。肿瘤可表现为散在的球形肿块，也可表现为巨大的肿瘤，表面呈多结

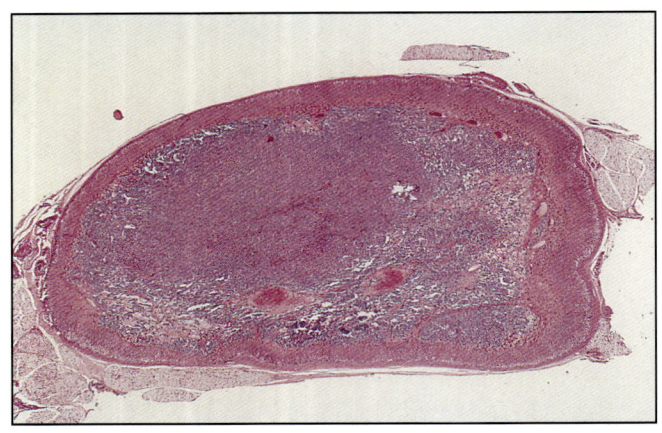

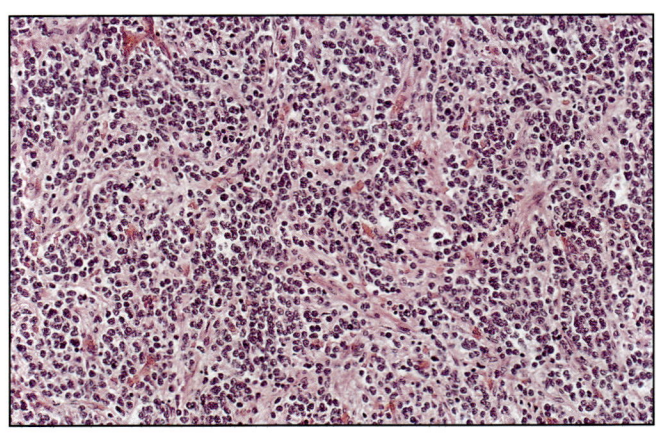

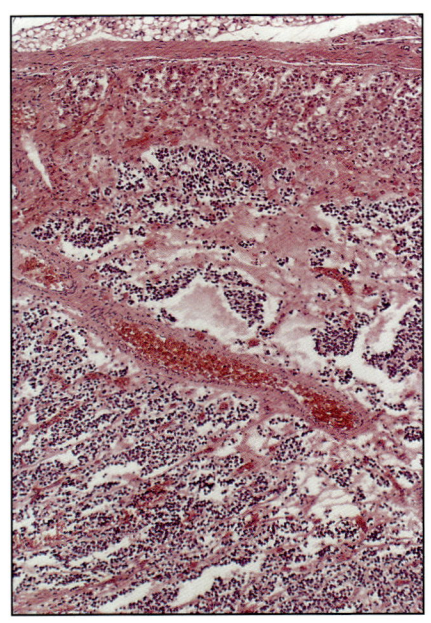

图28.25 （A）原位神经母细胞瘤，直径0.6 cm。这个肾上腺来自一个死于先天性心脏病的26天大的女孩。肿瘤造成肾上腺髓质部分膨胀，境界清楚，边缘呈推挤状。（B）原位神经母细胞瘤。视野顶端有完整的肾上腺包膜，其下残留薄的皮质。肿瘤有水肿和早期微囊性改变的区域。（C）原位神经母细胞瘤的具有代表性的视野，与典型的儿童期神经母细胞瘤难以区分。

节状[1,10]（图28.26）。它可能侵犯邻近器官或组织。神经母细胞瘤的横切面常常呈粗结节状，伴有出血和坏死区。大体表现可能类似于血肿伴囊性退变。肿瘤内钙化可以表现为白垩色或淡黄色的点状区域，标本的放射学检查可以更好地证实钙化。据报道，在肾上腺肿瘤的放射学检查、超声检查和CT检查中，钙化性肿块最常见于神经母细胞瘤[50]。囊性神经母细胞瘤已有报道，类似于血肿或肾上腺囊肿[1,10,47]（图28.27）。神经节母细胞瘤显示分化水平逐渐增高（见下文），大体检查时肿瘤横切面的外观均匀一致（图28.28）。

神经母细胞瘤（neuroblastoma）是儿童时期"小蓝细胞"肿瘤的典型类型，通常具有境界不清的分叶状或巢状生长方式，伴有纤细的纤维血管间隔（图28.29）。据说，具有显著巢状（"器官样"）结构的肿瘤患者预后较好[51]。细胞之间常有不同量的淡染的原纤维物质，是神经细胞突起。这种神经原纤维物质类似于中枢神经系统的神经纤维网，可以形成玫瑰花结的中心（图28.30A）或形成不规则的宽阔的丛状；少数情况下，玫瑰花结结构具有节律性或栅栏状构型（图28.30B）。在未分化的神经母细胞瘤中，神经原纤维物质可能完全缺失，以至于诊断困难（图28.31）。核染色质通常为细而

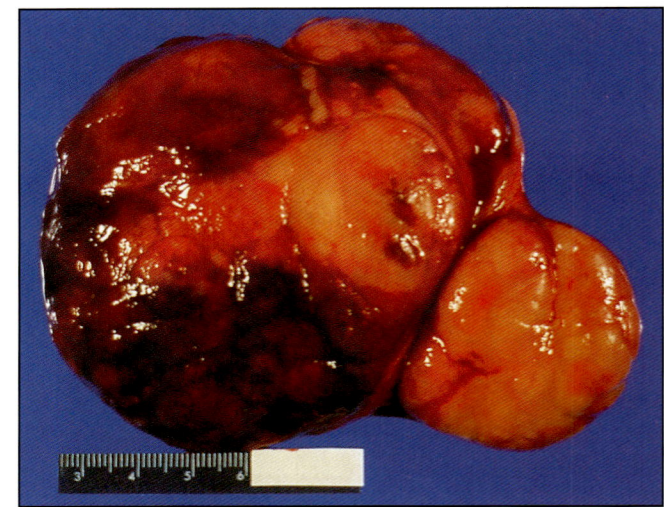

图28.26 肾上腺外神经母细胞瘤的横切面，呈现隆起的分叶状外观，伴有出血和坏死区。小部分区域的肿瘤细胞的分化相当于神经节母细胞瘤。

分散的小团块，呈现小斑点或"胡椒盐"表现；核仁一般不明显，但在伴有神经节细胞分化时可以变得突出。新近认识到（但是罕见），伴有核大、核仁明显的大细胞类型好像特别具有侵袭性[52]。间变性神经母细胞瘤（anaplastic neuroblastoma）也有报道[53]，但是它的意义

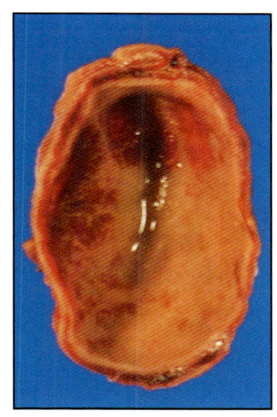
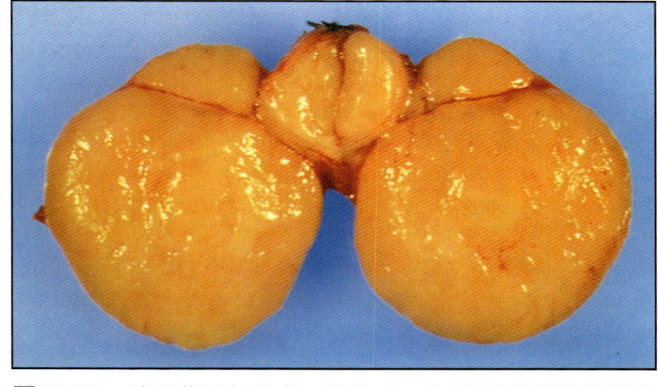

图28.27 先天性囊性神经母细胞瘤。(A)肿瘤是在宫内通过超声检查发现的,表现为一个囊性肾上腺肿块。囊肿周围为显著的残留的肾上腺皮质,囊内有血色液体。(B)病变(A)的代表性切片,显示神经母细胞瘤的不规则的巢状结构,被出血分隔开。这个囊性肿瘤的内面含有血液和较多的纤维素性渗出物,而视野上方可见残留的肾上腺皮质。

图28.28 神经节母细胞瘤,其位于一个3岁幼儿的腹部脊柱旁区域。肿块的绝大部分类似于神经节细胞瘤,伴有明显的梭形细胞(神经鞘)基质,但在几个区域有少量神经节母细胞瘤成分。应用Shimada分类,这个肿瘤应该属于混合性富于间质的神经节母细胞瘤。

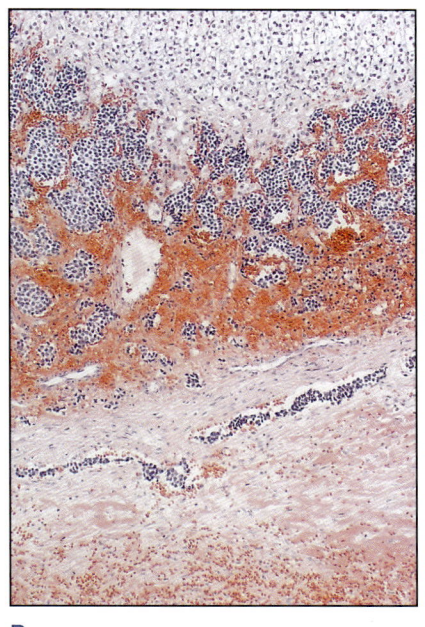

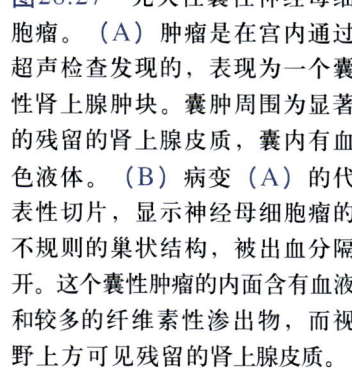

图28.29 神经母细胞瘤,伴有模糊的分叶状结构和纤细的微血管成分。在有些区域,小圆细胞被神经原纤维基质分开。这个视野没有明显的玫瑰花结。

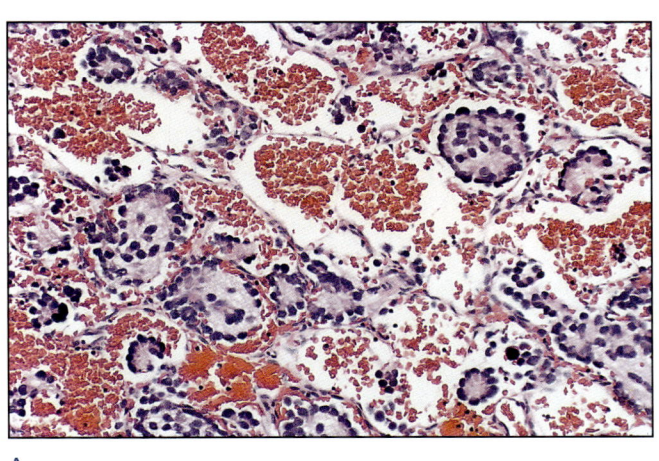
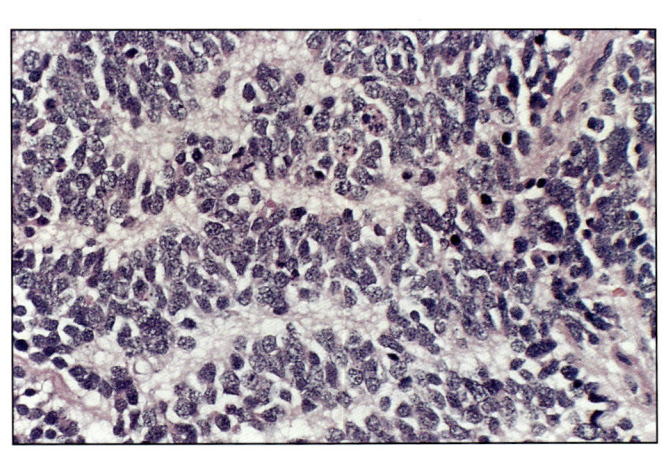

图28.30 (A)神经母细胞瘤,伴有明显的出血,小簇细胞形成Homer Wright玫瑰花结。(B)神经母细胞瘤的栅栏状玫瑰花结。注意点彩状染色质结构和突出的核仁缺失。

并不明确(图28.32)。其他少见的组织病理学特征也有报道，如硬化性改变、梭形神经母细胞、间质玻璃样变和致密的淋巴浆细胞浸润，其中有些特征可能与退化现象有关[54]。

神经节母细胞瘤（ganglioneuroblastoma）通常表现为有些细胞分化或成熟，伴有可辨认的神经节细胞或其前体细胞[1,10,55]。间质可能富含梭形细胞、神经鞘基质（图28.33）或神经原纤维（图28.34）。神经节细胞分化的证据包括：(1) 细胞核和胞浆扩增；(2) 细胞边界清楚；以及 (3) 胞浆嗜酸性增加。核的位置可能偏心，伴有染色质在边缘聚集，可以有明显的核仁。Stout认为，有弥漫性和混合性两种类型的神经节母细胞瘤[56]。混合性神经节母细胞瘤一部分是神经节细胞瘤，伴有一个或一个以上的神经母细胞瘤小灶[57,58]。

个别色素性神经节母细胞瘤病例也有报道，伴有前黑色素小体或黑色素小体[59]。多数色素被认为是神经黑色素（neuromelanin）。

神经节母细胞瘤的常用诊断标准不需要具备神经节细胞瘤成分。新近修订的神经节母细胞瘤诊断标准包括由较多神经节细胞瘤成分（即大于50%）和较少神经母细胞瘤成分组成的肿瘤[60]。归入神经母细胞瘤的病例应该分级，可分为预后相对好的肿瘤（1级和2级的5年生存率分别为90%和78%）和生存率低的肿瘤（3级，5年生存率为34%）。神经节母细胞瘤应该分为低度危险（中间性和交界性）和高度危险（结节性）两组。这些修订的标准给出了明确的肿瘤分类方法，并将神经节母细胞瘤与神经母细胞瘤区分开[60]。

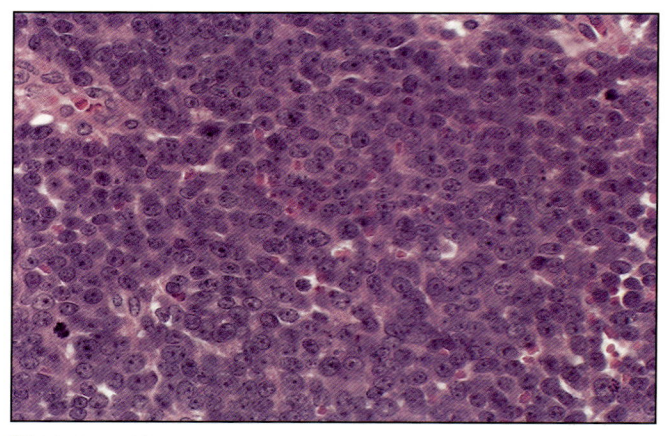

图28.31 神经母细胞瘤。由致密排列的肿瘤细胞组成，没有可辨认的玫瑰花结或神经原纤维基质。许多细胞核有小点状核仁，但没有神经节细胞分化的证据。肿瘤应用B-5溶液固定。

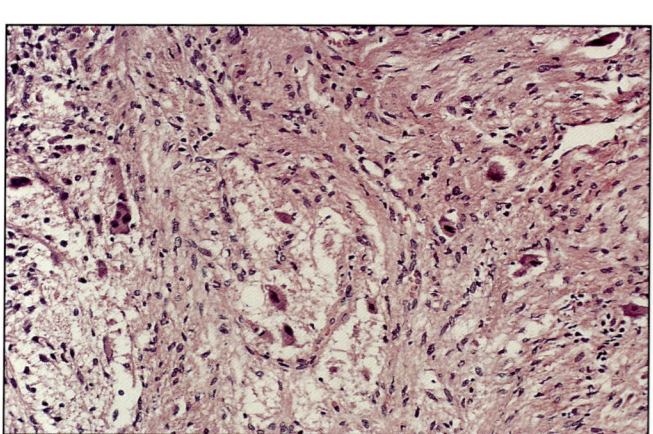

图28.33 神经节母细胞瘤。伴有大量突出的梭形细胞（神经鞘）基质以及小而不成熟细胞的原纤维基质的区域，有些区域显示神经节细胞分化。在Shimada分类中，这个肿瘤应该被称为富含间质的中间性神经节母细胞瘤。

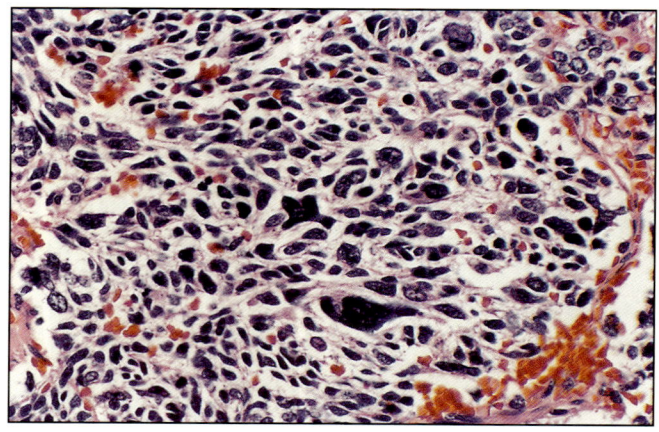

图28.32 间变性神经母细胞瘤。显示明显的多形性深染的细胞核。

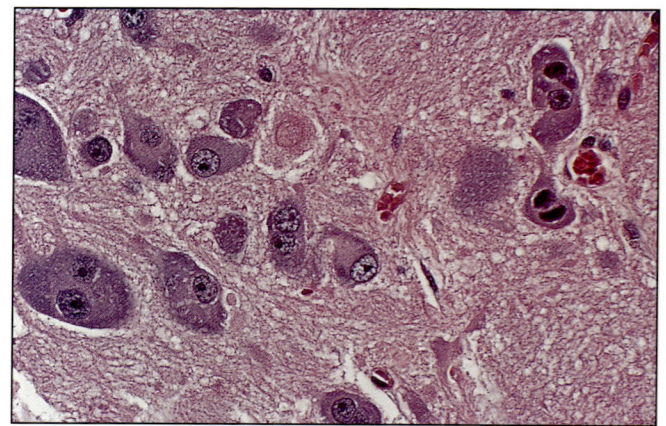

图28.34 神经节母细胞瘤。伴有神经节细胞分化，位于原纤维基质中。这个肿瘤应该归类为间质贫乏，伴有高比例的正在分化的细胞，核分裂象-核碎裂指数低；结合患儿年龄4岁，肿瘤应该属于预后好的间质贫乏的肿瘤（见表28.2）。

年龄相关的Shimada分类方法及其修订
Age-linked classification of Shimada and its modifications

对于儿童期神经母细胞瘤，有几种不同的分类方法，其中一个方案结合了年龄作为预后参数[61]，可将类似于神经纤维网的神经原纤维基质与富含细胞的梭形细胞（或神经鞘）基质区分开来。Shimada等提出了儿童期神经母细胞瘤的分类方法[61]，这种方法（图28.35）结合了分化成分（即神经节细胞）的比例、核分裂象-核碎裂指数（mitosis-karyorrhexis index, MKI）和患者年龄；患者年龄本身是儿童期神经母细胞瘤的一个重要的预后因素。

Shimada分类方法的切入点是：评估间质的"特性"，通常认为有两种类型：(1)富含间质的肿瘤(stroma-rich tumors)，伴有广泛的梭形细胞和神经鞘成分；以及(2)间质贫乏的肿瘤(stroma-poor tumors)，伴有大量的神经原纤维衬底。富含间质的肿瘤（表28.1）分为预后好的亚型（高分化和混合性；见图28.28和28.33）和预后不好的亚型（如结节型）。Stout描述的混合性神经节母细胞瘤可能相当于混合性和结节性亚型，取决于神经母细胞瘤是否出现大体可见的结节。表28.2列出了间质贫乏肿瘤的组织学特征。这些肿瘤也可分为预后好和预后不好两个亚型（表28.3）。这种分类方法已有一定的预后价值[62,63]，但仍需从其他可以获得的各种生物化学和细胞遗传学标记物来仔细分析其对预后的影响[64]。有趣

表28.1 富含间质肿瘤的预后良好和预后不好的组织学表现

广泛的神经鞘梭形细胞间质形成神经母细胞瘤或神经鞘瘤样结构：

预后良好的组织学表现
- 高分化：不成熟细胞以孤立的方式均匀一致分布
- 混合性：不成熟细胞呈孤立小簇状分布于整个肿瘤

预后不好的组织学表现
- 结节性：大体上肿瘤有一个（或多个）很不成熟的间质贫乏的部位（或者大体上一个在另一个之内，或者一个在原发性肿瘤，另一个在转移部位）

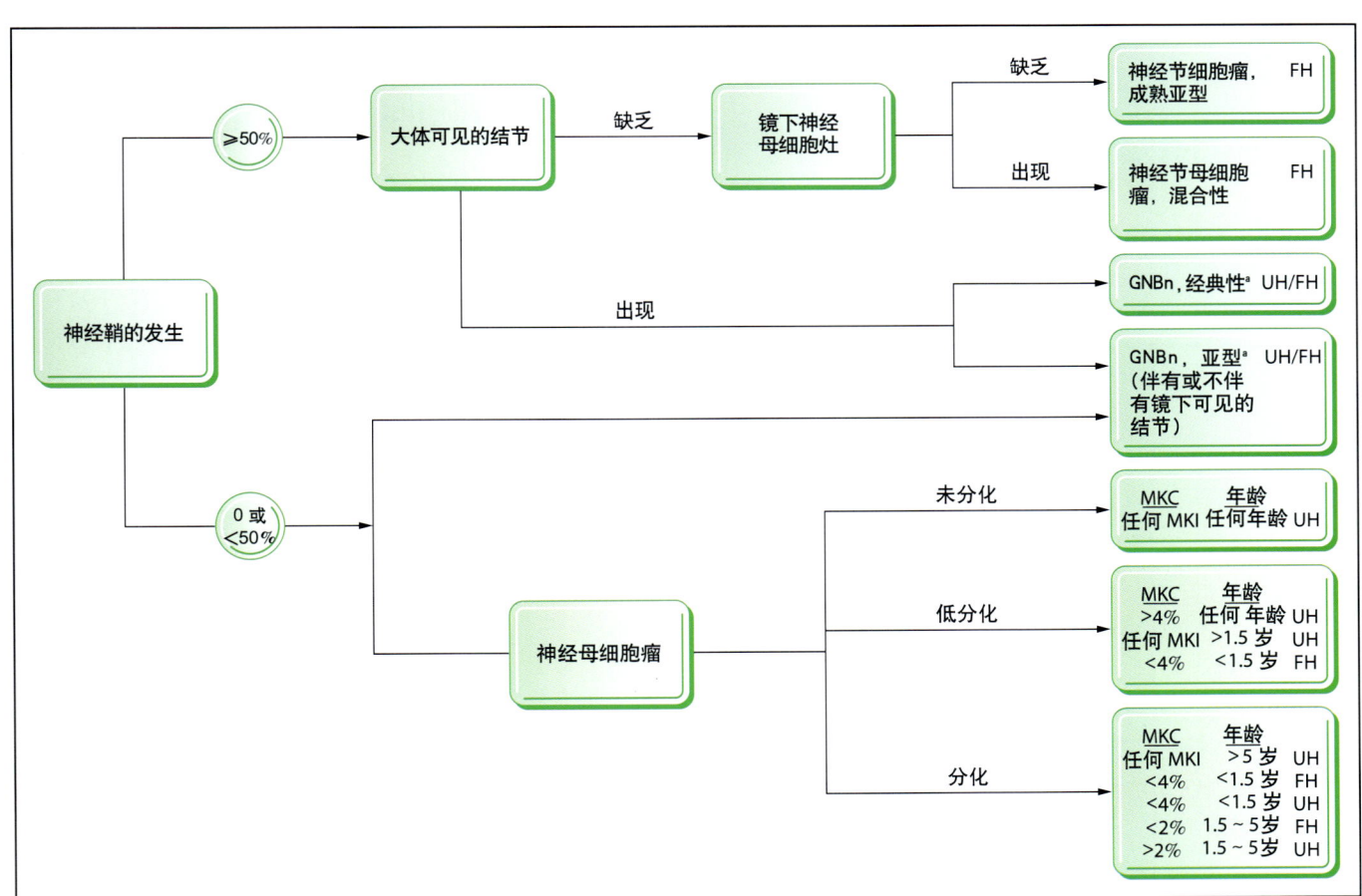

图28.35 国际神经母细胞瘤病理学分类。FH：组织学良好；UH：组织学不好；GNBn：神经节母细胞瘤，结节性；MKC：核分裂象和核碎裂细胞；MKI：核分裂象-核碎裂指数[a]，用于GNBn的预后评估，见文献[67,68]。
[a]核分裂象核碎裂细胞（MKC）：2%——5000个细胞中有100个，4%——5000个细胞中有200个。

表28.2 间质贫乏肿瘤的组织学分类，包括分化程度或分级以及核的形态学[72]

分化分级

未分化：分化成分<5%

分化中：分化成分≥5%

核的形态学

核分裂象-核碎裂指数（MKI）[a]

低：<100

中：<200

高：>200

[a] 根据在随机选取的视野中计数5000个细胞。

表28.3 根据分化成分，核分裂象-核碎裂指数（MKI）和诊断时年龄进行的预后不好和预后好的间质贫乏肿瘤的亚组分类[72]

预后不好的间质贫乏肿瘤亚型（生存率4.5%）

<1.5岁，高MKI，无论组织学分化成熟程度如何

1.5~5岁，伴有未分化组织学成分，无论MKI如何

1.5~5岁，伴有分化的组织学成分和高或中MKI

>5岁的所有患者

预后好的间质贫乏肿瘤亚型（生存率84%）

<1.5岁，伴有任何分化成熟和低或中MKI

1.5~5岁，伴有分化的组织学成分和低MKI

MKI包括核分裂细胞数目加畸形，分叶或固缩核以及坏死的单个细胞数目。应用MKI有助于减少观察者之间计数核分裂象的差异。

的是，应用这种方法，多数 IVS 期病例（预后好的特殊亚型，尽管有肝、皮肤或骨髓受累）显示出良好的组织学表现[65]。

神经母细胞瘤的另一种年龄相关的分类和预后分类是由来自儿科肿瘤学组的 Joshi 等提出的。儿科肿瘤学组定义的低危险组和高危险组与 Shimada 分类的组织学表现良好和组织学表现不好分组的生存曲线高度一致（84%）[66]。这种新的分级方法具有以下优点：应用熟悉的术语和组织学特征，而且因为不需要确定分化程度，所以评估相对容易。神经母细胞瘤被分为三个级别：1级，低核分裂率（每10个高倍视野核分裂象≤10个）和肿瘤内钙化；2级，低核分裂率或钙化；3级，肿瘤伴有高核分裂率（每10个高倍视野核分裂象>10）并缺乏钙化[67]。年龄分组（≤1岁和>1岁）与分级联系起来定义了两个危险组：（1）低危险组由年龄≤1岁和>1岁的1级肿瘤以及年龄<1岁的2级肿瘤患者组成；（2）高危险组由>1岁的2级肿瘤以及两个年龄组的3级肿瘤患者组成。重要的是要记住，根据 Joshi 等的定义[60]，神经母细胞瘤分级的组织学标准不能用于神经节母细胞瘤，因为后者多数是1级，而且根据生存不能进行适当分级[66]。

这些分级方法很复杂，需要进一步研究以提出更成熟的分类方法，如新近提出的神经母细胞瘤的分级方法，用 MKI 代替了核分裂率，并且删除了与年龄的关系[67]。新近包括所有主要首创者在内的国际神经母细胞瘤病理学委员会发表了统一分类方法，使这些不同的分类方法和伴随的争论多数得到了解决[68, 69]。这个分类非常类似于 Shimada 等的分类方法[61]，其与年龄相关，并根据分化、有无神经鞘间质以及 MKI 进行的分类。国际神经母细胞瘤病理学分类提出了四种类型的外周神经母细胞肿瘤：（1）神经母细胞瘤（神经鞘间质贫乏）；（2）神经节母细胞瘤，混合性（神经鞘间质丰富）；（3）神经节细胞瘤（神经鞘间质丰富）；以及（4）神经节母细胞瘤，结节性（混合性，神经鞘间质丰富/间质丰富和间质贫乏）[70]。根据结节性神经节母细胞瘤及其变种的形态学标准[71]，新近又提出了一个修订的分类方法[72]（图28.35）。

辅助技术 Ancillary techniques

神经母细胞瘤的 NSE 免疫染色呈阳性；S-100 蛋白染色可用于辨认分化的细胞，如神经鞘细胞。铁蛋白（ferritin）阳性细胞增加和 S-100 蛋白阳性细胞丧失与预后不好有关[58]。N-myc 癌基因扩增出现在大约25%的神经母细胞瘤[73]，并与进展期肿瘤和更强的侵袭行为有关[74]，但是其他因素也可能影响预后，尽管有些肿瘤并没有 N-myc 癌基因扩增。不过，一般说来 N-myc 扩增与肿瘤分化不好和 MKI 高有关，特别是在<1.5岁的患者更有意义[75]。应用免疫组化技术或聚合酶链反应（PCR）可以辨认癌基因产物、还有更新的技术能够迅速而直接地确定 N-myc 扩增、1号染色体复制数以及存在 1p 缺失，应用荧光原位杂交（在肿瘤印片和标准骨髓涂片）可检测倍体，这样有助于治疗的标准化[76]。多参数分析显示，染色体 1p 等位缺失、N-myc 扩增和额外的染色体 17q 复制与预后不好明显相关，一项研究显示，染色体 1p 缺失是最重要的预后因素[77]。这在新近一项大的研究中得到进一步的证实，这项研究显示，1p36 和 11q 杂合性缺失（LOH）是与预后较差相关的独立危险因素[77a]。

据报道，有些神经母细胞瘤和神经节母细胞瘤患儿会出现水样腹泻，且与肿瘤产生的血管活性肠多肽有关[1]

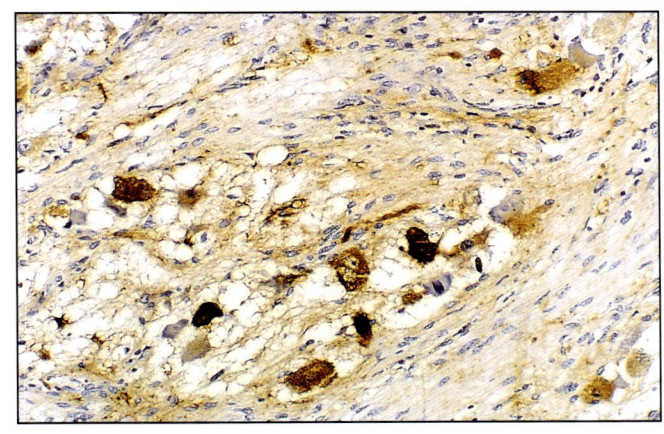

图28.36 神经节母细胞瘤,来自一个伴有大量水样腹泻的患儿。血清血管活性肠多肽（VIP）水平升高,许多分化中的神经节细胞显示VIP免疫染色阳性。在Shimada分类中,这个肿瘤应该是富含间质的混合性肿瘤。过氧化物酶-抗过氧化物酶染色。

（图28.36）。超微结构特征包括：神经突起伴有神经管和神经微丝（图28.37A）,以及致密轴心颗粒,后者通常规则,大小一致,直径小于200 nm[78]（图28.37B）。

神经节细胞瘤　Ganglioneuroma

多数神经节细胞瘤患者诊断时超过10岁,肿瘤常常位于后纵隔或腹膜后,只有相对少数的病例发生在肾上腺[1, 47]。一些研究报道其好发于女性。这种肿瘤境界通常清楚,质硬；切面常常光滑,淡黄色到灰白色或棕色,没有出血或坏死[1, 10, 47]。肿瘤切面可能有漩涡状或小梁状结构,类似于平滑肌瘤（图28.38）。常有丰富的梭形细胞基质,可能类似于神经鞘瘤或神经纤维瘤。存在成熟的神经节细胞,但是这些细胞的数目、密度和分

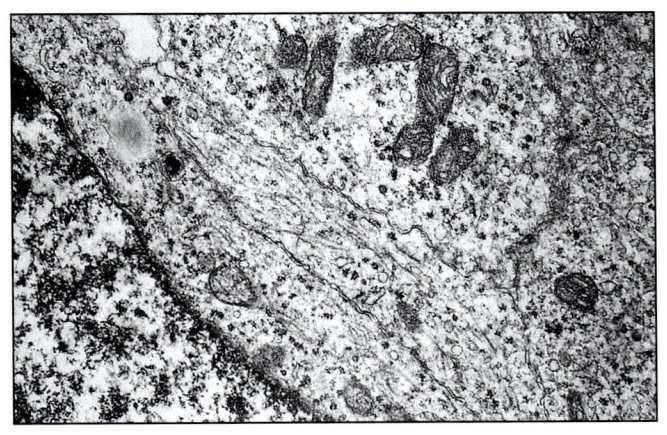

A

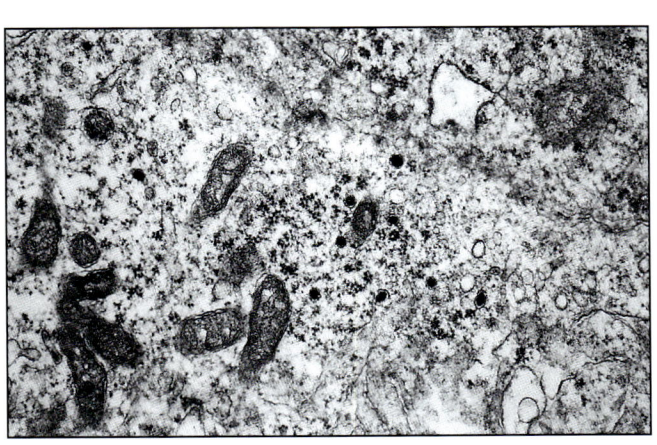

B

图28.37 神经母细胞瘤。（A）神经细胞突起伴有神经小管。神经微丝和致密轴心神经分泌颗粒出现在其他视野中。（B）几个致密轴心神经分泌型颗粒与游离多核糖体一起出现。颗粒常常呈圆形,规则,密度均匀,且被一界膜包绕。

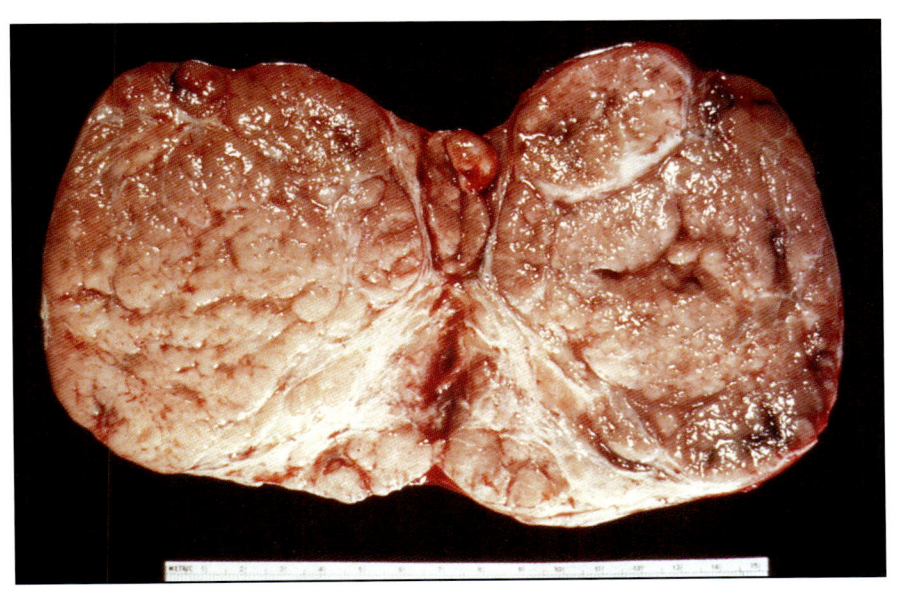

图28.38 神经节细胞瘤。切面隆起,色淡,呈粗小梁状表现,类似于"纤维瘤"或平滑肌瘤。其外表面相对光滑。

布可能差异很大（图 28.39）。有些病例可能有大量的细颗粒状棕色色素，类似于神经节细胞内的脂褐素或神经黑色素（图 28.40）。偶尔，有些神经节细胞周围可能有一层较小的细胞，提示为卫星细胞。有充分的证据表明，神经母细胞瘤可成熟变为神经节细胞瘤，但有证据表明，年龄较大和肾上腺外部位的多数肿瘤是原位来源的，至少在有些病例是这样的。少数几例神经节细胞瘤发展成恶性外周神经鞘肿瘤（恶性神经鞘瘤）已有报道[1,10,79]，有时发生在儿童期神经母细胞瘤放射治疗之后[1,80]。在个别情况下，有报道称神经节细胞瘤含有典型的伴有 Reinke 类晶体的 Leydig 细胞。1983 年，Aguirre 和 Scully 报道此种肿瘤可引起男性化[80]（图 28.41）。

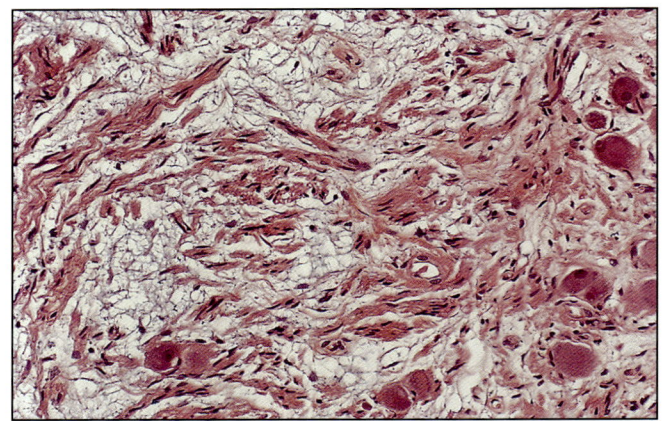

图 28.39　神经节细胞瘤。注意交错排列的类似于神经鞘细胞的梭形细胞束和分化的神经节细胞。

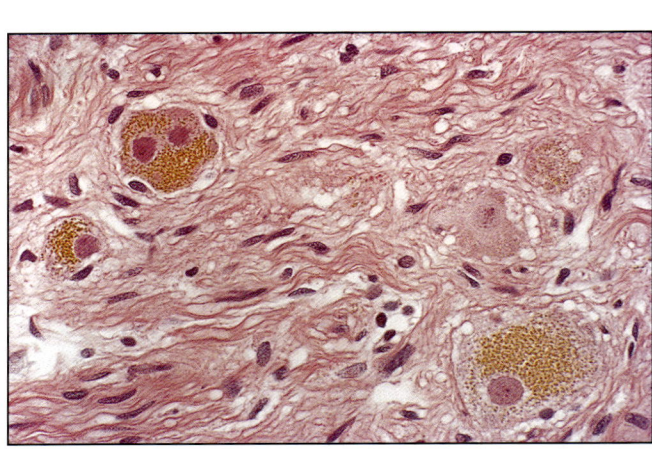

图 28.40　神经节细胞瘤。有些神经节细胞含有细颗粒状棕色色素。

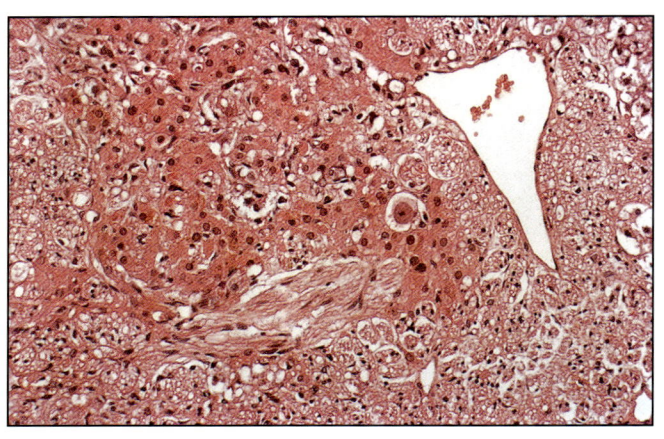

A   B

图 28.41　（A）这个男性化的肾上腺神经节细胞瘤含有增生的 Leydig 细胞巢，伴有具有确诊意义的 Reinke 类结晶。（B）高倍镜下显示 Reinke 类结晶。

参考文献

1. Lack E E 1997 Tumors of the adrenal gland and extra-adrenal paraganglia. Atlas of tumor pathology, series 3, fascicle 19. Armed Forces Institute of Pathology, Washington, DC
2. Arias-Stella J, Valcarcel J 1976 Chief cell hyperplasia in the human carotid body at high altitudes: physiologic and pathologic significance. Hum Pathol 7: 361–373
3. Heath D, Edwards C, Harris P 1970 Post-mortem size and structure of the human carotid body. Thorax 25: 129–140
4. Lack E E, Perez-Atayde A R, Young J B 1985 Carotid body hyperplasia in cystic fibrosis and cyanotic heart disease. A combined morphometric, ultrastructural and biochemical study. Am J Pathol 119: 301–314
5. Shamblin W R, ReMine W H, Sheps S G et al. 1971 Carotid body tumor (chemodectoma). Clinicopathologic analysis of ninety cases. Am J Surg 122: 732–739
6. Lack E E, Cubilla A L, Woodruff J M et al. 1977 Paragangliomas of the head and neck region. A clinical study of 69 patients. Cancer 39: 397–409
7. Lack E E, Cubilla A L, Woodruff J M 1979 Paragangliomas of the head and neck region. A pathologic study of tumors from 71 patients. Hum Pathol 10: 191–218
8. Nora J D, Hallett J W Jr, O'Brien P C et al. 1988 Surgical resection of carotid body tumors: long-term survival, recurrence, and metastasis. Mayo Clin Proc 63: 348–352
9. Hallett J W Jr, Nora J D, Hollier L H et al. 1988 Trends in neurovascular complications of surgical management for carotid body and cervical paragangliomas: a fifty-year experience with 153 tumors. J Vasc Surg 7: 284–291
10. Lack E E 1994 Pathology of adrenal and extra-adrenal paraganglia. Major problems in pathology, vol 29. W B Saunders, Philadelphia

11. Saldana M J, Salem L E, Travezan R 1973 High altitude hypoxia and chemodectomas. Hum Pathol 4: 251–263
12. Granger J K, Houn H-Y 1990 Head and neck paragangliomas: a pathologic study with DNA flow cytometric analysis. South Med J 83: 1407–1412
13. Granger J K, Houn H-Y 1990 Bilateral familial carotid body paragangliomas. Report of a case with DNA flow cytometric and cytogenetic analyses. Arch Pathol Lab Med 114: 1272–1275
14. van der Mey, Cornelisse C J, Hermans J et al. 1991 DNA flow cytometry of hereditary and sporadic paragangliomas (glomus tumours). Br J Cancer 63: 298–302
14a. Plaza J A, Wakely P E Jr, Moran C et al. 2006 Schlerosing paraganglioma: report of 19 cases of an unusual variant of neuroendocrine tumor that may be mistaken for an aggressive malignant neoplasm. Am J Surg Pathol 30: 7–12
15. Gallivan M V E, Chun B, Rowden G et al. 1979 Laryngeal paraganglioma. Case report with ultrastructural analysis and literature review. Am J Surg Pathol 3: 85–92
16. Barnes L 1991 Paraganglioma of the larynx. A critical review of the literature. ORL Otorhinolaryngol Relat Spec 53: 220–234
17. Fisher E R, Hazard J B 1952 Nonchromaffin paraganglioma of the orbit. Cancer 5: 521–524
18. Baysal B E, Ferrell R E, Willett-Brozick J E et al. 2000 Mutations in SDHD, a mitochondrial complex II gene, in hereditary paraganglioma. Science 287: 848–851
19. Astrom K, Cohen J E, Willett-Brozick J E et al. 2003 Altitude is a phenotypic modifier in hereditary paraganglioma type 1: evidence of an oxygen-sensing defect. Hum Genet 113: 228–237
20. Baysal B E 2003 On the association of succinate dehydrogenase mutations with hereditary paraganglioma. Trends Endocrinal Metab 14: 453–459
20a. Dannenberg H, van Nederveen F H, Abbou M et al. 2005 Clinical characteristics of pheochromocytoma patients with germline mutations in SDHD. J Clin Oncol 23: 1894–1901
21. Warren W H, Lee I, Gould V E et al. 1985 Paragangliomas of head and neck. Ultrastructural and immunohistochemical analysis. Ultrastruct Pathol 8: 333–343
22. Johnson T L, Zarbo R J, Lloyd R V et al. 1988 Paragangliomas of the head and neck: immunohistochemical neuroendocrine and intermediate filament typing. Mod Pathol 1: 216–223
23. Kliewer K E, Wen D-R, Cancilla P A et al. 1989 Paragangliomas: assessment of prognosis by histologic, immunohistochemical, and ultrastructural techniques. Hum Pathol 20: 29–39
24. Grimley P M, Glenner G G 1967 Histology and ultrastructure of carotid body paragangliomas: comparison with the normal gland. Cancer 20: 1473–1488
25. Lee J H, Barich F, Karnell L H et al. 2002 National Cancer data report on malignant paragangliomas of the head and neck. Cancer 94: 730–737
26. Zuckerkandl E 1901 Ueber nebenorgane des sympathicus im retroperitonaealraum des Menschen. Verh Dtsch Anat Ges 15: 95–107
27. Fries J G, Chamberlin J A 1968 Extra-adrenal pheochromocytoma: literature review and report of a cervical pheochromocytoma. Surgery 63: 268–279
28. Leestma J E, Price E B Jr 1971 Paragangliomas of the urinary bladder. Cancer 28: 1063–1072
29. Lack E E, Cubilla A L, Woodruff J M et al. 1980 Extra-adrenal paragangliomas of the retroperitoneum. A clinicopathologic study of 12 tumors. Am J Surg Pathol 4: 109–120
30. Moran C A, Rush W, Mena H 1997 Primary spinal paragangliomas: a clinicopathological and immunohistochemical study of 30 cases. Histopathology 31: 167–173
31. Sonneland P R L, Scheithauer B W, Lechago J et al. 1986 Paraganglioma of the cauda equina region. Clinicopathologic study of 31 cases with special reference to immunocytology and ultrastructure. Cancer 58: 1720–1735
32. Lack E E, Kim H, Reed K 1998 Pigmented ("black") extra-adrenal paragangliomas. Am J Surg Pathol 22: 265–269
33. Zhou M, Epstein J I, Young R H 2004 Paraganglioma of the urinary bladder. A lesion that may be misdiagnosed as urothelial carcinoma in transurethral resection specimens. Am J Surg Pathol 28: 94–100
34. Carney J A 1999 Gastric stromal sarcoma, pulmonary chondroma and extra-adrenal paraganglioma (Carney triad): natural history, adrenocortical component and possible familial occurence. Mayo Clin Proc 74: 543–552
35. Hamid Q, Varndell I M, Ibrahim N B et al. 1987 Extra-adrenal paragangliomas. An immunocytochemical and ultrastructural report. Cancer 60: 1776–1781
36. Kliewer K E, Cochran A J 1989 A review of the histology, ultrastructure, immunohistology, and molecular biology of extra-adrenal paragangliomas. Arch Pathol Lab Med 113: 1209–1218
37. Unger P, Hoffman K, Pertsemlidis D et al. 1991 S-100 protein-positive sustentacular cells in malignant and locally aggressive adrenal pheochromocytomas. Arch Pathol Lab Med 115: 484–487
38. Linnoila R I, Becker R L, Steinberg S M et al. 1993 The role of S-100 protein-containing cells in the prognosis of sympathoadrenal paragangliomas. Mod Pathol 6: 39A (abstract)
39. Taylor H B, Helwig E B 1962 Nonchromaffin paragangliomas of the duodenum. Virchow's Arch [A] 335: 356–366
40. Kepes J J, Zacharias D L 1971 Gangliocytic paragangliomas of the duodenum. A report of two cases with light and electron microscopic examination. Cancer 27: 61–70
41. Reed R J, Daroca P L Jr, Harkin J C 1977 Gangliocytic paraganglioma. Am J Surg Pathol 1: 207–216
42. Scheithauer B W, Nora F E, Lechago J et al. 1986 Duodenal gangliocytic paraganglioma: clinicopathologic and immunocytochemical study of 11 cases. Am J Clin Pathol 86: 559–565
43. Hamid Q A, Bishop A E, Rode J et al. 1986 Duodenal gangliocytic paragangliomas. A study of 10 cases with immunocytochemical neuroendocrine markers. Hum Pathol 17: 1151–1157
44. Burke A P, Helwig E B 1989 Gangliocytic paraganglioma. Am J Clin Pathol 92: 1–9
45. Beckwith J B, Perrin E V 1963 In-situ neuroblastomas: a contribution to the natural history of neural crest tumors. Am J Pathol 43: 1089–1104
46. Rosen E M, Cassady J R, Frantz C N et al. 1984 Neuroblastoma: The Joint Center for Radiation Therapy/Dana Farber Children's Hospital experience. J Clin Oncol 2: 719–732
47. Kozakewich H P W, Perez-Atayde A R, Donovan M J et al. 1998 Cystic neuroblastoma: emphasis on gene expression, morphology, and pathogenesis. Pediatr Dev Pathol 1: 17–28
48. Franks L M, Bollen A, Seeger R C et al. 1997 Neuroblastoma in adults and adolescents. An indolent course with poor survival. Cancer 79: 2028–2035
49. Argani P, Erlandson R A, Rosai J 1997 Thymic neuroblastoma in adults. Report of 3 cases with special emphasis on its association with the syndrome of inappropriate secretion of antidiuretic hormone. Am J Clin Pathol 108: 537–543
50. Kenney P J, Stanley R J 1987 Calcified adrenal masses. Urol Radiol 9: 9–15
51. Hachitanda Y, Tsuneyoshi M 1994 Neuroblastoma with a distinct organoid pattern: a clinicopathologic, immunohistochemical and ultrastructural study. Hum Pathol 25: 67–72
52. Tornoczky T, Kalman E, Kajtar P G et al. 2003 Large cell neuroblastoma. A distinct phenotype of neuroblastoma with aggressive clinical behavior. Cancer 100: 390–397
53. Cozzutto C, Carbone A 1988 Pleomorphic (anaplastic) neuroblastoma. Arch Pathol Lab Med 112: 621–625
54. Joshi V V, Silverman J F, Altshuler G et al. 1993 Systemization of primary histopathologic and fine-needle aspiration cytologic features and description of unusual histopathological features of neuroblastic tumors: a report from the Pediatric Oncology Group. Hum Pathol 24: 493–504
55. Adam A, Hochholzer L 1981 Ganglioneuroblastoma of the posterior mediastinum. Cancer 47: 373–381
56. Stout A P 1947 Ganglioneuroma of the sympathetic nervous system. Surg Gynecol Obstet 84: 101–110
57. Bove K E, McAdams A J 1981 Composite ganglioneuroblastoma. An assessment of the significance of histologic maturation in neuroblastoma diagnosed beyond infancy. Arch Pathol Lab Med 105: 325–330
58. Aoyama C, Qualman S J, Regan M et al. 1990 Histopathologic features of composite ganglioneuroblastoma. Immunohistochemical distinction of the stromal component is related to prognosis. Cancer 65: 255–264
59. Mullins J D 1980 A pigmented differentiating neuroblastoma. A light and ultrastructural study. Cancer 46: 522–528
60. Joshi V V, Cantor A B, Altshuler G et al. 1996 Conventional versus modified morphologic criteria for ganglioneuroblastoma. A review of cases from the Pediatric Oncology Group. Arch Pathol Lab Med 120: 859–865
61. Shimada H, Chatten J, Newton W A Jr et al. 1984 Histopathologic prognostic factors in neuroblastic tumors: definition of subtypes of ganglioneuroblastoma and an age-linked classification of neuroblastomas. J Natl Cancer Inst 73: 405–416
62. Chatten J, Shimada H, Sather H N et al. 1988 Prognostic value of histopathology in advanced neuroblastoma: a report from the Children's Cancer Study Group. Hum Pathol 19: 1187–1198
63. Joshi V V, Chatten J, Sather H N et al. 1991 Evaluation of the Shimada classification in advanced neuroblastoma with a special reference to the mitosis-karyorrhexis index: a report from the Children's Cancer Study Group. Mod Pathol 4: 139–147
64. Dehner L P 1988 Classic neuroblastoma: histopathologic grading as a prognostic indicator. The Shimada system and its progenitors. Am J Pediatr Hematol Oncol 10: 143–154
65. Hachitanda Y, Hata J-I 1996 Stage IVS neuroblastoma: a clinical, histological and biological analysis of 45 cases. Hum Pathol 27: 1135–1138
66. Joshi V V, Cantor A B, Altshuler G et al. 1992 Age-linked prognostic categorization based on a new histologic grading system of neuroblastoma. Cancer 69: 2197–2211
67. Joshi V V, Rao P V, Cantor A B et al. 1996 Modified histologic grading of neuroblastomas by replacement of mitotic rate with mitosis karyorrhexis index. A clinicopathologic study of 223 cases from the Pediatric Oncology Group. Cancer 77: 1582–1588
68. Shimada H, Ambros I M, Dehner L P et al. 1999 Terminology and morphologic criteria of neuroblastic tumors. Recommendations by the International Neuroblastoma Pathology Committee. Cancer 86: 349–363
69. Shimada H, Ambros I M, Dehner L P et al. 1999 The International Neuroblastoma Pathology Classification (the Shimada system). Cancer 86: 364–372
70. Shimada H, Umehara S, Monobe Y et al. 2001 International Neuroblastoma Pathology classification for prognostic evaluation of patients with peripheral neuroblastic tumors. A report from the Children's Cancer Group. Cancer 92: 2451–2461

71. Umehara S, Nakagawa A, Matthay K K et al. 2000 Histopathology defines prognostic subsets of ganglioneuroblastoma, nodular. A report from the Children's Cancer Group. Cancer 89: 1150–116
72. Peuchmour M, d'Amore E S G, Joshi V et al. 2003 Revision of the International Neuroblastoma Pathology Classification. Confirmation of favorable and unfavorable prognostic subsets in ganglioneuroblastoma, nodular. Cancer 98: 2274–2281
73. Raetz E A, Kim M K H, Moos P et al. 2003 Identification of genes that are regulated transcriptionally by *Myc* in childhood tumors. Cancer 98: 841–853
74. Brodeur G M, Seeger R C, Schwab M et al. 1984 Amplification of *N-myc* in untreated human neuroblastomas correlates with advanced disease stage. Science 224: 1121–1124
75. Goto S, Umehara S, Gerbing R B et al. 2001 Histopathology (International Neuroblastoma Pathology classification) and MYCN status in patients with peripheral neuroblastic tumors. A report from the Children's Cancer Group. Cancer 92: 2699–2708
76. Taylor C P, McGuckin A G, Bown N P et al. 1994 Rapid detection of prognostic genetic factors in neuroblastomas using fluorescence in situ hybridization on tumour imprints and bone marrow smears. United Kingdom Children's Cancer Study. Br J Cancer 69: 445–451
77. Caron H, Von Sluis P, de Kraker J et al. 1996 Allelic loss of chromosome 1p as a predictor of unfavorable outcome in patients with neuroblastoma. N Engl J Med 334: 225–230
77a. Attiyeh E F, London W B, Mosse Y P et al. 2005 Chromosome 1p and 11q deletions and outcome in neuroblastoma. N Engl J Med 353: 2243–2253
78. Triche T J 1990 Differential diagnosis of neuroblastoma and related tumors. In: Lack E E (ed) Pathology of the adrenal glands. Churchill Livingstone, New York, p 323–350
79. Fletcher C D M, Fernando I N, Braimbridge M V et al. 1988 Malignant nerve sheath tumour arising in a ganglioneuroma. Histopathology 12: 445–448
80. Ricci A Jr, Callihan T, Parham D M et al. 1984 Malignant peripheral nerve sheath tumors arising from ganglioneuromas. Am J Surg Pathol 8: 19–29
81. Aguirre P, Scully R E 1983 Testosterone-secreting adrenal ganglioneuroma containing Leydig cells. Am J Surg Pathol 7: 699–705

眼和眼附属器肿瘤
Tumors of the eye and ocular adnexa

Robert Folberg 著

回允中　韩桂萍 译

眼睑和眼周皮肤肿瘤	1781	眼眶肿瘤	1797
结膜肿瘤	1788	视神经的原发性肿瘤	1799
泪液排泄系统肿瘤	1796	眼内肿瘤	1801

评估眼和眼附属器的肿瘤性病变时，外科病理医生常常面临挑战。多数病理医生习惯于将其注意力集中于指导治疗的诊断和预后特征上。眼和眼附属器肿瘤的诊断还有额外的要求：病理医生还必须提供有助于外科医生保护视力的信息，这是治疗的目的，可能与肿瘤治疗本身同样重要。对于多数患者来说，惧怕丧失视力至少与惧怕失去生命同样强烈。多数眼科医生的确遇到过这样的患者，"大夫，我宁愿死也不愿成为一个盲人！"

治疗恶性肿瘤时，眼外科医生需要保护患者的视力，因此要求病理医生应用标准程序对组织进行大体检查并给出病理学报告。例如，为了保护视力，眼恶性肿瘤周围正常组织的切除一般很少。因此，虽然眼睑基底细胞癌或结膜鳞状上皮异型增生的组织病理学诊断可能并不困难，但是要提供有关切缘的准确信息则可能具有挑战性。另外一个例子是，结膜黑色素瘤及其前体病变的分类与皮肤黑色瘤不同[1,2]，这不是因为眼科病理医生培训不足，而是因为用于结膜的分类可以帮助眼科医生进行临床鉴别诊断和处理这些病变[3]。

在眼内和眼周，外科病理医生还可能见到熟悉的肿瘤，但是伴有不熟悉的行为。例如，在皮肤黑色素瘤，伴有大量淋巴细胞浸润的病例预后较好[4]，但在葡萄膜黑色素瘤，同样所见预后却不好[5,6]。皮肤和结膜黑色素瘤均来源于上皮成分，而葡萄膜黑色素瘤却来源于间叶成分，即脉络膜、睫状体和虹膜，因此，葡萄膜没有相对应的原位黑色素瘤。

有些肿瘤在普通外科病理学中很少遇到，但是如果病理医生为医务繁忙的眼科医生服务，却常常能够见到。眼睑含有人体内高度集中的皮脂腺，在我们的实验室中，皮脂腺癌比鳞状细胞癌常见得多。因此，提示眼睑Bowen样日光性角化症诊断的病理学变化，可能是皮脂腺癌的Paget样上皮内分布。

许多眼眶和眼睑肿瘤在本书其他章节讨论。本章集中讨论的是眼及其附属器的特有肿瘤，或那些病理医生在描述所见时需要考虑的对视力以及寿命有影响的肿瘤。本章是根据解剖部位组织编写的。每一个解剖部位的引言部分提供有关功能解剖的信息，以便病理医生了解理论基础，以便了解所用的切除技术。这种信息还能帮助病理医生进行大体组织检查，这是组织检查的第一步。

虽然多数眼部肿瘤的发生没有性别差异，但是这些肿瘤却有特殊的年龄分布。无论病理医生喜欢在阅读切片之前核对临床资料，还是喜欢"不偏不倚"地进行组织病理学鉴别诊断，最后的报告必须反映"确实核对"了临床状况。本章在讨论特殊类型的肿瘤时，讨论了眼部肿瘤的组织学鉴别诊断的陷阱，以及病理医生通过其病理报告可为眼外科医生治疗提供指导的技术。

眼睑和眼周皮肤肿瘤
Tumors of the eyelid and periocular skin

引言

眼睑的主要功能是保护角膜。肿瘤或手术干预造成的眼睑变形可能导致眼睑闭合不全、疼痛性角膜暴露及角膜感染和溃疡形成。

眼睑皮肤和沿着鼻梁内眦部位的邻近皮肤是不带毛发的（光秃的）皮肤。因此，大块切除眼睑的皮肤必须用对侧眼睑组织取代（例如，切除大量下睑组织可能需要从同一只眼的上睑"借用"组织），或用锁骨上或耳后皮肤做皮肤移植。大量切除眼睑组织和眼睑周围组织可能需要小心的重建，因此，眼科成形外科医生倾向于在切除肿瘤的同时，尽量减少病变周围正常组织的切除。

所幸的是，外科医生几乎能够切除下睑的 1/3 并无需植皮而达到保留原来闭合功能的目的。通过切断外侧眦韧带（一种普通的手术操作），外科医生也几乎能够切除下睑的 1/2 而可以保留原来的闭合功能。这个信息可能有助于引导病理医生和外科医生之间讨论有关伴有阳性切缘的肿瘤切除的管理问题。

多数眼睑肿瘤始发于眼睑的黏膜皮肤交界处（图 29.1）。眼睑的真皮只含有疏松排列的胶原，眼睑没有类似的网状真皮。而且，眼睑没有皮下脂肪。如果病理医生在眼睑的活检标本中见到了脂肪组织，则此脂肪组织或者是通过筋膜面（眼眶分隔）缺陷脱垂而来，或者是手术（和肿瘤）已经穿透了眼眶分隔，后者是分隔眼睑和眼眶的解剖学"防火墙"。眼睑内有顶浆分泌腺，可引起相对常见的单纯性囊肿（顶浆分泌腺汗腺囊瘤，apocrine hidrocystomas），或在少数情况下引起恶性肿瘤，包括黏液癌（mucinous carinoma）（图 29.2 和 29.3），一种局部浸润性肿瘤，很少转移，但是由于有局部浸润而需要完全切除[7]。接近眼睑的边缘可见皮脂腺，与睫毛（睑缘腺，Zeis gland）有关，或在睑板内（睑板腺，Meibomian gland）。皮脂腺癌可能来源于睑缘腺或睑板腺（图 29.4）。

泪点位于上下眼睑的内眦附近。眼泪是由埋在眼睑内的附属泪腺（类似于颊黏膜内的小涎腺，主泪腺对疼痛和情绪激动产生反应）连续分泌形成的，眼泪汇集在泪点，后者是一个隆起的小凹，通过泪管引流。手术可能损伤上睑的泪点，这对患者没有太多的影响，但是如果损伤了下睑的泪点或两个眼睑的泪点，则可能导致眼泪溢出到眼周组织。溢泪（epiphora）可令患者非常烦恼，可能妨碍他们的工作和娱乐活动。眼外科医生在切除肿瘤时应尽量避免损伤泪点和泪管。因此，在大体和镜下检查眼睑组织时，外科病理医生应该确认是否存在泪点和泪管（图 29.5 和 29.6）。

临床状况　Clinical context

虽然基底细胞癌、鳞状细胞癌和黑色素瘤可以发生在儿童期和年轻成人的眼睑，但在特别少见的情况下，这些眼睑肿瘤也可以发生在成人，例如着色性干皮病。因此，在儿童眼睑见到类似鳞状细胞癌的病变，在组织学上应该与假上皮瘤性增生（pseudoepitheliomatous hyperplasia）进行鉴别诊断。

这也有助于理解：虽然基底细胞癌是最常见的眼睑恶性肿瘤（倾向于发生在阳光暴露的下睑和内眦），眼睑鳞状细胞癌却可能比皮脂腺癌少见得多，这一点将在下面详细讨论。

眼睑肿瘤的大体检查
Gross examination of eyelid neoplasms

近年来，眼科医生一直被鼓励将眼周皮肤恶性肿瘤的患者转给皮肤外科医生进行 Mohs 显微外科手术[8-11]。这种手术的基本原理是基于接受了以下观

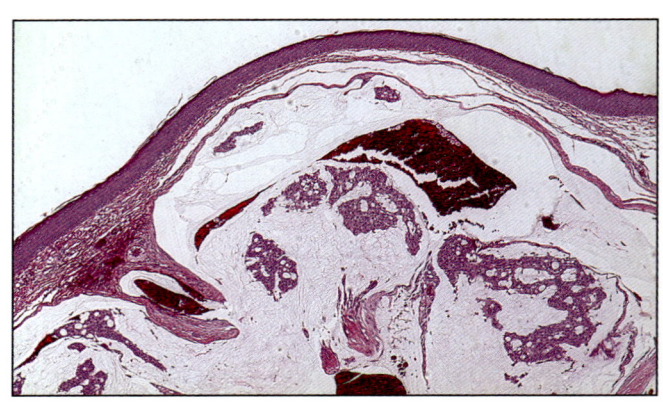

图 29.2　眼睑原发性黏液癌的低倍放大图像。注意肿瘤细胞明显地漂浮在黏液池中。

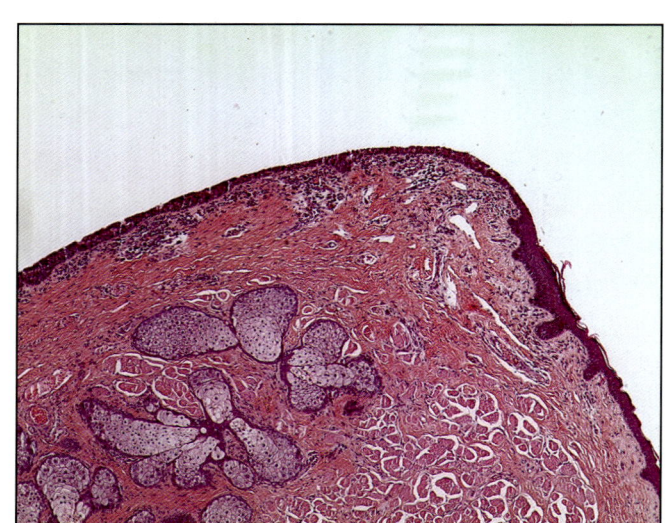

图 29.1　这幅显微照片显示了眼睑的黏膜皮肤边缘。因为多数眼睑肿瘤发生在此部位，当评估全层眼睑切除标本的边缘时，病理医生必须检查包括这个移行带在内的组织切片。注意正常眼睑皮肤缺乏皮下脂肪。

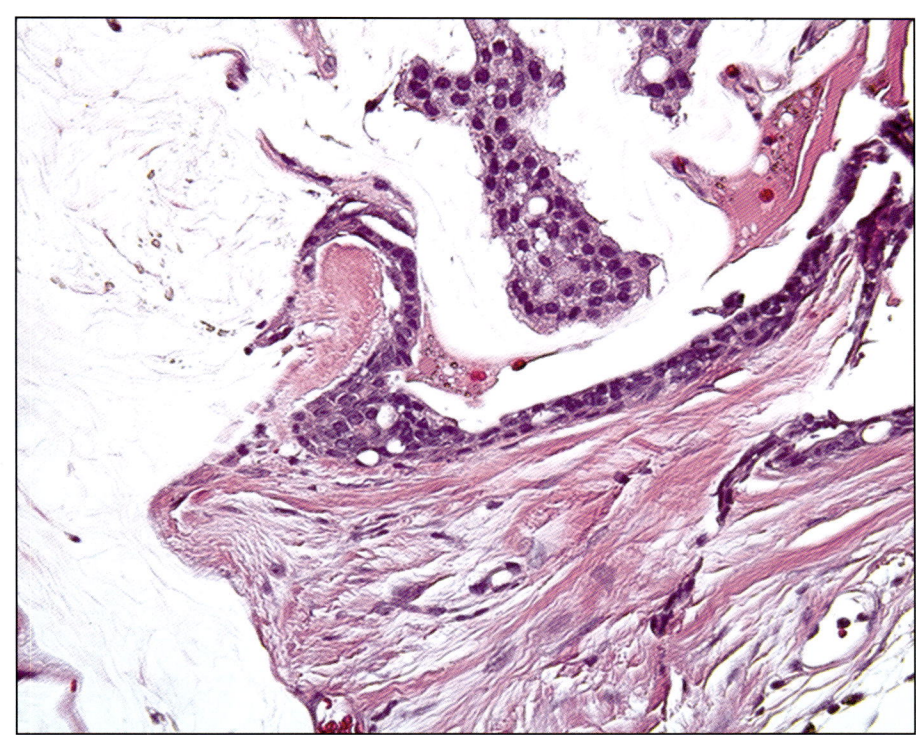

图29.3 为图29.2的高倍显微照片。一些肿瘤细胞衬附在增厚的胶原性小梁上。

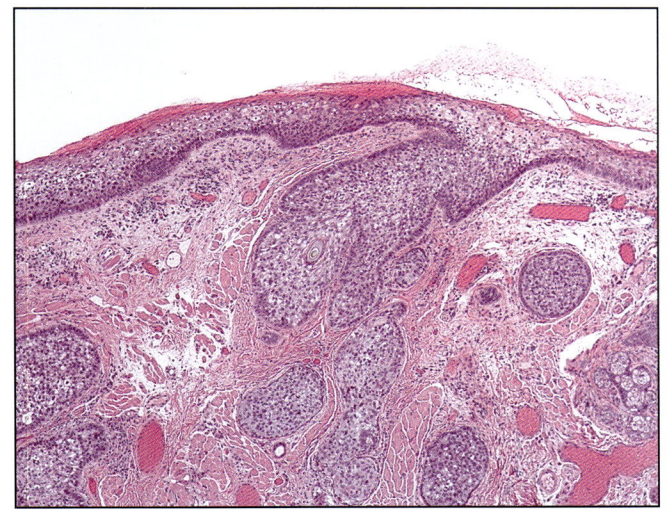

图29.4 来源于睑缘腺的皮脂腺癌，伴有一个睫毛。表皮增厚且结构紊乱，继发于肿瘤细胞的弥漫性Paget样生长。

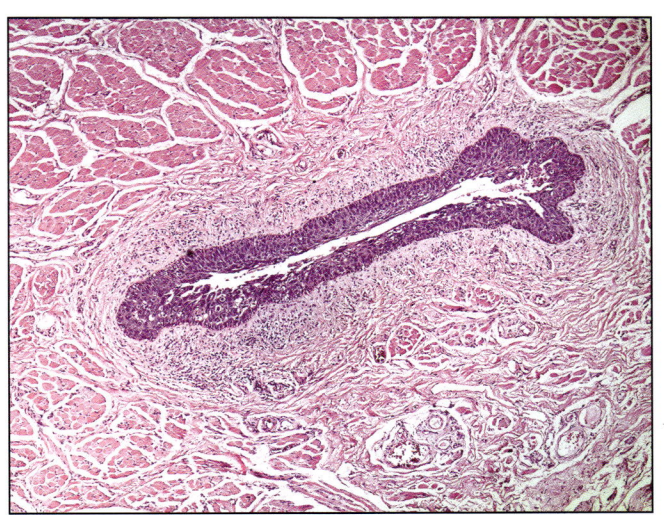

图29.5 泪管的低倍放大图像。正常泪管内衬非角化性复层鳞状上皮。在这张组织切片中，上皮的增厚和结构紊乱是由皮脂腺癌向泪管的Paget样扩散引起的。

点：在冰冻切片控制下切除眼周恶性肿瘤具有优点，可使切除的组织数量减少到最少。而一些眼成形外科医生认为，对患者而言，进行Mohs手术的外科医生与进行重建手术的外科医生不同才是最主要的，因为手术外科医生为了便于术后重建，恐怕会在切除组织的数量上做出妥协。最后，主张由Mohs外科医生切除肿瘤的人认为，这是唯一能够将整个切缘取样的技术。

病理医生需要知道这样一个事实，Mohs外科医生应用的切除眼睑边缘肿瘤的技术与眼科手术医生没有不同。因此，多数眼科医生有资格进行大多数眼睑肿瘤的切除和眼睑闭合手术。许多眼科医生坚持应用冰冻切片控制眼睑切缘的小肿瘤。因为手术技术涉及切除五边形的眼睑组织（图29.7），眼科医生可能需要检查每一个切面的四个切缘。几乎没有眼科医生了解做四张冰冻切

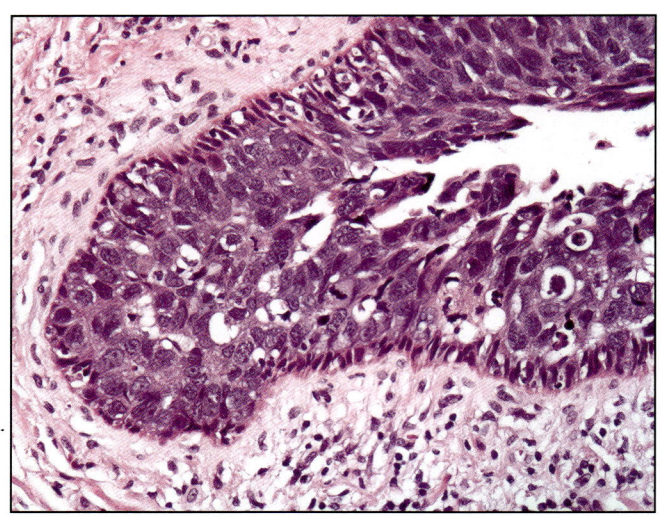

图29.6 为图29.5的高倍放大图像,显示泪管的皮脂腺癌。核的模糊特征是上皮内皮脂腺癌的特征。

片所需的时间。一些外科医生会预约冰冻切片,以便按标准方式进行手术,但在得知病理医生的检查结果之前也可能试图继续进行重建手术,这种方式常常造成外科医生和病理医生之间的不快。

一般来说,多数睑缘的眼周肿瘤可以安全切除,可用固定后的组织检查切缘[12]。手术医生可能愿意先行关闭眼睑缺损,而如果关闭缺损之后切缘检查结果呈阳性,一般切除瘢痕可能足以除掉残余的显微镜下肿瘤。因此,不管是检查冰冻切片还是检查固定后的组织,大体检查眼睑切除标本的原则是类似的。

多数眼睑肿瘤来源于黏膜皮肤边缘或其附近。因此,病理医生取材必须取得平行于手术切缘的组织(图29.7)。两个侧切缘应该分别送检(标记内侧或外侧,分别相当于眼科术语中的鼻侧和颞侧)。一些眼科手术医生切取减缩肿块体积手术的层面,并分别送检切缘。在

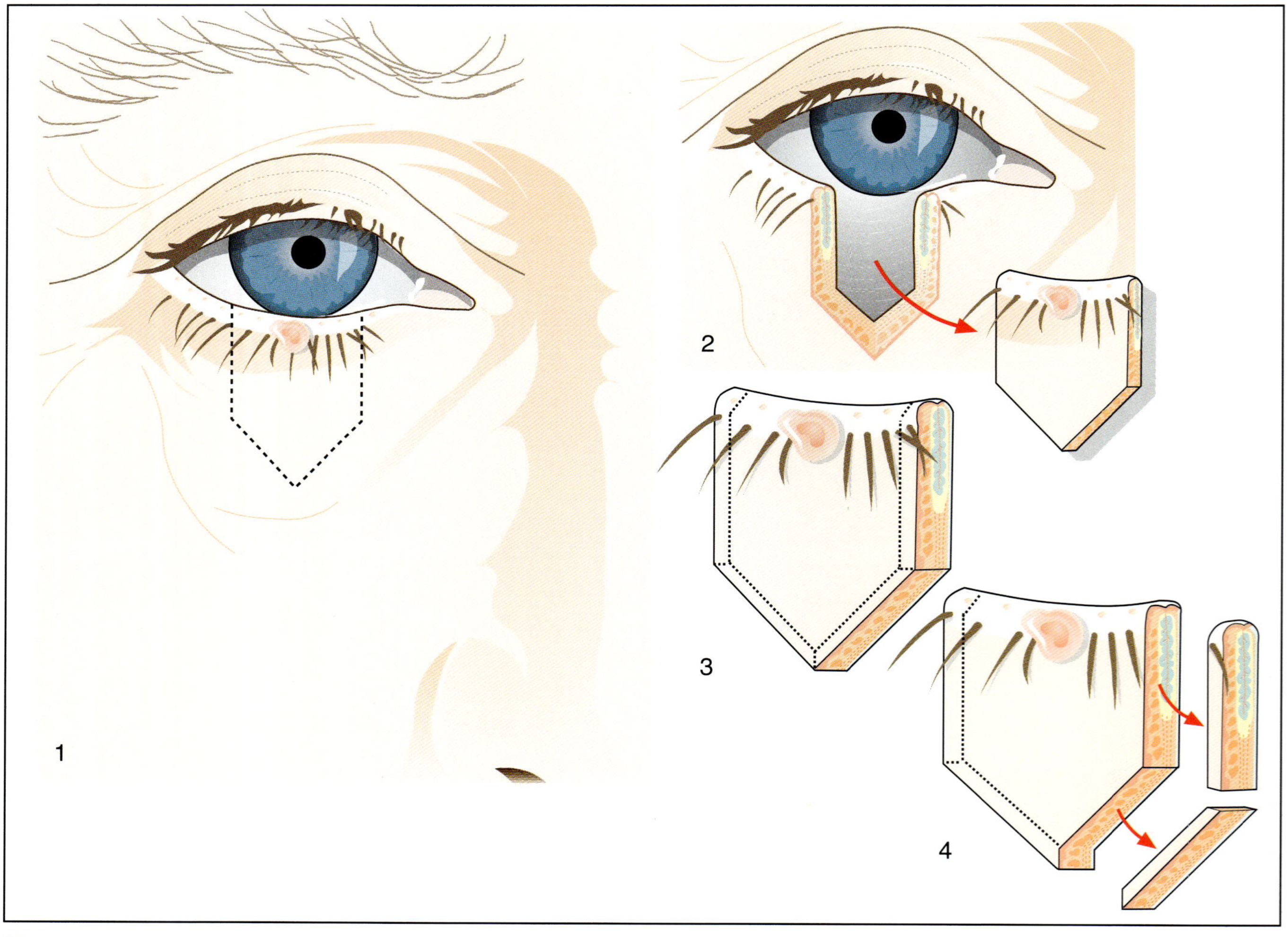

图29.7 图示睑缘肿瘤边缘取样步骤:(1)典型者切除一块五角形组织;(2)减缩肿块体积手术层面;(3)沿着四个切缘切除的一块组织,包括内缘、外缘和两个下缘。有些外科医生可能分别送检。如果分别送检的切缘没有包括减缩肿块体积手术层面,病理医生应该自行解剖这些切缘(3~4)。

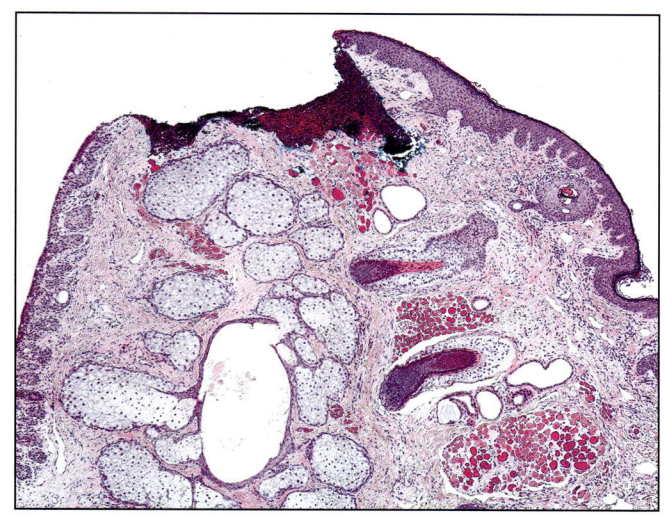

图29.8 在这张显微照片中,外科医生清除了眼睑黏膜皮肤交界,这个部位出现血液即可证明。有些时候,切片中可能没有黏膜皮肤交界,因为切片机没能切到包埋组织块中的这个重要部位。在这种情况下,应该要求组织学技术人员重新包埋或深切,直到可以见到黏膜皮肤交界并能评估。

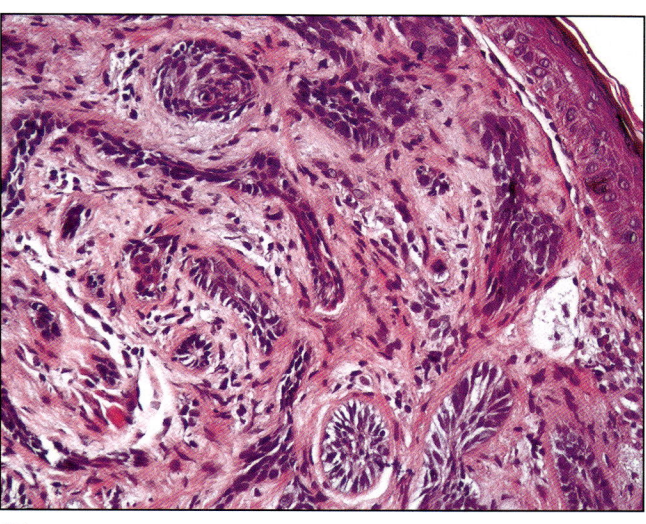

图29.9 基底细胞癌,硬化型。注意显著的胶原束之间有陷入的纤细的肿瘤条带。

做眼睑肿瘤的组织学切面时,不要使用常用于椭圆形皮肤癌的十字形取样方法。

重要的是,组织学切片应该包括眼睑的黏膜皮肤交界处。包埋组织块不正确可能导致重要标志取样不完全(图29.8),需要重新包埋并另取切面。

眼睑肿瘤对外科病理医生的重要性

外科病理医生熟悉多数眼睑肿瘤,并不需要特别考虑,因为它们累及眼周皮肤。然而,有些眼睑肿瘤在此值得特别提出。

基底细胞癌 Basal cell carcinoma

基底细胞癌的组织学诊断很少出问题。然而,当纤细的肿瘤条索陷入增厚的胶原束时(图29.9)——硬化型基底细胞癌(有时称为硬斑性基底细胞癌,morpheic basal cell carcinoma),病理医生在诊断时应该注意这种特征,或在病理学报告中加以评注。对于外科医生来说,通过临床检查确定肿瘤累及眼睑和眼周皮肤的范围可能非常困难。病理医生做出硬化性基底细胞癌诊断时,可能会促使手术医生广泛切除或在冰冻切片控制下切除,此时完全有理由应用冰冻切片。

皮脂腺癌 Sebaceous carcinoma

皮脂腺癌或者来源于睑缘腺,或者来源于睑板腺(图29.4)。临床上这些肿瘤可表现为散在的肿块(常常酷似一个睑板腺囊肿,一种局灶性脂质肉芽肿性炎症),或伴有弥漫的眼睑受累(常常酷似眼睑炎,blepharitis)。因此,许多眼科医生会给病理医生送检复发性睑板腺囊肿的标本,以"除外皮脂腺癌"的临床诊断;许多眼科医生还会怀疑伴有单侧眼睑增厚和睫毛丧失的患者有浸润性皮脂腺癌,典型的眼睑炎是一种双侧性的病变。

组织学检查,结节性皮脂腺癌类似于各种其他癌,甚至类似于某些良性病变[13]。典型的肿瘤小叶含有伴有泡沫样胞浆的细胞,胞浆空泡一般较小(图29.10)。肿瘤细胞核一般呈强嗜碱性,而且可能"模糊"。可以见到许多非典型性核分裂象。胞浆内空泡形成可能非常细微,小叶周围细胞集聚可能造成一种基底细胞癌的印象[14]。中心可以见到坏死区(粉刺形态)。在个别情况下,皮脂腺癌组织学上可能类似Merkel细胞瘤。有些肿瘤可见鳞状分化(图29.11),如果这种特征明显,病理医生可能会不加怀疑地将其错误诊断为鳞状细胞癌。虽然鳞状细胞癌的确可以发生在眼睑,但是在这个部位皮脂腺癌比较常见,认识到这一点可能有助于诊断。

几位研究者试图找出免疫组化谱,以区分皮脂腺癌与组织学检查类似于皮脂腺癌的其他肿瘤[15-17]。虽然通过免疫组化检查可以将部分病例区分开来,但是这些免疫组化标记物的敏感性和特异性尚不足以准确作出诊断,特别是对活检存在问题的患者。病理医生常常要求眼科医生提供新鲜组织进行油红O染色,以证实脂肪的

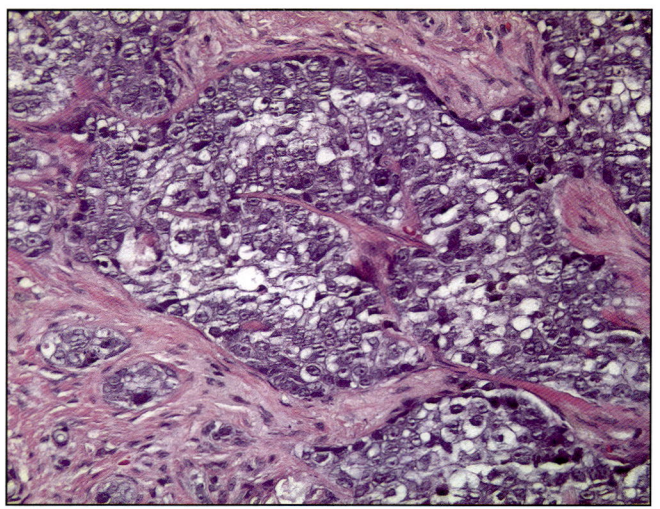

图29.10　皮脂腺癌，伴有典型的胞浆空泡形成。

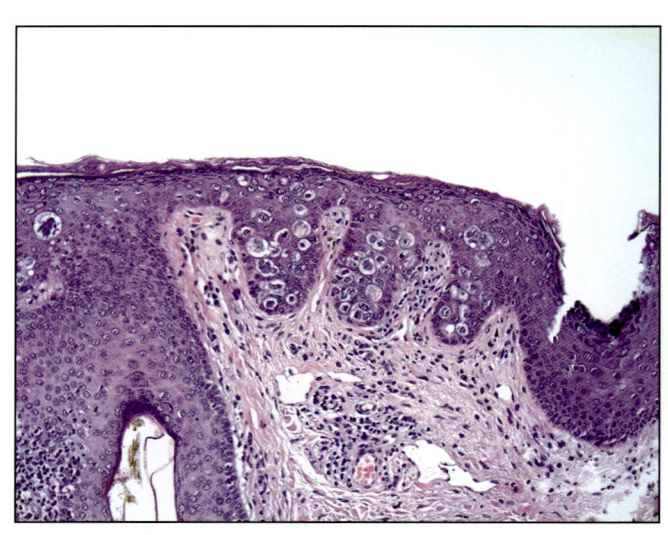

图29.12　上皮内皮脂腺癌。肿瘤呈显著的Paget样扩散。注意胞浆"透明"，这是典型的皮脂腺癌。

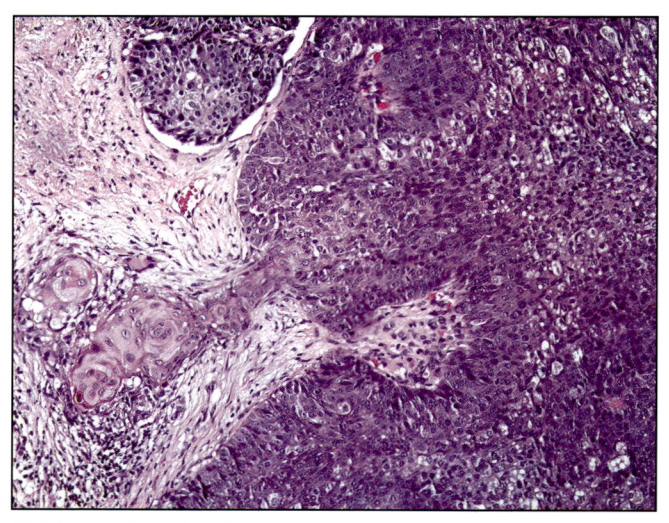

图29.11　皮脂腺癌伴有局灶性鳞状分化。皮脂腺癌可以类似各种皮肤肿瘤，包括基底细胞癌。

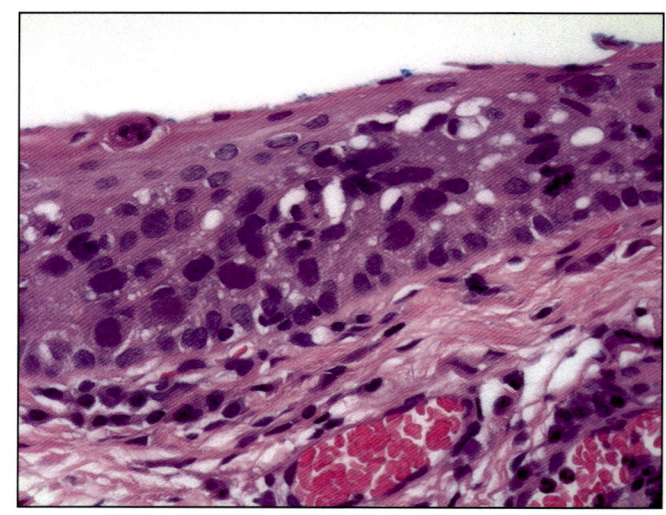

图29.13　结膜上皮内皮脂腺癌。虽然组织学可能提示鳞状上皮异型增生，出现胞浆空泡形成却是皮脂腺癌的特征。核的多形性程度以及核"模糊"对皮脂腺比对鳞状肿瘤形成更具特征性。

存在，为此目的，甚至可能坚持应用冰冻切片。一般来说，并不需要应用冰冻切片证实脂质，这在下面讨论，而且应用冰冻切片检查皮脂腺癌的边缘可能也无助于处理患者。

皮脂腺癌最具有挑战性的诊断问题或许是通过眼睑上皮（表皮和结膜上皮）弥漫扩散的肿瘤病例的诊断问题[18]。由于出现表皮内Paget样扩散（图29.12），病理医生在鉴别诊断时可能会考虑黑色素瘤，但是眼睑的原发性黑色素瘤非常少见，特别是浅表扩散性黑色素瘤。同上面提到的一样，通过表皮的Paget样扩散可能类似于Bowen样型日光性角化症，病理医生在鉴别诊断时开始可能考虑此病，值得牢记的是，沿着睑缘发生的皮脂腺癌比日光性角化症常见。

正常结膜表面缺乏角化层，皮脂腺癌可取代结膜上皮全层，以致被认为是见于表皮的Paget样扩散，而且可能见到比较类似于鳞状上皮异型增生或原位癌的形态（图29.13）。结膜上皮内皮脂腺癌与鳞状上皮内肿瘤形成有可能区分：上皮内皮脂腺癌的细胞一般为非粘着性的，彼此分开。虽然这种组织学特征可能与棘层松解性鳞状上皮异型增生和原位癌混淆，但是如果细胞具有轻微的胞浆内空泡形成以及呈强嗜碱性和有"模糊"的细胞核，则倾向于皮脂腺癌的诊断。结膜表皮被皮脂腺癌取代还可能类似乳头状结膜炎（图 29.14）。

被皮脂腺癌弥漫浸润的结膜上皮常常与基底膜分开（类似于眼瘢痕性类天疱疮的表皮下大疱）或脱落（图 29.15）。因为上皮下结缔组织的非特异性炎症常常伴随上皮内皮脂腺癌，免疫荧光检查可能发现免疫球蛋白和补体沉积。这样，当眼科医生取结膜活检以除外眼瘢痕性类天疱疮（ocular cicatricial pemphigoid）时，应该同时送检固定在甲醛溶液中的结膜组织以除外皮脂腺癌，并送检第二块组织进行免疫荧光检查。

皮脂腺癌浸润的结膜上皮可脱落，或者仅留下少数基底细胞粘连在基底膜上，呈"墓碑状"结构，或者显示一个剥光的基底膜。这样，在检查眼睑边缘时，病理医生应将眼睑上皮没有内衬这一特征记录在病理报告中，并附加一个评注，在综合诊断皮脂腺癌的情况下，缺乏上皮很可能代表此部位受累。

皮脂腺癌可通过眼睑扩散，并向下达到泪点进入泪管（图 29.5 和 29.6）、泪囊和鼻旁窦。皮脂腺癌还可通过结膜上皮扩散到泪腺小管，而后逆行进入眼眶。皮脂腺癌可以在睑板内的多个部位发生，形成"跳跃性病变"。因此，检查不存在 Paget 样扩散的眼睑结节性皮脂腺癌的切除标本时，病理医生可能需要评估切缘是否充分。然而，在有 Paget 样扩散的情况下，病理医生仍应小心，应该在报告中评估有关上皮剥落的区域，此处切缘可能为阳性，而且应该引起眼科医生的注意：有跳跃性病变的可能性，因此，"干净的"切缘可能并不是肿瘤扩散范围的限度。

有人建议，评估皮脂腺癌切除标本时，病理学报告中还应该特别提到一些组织学特征[19]。这些特征见表 29.1。与预后不好有关的组织学特征包括：肿瘤直径大于 10 mm，有 Paget 样扩散，有血管、淋巴管和眼眶软组织浸润，同时累及上下眼睑，分化不好，以及多中心性来源[13]。皮脂腺癌倾向于首先扩散到眼睑的局部淋巴结，即耳旁和颌下淋巴结。

治疗皮脂腺癌需要将肿瘤的浸润性和上皮内成分全部切除。为了测定疾病的整个范围，除了眼睑活检外，眼科手术医生还应该在结膜的多个部位取小的活检标本（"定位活检"，map biopsies）。如果结膜有上皮内肿瘤，眼科医生可切除眼睑肿瘤，并可选择应用滴眼药（丝裂霉素 C，Mitomycin C）对结膜病变进行化学治疗。

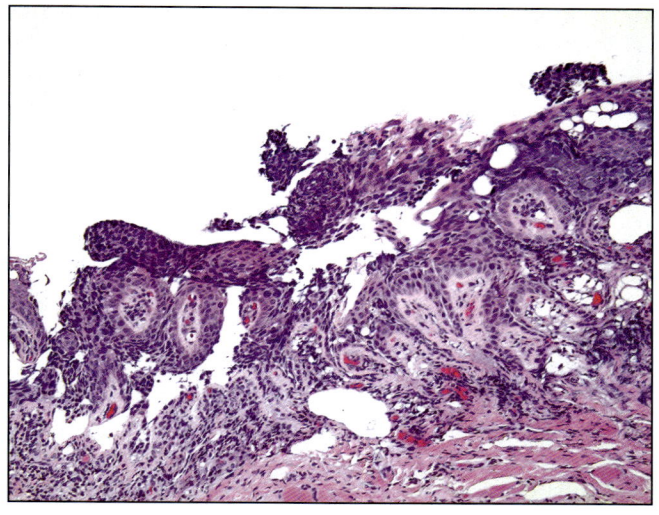

图29.14　上皮被皮脂腺癌弥漫性取代。肿瘤的乳头状生长方式在组织学上和临床上均有可能被误诊为乳头状结膜炎。

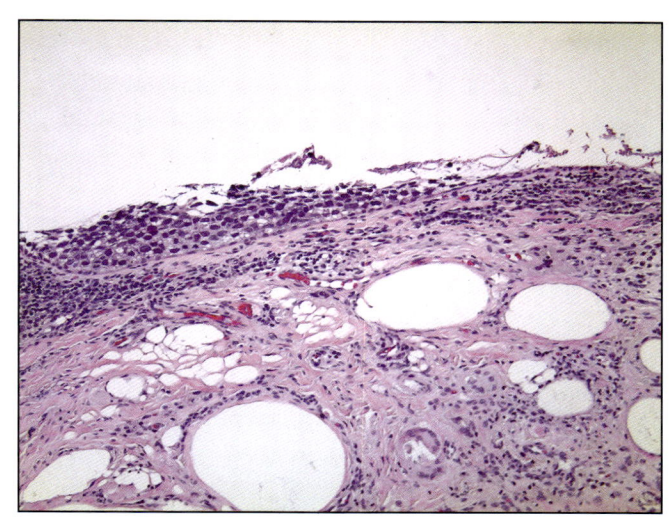

图29.15　在显微照片左侧，上皮增厚且结构紊乱，这是皮脂腺癌的特征。在显微照片右侧，上皮已经脱落。如果整个活检显示上皮脱落，则可能做出眼瘢痕性类天疱疮的诊断，临床上酷似皮脂腺癌。在临床怀疑皮脂腺癌的情况下，如果缺乏结膜上皮，在组织学诊断时应该慎重。

即使是在固定最好的石蜡包埋组织中，诊断肿瘤向表皮内和结膜上皮内扩散也是非常困难的，因此冰冻切片检测肿瘤边缘更具有挑战性。对于保证完全切除肿瘤，冰冻切片检测皮脂腺癌的边缘可能并不是一种可靠的方法[20]，因此有人提倡应用 Mohs 显微外科手术治疗这种肿瘤[21,22]。

表29.1	推荐报告的皮脂腺癌组织学特征
组织学特征	评注
肿瘤部位（上睑还是下睑）	一些病理医生认为，上睑肿瘤与侵袭性较强的临床经过有关
结节性成分（如果存在）的大小，mm	一些病理医生认为，这种测量是选择性的
腺体的来源	睑缘腺、睑板腺或两者。来源于睑缘腺的肿瘤常常伴有Paget样扩散
是否有浸润性生长方式或粉刺样坏死形态	这两种特征均与侵袭性临床经过有关
分化	
多中心程度	
Paget样扩散	
淋巴管受累	
脂肪组织受累	这种所见提示，肿瘤浸润眼眶，一种可能导致眶内容摘除的特征
切缘受累	切除的结膜缺乏上皮可能表示上皮已经被脱落的肿瘤细胞取代。这样的切缘可以解释为"阳性"，尽管缺乏上皮

Modified from Folberg et al.[19]

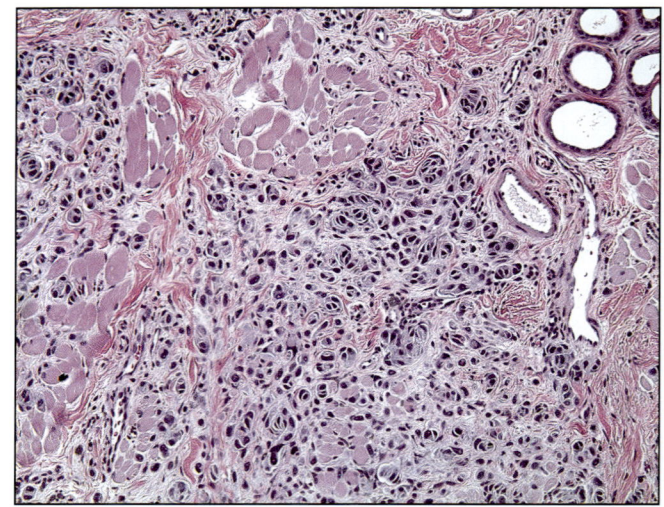

图29.16 眼睑部的小的先天性痣。眼环状骨骼肌附近和结膜睫腺（glands of Moll）（右上）附近可见痣细胞。

义无关紧要（图 29.16）。睑缘黑色素瘤不伴结膜受累者非常少见[24]。这些病变较典型的是伴有结膜黑色素瘤或结膜黑色素瘤前体病变，将在下面讨论。因为眼睑真皮没有乳头和网状结构，且这个部位没有皮下脂肪层，所以在这个部位难以应用黑色素瘤的 Clark 分级标准，病理学报告应该根据 Breslow 提出的方法判断浸润深度。

结膜肿瘤 Tumors of the conjunctiva

引言和大体检查

正常结膜的组织学随着其在眼的局部解剖部位的不同而不同。重要的是，外科病理医生要根据局部解剖部位正确评价结膜表现的差异。本章作者回想起一个会诊病例，当时病理医生错误地将正常的结膜穹窿诊断为结膜异型增生，结果导致了广泛而不必要的组织切除。

眼睑内面的结膜为睑结膜，其特征为伴有杯状细胞的假复层柱状上皮。睑结膜与其下的睑板关系非常紧密（图 29.17）。因此，睑结膜的黑色素细胞病变在临床上可以是扁平的，尽管可以向深部侵犯到眼睑的纤维性间质。相反，结膜穹窿的上皮下胶原排列疏松，在水肿的情况下，这种组织可以膨胀。穹窿上皮也是假复层柱状上皮，含大量杯状细胞（图 29.18）。副泪腺存在于穹窿和上下眼睑睑板的顶端，主泪腺的小管从上面和外侧穿入穹窿。正常情况下，穹窿有黏膜相关的淋巴组织集聚。杯状细胞散在分布于整个球结膜，球结膜是覆盖眼球的结膜，实际上正常角膜缘没有杯状细胞，角膜缘是角膜

眼睑痣和黑色素瘤
Nevi and melanomas of the eyelid

痣常出现在睑缘，一般通过削刮活检切除。痣可能在削刮活检部位复发，眼睑复发痣的组织学表现可能令人担忧，但是这种病变的生物学行为是良性的[23]。小的先天性痣的组织学证据可在睑板相当深的实质内发现，这种特征可能会进一步引起焦虑，尽管它的预后意

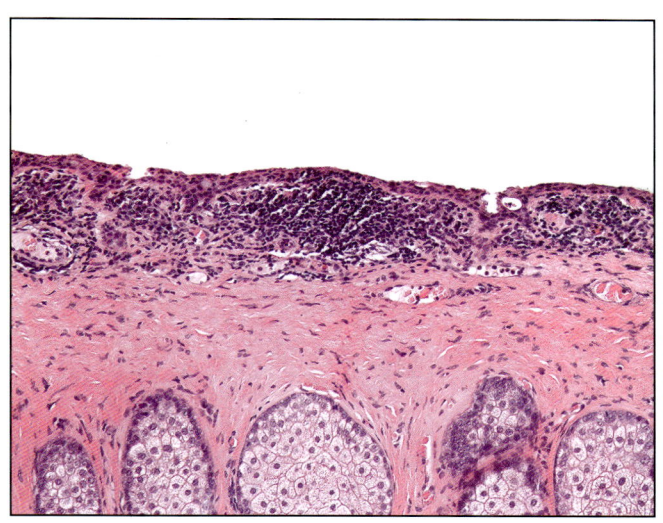

图29.17 睑结膜。注意上皮内出现杯状细胞。正常情况下,这个部位的上皮下存在淋巴细胞。注意在睑板致密排列的纤维结缔组织中含有睑板腺（Meibomian glands）。

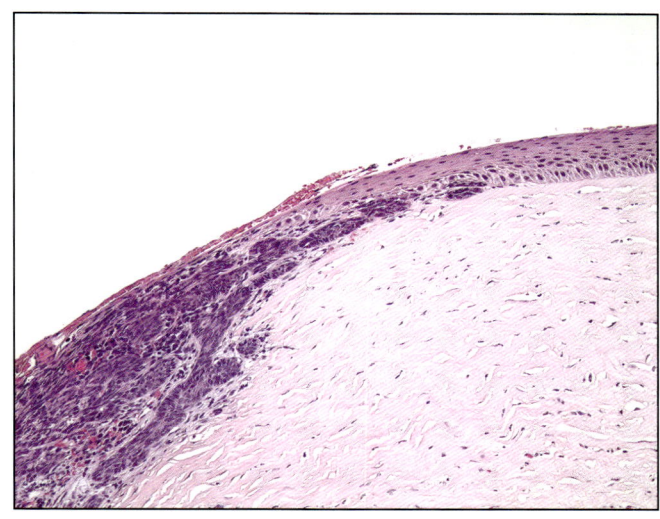

图29.19 角膜缘。在这张显微照片中,基底细胞癌已经侵及眼的表面（左侧）。注意上皮下肿瘤残留,肿瘤侵犯角膜,没有侵犯间质。上皮下的Bowman层是一个薄的无细胞的结缔组织带,它是肿瘤穿入角膜间质的有效屏障。

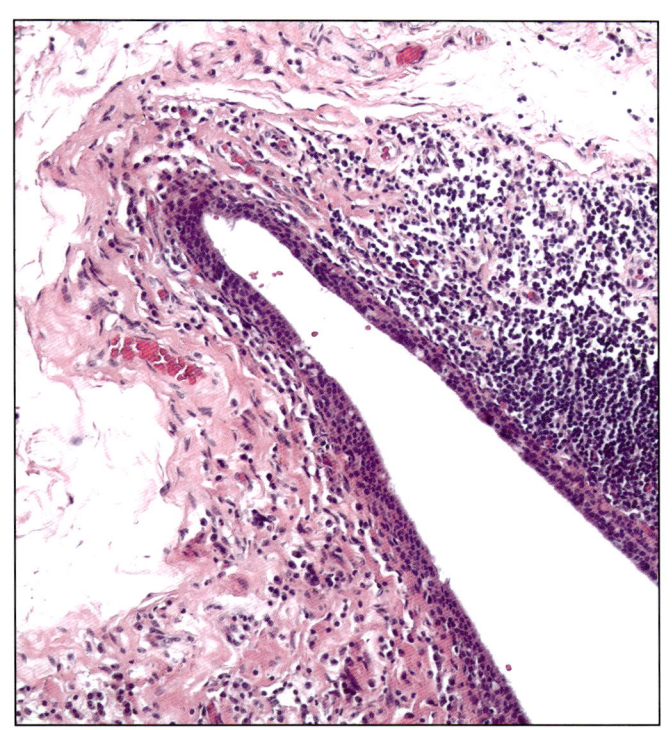

图29.18 结膜穹窿。上皮排列成假复层柱状结构,有许多杯状细胞。这个部位出现淋巴细胞是正常现象。

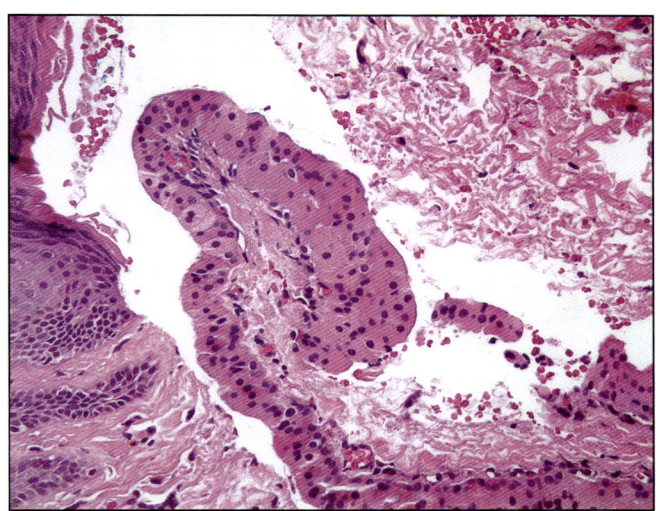

图29.20 结膜隆起的嗜酸细胞瘤。肿瘤来自正常存在于这个部位的顶浆分泌腺。

和巩膜的交界部位（图29.19）。

结膜隆起（conjunctival caruncle）和半月皱襞（plica semilunaris,为瞬膜在人类的类似结构）均位于结膜的内角,只有在组织学检查时才能发现。结膜隆起被覆非角化性鳞状上皮,常含有杯状细胞,但是上皮下结缔组织含有附件结构,如毛皮脂腺单位和汗腺。因此,结膜隆起的肿瘤可能不仅包括鳞状上皮乳头状瘤和癌、痣以及黑色素瘤,而且还包括皮脂腺瘤和皮脂腺癌（发生于结膜隆起的皮脂腺）以及发生于汗腺的嗜酸细胞瘤[25]（图29.20）。结膜半月皱襞有大量杯状细胞,这个部位的肿瘤与结膜其他部位的肿瘤相同。

不习惯检查眼科组织的外科病理医生无疑会对许多小的结膜活检感到困惑,甚至对许多侵袭性恶性肿瘤也是一样。鳞状细胞癌的切除活检，甚至黑色素瘤的切除活检，可包括最窄的边缘——或 1 mm 或更窄——在多数外科肿瘤学培训中，这样范围的癌周围正常组织切除被认为不够充分，边缘也不够安全。然而，眼科手术医生需要权衡，是完全切除结膜恶性肿瘤，还是保存结膜组织以维持眼表面的完整性和视力。较大的结膜切除，特别是涉及穹窿时，会减少杯状细胞的数量，从而损及表面黏液——对于眼泪中水的成分依附角膜上皮非常重要。经受大的结膜切除手术的患者多半患有眼干——严重时可疼痛，并且好发角膜浑浊和溃疡——因为杯状细胞医源性减少，副泪腺丧失，以及主泪腺小管可能受损。因此，病理医生在报告中说明所有结膜病变切缘是否均受累至关重要。对于切除结膜恶性肿瘤伴有狭窄切缘的患者，许多眼科医生采取非手术性辅助疗法（例如冷冻疗法或表面化疗），以确保完全根除这些病变。

眼表面的多数肿瘤均发生在角膜缘，不管是鳞状上皮来源还是黑色素细胞来源。手术切除这个部位的肿瘤非常困难，为了正确诊断这些活检标本并指导外科医生治疗，病理医生必须熟悉角膜缘的组织学。多数结膜恶性肿瘤不侵犯角膜间质，不管是鳞状上皮肿瘤还是黑色素细胞肿瘤。在典型的病例，肿瘤性鳞状上皮和黑色素细胞迁移到角膜上皮，但是仍然位于上皮基底膜之上，其下为 Bowman 层。Bowman 层是防止恶性肿瘤从上皮层向间质层穿透的有效屏障（图 29.19）。因此，进行角膜削刮活检（眼科术语为眼片角膜切除术，lamellar keratectomy）会损害此屏障。角膜缘肿瘤复发并不少见，这是医源性 Bowman 层缺乏为肿瘤细胞进入间质提供通道的结果。角膜间质恶性肿瘤通常是可以预防的，其手术处理可能需要角膜移植。

因此，眼科医生需要分两个阶段切除角膜缘恶性肿瘤。首先，眼科医生在结膜下注射麻醉药，使结膜组织从眼球表面膨胀如球状。之后，如果结膜组织粘连到眼球表面，通常说明肿瘤侵犯到巩膜外层结缔组织或巩膜。眼科医生可能会送检非常薄的浅表巩膜组织进行组织学检查。然后，眼科医生会切除肿瘤直到角膜缘而不切除任何角膜组织。在滴注表面麻醉剂之后，受累的角膜上皮通过化学机制清创术去除：用浸过纯酒精的棉签擦拭角膜表面，角膜上皮通常呈片块状脱落。多数眼科医生将这种凝胶状组织置于滤纸上并固定于中性甲醛缓冲液中。这种组织在外科病理检查台上可能难以辨认，在滤纸上滴加伊红通常容易辨认小而透明的组织标本。

角膜缘结膜减缩肿块体积手术层标本在大体检查台上需要准确定位。眼科医生用缝线标记标本切缘有助于病理医生定位。如果病理医生不能确定标本定

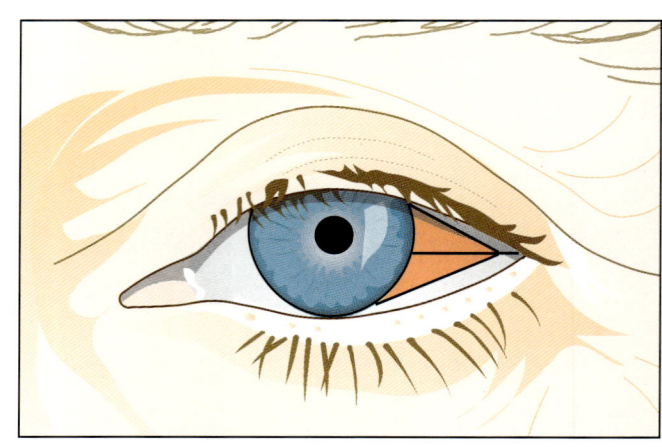

图29.21　切除的角膜缘结膜肿瘤的大体检查图解。切面应该与角膜缘垂直，并与上下切缘平行。

位，应该邀请手术医生到大体检查台前帮助定位。切面应该与角膜缘垂直，以便所有切缘均能充分取样（图 29.21）。

临床状况

多数结膜肿瘤发生于成人，虽然在儿童[26,27]和少年也有记录完整的结膜鳞状细胞肿瘤和黑色素瘤的报道。患者年龄有助于其与结膜色素性病变的鉴别诊断。例如，结膜淋巴瘤在儿童少见，儿童或少年结膜出现丰富的淋巴细胞浸润应该立即寻找痣的原因，亦即青春期炎症性结膜痣（inflamed conjunctival nevus of puberty，也叫炎症性幼年性痣，inflammatory juvenile nevus）[28]，将在下面讨论。病理医生很少遇到结膜交界痣，即使在儿童。无疑，确有记录完整的结膜交界痣病例，但是结膜痣发展的交界期必定非常之短：多数结膜痣有上皮下成分（用上皮下这一术语代替真皮下，是因为结膜结缔组织的显微镜下结构不同于真皮，在下面的结膜黑色素瘤的讨论中将强调这一点）。因此，在非幼儿患者的结膜上皮内出现黑色素细胞，无论是单个散在的还是成巢的，均应该诊断为伴有非典型性的原发性获得性黑变病（primary acquired melanosis with atypia），这是一种黑色素瘤的前体病变，不诊断为交界痣。

选择的对外科病理医生具有重要性的结膜肿瘤

鳞状上皮乳头状瘤和鳞状细胞癌
Squamous papilloma and squamous cell carcinoma

孤立性的有蒂鳞状上皮乳头状瘤（图29.22）和无蒂鳞状上皮乳头状瘤（图29.23）可以发生在泪阜、半月皱襞和穹窿。这些良性病变可以出现一定程度的反应性非典型性，继发于对脱垂眼睑组织的刺激或暴露。

鳞状细胞癌倾向于发生在睑间组织，即展开的眼睑之间的裂隙，或发生在穹窿。发生在睑间组织的鳞状细胞癌多半是日光损害的结果。发生在穹窿的肿瘤可能与HPV 16和18的存在有关[29]。不主张进行常规组织标本HPV试验，因为尚未有资料显示其与预后相关。

许多鳞状细胞癌由上皮内生长期发展而来，从不同程度的异型增生到原位癌，在此部位称为结膜上皮内肿瘤形成（conjunctival intraepithelial neoplasia, CIN）。多数鳞状细胞癌经过尚好，既不侵犯眼也不转移，除非在治疗明显延误病例和晚期病例。两种鳞状细胞癌的组织学亚型值得注意：黏液表皮样癌[30]和梭形细胞癌[31,32]，因为这两种亚型可能具有侵袭性的临床经过，伴有眼的浸润和转移（图29.24和29.25）。

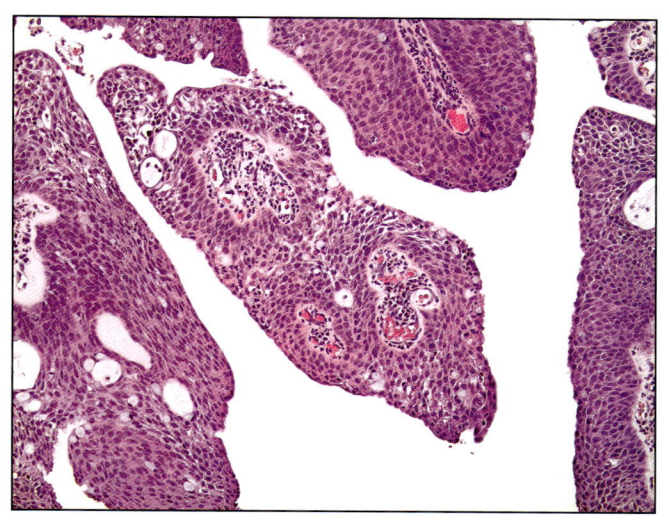

图29.22 结膜鳞状上皮乳头状瘤。上皮可能显示"反应性非典型性"特征。

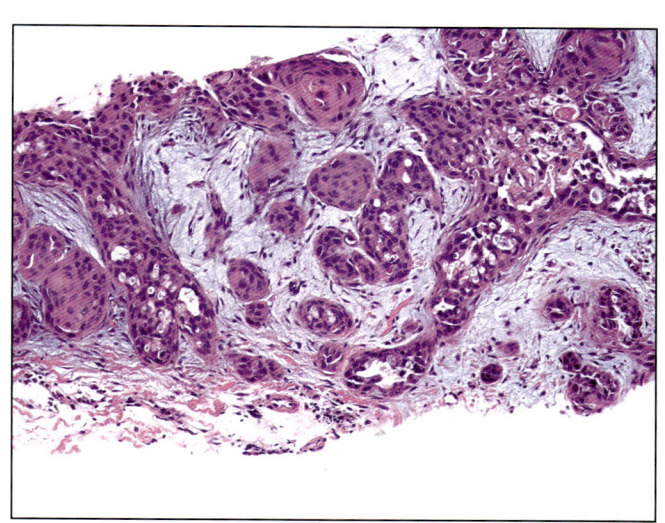

图29.24 结膜黏液表皮样癌。虽然这种病变表浅，类似于伴有鳞状分化的皮脂腺癌（图29.11），但是黏液样表皮样癌的空泡较大。通过黏液染色可以证实黏液表皮样癌的诊断。

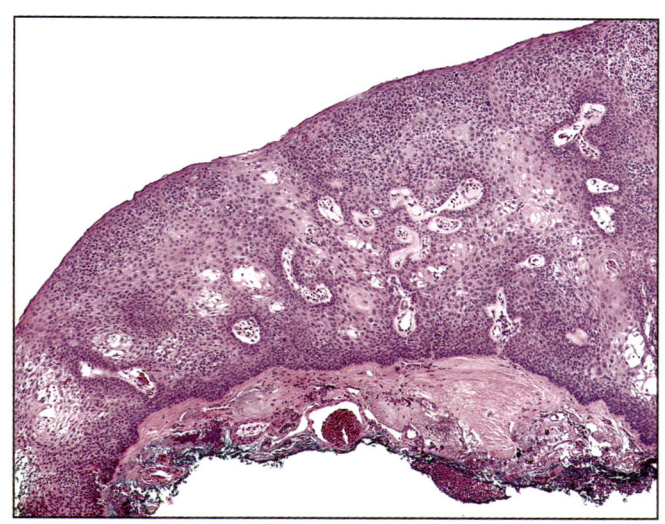

图29.23 结膜无蒂乳头状瘤。这种病变在临床上可能被误诊为鳞状细胞癌。

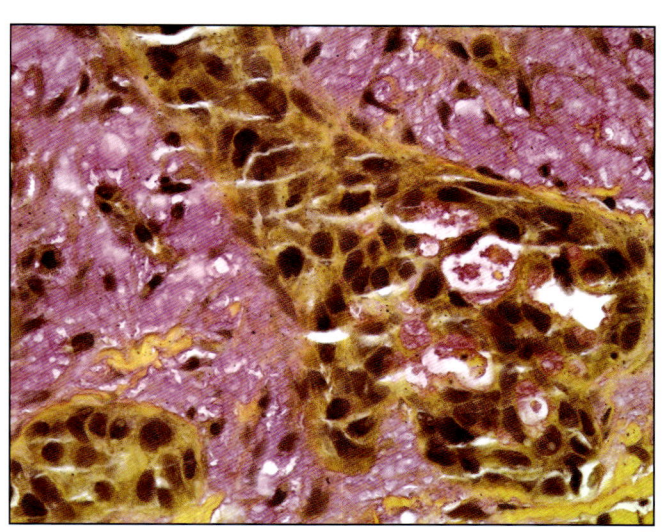

图29.25 黏液表皮样癌，黏液卡红染色。这是邻近图29.24所示切片的一张切片。

鳞状上皮肿瘤可能发生在有翼状胬肉（pterygium）的情况下，翼状胬肉是从结膜组织的角膜缘向角膜表层生长的良性病变。在翼状胬肉处还发现过无黑色素性黑色素瘤。因此，虽然多数翼状胬肉的组织学检查并不特殊，即在结膜固有膜的上方为良性上皮，特征为突出的日光性弹力组织变性和血管充血，但是所有翼状胬肉均应送检病理学检查，以除外临床上未能怀疑到的肿瘤的可能性。

结膜痣、黑色素瘤前体病变和黑色素瘤[2,23,33-35]
Conjunctival nevi, melanoma precursors, and melanoma

值得重复的是，外科病理医生很少遇到结膜痣，而且在超过青春期年龄的个体从不应该诊断交界痣。在外科病理学课本中很少应用"从不"（never）一词。但是在这种情况下，应用这个绝对的修饰词是有道理的：结膜上皮基底膜正上方出现单个或成巢的黑色素细胞，多半是黑色素瘤前体病变，除了在幼儿以外，这种病变在任何患者均称为伴有非典型性的原发性获得性黑变病，而不诊断交界痣。

组织学上复合痣和上皮下痣是不同的，因为不是存在实性上皮巢，就是存在上皮下囊性包涵体（图 29.26 和 29.27）。这些上皮下的残留部分和囊性包涵体被认为是来源于上皮的黑色素细胞脱落进入固有膜物质内（痣细胞团下移，Abtropfung），将上皮向下拉入疏松排列的上皮下胶原中。囊性包涵体可以表现为一个相当大的囊肿，且可以是主要的组织学图像，几乎掩盖了痣的存在。结膜痣很少侵犯角膜，仅仅在非常罕见的情况下见于穹窿和睑结膜。因此，任何推测是痣的病变累及这些解剖部位时，均应立即怀疑有无黑色素瘤。

青春期和青春期前后的儿童的复合痣内可能有相当多的淋巴细胞、浆细胞和嗜酸性粒细胞浸润。因为父母可能对眼表面病变的生长感到惊恐，也引起了病理医生的注意。临床上观察到的"肿物"多半是炎症浸润的结果，炎症浸润的表现可能掩盖其下的痣，导致病理医生将其误诊为淋巴组织增生或淋巴瘤，这两种疾病在儿童的结膜非常罕见。青春期前后的儿童的复合痣或上皮下痣内出现的慢性炎症，一般伴有嗜酸性粒细胞，或者诊断为青春期炎症性结膜痣（inflamed conjunctival nevus of puberty），或者诊断为炎症性幼年性结膜痣（inflamed juvenile conjunctival nevus）[23,28]（图 29.28）。这种病变完全是良性的，与晕痣（halo nevus）没有任何关系。有病理医生提出，这些病变与变异反应（atopy）有关。

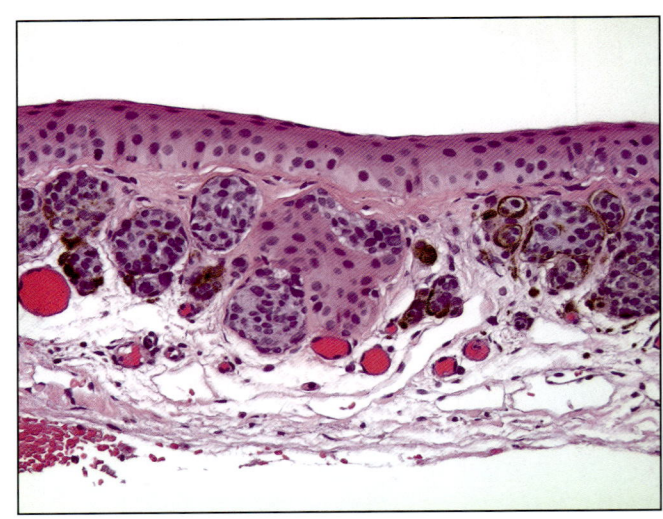

图29.27 结膜复合痣。有些复合痣的上皮下包涵体是实性的而不是囊性的。

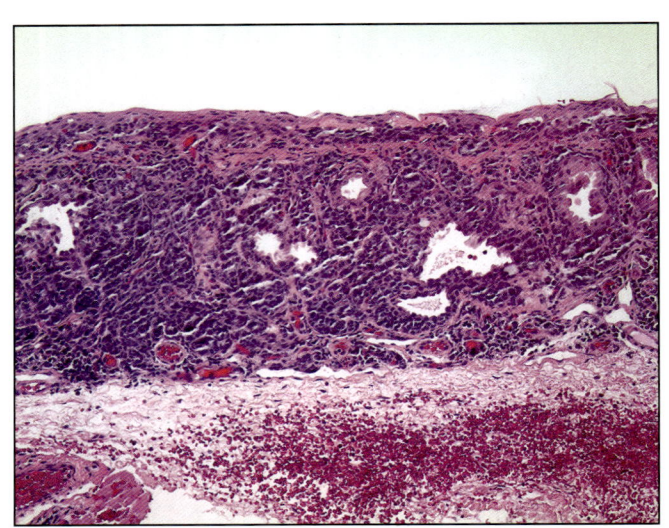

图29.26 结膜复合囊性痣。上皮下"囊肿"内衬表面上皮，可能含有杯状细胞。

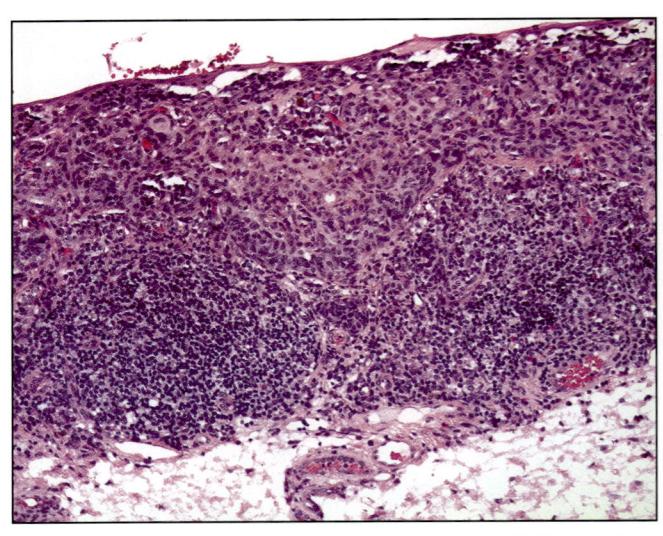

图29.28 青春期炎症性结膜痣。这个痣有明显的淋巴细胞反应，在有些病例，甚至可能遗漏痣的成分。原发性结膜淋巴瘤在儿童中非常罕见。

在结膜，几乎每一种在皮肤描述的痣均有描述[23]，包括蓝痣（图29.29）、细胞性蓝痣、Spitz痣和其他[36,37]。有作者提出有异型增生性结膜痣（dysplastic conjunctival nevi）存在，但是结膜上皮和固有膜并不形成网嵴，并且在结膜也没发现着色斑性黑色素细胞增生的特征。因此，没有固定的标准去辨认异型增生性结膜痣。

由于结膜缺乏出现在皮肤的组织学标志，组织学上难以区分雀斑（ephelis）和着色斑（lentigo）。因此，眼表面的色素性病变的命名不同于用于皮肤病学和皮肤病理学的命名，而是设计为帮助眼科医生决定哪些病变需要活检、哪些病变在治疗上可以忽略的命名。结膜黑色素瘤的总死亡率是25%[2]，本病最好的治疗是发现和切除任何结膜色素性病变，因为这些患者均处于发生黑色素瘤的危险之中。

一般来说，眼科医生对发生在面部的任何单侧性扁平色素性病变均应行活检。临床上这样的病变命名为原发性获得性黑变病（primary acquired melanosis, PAM）。这些病变被称为原发性是为了与继发性结膜色素沉着区分，后者的病例不存在任何发生结膜黑色素瘤的危险。继发性获得性黑变病（secondary acquired melanosis）的病例包括双侧性色素沉着，临床上见于皮肤颜色深的患者，色素沉着的发生与全身性疾病（Addison病或Peutz-Jeghers综合征）和局部用药（肾上腺素或含有银成分的滴眼剂）有关。获得性这一术语用作PAM的一个部分，是为了将这种病变与称为先天性眼黑变病（congenital melanosis oculi）的眼表面的先天性色素沉着区分开。先天性眼黑变病实际上是一种眼色素膜束（脉络膜、睫状体和虹膜）下方的弥漫性先天性痣，眼色素膜是将蓝色赋予巩膜，而不是结膜。患有先天性眼黑变病的高加索人种的患者可能处于发生色素膜黑色素瘤的危险中，而不是结膜黑色素瘤的危险中。

一旦眼科医生从鉴别诊断中排除了先天性眼黑变病和继发性获得性黑变病，而且可以确定病变不是痣——因为痣是扁平的，境界不清，而且缺乏囊肿——即可将这种病变诊断为PAM。因此，PAM这个临床术语是一个范围广泛的组织学病变。眼科医生应该学会辨认这些PAM患者，然后由病理医生对这些病变进行分类：确定其是几乎没有进展为黑色素瘤的危险的病变（没有非典型性的PAM），还是具有进展为黑色素瘤显著危险的病变（伴有非典型性的PAM）。组织学检查，没有非典型性的PAM（PAM without atypia）显示为结膜色素沉着，不伴有任何黑色素细胞增生（图29.30和29.31），可能类似于雀斑，或者是伴有或不伴有色素沉着的黑色素细胞增生。同预料的一样，没有非典型性的PAM没有进展为黑色素瘤的危险性。黑色素细胞增生伴有细胞学非典型性——伴有非典型性的PAM（PAM with atypia）（图29.32至29.34）——50%～90%有进展为黑色素瘤的危险性。

在伴有非典型性PAM中，非典型性黑色素细胞的多形性往往非常显著。当沿着上皮基底膜排列时，它们在形态学上类似于在窗台上摆放的一排坚果（花生、腰果、杏仁和胡桃）。典型者，不仅会忽略这些非典型性的黑色素细胞，而且会忽略上皮。痣内的黑色素细胞巢一般具有粘着力，并且常可发现其与邻近的上皮密切

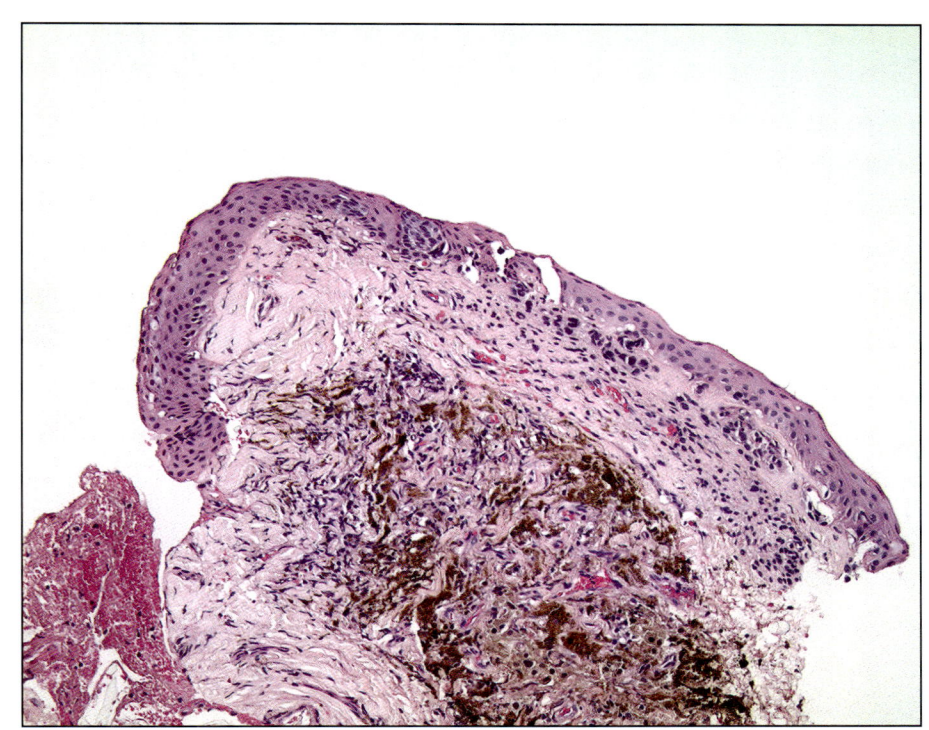

图29.29 结膜蓝痣。诊断皮肤蓝痣的组织学标准同样可以用于结膜蓝痣。

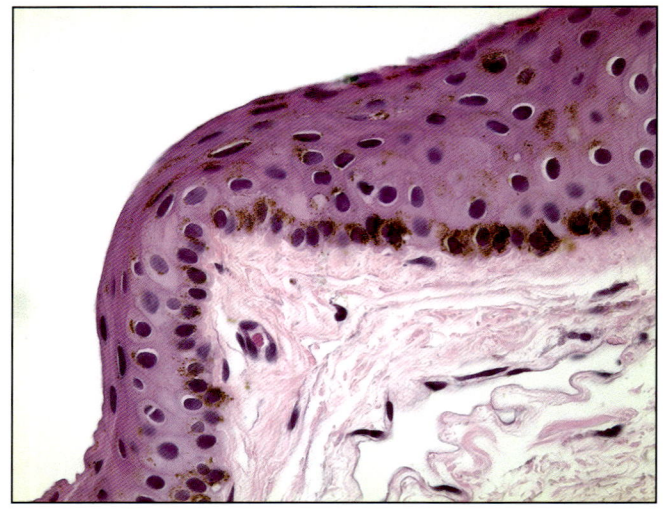

图29.30 球结膜没有非典型性的原发性获得性黑变病。黑色素出现在上皮基底层，并且在其上面的鳞状上皮细胞内也能发现。没有黑色素细胞增生或非典型性的证据。

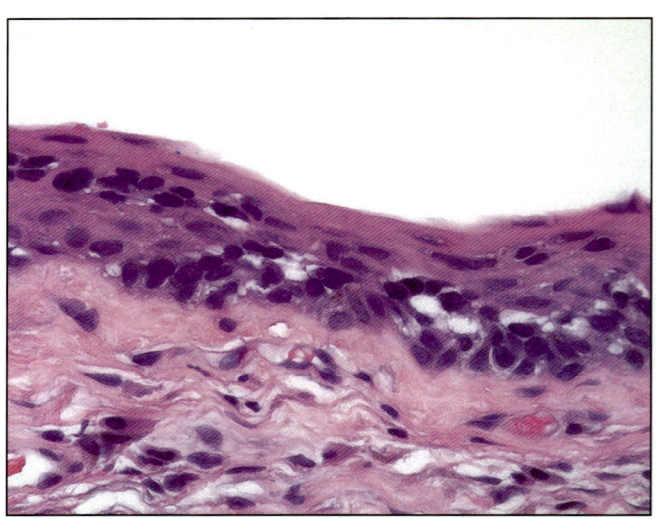

图29.32 伴有非典型性的原发性获得性黑变病。这张显微照片中的非典型性黑色素细胞沿着上皮基底层成簇分布。注意这些肿瘤性黑色素细胞"不顾"邻近的上皮细胞，表现为黑色素细胞与角化细胞分离。

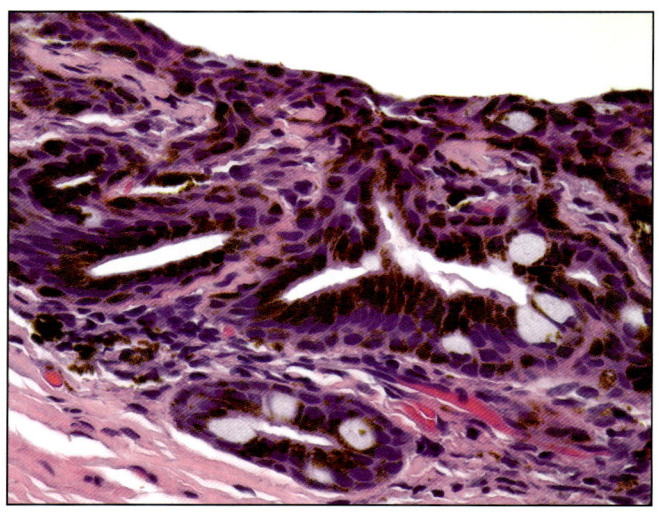

图29.31 穹窿结膜没有非典型性的原发性获得性黑变病。没有黑色素细胞增生或非典型性黑色素细胞延伸到Henle假腺体，上皮（伴有大量杯状细胞）突入其下的固有膜。

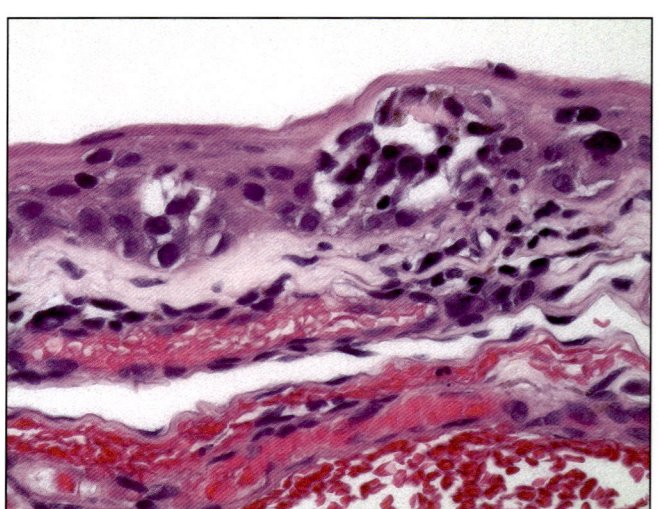

图29.33 伴有非典型性的原发性获得性黑变病。注意肿瘤性黑色素细胞成巢分布，而且"不顾"邻近的角化细胞。

相关。不管是单个的还是成巢的，黑色素细胞可向上扩散，形成Paget样分布。伴有非典型性的PAM可以扩散到痣的上皮下实性或囊性包涵体中，而且只要这种细胞与表面上皮有关，即使表面上皮位于固有膜内，都应该认为这种病变完全是上皮内的（图29.32至29.34）。对于病理医生来说，在穹窿的假复层柱状上皮内辨认非典型性黑色素细胞可能非常具有挑战性。有时，上皮基底的非典型性黑色素细胞可能向表面释放色素，并可能与其上的杯状细胞结合，此表现不应该与Paget样扩散混淆。

因为伴有非典型性的PAM可以出现在伴有痣的结膜内，所以许多病理医生发现，区分复合痣的交界性成分和与复合痣有关的伴有非典型性的PAM是困难的。表皮内黑色素细胞增生延伸超出真皮内3个网嵴就意味着是原位黑色素瘤，这种常常用于皮肤色素性病变的规则不能用于结膜。因为结膜缺乏网嵴，所以倾向于应用下面的原则：如果出现符合非典型性增生标准的黑色素细胞，而且病变两侧最大范围的上皮下成分一致，就可以诊断这个病变是伴有非典型性的PAM。

有人可能认为，伴有非典型性的原发性获得性黑变病与"原位黑色素瘤"一样，而且后一种命名应该用于病理学报告中[38]。虽然原位黑色素瘤生物学上相

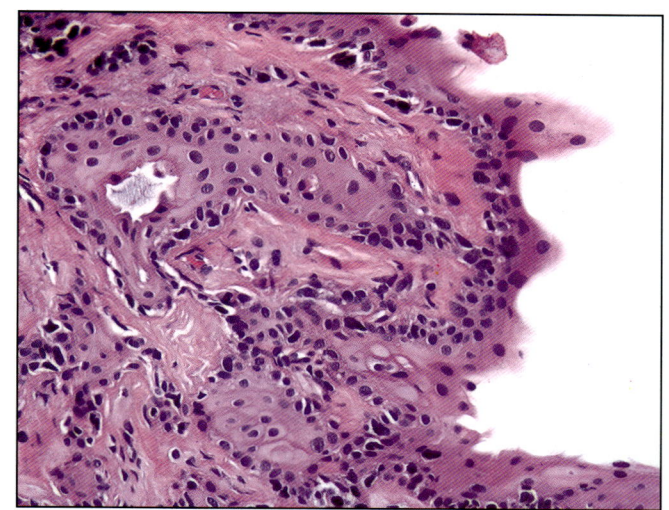

图 29.34 伴有非典型性的原发性获得性黑变病。非典型性黑色素细胞沿着基底层散在分布，没有堆积，同图 29.32，也没有形成细胞巢，同图 29.33。非典型性黑色素细胞沿着上皮下突起分布，进入固有膜。

当于伴有非典型性的 PAM，但是强烈推荐外科病理医生应用伴有非典型性的 PAM 这一术语来描述符合诊断标准的病变，因为这一术语对眼科医生有很大的帮助[3]。不要忘记，眼科医生确实没有有效的临床标准区分不伴有非典型性的 PAM 和伴有非典型性的 PAM 并做出 PAM 的诊断，而是留给病理医生去区分有无非典型性。改变病理学报告中的命名法会妨碍用于选择活检患者的临床逻辑思维（图 29.35）。外科病理医生应该努力帮助外科医生处理他们的患者，不应该把在生物学上可能是准确的分类方法强加给他们，应该避免造成临床上的混淆。

有人可能认为，主要沿着结膜基底层分布的、伴有非典型性的原发性获得性黑变病与恶性雀斑（lentigo maligna）类似，并且具有 Paget 样扩散特征的、伴有非典型性的 PAM 应该叫做 1 级浅表扩散性黑色素瘤。虽然最初有人非常积极地将皮肤黑色素瘤的组织学亚型应用于结膜黑色素瘤[39]，但是这种分类方法还是失败了，因为在多数情况下，在同一活检标本中可以发现恶性雀斑和 1 级浅表扩散性黑色素瘤[1]。奇怪的是，在结膜黏膜组织学检查时，人们很少遇到肢端雀斑性黑色素瘤（acral lentiginous melanoma）。

伴有非典型性的 PAM 可能非常弥漫，可累及眼表面的大部分，包括球结膜、穹窿、睑结膜、泪阜或半月皱襞。因为非典型性肿瘤性黑色素细胞可能不产生色素，所以伴有非典型性的 PAM 累及的结膜表面在临床上可能完全正常（无色素性 PAM，PAM sine pigmento）[40]。如果色素沉着片块小到足以能够局部切除，眼科医生可选择切除活检。如上所述，为了保留结膜组织，正常结

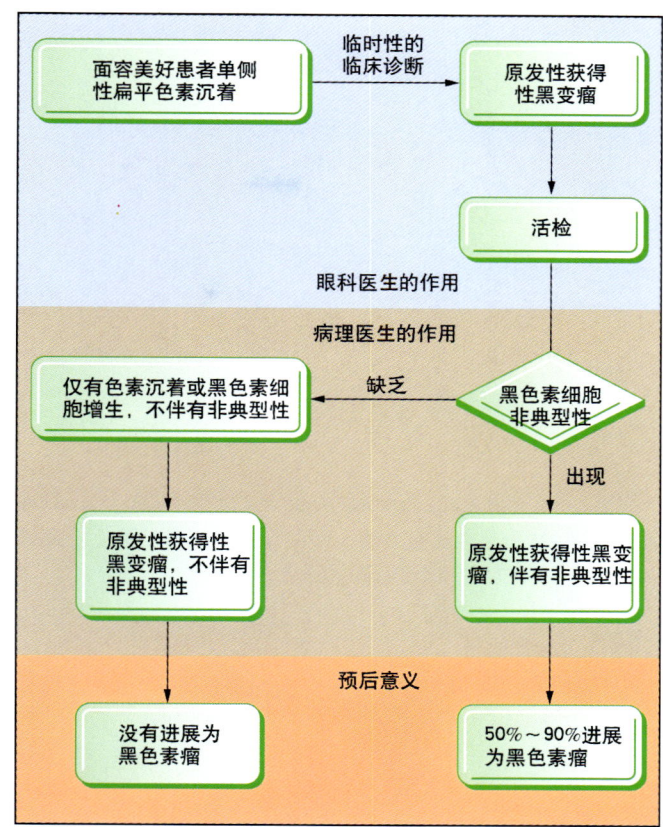

图 29.35 结膜的色素性病变的诊断流程图。它有助于眼科医生将任何新发现的扁平的单侧性结膜色素沉着认作"原发性获得性黑变病"。这样的病变应行活检并由病理医生分类。

膜切缘一般非常狭窄。因此，一些眼外科肿瘤医生会选择应用冷冻疗法治疗残留的结膜组织切缘，以期根除残余的非典型性黑色素细胞。

在治疗弥漫性结膜 PAM 患者时，眼科医生可进行许多小的切取活检，即"定位活检"（map biopsies），这是与测定结膜上皮内皮脂腺癌分布完全相同的一种策略。虽然在技术上手术切除整个受上皮内肿瘤累及的结膜组织是可行的，但是同上面说明的一样，这种方法很少应用。代替方法，弥漫性非典型性 PAM、弥漫性结膜上皮内肿瘤形成或弥漫性上皮内皮脂腺癌患者，现在可以通过局部应用丝裂霉素 C（Mitomycin C）治疗[41,42]。病理医生需要解释局部化疗后获取的活检，而且应该知道，化疗有引起上皮细胞非典型性的可能性[43]，类似于血管内应用丝裂霉素 C 治疗弥漫性浅表移行细胞癌的膀胱改变。化学治疗引起的这些变化不应解释为是残留的病变。患者的局部化疗可能需要多个疗程，为了评估疗效，每个疗程之后通常都取活检。

结膜黑色素瘤（conjunctival melanomas）可能是一个孤立性的结节，不伴有非典型性的 PAM 成分（类似于结节性皮肤黑色素瘤）。结节性结膜黑色素

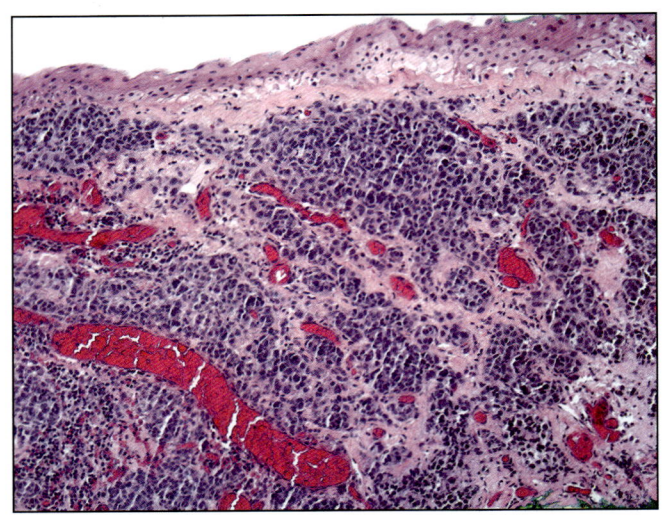

图29.36 结膜恶性黑色素瘤。浸润深度的测量是从上皮顶端（结膜没有颗粒层）到浸润的最深点。

表29.2	推荐报告的结膜黑色素瘤的组织学特征
组织学特征	**评注**
是否侵犯下方组织	
侧缘和深切缘有无肿瘤	
肿瘤厚度	从上皮顶端到浸润最深点以mm或分数进行测量。病变厚度小于0.8 mm，预后较好，而较厚的病变与转移性结膜黑色素瘤引起的死亡相关
在结膜内的部位	发生在睑结膜、穹窿结膜隆起或半月皱襞的黑色素瘤比发生在角膜缘或整个眼球（球结膜）的黑色素瘤具有更为明显的侵袭性临床经过
淋巴管内浸润	虽然从未证实是一项独立的预后特征，但是组织学检查出现淋巴管内浸润，应该切除前哨淋巴结
包括在报告中的可选择的特征	增生指数，肿瘤累及的侧向范围

Modified from Folberg et al.[19]

瘤少见，倾向于发生在角膜缘的附近。当肿瘤位于或靠近角膜缘时，不管病变的厚度如何，预后可能都非常好。然而，多数结膜黑色素瘤发生在伴有非典型性PAM的情况下（图29.36）[2,34,35]。有人认为，伴有非典型性的PAM是结膜黑色素瘤的径向生长期（radial growth phase），但是这种推理是不完善的：皮肤黑色素瘤的径向生长期在真皮乳头水平可能有一种浅表皮肤浸润的成分，而结膜上皮下胶原不能分出真皮乳头和网状结构，正常情况下也没有脂肪组织。因此，Clark分级不能用于结膜黑色素瘤。病变厚度是结膜黑色素瘤的预后因素，厚度测量是从上皮顶部（结膜没有颗粒层）到病变基底。多数研究显示，厚度小于0.8 mm的病变预后良好，而较厚的病变具有黑色素瘤转移的危险[2,44,45]。

有人提出，当评估结膜黑色素瘤切除标本时，在病理学报告中应该特别提到一些组织学特征[19]。这些特征总结在表29.2中。

结膜黑色素瘤倾向于首先扩散到局部淋巴结，即颌下淋巴结和腮腺淋巴结，虽然也有最初转移到内脏和脑的报道[46]。现在，一些眼科肿瘤医生推荐，对结膜黑色素瘤进行前哨淋巴结活检[47]，但是这项工作尚未推广，因为尚未有足够多的患者数据证实这个步骤有益。

其他结膜恶性肿瘤
Other conjunctival malignancies

淋巴瘤可以原发于结膜。可以单侧受累，也可以双侧受累，后者并不代表一种侵袭性临床经过。结膜淋巴瘤的分类与其他黏膜部位的淋巴瘤分类一样（这些病变常常但并不总是边缘带黏膜相关的淋巴组织淋巴瘤[47a]，见第21章）。结膜淋巴瘤一般通过针对眼附属器进行放射治疗[48,49]。结膜和眼睑可以发生Kaposi肉瘤[50,51]，特别是在获得性免疫缺陷综合征（AIDS）的患者。

泪液排泄系统肿瘤
Tumors of the lacrimal drainage system

泪点位于两侧上下眼睑的内侧，被覆非角化性复层鳞状上皮。泪管和泪小管同样内衬非角化性鳞状上皮。泪囊本身内衬假复层柱状上皮。泪囊原发性癌已有描述，可以为鳞状细胞癌或移行细胞癌。原发性淋巴瘤和腺癌（发生于与泪囊有关的小腺体）也有描述。手术标本可能包括眼睑或眼眶组织，这样切除的所有标本均应检查切缘[52-54]。泪液排泄系统肿瘤几乎全发生于成人。

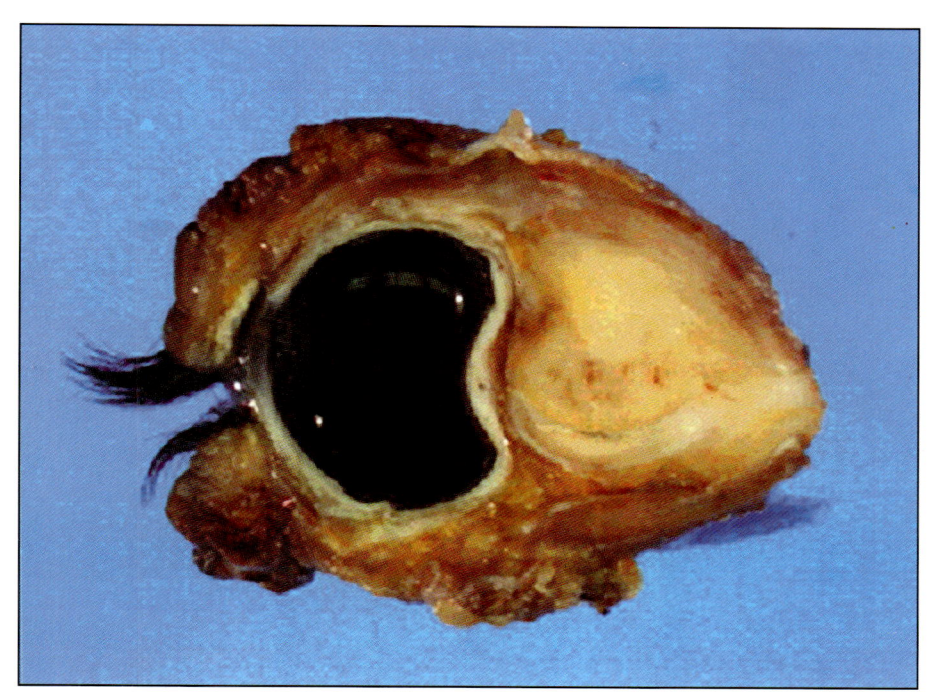

图29.37 发生于眼眶的未分化肉瘤,患者早在30年前就由于两侧视网膜母细胞瘤而行放射治疗。肿瘤侵犯眶底,如果不经治疗,可能延伸到脑。(Courtesy by Dr. David Abramson, Memorial Sloan-Kettering Hospital)

眼眶肿瘤 Tumors of the orbit

引言

眼眶占位性病变可能起因于炎症性疾病(Graves病和眼眶假瘤,也叫特发性眼眶炎症,idiopathic orbital inflammation)、原发性肿瘤、眼内恶性肿瘤的眼外蔓延(视网膜母细胞瘤和葡萄膜黑色素瘤),或来自眼睑、结膜和邻近鼻旁窦的肿瘤的浸润。眼眶内壁和下壁分别毗连筛窦和上颌窦,而眼眶的上壁和后壁通向颅腔内。因此,眼眶恶性肿瘤可能危及生命,因为有可能向颅内扩散(图29.37)。

儿童的主要造血系统肿瘤是白血病浸润。淋巴瘤——除了在特定位置Burkitt淋巴瘤累及鼻旁窦,继而累及眼眶以外——很少累及儿童眼眶。淋巴瘤累及眼眶确有发生,只是非常罕见。眼眶淋巴瘤主要发生于成人,典型者为B细胞淋巴瘤(虽然眼眶T细胞淋巴瘤的病例也有报道),这些淋巴瘤的组织学分类与用于人体其他部位的淋巴组织增生性疾病的分类相同(见第21章)[47a,48,49,55]。

在检查怀疑肿瘤的组织时,外科病理医生可能遇到眼眶炎症性假瘤(orbital inflammatory pseudotumor,眼科医生称为特发性眼眶炎症)。眼眶假瘤的组织学表现包括:慢性炎症,常伴有不同数量的嗜酸性粒细胞、纤维化,而且或许还有血管炎的成分(图29.38)[56,57]。偶尔可能遇到一种复合性病变,具有眼眶假瘤和黄瘤性甚或黄色肉芽肿性成分的组织病理

学特征(图29.39)[58]。这些病变与成年发作的哮喘有关。眼眶渐进性坏死性黄色肉芽肿(necrobiotic xanthogranuloma)的病例已有报道[59]。

Wegener肉芽肿病可以原发于眼眶,诊断时可无全身性疾病的证据。所谓的"局限性眼眶"(orbital-limited)Wegener肉芽肿病可类似眼眶转移癌的表现。相反,有些类型的眼眶转移癌,特别是转移性前列腺癌,可能类似于眼眶炎症性假瘤的临床表现。炎症性假瘤可能是广泛性的,累及所有眼眶组织,也可能是局限于一种或一

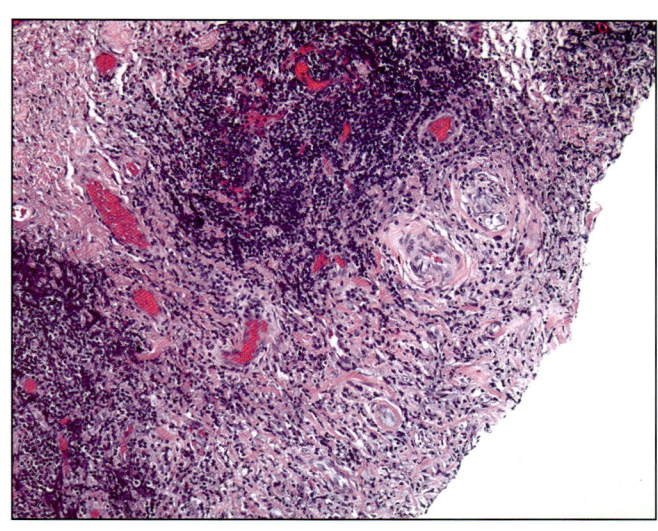

图29.38 特发性眼眶炎症(硬化性眼眶假瘤)。注意由于致密的慢性炎症,眼眶脂肪组织消失。这里见到的血管炎是一个可变的特征。本图左上方见到的纤维化可能是一些病例的组织学结构的主要成分。

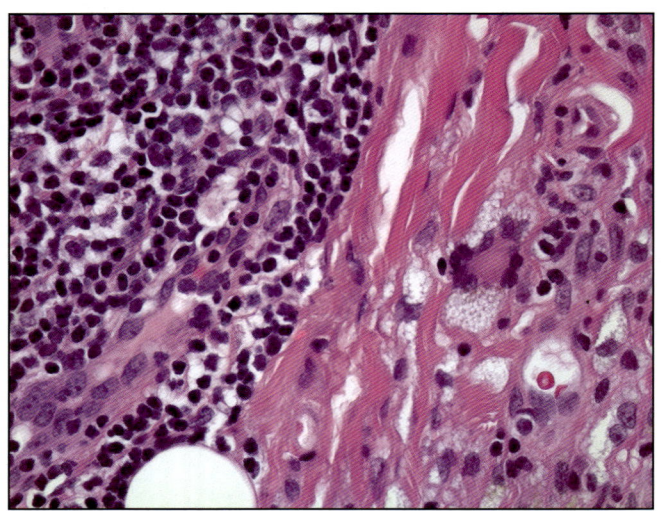

图29.39 慢性眼眶炎症伴有黄色瘤性或黄色肉芽肿性成分。这样的病变与成年发作的哮喘有关。

种以上眼眶组织。例如，眼外肌肉假瘤可能被归入眼眶肌炎（orbital myositis）。泪腺炎症性假瘤可能产生硬化性泪腺炎（sclerosing dacryoadenitis）的组织学图像。

同掌握一种外语一样，在探讨眼眶病理学时，外科病理医生将会遇到类似于"不规则动词"（irregular verbs）的情况。例如，尽管在眼眶有脂肪肉瘤的报道[60,61]，但却没有眼眶脂肪瘤病例的记录。一些眼科手术医生描述的眼眶脂肪瘤可能是从眼睑的眼眶隔脱垂而来的眼眶脂肪。

眼眶肿瘤的诊断通常是通过前路（通过眼睑切口）活检或侧路切除一段颧颞突（侧眶切开术）做出的。有些眼科医生提倡应用针吸活检确立眼眶肿瘤的诊断[62,63]。

良性眼眶肿瘤的治疗一般采取手术切除（如常常遇到的有包膜的海绵状血管瘤）。有些界限不清的眼眶良性肿瘤不能完全切除，如淋巴管瘤。对这种病例的手术策略是：切除足够的肿瘤组织以减轻眼眶占位病变引起的眼球前移（proptosis）这一主要症状。眼球前移不仅影响容颜，而且可能会使眼睑不能完全覆盖角膜。同前面讨论的一样，角膜暴露可引起疼痛，易于发生感染性角膜溃疡。

恶性眼眶肿瘤一般通过眼眶内容剜出术（exenteration）治疗。剜出眼球（enucleation）这一术语仅仅用于去除眼球，而不切除结膜和眼睑。眼球内容剜出术（evisceration）是指去除眼内容物而用占位性物质替代，以保留容颜上合意的假眼的活动性。当治疗眼内恶性肿瘤时，不一定进行眼球内容剜出术。然而，眼眶内容剜出术涉及切除眼、结膜、眼眶的整个软组织以及大部分眼睑，如果不是全部眼睑的话。因此，眼眶内容剜出术的患者要经受严重的功能和容颜损害的痛苦。考虑到通过前路或侧路眼眶切开术或针吸活检能够确立诊断，如果恶性诊断的后果是眼眶内容剜出术，那么病理医生应该怀疑通过冰冻切片确立眼眶原发性恶性肿瘤诊断的可能性。应该考虑到冰冻切片时晚期硬化性泪腺炎（泪腺假瘤）的组织学表现可能类似于腺样囊性癌的组织学表现，这种危险对于患者以及对于外科医生和病理医生都很明显。

当然，眼眶组织冰冻切片检查需要有明显的指征。这些指征包括：检测切缘确保完全切除了肿瘤、检查肿瘤组织使外科医生放心、对肿瘤组织已取样研究。例如，可能完全有理由对怀疑患有胚胎横纹肌肉瘤的儿童眼眶行冰冻切片检查，但这种病变的治疗是减小肿瘤体积，随后进行化疗或放疗，而不是行眼眶内容剜出术。病理医生应该知道，只有在非常少的情况下，冰冻切片诊断可改变眼眶手术过程。

临床状况

无论病理医生选择在阅读切片之前还是之后查阅临床资料，即了解眼眶肿瘤的临床状况，均有助于组织病理学的鉴别诊断。例如，只有几种眼眶肿瘤是真正有包膜的：泪腺多形性腺瘤、神经鞘瘤、皮样囊肿以及海绵状血管瘤（原发性视神经胶质瘤位于硬脑膜内，因此境界非常清楚）。只有几种眼眶肿瘤本质上是囊性的：皮样囊肿、眼眶先天性囊性畸胎瘤、变性的神经鞘瘤和一些原发性视神经胶质瘤。许多眼眶淋巴瘤倾向于影响眼的表面，而不影响眼球。

在眼眶疾病病理学研讨会上，Frederick A. Jakobiec医生根据肿瘤首先出现在眼眶的年龄提出了一种眼眶肿瘤的分类方法。这些眼眶肿瘤几乎都可以明显地分为两类，即首先出现在儿童期的肿瘤和首先出现在成人期的肿瘤。这种分类的修订方案列在表29.3中。虽然应用这种方法的确有例外，但是表29.3的分类可能有助于借助临床特征进行组织学鉴别诊断。

大体检查

大体检查应该从标本侧向定位开始——是右侧还是左侧眼眶。一些眼科病理医生倾向于将眼眶标本固定24～48小时之后延迟切开检查。然而，因为埋在眼眶脂肪中的肿瘤不会完全固定，即使用更长的时间固定，

表29.3 基于诊断时的年龄进行分类的眼眶肿瘤

组织类型	儿童	成人
炎症性		炎症性假瘤 Graves病
造血性	白血病	淋巴瘤
血管性	毛细血管瘤	海绵状血管瘤
神经性（外周神经）	神经纤维瘤	神经鞘瘤
骨	嗜酸性肉芽肿 骨化性纤维瘤 纤维性发育不良	骨瘤
间叶性	横纹肌肉瘤 恶性外周神经鞘瘤	非肌原性肉瘤（如多形性肉瘤、孤立性纤维性肿瘤、脂肪肉瘤、平滑肌肉瘤、腺泡状软组织肉瘤及其他）
泪腺		多形性腺瘤 腺样囊性癌 腺癌（直接形成或来自多形性腺瘤）
囊性病变	先天性囊性畸胎瘤	黏液囊肿 皮样囊肿
转移到眼眶	神经母细胞瘤 肾母细胞瘤	乳腺、肺、前列腺最常见

所以也许值得在切除之后立即开始解剖眼眶内容剜出术标本。而且，一些眼科病理医生倾向于在同一垂直切面上检查包括眼、视神经和上下眼睑的组织学标本（图29.37）。当这种做法可行时，标本适合用于教学。然而，需要检查的肿瘤的位置可能并不在这个平面（例如，泪囊的肿瘤从内下部位浸润到眼眶，或伴有浸润性肿块的眼睑弥漫性皮脂腺癌不在切除标本的中线）。另外，一些组织学实验室设备不完善，不能处理大尺寸的标本，导致载玻片难于在实验室存档的组织学设备中归档。

因此，病理医生可能希望尝试应用替代的大体病理学检查方法。测量标本并陈述眼睑组织的数量。在记录眼眶骨膜的完整性之后（大体上定为一种闪光的质地硬韧的组织，可能包围眼眶软组织），病理医生用墨水标记手术切缘。有些手术医生在进行眼眶内容剜出术时不切除骨膜（可能被称为眶骨膜，periorbita），所以缺乏这个解剖学标志并不一定代表肿瘤突破了这个主要的解剖面（图29.40）。后切缘为眶顶，应该与标本的其余部分分开，并送检组织学检查（除非手术医生已经单独送检标记为"眶顶"的组织进行评估）。通过在眼睑内侧和外侧皮肤的上下眼睑汇合处——即内眦和外眦——分别做一个切口，并向后延长这个切口，可以将上睑和眼眶软组织的上半部分与下睑和眼眶软组织的下半部分分开。然后，可以通过钝器和利器剥离，将眼球与眼眶软组织和眼睑分开。眼球的处理在下文描述。样本可取自眼睑组织和眼眶内容，它们可能涉及肿瘤或对于确定切缘是否充分非常重要。

这种替代方法有一些缺点。其操作需要精确地解剖和记录组织样本。眼眶组织取样的手绘图可能有帮助。这种方法的主要优点是：准确绘图和定位眼眶受累。

鼓励病理医生改变他们报告眼眶肿瘤的方式，如同这种肿瘤是从身体任何其他部位活检的一样。这样，一个泪腺多形性腺瘤的报告应该提到包膜的完整性，眼眶淋巴瘤的报告应该包括任何其他结外淋巴瘤报告中的同样特征。

视神经的原发性肿瘤
Primary tumors of the optic nerve

视神经是中枢神经系统的一束。完全被硬脑膜、蛛网膜和软脑膜包被，脑脊液围绕视神经循环、视网膜母细胞瘤倾向于侵犯视神经，因此可扩散到脑，移行并横跨视交叉到达对侧视神经，或种植于神经轴。

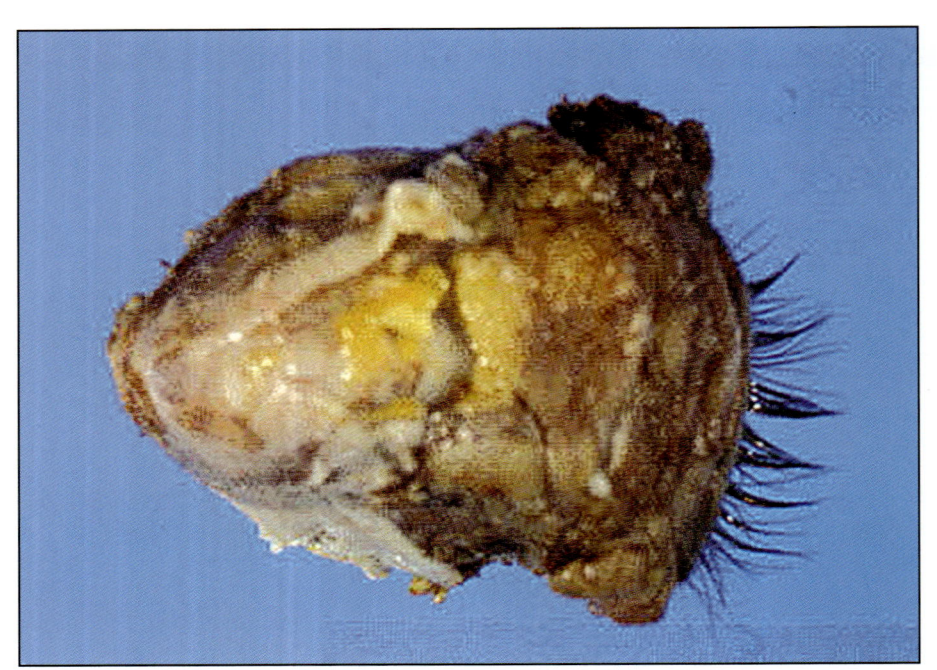

图29.40 眼眶内容剜出术标本显示骨膜缺陷。此图为图29.37病例的另一个视野。后面（左侧）闪光的白色组织已经破裂，是由下方的肿瘤膨出造成的。

神经胶质瘤（glioma）和脑膜瘤（meningioma）是视神经的主要原发性肿瘤，神经胶质瘤一般是毛细胞性星形细胞瘤（pilocytic astrocytoma），而脑膜瘤一般是脑膜瘤型脑膜瘤[64]。临床上两者均可造成视神经增大，通过影像检查可以发现，而且两种肿瘤均可能损害视力。将儿童和成人原发性视神经胶质瘤与原发性视神经脑膜瘤向后扩散到颅腔的可能性加以比较是有用的（表29.4）。虽然这种看法在概念上尚有例外[65]，在儿童，视神经毛细胞性星形细胞瘤的经过多数缓慢，在成人则经过加速；而在成人，原发性视神经脑膜瘤的经过多数缓慢，在儿童则有较为侵袭性的经过。

当用连续的影像记录视神经肿物的增长时，眼科医生与神经外科医生合作可以决定对病变进行活检，特别是如果视力严重受损或病变已经造成眼球突出时。此时，可能要求外科病理医生应用冰冻切片区分视神经胶质瘤和脑膜瘤，这项工作似乎很普通，但是如果视神经胶质瘤发生在合并有神经纤维瘤病的情况下，可能会有困难。脑膜增生在组织学上无法与脑膜瘤区分，在这种临床状况下，脑膜增生可能环绕胶质瘤，视神经浅表活检可能会导致误诊为脑膜瘤[66]，以致进行损害性的神经外科手术。视神经胶质瘤常是硬脑膜内的肿瘤，甚至在神经纤维瘤病的情况下，伴随胶质瘤的脑膜增生也完全是硬脑膜内的，了解这些对外科病理医生是有帮助的。另一方面，原发性视神经脑膜瘤可能在硬脑膜内，也可能在硬脑膜外。这样，病理医生和外科医生交流可以解决冰冻切片诊断中的模糊问题：如果组织学特征支持脑膜瘤的诊断，且外科医生保证活检的确来源于硬膜外，那么病理医生就可以明确做出脑膜瘤的诊断；如果组织学特征提示脑膜瘤的诊断，且外科医生陈述活检取自硬膜内的组织，那么病理医生可能有理由提示重复活检进行冰冻切片检查；如果视力已经损害，可选取视神经较深的切面。因此，在做出这个重要的术中诊断时，病理医生需要慎重，因为外科医生可能并不知道该儿童是否患有神经纤维瘤病。

一些视神经胶质瘤其特征是以囊性改变为主，这没有预后意义。这些囊肿融合可以解释眼球突出程度的突然加重，并使外科医生和患者放心：视神经没有恶性改变。视神经恶性胶质瘤非常罕见。

有些原发性视神经脑膜瘤可能出现钙化，影像检查时表现为有大量的沙粒体。这种特征缺乏预后意义。

病理医生对视神经胶质瘤和脑膜瘤活检的报告内容与对中枢神经系统其他部位活检的报告内容没有明显不同。这两种肿瘤的切缘是视神经后部的横切缘，即外科医生的视神经切缘。应该从手术切缘取视神经的横切面，并注意是否存在肿瘤。

表29.4	原发性视神经肿瘤的临床病理学框架	
	儿童	成人
神经胶质瘤	慢性经过	侵袭性经过
脑膜瘤	侵袭性经过	慢性经过

眼内肿瘤 Intraocular tumors

背景

许多眼内肿瘤从不引起外科病理医生的注意。正如本章引言部分讨论的一样，有充分的理由要求对患者的治疗不仅是消除癌，而且要保留视力。这样，如果一个视网膜母细胞瘤相对较小，而且不在损害视力的解剖学部位（例如在视神经上或在黄斑内，后者是提供高水平视觉分辨力的视网膜区），可以通过冷冻疗法或激光疗法消除肿瘤。在肿瘤较大的情况下，患者可以经由眼周注射化疗药物减小肿瘤体积（化学减灭）[67,68]。同样，目前对于葡萄膜黑色素瘤来说，放疗与剜出术具有相同的生存率[69]。淋巴瘤可以原发于眼，但是原发性视网膜淋巴瘤（几乎完全见于 65～70 岁以上的患者）的诊断一般是通过眼内穿刺活检细胞学检查或玻璃体液细胞学检查做出的[70]。眼的转移性肿瘤一般进行放射治疗。这样，显著降低了肿瘤性疾病眼球剜出术的发生率[71]。

临床状况

视网膜母细胞瘤是儿童最常见的眼内原发性肿瘤。髓上皮瘤（medulloepithelioma）是较大儿童和成人中罕见的原发性肿瘤，且存在非畸胎瘤性和畸胎瘤性两种类型，并有良性和恶性变型（恶性一般定义为肿瘤出现眼外扩散）[72,73]。这些肿瘤的特征是：视网膜上皮器官样增生，如果含有异源性的间叶成分，则标记为畸胎样。成人最常见的肿瘤是眼的转移性肿瘤，特别是来自乳腺和肺的原发性肿瘤的转移，而成人最常见的原发性眼内肿瘤是葡萄膜黑色素瘤。这些肿瘤的发生似乎无性别差异。

大体检查

当眼内肿瘤有手术指征时，视网膜母细胞瘤选择的手术是剜出术，即摘除眼球。局限于虹膜或睫状体的黑色素瘤可以单独整块切除虹膜，或切除虹膜和睫状体（虹膜睫状体切除术）。在欧洲，有些局灶性脉络膜黑色素瘤通过切除眼壁（eye-wall resection）治疗，这种手术在美国很少应用。大的不能切除的葡萄膜黑色素瘤和伴有明显视力丧失的葡萄膜黑色素瘤通过眼球摘除术治疗。

详细的大体检查程序可在别处找到[74,75]。简而言之，对于患有视网膜母细胞瘤或黑色素瘤的眼球，病理医生应该不依赖于外科医生的描述而确认标本侧别（是右眼还是左眼），要注意与视神经附着有关的下斜肌的附着。下斜肌在视神经的外侧（颞侧）。从视神经开始清理，病理医生应该见到长的上斜肌腱的附着。应该仔细检查眼的表面以寻找肿瘤向眼外扩散的证据，后者对预后有负面影响。一些病理医生认为，应该切除葡萄膜黑色素瘤的所有 4 个涡状静脉并进行组织学检查，但是尚无发表的资料提示这种做法有任何预后意义。

应该检查肿瘤是否累及视神经。虽然最好是在固定 24～48 小时之后切开眼球，但在大体检查室收到眼球时取一个视神经的切面可能是恰当的，特别是对视网膜母细胞瘤病例，因为视网膜母细胞瘤容易侵犯视神经（葡萄膜黑色素瘤侵犯视神经非常少见）。有些眼科肿瘤医生可能要求应用冰冻切片评估视神经。

因为眼科手术医生不是在直视下切取视神经，所以手术切缘（视神经的切端）常常被眼球摘出剪挤压。因此，在视神经附着于眼球的部位横切视神经，并检查这个视神经切面有无肿瘤浸润，对诊断是有帮助的。此切面没有肿瘤可以确保手术切缘没有肿瘤。如果在眼球和视神经的交界面见到肿瘤，可以切取另外一个切面，直到视神经没有受累，或肿瘤追踪到手术切缘。

对于患有视网膜母细胞瘤或黑色素瘤的眼球，重要的是，在切开眼球之前，病理医生要辨认眼内肿瘤的位置。在切开之前定位眼内肿瘤的最好方法是眼球透照检查。从任何经线上打开眼球几乎都是可行的，"标准"水平切面将会漏掉位于下面的肿瘤。有些病理医生怀疑：在切开眼球之前是否需要应用光线投照摘除的眼球来定位肿瘤。这些病理医生中有人赞成通过浆膜盲目切开结肠癌切除标本并希望这种切面通过肿瘤吗？所有病理医生都提倡将黑色素瘤皮肤切除标本表面向下放在取材板上并在没有直接见到肿瘤的情况下从皮下脂肪切开吗？

虽然已经发明了精心制作的装置帮助进行透光试验，但是只需要一种强烈的光源（一种非常亮的光笔或用作照相装备的一种纤维光学设备）。光源可以直对瞳孔，阴影痕迹在眼表面用标记铅笔标记。然后可以做包括阴影区域在内的切面。

因患视网膜母细胞瘤而切除的眼球一般含有大的肿瘤，或肿瘤具有弥漫性的玻璃体种植。一些外科医生在手术室切开眼球取出新鲜组织进行细胞遗传学研究、送组织库或建立细胞系。外科医生一般会切取一块巩膜，在眼球上开一个窗，并通过这个窗口引出组织。这种操作对病理医生具有几种挑战。首先，眼球软，难于做一个切面。其次，必须在一个不包括巩膜缺损的平面上切开眼球；是外科医生而不是病理医生决定如何切开眼球。最后，视网膜母细胞瘤脆而易碎，采集新鲜组织可能会使肿瘤细胞散布于整个眼球甚至眼外。有几个线索能够帮助病理医生识别是脉络膜浸润和眼外延伸，还是继发于在新鲜状态下打开眼球时的肿瘤的人为分散假象。

含有视网膜母细胞瘤的完整眼球一般是沿着前后径切开，包括瞳孔、肿瘤和视神经，这是切开眼球剜出标本的常规技术。这项技术的一个缺点是：肿瘤的最大轴可能并不包括在含有瞳孔和视神经的切面内。这一点对含有视网膜母细胞瘤的眼球并不重要，因为肿瘤大小不是预后指标。

然而，描述的肿瘤接触巩膜区带的最长尺寸，即"肿瘤生长的水平范围"，是葡萄膜黑色素瘤的最重要的预后指标。因此，因黑色素瘤而切除的眼球可以应用常规技术或通过一种替代方法切开。后者的目的是肿瘤能够包括在巩膜接触的最大面中。替代方法是通过睫状环的冠状切面打开后中纬线含有肿瘤的眼球，这样能将前段（角膜和晶体虹膜隔膜）和含有肿瘤的后极分开。然后可以将打开的眼球浸放在乙醇溶液中并照相以确定准确的临床病理关系，可以沿着最大的巩膜接触经线（在病理学报告的大体描述中应该记录）对切肿瘤；对切前段并分别送检。

环状黑色素瘤（ring melanoma）是围绕睫状体周围生长的肿瘤，含有环状黑色素瘤的眼球最好也用这种方式打开，因为肿瘤或许会完全位于前段内，可将前段切成馅饼形薄片，以定位前段受累的情况。如果黑色素瘤累及睫状体和脉络膜，最好与肿瘤轴平行切除眼帽（cap of the eye），沿着前后经线打开眼球。然后可以在直视下对切肿瘤。通过替代方法不能得到包括肿瘤和所有重要结构在内的整个眼球标本，但是与常规技术相比，它能较为准确地分析葡萄膜黑色素瘤的最大基底径。

切除位于虹膜的肿瘤时（虹膜切除术），病理医生需要评估边缘是否受累。这些组织标本一般非常小，并且虹膜组织易碎。在眼科医生绘制的草图指引下，在大体标本实验台上定位标本的方法是可取的。两个侧缘应该分别放在包埋盒内检查，按照组织在虹膜上的相应位置以钟点的形式表示。

当黑色素细胞肿瘤累及睫状体且或许累及虹膜而没有延伸到脉络膜时，外科医生可能会切除整个虹膜和睫状体，即行虹膜睫状体切除术。另外，病理医生对每一个切缘要分别取材，并且用钟点的形式标记虹膜上的两个侧缘是非常重要的。切面应该平行于睫状突的方向。通过在睫状突之间的凹陷处做切口采取切面是有帮助的。

因眼内肿瘤而切除的眼球的显微镜下描述：一般原则

对多数肿瘤的病理学报告，病理医生应该将重点放在能够提供预后信息和指导治疗的重要组织学特征上。报告的结构常常有固定的格式，以指导外科医生和肿瘤医生确定对患者的不同治疗方案。病理医生很少注重描述随同肿瘤一起切除的正常组织。然而，当检查因眼内肿瘤而切除的眼球时，病理医生不仅有责任描述能够提供预后信息的肿瘤状况，而且应该描述肿瘤对眼球其余部分的影响。对眼球的继发性影响可能包括青光眼、视网膜脱离和白内障。将诊断报告分为两个部分是有帮助的：具有预后意义的所见，以及肿瘤对眼球的继发性影响。

视网膜母细胞瘤　Retinoblastoma

为了挽救患儿视网膜母细胞瘤的眼球，已经进行了诸多的尝试，病理医生可能遇到的只是充满了肿瘤的眼球或玻璃体广泛种植的眼球，对保存视力的治疗没有效果的含有肿瘤的眼球，或在根除肿瘤时并发令人痛苦的视力丧失的眼球。

在准确的临床影像技术应用以前，由于临床误诊的视网膜母细胞瘤，切除了许多眼球。这些多数为类似视网膜母细胞瘤临床表现的良性病变（如持续性增生性原玻璃体、弓蛔虫眼内炎和视网膜大块神经胶质瘤病，这些病变在眼科专科病理学教科书中均有详细描述[75]）。所幸的是，这些病变是非常罕见的，组织学检查可能与视网膜母细胞瘤混淆。低倍镜下，视网膜母细胞瘤的典型改变是存活的与坏死的肿瘤组织交替出现，有显著的局灶性钙化（图29.41）。值得注意的是，病理医生的报告应该提到存在这种钙化，因为眼科医生常常通过影像学检查发现眼内钙化来区分视网膜母细胞瘤和临床上酷似视网膜母细胞瘤的病变。在视网膜母细胞瘤，血管增生显著，存活的肿瘤倾向于围绕着血管成簇生长（图29.42）。

有人提出，在评估视网膜母细胞瘤的眼球剜出标本时，病理学报告中要注明一些组织学特征[19]。这些特征列在表29.5中，其中还包括对见于此肿瘤的玫瑰花结的描述（图29.42和29.43）。同肺小细胞癌一样，视网膜母细胞瘤的血管可能常常出现嗜碱性改变（图29.44），推测是由于血管内衬坏死肿瘤细胞的DNA的集聚[77]，尚不清楚这种嗜碱性的血管改变是否具有预后意义。

许多研究显示，侵犯视神经与临床行为不好相关，而且侵犯的部位越靠后其临床经过越具有侵袭性[78,79]。

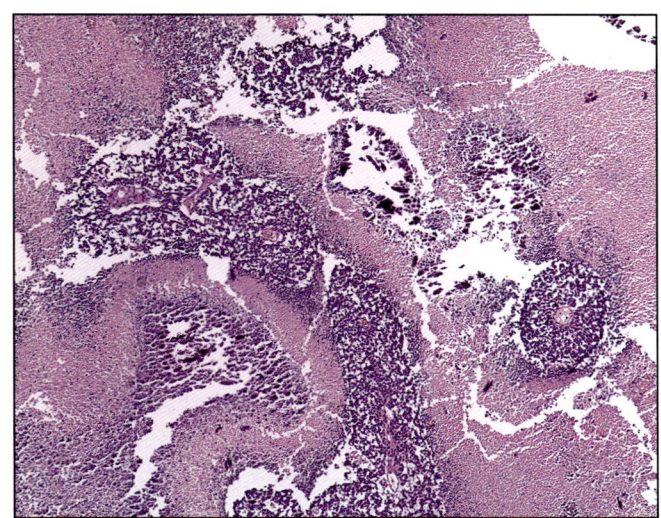

图29.41 视网膜母细胞瘤的低倍所见。存活的肿瘤一般集聚在血管的周围,出现交替坏死带。钙化灶可使肿瘤的组织学表现更加突出。

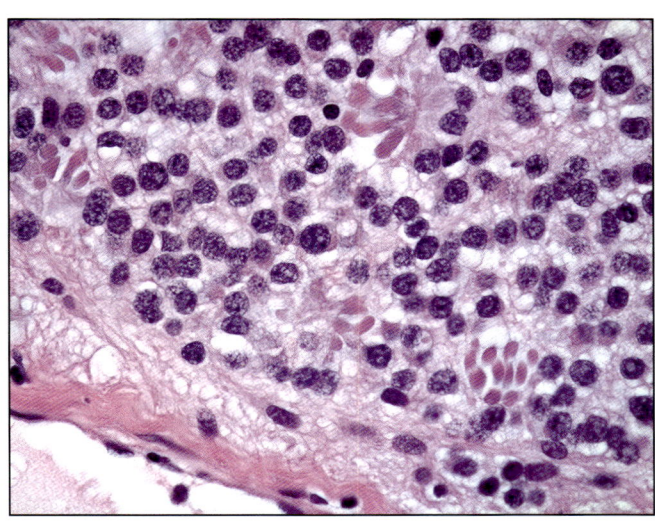

图29.43 伴有视细胞分化的高分化视网膜母细胞瘤。注意嗜酸性的"蒂"是视细胞。显微照片的中心可见一个菊形团,恰好在图的顶部之下。

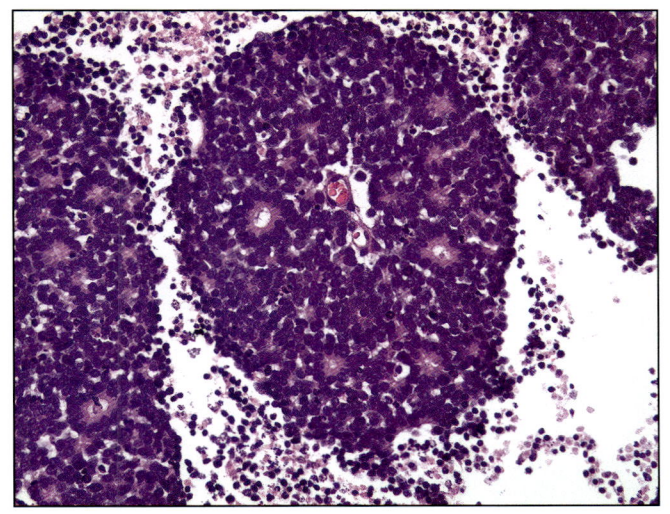

图29.42 视网膜母细胞瘤围绕着位于中心的血管生长。注意有许多伴有特征性中心腔隙的Flexner-Wintersteiner玫瑰花结。

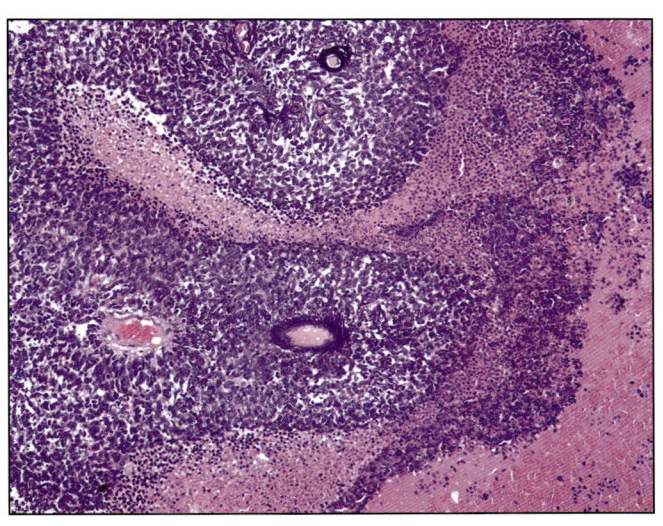

图29.44 视网膜母细胞瘤,肿瘤血管伴有嗜碱性改变。

事实上,许多外科医生都曾接受过获得一长段有附属物的视神经的训练,以确保完全切除肿瘤累及的视神经。然而,在不同的研究者之间,可影响视网膜母细胞瘤预后的独立特征,显然尚存在大的争论。一些病理医生认为,脉络膜浸润是侵袭性行为的一种特征,而另外的研究提示,脉络膜浸润与眼外扩散有关,是转移的主要危险因素[80]。最近的一项研究显示[81],在有孤立性脉络膜浸润和视神经后板浸润的患者,不经辅助化疗其预后也非常好。而肿瘤延伸到视神经切缘(手术切缘)的患者可辅助性化疗。有复合性脉络膜浸润、巩膜浸润以及视神经后板浸润的患者也可得益于辅助性化疗。

一些患有视网膜母细胞瘤的眼球可以在一个疗程的化疗之后切除。治疗早期,肿瘤可能出现坏死和局灶性钙化(图29.45)。长时间后,肿瘤可能有神经胶质增生(gliotic)[67]。

在新鲜状态下打开眼球采集细胞进行细胞遗传学研究时,肿瘤细胞可能涌出进入脉络膜、视神经膜以及整个眼的表面。一般来说,可以将这种人为造成的细胞弥散的假象与肿瘤浸润脉络膜和眼外扩散区别开来。切除眼球之后种植的细胞倾向于彼此分离,且显示与邻近的组织没有关联(图29.46和29.47)。在真正的脉络膜浸润,脉络膜的胶原一般会由于肿瘤膨胀而发生移位(图29.48),而在人为造成的种植假象,这种细胞并不是任

表29.5	推荐报告的视网膜母细胞瘤的组织学特征
组织学特征	**评注**
视神经浸润	许多研究显示，视神经浸润与预后不好相关。浅表浸润（前面的筛板）比后板浸润预后好，视神经切缘浸润被认为预后非常不好。眼外蔓延和视神经切缘蔓延均意味着"切缘阳性"。对于病理医生来说，重要的是要记住，视神经是一束中枢神经，与脑连续。这样，视网膜母细胞瘤可以沿着视神经直接蔓延到脑或通过围绕视神经循环的脑脊液种植到脑
眼外蔓延	眼外蔓延很少在患者容易得到医疗保健的地方见到，是易被忽视的晚期视网膜母细胞瘤的一个典型特征。眼外蔓延预后不好
脉络膜浸润，巩膜浸润	一些作者将脉络膜浸润和巩膜浸润与预后不好联系起来，虽然两者都不是普遍认为的预后不良的特征
前房种植	有些研究显示，视网膜母细胞瘤细胞前房种植伴有侵袭性的临床经过
生长方式	不形成孤立的肿块而是视网膜弥漫性增厚的视网膜母细胞瘤（弥漫性视网膜母细胞瘤）倾向于具有侵袭性的临床经过。弥漫性视网膜母细胞瘤少见，在报告中无需提到生长方式，除非肿瘤为弥漫性的。有些眼科医生会要求病理医生评估肿瘤是外生性的（主要在视网膜下方生长）还是内生性的（长入玻璃体），但是这些生长方式均不具有任何预后意义
分化	视网膜母细胞瘤有三种玫瑰花结。玫瑰花结反映神经元或视细胞分化。Flexner-Wintersteiner玫瑰花结的特征是：围绕中心腔隙的单层肿瘤细胞集聚（图29.43）。菊形团是由单层细胞组成的，细长的胞浆突起（类似于视细胞的外段）突入玫瑰花结的中心（图29.43）。Homer Wright玫瑰花结与在神经母细胞瘤和髓母细胞瘤中描述的一样。玫瑰花结出现时，一般仅占据肿瘤的一部分。在报告中值得提到玫瑰花结，但是肿瘤分化程度并不影响临床经过。高分化肿瘤放疗和化疗疗效不佳[100]。小的普遍高分化的视网膜肿瘤可能是视网膜细胞瘤（retinocytoma）[101]的实例，许多作者认为，它是视网膜母细胞瘤的良性病变（虽然视网膜细胞瘤也可能是处于类似于视网膜母细胞瘤分化过程中的"分化性视网膜母细胞瘤"。眼球很少因为视网膜细胞瘤而摘除。在同一个患者，同时发生视网膜细胞瘤和视网膜母细胞瘤，说明存在种系突变
包括在病理学报告中的可选择的特征	视网膜母细胞瘤的血管可见DNA沉积，但是这种所见与预后不好无关。虹膜出现新生血管形成时在报告中应予以描述。虽然它不影响预后，但是虹膜的这种组织学表现可能导致临床上虹膜颜色的变化，这对于眼科医生来说是一种重要表现。视网膜母细胞瘤的视网膜可能分离，晶状体可能有白内障。最近的两项研究提示，微血管密度增高可能是转移性行为的一个独立标志[102,103]

Modified from Folberg et al.[19]

何膨胀性病变的一部分。

过去，病理医生曾被鼓励评估是否存在多灶性视网膜受累；多灶性被认为是一种 *Rb* 种系突变的组织学标志，而不是 *Rb* 体细胞突变的组织学标志。现在并不主张病理医生评估多灶性，因为区分多灶性原发性视网膜肿瘤和肿瘤的视网膜种植非常困难。此外，现在有较为特异的方法确定 *Rb* 种系突变，眼科医生和肿瘤医生应该依赖这些试验。

众所周知，具有种系突变的患者容易发生其他肿瘤。有些患者可能发生松果体母细胞瘤（pinealoblastoma）——所谓的三侧性视网膜母细胞瘤（trilateral retinoblastoma）[82-84]。眼科肿瘤医生现在已意识到放射治疗对种系突变的视网膜母细胞瘤患者具有危险性。治疗多年之后放射野内可能发生肉瘤（图29.37）。

黑色素细胞眼内肿瘤：痣和黑色素瘤
Melanocytic intraocular tumors: nevi and melanomas

描述眼内黑色素细胞病变时，病理医生可以使用的诊断术语局限于痣和黑色素瘤。除葡萄膜的"普通"痣以外，只有两种特殊形式的葡萄膜痣：黑色素细胞

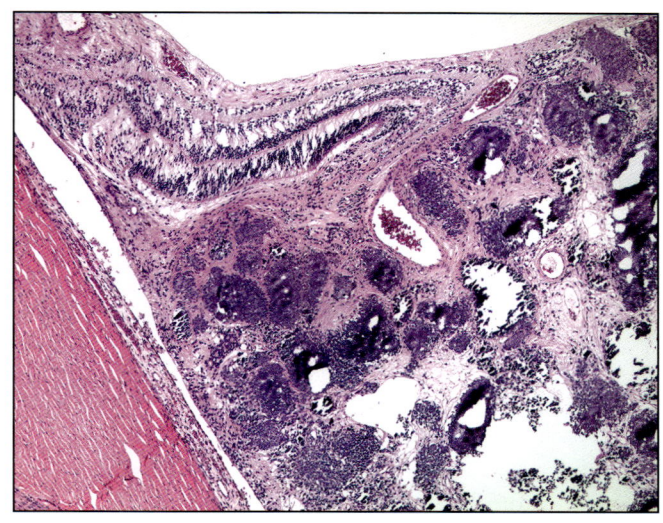
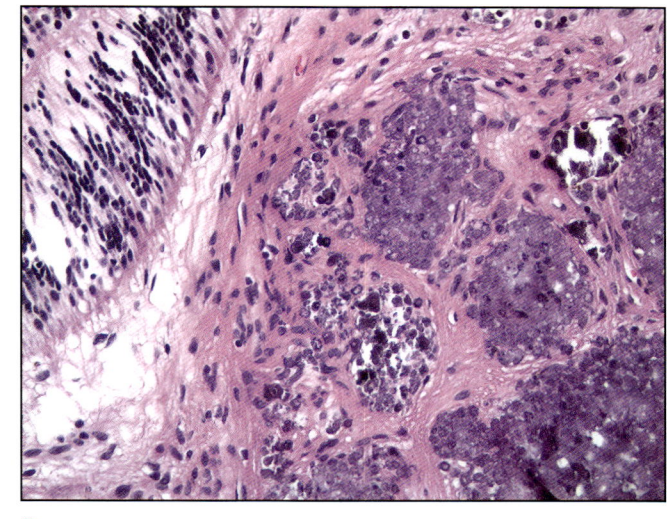

图29.45 视网膜母细胞瘤化疗之后的放大扫描所见。注意钙化和神经胶质增生。（A）较高的放大倍数；（B）"干尸化"肿瘤细胞。

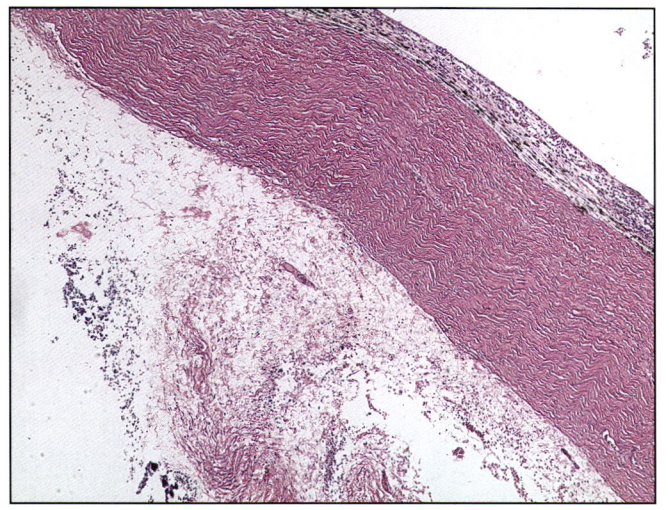
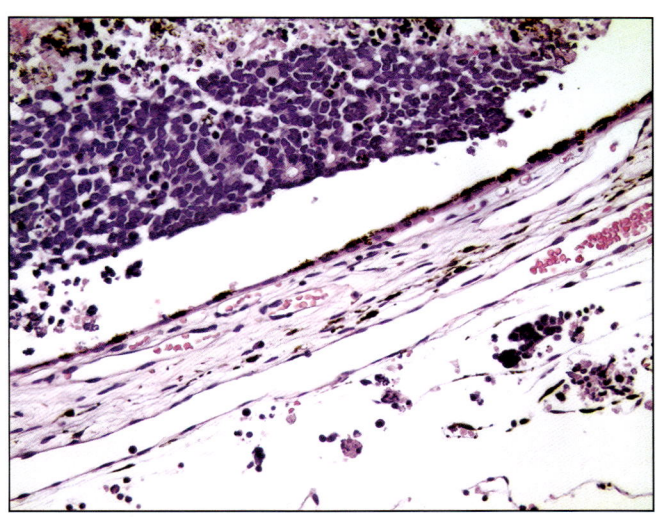

图29.46 注意照片左边散在的肿瘤细胞，在厚的纤维性巩膜附近的结缔组织外。这是眼外肿瘤细胞人为扩散的假象。眼外蔓延以粘着肿胀（cohesive tumefaction）为特征。

图29.47 脉络膜的人为种植假象。注意上方和左侧的完整的视网膜母细胞瘤。显微照片右下方散在的肿瘤细胞与脉络膜的胶原束无关。与图29.48进行比较。

（melanocytoma，或黑色素细胞痣，magnocellular nevus）和眼先天性黑变病（congenital melanosis oculi）。在葡萄膜黑色素细胞病变中，没有见到在皮肤中描述的特殊类型的痣，如Spitz痣、色素性梭形细胞肿瘤、异型增生性痣和其他，也没有描述黑色素瘤的前体病变，如恶性雀斑（lentigo maligna）。即使组织学检查，也从未将交界性黑色素细胞葡萄膜病变描述为"非典型性黑色素细胞增生"。将任何葡萄膜黑色素细胞病变称为"原位"都是不恰当的，因为这些病变发生在间叶而不是上皮组织。

眼科医生倾向于观察临床上认为是痣的眼内色素性病变。一些较大的痣在临床上常常被称为"非典型性痣"，

对这些病变可以进行观察而不治疗。如果病理医生有可能将这种病变描述为良性的话，眼科医生不希望使用破坏视力的操作切除临床上可疑的病变。"瞧，我们切除了肿瘤，所幸它是良性的！"，这样告诉患者对于眼科医生本人来说并不能从中得到安慰。另外，这种陈述可能减轻有其他部位疾病的患者的痛苦，但是却可能使眼科患者感到痛苦和失望："大夫，你是告诉我，因为不必要的治疗，我丧失了视力吗？"

虹膜痣和黑色素瘤 Iris nevi and melanomas

通过组织学检查鉴别虹膜痣和虹膜黑色素瘤非常困难。虹膜痣和虹膜黑色素瘤均容易造成虹膜间质扩张，

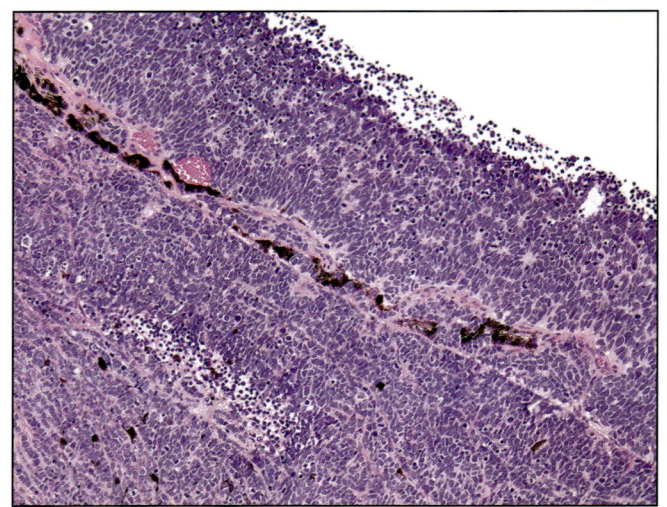

图29.48 视网膜母细胞瘤侵犯脉络膜。视网膜色素上皮明显，表现为从左上延伸到右下的色素沉积。脉络膜位于视网膜色素上皮下方。

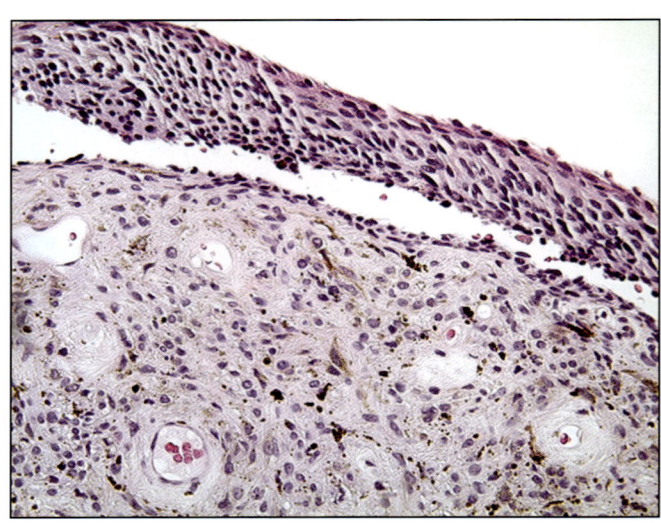

图29.49 伴有表面斑块的虹膜痣。表面斑块是由良性梭形细胞组成的。痣细胞弥漫分布于虹膜间质。

依靠结构特征不能可靠地将它们区分开。同其他部位的痣一样，虹膜痣细胞核容易出现"空心"（hollowed out）的特征。缺乏突出的核仁是虹膜良性黑色素病变的组织学特征，而发现突出的核仁则倾向于诊断为黑色素瘤。多数虹膜黑色素瘤缺乏侵袭性葡萄膜黑色素瘤的特征性的上皮样细胞、带状坏死、炎症和增生的证据（通过辨认核分裂特征或计数增生指数）。

部分痣的特征是虹膜表面出现痣细胞斑块，使得组织学检查区分痣和黑色素瘤更加复杂（图29.49）[85]。痣细胞表面斑块一般是由紧密排列的梭形细胞组成，细胞核具有良性的细胞学特征。表面斑块一般只有几层细胞厚度，因此眼科医生在临床上可能发现不了，而只能切除可以看见的痣的部分。病理医生应该报告斑块的存在，而且要特别提到侧缘出现斑块。痣的表面斑块可能散布于整个虹膜表面，如果虹膜角受到损害，可能导致青光眼。这样看来，虽然虹膜痣在生物学上是良性的，不至于危及患者的生命，但是伴有表面斑块成分的痣却有可能致盲。

睫状体和脉络膜痣
Nevi of the ciliary body and choroid

一般情况下，外科病理医生从未因为痣而切除眼球。在由于其他原因而切除的眼球中可能见到痣。据估计，葡萄膜痣见于10%的高加索人。脉络膜痣境界一般清楚，由梭形黑色素细胞组成，典型者缺乏核仁。在视网膜色素上皮和Bruch膜（脉络膜基底层）之间的嗜酸性和PAS阳性的脉络膜小疣，可见于脉络膜痣的上方。无黑色素性痣可能累及睫状体，如果虹膜角被弥漫痣取代，可能引起青光眼。这个部位的无黑色素性痣组

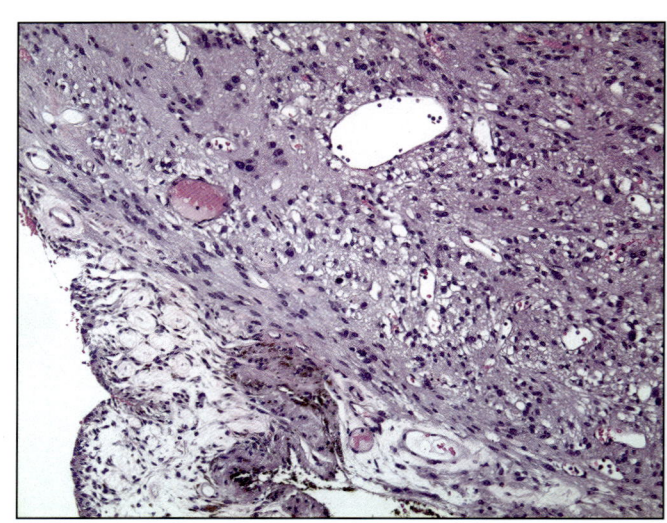

图29.50 中外胚层平滑肌瘤。显微照片上2/3的组织的形态学表现为"原纤维性"平滑肌，类似于神经的表现。前段的平滑肌在胚胎发生上来源于神经嵴。

织学检查可与睫状体中外胚层平滑肌瘤（mesectodermal leiomyomas）混淆[86]，睫状体的平滑肌在胚胎时来自神经外胚层而不是中胚层（图29.50和29.51）。弥漫性葡萄膜色素沉着伴有邻近巩膜受累，称为眼的先天性黑变病（congenital melanosis ocujli），实际上是虹膜、睫状体和脉络膜的先天性痑。这种病变可见于葡萄膜黑色素瘤的患者，特别是在高加索人。

一种特殊类型的葡萄膜痣可能引起外科病理医生的注意，即黑色素细胞瘤（melanocytoma），或巨细胞痣（magnocellular nevus）[87]。眼科医生了解这些病变是视网膜上的深黑色病变。在这个部位，他们不主张尝试任何外科治疗。然而，黑色素细胞瘤可能累及睫状体，而且可能与黑色素瘤混淆。偶尔这些肿瘤可能增大并压迫

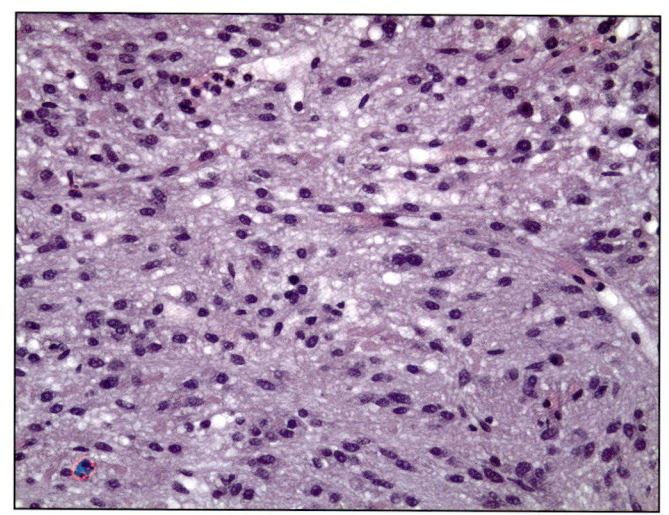

图29.51 中外胚层平滑肌瘤。图29.50的高倍放大图像。

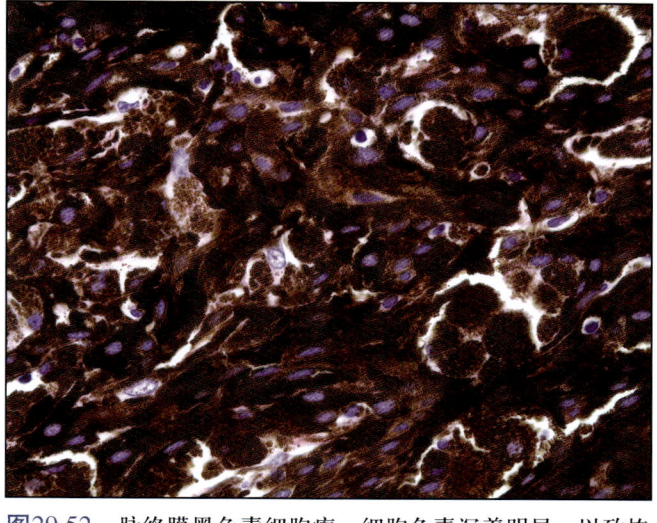

图29.52 脉络膜黑色素细胞瘤。细胞色素沉着明显，以致掩盖了多数的核仁。

晶状体，引起部分性白内障（sectoral cataract）。睫状体黑色素细胞瘤可引起眼压升高（通过浸润虹膜角，通过睫状体转动靠近虹膜角，或发生在自发性坏死和释放大量黑色素到眼房水中之后，即黑色素细胞瘤溶解性青光眼，melanocytomalytic glaucoma[88]）。有些情况下，良性的睫状体痣可侵蚀巩膜，这种行为并不代表恶性[89]。

组织学检查，黑色素细胞瘤是由均匀的大的富于色素的细胞组成，这种细胞为圆形到多角形或梭形。黑色素细胞瘤出现梭形细胞代表有局灶侵袭性倾向，即局灶浸润性，但是仍然认为这些病变是良性的。据报道，黑色素瘤与黑色素细胞瘤有关，但是一般来说，葡萄膜痣（眼的先天性黑变病除外）与黑色素瘤前体病变无关。许多黑色素细胞瘤的组织切片不经漂白不可能发现核仁。核为小圆形，大小一致，一般位于中心，可能含有小的核仁（图29.52和29.53），可能有许多噬黑色素细胞（melanophages）。相反，多数色素性葡萄膜黑色素瘤的细胞其大小和形状不同，同样，核和核仁的大小和形状也有不同。

睫状体和脉络膜黑色素瘤
Melanomas of the ciliary boby and choroid

这些病变可为无色素性的或有不同程度的色素沉着。多数肿瘤着染某种程度的S-100蛋白、HMB-45或Melan-A[90]，只有少数病例需要通过免疫组化染色证实诊断。临床上眼科医生鉴别葡萄膜黑色素瘤和类似于黑色素瘤的病变的准确性已经提高。倘若眼科医生把误诊为黑色素瘤的眼球切除，病理医生见到的可能是脉络膜出血、海绵状血管瘤或脉络膜转移性肿瘤，这些病变的组织学诊断不应该出现太多的困难。

因此，病理医生的注意力应该回到黑色素瘤的临床

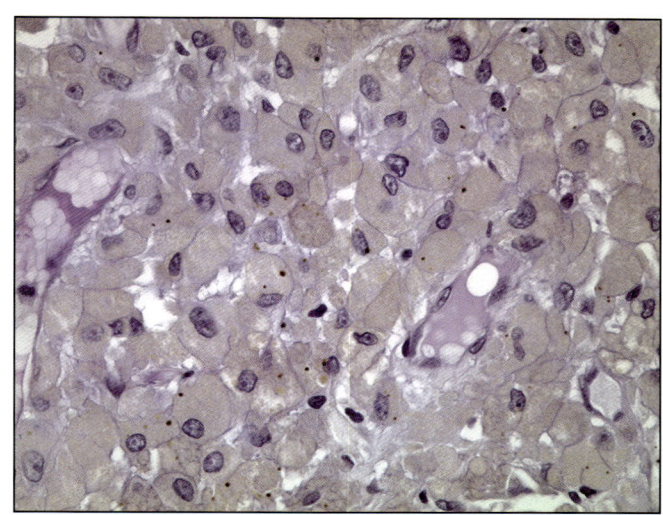

图29.53 与图29.52为同一肿瘤，为经过高锰酸钾漂白去除黑色素以后。注意细胞较大，核位于中心，细胞学呈良性表现。

诊断上。有人提出，当评估由于葡萄膜黑色素瘤而摘除的眼球标本时，病理学报告应该提到一些组织学特征[19]。这些特征总结在表29.6中，并将在下面展开讨论。

细胞类型 Cell type

实际上，Callender分类是一个形态学谱系（见表29.6）[911]。这种分类虽然有所帮助，但是在不同病理医生之间不具有可重复性。例如，将"混合细胞肿瘤"替换为"上皮样"黑色素瘤必须出现上皮样细胞，但是在计数上皮样细胞的数目上有很大的不一致性。梭形黑色素瘤细胞的横切面可能类似于小的上皮样细胞。一些研究摈弃了表29.6的分类方法，而只是记录有无上皮样细胞[92]。

表29.6	推荐报告的葡萄膜黑色素瘤的组织学特征
组织学特征	评注
部位	肿瘤局限于脉络膜者比蔓延至或局限于睫状体者预后好
眼外蔓延	一些肿瘤沿着导血管和神经浸润巩膜。通过连续或不连续切片追踪这种所见并寻找肿瘤是否蔓延至巩膜表面是可取的。出现眼外蔓延应记录在报告中。应用眼科测微计测量眼外蔓延的直径是有帮助的,因为一些肿瘤医生认为,微小眼外蔓延并不代表患者有危险。在病理医生的报告中,还应提到从睫状体蔓延到结膜的眼外延伸。眼内没有淋巴管,葡萄膜黑色素瘤一般是通过血行播散到肝。然而,当眼外蔓延累及结膜时,转移到局部淋巴结是有可能的
生长方式	相对扁平和弥漫的肿瘤(弥漫性黑色素瘤)倾向于与侵袭性的临床经过有关。累及虹膜主动脉环后,肿瘤在睫状体内呈环状生长(环状黑色素瘤),这种黑色素瘤也具有侵袭性的临床经过。如果这两种生长方式在报告中均未提到,眼科医生有理由认为肿瘤是局灶性的
大小	与皮肤和结膜黑色素瘤不同,肿瘤高度(垂直测量)不具预后意义。病理医生应该记录接触巩膜的最大尺寸。如果在大体检查时没有记录,可以从切片上测量
细胞类型	1931年,Callender首先描述了形态学(细胞类型)和预后的关系。尽管发现了许多分子学和细胞遗传学标记物,多数研究认为细胞类型仍然是一个独立的预后因素。Callender描述了三种类型的细胞。 1. A型梭形细胞细长,核的中心有皱褶(同卵巢的Brenner瘤)。A型梭形细胞一般缺乏核仁 2. B型梭形细胞核缺乏中心皱褶,其特征是有突出的核仁 3. 上皮样细胞一般含有丰富的胞浆、空泡状核以及大而多形性的核仁
增生	许多研究显示,在40倍高倍视野下计数的核分裂象的数目具有预后意义。Ki-67增生指数也有预后意义,而且可以代替核分裂计数
肿瘤中的淋巴细胞浸润	每20个高倍视野中淋巴细胞>100的肿瘤比<100个淋巴细胞的肿瘤预后差
血管原性类似形态	容易发现肿瘤的这种特征,而且在病理医生之间具有高度的可重复性。组织切片应用PAS染色,不用苏木素复染,应用绿色滤光片观察(如果PAS染色呈阳性,可将其转变为黑色)。PAS染色抗漂白可去除黑色素。这种形态层粘连蛋白(laminin)呈阳性,但是应用PAS染色比免疫组化检查容易发现。肿瘤细胞束周围出现PAS阳性物质构成的闭环或出现至少3个背靠背的闭环(称为网状结构)与肿瘤相关性死亡独立强相关
可选择的特征	有些葡萄膜黑色素瘤完全坏死,被归入坏死型黑色素瘤。将一个肿瘤命名为坏死型,代表预后处于中间状态。最近发现特异性细胞遗传学异常(尤其是3号染色体单体和8号染色体额外复制)与预后不良有关。一般是在新鲜组织进行这些检测。现在,在组织学切片上进行的检查是在研究实验室进行的,不提倡作为组织病理医生的常规检查。如果存在的话,病理医生应该提到视网膜脱落(几乎总是出现)、Bruch膜破裂、白内障或青光眼

Modified from Folberg et al.[19]

仅含有梭形A细胞的肿瘤不常见,这种肿瘤可能具有良性行为。梭形细胞黑色素瘤(spindle cell melanoma)或由梭形A细胞和梭形B细胞混合组成,或完全由梭形B细胞组成。多数葡萄膜黑色素瘤是由梭形细胞和上皮样细胞混合组成的肿瘤,称为混合细胞性黑色素瘤(mixed cell melanoma)。主要由上皮样细胞组成的肿瘤称为上皮样黑色素瘤(epithelioid melanoma)。一般来说,肿瘤出现的上皮样细胞越多,预后越差(图29.54和29.55)。

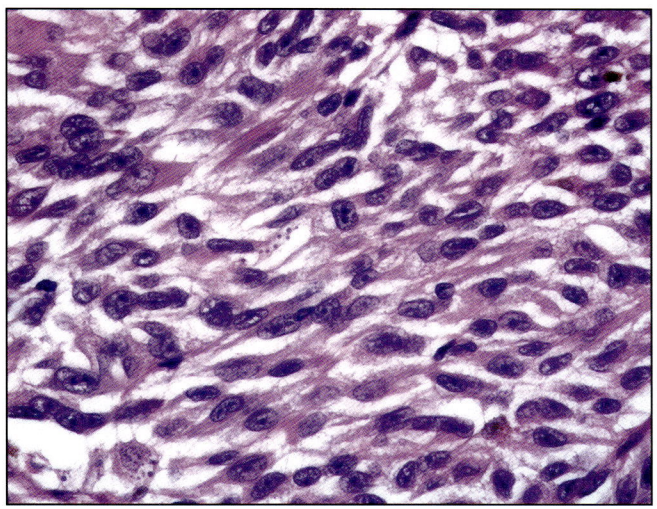

图29.54 脉络膜黑色素瘤的梭形B黑色素瘤细胞。细胞呈梭形，含有明显的核仁。还可见到少数具有"咖啡豆"核的梭形A细胞。

血管原性拟态模式
Vasculogenic mimicry patterns

肿瘤细胞束周围出现由PAS阳性物质构成的闭环或至少有3个背靠背的闭环（称为网状结构）是与肿瘤相关性死亡密切相关的独立因素（图29.56）[92]。虽然这些环层粘连蛋白染色阳性，但是用PAS染色容易发现它们[93]。PAS染色阳性的环比较薄，不同于出现在葡萄膜黑色素瘤的纤维血管间隙，后者缺乏独立的预后意义[94,94a]。PAS阳性结构是由高度浸润性的黑色素瘤细胞通过一种称为血管原性拟态的过程形成的[95-97]。这些形态可以见于其他癌症[94]，包括皮肤黑色素瘤[93,98]。认为这种模式是液体传导[99]，而且在肿瘤中或许可传导红细胞。

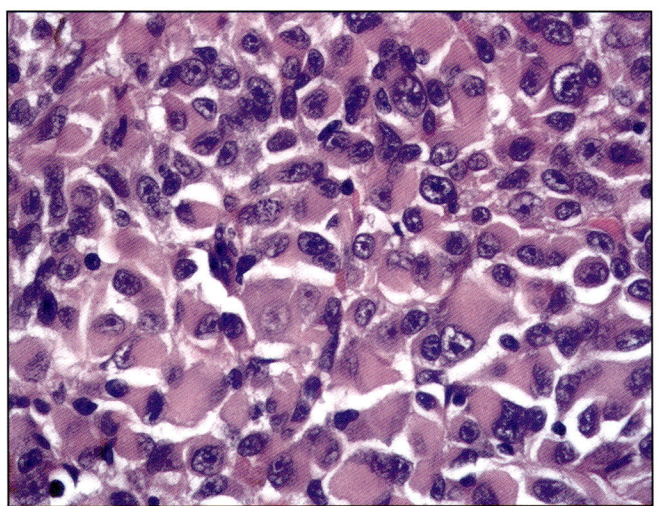

图29.55 上皮样黑色素瘤细胞。细胞为多角形，核多形性，核仁突出。

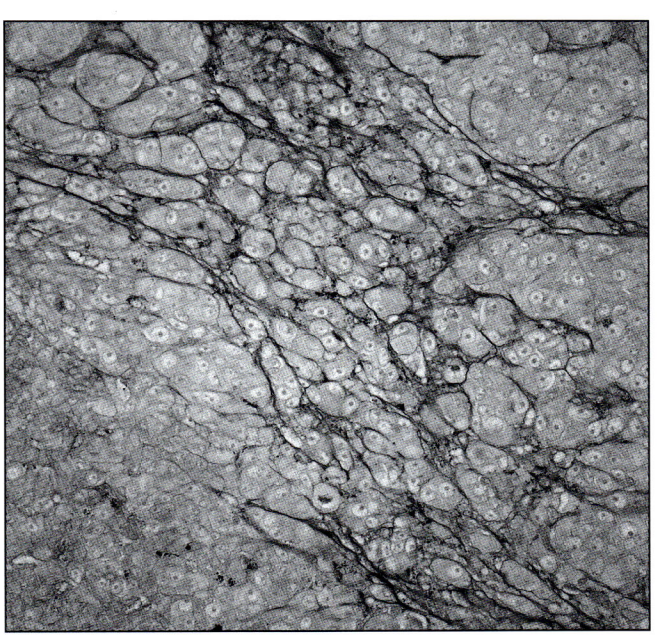

图29.56 脉络膜恶性黑色素瘤，PAS染色，未经苏木素复染。PAS阳性物质细环围绕着黑色素瘤细胞束。这种环层对粘连蛋白和肝素表面蛋白多醣呈阳性。它们形成血浆，而且可能形成红细胞，是高度浸润的肿瘤细胞通过血管原性拟态过程形成的。

参考文献

1. Folberg R, McLean I W, Zimmerman L E 1984 Conjunctival acquired melanosis and malignant melanoma. Ophthalmology 91: 673–678
2. Folberg R, McLean I W, Zimmerman L E 1985 Conjunctival malignant melanoma. Hum Pathol 16: 136–143
3. Folberg R, Jakobiec F A, McLean I W et al. 1992 Is primary acquired melanosis of the conjunctiva equivalent to melanoma in situ? Mod Pathol 5: 2–5
4. Tuthill R J, Unger J M, Liu P Y et al. 2002 Risk assessment in localized primary cutaneous melanoma – a Southwest Oncology Group study evaluating nine factors and a test of the Clark logistic regression prediction model. Am J Clin Pathol 118: 504–511
5. de la Cruz P O J, Specht C S, McLean I W 1990 Lymphocytic infiltration in uveal malignant melanoma. Cancer 65: 112–115
6. Folberg R, Rummelt V, Parys-Van Ginderdeuren R et al. 1993 The prognostic value of tumor blood vessel morphology in primary uveal melanoma. Ophthalmology 100: 1389–1398
7. Wright J D, Font R L 1979 Mucinous sweat gland adenocarcinoma of eyelid: a clinicopathologic study of 21 cases with histochemical and electron microscopic observations. Cancer 44: 1757–1768
8. Malhotra R, Huilgol S C, Huynh N T et al. 2004 The Australian Mohs database, part II: periocular basal cell carcinoma outcome at 5-year follow-up. Ophthalmology 111: 631–636
9. Malhotra R, Huilgol S C, Huynh N T et al. 2004 The Australian Mohs database, part I: periocular basal cell carcinoma experience over 7 years. Ophthalmology 111: 624–630
10. Malhotra R, Huilgol S C, Huynh N T et al. 2004 The Australian Mohs database: periocular squamous cell carcinoma. Ophthalmology 111: 617–623
11. Bartley G B 2004 Mohs surgery: proclamation, proof, principles, and promise. Ophthalmology 111: 615–616
12. Hsuan J D, Harrad R A, Potts M J et al. 2004 Small margin excision of periocular basal cell carcinoma: 5 year results. Br J Ophthalmol 88: 358–360

13. Rao N A, Hidayat A A, McLean I W et al. 1982 Sebaceous carcinomas of the ocular adnexa: a clinicopathologic study of 104 cases, with five-year follow-up data. Hum Pathol 13: 113–122
14. Wolfe J T III, Yeatts R P, Wick M R et al. 1984 Sebaceous carcinoma of the eyelid. Errors in clinical and pathologic diagnosis. Am J Surg Pathol 8: 597–606
15. Ansai S, Katagata Y, Yoshikawa K et al. 1994 An immunohistochemical study of sebaceous carcinoma with anti-keratin monoclonal antibodies: comparison with other skin cancers. J Dermatol 21: 553–559
16. Johnson J S, Lee J A, Cotton D W et al. 1999 Dimorphic immunohistochemical staining in ocular sebaceous neoplasms: a useful diagnostic aid. Eye 13: 104–108
17. Sinard J H 1999 Immunohistochemical distinction of ocular sebaceous carcinoma from basal cell and squamous cell carcinoma. Arch Ophthalmol 117: 776–783
18. Russell W G, Page D L, Hough A J et al. 1980 Sebaceous carcinoma of meibomian gland origin. The diagnostic importance of pagetoid spread of neoplastic cells. Am J Clin Pathol 73: 504–511
19. Folberg R, Salomao D, Grossniklaus H E et al. 2003 Recommendations for the reporting of tissues removed as part of the surgical treatment of common malignancies of the eye and its adnexa. Am J Surg Pathol 27: 999–1004
20. Folberg R, Whitaker D C, Tse D T et al. 1987 Recurrent and residual sebaceous carcinoma after Mohs' excision of the primary lesion. Am J Ophthalmol 103: 817–823
21. Dzubow L M 1985 Sebaceous carcinoma of the eyelid: treatment with Mohs surgery. J Dermatol Surg Oncol 11: 40–44
22. Yount A B, Bylund D, Pratt S G et al. 1994 Mohs micrographic excision of sebaceous carcinoma of the eyelids. J Dermatol Surg Oncol 20: 523–529
23. Folberg R, Jakobiec F A, Bernardino V B Jr et al. 1989 Benign conjunctival melanocytic lesions: clinicopathologic features. Ophthalmology 96: 436–461
24. Tahery D P, Goldberg R, Moy R L 1992 Malignant melanoma of the eyelid. A report of eight cases and a review of the literature. J Am Acad Dermatol 27: 17–21
25. Morgan M B, Truitt C A, Romer C et al. 1998 Ocular adnexal oncocytoma: a case series and clinicopathologic review of the literature. Am J Dermatopathol 20: 487–490
26. Lopansri S, Mihm M C Jr 1979 Clinical and pathological correlation of malignant melanoma. J Cutan Pathol 6: 180–194
27. McDonnell J M, Carpenter J D, Jacobs P et al. 1989 Conjunctival melanocytic lesions in children. Ophthalmology 96: 986–993
28. Zamir E, Mechoulam H, Micera A et al. 2002 Inflamed juvenile conjunctival naevus: clinicopathological characterisation. Br J Ophthalmol 86: 28–30
29. Scott I U, Karp C L, Nuovo G J 2002 Human papillomavirus 16 and 18 expression in conjunctival intraepithelial neoplasia. Ophthalmology 109: 542–547
30. Rao N A, Font R L 1976 Mucoepidermoid carcinoma of the conjunctiva: a clinicopathologic study of five cases. Cancer 38: 1699–1709
31. Cohen B H, Green W R, Iliff N T et al. 1980 Spindle cell carcinoma of the conjunctiva. Arch Ophthalmol 98: 1809–1813
32. Huntington A C, Langloss J M, Hidayat A A 1990 Spindle cell carcinoma of the conjunctiva. An immunohistochemical and ultrastructural study of six cases. Ophthalmology 97: 711–717
33. Folberg R, McLean I W, Zimmerman L E 1985 Primary acquired melanosis of the conjunctiva. Hum Pathol 16: 136–143
34. Folberg R, McLean I W 1986 Primary acquired melanosis and melanoma of the conjunctiva: terminology, classification and biologic behavior. Hum Pathol 17: 652–655
35. Jakobiec F A, Folberg R, Iwamoto T 1989 Clinicopathologic characteristics of premalignant and malignant melanocytic lesions of the conjunctiva. Ophthalmology 96: 147–166
36. Seregard S 2000 Pigmented spindle cell naevus of reed presenting in the conjunctiva. Acta Ophthalmol Scand 78: 104–106
37. Crawford J B, Howes E L Jr, Char D H 1999 Combined nevi of the conjunctiva. Arch Ophthalmol 117: 1121–1127
38. Ackerman A B, Sood R, Koenig M 1991 Primary acquired melanosis of the conjunctiva is melanoma in situ. Mod Pathol 4: 253–263
39. Bernardino V B, Naidoff M A, Clark W H 1976 Malignant melanomas of the conjunctiva. Am J Ophthalmol 82: 383–394
40. Griffith W R, Green W R, Weinstein G W 1971 Conjunctival malignant melanoma originating in acquired melanosis sine pigmento. Am J Ophthalmol 72: 595–599
41. Frucht-Pery J, Rozenman Y, Pe'er J 2002 Topical mitomycin-C for partially excised conjunctival squamous cell carcinoma. Ophthalmology 109: 548–552
42. Frucht-Pery J, Pe'er J 1996 Use of mitomycin C in the treatment of conjunctival primary acquired melanosis with atypia. Arch Ophthalmol 114: 1261–1264
43. Salomao D R, Mathers W D, Sutphin J E et al. 1999 Cytologic changes in the conjunctiva mimicking malignancy after topical mitomycin C chemotherapy. Ophthalmology 106: 1756–1760
44. Seregard S 1993 Cell proliferation as a prognostic indicator in conjunctival malignant melanoma. Am J Ophthalmol 116: 93–97
45. Paridaens A D A, Minassian D C, McCartney A C E et al. 1994 Prognostic factors in primary malignant melanoma of the conjunctiva – a clinicopathological study of 256 cases. Br J Ophthalmol 78: 252–259
46. De P P, Shields C L, Shields J A et al. 1993 Clinical predictive factors for development of recurrence and metastasis in conjunctival melanoma: a review of 68 cases. Br J Ophthalmol 77: 624–630
47. Esmaeli B, Eicher S, Popp J et al. 2001 Sentinel lymph node biopsy for conjunctival melanoma. Ophthalm Plast Reconstr Surg 17: 436–442
47a. Charlotte F, Doghmi K, Cassoux N et al. 2006 Ocular adnexal marginal zone B cell lymphoma: a clinical and pathologic study of 23 cases. Virchows Arch 448: 506–516
48. Knowles D M, Jakobiec F A, McNally L et al. 1990 Lymphoid hyperplasia and malignant lymphoma occurring in the ocular adnexa (orbit, conjunctiva, and eyelids): a prospective multiparametric analysis of 108 cases during 1977 to 1987. Hum Pathol 21: 959–973
49. Coupland S E, Krause L, Delecluse H J et al. 1998 Lymphoproliferative lesions of the ocular adnexa. Analysis of 112 cases. Ophthalmology 105: 1430–1441
50. Howard G M, Jakobiec F A, DeVoe A G 1975 Kaposi's sarcoma of the conjunctiva. Am J Ophthalmol 79: 420–423
51. Jaimovich L, Calb I, Kaminsky A 1986 Kaposi's sarcoma of the conjunctiva. J Am Acad Dermatol 14: 589–592
52. Pe'er J J, Stefanyszyn M, Hidayat A A 1994 Nonepithelial tumors of the lacrimal sac. Am J Ophthalmol 118: 650–658
53. Stefanyszyn M A, Hidayat A A, Pe'er J J et al. 1994 Lacrimal sac tumors. Ophthalm Plast Reconstr Surg 10: 169–184
54. Pe'er J, Hidayat A A, Ilsar M et al. 1996 Glandular tumors of the lacrimal sac. Their histopathologic patterns and possible origins. Ophthalmology 103: 1601–1605
55. White W L, Ferry J A, Harris N L et al. 1995 Ocular adnexal lymphoma. A clinicopathologic study with identification of lymphomas of mucosa-associated lymphoid tissue type. Ophthalmology 102: 1994–2006
56. Richards A B, Shalka H W, Roberts F J et al. 1980 Pseudotumor of the orbit and retroperitoneal fibrosis. A form of multifocal fibrosclerosis. Arch Ophthalmol 98: 1617–1620
57. Medeiros L J, Harmon D C, Linggood R M et al. 1989 Immunohistologic features predict clinical behavior of orbital and conjunctival lymphoid infiltrates. Blood 74: 2121–2129
58. Jakobiec F A, Mills M D, Hidayat A A et al. 1993 Periocular xanthogranulomas associated with severe adult-onset asthma. Trans Am Ophthalmol Soc 91: 99–125
59. Robertson D M, Winkelmann R K 1984 Ophthalmic features of necrobiotic xanthogranuloma with paraproteinemia. Am J Ophthalmol 97: 173–183
60. Jakobiec F A, Rini F, Char D et al. 1989 Primary liposarcoma of the orbit. Problems in the diagnosis and management of five cases. Ophthalmology 96: 180–191
61. Cai Y C, McMenamin M E, Rose G et al. 2001 Primary liposarcoma of the orbit: a clinicopathologic study of seven cases. Ann Diagn Pathol 5: 255–266
62. Kennerdell J S, Dekker A, Johnson B L et al. 1979 Fine-needle aspiration biopsy. Its use in orbital lesions. Arch Ophthalmol 97: 1315–1317
63. Gupta S, Sood B, Gulati M et al. 1999 Orbital mass lesions: US-guided fine-needle aspiration biopsy – experience in 37 patients. Radiology 213: 568–572
64. Marquardt M D, Zimmerman L E 1982 Histopathology of meningiomas and gliomas of the optic nerve. Hum Pathol 13: 226–235
65. Levin L A, Jakobiec F A 1992 Optic nerve tumors of childhood: a decision-analytical approach to their diagnosis. Int Ophthalmol Clin 32: 223–240
66. Stern J, Jakobiec F A, Housepian E M 1980 The architecture of optic nerve gliomas with and without neurofibromatosis. Arch Ophthalmol 98: 505–511
67. Dithmar S, Aabert T M Jr, Grossniklaus H E 2000 Histopathologic changes in retinoblastoma after chemoreduction. Retina 20: 33–36
68. Demirci H, Eagle R C Jr, Shields C L et al. 2003 Histopathologic findings in eyes with retinoblastoma treated only with chemoreduction. Arch Ophthalmol 121: 1125–1131
69. Diener-West M, Earle J D, Fine S L et al. 2001 The COMS randomized trial of iodine 125 brachytherapy for choroidal melanoma, III: Initial mortality findings. Arch Ophthalmol 119: 969–982
70. Akpek E K, Ahmed I, Hochberg F H et al. 1999 Intraocular-central nervous system lymphoma: clinical features, diagnosis, and outcomes. Ophthalmology 106: 1805–1810
71. Kitzmann A S, Weaver A L, Lohse C M et al. 2003 Clinicopathologic correlations in 646 consecutive surgical eye specimens, 1990–2000. Am J Clin Pathol 119: 594–601
72. Canning C R, McCartney A C E, Hungerford J 1988 Medulloepithelioma (diktyoma). Br J Ophthalmol 72: 764–767
73. Broughton W L, Zimmerman L E 1978 A clinicopathologic study of 56 cases of intraocular medulloepitheliomas. Am J Ophthalmol 85: 407–418
74. Folberg R, Verdick R E, Weingeist T A et al. 1986 Gross examination of eyes removed for ciliary body or choroidal melanoma. Ophthalmology 93: 1643–1647
75. Folberg R 1995 The Eye: in Spencer, W H 1995 Ophthalmic pathology: an atlas and textbook, 4th edn. W B Saunders, Philadelphia
76. Spencer W H 1996 Ophthalmic pathology: an atlas and textbook, 4th edn. W B Saunders, Philadelphia
77. Bunt A H, Tso M O 1981 Feulgen-positive deposits in retinoblastoma. Incidence, composition, and ultrastructure. Arch Ophthalmol 99: 144–150
78. Khelfaoui F, Validire P, Auperin A et al. 1996 Histopathologic risk factors in retinoblastoma: a retrospective study of 172 patients treated in a single institution. Cancer 77: 1206–1213

79. Stannard C, Lipper S, Sealy R et al. 1979 Retinoblastoma: correlation of invasion of the optic nerve and choroid with prognosis and metastases. Br J Ophthalmol 63: 560–570
80. Kopelman J E, McLean I W, Rosenberg S H 1987 Multivariate analysis of risk factors for metastasis in retinoblastoma treated by enucleation. Ophthalmology 94: 371–377
81. Chantada G L, Dunkel I J, de Davila M T et al. 2004 Retinoblastoma patients with high risk ocular pathological features: who needs adjuvant therapy? Br J Ophthalmol 88: 1069–1073
82. Bader J L, Meadows A T, Zimmerman L E et al. 1982 Bilateral retinoblastoma with ectopic intracranial retinoblastoma: trilateral retinoblastoma. Cancer Genet Cytogenet 5: 203–213
83. Marcus D M, Brooks S E, Leff G et al. 1998 Trilateral retinoblastoma: insights into histogenesis and management. Surv Ophthalmol 43: 59–70
84. Kivela T 1999 Trilateral retinoblastoma: a meta-analysis of hereditary retinoblastoma associated with primary ectopic intracranial retinoblastoma. J Clin Oncol 17: 1829–1837
85. Jakobiec F A, Silbert G 1981 Are most iris "melanomas" really nevi? A clinicopathologic study of 189 lesions. Arch Ophthalmol 99: 2117–2132
86. Jakobiec F A, Font R L, Tso M O et al. 1977 Mesectodermal leiomyoma of the ciliary body: a tumor of presumed neural crest origin. Cancer 39: 2102–2113
87. Juarez C P, Tso M O 1980 An ultrastructural study of melanocytomas (magnocellular nevi) of the optic disk and uvea. Am J Ophthalmol 90: 48–62
88. Fineman M S, Eagle R C Jr, Shields J A et al. 1998 Melanocytomalytic glaucoma in eyes with necrotic iris melanocytoma. Ophthalmology 105: 492–496
89. Rummelt V, Naumann G O, Folberg R et al. 1994 Surgical management of melanocytoma of the ciliary body with extrascleral extension. Am J Ophthalmol 117: 169–176
90. Heegaard S, Jensen O A, Prause J U 2000 Immunohistochemical diagnosis of malignant melanoma of the conjunctiva and uvea: comparison of the novel antibody against melan-A with S100 protein and HMB-45. Mel Res 10: 350–354
91. McLean I W, Foster W D, Zimmerman L E et al. 1983 Modifications of Callender's classification of uveal melanoma at the Armed Forces Institute of Pathology. Am J Ophthalmol 96: 502–509
92. Rummelt V, Folberg R, Rummelt C et al. 1994 Microcirculation architecture of melanocytic nevi and malignant melanomas of the ciliary body and choroid. A comparative histopathologic and ultrastructural study. Ophthalmology 101: 718–727
93. Thies A, Mangold U, Moll I et al. 2001 PAS-positive loops and networks as a prognostic indicator in cutaneous malignant melanoma. J Pathol 195: 537–542
94. Folberg R, Maniotis A J 2004 Vasculogenic mimicry. APMIS 112: 508–525
94a. Lin A Y, Maniotis A J, Valyi-Nagy K et al. 2005 Distinguishing fibrovascular septa from vasculogenic mimicry patterns. Arch Pathol Lab Med 129: 884–892
95. Maniotis A J, Folberg R, Hess A et al. 1999 Vascular channel formation by human melanoma cells in vivo and in vitro: vasculogenic mimicry. Am J Pathol 155: 739–752
96. Folberg R, Hendrix M J, Maniotis A J 2000 Vasculogenic mimicry and tumor angiogenesis. Am J Pathol 156: 361–381
97. Maniotis A J, Chen X, Garcia C et al. 2002 Control of melanoma morphogenesis, endothelial survival, and perfusion by extracellular matrix. Lab Invest 82: 1031–1043
98. Warso M A, Maniotis A J, Chen X et al. 2001 Prognostic significance of periodic acid–Schiff-positive patterns in primary cutaneous melanoma. Clin Cancer Res 7: 473–477
99. Clarijs R, Otte-Holler I, Ruiter D J et al. 2002 Presence of a fluid-conducting meshwork in xenografted cutaneous and primary human uveal melanoma. Invest Ophthalmol Vis Sci 43: 912–918
100. Singh, A D, Shields, C L, Shields, J A 2002 Lack of response to chemoreduction in presumed well differentiated retinoblastoma. J Pediatr Ophthalmol Strabismus 39: 107–109
101. Margo C, Hidayat A, Kopelman J et al. 1983 Retinocytoma. A benign variant of retinoblastoma. Arch Ophthalmol 101: 1519–1531
102. Marback E F, Arias V E A, Paranhos A et al. 2003 Tumour angiogenesis as a prognostic factor for disease dissemination in retinoblastoma. Br J Ophthalmol 87: 1224–1228
103. Rossler J, Dietrich T, Pavlakovic H et al. 2004 Higher vessel densities in retinoblastoma with local invasive growth and metastasis. Am J Pathol 164: 391–394

耳肿瘤
Tumors of the ear

Leslie Michaels 著

回允中　张艳梅 译

30

外耳肿瘤	1813	中耳肿瘤	1817
表皮肿瘤	1813	胆脂瘤	1817
黑色素细胞肿瘤	1816	发育性瘤样异常	1819
骨和软骨肿瘤	1816	真性肿瘤	1820
神经肿瘤	1816	内耳肿瘤	1824
肌肉肿瘤	1816	原发性肿瘤	1824
淋巴网状系统肿瘤	1816	耳的继发性肿瘤	1827

　　耳肿瘤并不常见，但是可造成病理医生的诊断困难。内耳由特殊类型的无活动力的骨和神经组织组成，无活动力的骨实际上是一个没有核分裂的感觉区。内耳的肿瘤主要是神经鞘细胞谱系的肿瘤，神经鞘细胞是该部位唯一相对不稳定的细胞。中耳内衬单层扁平上皮，能通过生成腺体对炎症产生明显的反应，这能够解释为什么腺瘤是中耳最常见的肿瘤。外耳是特化的皮肤附件，外耳肿瘤主要反映了可见于其他皮肤部位的各种肿瘤。

外耳肿瘤　Neoplasms of the external ear

表皮肿瘤　Epidermal neoplasms

基底细胞癌　Basal cell carcinoma

临床特征

　　虽然头颈部恶性上皮性肿瘤多数是基底细胞癌（见第23章），但是在外耳耳廓，基底细胞癌的发生率仅仅略多于鳞状细胞癌[1]。

　　基底细胞癌是一种生长缓慢的肿瘤，治愈率高，偶尔反复复发，可向深部延伸至中耳、乳突甚至延伸至颅内。几乎从不发生转移。

大体表现

　　基底细胞癌通常表现为珍珠色的蜡样结节，伴有溃疡形成。硬斑型（morpheic type）病例占25%，皮下边缘呈浸润性，因为肿瘤硬化显著，所以在临床或大体病理学检查时不能辨认（见下文）。

组织学表现

　　外耳基底细胞癌镜下表现类似于发生在其他皮肤部位的基底细胞癌（见第23章）。硬斑型基底细胞癌的特征是：肿瘤细胞被明显玻璃样变的间质胶原分成基底细胞条索。这些肿瘤倾向于潜行发生浸润，因此预后不好。溶基质素3（stromelysin 3）是金属蛋白酶家族的成员之一，它在硬斑型以及其他侵袭性基底细胞癌的间质中呈强阳性表达[2]。使用增生相关性抗原Ki-67（MIB-1）进行免疫组化染色时发现，复发性基底细胞癌中Ki-67阳性细胞的比例高于没有复发的肿瘤[3]。

鳞状细胞癌　Squamous cell carcinoma

临床特征

　　外耳鳞状细胞癌多数发生于耳廓，少数发生于外耳道。在个别情况下可出现两侧外耳受累[4]。在一项有52例患者的研究中，耳廓受累的部位见表30.1[5]。

　　耳廓作为显著的部位，其病变能够早期发现。外耳道病变的严重问题在于：延误诊断，因为很少出现症状。疼痛、听力丧失以及流血或流脓是外耳道鳞状细胞癌的主要症状。斑块样乃至息肉样肿块可以感觉到甚至看到（图30.1）。

表皮肿瘤

表30.1 52例耳廓鳞状细胞癌患者的受累部位[5]

部位	病例数
耳轮	27
后耳廓	11
对耳轮	6
三角窝	3
耳壳	3
小叶	2

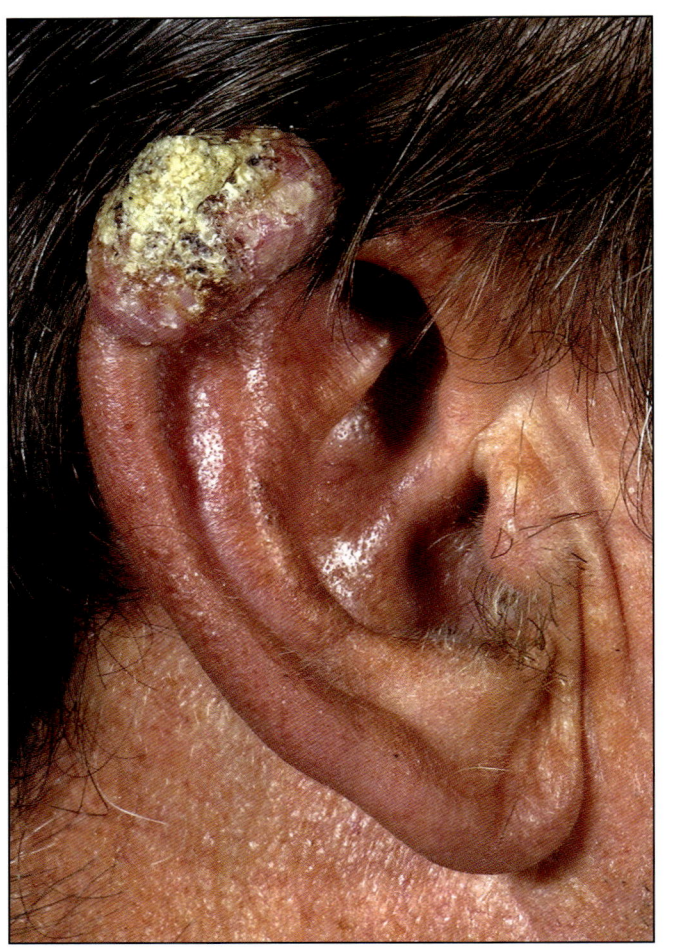

图30.1 位于耳廓耳轮的鳞状细胞癌的大体照片。

大体表现

发生在耳廓的鳞状细胞癌大体检查类似于其他部位皮肤的鳞状细胞癌。外耳道病变的表现是肿块，有时呈湿疣样，堵塞外耳道并向深部浸润周围的组织。可能有鼓膜破坏伴中耳浸润。可以转移到耳前或颈上淋巴结。

组织学表现

该部位的鳞状细胞癌通常为角化性的。通常存在来源于邻近表皮的证据。此外，发生于外耳道内部的病变常常是中耳上皮起源的，伴有鼓膜的破坏（见下文）。肿瘤可能是高分化的，以致与良性乳头状瘤混淆。在外耳道，高分化鳞状细胞癌伴有显著的纤维组织增生，也可能造成延误正确诊断（图30.2）。

疣状鳞状细胞癌
Verrucous Squamous cell carcinoma

外耳疣状鳞状细胞癌已有描述。这种肿瘤可能是局灶侵袭性的，广泛浸润甚至可直至后颅窝[6]。

耵聍腺肿瘤：良性（表30.2）
Neoplasms of ceruminous glands: benign

腺瘤（耵聍腺腺瘤）　　Adenoma (ceruminoma)

临床特征：耵聍腺腺瘤极其罕见。一般发生于老年人，男女均可受累[7]。通常表现为外耳道阻塞，而且常

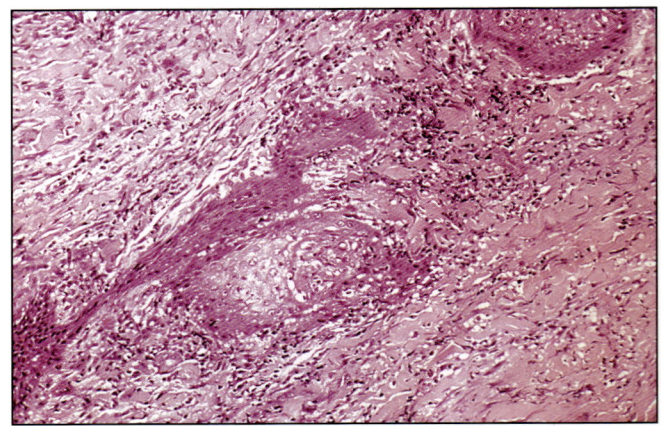

图30.2 外耳道鳞状细胞癌，显示小梁状肿瘤周围有广泛的胶原沉积，一些肿瘤小梁变细。

表30.2 耵聍腺肿瘤的分类

良性
腺瘤（耵聍腺腺瘤）
乳头状汗腺腺瘤
圆柱瘤

恶性
黏液表皮样癌
腺癌
腺样囊性癌

常伴有排液。外耳道的所有腺上皮肿瘤都必须除外腮腺或中耳来源的肿瘤。局部复发与切除不完全有关，但不常见。

大体表现：肿瘤为一个浅表的灰色肿块，一般小于 2 cm，但是直径可达 4 cm，被覆皮肤。

组织学表现：耵聍腺腺瘤缺乏明确的包膜。显示规则的腺体，常常有两层细胞，外层是肌上皮，但不是肿瘤的所有部分都能见到明显的肌上皮细胞。上皮常常显示腔内凸起，为顶浆分泌的特征（图 30.3）。腺体常常排列成群，周围绕以玻璃样变性的纤维组织。耐酸荧光色素可见于正常耵聍腺中，有时肿瘤细胞也可见耐酸荧光色素。

在一项有 36 例耵聍腺腺瘤的病例研究中，腺腔细胞 CK7 呈弥漫性强阳性，而基底（肌上皮）细胞 CK 5/6、S-100 蛋白和 p63 呈阳性[7]。

圆柱瘤 Cylindroma

圆柱瘤（也见第 23 章）是外耳的一种良性肿瘤[8]，可能与原发性腺样囊性癌混淆（见下文）。圆柱瘤为光滑的圆顶形隆起，常见于头皮，称为"缠头巾瘤"（turban tumor）（也见第 23 章）。有时可发生于耳廓（图 30.4）。组织学上，圆柱瘤是真皮内由小而深染的细胞构成的圆形团块物，肿瘤细胞排列成锯齿状结构，并且被粉染的玻璃样物质包围（图 30.5）。玻璃样小体常常出现在富于细胞的肿块中，这些细胞较大，伴有空泡状细胞核。圆柱瘤不同于腺样囊性癌，缺乏筛状结构，而且存在较大的细胞。多发性圆柱瘤是一种常染色体显性遗传性疾病，伴有毛上皮瘤（trichepitheliomas）的多发性圆柱瘤称为 Brooke-Spiegler 综合征。伴有腮腺腺瘤的 1 例 Brooke-Spiegler 综合征已有描述[9]。

耵聍腺肿瘤：恶性（表30.2） Neoplasms of ceruminous glands: malignant

恶性耵聍腺肿瘤发生于外耳道，最常见的是腺样囊性癌。这种肿瘤的大体和镜下特征类似于涎腺肿瘤，包

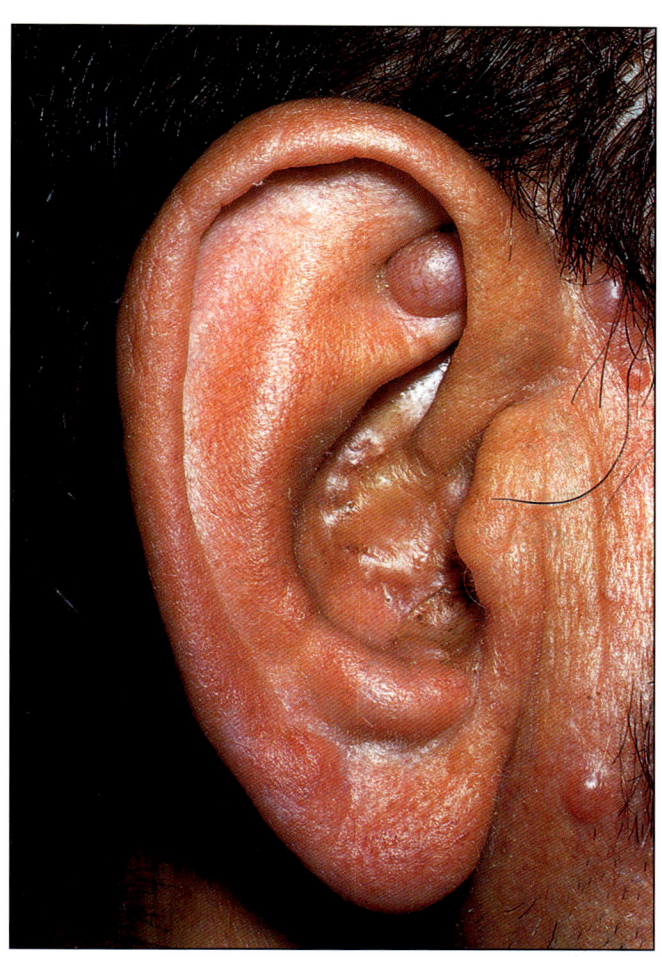

图30.4　耳廓圆柱瘤的大体照片。注意颊部和颞部类似的圆顶形隆起。

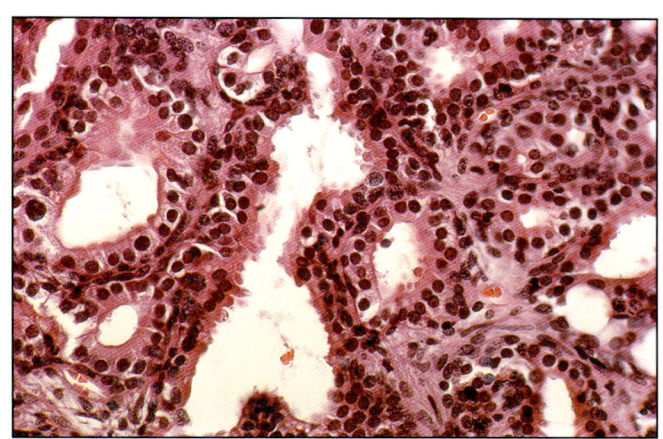

图30.3　耵聍腺腺瘤显示腺腔内凸起和两层上皮。

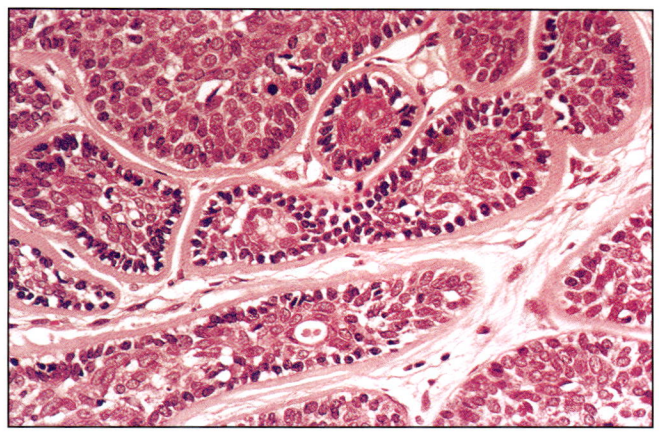

图30.5　为图30.4中圆柱瘤的组织学表现，显示紧密排列的小细胞周围绕以淡染的玻璃样物质。

括倾向于沿神经鞘浸润（见第7章）。常常局部复发且出现转移，特别是转移到肺，这也是这种肿瘤的特征。

黑色素细胞肿瘤（见第23章）
Melanocytic neoplasms

黑色素细胞痣（melanocytic nevi）常常发生在外耳道，但却罕见于耳廓。**恶性黑色素细胞肿瘤**（malignant melanocytic neoplasms）在外耳的任何部分均不常见。当发生恶性黑色素细胞肿瘤时，通常见于耳廓，33%的患者在诊断时已发生局部淋巴结转移[10]。

骨和软骨肿瘤
Neoplasms of bone and cartilage

巨细胞修复性肉芽肿
Ciant cell reparative granuloma

虽然在上颌和下颌并不少见，但是在外耳罕见，有人认为这种病变是反应性的，可以发生于颞骨。肿瘤来源于外耳周围的骨，可能由于堵塞外耳道的深部而被发现。组织学表现类似于颌骨的病变，由多核巨细胞和纤维母细胞组成[11]。

良性纤维-骨性病变（单骨性纤维结构不良或骨化性纤维瘤）[12]
Benign fibro-osseous lesion (monostotic fibrous dysplasia or ossifying fibroma)

由编织骨和纤维组织组成的孤立性良性肿瘤很难归入下列范畴：单骨性纤维结构不良或骨化性纤维瘤。多数情况下可以使用"良性纤维-骨性病变"这一命名，以防发生这种分类上的问题。

临床特征：多数患者有由于外耳道狭窄引起的传导性听力丧失，有些患者有显著的感音神经性听力丧失或因为累及颞骨的内部而造成面神经麻痹。该病常见于成人，特别是21～40岁的成人。

大体表现：颞骨良性纤维-骨性病变大体表现为黄白色的有弹性的组织，偶尔伴有充满琥珀色液体的小囊肿形成。可突然转化为正常骨。

组织学表现：镜下，不规则的编织骨小梁埋于纤维结缔组织间质内。通常认为在"纤维结构不良"间质中的骨小梁周围缺乏骨母细胞，但是这种征象没有实际意义。

骨瘤和外生骨疣 Osteoma and exostosis

外耳道深部的骨组织有两种类型的良性骨增生：骨瘤和外生骨疣。骨瘤是一个球形肿块，由鼓室鳞部或鼓室乳突缝发生，镶着独特的骨蒂（图30.6A）。偶尔其可能出现在中耳[13]（图30.6B）。外生骨疣与骨瘤不同，具有宽的基底，而且常常为双侧性的。外生骨疣在外耳道的位置通常比骨瘤的更深。骨瘤和外生骨疣均由板层骨组成，有时表面有编织骨附着（图30.6C）。组织学上这两种肿瘤不能区分[14]。

骨瘤的病因不明，但是有显著的证据表明：外生骨疣与在冷水中游泳有关。这种现象可以解释为，正常外耳道的骨的部分没有附件结构，皮下组织和骨膜结合形成薄层结缔组织。表皮表面到其下骨的距离自然较小，当水进入外耳道深部以后，似乎对骨的表面可产生冷效应并刺激新骨的形成。

神经肿瘤 Neural neoplasms

颞骨和耳的唯一常见的神经肿瘤是前庭神经鞘瘤（见下文）。面神经神经鞘瘤偶尔可见，而且伴有面神经麻痹。组织学上具有典型神经鞘瘤的特征（见第27章）。

肌肉肿瘤 Muscle neoplasms

横纹肌肉瘤 Rhabdomyosarcoma

横纹肌肉瘤（见第24章）偶尔见于幼儿的中耳[15]。个别情况下也见于成人的中耳[16]。鼓膜通常被向外耳道延伸的肿物侵蚀。肿瘤大体上呈分叶状、暗红色，切面有出血。几乎所有的颞骨横纹肌肉瘤均为胚胎性横纹肌肉瘤，主要为梭形或圆形的原始细胞，有些细胞胞浆透明，糖原染色阳性，而另一些细胞胞浆嗜酸性。这种肿瘤横纹不常见。针对结蛋白（desmin）和肌肉特异性肌动蛋白（muscle-specific actin）的免疫组化标记物有助于确定诊断。

颞骨横纹肌肉瘤通常不能切除，而且可能广泛播散到颅腔，或向外扩散到咽部。其患者经常发生淋巴结转移和血行转移。然而，经过现代多种方式的治疗，在过去的20年间，生存率有了显著的改善[17]。

淋巴网状系统肿瘤
Lymphoreticular neoplasms

Langerhans 细胞组织细胞增生症
Langerhans cell histiocytosis

Langerhans 细胞组织细胞增生症是网状内皮系统的

增生性疾病（见第21章），常常累及骨。颞骨可能是第一个受累的部位，通常发生于儿童的外耳道中部[18]。在小于3岁的患者，很可能是颅骨多灶性病变，预后不好。显微镜下，具有诊断意义的是出现许多S-100蛋白阳性的、伴有核沟的巨噬细胞。电子显微镜检查可见胞浆内存在Birbeck颗粒。

恶性淋巴瘤　Malignant lymphoma

恶性淋巴瘤可以出现在外耳，为全身性病变的一部分。偶尔可以原发于此部位。两侧对称性的耳淋巴瘤病变已有描述[19]。

中耳肿瘤　Neoplasms of the middle ear

肿瘤通常发生于中耳的相对不活跃的上皮。不过，最常见的是中耳腺瘤。在副神经节或蛛网膜绒毛附近，偶尔可以发生相应的肿瘤，分别为副神经节瘤或脑膜瘤，这些肿瘤可延伸到中耳裂，位置较深，主要围绕着骨，意味着中耳原发性恶性肿瘤本身通常没有症状，直到临床晚期。

表30.3列出了中耳最常见的肿瘤和类似病变。

胆脂瘤　Cholesteatoma

胆脂瘤是中耳复层鳞状上皮增生，通常伴有明显的角化。它不是肿瘤，但是具有一定的生长速度，而且容

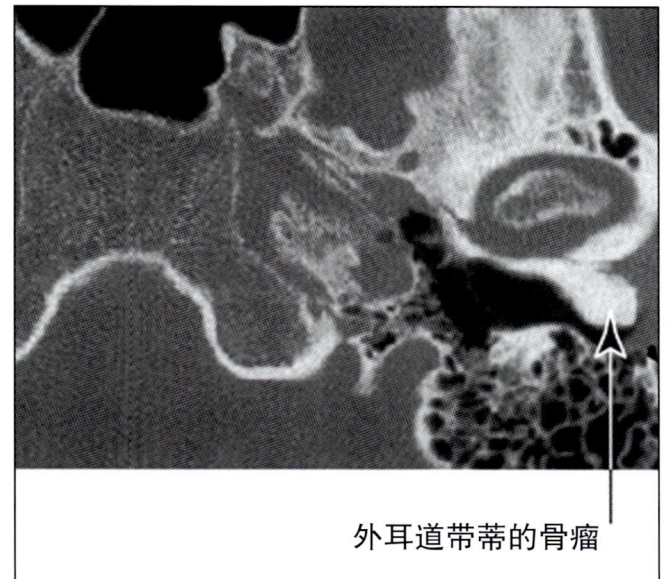

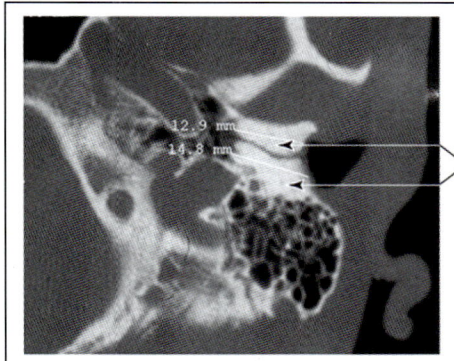

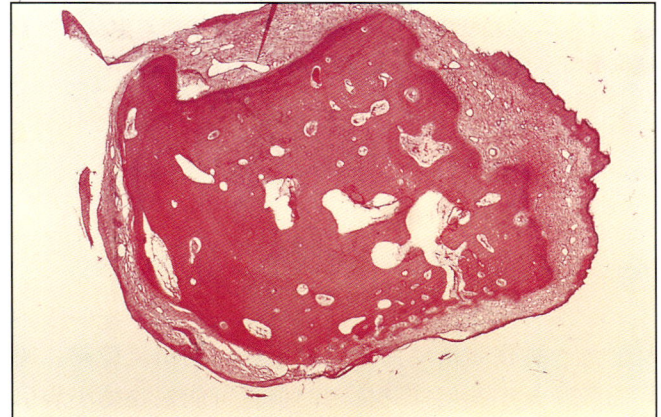

图30.6　CT扫描显示外耳道深部的两种类型的骨肿物的不同生长方式。（A）有蒂的骨瘤，发生在蒂上；（B）宽基的外生骨疣，具有围绕骨性耳道的广泛来源；（C）外耳骨瘤是由板层骨组成的。注意其被覆鳞状上皮。

表30.3	中耳肿瘤和类似病变
类似肿瘤的疾病	
胆脂瘤 • 先天性 • 获得性	
发育性瘤样异常 • 涎腺迷芽瘤 • 胶质沉积	
"真正的"肿瘤	
原发性 • 腺瘤 • 脑膜瘤 • 副神经节瘤 • 鳞状细胞癌 • 侵袭性乳头状肿瘤	
继发性	

易复发，类似肿瘤。近年来已经公认，中耳胆脂瘤有两种独特的类型：获得性和先天性。

获得性胆脂瘤　Acquired cholesteatoma

获得性胆脂瘤发生在广泛的年龄范围，表现为中耳裂后上部分的一个开放性珍珠白色的肿块。总是出现炎症性改变，包括显著的充血和脓肿。在多数病例，至少一个中耳小骨和一些骨壁严重破坏。多数病例有鼓膜穿孔，位于鼓膜弛缓部或接近紧张部的边缘。胆脂瘤的珍珠样物质是由坏死而无核的角化鳞屑组成的，即由复层鳞状上皮的角化层组成。这种鳞屑是由完全分化的鳞状上皮"基质"形成，这种鳞状上皮是由伴有明显核仁密集排列的球形细胞组成，其上为分化好的颗粒层，但是不存在皮肤附件结构（图30.7）。复层鳞状上皮向下生长，常常从基底层穿入其下的结缔组织（图30.8）。由胆脂瘤的复层鳞状上皮覆盖的小骨常常受到侵蚀。

免疫组化和其他技术可以提供胆脂瘤具有显著增生活性的证据。胆脂瘤的抗 Ki-67 抗原（MIB-1 用于石蜡切片）强表达[20-22]，而且嗜银核仁组成区（argyrophilic nucleolar organizer regions, AgNOR）增加[23]。

发病机制

根据提示，获得性胆脂瘤可以通过下面任何一种机制发生：中耳上皮化生、鼓膜外上皮游走移动到中耳、鼓膜内陷成一收缩小袋以及外伤（如冲击伤或鼓膜植入通气管）。尚无明确的证据支持化生，但有大量的资料支持其他三种机制。外耳复层鳞状上皮游走到中耳，常常推测是听道上皮游走功能迷乱的结果。这是具有很大活力的表皮从侧面移出，可能是控制机制的障碍，如凋亡、严重的中耳炎之后，可能会导致不受调控的上皮进入中耳，即胆脂瘤形成的过程[24]。

外耳道上皮通过鼓膜进入中耳并发生胆脂瘤已有动物模型，即首先将化学刺激物置入中耳腔诱导中耳炎。如将丙二醇溶液滴注到南美栗鼠的中耳[25,26]，中耳和鼓膜表面侧面的上皮被破坏，随后上皮化生，伴有表皮细胞增生，通过增厚的鼓膜纤维层穿入中耳腔，导致胆脂瘤。

收缩小袋是指鼓膜陷入中耳腔的部分，通过类似的过程可以引起胆脂瘤。收缩小袋常在面神经、镫骨或中耳岬的部位粘连到中耳的后壁。收缩小袋壁的组织学切片显示缺乏正常鼓膜的胶原层，后者已被炎症破坏，但在靠近中耳或中耳内部，常可见来自鼓膜表皮的带状复层鳞状上皮[27]。收缩小袋引起胆脂瘤可能

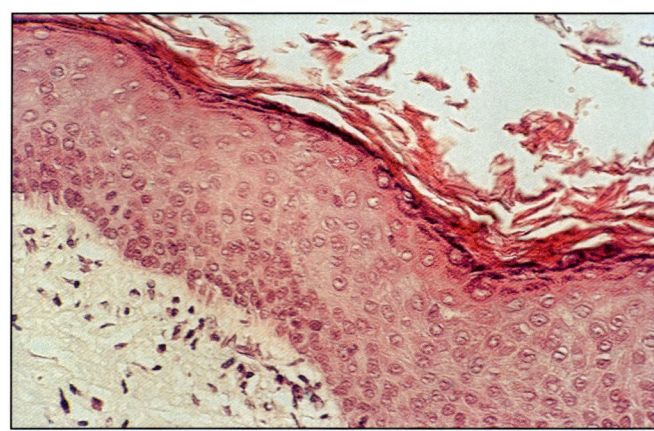

图30.7　中耳胆脂瘤由增厚的角化表皮组成，伴有密集排列的圆形角化（Malpighi）细胞。

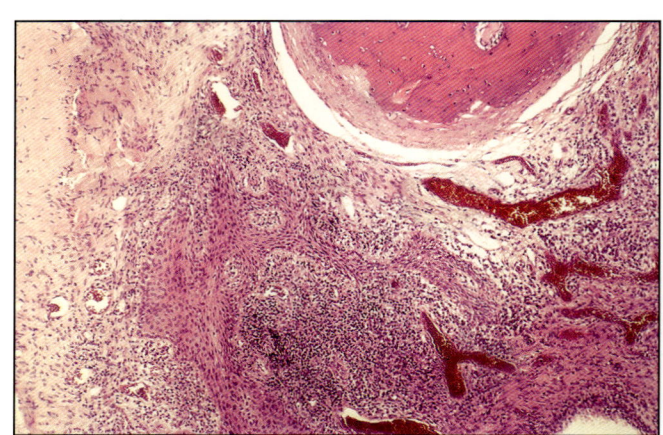

图30.8　复层鳞状上皮从中耳胆脂瘤的基质向下生长，胆脂瘤位于图片的右下角。右上方的小骨是砧骨。

是通过一种侵袭活动而不是由于任何的引流障碍。凋亡和鼓膜上皮其他抑制机制的损害可能是收缩小袋引起中耳炎的机制。

外伤有时是诱发获得性胆脂瘤的主要原因，通常发生在鼓膜冲击伤后，偶尔也见于通过鼓膜植入通气管之后。

先天性胆脂瘤　Congenital cholesteatoma

获得性胆脂瘤是一种已有一个世纪历史的临床病理疾病，而先天性胆脂瘤得到公认却是近来的事。现已发现，先天性胆脂瘤在北美和欧洲的幼儿中非常常见[28,29]。

多数先天性胆脂瘤病例表现为球形的白色病变，最常见于鼓室腔的前上部分，但有时发生在鼓室腔的其他部分，如完整鼓膜的后方（图30.9）。手术时，胆脂瘤通常为一囊肿，直径3 mm或以上，其部位与鼓膜密切相关。当胆脂瘤较小时，不出现骨的侵蚀，但是病变最终可能变大并侵蚀小骨，累及乳突，甚至长入中颅窝[29]。这样，有些先天性胆脂瘤的病变可变大，以致无法与获得性胆脂瘤区分。

发病机制

先天性胆脂瘤可能是由表皮样细胞残余造成的，即由表皮样瘤结构造成，后者可见于所有胎儿和幼婴的中耳，而且总是在上皮的同一部位，即咽鼓管和中耳的交界处，通常在鼓膜的前上象限，但有时可在鼓膜邻近骨环的其他部分[30]。免疫组化标记物染色显示，表皮样瘤结构是由妊娠15周时的鼓膜表皮发生的，并且在妊娠期间不断增大（图30.10）。因此，获得性和先天性胆脂瘤均来源于被覆鼓膜的表皮[30,31]。

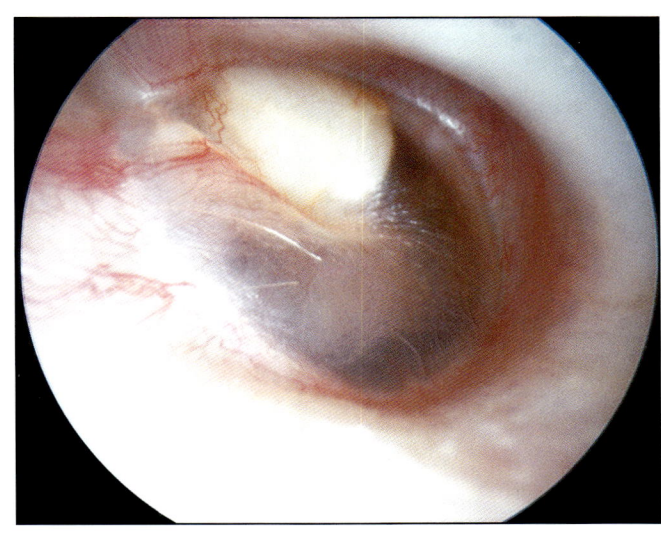

图30.9　中耳前上区域的先天性胆脂瘤的耳镜检查所见。

发育性瘤样异常
Developmental tumor-like anomalies

迷芽瘤　Choristomas

迷芽瘤一般较常见于女性，且中耳迷芽瘤常发生在左侧[32]。中耳迷芽瘤是由涎腺、神经胶质或皮脂腺组织组成的。涎腺迷芽瘤通常由黏液性和浆液性成分混合组成，如同正常的颌下腺或舌下腺，但是不同于腮腺[33]。可能存在一个新的综合征，包括中耳的涎腺迷芽瘤、第一和第二鳃弓以及耳囊和面神经的异常[34]。在1例中耳涎腺迷芽瘤新生儿患者，其咽部还有毛畸胎样（迷芽瘤性）息肉[32]。

异位的神经胶质肿块主要是由星形细胞组成的（图30.11），GFAP免疫组化染色可以确定星形细胞的存在。还可能出现神经元。确定中耳的神经胶质肿块是神经胶质迷芽瘤还是脑膨出（encephaloceles），必须进行影像学检查或结合手术所见，因为仅应用组织学检查不能做出准确的诊断[35]。

脑膨出是由于脑组织通过骨的缺陷疝出形成的。错构瘤（hamartoma）也可见到，是由正常见于中耳的组织形成的肿块。

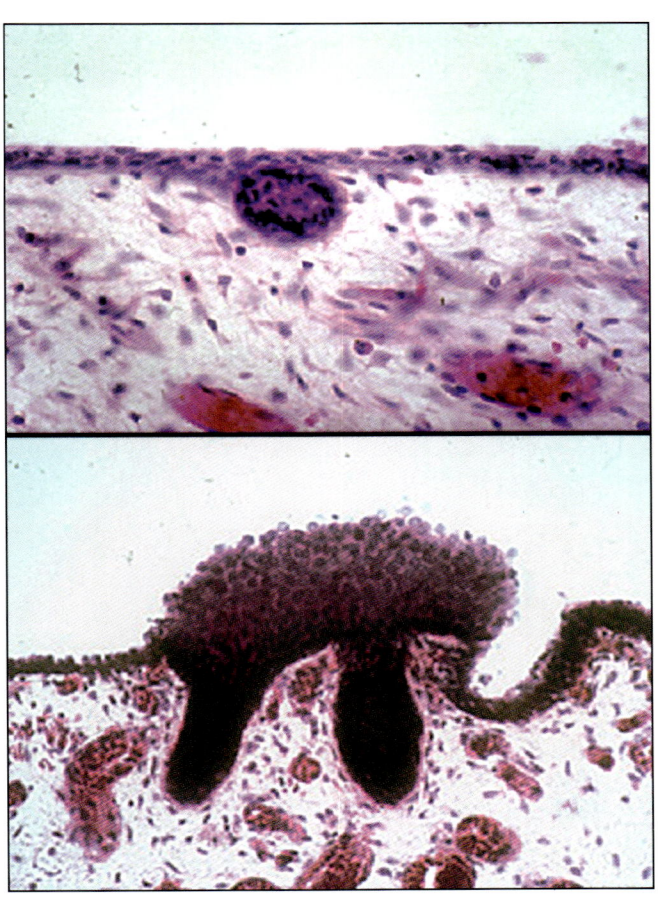

图30.10　胎儿咽鼓管交界处的中耳上皮。上：妊娠第17周时的上皮样瘤结构；下：妊娠第37周时同一放大倍数的上皮样瘤结构。

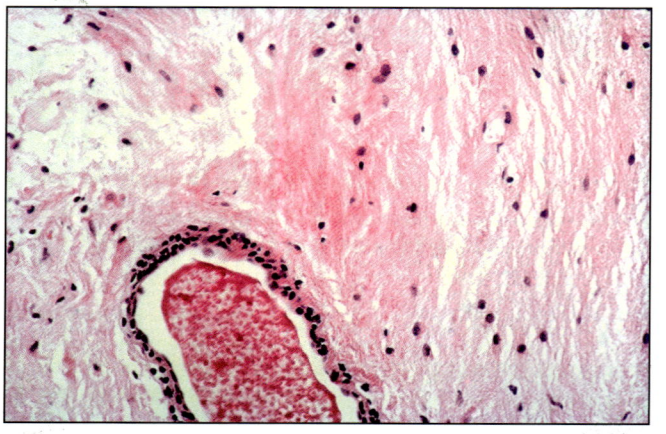

图30.11 中耳神经胶质迷芽瘤("胶质瘤")。其组织结构是由原纤维和少数星形细胞组成的。腺体是中耳上皮腺体化生的结果,为中耳胶质瘤的一种常见改变。

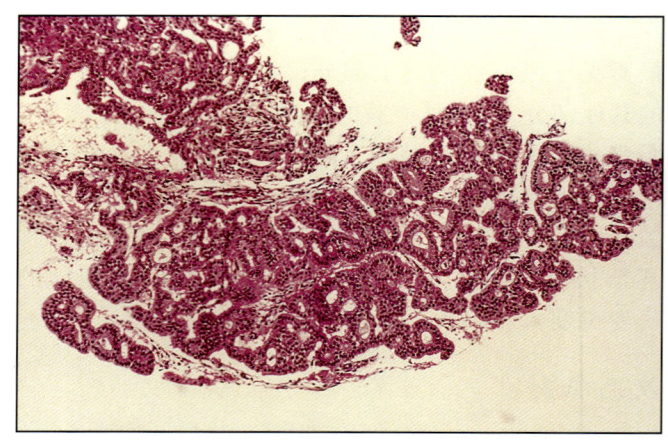

图30.12 中耳腺瘤的低倍观。

真性肿瘤 True neoplasms

腺瘤 Adenoma

来源于中耳上皮的良性腺体肿瘤最初于1976年描述[36,37]。腺体化生常见于中耳炎,而腺瘤似乎是这种化生的良性肿瘤的对应病变。

临床特征

这些不常见的病变最常见于中年成人,男女均可发生。多数患者出现传导性耳聋。鼓膜通常正常,肿瘤局限于中耳裂,有时累及乳突气室。有腺瘤穿孔可以延伸到外耳道的报道[36],甚至可以穿过完整鼓膜[38]。腺瘤是可以治愈的良性病变。少数病例复发[36,39,40],但是尚无转移的病例报告。

大体表现

手术时肿瘤表现为白色/灰色或棕红色,与副神经节瘤不同,血管并不丰富。腺瘤容易与周围的中耳壁分开,虽然小骨有时可能陷入腺瘤之中,甚至被其破坏。

组织学表现

腺瘤是由规则的小腺体组成,伴有"背靠背"现象(图30.12和30.13)。在一些部位出现实性或小梁状排列,当这种现象显著时,可能出现不含腺体结构的较大的结构破坏区域。这可能是人为假象,与活检损伤肿瘤的纤细结构有关。肿瘤细胞规则,呈立方形或柱状,可能显示腔内有分泌物,没有肌上皮层。PAS和Alcian染色可显示腺腔内以及肿瘤细胞胞浆内有黏蛋白分泌物。Grimelius染色可证实细胞基底部(腺泡周围)有颗粒状

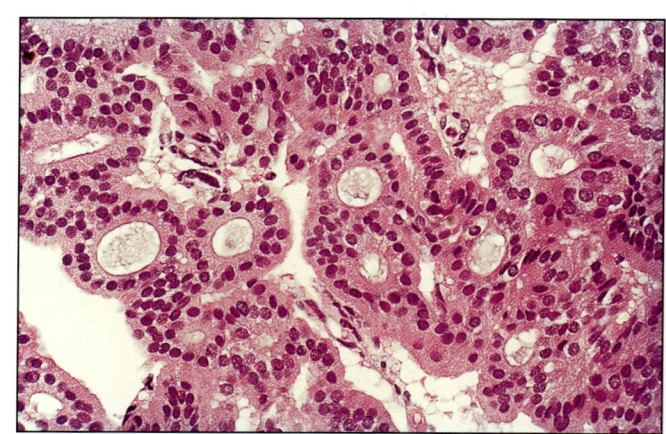

图30.13 中耳腺瘤的高倍观。腺体成单管状结构,由密集排列成"背靠背"表现的良性腺体组成。

胞浆阳性物质,电子显微镜检查显示,这是神经分泌颗粒的位置[41]。

免疫细胞化学

除了角蛋白之外,免疫细胞化学染色发现,所有中耳腺瘤均有神经分泌标记物的表达(见下文)。染色通常为阳性结果,包括神经元特异性烯醇化酶(NSE)和嗜铬素(chromogranin)。

电子显微镜检查

电子显微镜检查显示黏液分化,细胞的腺腔面有微绒毛突起,与其他细胞的接触点有基底桥粒,而且许多细胞的胞浆内有大的电子致密颗粒,可能是神经分泌颗粒[41]。在一项5例病例的超微结构研究中,每例均有黏液和神经内分泌双向分化,前者表现为顶端有微绒毛和

黏液颗粒的暗细胞，后者为基底具有神经分泌颗粒的透明细胞[42]。

"类癌" "Carcinoid tumor"

发生在中耳的"类癌"的报告是单纯基于免疫细胞化学检查出现神经内分泌特征以及电子显微镜检查肿瘤细胞内有神经内分泌颗粒做出的。与以前描述的伴有或不伴有这些神经内分泌特征的腺瘤相比，其临床行为没有不同。的确，如上所述，现在已经确定，所有的中耳腺瘤均显示神经内分泌特征。因此，分出"类癌"变型是没有理由的[43]。

脑膜瘤 Meningioma

脑膜瘤为良性肿瘤，通常发生在颅内，但有时也累及脑周围的骨结构，包括中耳。其来源于脑膜的蛛网膜细胞。肿瘤在颞骨的许多部位均可见到，包括内听道、颈静脉孔、膝状神经节部位以及咽鼓管顶部。这样，脑膜瘤可以从颞骨本身的不同部位发生[44]。原发性脑膜瘤在颞骨最常见的部位是中耳裂。最近一项有 36 例病例的研究发现，其中多数累及中耳，少数累及邻近结构，如外耳道或颞骨，仅有 2 例放射学检查显示与中枢神经系统连接[45]。

临床特征

中耳脑膜瘤女性比男性多见，年龄分布在 10～80 岁之间，平均年龄为 49.6 岁，女性患者年龄（平均 50.2 岁）大于男性患者（平均 44.8 岁）[45]。临床上患者表现为听力丧失、中耳炎、疼痛和眩晕。

大体表现

大体表现为颗粒状或砂砾状肿块。

组织学表现

显微镜下，肿瘤表现与任何描述完好的颅内脑膜瘤一样。中耳最常见的变型是脑膜上皮型脑膜瘤，肿瘤细胞形成规则的上皮样细胞团，常常倾向于漩涡状排列（图 30.14）。中耳有时还能见到纤维母细胞型和沙粒体型脑膜瘤。

免疫细胞化学

脑膜瘤的组织学诊断比较困难，因为上述特征模糊。在这种情况下，免疫细胞化学检查具有一些诊断价值。多数标记物呈阴性，包括细胞角蛋白（cytokeratins）。然而，多数脑膜瘤波形蛋白（vimentin）和 EMA 呈阳性。

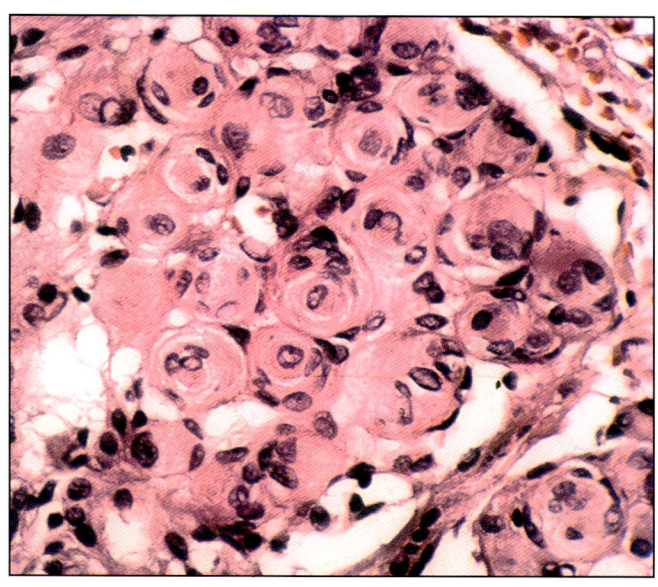

图30.14 中耳脑膜瘤显示细胞呈同心圆性漩涡状排列，伴有上皮（所谓的脑膜上皮）表现。

预后因素

20 世纪 60 年代，Nager 在有关脑膜瘤的综述中指出，30 例患者中只有 2 例生存期为 5 年[44]。最近有关中耳脑膜瘤的经验指出，经过彻底的局部切除后，预后较好。在最近的一项肿瘤主要位于中耳的 36 例患者的研究中，所有患者均进行了手术切除。10 例患者术后 5 个月到 2 年出现复发，5 例患者死于复发性疾病（平均 3.5 年），其余的 30 例患者存活（25 例，平均 19 年）或死于不相关的原因而没有疾病的证据（5 例，平均 9.5 年）[45]。中耳脑膜瘤是一种缓慢生长的肿瘤，总的预后很好（总的 5 年生存率为 83%）。手术切除的范围可能是影响预后的最重要的因素。28% 的病例发生复发。

颈静脉鼓室副神经节瘤 Jugulotympanic paraganglioma

颈静脉鼓室副神经节瘤也叫"血管球"瘤（"glomus" tumor）或化学感受器瘤（chemodectoma）（也见第 28 章）。

颈静脉鼓室副神经节瘤是一种具有不同侵袭性的肿瘤，但是很少转移，多数为颈静脉副神经节瘤，来源于颈静脉球附近的副神经节；少数为鼓室副神经节瘤，位于中耳内侧岬壁。通过现代影像学技术可将颈静脉副神经节瘤和鼓室副神经节瘤区分开来，颈静脉肿瘤被认为是来源于颈静脉球部，具有浸润岩骨的证据；而鼓室肿瘤却局限于中耳。然而，这两种类型的中耳肿瘤的大体和组织学表现是相同的。

颈静脉鼓室副神经节瘤也可能是多中心性的或与其他类型的肿瘤共存。在同一个患者，肿瘤可以是两侧性的，并与颈动脉体副神经节瘤共存，颈动脉体副神经节瘤也可以是两侧性的[46]。它们还可以与肾上腺嗜铬细胞瘤共存，后者可引起高血压。

临床特征

孤立性颈静脉鼓室副神经节瘤主要发生于女性，见于13～85岁之间的患者，平均年龄大约为50岁。家族性病例好发于男性。

多数患者表现为传导性听力丧失、耳痛、面神经麻痹、出血以及耳鸣。检查可见一个红色富于血管的肿块，或在完整的鼓膜后面，或通过鼓膜生长进入外耳道。活检时，手术探查肿块常常导致严重出血。

颈静脉鼓室副神经节瘤是一种缓慢生长的肿瘤。颈静脉副神经节瘤浸润岩骨，但是远处转移罕见。放射治疗以及手术治疗有较高的治愈率，经过这些治疗之后，预后依然不好的患者数目非常少。

孤立性副神经节瘤的病因尚不清楚。多发性家族性副神经节瘤有位于11号染色体上的 *SDHD* 基因种系突变的证据[46a]。

大体表现

这种肿瘤是外耳道表面的一种红色生芽的肿块。在颈静脉副神经节瘤，岩颞骨大部分被红色质硬的物质取代，中耳间隙被质软的肿块占据，直至鼓膜（图30.15）。副神经节瘤很少浸润耳囊。在解剖病例，通过颞骨薄切片方法检查副神经节瘤发现，颈静脉球的形状依然存在，但是腔内已完全被肿瘤充满。

组织学表现

肿瘤的组织学表现类似于颈动脉体瘤，伴有细颗粒状胞浆的小而一致的上皮样细胞被许多血管分开。肿瘤细胞常常成簇或形成"细胞球"（"Zellballen"），其周围为扁平细胞。细胞核通常小而一致（图30.16A），但是有时出现奇异或多核细胞，以致难以诊断（图30.16B）。这些表现并不代表恶性。肿瘤有时可见突出的纤维性间质。

免疫细胞化学

颈静脉鼓室副神经节瘤表达神经元特异性烯醇化酶（NSE）、嗜铬素A（chromogranin A）和其他神经

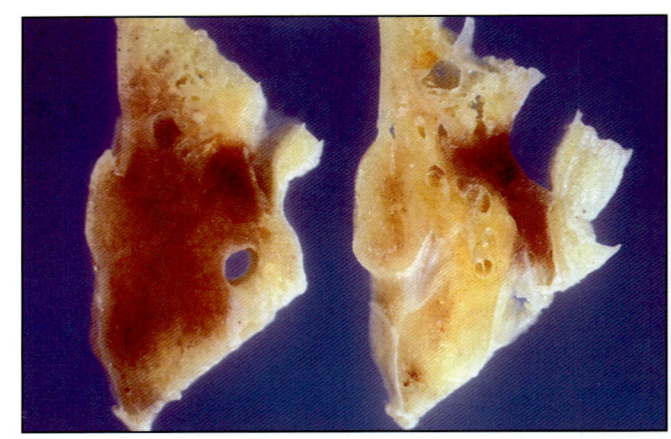

图30.15 尸解时取出的颈静脉副神经节瘤的薄片标本。可见肿瘤部位的两个颞骨薄片。左面的薄片显示淡红色的副神经节瘤从尖端侵蚀颞骨，直至鼓膜。右面的薄片取自较高水平，显示肿瘤没有侵犯耳蜗和骨迷路。

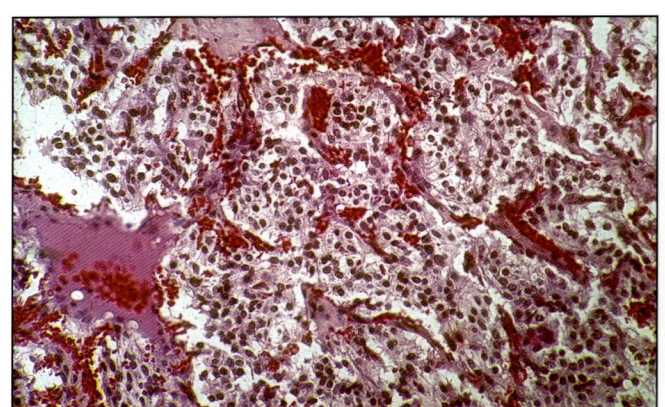

A

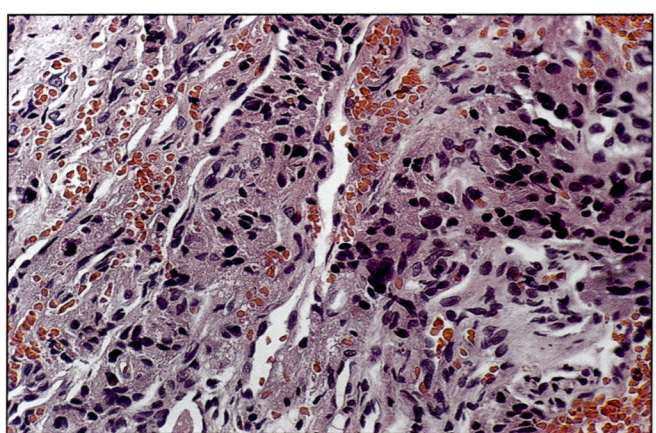

B

图30.16 颈静脉副神经节瘤。（A）肿瘤细胞形成小簇，伴有许多介入的血管；（B）一些区域显示有显著的核非典型性。

内分泌标记物，而细胞角蛋白总是呈阴性[47]。正常副神经节组织含有两型细胞：主细胞（chief cell）或称 I 型细胞，以及支持细胞（sustentacular cell）或称 II 型细胞。前者是神经内分泌细胞，后者不是神经内分泌细胞，但是含有 S-100 蛋白。在肾上腺髓质增生和肿瘤中，含有 S-100 蛋白的支持细胞减少，这种现象可用于研究其他部位副神经节组织良性和恶性肿瘤支持细胞的状况。S-100 蛋白和 GFAP 染色阳性可以确认支持细胞。在颈静脉鼓室副神经节瘤中，S-100 蛋白染色阳性的支持细胞通常稀疏，但不缺乏，提示肿瘤具有相当的侵袭性潜能，但不完全是恶性的。在使用抗 S-100 蛋白抗体免疫染色的切片中，后者明显呈阳性，相当于正常副神经节的支持或 II 型细胞。中等和恶性副神经节瘤，即伴有复发或局灶侵袭的肿瘤，几乎没有 II 型细胞，伴有 S-100 蛋白反应减少或缺乏[48]。

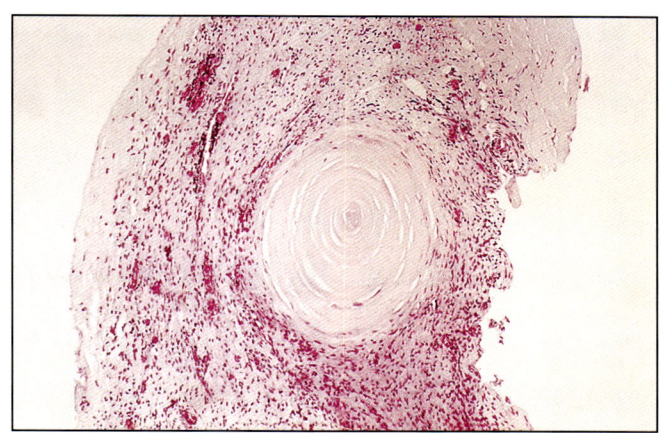

图30.17　在炎症细胞中的中耳小体。中耳小体是由同心圆性板层排列的胶原组成的，是中耳老化的正常特征。

鳞状细胞癌　Squamous cell carcinoma

临床特征

中耳鳞状细胞癌是为一种少见的肿瘤。常常有其与慢性中耳炎有关的提示，但是已有公开质疑。耳道排液和传导性听力丧失出现在所有的患者。常见耳痛、出血和面神经麻痹。没有发现伴发胆脂瘤[49]。

组织学表现

在其直接来源于中耳表面的复层鳞状上皮及其立方上皮的化生，可见肿瘤具有表皮样本质。在一些区域，显然其来源于立方或柱状上皮的基底层。在有些病例，肿瘤由外耳和中耳发生（见下文）。组织学检查可以证实，部分肿瘤来源于外耳道表面的复层鳞状上皮（通过其毛囊、皮脂腺和顶浆分泌腺确认）。在这种病例，癌的扩散无疑是通过外耳和中耳上皮的部位变化扩散的，而不是通过肿瘤在上皮下从一处到另一处扩散的。鳞状细胞癌是一种表皮样癌，它的角化和上皮分化程度类似于上呼吸道其他部位的同样组织学类型的肿瘤。在多数病例，靠近浸润癌的中耳上皮可出现局灶性原位癌。

中耳小体的同心圆性分层的嗜酸性团块，可与鳞状细胞癌的角化珠混淆，在冰冻切片检查时可能会令人烦恼（图 30.17）[50]。

扩散

肿瘤可以从中耳上皮扩散，这已经在尸检的颞骨切片上进行了分析[49]，并且随后又在中耳鳞状细胞癌患者的放射学检查上得到证实[51]。癌倾向于长入并侵蚀分隔中耳内壁的薄的骨间隔，在其与咽鼓管交界的部位，自颈动脉开始。穿透上述结构之后，肿瘤迅速沿着颈动脉的交感神经蔓延，此时通过手术切除已经不可能治愈。肿瘤进展的另外一种方式是：通过后乳突气室的骨壁直至颞骨后面的硬膜，由此向内侧延伸进入内听道，然后沿着第 8 颅神经的前庭支和耳蜗支侵犯耳蜗和前庭。另一方面，骨迷路的骨独具抵抗肿瘤从中耳直接扩散的能力。鼓膜圆窗似乎也能抵抗侵犯。肿瘤还可以向前播散，侵犯下颌骨髁。在后期，肿瘤广泛生长进入中颅窝，这种形式的扩散多半是致死性的。淋巴结转移少见，血行转移更少见。

中耳侵袭性乳头状肿瘤 Aggressive papillary tumor of middle ear

显示侵袭性行为的、具有乳头状非复层上皮形态的中耳肿瘤已有报道。从文献中大约可以搜集到 24 例这种中耳肿瘤。女性 17 例，男性 7 例。病例诊断时的年龄范围在 16～55 岁之间，平均年龄为 33 岁。然而，多数病例诊断时，患者已经有了痛苦的症状，随后归因于肿瘤，发病年龄可能比提示的要年轻的多[52]。

这种肿瘤可见于中耳的任何部位，包括乳突突起和气室，而且可能充满鼓室腔。除了 3 例以外，报道的所有病例均广泛侵犯到中耳以外，包括多数病例累及岩骨的顶部，少数病例肿瘤到达小脑脑桥角和小脑。

有人认为，广泛累及颞骨的中耳侵袭性乳头状肿瘤病例可能来源于内淋巴囊原发性乳头状腺癌 [内淋囊肿瘤，endolymphatic sac tumor (ELST)，见下文][53]。中耳乳头状肿瘤常常伴有同样类型的岩骨顶端肿瘤，这两个部位的肿瘤的组织学表现类似，而且这两个部位的一些乳头状肿瘤病例伴有 von Hippel-Lindau 病，但是这种肿瘤的一些病例尚未完全排除中耳起源。

中耳裂，包括乳突气室，通常充满了乳头状肿瘤。常见骨的侵犯。乳头状腺体结构表现为复杂的犬牙交错的乳头，位于疏松或浸润性的纤维结缔组织中。乳头被覆单层矮立方或柱状上皮细胞，核均匀一致、胞浆嗜酸性、细胞界限不清（图30.18）。可以出现类似于内淋巴囊肿瘤的甲状腺滤泡样的区域（见下文）。

Cytokeratin、EMA 和 S-100 蛋白等标记物阳性。缺乏甲状腺球蛋白（thyroglobulin）可以用于排除来自甲状腺的转移性乳头状癌。CK 7、CK20 和癌胚抗原（CEA）等标记物也可以用于排除来自肺和结肠的转移性肿瘤。

内耳肿瘤 Neoplasms of the inner ear

原发性肿瘤 Primary neoplasms

前庭神经鞘瘤 Vestibular schwannoma

前庭神经鞘瘤是一种常见的良性肿瘤，来源于内听道的前庭耳蜗神经分支，最终从听道延伸至小脑脑桥角。已经发现，大约0.8%的成人有前庭神经鞘瘤[54]。

临床特征

这种肿瘤最常见于41～60岁的患者，虽然总的年龄范围广泛。单侧前庭神经鞘瘤占所有颅内肿瘤的5%～15%，而且占小脑脑桥角肿瘤的绝大部分。

前庭神经鞘瘤通常是单侧性的，但也可以是双侧性的，双侧性病例的病变表现为神经纤维瘤病2（neurofibromatosis 2，NF-2；见下文）。

其临床特征通常是由耳蜗损伤引起的，表现为一侧耳的听力进行性丧失（90%的患者）和耳鸣（70%的患者）。不常见的症状是头痛、眩晕、面部疼痛和面部无力。肿瘤生长缓慢，可以持续多年不引起症状，而只在尸检时才首次得到诊断。通常是通过磁共振成像（MRI）扫描作出诊断。对于小而缓慢生长的肿瘤，治疗可能仅仅选择间断进行MRI扫描以观察肿物生长。可以进行手术切除，通过外耳道颞骨钻孔或通过颅骨切开术自中窝到达内听道，或通过立体定位指导下的伽马刀手术。

与神经纤维瘤病2不同，前庭神经鞘瘤与确定的基因突变无关，病因学基础还不清楚。

大体表现

前庭神经鞘瘤最常发生在第8颅神经的神经胶质-神经鞘交界处，后者通常位于内听道内，但是这样一来源部位是不大可能的。一项有5例颞骨小神经鞘瘤病例的研究显示，肿瘤发生的位置比通常的交界处靠外，在 Scarpa（前庭）神经节或其附近[55]。然而，手术或尸检时见到的多数前庭神经鞘瘤病例占据了神经的绝大部分。它通常是受累神经的前庭分支（图30.19）；少数病例肿瘤来源于耳蜗支。肿瘤从起源部位发生，既可以向着中心直达小脑脑桥角，又可以远侧沿着内耳道生长。

大体上，肿瘤大小不同，呈圆形或卵圆形。小的肿瘤并不造成内耳道扩大，或只在骨内形成一个小的切迹（图30.20）。较大的肿瘤常常呈蘑菇形，具有两种成分：蒂——管道内狭窄的细长部分——以及小脑脑桥角部位的膨大部分。当肿瘤生长时，内耳道的骨扩大呈漏斗形。肿瘤表面光滑，呈分叶状，切面黄色，常常伴有出血区域和囊肿。多囊性前庭神经鞘瘤已有报道[56]。肿瘤表面可见第8颅神经的前庭分支并附着其上，而耳蜗分支常常被肿瘤牵拉，但不附着其上。

组织学表现

前庭神经鞘瘤具有与软组织神经鞘瘤同样的双相成带现象（见第27章）。Antoni A 区显示梭形细胞彼此密集排列，伴有栅栏状排列的细胞核（图30.21）。Verocay 小体可能出现在 Antoni A 区，是栅栏状肿瘤细胞核形成的漩涡状结构。肿瘤细胞密集程度可高可低。梭形细胞常常显示退行性的核非典型性，但是核

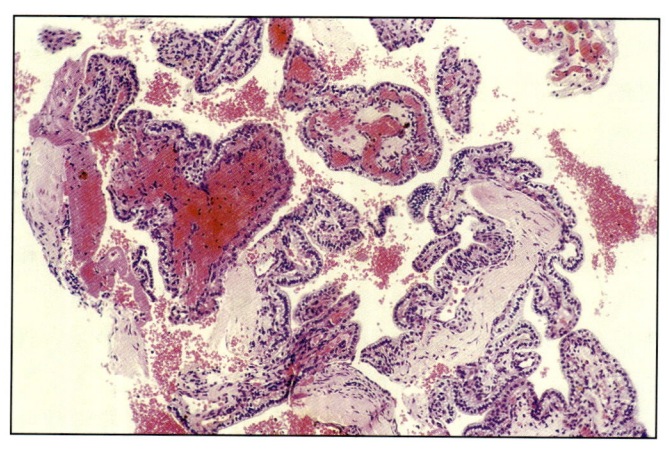

图30.18　中耳侵袭性乳头状肿瘤。

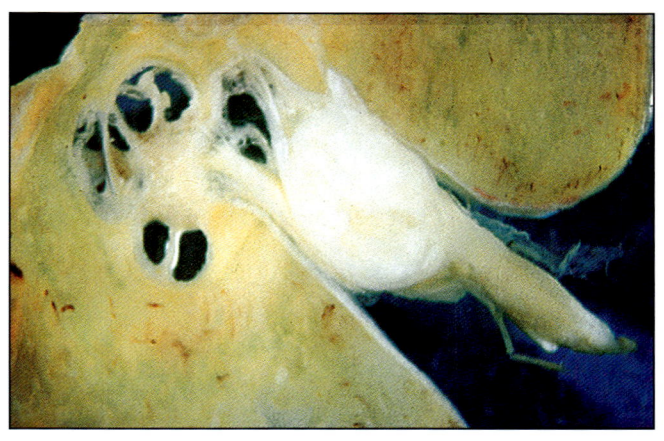

图30.19　经过特殊薄片操作的颞骨前庭神经鞘瘤。肿瘤发生于内听道第8颅神经的前庭支,而且压迫耳蜗支。注意内衬耳蜗的颗粒状沉积（渗出）。

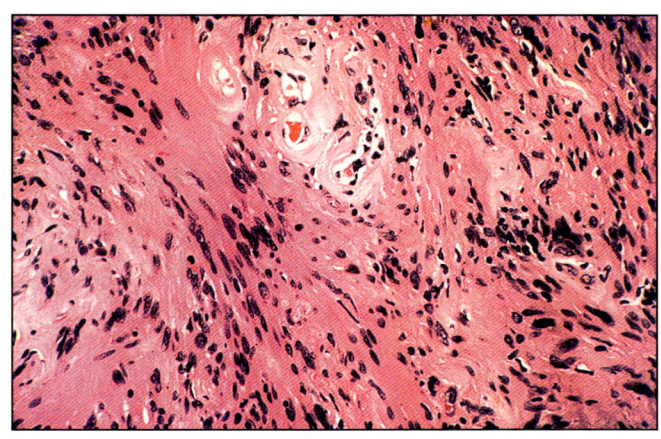

图30.21　前庭神经鞘瘤的Antoni A区,显示神经鞘细胞呈栅栏状排列。

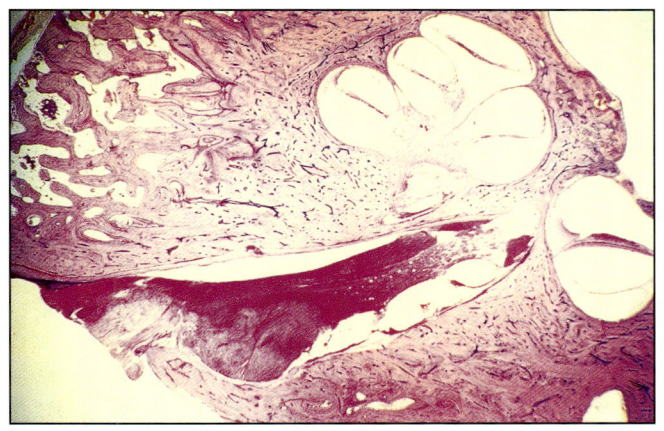

图30.20　小的前庭神经鞘瘤。它发生于第8颅神经的前庭支,而且仅仅在内耳道的骨壁形成一个小的切迹。前庭有渗出,而耳蜗没有渗出。

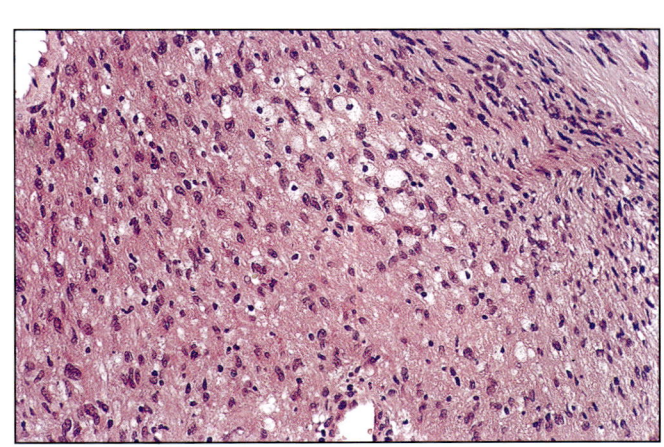

图30.22　前庭神经鞘瘤的Antoni B区,以泡沫细胞为特征。

分裂象罕见。出现非典型性并不意味着是恶性,但在非常罕见的病例,可以出现明确的恶性变,临床上伴有生长速度加快[57]。Antoni B区显示疏松的网状结构,伴有黏液样间质,有时伴有组织细胞增生（图30.22）。肿瘤的有些部分可出现血栓形成和坏死。沿着耳蜗或前庭神经分支可能出现轻度的耳蜗（modiolus）或前庭浸润,是孤立性前庭神经鞘瘤。耳蜗和前庭外淋巴间隙通常存在颗粒状或均匀一致液体渗出,在较大的肿瘤,这可能是肿瘤压迫内听道耳蜗和前庭引流静脉的结果。可以发生内淋巴系统积水,在较大的肿瘤,可有螺旋神经节和基底膜的神经纤维萎缩。

免疫细胞化学

对于所有的神经鞘瘤来说,最强烈和最一致的免疫组化反应是S-100蛋白呈阳性。标记物GFAP和NSE有时也阳性,CD34阳性可见于Antoni B区或退变明显的病变[58]。

抗Ki-67抗体（MIB-1）已经用于许多研究,以确定这种增生标记物的阳性程度是否与神经鞘瘤的临床行为有关。已经证实,与直径大于18 mm的肿瘤相比,直径小于或等于18 mm的肿瘤的增生指数和生长率较低[59]。在神经纤维瘤病2（NF-2）的病例,其增生标记物的阳性程度高于孤立性前庭神经鞘瘤的[60]。

电子显微镜检查

一般说来,神经鞘细胞的最重要的超微结构特征是:有犬牙交错的纤细的胞浆突起,被覆一层连续的外板,这也是前庭神经鞘瘤的主要超微结构特征[61]。

来自第8颅神经前庭分支的肿瘤的生长可侵袭感觉器官，即使是小的肿瘤，也能引起前庭感觉组织的广泛变性[62]。

神经纤维瘤病2　Neurofibromatosis 2

神经纤维瘤病2（NF-2）是一种常染色体显性遗传性疾病，其特征是双侧前庭神经鞘瘤、颅内和周围神经的其他神经鞘瘤以及其他良性颅内和脊柱内肿瘤的发生率高。本病临床上通常发生在1～20岁。

临床特征

最常见的表现是双侧前庭神经鞘瘤。此外，可能出现其他颅内和周围神经的神经鞘瘤，在疾病期间，可发生多种其他良性颅内和脊柱内肿瘤，包括脑膜瘤、室管膜瘤、脊柱神经纤维瘤和神经胶质瘤。还可发现幼年性后被膜下白内障。

在一个伴有遗传性涎腺神经内分泌癌和釉质生长不全（amelogenesis imperfesta）的家族（a family on the Isle of Man, UK）中，两个有血缘关系的男性显示有前庭神经鞘瘤，其中1例为双侧性[63]。这个家族的疾病过程在遗传学上可能与NF-2有关。

NF-2患者的前庭神经鞘瘤常常比散发性单侧性神经鞘瘤生长迅速。受累患者的亲属在有神经鞘瘤的情况下常常有正常的听力图和正常的听觉脑干反应，因此有人建议应用Gd-DTPA增强的核共振成像筛查NF-2患者的亲属[64]。

大体表现

肿瘤通常发生于第8颅神经的前庭上支。NF-2前庭神经鞘瘤的大体表现类似于散发性前庭神经鞘瘤，除了一些病例有内听道内的面神经浸润，以及耳蜗和前庭骨壁浸润的证据以外[65]。

组织学表现

NF-2前庭神经鞘瘤的组织学表现类似于散发性前庭神经鞘瘤（见上文），除了前者有较多的Verocay小体和较多的富于细胞的区域以外。

免疫细胞化学

NF-2相关性病例的增生标记物Ki-67的标记阳性程度比散发性前庭神经鞘瘤的高[60]。

遗传学

NF-2是一种常染色体显性遗传性疾病。大约50%的NF-2患者是新突变的结果，50%是从受累的双亲遗传而来。受累患者的子女有50%的机会遗传这种疾病，产前诊断有帮助。NF-2的基因是一种抑制基因，定位于22号染色体的长臂（22q12）。

内听道脂肪瘤　Lipoma of the internal auditory canal

内听道脂肪细胞良性肿瘤在这个部位是重要的，因为在临床上可能类似于前庭神经鞘瘤。为了正确诊断，应该进行冰冻切片检查，因为切除脂肪瘤有损害第7颅神经或第8颅神经或其分支的高度危险性，这些神经可以穿过脂肪瘤。这种肿瘤类似于其他部位的良性脂肪瘤，除了在脂肪细胞中可能存在第7颅神经或第8颅神经或其分支以外（图30.23）[66]。

微小神经瘤和骨的Paget病　Microneuromas and Paget's disease of bone

在耳膜部位，颞骨受累的骨Paget病病例，有时可以发现耳蜗或前庭内或其附近有小的肿瘤，这些肿瘤由相互缠结的神经纤维束和神经鞘细胞组成。这些小肿瘤产生的基础是：变性骨炎导致骨增大，压迫变性的神经纤维，从而形成创伤性神经瘤[67]。

内淋巴囊肿瘤（ELST）　Endolymphatic sac tumor (ELST)

ELST，过去被称为侵袭性乳头状肿瘤或Heffner瘤，是一种生长缓慢的非转移性腺癌，广泛侵犯岩骨，

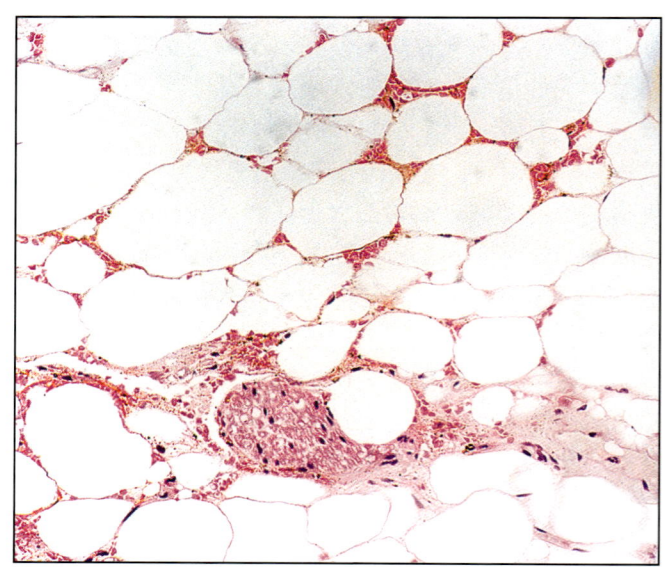

图30.23　内听道脂肪瘤，伴有小的神经从中穿过。

但是被认为来源于内淋巴囊[53,68]。它是一种仅见于成人的罕见的肿瘤。有些病例表现为两侧同样类型的肿瘤，有些病例还伴有 von Hippel-Lindau 病[69,70]。

在早期发现肿瘤时，肿瘤位于内淋巴囊内。在晚期阶段，肿瘤可占据岩骨的大部分，包括中耳[53]。

临床特征

耳鸣、听力丧失和眩晕出现在大约 1/3 的患者，类似于或与 Ménière 病的症状一样。推测是由于内淋巴囊早期梗阻导致迷路的内淋巴系统积水，以致发生 Ménière 综合征。当肿瘤蔓延时，可能发生面神经麻痹和小脑障碍。影像学检查显示颞骨溶骨性病变，来源于内听道和乙状窦之间的部位（大约是内淋巴囊的位置），或在早期阶段，来源于内淋巴囊本身。最后明显延伸到后颅腔并侵犯中耳。

组织学特征

多数 ELST 病例有乳头状腺体表现，乳头状增生被覆单层矮立方细胞，类似于内衬正常内淋巴囊的乳头状结构（图 30.24）。在一些病例，乳头的血管本质使其类似于脉络丛乳头状瘤的组织学特征。在另一些病例，肿瘤显示腺体扩张的区域，腺腔内含有类似于胶样物的分泌物（图 30.25），因此病变可能类似于甲状腺乳头状腺癌。甲状腺样区域甚至可能是主要的组织学形态。少数病例以透明细胞为主，类似于肾细胞癌。

所谓的侵袭性乳头状中耳肿瘤（见上文）大多可能是 ELST 伴有肿瘤蔓延至中耳。少数病例并不显示向颞骨顶端蔓延，因此可能原发于中耳。

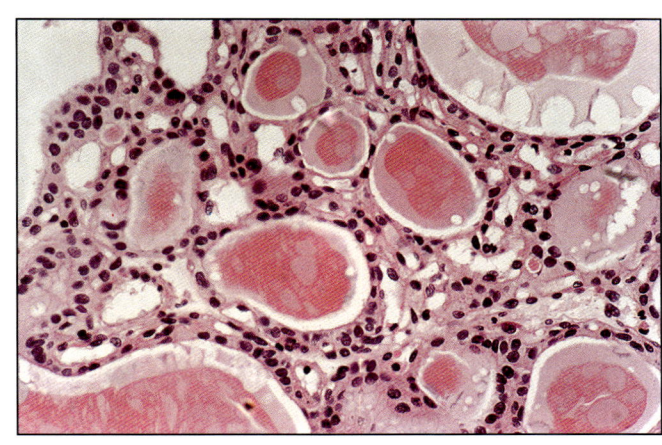

图30.25　内淋巴囊肿瘤，显示甲状腺样滤泡。

免疫细胞化学

免疫细胞化学检查显示，肿瘤的上皮细胞细胞角蛋白和 EMA 呈阳性，S-100 蛋白也常呈阳性[68]。一些肿瘤含有 GFAP。甲状腺球蛋白(thyroglobulin)总是呈阴性。

遗传学

虽然 ELST 在普通人群中非常罕见，但据报道，相当数量的病例伴有 von Hipple-Lindau 病[69,70]。*VHL* 肿瘤抑制基因是引起 von Hipple-Lindau 病的原因，其定位于 3 号染色体的短臂，能够控制氧感觉通路[71]。

预后

肿瘤生长过程可以延续多年而察觉不到已有转移。诊断时许多肿瘤已经较大。对于所有 von Hipple-Lindau 病患者，通过成像技术筛查有无 ELST 是非常重要的，这样可以手术切除肿瘤，预期预后很好[69]。

耳的继发性肿瘤
Secondary tumors of the ear

来源于耳和颞骨以外部位的肿瘤临床上虽然并不常见，但却常见于死于恶性肿瘤的患者。这种肿瘤可以由邻近部位的肿瘤通过浸润颞骨直接扩散而来，也可以经由血管或淋巴管转移而来。乳腺癌是最常见的转移到颞骨的恶性肿瘤，其次是肺和（或）支气管、前列腺、黑色素瘤和甲状腺的癌症。

内听道是常见的转移部位。恶性细胞一旦发生沉积，可以进一步扩散到耳蜗。

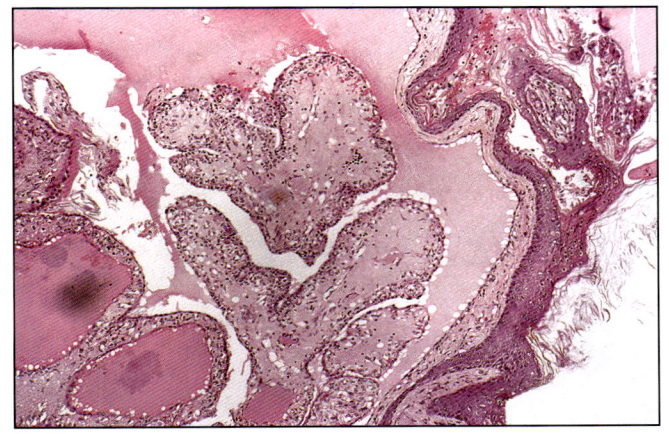

图30.24　内淋巴囊肿瘤，显示含有分泌物的囊腔内有乳头状突起。这部分肿瘤取自中耳。注意照片右侧可见伴有上皮向下生长的胆脂瘤。

白血病常常累及内耳，产生前庭和耳蜗两方面紊乱的症状。白血病患者的内耳出现的最常见的病理学改变是出血进入膜间隙内。血液可以单独进入外淋巴间隙，也可以同时进入外淋巴间隙和内淋巴间隙。白血病出现耳蜗内出血后，Corti 器和螺旋神经节可以变性，结缔组织和新骨可能长入耳蜗的各种通道[72]。另一种类型的受累发生于慢性淋巴细胞性白血病患者，表现为耳蜗外淋巴间隙严重的白血病浸润。白血病细胞可能是从脑脊液经由耳蜗小管进入的。

参考文献

1. Ahmad I, Das Gupta A R 2001 Epidemiology of basal cell carcinoma and squamous cell carcinoma of the pinna. J Laryngol Otol 115: 85–86
2. Cribier B, Noacco G, Peltre B et al. 2001 Expression of stromelysin 3 in basal cell carcinomas. Eur J Dermatol 11: 530–533
3. Healy E, Angus B, Lawrence C M et al. 1995 Prognostic value of Ki67 antigen expression in basal cell carcinomas. Br J Dermatol 133: 737–741
4. Wolfe S G, Lai S Y, Bigelow D C 2002 Bilateral squamous cell carcinoma of the external auditory canals. Laryngoscope. 112: 1003–1005
5. Shiffman N J 1975 Squamous cell carcinomas of the skin of the pinna. Can J Surg 18: 279–283
6. Hagiwara H, Kanazawa T, Ishikawa K et al. 2000 Invasive verrucous carcinoma: a temporal bone histopathology report. Auris Nasus Larynx 27: 179–183
7. Thompson L D, Nelson B L, Barnes E L 2004 Ceruminous adenomas: a clinicopathological study of 41 cases with a review of the literature. Am J Surg Pathol 28: 308–318
8. Wilson R S, Johnson J T 1980 Benign eccrine cylindroma of the external auditory canal. Laryngoscope 90: 379–382
9. Kakagia D, Alexiadis G, Kiziridou A et al. 2004 Brooke–Spiegler syndrome with parotid gland involvement. Eur J Dermatol 14: 139–141
10. Shah J P, Kraus D H, Dubner S et al. 1991 Patterns of regional lymph node metastases from cutaneous melanomas of the head and neck. Am J Surg 162: 320–323
11. Liu J, Zhong D R, Liu L F et al. 2001 Giant cell reparative granuloma of the temporal bone. Acta Otolaryngol 121: 523–528
12. Nager G T, Kennedy D W, Kopstein E 1982 Fibrous dysplasia: a review of the disease and its manifestations in the temporal bone. Ann Otol Rhinol Laryngol 92 (suppl): 1–52
13. Milroy C M, Phelps P D, Michaels L et al. 1989 Osteoma of the incus. J Otolaryngol 18: 226–228
14. Fenton J E, Turner J, Fagan P A 1996 A histopathologic review of temporal bone exostoses and osteomata. Laryngoscope 106: 624–628
15. Wiatrak B J, Pensak M L 1989 Rhabdomyosarcoma of the ear and temporal bone. Laryngoscope 99: 1188–1192
16. Nakhleh R E, Swanson P E, Dehner L P 1991 Juvenile (embryonal and alveolar) rhabdomyosarcoma of the head and neck in adults. A clinical, pathologic, and immunohistochemical study of 12 cases. Cancer 67: 1019–1024
17. Hawkins D S, Anderson J R, Paidas C N et al. 2001 Improved outcome for patients with middle ear rhabdomyosarcoma. A Children's Oncology Group study. J Clin Oncol 19: 3073–3079
18. Quesada P, Navarrete M L, Perrello E 1990 Eosinophilic granuloma of the temporal bone. Eur Arch Otorhinolaryngol 247: 194–195
19. Goudie R B, Soukop M, Dagg J H et al. 1990 Hypothesis: symmetrical cutaneous lymphoma. Lancet 335: 316–318
20. Bujia J, Schilling V, Holly A et al. 1993 Hyperproliferation-associated keratin expression in human middle ear cholesteatoma. Acta Otolaryngol 113: 364–368
21. Sudhoff H, Bujia J, Fisselereckhoff A et al. 1995 Expression of a cell-cycle-associated nuclear antigen (MIB1) in cholesteatoma and auditory meatal skin. Laryngoscope 105: 1227–1231
22. Maigot D, Bene M C, Perrin C et al. 1993 Restricted expression of Ki-67 in cholesteatoma epithelium. Arch Otolaryngol Head Neck Surg 119: 656–658
23. Sudhoff H, Fisseler-Eckhoff A, Stark F et al. 1997 Argyrophilic nucleolar organizer regions (AgNORs) in auditory meatal skin and middle ear cholesteatoma. Clin Otolaryngol 22: 545–548
24. Michaels L, Hellquist H B 2001 Ear, nose and throat histopathology, 2nd edn. Springer Verlag, London
25. Wright C G, Meyerhoff W L, Burns D K 1985 Middle ear cholesteatoma: an animal model. Am J Otolaryngol 6: 327–341
26. Masaki M, Wright C G, Lee D H et al. 1989 Experimental cholesteatoma. Epidermal ingrowth through tympanic membrane following middle ear application of propylene glycol. Acta Otolaryngol (Stockh) 108: 113–121
27. Wells M D, Michaels L 1983 Role of retraction pockets in cholesteatoma formation. Clin Otolaryngol 8: 39–45
28. Friedberg J 1994 Congenital cholesteatoma. Laryngoscope 104 (suppl 62): 1–24
29. Grundfast K M, Ahuja G S, Parisier S C et al. 1995 Delayed diagnosis and fate of congenital cholesteatoma (keratoma). Arch Otolaryngol Head Neck Surg 121: 903–907
30. Michaels L 1986 An epidermoid formation in the developing middle ear: possible source of cholesteatoma. J Otolaryngol 15: 169–174
31. Liang J, Michaels L, Wright A 2003 Immunohistochemical characterization of the epidermoid formation in the middle ear. Laryngoscope 113: 1007–1014
32. Simoni P, Wiatrak B J, Kelly D R 2003 Choristomatous polyps of the aural and pharyngeal regions: first simultaneous case. Int J Pediatr Otorhinolaryngol 67: 195–199
33. Quaranta A, Mininni F, Resta L 1981 Salivary gland choristoma of the middle ear. A case report. J Laryngol Otol 95: 953–956
34. Buckmiller L M, Brodie H A, Doyle K J et al. 2001 Choristoma of the middle ear: a component of a new syndrome? Otol Neurotol 22: 363–368
35. Gyure K A, Thompson L D, Morrison A L 2000 A clinicopathological study of 15 patients with neuroglial heterotopias and encephaloceles of the middle ear and mastoid region. Laryngoscope 110: 1731–1735
36. Hyams V J, Michaels L 1976 Benign adenomatous neoplasms (adenoma) of the middle ear. Clin Otolaryngol 1: 17–26
37. Derlacki E L, Barney P L 1976 Adenomatous tumors of the middle ear and mastoid. Laryngoscope 86: 1123–1135
38. Jahrdoerfer R A, Fechner R E, Selman J W et al. 1983 Adenoma of the middle ear. Laryngoscope 93: 1041–1044
39. Mills S E, Fechner R E 1984 Middle ear adenoma. A cytologically uniform neoplasm displaying a variety of architectural patterns. Am J Surg Pathol 8: 677–685
40. Stanley M W, Horwitz J, Levinson R M et al. 1987 Carcinoid tumors of the middle ear. Am J Clin Pathol 87: 592–600
41. Hale R S, McMahon R F T, Whittaker J S 1991 Middle ear adenoma: tumor of mixed mucinous and neuroendocrine differentiation. J Clin Pathol 44: 652–654
42. Wassef M, Panagiotis K, Polivka M et al. 1989 Middle ear adenoma. A tumor displaying mucinous and neuroendocrine differentiation. Am J Surg Pathol 13: 838–847
43. Torske K R, Thompson L D 2002 Adenoma versus carcinoid tumor of the middle ear: a study of 48 cases and review of the literature. Mod Pathol 15: 543–555
44. Nager G T 1963 Meningiomas involving the temporal bone. Charles C Thomas, Springfield, IL
45. Thompson L D, Bouffard J P, Sandberg G D et al. 2003 Primary ear and temporal bone meningiomas: a clinicopathologic study of 36 cases with a review of the literature. Mod Pathol 16: 236–245
46. Ophir D 1991 Familial multicentric paragangliomas in a child. J Laryngol Otol 105: 376–380
46a. Baysal B E, Ferrell R W, Willett-Brozick J E et al. 2000 Mutations in SDHD, a mitochondrial complex II gene, in hereditary paraganglioma. Science 287: 848–851
47. Martinez-Madrigal F, Bosq J, Micheau C et al. 1991 Paragangliomas of the head and neck. Immunohistochemical analysis of 16 cases in comparison with neuro-endocrine carcinomas. Pathol Res Pract 187: 814–823
48. Kliewer K E, Duan-Ren W, Pasquale A et al. 1989 Paragangliomas: assessment of prognosis by histologic, immunohistochemical and ultrastructural techniques. Hum Pathol 20: 29–39
49. Michaels L, Wells M 1980 Squamous cell carcinoma of the middle ear. Clin Otolaryngol 5: 235–248
50. Michaels L, Liang J 1993 Origin of middle ear corpuscles. Clin Otolaryngol 18: 257–262
51. Phelps P D, Lloyd G A S 1981 The radiology of carcinoma of the ear. Br J Radiol 54: 103–109
52. Michaels L 2006 The ear and temporal bone. In: Cardesa A, Slootweg P (eds) Head and neck pathology. Springer Verlag, Heidelberg, Ch. 8
53. Heffner D K 1989 Low-grade adenocarcinoma of probable endolymphatic sac origin. A clinicopathologic study of 20 cases. Cancer 64: 2292–2302

54. Leonard J, Talbot M 1970 Asymptomatic acoustic neurilemmoma. Arch Otolaryngol 91: 117–124
55. Xenellis J E, Linthicum F H Jr 2003 On the myth of the glial/schwann junction (Obersteiner–Redlich zone): origin of vestibular nerve schwannomas. Otol Neurotol 24: 1
56. Muzumdar D P, Goel A, Pakhmode C K 2002 Multicystic acoustic neurinoma: report of two cases. J Clin Neurosci 9: 453–455
57. Bari M E, Forster D M, Kemeny A A et al. 2002 Malignancy in a vestibular schwannoma. Report of a case with central neurofibromatosis, treated by both stereotactic radiosurgery and surgical excision, with a review of the literature. Br J Neurosurg 16: 284–289
58. Tosaka M, Hirato J, Miyagishima T et al. 2002 Calcified vestibular schwannoma with unusual histological characteristics – positive immunoreactivity for CD-34 antigen. Acta Neurochir (Wien) 144: 395–399
59. Bedavanija A, Brieger J, Lehr H A et al. 2003 Association of proliferative activity and size in acoustic neuroma: implications for timing of surgery. J Neurosurg 98: 807–811
60. Aguiar P H, Tatagiba M, Samii M et al. 1995 The comparison between the growth fraction of bilateral vestibular schwannomas in neurofibromatosis 2 (NF2) and unilateral vestibular schwannomas using the monoclonal antibody MIB 1. Acta Neurochir (Wien) 134: 40–45
61. Chitale A R, Murthy A K, Desai A P et al. 1991 Peripheral nerve sheath tumors: an ultrastructural study of 30 cases. Ind J Cancer 28: 1–8
62. Sans A, Bartolami S, Fraysse B 1996 Histopathology of the peripheral vestibular system in small vestibular schwannomas. Am J Otol 17: 326–324
63. Michaels L, Lee K, Manuja S L et al. 1999 Family with low-grade neuroendocrine carcinoma of salivary glands, severe sensorineural hearing loss and enamel hypoplasia. Am J Med Genet 83: 183–186
64. Kishore A, O'Reilly B F 2000 A clinical study of vestibular schwannomas in type 2 neurofibromatosis. Clin Otolaryngol 25: 561–565
65. Sidek D, Michaels L, Wright A 1996 Changes in the inner ear in vestibular schwannoma. In: Iurato S, Veldman J E (eds) Progress in human auditory and vestibular histopathology. Kugler Publications, Amsterdam, p 95–101
66. Singh S P, Cottingham S L, Slone W et al. 1996 Lipomas of the internal auditory canal. Arch Pathol Lab Med 120: 681–683
67. Schuknecht H F 1993 Pathology of the ear, 2nd edn. Lea & Febiger, Philadelphia, 1993
68. Devaney K O, Ferlito A, Rinaldo A 2003 Endolymphatic sac tumor (low grade papillary adenocarcinoma) of the temporal bone. Acta Otolaryngol 23: 1022–1026
69. Lonser R R, Kim H J, Butman J A et al. 2004 Tumors of the endolymphatic sac in von Hippel–Lindau disease. N Engl J Med 350: 2481–2486
70. Choo D, Shotland L, Mastroianni M et al. 2004 Endolymphatic sac tumors in von Hippel–Lindau disease. J Neurosurg 100: 480–487
71. Kim W Y, Kaelin W G 2004 Role of VHL gene mutation in human cancer. J Clin Oncol 22: 4991–5004
72. Smith N, Bain B, Michaels L et al. 1991 Atypical Ph negative chronic myeloid leukaemia presenting as sudden profound deafness. J Clin Pathol 44: 1033–1034

肿瘤诊断中的电子显微镜检查
Electron microscopy in tumor diagnosis

Bruce Mackay 著

回允中 姜 影 译

引言	1831
癌	1832
鳞状细胞癌	1832
腺癌	1834
间皮瘤	1838
黑色素瘤	1840
小圆细胞肿瘤	1842
软组织肿瘤	1842
纤维母细胞肿瘤	1842
脂肪肉瘤	1845
肌原性肿瘤	1845
成血管细胞肿瘤	1848
外周神经鞘细胞肿瘤	1848
其他肉瘤	1850
淋巴瘤/白血病	1852
中枢神经系统肿瘤	1855
结论	1857

引言

1939年，电子显微镜已可以买到[1]，当时对于它在医学上应用的潜能，有相当多的推测和争议[2]。若干年之后，其技术操作得到了发展，达到了能够制备合适的生物学标本进行研究的水平，1947年，首先应用其研究了来自鼠肉瘤的肿瘤细胞[3]。经过一段时间，尽管病理学系能够添置电子显微镜并将其用于研究标本并报告，但是其逐渐被用于分析。这之后发现，虽然电子显微镜在医学上的某些应用具有相当大的价值，但是对于多数病理医生来说，应用光学显微镜仍然可以胜任工作。随着免疫组织化学技术的发展，电子显微镜在诊断方面的应用有所减少，现在应用更少，只是选择性地用于外科病理学，而且主要是在大医院和医学院的医学中心。然而，超微结构研究彻底改变了有关细胞和组织结构的知识，而且其在医学研究中的作用依然无法估价。已有不止一种类型的电子显微镜在外科病理学中具有显著应用价值，其透射电子显微镜电子束能够通过标本薄切片。扫描或分析电子显微镜用于诊断的适用范围很小。在外科病理学中，透射电子显微镜的适用范围局限于少数几个领域，包括肾活检和其他非肿瘤性标本[4]。肿瘤研究证实，诊断电子显微镜具有最广泛而又最有价值的作用[5]，本章将对此进行简要的描述。

虽然电子显微镜常常能够揭示常规光学显微镜不能发现的肿瘤的有关信息[6]，但它并不总是具有实用价值。经济上的考虑也是一个原因。透射电子显微镜是一种复杂的仪器，购置和维修费用昂贵，需要特殊的辅助设备和熟练的技术支持，因而操作电子显微镜的实验室的费用会增加。必须进行大量的病例研究，得到足够的收入，以证明这样一种重大投资是值得的，但是即使是在大的病理系，这也基本上是不可行的，除非费用可以由科研基金支付。

虽然可以预期电子显微镜对特别的病例可提供有用的信息，但是如果检查所见不影响患者的治疗，这种操作也不会应用。如果将这种检查的费用与它所能提供信息的临床价值进行比较，其潜在的益处可能不能证明其费用具有合理性。应用电子显微镜对高级别多形性软组织肉瘤进行亚分类可能就是一个好的例证，越来越多的证据表明，这些肿瘤的亚分类对预后具有意义，从而可能改变这种认识[7]。

电子显微镜作为诊断工具有其局限性，主要是缺少经过诊断电子显微镜检查培训的外科病理医生。评估肿瘤的细微结构和得出可靠的诊断结论需要相当多的经验。超微结构特征非常容易被过度解释或误认，特别是当由于延误固定、挤压、坏死或其他人为假象造成提供的检查标本质量不佳时。应该由能将其观察所见与其他镜下所见联系起来、并能与临床状况联系起来的病理医生进行电子显微镜检查。

免疫组织化学检查的广泛应用已经极大地限制了电子显微镜在诊断方面的作用[8]。现在应用的抗体能够解决许多在该领域中曾经出现的问题。应用一组筛查免疫染色操作可以缩小鉴别诊断范围，这种筛查可以应用市售的抗体进行，而且在任何病理学实验室均能做到。与电子显微镜检查只能检查小样本不同，免疫组织化学检查的另外一个好处是：病理医生可以在光学显微镜切片中检查大量的肿瘤细胞。免疫电子显微镜检查是一种精致的研究工具，但是应用光学显微镜一般就可以得到必要的诊断信息[9]。

从这些评论中，电子显微镜不应该被理解为在诊断病理学中几乎没有价值。相反，它能提供有关各种标本的有用信息，对于某些肿瘤来说，它可能是获取重要信息的唯一手段。然而，在着手进行一个肿瘤的超微结构检查之前，预先要慎重考虑可能揭示的信息，如果尚未进行免疫组化染色，还要考虑免疫组化检查可能具有的作用。常规的做法是：在采取电子显微镜检查之前，进行一些免疫组化染色，只有当免疫染色结果含糊或提供的信息不充分时，才需要进行电子显微镜检查[10]。在一些情况下，应同时应用两种技术以便尽可能更多地获得信息而不延误适当的治疗。

用于诊断电子显微镜检查的组织标本应该具有好的质量。超微结构检查没有起到作用的最常见原因在于材料，或因不具有代表性或因保存不好。电子显微镜检查之前的常规是：制备并在光镜下检查塑料包埋的组织切片，这样可以选择最适合的部位。可以使用甲醛溶液固定甚或石蜡包埋的材料，而且当小片组织及时固定在缓冲戊二醛溶液中时，检查结果显然是满意的。用于电子显微镜检查的材料应该尽可能地在切除标本时采集，这就意味着，病理医生或细胞学医生必须提前知道可能需要电子显微镜检查。这可从先前的活检检查中了解或预测到，或在冰冻切片检查时觉察到。如果怀疑一个特殊的样本是否具有代表性，可以从实性肿瘤印片或冰冻切片或细针吸取快速涂片中得到答案。许多病理医生和多数临床医生还没有认识到获得保存好的组织对于电子显微镜检查的重要性。通常出现在常规光学显微镜切片或涂片中的人为假象造成的严重扭曲，在超微结构水平是不能接受的。从人体实性肿瘤的新鲜切面获取薄片组织并将其浸于缓冲戊二醛溶液中是一个快速而又简单的操作。每一个外科病理医生都应该知道如何正确操作，而且还必须知道，实性肿瘤以外的各种类型的标本进行电子显微镜检查时，必须以特别的方法处理[11]。细针吸取活检现在广泛应用于确立最初的诊断，而且提供的少量细胞已经足够用于电子显微镜检查，前提是对标本要进行正确的处理[12]。从实性肿瘤吸取的材料应该立即固定在缓冲戊二醛溶液中，轻轻振荡容器使细胞分散。在实验室将固定的标本通过细布滤网过滤，可以去除多数不可避免的外周血细胞[13,14]。这样得到的标本一般具有良好的质量（见图31.18，作为一个例子），可以提供有价值的诊断信息[15,16]。细胞学医生能够立即评估快速涂片，并能决定此病例是否具有诊断问题，由他进行浅表细针吸取活检是一个有利条件，可以获得另外的材料用于电子显微镜检查。多数深部吸取活检是由放射科医生操作的，但是只有当细胞学医生观察后，才可能知道进行快速涂片分析的细胞是否充分，同时才有可能获得较多的细胞。

加快电子显微镜诊断研究进程是重要的。电子显微镜检查可以在收到标本后几小时内完成，不过需要一种繁忙的快速处理技术[17]，在繁忙的实验室工作中，几乎总是倾向于选择这种技术作为常规操作。在收到组织后48小时之内应该出具一份电子显微镜报告。如果在收到标本后当天进行处理，可以在检查石蜡切片后，备好包埋的组织块，进行切片，并且可以在请求进行检查的几小时内提供有关电子显微镜检查的口头意见。为了适当评估一个特殊病例超微结构检查所见的意义，必须综合常规光学显微镜检查所见以得出结论，包括免疫组化检查，病理学报告用语应让临床医生易于理解。外科病理医生只不过是一个能够根据临床和放射学资料解释显微镜下所见的医生。

本章描述有关肿瘤超微结构中一些比较重要的问题。图例是由Texas大学M D Anderson癌症中心的、有30年以上电子显微镜诊断经验的医生选择的。

癌 Carcinomas

分化性人体肿瘤往往具有超微结构特征，可以用作诊断标准。当一个肿瘤变得不太分化时，这些典型的特征逐渐丧失，可能变成亚型，因此，当评估一个未知肿瘤时，电子显微镜学家必须扩大考虑范围。鳞状细胞癌可以作为一个例证。

鳞状细胞癌 Squamous cell carcinoma

不管解剖部位如何，分化性鳞状细胞癌具有一些共同的超微结构特征。最值得注意的是：常常出现成熟的桥粒[18]和大量的细胞角蛋白，桥粒连接邻近细胞，而细胞角蛋白倾向于形成致密成束的胞浆丝。这些特征也见于具有上皮分化的其他肿瘤，包括黏液表皮样癌和一些附件肿瘤。桥粒的数目和细胞角蛋白的量并不总是密切相关，但是典型者两者均很明显。桥粒连接相邻的细胞膜，但是交界处的细胞表面回缩，形成扇贝样外观，使桥粒的部位更加明显（图31.1），然后可以对比并描述，尽管光学显微镜学家会将其错误地称为"细胞间桥"。黏膜鳞状细胞癌的细胞膜常常紧密相对，虽然可能存在许多桥粒，但在石蜡切片中见不到这样的"间桥"。高分化腺癌也有桥粒，但比鳞状细胞癌少，而且也不显著。

鳞状细胞癌的细胞常常弥漫成片。存在棘层松解的肿瘤其细胞之间桥粒的凝集力丧失，形成裂隙，可能酷似腺体（甚至血管）结构。这种现象在超微结构检查时可能更加明显，细胞表面出现细长的突起，类似于微绒毛。这些小突起比较准确的称呼是丝状伪足（filopodia），常常出现在鳞状细胞癌的桥粒之间。线状伪足缺乏均匀一致的形态和多数微绒毛的内部结构。在HE染色的石蜡切片中，鳞状细胞癌的致密的细胞角蛋白团块可能表现为嗜酸性胞浆包涵体，这也可能提示为腺体结构。在鳞状细胞癌，真正的胞浆内腔罕见[19]，但是这种类

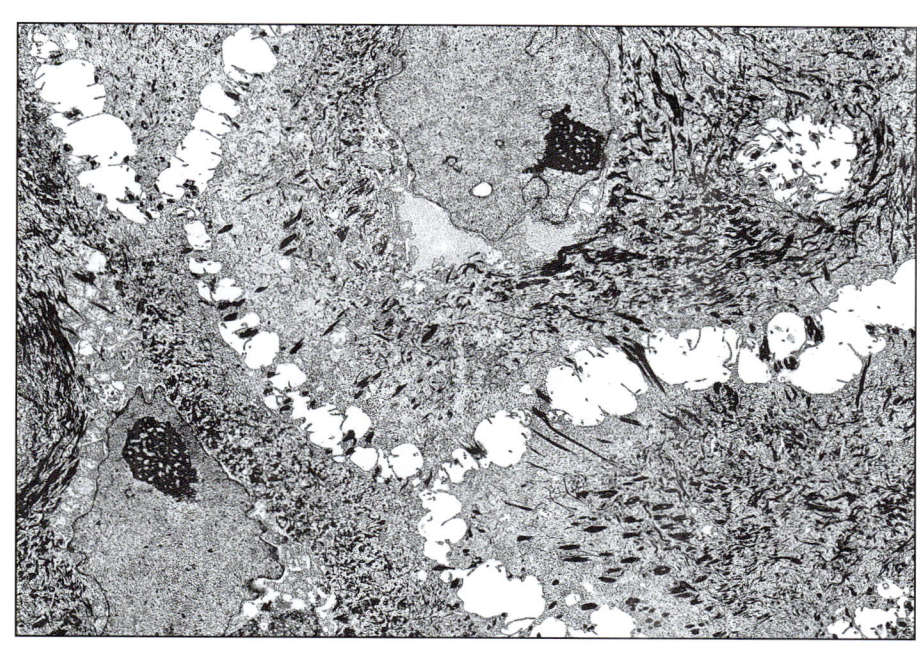

图31.1 图示皮肤高分化鳞状细胞癌具有丰富的细胞角蛋白细丝，而且在细胞之间的裂隙中常见桥粒。

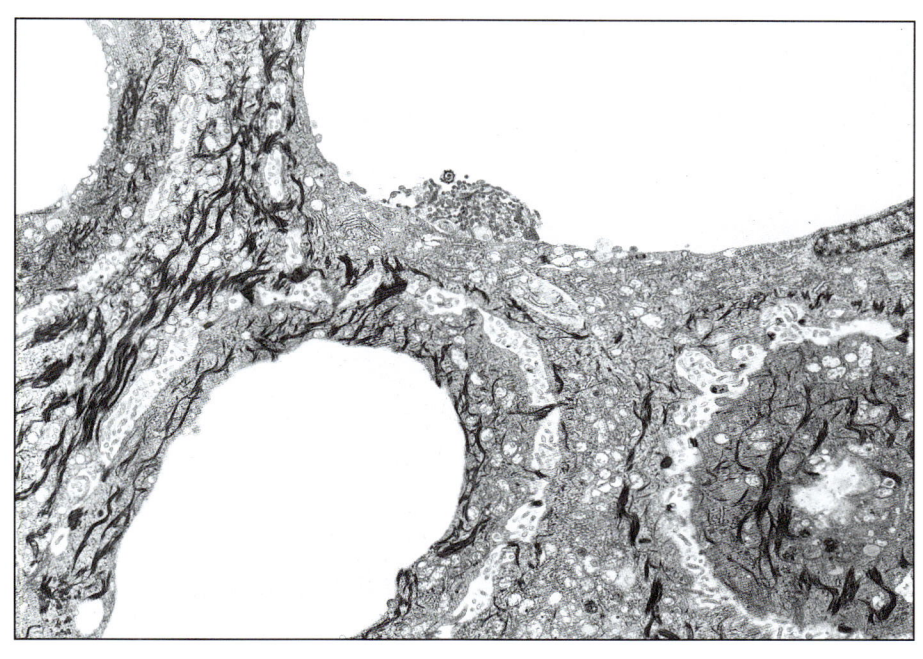

图31.2 鳞状细胞癌具有大的胞浆空泡，形成假腺体现象，但是有丰富的细胞角蛋白，表现为所谓的张力丝。

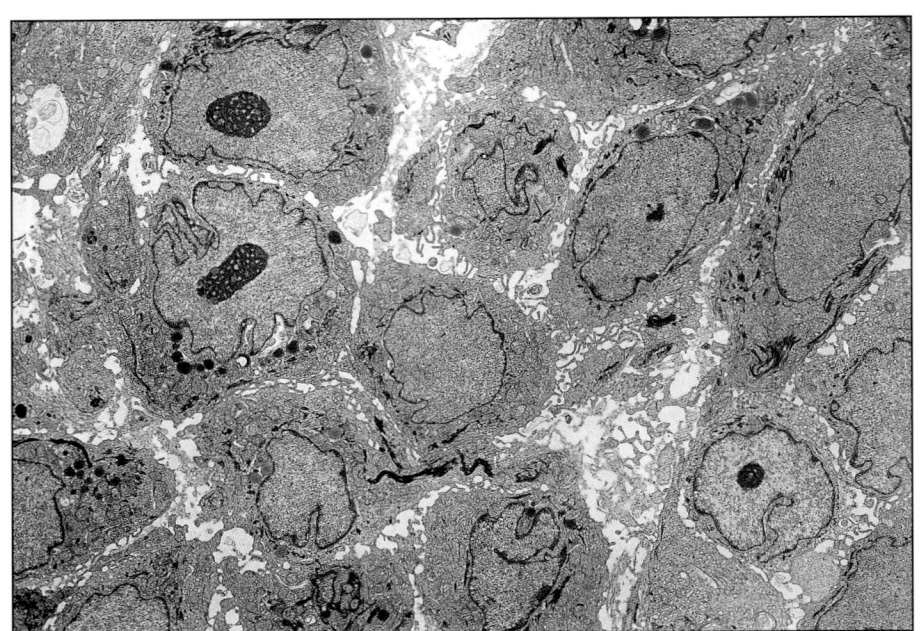

图31.3 多数低分化鳞状细胞癌的细胞之间彼此由不规则的裂隙分开。与图31.1的肿瘤相比，细胞连接和细胞角蛋白稀少。

型的大的间隙在光学显微镜检查时可能类似于印戒细胞（图31.2）。

肿瘤性鳞状细胞丧失分化伴桥粒数目逐渐减少，而且由于中心致密线消失以及胞膜下斑变薄和变短，其成熟结构模糊不清。最后，细胞附着减少，变成并列的细胞膜的散在的微小的致密体。这种变化伴有细胞角蛋白丝数目减少，最后消失（图31.3）。细胞角蛋白丝的数量并不总是与细胞角蛋白免疫反应程度相关。浸润性肿瘤的桥粒数目减少，但鳞状细胞癌在放疗之后可见到桥粒和细胞角蛋白丝增加[20]。伴随分化丧失的其他改变是细胞器数目减少和基底膜碎裂或丧失。对于光学显微镜学家所熟悉的变化而言，包括细胞和核的不规则性以及核浆比例增加，电子显微镜学家会观察的更好。

腺癌 Adenocarcinoma

在超微结构水平，腺体分化的特征是存在由肿瘤细胞围绕的腔隙，肿瘤细胞尖端具有微绒毛[21]。高分化腺癌形成腺泡，邻近的细胞膜一般在其腔隙端融合成紧密连接。在封闭膜的下方，细胞由桥粒连接。内衬正常胃肠道的柱状细胞的腔面有直而平行排列的密集的微绒毛，其中含有肌动蛋白丝轴心，胃肠道腺癌有类似的微绒毛（图31.4）。肌动蛋白丝延伸到胞浆顶端形成一个带，在紧密连接的下方插入旁边的细胞膜。微绒毛旁边可见糖萼体（glycocalyceal bodies）（图31.5）。在转移性腺癌出现这种类型的微绒毛时，提示肿瘤来源于胃肠道，但是这种表现并不完全具有特异性，因为在一些鼻咽癌、涎腺癌、肺癌和卵巢癌中也可以见到类似的微绒毛。许多腺癌的微绒毛不具有特异性，其长度和间隔不同，而且缺乏微丝轴心。分化较好的腺癌腺泡周围有基底膜围绕，但是随着分化降低，基底膜破碎并最终消失。因为腺癌细胞可以有桥粒和细胞角蛋白细丝，所以在分化较差的肿瘤，常不能与鳞状细胞癌鉴别开来。真正的腺鳞癌具有独特的鳞状和腺状成分，在一些分化较差的肿瘤，通过电子显微镜检查常常可以发现两种成分的混合存在，但是不可能挑选出优势的分化成分。非小细胞肺癌在超微结构水平常常是异源性的，但是电子显微镜检查肿瘤样本较小，不能发现光学显微镜检查见到的切除标本中的各种变化。因此，任何根据超微结构特征进行的癌的分类尝试必须与光学显微镜所见联系起来。

在腺癌细胞，有时可见真正的胞浆内腔[22]（图31.6），众所周知，这些胞浆内腔偶尔发生于乳腺肿瘤。少数不规则的微绒毛突入腔内。较大的胞浆内腔隙可见于一些胃腺癌（图31.7）和少数分化差的肿瘤（图31.8）。已经提到，在肿瘤性鳞状细胞内，偶尔可发现边缘为丝状伪足的腺样间隙，在少数移行细胞癌和个别黑色素瘤中也可见到[23]。

一些腺癌具有独特的超微结构特征，可能与组织来源有关。其中最值得注意的是见于胞浆内的细胞器的表现和分泌产物的出现。

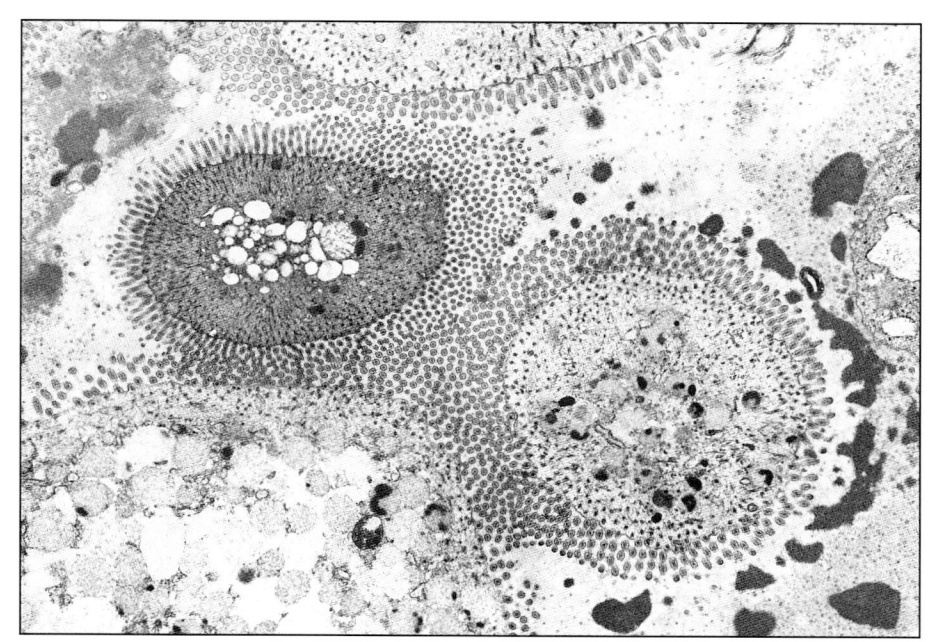

图31.4 鼻腔原发性腺癌显示肠的分化。它含有Paneth细胞和内分泌细胞、杯状细胞（在图示的细胞中，一个细胞可见一些黏液小滴）以及含有微丝轴心的微绒毛。这个切面穿过几个表面细胞，在这个切面上，许多微绒毛是横切的，位于中心的小点是肌动蛋白丝轴心。

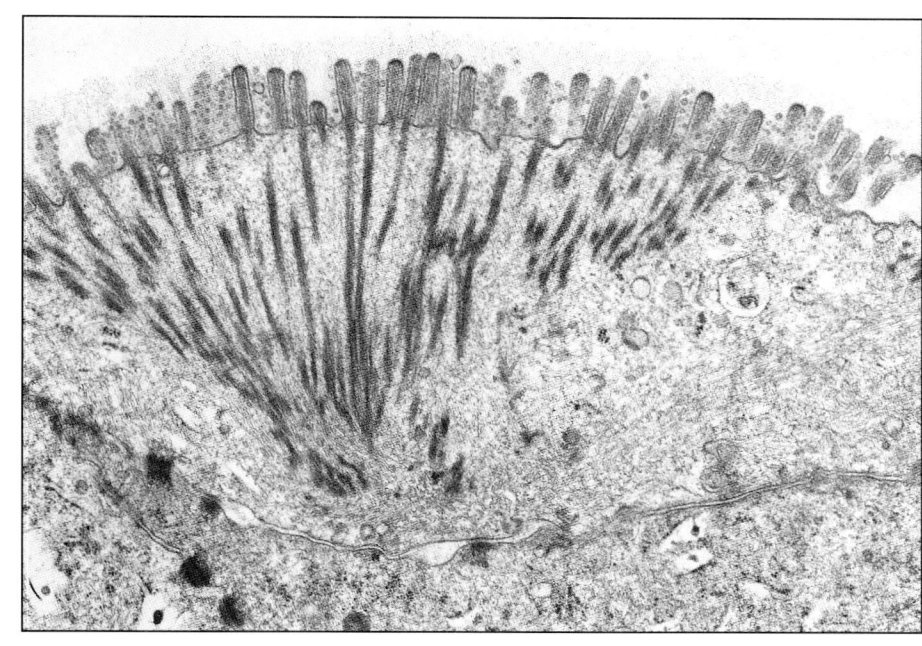

图31.5 这个来自胃腺癌细胞的微绒毛具有突出的微丝轴心，微绒毛之间有糖萼（glycocalyceal）空泡。

细胞器 Organelles

肿瘤细胞细胞器的数目、相对比例以及独特表现是有关肿瘤类型及其分化水平的信息来源，在转移性腺癌，细胞器还可提示原发部位[24]。内质网的数量、类型和结构水平可以提供信息。广泛的核糖体结合网是细胞正在形成蛋白的指征，蛋白将从细胞中排出，而分泌产物常常贮存在胞浆的致密轴心颗粒中（图31.9）。在增生性和良性肾上腺皮质病变中，滑面内质网发育良好，而在肾上腺皮质癌中却很难见到，这是一个重要的特征[25]（图31.10）。在肝细胞癌、一些卵巢肿瘤、睾丸间质细胞肿瘤和腺泡状软组织肿瘤，滑面内质网也可能明显。

在嗜酸性细胞中，线粒体数目明显增加（图31.11），而且线粒体嵴的形态往往异常[26,27]。在富于线粒体的肾肿瘤中，线粒体偶尔含有大的脂质包涵体，而在一些肾上腺皮质腺瘤，可见类似的致密小体。管状嵴出现在形成类固醇的细胞，有助于肾上腺皮质癌的确诊（图31.12），但这并不是特异性表现，偶尔可见于转移性黑色素瘤。横纹肌瘤和腺泡状软组织肉瘤可以见到奇异的线粒体；这是一个有趣的奇特现象，而在神经母细胞瘤，线粒体有时非常大。

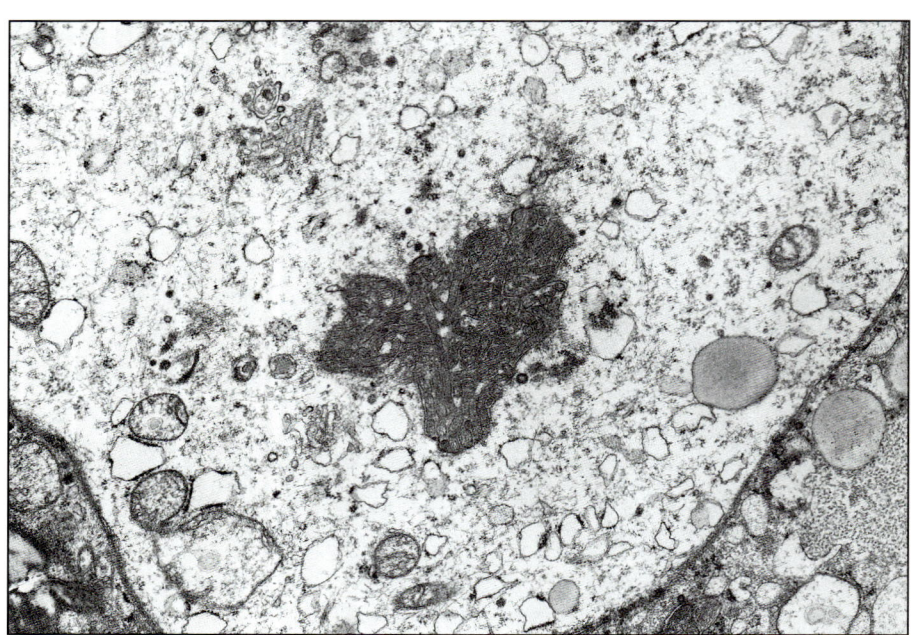

图31.6 转移性低分化腺癌。小的胞浆内腺泡内充满微绒毛。

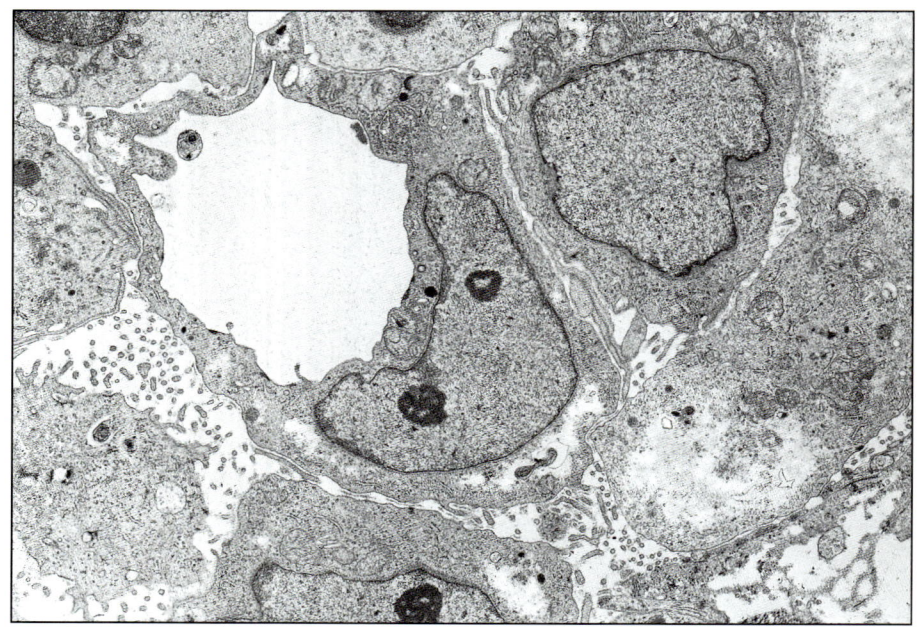

图31.7 锁骨上淋巴结转移性胃腺癌，一些细胞含有大的胞浆内腔。

分泌产物　Secretory products

许多分化性腺癌的细胞产生并贮存分泌物质，包括黏液、糖原和蛋白质产物。图31.13显示黏液小滴充满乳腺外Paget病的肿瘤细胞。石蜡切片的特殊染色不能发现的胞浆内糖原或黏液，通过电子显微镜检查可以发现。出现小量黏液或糖原可能无助于确定肿瘤类型，但是在转移癌中出现糖原和脂质小滴会提示：肾是原发部位。

细胞分泌出的蛋白在胞浆内形成圆形颗粒。颗粒的致密轴心周围围绕界膜，颗粒大小以及外观也可能提供信息。细胞浆内的致密小体不都是待分泌的蛋白产物。黏液小滴可能含有致密区域，而且内质网池内的物质也可能出现误导现象。Golgi复合体新产生的初级溶酶体似乎与次级颗粒相同。然而，存活的癌细胞中很少出现大量溶酶体，这些溶酶体的大小和形状各不相同，而且可能显示具有自体吞噬活性的特征，这反映在其异源性成分上。另一方面，许多肿瘤细胞中通常至少可以见到中等量的真正的次级颗粒，在一个特定的肿瘤中，其直径、形状和内部表现完全一致。具有混合性外分泌和内

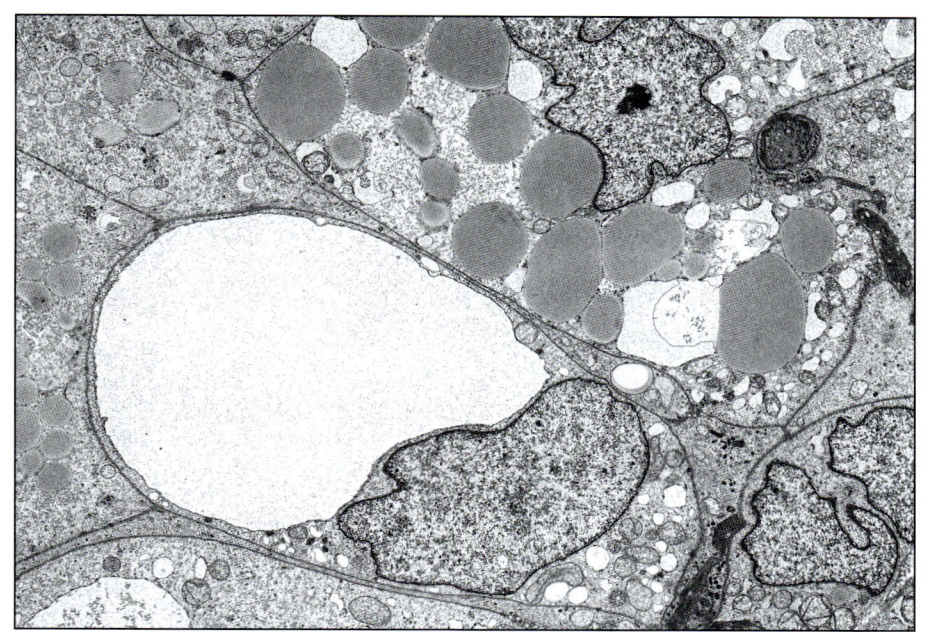

图31.8 来自肺的转移性肾细胞癌的细胞。许多脂质小滴具有特征性,而分化丧失的指征是缺乏微绒毛和出现形成具有单环结构的细胞的胞浆内腔。

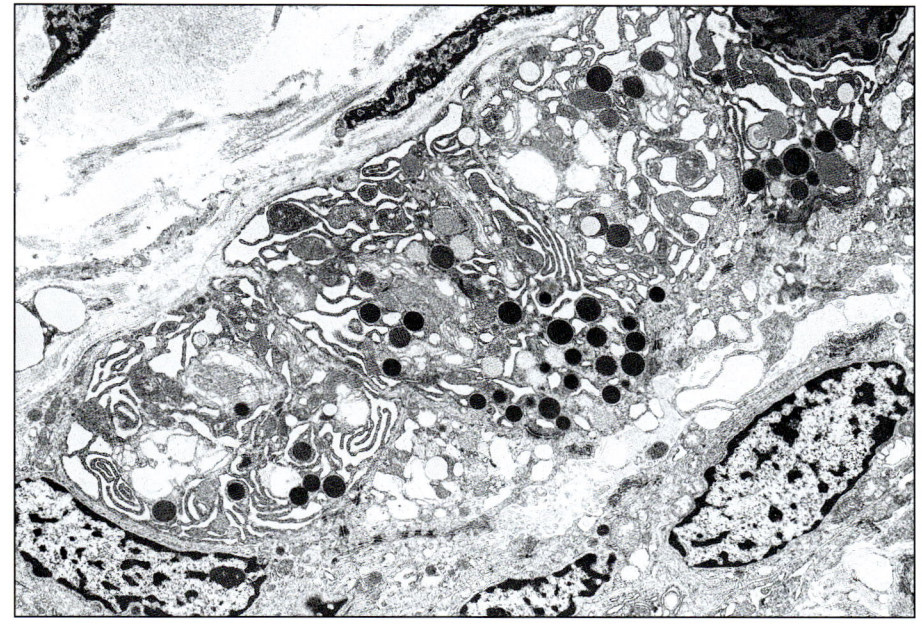

图31.9 胰腺腺泡细胞癌的两个显著的超微结构特征(本例是肝转移)是:广泛的内质网和顶端大的分泌颗粒。

分泌成分的肿瘤除外,如伴有肠分化的鼻腺癌[28]或腺类癌(adenocarcinoid)。黏液产物和内分泌分化偶尔见于同一个细胞内,这样就可以同时见到黏液小滴和内分泌型颗粒,有些黏液小滴可能有致密轴心[29]。内胚窦瘤和肝细胞癌可能出现比外分泌颗粒大的致密小体,可能是甲胎蛋白(alpha-fetoprotein)的集聚。

在不同类型的肿瘤中,颗粒大小可有不同。外分泌细胞及其肿瘤颗粒的直径在 600～900 nm 之间,在腺泡细胞涎腺癌中,这些颗粒可能充满胞浆,或集聚在胰腺腺泡细胞癌的胞浆顶端(图 31.9)[30]。细支气管肺泡腺癌的柱状细胞显示 Clara 细胞分化,颗粒集聚在隆起的顶冠内,其中可混有黏液小滴[31]。一些细支气管肺泡癌显示 II 型肺细胞分化,含有板层小体(表面活性)。

肿瘤性内分泌细胞(图 31.14)的多数颗粒的直径在 100～400 nm 之间。通过电子显微镜检查进行形态学分析可以高度精确地测量肿瘤细胞的结构细节。使用这种方法,50 例肺类癌分泌颗粒的平均直径在 93～383 nm 之间[32]。使用同样的技术,20 例非 β 胰岛细胞肿瘤的颗粒直径在 104～292 nm 之间[33]。根据颗粒大小可以区分胰岛细胞肿瘤和腺泡细胞癌[34]。内分

间皮瘤

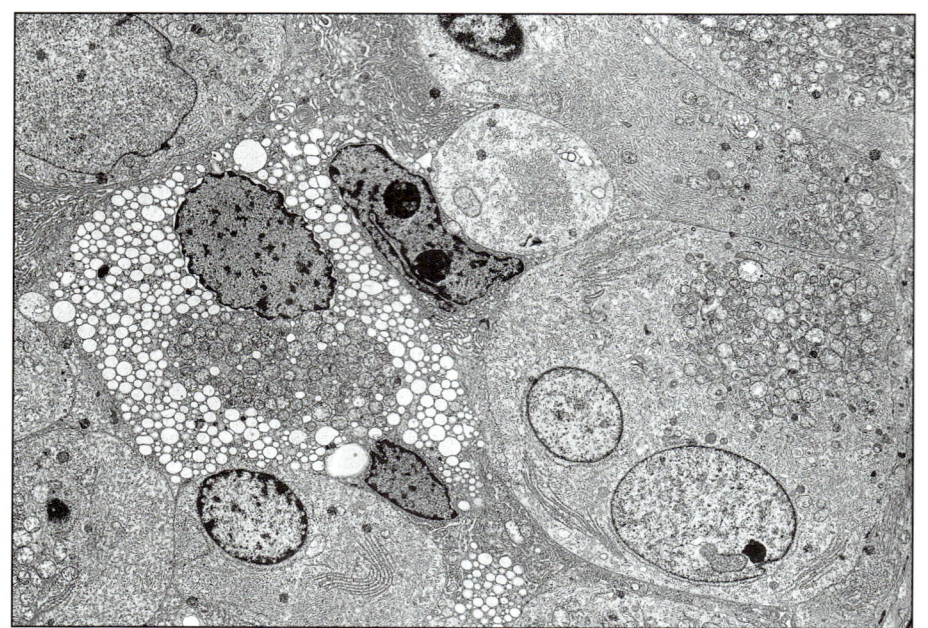

图31.10 肾上腺皮质癌。细胞内丰富的滑面内质网形成较细的小管和较大的空泡。

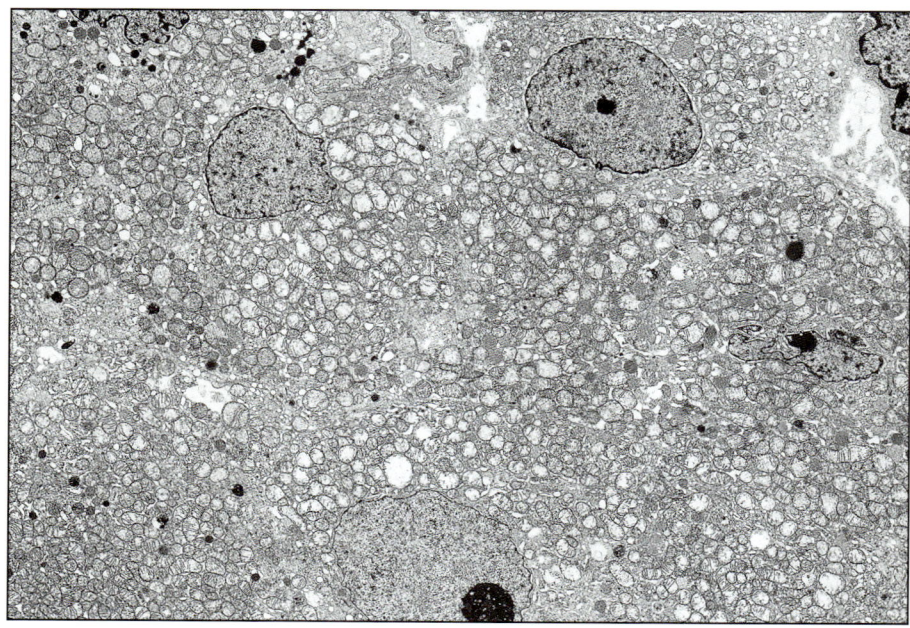

图31.11 肾上腺皮质癌。许多线粒体是嗜酸性细胞分化的证据。

泌颗粒一般为圆形，伴有同质性轴心。50例肺类癌中只有4例的肿瘤细胞含有多角形或多形性颗粒[32]。结晶状轴心可见于胰岛素瘤，而卵圆形界膜内的偏心轴则是嗜铬细胞瘤的特征。伴有后一种表现的颗粒常见于肾上腺的嗜铬细胞瘤，而在肾上腺外副神经节瘤则较少见[35]。

小细胞肿瘤颗粒直径通常较小。多年来公认，小细胞肺癌存在颗粒，而且可作为诊断标准。颗粒直径一般为100 nm，只是常常稀少或缺乏。由于肺类癌的颗粒也可能在100 nm左右，因此仅仅根据颗粒大小来区分类癌和小细胞肺癌是不恰当的，应该应用其他超微结构特征进行鉴别。电子显微镜检查没有识别小细胞肺癌亚型的标准[36]。神经母细胞瘤的颗粒直径为100 nm，类似的颗粒可见于显示有神经内分泌分化的肺外小细胞癌（图31.15）[37,38]。

间皮瘤 Mesothelioma

间皮瘤预后不良并牵涉到许多医学法律问题，提醒病理医生：胸膜肿瘤可能需要电子显微镜检查，不然通过常规光学显微镜检查会诊断为其他肿瘤。组织化学染色价值有限，因为间皮瘤和腺癌均可以含有糖原[39]或

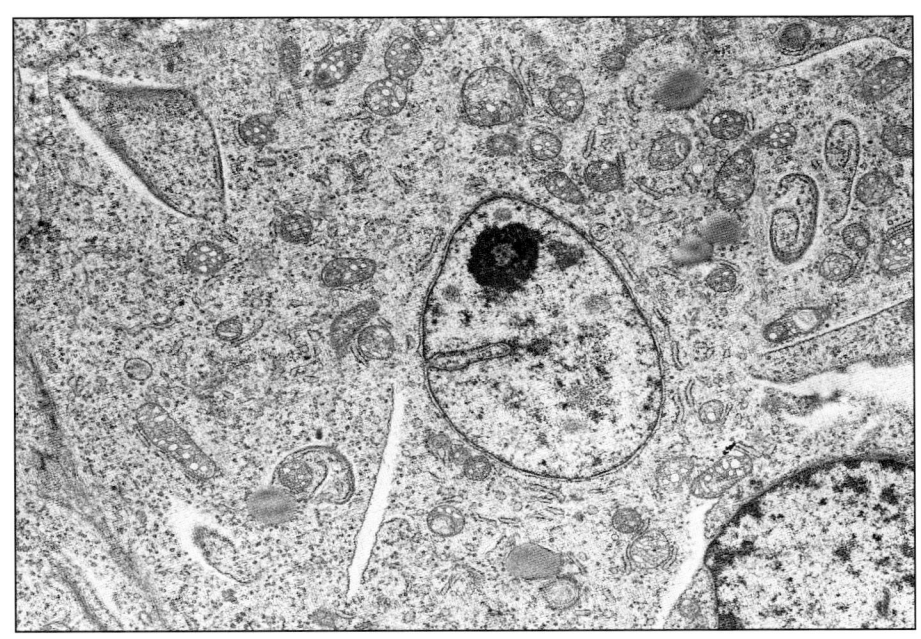

图31.12 当一个肿瘤的所有线粒体均具有显著的管状嵴时,必须怀疑它来源于产生类固醇的细胞。这个腹膜后癌来源于肾上腺皮质。

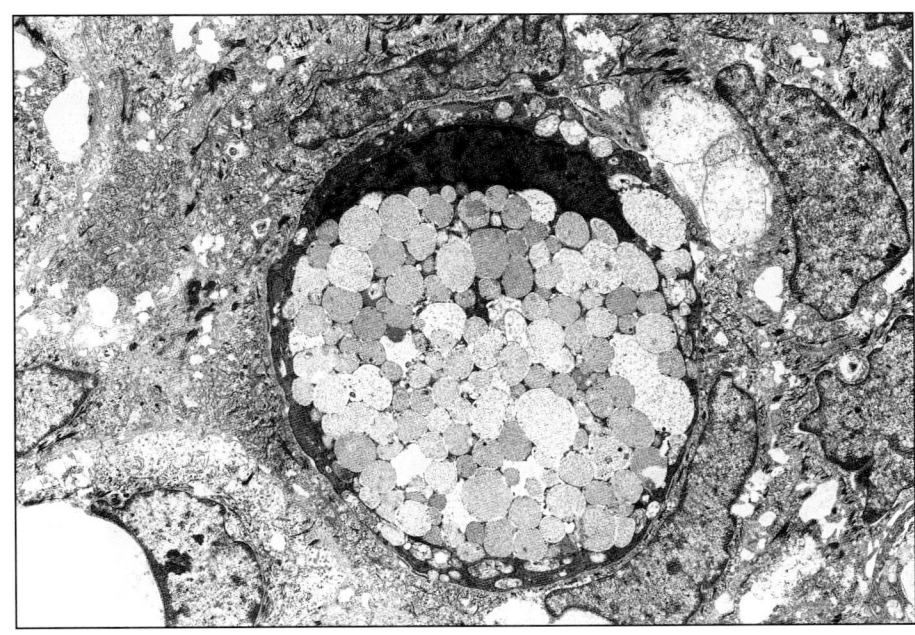

图31.13 黏液小滴可以充满乳腺外Paget病细胞的细胞浆内。

黏液[40],最好是结合光学显微镜所见以及细胞角蛋白和其他标记物的免疫染色结果,或应用电子显微镜检查来探讨这个问题[41,42]。超微结构研究发现,长而弯曲的微绒毛常可确诊,典型者细胞的游离面存在大量微绒毛(图31.16)。分化好的间皮瘤的细胞连接是成熟的桥粒。胞浆成分无特异性。多数间皮瘤细胞具有稀疏的细胞器,而且常常含有非特异性细丝,特别是在细胞核周围的部位。正常间皮的一个特征是:在邻近细胞的侧缘出现裂隙,这种特征常常见于分化好的间皮瘤。正常浆膜出现这些裂隙可使物质容易从浆膜腔进入基底膜下的毛细血管。腹膜间皮瘤具有与胸膜间皮瘤类似的超微结构特征。发生在腹膜的所谓的良性囊性间皮瘤[43]很少累及胸膜。当间皮瘤分化较差时[44],微绒毛变短变少,以致无法与低分化腺癌细胞区分。

浆膜下的梭形间充质细胞能够向间叶和上皮两个方向分化,实验研究显示,这些细胞受到刺激后增生,丧失了其对波形蛋白的免疫反应性而获得了细胞角蛋白的表达[45,46]。因此,梭形细胞间皮瘤可能显示片块状上皮

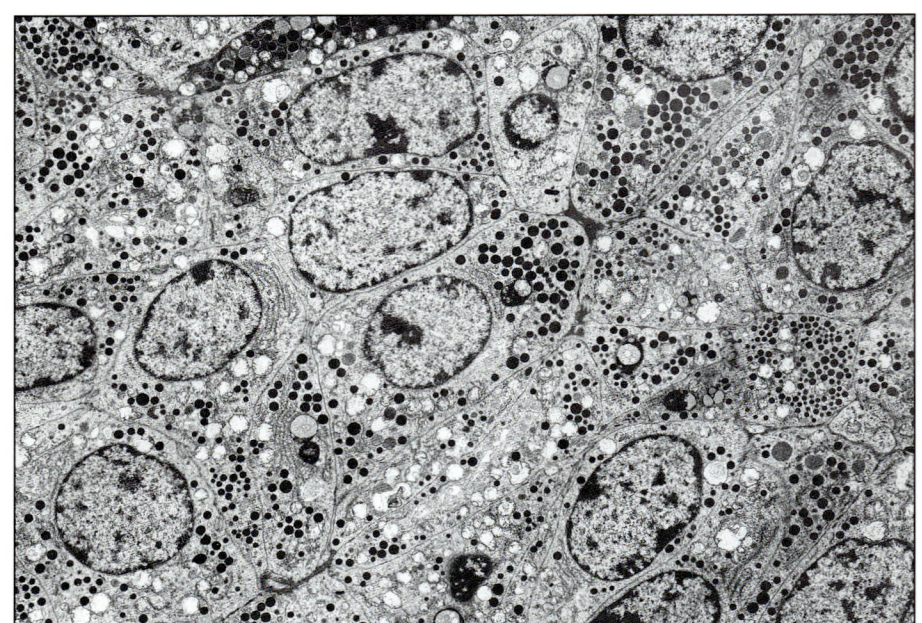

图31.14 图示支气管类癌细胞内有许多内分泌直径的分泌颗粒。

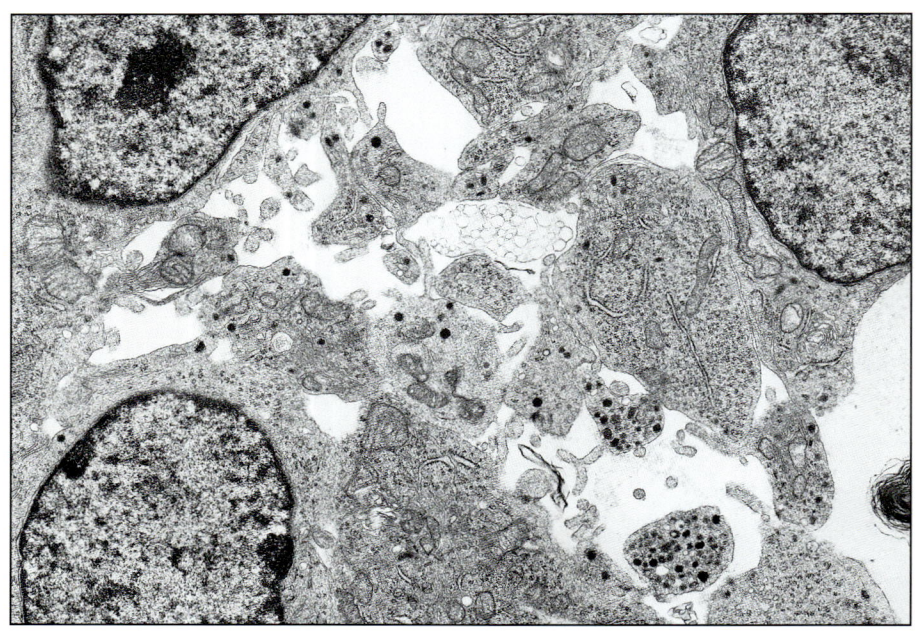

图31.15 皮肤小细胞肿瘤（Merkel细胞癌）的神经内分泌分化。在由肿瘤细胞围绕的一个小的腔隙内有几个树突状突起，其中含有小的有界膜的颗粒。

特征，虽然其细胞类似于纤维母细胞。真正的混合性间皮瘤含有类似于上皮性间皮瘤的分化性上皮成分和梭形细胞的间质样成分。

黑色素瘤 Melanoma

转移性黑色素瘤常常可以根据常规光学显微镜检查和选择性的免疫染色作出诊断。在超微结构水平，黑色素瘤细胞可有一系列的表现[23,47,48]，而且可能类似于其他类型的细胞，所以超微结构所见并不总是具有决定性，但是可用于缩小鉴别诊断的范围[49]。

黑色素细胞的特征是：沉积在黑色素小体内的黑色素产物，黑色素小体在胞浆空泡内成熟（图31.17）。这个过程可能停止，导致一些黑色素瘤细胞只含有前黑色素瘤小体。胞浆内的不规则致密小体支持黑色素瘤的诊断，但包括普遍存在的溶酶体在内的其他物体也可具有同样的表现，所以对 II 型前黑色素小体的条纹状物质进行辨认非常重要。池内排列的微管见于少数转移性黑色素瘤，但是无特异性。黑色素瘤以外的肿瘤可以含有成

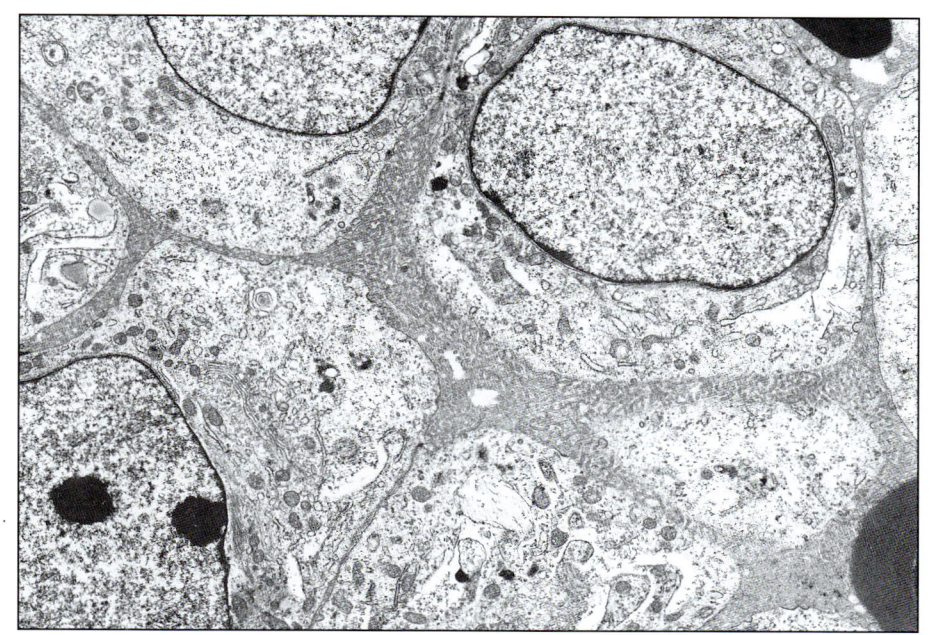

图31.16 这个胸膜肿瘤细胞之间的裂隙充满大量微绒毛，提示它是一个间皮瘤。

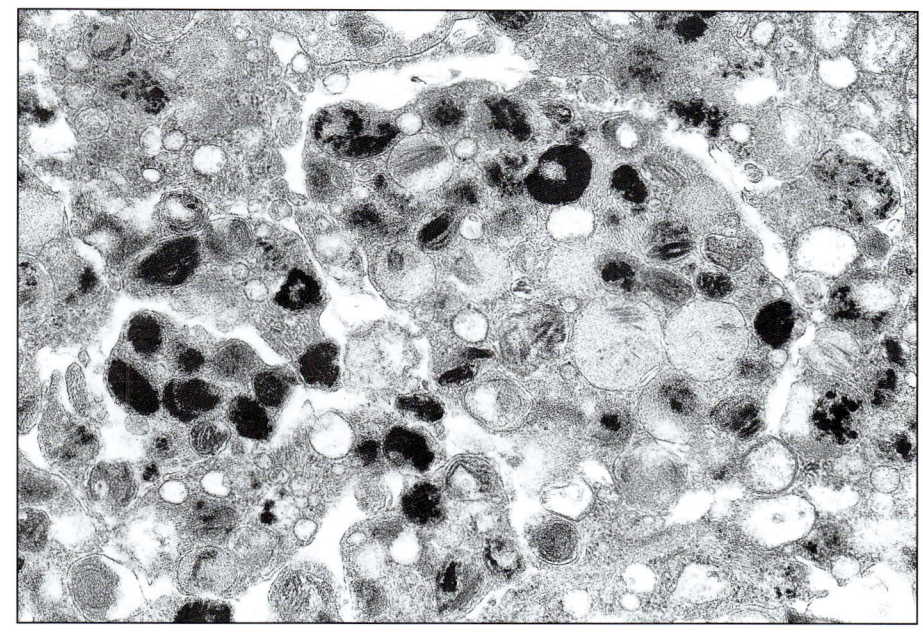

图31.17 这些黑色素瘤细胞的胞浆内有许多致密小体，显示黑色素小体成熟过程的不同阶段。

熟和不成熟的黑色素小体[50]，包括基底细胞癌[51]，而且有可能变成有继发性黑色素细胞存在的肿瘤[52,53]。

电子显微镜检查有助于辨认两种类型的黑色素瘤。软组织肿瘤最初被称为透明细胞肉瘤，现在认为是显示黑色素细胞分化的肿瘤，一些专家提出软组织恶性黑色素瘤这一术语[54]（见第27章），虽然有时这可能使临床医生的感到困扰。推测可能是胚胎期间多潜能前体细胞从神经嵴错位迁移到皮肤[55]。在石蜡切片中，黑色素瘤细胞常常可见大的核仁，这也是突出的超微结构特征[56]。多数病例可以发现黑色素小体，虽然通常比较稀少。

纤维组织增生性恶性黑色素瘤是一种不常见的类型，浸润性肿瘤中伴有纤维组织形成（fibroplasia）[57]，类似于光学显微镜检查中的纤维化。无黑色素性梭形黑色素细胞呈现神经鞘表现者被称为亲神经性黑色素瘤（neurotropic melanoma）[58]，但是已经能够恰当区分亲神经性（neurotropism）和神经转化（neural transformation），这些表现可以单独存在也可以合并出现[59]。神经鞘分化的超微结构证据[60]见于具有长的胞浆突起的梭形细胞细束中，胞浆突起出现在肿瘤的放射状生长期。神经鞘细胞和黑色素细胞彼此重叠的其他证据是：痣[61]和黑色素性外周神经鞘瘤[62]的长的胞浆突起被基底膜物质包绕。

小圆细胞肿瘤　Small round cell tumors

对于由均匀一致的弥漫性片状小圆形细胞组成的肿瘤，光学显微镜检查的分类尝试可能会失败，即使借助于特殊染色的帮助。异质性肿瘤标本的鉴别诊断，随着患者年龄和来源部位的不同而不同。对于成人，肿瘤通常是癌。对于儿科患者，神经母细胞瘤、横纹肌肉瘤和 Ewing 肉瘤均在考虑之中。

小细胞癌在许多肺外部位均有描述，其中包括皮肤[37]、胃肠道[63]和泌尿生殖道[64]。某些小细胞癌具有神经内分泌的特点，电子显微镜检查能够有效地显示这些肿瘤的特征性的树突状突起和小的致密轴心颗粒[65,66]。

一个典型的 Ewing 肉瘤的细胞及其细胞核都是小的，外形光滑[67,68]。细胞排列紧密，难以发现细胞连接。细胞器稀少，糖原显示不明显，通过电子显微镜检查才能发现，但是通常可以见到一些糖原，在胞浆内可形成大的糖原湖（图 31.18）。非常少数的骨的 Ewing 肉瘤中，可见神经外胚层特征[69-71]。对来自软组织 Ewing 肉瘤细胞系的超微结构观察中，描述了类似的形态学改变[72]。典型形态学的一些变异常见于 Ewing 肉瘤：不规则的细胞和核的外形，甚至中等量的细胞器仍然可以诊断为 Ewing 肉瘤[73]。骨 Ewing 肉瘤的鉴别诊断必须包括小细胞骨肉瘤和间叶性软骨肉瘤，前者的间质可能存在骨样结构的证据[74]。

神经母细胞瘤的小的卵圆形至圆形细胞有外形光滑的细胞核，染色质细，胞浆稀少，只含有少数细胞器。其树突状突起比神经内分泌癌多，而且长（图 31.19），成束排列。这些突起区域相当于光学显微镜检查所见到的原纤维物质。神经母细胞瘤的细胞突细长，并且含有纵行排列的微管和致密轴心颗粒。小的颗粒集中于突起内，只有少数见于细胞体内。玫瑰花结的中心由缠绕的突起组成。突起数目增加代表神经母细胞瘤成熟，突起可能缠绕在细胞周围，呈同心圆状排列（图 31.20），另外，胞浆增加引起细胞大小变化也代表神经母细胞瘤的成熟。真正的嗅神经母细胞瘤具有独特的超微结构特征[75]。

软组织肿瘤　Soft tissue tumors

间叶细胞的超微结构所见在软组织肿瘤中有不同程度的重现，通过电子显微镜可以发现这些特征，常常能够对一个肿瘤进行准确的亚型分类[76,77]。目前，电子显微镜检查的临床意义相对有限，因为亚型对于高级别肉瘤的治疗并无太大影响，横纹肌肉瘤就是一个例子。由于多种模式治疗方法的复杂性增加，肉瘤亚型和治疗之间的相互关系日益密切。主要类型的超微结构特征简要总结如下。

纤维母细胞肿瘤　Tumors of fibroblasts

从电子显微镜学家的主要观点来看，纤维母细胞肿瘤中可见到的形态学范围比光学显微镜学家认识到的广泛。多年来，这种亚型分类出现混淆的一个原因是：纤维母细胞具有显著的形态学柔韧性，这种柔韧性表现在

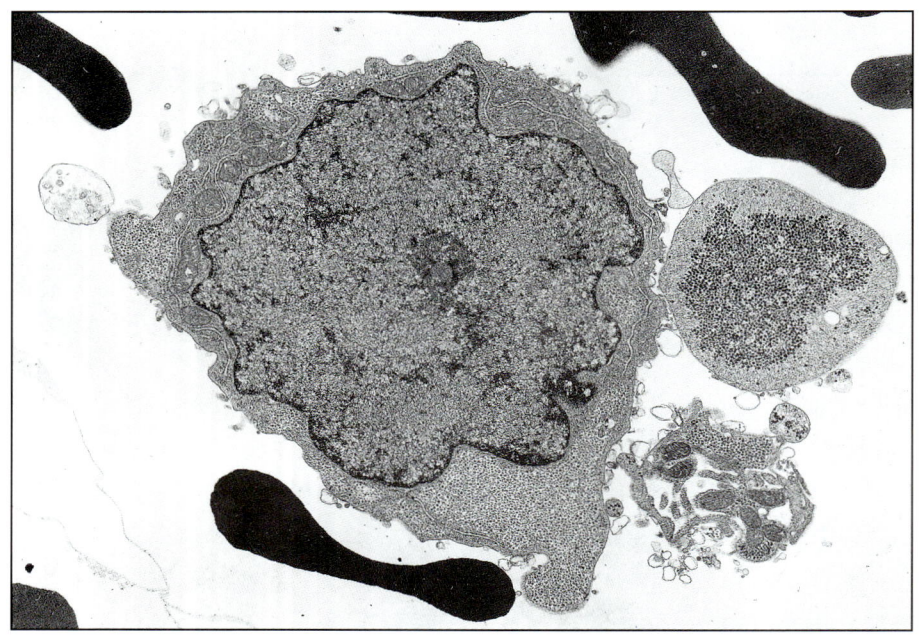

图 31.18　来自骨 Ewing 肉瘤的细针抽吸活检的一个细胞，含有明显的糖原湖。

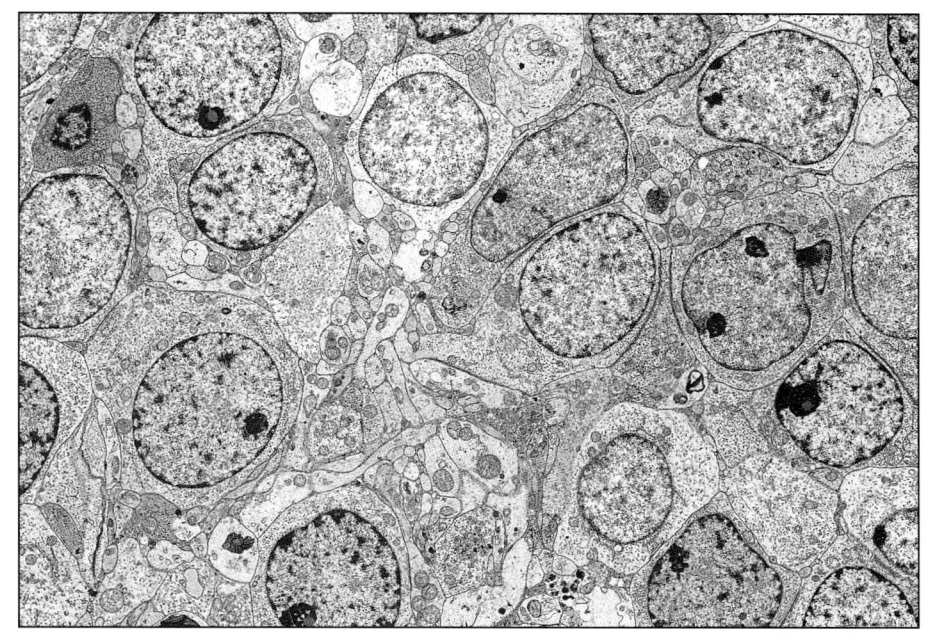

图31.19　图示神经母细胞瘤有许多树突状突起，突起成束，在石蜡切片中表现为原纤维。

反应性软组织病变、良性肿瘤和肉瘤上。纤维肉瘤的细胞一般是长形的，从细长到肥胖不等。梭形的细胞一般逐渐变细，而且常常具有分枝状的胞浆。明显变细的胞浆突起是隆凸性皮肤纤维肉瘤的一个特征。不要将长的突起误认为是神经鞘的特征；这种突起没有笔直的外形或均匀一致的直径，至多有少数微管出现在其中，而且没有基底膜包绕。低级别的肿瘤的间质含有交互排列的胶原纤维。当胶原纤维丰富时，相邻细胞之间接触少；而在较富于细胞的肿瘤，细胞膜有局灶接触，通过散在的原始附着位点连接。

在分化较好的纤维肉瘤，细胞浆类似于正常或反应性纤维母细胞[78]。最显著的特征是：广泛散布的核糖体内质网池，后者可能细长或扩张。内质网池一般充满胞浆，比其他软组织肉瘤细胞丰富。肿瘤中有时可见肌纤维母细胞分化，表现为胞浆周围有细长的平滑肌肌丝[79-81]。肌纤维母细胞分化常见于纤维瘤病，并发生于一些低级别的纤维肉瘤。正常肌纤维母细胞的肌丝将细胞固定在周围的胶原中[82]，这些连接可见于纤维瘤病，但在肉瘤中罕见。非特异性中间丝可能占据纤维肉瘤细胞胞浆的大部分区域（图31.21），细胞内偶尔含有胶原原

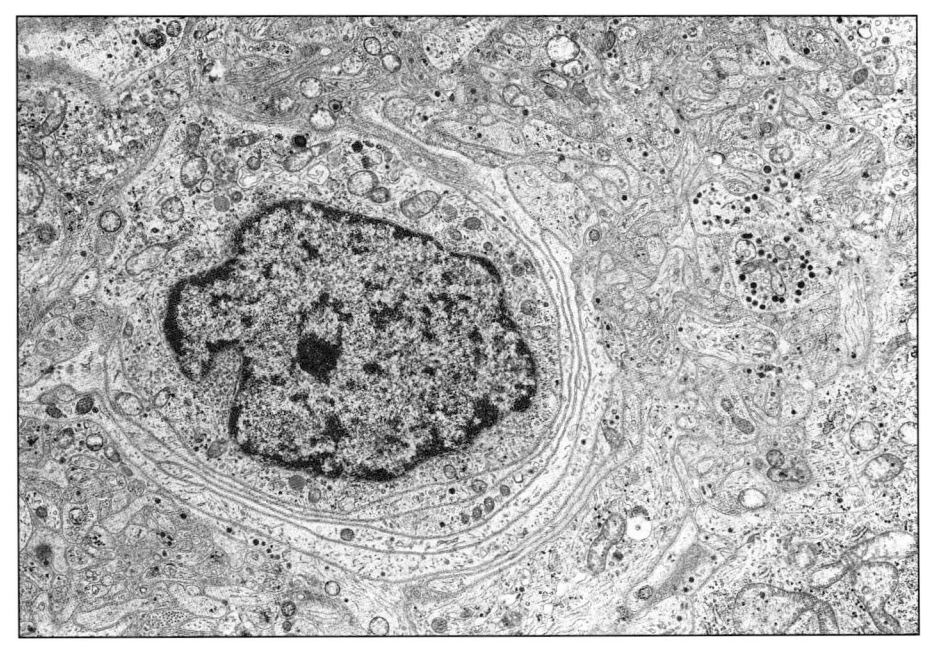

图31.20　缠绕在一个神经母细胞瘤细胞周围的胞浆突起是早期分化的线索。

纤维母细胞肿瘤

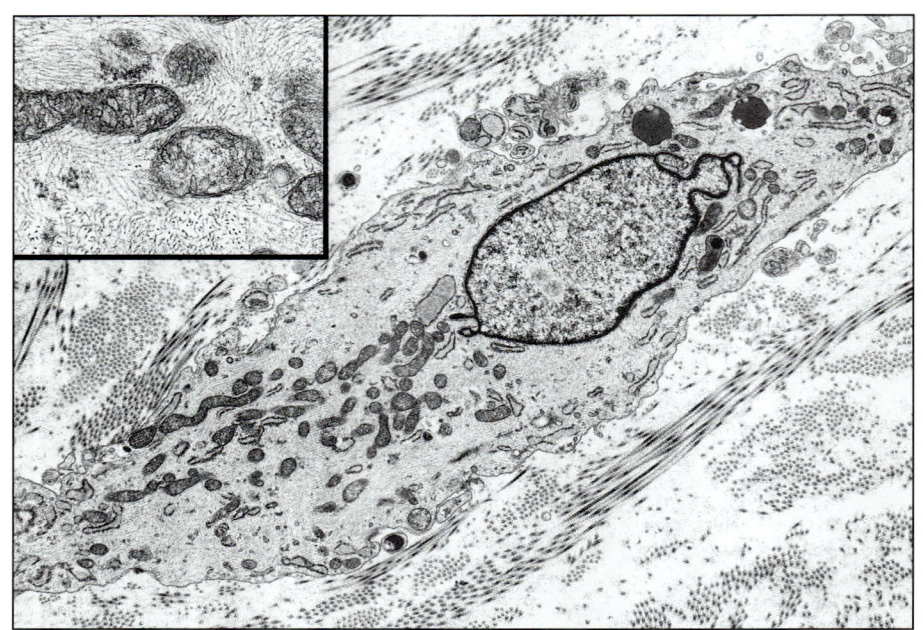

图31.21 肿瘤性纤维母细胞的弥漫性细丝在整个胞浆中形成了中等电子密度。只有局灶性的平滑肌分化。插图：多数细丝的表现是非特异性的。

纤维。至于这些胶原原纤维是从周围间质中吞噬而来，还是反映了原纤维合成异常，仍存在争论。这些典型的特征在高级别肉瘤中发育不好，难以决定是将其称为低分化纤维肉瘤，还是简单地称为原始的间叶性肿瘤。

鉴于常常做出恶性纤维组织细胞瘤的诊断（至少在前些年中），特别是在老年人，根据光学显微镜检查进行亚型分类或许并不奇怪。然而，正如预料的那样，这些多形性肉瘤的亚型在超微结构水平上有一些相似之处[83]，主要的差异和不断争论的来源是血管瘤样肿瘤[84-86]。对于高级别席纹状多形性肉瘤，梭形细胞可能无法与纤维肉瘤区分，但是肌纤维母细胞瘤分化少见。多形性细胞可能含有多个细胞核，但是胞浆非常类似于梭形细胞，支持它们属于同一种细胞类型的变异这种观点。同纤维肉瘤一样，胞浆内池可以细长或膨胀（图31.22）。在结构上，大部分胞浆常常被弥漫性的非特异性细丝占据，其表现类似于纤维肉瘤。在一些未分类的多形性肉瘤中，细胞呈圆形，排列紧密，形成一种上皮样外观。黏液纤维肉瘤（从前称为黏液样恶性纤维组织细胞瘤）的梭形细胞非常类似纤维母细胞。在所谓的巨细胞恶性纤维组织细胞瘤，单核和破骨细胞样多核细胞的胞浆非常类似

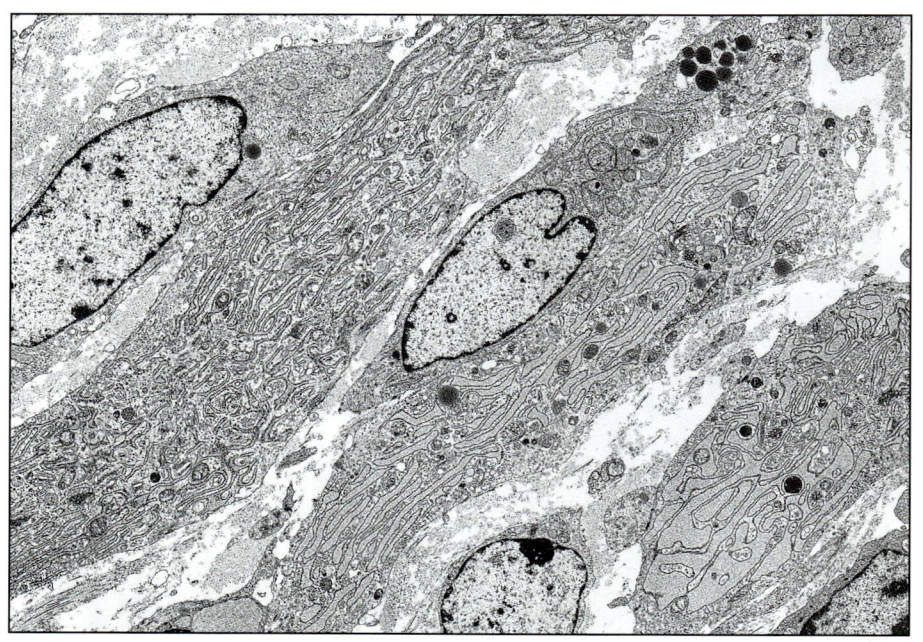

图31.22 纤维母细胞分化的特征是：胞浆中有许多池，图示的梭形细胞来自黏液纤维肉瘤。

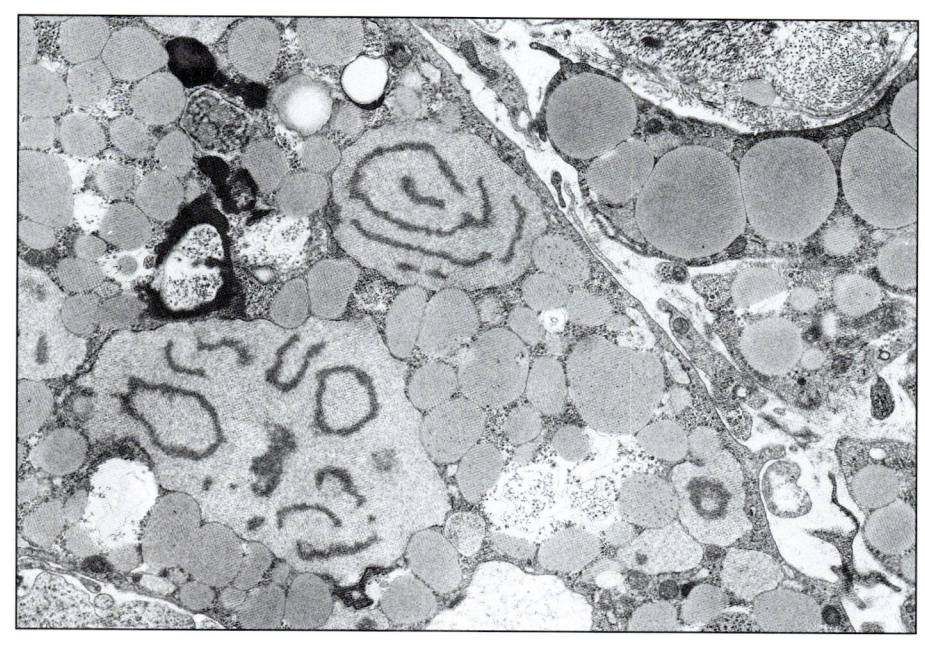

图31.23 在一个转移性多形性脂肪肉瘤，池内的电子致密物质形成线样条索。细胞含有许多直径不同的脂质小滴。

席纹状多形性病变的大细胞的胞浆，与其低分化本质是一致的，尤其是非特异性本质。

脂肪肉瘤　Liposarcoma

虽然脂肪肉瘤细胞最值得注意的特征是出现脂质小滴[87]，但是它们有时是稀少的。脂质小滴也可出现在纤维肉瘤和多形性肉瘤中，但数量较少，分布于散在的细胞中，它们的大小相当一致。在脂肪肉瘤细胞中，脂质小滴的直径是不同的，可以扩大或融合，最好出现印戒构型，此时细胞核和细胞器被单个的大的脂滴推挤到细胞周围。其他超微结构表现的诊断价值有限，虽然常常可见小而致密的线粒体。有些大的脂肪肉瘤细胞含有膨胀的池，池内有浓缩的电子致密物质，形成细丝状结构（图31.23），类似的表现有时也见于其他多形性肉瘤（图31.24）。

肌原性肿瘤　Myogenic tumors

多数肉瘤细胞至少含有一些胞浆细丝，但是如果这些细丝的结构是非特异性的，它们对于确定细胞类型仅能提供有限的帮助。相反，从超微结构可以辨认出肌丝是平滑肌还是骨骼肌，因此，电子显微镜是一个有用的

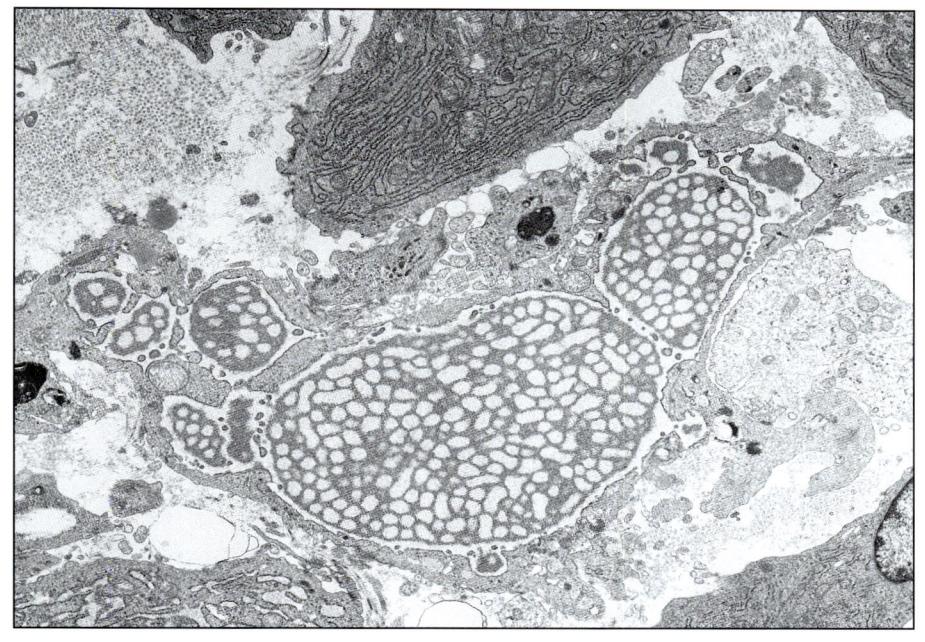

图31.24 许多多形性肉瘤细胞具有膨胀的池，其中的电子致密物质形成筛状结构。

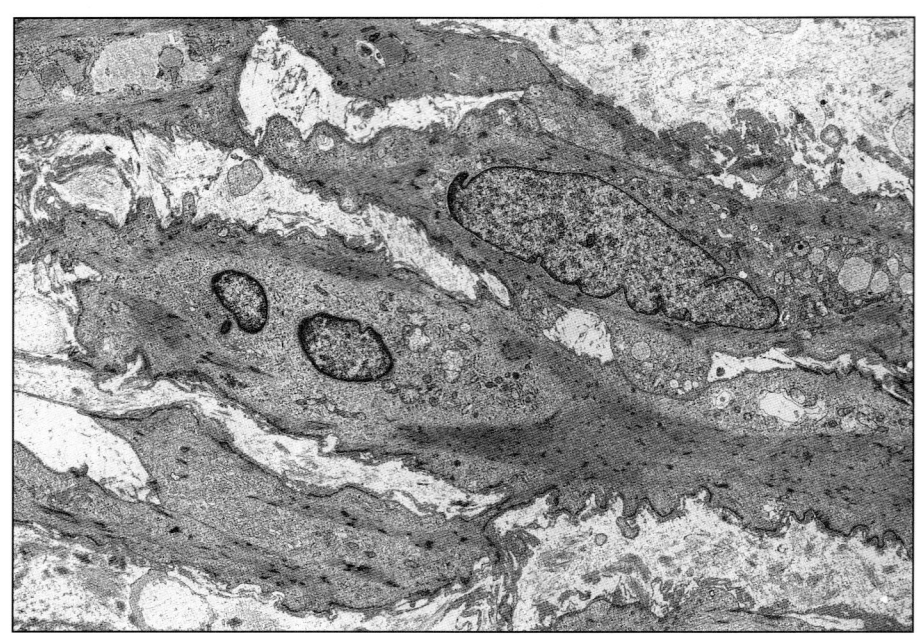

图31.25 这些平滑肌肉瘤细胞显示的平滑肌分化好,细胞和许多肌丝之间有接触。肿瘤发生于腹股沟,30年前由于转移性黑色素瘤而进行过放射治疗。

工具,它能确定或证实平滑肌肉瘤或横纹肌肉瘤的诊断,但是其应用也受到许多限制。并不是所有的平滑肌或骨骼肌肿瘤细胞都含有肌丝,或可能仅仅有少量肌丝出现在散在的细胞中,因而难以定位。同样,肌丝可以出现在其他一些肿瘤,而且当一个肉瘤浸润骨骼肌时,变性的肌纤维可能被误认为肿瘤细胞。在电子显微镜检查之前,常常尝试应用标记平滑肌或骨骼肌或两者的抗体进行免疫过氧化物酶检查,但并不总是能够见到免疫染色和电子显微镜检查之间的良好的相关性。当免疫染色呈强阳性时,细胞内常常有丰富的肌丝,但在有些病例,染色可疑或呈阴性,细胞却仍然含有足够的细丝,仍可以进行诊断。另一方面,免疫染色阳性并不能保证电子显微镜检查能够发现肌丝。

平滑肌肌丝束分布于许多平滑肌肉瘤的胞浆中[88](图31.25)。当肌丝稀少时,可能难以将这些肿瘤与伴有肌纤维母细胞分化的肿瘤区分,虽然出现胞浆膜下致密体和细胞接触表示为真正的平滑肌细胞。平滑肌肌丝还可见于少数伴有邻近细胞膜胞饮小泡的血管球瘤细胞中。肿瘤性肌上皮细胞也含有平滑肌肌丝[89],但是这种肌丝的表现常常是非特异性的,而且还可能出现致密的

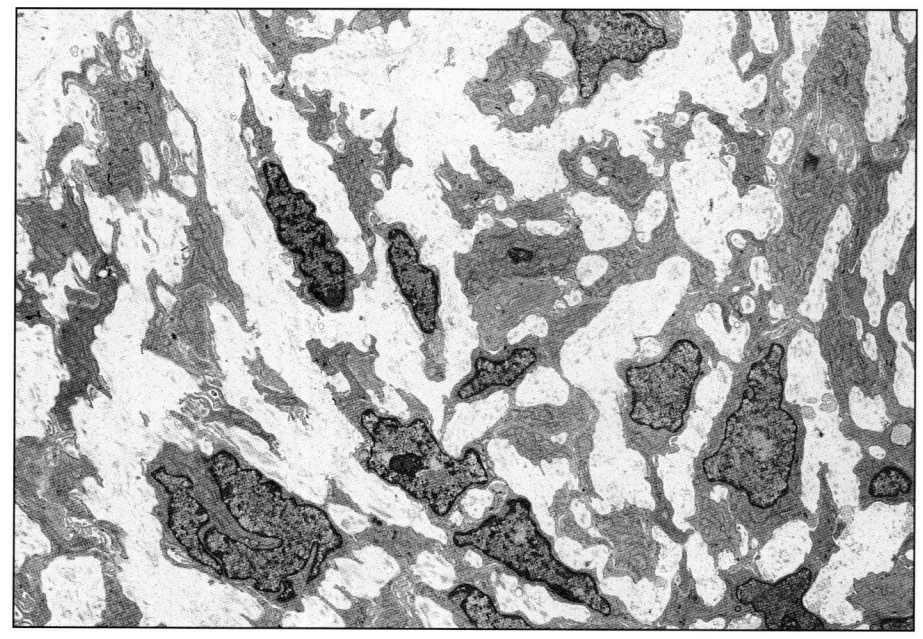

图31.26 光学显微镜检查看上去像一个平滑肌肉瘤的胃肿瘤,在超微结构水平没有平滑肌分化的指征。因此,其细胞学特征和结构比较符合胃间质瘤(GIST)。

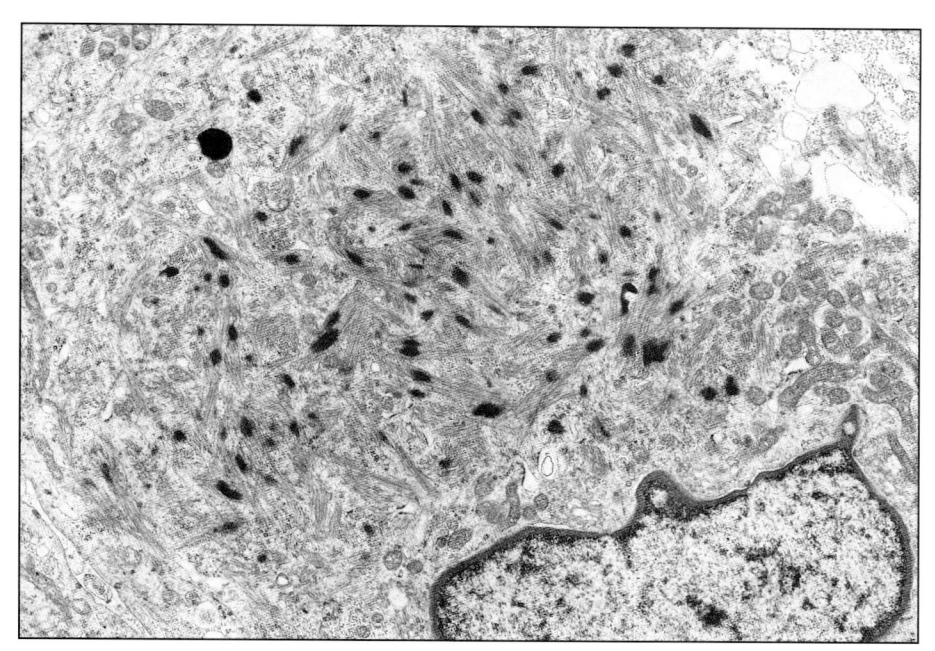

图31.27 这个肿瘤细胞有明显的横纹肌母细胞分化,可见许多肌纤维段,每个肌纤维段的中心都具有致密的Z带物质。

波浪状细胞角蛋白束[90]。

胃肠道恶性间叶性肿瘤通过常规光学显微镜检查通常被分类为平滑肌肉瘤,但是在电子显微镜检查时,多数并不显示平滑肌特征(图31.26),尤其当肿瘤具有上皮样形态学时[91]。现已公认,这样的病变多数是胃肠间质瘤(GIST)[92]。在胃肠道梭形细胞肿瘤中,偶尔可以见到神经鞘特性,在所谓的胃肠自主神经肿瘤中,还有向肠肌神经丛分化的描述[93,94],但是现在认为,这些属于GIST的形态学和分子遗传学范畴(见第9章)。许多横纹肌肉瘤具有丰富的骨骼肌肌丝[95](图31.27),但是肌丝可能稀少或缺乏。肌丝可形成几个肌节长度的肌纤维段(segments of myofibrils),类似葡萄状胚胎性横纹肌肉瘤的长细胞。较常见到杂乱分布的短而细长的肌纤维段。肌纤维段容易辨认,与肌动蛋白(actin)和肌浆球蛋白(myosin)共同存在,并且具有独特的空间分布。偶尔,Z带物质可能见于集聚的肌丝中,甚至缺乏显著的带状结构;Z带肌丝的内部结构显示它的本质(图31.28)。当仅有肌浆球蛋白肌丝形成时,可以从其直径和小束状排列辨认出来,平行肌丝的末端之间有短排的核糖体。这是肌浆球蛋白和肌动蛋白肌丝的有机

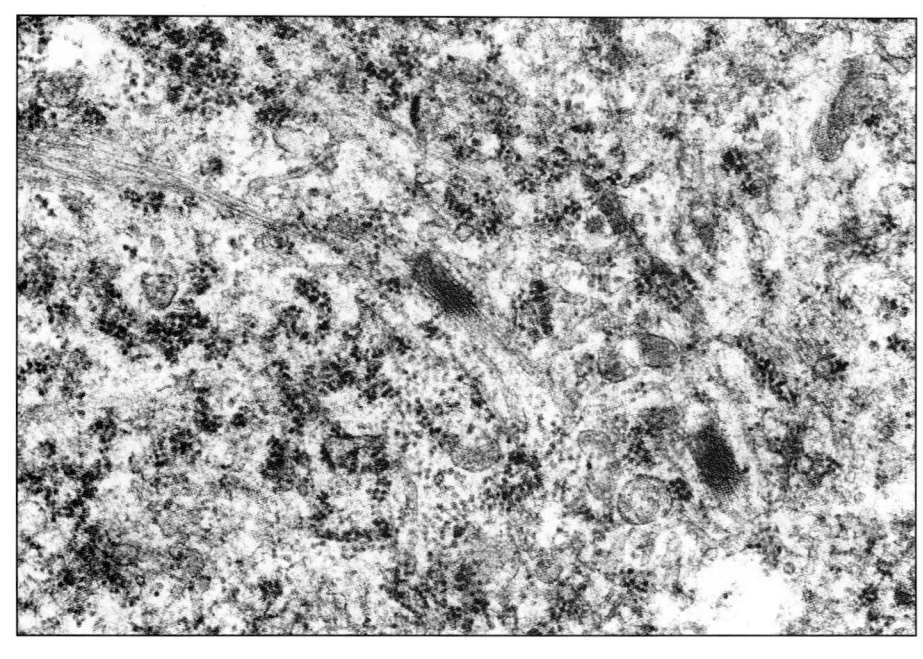

图31.28 当仅有少量骨骼肌肌丝存在时,因为具有致密的Z带肌动蛋白丝通过Z带延伸,仍可发现它们。

结构，而不是光学显微镜学家寻找的横纹表现；除非肌丝正在形成足够的整齐的肌纤维段，否则在石蜡切片中见不到横纹。横纹肌肉瘤中的骨骼肌肌丝可能形成阶梯样的斑马小体，或形成在低倍放大下无结构的致密包涵体，但是仔细检查其周围可以发现其是由紧密排列的肌丝组成。相反，所谓的"横纹肌样"肿瘤（"rhabdoid" tumors）含有核周的或呈弥漫分布的非特异性细丝[96,97]。

横纹肌肉瘤以外的可能含有骨骼肌肌丝的一些肿瘤，可以通过其临床表现和常规光学显微镜检查辨认出来。这些肿瘤包括肉瘤样Wilms瘤、混合性中胚层肉瘤、伴有横纹肌母细胞的恶性外周神经鞘肉瘤（蝾螈瘤，Triton tumors），以及伴有其他间叶成分的去分化软骨肉瘤。

成血管细胞肿瘤
Tumors of vasoformative cells

观察血管肉瘤的超微结构观察主要是学术上的事情。肿瘤性内皮细胞的用于辨认的超微结构特征并非是特异性的，所以电子显微镜研究不能提供信息。偶尔出现的Weibel-Palade小体，并不是一种可靠的或一致的标准。在石蜡切片中，一些血管肉瘤是实性的，电子显微镜检查能够发现自然管腔形成的证据和肿瘤细胞之间的明显的亲和力以及红细胞[98]。在Kaposi肉瘤，早期病变的梭形细胞类似于纤维母细胞，但是可以吞噬红细胞，而且应用内皮标记物可显示其成血管的潜能。肿瘤形成不良的管腔，常常缺乏基底膜或成熟的细胞连接，这些管腔含有红细胞（图31.29），这些自然血管壁内的裂口允许红细胞漏出而进入周围的间质。

光学显微镜检查常常倾向于诊断血管周细胞瘤，因为不同类型的软组织肿瘤可能含有相互吻合的血管灶，形同血管周细胞瘤的表现[99]。虽然血管周细胞瘤细胞的超微结构没有特异性，但是在超微结构水平见到的形态偶尔可能可给诊断提供支持证据。典型者，肿瘤细胞稀疏但均匀地分布在小的血管之间，纤细的胞浆突起与邻近的细胞连接。有些细胞中出现小的非特异性胞浆细丝集聚。鼻腔血管周细胞瘤样肿瘤显示较明显的肌样特征[100]（见第3章）。

骨外黏液样软骨肉瘤
Extraskeletal myxoid chondrosarcoma

一些骨外黏液样软骨肉瘤含有大量的微管，平行排列于内质网中[101]。池内微管的几何图形排列还可见于少数转移性黑色素瘤[102]。一种罕见类型的软组织肿瘤其光学显微镜检查有些类似于骨外黏液样软骨肉瘤，但是现在一般认为它是一种肌上皮肿瘤。它的细胞类似于真正的脊索瘤，S-100蛋白和上皮标记物染色呈阳性。应用电子显微镜可能发现上皮特征，包括基底膜片段、原始的细胞连接以及含有微绒毛的小间隙[103]。

外周神经鞘细胞肿瘤
Tumors of peripheral nerve sheath cells

虽然临床上神经鞘瘤和神经纤维瘤有所不同，但是增生细胞的超微结构却十分相似。多数神经纤维瘤中混有丰富的纤维母细胞和胶原。肿瘤性神经鞘细胞的主要特征是长而纤细的胞浆突起[104]（图31.30）。在良性肿瘤，

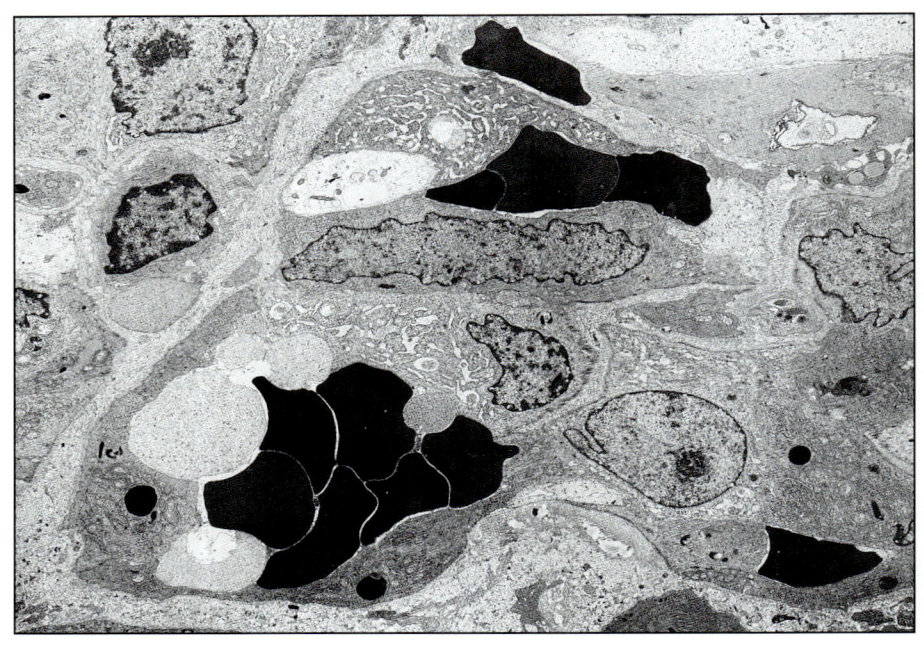

图31.29 含有红细胞的Kaposi肉瘤的不成熟血管腔。

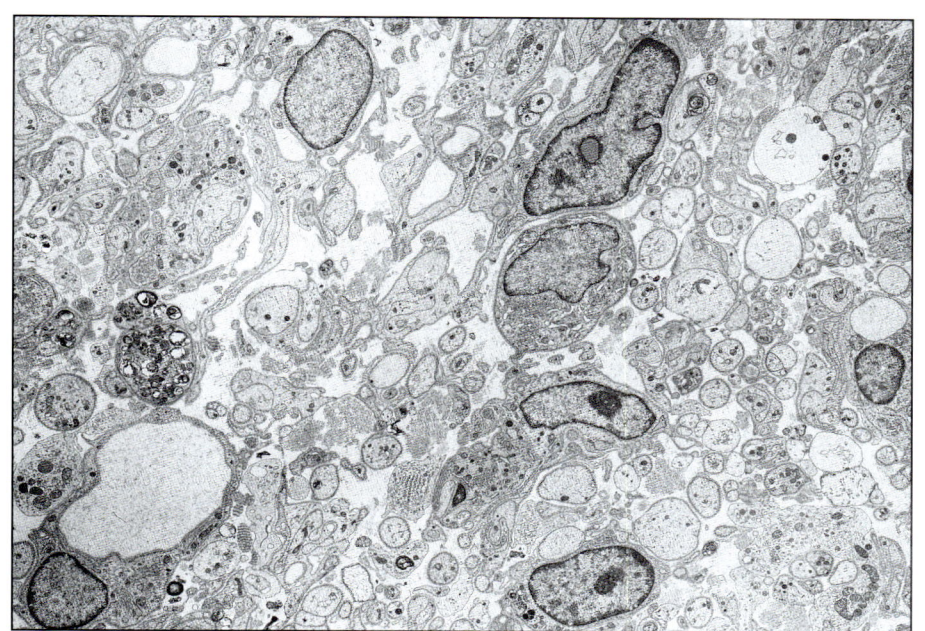

图31.30 分开神经鞘瘤细胞核的大量嗜酸性组织是由胞浆突起组成的,这里看到的是横切面。

胞浆突起直径完全一致,含有纵行排列的微管和细丝,并且被基底膜包绕。在两种类型的良性外周神经鞘肿瘤,胞浆突起呈分枝状并相互连接,而在神经鞘瘤,其形态则比较复杂。在良性和恶性肿瘤,偶尔可发现轴突系膜(mesaxon)结构,其中肿瘤细胞胞浆的螯样(pincer-like)突起围绕小的间隙(图31.31)。没有发现细的突起有卷入的轴索,突起可能围绕少量的胶原纤维,甚至内衬伴有基底膜的封闭间隙。神经鞘瘤有时可见间隙宽的胶原(所谓的Luse小体),但是这对于神经鞘肿瘤来说并不是特异性的。

虽然几乎所有的外周神经鞘肿瘤都是神经鞘瘤,但是少数神经束膜细胞谱系肿瘤已经得到公认[105,106]。这些肿瘤一般是良性的,上皮膜抗原(EMA)免疫反应呈阳性支持诊断。正常外周神经的神经束膜细胞围绕外周神经纤维束形成神经鞘,神经鞘与神经根离开脊髓处的脊膜相连续,肿瘤性神经束膜细胞具有长而细的突起,部分被基底膜覆盖,并含有许多胞饮小泡,平行的突起形成弯曲的束状结构(图31.32)。

恶性外周神经鞘肿瘤属于最难准确分类的软组织肉瘤。有些肿瘤可以通过其细胞结构特征辨认出来(见

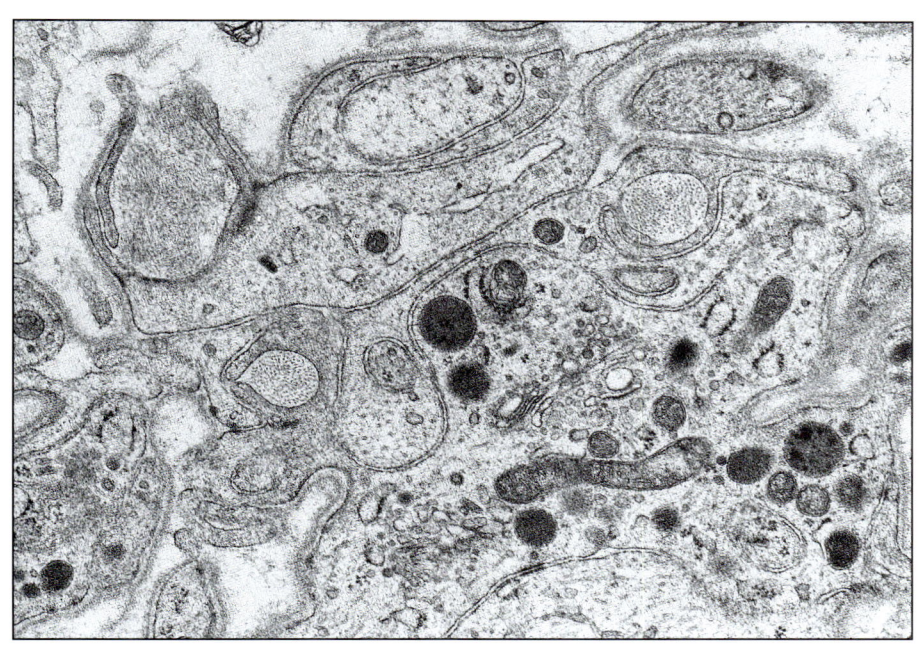

图31.31 显示神经鞘瘤有轴突系膜形成。螯样胞浆突起环绕小簇状胶原纤维。

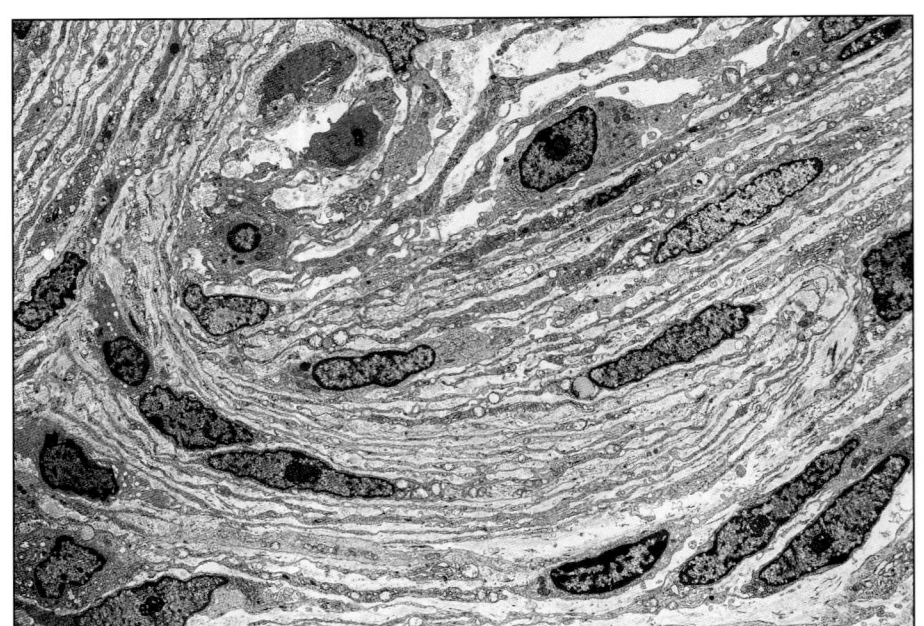

图31.32 来自神经束膜细胞瘤,有许多平行、弯曲、变细的胞浆突起。

第27章),但是多数难以辨认,部分具有非常类似于其他肉瘤的细胞学形态,包括所谓的恶性纤维组织细胞瘤[107]。只有大约半数病例S-100蛋白呈阳性,而且来自外周神经的公认标准或神经母细胞瘤病的特征仅仅见于部分病例,因此其价值有限。电子显微镜检查常常有助于诊断。同良性肿瘤一样,胞浆突起也能提供肉瘤神经鞘分化的线索。典型的胞浆突起长而并列,缺乏基底膜。在由短而密集排列的细胞组成的富于细胞的肿瘤,以及在上皮样恶性外周神经鞘肿瘤,胞浆突起短而弯曲,其神经鞘本质并不总是明显。少数肉瘤出现轴突系膜结构。通过光镜检查可能难以辨认的恶性外周神经鞘肿瘤的变型是上皮样型[108]和蝾螈瘤[109],而电子显微镜检查可以诊断两者。在偶尔出现在外周神经鞘肿瘤的腺体成分,柱状细胞的微绒毛具有微丝轴心,并有散在的内分泌细胞,代表有胃肠型分化[110]。

颗粒细胞瘤 Granular cell tumor

电子显微镜检查支持普遍存在的颗粒细胞瘤是由神经鞘衍化而来。每一个颗粒细胞都含有许多密集排列的有界膜的隔室[111](图31.33),在适当的切面显示长的间隔,有时其中可见少数微管。大量的溶酶体容易掩盖隔室周围的膜。多数颗粒细胞瘤是良性的,但少数为恶性,核可能表现为不规则的外形[112]。在恶性肿瘤中仍有许多溶酶体出现,但是无法区分良、恶性细胞。因为任何变性的肿瘤细胞都含有溶酶体,所以与光镜检查结合起来非常重要。

其他肉瘤 Other Sarcomas

腺泡状软组织肉瘤 Alveolar soft part sarcoma

应用电子显微镜检查来证实怀疑为腺泡状软组织肉瘤的诊断,有时是有用或必需的。在石蜡切片,腺泡状结构可能不很清楚,PAS阳性的晶体也不是总能发现。结晶是重要的超微结构特征(图31.34),但较稀少,甚至不能发现。伴有小而致密颗粒的广泛的Golgi复合体是一种比较一致的细胞所见[113]。这种颗粒小于多数内分泌颗粒且不同于副神经节瘤的颗粒,并不分布于整个胞浆中。在Golgi复合体附近,还可见到具有溶酶体表现的较大的致密小体,仔细观察其致密的内部结构,会发现细微的周期性,确立它们是早期的晶体形成灶。成熟的晶体常常有界膜。单个晶体成角,常常有长斜方形的轮廓,虽然与邻近的晶体粘着可以呈不规则的形状。结合免疫组织化学和超微结构所见,有时可提示肿瘤细胞可能具有骨骼肌表型[113,114],结晶偶尔可以见于横纹肌瘤,这种看法是恰当的,但是仍有争论。

滑膜肉瘤 Synovial sarcoma

在滑膜肉瘤的上皮性成分中,细胞为立方到柱状,位于基底膜之上,尖端有稀少的微绒毛,由紧密连接相连,与许多腺癌的腺泡无法区分[115]。正常或化生的滑

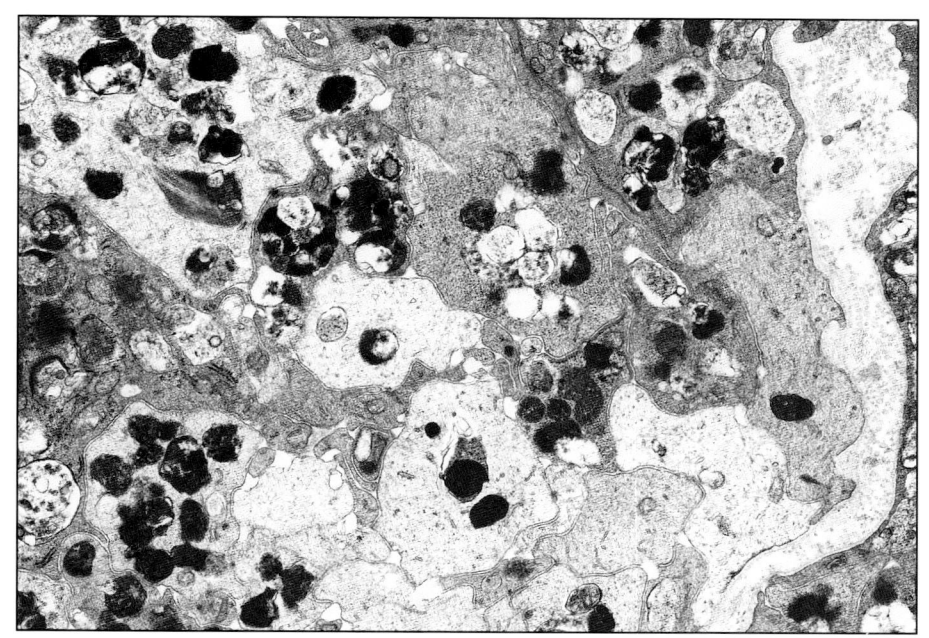

图31.33 在颗粒细胞瘤中，增生的细胞是由密集排列的、有界膜的隔室组成。这种细微结构常常被集聚的溶酶体掩盖，但是在这里尚可见到。

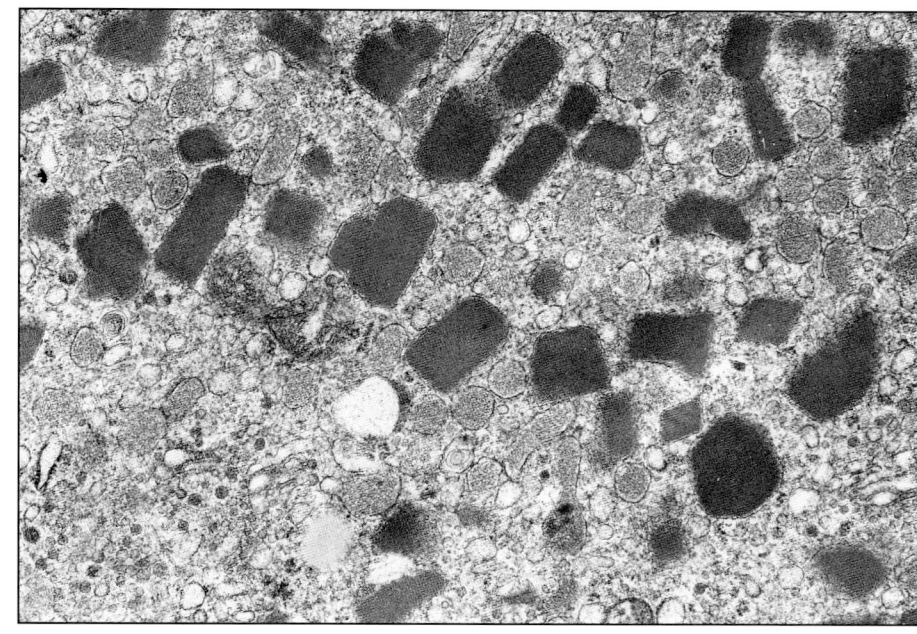

图31.34 横纹肌样结晶占据了这个腺泡状软组织肉瘤细胞的胞浆，但是还可见到许多溶酶体样小体和许多小的颗粒。后者局限于Golgi复合体的附近。

膜细胞并不显示这些上皮特征[116]。双相性或单相性滑膜肉瘤的间质细胞类似于伴有稀少细胞器的短的纤维母细胞。光学显微镜见到的细胞构成在超微结构水平是类似的，密集排列的梭形细胞末端短，逐渐变细，没有分叉，内质网比多数肿瘤性纤维母细胞的少。

上皮样肉瘤　Epithelioid sarcoma

当上皮样肉瘤发生在肢体远端以外部位时，以及如果细胞是形成弥漫性片状而不是明显的结节时，通过光学显微镜检查进行诊断可能具有挑战性。广泛的中间丝可使细胞核偏心移位[117,118]（图31.35）。细丝的表现一般不具有特异性。细胞之间的连接是原始的，它们在肿瘤细胞结节中心很难见到，因为此处细胞粘着丧失并有坏死灶，细丝难以定位。

纤维组织增生性小细胞肿瘤　Desmoplastic small cell tumor

各种表现通过光镜检查均可见于这种肿瘤，两个最常见的形态是：密集排列的实性细胞巢和以类似细胞为界的小腔隙，实性巢与纤维背景之间界限清楚。腹腔内纤维组织增生性小圆细胞肿瘤这一术语是在1991年提出的[119]。角蛋白和结蛋白免疫染色证实有异向分化。

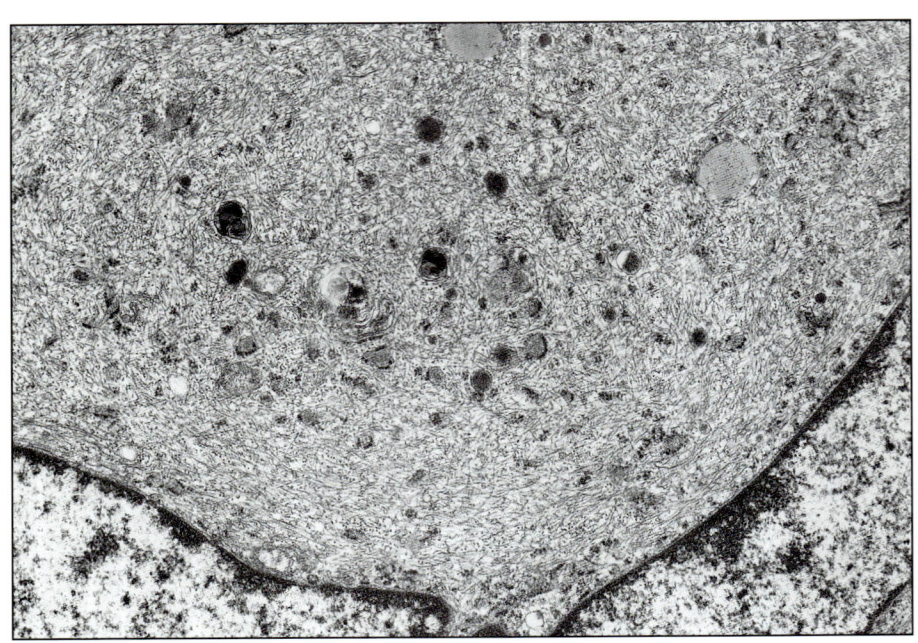

图31.35 上皮样肉瘤细胞的胞浆大部分被弥漫的中间丝占据，核有深凹痕。

电子显微镜检查尚未发现特异的细胞来源，而发现了包括神经内分泌在内的几个方面的分化，支持其是由多潜能细胞衍化而来[120]。

淋巴瘤/白血病　Lymphoma/leukemia

在淋巴瘤/白血病的范畴内，许多可疑的肿瘤可以应用一组简单的筛查染色来确认，并且这些肿瘤可以通过应用更多的染色程序进行分型。通常只有当染色模糊或呈阴性时，才需要进行电子显微镜检查，但是当常规光学显微镜检查没有异议时，其偶尔也能帮助诊断。光学显微镜检查下用于淋巴瘤或白血病再分类的重要的细胞核特征，在用于电子显微镜检查的塑料包埋组织的光学显微镜切片中清楚可辨，在低倍放大的电子显微镜照片上显得非常清楚。

常规光学显微镜检查可能会将粒细胞肉瘤误认为结缔组织中的小细胞癌，但在超微结构上，细胞或多或少有些圆，核位于中心，没有细胞连接，胞浆含有少量到中等量的致密小体，其大小和形状类似于原始的溶酶体（图 31.36）。电子显微镜检查已经用于研究非 Hodgkin 淋巴瘤的核仁，发现其形态学与肿瘤分级有关[121]。随

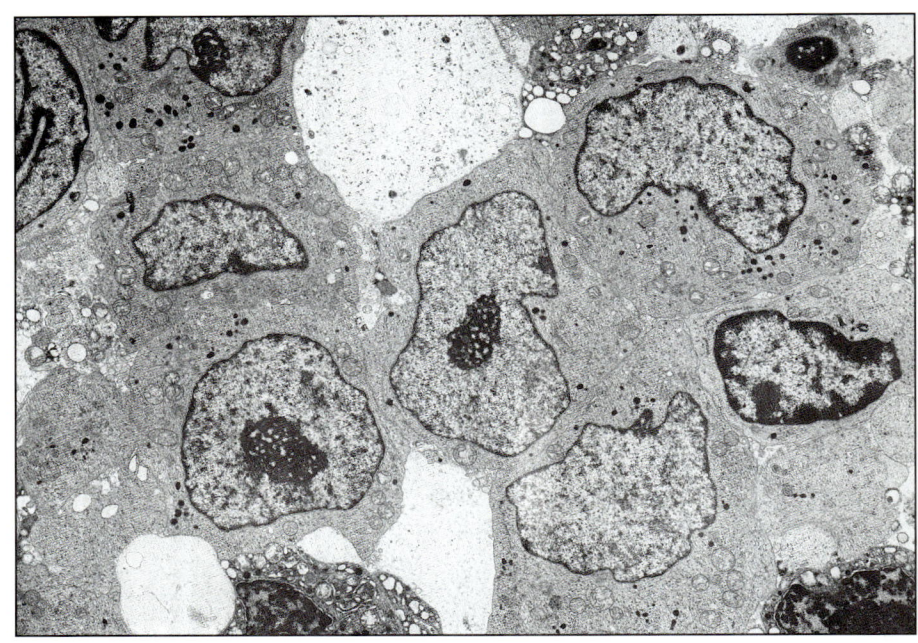

图31.36 在粒细胞肉瘤，细胞可能密集排列，但是没有连接形成；胞浆内的致密小体的数目和直径各不同，是特征性的。

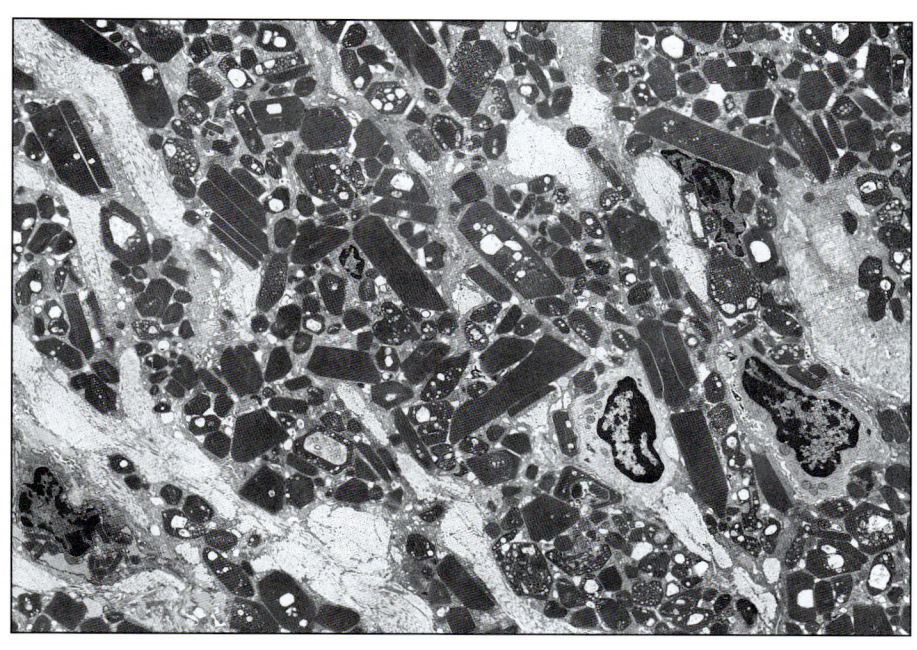

图31.37 一位成年女性由于弥漫性肺浸润而行开胸肺活检。图像中的多量结晶代表在一个伴有浆细胞分化特征的小细胞淋巴瘤中免疫球蛋白聚集。

着免疫母细胞的转化，淋巴瘤细胞内质网的数量有所增加。一些浆细胞肿瘤，特别是伴有原始细胞的浆细胞肿瘤，在常规染色的石蜡切片中不能辨认，而大量的内质网会提示细胞类型。结晶可能出现在伴有浆细胞样分化的淋巴瘤的间质组织细胞中（图 31.37）[122,123]。

一些网状内皮肿瘤的细胞含有独特的胞浆小体。毛细胞白血病的核糖体-层状复合体就是一个例子，虽然它们对于这个肿瘤并不特异。类似的胞浆小体也见于一些单核细胞性白血病（图 31.38）。这种复合体可能是由同心圆管组成的，或有一种螺旋状结构[124,125]。淋巴瘤细胞的大空泡可能产生印戒状结构，类似于转移性腺癌[126,127]。组织细胞增生症 X 的增生性组织细胞在低倍下具有独特的表现，为伴有稀疏的溶酶体和形状像蘑菇头的细胞核（图 31.39），它们含有 Birbeck 颗粒。这些颗粒呈杆状或盘形（图 31.40），它们好像具有细胞内吞细胞器的作用，在细胞表面形成（当难于发现时，应该在细胞表面寻找），并迁移至 Golgi 复合体。一旦一个颗粒与 Golgi 复合体的小囊融合，就会形成一个球拍样外形。

可以推测，在超微结构水平辨认大细胞淋巴瘤很容易，但也不总是这样。转化淋巴细胞的一般特征常见，包括圆形而有裂的核、细而散在的核染色质及明显的致

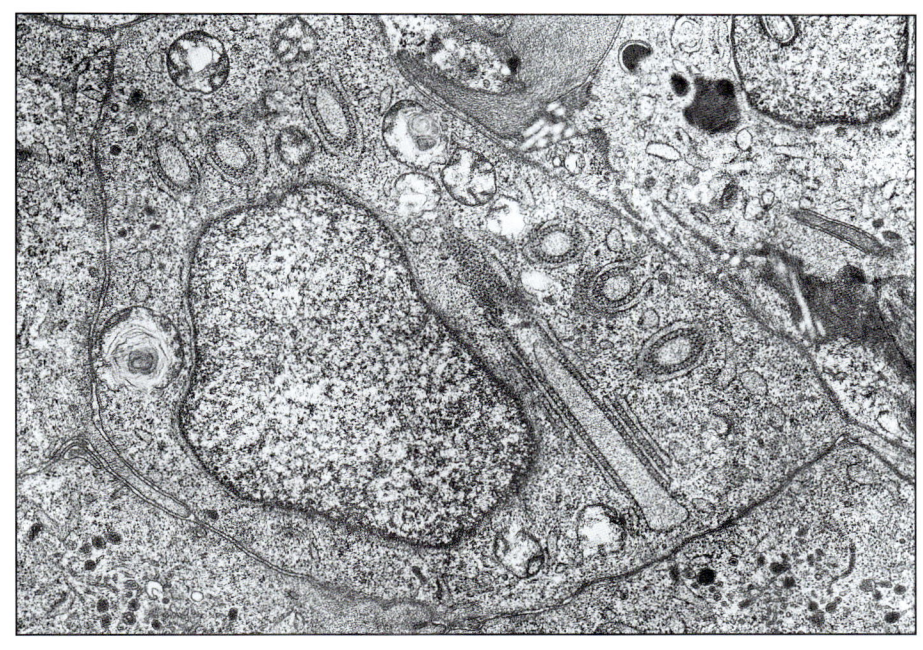

图31.38 在一些网状内皮肿瘤，可见不同寻常的内质网和核糖体结构。本例单核细胞性白血病伴有皮肤结节。

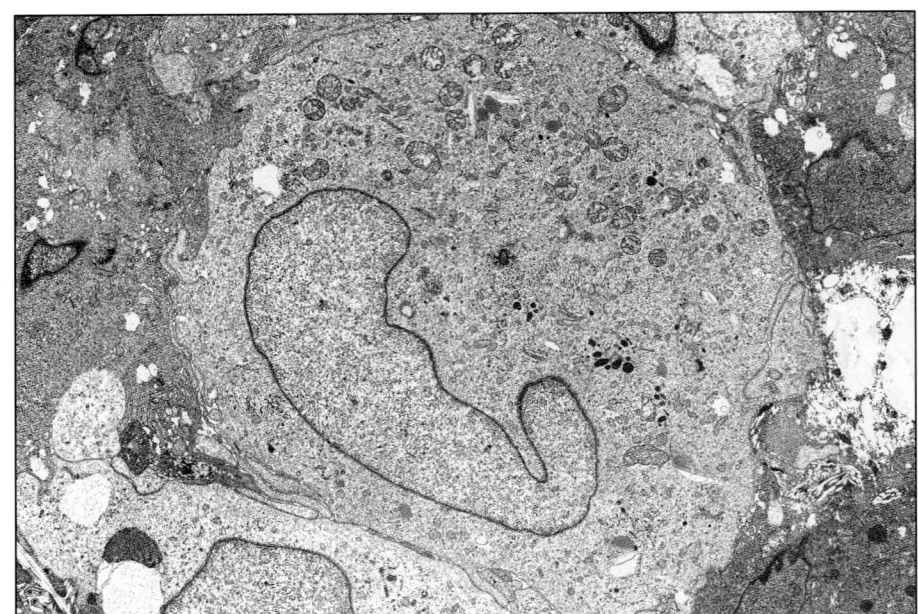

图31.39 这个组织细胞增生症X细胞核的横切面显示，它的形状像蘑菇头。胞浆内只有少数溶酶体。

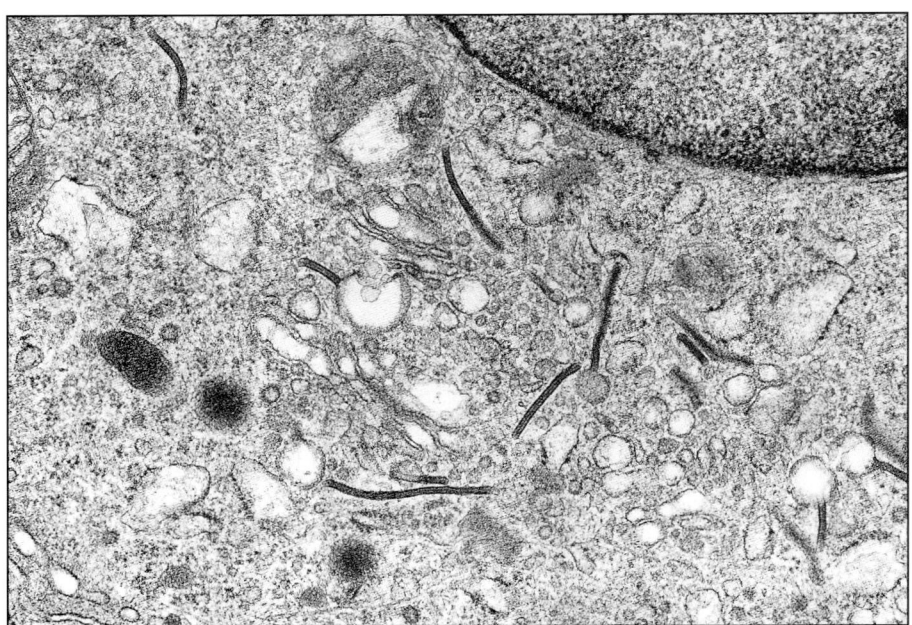

图31.40 组织细胞增生症X的杆状Birbeck颗粒。当与Golgi复合体的小囊融合时，形成球拍样外观。

密核仁；而典型的胞浆有许多自由核糖体、细长的池、少数线粒体以及一个或两个脂质小滴。核袋（图31.41）相当常见，但是没有特异性，淋巴瘤细胞之间从未见到成熟的细胞连接，但在并列的细胞膜上，偶尔可见细小而无结构的致密体。根据这些特征并不总是能够明确地将大细胞淋巴瘤与未分化癌区别开来；区分非角化性癌（淋巴上皮瘤）和大细胞淋巴瘤的唯一可靠标准是：出现细胞连接。偶尔，大细胞淋巴瘤细胞有许多类似于微绒毛的周围突起（图31.42），以致与腺癌混淆。淋巴瘤细胞的短而宽的突起常常缠结，而在滤泡性树突状细胞肿瘤，长的突起犬牙交错[128]。细长的胞浆突起形成迷宫样丛，广泛的滑面内质网[129]，粘着斑型连接，略微类似的突起和连接，这些表现均可见于具有犬牙交错的网状细胞特征的淋巴瘤[130]。

同过去描述的一样，组织细胞性恶性肿瘤构成了一组多变的临床病理疾病[131]，真正的组织细胞肉瘤和淋巴瘤的超微结构可能类似于未分化的上皮性肿瘤，特别是因为原始的细胞连接有时见于两种类型的细胞。免疫过氧化物酶方法[132]倾向于用于电子显微镜检查，以解决诊断这个难题。如果能够得到进行电子显微镜检查的

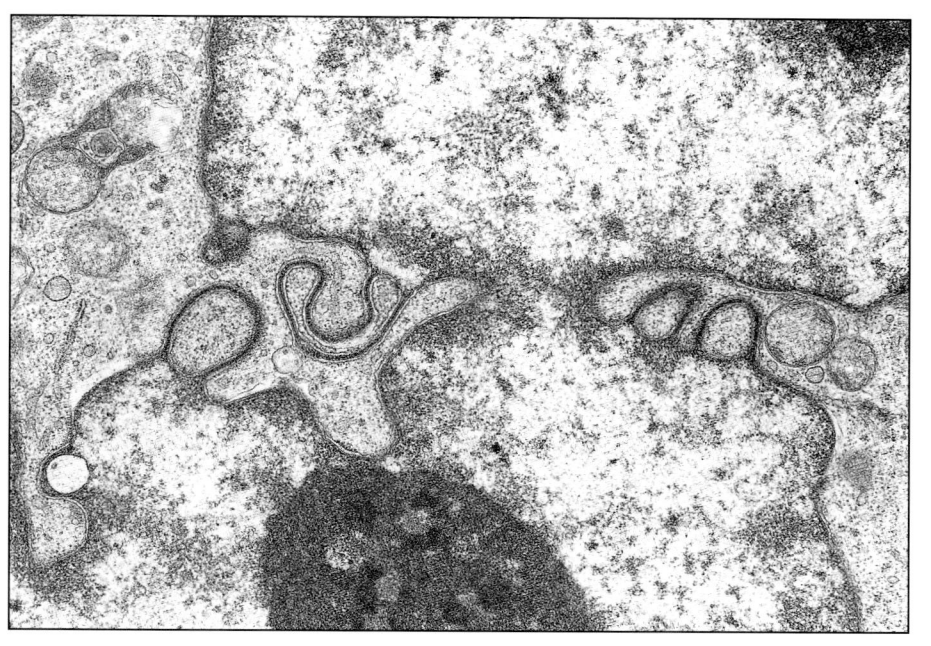

图31.41 大细胞淋巴瘤的核袋。

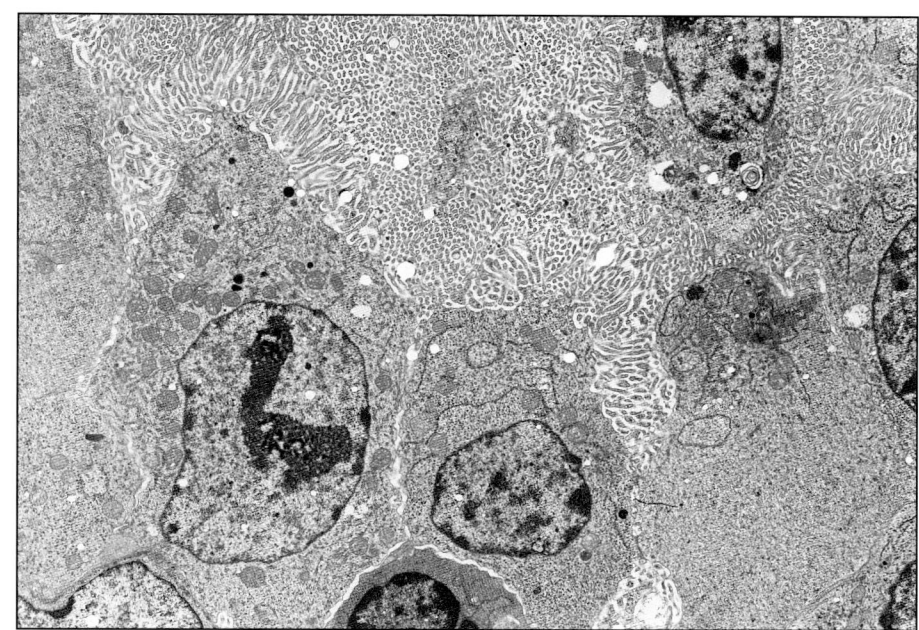

图31.42 这个肿瘤是大细胞淋巴瘤，但是其细胞具有许多细长的微绒毛样突起。

组织，可能有利于纵隔肿块的鉴别诊断。胸腺瘤的上皮和淋巴细胞的对比在低倍下是明显的（图 31.43），常常有几个连续突出的桥粒连接上皮细胞[133]。

中枢神经系统肿瘤
Central nervous system tumors

应用电子显微镜诊断中枢神经系统肿瘤的作用依然存在（见第 26 章）[134]。星形细胞瘤的形态学多样性已经得到公认，个别病例发生在诸如软脑膜、小脑脑桥角以及神经轴以外等不常见的部位[135]。有些肿瘤性星形细胞具有含有微管的长突起，而另外一些则充满了中间丝。见于毛细胞性和原纤维性星形细胞瘤的 Rosenthal 纤维，被认为是由变性的神经胶质原纤维衍化而来的。它们由嗜锇的颗粒状物质组成，在中间丝带中形成显著的致密小体。少突胶质细胞一般为圆形，核温和，位于中心，有中等量的线粒体，偶尔含有结晶样结构[136]。

室管膜瘤血管周围的无细胞区是由细长的细胞突起缠绕而成的，其中含有大量的中间丝[137]。在胞浆突起带和毛细血管周围的结缔组织之间，有波浪状的基底膜介入。在群集的室管膜细胞中，常见许多弯曲的微绒毛

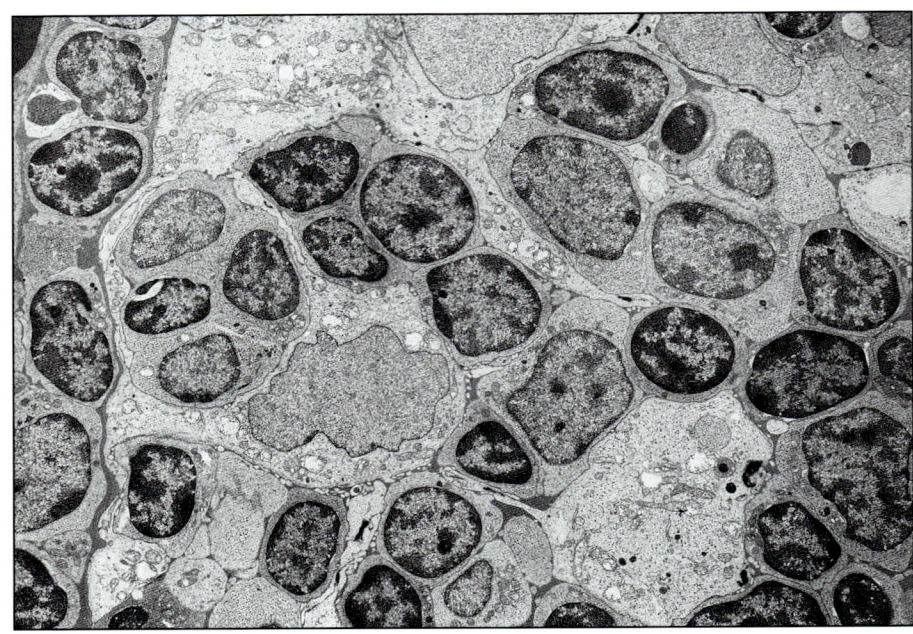

图31.43 胸腺瘤上皮细胞的大小和染色质结构与淋巴细胞的对比是明显的。

和一些纤毛的小间隙[138]，并有非常长的连接将周围的细胞联系起来。因此，电子显微镜检查在确定髓外室管膜瘤的诊断方面可能有价值。

脑膜瘤细胞的超微结构特征在鉴别诊断上可能有用[139]。除了比较类似于神经束膜细胞的脑膜瘤细胞之外，它们还有些像神经鞘细胞。脑膜瘤细胞的胞浆突起可能是长的，但是倾向于弯曲和分叉，形成复杂的结构，当细胞疏松排列时更加明显可见（图31.44）。并列的表面常常呈波浪形。有些脑膜瘤细胞是圆形的，其中充满细丝。发生在头皮和颈部软组织的颅外脑膜瘤的超微结构类似于颅内肿瘤的[140,141]。电子显微镜可用于辨认延伸到颈内静脉腔内的脑膜瘤，后者的临床表现和光学显微镜下表现类似于颈动脉体瘤[142]（图31.45）。

在超微结构水平，有时能够发现鉴别中枢神经系统的小细胞肿瘤的证据[143,144]。在一些视网膜母细胞瘤[145]和髓母细胞瘤[146]，可以见到短的突起和少数大小类似于神经母细胞瘤的致密轴心颗粒。髓母细胞瘤的早期神经元分化的主要表现为：Homer Wright 玫瑰花结和没有网状纤维的"苍白岛"（pale islanda）[147]。电子显微镜检查可以辨认存在间叶成分的细胞类型。

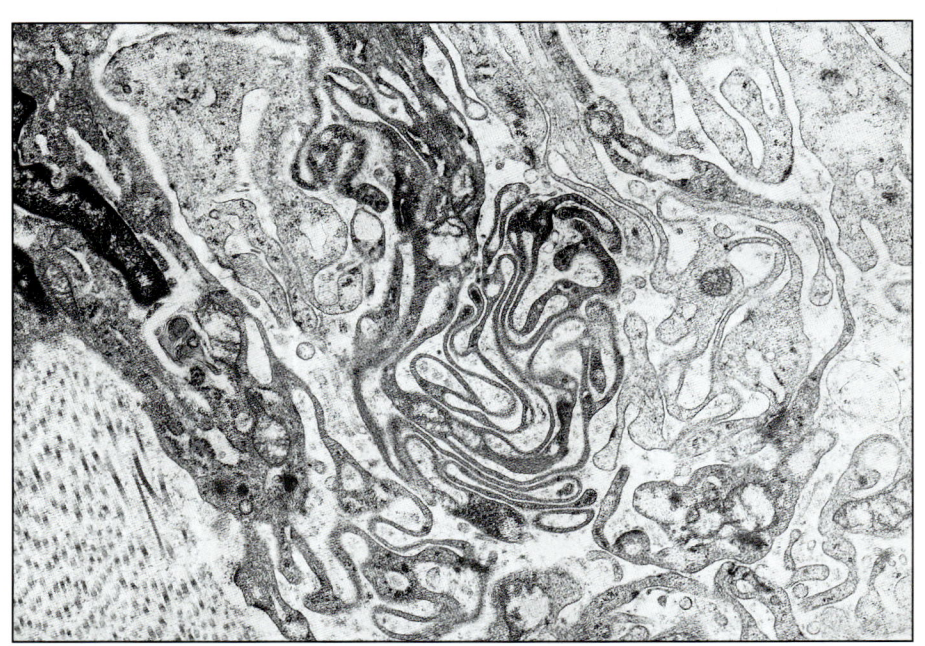

图31.44 颅外脑膜瘤细胞的弯曲及变细的胞浆条带，后者构成了丝状结构。

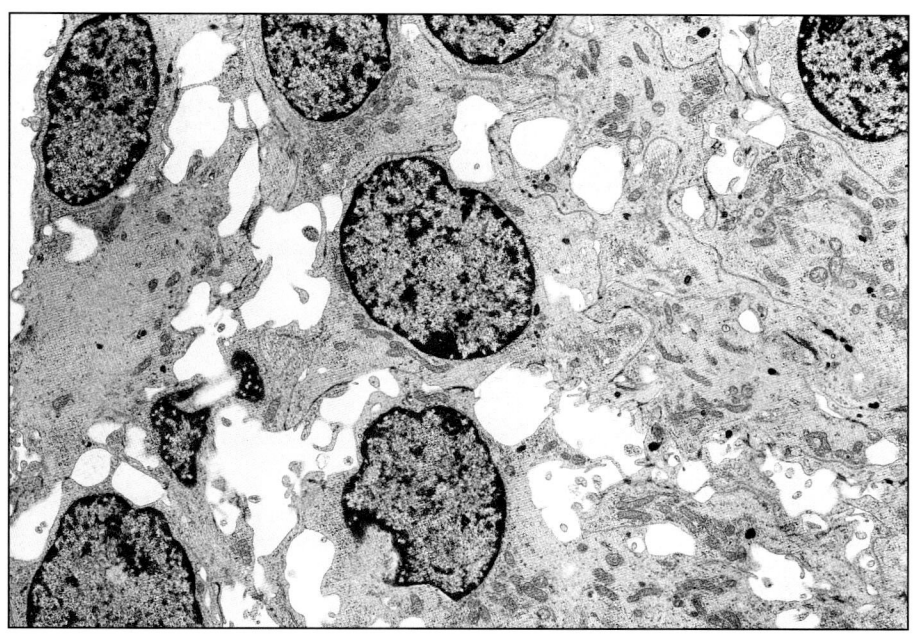

图31.45 脑膜瘤细胞表面呈波浪状，可以游离或密集排列。由于存在弥漫的细丝，胞浆呈中等致密程度。

结论

虽然透射电子显微镜现在应用很少，只是选择性地作为常规外科病理学的诊断工具，但是唯有它能透彻了解肿瘤细胞的结构。当将其用作诊断工具时，必须将超微结构所见与常规光学显微镜和免疫组织化学所见结合起来。

参考文献

1. Mulvey T 1962 Origins and historical development of the electron microscope. Br J Appl Phys 13: 197–207
2. Ruska E 1980 The early development of electron lenses and electron microscopy (translated by Thomas Mulvey). S. Hirzel Verlag, Stuttgart
3. Erlandson R A 1987 Application of transmission electron microscopy to human tumor diagnosis: an historical perspective. Cancer Invest 5: 487–505
4. Papadimitriou J M, Henderson D W, Spagnolo D V 1992 Diagnostic ultrastructure of non-neoplastic diseases. Churchill Livingstone, New York
5. Erlandson R A 1994 Diagnostic transmission electron microscopy of tumors. Raven Press, New York
6. Hammar S P, Bockus D, Remington F 1987 Metastatic tumors of unknown origin: an ultrastructural analysis of 265 cases. Ultrastruct Pathol 11: 209–250
7. Deyrup A T, Haydon R C, Huo D et al. 2003 Myoid differentiation and prognosis in adult pleomorphic sarcomas of the extremity: an analysis of 92 cases. Cancer 98: 805–813
8. Mackay B, Ordonez N G 1996 Electron microscopy in the immunocytochemical era. Adv Pathol 9: 277–310
9. Dardick I, Christensen H, Stratis M 1996 Immunoelectron microscopy for chromogranin A in small cell neuroendocrine carcinoma of the lung. Ultrastruct Pathol 20: 361–368
10. Mackay B, Ordonez N G 1993 Pathological evaluation of tumors with unknown primary site. Semin Oncol 20: 206
11. Mills A E, Emms M, Licata S G 1990 Techniques. A simple technique for preparation of bone marrow or peripheral blood buffy coat cells for electron microscopy. Ultrastruct Pathol 14: 173–176
12. Facundo D J, Quinonez G, Ravinsky E 2003 Transmission electron microscopy of fine needle aspiration biopsies of metastases. Accuracy of both techniques as established by biopsy diagnoses. Acta Cytol 47: 457–462
13. Akhtar M, Bakry M, Nash E J 1986 An improved technic for processing aspiration biopsy for electron microscopy. Am J Clin Pathol 85: 57–60
14. Mackay B, Fanning T, Bruner J M et al. 1987 Diagnostic electron microscopy using fine needle aspiration biopsies. Ultrastruct Pathol 11: 659–672
15. Dardick I, Yazdi H M, Brosko C et al. 1991 A quantitative comparison of light and electron microscopic diagnoses in specimens obtained by fine-needle aspiration biopsy. Ultrastruct Pathol 15: 105–109
16. Strausbauch P, Neill J, Dabbs D J et al. 1989 The impact of fine-needle aspiration biopsy on a diagnostic electron microscopy laboratory. Arch Pathol Lab Med 113: 1354–1356
17. Baic D, Baic B 1984 New techniques. A fast method for processing biopsy material for electron microscopy. Ultrastruct Pathol 6: 347–349
18. Kowalczyk A P, Bornslaeger E A, Norvell S M et al. 1999 Desmosomes: intercellular adhesive junctions specialized for attachment of intermediate filaments. Int Rev Cytol 185: 237–302
19. Cramer S F, Heggeness L M 1989 Signet-ring squamous cell carcinoma. Am J Clin Pathol 91: 488–491
20. Kellokumpu-Lehtinen P, Soderstrom K O, Kortekangas A et al. 1989 Ultrastructural effects of irradiation on squamous cell carcinoma of the head and neck. Cancer 63: 1108–1118
21. McGregor D H, Dixon A, McGregor D K 1988 Adenocarcinoma of the lung: a comparative diagnostic study using light and electron microscopy. Hum Pathol 19: 910–913
22. Sobrinho-Simoes M, Johannessen J V, Gould V E 1981 The diagnostic significance of intracytoplasmic lumina in metastatic neoplasms. Ultrastruct Pathol 2: 327–335
23. Yamashina M, Mackay B, Ordonez N G et al. 1987 Ultrastructural diagnosis of melanoma from an endoscopic biopsy. Ultrastruct Pathol 11: 465–472
24. Herrera G A, Reimann B E F 1984 Electron microscopy in determining origin of metastatic adenocarcinomas. South Med J 77: 1557–1566
25. Mackay B, El-Naggar A, Ordonez N G 1994 Ultrastructure of adrenal cortical carcinoma. Ultrastruct Pathol 18: 181–190
26. Kataoka R, Hyo Y, Hoshiya T et al. 1991 Ultrastructural study of mitochondria in oncocytes. Ultrastruct Pathol 15: 231–239
27. El-Naggar A K, Evans D B, Mackay B 1991 Oncocytic adrenal cortical carcinoma. Ultrastruct Pathol 15: 557
28. Batsakis J G, Mackay B, Ordonez N G 1984 Enteric-type adenocarcinoma of the nasal cavity: an electron-microscopic and immunocytochemical study. Cancer 54: 855–860
29. Ordonez N G, Balsaver A M, Mackay B 1988 Mucinous islet cell (amphicrine) carcinoma of the pancreas associated with watery diarrhea and hypokalemia syndrome. Hum Pathol 19: 1458–1461
30. Ordonez N G, Mackay B 2000 Acinar cell carcinoma of the pancreas. Ultrastruct Pathol 24: 227–241
31. Mackay B, Lukeman J N, Ordonez N G 1990 Tumors of the lung. W B Saunders, Philadelphia, p 146
32. Mackay B, Ordonez N G, Bennington J L et al. 1989 Ultrastructural and morphometric features of poorly differentiated and undifferentiated lung tumors. Ultrastruct Pathol 13: 561–571

33. Fitzpatrick B, Ordonez N G, Mackay B 1991 Islet cell tumor. Ultrastruct Pathol 15: 570–576
34. Mackay B, Franzini D A, Bennington J L et al. 1981 Retroperitoneal tumor with liver metastases in a 38-year-old female. Ultrastruct Pathol 2: 183–186
35. Gomez R, Osborne B M, Ordonez N G et al. 1991 Pheochromocytoma. Ultrastruct Pathol 15: 549–554
36. Hirsch F R, Matthews M J, Aisner S et al. 1988 Histopathologic classification of small cell lung cancer: changing concepts and terminology. Cancer 62: 973–977
37. Silva E G, Mackay B, Goepfert H et al. 1984 Endocrine carcinoma of the skin (Merkel cell carcinoma). Pathol Annu 19: 1–30
38. Kraemer B B, Mackay B, Batsakis J G 1983 Small cell carcinomas of the parotid gland: a clinicopathologic study of three cases. Cancer 52: 2115–2121
39. Ordonez N G, Mackay B 1999 Glycogen-rich mesothelioma. Ultrastruct Pathol 23: 401–406
40. Hammar S P, Bockus D E, Remington F L et al. 1996 Mucin-positive epithelial mesotheliomas: a histochemical, immunohistochemical, and ultrastructural comparison with mucin-producing pulmonary adenocarcinoma. Ultrastruct Pathol 20: 293–325
41. Ordonez N G, Mackay B The roles of immunohistochemistry and electron microscopy in distinguishing epithelial mesothelioma of the pleura from adenocarcinoma. Adv Anat Pathol 3: 273–293
42. Oury T D, Hammar S P, Roggli V L 1998 Ultrastructural features of diffuse malignant mesotheliomas. Hum Pathol 29: 1382–1392
43. Pelosi G, Zannoni M, Caprioli F et al. 1991 Benign multicystic mesothelial proliferation of the peritoneum: immunohistochemical and electron microscopic study of a case and review of the literature. Histol Histopathol 6: 575–683
44. Dardick I, Jabi M, McCaughey W T E et al. 1988 Diffuse epithelial mesothelioma: a review of the ultrastructural spectrum. Ultrastruct Pathol 11: 503–533
45. Bolen J W, Hammer S P, McNutt M A 1986 Reactive and neoplastic serosal tissue. A light-microscopic, ultrastructural, and immunocytochemical study. Am J Surg Pathol 10: 34–37
46. Bolen J W, Hammar S P, McNutt M A 1987 Serosal tissue: reactive tissue as a model for understanding mesotheliomas. Ultrastruct Pathol 11: 251–262
47. Mazur M T, Katzenstein A A 1980 Metastatic melanoma: the spectrum of ultrastructural morphology. Ultrastruct Pathol 1: 337–356
48. Mourad W A, Mackay B, Ordonez N G et al. 1993 Clear cell melanoma of the bladder. Ultrastruct Pathol 17: 463–468
49. Herrera G A, Turbat-Herrera E A 2003 Current role of electron microscopy in the diagnosis of pigmented tumors. Semin Diagn Pathol 20: 60–71
50. Szpak C A, Shelburne J, Linder J et al. 1988 The presence of stage II melanosomes (premelanosomes) in neoplasms other than melanomas. Mod Pathol 1: 35–43
51. Lao L M, Kumakiri M, Kiyohara T et al. 2001 Sub-populations of melanocytes in pigmented basal cell carcinoma: a quantitative, ultrastructural investigation. J Cutan Pathol 28: 34–43
52. Umlas J, Liteplo M, Ucci A 1999 Squamous carcinoma in situ of the skin containing premelanosomes, with melanocytic colonization of the tumor. Hum Pathol 30: 530–532
53. Lloreta-Trull J, Ordonez N G, Mackay B 2000 Pigmented carcinoma of the breast: an ultrastructural study. Ultrastruct Pathol 24: 109–113
54. Chung E B, Enzinger F M 1983 Malignant melanoma of soft parts. A reassessment of clear cell sarcoma. Am J Surg Pathol 7: 405–413
55. Cramer S F 1991 The origin of epidermal melanocytes. Implications for the histogenesis of nevi and melanomas. Arch Pathol Lab Med 115: 115–119
56. Benson J D, Kraemer B B, Mackay B 1985 Malignant melanoma of soft parts: an ultrastructural study of four cases. Ultrastruct Pathol 8: 57–70
57. Jain S, Allen P W 1989 Desmoplastic malignant melanoma and its variants. A study of 45 cases. Am J Surg Pathol 13: 358–373
58. Reed R J, Leonard D D 1979 Neurotropic melanoma: a variant of desmoplastic melanoma. Am J Surg Pathol 3: 301–312
59. Smithers B M, McLeod G R, Little J H 1990 Desmoplastic, neural transforming and neurotropic melanoma: a review of 45 cases. Aust NZ J Surg 60: 967–972
60. DiMaio S, Mackay B, Smith J L et al. 1982 Neurosarcomatous transformation in malignant melanoma. Cancer 50: 2345–2354
61. Van Paesschen M A, Goovaerts G, Buyssens N 1990 A study of the so-called neurotization of nevi. Am J Dermatopathol 12: 242–248
62. Mandybur T I 1974 Melanotic nerve sheath tumors. J Neurosurg 41: 187–192
63. Burke A B, Shekitka K M, Sobin L H 1991 Small cell carcinomas of the large intestine. Am J Clin Pathol 95: 315–321
64. Mills S E, Wolfe J T, Weiss M A et al. 1987 Small cell undifferentiated carcinoma of the urinary bladder: a light-microscopic, immunocytochemical, and ultrastructural study of 12 cases. Am J Surg Pathol 11: 606–617
65. Peydro-Olaya A, Llombart-Bosch A, Carda-Batalia C 2003 Electron microscopy and other ancillary techniques in the diagnosis of small round cell tumors. Semin Diagn Pathol 20: 25–45
66. Brahmi U, Srinivasan R, Komai H S et al. 2003 Comparative analysis of electron microscopy and immunocytochemistry in the cytologic diagnosis of malignant small round cell tumors. Acta Cytol 47: 443–449
67. Llombart-Bosch A, Contesso G, Peydro-Olaya A 1996 Histology, immunohistochemistry, and electron microscopy of small round cell tumors of bone. Semin Diagn Pathol 13: 153–170
68. Suh C-H, Ordonez N G, Hicks J et al. 2002 Ultrastructure of the Ewing's family of tumors. Ultrastruct Pathol 26: 67–76
69. Schmidt D, Mackay B, Ayala A G 1982 Ewing's sarcoma with neuroblastoma-like features. Ultrastruct Pathol 3: 143–151
70. Llombart-Bosch A, Lacombe M J, Contesso G et al. 1987 Small round blue cell sarcoma of bone mimicking atypical Ewing's sarcoma with neuroectodermal features. An analysis of five cases with immunohistochemical and electron microscopic support. Cancer 60: 1570–1582
71. Franchi A, Pasquinelli G, Cenacchi G et al. 2001 Immunohistochemical and ultrastructural investigation of neural differentiation in Ewing sarcoma/PNET of bone and soft tissues. Ultrastruct Pathol 25: 219–225
72. Llombart-Bosch A, Carda C, Peydro-Olaya A et al. 1990 Soft tissue Ewing's sarcoma. Characterization in established cultures and xenografts with evidence of a neuroectodermic phenotype. Cancer 66: 2589–2601
73. Llombart-Bosch A, Blache R, Peydro-Olaya A 1978 Ultrastructural study of 28 cases of Ewing's sarcoma: typical and atypical forms. Cancer 41: 1362–1373
74. Dickersin G R, Rosenberg A E 1991 The ultrastructure of small-cell osteosarcoma, with a review of the light microscopy and differential diagnosis. Hum Pathol 22: 267–275
75. Griego J E, Mackay B, Ordonez N G et al. 1996 Olfactory neuroblastoma. A case report. Ultrastruct Pathol 20: 399–406
76. Kandel R, Bedard Y C, Fan Q H 1998 Value of electron microscopy and immunohistochemistry in the diagnosis of soft tissue tumors. Ultrastruct Pathol 22: 141–146
77. Kindblom L G, Widehn S, Meis-Kindblom J M 2003 The role of electron microscopy in the diagnosis of pleomorphic sarcomas of soft tissue. Semin Diagn Pathol 20: 72–81
78. Suh C-H, Ordonez N G, Mackay B 1993 Fibrosarcoma. Observations on the ultrastructure. Ultrastruct Pathol 17: 221–229
79. Biselli R M, Boldrini R, Ferlini C et al. 1999 Myofibroblastic tumours: neoplasias with divergent behavior. Ultrastructural and flow cytometric analysis. Pathol Res Pract 195: 619–632
80. Gonzalez-Campora R, Escudero A G, Rios Martin J J et al. 2003 Myofibrosarcoma (low-grade myofibroblastic sarcoma) with intracytoplasmic hyaline (fibroma-like) inclusion bodies. Ultrastruct Pathol 27: 7–11
81. Roth T M, Fratkin J, Woodring T C et al. 2004 Low-grade myofibroblastic sarcoma of the vulva. Gynecol Oncol 92: 361–364
82. Singer I I 1979 The fibronexus: a transmembrane association of fibronectin-containing fibers and bundles of 5 nm microfilaments in hamster and human fibroblasts. Cell 16: 675–685
83. Suh C-H, Ordonez N G, Mackay B 2000 Malignant fibrous histiocytoma: an ultrastructural perspective. Ultrastruct Pathol 24: 243–250
84. Pettinato G, Manivel J C, De Rosa G et al. 1990 Angiomatoid malignant fibrous histiocytoma: cytologic, immunohistochemical, ultrastructural, and flow cytometric study of 20 cases. Mod Pathol 3: 479–487
85. Fletcher C D M 1991 Angiomatoid "malignant fibrous histiocytoma." Hum Pathol 22: 563–568
86. Fanburg-Smith J C, Miettinen M 1999 Angiomatoid "malignant" fibrous histiocytoma: a clinicopathologic study of 158 cases and further exploration of the myoid phenotype. Hum Pathol 30: 1336–1343
87. Rossouw D J, Cinti S, Dickersin G R 1986 Liposarcoma. An ultrastructural study of 15 cases. Am J Clin Pathol 85: 649–667
88. Mackay B, Ro J, Floyd C et al. 1987 Ultrastructural observations on smooth muscle tumors. Ultrastruct Pathol 11: 593–608
89. Dekmezian R, Ordonez N G, Mackay B 1991 Bronchioloalveolar adenocarcinoma with myoepithelial cells. Cancer 67: 2356–2360
90. Mackay B, Ordonez N G, Batsakis J G et al. 1988 Pleomorphic adenoma of parotid with myoepithelial cell predominance. Ultrastruct Pathol 12: 461–468
91. Weiss R A, Mackay B 1981 Malignant smooth muscle tumors of the gastrointestinal tract: an ultrastructural study of 20 cases. Ultrastruct Pathol 2: 231–240
92. Fletcher C D M, Berman J J, Corless C et al. 2002 Diagnosis of gastrointestinal stromal tumors. A consensus approach. Hum Pathol 33: 459–465
93. Herrera G A, Cerenzo L, Jones J E et al. 1989 Gastrointestinal autonomic nerve tumors: plexosarcomas. Arch Pathol Lab Med 113: 846–853
94. Lauwers G Y, Erlandson R A, Casper E S et al. 1993 Gastrointestinal autonomic nerve tumors. A clinicopathological, immunohistochemical, and ultrastructural study of 12 cases. Am J Surg Pathol 17: 887–897
95. Erlandson RA 1987 The ultrastructural distinction between rhabdomyosarcoma and other undifferentiated "sarcomas." Ultrastruct Pathol 11: 83–101
96. Kodet R, Newton W A Jr, Hamoudi A B et al. 1991 Rhabdomyosarcomas with intermediate-filament inclusions and features of rhabdoid tumors. Light microscopic and immunohistochemical study. Am J Surg Pathol 15: 257–267
97. Weeks D A, Beckwith J B, Mierau G W et al. 1989 Rhabdoid tumor of kidney. A report of 111 cases from the National Wilms' Tumor Study Pathology Center. Am J Surg Pathol 13: 439–458
98. Mackay B, Ordonez N G, Huang W L 1989 Ultrastructural and immunocytochemical observations on angiosarcomas. Ultrastruct Pathol 13: 97–110
99. Nappi O, Ritter J H, Pettinato G et al. 1995 Hemangiopericytoma: histopathological pattern or clinical entity? Semin Diagn Pathol 12: 221–232

100. Eichhorn J H, Dickersin G R, Bhan A K et al. 1990 Sinonasal hemangiopericytoma: a reassessment with electron microscopy, immunohistochemistry, and long-term follow-up. Am J Surg Pathol 14: 856
101. Payne C, Dardick I, Mackay B 1994 Extraskeletal myxoid chondrosarcoma with intracisternal microtubules. Ultrastruct Pathol 18: 257–261
102. Mackay B, Ayala A G 1980 Intracisternal tubules in human melanoma cells. Ultrastruct Pathol 1: 1–6
103. Shin H C, Mackay B 1994 Parachordoma. Ultrastruct Pathol 18: 249–256
104. Dickersin G R 1987 The electron microscopic spectrum of nerve sheath tumors. Ultrastruct Pathol 11: 103–146
105. Mentzel T, Dei Tos A P, Fletcher C D M 1994 Perineurioma (storiform perineurial fibroma): clinicopathological analysis of 4 cases. Histopathology 25: 261–268
106. Hornick J L, Fletcher C D M 2005 Soft tissue perineurioma: clinicopathologic analysis of 81 cases including those with atypical histologic features. Am J Surg Pathol 29: 845–858
107. Goodlad J R, Fletcher C D M 1991 Malignant peripheral nerve sheath tumor with annulate lamellae mimicking pleomorphic malignant fibrous histiocytoma. J Pathol 164: 23–29
108. Mackay B, Bruner J M, Ordonez N G 1985 Soft tissue sarcoma with neural differentiation. Ultrastruct Pathol 9: 181–188
109. Lagace R 1988 Triton tumor (malignant schwannoma with rhabdomyoblastic differentiation). Ultrastruct Pathol 11: 777–780
110. Wong S Y, Teh M, Tan Y O et al. 1991 Malignant glandular triton tumor. Cancer 67: 1076–1083
111. Ordonez N G, Mackay B 1999 Granular cell tumor: a review of the pathology and histogenesis. Ultrastruct Pathol 23: 207–222
112. Troncoso P, Ordonez N G, Raymond A K et al. 1988 Malignant granular cell tumor: immunohistochemical and ultrastructural observations. Ultrastruct Pathol 12: 137–144
113. Ordonez N G, Mackay B 1998 Alveolar soft part sarcoma: a review of the pathology and histogenesis. Ultrastruct Pathol 22: 275–292
114. Miettinen M, Ekfors T 1990 Alveolar soft part sarcoma: immunohistochemical evidence for muscle cell differentiation. Am J Clin Pathol 93: 32–38
115. Ordonez N G, Mahfouz S M, Mackay B 1990 Synovial sarcoma: an immunohistochemical and ultrastructural study. Hum Pathol 21: 733
116. Bui H X, Petrocine S, Sheehan C et al. 1995 True synovial metaplasia of breast implant capsules: a light and electron microscopic study. Ultrastruct Pathol 19: 83–93
117. Fisher C 1988 Epithelioid sarcoma: the spectrum of ultrastructural differentiation in seven immunohistochemically defined cases. Hum Pathol 19: 265–275
118. Meis J M, Mackay B, Ordonez N G 1988 Epithelioid sarcoma: an immunohistochemical and ultrastructural study. Surg Pathol 1: 13–31
119. Gerald W I, Miller H K, Battifora H et al. 1991 Intra-abdominal desmoplastic small round cell tumor. Report of 19 cases of a distinctive type of high-grade polyphenotypic malignancy affecting young individuals. Am J Surg Pathol 15: 499–513
120. Ordonez N G 1998 Desmoplastic small round cell tumor: II: an ultrastructural and immunohistochemical study with emphasis on new immunohistochemical markers. Am J Surg Pathol 22: 1314–1327
121. Goodlad J R, Crocker J, Macartney J C 1991 Nucleolar ultrastructure in low- and high-grade non-Hodgkin's lymphomas. J Pathol 163: 233–237
122. Kapadia S B, Enzinger F M, Heffner D K et al. 1993 Crystal-storing histiocytosis associated with lymphoplasmacytic neoplasms. Am J Surg Pathol 17: 461–467
123. Harada M, Shimada M, Fukuyama M et al. 1996 Crystal-storing histiocytosis associated with lymphoplasmacytic lymphoma mimicking Weber–Christian disease: immunohistochemical, ultrastructural and gene-rearrangement studies. Hum Pathol 27: 84–87
124. Begin L Y, Osborne B M, Mackay B 1981 Monocytic leukemia with cutaneous involvement: ultrastructural observations on unusual cytoplasmic complexes. Ultrastruct Pathol 2: 11–18
125. Font R L, Mackay B, Tang R 1985 Acute monocytic leukemia recurring as bilateral perilimbal infiltrates. Immunocytochemical and ultrastructural confirmation. Ophthalmology 92: 1681–1685
126. Grogan T M, Payne C M, Richter L C et al. 1985 Case report. Signet-ring cell lymphoma of T-cell origin. An immunocytochemical and ultrastructural study relating giant vacuole formation to cytoplasmic sequestration of surface membrane. Am J Surg Pathol 9: 684–692
127. Weiss L M, Wood G S, Dorfman R F 1985 T-cell signet-ring cell lymphoma. A histologic, ultrastructural, and immunohistochemical study of two cases. Am J Surg Pathol 9: 273–280
128. Hollowood K, Pease C, Mackay A M et al. 1991 Sarcomatoid tumours of lymph nodes showing follicular dendritic cell differentiation. J Pathol 163: 205–216
129. Poblete M T, Figueroa C D, Caorsi I 1987 Ultrastructural characteristics of the interdigitating dendritic cell in dermatopathic lymphadenopathy of mycosis fungoides patients. J Pathol 151: 263–269
130. Rabkin M S, Kjeldsberg C R, Hammond M E et al. 1988 Clinical, ultrastructural, immunohistochemical and DNA content analysis of lymphomas having features of interdigitating reticulum cells. Cancer 61: 1594–1601
131. Turner R R, Colby T V, Wood G S et al. 1984 Histiocytic malignancies. Morphologic, immunologic, and enzymatic heterogeneity. Am J Surg Pathol 8: 485–500
132. Hornick J L, Jaffe E S, Fletcher C D M 2004 Extranodal histiocytic sarcoma: clinicopathologic analysis of 14 cases of a rare epithelioid malignancy. Am J Surg Pathol 28: 1133–1144
133. Osborne B M, Mackay B, Battifora H 1985 Thymoma: a clinicopathologic study of 23 cases. Pathol Annu 20: 289–316
134. Langford L 1996 Central nervous system neoplasms. Indications for electron microscopy. Ultrastruct Pathol 20: 35–46
135. Scheithauer B W, Bruner J M 1987 The ultrastructural spectrum of astrocytic neoplasms. Ultrastruct Pathol 11: 535–581
136. Sarasa J L, Agueras S R, Burzaco J 1990 Crystals in an oligodendroglioma: an optical, histochemical, and ultrastructural study. Ultrastruct Pathol 14: 151–159
137. Sara A, Bruner J M, Mackay B 1994 Ultrastructure of ependymoma. Ultrastruct Pathol 18: 33–42
138. Kawano N, Ohba Y, Nagashima K 2000 Eosinophilic inclusions in ependymoma represent microlumina: a light and electron microscopic study. Acta Neuropathol 99: 214–218
139. Al-Sarraj S, King A, Martin A J et al. 2001 Ultrastructural examination is essential for diagnosis of papillary meningioma. Histopathology 38: 318–324
140. Mackay B, Osborne B M, Guillamondegui O M 1983 Extracranial meningioma: case report. Ultrastruct Pathol 5: 353–357
141. Mackay B, Bruner J M, Luna M A 1994 Malignant meningioma of the scalp. Ultrastruct Pathol 18: 235–240
142. Schmidt D, Mackay B, Luna M A et al. 1981 Aggressive meningioma with jugular vein extension. Arch Otolaryngol 107: 635–637
143. Cruz-Sanchez F F, Rossi M L, Hughes J T et al. 1991 Differentiation in embryonal neuroepithelial tumors of the central nervous system. Cancer 67: 965–976
144. Dehner L P, Abenoza P, Sibley R K 1988 Primary cerebral neuroectodermal tumors: neuroblastoma, differentiated neuroblastoma, and composite neuroectodermal tumor. Ultrastruct Pathol 12: 479–494
145. Utsuki S, Kawano N, Oka H et al. 2003 Pineal parenchymal tumor with marked retinoblastic differentiation: case report. Brain Tumor Pathol 20: 33–37
146. Weeks D A, Malott R L, Goin L et al. 2003 Ultrastructural spectrum of medulloblastoma with immunocytochemical correlations. Ultrastruct Pathol 27: 101–107
147. Katsetos C D, Liu H M, Zacks S I 1988 Immunohistochemical and ultrastructural observations on Homer Wright (neuroblastic) rosettes and the "pale islands" of human cerebellar medulloblastomas. Hum Pathol 19: 1219–1227

分子遗传学技术在诊断和预后中的应用

Molecular genetic techniques in diagnosis and prognosis

Janina A. Longtine 和 Jonathan A. Fletcher 著

刘芳芳 译　回允中 校

引言	1861
应用体细胞突变作为肿瘤诊断和分类的标记物	1862
抗原受体重排	1872
肿瘤标本的转录谱	1874
分子生物学标记物在诊断和预后方面的特殊应用	1875
癌症治疗的药物基因组学	1878
结语	1878

引言

传统上外科病理学实践依赖于大体上和显微镜下评价组织标本的特征，并结合临床病史和其他实验室资料做出一个明确的诊断，预测预后，帮助临床医生并最终帮助患者选择最合适的治疗方式。几十年来，在确定恶性肿瘤、肿瘤分类、肿瘤分级以及（在大多数情况下）疾病分期方面，组织标本的组织学检查具有重要的作用。长期以来，这种诊断方法的价值通过其与治疗反应和临床结局的相关性已得到证实。另外，这种诊断程序十分完备，可以迅速获得诊断资料，特别是在应用冰冻切片时，而且全部诊断的花费相对便宜。

然而，形态学有其一定的局限性。在美国，有13.2%的妇女在其生命的某个阶段被诊断患有乳腺癌[1]；2005年，超过40 000名妇女死于乳腺癌[2]。辅助性激素疗法和多种化学疗法通过根除远处微小转移而降低了乳腺癌复发和死亡的危险性。肿瘤大小、淋巴结状况、雌激素/孕激素受体状况、肿瘤分级和出现淋巴管血管浸润[3]都可用于确定哪些患者最可能从这些潜在的毒性治疗方案中受益。不过，由于传统标准的预测能力有限，所以没有必要进行治疗的妇女可能也接受了系统的治疗。类似的问题也适用于其他许多恶性肿瘤，虽然同过去一样，外科病理学专业医生在优化患者的处理和组织切片的组织学检查方面能够做很多的工作，但却常常不能对患者进行分层次优化的肿瘤特异性治疗。显然，需要改进生物学标志物，以便确定需要进行特异性辅助治疗的患者。

除了经常缺乏形态学特征来区分具有不同临床行为方式的肿瘤亚型之外，组织的组织学检查还受到其他诸多限制。有些是技术性的，牵涉到由于标本保存、固定或染色不好而引起的人工假象或问题。其他一些困难则来自分析的主观性，后者主要受医生经验、偏爱和培训状况的影响。由于有困难，一些"低分化"或罕见肿瘤在观察者之间或观察者内的差异可能很高[4]。即使是在一些诊断相对容易的常见疾病中，由于缺乏规格化的诊断标准，意见也可能不一[5,6]。为了克服组织学检查的局限性，已经采用了一些较新的基于组织的方法，其总体目标是将肿瘤按照生物学同源性分组。

在过去几十年中，有三次革新对外科病理学具有影响。电子显微镜（见第31章）首先揭示了一系列亚细胞细胞器的存在，很快被外科病理医生接受，并将分化的超微结构特征用于疑难肿瘤的诊断，如桥粒、黑色素小体和Birbeck颗粒。随后，免疫组化和单克隆抗体被用于常规外科病理学中，并在引入到病理学这个领域之后不久很快就起到了作用。现在，癌可以容易而可靠地与淋巴瘤和黑色素瘤区分开来，从前的分类可用一系列的细胞分化标记物的抗体进行重新评估。这与淋巴瘤和白血病分类的关系尤其密切。应用免疫组化检查，常规组织学检查常常认为是癌的间变性大细胞淋巴瘤，可以通过其CD30和ALK1表达来确认。富于T细胞的B细胞淋巴瘤是弥散性大B细胞淋巴瘤的一个亚型，通过在大量良性T细胞的背景中突出大B细胞可以较容易地确认。套细胞淋巴瘤是一种不能治愈的中级别淋巴瘤，通过其免疫表达谱（$CD20^+$、$CD5^+$、$CD10^{-/+}$、$CD23^-$、 cyclin D1⁺）可与诸如滤泡性和小淋巴细胞性淋巴瘤等低级别淋巴瘤鉴别[7]。

组织标本分子遗传学分析是对外科病理学产生影响的最新方法。这个领域的一些技术已经用于诊断外科病理学，而另外一些技术则为发现新的标记物以及新的诊断程序提供了可能性。本章将概括描述可能用于评估组织标本的现有的分子生物学标记物和技术，还将总结在未来几年内这个领域可能影响外科病理学的研究方向。

组织标本分子遗传学分析的通用靶点是核酸或DNA或RNA。诊断标记物通常是某种形式的DNA突变，后者它可能表现为由突变基因转录而来的RNA结构的改变。癌症是一种遗传性疾病，从这个意义上讲，获得性的所谓的"体细胞"DNA突变（也就是在患者一生中发生在种系以外的突变）在肿瘤的发生过程中占据核心地位。实际上，细胞完全转化为恶性可能需要关键基因的不同形式的突变。这些突变表现为肿瘤前体细胞DNA的缺失、复制、易位和（或）点突变。最终，这些突变影响细胞周期的调节、凋亡或细胞-细胞之间以及细胞-基质之间的相互作用。不同的肿瘤具有不同的遗传学改变的组合，正是这些组合导致了细胞的克隆性增生。癌症的遗传学改变已经为诊断提供了标记物，因为它们可用作恶性表型的独立而又客观的信号。用于检测这些标记物的方法差别很大，取决于需要寻找的突变的类型。

除了DNA或RNA突变以外，表观遗传学改变（epigenetic changes，即基因活性改变，其结构没有改变）也是细胞恶性转化的原因，其中的DNA核苷酸序列不受影响[8-10]。这些改变包括DNA甲基化的改变、基因组特定区域染色质结构的修饰以及异常基因表达，常常是其他基因突变的继发效应。其中某些表遗传学核酸的干扰作为肿瘤诊断、预后和治疗的标记物已越来越受到关注。起决定性作用的分子生物学标记物是来自感染因子的外源性核酸，主要是与癌症起因有关的病毒，在引起癌症的过程中复制。迄今只有少数这类因子，但是在特殊的情况下，这些因子基因组的核酸序列也可以作为肿瘤诊断的有用标记物。

应用体细胞突变作为肿瘤诊断和分类的标记物
Utilization of somatic mutations as markers for the diagnosis or classification of neoplasms

染色体易位　Chromosomal translocations

自从20世纪早期Boveri的研究以来，人们就已经知道，肿瘤可以发生染色体畸变[11]，但是，直到1960年才首次报道了特异性的反复发生的染色体结构异常，当时描述在慢性髓性白血病的细胞中有费城染色体（Philadelphia chromosome，染色体易位的一个实例，见下文）[12,13]。从那之后，在肿瘤中又发现了其他类型的特异性染色体异常，包括倒位（inversions）、缺失（deletions）和扩增（amplifications）。然而，在诊断方面，染色体易位（chromosomal translocations）是最重要的染色体异常，在造血系统肿瘤和软组织肉瘤中特别常见。在癌几乎见不到易位，这可能部分地反映了这些肿瘤细胞遗传学分析存在较大的技术上的困难。染色体易位是不同染色体区域之间的非同源性DNA重组，通常是交互易位以及平衡或接近平衡的易位，意味着两个染色体之间的染色体物质发生了交换，并不伴有真正的DNA丢失。

染色体易位的分子分析表明，重组相关性染色体断裂可导致基因表达的改变，或通过邻近基因表达调节障碍，或通过基因的1个或2个断裂点的直接破坏。后者的一个实例是费城染色体，可以缩写为Ph'，应用正规的细胞遗传学命名法称为t（9；22）(q34；q11)（第一个括弧表示参与易位的两个染色体；第二个括弧表示含有断裂点的每个染色体的臂和条带，q代表长臂，p代表短臂）。这种易位的断裂点位于两个基因内，*ABL1*基因位于9号染色体，而*BCR*基因位于22号染色体（图32.1）。作为断裂点重组的结果是，编码BCR蛋白氨基末端部分的*BCR*基因的5'端，与编码ABL蛋白碳基末端的*ABL1*基因的3'端相连，形成了一个新的*BCR-ABL*嵌合基因。断裂点发生在两个基因的内含子（introns）（DNA的非编码且可能是非功能的片段，散在分布于基因编码区域之间）。因此，基因的编码区，或称之为外显子（exons），仍然保持完整，而且可以被转录和翻译形成一种融合蛋白。这种融合蛋白正是造血细胞的癌基因。

在*BCR*基因中已经鉴定了两个不同的断裂点区域，它们只能在分子水平进行区分，而在常规核型分析（显微镜下）水平不能区分（图32.1）。最常见的断裂点发生在*BCR*基因5.8kb的主要断裂点聚集区域（major breakpoint cluster region，M-bcr），导致210 kDa的融合蛋白（p210），它能增强酪氨酸激酶活性。Ph'在髓细胞恶性行为中具有重要作用，通过显示小鼠骨髓表达p210 BCR-ABL蛋白可导致一种类似于CML的疾病可得到证实[14,15]。另外，原发性慢性期CML细胞中的髓前体细胞的增生可能由*BCR-ABL*融合序列导致的RNA干扰（RNA interference，RNAi）而减少[16]。而且，一种选择性的蛋白激酶抑制剂甲磺酸伊马替尼（imatinib mesylate），在体内和体外均能抑制表达p210蛋白的细胞增生。I/II期临床试验显示，甲磺酸伊马替尼可在抗

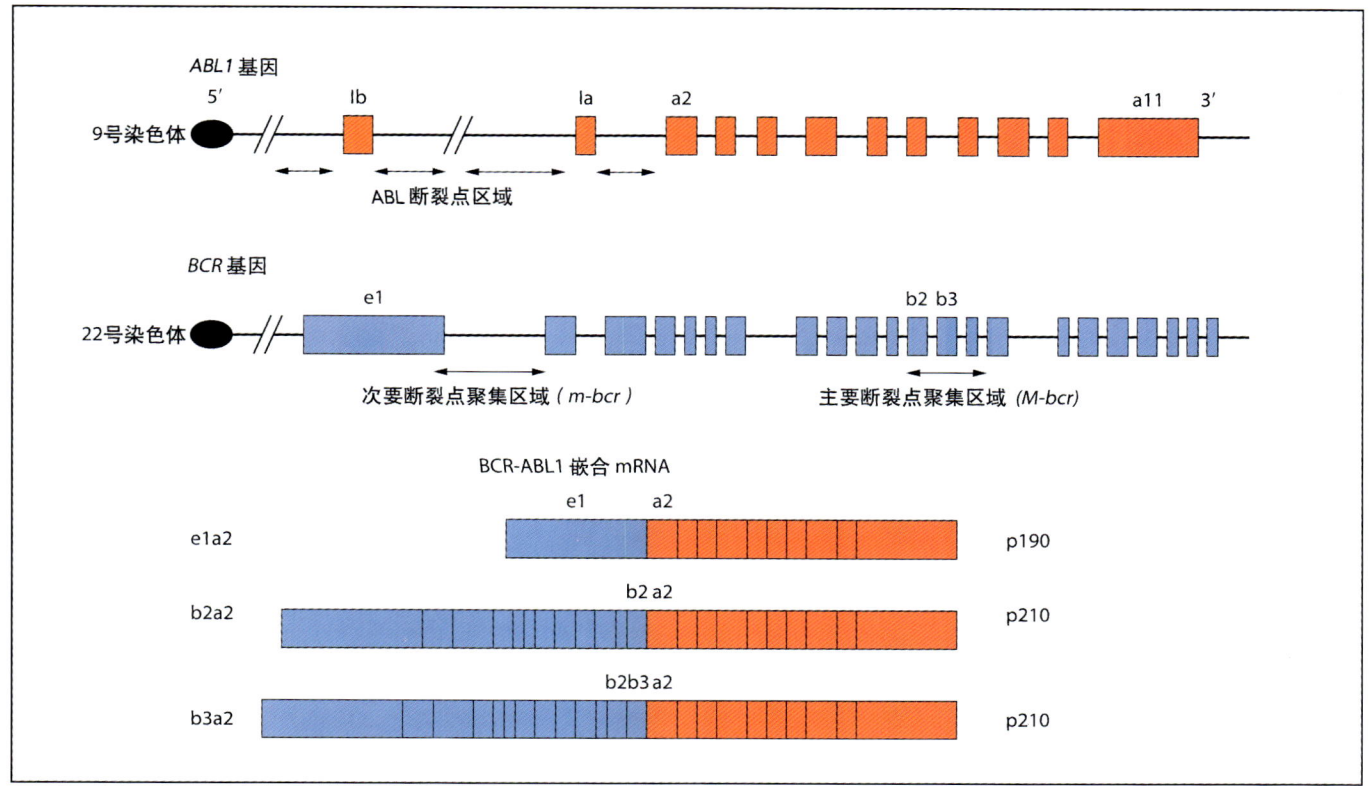

图32.1 慢性髓性白血病（CML）和急性淋巴母细胞性白血病（ALL）的参与t(9;22)(q34;q11)（Ph'染色体）形成的ABL和BCR基因结构。方框代表外显子。在两种白血病中，ABL断裂点散在分布于整个大的第一内含子。在CML，BCR断裂点也在内含子内，且发生在主要断裂点聚集区域（M-bcr）内，形成8.5kb的嵌合mRNA，编码210kd的融合蛋白。在ALL，BCR断裂点可发生在M-bcr，或较常见的是发生在第一内含子的5'端（次要断裂点区域；m-bcr）。后者产生一个7.0kb的嵌合mRNA，编码190kd融合蛋白的。

干扰素治疗的患者中引起全面的血液反应，进一步支持了这种易位在疾病临床表现中的重要性[17]。一项III期随机临床试验表明，甲磺酸伊马替尼远远优于干扰素加阿糖胞苷[18]，因此，甲磺酸伊马替尼（Gleevec, Novartis Pharma AG, Basel, Switzerland）作被允许为治疗CML的一线药物。这是第一个被批准的分子靶向药物，它能直接关闭已知的引起癌症的蛋白信号。实际上，在所有的CML病例以及10%的成人急性淋巴母细胞白血病（ALL）病例和5%的成人急性髓细胞性白血病（AML）病例中，均可检测到与p210蛋白相关的BCR-ABL易位。

其次，Ph'的不常见的断裂点区域位于第一内含子BCR的5'端，形成一个190kDa的BCR-ABL融合蛋白。这个断裂点见于大约10%的成人ALL病例和5%～10%的儿童ALL病例[19,20]。在急性白血病病例中，出现Ph'，不管其BCR断裂点的部位如何，单单接受标准化疗患者预后不好，提示在首次临床缓解后要考虑骨髓移植[21,22]。因此，Ph'及其新的基因产物可以用作骨髓增生紊乱的诊断标记物，而且可以用作急性白血病的预后标记物。染色体易位，BCR-ABL基因重组，其嵌合的mRNA转录以及融合蛋白产物都已经被用作一种或另外一种形式的临床分析的靶点。

嵌合产物，癌基因蛋白常常是肿瘤染色体易位的结果；然而，还有其他一些机制，通过这些机制接近（或在）断裂点的基因产物发生改变。例如，弱表达基因或不表达基因的mRNA和蛋白产物，可以通过邻近活跃启动子区域成分的基因易位而明显上调为一个强表达的基因。在非Hodgkin淋巴瘤，染色体易位常常累及一个抗原受体基因，例如位于14号染色体长臂32条带上的免疫球蛋白重链基因（IGH）。这个位点，正常情况下在B细胞的发育中发生基因内重组，是合成免疫球蛋白的一个步骤（见下文），偶尔这个位点也参与异常重组，从而导致免疫球蛋白基因的一部分与另外一个染色体上的DNA相连。其他染色体的重组位点可能接近或位于某一基因内部，其近端的IGH强化因子可造成转录调节障碍，这是一个激发转录的调节序列。因此，易位的并列IGH强化因子可导致B细胞淋巴瘤中编码各种癌基因序列的特异蛋白的过度表达。这种类型的易位的一个实例是滤泡性淋巴瘤的t(14;18)(q32;q21)，其中位于18号染色体上的抗凋亡基因BCL2（B-cell leukemia/lymphoma 2）持续表达[23]。作为染色体易位的结果，BCL2过度表达本身并不足以导致肿瘤转化，但其抗凋亡功能可能是B

细胞长期存活的原因。在转基因小鼠中植入调节障碍的 *BCL2*，这种基因的过度表达可导致滤泡增生，但并不发生淋巴瘤，除非同时植入癌基因 *CMYC* 或通过自发性突变事件激活[24,25]。还有证据表明，t(14;18)(q32;q21) 易位以及随之改变的 *BCL2* 基因表达不足以引起人类的肿瘤性转化。应用敏感的聚合酶链反应（PCR）技术偶尔可以在反应性淋巴结、扁桃体或血液中检测到非常低水平的 t(14;18)(q32;q21) 易位[26,27]。随后发生的遗传学和（或）表遗传学改变目前尚不清楚，后者在滤泡性淋巴瘤细胞和正常淋巴组织的少数细胞中是不同的。然而少数非肿瘤性细胞出现易位提示，除了增强恶性 B 细胞的存活之外，*BCL2* 表达改变也有可能会使非恶性淋巴瘤前体细胞的生存期延长，而在此期间其他转化突变也可能发生。其他最近的研究认为，非恶性细胞基因表达与淋巴瘤预后之间有相关性。例如，基因表达数据表明，滤泡性淋巴瘤的生存期[28]或对治疗的反应[29]可用非恶性细胞的表达信号来解释，特别是 T 细胞、巨噬细胞或树突状细胞，提示淋巴瘤细胞微环境的重要性。不过从诊断的角度来看，t(14;18)(q32;q21) 易位是一贯的遗传学改变，与滤泡性淋巴瘤的特殊肿瘤表型有关。染色体易位可以通过多种技术来检测，包括细胞遗传学、荧光原位杂交、Southern 印迹杂交或 PCR。因为易位可导致正常 *BCL2* 编码序列的过度表达，检测蛋白增加可以辅助组织学诊断。正常淋巴结的反应性滤泡 BCL2 蛋白表达水平低。因此，反应性滤泡增生和滤泡性淋巴瘤（见第 21 章）的形态学鉴别诊断可通过免疫组织化学证实组织切片中的滤泡 BCL2 表达来区分（图 32.2）。

染色体易位是以不同的生物化学途径影响基因，但是参与染色体易位的各种类型的基因的形态好像与某些肿瘤有关。编码转录因子的基因在急性白血病和肉瘤的易位中特别常见。异源二体造血转录因子，核心结合因子（CBF），由 RUNX1 和 CBFβ 亚单位组成，对于造血来说是必需的，也是急性白血病易位重组的已知的最常见的靶点[30]。CBF 是造血的一种转录调节因子，许多易位可生成嵌合蛋白，似乎具有 CBF 功能抑制作用，因此可影响造血细胞的生长和分化途径。涉及这些基因的易位发生在 30% 的 AML 和 25% 的 ALL 病例[31]。*RUNX1* 基因在 AML M2 的 t(8;21)(q22;q22)[32-34] 被破坏，在儿童 B ALL 前体的 t(12;21)(p13;q22)[35-38] 被破坏。编码非 DNA 结合亚单位 CBFβ 的基因在 AML-M4Eo 的 inv16 中被破坏[39,40]。

肉瘤的染色体易位同样涉及编码转录因子的基因（也见第 24 章）。*EWSR1* 基因编码一个 RNA 结合分子，EWS，即当其与一个异源的 DNA 结合区融合时，可以刺激基因转录[41]。*EWSR1* 是由 Ewing 肉瘤 / 外周原始神经外胚层肿瘤（PNET）的 t(11;22)(q24;q12) 断裂点的分子克隆分离出来的，这是第一个具有易位分子特征的肉瘤[42,43]。*EWSR1* 位于 22 号染色体长臂，而 11 号染色体重组位点位于 *FLI1*（Friend 白血病病毒整合位点 1，Friend leukemia virus integration site 1）。*FLI1* 基因属于 *ETS*（成红细胞增多症病毒转化序列，erythroblastosis virus transforming sequence）家族相关基因，这些基因全都含有序列特异性 DNA 结合区[44,45]。融合 EWS-FLI1 癌基因蛋白将 EWS 的 N 末端反式激活区与 FLI1 的 C 末端 DNA 结合区连接起来，是有效的转录激活蛋白[46,47]。包含这些区域对于蛋白致癌性的重要性是显而易见的，因为尽管 Ewing 肉瘤 /PNET 肿瘤的断裂点存在个体变异性，但是 EWS-FLI1 的所有类型都包括完整的 *EWS N* 末端区域（在前七个外显子编码）和完整的 *FLI1* 的 *DNA* 结合区。在大约 10% 的 Ewing 肉瘤 /PNET 中，可见所谓的"变异易位"，如 t(21;22)(q22;q12) 和 t(7;22)(q22;q12)[48-51]。其中 *EWS* 和 ETS 蛋白家族的其他成员（21 号染色体的 *ERG* 和 7 号染色体的 *ETV1*）相连，这些嵌合蛋白在结构上与 *EWS-FLI1* 类似。在其他肉瘤中也可见到 *EWS* 基因重排，如透明细胞肉瘤[52]、腹内纤维组织增生性小圆细胞肿瘤[53,54]和骨外黏液性软骨肉瘤[55]。在每一种融合蛋白中，据推测 *EWS* 的 N 末端区都具有转录活性和其他调节功能，而第二个基因可产生序列特异性 C 末端 DNA 结合区。在不同类型的肉瘤中，这些蛋白的谱系特异性似乎是通过 DNA 结合区的特异性来表现的。新近，ETS 转录因子 ERG 和 ETV1 在前列腺癌反复发生中的易位已被发现，提示在一某些上皮性肿瘤中，癌发生可能具有类似的机制[56]。

应用染色体易位作为诊断标记物改善了各种恶性肿瘤的分类。仅仅在过去十年里，套细胞淋巴瘤才

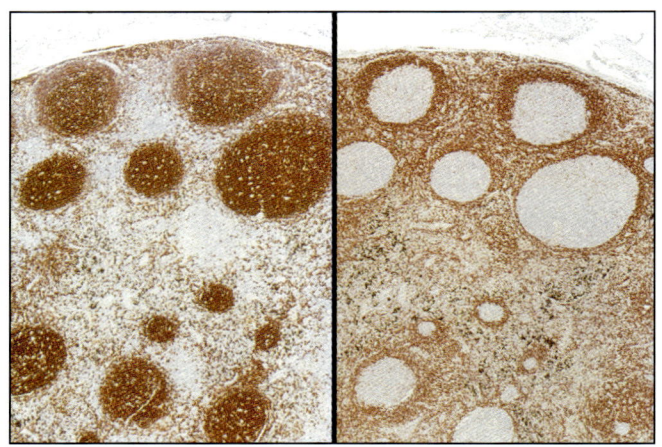

图32.2 显示反应性滤泡增生的淋巴结。连续切片显示滤泡 CD20 免疫反应呈强阳性（左），而滤泡bcl-2染色呈阴性（右）。

被广泛认为是明确的临床病理疾病[57-59]。对特征性的 t(11;14)(q13;q32) 的识别导致了这种疾病诊断标准的细化[60-62]，从前通过形态学标准认为其为低级别肿瘤，而现在认为其预后不好，平均生存期仅为 3～5 年（见第 21 章）。t(11;14) 易位是 11 号染色体长臂 13 条带上的 DNA 与 14 号染色体长臂 32 条带上 IGH 基因中的 DNA 相连。细胞周期调节蛋白 cyclin D1 的转录由接近 11 号染色体重组位点的 CCND1 基因编码，由于与 IgH 增强因子并列而被下调，由此 cyclin D1 蛋白在这些淋巴瘤中过度表达。cyclin D1 的过度表达可通过免疫组化来检测，在诊断上用于区分套细胞淋巴瘤和其他 B 细胞淋巴瘤。另一个在诊断上具有重要意义的染色体易位的例子是：急性前髓细胞白血病（ALM M3）的 t(15;17)(q22;q21)（见第 22 章）。这种易位是 PML 和 RARA 两个基因的连接，具有特殊的治疗意义，因为出现易位是应用维甲酸（ATRA）治疗敏感的特异性标记物，ATRA 可诱导组成这种肿瘤恶性细胞的未成熟性髓细胞的最终分化[63,64]。

认识到这些染色体易位和其他染色体畸变在诊断中的作用，世界卫生组织（WHO）血液淋巴系统肿瘤分类方案[65]主要根据特殊的细胞遗传学异常来区分一些 AML 和 ALL 的亚型，这些异常与形态学和（或）独特的临床特征有关（见表 32.1）。细胞遗传学异常起主要作用的类似分类方案也出现在实体肿瘤，尤其是肾细胞癌（见第 12 章）[66]。此外，除了在肿瘤分类中的作用之外，易位和其他细胞遗传学异常也可用于评估许多肿瘤的预后或对治疗的反应，见下文。

检测染色体易位的技术
Techniques for detecting chromosomal translocations

有多种技术可以用于检测肿瘤中的染色体易位。细胞遗传学分析是染色体分析的常规方法，这种方法与严格的分子学方法相比是更为形态学的分析，可以检测所有的染色体改变，但要求有新鲜的组织、细胞培养、特殊的实验室和受过培训的技师和专业人员。为了进行细胞遗传学分析，从肿瘤标本中获得的细胞悬液培养数天，并且添加有丝分裂纺锤体抑制剂，如秋水仙碱和长春新碱，使分离的细胞停止在分裂中期。浓缩的分裂中期染色体应用 Giemsa 染料染色显示特征性的条带结构（G 带），用于辨认单个染色体以及其中结构或数目的畸变。这种技术劳动强度大且费用昂贵，最好用于需要进行多种潜在异常分析的诊断或有预后预测目的时，例如 AML 的亚分类。在分辨所谓的"隐蔽性易位"和小的缺失（碱基少于 5 兆）时，细胞遗传学分析也有其局限性[67]。然而，这个技术的最大缺点是：其依赖于在体外成功的肿瘤细胞增殖以获得分裂中期的染色体标本。当培养的肿瘤细胞生长不良时，细胞遗传学分析常常失败；这可能是由预先处理不当、固有坏死造成了生长不好或非肿瘤性间质成分过度生长造成的。

其他更多的分子技术也可以用于检测特异性的染色体易位，但不能像常规细胞遗传学分析那样观察的细胞的整个染色体结构。在荧光原位杂交（fluorescence in situ hybridization，FISH）中，荧光标记的 DNA 探针与整个染色体（是指染色体图）或更常见的是与染色体的特定区域杂交。这些探针含有的核酸序列碱基对通常在 10 个至数百个之间。这些探针可以用于分裂中期染色体，作为确定细胞遗传学分析的有用方法（图 32.3），如当怀疑两个以上的染色体有复杂的交换时，或作为一种寻找常规细胞遗传学分析不能检测到的少量染色体物质交换的方法。然而，这是一种直接在完整的非分离的肿瘤细胞核上进行分析的机会，因而可使 FISH 技术极具价值。这些细胞核可从印片[68]、吸取涂片[69]、细胞学标本[68]或石蜡切片解聚的细胞核中获得[70-72]。通过选择可与断裂点相邻区域杂交的 DNA 探针，细胞核 DNA 信号的模式（位于正常染色体侧翼断裂点的分离信号，或正常染色体两个断裂点附近的杂交融合信号）将表明染色体易位的存在。FISH 也可检测染色体缺失。FISH 比标准的细胞遗传学分析便宜，不需要新鲜的组织，并且相对快速。然而，FISH 需要荧光显微镜以及特殊的计算机软件来优化荧光信号。此外，常规 FISH 只能用来鉴定特异的染色体改变，不能进行肿瘤细胞遗传学的全面观察。

基因座特异性原位杂交（locus-specific in situ hybridization）也可用于组织学切片，而不是从石蜡包埋组织中提取完整的细胞核[73]。应用组织学切片的优点

表 32.1　急性白血病中经常发生的染色体易位

染色体易位	受累基因	危险分组
急性髓性白血病		
t(8;21)(q22;q22)	RUNX1-1/ETO	良好
inv16(p13;q22)	CBFB-MYH11	良好
t(15;17)(q22;q21)	PML-RARA	良好
t(9;11)(p21-22;q23)	MLL-AF9	不良
急性淋巴母细胞性白血病		
t(12;21)(p12;q22)	TEL-RUNX1	良好
t(9;22)(q34;q11)	BCR-ABL1	不良
t(1;19)(q23;p13)	E2A-PBX1	不良
t(4;11)(q21;q23)	MLL-AF4	不良

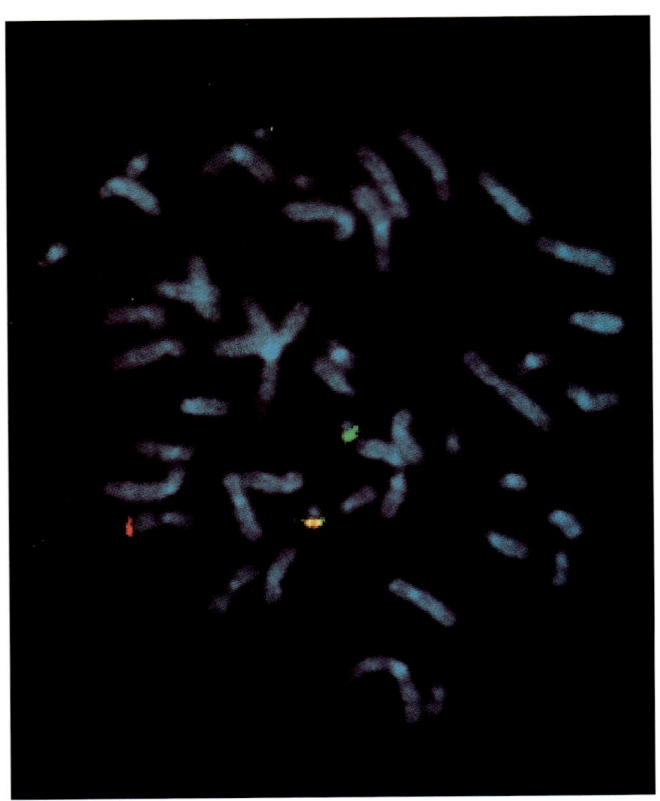

图32.3 Ewing肉瘤分裂中期细胞双色荧光原位杂交,应用着丝粒[异硫氰酸荧光素(FITC)检测为绿色]和端粒（罗丹明检测为红色）探针检测位于22号染色体上的EWS基因位点。正常22号染色体具有完整的绿-红探针对,生成物光谱重叠,发出黄色信号。另一个22号染色体复制具有EWS位点易位,导致侧翼红-绿探针对分开。

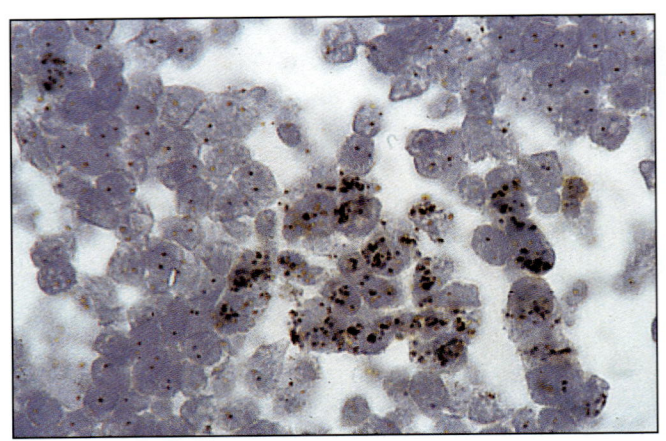

图32.4 乳腺癌石蜡切片ERBB2（HER2/NEU）探针（Zymed实验室）比色原位杂交。通过过氧化物酶/DAB进行探针检测。单个棕色小点相当于ERBB2位点,癌显示异原性的扩增结构。有些细胞具有ERBB2扩增（成簇的棕色小点）,而其他细胞为非扩增性的（1或2个单独的棕色小点）。

是：肿瘤的结构和细胞学特征是完整的,可以与染色体的改变相互联系。然而,由于细胞核的切割和重叠,杂交信号比较难以解释。完整的细胞核或组织学切片中的染色体或染色体位点的基因座特异性原位杂交,可以应用酶检测方法和明视野显微镜而不是荧光来进行（所谓的"比色原位杂交", colorimetric in situ hybridization, CISH）。虽然不如荧光敏感,但是CISH不需要FISH所需要的荧光显微镜、影像设备和软件。CISH最易于用于基因扩增的评估[74-77],如乳腺癌中的HER-2/NEU（也叫ERBB2）（图32.4）。

FISH处于常规细胞遗传学分析和纯粹的分子技术之间的中间位置,下面予以讨论；也就是说,FISH能够检测常规细胞遗传学技术不能检测的染色体重排,但不能检测DNA中一些小的改变（特别是10kb以下的序列）,这些小的变化可能具有如同易位一样的遗传学重要性,只能通过分子技术来检测。相反,当试图检测异源性的和广泛分布于大的DNA序列的易位断裂点时,可以选择FISH这项技术,例如在Burkitt淋巴瘤中环绕MYC基因的易位[78,79]。

染色体易位还可以通过Southern印迹杂交(Southern blot hybridization)来检测,条件是一个或另外一个参与的染色体的断裂点集中在DNA的15～20kb的区域。然而,在大多数临床情况下,这种实验室技术已经被更快速的技术所取代,例如FISH和PCR（见下文）。

聚合酶链反应（PCR）的敏感性、通用性和速度对于检测染色体易位具有重要的影响,就像它对整个分子病理学领域具有影响一样。这种技术常规上可以用于检测多达大约1000bp的DNA片段,应用改良的条件在体外可以成指数地扩增更长的片段。然而必须知道,其仅靠要扩增的侧翼区域的DNA序列（虽然有可以达到这一要求的操作方法）。为复制模板DNA, PCR应用纯化的细菌DNA多聚酶,利用这些多聚酶不能从头合成DNA、只能延长先前存在的DNA链的3'端这一特性。加到这个DNA 3'端的核酸或引物链,是与引物退火的模板链互补的核酸；换句话说,鸟核苷酸（Gs）加至相反的胞核苷酸（Cs）延长的引物链,而腺核苷酸（As）总是加至相反的胸腺苷（Ts）。同样, Cs加至相反的Gs,而Ts加至相反的As。多聚酶从而产生了原始单链模板的一个互补的复制。如果引物在这个合成的DNA链上退火,多聚酶的第二次循环将复制原始的模板链（图32.5）。

实际上, PCR最常用于扩增双链DNA模板,引物是寡核苷酸,或是在DNA自动合成仪上化学合成的大约20～40bp长度的DNA小片段。PCR引物与要扩增的模板DNA的双链侧翼序列是互补的。引物退火位点之间的DNA在重复的DNA合成循环中被扩增,其中,

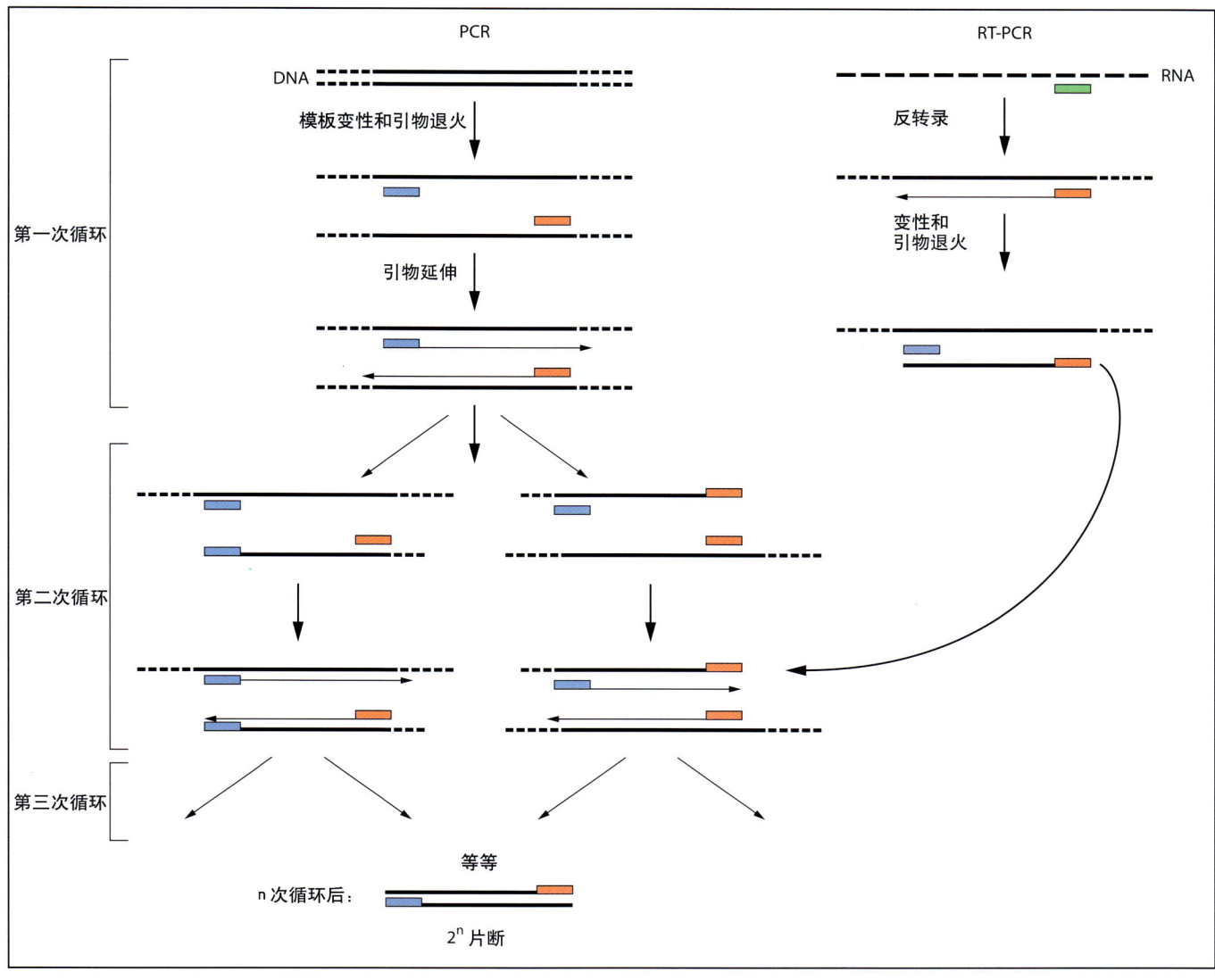

图32.5 图示 DNA 的 PCR 和 RNA 的 RT-PCR 扩增。

通过加热反应混合物中的模板链首先分离，随后降低温度，允许引物与摩尔成比例过量的模板发生退火，最后将温度调整至适合引物的延伸。已经发明了特殊的称为热循环仪的孵育器，以适应不同温度的频繁切换，从嗜热细菌中分离出的耐热 DNA 聚合酶也已被采纳应用，因此，这种酶只需要在反应开始时加入。原则上，在每一次循环中被扩增的 DNA 都加倍，所以大约在 20 个循环后，每一个模板可有一百万个 DNA 片段聚积在反应开始的部位。尽管实际的 PCR 扩增很少有这么高的效率，但是通常能够产生足够数量的片段产物，这些产物可在凝胶电泳中以条带的形式出现，应用荧光染料溴化乙啶 DNA 染色后可在紫外灯下检测出来。

PCR 技术可以检测染色体易位，其中参与易位的两个染色体的断裂点重复地集中在明确的狭窄的 DNA 区域，倘若知道这些区域周围的准确 DNA 序列。需要合成一对引物，使得其中一条特异地与每一个断裂点以外的 DNA 退火。如果易位存在于从组织标本中提取的全细胞的 DNA 中，将会从横越重组位点的 DNA 产生一个 PCR 产物。然而，在正常 DNA，寡核苷酸引物将会与分开的染色体中的 DNA 退火，或与单一染色体中广泛分离的区域退火，而且没有 PCR 产物产生。在某些易位中，断裂点可能散在分布于 DNA 的很大的区域（几十万个碱基），就像上面提到的涉及 MYC 的易位。在这种情况下，设计引物通过 DNA 的 PCR 来检测所有可能的易位产物用于诊断目的是不实际的。然而，如果断裂点分布在大的内含子内且产生了嵌合的 RNA，PCR 技术的变异，即反转录聚合酶链反应（reverse transcription PCR，RT-PCR），则可以用于检测这些易位。在 RT-PCR 中，从标本中提取的 RNA 作为模板，其基本原理是，虽然不同病例的易位的 DNA 产物差异可能很大，但从融合基因转录而来的嵌合 RNA 在不同病例之间是恒定的。RT-PCR 与 PCR 的不同之处在于：其起始步骤应用的是最初从反转录病毒获得的 RNA 依赖性 DNA 多聚酶（反转录酶），通过延伸引物与 RNA 退火，将 RNA 转录成单链 cDNA（复制 DNA）。cDNA 内的核苷酸核序列随后按照标准 PCR 程序扩增。例如，在 CML 的 Ph'，*BCR* 基因的断裂点集中在断裂点聚集区的几个不同的内含子内，而 *ABL1* 基因的断裂点位于非常大的第一个内含子内。一些不同的嵌合 RNA 是由这些易位产生的，取决于断裂点位于 *BCR* 的部位。因此，RT-PCR 应用少数几个 PCR 引物覆盖不同部位的 *BCR* 断裂点，可以用来检测 CML 的 mRNA 易位。

对于检测组织活检标本中的染色体易位，PCR 和 RT-PCR 比其他技术具有几个方面的优点。由于在反应过程中序列呈指数扩增，只需要很少数量的肿瘤细胞，因此，当仅能获得有限的活检标本时，PCR 对于主要的诊断可能是一个有价值的辅助技术。从甲醛溶液固定的石蜡包埋组织中分离出来的 DNA 也能进行 PCR 扩增。此外，从这些组织中提取的 RNA 常常可以用于 RT-PCR 检查。然而，PCR 的最大优点或许是其高度的敏感性。染色体易位重组位点 DNA 的 PCR 扩增可以常规检测数十万个肿瘤细胞中的一个细胞。而嵌合 RNA 的 RT-PCR 能检测一百万个肿瘤细胞中的一个细胞（检测阈值只保留在一个反应中可以被常规分析的全部细胞核酸的量）。相反，组织学分析或细胞遗传学分析和 FISH 的敏感性的下限大约是 1/100。考虑到以 PCR 为基础检测染色体易位的敏感性，在对病人的微小残留病变进行治疗后，现在可在亚显微水平进行随访，这种检测水平可能远远低于常规组织学分析（见 1875 页）。

实时 PCR（real time PCR）技术的出现，可使反应过程中的 PCR 反应动力学受到监控，在微小残留病变的检测方面明显优于终点检测。在 PCR 反应开始时，所有的反应物充足而又新鲜，反应动力学有利于精确的双倍扩增（指数扩增），反应特异且准确。随着反应物的消耗，反应减慢，产物开始降解。常规的终点 PCR 检测是通过 PCR 产物凝胶分析终点或平台期的反应结果。实时 PCR 技术将荧光纳入反应，能够评价反应的指数扩增期。在"Taq-man"（应用生物系统，Applied Biosystems）实时 PCR，设计的探针与位于正向和反向两个引物之间的特异性靶基因序列退火。探针的 5'端具有高能呈报（reporter）染料，而 3'端具有低能"猝灭"（quencher）染料。在完整的探针中，呈报和猝灭靠得很近。当被光源激活后，呈报染料的散发被转移至猝灭染料，而能量释放受到抑制。DNA 多聚酶具有 5'端外切核酸酶活性，可以切除 Taq-man 探针，因为探针向 5'端引物的下游退火，并被 DNA 多聚酶的 5'端核酸酶活性切割。这就从猝灭剂中释放出呈报染料，并增加了呈报染料的荧光发射。荧光信号被仪器捕获并反复呈报。呈报信号数量的增加与样本产生的产物的数量成比例。在指数期开始时，起始模板的量越大，产生的荧光量也越大。因此，这项技术可以定量测量靶 DNA 或 RNA。光循环控制装置系统（Lightcycler system）（Roche）是一种实时 PCR 的替代技术，同样依赖于荧光共振能量传递。在这项技术中，设计了两个用不同荧光染料标记的寡核苷酸，用于与彼此相邻的靶点退火。当被光源激发后，能量从一种染料传递至另一种染料，产生能或光，可被仪器监测。这两种技术已经用于检测具有染色体易位的肿瘤细胞和监测治疗后的肿瘤负荷（见微小残留病变一节）。

染色体易位以外的染色体异常
Chromosomal abnormalities other than chromosomal translocations

虽然不常见，并且一般很少经得起纯粹的分子诊断技术的检验，但是易位以外的反复发生的染色体异常也是不同肿瘤恶性表型的原因，而且可以用作诊断标记物。染色体倒位（chromosomal inversions）涉及一小段染色体内的断裂，伴有 180° 的重排，以致出现染色体片段方向上的颠倒。这些片段可能是染色体臂的任何部位，或可能是它们在着丝粒的任何一端的伴有断裂点的臂间倒位，就像 M4Eo 的 inv16（伴有嗜酸性细胞增多的急性髓性单核细胞白血病）一样。倒位在功能上与易位类似，表现在其变化发生在某一断裂点附近基因的结构或活性上。染色体缺失（chromosomal deletions）可能来自整个染色体的丢失，仅仅留下一个同系物（单体性，monosomy），或是整个染色体臂的丢失，或是一个染色体臂中间隙片段的丢失，就像与脊髓发育不良相关的 5q 综合征一样。缺失经常有不同的断裂点，通常导致缺失片段内肿瘤抑制基因丢失而致癌的后果。整个染色体的复制（如 12 三体，大约见于 15% 的慢性淋巴细胞白血病）[80] 或染色体内不同区域的复制也是某些肿瘤的特征。等臂染色体（isochromosomes）是复制和缺失的组合。在这些染色体中，一个臂缺失，另一个臂则复制，导致一个染色体臂的三体伴另外一个臂的单体，例如肝脾 γδT 细胞淋巴瘤的 7q 等臂染色体[81]。环状染色体（ring chromosomes）是缺失和易位的组合，其中断裂和重接发生于一个染色体的两个臂之间，接近染色体的两端（或端粒）。额外环状染色体（supernumerary ring chromosomes）是高分化脂肪肉瘤或非典型性脂肪瘤性肿瘤的特征，含有 12 号染色体长臂的扩增[82,83]。扩增，或染色体片段的串联重复，可能在染色体内发现，表现为均匀着色区（homogeneously stainingregions，HSR）或许多自由复制的染色体外片段（所谓的"双微染色体"，double minute chromosomes）。临床上应用扩增突出的例子是证明神经母细胞瘤累及 *MYCN* 基因的 HSR 或双微染色体扩增，以及证明乳腺浸润性导管癌的 *HER2/NEU*（*ERBB2*）扩增，将在下文讨论。

已经描述的许多类型的染色体异常，或多数病例的一种特殊类型的异常，可以共同出现在一个肿瘤中；而且，不同寻常的组合作为某些肿瘤亚型的特征已经日益得到公认，而不是出现任何单一的异常。肾上皮性肿瘤的 Heidelberg 分类阐明了细胞遗传学分析如何精炼和增强了旧的形态学分类体系[84]。多年以来，具有颗粒状胞浆的肾肿瘤被归类为透明细胞癌的颗粒性变型。临床病理学研究、免疫组织化学和细胞遗传学分析表明，这一组肿瘤实际上是由嗜酸细胞瘤、某些嫌色细胞瘤、透明细胞癌、集合管癌、乳头状肾细胞癌和上皮样血管肌肉脂肪瘤组成的[85]（也见第12章）。同样，乳头状肾肿瘤被归类为常见的肾（透明）细胞肿瘤，尽管其具有独特的形态学特征。细胞遗传学研究已证实这样一个概念，即这些肿瘤在生物学上是独特的肿瘤，并且已经证实它们之中存在一贯的不同方式的染色体异常[86]。90% 以上的透明细胞癌有染色体 3p 缺失以及其他异常[87-89]，乳头状肾细胞癌有 7 号、17 号和 20 号染色体三体而没有 3p 缺失[90]（图 32.6）。嫌色细胞癌是亚二倍体（不足染色体的全部补体）肿瘤，伴有 1、2、6、10、13、17 和 21 号染色体杂合性缺失[91,92]。最近，根据 *TFE* 基因家族融合已经确定了易位相关性儿童肾细胞癌的新的亚型[92a]。通过细胞遗传学种类归类的肾细胞肿瘤已经阐明了这些肿瘤的诊断形态学特征[93]，而且这种分类方式正在得以澄清，在常规切片中见到的严格的形态学标准通常足以能够将这些肿瘤在生物学上分为相关的组别[66]。

除易位以外的检测染色体异常的技术
Techniques to detect chromosomal abnormalities other than translocations

常规细胞遗传学分析或 FISH 通常是检测总的染色体异常而不是易位，如扩增、缺失和复制。FISH 应用于扩增相对容易，并且已得到广泛应用。检测缺失和复制需要小心，因为非常可能出现假阴性和假阳性的人工假象，后者由于探针未能进入靶序列或由于假的背景信号造成的。通过在杂交中加入额外的探针作为内对照，这个问题可以得到部分解决，如设计一个辨认与缺失位点相邻区域的探针或着丝粒探针。FISH 技术的改良版本也可用来检测这些异常。光谱核型分析（spectral karyotyping，SKY）是一项可以进行综合细胞遗传学分析的技术。除了几个荧光标记的 FISH 探针以外，还混合有许多对每一个染色体特异的探针来与细胞分裂中期的染色体杂交。这些探针应用不同比例的荧光标记物分别进行标记[94]。组合的杂交标记物赋予 24 个染色体中每个染色体以独特的颜色。这项技术对于检查复杂的染色体异常特别有用，包括多个染色体之间的易位，而这些易位通过 G 带技术（Giemsa-banding techniques）却难以描绘[95,96]。多重 FISH（multiplexer FISH，M-FISH）[97] 和复合二元比例标记（combined binary ratio labeling，COBRA）[98] 是类似的技术，应用组合的荧光进行不同的标记。这些技术昂贵，花费时间，需要活的细胞，因而主要是作为研究工具而不是诊断方法。

比较基因组杂交（comparative genomic hybridization，CGH）是另外一项用来检测缺失和复制的技术[99-101]，它的优点是可以用于冰冻和石蜡包埋的肿瘤组织以及新鲜组织[102]。在 CGH 中，DNA 是从组织样本和非肿瘤细胞群中提取出来的。将这两种 DNA 分别标记，并与来自任何正常人体细胞的分裂中期染色体一起杂交。肿瘤的染色体复制或扩增区域将会通过切片上的颜色转变来显示，即在正常分裂中期染色体的相应区域染色转变成肿瘤 DNA 荧光标记物的染色。肿瘤染色体缺失可以得到相反的结果：分裂中期染色体相应区域的颜色转变为从正常 DNA 制备的探针标记物的颜色。这项技术可以用于从组织微切割中获得的少量细胞，以及通过 PCR 扩增的无偏的整个基因组[103-105]。CGH 对于基因组不平衡来说是一个有用的检测工具，但是对于易位、倒位或倍体改变等应用价值有限。

在 CGH 阵列（array CGH）中，标记的肿瘤和非

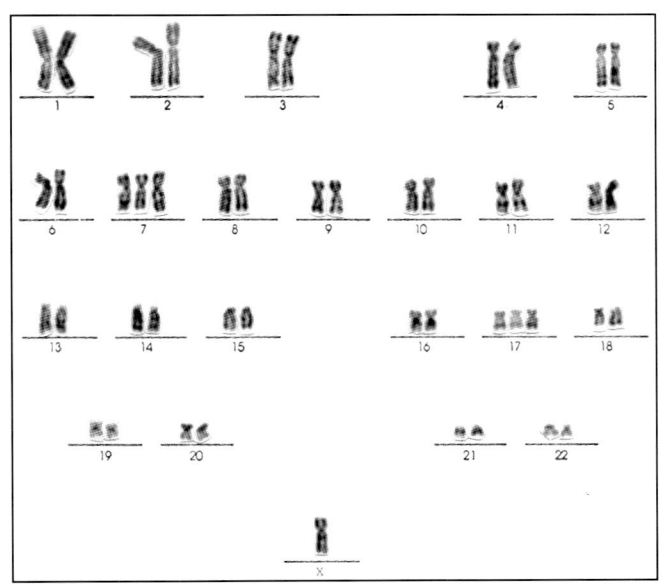

图32.6 乳头状肾细胞癌的G带（Giemsa-banded）显著核型，显示7号和17号染色体三体以及一个性染色体丢失。

肿瘤细胞 DNA 是杂交的 DNA 微阵列，而不是分裂中期的延伸。每一点相应的荧光强度是通过图像分析计算出来的，反映了 DNA 复制数的不同。分辨率是由克隆大小和阵列密度决定的。在细菌人工染色体（bacterial artificial chromosome，BAC）阵列中，克隆呈点状分布于载玻片上，分辨可达 1 个兆碱基（megabase）。在寡核苷酸阵列中，寡核苷酸呈点状分布于载玻片上或原位直接合成，分辨率可以增加至 1 kb。除了肿瘤染色体位点的明确丢失和获得外[106]，CGH 阵列已经证明，人类基因组基因复制数量的差异比预期的要大得多[107-109]。复制数量的差异可能与基因表达有关，也可能与人类表型的变异和对疾病的易感性有关。将来，诊断细胞遗传学实验室有可能将常规的核型分析与分子细胞遗传学技术结合起来，以增强分辨率和细化疾病的分类。

作为诊断性肿瘤标记物的亚显微突变
Submicroscopic mutations as diagnostic tumor markers

微卫星重复或短的串联重复是单核苷酸、双核苷酸、三核苷酸或四核苷酸序列的串联重复（例如 CA 在 DNA 的一条链上，而相反的 GT 在 DNA 另外一条链上）散在分布于整个基因组，它们没有已知的功能[110]。这些重复序列的位置在不同的个体中是保守的，但在特定位点上重复的数目是不同的，可从几个到数百个。微卫星一般稳定地由父母遗传给孩子，而个体在任何特殊位点重复的数目一般是杂合的。在人体一生中，所有正常细胞是否能够保持同样数目的重复尚不清楚。微卫星重复的两种改变与肿瘤相关。在肿瘤中特别常见的一种改变是：由于含有重复序列的 DNA 位点缺失而造成整个位点的丢失。这类丢失只能可靠地评估患者可疑位点重复数目是否是杂合的，在这个过程中，一个染色体上的一组重复丢失，因此称为杂合性丢失（loss of heterozygosity，LOH）。从功能的角度来看，肿瘤中 LOH（以及较大的缺失，就此而言）的多数例子似乎是指与肿瘤抑制基因紧密连锁的基因缺失，其编码蛋白通过某种方式帮助抑制的细胞生长。其次，这些病例中的非缺失性肿瘤抑制等位基因还必须被灭活，常常通过基因的小的突变来完成。这些突变包含一个或两个碱基对的缺失，后者可改变编码序列的阅读框架，或包含可产生无义突变的碱基取代（点突变），导致蛋白合成提前终止，或可产生有缺陷蛋白的错义突变。缺失和肿瘤抑制基因失活的复合效应与其他促癌突变和表遗传学改变共同作用，导致肿瘤细胞的无控制性生长。

微卫星重复的改变可以通过 DNA 的 PCR 扩增来检测，应用的引物与侧翼重复的独特序列互补。PCR 产物通过凝胶电泳分析，在普通凝胶的相应位置上出现不同大小片段的条带（或在毛细管凝胶上显示为峰值）。假如病人是杂合性的，杂合性缺失的主要所见是一个条带缺失，而另外一个条带保留，与出现在正常组织分析中的两个条带形成对此。杂合性缺失分析被用作辨认预后标记物的一种工具，例如间变性少突胶质细胞瘤的 1p 和 19q 丢失[111,112]，或结肠癌的 18q 丢失[113,114]。

在肿瘤细胞微卫星重复中可能发现的第二个改变是：出现重复成分的数目增加或减少，这种数目的增加或减少与在患者正常细胞同一位点检测到的重复数目有关，称为微卫星不稳定性（microsatellite instability，MSI）。这种改变最先在遗传突变的患者中发现，表现为 DNA 错配修复基因 hMSH2、hMLH1、hMSH6 和 hPMS2，这些错配修复基因与遗传性非息肉病结肠癌（hereditary non-polyposis colon carcinoma，HNPCC）有关，后者也叫 Lynch 综合征[115]。Lynch 综合征是一种常染色体显性综合征，其特征是肿瘤（结直肠、子宫内膜、胃、卵巢、肾和皮肤）早期发作（45 岁以前），各部位肿瘤同时或异时发生，并有微卫星不稳定性。没有正常 DNA 修复蛋白，DNA 序列的复制错误在每一次复制循环后没有得到校正，而且错误复制的 DNA 模板被固定于基因组上。微卫星重复特别容易重现扩大或减少重复数目的错误，因为生长的 DNA 链上的核苷酸可能与整个重复区域模板链上的互补核苷酸错配，于是在模板链（导致重复数目的减少）或在生长链（导致重复数目的增多）上产生了非配对重复的小环。重复数目的改变不是肿瘤形成的直接原因，但是错配修复基因的缺陷易于获得癌基因和肿瘤抑制基因的突变，这在肿瘤的转化中具有直接的作用[116]。

错配修复基因突变的种系检测昂贵而又费力。辨认 Lynch 综合征危险家族的标准已经确立，包括微卫星不稳定性检测[117,118]。为了筛选微卫星不稳定性表型的癌组织，应从肿瘤和非肿瘤组织（冰冻或石蜡包埋组织）中分别提取 DNA。美国国家癌症研究所[119]推荐至少在 5 个不同的微卫星位点进行 PCR 扩增。与正常组织 DNA 比较时，肿瘤 DNA 的 PCR 产物出现额外的条带是不稳定性的标记（图 32.7）。推荐的微卫星重复位点出现 40% 或 40% 以上的不稳定性肿瘤被分类为高频微卫星不稳定表型（MSI-high）。这些患者要求助于种系突变分析。对于检测错配修复基因表达的丢失，免疫组化分析与 MSI PCR 分析可能有互补作用[117]。

一个或更多位点微卫星重复不稳定性也可在少部分（10%～20%）各种不同类型的肿瘤中见到，这些患者并不知道他们具有 DNA 错配修复种系缺陷[120]。例如，大约 15% 的结肠癌具有 MSI-high 表型。MSI-high 癌较常位于脾曲近侧，而且组织学表现为低分化黏液性癌，伴有致密的淋巴细胞浸润（也见第 9 章）[121]。这些肿瘤

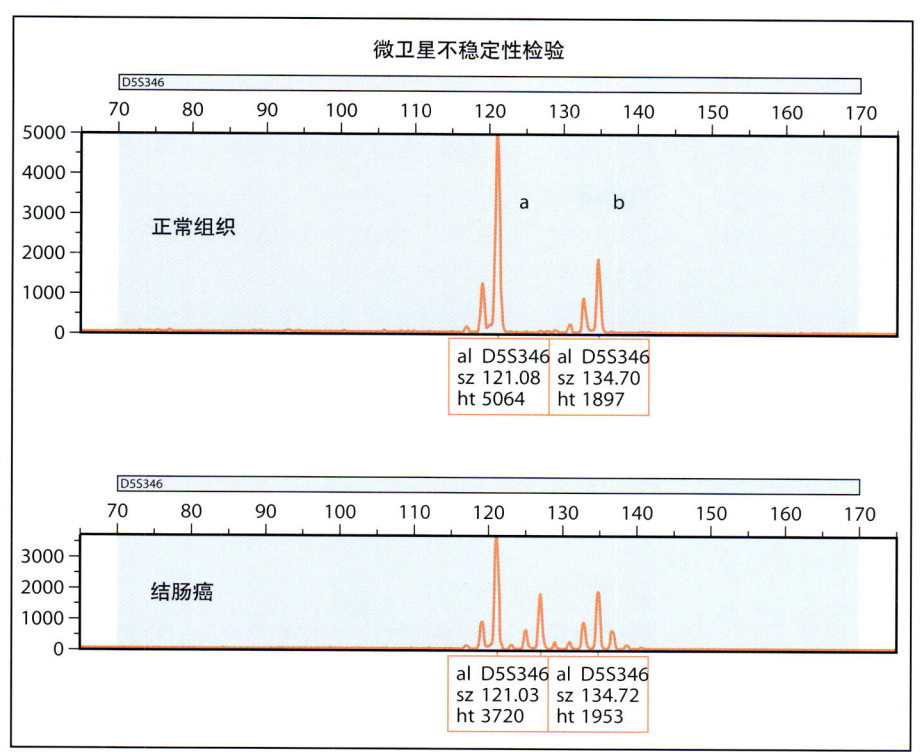

图32.7 来自结肠癌和邻近正常组织DNA的PCR扩增,应用荧光标记的二核苷酸微卫星重复(D5S346)引物,并用毛细管凝胶电泳分析。从正常组织获得的峰的模式来自两个等位基因a和b。结肠癌,在127和137碱基对有等位基因替换,很可能分别代表等位基因a和b的扩展。

大多数与HNPCC/Lynch的综合征的特征性种系突变无关,而是代之以由于启动子甲基化基因沉默而形成的错配修复蛋白缺陷[122]。MSI-high结直肠癌患者的生存期比分期相配的MSI稳定(MSI-stable)的结直肠癌患者的生存期长[123],但对以5-氟尿嘧啶为基础的辅助化疗无效[124, 25]。

少量核苷酸的点突变、缺失和插入是癌基因活化和肿瘤抑制基因失活的主要机制。在某些突变的例子中,在具有这种突变的个别肿瘤中,突变局限于几个部位,例如在原癌基因 *RAS* 家族3个成员中是12、13和61号密码子[126]。较常见的是,突变集中在一个基因的特殊位点,例如在肿瘤抑制基因 *p53* 的5～8号外显子[127]。小的核苷酸改变是酪氨酸激酶基因激活突变的特征,几种不同类型的肿瘤标记已经被用于靶向小分子治疗的发展过程[128]。酪氨酸激酶是催化来自携能ATP分子的γ磷酸基团向多肽内的酪氨酸残基转化的酶,而且与关键信号机制有关[129]。受体蛋白酪氨酸激酶是跨膜受体,由一个细胞外配体结合区、一个跨膜区和一个细胞内激酶区组成,例如KIT和PDGFRA。配体结合导致受体同源二聚体化、酪氨酸激酶的自动磷酸化激活以及下游基质的磷酸化。这些激酶的致癌突变包括点突变、读框内缺失(in-frame deletion)和插入,并且在缺乏配子的情况下,所有这些突变一般均可诱导激酶活性,产生活化激酶的癌蛋白。

KIT 突变大约发生于85%～90%的胃肠道间质瘤(GIST),在这些肿瘤的生长和存活中起着重要的作用[130-137]。*KIT* 突变最常集中于近膜区(11号外显子)(图32.8)或在细胞外区域的9号外显子。后者的特征是与小肠GIST有关。不到10%的GIST具有 *PDGFRA* 替代性突变,*PDGFRA* 是与 *KIT* 密切相关的受体酪氨酸激酶基因。致癌性 *PDGFRA* 突变常常发生于激酶区,但是如同KIT近膜区和细胞外区的突变一样,可导致配体非依赖性酶的活性以及MAP激酶、AKT和STAT3信号通路

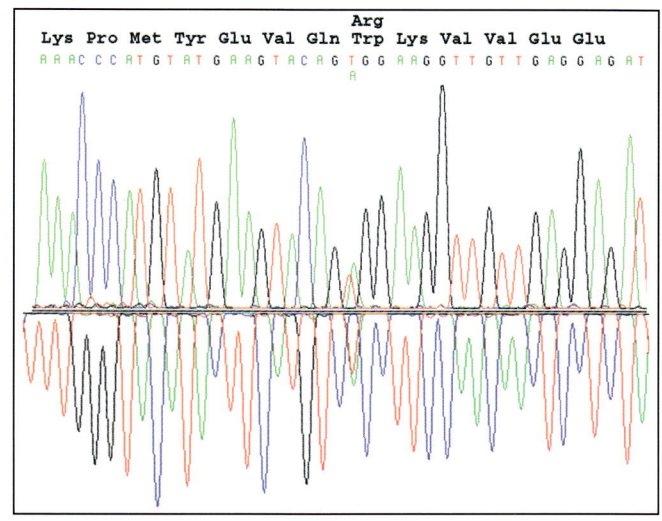

图32.8 自动序列分析。胃肠间质瘤KIT 11号外显子序列电泳图。正向和反向序列分别位于基线上方和下方。*KIT* 基因从T到A的错义突变导致精氨酸替代色氨酸。

的下游激活[138]。*PDGFRA* 突变的 GIST 发生于胃、肠系膜或网膜，与以梭形细胞形态学为主的 *KIT* 突变的 GIST 相比，较常出现上皮样细胞形态学[138-141]。重要的是，酪氨酸激酶抑制剂甲磺酸伊马替尼，通过抑制 ATP 与 ABL 酪氨酸激酶的结合，可以有效地治疗慢性髓性白血病，它还具有抑制 KIT 和 PDGFRA 活性的作用。然而，GIST 突变对甲磺酸伊马替尼具有不同的反应。一项伊马替尼治疗转移性 GIST 的 II 期随机试验发现，伴有 11 号外显子 *KIT* 突变的患者比那些 9 号外显子突变或没有突变的患者具有较好的部分反应率 [83.5% (n = 85) 对 48.7% (n = 23, p = 0.0006) 对 0% (n = 9, p < 0.0001)]，而伴有 D842V 激酶活性环状突变的 *PDGFRA* 反应患者没有反应，GIST 的分子亚分类尚有争论[136]。

表皮生长因子受体（EGFR）是另外一种酪氨酸激酶受体，通过 EGFR 配体的过度表达、EGFR 的扩增或突变激活而与肿瘤形成有关[142]。许多非小细胞性肺癌中有 EGFR 过度表达，促使应用酪氨酸激酶抑制剂吉非替尼（gefitinib）或埃洛替尼（erlotinib）进行临床试验[143-147]。

只有 10%～20% 的患者出现明显的肿瘤消退，倾向于发生在女性、从不吸烟者、东亚人以及有腺癌而不是其他非小细胞性癌组织学改变的患者。随后，*EGFR* 基因测序显示：81% 伴有临床反应的患者具有错义点突变、小的缺失或酪氨酸激酶的框内缺失[142,148-150]。因此认为 *EGFR* 突变可以导致结构的变化，从而引起致癌活性的增加以及对于酪氨酸激酶抑制剂敏感性的增加。在癌症发病机制中，突变激酶具有重要性的其他例子包括真性红细胞增多症、原发性血小板增多症和特发性骨髓纤维化的非受体酪氨酸激酶 *JAK2* V617F 突变[151-153]、系统性肥大细胞增多症的 *KIT* 点突变[154-158] 以及 *BRAF* 的 T1799A（V600E）点突变，*BRAF* 是一种见于恶性黑色素瘤和甲状腺乳头状癌的 seronine/threonine 激酶[159-162]。实验室检测的这些突变在临床上可以用于诊断和（或）做出治疗决定。

小的突变可以通过多种技术检测。由整个基因扩增而来的 PCR 产物的序列分析有可能比较容易得到高通量的序列。肿瘤常常是特定突变的杂合，因此，实际上分析的是肿瘤中正常和突变 DNA 片段的混合物。此外，多数肿瘤组织混有不同数量的正常细胞，这就进一步地遮盖了突变的证据，并且降低了序列分析的敏感性。热测序（pyrosequencing）是一种较为敏感的测序方法，可以用于短 DNA 序列[163]。这项技术用于串联酶反应，将在 DNA 合成过程中释放的焦磷酸盐转换成可见光，这与结合的核苷酸数目成比例。将四种核苷酸的一种加于测序反应中。如果这种核苷酸与引物核酸链上的下一个碱基互补，就可释放出焦磷酸盐分子，并在 ATP 硫酸化酶的作用下转化成 ATP。这个反应可为荧光素酶转化为荧光素乃至氧化荧光素提供能量，并产生与 ATP 数量成比例的可见光。光信号被电荷耦合装置（CCD）相机捕获，在"热解图"中表现为峰值。在反应中加入两个胞嘧啶可以产生两倍于加入一个胞嘧啶的光，并且成比例地反映在相应的峰值上。随着热测序的继续，互补 DNA 链延伸，并且序列可通过一系列的峰值来读取。筛查基因片段突变和检测许多（但不是全部）小的突变的替代技术包括单链构象多态性（SSCP）[164]，变性梯度凝胶电泳（DGGE）[165] 和变性高效液相色谱（DHPLC）[166]。这些技术是建立在突变 PCR 产物在分离矩阵上的迁移率改变的基础之上。

抗原受体重排
Antigen receptor rearrangements

非 Hodgkin 淋巴瘤和淋巴细胞性白血病的原始诊断取决于将肿瘤性 B 细胞、T 细胞或少见的 NK 细胞的克隆性增生与正常淋巴细胞的反应性多克隆性扩展区分开来。抗原受体基因内的 DNA 重组可被用作检测组织标本中淋巴细胞克隆性的标记物。抗原受体基因含有组成免疫球蛋白和 T 细胞受体的 7 个多肽亚单位编码序列[167,168]。其中三个亚单位，即重链（IgH）、κ 轻链（Igκ）和 λ 轻链（Igλ），结合形成由 B 细胞合成的免疫球蛋白。剩下的 4 个亚单位，即 α、β、γ 和 δ 亚单位，成对结合形成 T 细胞表达的 αβ 或 γδ T 细胞受体。真正的 NK 细胞并不表达抗原受体，其抗原受体基因也不进行重组。

抗原受体基因拥有共同的整体结构。除了 B 细胞和 T 细胞外，种系细胞和所有体细胞的每一个基因都含有被称之为可变区（V 区，variable）、连接区（J 区，joining）和恒定区（C 区，constant）的多套基因片段，某些基因具有额外的非常短的片段，称之为差异区（D 区，diversity）。在早期 B 或 T 细胞分化中，这些基因片段发生染色体内重组，伴有插入序列的切除，因此，每一个 V、D 和 J 区的一个成员在基因内连接成一体（图 32.9A）。由这种 DNA 重排产生的序列与下游 C 片段一起转录成 mRNA。RNA 的剪接产生一个连续的 V-（D）-J-C 编码序列，从而形成翻译成蛋白质的模板。V-（D）-J 连接的组合多样性是诸多抗原受体结构变异的原因，因此，这些受体对于不同抗原具有特异性。V、D 和 J 片段末端不同数目核苷酸对的缺失进一步增加了这种多样性，随后将随机的核苷酸对在连接前加入到这些末端内[169,170]。这些附加的核苷酸组成了所谓的"N 区域"，其长度可以是 0 到大约 30 个核苷酸。其结果是，V-N-

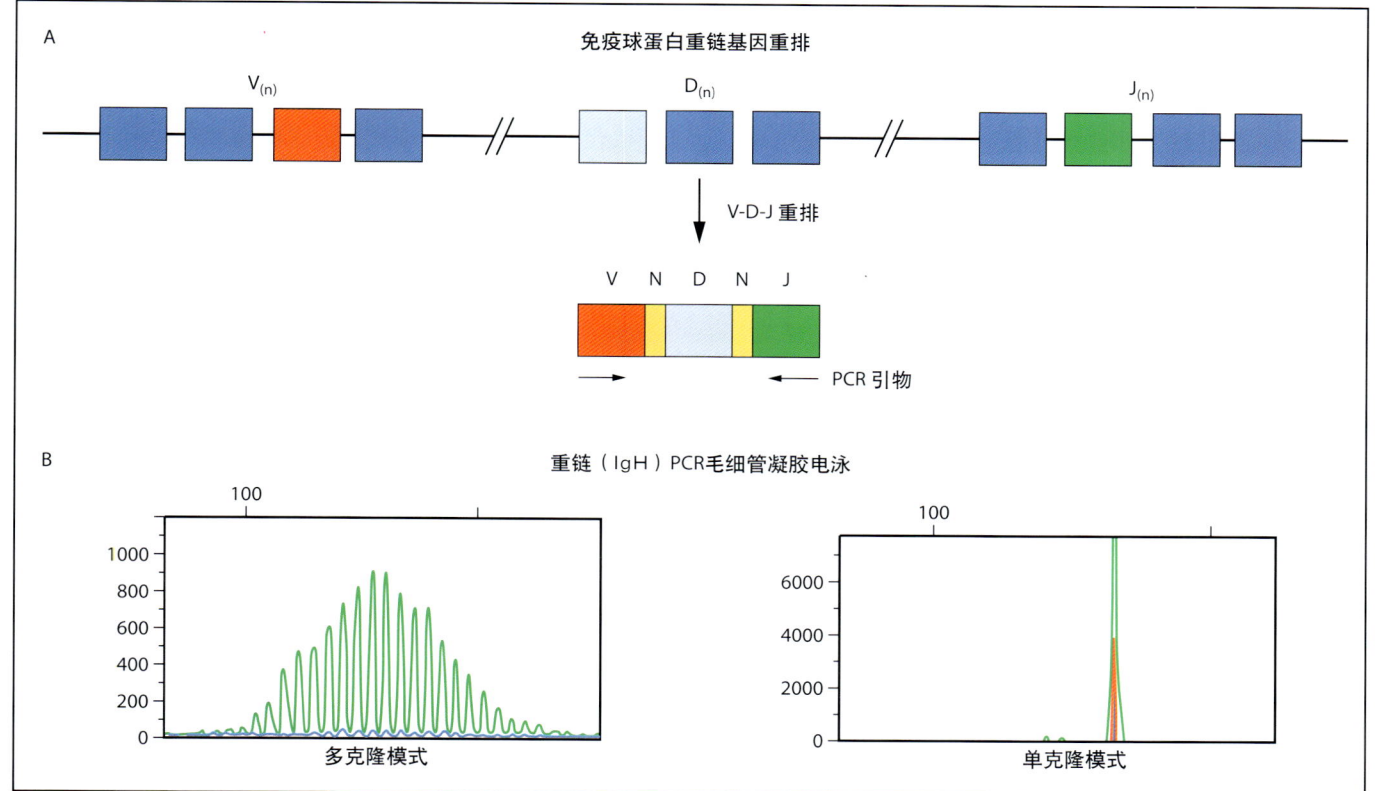

图32.9 （A）免疫球蛋白重链基因图解,显示V区、D区和J区基因片段的种系位置。基因重排后片段的结构和PCR引物的位置在下面显示。（B）应用荧光标记的PCR引物进行重链（IgH）PCR检查,并用毛细管凝胶电泳分析。X轴是PCR产物的大小,用碱基对表示。Y轴是荧光单位。含有多克隆B细胞的反应性组织产生了正态分布的PCR产物。B细胞淋巴瘤产生一个突出的单峰。

(D-N)-J连接成为重排抗原受体基因和相应蛋白区域的高度变异区域。这些高度变异的蛋白区域位于组装受体的抗原结合袋内,对于确定抗原特异性非常重要。此外,当B细胞通过淋巴结的生发中心时,免疫球蛋白基因(但不是T细胞受体)在重排的V片段内积聚点突变,这也是造成免疫球蛋白结构多样化的过程。不过,在重排发生后抗原受体内总的DNA序列是相对稳定的。

抗原受体基因重排是一种高度易错的过程。核苷酸的随机获得或丢失是不受精确控制的,可能引起V-N-(D-N)-J连接部位密码突变的终止,或超出时相的移动下游阅读框,以至于终止的密码相遇或生成无功能的C片段序列。因此,许多重排的抗原受体基因是无效的。然而,每一个淋巴细胞在完成有效抗原受体基因重排时具有两次机会,由于每个基因的两个等位基因都能重排,尽管如果第一个等位基因有效的话,第二个等位基因重排受到抑制。两个等位基因重排都不成功将导致凋亡。

抗原受体重排还有层次。在B细胞的发育中,*IGH*基因是最先重排的,随后是*IGK*。如果*IGK*等位基因重排无效,则*IGL*基因发生重排[171,172]。T细胞受体基因重排的层次尚不清楚,但δ似乎最先重排,接着是γ、β,最后是α重排[173-175]。

虽然当为诊断目的而分析这些基因时,上述抗原受体基因重排细节可以解释许多现象,而且对于解释结果来说也是重要的,但是这些基因用于诊断的基本原理是：重排抗原受体基因的DNA序列标记已经发生重排的淋巴细胞。这个标记物可传递给这种细胞的子代,因此,其对于含有重排的由原来淋巴细胞形成的任何B细胞或T细胞的克隆都是高度特异的。

检测抗原受体重排的技术
Techniques to detect antigen receptor rearrangements

Southern印迹杂交（blot hybridization）是通过抗原受体重排检测淋巴细胞克隆性的提供信息最多的方法,依赖于分析重排基因内V和J片段的结构（也就是哪一个V片段与哪一个J片段相连）。由于重排,位于种系形式基因V和J片段重组之间的限制性位点将会丢失,在重组J片段的附近将会出现一个新的限制性位点,取决于哪一个 V 片段与其相连（D 片段较小，很少含有用于分析的限制性核酸内切酶的限制性位点）。这些变化意味着来自重排基因的限制性片段（通过限制性核酸内切酶消化而产生）的长度与非重排种系 DNA 片段不同，而且对于一个特定的重排来讲，其片段长度也有不同。这些不同通过应用一个和有时两个限制性核酸内切酶消化从标本中提取的总 DNA 来评估，选择的核酸内切酶可以剪切在 J 片段侧翼位点的 DNA。消化及转移到膜上的 DNA 经过凝胶电泳后，分布于膜上的 DNA 片段与含有 J 片段内和附近序列的探针杂交，适合检测一个或另外一个抗原受体基因。对于非淋巴组织，在杂交膜的放射自显影图像中将会见到一个代表未重排抗原受体 DNA 的条带。如果在起始的物质中有一个足够大的淋巴细胞克隆，在放射性自显影图像中将会出现一个位置有些不同的条带，表示在这个克隆中有一致的基因重排。此外，反应性淋巴组织分析只能在未重排的位置产生一个条带，尽管在标本内含有许多淋巴细胞。这个条带由间质细胞、内皮细胞、巨噬细胞和各种 T 细胞或 B 淋巴细胞的未重排的等位基因衍生而来。多克隆淋巴细胞中个别抗原受体基因的形形色色的重排通常并不足以在放射自显影图像中发现。至少 1%~5% 的细胞有同样的 V 和 J 片段的构象才能应用这种方法检测[176]。

为了评估 B 细胞淋巴瘤或白血病的标本，通常要分析 DNA 的 *IGH* 和 *IGK* 基因的重排，因为能够检测到最无效的重排，即使已有 *IGL* 基因重排的细胞也会携带与其他轻链未能成功重排的痕迹。某些 B 细胞肿瘤，值得注意的是 B 系 ALL，起源于 *IGK* 基因重排之前的细胞，因此，将会只有 *IGH* 重排。已经有少数肿瘤病例具有轻链基因重排而没有 *IGH* 重排的报道。

同多数 T 细胞一样，绝大多数 T 细胞肿瘤含有 α 和 β T 细胞受体基因重排。α 基因 J 片段在 DNA 内分布的距离太大，不能方便地应用常规 Southern 印迹杂交方法分析。β 基因可以分析，当怀疑 T 淋巴细胞增生性病变时，应该常规检测克隆重排。在罕见的表达 γδ 受体的肿瘤中可以分析 δ 基因。后者在表达 αβ 受体的肿瘤中没有作用，因为 δ 基因位于 α 基因内，当 α 基因重排时，δ 基因有缺失。在 γδ T 细胞肿瘤中可以分析 γ T 细胞受体。后者在表达 αβ 的肿瘤中也经常发生重排。然而，至少在肿瘤细胞中，任何抗原受体基因的重排可能都不具有谱系特异性，以致重排可见于一个特定谱系细胞正常情况下并不表达的受体基因[177-179]。在 B 系 ALL 中，γ T 细胞受体基因尤其是这样。

Southern 印迹检测抗原受体基因费力且较慢。其主要优点在于：原则上可以检测所有应用的抗原受体基因重排。PCR 是一种快速的替代方法，与 Southern 印迹杂交不同，它可以用于从固定组织中提取的 DNA 片段[180-182]。这些是显著的优点，因此，在多数临床实验室，PCR 已经取代了 Southern 印迹。用于这项技术的克隆标记是在 V-N-(D-N)-J 连接处的序列，而不是用于 Southern 印迹杂交的 V 和 J 片段的构象。序列扩增是应用成对的引物完成的，构建的引物与特殊基因内 V 片段和 J 片段中保留的核苷酸序列互补（图 32.9B）。PCR 产物通过凝胶电泳分析评估产物的大小（主要在诸如伴有 D 片段的 *IGH* 基因内，以及 V 和 J 片段末端的长而高度变异的序列）[183,84]或筛查序列（主要在诸如 *TCRG* 的基因内，其中没有 D 片段，而且 V 和 J 片段末端之间的序列少有变异）[182,185-187]。从多克隆群中扩增而来的 PCR 产物[188]在凝胶中表现为不清楚的成片的条带，而来自单克隆群的产物却表现为分散的条带。PCR 分析的缺点是：某些 V 片段经常缺乏引物与之退火的保留的序列。例如，应用一组引物在 *IGH* 基因中只能检测到大约 60% 的重排。欧洲实验室联盟已经设计并优化了伴有单个共有序列 J 引物的多个 V 区的引物，能够检测通过 Southern 印迹分析而被克隆的 86% 的样本，此时 PCR 产物可以通过凝胶毛细管凝胶电泳分析[188]。PCR 在方便、花费和速度上优于 Southern 印迹杂交，但受假阴性率限制。

肿瘤标本的转录谱
Transcriptional profiling of tumor specimens

肿瘤的转录谱或 mRNA 水平的基因组广度测量最近受到了广泛的关注，它作为一种单独分析的平台，能够评估受肿瘤转化影响的大量细胞通路。与本章描述的所有其他标记物不同，这个方法应用的标记物不是 DNA 的突变或其他改变，而实际上是来自任何基因的 RNA 转录水平的差异。这种研究的依据是：细胞和组织的所有特征最终都是基因表达的产物。因此基因表达的综合性描述应该可以提供非常正确的方法用于肿瘤分类及预测治疗反应，并且应该可以确定治疗干预的生物学通路。有许多种方法可以用于鉴定 RNA 水平的不同。最受关注的方法涉及 DNA 芯片（DNA microarrays）的杂交。已经发明了两种形式的芯片。一种是高密度寡核苷酸芯片（high-density oligonucleotide chip），类似于用来检测基因点突变的芯片，只是寡核苷酸代表不同的基因。长度为 25~60 个核苷酸的寡核苷酸被点布于玻片上或在聚硅氧烷胶片上原位合成。基因组广度高密度芯片是比较聚焦的芯片或定做的芯片，可从 Affymetrix、Santa Clara、CA 买到（www.affymetrix.com）。第二种类型的芯片是由 cDNA 构建的，由 cDNA 克隆插入的 PCR 扩增产物组成，可以点布于载玻片上（图 32.10）。几家公司出售能执行点样的机器人，允许研究者设计和建立他们自己的芯片。这个平台相对便宜，但在技术上可能具有挑战性。

应用寡核苷酸芯片（oligonucleotide chips）或 cDNA 芯片（cDNA microarrays），RNA 是从组织标本中提取的，转化成用生物素和（或）荧光染料标记的 cDNA 或 cRNA，然后在芯片上杂交。共聚焦激光扫描仪测量每一个寡核苷酸或 cDNA 位置的荧光强度。管理和处理成千上万的寡核苷酸和 cDNA 杂交数据是令人畏缩的问题（图 32.11），而围绕处理和解释芯片杂交原始结果而设计的计算机软件这项任务，则正在形成生物信息学领域的一个特殊分支。当这些结果与临床情况联系起来时，这项分析工作会变得更加复杂，要求患者和组织相对同源，评价组织，并独立验证上述所见。

作为原理的证据，基因表达芯片数据容易区分急性髓性白血病和急性淋巴母细胞性白血病[189]。在另一项研究中，未经指导（并不知道临床终点）的一组基因表达数据与儿科急性淋巴细胞性白血病的细胞遗传学亚分类相关（T-ALL、E2A-PBX1、BCR-ABL1、TEL-RUNX1、MLL 重排和超二倍体 > 50 染色体），并通过其独特的表达谱鉴定了另外一个亚群[190]。而且，在个别白血病亚型中，特殊的表达谱可以用于预测复发。基因表达谱可将弥漫性大 B 细胞淋巴瘤在分子学和临床上分为两个独特的亚型：一个亚型类似于正常生发中心 B 细胞（生发中心 B 细胞样），一个亚型类似于体外活化的外周血 B 细胞（活化 B 细胞样）[191-194]。未经治疗的滤泡性淋巴瘤的基因表达谱可以预测这个临床上异源性疾病的生存[28]。令人惊奇的发现是，预测信号通过非恶性肿瘤浸润性免疫细胞可以反映基因表达。在实体肿瘤，未经指导的分析转录谱已经确定了临床上独特的五种亚型的乳腺癌[195-200]。能够预测没有转移的生存和总体生存的乳腺癌的基因表达信号也已确定，并且已进行了进一步的验证[201,202]。

从最近相关文献中的大量小样本研究中可以清楚地看到，转录谱可以明显改变人类癌症的分类以及我们对其基本生物学的理解。然而，由于组织需要特殊处理，缺乏标准化，以及费用问题，转录谱技术进入实验室的速度缓慢，替代的结合这些发现的方法已经可行。例如，在弥漫性大 B 细胞淋巴瘤，RT-PCR 能够定量测量从前通过转录谱鉴定的 6 个基因的表达[203]，或应用小量免疫组化组合[204] 就足以能够预测总体生存。同样，应用有限数量的、根据基因表达资料选择的生物标记物进行免疫组化检查，能够确定乳腺癌的亚型[205-208]。这些方法多半可行，从长远观点看一般可以应用。

分子生物学标记物在诊断和预后方面的特殊应用
Special applications of molecular biologic markers in diagnosis and prognosis

微小残留疾病　Minimal residual disease

临床完全缓解的患者可能有多达 10^{10} 个残留的细胞，通过常规细胞形态学无法检测，有时候可能导致复发。确认有隐匿肿瘤细胞、随后有复发危险的患者，有助于早期进行毒性较低的治疗。PCR 或 RT-PCR 是用于检测

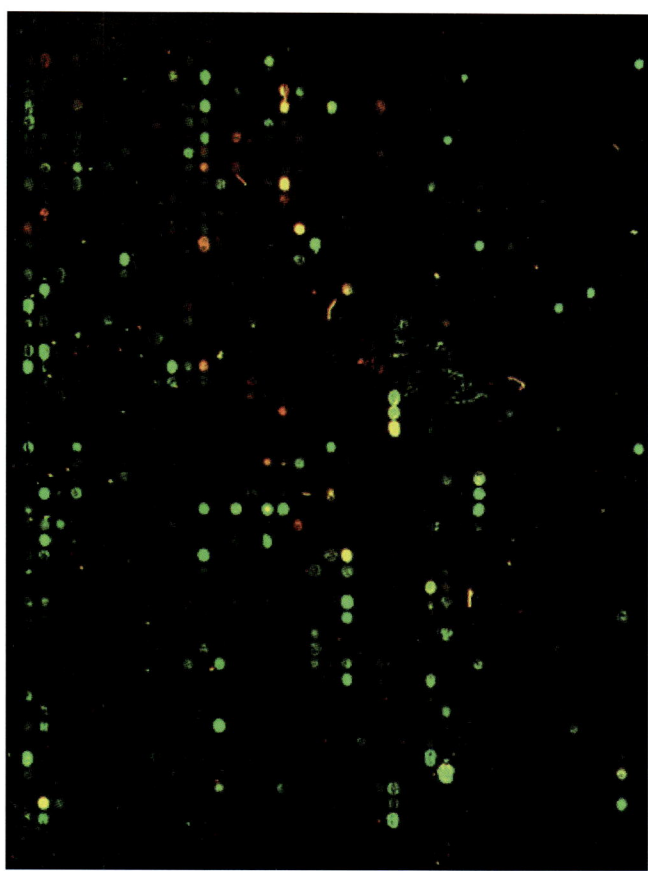

图 32.10　扫描 cDNA 芯片图像。从正常脂肪和高分化脂肪肉瘤中分离的 RNA 分别用红色和绿色荧光标记，并与自动点布于预装芯片玻片上的 cDNA 杂交。出现在正常脂肪而不是高分化脂肪肉瘤的高表达的基因显示为红点，而出现在脂肪肉瘤而不是正常脂肪的高表达的基因显示为绿点。基因表达程度相对同等时显示为黄点。芯片上的空白点表明这些组织不表达这些 cDNA。（Image courtesy of Dr Frank Kuo, Department of Pathology, Brigham & Women's Hospital, Boston, Massachusetts.）

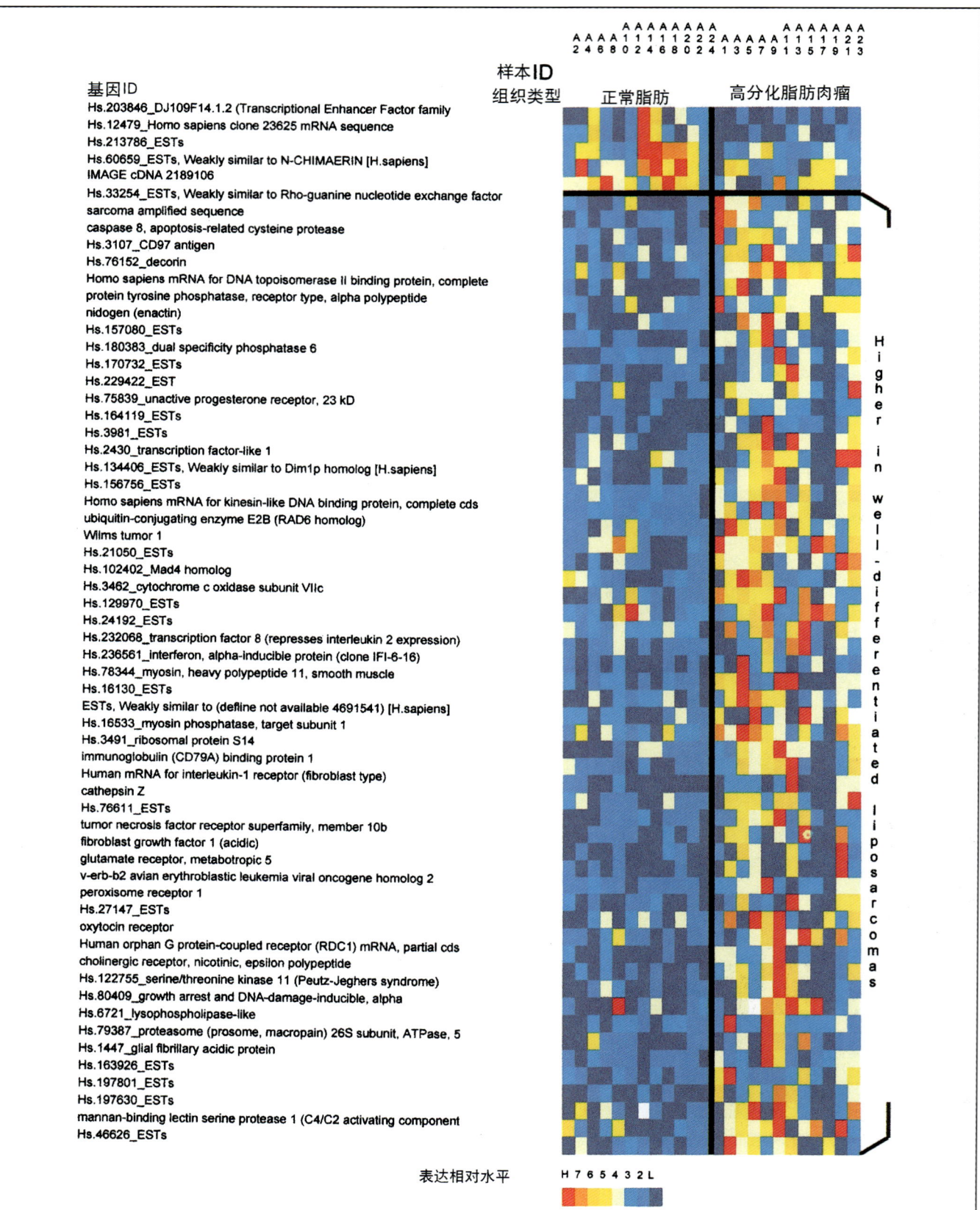

图32.11 彩色编码显示相应的基因表达。从图32.10 cDNA芯片中得到的数据，比较正常脂肪和高分化脂肪肉瘤，表达为一种彩色梯度，与测试的编码序列并列。（Image courtesy of Dr Frank Kuo, Department of Pathology, Brigham & Women's Hospital, Boston, Massachusetts.）

微小残留疾病的主要技术，因为它们对于检测罕见的肿瘤细胞高度敏感。然而，这种敏感性也带来了技术上的问题和解释结果的困难。主要的技术问题是试验假阳性，大概是由于来自从前扩增的少量产物对 PCR 反应的污染。另一个问题是：标准的 PCR 本身缺乏精确的定量。在反应进行时应用测量反应过程中产物累积的仪器进行 PCR 的实时分析会出现这些问题，现在已有革命化的 MRD 试验。伴随每一轮或每一次循环的扩增，通过监测荧光染料可以对 DNA 进行定量，即将荧光染料中插入 DNA，或用与靶 DNA 特异性杂交的荧光标记的寡核苷酸探针。反应发生于密闭的反应性试管内，不再需要随后的凝胶电泳，且减少了污染的机会。实时 PCR 常常与肿瘤特异性 mRNA 反转录结合应用，这样基因表达可以敏感地定量，即所谓的定量 RT-PCR。PCR 用于诊断残留疾病的主要问题是：DNA 或 RNA 的标记物的检测代表非常少量的细胞，并不一定意味肿瘤细胞生存或有致瘤的可能。通过血清监测来确定残留疾病的动力学，有助于解释一个单个分子结果的临床重要性。

迄今为止，最小残留疾病的多数研究集中于造血系统肿瘤。CML 的 Ph' 染色体及其相关的 *BCR-ABL1* RNA 转录已被广泛用于评估肿瘤对治疗的反应。白细胞计数和脾的大小正常是治疗反应的第一个征象。细胞遗传学反应能够进一步揭示肿瘤抑制的指征，例如通过测量 20 个分裂中期细胞中 Ph' 染色体的百分比。一旦细胞遗传学缓解，患者就可以通过定量 RT-PCR 方法进一步跟踪标准化的 *BCR-ABL1* RNA 转录，以管家基因作为对照。在慢性期 CML 将伊马替尼与 α-干扰素和阿糖胞苷进行比较的 IRIS 试验不仅表明，伊马替尼是较好的疗法，并且确定了 *BCR-ABL1* RNA 转录的最小残留水平的靶向，这与没有进展的生存有关[18,209]。这些相同的方法可用来连续监测伊马替尼或干细胞移植治疗的 CML 患者。*BCR-ABL1* RNA 水平上升表明分子复发，需要增加或改变治疗方法。然而，方法学的标准化仍然是一种挑战，并且是需要的，以便不管在哪里进行分析，分子监测值都具有类似的生物学意义。

RT-PCR 分析也被用来评估急性前髓细胞性白血病对治疗的反应，大约 30% 的前髓细胞性白血病的患者在应用全反式视黄酸治疗和化疗后将会复发。研究显示，加强治疗后，90% 以上的 RT-PCR 检查中骨髓 *PML-RARA* 融合转录呈阴性的患者将保持临床缓解，即使其骨髓 RT-PCR 持续阴性，每 3~6 个月也要进行监测[210,211]。相反，95% 的治疗后从 PCR 阴性转为 PCR 阳性的患者将在第一个阳性结果出现 3 个月内发生血液学复发[212]。因而，急性前髓细胞性白血病患者在诱导治疗后要通过 RT-PCR 进行监测。在分子复发而不是血液学复发时进行超前治疗，可使生存率改善[213]。

接受治疗的 ALL 患者可用重排的 *TCRG* 和 *IGH* 基因的 PCR 监测残留的疾病。这些研究的策略是：在具有大量 ALL 的骨髓诊断样本中，确定 *TCRG* 或 *IGH* 基因中克隆性 V-N-（D-N）-J 连接中的核苷酸序列。构建与这个区域特异序列互补的寡核苷酸可检测治疗后血液或骨髓标本中残留的 ALL。这个寡核苷酸可以同 V 区探针一起用作引物，或作为探针与从治疗后标本扩增而来的 *TCRG* 或 *IGH* DNA 杂交。这种方法的敏感性大致相当于或略低于嵌合 RNA 的 RT-PCR 检测。然而，与嵌合 RNA 的 RT-PCR 不同，不同患者之间其白血病 RNA 靶相似，这项技术要求患者产生特异性的引物，这样一来对于常规临床应用来过于昂贵且费力。

预后标记物 Prognostic markers

如今癌症研究者对辨认分子遗传学标记物有着较高的期望，期望这些标记物可以用于预测治疗反应、临床经过以及组织学分类同源而可能伴有异源性临床行为的个别肿瘤的结果。这种热情主要集中在：这些标记物提供的信息可被用于每一个肿瘤患者的个性化治疗。大多数类型的肿瘤的临床研究不充分，至今尚无这样的分子遗传学标记物可用作决定治疗的根据。这些期望是否能够满足尚有待于确定。个别病例的行为和结果不依赖于：肿瘤的免疫反应，并发的疾病，正常血管对来自肿瘤的血管生成性刺激的反应，周围组织对肿瘤侵袭的抵抗，以及其他不能通过检查肿瘤本身来评估的因素。然而，肿瘤的行为和结果似乎明显受到肿瘤内分子遗传标记物的影响，一些与预后相关的标记物已经被确定。

某些肿瘤的染色体异常具有明确的预后价值，已被纳入分类方案，特别是 AML 和 ALL 的分类[65,214,215]（表 32.1）。超二倍体（> 50 染色体）被认为是儿童 ALL 的一个有利的预后指征[216]。

染色体异常还能确定多发性骨髓瘤的预后[217,218]。在多发性骨髓瘤，10%~20% 的病例通过间期 FISH 检查可以检测到受体激酶 *FGFR3* 的核型隐蔽 t(4;14)(p16.3;q32) 易位到 IgH 开关部位。*FGFR3* 和一个邻近的基因 *MMSET* 均受免疫球蛋白增强子的影响，可导致调节障碍。对于应用常规疗法或高剂量化疗的骨髓瘤患者来说，t(4;14) 是一个不良的预后因素。同样，t(11;14)(q13;q32) 可见于大约 15%~20% 的骨髓瘤患者，还涉及免疫球蛋白位点，但是与应用高剂量化疗患者的生存或中位生存期改善有关。相反，13q 或 17p13（p53 位点）的染色体缺失具有不良的预后。高危险度的患者应该避免常规的高剂量美法兰（melphalan）治疗，已经

结语

证明后者在调查的疗法中相对无效。

　　癌基因和细胞周期基因的扩增显示对几种肿瘤具有预后意义。这些扩增包括神经母细胞瘤的 *MYCN*、乳腺癌的 *HER2/NEU*（*ERBB2*）和细胞周期蛋白 D1（cyclin D1）。在神经母细胞瘤的 *MYCN* 和乳腺癌的 *HER2*/NEU（*ERBB2*）的例子中，FISH 或免疫组化检测扩增已经成为组织活检标本常规诊断评估的一部分。总体上，*MYCN* 扩增发生于大约 25% 的神经母细胞瘤，*MYCN* 是位于 2 号染色体短臂 23-24 条带的一个编码一种转录因子的基因。*MYCN* 扩增好像是这一小部分神经母细胞瘤最初的稳定的特征，而不是在肿瘤进展过程中发生的一种改变。这个基因的扩增与侵袭性临床行为和不良结局有关，随着基因复制数目的增加，预后更差[219]。*MYCN* 扩增见于 30%～40% 的晚期患者，而仅见于 5%～10% 的分期低或 IV-S 期患者。具有 *MYCN* 扩增的分期低的患者预期结局不好。

　　位于 17 号染色体长臂 11-12 条带上的 *HER2* 基因编码跨膜酪氨酸激酶生长因子受体。*HER2* 扩增或 *HER2/NEU* 蛋白过度表达见于 25%～30% 的乳腺癌（也见第 16 章）。研究指出，*HER2/NEU*（*ERBB2*）基因扩增和蛋白过度表达与淋巴结阴性患者预后不良有关[220,221]。应用直接针对 HER2/NEU 蛋白的人工合成的单克隆抗体 [trastuzumab（Herceptin, Genentech, South San Francisco, CA）] 治疗 HER2/NEU 过度表达的转移性乳腺癌患者后发现，疾病进展时间明显延长，反应率较高较长，而且总体生存得到改善[222]。*HER2* 基因扩增或蛋白过度表达可以通过（美国）食品与药品管理局（Food and Drug Administrtion, FDA）批准的试剂盒测定 [FISH：Path Vysion Her2 DNA 探针试剂盒（Vysis/Abbott 实验室，Des Plaines, IL）；免疫组化：Hercep 检验（DAKO, Carpinteria, CA）]。

　　从历史上看，慢性淋巴细胞性白血病被认为是来源于幼稚的 B 淋巴细胞，这种淋巴细胞尚未接触生发中心的抗原。然而，研究者们已经发现，基于有无明显数目的 IgV$_H$ 基因突变可将 CLL 分为两个亚组[223,224]，例如体细胞超突变，一种生发中心后 B 淋巴细胞标记物。通过 IgV$_H$ 突变状态可将分期低的 CLL 患者（Binet A 期）分层，具有明显不同的生存期[225,226]。伴有种系非突变 IgV$_H$ 基因的患者的中位生存期为 8～9 年，与之相比，伴有体细胞突变 IgV$_H$ 基因的患者的生存期超过 24 年。IgV$_H$ 基因突变检测在技术上存在困难，昂贵，没有得到广泛应用。已经找到替代的标记物，如 CD38 和 ZAP70 的表达，好像对预后有用[226a]。

癌症治疗的药物基因组学
Pharmacogenomics of cancer therapy

　　个体化用药时代预示着药物的靶点接近癌症的特殊生物学亚类，并且癌症化疗的个体化能使毒性降至最低并增加疗效。种系多态性（germline polymorphisms）能够改变药物代谢酶或药物运输蛋白的表达。最近在癌症化疗中有两个药物基因组学实例，均涉及编码参与化疗药物失活的酶的单一基因的多态性。硫代嘌呤甲基转移酶（TMPT）催化巯嘌呤和其他硫代嘌呤药物（例如硫代鸟嘌呤）的 S-甲基化，可以用于 ALL 的治疗。TMPT 基因多形性等位基因变异可导致氨基酸替换，可改变 *TMPT* 的活性[227,228]。三个变异的等位基因 [*TMPT*2*，密码子 18（Ala>Pro）；*TMPT*3A*，密码子 254（Ala > Thr），以及密码子 240（Try > Cys）；*TMPT*3C*，只有密码子 240（Try > Cys）] 占低或中等酶活性的 95% 以上。TMPT 等位基因是共显性遗传，以便伴有两个野生型等位基因者（*TMPT*1*）具有最大的酶活性，野生型/变异型杂合者具有中等酶活性，而纯合性变异等位基因具有最小的酶活性。大约 10% 的个体是杂合性的，而每 300 个个体中有 1 个具有纯合性变异，而且是 TMPT 不足。TMPT 不足的患者积聚了过高浓度的硫代鸟嘌呤核苷酸，容易产生严重的造血毒性，可以致命。此外，骨髓抑制需要停止使用其他化疗药物，直至骨髓和中性粒细胞计数恢复，这有可能导致总体化疗效果下降。可调整并降低 *TMPT* 杂合性或纯合性患者巯嘌呤的剂量能够降低毒性并使治疗最佳化。

　　拓扑异构酶 I 抑制剂伊立替康（irinotecan）被用于转移性结肠癌患者的联合化疗。伊立替康活跃的代谢产物，SN38，在肝通过尿苷二磷酸葡萄糖醛酸基转移酶 1A1（UGT1A1）被葡萄糖醛酸结合而灭活。UGT1A1 启动子的 TATA 盒内 TA 重复的数目与酶的表达呈负相关。大约 10% 的北美人的 *UGT1A1*28* 等位基因是纯合的，它具有 7 个 TA 重复，不同于最常见的野生型等位基因的 6 个 TA 重复。对具有 *UGT1A1*28* 等位基因的患者用标准剂量的伊立替康治疗时，会发生严重的中性粒细胞减少症和贫腹泻[229-231]。FDA 认为，对 *UGT1A1*28* 等位基因纯合性个体的治疗应有所改变。

结语

　　所有的癌症都是由于基因突变连续积累引起的克隆性疾病。这些突变中的一小部分可以用于诊断或用于确定预后和选择理想的治疗方案。由平衡的染色体重排引起的突变，特别是易位，最适合用作诊断的标记物：它们可以通过传统的核型方法来证实，需要新鲜的肿瘤材料，整个的基因组在形态学上均应进行评估，与分子细胞遗传学和分子方法相比处在较低的分辨水平。另外，应用 FISH 或 PCR 可以更集中和更有效地评估易位。FISH 可在新鲜、冰冻或石蜡包埋材料中进行，检测敏感性可达每 100 个细胞可发现一个异常细胞，而 PCR 可在数千个细胞中检测到一个异常细胞，因此，在诊断和监测微小残留疾病中均可应用。其他类型的体细胞突变，包括基因扩增、缺失和点突变，在诊断的特异性方面不如易位，但可用于确定预后和辨认必需治疗的靶点。基因扩增通过 FISH 容易证实，但也可以通过免疫组化检测扩增基因过度表达的蛋白产物间接显示，例如乳腺癌的 HER2/NEU（ERBB2）扩增。基因缺失通过 FISH 可以有效证实，如预示预后不良的多发骨髓瘤的 p53 缺失，在许多病例中也能通过分析杂合性缺失来证实，其中局部单一核苷酸多态性或微卫星可以通过 PCR 方法检测。基因内的突变，不管是导致癌基因的活化还是导致肿瘤抑制基因的失活，均可以通过 PCR 分析突变"热点"基因组的部位来证实，并随后应用 HPLC 或序列分析使突变等位基因可视化。本章中所讨论的例子强调了细胞遗传学和分子分析方法是互补的，每一种方法都有其独特的优点和局限性，当选择性使用时，其提供的诊断和预后的内涵能够增强外科病理学的评估。

参考文献

1. National Cancer Institute 2005 Probability of Breast Cancer in American Women. Online. Available: http://www.cancer.gov/cancertopics/factsheet/Detection/probability-breast-cancer
2. American Cancer Society 2005 Cancer Facts and Figures. Online. Available http://www.cancer.org/docroot/STT/stt_0.as
3. Tavassoli F A, Devilee P (ed) 2003 World Health Organization Classification of Tumours. Pathology and genetics of tumours of the breast and female genital organs. IARC Press, Lyon
4. Fukunaga M, Katabuchi H, Nagasaka T et al. 2005 Interobserver and intraobserver variability in the diagnosis of hydatidiform mole. Am J Surg Pathol 29: 942–947
5. Rosai J 1991 Borderline epithelial lesions of the breast. Am J Surg Pathol 15: 209–221
6. Schnitt S J, Connolly J L, Tavassoli F A et al. 1992 Interobserver reproducibility in the diagnosis of ductal proliferative breast lesions using standardized criteria. Am J Surg Pathol 16: 1133–1143
7. Campo E, Raffeld M, Jaffe E S 1999 Mantle-cell lymphoma. Semin Hematol 36: 115–127
8. Toyota M, Issa J P 2005 Epigenetic changes in solid and hematopoietic tumors. Semin Oncol 32: 521–530
9. Baylin S B, Herman J G 2000 DNA hypermethylation in tumorigenesis: epigenetics joins genetics. Trends Genet 16: 168–174
10. Lund A H, van Lohuizen M 2004 Epigenetics and cancer. Genes Dev 18: 2315–2335
11. Boveri T 1914 Zur Frage der Entstehung maligner Tumoren. Gustave Fischer, Jena
12. Rowley J D 1973 Letter: A new consistent chromosomal abnormality in chronic myelogenous leukaemia identified by quinacrine fluorescence and Giemsa staining. Nature 243: 290–293
13. Nowell P C, Hungerford D A 1960 A minute chromosome in human granulocytic leukemia. Science 132: 1497
14. Kelliher M A, McLaughlin J, Witte O N et al. 1990 Induction of a chronic myelogenous leukemia-like syndrome in mice with v-abl and BCR/ABL. Proc Natl Acad Sci USA 87: 6649–6653
15. Daley G Q, Van Etten R A, Baltimore D 1990 Induction of chronic myelogenous leukemia in mice by the P210bcr/abl gene of the Philadelphia chromosome. Science 247: 824–830
16. Withey J M, Marley S B, Kaeda J et al. 2005 Targeting primary human leukaemia cells with RNA interference: Bcr-Abl targeting inhibits myeloid progenitor self-renewal in chronic myeloid leukaemia cells. Br J Haematol 129: 377–380
17. Druker B J, Lydon N B 2000 Lessons learned from the development of an abl tyrosine kinase inhibitor for chronic myelogenous leukemia. J Clin Invest 105: 3–7
18. O'Brien S G, Guilhot F, Larson R A et al. 2003 Imatinib compared with interferon and low-dose cytarabine for newly diagnosed chronic-phase chronic myeloid leukemia. N Engl J Med 348: 994–1004
19. Clark S S, McLaughlin J, Timmons M et al. 1988 Expression of a distinctive BCR-ABL oncogene in Ph1-positive acute lymphocytic leukemia (ALL). Science 239: 775–777
20. Hermans A, Heisterkamp N, von Linden M et al. 1987 Unique fusion of bcr and c-abl genes in Philadelphia chromosome positive acute lymphoblastic leukemia. Cell 51: 33–40
21. Snyder D S, Nademanee A P, O'Donnell M R et al. 1999 Long-term follow-up of 23 patients with Philadelphia chromosome-positive acute lymphoblastic leukemia treated with allogeneic bone marrow transplant in first complete remission. Leukemia 13: 2053–2058
22. Thomas X, Boiron J M, Huguet F et al. 2004 Outcome of treatment in adults with acute lymphoblastic leukemia: analysis of the LALA-94 trial. J Clin Oncol 22: 4075–4086
23. De Jong D 2005 Molecular pathogenesis of follicular lymphoma: a cross talk of genetic and immunologic factors. J Clin Oncol 23: 6358–6363
24. McDonnell T J, Korsmeyer S J 1991 Progression from lymphoid hyperplasia to high-grade malignant lymphoma in mice transgenic for the t(14; 18). Nature 349: 254–256
25. Strasser A, Harris A W, Bath M L et al. 1990 Novel primitive lymphoid tumours induced in transgenic mice by cooperation between myc and bcl-2. Nature 348: 331–333
26. Limpens J, Stad R, Vos C et al. 1995 Lymphoma-associated translocation t(14;18) in blood B cells of normal individuals. Blood 85: 2528–2536
27. Aster J C, Kobayashi Y, Shiota M et al. 1992 Detection of the t(14;18) at similar frequencies in hyperplastic lymphoid tissues from American and Japanese patients. Am J Pathol 141: 291–299
28. Dave S S, Wright G, Tan B et al. 2004 Prediction of survival in follicular lymphoma based on molecular features of tumor-infiltrating immune cells. N Engl J Med 351: 2159–2169
29. Bohen S P, Troyanskaya O G, Alter O et al. 2003 Variation in gene expression patterns in follicular lymphoma and the response to rituximab. Proc Natl Acad Sci USA 100: 1926–1930
30. Speck N A, Gilliland D G 2002 Core-binding factors in haematopoiesis and leukaemia. Nat Rev Cancer 2: 502–513
31. Rubnitz J E, Look A T 1998 Molecular genetics of childhood leukemias. J Pediatr Hematol Oncol 20: 1–11
32. Miyoshi H, Shimizu K, Kozu T et al. 1991 t(8;21) breakpoints on chromosome 21 in acute myeloid leukemia are clustered within a limited region of a single gene, AML1. Proc Natl Acad Sci USA 88: 10431–10434
33. Erickson P, Gao J, Chang K S et al. 1992 Identification of breakpoints in t(8;21) acute myelogenous leukemia and isolation of a fusion transcript, AML1/ETO, with similarity to Drosophila segmentation gene, runt. Blood 80: 1825–1831
34. Meyers S, Downing J R, Hiebert S W 1993 Identification of AML-1 and the (8;21) translocation protein (AML-1/ETO) as sequence-specific DNA-binding proteins: the runt homology domain is required for DNA binding and protein–protein interactions. Mol Cell Biol 13: 6336–6345
35. Golub T R, Barker G F, Bohlander S K et al. 1995 Fusion of the TEL gene on 12p13 to the AML1 gene on 21q22 in acute lymphoblastic leukemia. Proc Natl Acad Sci USA 92: 4917–4921
36. Romana S P, Mauchauffe M, Le Coniat M et al. 1995 The t(12;21) of acute lymphoblastic leukemia results in a tel-AML1 gene fusion. Blood 85: 3662–3670
37. Romana S P, Poirel H, Leconiat M et al. 1995 High frequency of t(12;21) in childhood B-lineage acute lymphoblastic leukemia. Blood 86: 4263–4269
38. Shurtleff S A, Buijs A, Behm F G et al. 1995 TEL/AML1 fusion resulting from a cryptic t(12;21) is the most common genetic lesion in pediatric ALL and defines a subgroup of patients with an excellent prognosis. Leukemia 9: 1985–1989
39. Liu P, Tarle S A, Hajra A et al. 1993 Fusion between transcription factor CBF beta/PEBP2 beta and a myosin heavy chain in acute myeloid leukemia. Science 261:1041–104
40. Le Beau M M, Larson R A, Bitter M A et al. 1983 Association of an inversion of chromosome 16 with abnormal marrow eosinophils in acute myelomonocytic leukemia. A unique cytogenetic–clinicopathological association. N Engl J Med 309: 630–636
41. Janknecht R 2005 EWS-ETS oncoproteins: The linchpins of Ewing tumors. Gene 363:1–14
42. Delattre O, Zucman J, Plougastel B et al. 1992 Gene fusion with an ETS DNA-binding domain caused by chromosome translocation in human tumours. Nature 359: 162–165

43. Zucman J, Delattre O, Desmaze C et al. 1992 Cloning and characterization of the Ewing's sarcoma and peripheral neuroepithelioma t(11;22) translocation breakpoints. Genes Chromos Cancer 5: 271–277
44. Rao V N, Ohno T, Prasad D D et al. 1993 Analysis of the DNA-binding and transcriptional activation functions of human Fli-1 protein. Oncogene 8: 2167–2173
45. Zhang L, Lemarchandel V, Romeo P H et al. 1993 The Fli-1 proto-oncogene, involved in erythroleukemia and Ewing's sarcoma, encodes a transcriptional activator with DNA-binding specificities distinct from other Ets family members. Oncogene 8: 1621–1630
46. May W A, Gishizky M L, Lessnick S L et al. 1993 Ewing sarcoma 11;22 translocation produces a chimeric transcription factor that requires the DNA-binding domain encoded by FLI1 for transformation. Proc Natl Acad Sci USA 90: 5752–5756
47. Ohno T, Rao V N, Reddy E S 1993 EWS/Fli-1 chimeric protein is a transcriptional activator. Cancer Res 53: 5859–5863
48. Zucman J, Melot T, Desmaze C et al. 1993 Combinatorial generation of variable fusion proteins in the Ewing family of tumours. EMBO J 12: 4481–4487
49. Giovannini M, Biegel J A, Serra M et al. 1994 EWS-erg and EWS-Fli1 fusion transcripts in Ewing's sarcoma and primitive neuroectodermal tumors with variant translocations. J Clin Invest 94: 489–496
50. Jeon I S, Davis J N, Braun B S et al. 1995 A variant Ewing's sarcoma translocation (7;22) fuses the EWS gene to the ETS gene ETV1. Oncogene 10: 1229–1234
51. Sorensen P H, Lessnick S L, Lopez-Terrada D et al. 1994 A second Ewing's sarcoma translocation, t(21;22), fuses the EWS gene to another ETS-family transcription factor, ERG. Nature Genet 6: 146–151
52. Fujimura Y, Ohno T, Siddique H et al. 1996 The EWS-ATF-1 gene involved in malignant melanoma of soft parts with t(12;22) chromosome translocation, encodes a constitutive transcriptional activator. Oncogene 12: 159–167
53. Ladanyi M, Gerald W 1994 Fusion of the EWS and WT1 genes in the desmoplastic small round cell tumor. Cancer Res 54: 2837–2840
54. Gerald W L, Ladanyi M, de Alava E et al. 1998 Clinical, pathologic, and molecular spectrum of tumors associated with t(11;22)(p13;q12): desmoplastic small round-cell tumor and its variants. J Clin Oncol 16: 3028–3036
55. Brody R I, Ueda T, Hamelin R et al.1997 Molecular analysis of the fusion of EWS to an orphan nuclear receptor gene in extraskeletal myxoid chondrosarcoma. Am J Pathol 150: 1049–1058
56. Tomlins S A, Rhodes D R, Perner S et al. 2005 Recurrent fusion of TMPRSS2 and ETS transcription factor genes in prostate cancer. Science 310: 644–648
57. Bertoni F, Zucca E, Cotter F E 2004 Molecular basis of mantle cell lymphoma. Br J Haematol 124: 130–140
58. Banks P M, Chan J, Cleary M L et al. 1992 Mantle cell lymphoma. A proposal for unification of morphologic, immunologic, and molecular data. Am J Surg Pathol 16: 637–640
59. Weisenburger D D, Armitage J O 1996 Mantle cell lymphoma – an entity comes of age. Blood 87: 4483–4494
60. Leroux D, Le Marc'Hadour F, Gressin R et al. 1991 Non-Hodgkin's lymphomas with t(11;14)(q13;q32): a subset of mantle zone/intermediate lymphocytic lymphoma? Br J Haematol 77: 346–353
61. Raffeld M, Sander C A, Yano T et al. 1992 Mantle cell lymphoma: an update. Leuk Lymphoma 8: 161–166
62. Shivdasani R A, Hess J L, Skarin A T, Pinkus G S 1993 Intermediate lymphocytic lymphoma: clinical and pathologic features of a recently characterized subtype of non-Hodgkin's lymphoma. J Clin Oncol 11: 802–111
63. Sanz M A, Tallman M S, Lo-Coco F 2005 Tricks of the trade for the appropriate management of newly diagnosed acute promyelocytic leukemia. Blood 105: 3019–3025
64. Tallman M S, Andersen J W, Schiffer C A et al. 1997 All-*trans*-retinoic acid in acute promyelocytic leukemia. N Engl J Med 337: 1021–1028
65. Jaffe E S, Stein H, Vardiman J W (eds) 2001 World Health Organization Classification of Tumours. Pathology and genetics of tumours of haematopoietic and lymphoid tissues. IARC Press, Lyon
66. Eble J N, Epstein J I, Sesterhenn I A (eds) 2004 World Health Organization Classification of Tumors. Pathology and genetics of tumours of the urinary system and male genital organs. IARC Press, Lyon
67. Wang N 2002 Methodologies in cancer cytogenetics and molecular cytogenetics. Am J Med Genet 115: 118–124
68. Xiao S, Renshaw A, Cibas E S et al. 1995 Novel fluorescence in situ hybridization approaches in solid tumors. Characterization of frozen specimens, touch preparations, and cytological preparations. Am J Pathol 147: 896–904
69. Anastasi J, Le Beau M M, Vardiman J W et al. 1992 Detection of trisomy 12 in chronic lymphocytic leukemia by fluorescence in situ hybridization to interphase cells: a simple and sensitive method. Blood 79: 1796–1801
70. Schofield D E, Fletcher J A 1992 Trisomy 12 in pediatric granulosa–stromal cell tumors. Demonstration by a modified method of fluorescence in situ hybridization on paraffin-embedded material. Am J Pathol 141: 1265–1269
71. Wolman S R, Waldman F M, Balazs M 1993 Complementarity of interphase and metaphase chromosome analysis in human renal tumors. Genes Chromos Cancer 6: 17–23
72. Qian J, Bostwick D G, Takahashi S et al. 1996 Comparison of fluorescence in situ hybridization analysis of isolated nuclei and routine histological sections from paraffin-embedded prostatic adenocarcinoma specimens. Am J Pathol 149: 1193–1199
73. Fletcher J A 1999 DNA in situ hybridization as an adjunct in tumor diagnosis. Am J Clin Pathol 112: S11–18
74. Gong Y, Gilcrease M, Sneige N 2005 Reliability of chromogenic in situ hybridization for detecting HER-2 gene status in breast cancer: comparison with fluorescence in situ hybridization and assessment of interobserver reproducibility. Mod Pathol 18: 1015–1021
75. Bhargava R, Lal P, Chen B 2005 Chromogenic in situ hybridization for the detection of HER-2/neu gene amplification in breast cancer with an emphasis on tumors with borderline and low-level amplification: does it measure up to fluorescence in situ hybridization? Am J Clin Pathol 123: 237–243
76. Bhargava R, Oppenheimer O, Gerald W et al. 2005 Identification of MYCN gene amplification in neuroblastoma using chromogenic in situ hybridization (CISH): an alternative and practical method. Diagn Mol Pathol 14: 72–76
77. Quezado M, Ronchetti R, Rapkiewicz A et al. 2005 Chromogenic in situ hybridization accurately identifies EGFR amplification in small cell glioblastoma multiforme, a common subtype of primary GBM. Clin Neuropathol 24: 163–169
78. Siebert R, Matthiesen P, Harder S et al. 1998 Application of interphase fluorescence in situ hybridization for the detection of the Burkitt translocation t(8;14)(q24;q32) in B-cell lymphomas. Blood 91: 984–990
79. Haralambieva E, Banham A H, Bastard C et al. 2003 Detection by the fluorescence in situ hybridization technique of MYC translocations in paraffin-embedded lymphoma biopsy samples. Br J Haematol 121: 49–56
80. Sindelarova L, Michalova K, Zemanova Z et al. 2005 Incidence of chromosomal anomalies detected with FISH and their clinical correlations in B-chronic lymphocytic leukemia. Cancer Genet Cytogenet 160: 27–34
81. Belhadj K, Reyes F, Farcet J-P et al. 2003 Hepatosplenic (gamma)(delta) T-cell lymphoma is a rare clinicopathologic entity with poor outcome: report on a series of 21 patients. Blood 102: 4261–4269
82. Micci F, Teixeira M R, Bjerkehagen B et al. 2002 Characterization of supernumerary rings and giant marker chromosomes in well-differentiated lipomatous tumors by a combination of G-banding, CGH, M-FISH, and chromosome- and locus-specific FISH. Cytogenet Genome Res 97: 13–19
83. Mertens F, Panagopoulos I, Jonson T et al. 2004 Retained heterodisomy for chromosome 12 in atypical lipomatous tumors: implications for ring chromosome formation. Cytogenet Genome Res 106: 33–38
84. Kovacs G, Akhtar M, Beckwith B J et al. 1997 The Heidelberg classification of renal cell tumours. J Pathol 183: 131–133
85. Storkel S, Eble J N, Adlakha K et al. 1997 Classification of renal cell carcinoma: Workgroup No. 1. Union Internationale Contre le Cancer (UICC) and the American Joint Committee on Cancer (AJCC). Cancer 80: 987–989
86. Kovacs G 1993 Molecular differential pathology of renal cell tumours. Histopathology 22: 1–8
87. Zbar B, Brauch H, Talmadge C et al. 1987 Loss of alleles of loci on the short arm of chromosome 3 in renal cell carcinoma. Nature 327: 721–724
88. Shuin T, Kondo K, Torigoe S et al. 1994 Frequent somatic mutations and loss of heterozygosity of the von Hippel–Lindau tumor suppressor gene in primary human renal cell carcinomas. Cancer Res 54: 2852–2855
89. Gnarra J R, Lerman M I, Zbar B et al. 1995 Genetics of renal-cell carcinoma and evidence for a critical role for von Hippel–Lindau in renal tumorigenesis. Semin Oncol 22: 3–8
90. Corless C L, Aburatani H, Fletcher J A et al. 1996 Papillary renal cell carcinoma: quantitation of chromosomes 7 and 17 by FISH, analysis of chromosome 3p for LOH, and DNA ploidy. Diagn Mol Pathol 5: 53–64
91. Kovacs A, Kovacs G 1992 Low chromosome number in chromophobe renal cell carcinomas. Genes Chromos Cancer 4: 267–268
92. Speicher M R, Schoell B, du Manoir S et al. 1994 Specific loss of chromosomes 1, 2, 6, 10, 13, 17, and 21 in chromophobe renal cell carcinomas revealed by comparative genomic hybridization. Am J Pathol 145: 356–364
92a. Argani P, Ladanyi M 2005 Translocation carcinomas of the kidney. Clin Lab Med 25: 363–378
93. Van den Berg E, Dijkhuizen T, Oosterhuis J W et al. 1997 Cytogenetic classification of renal cell cancer. Cancer Genet Cytogenet 95: 103–107
94. Speicher M R, Carter N P 2005 The new cytogenetics: blurring the boundaries with molecular biology. Nature Rev Genet 6: 782–792
95. Veldman T, Vignon C, Schrock E et al. 1997 Hidden chromosome abnormalities in haematological malignancies detected by multicolour spectral karyotyping. Nature Genet 15: 406–410
96. Macville M, Schrock E, Padilla-Nash H et al. 1999 Comprehensive and definitive molecular cytogenetic characterization of HeLa cells by spectral karyotyping. Cancer Res 59: 141–150
97. Speicher M R, Gwyn Ballard S, Ward D C 1996 Karyotyping human chromosomes by combinatorial multi-fluor FISH. Nature Genet 12: 368–375
98. Tanke H J, Wiegant J, van Gijlswijk R P et al. 1999 New strategy for multicolour fluorescence in situ hybridisation: COBRA: COmbined Binary RAtio labelling. Eur J Hum Genet 7: 2–11
99. Kallioniemi A, Kallioniemi O P, Sudar D et al. 1992 Comparative genomic hybridization for molecular cytogenetic analysis of solid tumors. Science 258: 818–821
100. Kallioniemi O P, Kallioniemi A, Piper J et al. 1994 Optimizing comparative genomic hybridization for analysis of DNA sequence copy number changes in solid tumors. Genes Chromosomes Cancer 10: 231–243
101. Knuutila S, Bjorkqvist A M, Autio K et al. 1998 DNA copy number amplifications in human neoplasms: review of comparative genomic hybridization studies. Am J Pathol 152: 1107–1123

102. Ried T, Just K E, Holtgreve-Grez H et al. 1995 Comparative genomic hybridization of formalin-fixed, paraffin-embedded breast tumors reveals different patterns of chromosomal gains and losses in fibroadenomas and diploid and aneuploid carcinomas. Cancer Res 55: 5415–5423
103. Speicher M R, du Manoir S, Schrock E et al. 1993 Molecular cytogenetic analysis of formalin-fixed, paraffin-embedded solid tumors by comparative genomic hybridization after universal DNA amplification. Hum Mol Genet 2: 1907–1914
104. Speicher M R, Jauch A, Walt H et al. 1995 Correlation of microscopic phenotype with genotype in a formalin-fixed, paraffin-embedded testicular germ cell tumor with universal DNA amplification, comparative genomic hybridization, and interphase cytogenetics. Am J Pathol 146: 1332–1340
105. Wiltshire R N, Duray P, Bittner M L et al. 1995 Direct visualization of the clonal progression of primary cutaneous melanoma: application of tissue microdissection and comparative genomic hybridization. Cancer Res 55: 3954–3957
106. Schwaenen C, Nessling M, Wessendorf S et al. 2004 Automated array-based genomic profiling in chronic lymphocytic leukemia: development of a clinical tool and discovery of recurrent genomic alterations. Proc Natl Acad Sci USA 101: 1039–1044
107. Iafrate A J, Feuk L, Rivera M N et al. 2004 Detection of large-scale variation in the human genome. Nature Genet 36: 949–951
108. Sebat J, Lakshmi B, Troge J et al. 2004 Large-scale copy number polymorphism in the human genome. Science 305: 525–528
109. Sharp A J, Locke D P, McGrath S D et al. 2005 Segmental duplications and copy-number variation in the human genome. Am J Hum Genet 77: 78–88
110. Weber J L, May P E 1989 Abundant class of human DNA polymorphisms which can be typed using the polymerase chain reaction. Am J Hum Genet 44: 388–396
111. Ino Y, Betensky R A, Zlatescu M C et al. 2001 Molecular subtypes of anaplastic oligodendroglioma: implications for patient management at diagnosis. Clin Cancer Res 7: 839–845
112. McDonald J M, See S J, Tremont I W et al. 2005 The prognostic impact of histology and 1p/19q status in anaplastic oligodendroglial tumors. Cancer 104: 1468–1477
113. Watanabe T, Wu T T, Catalano P J et al. 2001 Molecular predictors of survival after adjuvant chemotherapy for colon cancer. N Engl J Med 344: 1196–206
114. Sarli L, Bottarelli L, Bader G et al. 2004 Association between recurrence of sporadic colorectal cancer, high level of microsatellite instability, and loss of heterozygosity at chromosome 18q. Dis Colon Rectum 47: 1467–1482
115. Lynch H T, de la Chapelle A 1999 Genetic susceptibility to non-polyposis colorectal cancer. J Med Genet 36: 801–818
116. Lengauer C, Kinzler K W, Vogelstein B 1998 Genetic instabilities in human cancers. Nature 396: 643–649
117. Umar A, Boland C R, Terdiman J P et al. 2004 Revised Bethesda Guidelines for hereditary nonpolyposis colorectal cancer (Lynch syndrome) and microsatellite instability. J Natl Cancer Inst 96: 261–268
118. Umar A, Risinger J I, Hawk E T et al. 2004 Testing guidelines for hereditary non-polyposis colorectal cancer. Nat Rev Cancer 4: 153–158
119. Boland C R, Thibodeau S N, Hamilton S R et al. 1998 A National Cancer Institute Workshop on Microsatellite Instability for cancer detection and familial predisposition: development of international criteria for the determination of microsatellite instability in colorectal cancer. Cancer Res 58: 5248–5257
120. Arzimanoglou II, Gilbert F, Barber H R 1998 Microsatellite instability in human solid tumors. Cancer 82: 1808–1820
121. Kim H, Jen J, Vogelstein B et al. 1994 Clinical and pathological characteristics of sporadic colorectal carcinomas with DNA replication errors in microsatellite sequences. Am J Pathol 145: 148–156
122. Cunningham J M, Kim C Y, Christensen E R et al. 2001 The frequency of hereditary defective mismatch repair in a prospective series of unselected colorectal carcinomas. Am J Hum Genet 69: 780–790
123. Wright C M, Dent O F, Barker M et al. 2000 Prognostic significance of extensive microsatellite instability in sporadic clinicopathological stage C colorectal cancer. Br J Surg 87: 1197–1202
124. Ribic C M, Sargent D J, Moore M J et al. 2003 Tumor microsatellite-instability status as a predictor of benefit from fluorouracil-based adjuvant chemotherapy for colon cancer. N Engl J Med 349: 247–257
125. Benatti P, Gafa R, Barana D et al. 2005 Microsatellite instability and colorectal cancer prognosis. Clin Cancer Res 11: 8332–8340
126. Bos J L 1989 ras oncogenes in human cancer: a review. Cancer Res 49:4682–4689
127. Levine A J, Momand J, Finlay C A 1991 The p53 tumour suppressor gene. Nature 351: 453–456
128. Krause D S, Van Etten R A 2005 Tyrosine kinases as targets for cancer therapy. N Engl J Med 353: 172–187
129. Arena S, Benvenuti S, Bardelli A 2005 Genetic analysis of the kinome and phosphatome in cancer. Cell Mol Life Sci 62: 2092–2099
130. Hirota S, Isozaki K, Moriyama Y et al. 1998 Gain-of-function mutations of c-kit in human gastrointestinal stromal tumors. Science 279: 577–580
131. Taniguchi M, Nishida T, Hirota S et al.1999 Effect of c-kit mutation on prognosis of gastrointestinal stromal tumors. Cancer Res 59: 4297–4300
132. Moskaluk C A, Tian Q, Marshall C R et al. 1999 Mutations of c-kit JM domain are found in a minority of human gastrointestinal stromal tumors. Oncogene 18: 1897–902
133. Corless C L, McGreevey L, Haley A et al. 2002. KIT mutations are common in incidental gastrointestinal stromal tumors one centimeter or less in size. Am J Pathol 160: 1567–1572
134. Lux M L, Rubin B P, Biase TL et al. 2000 KIT extracellular and kinase domain mutations in gastrointestinal stromal tumors. Am J Pathol 156: 791–795
135. Lasota J, Wozniak A, Sarlomo-Rikala M et al. 2000 Mutations in exons 9 and 13 of KIT gene are rare events in gastrointestinal stromal tumors. A study of 200 cases. Am J Pathol 157: 1091–1095
136. Heinrich M C, Corless C L, Demetri G D et al. 2003 Kinase mutations and imatinib response in patients with metastatic gastrointestinal stromal tumor. J Clin Oncol 21: 4342–4349
137. Corless C L, Fletcher J A, Heinrich M C 2004 Biology of gastrointestinal stromal tumors. J Clin Oncol 22: 3813–3825
138. Corless C L, Schroeder A, Griffith D et al. 2005 PDGFRA mutations in gastrointestinal stromal tumors: frequency, spectrum and in vitro sensitivity to imatinib. J Clin Oncol 23: 5357–5364
139. Lasota J, Dansonka-Mieszkowska A, Sobin L H et al. 2004 A great majority of GISTs with PDGFRA mutations represent gastric tumors of low or no malignant potential. Lab Invest 84: 874–883
140. Medeiros F, Corless C L, Duensing A et al. 2004 KIT-negative gastrointestinal stromal tumors: proof of concept and therapeutic implications. Am J Surg Pathol 28: 889–894
141. Wardelmann E, Hrychyk A, Merkelbach-Bruse S et al. 2004 Association of platelet-derived growth factor receptor alpha mutations with gastric primary site and epithelioid or mixed cell morphology in gastrointestinal stromal tumors. J Mol Diagn 6: 197–204
142. Pao W, Miller V A 2005 Epidermal growth factor receptor mutations, small-molecule kinase inhibitors, and non-small-cell lung cancer: current knowledge and future directions. J Clin Oncol 23: 2556–2568
143. Kris M G, Natale R B, Herbst R S et al. 2003 Efficacy of gefitinib, an inhibitor of the epidermal growth factor receptor tyrosine kinase, in symptomatic patients with non-small cell lung cancer: a randomized trial. JAMA 290: 2149–2158
144. Fukuoka M, Yano S, Giaccone G et al. 2003 Multi-institutional randomized phase II trial of gefitinib for previously treated patients with advanced non-small-cell lung cancer (The IDEAL 1 Trial) [corrected]. J Clin Oncol 21: 2237–2246
145. Perez-Soler R, Chachoua A, Hammond L A et al. 2004 Determinants of tumor response and survival with erlotinib in patients with non-small-cell lung cancer. J Clin Oncol 22: 3238–3247
146. Shepherd F A, Rodrigues Pereira J, Ciuleanu T et al. 2005 Erlotinib in previously treated non-small-cell lung cancer. N Engl J Med 353: 123–132
147. Janne P A, Engelman J A, Johnson B E 2005 Epidermal growth factor receptor mutations in non-small-cell lung cancer: implications for treatment and tumor biology. J Clin Oncol 23: 3227–3234
148. Paez J G, Janne P A, Lee J C et al. 2004 EGFR mutations in lung cancer: correlation with clinical response to gefitinib therapy. Science 304: 1497–1500
149. Lynch T J, Bell D W, Sordella R et al. 2004 Activating mutations in the epidermal growth factor receptor underlying responsiveness of non-small-cell lung cancer to gefitinib. N Engl J Med 350: 2129–2139
150. Pao W, Miller V, Zakowski M et al. 2004 EGF receptor gene mutations are common in lung cancers from 'never smokers' and are associated with sensitivity of tumors to gefitinib and erlotinib. Proc Natl Acad Sci USA 101: 13306–13311
151. Baxter E J, Scott L M, Campbell P J et al. 2005 Acquired mutation of the tyrosine kinase JAK2 in human myeloproliferative disorders. Lancet 365: 1054–1061
152. James C, Ugo V, Le Couedic J P et al. 2005 A unique clonal JAK2 mutation leading to constitutive signalling causes polycythaemia vera. Nature 434: 1144–1148
153. Levine R L, Wadleigh M, Cools J et al. 2005 Activating mutation in the tyrosine kinase JAK2 in polycythemia vera, essential thrombocythemia, and myeloid metaplasia with myelofibrosis. Cancer Cell 7: 387–397
154. Nagata H, Worobec A S, Oh C K et al. 1995 Identification of a point mutation in the catalytic domain of the protooncogene c-kit in peripheral blood mononuclear cells of patients who have mastocytosis with an associated hematological disorder. Proc Natl Acad Sci USA 92: 10560–10564
155. Pardanani A, Reeder T L, Kimlinger T K et al. 2003 Flt-3 and c-kit mutation studies in a spectrum of chronic myeloid disorders including systemic mast cell disease. Leuk Res 27: 739–742
156. Longley B J, Tyrrell L, Lu S Z et al. 1996 Somatic c-kit activating mutation in urticaria pigmentosa and aggressive mastocytosis: establishment of clonality in a human mast cell neoplasm. Nature Genet 12: 312–314
157. Pignon J M 1997 C-kit mutations and mast cell disorders. A model of activating mutations of growth factor receptors. Hematol Cell Ther 39: 114–116
158. Buttner C, Henz B M, Welker P et al. 1998 Identification of activating c-kit mutations in adult-, but not in childhood-onset indolent mastocytosis: a possible explanation for divergent clinical behavior. J Invest Dermatol 111: 1227–1231
159. Davies H, Bignell G R, Cox C et al. 2002 Mutations of the BRAF gene in human cancer. Nature 417: 949–954
160. Namba H, Nakashima M, Hayashi T et al. 2003 Clinical implication of hot spot BRAF mutation, V599E, in papillary thyroid cancers. J Clin Endocrinol Metab 88: 4393–4397

161. Kimura ET, Nikiforova M N, Zhu Z et al. 2003 High prevalence of BRAF mutations in thyroid cancer: genetic evidence for constitutive activation of the RET/PTC-RAS-BRAF signaling pathway in papillary thyroid carcinoma. Cancer Res 63: 1454–1457
162. Xing M 2005 BRAF mutation in thyroid cancer. Endocr Relat Cancer 12: 245–262
163. Ronaghi M 2001 Pyrosequencing sheds light on DNA sequencing. Genome Res 11: 3–11
164. Dong Y, Zhu H 2005 Single-strand conformational polymorphism analysis: basic principles and routine practice. Methods Mol Med 108: 149–157
165. Fodde R, Losekoot M 1994 Mutation detection by denaturing gradient gel electrophoresis (DGGE). Hum Mutat 3L: 83–94
166. Xiao W, Oefner P J 2001 Denaturing high-performance liquid chromatography: A review. Hum Mutat 17: 439–474
167. Tonegawa S 1983 Somatic generation of antibody diversity. Nature 302: 575–581
168. Alt F W, Blackwell T K, DePinho R A et al. 1986 Regulation of genome rearrangement events during lymphocyte differentiation. Immunol Rev 89: 5–30
169. Alt F W, Baltimore D 1982 Joining of immunoglobulin heavy chain gene segments: implications from a chromosome with evidence of three D–JH fusions. Proc Natl Acad Sci USA 79: 4118–4122
170. Desiderio S V, Yancopoulos G D, Paskind M et al. 1984 Insertion of N regions into heavy-chain genes is correlated with expression of terminal deoxytransferase in B cells. Nature 311: 752–755
171. Hieter P A, Korsmeyer S J, Waldmann T A et al. 1981 Human immunoglobulin kappa light-chain genes are deleted or rearranged in lambda-producing B cells. Nature 290: 368–372
172. Korsmeyer S J, Hieter P A, Ravetch J V et al. 1981 Developmental hierarchy of immunoglobulin gene rearrangements in human leukemic pre-B cells. Proc Natl Acad Sci USA 78: 7096–7100
173. Bassing C H, Swat W, Alt F W 2002 The mechanism and regulation of chromosomal V(D)J recombination. Cell 109(Suppl): S45–55
174. Blom B, Verschuren M C, Heemskerk M H et al. 1999 TCR gene rearrangements and expression of the pre-T-cell receptor complex during human T-cell differentiation. Blood 93: 3033–3043
175. Hawwari A, Bock C, Krangel M S 2005 Regulation of T cell receptor alpha gene assembly by a complex hierarchy of germline J alpha promoters. Nature Immunol 6: 481–489
176. Cleary M L, Chao J, Warnke R et al. 1984 Immunoglobulin gene rearrangement as a diagnostic criterion of B-cell lymphoma. Proc Natl Acad Sci USA 81: 593–597
177. Greaves M F, Chan L C, Furley A J et al. 1986 Lineage promiscuity in hemopoietic differentiation and leukemia. Blood 67: 1–11
178. Kitchingman G R, Rovigatti U, Mauer A M et al. 1985 Rearrangement of immunoglobulin heavy chain genes in T cell acute lymphoblastic leukemia. Blood 65: 725–729
179. Schmidt C A, Przybylski G K 2001 What can we learn from leukemia as for the process of lineage commitment in hematopoiesis? Int Rev Immunol 20: 107–115
180. Inghirami G, Szabolcs M J, Yee H T et al. 1993 Detection of immunoglobulin gene rearrangement of B cell non-Hodgkin's lymphomas and leukemias in fresh, unfixed and formalin-fixed, paraffin-embedded tissue by polymerase chain reaction. Lab Invest 68: 746–757
181. Wan J H, Trainor K J, Brisco M J et al. 1990 Monoclonality in B cell lymphoma detected in paraffin wax embedded sections using the polymerase chain reaction. J Clin Pathol 43: 888–890
182. Signoretti S, Murphy M, Cangi M G et al. 1999 Detection of clonal T-cell receptor gamma gene rearrangements in paraffin-embedded tissue by polymerase chain reaction and nonradioactive single-strand conformational polymorphism analysis. Am J Pathol 154: 67–75
183. McCarthy K P, Sloane J P, Wiedemann L M 1990 Rapid method for distinguishing clonal from polyclonal B cell populations in surgical biopsy specimens. J Clin Pathol 43: 429–432
184. Trainor K J, Brisco M J, Story C J et al. 1990 Monoclonality in B-lymphoproliferative disorders detected at the DNA level. Blood 75: 2220–2222
185. Bourguin A, Tung R, Galili N et al. 1990 Rapid, nonradioactive detection of clonal T-cell receptor gene rearrangements in lymphoid neoplasms. Proc Natl Acad Sci USA 87: 8536–8540
186. Greiner T C, Raffeld M, Lutz C et al. 1995 Analysis of T cell receptor-gamma gene rearrangements by denaturing gradient gel electrophoresis of GC-clamped polymerase chain reaction products. Correlation with tumor-specific sequences. Am J Pathol 146: 46–55
187. Kaul K, Petrick M, Herz B et al. 1996 Detection of clonal rearrangement of the T-cell receptor gamma gene by polymerase chain reaction and single-strand conformation polymorphism (PCR–SSCP). Mol Diagn 1: 131–137
188. Van Dongen J J, Langerak A W, Bruggemann M et al. 2003 Design and standardization of PCR primers and protocols for detection of clonal immunoglobulin and T-cell receptor gene recombinations in suspect lymphoproliferations: report of the BIOMED-2 Concerted Action BMH4-CT98-3936. Leukemia 17: 2257–2317
189. Golub T R, Slonim D K, Tamayo P et al. 1999 Molecular classification of cancer: class discovery and class prediction by gene expression monitoring. Science 286: 531–537
190. Yeoh E J, Ross M E, Shurtleff S A et al. 2002 Classification, subtype discovery, and prediction of outcome in pediatric acute lymphoblastic leukemia by gene expression profiling. Cancer Cell 1: 133–143
191. Alizadeh A A, Eisen M B, Davis R E et al. 2000 Distinct types of diffuse large B-cell lymphoma identified by gene expression profiling. Nature 403: 503–511
192. Rosenwald A, Wright G, Chan W C et al. 2002 The use of molecular profiling to predict survival after chemotherapy for diffuse large B-cell lymphoma. N Engl J Med 346: 1937–1947
193. Wright G, Tan B, Rosenwald A et al. 2003 A gene expression-based method to diagnose clinically distinct subgroups of diffuse large B cell lymphoma. Proc Natl Acad Sci USA 100: 9991–9996
194. Staudt L M, Dave S 2005 The biology of human lymphoid malignancies revealed by gene expression profiling. Adv Immunol 87: 163–208
195. Perou C M, Jeffrey S S, van de Rijn M et al. 1999 Distinctive gene expression patterns in human mammary epithelial cells and breast cancers. Proc Natl Acad Sci USA 96: 9212–9217
196. Perou C M, Sorlie T, Eisen M B et al. 2000 Molecular portraits of human breast tumours. Nature 406: 747–752
197. Sorlie T, Perou C M, Tibshirani R et al. 2001 Gene expression patterns of breast carcinomas distinguish tumor subclasses with clinical implications. Proc Natl Acad Sci USA 98: 10869–10874
198. Sorlie T, Tibshirani R, Parker J et al. 2003 Repeated observation of breast tumor subtypes in independent gene expression data sets. Proc Natl Acad Sci USA 100: 8418–8423
199. Sotiriou C, Neo S Y, McShane L M et al. 2003 Breast cancer classification and prognosis based on gene expression profiles from a population-based study. Proc Natl Acad Sci USA 100: 10393–10398
200. Brenton J D, Carey L A, Ahmed A A et al. 2005 Molecular classification and molecular forecasting of breast cancer: ready for clinical application? J Clin Oncol 23: 7350–7360
201. Van 't Veer L J, Dai H, van de Vijver M J et al. 2002 Gene expression profiling predicts clinical outcome of breast cancer. Nature 415: 530–536
202. Wang Y, Klijn J G, Zhang Y et al. 2005 Gene-expression profiles to predict distant metastasis of lymph-node-negative primary breast cancer. Lancet 365: 671–679
203. Lossos I S, Czerwinski D K, Alizadeh A A et al. 2004 Prediction of survival in diffuse large-B-cell lymphoma based on the expression of six genes. N Engl J Med 350: 1828–1837
204. Hans C P, Weisenburger D D, Greiner T C et al. 2004 Confirmation of the molecular classification of diffuse large B-cell lymphoma by immunohistochemistry using a tissue microarray. Blood 103: 275–282
205. Callagy G, Cattaneo E, Daigo Y et al. 2003 Molecular classification of breast carcinomas using tissue microarrays. Diagn Mol Pathol 12: 27–34
206. Abd El-Rehim D M, Pinder S E, Paish C E et al. 2004 Expression of luminal and basal cytokeratins in human breast carcinoma. J Pathol 203: 661–671
207. Nielsen T O, Hsu F D, Jensen K et al. 2004 Immunohistochemical and clinical characterization of the basal-like subtype of invasive breast carcinoma. Clin Cancer Res 10: 5367–5374
208. Jacquemier J, Ginestier C, Rougemont J et al. 2005 Protein expression profiling identifies subclasses of breast cancer and predicts prognosis. Cancer Res 65: 767–779
209. Hughes T P, Kaeda J, Branford S et al. 2003 Frequency of major molecular responses to imatinib or interferon alfa plus cytarabine in newly diagnosed chronic myeloid leukemia. N Engl J Med 349: 1423–1432
210. Mandelli F, Diverio D, Avvisati G et al. 1997 Molecular remission in PML/RAR alpha-positive acute promyelocytic leukemia by combined all-trans-retinoic acid and idarubicin (AIDA) therapy. Gruppo Italiano–Malattie Ematologiche Maligne dell'Adulto and Associazione Italiana di Ematologia ed Oncologia Pediatrica Cooperative Groups. Blood 90: 1014–1021
211. Sanz M A, Martin G, Rayon C et al. 1999 A modified AIDA protocol with anthracycline-based consolidation results in high antileukemic efficacy and reduced toxicity in newly diagnosed PML/RARalpha-positive acute promyelocytic leukemia. PETHEMA group. Blood 94: 3015–3021
212. Diverio D, Rossi V, Avvisati G et al. 1998 Early detection of relapse by prospective reverse transcriptase–polymerase chain reaction analysis of the PML/RARalpha fusion gene in patients with acute promyelocytic leukemia enrolled in the GIMEMA–AIEOP multicenter 'AIDA' trial. GIMEMA–AIEOP Multicenter 'AIDA' Trial. Blood 92: 784–789
213. Reiter A, Lengfelder E, Grimwade D 2004 Pathogenesis, diagnosis and monitoring of residual disease in acute promyelocytic leukaemia. Acta Haematol 112: 55–67
214. Mrozek K, Heerema N A, Bloomfield C D 2004 Cytogenetics in acute leukemia. Blood Rev 18: 115–136
215. Mancini M, Scappaticci D, Cimino G et al. 2005 A comprehensive genetic classification of adult acute lymphoblastic leukemia (ALL): analysis of the GIMEMA 0496 protocol. Blood 105: 3434–3441
216. Harrison C J, Foroni L 2002 Cytogenetics and molecular genetics of acute lymphoblastic leukemia. Rev Clin Exp Hematol 6: 91–113
217. Fonseca R, Barlogie B, Bataille R et al. 2004 Genetics and cytogenetics of multiple myeloma: a workshop report. Cancer Res 64: 1546–1558
218. Stewart A K, Fonseca R 2005 Prognostic and therapeutic significance of myeloma genetics and gene expression profiling. J Clin Oncol 23: 6339–6344
219. Brodeur G M 2003 Neuroblastoma: biological insights into a clinical enigma. Nat Rev Cancer 3: 203–216
220. Slamon D J, Clark G M, Wong S G et al. 1987 Human breast cancer: correlation of relapse and survival with amplification of the HER-2/neu oncogene. Science 235: 177–182

221. Press M F, Pike M C, Chazin V R et al. 1993 Her-2/neu expression in node-negative breast cancer: direct tissue quantitation by computerized image analysis and association of overexpression with increased risk of recurrent disease. Cancer Res 53: 4960–4970
222. Slamon D J, Leyland-Jones B, Shak S et al. 2001 Use of chemotherapy plus a monoclonal antibody against HER2 for metastatic breast cancer that overexpresses HER2. N Engl J Med 344: 783–792
223. Schroeder H W Jr, Dighiero G. 1994 The pathogenesis of chronic lymphocytic leukemia: analysis of the antibody repertoire. Immunol Today 15:, 288–294
224. Fais F, Ghiotto F, Hashimoto S et al. Chronic lymphocytic leukemia B cells express restricted sets of mutated and unmutated antigen receptors. J Clin Invest 102: 1515–1525
225. Damle R N, Wasil T, Fais F et al. 1999 Ig V gene mutation status and CD38 expression as novel prognostic indicators in chronic lymphocytic leukemia. Blood 94: 1840–1847
226. Hamblin T J, Davis Z, Gardiner A et al. 1999 Unmutated Ig V(H) genes are associated with a more aggressive form of chronic lymphocytic leukemia. Blood 94: 1848–1854
226a. Del Gindice I, Morilla A, Dsuji N et al. 2005. Zeta-chain associated protein 70 and CD38 combined predict the time to first treatment in patients with chronic lymphocytic leukemia. Cancer 104: 2124–2132
227. Schaeffeler E, Fischer C, Brockmeier D et al. 2004 Comprehensive analysis of thiopurine S-methyltransferase phenotype–genotype correlation in a large population of German Caucasians and identification of novel TPMT variants. Pharmacogenetics 14: 407–417
228. Cheok M H, Evans W E 2006 Acute lymphoblastic leukaemia: a model for the pharmacogenomics of cancer therapy. Nat Rev Cancer 6: 117–129
229. Ando Y, Saka H, Ando M et al. 2000 Polymorphisms of UDP-glucuronosyltransferase gene and irinotecan toxicity: a pharmacogenetic analysis. Cancer Res 60: 6921–6926
230. Iyer L, Das S, Janisch L et al. 2002 UGT1A1*28 polymorphism as a determinant of irinotecan disposition and toxicity. Pharmacogenomics J 2: 43–47
231. Innocenti F, Undevia S D, Iyer L et al. 2004 Genetic variants in the UDP-glucuronosyltransferase 1A1 gene predict the risk of severe neutropenia of irinotecan. J Clin Oncol 22: 1382–1388

索引

AA protein, 128
ABL gene, 1862–3
Abrikossof tumor *see* Granular cell tumor
Abtropfung, 1792
Acantholytic acanthoma, 1427
Acantholytic carcinoma, larynx, 167
Acantholytic squamous carcinoma *see* Adenoid squamous carcinoma
Acanthoma
  acantholytic, 1427
  epidermolytic, 1428–9
  large cell, 1435
  pale (clear) cell, 1427–8
  pilar sheath, 1446
  see also Adenoacanthoma; Keratoacanthoma
Acanthomatous ameloblastoma, 224, 225
Acinic cell carcinoma, 476–7
  breast, 954–5
  lung (Fechner tumor), 191
  pleura, 191
  salivary gland, 263, 284–8
    clinical features, 284–5
    definition, 284
    differential diagnosis, 288
    electron microscopy, 287
    immunohistochemistry, 287
    macroscopic appearances, 285
    microscopic appearances, 285–7
    prognostic factors, 287
Acinic cell cystadenocarcinoma, 477
Acoustic neuroma/neurilemmoma/neurinoma/neurofibroma *see* Vestibular schwannoma
Acquired immunodeficiency syndrome *see* AIDS
Acquired retention cyst, esophagus, 339
Acral lentiginous melanoma, 1469, 1482
Acral melanocytic nevus, 1471
  intradermal, 1469
  junctional, 1468
Acral myxoinflammatory fibroblastic sarcoma, 1557
Acroangiodermatitis, 49, 61
Acromegaly, 16, 182, 836, 980–3, 989, 1124, 1132–3
Acrospirocarcinoma (malignant acrospiroma), 1463–4

Acrospiroma (poroma), 1457–9
  malignant, 1463–4
Acrosyringeal nevus (syringofibroadenoma), 1456–7
ACTH, 1132
  pheochromocytoma, 1112
ACTH-secreting pituitary adenoma, 984–5
  Crook's hyaline change, 984
  silent "corticotroph" adenoma, 985
Actin
  adenoid cystic carcinoma, 190
  adenomyoepithelioma, 951
  capillary hemangioma, 45
  cardiac myxoma, 13
  cardiac rhabdomyoma, 19
  cavernous hemangioma, 48
  desmoid fibromatosis, 1552
  epithelial-myoepithelial carcinoma, 192
  fibroblastic dendritic cell tumors, 1242
  fibroepithelial stromal polyp, 722
  fibrosarcoma, 196
  follicular dendritic cell sarcoma, 129, 1242
  Gardner fibroma, 1547
  hemangiopericytoma, 72
  Kaposiform hemangioendothelioma, 56
  keloid scar, 1539
  leiomyoma, 93
  leiomyosarcoma, 194
  malignant mesothelioma, 206
  mucinous carcinoma, 579
  myoepithelial carcinoma, 261
  nasopharyngeal angiofibroma, 91
  oral cavity tumors, 296
  papillary adenoma, 204
  postoperative spindle cell nodule, 723
  salivary gland tumors, 239
  sarcomatoid carcinoma, 534
  Sertoli cell tumor, 598
  sinusoidal-type hemangioma, 100
  solitary fibrous tumor, 92
  spindle cell hemangioma, 53
  spindle cell squamous carcinoma, 105
Actin, muscle-specific
  adenoid cystic carcinoma, 710
  adrenal leiomyosarcoma, 1119
  basal cell hyperplasia, 780
  glomus tumor, 71

Actin, muscle-specific (*Cont'd*)
  leiomyoma, 93
  micropapillary carcinoma, 534
  oral cavity tumors, 296
  rhabdomyosarcoma, 131, 851, 1816
  sclerosing adenosis, 783
  sinonasal-type hemangiopericytoma, 100
  solitary fibrous tumor, 1714
  splenic hamartoma, 1308
  xanthogranuloma, 1493
Actin, smooth muscle
  adenoid cystic carcinoma, 123, 191, 954
  adenosquamous carcinoma, 939
  adult granulosa cell tumor, 591
  angiomyolipoma, 430, 504
  atypical teratoid/rhabdoid tumor, 1705
  cardiac leiomyosarcoma, 35
  cardiac sarcoma, 34
  cellular angiofibroma, 740
  ductal papilloma, 915
  endometrial stromal tumor, 667
  epithelioid hemangioendothelioma, 63
  fibroma-thecoma, 837
  fibrous histiocytoma, 1558
  gastrointestinal stromal tumors, 358
  genital leiomyoma, 1564
  glomus tumor, 71, 200
  gonadal stromal tumor, 838
  hemangiopericytoma, 72, 73, 100
  hyalinizing clear cell carcinoma, 296
  intimal sarcoma, 67
  keloid scar, 1540
  leiomyoma, 93
  leiomyosarcoma, 194, 744
  lymphangioleiomyomatosis, 197
  malignant teratoma, 134
  mesothelioma, 207
  molluscum contagiosum, 862
  mucinous cystic tumors, 474
  myeloepithelioma, 88
  myofibroblastic sarcoma, 1554
  myofibroblastoma, 958
  nasopharyngeal angiofibroma (juvenile angiofibroma), 91
  neural tumors, 1495
  ossifying fibromyxoid tumor, 1573
  papillary carcinoma, 929
  peritoneal fibrosis, 884

Actin, smooth muscle (Cont'd)
  pleomorphic adenoma, 736
  polymorphous low-grade
      adenocarcinoma, 290
  postoperative spindle cell nodule, 796
  pseudosarcomatous fibromyxoid tumor, 797
  radial scar/complex sclerosing lesion, 914
  salivary gland neoplasms, 88
  sclerosing stromal tumor, 602
  smooth muscle tumors, 337
  spindle cell epithelioma, 725
  spindle cell squamous carcinoma, 106
  stromal sarcoma, 799
  undifferentiated sarcoma, 34
Actinic (solar) keratosis, 1434–42
Actinomycosis, larynx, 156
Adamantinoma, long bones, 1594, 1625–7
Addison's disease, 1120
Adenoacanthoma, pancreas, 662
Adenocarcinoma
  anal canal, 410
  apocrine, 1460–1
  appendix, 390–1
  bladder, 539–43
  cervix, 704–9
    early, 704
    endocervical, 704–5
    endometrioid, 707
    enteric, 707
    mesonephric, 708–9
    minimal-deviation, 705–6
    papillary serous, 708
    villoglandular, 706
  clear cell see Clear cell adenocarcinoma
  digital papillary, 1464–5
  eccrine/apocrine glands, 1460–1
  electron microscopy, 1834–8
  endolymphatic sar origin, low grade
      (aggressive papillary tumor of
      middle ear), 1827
  endometrioid, 581, 661–2
  endometrium, 660
    exclusion of, 657–8
  enteric, 707
  epididymis, 849–50
  esophagus, 333–4
  fallopian tube, 625–7
  gallbladder, 445–8
  intestinal-type, 120–2
    vagina, 721
  larynx, 172–3
  lung and pleura, 183
  mammary-type, 737
  mucinous see Mucinous adenocarcinoma
  orbit, 1799
  ovary, 582–3
  pancreas, 463–8
  prostate, 755–74
    crystalloids, 757
    differential diagnosis, 759–60
    grading systems, 763–7
    immunohistochemistry, 760–2
    nerve invasion, 762

Adenocarcinoma (Cont'd)
    staging systems, 762–3
    transition-zone cancer, 758–9
    treatment effect, 768–71
  renal pelvis/ureter, 522
  rete testis, 843
  salivary gland, 301–2
  seminal vesicles, 802–3
  Skene's gland, 737–8
  small intestine, 380
  stomach, 344–50
  thymus, 1334, 1351
  tongue, 290–1
  trachea, 172–3
  villoglandular
    cervix, 706
    vulva, 738
  see also Cystadenocarcinoma
Adenocarcinoma in-situ
  cervical glandular intraepithelial
      neoplasia (CGIN), 699–702
  vulvar Paget's diseaes, 736–7
Adenofibroma
  biliary, 451
  cervix, 712
  lung, 204
  metanephric, 488–90
  salivary gland, 275
Adenofibromatous borderline tumor, ovary,
    570, 580, 581, 619
Adenohypophysis (anterior pituitary), 971
Adenoid basal carcinoma see Basaloid
    carcinoma
Adenoid basal cell tumor, prostate, 781,
    781–2
Adenoid carcinoma, oral cavity, 216–17
Adenoid cystic carcinoma, 107, 172, 190–1,
    1464
  breast, 953–4
  cervix, 710
  esophagus, 334
  lung and pleura, 190–1
  orbit, 1799
  prostate, 781–2
  salivary gland, 123, 280–4
    dedifferentiated type, 282
Adenoid squamous carcinoma, larynx, 167
Adenolymphoma of salivary gland see
    Warthin's tumor
Adenoma
  acidophilic stem cell, 983–4
  ACTH-secreting, 984–5
  adrenal cortical, 1100–3
    in Cushing's syndrome, 1100
    function pigmented ("black"), 1102–3
    in primary hyperaldosteronism,
        1100–2
  appendix, 390
  bile duct, 449–50
  breast, 916, 1454–5
    lactational, 908
    tubular, 907–8
  ceruminous gland (ceruminoma),
      1814–15

Adenoma (Cont'd)
  cervical, in situ, 699–702
  ductal, of breast, 917
  esophagus, 327
  external ear, 1814–15
  fallopian tube, 624–5
  gallbladder, 443–4
  gonadotropin-secreting, 985–7
  growth hormone-producing, 980–2
  kidney, 485–6
  large intestine, 393–5
    see also Familial adenomatous
        polyposis
  liver cell (hepatocellular), 417–19
  malignum, 705–6
  metanephric, 488–90
  middle ear, 1820–1
  minor vestibular gland, 736
  nephrogenic, 519, 553
  nipple, 916
  Paneth cell, 341
  papillar see Papillary adenoma
  parathyroid glands, 1081–7
    atypical, 1091–2
    follicular variant, 1086
    lipoadenoma, 1086
    oxyphil, 1086
    papillary variant, 1086
    water-clear variant, 1086
  pituitary, 88–9, 973–4
    null-cell, 987
    pathogenesis, 975–7
    pituitary apoplexy, 988–9
    plurihormonal, 988
    prolactin-secreting, 978–80, 982–4
  prostate, 783–4
  sebaceous see Sebaceous adenoma
  small intestine, 379–80
  stomach, 340–2
  thyroid see Follicular adenoma
  TSH-secreting, 987–8
  tubular apocrine, 1454
  villous see Villous adenoma
  see also Cystadenoma; Fibroadenoma;
      Hidradenoma; L:ipoadenoma;
      Lymphadenoma; Microadenoma;
      Spiradenoma; Syringocystadenoma
      papilliferum
Adenomatoid tumor
  fallopian tumor, 624–5
  myometrium, 688
  odeontogenic, 227–8
  ovary, 618
  paratesticular tissues, 846–7
  peritoneum, 886
  pleura, 219
  prostate (sclerosing adenosis), 783–4
Adenomatosis, renal, 486
Adenomatous (colloid) thyroid nodule,
    1010, 1029
Adenomatous hyperplasia
  liver, 419–21
  prostate, 778–9
  rete testis, 842

Adenomucinosis, peritoneal disseminated, 621, 622
Adenomyoepithelioma, breast, 951–2
Adenomyoma
  bile duct, 451
  cervix, 712–13
  endocervical, 712–13
  myometrium, 687–8
  polypoid, 666
Adenomyomatous polyps, 666
Adenosarcoma
  bladder, 547–8
  endometrium, 665–7
  fallopian tube, 627–8
  Müllerian, 713
  ovary, 583
  vagina, 726
Adenosis
  breast
    blunt duct, 904–5
    microglandular, 912–13
    sclerosing, 911–12
  prostate, 783–4
  salivary gland, 273
Adenosquamous carcinoma, 107–8, 166, 167–8
  Bartholin's gland, 737
  breast, 939
  cervix, 709–10
  endometrioid, 720, 721
  esophagus, 334
  fallopian tube, 624–5
  gallbladder, 447
  lung and pleura, 186–7
  pancreas, 469
  penis, 872–3
  prostate, 775–6
  stomach, 351–2
  thyroid, 1031
Adipocytic liposarcoma, 1534–9
Adipocytic tumors, 1528–39
Adnexal tumors, 1442–65
  eyelids, 1456–7
  folliculosebaceous, 1443
  hair follicle, 1442–51
  ovary, 617–18, 627
  sebaceous, 1451–3
  skin, 1442–65
  of Wolffian origin, 628–9
Adrenal cortical tumors
  adenomas, 1100–3
  carcinomas, 1104–9
  virilizing/feminizing, 1103–4
Adrenal gland, 1099
  metastatic tumors, 1118–19, 1120
Adrenal hyperplasia, congenital (adrenogenital syndrome), 838–9
Adrenal medullary hyperplasia, 1110, 1114–15
Adrenal rests, 628
  paratesticular, 844
  placenta, 672
Adrenal tumefactive spindle cell lesion, 1118

Adrenocorticotrophic hormone see ACTH
Adrenogenital syndrome (cortical adrenal hyperplasia), 838–9
Adult T-cell leukemia/lymphoma, 1229, 1405–6, 1496
  splenic involvement, 1292
Aflatoxin, 425, 431
Aggressive fibromatosis, 92–3
Aggressive NK-cell leukemia, 1233, 1413
  splenic involvement, 1292
Agnogenic myeloid metaplasia, 421, 1291, 1295, 1302, 1399
AgNor counts
  central nervous system tumors, 1655
  cholesteatoma, 1818
  pancreatic tumors, 1128
  prostate tumors, 753
AIDS, 1234–6
  adrenal tumors, 1118
  bacillary angiomatosis, 1250
  diffuse BALT hyperplasia (lymphoid interstitial pneumonia), 198
  Kaposi sarcoma see Kaposi sarcoma
  lymphoma
    Burkitt's, 1211
    central nervous system, 1173, 1715
    Hodgkin, 1152, 1159
    MALT, 307
    plasmablastic, 1208
    primary effusion (body cavity), 1207
    primary hepatic, 443
  molluscum contagiosum, 862
  myobacterial spindle cell pseudotumor, 1303
  plasmacytoma, 840
  pyogenic granuloma, 47
  see also HIV
Albright syndrome, 96, 97, 1636
Albumin ISH, 430
Aldosteronoma, 1100–2
ALK+ histiocytosis, 1238
ALK+ large B-cell lymphoma, 1208
ALK see Anaplastic lymphoma kinase
ALKoma, 1224
Allergic granulomatosis and vasculitis, 126, 127
Alpha chain disease, 386
Alpha-antichymotrypsin
  breast tumors, 954
  skin tumors, 1490
  vimentin-positive gastric carcinoma, 352
Alpha-antitrypsin
  dermatofibrosarcoma protruberans, 1490
  embryonal sarcoma, 442
  hepatocellular carcinoma, 427
  liver cirrhosis, 423
  pancreatoblastoma, 479
  papillary adenoma, 486
  yolk sac tumor, 825
Alpha-antitrypsin deficiency, 423, 425
Alpha-fetoprotein
  dysgerminoma, 605
  embryonal carcinoma, 1718

Alpha-fetoprotein (Cont'd)
  germ cell tumors, 604, 816, 1340
    malignant, 819
  hepatic adenoma, 417, 419
  hepatoid tumors, 352
  immature teratoma, 610
  pancreatoblastoma, 478
  seminoma, 818
  Sertoli-Leydig cell tumors, 596
  yolk sac tumor, 551, 605
Alpha-fetoprotein-producing carcinoma, 352
Alveolar adenoma, 203
Alveolar rhabdomyosarcoma, 1528, 1568–9
  nasopharynx, 131
Alveolar soft part sarcoma, 1528, 1579–80
  cervix, 714
  electron microscopy, 1850
  endometrium, 669
  sinonasal tract/nasopharynx, 134
  thymus, 1351
  vulva, 745
Alveolar soft-part sarcoma, 669
Ameloblastic carcinoma, 231
Ameloblastic fibro-odontoma, 227
Ameloblastic fibrodentinoma, 227
Ameloblastic fibroma, 227
Ameloblastoma, 98
  acanthomatous, 224, 225
  malignant, 231–2
  oral cavity, 224–5, 231–2
  unicystic, 225–6
Amianthoid fibers, 209
AML1-ETO fusion protein, 1375
Amputation (traumatic) neuroma, 1733
Amylase
  acinic cell carcinoma of pancreas, 477
  salivary gland tumors, 240, 263, 265, 287
Amylin (islet cell amyloid polypeptide), insulinoma, 1129
Amyloid
  esophagus, 339
  larynx and trachea, 156–7
  seminal vesicles, 801
  stomach, 370
Amyloid tumor, stomach, 370
Amyloidoma of spleen, 1309
Amyloidosis, laryngeal, 156–7
Anal canal tumors, 409–11
  adenocarcinoma, 410
  cyst hamartoma, 411
  giant condyloma and verrucous carcinoma, 410
  malignant melanoma, 410–11
  squamous carcinoma, 409–10
Anal margin tumors, 411–12
Analgesic abuse, capillarosclerosis, 521
Anaplastic lymphoma kinase (ALK), 1149, 1224
Anaplastic variants
  astrocytic tumors, 1658–9
  astrocytoma, 1662–3
  carcinoma see Undifferentiated carcinoma
  ependymoma, 1680–1

Anaplastic variants (Cont'd)
  ganglioglioma, 1694–5
  lymphoma
    diffuse large B-cell, 1201
    follicular, 1189
    large cell, 1223–8
  medullary thyroid carcinoma, 1041
  medulloblastoma, 1705
  meningioma, 1710–12
  neuroblastoma, 1774
  oligoastrocytoma, 1677–8
  oligodendroglioma, 1675–6
  rhabdomyosarcoma, 1568
Androgen receptors, nasopharyngeal angiofibroma, 91
Androgenic/anabolic steroids, 417, 418, 439, 1305
Anemia
  refractory
    with excess blasts, 1368–9
    pure dyserythropoietic, 1366
    with ringed sideroblasts, 1367
Anemone cell large cell lymphoma, 1201
Aneurysmal (angiomatoid) fibrous histiocytoma, 1486
Aneurysmal bone cyst, 1570, 1634–6
  larynx and trachea, 158
  solid (giant cell reparative granuloma), 97–8, 1816
Angioblastoma
  giant cell, 56–7
  of Nakagawa (tufted), 46
Angiocentric natural killer/T-cell lymphoma, 126, 127
Angioendotheliomatosis, reactive, 43
Angiofibroma
  cellular, 1548–9
  nasopharyngeal (juvenile), 91–2
  thymus, 1351
  vulva, 740–1
Angioimmunoblastic lymphadenopathy with dysproteinemia, 1220–1
Angioimmunoblastic T-cell lymphoma, 1219–21
  genetic features, 1220
  histologic features, 1219
  immunocytochemistry, 1220
  splenic involvement, 1292
Angioimmunoproliferative lesion (lymphomatoid granulomatosis), lung, 198, 1205–6
Angiokeratoma, 44–5
  corporis diffusum, 44
  Fordyce, 44
  Mibelli, 44
  penis, 866
  solitary, 44
  vulva, 742
Angioleiomyoma
  larynx and trachea, 154
  smooth muscle, 1563
Angiolipoma, 1531
  intramuscular, 54
  stomach, 360

Angiolymphoid hyperplasia with eosinophilia (epithelioid hemangioma), 51–2
Angioma
  cherry (senile; Campbell de Morgan spot), 46
  littoral cell, 1305
  serpiginosum, 44
  tufted (angioblastoma of Nakagawa), 46
Angiomatoid variant
  malignant fibrous histiocytoma, 1486, 1574–5
  thymic carcinoid tumor, 1337–9
  thyroid undifferentiated tumors, 1031
Angiomatosis, 55
  breast, 956
Angiomyofibroblastoma, 1547–8
  vagina, 723
  vulva, 740
Angiomyolipoma, 1245
  extrarenal, 1532
  kidney, 502–4
  liver, 437–8
  spleen, 1310
Angiomyoma, larynx and trachea, 154
Angiomyomatous hamartoma, 1247
Angiomyxoma
  placenta (chorangioma), 672
  soft tissue, 1571–2
  superficial, 1571–2
  vagina, 724
  vulva, 742–3
Angiosarcoma, 63–7
  adrenal gland, 1119
  bone, 1594, 1628–9
  breast, 956–7
    post-radiation, 957
  cardiac, 7, 32–3
  epithelioid, 66–7, 1629
  heart, 7, 32–3
  idiopathic of face, neck and scalp, 64
  intimal, 67
  large intestine, 405
  larynx, 174
  littoral cell, 1305–7
  liver, 439–40
  lung and pleura, 196
  lymphedema-associated, 64
  ovary, 603
  postradiation, 64
  sinonasal tract/nasopharynx, 131
  small intestine, 383
  soft-tissue, 64–6
  spleen, 1305–7
  thyroid, 1052–3
  vulva, 745
Angiotropic lymphoma (intravascular large B-cell lymphoma), 1497, 1499, 1505
Anlage tumor
  retinal, 669, 1754–6
  salivary gland, 272
Ann Arbor staging system, Hodgkin's lymphoma, 1153
Anogenital melanoma, 1483

Antibodies
  lymphoproliferative lesions, 1144–50
  metastatic lymph node carcinoma, 1246
Antigen receptor gene rearrangements, 1872–4
Antimüllerian hormone (Müllerian inhibiting substance)
  granulosa cell tumor, 589
  sex cord tumor with annular tubules, 599
Antineutrophil cytoplasmic antibodies (ANCA), 126
Antrochoanal polyps, 134
Aortic bodies, 1769
Aortic bodies (organs of Zuckerkandl), 1769
APC mutation, 91
  familial adenomatous polyposis, 396
  gastric carcinoma, 345
  hepatoblastoma, 435
  squamous carcinoma, esophagus, 328
  thyroid tumors, 1010
Apocrine adenocarcinoma, 1460–1
Apocrine ductal carcinoma in-situ, breast, 927
Apocrine hidrocystoma/cystadenoma, 1453
  eyelid, 1782
Apocrine metaplasia of breast, 904
Apoplectic leiomyoma of myometrium, 685
Appendix epiploica infarction, 886
Appendix tumors, 390–3
  endocrine, 391–2
  epithelial, 390–1
Argyrophilia, 118, 578
Arsenic toxicity, 1436
Arteriovenous hemangioma, 49–50
  breast, 955–6
Asbestos exposure, 205, 849, 884
Askanazy adenoma/carcinoma *see* Hurthle cell adenoma/carcinoma
Askin tumor, 1750–2
Aspergillosis, 137, 156
Astroblastoma, 1687
Astrocytic tumors, 1655–72
  anaplastic progression, 1658–9
  grading, 1657–8
  invasiveness, 1658
  see also individual types
Astrocytoma, 1659–62
  anaplastic, 1662–3
  desmoplastic infantile, 1689–90
  fibrillary, 1661–2
  monomorphous pilomyxoid, 1668
  pilocytic, 1667–70
  posterior pituitary, 990
  protoplasmic, 1662
  small cell, 1663
  subependymal giant cell, 1672
  see also Oligoastrocytoma
Ataxia-telangiectasia, 1236
ATM mutations
  B-cell chronic lymphocytic leukemia, 1178
  mantle cell lymphoma, 1184

Atrial, malignant fibrous histiocytoma, 33–4
Atrial tumors
　myxoma, 7
　rhabdomoma, 17–18
　septum lipomatous hypertrophy, 2, 22, 23
Atrioventricular node mesothelioma, 7, 30–1
Atrophy, prostate, 790–2
Atypia (dysplasia)
　anal margin, 411–12
　breast, 920–2
　esophagus, 327
　gastric flat, 342–4
　liver cell, 422–4
　oral premalignancy, 219–20
Atypical adenomatous hyperplasia, prostate, 778–9
Atypical ductal hyperplasia, breast, 295, 296
Atypical fibroxanthoma, 1491–2
Atypical lobular hyperplasia, breast, 919, 922
Atypical mole syndrome, 1468, 1478, 1478–9
Atypical variants
　carcinoid tumor, cervix, 711
　endometrial polypoid adenomyoma, 666
　fibroxanthoma, 1491–2
　leiomyoma, 684–5
　lipoma, 1528
　meningioma, 1710
　parathyroid gland adenoma, 1091–2
　prostate adenoma, 762
　stromal hyperplasia of prostate, 793–4
　teratoid/rhabdoid tumor, 1705–6
　thyomoma, 1336
　thyroid gland follicular gland, 1026
Auer rods, 1364
Autoimmune lymphoproliferative syndrome, 1215, 1254, 1256
Autoimmune thyroiditis, 1060
Autoimplants, 571
Autonomic nerve tumor (plexosarcoma; GANT), 358, 381, 383
Autonomic nervous system, 1763–78
　extra-adrenal paraganglia
　　head and neck, 1763–4
　　sympathoadrenal neuroendocrine system, 1769–70
　gangliocytic paraganglioma, 1770–1
　ganglioneuroma, 1777–8
　neuroblastoma, 1771–7
　paragangliomas of head and neck, 1764–9
Azzopardi phenomenon (nuclear encrustation), 189

B lymphocytes, 1140
　antigen receptor gene rearrangements, 1872–4
　development, 1141
　immunophenotypes, 1156–7
B-72.3, 430
　intestinal-type adenocarcinoma, 121
　liver tumors, 453
　mesothelioma, 207, 208
　ovarian tumors, 587, 625
　paratesticular tumors, 849
　peritoneal tumors, 889
B-cell lymphoma
　antigen receptor gene rearrangements, 1872–4
　Burkitt, 120, 1169
　Burkitt-like, 1169
　cutaneous, 1503–5
　diffuse large cell, 126, 127, 307–8, 1169, 1198–209
　diffuse small cell, 1256–8
　esophagus, 338–9
　extranodal marginal zone B-cell lymphoma of MALT type, 1152, 1169, 1193–6
　follicular, 1152, 1169, 1175, 1184–93
　hairy cell leukemia, 1406–8
　Hodgkin's disease, 198–9, 1152–68
　lymphoblastic see B-lymphoblastic lymphoma
　mantle cell, 1152, 1169, 1181–4
　nodal marginal zone, 1169
　plasmacytoma, 1209–10
　sinonasal tract/nasopharynx, 127
　small intestine, 384–7
　spleen, 1295–7
　stomach, 360–3
　Waldeyer's tonsillar tissues, 127–8
B-K mole and syndrome (lentiginous melanocytic nevus), 1468, 1478–9
B-lymphoblastic lymphoma, 1172, 1174, 1175
B-prolymphocytic leukemia, 1410–11
Bacillary angiomatosis, 1250, 1307
Balanitis xerotica obliterans (lichen sclerosus et atrophicus), 863–4
Balkan nephropathy, 520
Balloon cell melanoma, 1484
Balloon cell nevus of vulva, 1471
BALT (bronchus-associated lymphoid tissue) diffuse hyperplasia (lymphoid interstitial pneumonia), 198
　lymphoma, lung, 197
Barrett's esophagus, 328, 333, 334, 340, 343, 345, 348
Bartholin's gland
　adenoma, 735
　carcinoma, 737
Bartonella henselae, 1250
Basal cell adenocarcinoma, salivary gland, 257–8
Basal cell adenoma, salivary gland, 255–7
　congenital (sialoblastoma), 302–3
Basal cell carcinoma
　breast, 937–8
　external ear, 1813
　eyelid, 1785
　penis, 873
　scrotum, 875
Basal cell carcinoma (*Cont'd*)
　skin, 1425
　vulva, 735
Basal cell hyperplasia of prostate, 779–81
Basaloid carcinoma, 185
　anal canal, 410
　cervix, 710
　lung and pleura, 185
　penis, 871
　prostate, 781–2
　thymus, 1333
Basaloid squamous carcinoma
　cervix, 703
　larynx/trachea, 166–7
　oral cavity, 218
　sinonasal tract/nasopharynx, 101, 106–7
Basaloid vulvar intraepithelial neoplasia (VIN), 732–3
Basophils, 1392
Bcl-1, lymphoma, 405, 1151, 1152
Bcl-10
　lymphoma
　　extranodal marginal zone B-cell, 1152
　　follicular, 386
Bcl-2, 1148, 1151, 1202
　basaloid carcinoma, prostate, 782
　ductal carcinoma in-situ, breast, 925
　embryonal sarcoma, 442
　gastric carcinoma, 345
　keratoacanthoma, 1434
　lymphoma, 1151
　　Burkitt, 1148
　　diffuse large B-cell, 1202, 1213
　　extranodal marginal zone B-cell, 1195, 1197
　　follicular, 386, 1050, 1151, 1152, 1185, 1190, 1191, 1252
　　splenic marginal zone, 1298
　melanoma, 200
　pleomorphic low-grade adenocarcinoma of salivary gland, 290
　solitary fibrous tumor
　　lung, 209
　　sinonasal tract/nasopharynx, 92, 100
　　thyroid, 1053
　synovial sarcoma, 195, 196
　thyroid tumors, 1044
Bcl-6, 1148, 1157, 1202
　lymphoma
　　Burkitt's, 386
　　diffuse large B-cell, 362, 1152
　　follicular, 840, 1050, 1148
　　Hodgkin, 1157, 1158
BCR gene, 1862–3
BCR-ABL fusion gene, 1391
Becker's nevus, 1562
Beckwith-Wiedemann syndrome, 433, 511
Bednar tumor, 1488, 1490
Bence-Jones protein, 1402
Benign fibro-osseous lesions, 95–9
　ameloblastoma, 98
　benign teratoma, 98–9
　chondroma, 98
　craniopharyngioma, 98

Benign fibro-osseous lesions (Cont'd)
  fibrous dysplasia, 96–7
  giant cell reparative granuloma, 97–8
  ossifying fibroma, 95
  psammomatoid (active) ossifying, 95–6
Benign lipoma, 1529
Benign lymphangioendothelioma, 68–9
Benign myxoma, cardiac, 7, 9–17
Benign neuroectodermal tumors, 88–90
  meningioma, 89–90
  paraganglioma, 89
  pituitary adenoma, 88–9
Benign synovioma, 1558
3',4'-Benzpyrene exposure, 875
Ber-EP4
  adenocarcinoma, 625
  basal cell carcinoma, 1442
  mesothelioma, 207, 889
  squamous carcinoma, 1439
Ber-H2 see CD30
Beta-catenin gene mutations, 91, 366, 431, 1010
Beta-endorphin, 984, 1043, 1339
Beta-tubulin, olfactory neuroblastoma, 117
Bile duct adenoma, 449–50
Bile duct adenomyoma, 451
Bile duct carcinoma, 453–4
Bile duct neuroma, 451
Bile duct papillomatosis, 454–5
Bile duct tumors
  benign, 449–51
  precursor intraductal lesions, 454–5
Biliary adenofibroma, 451
Biliary dysplasia, 454
Biliary hamartoma, 449
Biliary (hepatobiliary) cystadenoma/cystadenocarcinoma, 450–1
Birbeck granules, 1853, 1854
Bizarre parosteal osteochondromatous proliferation, 1641
Bladder tumors, 523–52
  epithelial
    benign, 523–6
    malignant, 526–37
  mesenchymal, 545–7
    benign, 545
    malignant, 545–6
  mixed, 547–8
  paraganglioma, 549–50
  secondary, 551–2
  transitional cell carcinoma, 526–37
Blastema, 513
Blastic (blastoid) NK-cell lymphoma, 1233–4
Blastoma
  lung, 193
  Wilms' tumor (nephroblastoma), 511–15
Blastomycosis, larynx, 156
Blue nevus, 1469, 1476–7
  cervix, 714
  conjunctiva, 1793
  epithelioid type, 1469
  prostate, 794–6
  vagina, 726–7

Blue nevus-like melanoma, 1484
Blue rubber bleb nevus syndrome, 48, 70
Blunt duct adenosis of breast, 904–5
Bob.1, 1145
Body cavity (primary effusion) lymphoma, 1207
Bombesin
  adenocarcinoma, 380
  medullary thyroid carcinoma, 1043
  neuroendocrine carcinomas, 187
  paragangliomas, 1112
  pheochromocytoma, 1112
Bombesin-producing tumor, 1132
Bone lesions
  cystic, 1634–6
  fibrous non-neoplastic, 1636–7
  reactive new bone formation, 1639–41
Bone surface osteosarcoma, 1620–3
Bone tumors, 1593–647
  biopsy
    fine-needle aspiration, 1595–6
    needle, 1596
    open, 1596–7
  chondroid, 1602–13
  classification, 1594–5
  external ear, 1816
  fibrogenic, 1631–2
  fibrohistiocytic, 1630
  grading and staging, 1595
  lipogenic, 1634
  neural, 1634
  notochordal, 1632–4
  osteogenic, 1613–23
  small cell, 1597–602
  unknown origin, 1623–7
  vascular, 1627–30
Borderline tumors
  broad ligament, 628
  fibrogenic, of bone, 1631–2
  ovary
    adenofibromatous, 570, 580, 581, 619
    Brenner, 586
    clear cell, 584
    endometrioid, 579–80
    mucinous, 577
    serous, 570–3
Borrelia burgdorferi, 1173
Botryoid odontogenic cysts, 235
Botryoid rhabdomyosarcoma, 1567–8
Botryomycosis, sinonasal tract/nasopharynx, 137
Bowenoid actinic (solar) keratosis, 1437
Bowenoid papulosis, 1437–8
  anal margin, 411
  penis, 865–6
  vulva, 731
Bowen's disease
  anal margin, 411
  penis, 865
  skin, 1425, 1436–8
  vulva, 732
Bowman's layer, 1790
Branchial pouch tumors, 1047–9
  see also Thymus

BRCA1, breast cancer, 574, 937
BRCA2, breast cancer, 574, 937
Breast tumors, 903–60
  adenoma of nipple, 916
  adenomyoepithelioma, 951–2
  carcinoma, 924
  chemotherapy, 950–1
  classification, 903
  epithelial, 951–5
  estrogen receptor in, 946–50
  familial breast cancer, 937
  hormone therapy, 951
  lymphoma, 90
  malignant, 924–51
  metastatic, 619, 620, 960
  Nottingham Prognostic Index, 950
  Paget's disease of nipple, 928
  phyllodes, 909–11
  prognostic factors, 939–46
  salivary gland type, 953–5
  stromal, 955–9
Brenner tumor, 585–7
  broad ligament, 628
  endometrium, 669
  ovary, 585–7
    benign, 585–6
    borderline, 586
    malignant, 586–7
  paratesticular, 848
Broad ligament tumors, 628–30
  see also Fallopian tube; Ovary
Brodie abscess, 1614
Bronchial mucous gland adenoma, 203–4
Bronchiectasis, 182
Bronchioalveolar carcinoma, 183–4
Bronchogenic (non-small cell) carcinoma, 181–3
Bronchus
  granular cell tumor, 201
  melanoma, 200
Brooke-Spiegler syndrome, 1815
BRST-2, 1246
Brunner's adenoma, 368
Brunner's gland hamartoma, 387
Budd-Chiari syndrome, 420
Burkitt lymphoma, 120, 1169, 1175, 1210–13
  AIDS-associated, 1211
  B-cell, 120, 1169
  definition, 1210
  differential diagnosis, 1213
  gene expression profiling, 1212–13
  genetic features, 1212
  immunocytochemistry, 1212
  ovary, 603
  pathology, 1211–12
  prostate, 800
  splenic involvement, 1292
  stomach, 360–4
  testis, 839–40
Burkitt-like lymphoma, 1169, 1212
Buschke-Lowenstein giant condyloma, 410, 870
Buttock cells, 1184

C-ANCA, 138
C-cell tumors, 1041
C-erbB2 (HER-2/neu), 948–50
   breast carcinoma prognosis, 948
   breast ductal carcinoma in situ, 946
   nasopharnygeal tumors, 112
   Paget's disease of penis, 875
   pleomorphia adenoma, malignant transformation, 254
   salivary gland tumors, 244
C-kit see CD117
C-met
   cholangiocarcinoma, 453
   thyroid papillary carcinoma, 1009
C-myc
   Burkitt lymphoma, 386, 1152, 1212
   diffuse large B-cell lymphoma, 1202, 1213
   Hodgkin's lymphoma, 1157, 1162
   medulloblastoma, 1705
   primary effusion lymphoma, 1208
   prostatic intraepithelial neoplasia, 753
   thyroid follicular tumors, 1028
CA125, 1246
   fallopian tube tumors, 625
   ovarian tumors
      adenocarcinoma, 620
      carcinoma, 574
   peritoneal malignant mesothelioma, 887
   seminal vesicle adenoma, 802
   testicular/paratesticular tumors, 849
CA19-9
   biliary carcinoma, 453
   biliary cystadenoma, 450
   Brenner tumor, 587
   gallbladder adenocarcinoma, 445
   gastric adenocarcinoma, 346
   intrahepatic cholangiosarcoma, 452
   malignant mesothelioma, 889
   pancreatic ductal adenocarcinoma, 466
Cadherin, 1148
   malignant mesothelioma, 207
Calcifying aponeurotic fibroma, 1549
Calcifying epithelioma of Malherbe (pilomatrixoma), 1449–50
Calcifying fibrous tumor, 1549
   peritoneum, 885
Calcifying odontogenic tumor (Pindborg tumor), 226–7
Calcitonin, 1001, 1246
   carcinoid tumors, 355, 380, 614
      atypical (large cell neuroendocrine carcinoma), 170, 430
   medullary thyroid carcinoma, 1246
   pancreatic tumors, 1131
   pheochromocytoma, 1112
   thyroid tumors, 1001, 1007, 1024, 1044
Calcitonin gene-related peptide, medullary thyroid carcinoma, 1043
Calcitoninoma, 1132
Caldwell-Luc procedure, 135
Call-Exner bodies, 590, 830, 831
Calponin, 123
   adenoid cystic carcinoma, 283

Calponin (Cont'd)
   basal cell adenoma, 257
   clear cell carcinoma, 263
   epithelial-myoepithelial carcinoma, 263, 292
   hyalinizing clear cell carcinoma, 296
   myoepithelioma, 259, 260
   myoepithelioma/mixed tumor, soft tissue, 1574
   pleomorphic adenoma, 88, 251
   salivary gland tumors, 123, 240, 241
Calretinin
   endometrioid carcinoma, 581
   granulosa cell tumor, 591
   Leydig tumors, 601
   metastatic carcinoma, 1246
   thecoma, 594
CAM 5.2
   adenocarcinoma of epididymis, 849
   chondroid syringoma (benign mixed tumor), 1456
   extramammary Paget's disease, 1461, 1462
   female adnexal tumor of Wolffian origin, 629
   granulosa cell tumor, 591
   intra-abdominal desmoplastic small round cell tumor, 891
   Merkel cell (neuroendocrine) carcinoma, 1466
   phyllodes tumor, 911
   renal carcinoma, 500
Campbell de Morgan spot, 46
Campylobacter jejuni, 1173
Canalicular adenoma of salivary gland, 266
Candida albicans, 215, 216
Capillary hemangioma, 45–6
   heart, 28
   intramuscular, 55
   orbit, 1799
   salivary gland, 303
   sinonasal cavity, 84, 90
   variants of, 46–53
      cherry angioma, 46
      lobular capillary hemangioma, 47–8
      tufted angioma, 46
      verrucous hemangioma, 46
Carcinoembryonic antigen, 191
   adenocarcinoma
      cervix, 705
      pancreatic ductal, 466
      stomach, 344
   adrenal cortical carcinoma, 1108
   basaloid squamous carcinoma, 106
   Brenner tumor, 587
   carcinoid tumor, 355
   colorectal cancer, 403
   endocervical-like borderline mucinous tumors, 577
   esophageal Paget's diseaes, 335
   granular cell tumor, 1745
   hepatic adenoma, 418
   hepatocellular carcinoma, 430

Carcinoembryonic antigen (Cont'd)
   medullary thyroid carcinoma, 1043
   mesothelioma, 30, 889
   ovarian carcinoma, 574
   pancreatic endocrine tumors, 1133
   renal carcinoma, 494
   salivary gland tumors, 191
   salivary glands, 240
   thymus, 1334
Carcinoid syndrome, 187, 380, 502
   atypical, 354
   ovarian carcinoids, 613
Carcinoid tumor, 169–70
   appendix, 391
   bile duct, 455
   bladder, 550–1
   cervix, 711
   gallbladder, 448
   goblet cell, 391–2
   lung and pleura, 187–8
   middle ear, 1821
   ovary, 613–14
   pigmented, 187
   small intestine, 380–1
   stomach, 353–6
   testis, 841–2, 841–4
   thymus, 1337–9
Carcinoid-like medullarythyroid carcinoma, 1043
Carcinoma
   acinar cell, 476–7
   acinic cell see Acinic cell carcinoma
   adenoid cystic see Adenoid cystic carcinoma
   adenoid squamous see Adenoid squamous carcinoma
   adenosquamous see Adenosquamous carcinoma
   adrenal cortex, 1104–9
   ameloblastic, 231
   Bartholin's gland, 737
   basal cell see Basal cell carcinoma
   basaloid see Basaloid carcinoma; Basaloid squamous carcinoma
   bile duct, 453–4
   bladder, 526–37
   breast, 903–60
      chemotherapy, 950–1
      classification, 903
      hormone therapy, 951
      metastatic, 619, 620, 960
      Nottingham Prognostic Index, 950
      prognostic factors, 939–46
      stromal features, 955–9
   bronchogenic (non-small cell), 181–3
   cervix, 702–4
   choroid plexus, 1685–6
   clear cell see Clear cell carcinoma
   clinging, 917
   collecting duct, 498–9
   colloid see Colloid carcinoma
   colorectal, 397–402
   conjunctiva, 1791–2
   embryonal see Embryonal carcinoma

Carcinoma (Cont'd)
   endometrial, 580–1
   external ear, 1813–17
   gallbladder, 447
   hair/hair follicle, 1450–1
   hepatocellular, 424–33
   intraosseous, 232
   large cell *see* Large cell neuroendocrine carcinoma; Large cell (undifferentiated) large cell) carcinoma
   larynx, 167
   lymphoepithelial *see* Lymphoeithelial carcinoma
   Merkel cell *see* Merkel cell carcinoma
   middle ear, 1478
   mucinous *see* Mucinous carcinoma
   myoepithelial *see* Myoepithelial carcinoma
   nasal vestibule, 101
   nasopharyngeal, 108–12
   neuroendocrine *see* Neuroendocrine carcinoma
   ovary, 587
   papillary *see* Papillary carcinoma
   parathyroid glands, 1087–91
   penis, 871, 873
   pituitary gland, 974–5
   prostate, 773–4
   renal cell, 263
   sarcomatoid *see* Sarcomatoid carcinoma
   sebaceous *see* Sebaceous carcinoma
   serous *see* Serous carcinoma
   showing thymus-like element (CASTLE), 1048–9, 1337
   small cell *see* Small cell carcinoma
   squamous cell *see* Squamous carcinoma
   thymus, 1331–6
      arising in thmyoma, 1317–31
   thyroid
      follicular, 1040–1
      medullary, 1043
   transitional cell *see* Transitional cell carcinoma
   tricholemmal, 1425, 1446–7
   tubular *see* Tubular carcinoma
   urethral, 554–5
   vagina, 720
   verrucous *see* Verrucous carcinoma
   vulva, 734–5
   Zeis gland, 1782, 1785
Carcinoma ex pleomorphic adenoma, 252–4
Carcinoma in-situ
   breast, ductal, 946
   cervix, 699–702
   gallbladder, 444–5
   see also Adenocarcinoma in-situ; Intraductal carcinoma
Carcinoma showing thymus-like element (CASTLE), 1048–9, 1337
Carcinosarcoma
   breast, 938
   cervix, 713

Carcinosarcoma (Cont'd)
   endometrium, 663–5
   esophagus, 332–3
   fallopian tube, 627–8
   lung and pleura, 185
   odontogenic, 233
   salivary gland, 254–5
   spleen, 1310
   thymus, 1332–3
   thyroid, 1031
   vagina, 726
Cardiac arrhythmias
   cardiac tumors, 17, 20, 22
   lipomatous hypertrophy of interatrial septum, 22, 23, 24
   Purkinje cell tumor, 7, 26–7
Cardiac transplantation, lymphocytic proliferations, 36
Cardiac tumors, 7–36
   benign, 9–32
   children, 7
   clinical aspects, 8–9
   malignant, 32–4
   pathology, 9
   surgical treatment, 8
Cardiac valves
   lipomatous hamartoma, 23
   myxoma, 9, 16
   papillary tumor (papillary fibroelastoma), 17
Carney's syndrome *see* Myxoma syndrome
Carney's triad, 1770
Caroli's disease, 452
Carotid body, 1764
   tumors of, 152
Carotid body paraganglioma, 31, 1764–7
   familial, 1767
   minute pulmonary, 204
   vagal, 1767
Cartilaginous nodules of peritoneum, 886
Cartilaginous tumors, 1608–10
   larynx and trachea, 173–4
   lung, 203
   sinonasal tract/nasopharynx, 95
Caruncle
   conjunctival, 1789
   prostatic, 787
   urethral, 552
CASTLE (carcinoma showing thymus-like element), 1048–9, 1337
Castleman disease, 58, 129
   differential diagnosis, 1210
   esophagus, 338
   hyaline-vascular, 1248–9
   multicentric, 58
   spleen, 1290
Castleman disease-like follicular lymphoma, 1190
Cat-scratch disease, 1165
Cathepsin B
   atypical fibroxanthoma, 1492
   xanthogranuloma, 1493
Cavernous hemangioma, 48–9
   liver, 435

Cavernous hemangioma (Cont'd)
   orbit, 1799
   salivary gland, 303–4
   sinonasal cavity, 91
   vulva, 742
Cavernous lymphangioma, 67–8
CCD22, 1388
CCD79a, 1388
CD10
   B-cell lymphoma, gastric, 362
   Burkitt lymphoma, 386, 1151
   female adnexal tumor of Wolffian origin, 629
   follicular lymphoma, 1050, 1139, 1190
   gynandroblastoma, 602
   lymphomas, 1148, 1151, 1376, 1388, 1409
   solid pseudopapillary tumor of pancreas, 479
   splenic marginal zone B-cell lymphoma, 1298
CD103, 387, 1148
   splenic marginal zone B-cell lymphoma, 1298
CD106, 1204
CD117 (c-kit), 1302, 1376
CD11c
   hairy cell leukemia, 1301, 1407
   histiocytic sarcoma, 1238
   Langerhans cell histiocytosis, 1240
CD123, 1150
CD13, 1376
CD134, 1218
CD138
   ALK+ large B-cell lymphoma, 1208
   diffuse large B-cell lymphoma, 1202
   lymphomas, 1148, 1151, 1376, 1404
   plasmacytoma, 128
CD14, 1376
CD15
   apocrine adenocarcinoma, 1460–1
   Hodgkin's lymphoma, 198
   lymphomas, 1150, 1151, 1157, 1376, 1388
   pseudomesotheliomatous adenoma, 207–8
CD16
   extranodal NK/T-cell lymphoma, 1233
   T-cell granular lymphocytic leukemia, 1175
CD163, 1149
CD19, 1376, 1404, 1409
   acute myelogenous leukemia, 1371
   acute myeloid leukemia, 1382
   B-cell lymphoblastic (precursor lymphoblastic) lymphoma, 1175, 1388
   Burkitt lymphoma, 1212
   hairy cell leukemia, 1301
   lymphomas, 1144
CD1a, 1149, 1376
   Langerhans cell histiocytosis, 1052, 1237, 1239, 1493
   thymocytes, 1315, 1376
   thymoma, 1330

CD2, 1145, 1376
  acute myelogenous leukemia, 1371
  adult T-cell leukemia/lymphoma, 1229
  extranodal NK/T-cell lymphoma, 1231
  hepatosplenic T-cell lymphoma, 1299
  nasal/nasal-type NK/T-cell lymphoma, 126, 1231
  Sézary syndrome, 1214
  T-cell lymphoblastic (precursor lymphoblastic) lymphoma, 1174
  T-cell lymphoma, peripheral, unspecified, 1218
  T-cell prolymphocytic leukemia, 1214
CD20 (L-26), 1376, 1404, 1409, 1598
  B-cell lymphoblastic (precursor lymphoblastic) lymphoma, 1175, 1388
  Burkitt lymphoma, 1212
  chronic lymphocytic leukemia/small lymphocytic lymphoma, 1175, 1176–9
  hairy cell leukemia, 1301
  Hodgkin's lymphoma, 1157
  large B-cell lymphoma of leg, 1499, 1505
  lymphomas, 1144, 1151
  Reed-Sternberg cells, 1152, 1155
  Waldeyer's tonsillar tissue lymphoma, 127–8
CD21/C3d receptor
  follicular dendritic cell sarcoma, 1240–2
  gastric B-cell lymphoma, 360
  inflammatory pseudotumor, 439
  lymphomas, 1150, 1151
  splenic marginal zone B-cell lymphoma, 1298
CD22
  Burkitt lymphoma, 386, 1151
  chronic lymphocytic leukemia/small lymphocytic lymphoma, 1175, 1176–9
  hairy cell leukemia, 1301
  lymphomas, 1144
  splenic marginal zone B-cell lymphoma, 1298
CD23
  chronic lymphocytic leukemia/small lymphocytic lymphoma, 1175, 1176–9
  follicular dendritic cell sarcoma, 129
  follicular lymphoma, 1050, 1139, 1190
  lymphomas, 1144, 1151, 1409
CD24, acute lymphoblastic leukemia, 1388
CD25
  adult T-cell leukemia/lymphoma, 1229, 1405
  anaplastic large lymphoma, 1223–8
  hairy cell leukemia, 1301
  lymphomas, 1147
  nasal/nasal-type NK/T-cell lymphoma, 126, 1231
  Reed-Sternberg cells, 1152, 1155
CD3
  adult T-cell leukemia/lymphoma, 1229, 1405

CD3 (Cont'd)
  angiocentric natural killer/T-cell lymphoma, 126, 127
  enteropathy-type T-cell lymphoma, 1221–2
  hepatosplenic T-cell lymphoma, 1299
  Hodgkin's lymphoma, 1157, 1162, 1259
  Langerhans cell histiocytosis, 1643
  lymphocytic hypophysitis, 992
  lymphomas, 1145, 1151, 1376
  nasal/nasal-type NK/T-cell lymphoma, 126, 1231
  pagetoid reticulosis (Woringer-Kolopp disease), 1498, 1501
  Sézary syndrome, 1214
  skin tumors, 1498
  T-cell granular lymphocytic leukemia, 1214
  T-cell lymphoblastic (precursor lymphoblastic) lymphoma, 1174
  T-cell prolymphocytic leukemia, 1214
  T-cell subcutaneous panniculitis-like lymphoma, 1222–3
  thymocytes, 1315
CD30 (Ber-H2; Ki-1)
  adult T-cell leukemia/lymphoma, 1229, 1405
  anaplastic large lymphoma, 1151, 1223
  diffuse large B-cell lymphoma, 1192
  embryonal carcinoma, 608, 816, 819, 823
  enteropathy-type T-cell lymphoma, 1221–2
  Hodgkin's lymphoma, 198, 1151, 1156, 1164, 1235
  large T-cell lymphoma, 1498, 1499, 1501–2
  lymphomas, 1147, 1151, 1157, 1246
  lymphomatoid papulosis, 1229
  mediastinal large B-cell lymphoma, 1346
  Reed-Sternberg cells, 1152, 1155
CD31, 63, 1289
  angiosarcoma, 65, 131, 1052, 1629
    epithelioid, 67
  cardiac myxoma, 13
  epithelioid hemangioendothelioma, 63, 197
  Kaposi sarcoma, 56, 196, 1248
CD33, 1376
CD34, 63, 1289, 1376, 1388
  acute myelogenous leukemia, 1371
  angiofibroma, cellular, 740
  angiosarcoma, 33, 65, 131, 196, 440, 1052
  B-cell lymphoblastic (precursor lymphoblastic) lymphoma, 1175
  chronic lymphocytic leukemia/small lymphocytic lymphoma, 1175, 1176–9
  clear cell (sugar) tumor, lung, 202
  dermatofibrosarcoma protruberans, 744
  eccrine angiomatous hamartoma, 1456
  epithelioid hemangioendothelioma, 62, 440
  epithelioid sarcoma, 1578–9

CD34 (Cont'd)
  gastrointestinal stromal tumors, 382
  hemangiopericytoma, 100
  hepatic adenoma, 418
  hepatocellular neoplasms, 428
  Kaposi sarcoma, 56, 61, 132, 196, 1248
  phyllodes tumor, 911
  sclerosing angiomatoid nodular transformation (SANT), 1307
  soft tissue perineurioma, 1743–4
  solitary fibrous tumor, 92, 305, 886, 1053
CD35
  extranodal NK/T-cell lymphoma, 1231–2
  follicular dendritic cell sarcoma, 1240–2
  lymphomas, 1150, 1151
  splenic marginal zone B-cell lymphoma, 1298
CD38, 1404
CD4
  adult T-cell leukemia/lymphoma, 1229, 1405
  anaplastic large lymphoma, 1223–8
  angioimmunoblastic T-cell lymphoma, 1220
  hepatosplenic T-cell lymphoma, 1299
  interdigitating dendritic cell sarcoma, 1242
  lymphoma, 1146, 1234–5, 1376
  pagetoid reticulosis (Woringer-Kolopp disease), 1498, 1501
  Sézary syndrome, 1214
  T-cell lymphoblastic (precursor lymphoblastic) lymphoma, 1174
  T-cell prolymphocytic leukemia, 1214
  T-cell subcutaneous panniculitis-like lymphoma, 1222–3
CD40
  Hodgkin's lymphoma, 1157, 1161
  splenic marginal zone lymphoma, 1298
CD41, 1376
CD42, 1376
CD43
  Burkitt lymphoma, 1212
  extranodal NK/T-cell lymphoma, 1231–2
  follicular lymphoma, 1051
  histiocytic sarcoma, 1238
  lymphomas, 603, 1146, 1409
  mantle cell lymphoma, 1183
  plasmacytoma, 1209
CD44
  adenocarcinoma, 345
  papillary carcinoma of thyroid gland, 1013
  sarcomatoid mesothelioma, 207
CD45 (leukocyte common antigen)
  diffuse large B-cell lymphoma, 127
  extramedullary plasmocytoma, 128
  Hodgkin's lymphoma, 1235, 1344
  lymphomas, 603, 1144, 1146, 1376, 1404, 1598
  malignant lymphoma of Waldeyer's tonsillar tissues, 129
  myeloma, 1598
  thyroid tumors, 1001

CD45RB, 1157
　ALK+ large B-cell lymphoma, 1208
　Hodgkin's lymphoma, 1157
　lymphoma, 1144
　mediastinal large B-cell lymphoma, 1346
　plasmacytoma, 1209
　primary effusion lymphoma, 1207
CD45RO, 126
　lymphomas, 603, 1146
　Sézary syndrome, 1500, 1501
　T-cell lymphomas, 387
CD49a, 1204
CD5
　adult T-cell leukemia/lymphoma, 1229, 1405
　carcinoma showing thymus-like element (CASTLE), 1048–9
　chronic lymphocytic leukemia/small lymphocytic lymphoma, 1175, 1176–9
　hepatosplenic T-cell lymphoma, 1299
　lymphomas, 1151, 1246, 1376, 1409
　malignant lymphomatous polyposis of stomach, 363
　mantle cell lymphoma, 1183
　Sézary syndrome, 1214
CD54, 1204
CD56
　angiocentric NK/T-cell lymphoma, 126, 127
　carcinoid tumors, 381
　enteropathy-type T-cell lymphoma, 1221–2
　Ewing's sarcoma, 115
　hepatosplenic T-cell lymphoma, 1299
　lymphomas, 1146, 1151, 1234–5, 1598
　Merkel cell (trabecular) carcinoma, 298
　nasal/nasal-type NK/T-cell lymphoma, 126, 1231
　T-cell granular lymphocytic leukemia, 1214
　T-cell subcutaneous panniculitis-like lymphoma, 1222–3
CD57
　adult T-cell leukemia/lymphoma, 1229
　anaplastic large lymphoma, 1223–8
　clear cell (sugar) tumor, lung, 202
　follicular lymphoma, 1216
　Hodgkin's lymphoma, 1157, 1166
　lymphomas, 1146
　papillary carcinoma of thyroid, 1013
　prostatic intraepithelial neoplasia, 753
　T-cell granular lymphocytic leukemia, 1214, 1413
　thymoma, 1319
CD61, 1376
CD68, 1149, 1151, 1289, 1376
　ALK+ histiocytosis, 1238
　follicular dendritic cell sarcoma, 129
　granular cell tumor, 959, 990
　hemangiopericytoma, 99
　histiocytic lymphoma, 1149, 1237
　histiocytic sarcoma, 1237
　inflammatory pseudotumor, 305

CD68 (Cont'd)
　interdigitating dendritic cell sarcoma, 1242
　leukemia, 727
　plasmacytoid monocytic lymphoma, 1243
　splenic non-hematolymphoid tumors, 1289, 1297, 1301, 1304, 1305
　tendon sheath giant cell tumor (benign synovioma), 1558
　xanthogranuloma, 1493
CD7
　enteropathy-type T-cell lymphoma, 1221–2
　hepatosplenic T-cell lymphoma, 1299
　lymphomas, 1146
　nasal/nasal-type NK/T-cell lymphoma, 126, 1231
　Sézary syndrome, 1214
　T-cell lymphoblastic (precursor lymphoblastic) lymphoma, 1174
CD79a, 1144, 1157, 1404, 1409
　ALK+ large B-cell lymphoma, 1208
　B-cell lymphoblastic leukemia/lymphoblastic lymphoma, 1388
　Burkitt's lymphoma, 386
　chronic lymphocytic leukemia/ small lymphocytic lymphoma, 1177
　diffuse large B-cell lymphoma, 127
　gastric lymphoma, MALT type, 362
　hairy cell leukemia, 1301
　HHV8+ germinotropic large B-cell lymphoma, 1208
　Hodgkin's lymphoma, 1157, 1235
　lymphoblastic lymphoma, 1174–5
　lymphomas, 405, 603, 1144, 1151, 1259, 1499
　mediastinal large B-cell lymphoma, 1346
　plasmacytoma, 1209
　senile EBV+ B-cell lymphoproliferative disorder, 1207
CD8
　anaplastic large lymphoma, 1223–8
　hepatosplenic T-cell lymphoma, 1299
　lymphomas, 1146, 1289, 1376
　pagetoid reticulosis (Woringer-Kolopp disease), 1498, 1501
　T-cell granular lymphocytic leukemia, 1214
　T-cell lymphoblastic (precursor lymphoblastic) lymphoma, 1174
　T-cell prolymphocytic leukemia, 1214
　T-cell subcutaneous panniculitis-like lymphoma, 1222–3
CD95 (Fas)
　central nervous system lymphomas, 1717
　extranodal NK/T-cell lymphoma, 1232
　T-cell large granular lymphocyte leukemia, 1413
CD99
　angiofibroma, nasopharyngeal, 92
　desmoplastic small round cell tumor, 617
　Ewing's sarcoma, 115, 1148, 1601
　fibroma-thecoma, 837

CD99 (Cont'd)
　granulosa cell tumors, 591, 593
　lymphomas, 1148
　Sertoli-Leydig cell tumor, 597, 598, 836
　sinonasal undifferentiated carcinoma, 113
　sinonasal-type hemangiopericytoma, 100
　solitary fibrous tumors, 209, 1053
　synovial sarcoma, 1577
　teratoma, 612
　thymocytes, 1317
CD99a
　Ewing's sarcoma, 1148, 1174
　lymphomas, 1148
　thymocytes, 1317, 1330
CDKN2A, 295
　anaplastic oligoastrocytoma, 1677
　astrocytic tumors, 1659
　giant cell glioblastoma, 1666
　precursor T-cell lymphoblastic leukemia/lymphoblastic lymphoma, 1390
CDX-2, 1246
Celiac disease, 328, 380, 384, 385, 387, 1221, 1222
Cellular angiofibroma, 1548–9
　vulva, 740–1
Cellular ependymoma, 1679
Cellular fibrous histiocytoma, 1486–7
Cellular leiomyoma, 683–4
Cellular neurothekeoma, 1745
Cementifying/cemento-ossifying fibroma, 95–6
Cemento-osseous dysplasia, 230–1
Cementoblastoma, 230
Central nervous system tumors, 1653–721
　electron microscopy, 1855–7
　germ cell, 1717–19
　intraoperative diagnostic techniques, 1653–4
　meninges, 1707–14
　neuroepithelial, 1655–707
　　astrocytic tumors, 1655–72
　　choroid plexus tumors, 1684–6
　　embryonal tumors, 1700–7
　　ependymal tumors, 1678–84
　　neuronal and mixed neuronal-glial tumors, 1688–97
　　oligodendroglial tumors and mixed gliomas, 1673–8
　　pineal parenchymal tumors, 1697–700
　　of uncertain origin, 1686–8
　non-neuroepithelial neoplasms/cysts, 1720–1
　stains and immunohistochemistry, 1654–5
　tissue processing, 1654
　of uncertain histogenesis, 1714–17
Cerebriform nuclei, 1190
Ceruminoma, 1814–15
Ceruminous carcinoma, 1460–1
Ceruminous gland tumors, 1814–16
Cervical glandular intraepithelial neoplasia (CGIN), 699–702
　ciliated, 700

Cervical glandular intraepithelial neoplasia
    (CGIN) (Cont'd)
  clinical features, 699
  early-stage, 700–2
  endocervical, 700
  endometrioid, 700
  intestinal, 700
  stratified/squamomucinous, 700
Cervical (squamous) intraepithelial
    neoplasia (CIN), 697–8
Cervical tumors, 697–715
  extrarenal Wilms' tumor, 715
  hematopoietic tumors, 715
  invasive adenocarcinoma, 704–9
  invasive squamous carcinoma, 702–4
  mature cystic teratoma, 715
  melanocytic tumors, 714–15
  mesenchymal tumors, 713–14
  mixed epithelial and mesenchymal
      tumors, 711–13
  mixed tumors, 709–10
  neuroendocrine carcinoma, 710–11
Charcot-Böttcher filaments, 600
Chemodectoma see Carotid body
    paraganglioma
Chernobyl-associated thyroid cancer,
    999–1000
Cherry angioma (Campbell de Morgan
    spot), 46
Chest wall hamartoma, 1643–4
Chicken-wire pattern, 1673, 1674
Children
  granulosa cell tumor, 591–3
  heart and pericardial tumors
    benign, 7
    malignant, 7
  pancreatic tumors, 480
  renal tumors, 510–19
    clear cell sarcoma, 515–16
    congenital mesoblastic nephroma,
        518–19
    germ cell neoplasms, 519
    rhabdoid tumor, 516–18
    Wilms' tumor, 511–15
  thymoma, 1317
  thyroid cancers, 998–9
Chinese characters, 97
Chlamydia psittaci, 1173
Chloroma see Granulocytic sarcoma
Cholangiocarcinoma, 451–2
  intrahepatic, 452–3
Cholecystokinin, 121, 380
Choledochal cyst, 452
Cholesteatoma, 1817–19
  acquired, 1818
  congenital, 1819
Cholesterol polyp, 449
Chondro-osseous tumors, 1570
Chondroblastoma, 1606–7
  bone, 1594, 1606–7
Chondroid lipoma, 1531–2
Chondroid syringoma (benign mixed
    tumor), 1455–6
  vulva, 736

Chondroid tumors
  benign, 1602–7
  bone, 1602–13
  malignant, 1608–10
Chondrolipoangioma, 1529
Chondrolipoma, thymus, 1351
Chondroma, 1604–6
  enchondroma, 1604–5
  fallopian tube, 625
  liver, 439
  periosteal, 1605
  prostate, 750
  sellar region, 971
  sinonasal tract/nasopharynx, 98
  soft tissue, 1605
Chondromatosis, synovial, 1646–7
Chondromatous hamartoma of thyroid
    gland, 1054
Chondromyxoid fibroma, 1594, 1607
Chondrosarcoma, 35, 1608–10
  clear cell, 1610–11
  dedifferentiated, 1611–12
  head and neck, 132–3
  heart, 35
  mesenchymal, 1612–13
  myxoid, 1528, 1580–1, 1848
  ovary, 603
  periosteal, 1610
  secondary, 1610
  sellar region, 971
  vulva, 745
Chorangioma, 672
Chordoid glioma of third ventricle, 1686–7
Chordoma
  bone, 1594, 1632–4
  head and neck, 84, 133
  notochord, 1632–3
  peripheral (parachordoma), 1574
  sellar region, 971
Choriocarcinoma
  bladder, 551
  central nervous system, 1719
  esophagus, 335
  gestational, 677–9
  intraplacental, 679
  kidney, 519
  lung, 201
  ovary, 588, 608
  stomach, 352
  testis, 827–8
  thymus, 1342
Choristoma
  bronchogenic, 1465
  middle ear, 1819–20
  pituitary adenoma-adenohypophyseal
      neuronal (PANCH), 989
Choroid
  melanoma, 1807, 1809
  nevus, 1806–7
Choroid plexus tumors, 1684–6
Chromogranin, 1001
  carcinoid tumors, 381
  Ewing's sarcoma, 115
  Merkel cell (trabecular) carcinoma, 298

Chromogranin (Cont'd)
  mucosal malignant melanoma, 115
  nasal-type natural killer/T-cell
      lymphoma, 115
  neuroendocrine tumors, 430
  olfactory neuroblastoma, 115
  pancreatic endocrine tumors, 1126
  paraganglioma, 32
  pheochromocytoma, 1112
  rhabdomyosarcoma, 115
  sinonasal undifferentiated carcinoma,
      115
  small cell neuroendocrine undifferentiated
      carcinoma, 115
  squamous carcinoma, 115
  thyroid tumors, 1001
Chromophobe carcinoma, renal cell,
    496–8
Chromosomal deletions, 1865, 1868, 1869,
    1878
Chromosomal duplications, 1868, 1869
Chromosomal inversions, 1013, 1377, 1868
Chromosomal translocations, 1862–8
  detection of, 1865–8
Chronic lymphocytic leukemia/small
    lymphocytic lymphoma (Richter's
    syndrome), 1175, 1176–9, 1408–10
Church-spire keratosis, 104
Churg-Strauss disease, 126, 127, 139
Chymotrypsin
  acinar cell carcinoma, 477
  pancreatoblastoma, 478
Cicatricial fibromatosis, 1552
Ciliary body tumors, 1806–7
Ciliated glandular intraepithelial neoplasia,
    700
Ciliated hepatic foregut cyst, 451
CIN see cervical (squamous) intraepithelial
    neoplasia
Cirrhosis, 43, 309, 421–4
  hepatocellular carcinoma, 419
Clear cell acanthoma, 1427–8
Clear cell adenocarcinoma
  cervix, 707–8, 709–10
  urethra, 554
  vagina, 720–1
Clear cell adenoma, thyroid, 1023–4
Clear cell carcinoma
  endometrium, 662–3
  kidney, 490–5
  odontogenic, 232–3
  ovary, 584, 584–5
  prostate, 758–9
  salivary gland, 263, 296–7
    hyalinizing variant, 296–7
  thymus, 1333–4
Clear cell chondrosarcoma, 1610–11
Clear cell cribriform hyperplasia of
    prostate, 782–3
Clear cell ependymoma, 1679
Clear cell hidradenocarcinoma, 1463–4
Clear cell lymphoma, 1200
Clear cell oncocytoma, salivary gland, 263
Clear cell papillary cystadenoma, 629

索引

Clear cell sarcoma, 1528
  kidney, 515–16
Clear cell (sugar) tumor
  larynx, 154
  lung, 202
  ovary, 583–5, 584
Clinging carcinoma, 917
Cloacogenic carcinoma see Basaloid
    carcinoma
Clonorchis sinensis, 452
Clusterin, 1150
Cμ-Ig, 1388
Coccidioidomycosis, 156
Collagenoma, storiform (sclerotic fibroma),
    1546
Collagenous fibroma (desmoplastic
    fibroma), 1546
Collecting duct carcinoma, 498–9
Collision tumor of thyroid, 1046–7
Colloid (adenomatous) thyroid nodule,
    1010, 1029
Colloid carcinoma
  lung, 184
  pancreas, 469
Colorectal carcinoma, 397–402, 403
  Dukes classification, 402
  early cancer, 402
Columnar cell carcinoma, thyroid gland,
    1036–7
Columnar cell lesions, breast, 917–19
Combined nevus, 1472–3
Common variable immunodeficiency, 1236,
    1469
Complex sclerosing lesion (radial scar),
    breast, 911, 912
Composite hemangioendothelioma, 58
Compound melanocytic nevus, 1467, 1468,
    1470
Condylomata
  acuminata, 697–8, 1430
    anal canal, 410
    oral cavity, 215
    urethral, 552
    vulva, 731–2
    penis, 861–2
  planum, 1430
Condylomatous (warty) carcinoma
  cervix, 703
  penis, 870
Congenital basal cell adenoma/carcinoma
    of salivary gland see Sialoblastoma
Congenital (granular cell) epulis, 222
Congenital mesoblastic nephroma, 518–19
Conjunctival intraepithelial neoplasia, 1791
Conjunctival tumors, 1788–96
  melanocytic, 1792–6
Connective tissue tumors, 1492
Contact ulcer/granuloma of larynx, 154–5
Coronary glomera, 31
Cowden's syndrome, 406, 1447
Cowper's glands, 789–90
Craniopharyngioma, 98, 991, 1720
Cribriform pattern
  cystadenocarcinoma, 271

Cribriform pattern (Cont'd)
  invasive breast carcinoma, 934
  prostate hyperplasia, 782–3
  thyroid papillary carcinoma, 1010
  tongue adenoma, 290–1
Crohn's disease, 363, 380, 387, 398, 404,
    408, 410
Cronkhite-Canada syndrome, 365, 367, 407
Crooke's cell adenoma, 984
Crook's hyaline change, 984
Cryoglobulinemia, 43, 1173
Crystalloids of Reinke, 601, 757
  Sertoli-Leydig cell tumor, 594, 596, 600,
    834
Cushing's syndrome, 187, 189, 1099–100
  adenomas in, 1100
Cutaneous cysts, 1465
Cutaneous epithelioid angiomatous nodule,
    50–1
Cutaneous lymphadenoma, 1445
Cutaneous T-cell lymphoma, 1223, 1497
Cyclin D1, 1149, 1151, 1409
  adenoid cystic carcinoma, 282
  esophageal squamous carcinoma, 328
  laryngeal squamous carcinoma, 161
  lymphomas, 405, 1149
  malignant lymphomatous polyposis, 363
  mantle cell lymphoma, 1183, 1252, 1299
Cyclin E, 345
Cylindrocarcinoma, cutaneous adnexa,
    1465
Cylindroma, 1459
  ear, 1815
Cyst
  acquired retention cyst of esophagus,
    339
  aneurysmal bone, 1570, 1634–6
    larynx and tracheal, 158
  bile duct, 451
  bone, 1636
    aneurysmal, 1570, 1634–6
    ganglion, 1636
  breast, 904
  choledochal, 452
  ciliated, 451
  cutaneous, 1465
  dermoid, 1465
    bladder, 551
    central nervous system, 1721
    orbit, 1799
  epidermal inclusion
    penis, 863
    scrotum, 874
  epidermoid, 843–4, 1447–8, 1721
  eruptive vellus hair, 1448–9
  esophagus, 339
  hybrid follicular, 1448
  inclusion of peritoneum, 882–4
  infundibular, 1447–8
  iris, 1805
  larynx and trachea, 155–6
  lymphoepithelial, 309
  penile, 863
  pigmented follicular, 1448

Cyst (Cont'd)
  primordial (odontogenic keratocyst),
    234–5
  Rathke's cleft, 971, 991
  saccular, 155–6
  sebaceous duct (steatocystoma), 1449
  seminal vesicles, 801
  spleen, 1309
  tricholemmal, 1448
  umbilical (omphalomesenteric duct),
    1465
Cystadenocarcinoma
  biliary (hepatobiliary), 450–1
  salivary gland, 271
Cystadenofibroma
  endometrioid, 896
  fallopian tube, 624, 625
  ovary, 570, 575, 576, 580
Cystadenoma, 1453
  apocrine, 1453
  bile duct, 451
  biliary (hepatobiliary), 450–1
  bladder, 526
  clear cell papillary, 629
  prostate, 792
  salivary gland, 270–1
    clinical features, 270
    definition, 270
    differential diagnosis, 271
    pathologic features, 270–1
Cystic granuloma cell tumor, 590
Cystic hamartoma, anal canal, 411
Cystic hygroma, 67–8
Cystic hypersecretory DCIS, 927
Cystic nephroma (multilocular cyst), 508–9
Cystic thymoma, 1328
Cystomyoma, seminoma vesicles, 801–3
Cytokeratin, 581, 1001, 1032, 1246
  acinic cell carcinoma, 287
  acinic cell tumor, salivary gland, 287
  acrospiroma, 1457–9
  adenocarcinoma, 1834
  adenoepithelioma, 951, 952
  adenoid cystic carcinoma, 123
  adenosquamous carcinoma, 107
  basal cell hyperplasia, 780
  basaloid squamous carcinoma, 106
  benign schwannoma, 93
  borderline serous tumor, 572
  breast tumors, 937, 939
  Brenner tumor, 587
  choriocarcinoma, 678
  clear cell carcinoma, 585
  collecting duct carcinoma, 499
  dermatofibrosarcoma protuberans, 1488
  embryonal carcinoma, 608
  endometrioid carcinoma, 581
  epithelioid angiosarcoma, 66
  epithelioid hemangioendothelioma, 63
  Ewing's sarcoma, 115
  fallopian tube tumors, 625
  familial paraganglioma, 1767
  female adnexal tumor of Wolffian origin,
    629

Cytokeratin (*Cont'd*)
  fibrous histiocytoma, 1488
  foamy cell carcinoma, 761
  follicular dendritic cell sarcoma, 1242, 1243
  gastric stromal tumor, 351
  gonadoblastoma, 616
  hepatic adenoma, 418
  hepatocellular carcinoma, 429
  inflammatory pseudotumor, 305
  leiomyosarcoma, 1565
  lymphoepithelial carcinoma, 108
  lymphomas, 1139
  melanocytic lesions, 1468, 1469
  meningioma, 90, 1821
  Merkel cell (trabecular) carcinoma, 298, 1465
  mesonephric adenocarcinoma, 708
  mesothelial hyperplasia, 882
  microcystic adnexal carcinoma, 1462
  mucinous carcinoma, 1463
  mucoepidermoid carcinoma, 278
  myoepithelioma, 260
  myxoma, 14
  nasopharyngeal carcinoma, 111, 112, 115
  neuroendocrine carcinoma, 118
  neurothekeoma, 1495
  oncocytoma, 488
  ovarian tumors, 574, 577, 591, 620
  Paget's disease
    extramammary, 1461
    vulva, 737
  pancreatic tumors, 467
  plasmacytoma, 1209
  pleomorphic adenoma, 88
  prostate tumors, 784
  prostatic hyperplasia, 779
  renal carcinoma, 494
  salivary gland tumors, 240, 263, 294
  sarcomatoid carcinoma, 534, 579
  sclerosing mucoepidermoid carcinoma with eosinophilia, 1038
  serous carcinoma, 573
  Sertoli cell tumors, 598
  small cell carcinoma, 298, 588
  solitary fibrous tumor, 886, 1053
  spindle cell carcinoma, 105, 106, 216, 1061
  squamous carcinoma, 1833
  steroid cell tumor, 601
  thymus tumors, 1316, 1326, 1327, 1330
  thyroid tumors, 1001
  verumontanum mucosal gland hyperplasia, 785
  yolk sac tumor, 607
Cytomegalovirus, 137

Dabska endovascular papillary angioendothelioma, 57–8, 1310
Darier's disease, 1427, 1447
DCIS *see* ductal carcinoma in situ
Decidua, ectopic, 897–8
Deciduosis, intra-abdominal lymph nodes, 1248
Dedifferentiated chondrosarcoma, 1611–12
Del(17p), 1369
Del(20q), 1369
Dendritic cell proliferation, 1303
Dendritic cell tumors, 1236–43
  ALK+ histiocytosis, 1238
  classification, 1237
  fibroblastic, 1242–3
  follicular sarcoma, 1240–2
  histiocytic sarcoma, 1237–8
  interdigitating sarcoma, 1242
  Langerhans cell histiocytosis, 1238–40
  malignant histiocytosis, 1238
  neurofibroma, 1742
  plasmacytoid monocytic lymphoma, 1243
  thymus, 1349
Dentigerous odontogenic cyst, 233–4
Denture granuloma (denture-induced hyperplasia; epulis fissarum), 222–3
Dermal fasciitis, 1492
Dermal lipoma, 1529–30
Dermal tumors
  melanocytic nevus, 1469
  nerve sheath myxoma, 1494–5, 1744–5
Dermatofibroma
  with monster cells, 1486
  vulva, 741
  see also Fibrous histiocytoma
Dermatofibrosarcoma protuberans, 743–4, 1489–91, 1528
Dermatomyofibroma, 1492, 1546–7
Dermatopathic lymphadenopathy, 1240
Dermoid cysts, 1465
  bladder, 551
  central nervous system, 1721
  orbit, 1799
Desmin, 105
  angiomyolipoma, 430, 504
  desmoplastic small cell tumor, 1852
  endometrial stromal tumor, 667
  Ewing's sarcoma, 115
  fibrous histiocytoma, 1485
  gastrointestinal stromal tumor, 358, 359, 382
  Kaposi sarcoma, 196
  leiomyoma, 684
  leiomyosarcoma, 194, 691, 1561
  low-grade myofibroblastic sarcoma, 1554
  mesothelioma, 207
  mucinous carcinoma, 579
  mucosal malignant melanoma, 115
  myobacterial spindle cell tumor, 1304
  myofibroblastoma, 958
  myxoma, 13
  nasal-type natural killer/T-cell lymphoma, 115
  olfactory neuroblastoma, 115
  ossifying fibromyxoid tumor, 1573
  pleomorphic rhabdomyosarcoma, 1569
  postoperative spindle cell nodule, 796
  pseudosarcomatous fibromyxoid tumor, 797
  rhabdomyosarcoma, 115, 1816

Desmin (*Cont'd*)
  schwannoma, 1739
  sinonasal undifferentiated carcinoma, 113, 115
  small cell neuroendocrine undifferentiated carcinoma, 115
  spindle cell hemangioma, 53
  spindle cell squamous carcinoma, 105, 106
  squamous carcinoma, 115
Desmoid fibromatosis, 1551–3
Desmoid-type fibromatosis, 92–3
Desmoplakin, 1242
Desmoplastic cerebral astrocytoma of infancy, 1689–90
Desmoplastic fibroma, 1546
  bone, 1594, 1631
Desmoplastic infantile ganglioglioma, 1689–90
Desmoplastic melanoma, 1469, 1483
Desmoplastic small cell tumor, 617, 1528
  electron microscopy, 1851–2
Desmoplastic trichoepithelioma, 1444
Diabetes insipidus, 990
Diabetes mellitus, 417
Diffuse BALT hyperplasia (lymphoid interstitial pneumonia), 198
Diffuse ganglioneuromatosis, 404
Diffuse large B-cell lymphoma, 126, 127, 307–8, 1169, 1198–209
  ALK+ form, 1208
  clinical features, 1198–9
  definition, 1198
  differential diagnosis, 1203
  genetic features, 1202–3
  HHV8+ germinotropic form, 1208
  histogenetic groups, 1203
  immunocytochemistry, 1202
  intravascular, 1204
  lymphomatoid granulomatosis-type, 1205–6
  malignant histiocytosis-like, 1204
  pathology, 1199
  plasmablastic, 1208–9
  primary effusion, 1207–8
  prognostic factors, 1203
  pyothorax-associated, 1207
  T-cell rich, 1204–5
Digital fibroma of childhood, 1493
Digital fibromyxoma, 1571
Digital papillary adenocarcinoma, 1464–5
Dilated pore (Winer), 1446
Disseminated peritoneal leiomyomatosis, 693
Duct papilloma, breast, 914–16
Ductal adenocarcinoma of pancreas, 463–8
  genetics, 466–7
  immunohistology, 466
  tumor spread, staging and grading, 468
  variants, 468–70
Ductal adenoma
  breast, 917
  salivary gland, 271–2

Ductal carcinoma, breast, 924–8
    grading, 926
    rare variants, 926
Ductal cyst, larynx, 155–6
Ductal papilloma, 272
Ductal-endometrioid carcinoma, prostate, 773–4
Dukes classification, colorectal carcinoma, 402
Duplication cyst, esophagus, 339
Dupuytren's contracture (palmar fibromatosis), 1150–1
Dutcher bodies, 1254, 1403
Dysembryoplastic neuroepithelial tumor, 1690–2
Dysgerminoma, 604–5
    clinical features, 604
    pathology, 604–5
Dyskeratoma, warty, 1427
    larynx and trachea, 158
Dyskeratosis, 101–2
Dysplasia
    biliary, 454
    cemento-osseous, 230–1
    esophagus, 327–8
    fibrous, 96–7
    gallbladder, 444–5
    liver, 422–4
Dysplastic angiopathy, congenital (Klippel-Trenaunay syndrome), 44, 53, 420, 504
Dysplastic gangliocytoma of cerebellum, 1688–9
Dysplastic nevus, 1468, 1478–9

Ear tumors
    external ear, 1813–17
    inner ear, 1824–7
    middle ear, 1817–24
    secondary, 1827–8
Early cervical adenoma, 704
Early colorectal carcinoma, 402
Early esophageal cancer, 328
Eaton-Lambert syndrome, 189
EBV see Epstein-Barr virus
EBV LMP-1, 1157
EBV nuclear antigens, 109
EBV-associated post-transplant smooth muscle tumor of spleen, 1310
Eccrine angiomatous hamartoma, 1456
Eccrine hidrocystoma, 1453–4
Eccrine nevi, 1456–7
Eccrine porocarcinoma (malignant eccrine poroma), 1456
Ectomesenchymal chondromyxoid tumor, 1574
    tongue, 314
Ectomesenchymoma, 1752–3
Ectopic decidua, 897–8
Ectopic hamartomatous thymoma, 1572
Ectopic thymoma, 1047, 1336, 1350
Edema, massive ovarian, 624

EGFR (epidermal growth factor receptor), 182, 1872
    squamous carcinoma, 328, 1032
Ejaculatory duct tissue in prostate specimens, 788–9
Elastofibrolipoma, thymus, 1351
Elastofibroma, 1542
Electron microscopy, 1831–57
    adenocarcinoma, 1834–8
    alveolar soft part sarcoma, 1850
    central nervous system tumors, 1855–7
    desmoplastic small cell tumor, 1851–2
    epithelioid sarcoma, 1851
    fibroblast tumors, 1842–5
    granular cell tumor, 1850
    leukemia/lymphoma, 1852–5
    liposarcoma, 1845
    melanoma, 1840–1
    mesothelioma, 1838–40
    myogenic tumors, 1845–8
    peripheral nerve sheath cell tumors, 1848–50
    small round cell tumors, 1842
    squamous carcinoma, 1832–4
    synovial sarcoma, 1850–1
    tumors of vasoformative cells, 1848
Embryoma see Sialoblastoma
Embryonal carcinoma, 607–8
    central nervous system, 1718
    ovary, 607–8
    testis, 822–4
    thymus, 1342
Embryonal rhabdomyosarcoma (sarcoma botryoides), 1567
    bile duct, 455
    cervix, 714
    vagina, 724
Embryonal sarcoma, undifferentiated, 442
Embryonal tumors, 1700–7
Encephalocele, 135
Enchondroma, 1604–5
Endobronchial lipoma, 203
Endocervical adenocarcinoma, 704–5
Endocervical adenomyoma, 712–13
Endocervical glandular intraepithelial neoplasia, 700
Endocervical polyp, 712
Endocervical-like borderline mucinous tumor, ovary, 577
Endocervicosis
    bladder, 542
    peritoneum, 896
Endodermal sinus tumor see Yolk sac tumor
Endolymphatic sac tumor, 1827
Endometrial glandular neoplasia, 652–3
Endometrial intraepithelial neoplasia (EIN), 654–5
    architectural changes, 655–7
Endometrial stromal tumors, 667–9
Endometrial tumors
    adenocarcinoma, 660
    keratin granuloma of peritoneum, 884
    metastatic, 669
    non-Müllerian, 669

Endometrial tumors (Cont'd)
    precancer, 653–4
    staging, 656
    stromal, 583, 667–9
    tamoxifen therapy, 669
Endometrioid adenocarcinoma, 661–2
    cervix, 707
    vagina, 721
Endometrioid adenofibroma, ovary, 579
Endometrioid carcinoma
    endometrium, 580–1
    fallopian tube, 627
    ovary, 567, 579
    prostate (ductal), 753
Endometrioid cystadenofibroma, 896
Endometrioid glandular intraepithelial neoplasia, 700
Endometrioid stromal sarcoma, 583, 714
    ovary, 582
    peritoneum, 896
Endometrioid tumors
    ovary, 579–82
        benign, 579
        borderline, 579–80
        carcinoma, 580–1
    peritoneum, 896
Endometriosis, 701
    appendix, 393
    bladder, 541
    cutaneous, 1465
    large intestine, 408
    lymph node, 1250
    peritoneal inclusion cysts, 883
Endosalpingiosis, 893–4
Endothelioma
    malignant endovascular papillary (Dabska's tumor), 57–8
    spleen, 1307
Endovascular papillary angioendothelioma, 57–8
[Leu5]-Enkephalin, pheochromocytoma, 1112
[Met5]-Enkephalin, pheochromocytoma, 1112
Enteric adenocarcinoma, 707
Enteropathy-type intestinal T-cell lymphoma, 1221–2
EORTC cutaneous lymphoma classification, 1495–6
Eosinophilia, 1395, 1415
Eosinophilic granuloma see Langerhans cell histiocytosis
Ependymal soft tissue lesions, 1754
Ependymoblastoma, 1702
Ependymoblastomatous rosettes, 1702
Ependymoma, 612
    anaplastic, 1680–1
    broad/round ligament, 630
    cellular, 1679
    clear cell, 1679
    myxopapillary, 1681–4
    papillary, 1679
    tanycytic, 1679
    thymus, 1350

Epicardial fat deposition, 23
Epidermal inclusion cyst
  penis, 863
  scrotum, 874
Epidermal tumors, 1423–42
  actinic keratoses, 1434–42
  benign, 1423–9
  virally-induced, 1429–34
Epidermodysplasia verruciformis, 1430
Epidermoid cyst, 1447–8
  central nervous system, 1721
  testis, 843–4
Epidermolytic acanthoma, 1428–9
Epididymal tumors *see* Paratesticular tissue tumors
Epididymis
  adenocarcinoma, 849–50
  papillary cystadenoma, 847–8
  retinal anlage tumor, 848
Epithelial dysplasia, esophagus, 327
Epithelial hyperplasia
  breast, 919–24
  oral cavity (Heck's disease), 216
Epithelial membrane antigen, 1148, 1157
  ALK+ large B-cell lymphoma, 1208
  apocrine adenocarcinoma, 1460–1
  bile duct carcinoma, 453–4
  Brenner tumor, 587
  canalicular adenoma of salivary gland, 266
  central nervous system tumors, 1654–5
  desmoplastic small cell tumor, 1528
  endometrioid carcinoma, 581
  extramammary Paget's disease, 1460–2
  extrarenal rhabdoid tumor, 1581
  follicular dendritic cell sarcoma, 1240–2
  gallbladder carcinoma, 447
  granulosa cell tumor, 591
  hepatoblastoma, 435
  Hodgkin's lymphoma, 1157
  malignant peripheral nerve sheath tumor, 129
  Merkel cell (trabecular) carcinoma, 298
  micropapillary carcinoma, breast, 936–7
  minute pulmonary chemodectoma, 204
  mucoepidermoid carcinoma, 278
  myoepithelioma, 260
  nasopharyngeal papillary adenocarcinoma, 124
  papillary adenoma, lung, 204
  perineurioma, 1743–4
  plasmacytoma, 1209
  pleomorphic adenoma, salivary gland, 251–2
  polymorphous low-grade adenocarcinoma, salivary gland, 290
  pulmonary adenofibroma, 204
  pulmonary blastoma, 193
  salivary gland adenocarcinoma, 301–2
  sclerosing hemangioma, 201–2
  serous cystic tumors, pancreas, 474–6
  sinonasal cavity capillary hemangioma, 90

Epithelial membrane antigen (*Cont'd*)
  sinonasal undifferentiated carcinoma, 115
  sinonasal-type hemangiopericytoma, 99–101
  solitary circumscribed (palisaded encapsulated) neuroma, 1735–6
  syringoma, 1457
  third ventricle choroid glioma, 1686–7
  transitional cell carcinoma, ovary, 586–7
  vulvar Paget's disease, 736–7
Epithelial-myoepithelial carcinoma
  pleura, 192
  salivary gland, 263, 291–2
Epithelioid angiosarcoma, 66–7
  bone, 1629
Epithelioid fibrous histiocytoma, 1486
Epithelioid granuloma, 1303
Epithelioid hemangioendothelioma, 1628–9
  liver, 440–2
  lung and pleura, 196–7
  vascular, 62–7
Epithelioid hemangioma (angiolymphoid hyperplasia with eosinophilia), 51–2
  salivary gland, 304
  vascular, 51–2
Epithelioid leiomyoma, 686
Epithelioid leiomyosarcoma, myometrium, 691–2
Epithelioid mesothelioma, 206
Epithelioid neurofibroma, 1742
Epithelioid sarcoma, 1578–9
  electron microscopy, 1851
Epithelioma
  adenoides cysticum (trichoepithelioma), 1443–5
  calcifying (trichomatricoma; pilomatrixoma), 1449–50
Epitheliotropism, 125
Epstein-Barr virus, 108, 109, 186, 1173
  adrenal gland lymphoma, 1117
  angioimmunoblastic T-cell lymphoma, 1220
  Burkitt lymphoma, 385
  gastric carcinoma, 345, 351
  hairy leukoplakia, 220
  iintrahepatic cholangiocarcinoma, 1299
  inflammatory pseudotumor, 439
  intrahepatic cholangiocarcinoma, 452
  inverted papilloma, 85
  leiomyosarcoma, 1053, 1564
  lymphoepithelioma-like carcinoma, 186, 300, 479
  malignant lymphoma, 1117
  nasopharyngeal carcinoma, 109
  non-Hodgkin's lymphoma, 1173
  plasmacytoma, 1117
Epulides, 221–2
  congenital, 222
  denture-induced hyperplasia, 222–3
  fibrous, 221–2
  giant cell, 222
Erythrophagocytic Tγ lymphoma, 1215
Erythroplakia, oral cavity, 219
Erythroplasia of Queyrat, 865, 866

Esophageal tumors, 327–40
  secondary tumors, 339
Essential thrombocythemia, 1398–9
Esthesioneuroblastoma, 114, 1602
Esthesioneuroepithelioma, 114
Esthesioneuroma, 114
Estrogen receptor, 946–50
  assay methods, 947
  breast carcinoma, 946–50
  clinical application, 948–50
  controls, 947
  immunocytochemical assay, 947
  staining assessment, 947–8
Ewing's sarcoma, 1528, 1600–2
  cytogenetic aberrations, 1528
  electron microscopy, 1842
  extraosseous, 1750–2
  larynx, 174
  sinonasal tract/nasopharynx, 84, 115
  vagina, 725
  see also Primitive neuroectodermal tumor
EWS rearrangements
  desmoplastic small round cell tumor, 889
  extraosseous Ewing's sarcoma, 1750
  kidney tumors, 502
  olfactory neuroblastoma, 114
  sarcoma, 1864
EWS-ERG fusion, 1602
EWS-FLI1 fusion, 1602, 1864
EWS/WT1 fusion, 889
Exophytic squamous carcinoma
  lung, 185
  sinonasal tract, 102–3
Exostosis
  external ear, 1816
  subungual, 1640–1
External ear tumors, 1813–17
  basal cell carcinoma, 1813
  bone and cartilage, 1816
  ceruminous gland, 1814–15
  cylindroma, 1815
  lymphoreticular, 1816–17
  melanocytic, 1816
  muscle, 1816
  neural, 1816
  squamous carcinoma, 1813–14
Extra-abdominal desmoid, 92–3
Extra-adrenal myelolipoma, 1532–3
Extra-adrenal paraganglia, 1763–4, 1769
  head and neck, 1763–4
  sympathoadrenal neuroendocrine system, 1769
Extramammary Paget's disease, 1460–2
Extramedullary plasmacytoma, 128–9
Extranodal marginal zone B-cell lymphoma, 1169, 1499
  anti-*Helicobacter* therapy response, 1195
  clinical features, 1193
  differential diagnosis, 1196
  genetic features, 1195–6
  immunocytochemistry, 1195
  large cell transformation, 1196
  pathology, 1194–5
  splenic involvement, 1292, 1297–9

Extranodal NK/T-cell lymphoma, 1229–33, 1496
  clinical features and behavior, 1230
  definition, 1229–30
  diagnosis, 1232
  differential diagnosis, 1232–3
  genetic studies, 1232
  immunocytochemistry, 1231–2
  pathologic findings, 1230–1
  splenic involvement, 1292
Extranodal sinus histiocytosis with massive lymphadenopathy, 139–40
Extrarenal angiomyolipoma, 1532
Extrarenal rhabdoid tumor, 1581–2
Extraskeletal myxoid chondrosarcoma, 1528, 1580–1, 1848
Eye tumors, 1781–809
  conjunctiva, 1788–96
  eyelid and periocular skin, 1781–8
  intraocular, 1801–9
  lacrimal drainage system, 1796–7
  optic nerve, 1799–800
  orbit, 1797–9
Eyelid tumors, 1781–8
  basal cell carcinoma, 1785
  melanoma, 1788
  nevi, 1788
  sebaceous carcinoma, 1785–8

FAB classification, myelodysplastic syndromes, 1364
Fabry's disease, 44, 45
Factor VIII-related antigen, 1289
  angiosarcoma, 131, 196
    epithelioid, 209
  epithelioid hemangioendothelioma, 197
  infantile hemangioendothelioma, 436
  Kaposi sarcoma, 60
Factor XIIIa
  cardiac myxoma, 17
  fibrous histiocytoma, 1485
  sinonasal-type hemangiopericytoma, 100
  verruciform xanthoma, 864
Fallopian tube, 624–8
  benign, 624–5
  gestational trophoblastic disease, 628
  malignant, 625–8
Familial adenomatous polyposis, 91, 340, 365, 379, 396, 396–7, 417
Familial atypical multiple mole-melanoma syndrome, 1468, 1478–9
Familial breast cancer, 937–8
Familial carotid body paraganglioma, 1767
Familial endocrine myxolentiginosis see Myxoma syndrome
Familial paraganglioma, 1767, 1767–8
Familial pheochromocytoma, 1114–15
Fasciitis
  dermal, 1492
  ischemic, 1541–2
  nodular, 305
  ossificans, 1540
  proliferative, 1540–1
Fat necrosis, scrotum, 874

Fechner tumor (acinic cell carcinoma), 191
Female adnexal tumor of Wolffian origin
  broad/round ligament tumors, 628–9
  ovary, 617–18, 627
Female genital tract tumors, 567–630
  broad ligament, 628–30
  cervix, 697–715
  endometrium, 652–69
  fallopian tube, 624–8
  myometrium, 683–95
  ovary, 567–624
  placenta, 672–80
  sex cord-stromal tumors, 588–603
  vagina, 719–27
  vulva, 730–45
Feminizing adrenal cortical tumors, 1103–4
Ferritin
  hepatocellular carcinoma, 427
  neuroblastoma, 1776
Fetal malignancies of placenta, 673
FHIT, 816
Fibrillary astrocytoma, 1661–2
Fibro-odontoma, ameloblastic, 227
Fibro-osseous pseudotumor, 1541
Fibro-osseous tumor, sinonasal tract/nasopharynx, 95–9
Fibroadenoma
  breast, 906–7
    juvenile, 907
  prostate, 795
Fibroblastic tumors
  acral myxoinflammatory fibroblastic sarcoma, 1557
  dendritic cell, 1242–3
  electron microscopy, 1842–5
  sarcomas, 1554–7
Fibroblastoma
  desmoplastic, 1546
  giant cell, 1487–9, 1528
Fibrocartilaginous mesenchymoma, 1644
Fibrocystic change, breast, 903
Fibroelastic hamartoma, 20
Fibroelastic papilloma (papillary fibroelastoma), 7, 24–6
Fibroepithelial polyp, 862, 1492
  penis, 862
  renal pelvis/ureter, 520
  urethra, 552
  vagina, 722–3
  vulva, 739–40
Fibroepithelioma (Pinkus), 1444–5
Fibrogenic tumors, bone, 1631–2
Fibrohistiocytic tumors, 1630
Fibroids see leiomyoma
Fibrokeratoma, acquired (digital), 1493
Fibrolipoma
  larynx/trachea, 154
  neural (fibrolipomatous hamartoma), 1734
Fibroma
  ameloblastic, 227
  calcifying aponeurotic, 1549
  cementifying/cemento-ossifying, 95–6
  chondromyxoid, 1594

Fibroma (Cont'd)
  desmoplastic, 1546
  Gardner, 1547
  heart, 7, 19–21
  inclusion body (infantile digital), 1493
  metaphyseal fibrous defect (non-ossifying), 1638–9
  nuchal-type, 1547
  odontogenic, 230
  ossifying, 95
  ovary, 595
  pleomorphic, 1486, 1492
  psammomatoid (active) ossifying, 95–6
  sclerotic (storiform collagenoma), 1492
  sex cord-stromal, 595
  spleen, 1309–10
  tendon sheath, 1492, 1545
  trichoblastic, 1443, 1444
  vulva, 740–1
Fibroma-thecoma of testis, 837
Fibromatosis, 92–3
  aggressive, 92–3
  breast, 959
  cicatricial, 1552
  coli, 1544–5
  desmoid, 1551–3
  inclusion body, 1547
  juvenile hyaline, 1493, 1545
  ovary, 624
  palmar (Dupuytren's contracture), 1150–1
  penile see Peyronie's disease
  penis (Peyronie's disease), 863, 1551
  plantar (Ledderhose's disease), 1151
  sinonasal tract/nasopharynx, 92–3
  thymus, 1351
Fibromyxoid sarcoma, 1528, 1556
Fibromyxoid tumor
  ossifying, 1573
  pseudosarcomatous, 797
Fibromyxoma
  digital, 1571
  trachea, 154
Fibromyxosarcoma, 32, 442
Fibrosarcoma, 1554–5
  bone, 1631–2
  cardiac, 7, 34
  infantile, 1528, 1554
  lung, 195–6
  ovary, 595, 603
  sinonasal, 129–30
  spleen, 1310
Fibrosis
  nodular subepidermal see Fibrous histiocytoma
  peritoneal, 884–5
Fibrothecoma, 594
Fibrous dysplasia
  bone, 1636–7
  monostotic, 1816
  orbit, 1799
  sinonasal tract/nasopharynx, 96–7
Fibrous epulis, 221–2
Fibrous hamartoma of infancy, 1493, 1543

Fibrous histiocytoma
  aneurysmal (angiomatoid), 1486
  bone, 1594, 1630
  cellular, 1486–7
  deep benign, 1558–9
  endometrium, 669
  epithelioid, 1486
  malignant, 7, 33–4, 129–30, 1560
    angiomatoid, 1486, 1574–5
    atrial, 33–4
    endometrium, 669
    giant cell, 1561
    inflammatory, 1561–2
    kidney, 506
    larynx, 174
    lung, 195–6
    pleomorphic, 1560–1
    spleen, 1310
    thymus, 1351
  pseudosarcomatous, 1486
  skin, 1485–6
  trachea, 154
  vulva, 741
Fibrous periorchitis, 846
Fibrovascular (fibrous) polyp, 339
Fibroxanthoma, atypical, 1491–2
FIGO staging
  endometrial carcinoma, 656
  ovarian cancer, 569
Filiform large cell lymphoma, 1201
Fine needle biopsy
  bone tumors, 1595–6
  pancreatic endocrine tumors, 1126
  thyroid lesions, 1061–2
Flame cells, 1403
Flexner-Wintersteiner rosettes, 1703, 1803
Flow cytometry, 1142–3
Fluorescence in situ hybridization (FISH), 1151
Focal epithelial hyperplasia, oral cavity (Heck's disease), 216
Focal lymphoid hyperplasia, esophagus, 338
Focal nodular hyperplasia, liver, 419–21
Follicle center cell lymphoma, primary cutaneous, 1499
  see also Follicular lymphoma
Follicular adenoma, 1017–19, 1028
  atypical, 1026
  with bizarre nuclei, 1026
  hot, 1024
  hyalinizing trabecular, 1021–3
  with papillary hyperplasia, 1024
  signet-ring cell, 1023
  with spindle cell metaplasia, 1026
Follicular carcinoma, thyroid gland, 1017–19, 1028
  categories of, 1019–21
  clinical features, 1015–16
  prognostic factors, 1028–9
  signet-ring cell, 1023
Follicular cysts
  hybrid, 1448
  pigmented, 1448
Follicular dendritic cell sarcoma, 1240–2

Follicular dendritic cell tumor, 129
Follicular infundibular tumor, 1445–6
Follicular keratosis, inverted, 1425–7
Follicular lymphoma, 1050–1
  Castleman disease-like, 1190
  differential diagnosis, 1051
  large B-cell lymphoma transformation, 1196
  prognostic factors, 1050–1
  T-cell, 1216
Follicular-parafollicular thyroid carcinoma, 1046–7
Fracture callus, 1639
Fried egg appearance, 1673
Frozen sections
  lymphoma, 1142–3
  parathyroid glands, 1092–3
  thyroid gland, 1062–3
Fundic gland (cystic hamartomous) polyps, 365–6
Fungal disease
  larynx, 156
  sinonasal tract/nasopharynx, 137

Gallbladder tumors
  benign, 443–4
  malignant, 445–8
Gamna-Gandy bodies, 14, 15
Gangliocytic paraganglioma, 384
Gangliocytoma
  dysplastic, of cerebellum, 1688–9
  posterior pituitary, 989–90
Ganglioglioma, 692–4
  anaplastic (malignant), 1694–5
  desmoplastic infantile, 1689–90
Ganglion cyst, bone, 1636
Ganglioneuroblastoma, 1771–4
  cerebral, 1701
  composite pheochromocytoma, 1113
  lung, 201
  thymus, 1351
Ganglioneuroma, 404, 1777–8
  autonomic nervous system, 1777–8
  composite pheochromocytoma, 1113
  large intestine, 404
  small intestine, 384
Ganglioneuromatosis, 384
  large intestine, 404
Gardner fibroma, 1547
Gardner's syndrome, 95, 1449, 1450
Gastric carcinoma
  with extensive neutrophilic infiltration, 351
  with lymphoid stroma, 351
  vimentin-positive with rhabdoid features, 352
Gastric cystica polyposa or profunda, 350, 369–70
Gastric heterotopia, 406
Gastric stump carcinoma, 350–1, 370
Gastrin
  adenocarcinoma, 380
  carcinoid tumor, 353, 354
  mucinous tumors, 577

Gastrin-releasing peptide, 1040
  pancreatic tumors, 1123
Gastrinoma, 1130–1
Gastritis, 353
  atrophic, 340
  chronic, 342, 345, 347
  reactive, 344
Gastroesophageal junction, hyperplastic polyps, 340
Gastrointestinal autonomic nerve tumor (GANT), 381
Gastrointestinal stromal tumors, 338, 356–9
  electron microscopy, 1847
  small intestine, 381–3
Gaucher disease, 1303
GCDFP-15
  breast tumors, 955
  extramammary Paget's disease, 875, 1461, 1462
  ovarian tumors, 620
  salivary duct carcinoma, 294
  vulvar Paget's disease, 737
Genetic features
  angioimmunoblastic T-cell lymphoma, 1220
  Burkitt lymphoma, 1212
  diffuse large B-cell lymphoma, 1202–3
  ductal adenocarcinoma of pancreas, 466–7
  extranodal marginal zone B-cell lymphoma, 1195–6
  hepatocellular carcinoma, 431
  Hodgkin's lymphoma, 1162
  leiomyoma, 683
  leioyosarcoma, 689
  lymphoblastic lymphoma, 1175
  lymphoplasmacytic lymphoma, 1181
  modal marginal zone B-cell lymphoma, 1197
  mucoepidermoid carcinoma, salivary gland, 278
  myometrial tumors, 683
  nodular lymphocyte-predominant Hodgkin's lymphoma, 1157–8
  pancreatic ductal adenocarcinoma, 466–7
  plasma cell myeloma, 1404
  pleomorphic adenoma, salivary gland, 252
  polycythemia vera, 1397–8
  rhabdomyosarcoma, 131
  salivary duct carcinoma, 294–5
  sinonasal tract tumours, 108
  splenic marginal zone B-cell lymphoma, 1298
  systemic mastocytosis, 1302
  thymoma, 1330
  see also Molecular genetics
Genital rhabdomyoma
  cervix, 714
  vagina, 723
  vulva, 742
Genital tract tumors
  female, 567–630
  male, 749–879

Germ cell tumors, 812–41
  broad ligament, 628–30
  central nervous system, 1717–19
  kidney, 519
  lung and pleura, 201
  ovary, 604–16
    malignant mixed, 614–15
  prostate, 800–1
  testis, 812–41
    classification, 815
    intratubular, 812–16
    mixed, 829–30
    mixed germ cell and sex cord tumors, 830–3
    non-seminomatous, 822–6
    seminomatous, 816–22
  thymus, 1340–3
Germinoma
  central nervous system, 1718
  thymus, 1341
Gestational choriocarcinoma, 677–9
Gestational trophoblastic disease, 628, 674–80
  invasive and metastatic mole, 677
  trophoblastic origins, 674–5
Giant cell angioblastoma, 56–7
Giant cell angiofibroma, thymus, 1351
Giant cell carcinoma, bladder, 544
Giant cell epulis, 222
Giant cell fibroblastoma, 1487–9, 1528
Giant cell glioblastoma, 1665–6
Giant cell malignant fibrous histiocytoma, 1561
Giant cell reparative granuloma, 97–8
  ear, 1816
Giant cell tumor
  benign, 1623–5
  bone, 1594
  endometrium, 669
  malignant, 1625
  salivary gland, 305
  soft tissue, 1560
  tendon sheath (benign synovioma), 1558
Giant condyloma
  anal canal, 410
  Buschke-Lowenstein, 410, 870
Giant Lambl's excrescence, 24
Glandular dysplasia, esophagus, 328
Glandular intraepithelial neoplasia, cervix (CGIN), 699–702
  intestinal, 700
Glandular medullary thyroid carcinoma, 1040–1
Glandular schwannoma (neurilemmoma), 1740
Glandular (sialo-odontogenic) odontogenic cysts, 235
Glassy cell carcinoma, 709
Gleason prostate cancer grading system, 763–7
Glial fibrillary acidic protein (GFAP), 106, 191, 612, 1686, 1702, 1768
  astroblastoma, 1687
  atypical meningioma, 1710

Glial fibrillary acidic protein (GFAP) (Cont'd)
  atypical teratoid/rhabdoid tumor, 1705–6
  basal cell adenoma, salivary gland, 255–7
  central neurocytoma, 1695–7
  ectomesenchymal chondromyxoid tumor, 1574
  ependymoblastoma, 1702
  ganglioneuroblastoma, 1771–4
  gliomatosis cerebri, 1687–8
  gliosarcoma, 1666–7
  heterotopic glial nodules, 1754
  immature teratoma, 610
  malignant ganglioglioma, 1694–5
  malignant peripheral nerve sheath tumor, 1747–50
  oligodendroglioma, 1673–4
  pleomorphic adenoma, salivary gland, 251–2
  retinoblastoma, 1702–3
  third ventricle chordoid glioma, 1686–7
Glial heterotopias, 135
Glioblastoma, 1655
  diagnostic molecular analyses, 1665–6
  giant cell, 1665–6
  multiforme, 612, 1663–7
Glioma
  mixed, 1673–8
  optic nerve, 1800
  third ventricle choroid, 1686–7
  WHO grading, 1657
Gliomatosis cerebri, 1687–8
Gliosarcoma, 1666–7
Glomangioma, 71
  trachea, 154
Glomangiomyoma, 71
Glomangiopericytoma, 72, 73, 100
Glomeruloid hemangioma, 43
Glomus tumor, 70–2
  bone, 1628
  gastric, 360
  infiltrating, 71
  lung, 200
  middle ear see Jugulotympanic paraganglioma
  ovary, 612
  trachea, 154
Glucagon
  adenocarcinoma, 380
  carcinoid tumor, 355, 614
Glucagonoma, 1131
Glucagonoma syndrome, 1131, 1132, 1133
Glycogen storage disease, 18, 19, 425
Glycogenic acanthosis, 339
Glycophorin A, 1376
Goblet cell carcinoid, appendix, 391–2
Goblet cells, 578
Goiter
  dyshormonogenetic, 1060
  nodular, 1059
Goltz syndrome, 327
Gonadal dysgenesis, 604, 837

Gonadoblastoma, 615–16
  clinical features, 615
  pathology, 615–16
  testis, 830
Gonadotropin-secreting pituitary adenoma, 985–7
Gonocytoma in-situ see Intratubular germ cell neoplasia
Gorham disease, 1628
Gorlin syndrome, 21
Gout, larynx and trachea, 158
Granular cell (congenital) epulis, 221–2
Granular cell neurofibroma, 1742
Granular cell tumor
  bile duct, 451
  breast, 959
  bronchus, 201
  cardiac, 32
  electron microscopy, 1850
  esophagus, 338
  gallbladder, 444
  gingival, of newborn infants, 1746
  larynx and trachea, 152
  malignant, 1747
  neuroectodermal, 1745–7
  pituitary gland, 990–1
  primitive polypoid, 1746–7
  vulva, 741
Granular cell tumors, bile duct, 451
Granulocytic sarcoma (chloroma)
  cervix, 715
  thymus, 1350
Granuloma, 154–5
  denture (denture-induced hyperplasia; epulis fissarum), 222–3
  eosinophilic, 364, 1238–40, 1642–3
  epithelioid, 1303
  giant cell reparative (solid aneurysmal bone cyst), 97–8, 1816
  keratin, peritoneum, 884
  larynx, 154–5
  lethal midline, 124, 1230
  pyogenic, 47
  sperm, 845
  vocal cord Teflon, 158
Granulomatous slack skin, 1498, 1503
Granulosa cell tumor, 589–93
  adult, 589–91
  juvenile, 591–3
  testis, 836–7
Granulosa theca cell tumor, 1118
Granzyme B, 70
  adult T-cell leukemia/lymphoma, 1405
  lymphoma, 1147
Graves disease, 1799
Gritty necrosis, 125
Grover's disease, 1427
Growth hormone-secreting pituitary adenoma, 980–2
Gynandroblastoma, 601–2

Hailey-Hailey disease, 1427
Hair cyst, vellus eruptive, 1448–9
Hair nevus, 1442

Hair/hair follicle tumors, 1442–51
  complex follicular, 1450
  eyelid, 1781–8
Hairy cell leukemia, 1406–8
  clinical and laboratory features, 1406
  cytochemical and immunophenotypic findings, 1407
  definition, 1406
  differential diagnosis, 1198, 1407–8
  molecular genetic findings, 1407
  peripheral blood, bone marrow and aspirate, 1406–7
  splenic involvement, 1292, 1300–1, 1407
Hairy leukoplakia, 220
Hairy polyp, nasopharyngeal, 99
Hallmark cells, 1224
Halo nevus, 1472
Hamartoma
  anal canal, 411
  angiomyomatous, 1247
  appendix, 392
  biliary, 449
  Brunner's gland, 387
  chest wall, 1643–4
  congenital smooth muscle, 1562, 1562–3
  Cowden's syndrome, 406
  eccrine angiomatous, 1456
  fibroelastic, 20
  fibrolipomatous, 1734
  fibrous of infancy, 1493, 1543
  heart, 23
  larynx and trachea, 158
  liver, 437
  lung, 203
  mammary, 908–9
  nasal choncromesenchymal, 136
  neuromuscular, 1735
  omental-mesenteric myxoid, 891
  parathyroid glands, 1086
  respiratory adenomatoid, 135
  rhabdomyomatous mesenchymal, 1566
  spleen, 1308–9
  thyroid gland, 1054
Hand mirror cells, 1386
Hand-Schüller-Christian disease, 1642
Hashimoto thyroiditis, 1060
HBME1, 1309
Head and neck
  paraganglia, 1763–4
  paragangliomas, 1764–9
Heck's disease, 216
Helicobacter pylori, 1173
Hemangioblastoma, meninges, 1714–15
Hemangioendothelioma
  composite, 58
  epithelioid, 63
  infantile, 436
  kaposiform, 56
  retiform, 57
  spleen, 1307
Hemangioma
  acquired elastotic, 50
  arteriovenous, 49–50, 955–6

Hemangioma (Cont'd)
  bone, 1594, 1627–8
  breast, 956
  capillary *see* Capillary hemangioma
  cardiac, 7, 28–30
    biologic behavior, 29
    differential diagnosis, 29–30
    gross pathology, 28
    histopathology, 28–9
  cavernous *see* Cavernous hemangioma
  epithelioid, 51–2
  epithelioid *see* Epithelioid hemangioma
  glomeruloid, 43
  hobnail (targetoid hemosiderotic), 50
  hystiocytoid, 28, 29
  intraneural, 55
  kidney, 504
  larynx, 153–4
  liver, 435
  lobular capillary, 47–8, 90–1
  microvenular, 50
  renal pelvis/ureter, 520
  sclerosing, 201–2
  sinonasal cavity/nasopharynx, 90
  sinusoidal, 48–9
  small intestine, 383
  spindle cell, 52–3
  spleen, 1305
  synovial, 55, 1647
  venous, 52
  verrucous, 46
Hemangiomatosis, spleen, 1305
Hemangiopericytoma, 72–4
  adult, 72, 73
  bone, 1594, 1629–30
  clinical features, 72–3
  differential diagnosis, 74
  histologic appearances, 73–4
  infantile, 72, 73
  malignant, 174
  meningeal, 1712–13
  sinonasal, 72, 100
  spleen, 1310
  trachea, 154
Hematoopoietic system tumors, 1363–415
Hemochromatosis, 422, 424, 425
Hemoglobin, 1376
Hemophagocytic syndrome, 127, 1215, 1303
Hemorrhagic spindle cell tumor, 1245
Hemosiderotic fibrolipomatous tumor, 1572–3
Henderson-Patterson bodies, 863, 1431
HEP-PAR1, 429, 1246
Hepatic adenoma, 417–19
  clinical features, 417
  differential diagnosis, 418
  pathologic features, 417–18
  placenta, 672
  prognosis and outcome, 418–19
Hepatitis B surface antigen, 428
Hepatitis C, 1173
Hepatoblastoma, 433–5
  clinical features, 424–5, 433

Hepatoblastoma (Cont'd)
  differential diagnosis, 434–5
  molecular genetic changes, 435
  pathologic features, 433–4
  prognosis and therapy, 435
Hepatocellular carcinoma, 424–33
  acinar, pseudoglandular or adenoid pattern, 426
  clinical features, 424–5
  combined hepatocellular-cholangiocarcinoma, 432–3
  cytologic features, 427
  differential diagnosis, 428–31
  fibrolamellar variant, 431–2
  molecular genetics, 431
  pathologic features, 425–8
  scirrhous pattern, 426, 427
  solid or compact pattern, 426
  trabecular pattern, 425, 426
Hepatoid carcinoma, 352, 588
Hepatosplenic γδT-cell lymphoma, 1292, 1299–300
HER-2, 948–50
Hereditary C-cell differentiated thyroid tumors, 1044–5
Hereditary hemorrhagic telangiectasia (Osler-Weber-Rendu), 44
Hereditary medullary thyroid carcinoma, 1044–5
Herpes simplex, sinonasal tract/nasopharynx, 137
Herringbone pattern, 129, 194, 195, 196
Heterotopia/heterotopic tissue
  central nervous system, 135
  esophagus, 340
  gallbladder, 449
  gastric, 406
  glial, 135, 1754
  pancreas, 388
  stomach, 367–8
Hibernoma, 1534
Hidradenoma
  papillary
    perianal, 1454
    vulva, 735–6
  papilliferum, 411
Hidrocystoma
  apocrine, 1453
  eccrine, 1453–4
  eyelid, 1782
High-grade surface osteosarcoma, 1623
Hilus cell tumor *see* Leydig cell tumor
Hirschsprung's disease, 404
Hirsutoid papilloma, penis (pearly penile papules), 862
Histiocyte tumors, 1236–43
Histiocytic cytophagic panniculitis *see* Subcutaneous panniculitis-like T-cell lymphoma
Histiocytic lymphoma, 1149, 1237
Histiocytic proliferation, 1303
Histiocytic sarcoma, 1237–8
  differential diagnosis, 1228
Histiocytoid hemangioma, 28, 29

Histiocytoma
  aneurysmal (angiomatoid) fibrous, 1486
  angiomatoid fibrous, 1351
  atypical fibrous, 1486
  cellular fibrous, 1486–7
  deep benign fibrous, 1558–9
  epithelioid fibrous, 1486
  fibrous
    bone, 1630
    endometrium, 669
    skin, 1485–6
    trachea, 154
    vulva, 741
  malignant fibrous see Malignant fibrous histiocytoma
Histiocytosis X see Langerhans histiocytosis
Histoplasmosis, 156, 1303
HIV, 137
  central nervous system lymphoma, 1715–17
  hairy cell leukemia, 1406–8
  infection of Waldeyer's tonsillar tissues, 137–8
  lymphoma, 1153
  see also AIDS
HLA-DR, 1376, 1388
HMB-45, 106
  angiomyolipoma, 430, 1245, 1532
  atypical fibroxanthoma, 1491–2
  basaloid squamous carcinoma, 106
  blue nevus, 1477
  clear cell (sugar) tumor, lung, 202
  dermatofibrosarcoma protuberans, 1488
  extramammary Paget's disease, 1462
  fibrous histiocytoma, 1488
  lymphangiomyomatosis, 70, 197
  melanoma, 431
    bladder, 551
    esophagus, 336
  peripheral nerve sheath tumor, 1750
  placenta, 673
  sinonasal tumors, 115
  uterine perivascular epithelioid tumor, 694
HMB-50, clear cell tumor, lung, 202
Hobnail configuration, 184
Hobnail (targetoid hemosiderotic) hemangioma, 50
Hodgkin's lymphoma, 198–9, 1152–68
  AIDS associated, 1152, 1153, 1159
  Ann Arbor staging system, 1153
  chronic lymphocytic leukemia/small lymphocytic lymphoma, 1175, 1176–9, 1408–10
  classical, 1159–68
    EBV association, 1162–3
    genetic features, 1162
    immunocytochemistry, 1161–2
    morphologic features, 1167
    prognostic factors, 1168
    Reed-Sternberg cells, 1159–61
  classification, 1152–3
  composite non-Hodgkin's lymphoma, 1153

Hodgkin's lymphoma (Cont'd)
  definition, 1152
  differential diagnosis, 1228
  liver, 443
  lung, 198–9
  nodular lymphocyte-predominant, 1154–9
  staging, 1153
  thymus, 1344
Homer Wright rosettes, 114, 1701, 1703, 1856
Hormone therapy, breast tumors, 951
HTLV-1
  adult T-cell leukemia/lymphoma, 1229, 1405
  dysgerminoma, 604–5
  Waldeyer's ring lymphoma, 128
Human chorionic gonadotrophin
  atypical teratoid/rhabdoid tumor, 1706
  carcinoid tumor, 355
  choriocarcinoma, 608, 1719
  embryonal carcinoma, 607, 1718
  germ cell tumors, 614, 1343
  germinoma, 1718
  luteoma of pregnancy, 623
  ovarian tumors, 588
  seminoma, 818
Human herpesvirus 8 (HHV-8)
  angiosarcoma, 64
  epithelioid hemangioma, 51
  germinotropic large B-cell lymphoma, 1208
  glomeruloid hemangioma, 43
  hemangioma, 91
  Kaposi's sarcoma, 106
  non-Hodgkin's lymphoma, 1173
Human immunodeficiency virus see HIV
Human leukocyte antigen, 109
Human papillomavirus, 697, 1429
  bowenoid papulosis, 1438
  condyloma, 861
  focal epithelial hyperplasia, 216
  laryngeal squamous papilloma, 150
  seborrheic keratosis, 1425
  squamous intraepithelial neoplasia, 697
  squamous papilloma, 1791
Human T-lymphotropic virus 1, 1173
Hurthle cell adenoma/carcinoma, 1026–8
Hyalinizing clear cell carcinoma, salivary gland, 296–7
Hyalinizing spindle cell tumor with giant rosettes, 1556
Hybrid follicular cyst, 1448
Hydatidiform mole, 675–7
  invasive, 677
  metastatic, 677
  partial, 676–7
Hydropic leiomyoma, 685–6
21-Hydroxylase deficiency, 1104
5-Hydroxytryptamine see Serotonin
Hyper-IgM syndrome, 1236
Hypercalcemia
  clear cell carcinoma, 584, 1334
  dysgerminoma, 604
  hepatocellular carcinoma, 426

Hypercalcemia (Cont'd)
  hyperparathyroidism, 1080, 1082, 1087
  myeloma, 1597
  plasma cell myeloma, 1402
  renal cell carcinoma, 490
  small cell carcinoma, 616, 774
  squamous carcinoma, 182
  thymic carcinoma, 1331
  urethral carcinoma, 554
Hypergastrinemia, 353, 354, 1131
Hyperparathyroidism, 1080–1
  forms of, 1082
  intraoperative diagnosis, 1092–4
  parathyroid adenoma, 1081–7
  syndromes associated with, 1083
Hyperparathyroidism-jaw tumor syndrome, 1081
Hyperplasia
  adenomatous, rete testis, 842
  adrenal, 838–9
  angiolymphoid with eosinophilia, 51–2
  breast
    ductal, 295, 296
    epithelial, 919–24
    lobular, 919, 922
    stromal, 956
  denture-induced, 222–3
  epithelial
    breast, 919–24
    oral cavity (Heck's disease), 216
  esophagus, 338
  liver, adenomatous, 419–21
  lymphoid, 1228
    skin, 1496–7
    small intestine, 384
  mantle zone, 1184
  Masson's tumor, 41–3
  monocytoid B-cell, 1198
  papillary, 1024
  peritoneal, 881–2
  prostate, 793–4
    adenomatous, 778–9
    cribriform, 782–3
    stromal, 793
    verumontanum muocosal gland, 785–6
Hyperplasiogenous polyp see Hyperplastic polyp
Hyperplastic polyp, 364–5
Hyperprolactinemia, 978–80
Hyperreactio luteinalis, 622–3
Hypertrophic scar, 1492, 1539
Hypogammaglobulinemia, 384, 1317

Idiopathic calcinosis of scrotum, 874
Idiopathic laryngotracheal stenosis, 155
Imatinib mesylate, 1392, 1394
Immunoblastic lymphoma, 128, 1203, 1214
Immunocytoma, primary cutaneous (marginal zone B-cell lymphoma), 1499
Immunodeficiency-associated lymphoproliferative disorders
  AIDS patients see AIDS
  congenital, 1236

Immunoglobulin, 1145, 1151
   angioimmunoblastic T-cell lymphoma, 1219–21
   Burkitt lymphoma, immunocytochemistry, 1212
   cytoplasmic, 1376
   extranodal marginal zone B-cell lymphoma, 1195
   surface, 1376
Immunophenotype
   adult T-cell leukemia/lymphoma, 1405–6
   angioimmunoblastic T-cell lymphoma, 1220
   Burkitt lymphoma, 1212
   capillary hemangioma, 45
   diffuse large B-cell lymphoma
      ALK+ form, 1208
      intravascular, 1204
      lymphomatoid granulomatosis-type, 1205–6
      plasmablastic, 1208–9
      splenic marginal zone B-cell lymphoma, 1298
   extranodal marginal zone B-cell lymphoma immunocytochemistry, 1195
   hepatosplenic γδT-cell lymphoma, 1299–300
   Hodgkin's lymphoma
      classical, 1161–2
      nodular lymphocyte-predominant, 1156–7
   lymphoblastic lymphoma, 1174–5
   lymphoplasmacytic lymphoma, 1180–1
   mantle cell lymphoma, 1183
   modal marginal zone B-cell lymphoma, 1197, 1198
   non-Hodgkin's lymphoma, 125, 1170–2
   peripheral T-cell lymphoma, 1218
   splenic marginal zone B-cell lymphoma, 1298
   thymoma, 1330
   thymus, 1315–17
Immunosuppression-associated Kaposi sarcoma, 59
Inclusion body (infantile digital) fibromatosis, 1547
Indolent myeloma, 1401
Indolent NK lymphoproliferative disease, 1233, 1413
Infantile fibrosarcoma, 1528, 1554
Infantile hemangioendothelioma, 435–7
Infantile hemangiopericytoma, 72, 73
Infantile myofibromatosis, 1543–4, 1639
Infants, pancreatic tumors, 480
Infection
   larynx and trachea, 156
   nasopharyngeal, 137
   sinonasal, 137
Infectious mononucleosis, 1260
Infiltrating glomus tumor, 71
Inflammatory breast fibrocystic change, 903
Inflammatory fibroid polyp, 339, 366–7

Inflammatory hypophysitis, 991–3
   giant-cell granulomatous, 992–3
   lymphocytic, 992
Inflammatory juvenile nevus, 1790
Inflammatory malignant fibrous histiocytoma, 1561–2
Inflammatory myofibroblastic tumor, 1553–4
   lung and pleura, 202–3
   peritoneum, 891
Inflammatory myxohyaline tumor, 1557
Inflammatory nevus, 1790
Inflammatory pseudotumor, 439
   larynx and trachea, 158
   liver, 439
   lymph nodes, 1247
   salivary glands, 158, 305
   spleen, 1307–8
   thymus, 1350
   see also Inflammatory myofibroblastic tumor; Plasma cell granuloma
Inflammatory pseudotumor-like follicular dendritic cell tumor, 1304
Infundibular cyst see Epidermoid cyst
Inhibin, 100, 106, 113, 123, 191, 581, 591, 594
Inner ear tumors, 1824–7
Insulinoma, 1124, 1128–9
Interdigitating dendritic cell sarcoma, 1242
Interfollicular large B-cell lymphoma, 1201
Intermediate cells, 151
Intestinal glandular intraepithelial neoplasia, 700
Intestinal-type adenocarcinoma, 120–2
   vagina, 721
Intimal angiosarcoma, 67
Intra-abdominal desmoplastic small round cell tumor, 889–90
Intradermal melanocytic nevus, 1469
Intraductal carcinoma of salivary gland, 295–6
   clinical features, 295
   diagnosis, 295–6
   pathologic features, 295
Intraductal papillary bile duct neoplasia, 454–5
Intraductal papillary mucinous pancreatic neoplasms, 470–3
Intraductal papilloma, 272
Intraepithelial neoplasia
   cervical (CIN), 697–8
   cervical glandular (CGIN), 699–702
   conjunctival, 1791
   endometrial (EIN), 654–5
   intestinal glandular, 700
   prostatic (PIN), 750–5
   vulva (VIN), 732–3
Intrahepatic cholangiocarcinoma, 452–3
Intramuscular angiolipoma, 54
Intramuscular angioma, 54–5
Intramuscular lipoma, 1530
Intramuscular myxoma, 1570–1
Intraneural hemangioma, 55

Intraocular tumors, 1801–9
Intraplacental choriocarcinoma, 679
Intrapulmonary thymoma, 199–200
Intrathyroid parathyroid tumor, 1054
Intratubular germ cell neoplasia, 812–16
   immunohistochemistry, 815–16
   pathology, 813–15
Intrauterine diffuse leiomyomatosis, 693–4
Intravascular large B-cell lymphoma, 1497, 1499, 1505
Intravascular papillary endothelial hyperplasia (Masson's tumor), 41–3
Intravenous (intravascular) leiomyomatosis, 692–3
Invasive papillomatosis, 152
Inverted ductal papilloma, 271–2
Inverted follicular keratosis, 1425–7
Inverted papilloma
   bladder, 524–6
   renal pelvis/ureter, 519–20
Iridocyclectomy, 1801
Iris tumors, 1805–6
Ischemic fasciitis, 1541–2
Islet amyloid polypeptide, 1129
Isthmus-catagen cyst, 1448

J-chain, Hodgkin's lymphoma, 1157
Joint tumors, 1644–7
Jugulotympanic paraganglioma, 1821–2, 1821–3
Junctional melanocytic nevus, 1467, 1468
Juvenile angiofibroma, 91
Juvenile fibroadenoma, breast, 907
Juvenile granulosa cell tumor, 591–3
Juvenile hyaline fibromatosis, 1493, 1545
Juvenile inflammatory nevus, 1790
Juvenile polyposis, 405–6
Juxta-articular myxoma, 1571
Juxtaglomerular cell tumor (reninoma), 506–7

Kamino bodies, 1474
Kaposi sarcoma, 58–62
   adrenal gland, 1120
   African, 59–61
   AIDS-related, 59
   classic endemic, 59
   clinical features, 59–62
   immunosuppression-associated, 59
   large intestine, 405
   liver, 442
   lung and pleura, 196
   lymph nodes, 1248
   promontory sign, 60
   sinonasal, 131–2
   spleen, 1310
   vulva, 745
Kaposi-like hemangioendothelioma, 56
Kasabach-Merritt syndrome, 48, 56, 435
Keloid scar, 1492, 1539
Keratin, 102
   adenoid cystic carcinoma, 123
   desmoplastic small cell tumor, 1852
   epithelial-myoepithelial carcinoma, 192

Keratin (Cont'd)
　　epithelioid hemangioendothelioma, 1628–9
　　fibrosarcoma, 1554–5
　　inflammatory myofibroblastic tumor, 1553–4
　　pulmonary adenofibroma, 204
　　pulmonary blastoma, 193
　　see also Cytokeratin
Keratin granuloma, peritoneum, 884
Keratin pearls, 702
Keratinizing invasive squamous carcinoma of cervix, 702
Keratinizing papilloma, 151
Keratoacanthoma, 1425, 1431–4
　　marginatum centrifugum, 1432
　　squamous carcinoma differentiation, 1433
　　subungual, 1432
Keratocyst, odontogenic, 234–5
Keratocystoma, salivary gland, 272
Keratohyaline granules, 702
Keratosis
　　actinic (solar), 1435–6
　　church-spire, 104
　　inverted follicular, 1425–7
　　lichenoid actinic, 1436
　　seborrheic, 1423–7
Ki-1 see CD30
Ki-67 index, 1147, 1151, 1655
　　adenoid basal cell tumor, 782
　　anaplastic olicogendroglioma, 1675
　　B-cell chronic lymphocytic leukemia/small lymphocytic lymphoma, 1177
　　basal carcinoma, 1813
　　Burkitt's lymphoma, 1176, 1212
　　choroid plexus papilloma, 1684
　　follicular lymphoma, 1191, 1252
　　ganglioglioma, 1694
　　keratoacanthoma, 1434
　　lymphoblastic lymphoma, 1176
　　lymphomas, 1147
　　meningioma, 1710
　　myoepithelial carcinoma, 261
　　neurocytoma, 1696
　　pancreatic endocrine tumors, 1124
　　pituitary tumors, 974
　　pleomorphic adenoma, 251
　　squamous intraepithelial lesion, 698
　　uveal melanoma, 1808
Kidney tumors, 485–523
　　children, 510–19
　　epithelial, 485–502
　　　staging and grading, 501–2
　　mesenchymal, 502–10
　　neuroendocrine, 502
　　renal pelvis/ureter, 519–23
Kiel classification, non-Hodgkin's lymphoma, 840, 1177
Kikuchi lymphadenitis, 1203, 1261
Kimura's disease
　　larynx and trachea, 158
　　salivary gland, 304–5
Klippel-Trenaunay syndrome, 44, 53, 420, 504

Klippel-Trenaunay-Weber syndrome, 420
Köbner phenomenon, 1449
Koilocytosis, 104
Krukenberg tumor, 621
Kuttner tumor (chronic sclerosing sialadenitis), 309–10

L-26 see CD20
Lacrimal drainage system tumors, 1796–7
Lactational adenoma, 908
LAMB syndrome see Myxoma syndrome
Langerhans cell histiocytosis (histiocytosis X), 364, 1238–40, 1642–3
　　bone, 1642–3
　　ear, 1816–17
　　orbit, 1799
　　sarcomatous, 1240
　　thyroid, 1051–2
Langerin, 1149
Langhans giant cells, 605
Large B-cell lymphoma
　　ALK+, 1208
　　anaplastic, 1201
　　chronic lymphocytic leukemia/small lymphocytic lymphoma (Richter's syndrome), 1175, 1176–9, 1408–10
　　cutaneous of leg, 1499, 1505
　　follicular lymphoma transformation, 1196
　　intravascular, 1497, 1499, 1505
　　see also Diffuse large B-cell lymphoma
Large cell acanthoma, 1435
Large cell calcifying Sertoli cell tumor, 836
Large cell lymphoma, 1238
　　anaplastic, 120, 1152, 1169, 1201, 1223–8
　　　cutaneous, 1228–9
　　anemone cell, 1201
　　filiform, 1201
　　microvillous, 1201
　　sinusoidal, 1201
　　see also Large B-cell lymphoma; T-cell/null cell anaplastic large cell lymphoma
Large cell medulloblastoma, 1705
Large cell neuroendocrine carcinoma
　　salivary gland, 299–300
　　thymus, 1340
Large cell non-keratinizing invasive squamous carcinoma of cervix, 702
Large cell (undifferentiated large cell) carcinoma
　　cervix, 711
　　lung and pleura, 186
　　salivary gland, 298
Large intestinal tumors, 393–409
　　epithelial, 393–403
　　　precancerous, 408–9
　　lymphoid, 404–5
　　non-epithelial, 404–5
　　secondary, 405
　　tumor-like lesions, 405–9
Laryngeal tumors, 150–74
　　benign, 150–8
　　chronic infections, 156

Laryngeal tumors (Cont'd)
　　malignant, 158–74
　　TNM staging, 162
Laryngocele, 155
Laryngotracheal stenosis, idiopathic, 155
LAT, 1146
Launois-Bensaude adenolipomatosis, 1530
Ledderhose's disease, 1551
Leiomyoma, 93–4, 683–8
　　atypical, 684–5
　　benign metastasizing, 694
　　broad/round ligament, 630
　　cellular, 683–4
　　cervix, 713–14
　　deep, 1563
　　epithelioid, 686
　　fallopian tube, 625
　　genital, 1563–4
　　kidney, 504–5
　　larynx and trachea, 154
　　lymph node, 1247
　　mitotically active, 684
　　molecular genetics, 683
　　myometrium
　　　apoplectic, 685
　　　benign metastasizing, 694
　　myxoid, 686
　　neurilemmoma-like, 687
　　ovary, 603
　　pathologic features, 683–8
　　pilar, 1562–3
　　plexiform, 686
　　prostate, 794
　　seminal vesicles, 801
　　sinonasal tract/nasopharynx, 93–4
　　thymus, 1351
　　vagina, 723
　　vascular, 1563
　　vulva, 741–2
　　see also Lipoleiomyoma
Leiomyomatosis
　　disseminated peritoneal, 693
　　esophagus, 339–40
　　intrauterine diffuse, 693–4
　　intravenous (intravascular), 692–3
　　lymph node, 1247
　　peritoneum, 898–9
　　vulva, 742
Leiomyosarcoma, 194, 688–92
　　adrenal gland, 1119
　　bladder, 545–6
　　bone, 1632
　　broad/round ligament, 630
　　cardiac, 7, 35
　　cervix, 714
　　clinical features, 688–9
　　electron microscopy, 1846
　　epithelioid, 691–2
　　kidney, 505
　　larynx, 174
　　lung and pleura, 193–4
　　molecular genetics, 689
　　myxoid, 691
　　pathologic features, 689–92

Leiomyosarcoma (Cont'd)
  prostate, 799
  sinonasal, 132
  soft tissue, 1564–5
  spindle cell, 689–91
  spleen, 1310
  thymus, 1351
  vagina, 724
  vulva, 744
  see also Lipoleiomyosarcoma; Xanthomatous leiomyosarcoma
Leishmaniasis, 1303
Lennert's (lymphoepithelioid) lymphoma, 1181, 1215
Lentiginous melanocytic nevus, 1468, 1478–9
Lentiginous melanoma, 1469, 1482
Lentigo (lentigo simplex), 1466–7, 1468
  vulva, 738
Lentigo maligna, 1795
Lepidic cell pattern, 11, 12, 13, 183
Leprosy, sinonasal tract/nasopharynx, 137
Lethal midline granuloma, 124, 1230
Letterer-Siwe disease, 1641, 1642
Leu-7 see CD57
Leu-M1 see CD15
Leukemia, 1243–4
  acute basophilic, 1382
  acute erythroid, 1382
  acute lymphoblastic (AL)
    B-lineage, 1386, 1387, 1388
    chromosomal translocations, 1865
    cytogenic features, 1175
    differential diagnosis, 1875
    Philadelphia chromosome, 1863
    T-cell, 1172
    testis, 840
  acute megakaryoblastic, 1382
  acute myeloid (AML), 1370–86
    classification, 1371, 1372
    clinical and laboratory features, 1371–2
    cytochemical findings, 1374
    cytochemical stains, 1375
    definition and classification, 1370–1
    immunophenotypic findings, 1374
    molecular genetic findings, 1374
    morphologic features, 1372–4
    with multilineage dysplasia, 1381
    with recurrent genetic abnormalities, 1375–81
    therapy-related myelodysplastic syndromes, 1381
  acute panmyelosis with myelofibrosis, 1382
  adult T-cell leukemia/lymphoma, 1229, 1405–6, 1496
    splenic involvement, 1292
  aggressive NK-cell, 1233, 1413
  B-prolymphocytic, 1410–11
  bile duct, 455
  bladder, 548–9
  chronic eosinophilic leukemia/ hypereosinophilic syndrome, 1394–6

Leukemia (Cont'd)
  chronic lymphocytic leukemia/small lymphocytic lymphoma (Richter's syndrome), 1175, 1176–9, 1408–10
  chronic myelogenous, 1391–4
  chronic myeloid (CML)
    differential diagnosis, 1370
    splenic involvement, 1295, 1296
  chronic myelomonocytic, 1364, 1370, 1395
  electron microscopy, 1852–5
  endometrial involvement, 669
  esophagus, 338–9
  liver, 443
  myelomonocytic, 1382
  orbit, 1799
  ovary, 603–4
  prostate, 800
  splenic involvement, 1289–95
  T-cell granular lymphocytic, 1214
    differential diagnosis, 1233
    splenic involvement, 1292
  T-cell prolymphocytic, 1213–14, 1411–12
    splenic involvement, 1292
  testis, 840
  vagina, 727
Leukocyte common antigen see CD45
Leukoplakia, 219
Lex, 430
Leydig cell tumor
  ovary, 600–1
  testis, 333–5
Lichen sclerosus et atrophicus (balanitis xerotica obliterans), 863–4
Lichenoid actinic keratosis, 1436
Linitis plastica, 329, 345, 346, 364
Linkage analysis, 110
Lipoadenoma
  parathyroid glands, 1086
  salivary gland, 274–5
Lipoblastoma, 1530–1
Lipoblastoma-like tumor of vulva, 742
Lipoblastomatosis, thymus, 1351
Lipofibromatosis, 1553
Lipogenic neoplasms, bone, 1634
Lipogranuloma
  penis, 863
  scrotum, 874
Lipohyperplasia of ileocecal valve, 389
Lipoleiomyoma, 686–7
  myometrium, 686–7
  ovary, 603
Lipoleiomyosarcoma, thymus, 1351
Lipoma
  atypical, 1528
  benign, 1529
  bone, 1594, 1634
  cardiac, 7, 21–4
    clinical correlates, 23
    gross pathology, 22
    histopathology, 22–4
  chondroid, 1531–2
  dermal, 1529–30
  inner ear, 1826

Lipoma (Cont'd)
  intramuscular, 1530
  kidney, 505
  large intestine, 404
  lung, 203
  small intestine, 383
  spleen, 1309
  synovial, 1530, 1647
  thymus, 1349
Lipomatosis, 1530
  large intestine, 404
  nerve, 1734
Lipomatous hamartoma of heart, 22
Lipomatous hypertrophy, interatrial septum, 22, 23, 24
Liponeurocytoma, cerebellar, 1697
Liposarcoma, 1534–9
  adipocytic, 1534–9
  bone, 1594, 1634
  cardiac, 7, 35
  electron microscopy, 1845
  kidney, 505–6
  larynx, 174
  myxoid/round cell, 1528
  thymus, 1349
  vulva, 744
  well-differentiated, 1528
Lisch nodules, 1741
Littoral cell angioma, 1305
Littoral cell angiosarcoma, 1305–7
Littoral cells, 1289
Liver tumors
  hepatocellular
    benign, 417–21, 421–4
    malignant, 424–35
  mesenchymal
    benign, 435–9
    malignant, 439–43
Lobular capillary hemangioma (pyogenic granuloma), 47–8
Lobular panniculitis, 1223
Loss of heterozygosity, 109
Low-grade fibromyxoid sarcoma, 1528, 1556
Low-grade myofibroblastic sarcoma, 1554
Lung tumors, 181–210
  benign, 203–4
  biphasic epithelial/mesenchymal neoplasms, 192–3
  bronchogenic (non-small cell), 181–7
  classification, 181
  embryonically displaced/ectopic tissues, 199–201
  lymphoproliferative disorders, 197–9
  mesenchymal neoplasia, 193–7
  metastases, 204–5
  mixed, 186–7
  neuroendocrine, 187–90
  pleural tumors, 205–10
  pulmonary adenofibroma, 204
  pulmonary mesenchymal neoplasia, 193–7
  salivary gland-type tumors, 190–2
  uncertain histogenesis, 201–3

Luteoma of pregnancy, 623
Lymph node tumors, 67–70
　atypical lesions after radiotherapy, 69–70
　benign lymphangioendothelioma, 68–9
　benign schwannoma, 1740
　cavernous lymphangioma and cystic hygroma, 67–8
　inflammatory pseudotumor, 1247
　Kaposi sarcoma, 1248
　lymphangioma circumscriptum, 68
　lymphangiomatosis, 69
　lymphangiomyomatosis, 70
　metastatic, 1244–5
　primary vascular, 1248
　smooth muscle proliferations, 1245–6
　tumor-like lesions, 1245–50
Lymph nodes, 1139–40
　capsule and sinuses, 1139
　cortex, 1139
　deciduosis, 1248
　epithelial/mesothelial inclusions, 1250
　medulla and hilum, 1140
　nevus cells, 1250
　paracortex, 1140
　sinus vascular transformation, 1249–50
Lymphadenoma
　cutaneous, 1445
　salivary gland, 269, 273–4
Lymphadenopathy, massive with sinus histiocytosis see Rosai-Dorfman disease
Lymphangioendothelioma, benign, 68–9
Lymphangioleiomyomatosis, lung, 197
Lymphangioma, 28
　acquired progressive, 68–9
　cavernous, 67–8
　circumscriptum, 68, 742
　kidney, 504
　small intestine, 383
　spleen, 1305
　vulva, 742
Lymphangiomatosis, 69
　spleen, 1305
Lymphangiomyomatosis, 70, 709, 1246
Lymphangiosarcoma, breast, 957–8
Lymphedema-associated angiosarcoma, 64
Lymphoblastic leukemia see Leukemia, acute lymphoblastic
Lymphoblastic (precursor lymphoblastic) lymphoma, 1172–6, 1210
　B-cell type, 1172
　clinical features, 1172
　definition, 1172
　differential diagnosis, 1175–6, 1184, 1213
　genetic features, 1175
　immunocytochemistry, 1174–5
　NK cell type, 1172
　pathology, 1172–4
　T-cell type, 1172
Lymphocyte development, 1140–1
Lymphocytic leukemia see Chronic lymphocytic leukemia/small lymphocytic lymphoma

Lymphocytic lobulitis, breast, sclerosing, 905–6
Lymphocytoma cutis see Lymphoid hyperplasia
Lymphoepithelial carcinoma see Lymphoepithelial-like carcinoma
Lymphoepithelial cyst, 309
Lymphoepithelial sialadenitis, 305–6
Lymphoepithelial-like invasive squamous carcinoma of cervix, 703–4
Lymphoepithelioid (Lennert's) lymphoma, 1181, 1215
Lymphoepithelioma, 108–12
Lymphoepithelioma-like carcinoma, 108, 167
　bladder, 544–5
　lung, 185–6
　salivary gland, 299–300
　thymus, 1332
Lymphohistiocytic variant, mesothelioma, 206
Lymphoid hyperplasia
　skin, 1496–7
　small intestine, 384
Lymphoid interstitial pneumonia (diffuse BALT hyperplasia), 198
Lymphoid polyps, small intestine, 384
Lymphoma
　adrenal gland, 1117
　AIDS-related see AIDS
　angiotropic, 1497, 1499, 1505
　B-cell see B-cell lymphoma; B-lymphoblastic lymphoma; Diffuse large B-cell lymphoma; Large B-cell lymphoma
　bladder, 548–9
　bone, 1594, 1598–600
　breast, 90
　cardiac, 36
　central nervous system, 1715–17
　composite, 1153
　conjunctiva, 1796
　cutaneous, 1495–505
　diagnosis, 1142–52
　　cytogenetic studies, 1143
　　immunohistochemistry, 1142–3
　　molecular studies, 1143–52
　　morphologic evaluation, 1142
　　technical factors, 1142
　electron microscopy, 1852–5
　endometrium, 669
　external ear, 1817
　gray zone, 1153
　Hodgkin, 1152–68
　immunoblastic, 128, 1203, 1214
　kidney, 509–10
　large cell see Large B-cell lymphoma; Large cell lymphoma; T-cell lymphoma
　large intestine, 405
　Lennert, 1181
　lymphoplasmacytic, 1169, 1179–81
　mantle cell, 1152, 1169, 1181–4
　mediastinal large B-cell, 1169

Lymphoma (Cont'd)
　nasal-type natural killer/T-cell, 115, 125–7
　NK cell see NK-cell lymphoma
　non-Hodgkin's see Non-Hodgkin's lymphoma
　orbit, 1799
　ovary, 603
　peripheral B-cell, 1176–213
　peripheral T-cell/NK-cell, 1169, 1198, 1213–34
　plasmablastic, 1208–9
　precursor lymphoblastic, 1172–6
　prostate, 800
　salivary glands, 306–9
　splenic involvement, 1289–95
　stomach, 360–4
　　malignant lymphomatous polyposis, 363
　T-cell see T-cell lymphoma; T-cell/null cell anaplastic large cell lymphoma
　testis, 839–40
　thyroid, 1049–51
　　diffuse large B-cell, 1050
　　follicular, 1050
　　MALT type, 1049–50
　vagina, 727
Lymphomatoid granulomatosis, 198, 1205–6
Lymphomatoid papulosis, 1229, 1498
Lymphoplasmacytic lymphoma, 1169, 1179–81
　clinical features, 1179–80
　definition, 1179
　differential diagnosis, 1181
　genetic features, 1181
　immunocytochemistry, 1180–1
　pathology, 1180
Lymphoproliferative disorders, 197–9
　diagnosis, 1250–62
　　diffuse large lymphoid cell proliferations, 1260–2
　　diffuse medium-sized lymphoid cell proliferations, 1260
　　diffuse small B-cell lymphomas, 1256–8
　　diffuse small cell/mixed cell lymphoid infiltrate, 1254–6
　　large lymphoid nodules, 1253–4
　　medium-sized follicles, 1250–2
　　scattered large cells, 1258–60
　histiocyte and dendritic cell tumors, 1236–43
　Hodgkin's disease, 198–9
　iatrogenic, 1236
　and immunodeficiency, 1234–6
　leukemia, 1243–4
　lymphomatoid granulomatosis/ angioimmunoproliferative lesion, 198
　malignant non-Hodgkin's lymphoma, 197–8
　post-transplant, 1234
　see also Lymph nodes

Lymphoreticular system, 1139–262
    extranodal lymphoid tissues, 1140
    lymph nodes, 1139–40
    lymphocyte development, 1140–1
    lymphoma see Lymphoma
Lymphoreticular tumors, external ear, 1816–17
Lysozyme, 1150, 1376

McCune-Albright syndrome, 97
Madelung's disease, 1530
Maffucci syndrome, 48, 53, 1606
Malakoplakia
    large intestine, 408
    larynx and trachea, 158
    testis, 844
Malaria, 1303
Male genital tract tumors, 749–879
    paratesticular tumors, 841–52
    penis, 861–76
    prostate, 749–801
    scrotum, 874–6
    seminal vesicles, 801–3
MALT lymphoma, 1152, 1169, 1193–6
    AIDS-related, 307
    breast, 90
    salivary gland, 306–9
    stomach, 362
    thymus, 1348–9
    thyroid, 1049–50
    see also Extranodal marginal zone B-cell lymphoma
Mantle cell lymphoma, 1152, 1169, 1181–4
    blastoid variant, 1175, 1182
    clinical features, 1181
    cyclin D1 expression, 1183
    definition, 1181
    differential diagnosis, 1184, 1299
    genetic studies, 1183–4
    immunocytochemistry, 1183
    in-situ, 1183
    pathology, 1181–3
    pleomorphic variant, 1183
    prognostic factors, 1184
    splenic involvement, 1292
Mantle zone hyperplasia, 1184
Map biopsy, 1787
Marginal zone B-cell lymphoma, cutaneous (primary immunocytoma), 1504–5
Marginatum centrifugum, 1432
Masson's tumor, 41–3
Mast cell disease, 1413–14
Mast cell leukemia, 1415
Mastocytosis, 1643
    bone, 1643
    systemic, 1198, 1301–3
        classification, 1301–2
        genetic features, 1302
        pathology, 1302
        systemoic, 1414–15
Mediastinal gray zone lymphoma of thymus, 1347
Mediastinal large B-cell lymphoma, 1169
    thymus, 1345–7

Medullary carcinoma
    breast, invasive, 935–6
    stomach (lymphoid stroma), 351
    thyroid, 1038–46
        clinical behavior, 1040
        clinical features, 1038–40
        differential diagnosis, 1044
        electron microscopy, 1043
        hereditary form, 1044–5
        immunohistochemistry, 1043
        molecular features, 1043
        prognostic factors, 1044
        variants, 1040–3
Medulloblastoma, 1703–5
    anaplastic, 1705
    large cell, 1705
    melanotic, 1705
Medulloepithelioma, 1700–1
    intraocular, 1801
Medullomyoblastoma, 1705
Megakaryocytes, 1392, 1400
Meibomian glands, 1782
Melanocanthoma, 1423, 1425
Melanocytic nevus, 673, 1425, 1466
    cervix, 714
    compound, 1467, 1468, 1470
    congenital, 1471
    deep penetrating, 1469
    ear, 1816
    intradermal, 1469, 1470–1
    junctional, 1467, 1468
    vulva, 1471
Melanocytic tumors, 1466–84
    blue nevus see Blue nevus
    cervix, 714–15
        blue nevus, 714
        melanoma, 715
    external ear, 1816
    lentiginous melanocytic nevus, 1468, 1478–9
    lentigo simplex, 1466–7, 1468
    mucosal melanotic macule, 1467
    pigmented spindle cell nevus, 1475–6
    Spitz nevus, 1468, 1469, 1473–5
    vagina, 726–7
        blue nevus, 726–7
        melanoma, 727
    vulva, 738–9
        genital-type nevi, 738–9
        lentigo, 738
        melanoma, 739
Melanoma, 1479–84
    acral, 1469, 1482
    adrenal gland, 1117
    anal canal, 410–11
    anogenital, 1483
    balloon cell, 1484
    benign juvenile (Spitz nevus), 1473–5
    bile duct, 455
    bladder, 551
    blue nevus-like, 1484
    bronchus, 200
    cervix, 715
    choroid, 1807, 1809

Melanoma (Cont'd)
    ciliary body, 1807
    conjunctival, 1792–6
    desmoplastic, 1469, 1483
    electron microscopy, 1840–1
    esophagus, 336–7
    eyelid, 1788
    intraocular, 1804–9
    invasive, 1479–83
    iris, 1805–6
    lentiginous, 1469, 1482
    malignant in situ, 1479
    mucosal, 115, 118–20
    neurotropic, 1483
    nevoid, 1469
    nodular, 1469, 1482–3
    nurotropic, 1469
    pagetoid, 1469
    penis, 873
    placenta, 673
    rhabdoid, 1484
    signet-ring cell, 1484
    in situ, 1469
    soft tissue, 1756–7
    superficial spreading, 1482
    urethra, 555
    vagina, 727
    vulva, 739
Melanosis
    peritoneum, 885–6
    primary acquired, 1794, 1795
    prostate, 794–6
Melanosis oculi, 1793–4
Melanotic hamartoma see Retinal anlage tumor
Melanotic medulloblastoma, 1705
Melanotic neuroectodermal tumor see Retinal anlage tumor
Melanotic progonoma see Retinal anlage tumor
Melanotic schwannoma, 1739–40
Membrane antigen, 109
MEN1 see multiple endocrine neoplasia type 1
Ménétrier's disease, 342, 368–9
Meningeal hemangiopericytoma, 1712–13
Meningeal tumors, 1707–14
Meningioma, 89–90, 1707–10
    anaplastic (malignant), 1710–12
    atypical, 1710
    lung, 199
    middle ear, 1821
    optic nerve, 1800
    rhabdoid, 1711–12
    sinonasal tract/nasopharynx, 89–90
Meningothelial-like nodule (minute pulmonary chemodectoma), 204
Merkel cell (neuroendocrine) carcinoma, 118, 1465–6
    skin, 1465–6
    vulva, 745
Mesenchymal chondrosarcoma, 1612–13
Mesenchymal tumors
    broad/round ligament, 630

Mesenchymal tumors (Cont'd)
   cervix, 713–14
   fallopian tube, 628
   kidney, 502–10
   ovary, 603
   pleural, 208–9
   salivary gland, 303–5
   skin, 1484–95
   spleen, 1304–9
   thymus, 1349–50
   thyroid, 1052–4
   vagina, 722–5
   vulva, 739–45
Mesenchymoma
   fibrocartilaginous, 1644
   malignant, 1582
   thymus, 1351
Mesonephric adenocarcinoma, cervix, 708–9
Mesonephric remnant hyperplasia, prostate, 784–5
Mesothelial hyperplasia of peritoneum, 881–2
Mesothelioma, 36
   atrioventricular node, 7, 30–1
   biphasic, 207
   cardiac, 36
   electron microscopy, 1838–40
   epithelioid, 206
   heart and pericardium, 36
   lung and pleura, 205–7
   lymphohistiocytoid, 206
   peritoneum, 887–9
   sarcomatoid, 206
   tunica vaginalis, 850
Mesothelioma of atrioventricular node, 7, 30–1
Metamyelocytes, 1392
Metaphyseal fibrous defect, 1638–9
Metaplastic carcinoma, breast, invasive, 938–9
Metastatic tumors
   adrenal gland, 1118–19, 1120
   bladder, 551–2
   breast, 619, 620, 960
   ear, 1827–8
   endometrium, 669
   esophagus, 339
   fallopian tube, 628
   hydatidiform mole, 677
   kidney, 263
   large intestine, 405
   lymph node, 1244–5
   ovary, 612, 618–22
   pancreas, 480
   penis, 873–4
   peritoneum, 891–2
   placenta
      fetal, 673
      maternal, 673–4
   prostate, 801
   skin, 1505–6
   small intestine, 387
   spleen, 1310

Metastatic tumors (Cont'd)
   stomach, 364
   testis, 840–1
   thymus, 1328, 1351
   vagina, 727
   vulva, 745
Meylocytes, 1392
Meyloperoxidase, 1150
MIBI see Ki-67 index
Michaelis-Gutmann bodies, 844
Microadenoma, adrenal, 16
Microarray analysis, 1151–2
Microcarcinoma (latent carcinoma), thyroid medullary, 1011–12
Microcystic carcinoma, 533–7
   adnexal, 1462–3
Microgemistocytes, 1674
Microglandular adenocarcinoma, pancreas, 480
Microglandular adenosis of breast, 912–13
Microneuroma, 1826–7
   inner ear, 1826–7
Micropapillary carcinoma
   breast, 936–7
   pancreas, 479
Micropapillomatosis labialis, 730
Microsatellite instability, 1870, 1871
Microsatellite repeats, 1870
Microsporidiosis, 137
Microthymoma, 1329
Microvenular hemangioma, 50
Microvillous large cell lymphoma, 1201
Middle ear tumors, 1817–24
   aggressive papillary tumor, 1823–4
   cholesteatoma, 1817–19
   developmental anomalies, 1819–20
Minor salivary gland tumor, 88
Minor vestibular gland adenoma, 736
Minute pulmonary chemodectoma, 204
Mitosis-karyorrhexis index, 1775–6
Mitotically active leiomyoma, 684
Mixed ductal-endocrine carcinoma, 470
Mixed epithelial-mesenchymal tumors
   cervix, 711–13
      adenofibroma, 712
      adenomyoma of endocervical type, 712–13
      carcinosarcoma, 713
      endocervical polyp, 712
      Müllerian adenosarcoma, 713
      Müllerian papilloma, 711–12
   vagina, 725–6
      adenosarcoma, 726
      carcinosarcoma, 726
      Müllerian papilloma, 725
      spindle cell epithelioma, 725–6
Mixed germ cell tumors
   ovary, 614–15
   testis, 829–30
Mixed GH/PRL-secreting pituitary adenoma, 982–4
   acidophilic stem cell adenoma, 983–4
   mammosomatotrophic cell adenoma, 983
   mixed GH-cell/PRL-cell adenoma, 982

Mixed neuroglial tumors, 1688–97
Mixed tumors
   bladder, 547–8
   cervix, 709–10
      adenoid basal carcinoma, 710
      adenoid cystic carcinoma, 710
      adenosquamous carcinoma, 709–10
   endometrium, 663–7
   kidney, 509
   lung and pleura, 186–7, 191
   ovarian mesodermal, 582–3
   pancreas, 470
   vulva, 736
MOC-31, 430
Molecular genetics, 1861–79
   antigen receptor rearrangements, 1872–4
   chromosomal abnormalities, 1869–70
   chromosomal translocations, 1862–8
   diagnostic and prognostic applications
      minimal residual disease, 1875–7
      prognostic markers, 1877–8
   pharmacogenomics of cancer therapy, 1878
   submicroscopic mutations, 1870–2
   transcriptional profiling, 1874–5
Molluscum contagiosum, 1431
   penis, 862
Mongolian spot, 1476
Monoclonal gammopathy of uncertain significance, 1401
Monocytic sarcoma, 1238
Monocytoid B-cell hyperplasia, 1198
Monomorphous pilomyxoid astrocytoma, 1668
Monophasic synovial sarcoma, 194–5
Monostotic fibrous dysplasia, 1816
Morton's neuroma (metatarsalgia), 1733–4
Mott cells, 1403
Mucin, 757
Mucinous adenocarcinoma
   ovary, 577–9
   prostate, 771–2
   salivary gland, 301
   vagina, 721
Mucinous carcinoma, 1463
   breast, 934–5
   eyelid, 1782
   kidney, 500
   lung, 184
   ovary, 577–9
   pancreas, 470–4
   peritoneum, 896
   thyroid, 1038
Mucinous cystadenoma, bladder, 526
Mucinous fibroplasia, 757–8
Mucocele
   appendix, 392
   orbit, 1799
Mucocutaneous γδ T-cell lymphoma, 1218
Mucoepidermoid carcinoma
   breast, 955
   esophagus, 334
   lung, 172, 191–2
   pleura, 219

Mucoepidermoid carcinoma (Cont'd)
  salivary gland, 263, 275–9
    genetic features, 278
    immunohistochemistry, 278
    prognostic factors, 278–9
  thymus, 1333
  thyroid, 1037
Mucormycosis, 137
Mucosal malignant melanoma, 118–20
  immunohistochemical reactivity, 115
Mucosal melanotic macule, 1467
Mucosal neuroma, 1735
Mucosal-associated lymphoid tissue lymphoma see MALT lymphoma
Muir-Torre syndrome, 398, 1451
Muller-Hermelink classification of thymoma, 1319–20
Müllerian adenosarcoma
  cervix, 713
  vagina, 713
Müllerian inhibiting substance, 589
Müllerian papilloma
  cervix, 712–13
  vagina, 725
Müllerian type tumors, testicular/paratesticular, 848–9
Müllerianosis, 893
Multilobulated large cell lymphoma, 1201
Multilobulated T-cell lymphoma, 1215
Multilocular cyst, 508–9
Multiple endocrine neoplasia type 1, 977, 1124
  pancreatic endocrine tumors in, 1132–3
Multiple endocrine neoplasia type 1 (MEN-1)
  gastrinoma, 1130–1
  glucagonoma, 1131
  insulinoma, 1124, 1128–9
  pancreatic endocrine tumors, 1123–33
  Zollinger-Ellison syndrome, 354, 369, 380, 1130
Multiple endocrine neoplasia type 2a (MEN-2a), pheochromocytoma, 31, 1109–15
  ganglioneuroneuroma composite tumor, 1113
MUM-1, 1149
Muscle tumors, 1495
  see also Skeletal muscle tumors; Smooth muscle tumors
Myc, 182
MYC proto-oncogene, 1202
Mycobacterial spindle cell pseudotumor, 1303–4
Mycobacterium avium intracellulare, 1303
Mycosis fungoides, 1214, 1496, 1497, 1500–1
  large cell transformation, 1229
  splenic involvement, 1292
Mycosis fungoides-associated follicular mucinosis, 1498, 1500
Myelodysplastic syndromes, 1363–70
  clinical and laboratory features, 1365
  cytogenetic findings, 1369–70

Myelodysplastic syndromes (Cont'd)
  definition and classification, 1363–5
  differential diagnosis, 1370
  dyserythropoietic abnormalities, 1365
  dysgranulopoietic abnormalities, 1365–6
  dysmegakaryopoietic abnormalities, 1466
  with isolated del(5q)(5q-syndrome), 1369
  refractory anemia
    with excess blasts, 1368–9
    pure dyserythropoietic refractory, 1366
    with ringed sideroblasts, 1367
  refractory cytopenia with multilineage dysplasia, 1367–8
Myelofibrosis, chronic idiopathic, 1399–401
Myeloid leukemia see Leukemia, acute myeloid
Myeloid sarcoma, 1175, 1243–4
Myelolipoma
  adrenal gland, 1115–17
  extra-adrenal, 1532–3
Myeloma
  bone, 1594, 1597–8
  indolent, 1401
  non-secretory, 1401
  plasma cell, 1404
  smoldering, 1401
Myelomonocytic leukemia see Leukemia, chronic myelomonocytic
Myeloperoxidase, 1151, 1376
Myeloproliferative disease, stomach, 364
Myelosarcoma see Granulocytic sarcoma
Myoepithelial carcinoma
  salivary gland, 260–2
    differential diagnoses, 262, 263
    immunohistochemistry, 261–2
Myoepithelial sialadenitis, 309–10
Myoepithelioma
  breast, 951–2
  salivary gland, 258–60
    clinical features, 258
    definition, 258
    differential diagnoses, 260
    immunohistochemistry, 260
    pathological features, 258–60
    ultrastructural studies, 260
  soft tissue, 1573–4
Myofibroblastic sarcoma, low-grade, 1554
Myofibroblastoma, breast, 958–9
Myofibroma, 1492
  solitary, 1547
Myofibromatosis, 1492
  infantile, 1543–4, 1639
Myogenic tumors, electron microscopy, 1845–8
Myogenin, 105
Myoglobin, rhabdomyoma, 18, 1566
Myointimoma of penis, 867
Myolipoma, 1531
Myometrial tumors, 683–95
  benign, 683–8
  malignant, 688–92
  smooth muscle proliferations with unusual features, 692–4

Myometrial tumors (Cont'd)
  smooth muscle tumors of uncertain malignant potential, 692
Myopericytoma, 72–3, 73–4
Myositis ossificans, 1541, 1639–40
Myospherulosis, 137
Myrmecia, 1430
Myxofibrosarcoma, 33, 1555–7
Myxoid chondrosarcoma, extraskeletal, 1528, 1580–1
Myxoid leiomyoma, 686
Myxoid leiomyosarcoma, 691
Myxoid/round cell liposarcoma, 1528
Myxoma
  atrial, 7
  cardiac, 7, 9–17
    cyst-like formations, 15
    gross pathology, 10–11
    heart valve origin, 16–17
    histogenesis, 17
    histopathology, 11–15
    macrophages, 13–14
    petrified, 10, 11
    recurrent and "malignant", 15–16
  intramuscular, 1570–1
  juxta-articular, 1571
  lymphocytes, 14
  moth-eaten appearance of arteries, 14
  nerve sheath, 1494–5, 1744–5
  ovary, 603
  soft tissue, 1570–2
Myxoma syndrome, 15, 16
Myxopapillary ependymoma, 1681–4
Myxosarcoma, cardiac, 7

NAME syndrome see Myxoma syndrome
Nasal cavity tumors, 83–140
  benign
    epithelial and neuroectodermal, 83–90
    fibro-osseous, 95–9
    mesenchymal, 90–5
    neuroectodermal, 89–90
  cartilaginous, 95
  classification, 84
  malignant
    epithelial/neuroectodermal, 101–23
    mesenchymal, 129–34
    non-epithelial, 124–9
    salivary gland tumors, 123–4
  osseous, fibro-osseous, 95
Nasal chondromesenchymal hamartoma, 136
Nasal glioma, 135
Nasal NK/T-cell lymphoma, 125–7, 1230
  immunohistochemical reactivity, 115
Nasal vestibule, carcinoma, 101
Nasopharyngeal angiofibroma, 91–2
Nasopharyngeal carcinoma, 108–12
  keratinizing, 109
  non-keratinizing, 109
  undifferentiated, 109
Nasopharyngeal dermoid, 135–6
Nasopharyngeal hairy polyp, 135–6

Nasopharyngeal papillary adenocarcinoma, low-grade, 124
Nasopharynx, squamous carcinoma, 1012
Needle biopsy, bone tumors, 1596
Nelson's syndrome, 1104
Neoplastic angioendotheliomatosis (intravascular large B-cell lymphoma), 1497, 1499, 1505
Nephroblastoma see Wilms' tumor
Nephroblastomatosis, 511–12
Nephrogenic adenoma, 519, 553
    prostate, 786–7
Nephrogenic rests, 511–12
Nephroma
    congenital mesoblastic, 518–19
    cystic (multilocular cyst), 508–9
Nerve sheath tumors
    appendix, 392–3
    cardiac, 35–6
    head and neck, 93
    heart, 35–6
    large intestine, 404
    lung, 194
    thymus, 1350
Neural cell adhesion molecule, 1126
Neural fibrolipoma (fibrolipomatous hamartoma), 1734
Neural hemangioma, 55
Neural tumors
    bone, 1634
    external ear, 1816
Neurenteric cyst, esophagus, 339
Neurilemmoma see Schwannoma
Neurilemmoma-like leiomyoma, 687
Neurinoma, acoustic see Vestibular schwannoma
Neuroblastoma, 1771–4, 1771–7
    anaplastic, 1774
    cerebral, 1701–2
    congenital, 673
    congenital cystic, 1773
    in-situ, 1771
    olfactory, 114
    orbit, 1799
    and renal carcinoma, 499–500
    thymus, 1350–1
Neuroblastoma-like medullary thyroid carcinoma, 1043
Neurocytoma, central, 1695–7
Neuroectodermal tumor
    benign, 88–90
    granular cell, 1745–7
    melanotic see Retinal anlage tumor
    nasal cavity, 83–90
    primitive, 1706–7
Neuroendocrine carcinoma, 113, 118
    cervix, 710–11
        atypical carcinoid, 711
        carcinoid, 711
    larynx, 168–72
    lung and pleura, 187–90
    moderately differentiated, 170–1
    poorly differentiated, 171–2
    renal, 502

Neuroendocrine carcinoma (Cont'd)
    well-differentiated, 169–70
    see also Large cell neuroendocrine carcinoma; Small cell carcinoma
Neuroepithelial tissue tumors, 1655–707
    astrocytic, 1655–72
    choroid plexus, 1684–6
    embryonal, 1700–7
    ependymal, 1678–84
    neuronal and mixed neuronal-glial, 1688–97
    oligodendroglial tumors and mixed gliomas, 1673–8
    pineal parenchymal, 1697–700
    uncertain origin, 1686–8
Neuroepithelioma, peripheral see Primitive neuroectodermal tumor
Neurofibroma, 93
    adrenal gland, 1118
    cardiac, 32
    dendritic cell, 1742
    diffuse, 1742
    epithelioid, 1742
    granular cell, 1742
    larynx and trachea, 154
    multiple, 1741–2
    pacinian, 1742
    plexiform, 1742–3
    small intestine, 384
    solitary, 1740–1
Neurofibromatosis, 384
Neurofibromatosis 1 (von Recklinghausen's disease), 495, 1124, 1827
    Lisch nodules, 1741
Neurofibromatosis 2, 1826
Neurofibrosarcoma see Peripheral nerve sheath tumor
Neurofilament protein
    adrenal cortical carcinoma, 1108
    ganglioneuroblastoma, 201
    gastrointestinal stromal tumor, 382
    neuroendocrine carcinoma, 1466
    olfactory neuroblastoma, 117
    teratoid/rhabdoid tumor, 1706
Neuroma
    acoustic, 1824–6
    amputation (traumatic), 1733
    bile duct, 451
    Morton's, 1733–4
    mucosal, 1735
    pacinian, 1734
    solitary circumscribed, 1735–6
    traumatic (amputation), 1733
Neuron-specific enolase, 1126
    adenoma, 1820
    adrenal carcinoma, 1107
    astrocytoma, 1661
    carcinoid tumor, goblet cell, 392
    desmoplastic small round cell tumor, 889
    ganglioneuroma, 404
    gastric carcinoma, 352
    granular cell tumor, 990
    hemangioblastoma, 1715
    hemangiopericytoma, 100

Neuron-specific enolase (Cont'd)
    intratubular germ cell neoplasia, 815, 819
    myxoma syndrome, 16
    neuroendocrine carcinoma, 188
    pancreatic tumors, 467, 1126
    papillary adenoma, 486
    paraganglioma, 1768, 1823
    sinonasal tract tumors, 115
    small cell (oat cell) carcinoma, 447
Neurotensin, pheochromocytoma, 1112
Neurothekeoma (dermal nerve sheath myxoma), 1494–5, 1744–5
    cellular, 1745
Neurotropic melanoma, 1483
Neutrophils, 1392
Nevus
    acrosyringeal, 1456–7
    apocrine, 1453
    araneus (spider), 44
    Becker's, 1562
    blue (Jadassohn-Tièche), 1469, 1476–7
        cervix, 714
        conjunctiva, 1793
        epithelioid type, 1469
        prostate, 794–6
        vagina, 726–7
    choroid, 1806–7
    ciliary body, 1806–7
    combined, 1472–3
    connective tissue, 1492
    eccrine, 1456–7
    eyelid, 1788
    hair, 1442
    inflammatory juvenile, 1790
    intraocular, 1804–9
    iris, 1805–6
    of Ito, 1476
    melanocytic, 673, 1425, 1466
        acral, 1471
        balloon cell, 1471
        cervix, 714
        compound, 1467, 1468, 1470
        congenital, 1471
        conjunctiva, 1792–6
        deep penetrating, 1469, 1472
        ear, 1816
        halo, 1472
        intradermal, 1469, 1470–1
        junctional, 1467, 1468
        lentiginous, 1181, 1215
        pigmented junctional spindle-cell, 1468
        pigmented spindle cell, 1475–6
        recurrent/persistent, 1473
        Spitz, 1473–5
        vulva, 1471
    of Ota, 1476
    porokeratotic "eccrine" ostial and dermal duct, 1456
    strawberry, 45, 46
Nevus cells, lymph node, 1250
Nevus flammeus, 44
Nevus sebaceus of Jadassohn, 1452–3
Niemann-Pick disease, 1303

Nipple
  adenoma, 916, 1454–5
  Paget's disease, 928
  see also Breast
NK cell lymphoblastic lymphoma, 1172, 1175
NK cell lymphoma see Peripheral T-cell/NK-cell lymphoma
NK (natural killer) cells, 1140
NK-cell lymphoma, 1169, 1213–34
  aggressive NK-cell leukemia, 1233
  blastic, 1233–4
  differential diagnosis, 1198
  nasal/nasal-type NK/T-cell, 1230
Nodal cytotoxic T-cell lymphoma, 1218
Nodal marginal zone B-cell lymphoma, 1196–8
  clinical features, 1196–7
  definition, 1196
  differential diagnosis, 1198
  genetic features, 1197
  immunocytochemistry, 1197, 1198
  pathology, 1197
  splenic variant, 1198
Nodular BALT hyperplasia, lung, 198
Nodular fasciitis, 1539–40
  salivary glands, 305
  vulva, 740
Nodular goiter, 1059
Nodular lymphocyte-predominant Hodgkin's lymphoma, 1154–9
  differential diagnosis, 1158–9
  genetic features, 1157–8
  immunocytochemistry, 1156–7
  immunohistochemical studies, 1156
  non-Hodgkin's lymphoma transformation, 1158
Nodular T-cell lymphoma, 1216
Non-Burkitt lymphoma see Burkitt-like lymphoma
Non-hematolymphoid tumors, 1245–50
Non-Hodgkin's lymphoma, 124–7, 1168–72
  bile duct, 455
  cervix, 715
  classification, 1168
  etiology, 1169–70
  immunocytochemistry, 1170–2
  International Prognostic Index, 1169, 1172
  liver, 443
  lung and pleura, 197–8
  REAL/WHO classification, 1168
  sinonasal tract
    diffuse large B-cell lymphoma, 127
    NK/T-cell lymphoma of nasal type, 125–7
  sinonasal tract/nasopharynx, 124–7
  survival, 1170
  types of, 1168–9
  unclassified/unclassifiable, 1172
  vulva, 745
Non-secretory myeloma, 1401
NOTCH1, 1222, 1390
Notochordal tumors of bone, 1632–4

Nottingham Prognostic Index, breast tumors, 950
Nuchal-type fibroma, 1547
Nuclear encrustation, 189
Null-cell pituitary adenoma, 987

Oat cell carcinoma see Small cell carcinoma
Oct-2, 1145
Oct-3/4, 1246
Ocular cicatricial pemphigoid, 1787
Odontoameloblastoma, 223
Odontogenic cysts, 223, 233–5
  botryoid, 235
  dentigerous, 233–4
  glandular, 235
  malignant change in, 233
  odontogenic keratocyst, 234–5
  radicular cyst, 233
Odontogenic fibroma, 230
Odontogenic ghost cell lesions, 228–9
Odontogenic keratocyst, 234–5
Odontogenic myxoma, 229–30
Odontogenic sarcoma, 233
Odontoma, 229
Olfactory neuroblastoma, 114–17
  clinical staging, 117
  Hymans' histologic grading system, 116
  immunohistochemical reactivity, 115
Oligoastrocytoma, 1676
  anaplastic, 1677–8
Oligodendroglioma, 1673–4
  anaplastic, 1675–6
Ollier disease, 1605–6
Omental-mesenteric myxoid hamartoma, 891
Omphalomesenteric duct cyst, 1465
Oncocytic adenoma
  adrenal cortex, 1104
  thyroid gland (Hurthle cell), 1026–8
  see also Oncocytoma
Oncocytic carcinoma
  adrenal cortex, 1103–4
  pleura, 187
  salivary gland, 265–6
    clinical features, 265
    metastasizing, 265
    pathologic features, 265
Oncocytic salivary gland neoplasm of uncertain malignant potential, 265
Oncocytoma
  caruncular, 1789
  clear cell, 264
  parathyroid glands, 1086
  pituitary, 987
  pleura, 192
  renal, 486–8
  salivary gland, 262–5
Oncocytomatosis (oncocytosis), 486
Opisthorchis viverrini, 452
Optic nerve tumors, 1799–800
Oral cavity tumors, 215–35
  denture-associated fibrous overgrowths, 222–3
  malignant odontogenic, 231–3

Oral cavity tumors (Cont'd)
  mesenchymal neoplasms/tumor-like lesions, 220–3
  odontogenic, 227–31
  odontogenic cysts, 223, 233–5
  oral epithelium, 215–20
Oral erythroplakia, 219
Oral leukoplakia, 219
Orbital enucleation, 1798
Orbital inflammation, 1797, 1798
Orbital myositis, 1798
Orbital tumors, 1797–9
  classification, 1799
Organoid nevus, 1452–3
Organs of Zuckerkandl, 1769
Osler-Weber-Rendu syndrome, 44, 420
Ossifying fibroma, 95
  ear, 1816
  orbit, 1799
Ossifying fibromyxoid tumor, 1573
Osteoarticular system tumors, 1593–647
  biopsy, 1595–7
  chondroid, 1602–13
  classification, 1594–5
  fibrogenic, 1631–2
  fibrohistiocytic, 1630
  lipogenic, 1634
  neural, 1634
  notochordal, 1632–4
  osteogenic, 1613–23
  small cell, 1597–602
  unknown origin
    benign, 1623–5
    malignant, 1625–7
  vascular, 1627–30
Osteoblastoma, 1594, 1614–15
Osteochondroma, 1602–4
  bone, 1594, 1602–4
Osteofibrous dysplasia, 1638
Osteogenic sarcoma see Osteosarcoma
Osteogenic tumors, 1613–23
  benign, 1613–15
  malignant, 1615–18
  Paget sarcoma, 1618–19
  postirradiation sarcoma, 1618
Osteoid osteoma, 1594, 1613–14
Osteoma, 95, 1615
  cutis, 1570
  ear, 1816
  orbit, 1799
  osteoid, 1594, 1613–14
Osteomyelitis, 1641–2
Osteosarcoma, 35
  bone, 1594
  bone surface, 1620–3
    high-grade surface, 1623
    parosteal, 1620–2
    periosteal, 1622–3
  cardiac, 35
  central low-grade, 1620
  conventional, 1616–18
  extraskeletal, 1570
  head and neck, 132
  larynx, 174

Osteosarcoma (Cont'd)
  ovary, 603
  small cell, 1620
  telangiectatic, 1619–20
  within bone, 1615–16
Ovarian tumors, 567–624
  adenomatoid, 618
  benign, 622–4
  desmoplastic small round cell tumor, 617
  epithelial, 567–88
  female adnexal tumor of probable Wolffian origin, 617–18
  germ cell, 604–16
  metastatic, 618–22
  non-specific, 603
  sclerosing peritonitis, 593, 884–5
  sex cord-stromal, 588–603
Oxyphil adenoma
  parathyroid glands, 1029
  thyroid gland (Hurthle cell), 1026–8
Oxyphilic carcinoma, thyroid gland (Hurthle cell), 1026–8

P-ANCA, 138
P16 expression mutations/mutations
  adenoid cystic carcinoma, 283
  astrocytoma, 1659
  cholangiocarcinoma, 453
  esophageal adenocarcinoma, 333
  follicular lymphoma, 1192
  hepatocellular carcinoma, 431
  mantle cell lymphoma, 1184
  nasopharyngeal carcinoma, 110
  pancreatic ductal carcinoma, 466
  small cell (oat cell) carcinoma, 447
P21 expression/mutations, spindle cell carcinoma, 165
P27 expression/mutations
  anaplastic ependymoma, 1680
  hepatocellular carcinoma, 431
P53 expression/mutations
  adenoid cystic carcinoma, 282
  adrenal tumors, 1109
  astrocytoma, 1659, 1661
  biliary adenofibroma, 451
  breast
    ductal hyperplasia, 921
    familial cancer, 937
  bronchogenic carcinoma, 181
  cholangiocarcinoma, 453
  dermatofibrosarcoma protruberans, 1488
  endometrial tumors, 660
  esophageal adenocarcinoma, 333
  fallopian tube tumors, 626
  fibrous histiocytoma, 1488
  gallbladder tumors, 447
  gastric adenocarcinoma, 345
  hepatic angiosarcoma, 440
  hepatocellular carcinoma, 431
  keratoacanthoma, 1434
  lymphomas, 1178, 1184, 1202
  mesothelial hyperplasia, 882
  pancreatic ductal adenocarcinoma, 466
  pancreatic endocrine tumors, 1124

P53 expression/mutations (Cont'd)
  pituitary adenoma, 977
  pleomorphic adenoma, 251, 254
  salivary gland carcinoma, 241
  spleen tumors, 1298
  squamous carcinoma, 328
  thyroid tumors, 1009
Pacinian neurofibroma, 1742
Pacinian neuroma, 1734
Pacinian schwannoma (neurilemmoma), 1740
Paget sarcoma, 1618–19
Pagetoid reticulosis (Woringer-Kolopp disease), 1498, 1501
Paget's disease
  esophagus, 335
  extramammary, 1460–2
  inner ear, 1826–7
  nipple, 928
  scrotum, 875
  vulva, 736–7
Palate, papillary hyperplasia, 223
Pale (clear) cell acanthoma, 1427–8
Palisaded encapsulated neuroma, 1494, 1735–6
Palmar fibromatosis (Dupuytren's contracture), 1150–1
Palmoplantar wart, 1430
Pancoast tumor, 182
Pancreatic endocrine tumors, 1123–33
  biologic behavior, 1125
  differential diagnosis, 1133
  epidemiology, 1124–5
  etiology and pathogenesis, 1123–4
  gastrinomas, 1130–1
  glucagonomas, 1131
  insulinomas, 1128–9
  in MEN1, 1132–3
  mixed endocrine-exocrine tumors, 1133
  morphologic features, 1125–8
    criteria for malignancy, 1127–8
    cytology, 1126
    electron microscopy, 1127
    histology, 1125–6
    immunophenotyping, 1126–7
    macroscopy, 1125
  non-functioning tumors, 1132
  somatostainomas, 1131–2
  terminology and classification, 1123
  tumors producing ectopic hormones, 1132
  vipomas, 1131
Pancreatic exocrine tumors, 463–81
  children, 480
  classification, 463
  ductal adenocarcinoma, 463–8
    differential diagnosis, 467–8
    genetics, 466–7
    immunohistology, 466
    prognosis, 468
    staging and grading, 468
    variants, 468–70
  non-epithelial tumors, 480
  secondary, 480

Pancreatic heterotopia, 388
  stomach, 406
Pancreatic polypeptide, pheochromocytoma, 1112
Pancreatoblastoma, 478
Paneth cell adenoma, 341
Papillary adenocarcinoma
  cervix, 708
  digital, 1464–5
  nasopharyngeal, 124
  thymus, 1334
Papillary adenoma
  apocrine, 1457
  eccrine, 1457
  kidney, 485–6
  lung, 204
  parathyroid, 1086
Papillary angioendothelioma, 57–8
  malignant endovascular (Dabska's tumor), 57–8, 1310
Papillary carcinoma, 184
  breast, 929
    invasive, 936
  penis, 871
  renal, 495–6
  thyroid, 1000–15
    clear cell variant, 1009
    clinical behavior and treatment, 1003
    clinical features, 1001–2
    cribriform-morular variant, 1010
    cytogenic and molecular features, 1013–14
    dedifferentiated, 1011
    differential diagnosis, 1015
    diffuse follicular variant, 1008
    diffuse sclerosing variant, 1007–8
    encapsulated variant, 1007
    with exuberant nodular fasciitis-like stroma, 1011
    follicular variant, 1006–7
    histologic appearances, 1003–6
    immunohistochemistry, 1012–13
    with lipomatous stroma, 1010
    macrofollicular variant, 1010
    macroscopic appearances, 1003
    microcarcinoma, 1011–12
    oxyphilic variant, 1009
    prognostic factors, 1014–15
    solid variant, 1007
    with spindle cell metaplasia, 1011
    tall cell variant, 1008–9
    trabecular variant, 1010
    Warthin tumor-like variant, 1009
Papillary cystadenoma, 629
  epididymis, 847–8
Papillary ependymoma, 1679
Papillary fibroelastoma, 7, 24–6
Papillary glioneuronal tumor, 1694–5
Papillary hidradenoma, 735–6
  perianal, 1454
  vulva, 735–6
Papillary hyperplasia, palate, 223
Papillary intralymphatic angioendothelioma, 57–8

Papillary invasive squamous carcinoma of cervix, 703
Papillary mesothelioma of peritoneum, 886–7
Papillary serous adenocarcinoma
  cervix, 708
  endometrium, 660
Papillary serous carcinoma, 662–3
Papillary serous tumors
  cervix, 708
  endometrium, 662–3
Papillary squamous carcinoma, 102–3, 151–2, 167
  oral cavity, 219
Papillary syringadenoma (syringocystadenoma papilliferum), 1454
Papilloma
  bladder, 523–6
  choroid plexus, 1684–5
  ductal, of breast, 914–16
  esophagus, 327
  intraductal, 272
  inverted
    bladder, 524–6
    renal pelvis/ureter, 519–20
  keratinizing, 151
  larynx, 150
  Müllerian, 712–13
  nasal cavity, 87
  oral cavity, 215
  schneiderian, 108
  solitary adult, 151
  squamous cell see Squamous cell papilloma
  urothelial, 553
  vulva, 730
Papillomatosis
  bile duct, 454–5
  esophagus, 327
  invasive, 152
  nipple duct, 916, 1454–5
Parachordoma, 1574
Paracoccidioidomycosis, 156
Paraffin section immunohistochemistry, 1142–3
Paraffinoma (lipogranuloma), penis, 863
Paraganglioma
  bile duct, 455
  bladder, 549–50
  cardiac, 7, 31–2
  carotid body, 31, 1764–7
  familial, 1767, 1767–8
  gangliocytic, 384
  head and neck, 89, 1764–9
  jugulotympanic, 1821–2, 1821–3
  larynx, 152–3
  malignant, 1768–9
  paraganglioma, 1770–1
  thymus, 1350
  thyroid, 1053–4
  trachea, 152–3
  vagal, 1767

Paraganglioma-like medullary thyroid carcinoma, 1043
Paraneoplastic syndromes
  bronchogenic (non-small cell) carcinoma, 181–3
  cervical neuroendocrine tumors, 710–11
  hepatocellular carcinoma, 424–33
  neuroendocrine carcinoma, 113, 118
  small cell prostate carcinoma, 774–5
  thymic carcinoid, 1337–9
Paraproteinemia, 1179
Paratesticular tumors, 841–52
  benign, 844–9
  malignant, 849–52
Parathyroid gland, 1080
Parathyroid gland tumors, 1080–94
  adenoma, 1091–2
  carcinoma, 1087–91
  intraoperative diagnosis, 1092–4
Parathyroid hormone, 1001
Parke-Weber syndrome, 44
Parosteal osteosarcoma, 1620–2
Parotid gland, polycystic disease, 271–2
Paterson-Kelly (Plummer-Vinson) syndrome, 328
Pawn ball nuclei, 1366
PAX5 proto-oncogene, 1145, 1202
Pearly penile papules (hirsutoid papilloma), 862
PEComa, 1575–6
Pelger-Huet anomaly, 1345
Peliosis
  hepatic adenoma, 417
  spleen, 1305
Peliosis hepatis, 418, 420, 428, 432
Peliosis thymomis, 1321
Penile fibromatosis see Peyronie's disease
Penile tumors, 861–76
  benign, 861–2, 866–7
  malignant, 867–70
  metastatic, 873–4
  premalignant, 864–7
Perforin, 1147, 1299, 1413
Pericardium, mesothelioma, 36
Perifollicular T-cell lymphoma, 1216–17
Perilobular hemangioma of breast, 956
Perineuroma, 1743–4
Periosteal chondroma, 1605
Periosteal chondrosarcoma, 1610
Periosteal osteosarcoma, 1622–3
Peripheral nerve sheath tumor
  benign see Schwannoma
  bone, 1632
  cardiac, 35–6
  electron microscopy, 1848–50
  malignant, 1747–50
  orbit, 1799
  pheochromocytoma composite, 1113
  thyroid, 1053
  Triton tumor, 194
Peripheral neuroectodermal tumors, 1733–57
  benign, 1735–47
  hamartomatous lesions, 1734–5

Peripheral neuroectodermal tumors (Cont'd)
  heterotopic meningeal lesions, 1753–6
  malignant, 1747–53
  reactive lesions, 1733–4
Peripheral neuroepithelioma, 1750–2
Peripheral T-cell lymphoma
  clinicopathologic variants, 1218
  differential diagnosis, 1223
  genetic studies, 1218
  immunocytochemistry, 1218
  morphologic variants, 1215–17
  with rosettes, 1215
  splenic involvement, 1292
  unspecified, 1214–18
Peritoneal fibrosis, 884–5
Peritoneal tumors, 881–99
  malignant vascular, 891
  mesothelial, 886–9
  metastatic, 891–2
  secondary Müllerian system, 893–9
  tumor-like lesions, 881–6
Perivascular cell tumors, 70–4
Peutz-Jeghers syndrome, 367, 387–8, 405, 599
  adenocarcinoma, cervix, 704–9
  adenoma malignum, 705
  gastric polyps, 367
  Sertoli cell tumor, 598, 835
  sex-cord tumors, 598–9
  small intestinal polyps, 387
Peyronie's disease, 863, 1551
Pharmacogenomics, 1878
Pheochromocytoma, 31, 1109–15
  cardiac, 31
  composite, 1113–14
  familial, 1114–15
  liver, 443
  malignant, 1115
  neuropeptide expression, 1112
  pigmented, 1114
  prostate, 797
  thyroid, 1039
Philadelphia chromosome, 1391, 1862
Phosphaturic mesenchymal tumor, 1572
Phyllodes tumor
  breast, 909–11
  prostate, 795
Pigmented (black) adrenal cortical adenomas, 1102–3
Pigmented carcinoid, 187
Pigmented follicular cyst, 1448
Pigmented junctional spindle-cell nevus, 1468
Pigmented spindle cell (Reed) melanocytic nevus, 1475–6
Pigmented villonodular synovitis (diffuse-type giant cell tumor), 1644–6
Pilar leiomyoma, 1562–3
Pilar sheath acanthoma, 1446
Pilocytic astrocytoma, 1667–70
Pilomatrixcoma, 1449–50
PIM1 proto-oncogene, 1202
Pindborg tumor, 226

Pineal parenchymal tumors, 1697–700
  intermediate differentiation, 1699–700
Pineoblastoma, 1698–9
Pineocytoma, 1697–8
Pituicytoma, 990
Pituitary apoplexy, 988–9
Pituitary gland, 972–3
Pituitary gland tumors, 971–94
  adenomas, 973–4
    pathogenesis, 975–6
    types of, 978–89
  carcinomas, 974–5
  inflammatory lesions, 989–93
  intraoperative consultation, 977–8
  specimen handling, 977–8
Placental alkaline phosphatase, 1246
  desmoplastic small round tumor, 617
  dysgerminoma, 605
  germ cell tumors, 815, 819, 1343
  germinoma, 1718
  malignant mesothelioma, 889
  seminoma, 815
  yolk sac tumor, 607
Placental site trophoblastic tumor, 624, 628, 679–80
Placental tumors, 672–80
  benign, 672–3
  chorangioma, 672
  metastatic
    fetal, 673
    maternal, 673–4
Plane wart (verruca plana), 1430
Plantar fibromatosis (Ledderhose's disease), 1151
Plasma cell bodies, 1199
Plasma cell granuloma
  abdominal, 891
  lung, 202
  ovary, 885
  thyroid, 1054
  see also Inflammatory myofibroblastic tumor; Inflammatory pseudotumor
Plasma cell myeloma, 1401–5
Plasmablastic lymphoma, 1208–9, 1210
Plasmacytoid monocytic lymphoma, 1243
Plasmacytoma, 1209–10
  adrenal gland, 1117
  AIDS-associated, 840
  bladder, 549
  clinical features, 1209
  cutaneous, 1497, 1498, 1499, 1505
  differential diagnosis, 1210
  extramedullary, 128–9
  genetic features, 1209
  immunocytochemistry, 1209
  kidney, 509
  liver, 443
  myeloma, 1597
  pathology, 1209
  prostate, 800
  skin, 1499, 1505
  testis, 840
  thymus, 1350
  thyroid, 1051

Plasmacytosis, reactive, 1210
Pleomorphic adenoma
  Bartholin's gland, 735
  breast, 953
  esophagus, 327
  lacrimal gland, 1799
  larynx, 152
  orbit, 1799
  salivary gland, 244–52
    differential diagnosis, 252
    genetic features, 252
    immunohistochemistry, 251–2
  thyroid, 1054
  vulva, 736
Pleomorphic carcinoma, lung, 186
Pleomorphic fibroma, 1486, 1492
Pleomorphic follicular lymphoma, 1503
Pleomorphic hyalinizing angiectatic tumor, 1575
Pleomorphic Reed-Sternberg cells, 1160
Pleomorphic rhabdomyosarcoma, 1569
Pleomorphic sarcoma, 1560–1
  with giant cells, 1561
  with prominent inflammation, 1561–2
Pleomorphic xanthoastrocytoma, 1680–2
Pleural tumors, 205–10
  mesenchymal, 208–9
  rare, 209–10
Pleuropulmonary blastoma, 210
Plexiform fibrohistiocytic tumor, 1559–60
Plexiform leiomyoma, 686
Plexiform neurofibroma, 1742–3
Plexiform schwannoma (neurilemmoma), 1739
Plexosarcoma, 358, 381, 383
Plummer-Vinson (Patterson-Kelly) syndrome, 328
Plurihormonal pituitary adenoma, 988
Pneumocytoma, 201–2
POEMS syndrome, 43
Polycystic kidney disease, 490
Polycystic liver disease, 451
Polycythemia vera, 1396–8
  molecular genetics, 1397–8
Polyembryoma
  ovary, 608
  testis, 825–6
Polymerase chain reaction, 1150–1, 1866, 1871
Polymorphous low-grade adenocarcinoma
  salivary gland, 288–91
    differential diagnosis, 290
    immunohistochemistry and special studies, 290
Polyp
  adenomyomatous, 666
  antrochoanal, 134
  benign lymphoid, 405
  cholesterol, 449
  endocervical, 712
  esophageal, 340
  fibroepithelial, 1492
    penis, 862
    renal pelvis/ureter, 520

Polyp (Cont'd)
  urethra, 552
  vagina, 722–3
  vulva, 739–40
  fibrovascular (fibrous), 339
  fundic gland, 365–6
  gallbladder
    cholesterol, 449
    inflammatory, 449
  gastric, 367
  hyperplastic, 364–5
    gastroesophageal junction, 340
    stomach, 364–5
  inflammatory fibroid, 339, 366–7, 388–9
  large intestine, 395–6
    hyperplastic, 407
    inflammatory, 407
    juvenile, 405–6
  sinonasal tract/nasopharynx, 99
  small intestine, 384
  ureter, 520
  urethra, 787–8
  vocal cord, 154, 155
  vulva, 739–40
Polypoid adenomyoma, 666
Polypoid granular cell tumor, 1746–7
Polyposis
  large intestine, 405
  small intestine, 384
Poorly differentiated carcinoma
  neuroendocrine, 171–2
  thyroid, 1033–6
Porocarcinoma, 1463–4
Porokeratotic "eccrine" ostial and dermal duct nevus, 1456
Poroma (acrospiroma), 1457–9
Port-wine stain see Nevus flammeus
Post-transplant lymphocytic proliferations, 36
Post-transplant lymphoproliferative disorders, 1234
Post-transplant smooth muscle tumor, spleen, 1310
Postirradiation sarcoma, 1618
Postoperative spindle cell nodule, 796
  prostate, 796
  vagina, 723
Postradiation angiosarcoma, 64
Pox virus, 1431
Precancer see Premalignant lesions
Precursor B-cell lymphoblastic leukemia/lymphoblastic lymphoma, 1386–9
  cytochemical and immunophenotypic findings, 1387
  differential diagnosis, 1388–9
  molecular genetic findings, 1387–8
Precursor lymphoblastic lymphoma, 1172–6
Precursor NK-cell lymphoblastic leukemia/lymphoma, 1234
Precursor T-cell lymmphoblastic leukemia/lymphoblastic lymphoma, 1389–90
Precursor T-lymphoblastic leukemia/lymphoma, 1152

Precursor T-lymphoblastic lymphoma, 1347–8
Pregnancy
  luteoma, 623
  microscopic granulosa cell proliferations, 623
  peritoneal leiomyomatosis, 898–9
Premalignant lesions
  endometrium, 653–4
  large intestine, 408–9
  larynx, 158–9
  penis, 864–7
  prostate, 749–55
  vulva, 732–3
  see also Intraepithelial neoplasia
Primary acquired melanosis, 1794, 1795
Primary cutaneous anaplastic large cell lymphoma, 1228–9
Primary cutaneous diffuse large B-cell lymphoma, 1497
Primary cutaneous follicle center lymphoma, 1497, 1504
Primary cutaneous marginal zone B-cell lymphoma, 1497
Primary cutaneous peripheral T-cell lymphoma, 1496
Primary effusion (body cavity) lymphoma, 1207–8
Primary immunocytoma, 1504–5
Primitive neuroectodermal tumor
  Askin tumor, 1750–2
  cytogenetic changes, 1528
  kidney, 502
  pancreas, 480
  sinonasal tract/nasopharynx, 115
  supratentorial, 1706–7
Primordial cyst (odontogenic keratocyst), 234–5
Progesterone receptors
  acrospiroma, 1463–4
  angiomyolipoma of kidney, 502–4
  peritoneal leiomyomatosis, 898–9
  prostatic stromal sarcoma, 799
  solid pseudopapillary neoplasm, 479
Prognostic factors
  acinic cell carcinoma, 287
  breast tumors, 939–46
  diffuse large B-cell lymphoma, 1203
  follicular carcinoma, thyroid gland, 1028–9
  follicular lymphoma, 1050–1
  Hodgkin's lymphoma, 1168
  mantle cell lymphoma, 1184
  medullary carcinoma, thyroid gland, 1044
  papillary carcinoma, thyroid gland, 1014–15
  salivary duct carcinoma, 294
  thymoma, 1330–1
  Wilms' tumor, 514–15
Prognostic markers, 1877–8
Prolactin-secreting pituitary adenoma (prolactinoma), 978–80
Proliferative breast disease/epithelial hyperplasia, 919–24

Proliferative fasciitis, 1540–1
Proliferative myositis, 1541
Proliferative verrucous leukoplakia, 220
Prolymphocytic leukemia, 1213–14, 1411–12
Promontory sign, 60
Promyelocytes, 1392
Promyelocytic leukemia see Leukemia, acute promyelocytic
Proprotein convertases, 1126
Proptosis, 1798
Prostate tumors, 749–801
  adenocarcinoma, 755–74
  carcinoma mimics, 778–88
  germ cell tumors, 800–1
  malignant, 798–800
  metastatic, 801
  premalignant lesions, 749–55
  stromal lesions, 792–8
Prostate-specific antigen, 542, 555, 738, 753, 772, 775, 780, 1246
Prostatic atrophy, 790–2
  benign glands in perineural space, 791–2
  prostatrophic hyperplasia, 791
  skeletal muscle within prostate gland, 791–2
Prostatic intraepithelial neoplasia (PIN), 750–5
  clinical significance, 754–5
  differential diagnosis, 753–4
  distribution, 751–2
  histologic features, 751
  immunohistochemistry, 752–3
  multifocality and precursor of malignancy, 752
Protein YY, 353, 613, 614
Protoplasmic astrocytoma, 1662
Psammocarcinoma
  ovary, 575
  peritoneum, 895–6
Psammoma bodies, 124, 208, 575
  calcifying fibrous (pseudo) tumor, 885
  collecting duct carcinoma, 499
  endosalpingiosis, 893
  lung, papillary carcinoma, 184
  meningioma, 89, 90, 1708, 1800
  mesothelial hyperplasia, 881
  metanephric adenoma, 489
  papillary adenocarcinoma, 1334
  papillary adenoma, 486
  papillary carcinoma, thyroid, 1003, 1004, 1005–6
  papillary renal cell carcinoma, 495
  peritoneal mesothelioma, 888
  peritoneum, 882
  serous carcinoma, 575
  thyroid cancer, 1005
Psammomatoid (cementifying) ossifying fibroma, 95–6
Pseudo-Gaucher cells, 1392
Pseudo-Meigs' syndrome, 612
Pseudoadenomatoid tumor of prostate, 783
Pseudoangiomatous stromal hyperplasia of breast, 956

Pseudoepitheliomatous hyperplasia, 1431, 1432
  eyelid, 1782
Pseudoepitheliomatous keratotic and micaceous balanitis, 864
Pseudohyperplastic non-verruciform squamous carcinoma, 871
Pseudolipoma, liver, 421
Pseudolymphoma see Lymphoid hyperplasia
Pseudomesotheliomatous adenoma, 207–8
Pseudomesotheliomatous (epithelioid) angiosarcoma of pleura, 209
Pseudomonas aeruginosa, 137
Pseudomyxoma ovarii, 576
Pseudomyxoma peritonei, 621–2, 891–2
Pseudosarcomatous fibrous histiocytoma, 1486
Pseudosarcomatous myofibroblastic proliferation, 723
Pseudotumor
  fibro-osseous, 1541
  mycobacterial spindle cell, 1303–4
  paratesticular tissues (fibrous periorchitis), 846
  see also Inflammatory pseudotumor
Pseudovascular squamous carcinoma see Adenoid squamous carcinoma
Pterygium, 1792
Purkinje cell tumor, 7, 26–7
  gross pathology, 27
  histopathology, 27
  special interest, 27
Pyogenic granuloma, 47, 221
Pyothorax-associated large B-cell lymphoma, 1207
Pyothorax-related lymphoma, 205

5Q-syndrome, 1369

Radial scar (complex sclerosing lesion), breast, 911, 912
Radiation-induced angiosarcoma, 64
Radicular cyst, 233
Radiotherapy, atypical vascular lesions, 69–70
Ras mutations/expression, 182
  acinar cell carcinoma, 477
  cholangiocarcinoma, 453
  colorectal cancer, 403
  gallbladder adenocarcinoma, 447
  hepatic angiosarcoma, 440
  lung tumors, 182
  pancreatic ductal adenocarcinoma, 466
  papillary carcinoma of thyroid, 1014, 1028
  pituitary adenoma, 977
  serrated adenoma, 396
  squamous carcinoma, 159
Rathke's cleft cyst, 971, 991
Reactive angioendotheliomatosis, 43
Reactive gastritis, 344
Reactive lymphoid hyperplasia, 1228
Reactive new bone formation, 1639–41

Reactive plasmacytosis, 1210
Reactive vascular proliferations, 43
Reed-Sternberg cells, 1144, 1145, 1152, 1155
  diagnostic, 1159–60
  histogenesis, 1161
  Hodgkin's lymphoma, 1159–61
  mononuclear, 1160
  pleomorphic, 1160
Reed-Sternberg-like cells, 198, 1179
Refractory anemia with excess blasts, 1368–9
Refractory anemia, pure dyserythropoietic, 1366
Refractory anemia, with ringed sideroblasts, 1367
Refractory polyp *see* Hyperplastic polyp
Refractory sprue, 1222
Reinke crystalloids, 1778
REL proto-oncogene, 1202
Renal cell carcinoma, metastatic, 263
Renal pelvis tumors, 519–23
  benign tumors/tumor-like lesions, 519–20
  transitional cell carcinoma, 520–3
Renomedullary interstitial cell tumor, 507–8
Respiratory epithelial adenomatoid hamartoma, 135
Rete testis
  adenocarcinoma, 843
  adenomatous hyperplasia, 842
  microlithiasis and epididymis, 842–3
Reticulohistiocytoma, 1493–4
Retiform hemangioendothelioma, 57
Retinal anlage tumor, 669, 1754–6
  endometrium, 669
Retinoblastoma, 1702–3
Rhabdoid melanoma, 1484
Rhabdoid meningioma, 1711–12
Rhabdoid tumor
  atypical, 1705–6
  extrarenal, 1581
  renal, 516–18
Rhabdomyoma
  cardiac, 7, 17–18
  cervix, 714
  differential diagnosis, 19
  genital, 1567
  nasal, 94
  skeletal muscle
    adult, 1566
    fetal, 1566
  thymus, 1351
  vagina, 723
  vulva, 742
Rhabdomyomatous mesenchymal hamartoma, 1566
Rhabdomyosarcoma
  alveolar, 1528, 1568–9
  anaplastic, 1568
  bladder, 546–7
  botryoid, 1567–8
  cardiac, 7, 34
  cytogenetics, 131

Rhabdomyosarcoma (*Cont'd*)
  ear, 1816
  embryonal, 1567
    bile duct, 455
    cervix, 714
    vagina, 724
  kidney, 506
  larynx, 174
  lung and pleura, 194
  myometrium, 694
  orbit, 1799
  ovary, 603
  paratesticular, 851
  pleomorphic, 1569
  prostate, 798
  sclerosing, 1569–70
  sinonasal tract/nasopharynx, 115, 130–1
  skeletal muscle, 1567–70
  spindle cell, 1569
  spleen, 1310
  thymus, 1350
  vulva, 744
Rheumatoid arthritis, 43, 306, 371, 421, 1173
Rhinosporidiosis, 137
RhoH/TTF proto-oncogene, 1202
Richter's syndrome *see* Chronic lymphocytic leukemia/small lymphocytic lymphoma
Rosai-Dorfman disease, 139–40
  larynx and trachea, 158
Rosenthal fibers, 1686
Rosette-forming glioneuronal tumor of fourth ventricle, 1695
Round ligament tumors, 628–30
Russell bodies, 1180, 1403, 1686

S-100 protein, 105, 123, 191, 1001, 1149, 1151
  acinic cell carcinoma, 191
  acrospiroma (poroma), 1457–9
  adenoid cystic carcinoma, 107, 123, 172, 190–1, 290, 710, 1464
  adenomyoepithelioma, 951–2, 952
  basal cell adenoma, 256
  benign schwannoma (neurilemmoma), 93
  blue nevus, 1477
  cardiac myxoma, 17
  chordoma, 133, 1633
  clear cell (sugar) tumor of lung, 202
  congenital epulis, 222
  cutaneous lymphadenoma, 1445
  desmoid fibromatosis, 1552
  desmoplastic melanoma, 1483
  digital papillary adenocarcinoma, 1464
  eccrine hidrocystoma, 1454
  epithelial-myoepithelial carcinoma, 192
  epithelioid fibrous histiocytoma, 1486
  extraskeletal myxoid chondrosarcoma, 1848
  gangliocytic paraganglioma, 384
  ganglioneuroblastoma, 201
  glomus tumor, 70, 200
  granulosa cell tumor, 591

S-100 protein (*Cont'd*)
  jugulotympanic paraganglioma, 1823
  keratocystoma, 272
  Langerhans cell histiocytosis, 1642
  liposarcoma, 1534
  malignant fibrous histiocytoma, 129
  malignant periperipheral nerve sheath tumor, 714
  melanoma, 1807
  microglandular adenosis, 912
  mucinous carcinoma, 1463
  mucosal malignant melanoma, 115
  myoepithelial carcinoma, 262
  myoepithelioma, 88
  nasal type NK/T-cell lymphoma, 115
  neuroblastoma, 1776
  ossifying fibromyxoid tumor, 1573
  Paget's disease, 335
  paraganglioma, 1763
  pheochromocytoma, 1112
  pituicytoma, 990
  pleomorphic adenoma, 251
  pleomorphic hyalinizing angiectatic tumor, 1575
  primitive neuroectodermal tumor, 115
  pulmonary adenofibroma, 204
  pulmonary meningioma, 199
  rhabdomyosarcoma, 115, 194
  salivary gland tumors, 953
  schwannoma, 1738, 1739, 1740
  sinonasal undifferentiated carcinoma, 115
  small oat cell undifferentiated neuroendocrine carcinoma, 115
  soft tissue perineuroma, 1744
  squamous carcinoma, 115, 1439
  T-cell lymphoma, 1217
  thyroid tumors, 1001, 1008
Saccular cyst, 155–6
Salivary duct carcinoma, 292–5
  clinical features, 293
  definition, 292
  differential diagnosis, 295
  genetic features, 294–5
  immunohistochemistry, 294
  pathologic features, 293–4
  prognostic factors, 294
Salivary gland tumors, 88, 239–316
  behavior of, 241–2
  diagnosis, 242–4, 310–16
    genetic studies, 244
    histochemistry, 243–4
    immunohistochemistry, 244
    morphologic assessment, 310–16
  epithelial tumors/tumor-like lesions, 244–303
  general features, 240–1
  hematolymphoid tumors, 305–10
  hybrid tumor, 244
  malignant, 123–4
  mesenchymal lesions, 303–5
  overdiagnosis, 311
  progression, 244
  TNM staging, 243
  underdiagnosis, 312

Salivary gland-type tumors, 152
  breast, 953–5
  lung and pleura, 190–2
Salivary glands, 239–40
  applied anatomy, 239
  histology, 239–40
Salmonella typhi, 1303
Salt-and-pepper stippling, 187
Sarcoidosis, larynx and trachea, 158
Sarcoma
  alveolar soft part *see* Alveolar soft part sarcoma
  bone- and cartilage-forming, 196
  clear cell, 515–16
  embryonal, 442
  epithelioid, 1578–9
  Ewing's, 174, 1528
  fibroblastic, 1554–7
  fibroblastic *see* Fibrosarcoma
  follicular dendritic cell, 1240–2
  granulocytic, 715, 1350
  histiocytic, 1237–8
  interdigitating dendritic cell, 1242
  Kaposi *see* Kaposi sarcoma
  low-grade fibromyxoid, 1528, 1556
  low-grade myofibroblastic, 1554
  monocytic, 1238
  monophasic synovial, 194–5
  myeloid, 1175, 1243–4
  odontogenic, 233
  osteogenic, 35, 132, 184, 603
  penis, 873
  pleomorphic, 1560–1
  postirradiation, 1618
  renal, 515–16
  scrotum, 875–6
  stromal, 583
  synovial, 7, 35
  see also Adenosarcoma; Angiosarcoma; Carcinosarcoma; Chondrosarcoma; Dermatofibrosarcoma protruberans; Fibrosarcoma; Gliosarcoma; Leiomyosarcoma; Liposarcoma; Malignant fibrous histiocytoma; Myofibrosarcoma; Myxofibrosarcoma; Osteosarcoma; Rhabdomyosarcoma
Sarcoma botryoides, 130
Sarcomatoid carcinoma, 104–6
  penis, 871–2
  prostate, 777–8
  thymus, 1332–3
Sarcomatoid mesothelioma, 206
Scar
  cancer, 183
  hypertrophic, 1492, 1539
  keloid, 1492, 1539
  radial (complex sclerosing lesion), 911, 912
Schiller-Duval bodies, 606
Schistosomiasis, larynx and trachea, 158
Schneiderian (sinonasal-type) papillomas, 108

Schwannoma (neurilemmoma)
  ancient, 1738
  benign, 93
  bone, 1594, 1634
  cardiac, 7, 35–6
  cellular, 1738–9
  clinical features, 1736
  epithelioid, 1740
  glandular, 1740
  histologic features, 1736–8
  hybrid, 1740
  lymph node, 1740
  malignant
    cervix, 714
    larynx and trachea, 154, 174
    ovary, 603
  melanotic, 1739–40
  neuroectodermal, 1736–40
  orbit, 1799
  pacinian, 1740
  plexiform, 1739
  small intestine, 384
  stomach, 359
  vestibular, 1824–6
Sclerosing adenosis, 783
  breast, 911–12
  prostate, 783–4
  salivary gland, 273
Sclerosing angiomatoid nodular transformation, 1307
Sclerosing dacryoadenitis, 1798
Sclerosing hemangioma, 201–2
Sclerosing lipogranuloma of testis, 845–6
Sclerosing lymphocytic lobulitis, 905–6
Sclerosing mediastinitis, thymus, 1350
Sclerosing mesenteritis, 884–5
Sclerosing mucoepidermoid carcinoma with eosinophilia, 1038
Sclerosing peritonitis, 593, 884–5
Sclerosing rhabdomyosarcoma, 1569–70
Sclerosing stroma tumor, 602
Sclerotic fibroma, 1492
Scrotal tumors, 874–6
  neoplastic lesions, 874–6
  non-neoplastic lesions, 874
SDHD gene, 1767
Sebaceous adenoma, 1451
  salivary gland, 269, 2659
Sebaceous carcinoma, 1451–2
  eyelid, 1785–8
  salivary gland, 270
  vulva, 745
Sebaceous duct cyst (steatocystoma), 1449
Sebaceous lymphadenocarcinoma, salivary gland, 270
Sebaceous lymphadenoma, salivary gland, 269
Seborrheic keratosis, 1423–7
  vulva, 731
Secondary tumors *see* Metastatic tumors
Secretory carcinoma, breast, invasive, 938
Sellar region tumors *see* Pituitary gland tumors
Seminal vesicle cysts, 801

Seminal vesicle tissue remnants, 788–9
Seminal vesicle tumors
  benign, 801
  malignant, 802–3
Seminal vesicles, 801–3
  amyloid deposition, 801
Seminoma
  classic, 816–82
    clinical presentation, 816
    cytogenetic findings, 819
    differential diagnosis, 819
    histochemistry and immunohistochemistry, 818
  spermatocytic, 820–2
    immunohistochemistry, 821
Senile angioma (Campbell de Morgan spot), 46
Serous cystadenoma, bile duct, 451
Serous tumors
  bile duct cystadenoma, 451
  ovary, 569–75
    benign, 570
    borderline, 570–3
    carcinoma, 573–5
  pancreas, 474–6
  peritoneum, 895–6
Sertoli cell tumor
  ovary, 598
  testis, 835–6
Sertoli-Leydig cell tumor, 595–8
  clinical findings, 595–6
  pathology, 596–8
Sex cord tumor with annular tubules, 598–600
  clinical features, 598–9
  pathology, 599–600
Sex cord-stromal tumors
  ovary, 588–603
  testis, 833–8
    mixed/unclassified, 837–8
Sézary cells, 1214
Sézary syndrome, 1214, 1496, 1499, 1500–1
Short tandem repeats, 1870
Sialadenitis, chronic sclerosing (Kuttner tumor), 309–10
Sialadenoma papilliferum, 271
Sialo-odontogenic cyst, 235
Sialoblastoma, 302–3
Signet-ring cell adenocarcinoma, salivary gland, 301
Signet-ring cell adenoma, thyroid follicular, 1023
Signet-ring cell carcinoma
  pancreas, 470
  prostate, 772–3
Signet-ring cell DCIS, breast, 927
Signet-ring cell melanoma, 1484
Signet-ring cell-type lymphoma, 1200
  follicular, 1188–9
  T-cell, 1215
Signet-ring cells, 206
Sinonasal hemangiopericytoma, 72
Sinonasal (inflammatory) polyps, 134–5

Sinonasal (mucosal) adenocarcinoma, 120–3
  intestinal-type, 120–2
  non-intestinal, 122–3
Sinonasal myxoma/fibromyxoma, 94–5
Sinonasal tract, squamous carcinoma, 101
  immunohistochemical reactivity, 115
  molecular genetics, 108
  precursor lesions, 108
Sinonasal undifferentiated carcinoma, 112–14
  immunohistochemical reactivity, 115
Sinonasal-type hemangiopericytoma, 99–101
Sinonasal-type (Schneiderian) papillomas, 83–7
Sinus histiocytosis with massive lymphadenopathy (Rosai-Dorfman disease), 1240, 1643
Sinusoidal hemangioma, 48–9
Sinusoidal large cell lymphoma, 1201
Sjögren syndrome, 299, 306, 307, 309, 1193
Skeletal muscle tumors, 1566–70
Skene's gland adenocarcinoma, 737–8
Skin tumors, 1423–506
  adnexal tumors, 1442–65
  cysts, 1465
  eyelid *see* Eyelid tumors
  lymphoid, 1495–505
  melanocytic, 1466–84
  Merkel cell (neuroendocrine) carcinoma, 1465–6
  mesenchymal, 1484–95
  metastatic, 1505–6
Slg, 1388
Small cell astrocytoma, 1663
Small cell carcinoma
  bladder, 544
  cervix, 711
  esophagus, 334–5
  gallbladder, 447
  Merkel cell subtype, 297–8
  ovary, 587–8
    hypercalcemic type, 616–17
  pancreas, 480
  prostate, 774–5
  salivary gland, 297–8
  stomach, 352–3
  thymus, 1339–40
Small cell non-keratinizing invasive squamous carcinoma of cervix, 702–3
Small cell osteosarcoma, 1620
Small cell undifferentiated neuroendocrine carcinoma (SCUNC), 118
Small intestinal tumors, 379–89
  epithelial, 379–81
  lymphoid, 384–7
  non-epithelial, 381–3
  secondary tumors, 387
  tumor-like lesions, 387–9
  vascular, 383–4

Small "oat" cell undifferentiated neuroendocrine carcinoma
  immunohistochemical reactivity, 115
  larynx and trachea, 171–2
Small round cell tumor
  desmoplastic *see* Desmoplastic small round cell tumor
  electron microscopy, 1842
Smoldering myeloma, 1401
Smooth muscle tumors, 1562–6
  esophagus, 337
  myometrium
    benign, 683–8
    malignant, 688–92
  pleura, 209
  stomach, 359
  thyroid, 1053
  of uncertain malignant potential, 93
    myometrium, 692
Soft tissue angiosarcoma, 64–6
  differential diagnosis, 66
  histological appearances, 64
Soft tissue chondroma, 1605
Soft tissue tumors, 1527–82
  adipocytic, 1528–39
  chondro-osseous, 1570
  electron microscopy, 1842–57
  fibrohistiocytic, 1557–62
  fibrous, 1539–57
  skeletal muscle, 1566–70
  smooth muscle, 1562–6
Solar (actinic) keratosis, 1434–42
Solar lentigo, 1434
Solid aneurysmal bone cyst, 97–8, 1816
Solid pseudopapillary tumor of pancreas, 479
Solitary adult papilloma, 151
Solitary angiokeratoma, 44
Solitary circumscribed (palisaded encapsulated) neuroma, 1735–6
Solitary fibrous tumor, 92, 1549–50
  central nervous system, 1713–14
  lung, 195–6, 209
  meninges, 1713–14
  peritoneum, 886
  pleura, 208
  salivary glands, 305
  sinonasal tract/nasopharynx, 92, 100
  thymus, 1350
  thyroid, 1053
Solitary myofibroma, 1547
Solitary neurofibroma, 1740–1
Somatostatin
  adenocarcinoma, 380
  carcinoid tumor, 391
    goblet cell, 392
  familial paraganglioma, 1768
  gallbladder adenomyoma, 448
    carcinoid tumor, 614
  neuroendocrine tumors, 1125
  neurofibroma, 384
  pheochromocytoma, 1112
  small cell carcinoma, 352
  thyroid medullary carcinoma, 1043

Somatostatinomas, 1131–2
Southern blot analysis, 1150
Sperm granuloma, 845
Spermatocytic seminoma, 820–2
  clinical features, 820
  differential diagnosis, 821
  immunohistochemistry, 821
  management, 822
  pathologic features, 820–1
Spider cells, 18, 19
Spider nevus (nevus araneus), 44
Spindle cell carcinoma, 104–6, 163–6
  differential diagnosis, 165–6
  esophagus, 332–3
  gallbladder, 447
  kidney, 500
  oral cavity, 216
  penis, 871–2
  vagina, 726
Spindle cell hemangioma, 53
Spindle cell nevus
  pigmented (Reed), 1468
  Spitz (benign juvenile melanoma), 1473–5
Spindle cell nodule, postoperative, 796
  prostate, 796
  vagina, 723
Spindle cell pseudotumor, mycobacterial, 1303–4
Spindle cell rhabdomyosarcoma, 1569
Spindle cell tumor
  epithelial with thymus-like differentiation, 1047–8, 1337
  hemangioma, 52–3
  hemorrhagic, 1245
  hyalinizing with giant rosettes, 1556
  thymic carcinoid tumor, 1337–9
  thyroid, 1011
Spindle epithelial tumor with thymus-like element (SETTLE), 1337
Spiradenoma, 1459–60
Spironolactone bodies, 1102
Spitz nevus, 1473–5
  intradermal, 1469
  junctional, 1468
Spleen, 1289–310
  histiocytic/dendritic cell proliferations, 1303
  leukemia/lymphoma involvement, 1289–95
    beefy-red appearance, 1290
    miliary small modules, 1292–3
    solitary/multiple large fleshy nodules, 1295
    solitary/multiple small clustered nodules, 1293–5
  lymphoma
    B-cell lymphoma, 1292, 1297–9
    prominent splenic involvement, 1289–95
  mesenchymal tumors and tumor-like lesions, 1304–9
  metastatic tumors, 1310
  mycobacterial spindle cell pseudotumor, 1303–4

Spleen (*Cont'd*)
  normal, 1289
  systemic mastocytosis, 1301–3
Splenic-gonadal fusion, 844–5
Splenosis, 885
Sporotrichosis, 156
Sprue, refractory, 1222
Squamous carcinoma, 1432, 1433, 1438–40
  anal canal, 409–10
  anal margin, 411–12
  basaloid *see* Basaloid squamous carcinoma
  bladder, 537–9
  cervix, 702
  conjunctiva, 1791–2
  electron microscopy, 1832–4
  esophagus, 328–32
  external ear, 1813–14
  larynx and trachea, 158–61
    invasive, 159–61
    premalignant/preinvasive lesions, 158–9
  lung, 184–5
    spindle cell, 185
  middle ear, 1823
  oral cavity, 216–19
  ovary, 588
  penis, 867–9
  prostate, 775–6
  renal pelvis/ureter, 522–3
  salivary gland, 300–1
    clinical features, 300–1
    definition, 300
    differential diagnosis, 301
    pathology, 301
  scrotum, 875
  sinonasal tract/nasopharynx, 102–3
  stomach, 351–2
  thymus, 1331–2
  thyroid, 1031–2
  vagina, 720
  vulva, 734–5
  see also Adenosquamous carcinoma
Squamous dysplasia, esophagus, 327–8
Squamous intraepithelial neoplasia
  cervix, 697–8
    high-grade, 698–9
    low-grade, 697–8
  vagina, 719–20
Squamous odontogenic tumor, 226
Squamous papilloma
  bladder, 523–6
  conjunctiva, 1791–2
  esophagus, 327
  larynx, 150–4
  nasal cavity, 87
  oral cavity, 215
Stains, central nervous system, 1654–5
Starry-sky appearance, 128
Steatocystoma, 1449
Sternomastoid tumor (fibromatosis coli), 1544–5
Steroid (lipid) cell tumors, ovary, 601
Stewart-Treves syndrome, 64, 957–8

Stomach tumors, 340–71
  epithelial, 340–56
  non-epithelial, 356–64
  tumor-like lesions, 364–71
Storiform collagenoma, 1546
Stratified/squamomucinous glandular intraepithelial neoplasia, 700
Strawberry nevus, 45, 46
Stromal hyperplasia of prostate, 793
Stromal luteoma, 602
Stromal tumors
  breast, 955–9
  endometrium, 667–9
  esophagus, 338
  gastrointestinal, 338, 356–9
  kidney, 509
  prostate, 792–8, 799
  sex cord-stromal tumors, 588–603
Struma ovarii, 612–13
Strumosis, 613
Sturge-Weber syndrome, 504
Subcutaneous panniculitis-like T-cell lymphoma, 1222–3, 1496, 1498, 1503
Subependymal giant cell astrocytoma, 1672
Subependymoma, 1681–2
Subglottic hemangioma, 153–4
Substance P, pheochromocytoma, 1112
Subungual exostosis, 1640–1
Subungual keratoacanthoma, 1432
Sugar tumor *see* Clear cell tumor
Superficial angiomyxoma, 1571–2
Superior vena cava syndrome, 182, 189
Supratentorial primitive neuroectodermal tumors, 1706–7
Surfactant, 1246
Suster-Moran classification of thymic epithelial tumors, 1320
Swiss cheese appearance, 123
Swiss syndrome, 15, 16
Synaptophysin, 1001
  adrenal tumors, 1107, 1108
  basaloid squamous cell carcinoma, 106
  borderline mucinous tumors, 577
  carcinoid tumors, 381, 614, 841, 1339
  central neurocytoma, 1696, 1697
  desmoplastic infantile astrocytoma, 1690
  Ewing's sarcoma, 115
  gastrointestinal stromal tumors, 382
  hyalinizing trabecular tumor, 1023
  medulloblastoma, 1703
  meningioma, 90
  Merkel cell (trabecular) carcinoma, 298
  mucosal malignant melanoma, 115
  nasal-type NK/T-cell lymphoma, 115
  neuroendocrine carcinoma, 430, 579
    large cell, 190, 299
    lung, 187, 188
    small cell undifferentiated, 115, 118
  olfactory neuroblastoma, 115, 117
  Paget's disease, 1462
  pancreatic endocrine tumors, 1126
  pancreatic tumors, 467, 1126, 1127
  paraganglioma, 200

Synaptophysin (*Cont'd*)
  pheochromocytoma, 1112
  pituitary tumors, 989
  primitive neuroectodermal tumor, 115
  rhabdomyosarcoma, 115
  Sertoli-Leydig tumor, 598
  sinonasal intestinal-type adenocarcinoma, 121
  sinonasal undifferentiated carcinoma, 113, 115
  small cell carcinoma, 298
  squamous cell carcinoma, 115
  thyroid tumors, 1001
  undifferentiated carcinoma, 1031, 1033
Synovial chondromatosis, 1646–7
Synovial hemangioma, 55, 1647
Synovial lipoma, 1530, 1647, 1647–8
Synovial sarcoma, 35, 1528
  cardiac, 7, 35
  electron microscopy, 1850–1
  larynx, 174
  pleura, 209
  soft tissue, 1576–8
  thymus, 1315–17
  vulva, 745
Synovioma, 1558
Syringocystadenoma papilliferum, 1454
Syringofibroadenoma (acrosyringeal nevus), 1456–7
Syringoma, 1457
  chondroid, 736, 1455–6
  vulva, 736
Systemic mastocytosis, 1198, 1301–3

T lymphocytes, 1140
  development, 1141
T-cell granular lymphocytic leukemia, 1214, 1412–13
  differential diagnosis, 1233
  splenic involvement, 1292
T-cell lymphoma
  adult T-cell leukemia/lymphoma, 1229, 1405–6, 1496
  angioimmunoblastic, 1219–21
  cutaneous, 1223, 1497
  enteropathy-type intestinal, 1221–2
  erythrophagocytic Tγ, 1215
  hepatosplenic γδT-cell, 1292, 1299–300
  Lennert's (lymphoepithelioid), 1181, 1215
  multilobulated, 1215
  nasal NK/T-cell, 125–7, 1230
  nodular, 1216
  perifollicular, 1216–17
  peripheral
    clinicopathologic variants, 1218
    differential diagnosis, 1223
    genetic studies, 1218
    immunocytochemistry, 1218
    morphologic variants, 1215–17
    with rosettes, 1215
    splenic involvement, 1292
    unspecified, 1214–18
  plasmacytoid, 1243

T-cell lymphoma (Cont'd)
  signet-ring type, 1215
  subcutaneous panniculitis-like, 1222–3, 1496, 1498, 1503
  T-zone, 1215
  see also T-cell/null-cell anaplastic large cell lymphoma
T-cell receptors
  anaplastic large cell lymphoma, T-cell/null-cell type, 1223
  blastic (blastoid) NK-cell lymphoma, 1233–4
  gene rearrangements, 1150
  αβ versus γδ in lymphomas, 1146
  subcutaneous panniculitis-like T-cell lymphoma, 1223
  T-cell granular lymphocytic leukemia, 1214
  T-lymphoblastic lymphoma, 1175
T-cell type lymphoblastic lymphoma, 1172, 1174–5
T-cell/null-cell anaplastic large cell lymphoma, 1149, 1201, 1223–8
  anaplastic lymphoma kinase expression, 1224
  clinical features, 1223
  common type, 1225
  cutaneous type, 1228–9
  differential diagnosis, 1228
  genetic features, 1227–8
  giant cell variant, 1227
  hypocellular variant, 1226–7
  immunocytochemistry, 1227
  mixed cell variant, 1226
  monomorphic variant, 1225
  pathology, 1224–5
  small cell variant, 1225–6
T-lymphoblastic lymphoma, 1172
T-prolymphocytic leukemia, 1213–14, 1411–12
  splenic involvement, 1292
Tamoxifen, 669
Tancho's nodule, 863
Tanycytic ependymoma, 1679
Targetoid hemosiderotic (hobnail) hemangioma, 184
Tartrate-resistant acid phosphatase (TRAP) reaction, 1301, 1407
TdT (terminal deoxynucleotidyl transferase), 1376, 1388
Teflon granuloma, vocal cord, 158
Telangiectatic osteosarcoma, 1619–20
Tendon sheath fibroma, 1492, 1545
Tendon sheath giant cell tumor, 1492, 1558
Teratocarcinoma, testis, 815
Teratocarcinosarcoma, sinonasal tract/nasopharynx, 133–4
Teratoid tumor, atypical of central nervous system, 1705–6
Teratoma
  cardiac
    benign, 7, 27
    malignant, 36
  central nervous system, 1718

Teratoma (Cont'd)
  cervix, 715
  endometrium, 669
  fallopian tube, 625
  head and neck
    benign, 98–9
    malignant, 133–4
  immature, 610, 827
  kidney, 519
  larynx, 154
  lung and pleura, 201
  mature, 715, 826–7
  ovary, 608–14
    carcinoid tumor, 613–14
    immature, 609–12
    mature (benign), 609
    secondary neoplasms in, 612
    struma ovarii, 612–13
  placenta, 672
  spleen, 1310
  struma ovarii, 612–13
  testis, 826–7
    immature, 827
    mature, 826–7
  thymus, 1341–2
  thyroid, 1054
  trachea, 154
Terminal deoxynucleotidyl transferase, 1147, 1151
Testicular feminization syndrome, 812
Testicular tumors
  adrenogenital syndrome, 838–9
  classification, 813
  germ cell, 812–41
  paratesticular, 841–52
  sex cord-stroma, 833–8
Thecoma, 593–4
  clinical findings, 593
  pathology, 593–4
Third ventricle choroid glioma, 1686–7
Thrombomodulin, 1246
Thymic carcinoma, 1331–4
  arising in thymoma or cyst, 1334–5
  differential diagnosis, 1335–6
  immunocytochemistry, 1134–5
  prognostic factors, 1335
Thymic tumors
  epithelial, 1317–37
    borderline (atypical thymoma), 1336
    ectopic, 1350
  germ cell, 1340–3
  histiocytic and dendritic cell, 1349
  histologic/ultrastructural features, 1315
  lymphomas, 1343–9
  mesenchymal, 1349–50
  metastatic, 1351
  neuroendocrine, 1337–40
  rare, 1350–1
  T-lineage acute lymphoblastic leukemia, 1172
  vascular, 1350
Thymolipoma, 1349–50
Thymoma, 1317–31
  atypical, 1336

Thymoma (Cont'd)
  children, 1317
  classification, 1318, 1319–21
  clinical behavior and treatment, 1317–19
  clinical features, 1317
  cystic, 1328
  differential diagnosis, 1331
  ectopic, 1047, 1336, 1350
    hamartomatous, 1336–7, 1572
    pleura, 209
  electron microscopy, 1330
  genetic features, 1330
  immunocytochemistry, 1330
  invasion potential, 1329–30
  prognostic factors, 1330–1
  secondary changes, 1328
  staging, 1319
  types of, 1323–6
Thymus, 1315–53
  anatomy, 1315
  immunocytochemistry, 1315–17
Thyroglobulin, 124, 1001, 1246
  columnar cell carcinoma, 1036
  follicular thyroid neoplasms, 1024, 1028
  follicular-parafollicular thyroid carcinoma, 1046
  metastatic thyroid tumors, 1055
  mucinous carcinoma, 1038
  mucoepidermoid carcinoma, 1037
  poorly differentiated thyroid carcinoma (insular carcinoma), 1033
Thyroid gland, 997
Thyroid gland tumor-like lesions, 1054–5
Thyroid gland tumors, 997–1063
  C-cell differentiated, 1038–46
  Chernobyl nuclear-accident-associated cancer, 999–1000
  children, 998–9
  diagnosis, 1000, 1055–61
  differentiated, 1046–7
  fine needle aspiration cytology, 1061–2
  follicular/metaplastic epithelial, 1000–38
  hematolymphoid cell, 1049–52
  immunohistochemistry, 1055
  intraoperative frozen section diagnosis, 1062–3
  invasive tumor with solid growth, 1060
  mesenchymal, 1052–4
  metastatic, 1055
  mixed follicular/C-cell, 1046–7
  staging, 999
  thymic/branchial pouch, 1047–9
Thyroid transcription factor-1, 1246
Thyrolipoma, 1024
TIA-1, 1147
  adult T-cell leukemia/lymphoma, 1406
  hepatosplenic T-cell lymphoma, 1299
  Hodgkin's lymphoma, 1223
  lymphomatoid granulomatosis, 1223
  subcutaneous panniculitis-like T-cell lymphoma, 1222, 1223
  T-cell rich large B-cell lymphoma, 1223
TNM staging
  colorectal cancer, 402

TNM staging (Cont'd)
  esophageal carcinoma, 335, 521
  gastric carcinoma, 348
  laryngeal tumors, 162
  pancreatic ductal adenocarcinoma, 468, 469
  prostate cancer, 764
  renal cell carcinoma, 501
  salivary gland carcinomas, 241
  thyroid tumors, 999
Tongue, cribriform adenocardinoma, 290–1
Tonsil
  lymphangiomatous polyp, 136–7
  Waldeyer's tonsillar tissues
    HIV infection, 137–8
    malignant lymphoma, 127–8
TP53, 181
Trabecular carcinoma see Merkel cell carcinoma
Trabecular pattern
  follicular adenoma, 1021–3
  hepatocellular carcinoma, 425, 426
  thyroid papillary carcinoma, 1010
Tracheal tumors, 150–74
  benign, 150–8
  malignant, 158–74
Tracheobronchopathia osteochondroplastica, 157–8
Tracheopathia osteoplastica, 157–8
Transcriptional profiling, 1874–5
Transitional cell carcinoma
  bladder, 526–37
    microcystic carcinoma, 533–7
    non-papillary, 529–33
    papillary, 526–9
    variants of, 533
  cervix, 703
  endometrium, 652
  kidney, 517
  ovary, 586–7
  prostate, 776–7
  renal pelvis/ureter, 520–3
Traumatic (amputation) neuroma, 1733
Trichoadenoma of Nikolowski, 1444
Trichoblastic fibroma, vulva, 1443, 1444
Trichoblastoma, 1443
Trichoepithelioma, 1443–5
Trichofolliculoma, 1442–3
Trichogenic trichoblastoma, 1444
Tricholemmal cyst, 1448
Tricholemmoma, 1425, 1446–7
Trisomy 8, 1369
Triton tumor, 194
  neuromuscular, 1735
  thymus, 1350
Trophoblast, origins of, 674–5
Trophoblastic tumor
  epithelioid, 624, 628
  placental site, 624, 628, 679
TSH-secreting pituitary adenoma, 987–8
TTF-1, 1001
Tuberculosis, 182
  laryngeal, 156
  sinonasal tract/nasopharynx, 137

Tuberous sclerosis, 18–19
Tubular adenocarcinoma, stomach, 346
Tubular adenoma
  breast, 907–8
  gallbladder, 444
  large intestine, 393
  pancreas, 473
Tubular apocrine adenoma, 1454
Tubular carcinoma
  breast
    invasive, 933
    mixed, 933–4
Tubulin
  medulloblastoma, 1704
  melanocytic nevus, 1470
  neuroblastoma, 1702
  retinoblastoma, 1703
  subependymal giant cell astrocytoma, 1672
Tubulo-lobular carcinoma, breast, 931
Tufted angioma (angioblastoma of Nakagawa), 46
Turban tumor, 1815
Tylosis, 328
Tyndall effect, 1476

UCHL1 see CD45RO
Ulcer, laryngeal contact (granuloma), 154–5
Ulcer-cancer, 350
Ulcerative colitis, 398, 399, 403
Ulex europaeus agglutin
  cardiac myxoma, 13
  collecting duct carcinoma, 498
  mixed tumor, 1455
  prostatic intraepithelial neoplasia, 753
  pseudomesotheliomatous (epithelioid) angiosarcoma, 209
  soft tissue angiosarcoma, 66
Umbilical cyst (omphalomesenteric duct cyst), 1465
Undifferentiated carcinoma
  bladder, 544–5
    giant cell carcinoma, 544
    lymphoepithelioma-like cancers, 544–5
    small cell carcinoma, 544
  heart, 34
  liver, 442
  ovary, 587
  pancreas, 469–70
  salivary gland, 297–300
  sinonasal, 109, 112–14
  thymus, 1334
  thyroid, 1029–33
    adenosquamous carcinoma, 1031
    angiomatoid variant, 1031
    carcinosarcoma, 1031
    clinical features, 1029
    cytogenetic and molecular features, 1032
    differential diagnosis, 1032
    histologic appearances, 1030–1
    immunohistochemistry, 1032
    lymphoepithelioma-like carcinoma, 1031

Undifferentiated carcinoma (Cont'd)
    macroscopic features, 1029–30
    osteoclastic variant, 1031
    paucicellular variant, 1031
    rhabdoid variant, 1031
    squamous carcinoma, 1031–2
    versus angiosarcoma, 1032–3
  see also Small cell undifferentiated neuroendocrine carcinoma
Undifferentiated sarcoma
  cardiac, 32
  embryonal, 442
Unicystic ameloblastoma, 225–6
Upper respiratory tract tumors, 83–174
  larynx and trachea, 150–74
  nasal cavity, paranasal sinuses and nasopharynx, 83–140
Ureter see renal pelvis/ureter
Ureteric tumors, 519–23
  benign tumors/tumor-like lesions, 519–20
  transitional cell carcinoma, 520–3
Urethral polyp, prostatic-type, 787–8
Urethral tumors, 552–5
  benign tumors and tumor-like lesions, 552–4
  malignant tumors, 554–5
Urethritis glandularis, 554
Urinary tract tumors, 485–555
Urothelial papilloma, 553
Urticaria pigmentosa, 1301
Uterine perivascular epithelioid cell tumor, 694–5
Uterus see cervix; endometrium; myometrium
Uveal melanoma, 1781, 1793, 1801, 1807

V-(D)-J rearrangements, 1872
Vagal paraganglioma, 1767
Vagina, yolk sac tumor, 727
Vagina tumors, mixed epithelial-mesenchymal, 725–6
Vaginal intraepithelial neoplasia, 719–20
Vaginal tumors, 719–27
  melanocytic lesions, 726–7
  mesenchymal neoplasia and tumor-like conditions, 722–5
  metastatic, 727
  squamous neoplasia, 719–20
Van Nuys grading system for ductal carcinoma in-situ of breast, 925
Vascular ectasias, 43–4
Vascular endothelial growth factor, 100
Vascular epulides, 222
Vascular leiomyoma, 687
Vascular tumors, 41–74
  benign, 41–55
  bone
    benign, 1627–8
    malignant, 1628–30
  breast, 955–6
  classification, 42
  endometrium, 669
  eyelid, 45, 46
  intermediate malignancy, 55–6

Vascular tumors (Cont'd)
  lymph nodes, 1248
  malignant, 62–7
    angiosarcoma, 63–7
    epithelioid hemangioendothelioma, 62–3
  peritoneum, 891
  perivascular cells, 70–4
  skin, 1495
  small intestine, 383–4
  stomach, 359–60
  thymus, 1315
Vasoactive intestinal polypeptide
  neuroendocrine tumors, 430
  pancreatic tumors, 1123
  pheochromocytoma, 1112
Venous hemangioma, 52
  breast, 956
Venous lake, 44
Verner-Morrison syndrome, 1131
Verruca palmaris/plantaris (myrmecia; plamoplantar wart), 1430
Verruca plana (plane wart), 1430
Verruca senilis, 1423–7
Verruca vulgaris, 1429–30
Verruciform xanthoma of penis, 864
Verrucous carcinoma, 151, 162–3
  anal canal, 410
  bladder, 538
  cervix, 703
  esophagus, 331
  external ear, 1814
  larynx/trachea, 103–4
  oral cavity, 218–19
  penis, 870
  skin, 1439–40
  vulva, 735
Verrucous hemangioma, 46
Verrucous leukoplakia, proliferative, 220
Verumontanum mucosal gland hyperplasia, 785–6
Vestibular papilloma of vulva, 730
Vestibular schwannoma, 1824–6
Villoglandular adenocarcinoma
  cervix, 706
  vulva, 738
Villous adenoma
  appendix, 392
  bladder, 524, 526
  large intestine, 393–4
Vimentin, 100, 106, 113, 123, 191, 594, 1654
  adenoid cystic carcinoma, 123, 191
  adenomatous hyperplasia of rete testis, 842
  adrenal tumors, 1108
  angiomatosis, 956
  basal cell hyperplasia, 780
  basaloid squamous cell carcinoma, 106
  cardiac myxoma, 13
  dermatofibrosarcoma protuberans, 1488
  desmoplastic small round cell tumor, 891
  embryonal sarcoma, 442
  endometrial tumors, 707

Vimentin (Cont'd)
  epithelial-myoepithelial carcinoma, 192
  epithelioid fibrous histiocytoma, 1486
  epithelioid sarcoma, 1578
  Ewing's sarcoma, 115
  extrarenal rhabdoid tumor, 1582
  female adnexal tumor of probable Wolffian origin, 618
  fibroepithelial stromal polyp, 772
  fibroma-thecoma tumors, 837
  fibrous histiocytoma, 1485
  fibroxanthoma, 1492
  gallbladder adenocarcinoma, 447
  gastric carcinoma, 352
  germ cell tumors, 819
  granulosa cell tumor, 837
  gynandroblastoma, 602
  hemangiopericytoma, 72
  infantile hemangioendothelioma, 436
  intimal sarcoma, 67
  malignant teratoma, 133
  meningioma, 1821
  mesenchymal pleural tumors, 209
  metaplastic thymoma, 1328
  minute pulmonary chemodectoma, 204
  monophasic synovial carcinoma, 195
  mucinous carcinoma, 579
  mucinous cystic tumors, 474
  mucosal malignant melanoma, 115, 119
  myxofibrosarcoma, 1556
  nasal-type natural killer/T-cell lymphoma, 115
  nasopharyngeal angioma, 91
  neural tumors, 1495
  olfactory neuroblastoma, 115
  ovarian tumors, 574, 578, 579, 594
  pancreatic endocrine tumors, 1133
  pancreatic tumors, 467, 470
  peritoneal fibrosis, 884
  pituicytoma, 990
  postoperative spindle cell nodule, 796
  prostatic intraepithelial neoplasia, 753
  pulmonary meningioma, 195
  renal cell tumors, 494, 499
  retinal anlage tumor, 848
  rhabdoid tumor of kidney, 517
  rhabdomyosarcoma, 115
  salivary gland tumors, 266, 272, 283
  sclerosing hemangioma, 202
  seminoma, 818
  Sertoli cell tumor, 598, 835
  sex cord-stromal tumor, 831
  sinonasal undifferentiated carcinoma, 113, 115
  small cell neuroendocrine undifferentiated carcinoma, 115
  solid pseudopapillary neoplasm, 479
  solitary fibrous tumor, 886
  spindle cell hemangioma, 53
  spindle cell squamous carcinoma, 105, 106
  squamous carcinoma, 115
  steroid cell tumors, 601
  stromal sarcoma, 958

Vimentin (Cont'd)
  tricholemma, 1447
  undifferentiated thyroid carcinoma, 1033, 1034
  yolk sac (embryonal mesenchymal) sarcoma, 607
Vinyl chloride exposure, 63
Vipoma, 1123, 1131
Viral capsid antigen, 109
Virilizing tumors
  adrenal cortical, 1103–4
  ovary, 602, 628
Vocal cord polyps, 154, 155
Vocal cord Teflon granuloma, 158
Von Hippel-Lindau disease, 495, 1124, 1827
Von Meyenburg complex (biliary hamartoma), 449
Von Recklinghausen's disease, 70
Von Willebrand factor, 63, 1376
Vulvar intraepithelial neoplasia, 732–3
  classic type, 732–3
  differentiated (simplex) type, 733
Vulvar tumors, 730–45
  glandular, 735–9
    benign, 735–6
    malignant, 736–8
  melanocytic lesions, 738–9
  mesenchymal, 739–45
  premalignant, 732–3
  squamous, 730–5

Waldenström macroglobulinemia, 1179, 1405
Waldeyer's ring, 1140
  malignant lymphoma, 120
Waldeyer's tonsillar tissues
  HIV infection, 137–8
  malignant lymphoma, 127–8
Walthard nests, 848, 896, 897
Warthin's tumor, 156, 262, 266–9
  clinical features, 266–7
  definition, 266
  differential diagnosis, 269
  macroscopic appearances, 267
  malignant change, 269
  microscopic appearances, 267–9
Warty (condylomatous) carcinoma
  cervix, 703
  penis, 870
Warty dyskeratoma, 1427
  larynx and trachea, 158
Wegener's granulomatosis, 1797
  larynx and trachea, 158
  sinonasal tract/nasopharynx, 126, 127, 138–9
Weibel-Palade bodies, 197
Well-differentiated liposarcoma, 1528
Well-differentiated neuroendocrine carcinoma see Carcinoid tumor
Whipple triad, 1128
White fibrous papulosis, 1493
Whitmore-Jewett staging system for prostate cancer, 763

Wilms' tumor, 511–15
  cervix, 715
  differential diagnosis, 513–14
  endometrium, 669
  grading, staging and prognostic factors, 514–15
  histologic appearances, 513
  macroscopic appearances, 512–13
  nephrogenic rests and nephroblastomatosis, 511–12
  orbit, 1799
Wilson's disease, 425
Winer (dilated pore), 1446
Wiskott-Aldrich syndrome, 1236
Woringer-Kolopp disease (pagetoid reticulosis), 1498, 1501
Wry neck deformity, 1544
WT1, mesothelioma, 1246

X-linked lymphoproliferative disorder, 1236
Xanthelasma, 370, 371
Xanthogranuloma, 1493
Xanthogranulomatous pyelonephritis, 494
Xanthoma, 370, 371
Xanthomatous cardiomyopathy, infantile, 26
Xeroderma pigmentosum, 64
Xp11 translocation carcinoma, 499
Xp11 translocation carcinomas, 499

Yolk sac (endodermal sinus) tumor
  bladder, 551
  central nervous system, 1718
  cervix, 715
  endometrium, 669
  ovary, 605–7
    clinical features, 605–6

Yolk sac (endodermal sinus) tumor (*Cont'd*)
    pathology, 606–7
  testis, 824–5
  thymus, 1342
  vagina, 727
  vulva, 745
Yolk sac tumor, 669

Zeis gland carcinoma, 1782, 1785
Zellballen, 31, 89, 153, 187, 1477, 1764, 1765, 1769, 1822
Zollinger-Ellison syndrome, 354, 369, 380, 1130